Mechanisms Of Disease In Small Animal Surgery

3rd Edition

Mechanisms Of Disease In Small Animal Surgery

3rd Edition

Editor:

M. Joseph Bojrab, DVM, MS, PhD
Diplomate, American College of Veterinary Surgeons
Private Consulting Practitioner
Las Vegas, Nevada

Associate Editor:

Eric Monnet, DVM, PhD
Professor, Small Animal Surgery
Colorado State University
College of Veterinary Medicine and Biomedical Sciences

TETON NEWMEDIA
INNOVATIVE PUBLISHING OF VETERINARY & HUMAN MEDICINE

Executive Editor: Carroll C. Cann
Developement Editor: Tanya Lazar
Design and Production: www.fiftysixforty.com

Teton NewMedia
P.O. Box 4833
Jackson, WY 83001
1-888-770-3165
www.tetonnm.com

The authors and publisher have made every effort to provide an accurate reference text. However, they shall not be held responsible for problems arising from errors or omissions, or from misunderstandings on the part of the reader.

Note: Although the authors and the publisher have taken reasonable steps to ensure accuracy of the drug information included in this text before publication, drug information may change without notice and readers arc advised to consult the manufacturer's packaging inserts before prescribing medications.

PRINTED IN THE UNITED STATES OF AMERICA

ISBN # 1-59161-038-9

Library of Congress Cataloging-in-Publication Data on file.

Preface

Disease Mechanisms is a textbook designed to explain, in understandable language, how individual organs and organ systems are affected by disease processes. It defines the principles upon which surgical procedures are based and is therefore an ideal companion volume for CURRENT TECHNIQUES IN SMALL ANIMAL SURGERY. It not only helps the Practicing Veterinarian better understand the function of specific organs effected by disease; it also helps explain it and the selected surgical treatment to an ever more demanding client. It will be enormously helpful to the veterinary student, intern and resident studying for boards. This book assembled the most qualified experts in the fields of surgery and pathophysiology to present the mechanisms by which disease affects each organ system in practical and understandable terms. This book is an update of the highly successful second edition which was sold out and is no longer available. This book is also very helpful for the veterinary Technician because of its practical focus, consistent presentation and clear explanation of disease mechanisms in all body regions. One of the reasons the previous editions of this book were so extremely successful is because the practicing veterinarian can use it effectively for client information. In other words this book served as the veterinarians "second opinion" backing up his information to the client.

I know you will enjoy reading this book and learning the wealth of usable knowledge which will help you in all future cases. I believe that it will become the number one reference in your library.

M. Joseph Bojrab DVM, MS, PhD.

Acknowledgements

I would like to thank Dr. Eric Monnet and all of his residents for their many hours of hard work to ensure the accuracy and completeness of these manuscripts. It is due to them that this book is one of the most outstanding works on disease mechanisms every published.

Dr. M. Joseph Bojrab

Dedication

I would like to dedicate this book to my 94 year old Mother Julia Bojrab. She is still sharp as a tack and drives herself around Ft. Wayne, IN. She has been an inspiration for all 3 of her children to work hard, be the best you can be and be kind to others. Everyone is a creature of God. Thank you Mom!

Dr. M. Joseph Bojrab

Contributors

Tannaz Amalsadvala, DVM, MS
Clinical Instructor
Dept. of Clinical Sciences
Auburn University College of Veterinary Medicine
Alabama 36849

Pierre M. Amsellem, Docteur Vétérinaire, Dip ACVS
Colorado State University
Fort Collins, CO

André Autefage, DMV, PhD
Diplomate, European College of Veterinary Surgeons
Professor and Head of Small Animal Surgery
Department of Small Animal Clinical Sciences
School of Veterinary Medicine – University of Toulouse
Toulouse, France

Rodney S. Bagley, DVM, DACVIM
(Neurology and Internal Medicine)
Professor, Neurology and Neurosurgery
Department of Clinical Sciences
Washington State University
College of Veterinary Medicine
Pullman, WA

Jean-François Bardet, DVM, MS
Diplomate ECVS
Neuilly Sur Seine, France

Daniel P. Beaver, DVM, DACVS
Surgical Specialist in Practice
Chiron Veterinary Surgery
Baton Rouge, LA

Jamie R. Bellah, DVM
Diplomate, American College of Veterinary Surgeons
Professor, Small Animal Surgery
Director, Southeastern Raptor Center
Department of Clinical Sciences
College of Veterinary Medicine
Auburn University
Auburn, AL

RA Bennett, DVM, MS, DACVS
Department of Veterinary Clinical Medicine
Veterinary Medicine Teaching Hospital
University of Illinois
Urbana, IL

David Biller, DVM
Kansas State University
Manhattan, KS

Mark W. Bohling, DVM
Department of Small Animal Clinical Sciences
Veterinary Teaching Hospital
College of Veterinary Medicine
University of Tennessee
Knoxville, TN

Janice McIntosh Bright, BSN, MS, DVM
Diplomate ACVIM (Internal Medicine & Cardiology)
Professor of Cardiology
Department of Clinical Sciences
College of Veterinary Medicine and Biomedical Sciences
Colorado State University
Fort Collins, CO

Ronald M. Bright, DVM, MS, Dip ACVS
Staff Surgeon
VCA-Veterinary Specialists of Northern Colorado
Loveland, CO

Brigitte A. Brisson, DMV, DVSc
Diplomate ACVS
Associate Professor, Small Animal Surgery
Department of Clinical Studies
Ontario Veterinary College
University of Guelph
Guelph, Ontario, Canada

Hervé Brissot, DVM, DECVS, MRCVS
Station Farm
London Road
Six Mile Bottom
Suffolk CB8 0UH
United Kingdom

Daniel J. Brockman, BVSc, CVR, CSAO
Diplomate ACVS/ECVS ILTM MRCVS
Senior Lecturer in Small Animal Surgery
Royal Veterinary College
University of London
Hatfield, Hertfordshire, United Kingdom

Loretta J. Bubenik, DVM, MS
Diplomate ACVS
Assistant Professor
Companion Animal Surgery
Louisiana State University
School of Veterinary Medicine
Veterinary Clinical Sciences
Baton Rouge, LA

Stéphane Bureau, DVM
Diplomate ECVS
Bordeaux, France

Colin F. Burrows, PhD, BVetMed
Diplomate ACVIM
University of Florida
College of Veterinary Medicine
Department of Small Animal Clinical Sciences
Gainesville, FL

Laurent Cauzinille, DMV, Diplomate ACVIM (N) & ECVN
East Ipswich Queensland, Australia

Scott J. Campbell, BVSc, MACVSc, DACVN
Clinique Fregis
Arcueil, FRANCE

Daniel L. Chan, DVM, DACVECC, DACVN, MRCVS
Lecturer in Emergency and Critical Care
Department of Veterinary Clinical Sciences
Queen Mother Hospital for Animals
Royal Veterinary College
Hawkshead Lane
North Mymms, Hatfield
Hertfordshire, United Kingdom

Annie V. Chen, DVM
Resident, Neurology and Neurosurgery
Department of Clinical Sciences
Washington State University
College of Veterinary Medicine
Pullman, WA

Joan R. Coates, DVM, MS
Diplomate ACVIM (Neurology)
Associate Professor Veterinary Neurology/Neurosurgery
Department of Veterinary Medicine and Surgery
University of Missouri
Veterinary Medical Teaching Hospital
Columbia, MO

Michael G. Conzemius, DVM, PhD
Diplomate ACVS
Associate Professor
Department of Veterinary Clinical Sciences
College of Veterinary Medicine
Iowa State University
Ames, IA

James L. Cook, DVM, PhD
Diplomate ACVS
Associate Professor, Small Animal Surgery
Director, Comparative Orthopaedic Laboratory
University of Missouri – Columbia
Veterinary Medical Teaching Hospital
Columbia, MO

Bronwyn Crane, DVM, MS
College of Veterinary Medicine
Oregon State University
Corvallis, OR

Autumn P. Davidson, DVM, MS
Diplomate ACVIM
Clinical Professor
Department of Medicine and Epidemiology
School of Veterinary Medicine
SAC VMTH
University of California, Davis
Davis, CA

Charles E. DeCamp, DVM, MS
Diplomate, ACVS
Department of Small Animal Clinical Sciences
Michigan State University
East Lansing, MI

Loïc M. Dejardin, DVM, MS
Diplomate, American College of Veterinary Surgeons
Assistant Professor of Orthopaedic Surgery
College of Veterinary Medicine
Michigan State University
East Lansing, MI

Dianne Dunning, DVM, MS, DACVS
Clinical Associate Professor
College of Veterinary Medicine
North Carolina State University
Raleigh, NC

Gilles P. Dupré, Doctor Veterinary Medicine
Diplomate ECVS
Department of Small Animal Surgery
Clinical Department of Small Animals and Horses
Veterinary University Vienna,
Vienna, AUSTRIA

Erick Egger, DVM
Diplomate ACVS
Associate Professor of Surgery
College of Veterinary Medicine
Colorado State University
Ft. Collins, CO

Gary W. Ellison, DVM, MS
Diplomate ACVS
Professor and Service Chief
Department of Small Animal Clinical Sciences
Health Science Center
University of Florida
Gainesville, FL

Meredith Esterline
South Texas Veterinary Specialists
San Antonio, TX

Richard Evans, PhD
Assistant Professor
College of Veterinary Medicine
Iowa State University
Ames, IA

Catharina Linde Forsberg, DVM, PhD, Diplomate ECAR
Specialist in Dog and Cat Reproduction,
Professor of Small Animal Reproduction
Department of Clinical Sciences
Division of Comparative Reproduction
Obstetrics and Udder Health
Swedish University of Agricultural Sciences
Uppsala, Sweden

Derek B. Fox, DVM, PhD
Diplomate ACVS
Assistant Professor, Small Animal Surgery
Associate Director, Comparative Orthopaedic Laboratory
University of Missouri – Columbia
Veterinary Medical Teaching Hospital
Columbia, MO

Trent Gall, DVM
Small Animal Surgery Resident
Colorado State University
College of Veterinary Medicine and Biomedical Sciences
Fort Collins, CO

James S. Gaynor, DVM, MS
Diplomate, American College of Veterinary Anesthesiologists
Diplomate, American Academy of Pain Management
Medical Director
Animal Anesthesia and Pain Management Center
Colorado Springs, CO

Clare R. Gregory, DVM
Diplomate ACVS
Department of Surgical and Radiological Sciences
School of Veterinary Medicine,
University of California, Davis
Davis, CA

D.J. Griffon, DVM
Department of Veterinary Clinical Medicine
Veterinary Medicine Teaching Hospital
University of Illinois
Urbana IL

Tim Hackett, DVM MS DACVECC
Associate Professor
Small Animal Medical Chief of Staff
James L. Voss Veterinary Teaching Hospital
Colorado State University
Fort Collins, CO

Colin E. Harvey, BVSc, FRCVS
Diplomate ACVS, AVDC
Professor of Surgery and Dentistry
University of Pennsylvania School of Veterinary Medicine
Philadelphia, PA

Kei Hayashi, DVM, PhD, DACVS
Assistant Professor of Orthopedic Surgery
Department of Surgical and Radiological Sciences
School of Veterinary Medicine
University of California, Davis
Davis, CA

Herman A.W. Hazewinkel, DVM, PhD
Diplomate European College of Veterinary Surgeons
Diplomate European College of Veterinary and
Comparative Nutrition
Head, Section of Orthopedics-Neurosurgery-Dentistry
Department of Clinical Sciences of Companion Animals
Faculty of Veterinary Medicine
Utrecht University
Utrecht, The Netherlands

Cheryl S. Hedlund, DVM, MS
Diplomate, American College of Veterinary Surgeons
Professor of Surgery
Veterinary Clinical Sciences
School of Veterinary Medicine
Louisiana State University
Baton Rouge, LA

Peter E. Holt, BVMS, PhD, ILTM, DECVS, CBiol, FIBiol, FRCVS
Professor of Veterinary Surgery
University of Bristol
Division of Companion Animals
Department of Clinical Veterinary Science
School of Veterinary Science
University of Bristol
Langford House, Langford
Bristol, United Kingdom

Giselle Hosgood, BVSc, MS, PhD
Diplomate, American College of Veterinary Surgeons
Professor of Surgery
Veterinary Clinical Sciences
School of Veterinary Medicine
Louisiana State University
Baton Rouge, LA

Dr. DA Hulse
Texas A&M University
College of Veterinary Med
Veterinary Teaching Hospital
College Station, TX

Geraldine B. Hunt
Associate Professor in Small Animal Surgery
Faculty of Veterinary Science
University Veterinary Centre
University of Sydney, Australia

Susan P. James, PhD
Professor
Director, School of Biomedical Engineering
Colorado State University
Fort Collins, CO

Cheri A. Johnson, DVM, MS
Diplomate, ACVIM (SAIM)
Professor and Chief of Staff
College of Veterinary Medicine
Department of Small Animal Clinical Sciences
Michigan State University
Veterinary Medical Center
East Lansing, MI

Michael D. King, BVSc, MS
Chief Resident, Small Animal Surgery
Department of Small Animal Clinical Sciences
Virginia-Maryland Regional College of Veterinary Medicine
Virginia Polytechnic Institute and State University
Blacksburg, VA

Lisa Klopp, DVM, MS
Diplomate ACVIM (Neurology)
Assistant Professor of Neurology/Neurosurgery
Colorado State University
Fort Collins, CO

Kara A. Kolster, DVM
Resident in Theriogenology
Department of Large Animal Clinical Sciences
Virginia-Maryland Regional College of Veterinary Medicine
Virginia Tech
Blacksburg, VA

Janet R. Kovak, DVM, DACVS
Staff Surgeon
The Animal Medical Center
New York, NY

Dr. U. Krotscheck
Department of Clinical Sciences
College of Veterinary Medicine
Ithaca, NY

Jon M. Kruger, DVM PhD DACVIM
Department of Small Animal Clinical Sciences
College of Veterinary Medicine
Michigan State University
East Lansing, MI

Simon Timothy Kudnig, DVM MS DACVS
Staff Surgeon
Melbourne Veterinary Referral Centre
Glen Waverley, Victoria, Australia

Michelle Anne Kutzler, DVM, PhD, DACT
Assistant Professor of Theriogenology
Department of Clinical Sciences
College of Veterinary Medicine
Oregon State University
Corvallis, OR

Andrew E. Kyles, BVMS, PhD, Diplomate ACVS, ECVS
Associate Professor, Small Animal Surgery
Department of Surgical and Radiological Sciences
School of Veterinary Medicine
University of California, Davis
Davis, CA

Susan E. Lana, DVM, MS, DACVIM
Assistant Professor- Medical Oncology
Department of Clinical Sciences
College of Veterinary Medicine and Biological Sciences
Colorado State University
Ft Collins, CO

Jennifer L. Lansdowne, DVM, MSc
Resident in Small Animal Surgery
Department of Small Animal Clinical Sciences
College of Veterinary Medicine
Michigan State University
East Lansing, MI

Gerald V. Ling, DVM
Urinary Stone Laboratory Analysis
Department of Medicine and Epidemiology
University of California
Davis, CA

Peter Lotsikas, DVM
Surgical Resident
Department of Veterinary Clinical Sciences
College of Veterinary Medicine
Iowa State University
Ames, IA

Jody P. Lulich, DVM PhD DACVIM
Veterinary Clinical Sciences Department
College of Veterinary Medicine
University of Minnesota
St. Paul, MN

Catriona MacPhail, DVM
Diplomate ACVS
Assistant Professor, Small Animal Surgery
Department of Clinical Sciences
Colorado State University
Fort Collins, CO

Denis Marcellin-Little, DEDV, Diplomate ACVS
Diplomate ECVS
Associate Professor, Orthopedic Surgery
College of Veterinary Medicine
North Carolina State University
Raleigh, NC

Robert A. Martin, DVM, DACVS/DABVP
Professor, Small Animal Surgery
Department of Small Animal Clinical Sciences
Virginia-Maryland Regional College of Veterinary Medicine
Virginia Polytechnic Institute and State University
Blacksburg, VA

Elisa M. Mazzaferro, MS, DVM, PhD
Diplomate ACVECC
Director of Emergency Services
Wheat Ridge Veterinary Specialists
Wheat Ridge, CO

C. Wayne McIlwraith, BVSc, PhD, DSc, FRCVS
Diplomate ACVS
Professor of Surgery
Director of Orthopedic Research
Barbara Cox Anthony University Chair
Colorado State University
Ft. Collins, CO

Mary A. McLoughlin, DVM, MS
Diplomate ACVS
Associate Professor
Department of Veterinary Clinical Sciences
The Ohio State University
Columbus, OH

Margo Mehl, DVM
Diplomate ACVS
The Comparative Transplantation Laboratory
Department of Surgical and Radiological Sciences
School of Veterinary Medicine
University of California, Davis
Davis, CA

SJ Mehler, DVM
Veterinary Hospital of the University of Pennsylvania
Department of Clinical Studies
School of Veterinary Medicine
Philadelphia, PA

Eric Monnet, DVM, PhD, FAHA
Diplomate ACVS, ECVS
Professor
Colorado State University
College of Veterinary Medicine
Department of Clinical Sciences
Fort Collins, CO

Ron Montgomery, DVM, MS
Diplomate, American College of Veterinary Surgeons
Professor of Orthopaedics
Veterinary Teaching Hospital
Department of Clinical Sciences
College of Veterinary Medicine
Auburn University
Auburn, AL

Prudence J. Neath, BSc(Hons), BVetMed,
Diplomate ACVS, Diplomate ECVS, MRCVS
Northwest Surgeons
Delamere House
Ashville Point
Sutton Weaver
Cheshire, England

Dennis Olsen, DVM, MS
Diplomate, American College of Veterinary Surgeons
Program Director, Veterinary Technology
Community College of Southern Nevada
Las Vegas, NV

E. Christopher Orton, DVM, PhD, DACVS
Professor
Department of Clinical Sciences
James L. Voss Veterinary Teaching Hospital
Veterinary Medical Center
College of Veterinary Medicine and Biomedical Sciences
Colorado State University
Fort Collins, CO

Carl A. Osborne, DVM PhD DACVIM
Veterinary Clinical Sciences Department
College of Veterinary Medicine
University of Minnesota
St. Paul, MN

Ross H. Palmer, DVM, MS, DACVS
Associate Professor
Affilate faculty, School of Biomedical Engineering
Colorado State University
Fort Collins, CO

Laurie Pearce, DVM
Diplomate ACVIM (Neurology)
Assistant Professor
College of Veterinary Medicine
Colorado State University
Fort Collins, CO

Elizabeth Pluhar, DVM PhD
Diplomate ACVS
Associate Professor of Surgery
College of Veterinary Medicine
University of Minnesota
Saint Paul, MN

Cyrill Poncet
Centre Hospitalier Veterinaire Frégis
Arcueil, FRANCE

Curtis W. Probst, DVM
Diplomate, American College of Veterinary Surgeons
Professor of Orthopedic Surgery
Department of Small Animal Clinical Sciences
College of Veterinary Medicine
Michigan State University
East Lansing, MI

David A. Puerto, DVM
Diplomate American College of Veterinary Surgeons
Chief of Surgery
Center for Animal Referral and Emergency Services
Langhorne, PA

Beverly J. Purswell, DVM, PhD, DACT
Professor and Interim Head
Department of Large Animal Clinical Sciences
Virginia-Maryland Regional College of Veterinary Medicine
Virginia Tech
Blacksburg, VA

MaryAnn G. Radlinsky, DVM, MS
Diplomate, ACVS
Associate Professor
Department of Small Animal Medicine & Surgery
University of Georgia
Athens, GA

Alexander M. Reiter, Diplomate Tzt.,
Dr. med. vet., Diplomate AVDC, EVDC
Assistant Professor of Dentistry and Oral Surgery
University of Pennsylvania School of Veterinary Medicine
Philadelphia, PA

Mitch Robbins, DVM, DACVS
Veterinary Specialty Center
Buffalo Grove, IL

Mark P. Rondeau, DVM, DACVIM (SA-IM)
Department of Clinical Studies
Matthew J. Ryan Veterinary Hospital
University of Pennsylvania
Philadelphia, PA

Matthew Rooney, DVM, MS DACVS
Mountain State Veterinary Specialist
Longmont, CO

Rod A.W. Rosychuk, DVM, DACVIM
Associate Professor
Dept. of Clinical Sciences
Colorado State University
Ft. Collins, CO

Elizabeth Rozanski, DVM, DACVIM (SA-IM) DACVECC
Department of Clinical Sciences
Cummings School of Veterinary Medicine
Tufts University
North Grafton, MA

Annette L. Ruby, BA
Urinary Stone Laboratory Analysis
Department of Medicine and Epidemiology
University of California
Davis, CA

S. Kathleen Salisbury, DVM, MS, Dipl ACVS
Professor, Small Animal Surgery
Purdue University
Veterinary Clinical Sciences
West Lafayette, IN

G. Diane Shelton, DVM, PhD,
Diplomate ACVIM (Internal Medicine)
Adjunct Professor
Department of Pathology
School of Medicine
University of California, San Diego
La Jolla, CA,

Andy Shores, DVM, MS, PhD
Diplomate, ACVIM (Neurology)
Associate Clinical Professor, Surgery/Neurology
Mississippi State University
College of Veterinary Medicine
Mississippi State, MS

Brenda Austin Simmons, DVM, MS
Chief Resident, Surgery
Veterinary Teaching Hospital
Department of Clinical Sciences
College of Veterinary Medicine
Auburn University
Auburn, AL

Daniel D. Smeak, DVM, Diplomate, ACVS
Professor of Small Animal Surgery
Department of Veterinary Clinical Sciences
The Ohio State University
Columbus, OH

Emily Soiderer, DVM, Dipl ACVS
Assistant Professor, Small Animal Surgery
Kansas State University
Veterinary Medical Teaching Hospital
Manhattan, KS

Michele A. Steffey,
Department of Clinical Sciences
College of Veterinary Medicine
Cornell University
Ithaca, NY

Steven F. Swaim, DVM, MS
Professor Emeritus
Dept of Clinical Sciences and
Scott-Ritchey Research Center
Auburn University
College of Veterinary Medicine
Auburn, AL

Karen Tobias, DVM, MS
Diplomate ACVS
Professor, Small Animal Surgery
Department of Veterinary Clinical Sciences
University of Tennessee College of Veterinary Medicine
Veterinary Teaching Hospital
Knoxville TN

Rory J. Todhunter
Department of Clinical Sciences
College of Veterinary Medicine
Cornell University
Ithaca, NY

Dr. T. Tohundter
Department of Clinical Sciences
College of Veterinary Medicine
Ithaca, NY

David C. Twedt, DVM, Diplomate ACVIM
Professor
Small Animal Internal Medicine
Colorado State University
Fort Collins, CO

Susan W. Volk, VMD, PhD
Diplomate American College of Veterinary Surgeons
Staff Veterinarian in Small Animal Surgery
Department of Clinical Studies
Matthew J. Ryan Veterinary Hospital
School of Veterinary Medicine
University of Pennsylvania
Philadelphia, PA

Dirsko von Pfeil, Dr.med.vet
Assistant Professor, Small Animal Surgery
Kansas State University
Veterinary Teaching Hospital
1800 Denison Avenue
Manhattan, KS

Don R. Waldron
Diplomate, American College of Veterinary Surgeons
Professor of Surgery
Virginia-Maryland Regional College of Veterinary Medicine
Virginia Polytechnic Institute and State University
Blacksburg, VA

Craig B. Webb, PhD, DVM, DACVIM (SAM)
Assistant Professor
Clinical Sciences Department
Colorado State University
Fort Collins, CO

Chadwick R. West, DVM
Clinical Neurology and Neurosurgery
Animal Medical Center
New York, NY

Jodi L. Westropp, DVM, PhD, DACVIM
Department of Medicine and Epidemiology
School of Veterinary Medicine
University of California
Davis, CA

Richard Wheeler, DVM
Diplomate ACT
Affiliate Faculty
Small Animal Medicine, Reproduction
Colorado State University
James L. Voss Veterinary Teaching Hospital
Fort Collins, CO

Jacqueline Whittemore, C. DVM, DACVIM (SAM), PhD
Clinical Sciences Department
Colorado State University
Fort Collins, CO

Michael Willard, DVM, MS, Dipl ACVIM
College of Veterinary Medicine
Texas A&M University
College Station, TX

Amy Zalcman
Orthopaedic Fellow
College of Veterinary Medicine
The Ohio State University
Columbus, OH

Contents

Part V: Neurology

Part VI: Respiratory System

Part VII: Special Senses

Part VIII: Skin/Integument

Part IX: Urinary System

Part XIV: Exotics

Part I

General

Chapter 1

The Systemic Inflammatory Response Syndrome

Tim Hackett

Inflammation is good. A protective series of events, the inflammatory response is – under normal circumstances – an amazing dance. Infectious agents, external stimuli, even intrinsic disease can stimulate a cascade of events resulting in inflammation. The four signs of inflammation were recorded in Latin by Cornelius Celsus in first century Rome: *Rubor* (redness), *calor* (heat), *tumor* (swelling), and *dolor* (pain). It was understood later that the increased circulation, fever, and swelling were the results of potentially beneficial physiologic responses. In the 19th century, Rudolf Virchow added a fifth sign of inflammation: *Functio laesa* (loss of function), a suggestion that the temporary loss of function may be an adaptive response to limit use and allow healing.

This response is due to locally produced mediators that recruit and activate cells of the immune system (***recognition, release,*** and ***recruitment***). As these defenders arrive, they recruit and activate other proteins and chemical messengers. Some of these messengers are pyrogens. Others act on local vasculature, increasing circulation; the cause of redness. Circulation to the area brings oxygen, nutrients, and primarily neutrophilic cellular infiltrate. Some factors increase vascular permeability; the cause of local swelling. Increased permeability allows agents of the immune system to enter damaged tissues. As these cellular, chemical, and protein messengers stimulate the proinflammatory cascade, a simultaneous anti-inflammatory cascade acts to limit the process to the affected area. If it all works, the infection is vanquished, the damaged tissues heal, the inflammatory response is confined to the local area, and the organism survives (***removal, resolution,*** and ***restoration***).

When the inflammatory stimulus is extensive, or for other reasons the proinflammatory forces are not contained, this protective process can lead to systemic manifestations. When the inflammatory cascade results in systemic signs of infla mmation the process is called the **systemic inflammatory response syndrome** (SIRS). Clinical criteria of SIRS in veterinary patients are listed in Table 1-1. SIRS can be caused by invasion of normally sterile host tissues by microorganisms. **Septicemia** occurs when bacteria are found in the blood stream. When the systemic inflammatory response is associated with bacterial infection of normally sterile host tissues, the process is called **sepsis**. **Septic shock** is a state of inadequate oxygen delivery and organ dysfunction. Unlike other causes of circulatory shock, septic shock is characterized by hypotension often unresponsive to fluid and vasoactive therapies. While infection is a common cause of SIRS, there are many noninfectious causes. Any stimulus that initiates the production and release of circulating inflammatory mediators can cause systemic inflammatory changes. Examples of noninfectious causes of SIRS include pancreatitis, heat stroke, multiple trauma, rattlesnake envenomation, and neoplasia.

SIRS can occur preoperatively and may, in fact, be an indication for emergency surgery. SIRS can also result from the trauma of surgery itself. The inclusion criteria for SIRS have been criticized as being too sensitive and insufficiently specific. This is especially true in surgical patients. SIRS may also be mimicked by certain events that are commonplace in the immediate postoperative period. These signs will likely subside in the hours following surgery and are not caused by underlying physiologic derangements.

Table 1-1. Definitions Related to the Inflammatory Response and Related Disorders.

Definitions

Infection: Microbial invasion characterized by an inflammatory response to the presence of microorganisms or to the invasion of normally sterile host tissue by those organisms.

Systemic Inflammatory Response (SIRS): The systemic response to infection characterized by two or more of the following criteria:

1) Temperature > 103.5° or < 100° F
2) Heart rate > 160 bpm (dogs) and > 250 bpm (cats)
3) Respiratory rate > 20 bpm or $PaCO_2$ < 32 (28 at high altitude)
4) White blood cell count > 12,000 cells/ μl, < 4,000 cells/μl or <> 10% bands

Sepsis: The systemic response to confirmed infection characterized by two or more of the criteria above.

Septic shock: Sepsis with hypotension, despite adequate fluid resuscitation, along with the presence of perfusion abnormalities that may include, but are not limited to, lactic acidosis, oliguria, or acute changes in mental status.

Multiple Organ Dysfunction Syndrome (MODS): The presence of altered organ function in the acutely ill patient such that homeostasis cannot be maintained without intervention. Examples include hepatic, renal, and cardiac failure, stupor and coma, acute respiratory distress syndrome (ARDS), cardiac arrhythmias, and disseminated intravascular coagulopathy (DIC).

Compensatory Anti-inflammatory Response Syndrome (CARS): A severe reaction of anti-inflammatory mediators characterized by immune system depression.

Epidemiology

In the United States it is estimated that 750,000 patients suffer annually from sepsis and septic shock. Sixty percent of people suffering from severe sepsis and septic shock will develop circulatory shock with hypotension and organ failure. Traditionally, septic shock has been closely associated with gram-negative bacteria. The incidence of gram-negative sepsis in the United States has steadily increased. The endotoxin produced by gram-negative bacteria has long been known to cause many of the signs associated with SIRS. Since the late 1980s, however, the incidence of gram-positive and fungal sepsis has increased.

Reasons given for the increased incidence include an aging of the population and a rise in the incidence of geriatric diseases. With better medical care, patients live longer and succumb to the effects of chronic organ failure.

The incidence of sepsis in veterinary medicine also appears to be increasing. As in people, this may be a result of good preventative medicine and better medical care. Pets surviving into their golden years face chronic dysfunction of vital organs. When these animals present with surgical disease they may not have the physiologic reserve to mount an appropriate inflammatory response. Septicemia is found in critically ill veterinary patients. One study of 100 critically ill dogs and cats found 49 had bacteremia (positive blood cultures). Bacteremic patients in this study also had an increased mortality rate.

Patients with SIRS may experience dysfunction of one or more organ systems. This process is termed the **multiple organ dsyfunction syndrome (MODS).** Human patients with sepsis experience dysfunction of at least one organ, with multiple organ dysfunction occurring in 30% of such patients. MODS can also be found in more than 30% of trauma patients, 24% of patients with acute pancreatitis, and 33% of burn victims. A massive inflammatory reaction resulting from systemic cytokine release is the common pathway underlying multiple organ dysfunction. Despite the availability of more potent antibiotic and sophisticated critical care, mortality rates from sepsis still range from 20% to 75%.

Pathophysiology

Several factors have been identified that increase the risk of SIRS. These include the presence of infectious diseases or debilitating conditions (trauma, neoplasia, diabetes mellitus), immunosuppression (viral diseases, chemotherapy or other immunosuppressive treatments), advanced age, and malnutrition. Invasive therapeutic and diagnostic procedures can also increase the risk of acquiring a serious infection. Indwelling vascular and urinary catheters or chest tubes can let pathogens past natural protective mechanisms. General anesthesia can depress normal defenses directly by inhibiting the reticuloendothelial system. Anesthesia can also result in systemic hypotension, further depressing host defenses. A controlled inflammatory response can increase the risk of developing an exaggerated response to a second event. Called the "two hit" phenomenon this is of particular concern to the veterinary surgeon who may unwittingly supply the second "hit" when the patient is taken to surgery.

Surgical Stress and the Neurohormonal Response

Tissue injury is injury whether the cause is the front end of an automobile or the surgeon's knife. The neurohormonal response to tissue injury begins with adrenocorticotropin release by the anterior pituitary gland. The anterior pituitary also secretes growth hormone, prolactin, and endorphin. Arginine vasopressin is released by the posterior pituitary while the adrenal gland responds with cortisol and epinephrine. This fight-or-flight response is basic to survival and results in a variety of physiologic effects including tachycardia, tachyarrhythmias, hypertension, myocardial ischemia, congestive heart failure, hypokalemia, hypomagnesemia, hyperglycemia, altered immune function, and hypercoagulability.

Biochemical Mediators of SIRS

Mediators of the inflammatory response include endotoxin, cytokines, complement, kinins, endorphins, and myocardial depressant factor. These products contribute to hemodynamic changes, cardiopulmonary dysfunction, and multiple organ dysfunction associated with SIRS. Cellular messengers initiate a complex signaling sequence involving the release of secondary mediators (Figure 1-1). Surface receptors on macrophages recognize a variety of pathogens. While acquired immunity helps to fight a previously encountered pathogen, there are primitive, innate Toll-like receptors (TLRs) conserved across species that can also mount an immune response. Secondary mediators include platelet activating factor and metabolites of the arachidonic acid, cyclooxygenase, and lipoxygenase pathways. Induction of inducible nitric oxide synthetase, endothelial tissue factor expression, microvascular coagulation, and cell-adhesion molecule up-regulation are also considered secondary events.

Intercellular Communication

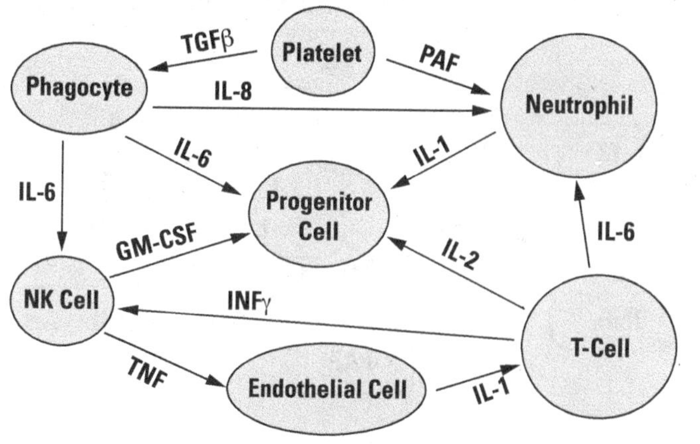

Figure 1-1. Some of the cells and mediators involved in the inflammatory response. Direction of the arrow indicates which cells activate other cells of the immune system and the mediators involved. GM-CSF = Granulocyte monocyte-colony stimulating factor, IL = Interleukin, INF = Interferon, NK = Natural killer cell, PAF = Platelet activating factor, TGF = Tissue growth factor, TNF = Tumor necrosis factor.

The substance most extensively investigated has been endotoxin, the lipopolysaccharide (LPS) moiety of the gram-negative bacterial cell wall. Endotoxin is detectable in the serum of nearly half the patients with septic shock. When endotoxin is given to experimental animals or to normal human volunteers, it can produce the same cardiovascular abnormalities as those seen in human septic shock. These and other observations lent support to the hypothesis that endotoxin represented the "Final Common Pathway" of sepsis. However, recent experiments have proven that endotoxin is not essential to the development of SIRS. Studies in dogs have demonstrated that *Staphylococcus aureus*, an organism without endotoxin, produces the same cardiovascular abnormalities as does *E. coli*.

LPS is delivered to immune cells and the CD14 cell surface receptor. Acute phase proteins and specific LPS binding proteins play a roll in presenting the LPS to the macrophage. Along with a Toll-like receptor, the LPS binding to the CD14 receptor signals the activation of the nuclear transcription factor NF-Kb, a transcription factor for many of the proinflammatory cellular glycoproteins or **cytokines**.

Cytokines, released from activated white blood cells, include tumor necrosis factor (TNF) alpha; interleukin (IL)-1, IL-6, IL-8; and platelet activating factor (PAF) (Figure 1-2). TNF is detectable in the serum of septic shock patients, as well as in healthy animals given endotoxin. TNF is now thought to be one of the primary mediators because the levels peak very early in sepsis and SIRS. TNF given experimentally to healthy animals produces fever, hypotension, anorexia, leukopenia, increased capillary permeability, and granulocyte colony-stimulating factor release.

Resolution occurs when soluble receptors contain TNF, and IL-1 or specific anti-inflammatory cytokines (IL-4, IL-10, IL-11, IL-13, and some of the colony-stimulating factors) counteract the effects of proinflammatory cytokines (Figure 1-2). Other mechanisms include an intracellular suppressor of cytokine signaling and elimination of circulating cytokines through normal systemic metabolic pathways.

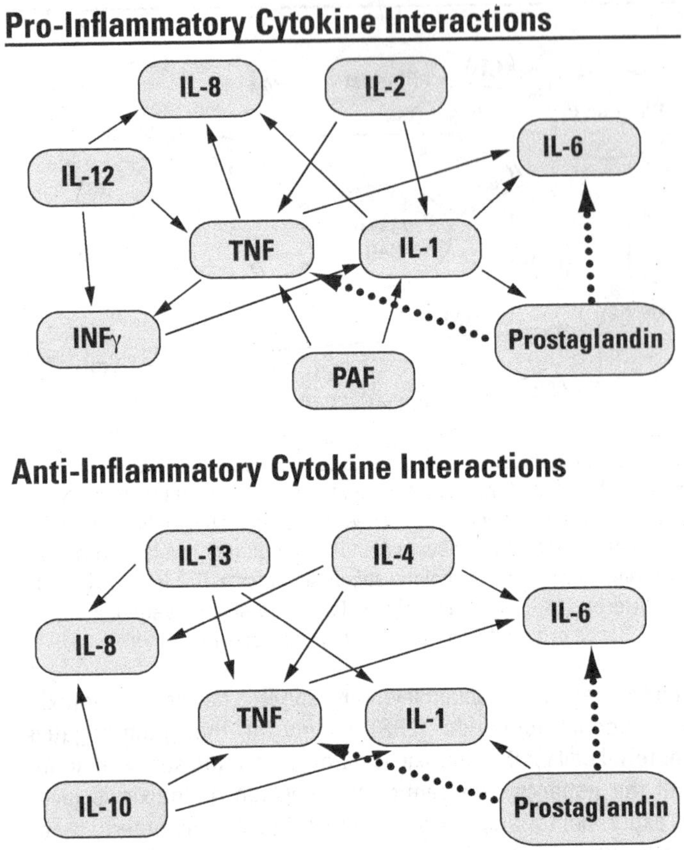

Figure 1-2. Pro- and anti-inflammatory cytokine-cytokine interactions. Arrow direction indicates which cytokines activate (in proinflammatory cascade) or inhibit (in the anti-inflammatory cascade) other cytokines. Dashed lines indicate stimulating and suppressing functions. GM-CSF = Granulocyte monocyte-colony stimulating factor, IL = Interleukin, INF = Interferon, PAF = Platelet activating factor, TGF = Tissue growth factor, TNF = Tumor necrosis factor.

Clinical Features

SIRS becomes detrimental with arterial hypotension and evidence of inadequate perfusion in the setting of a systemic insult. Patients with SIRS experience three types of circulatory shock. Hypovolemia as a result of increased vascular permeability and fluid loss into the tissues, distributive shock because of inappropriate vasodilatation and shunting of blood from vital areas, and a cardiogenic component due to depressed cardiac function. Many features, such as tachycardia, depressed mentation, and oliguria, are nonspecific: presentations vary from hypothermia with cold extremities and weak pulses to hyperthermia with warm extremities and bounding pulses. Cardiovascular instability may last from hours to days, but typically it will respond to therapy within 1 to 4 days in patients destined to survive the acute phase of the illness. An early change in septic shock and uncompensated SIRS is altered blood flow regulation. The coagulation cascade may also play a role in this response. Overexpression of proinflammatory cytokines is thought to upset the balance toward procoagulation. Decreased circulating levels of protein C and antithrombin are found in patients with severe sepsis and septic shock. Capillaries become blocked with activated white blood cells and microthrombi. Systemic release of inflammatory mediators also contributes to inappropriate shunting of blood around important vascular beds. Many systems are affected, and signs of progressive multiple organ system dysfunction may begin to appear.

Diagnosis

Suspicion of infectious causes of SIRS requires that diagnostic material be collected early while appropriate therapy and monitoring are instituted. SIRS is not a diagnosis but a syndrome with multiple causes. Possible causes must be excluded through history, physical examination, and diagnostic testing. Patients should be expected to do better if the source of the inflammation can be quickly identified and removed or drained. This means surgical disease should be ruled out first. Imaging of the abdomen may reveal mass lesions, organomegally, or local fluid accumulation. Loss of abdominal detail on plain radiographs would suggest abdominal fluid. Ultrasound may be more sensitive for abnormal fluid and useful for sampling. Radiographs of the chest and echocardiography help to evaluate the heart and lungs. When fluid is suspected in the chest or abdomen, sterile collection (either thoracocentesis, abdominocentesis, or diagnostic peritoneal lavage) for fluid analysis should be performed. It should be noted that abdominocentesis alone is relatively insensitive and a diagnostic peritoneal lavage with 10 to 20 ml/kg of sterile physiologic crystalloid fluid can increase sensitivity. Nonsurgical infectious and noninfectious causes of SIRS require intensive reassessment of therapy. Where (as with bacterial culture) a positive diagnosis may take days, therapy should be directed at likely pathogens. Areas of particular concern include the urinary tract, reproductive tract, abdominal cavity, respiratory tract, teeth and gums, and the heart valves. A thorough physical examination is performed with attention to oral examination, cardiac and thoracic auscultation, and abdominal palpation. Blood samples are drawn for CBC, serum biochemical profile, coagulation testing, rickettsial, fungal, and immune testing if indicated. Urine is collected for analysis and culture. Blood cultures should be taken from the jugular vein after surgically preparing the skin. Because blood cultures can have a relatively low yield, multiple samples should be taken 15 minutes to 1 hour apart, ideally during peak rises in body temperature. Antibiotic administration should be withheld until samples are collected but no significant delay should occur in starting therapy. If interstitial changes in the lung fields and clinical findings support possible pulmonary disease, bronchoscopy or a transtracheal wash may provide samples for a diagnosis.

Treatment/Monitoring

Standard sepsis treatment strategies include volume support to maintain cardiac output, the use of antibiotics to kill invading bacteria, surgical procedures to eradicate the nidus of infection, and intensive life-support procedures such as dialysis, mechanical ventilation, and the use of vasoactive drugs. Despite these approaches the mortality rate from septic shock is high, ranging form 25% to 75%. In addition, the incidence of sepsis syndrome in hospitals in the United States increased 139% between 1979 and 1987. This increase may be caused by several medical trends: improved life-support technology that keeps patients who have a high risk for infection alive at the extremes of age; increased use of invasive medical procedures; advances in cancer chemotherapy and immunotherapy; and the prevalence of acquired immunodeficiency syndrome. The increasing incidence of sepsis and its high mortality rate have charged the search for additional therapies.

Advances in cytokine biology have stimulated research to mitigate the biologic activity of cytokines on target cells. Binding cytokines with neutralizing molecules in circulation and blocking the interaction between cytokines and their cell-surface receptors in the target tissues are the two strategies employed. Repeating experiments performed on anti-endotoxin antibody, researchers used anti-TNF antibodies with significant success in protecting mice against lethal doses of endotoxin. However to date no convincing studies exist that anti-TNF antibodies are effective in clinical SIRS. The same can be said for similar work with other proinflammatory cytokines. All of these studies have failed to take into account the natural anti-inflammatory counterpart to these cytokines and other mediators. Interleukin-4, 10, 11, and 13 as well as the colony-stimulating factors and natural receptor antagonists are induced by TNF, IL-1, and other proinflammatory compounds. These anti-inflammatory mediators suppress many of the inflammatory effects of TNF and cytokines. New therapies for sepsis and SIRS should be directed at restoring homeostasis and not simply suppressing inflammation.

The management of patients with life-threatening infections and systemic inflammation still largely consists of hemodynamic and pulmonary support, appropriate antibiotics, and timely surgical intervention. Despite the exponential growth in our understanding of the basic biology of inflammation, our arsenal does not yet include a magic bullet to normalize the mediators of the proinflammatory and anti-inflammatory response.

Chapter 2

Shock

Tim Hackett

Oxygen delivery to tissues is one of the primary functions of the cardiopulmonary system and of primary importance to the patient manifesting signs of circulatory failure. Oxygen delivery is a function of cardiac output and oxygen content of arterial blood (Figure 2-1). In health, blood flow (cardiac output) is adjusted to meet the oxygen demands of the individual. This occurs primarily through changes in heart rate and vasomotor control of perfusion to maintain oxygenation of active tissues. Many acute disease states result in inadequate oxygen delivery to the tissues and tissue hypoxia. Initially, this drop in oxygen delivery can be overcome by compensatory increases in oxygen delivery variables and increases in oxygen extraction. When these mechanisms fail to restore oxygen homeostasis, global tissue hypoxia (shock) results.[1] If the defect in the transport of oxygen to the vital tissues can be identified and corrected while the patient is undergoing supportive care, recovery is possible. Failure to correct poor perfusion will lead to decreased oxygen consumption in the tissues, organ dysfunction, and death.

$$DO_2 \text{ (oxygen delivery)} = CaO_2 \text{ (oxygen content)} \times CO \text{ (cardiac output)}$$
$$CO = \text{Heart rate} \times \text{Stroke volume}$$
$$CaO_2 = Hgb \times SaO_2 \times 1.34 + (PaO_2 \times 0.003)$$

Figure 2-1. Variables determining oxygen delivery. SaO_2 = Arterial oxygen saturation; Hgb = Hemoglobin concentration; PaO_2 = Partial pressure of oxygen in arterial blood. Each gram of hemoglobin carries 1.34 ml of oxygen when fully saturated. Dissolved oxygen is equal to 0.003 ml of O_2 per 100 ml of blood per mm of Hg PO_2.

Classification of Shock

Shock may be classified in many ways, including by common pathway or specific cause. It is helpful to think of shock in terms of broad categories before further defining the type of shock within each category. The broadest classification system includes three major and exceedingly different causes of shock: cardiogenic shock, hypovolemic shock, and distributive shock.[2] Each results in reduced oxygen delivery to tissues through low blood flow or uneven distribution of flow. In practice, each primary event can lead to a cascade of complex physiologic problems, neurohormonal compensations, and activation of various biochemical mediators and inflammatory responses integral to the shock syndromes. A single patient may have several pathologic processes simultaneously resulting in reduced perfusion of tissues.

Hypovolemic Shock

The primary defect in hypovolemic shock is an inadequate circulating volume. This can be from sudden massive blood loss as in surgery or trauma, or fluid loss from vomiting, diarrhea, or renal disease. Neurohormonal pathways detecting a drop in blood pressure will stimulate the renin-angiotensin-aldosterone system to conserve water through the action of antidiuretic hormone. Stimulation of the sympathetic nervous system leads to epinephrine and norepinephrine release from the adrenal gland. These hormones increase vascular tone in an attempt to shunt circulation from the periphery to vital tissue beds and result in cool extremities and prolonged capillary refill time. Myocardial contractility is also increased through their action. As the patient begins to decompensate, tachycardia is a common finding, allowing maintenance of oxygen delivery in the face of diminished stroke volume. Concurrently, fluid shifts from interstitial fluid reserves in an attempt to preserve vital perfusion of the brain, heart, and kidneys while stealing supplies from other organs and tissues such as skeletal muscle and the gastrointestinal tract.[3]

Cardiogenic Shock

Cardiogenic shock occurs when the pumping function of the heart is severely impaired, leading to circulatory failure. As with hypovolemic shock, the patient will be tachycardic, weak, oliguric, have cool extremities and weak pulses. The patient with cardiac failure may also have evidence of primary cardiac disease such as an auscultable murmur, ascites, jugular venous distention, pulmonary edema, or cardiac arrhythmias. The primary defect in oxygen delivery is a reduced cardiac output.[4]

CO = Heart Rate x Stroke Volume

Stroke volume is determined by preload, afterload, and contractility. Within limits, cardiac output increases as heart rate increases. High heart rates will eventually decrease cardiac output by impairing cardiac filling and subsequent stroke volume. Tachycardia may be the result of cardiac arrhythmia or simply a physiologic response to low volume. Specific antiarrhythmic therapy and correction of underlying causes of tachycardia should be used to normalize heart rate. Clinically significant bradyarrhythmias are less common. Hyperkalemia or decompensated shock (especially in the feline) can result in clinical bradycardia. Specific arrhythmias include sick sinus syndrome, second- and third-degree atrioventricular block. It is uncommon for these slow heart rates to require emergency treatment. Often these patients have already compensated with increased stroke volume and can be referred for pacemaker treatment.[5]

Stroke volume is dependent on three determinants of cardiac function: preload, afterload, and contractility. With congestive heart failure, the pump is failing because of decreased contractility. The body attempts to compensate by increasing preload (sodium and fluid retention). Normally, the heart is able to pump the fluid presented to it through increased stretch of myocardial muscle fiber, resulting in increased contractility. Therefore, by increasing preload, the heart will increase stroke volume. In cardiac failure, the excess fluid cannot be moved and it accumulates downstream of the failing ventricle. This results in pulmonary edema in left-ventricular failure and ascites, pleural effusion, and hepatic congestion in right-ventricular failure.[6]

Maximize stroke volume (and cardiac output) by recognizing and treating the primary defect. In congestive failure, preload can be optimized by monitoring central venous pressure, administering diuretics such as furosemide, and venodilators such as nitroglycerine. With obstructive failure, as is seen with pericardial effusion, removal of even a small amount of pericardial fluid will relieve the pressure on the right ventricle and allow more normal filling.[7] Cardiac output can also be enhanced by decreasing afterload with calcium channel blockers or ACE inhibitors. These are especially useful in treating failure caused by mitral insufficiency where contractility may be normal to increased but a portion of the cardiac output is going backwards into the left atrium instead of out and into systemic circulation. In documented myocardial failure, contractility can be enhanced with positive inotropic drugs such as dobutamine, digoxin, or pimobendan.[8]

Distributive Shock

Distributive shock is probably the most challenging of the shock syndromes and one of the most difficult to reverse. The primary defect with distributive shock is an abnormal systemic vasomotor response leading to peripheral vasodilation and maldistribution of blood flow.[9] Increases in vascular permeability can further exacerbate this shock syndrome. Both peripheral vasodilation and increased vascular permeability result in decreased perfusion of vital tissues. The many causes of distributive shock are summarized in Table 2-1.

Table 2-1. Causes of Distributive Shock

Sepsis and endotoxemia
Metabolic (renal or hepatic failure or severe acid base imbalances
Toxic (anesthetic overdose, heavy metal toxicosis)
Endocrinologic (adrenocortical insufficiency, diabetic ketoacidosis)
Neurogenic (cerebral and spinal disease)

Components of other forms of shock may contribute to poor tissue oxygenation in distributive shock. Fluid loss into body cavities and interstitial spaces results in relative hypovolemia. The release of inflammatory mediators in septic shock can depress the myocardium, resulting in a cardiogenic component. Therapy must be directed at the underlying systemic defect. In sepsis, therapy consists of drainage and control of the infected focus. Because systemic inflammation resulting from sepsis and other inflammatory disease can affect oxygen delivery in many vital tissues, serial monitoring of many variables becomes necessary to treat the variety of problems an individual may face.[10]

Treatment and Monitoring

Treatment of shock should be directed at the primary problem(s) while correcting the fluid deficit. Crystalloid fluids can be used initially to restore circulating volume. Crystalloids improve cardiac output and should not be withheld for fear of diluting the red blood cell mass.[11] Oxygen delivery is a function not only of oxygen content, but also of cardiac output. Improved stroke volume should offset the initial drop in packed cell volume as the patient's true level of anemia becomes apparent. If signs of shock persist as the patient becomes more anemic, a hemoglobin-containing fluid (whole blood, packed red blood cells, or Oxyglobin®) should be administered.[12,13]

With a treatment goal of improving oxygen delivery to the tissues, we can increase cardiac output by increasing stroke volume (appropriate fluids). Oxygen content can be increased by increasing the hemoglobin concentration (hemoglobin transfusion) and by increasing oxygen saturation (oxygen supplementation).

Volumes of fluid for resuscitation should be tailored to the individual patient. It has long been recommended that the initial goal with crystalloid fluids is to give a blood volume (approximately 90 ml/kg dog, 60 ml/kg cat) in an hour.[14] This is often more than enough fluid, and in extremely debilitated patients may lead to fluid overload (pulmonary and cerebral edema).[15] Patients with systemic inflammatory conditions may also be prone to vascular leakage. Excessive fluids can affect electrolytes, dilute clotting factors, and lead to accumulations of fluid in interstitial spaces and body cavities. It may be more practical to titrate this dose in smaller increments. Smaller boluses of 22 ml/kg in dogs or 10 ml/kg in cats (approximately 25% of the total shock volume) of crystalloid fluids should be given intravenously followed by repeated doses if the patient's clinical signs fail to improve.[16] Endpoints of resuscitation should be evaluated closely and the rapid administration of fluids should be discontinued when the patient is improving.[17] Questions to ask: Are the pulses stronger? Slower? Is the patient more alert? If the answer is "no," more fluids are administered while alternate mechanisms of shock are investigated.

Following the administration of a bolus of 25% shock dose of crystalloid fluids, the packed cell volume and total solids should be compared to pre-fluid values. If a patient receiving large quantities of crystalloids becomes anemic or hypoproteinemic, the fluid should be switched to an appropriate colloid such as whole blood, packed red blood cells, plasma, or a synthetic colloid. If the total solids drop to less than 50% of pretreatment values, a colloid should be considered for further resuscitation. If the PCV has dropped precipitously, administer whole blood and search for the source of blood loss. Often, in traumatic hemorrhage, correction of blood loss volume and pressure facilitates repeated hemorrhage in areas of vascular trauma, while simultaneously diluting available clotting factors. Therefore, close attention during initial fluid resuscitation is important.

Heart and respiratory rates are useful objective variables to monitor in critical patients. Capillary refill, peripheral pulse quality, and mentation are subjective but still valuable parameters to help assess perfusion when used by experienced professionals. Blood pressure and pulse oximetry are gaining wider use in veterinary medicine and may provide additional information on cardiopulmonary function so long as limitations of the equipment are understood.

Blood pressure is the lateral force per unit area of vascular wall. Blood flow is the amount of motion provided by blood pressure working against vascular resistance. Throughout the cardiac cycle, the blood pressure oscillates about a mean pressure. Pulse pressure, which determines pulse quality or strength, is the difference between systolic and diastolic pressure. Systolic pressure is determined by stroke volume, peak rate of ejection, and arterial compliance. Diastolic pressure is a function of end-systolic arterial pressure, diastolic duration, peripheral vascular resistance, and blood volume.[18]

Indirect blood pressure measurement involves the occlusion of a peripheral artery by inflation of a pneumatic cuff. The closing and opening of the artery is detected through palpation, auscultation, or oscillometric or ultrasonic means. Diastolic pressure, which is much more important in the critically ill animal, unfortunately is much more difficult to establish. Limitations to the use of indirect blood pressure monitoring include the expense of the equipment and the inability to reliably detect blood pressure in smaller animals or those critically ill patients with low-pressure readings.

Oscillometric indirect blood pressure measurement senses amplitude of oscillations in a pressurized cuff. These oscillations are produced by changes in arterial diameter caused by changes in pulse pressure. A sudden increase in the amplitude of oscillations corresponds to systolic pressure and a low point of maximum oscillations corresponds to the diastolic pressure. The mean arterial pressure is measured directly as the lowest cuff pressure at which the oscillations are at their highest amplitude. Appropriate cuff size should be 40% of limb circumference. If the cuff is too narrow it may lead to a falsely high blood pressure. If it is too wide the blood pressure will be falsely low.[18, 19]

Ultrasonic pulse detectors use ultrasound kinetoarteriography to detect arterial wall motion using ultrasonic waves to amplify the sound of pulsating blood. Gradual deflation of cuff pressure allows blood flow as pressures drop below systolic blood pressure. Systolic pressure is recorded as the first audible sound as blood begins to flow through the artery.[18] Diastolic pressure is much more subjective and is recorded when the sound quality changes dramatically and becomes muffled. The advantage of ultrasonic sphygmomanometry is its adaptability to many animals. Also, the equipment is relatively inexpensive. Disadvantages and limitations are similar to those of the oscillometric devices. Because determination of actual pressure cutoff points is operator dependent, fluctuation in reported values can be greater. Mean arterial pressure cannot be determined directly by this method but can be calculated if systolic and diastolic pressures are recorded.

Pulse oximetry allows the estimation of arterial oxyhemoglobin saturation by transmitting light through a skin fold and sensing the difference between light absorption during pulsation (arterial flow) and background absorption. Although oxyhemoglobin (SaO_2) saturation is not directly related to arterial PO_2, it provides information about tissue delivery of oxygen. The advantage of measuring SaO_2 is the continuous, immediate noninvasive estimate of oxygenation. Disadvantages include the difficulty in maintaining the transducer in small conscious patients, interference in pigmented skin, and the inability to detect adequate signals with certain diseases (low cardiac output states, icterus, anemia, and hypothermia).[20]

An important clinical question is how to determine when the shock state is controlled. With goal-directed therapy, fluid rates can be lowered to deficit replacement, maintenance volumes, and ongoing losses when clinical signs of shock resolve. It is important to note that traditional endpoints of resuscitation (capillary refill time, heart rate, peripheral pulse quality, blood pressure, level of mentation, and urine output) may be normal in early, compensated shock and altered only when the patient decompensates. However, the opposite is also a problem: In animals in which the above endpoints are successfully corrected but that still have ongoing evidence of tissue hypoxia, more sensitive markers of oxygen transport must be evaluated.[17]

Intensive oxygen transport monitoring gives greater importance to detecting oxygen delivery. Researchers in the 1980s hypothesized that oxygen delivery and oxygen consumption were the best means of assessing adequate tissue oxygenation. Their research led to the idea that supranormal oxygen delivery in acute perioperative shock would lead to reduced mortality.[21]

This led to the routine use of pulmonary artery catheters and measurement of variables such as cardiac index (cardiac output standardized to body weight), central venous pressure, and pulmonary capillary wedge pressure. By sampling mixed venous (pulmonary arterial) blood and comparing it with arterial blood, oxygen extraction and utilization could be measured and monitored. Unfortunately many studies performed since have led to conflicting results and routine placement of pulmonary artery catheters has been associated with technical problems and catastrophic complications.[22] Even so, decreases in oxygen utilization have been shown to negatively affect prognosis in patients that fail to achieve normal oxygen utilization within 12 hours of resuscitation.[23] For this reason, alternative means to assess patients' relative oxygen debt continue to be investigated. Blood lactate, serum base excess (or deficit), gastric tonometry, and organ-specific cellular oxygen utilization techniques have provided new means to assess oxygen debt.[17]

Lactate is produced from pyruvate (via lactate dehydrogenase) during periods of tissue hypoxia. Normally less than 2 mmol/L, arterial lactate climbs with anaerobic metabolism. Tissue hypoxia causes lactate levels to climb beyond the ability of normal clearance mechanisms.[24] While it can indicate poor perfusion, tissue hypoxia, and lactic acidosis, lactate can be normal during periods of deranged cardiac output (before clearance mechanisms have become saturated). Hemorrhagic shock in a canine model found lactic acidosis more predictive of the severity of oxygen debt than blood pressure or cardiac output.[25] Lactate can be used to monitor resuscitative efforts, as levels should drop quickly with improved perfusion. Lactate measurement has limitations because other forms of lactic acidosis exist that are not specific for global oxygen debt. An example of this occurs with sepsis and catecholamine administration in which altered lactate metabolism can overestimate the severity of tissue hypoxia.[24]

Determination of base deficit has been favored over that of blood lactate in human critical care. Base deficit is calculated by most blood gas analysis equipment as the amount of a base required to titrate a set volume of the patient's blood to a normal pH (7.40). Base deficit is a measure of the amount of excess fixed acid (metabolic acidosis) in the patient. Clinical and experimental studies have shown that high base deficit is inversely related to outcome.[26, 27] Compared with lactate, mean arterial blood pressure, and cardiac output in another canine model of hemorrhagic shock, base deficit correlated the most closely with oxygen debt and mortality.[27]

Although technically demanding, direct analysis of organ-specific oxygenation is becoming available. Gastric tonometry allows the measurement of gastric pH and with it, evaluation of gastric perfusion.[28] Transcellular probes applied to skin, inserted into muscle, or attached directly to the surface of organs can evaluate tissue oxygenation of specific vascular beds. These newer techniques may take some of the subjective guesswork out of treating shock. Each deserves objective evaluation and further research in evaluation of the ability to monitor the effectiveness of shock therapy.

Conclusions

New technology is providing interesting new choices in the diagnosis and management of shock. Each intervention deserves investigation and, if proven practical and effective, will help clinicians manage this devastating syndrome. In the meantime, circulatory shock needs multimodal treatment with a basic goal: to improve oxygen delivery (DO_2) (Table 2-2). Improved oxygen delivery is achieved by optimizing oxygen content (CaO_2) and increasing oxygen saturation (SaO_2). If the packed cell volume is limiting DO_2, we can increase hemoglobin concentration with whole blood transfusion, packed red blood cell transfusion, or hemoglobin-based oxygen-carrying fluids (HBOC). We may also improve DO_2 by optimizing cardiac output (CO). This is done by optimizing heart rate (monitor pulse rate, quality, electrocardiogram), treating specific arrhythmias, and optimizing stroke volume. The goal of shock stabilization is to give the clinician time to treat the primary problem and improve the chance of a successful outcome.

Table 2-2. Monitoring Variables, Goals, and Therapeutic Interventions used to Address Impaired Oxygen Delivery and Circulatory Shock.

Physiologic Variable	Optimal Values	Therapeutic Interventions
Systolic arterial pressure	> 90 mmHg	Fluids, vasoactive/inotropic
Mean arterial pressure	> 70 mmHg	Fluids, vasoactive/inotropic
Central venous pressure	< 3 cm H_2O – normal 5-10 cm H_2O when loading	Fluids when low, diuretics and venodilators when high
Urine output	> 1 ml/kg/hr	Fluids, diuretics, dopamine
Blood glucose	70-200 gm/dL	Nutrition, dextrose if low Regular Insulin if high
Total serum solids	3.5-5.5 gm/dL	Plasma, colloids, nutrition
Albumin	> 1.5 g/dL	Plasma, 25% HSA, nutrition
Arterial blood gasses	Pa02 > 70 mmHg	Supplemental oxygen
	PaC02 < 35 mmHg	Ventilatory support
	HC03 14-24	Fluids, bicarbonate
	pH 7.35-7.45	Fluids, ventilator therapy, bicarbonate
	Base deficit -2 to 2 mEq/L	Fluids, vasoactive/inotropic
	Lactate < 2 mmol/L	Fluids, vasoactive/inotropic
Heart rate	70-150 BPM	Fluids, analgesics, antiarrhythmics

References

1. Muir WW: Shock. Comp Cont Ed Pract Vet 20(5):549-567,1998.

2. Shoemaker WC: Diagnosis and treatment of shock and circulatory failure. *In* Shoemaker WC, Ayres SM, Grenjvik A, Holbrook PR, eds. Textbook of Critical Care, 4th ed. Philadelphia: WB Saunders, 2000, pp. 92-113.

3. Marino PL: Tissue oxygenation. *In* Marino PL: The ICU Book, 3rd ed. Philadelphia: Lippincott Williams & Wilkins; 2007, p 193-205.

4. Côté E: Cardiogenic shock and cardiac arrest. Vet Clin North Am Small Anim Pract 31(6):1129-1145, 2001.

5. MA Oyama, DD Sisson, LB Lehmkuhl: Practices and outcome of artificial cardiac pacing in 154 dogs. J Vet Intern Med 15(3):229-239, 2001.

6. Barry WL, Sarembock IJ: Cardiogenic shock: therapy and prevention. Clin Cardiol 21: 72-80, 1998.

7. Braunwald E (ed): Heart Disease: A Textbook of Cardiovascular Medicine. Philadelphia: WB Saunders Company; 1997, pp. 1478-1496.

8. Gordon SG, Miller MW, Saunders AB: Pimobendan in heart failure therapy - a silver bullet? J Am Anim Hosp Assoc 42(2):90-93, 2006.

9. Landrỳ DW, Oliver JA: The pathogenesis of vasodilatory shock. N Engl J Med 345(8): 588-595, 2001.

10. Boag AK, Hughes D: Assessment and treatment of perfusion abnormalities in the emergency patient. Vet Clin North Am Small Anim Pract 35(2):319-342, 2005.

11. Manning JE: Fluid and blood resuscitation. *In* Emergency Medicine: A Comprehensive Study Guide, 6th ed. New York: McGraw-Hill; 2004, pp. 225-231.

12. Gutierrez G, Reines HD, Wulf-Gutierrez ME: Clinical review: hemorrhagic shock. Crit Care 8(5):373-381, 2004.

13. Drieseen B, Jahr JS, Lurie F, et al: Arterial oxygenation and oxygen delivery after hemoglobin-based oxygen carrier infusion in canine hypovolemic shock: a dose-response study. Crit Care Med 31(6):1771-1779, 2003.

14. Rozanski E, Rondeau M: Choosing fluids in traumatic hypovolemic shock: the role of crystalloids, colloids, and hypertonic saline. J Am Anim Hosp Assoc 38(6):499-501, 2002.

15. Kreimerier U: Pathophysiology of fluid imbalance. Critical Care 4(Suppl 2):S3-S7, 2000.

16. Wingfield WE: Fluid and electrolyte therapy. In Wingfield WE, Raffe MR, eds. The Veterinary ICU Book. Jackson Hole, WY: Teton NewMedia; 2002, pp. 166-188.

17. Prittie J: Optimal endpoints of resuscitation in early goal-directed therapy. JVECCS 16(4):329-339, 2006.

18. Henik RA, Dolson MK, Wenholz LJ: How to obtain a blood pressure measurement Clin Tech Small Anim Pract 20(3):144-150, 2005.

19. Haberman CE, Kang CW, Morgan JD, Brown SA: Evaluation of oscillometric and Doppler ultrasonic methods of indirect blood pressure estimation in conscious dogs. Can J Vet Res 70(3):211-217, 2006.

20. Hackett TB: Pulse oximetry and end-tidal carbon dioxide monitoring. Vet Clin North Am Small Anim Pract 32(5):1021-1029, 2002.

21. Shoemaker WC, Appel PL, Kram HB, et al: Prospective trial of supranormal values of survivors as therapeutic goals in high-risk surgical patients. Chest 94:1176-1186, 1988.

22. Bernard GR, Sopko G, Cerra F: Pulmonary artery catheterization and clinical outcomes: National Heart, Lung, and Blood Institute and Food and Drug Administration Workshop Report. Consensus Statement. JAMA 283(19):2568-2572, 2000.

23. Shoemaker WC, Montgomery ES, Kaplan E, Elwyn DH: Physiologic patterns in surviving and nonsurviving shock patients. Use of sequential cardiorespiratory variables in defining criteria for therapeutic goals and early warning of death. Arch Surg 106(5):630-636. 1973.

24. Lagutchik MS, Ogilvie GK, Wingfield WE, Hackett TB: Lactate kinetics in veterinary critical care: A review. JVECCS, 6:81-95, 1996.

25. Dunham M, Siegel JH, Weireter L, et al: Oxygen debt and metabolic acidemia as quantitative predictors of mortality and the severity of the ischemic insult in hemorrhagic shock. Crit Care Med 19(2):231-243, 1991.

26. Davis JW, Shackford SR, Holbrook TL: Base deficit as a sensitive indicator of compensated shock and tissue oxygen utilization. Surgery 173:473-476, 1991.

27. Waisman Y, Eichacher PQ, Banks SM, et al: Acute hemorrhage in dogs: construction and validation of models to quantify blood loss. J Appl Physiol 74:510-519, 1993.

28. Kolkman JJ, Otte JA, Groeneveld ABJ: Gastrointestinal luminal PCO2 tonometry: an update on physiology, methodology and clinical applications. Br J Anaesth 84(1):74-86, 2000.

Chapter 3

Transfusion Medicine

Elizabeth Rozanski
Mark P. Rondeau

Over the last 25 years, blood transfusions given to ill or injured patients in veterinary medicine have evolved from a relatively rare occurrence to a routine and frequently life-saving practice.[1-6] It is impossible to contemplate a successful surgeon and surgery team not having a strong knowledge base in transfusion medicine and easy access to blood products. The purposes of this chapter are to outline the physiology of blood and plasma, and to describe blood groups, methods of collection, blood components, indications for transfusion, methods of administration and monitoring during transfusions, and transfusion reactions.

Physiology of Blood and Plasma

The purpose of red blood cells is efficiently to carry oxygen to support oxygen delivery to the tissues. Red blood cells are highly evolved to be exceedingly efficient at oxygen transport by saturation of the hemoglobin (Hb) molecule with oxygen absorbed at the interface between the alveolar and pulmonary capillaries. Oxygenated hemoglobin contains approximately 1.34 ml of oxygen per gram of Hb. The oxygen content of the blood is dependant primarily on the oxygen saturation of Hb, but also, to a far lesser extent, on the dissolved partial pressure of oxygen. The oxygen content of blood can be calculated (Table 3-1).

Table 3-1. Calculation of the Oxygen Content of Blood. This Formula may be used for Arterial or Venous Blood. Each mg of Hemoglobin may carry 1.34 grams of Oxygen.

Oxygen content = [Hemoglobin (g/dl) x % saturation x 1.34] + [PaO_2 (in mm Hg) x 0.003]
For example = (15 x 0.98 x 1.34) + (100 x 0.003) = 20 ml O_2/g Hb/dl

However, the oxygen content alone is only part of the equation of successful oxygen delivery. Oxygen delivery to the tissues is also dependant on cardiac output (CO) which is the product of stroke volume (SV) and heart rate. Thus, in an anemic animal the attempt to improve oxygen delivery by increasing cardiac output is by increasing rate and/or stroke volume. This can result in tachycardia and "bounding pulses." Bounding pulses associated with anemia are a result of a greater pulse pressure (systolic – diastolic), which is usually associated with either increased systolic pressures because of increased stroke volume or from diastolic run-off if concurrent hypovolemia is present. Tachycardia becomes an important branch in decision-making about a transfused pet. In some cases, dogs will have a normal heart rate while resting, but develop a marked tachycardia (e.g., 80 bpm to 180 bpm) upon standing or being encouraged to walk, because oxygen delivery to the tissues is limited and the cardiovascular system attempts to compensate for tissue hypoxemia.

The cellular components of the blood also include white blood cells and platelets. White blood cells have a variety of roles, primarily involving modulation of the immune response and defense against infection. Because of the limited survival times of white blood cells, low white blood cell counts are not treated with transfusion and, in some cases, removal of the white cells (leukoreduction) has been advocated as a method of limiting immune response associated with transfusion.[7]

Platelets are involved in primary hemostasis. Thrombocytopenia is common in animals with anemia. Platelet-rich plasma or platelet concentrates may be transfused in dogs. However, if thrombocytopenia is secondary to immune-mediated destruction, the transfused platelets will be destroyed within a matter of minutes.[8] The plasma component of blood acts to reduce overall viscosity in addition to containing plasma proteins (albumin and globulin), antithrombin, electrolytes and glucose, pro- and anticoagulant factors, hormones, and a multitude of other factors.

Blood Groups and Blood Type

Dogs have many different blood groups, which are defined by glycolipid and glycoprotein antigens found on the red blood cell surface.[9] These are named dog erythrocyte antigens (DEA). Up to 9 antigens have been recognized within this system (DEA 1.1, 1.2, 1.3, 3, 4, 5, 6, 7, and 8). Not all antigens are considered equally important in regard to their ability to trigger a transfusion reaction. DEA 1.1 is the most likely to trigger an acute hemolytic transfusion reaction in dogs. Forty to 50 % of dogs are positive for DEA 1.1. A DEA 1.1-negative dog that has been previously sensitized with DEA 1.1 positive red blood cells may develop an acute hemolytic transfusion reaction on subsequent exposure to DEA 1.1-positive red blood cells. DEA 1.2 is also capable of eliciting an acute reaction in sensitized dogs. DEA 4 is the most prevalent of canine blood types, occurring in up to 98% of dogs. While it was previously believed that DEA 4 did not play a role in transfusion reactions, severe hemolytic reactions have been described.[10] Fortunately, transfusion reactions are rare in dogs that have not previously been transfused or that have had puppies. Dogs are unlikely to have preformed antibodies against other determinants. It has been suggested that some DEA 7-negative dogs have preformed antibodies against the DEA 7 antigen, although the antibody is weak. Sensitized DEA 7-negative dogs that are transfused with DEA 7-positive blood experience a delayed transfusion reaction where the transfused red blood cells are lost in 72 hours. Blood typing of both the recipient and the donor dog can be performed at a variety of laboratories and also with commercial blood typing cards (Appendix 3-1). Although blood typing of a recipient dog prior to transfusion is ideal, in an emergency situation it is unlikely that a transfusion will result in a reaction for the first-time recipient, because of the lack of preformed antibodies. Blood typing of both the donors and the recipients helps to maintain a better blood bank by controlling the resources. Blood typing antisera are available for DEA 1.1, 1.2, 3, 4, 5, and 7, although most commercial blood banks and laboratories type for DEA 1.1 only, as it is the most antigenic.

In an animal that has been previously transfused or in which the transfusion history is unknown, cross-matching prior to the initial transfusion is prudent to reduce the risk of a reaction.

The cat blood group system has classically been made up of A, B, and AB types;[2,11] however, the existence of a new red blood cell antigen (MIK) has been described in a domestic short hair cat.[12] Cats, unlike dogs, have naturally occurring alloantibodies to blood groups other than their own, even without previous transfusion. Type A is the overwhelmingly prevalent type in domestic mixed-breed cats in the United States. Some purebred cats (notably the Devon Rex and British Shorthair) have a high incidence of type B blood. If a cat with type A is given type B blood, the transfusion will typically be hemolyzed within 48 hours; however, if a cat with type B is given type A blood, a fatal transfusion reaction is likely to occur. Thus, **all** recipient cats should be typed or cross-matched prior to transfusion. In cats requiring multiple transfusions, cross-matching may be warranted each time, particularly in cats that have had prior transfusion reactions.

Blood Collection and Processing

Although historically in veterinary medicine, fresh whole blood was collected as needed from either clinic animals or pets belonging to the staff of veterinary hospitals, this is considered antiquated and is not advised if it is possible to avoid. Blood banking is commonly performed in the larger veterinary hospitals. Several large commercial blood banks for animals also exist (Appendix 3-1). The purpose of a blood bank is to provide a readily available source of packed red blood cells or plasma for use in hospitalized patients. Most veterinary blood banks rely on client and staff-owned animals. Pre-donation screening is strongly recommended for the donors. Typically, screening involves a physical examination, a complete blood count, and chemistry profile. Species-specific screening for cats includes testing for feline leukemia and feline immunodeficiency viruses, and for dogs, heartworm testing. In some geographic locations, testing for exposure to tick-borne diseases such as Erhlichia is also recommended. The American College of Veterinary Internal Medicine has published a consensus statement concerning the recommended pre-testing of animal donors.[13]

The ideal feline donor is a large (more than 8- to 10-pound) well mannered adult cat. Most if not all cats require some sedation for donation. Frequently used sedatives include ketamine, narcotics, and diazepam. Feline blood donors should be carefully ausculted prior to sedation, as occult cardiomyopathies are not rare and could contribute to morbidity or mortality for the donor cat. Approximately 50 ml of whole blood may be collected from a donor cat. Blood may be collected as frequently as every 4 weeks, although with pet cats the donation interval is typically 2 to 3 months. The blood may be anticoagulated with heparin if it is to be used immediately, or with citrate-phosphate-dextrose-adenine (CPDA-1) for storage. Cat blood is often transfused as either fresh or stored whole blood, although interest has been growing in the use of components in cats as well (Figure 3-1).

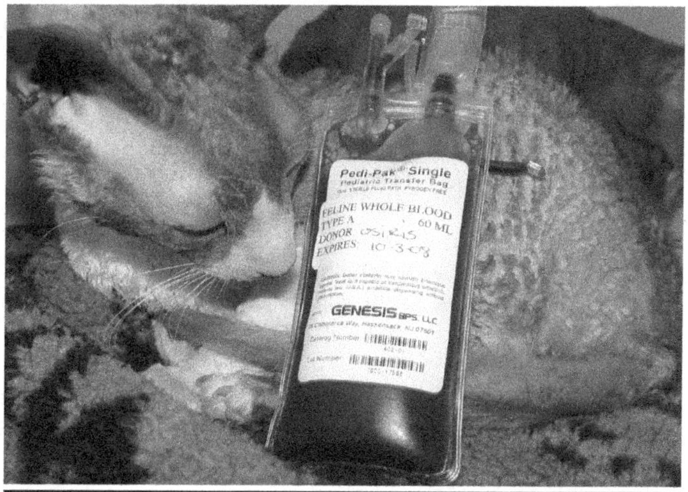

Figure 3-1. A cat following collection of one unit of fresh whole blood.

The canine blood donor is typically a large breed (more than than 50 pounds) well mannered adult dog. Unlike cats, typically dogs do not require any sedation (Figure 3-2). Approximately 1 unit (450 ml) may be collected from each donor. Generally, canine blood is collected into bags containing CPDA-1 designed for human blood donation. Canine blood is almost always divided into components to best utilize the available resources.[3] The different blood products that are available include fresh and stored whole blood, packed red blood cells, platelet-rich plasma, fresh frozen plasma, stored frozen plasma, cryoprecipitate, and cryo-poor plasma. (Table 3-2) The most widely used components are packed red blood cells and fresh frozen plasma. The blood components are prepared by separating and processing the units after collection.

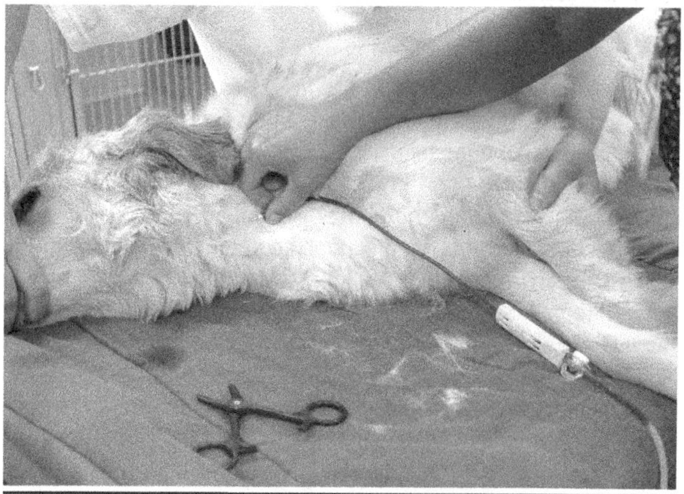

Figure 3-2. A golden retriever donating a unit of blood.

Fresh whole blood (FWB) contains red blood cells, platelets, leukocytes and plasma. Fresh whole blood is blood that is transfused within 8 hours of collection. The primary indications for transfusion with fresh whole blood include hemorrhage (resulting in loss of both red cells and plasma), thrombocytopenia with active hemorrhage, and lack of other available blood components. If a freshly collected unit of whole blood is not to be used within 8 hours, it should be separated into components or refrigerated at 4°C. Whole blood may be stored for up to 35 days, depending on the anticoagulant-preservative used. Stored whole blood contains viable red blood cells and plasma proteins such as

Table 3-2. Characteristics of Blood and Blood Components Available for Transfusion for Dogs.

Product	Contents	Advantages	Disadvantages
Fresh whole blood	Red blood cells, white cells, platelets and plasma	No processing, replaces shed blood	Potential waste of resources, volume overload, short shelf life (8 hours)
Stored whole blood	Red blood cells and plasma	No processing	Potential waste of resources, volume overload
Fresh frozen plasma	Clotting factors, including V, VIII, von Willebrand factor, albumin and antithrombin	Rich in clotting factors, useful in some coagulopathies	Limited source of albumin, stable for 1 year; if thawed and not used, may be re-frozen as stored plasma
Stored plasma	Some clotting factors (II, VII, IX, X), albumin, antithrombin	Useful in some coagulopathies (e.g., anticoagulant rodenticide), source of plasma proteins	Stable for 5 years
Cryoprecipitate	Concentrated form of clotting factors (specifically VIII, von Willebrand factor and fibrinogen)	Useful if volume overload from fresh frozen plasma a concern; cryo-poor component may be used for albumin and other plasma proteins	Extra step to prepare from fresh frozen plasma

albumin and globulin (although labile coagulation factors V and VIII will lose their activity). The primary indication for the use of stored whole blood is hemorrhage or the lack of other readily available components.

Commonly, individual units of canine whole blood are processed into components. The red cell portion of the unit is called packed red blood cells (pRBC). Packed red blood cells are prepared by spinning a unit of fresh whole blood at 4°C at 5000 rpm for 15 minutes and removing the majority of the plasma. A unit of pRBC may be stored for approximately 35 days at 4°C, depending on the anticoagulant-preservative used. The average hematocrit of a unit of pRBC is 70 to 80%. Typically, a unit of packed red cells is re-suspended in saline (0.9%) prior to transfusion. The ammonia levels will increase in stored red cells and the glucose level (because of the preservatives) will be high (> 500 mg/dl).[14] However, the clinical significance of this effect is unknown at this time, and packed red blood cells are indicated to provide oxygen-carrying support to anemic animals requiring such support regardless of underlying cause. In a patient with suspected severe hepatic encephalopathy, it may be prudent to avoid packed cells at the end of their shelf life.

Plasma may be classified as fresh frozen plasma, stored plasma, platelet-rich plasma, cryoprecipate, or cryo-poor plasma, depending on how the unit of whole blood is processed. The types of plasma differ in their relative number and efficacy of the clotting factors. Fresh frozen plasma (FFP) is prepared by separating a unit of fresh whole blood within 6 hours of collection. Fresh frozen plasma is a good source of all the clotting factors including V, VIII, and von Willebrand factor. Fresh frozen plasma is stable for up to 1 year if stored at -40°C. After 1 year, the more labile factor activity is diminished and the unit is termed stored plasma. Stored plasma may also be produced at any point from a unit of stored whole blood or if FFP is inadvertently thawed and then refrozen. Stored plasma has adequate amounts of factors II, VII, IX, and X (the vitamin K-dependant factors), and also albumin.

Platelet-rich plasma may be made by centrifugation of fresh whole blood at lower than normal speeds (2000 rpm). Platelet concentrates have also been described in dogs. Practically, transfusions of platelet-rich plasma or platelet concentrates is rarely performed in veterinary medicine because of the technical requirements for preparation of the products.[15,16]

Cryoprecipitate may be prepared by thawing and centrifuging partially thawed fresh frozen plasma. Cryoprecipate is rich in clotting factors VIII, von Willebrand factor, and fibrinogen. It also contains clotting factors IX, XI, and XIII. It is stable for 1 year after the initial collection of the plasma. The cryo-poor component may also be used for some clotting factors and albumin. Cryoprecipitate was initially created for use in people with congenital coagulopathies requiring multiple transfusions in whom volume overload with plasma products was a concern.

Indications for Transfusion

Indications for transfusion are plentiful in injured or ill animals. It is helpful to divide the indications for transfusion into absolutely indicated and potentially indicated. Transfusions carry the risk of reaction or possibly even disease transmission and certainly can add extra expense. Transfusions are considered primarily indicated to treat anemia and coagulopathy. In surgical patients, transfusions may be particularly warranted prior to anesthesia to improve the oxygen-carrying capacity and decrease the potential for anesthetic complications.

Anemia

Anemia should be divided into normovolemic anemia and hypovolemic anemia. Animals that are anemic with a normal volume status typically have either nonregenerative or hemolytic anemias. In these animals the anemia may have been longstanding and/or accompanied by a relative increase in plasma volume. Normovolemic anemic patients appear relatively bright, have normal to slightly elevated total solids, and have pale rather than white mucous membranes.

Normovolemic anemic patients require slow administration of packed red cells to avoid volume overload. In comparison, hypovolemic anemic patients have typically suffered from catastrophic blood loss within the last 12 to 24 hours. These patients are very weak, have rapid and faint pulses, and mucous membranes that appear more pale than their hematocrit might suggest. Their total solids are almost invariably low. These patients require aggressive volume resuscitation as well as blood transfusion. It is not uncommon to find that the post transfusion hematocrit may be lower that the starting point as a result of dilution of the circulating volume with crystalloids or colloids. It is crucial for the clinician to remember that oxygen delivery may be improved dramatically by increasing blood volume (and thereby letting cardiac output improve) even in the face of a lower number for the hematocrit. Massive transfusion, defined as one entire blood volume (90 ml/kg over 24 hours or half a blood volume over 3 hours) has been described in dogs.[17]

Packed red cells are usually transfused at either a dose of 1 ml per pound of body weight x the desired increase in hematocrit (Table 3-3) or simply in increments of 1/4, 1/2, or 1 unit. Each unit of packed red cells contains approximately 225 to 250 ml.

Table 3-3. Calculation of the Volume of Blood to Transfuse. This formula assumes lack of active Hemorrhage and stable Intravascular Volume. In Hemorrhaging Animals, Blood should be Transfused to an acceptable Cardiovascular End-point.

Need to know:
Recipent's PCV and body weight
Desired PCV
Hematocrit of transfusate- Assume 75% for packed red blood cells (pRBCs)
Each 1 ml/ pound of body weight (2.2 ml/kg) will raise the PCV by 1%: e.g., in a 44 # dog, PCV is 15%, you want to make it 25%.
10 (% increase) x 44 (bw) = 440 ml of packed red cell required.

Coagulopathy

Blood or plasma transfusions are also considered indicated to treat coagulopathy from decreased coagulation factors. (Tables 3-4 and 3-5) This may be inherited or acquired. Coagulopathy may be a difficult term to completely define. The normal coagulation system has a relatively large pool of circulating inactive coagulation factors, which are available if massive hemorrhage ensues. The methods of routinely assessing coagulation (prothrombin time, activated partial thromboplastin time, activated clotting time) typically rely on the detection of the formation of a fibrin clot. By the time these assays are abnormal, much of the coagulation ability is lost. Inherited coagulopathies that may benefit from plasma transfusion include hemophilia A or B, von Willebrand disease, and other specific coagulation factor deficiencies. Acquired coagulopathies are common in critically ill animals and include anticoagulant rodenticide toxicities, liver failure, and possibly disseminated intravascular coagulation (DIC). Coagulopathy is markedly worsened by hypothermia and acidosis. Plasma is usually given at a dose of 8 to15 ml/kg, repeated every 12 hours as needed until normalization of the coagulation times. Plasma is also commonly transfused at 1/4, 1/2, or full unit volumes. A full unit of plasma is approximately 225 to 250 ml.

Table 3-4. Criteria for Transfusion of packed Red Blood Cells.

Packed cell volume < 15%
Packed cell volume < 21% and surgical or anesthetic procedure planned
Acute blood loss, packed cell volume < 30% and heart rate > 150 bpm

Table 3-5. Criteria for Transfusion of Plasma

Documented acquired coagulopathy, with prolongation of prothrombin time and activated partial thromboplastin times
Inherited coagulopathy and planned surgical intervention (Evaluate on a case by case basis)
Very small [< 5 kg (11 lbs)] patient with profound hypoproteinemia

Other Indications

Transfusions are also potentially indicated with therapy of sepsis/multiple organ dysfunction syndrome, pancreatitis, hypoalbuminemia, and DIC without associated laboratory-proven coagulopathy. It appears commonplace among clinicians to want to give plasma when animals appear critically ill. However, it is prudent to try to determine what the end-point of transfusion is (i.e., normalization of a specific laboratory parameter versus cardiovascular parameter versus other). Correction of an albumin deficit is usually impractical in all but very small patients as much of the patient's albumin is actually extravascular.

Thrombocytopenia

In patients with severe thrombocytopenia that require surgical intervention, attention to meticulous hemostasis is mandatory. In these specific cases, transfusion with platelets in the form of fresh whole blood, platelet-rich plasma, or platelet concentrates may be appropriate. Practically, it is essential that the surgical team recognizes the time constraints (45-60 minutes) of either collection of fresh whole blood and/or processing into platelet-rich plasma or platelet concentrates.

Thus, while transfusions may be beneficial for a variety of reasons, it is wise to carefully consider the predicted benefit in each patient and post-transfusion to try to assess whether that benefit was reached.

Transfusion Administration and Reactions

Transfusions of both plasma and pRBC should be completed within 4 hours. Transfusions should be administered through filters and may be allow to either flow in by gravity or through the use of specific fluid pumps. If concurrent fluid therapy is warranted, the transfusate should not be allowed to mix with a crystalloid solution that contains calcium (e.g., lactated Ringer's solution) as the calcium may interfere with the action of the anticoagulant citrate.

Complications are possible with blood transfusions and deserve mention. (Table 3-6) Transfusion reactions occur from time to time, but the actual incidence is not well established in dogs and cats. Studies in dogs have reported transfusion reactions occurring in 2.9 to 13% of cases, with the majority of reactions being mild.[6,18] Transfusion reactions are usually classified as immune- or nonimmune-mediated and acute (within 48 hours) or delayed. Immunologic reactions may include hemolysis or hypersensitivity reactions (such as urticaria or facial swelling). Nonimmunologic reactions may include circulatory overload, bacterial contamination, hyperammonemia, or infectious disease transmission. It is important to monitor the patient carefully for any signs of problems (vomiting, fever, hemoglobinuria/hemoglobinemia). Delayed transfusion reactions, when they occur, are likely due to the development of alloantibodies.[19] Rarely, transfusion-related acute lung injury (TRALI) may occur, although the syndrome has been much better described in people.[20]

Table 3-6. Clinical signs Associated with Acute and Delayed Transfusion Reactions.

Acute reaction
Fever
Vomiting
Hypersensitivity (Urticaria)
Hemoglobinuria and hemoglobinemia (e.g., intravascular hemolysis)
Cardiovascular collapse
Delayed reaction
Bilirubinemia and bilirubinuria (e.g., Extravascular hemolysis)
Development of a positive Coombs test
Shortened transfusate survival

The standard monitoring during a transfusion should include measurement of temperature, pulse, and respiration every 15 minutes for the first hour, then hourly, and monitoring for increased respiratory effort, vomiting, pigmentuia or signs of facial swelling. The most life-threatening type of transfusion reaction is the acute hemolytic transfusion reaction. This occurs most commonly when a previously sensitized DEA 1.1-or 1.2-negative recipient is given DEA 1.1- or 1.2-positive blood. The severity of these reactions varies, but the reactions are most severe when complement is activated by IgM antibody. The release of vasoactive mediators during an acute hemolytic transfusion reaction can lead to shock, DIC, and multiple organ failure. Diagnosis of an acute hemolytic transfusion reaction is usually based on suspicious clinical findings such as development of hemoglobinuria, hemoglobinemia, and fever shortly after blood transfusion in an animal that may have been transfused 4 or more days earlier. If an acute hemolytic transfusion reaction is suspected, the transfusion should be stopped immediately and supportive care to maintain vital organ perfusion should begin. Supportive care may include IV fluid administration, furosemide, dopamine, or mannitol to prevent or treat acute renal failure. It may include fresh frozen plasma administration if DIC is suspected. Monitoring should include careful measurement of systemic arterial pressure, central venous pressure, and urine output.

Delayed hemolytic transfusion reactions may occur 3 to 21 days after a blood transfusion. These reactions usually involve extravascular hemolysis and are mediated by IgG antibody. These reactions are typically mild. Fever is common, and anorexia or icterus has been reported.[18] A positive Coombs test provides strong support for the suspicion of a delayed hemolytic reaction in a patient that was previously Coombs negative. Specific treatment is not usually required. The lifespan of transfused red blood cells may be shortened, resulting in the need for further transfusion.

Conclusions

Transfusion medicine represents a vital adjuvant to clinical practice. Basic tenets of transfusion medicine include knowledge of benefits and risks surrounding transfusion and concepts associated with practical transfusion. For surgical patients in particular, careful planning is advisable to avoid emergent crisis.

Appendix 3-1. Resources for Transfusion Medicine (Current as of 8/2008)

Collection bags
BAXTER/FENWAL Product 4R-34-20NM
3 bag system for pRBCS, and plasma- Contains ADSOL as a preservative

Blood typing cards
RapidVet-H
DMS Laboratories, Inc.
2 Darts Mill Road
Flemington, NJ 08822
Tel: (800) 567-4DMS

Animal Blood banks
Eastern Veterinary Blood Bank
808 Bestgate Rd. Suite 111
Annapolis, MD 21401
1-800-949-EVBB
www.evbb.com

Animal Blood Bank
1-800-243-5759
www.animalbloodbank.com
California

The Pet Blood Bank
1-800-906-7059/1-877-212-4134
www.PetsHelpingPets.com
3610 Lohman Ford Road Suite 100
LagoVista, TX 78645

Midwest Animal Blood Services Inc.
4983 Bird Drive, Stockbridge, Michigan 49285
Toll Free: 877-517-MABS
Office: 517-851-8244
Fax: 517-851-7762
http://www.midwestabs.com

Hemopet- California
http://hemopet.free.fr/index.html

References

1. Klaser Da, Reine NJ, Hohenhaus AE: Red blood cell transfusion in cats: 126 cases (1999). J Am Vet Med Assoc 226:920-923, 2005.

2. Castellanos I, Couto CG, Gray TL: Clinical use of blood products in cats: a retrospective study (1997-2000). J Vet Intern Med 18:529-532, 2004.

3. Lucas RL, Lentz KD, Hale AS: Collection and preparation of blood products. Clin Tech Small Anim Pract 19:55-62, 2004.

4. Logan JC, Callan MB, Drew K, et al: Clinical indications for use of fresh frozen plasma in dogs: 74 cases (October through December 1999). J Am Vet Med Assoc 218:1449-1455, 2001.

5. Callan MB, Oakley DA, Shofer FS, et al: Canine red blood cell transfusion practice. J Ann Anim Hosp Assoc 32:303-311, 1996.

6. Kerl ME, Hohenhaus AE: Packed red cell transfusions in dogs: 131 cases, J Am Vet Med Assoc 202:1495-1499, 1993.

7. Brownlee L, Waldrop KJ, Sellon RK, et al: Use of prestorage leukoreduction filter effectively removes leukocytes from canine whole blood while preserving red blood cell viability. J Vet Intern Med 14:412-417, 2000.

8. Gopegui RR, Feldman BF: Use of blood and blood components in canine and feline patients with hemostatic disorders. Vet Clin North Am Small Anim Pract 25:1387-1402, 1995.

9. Hale AS: Canine blood groups and their importance in veterinary transfusion medicine. Vet Clin North Am Small Anim Pract. 25:1323-1332, 1995.

10. Melzer KJ, Waldrop KJ, Hale AS, et al: A hemolytic transfusion reaction due to DEA 4 alloantibodies in a dog. J Vet Intern Med 17:931-933, 2003.

11. Griot-Wenk ME, Giger U: Feline transfusion medicine. Blood types and their clinical importance. Vet Clin North Am Small Anim Pract 25:1305-1322, 1995.

12. Weinstein NM, Blais MC, Greiner K, et al: A new blood group antigen in domestic shorthair cats: the feline MIK red cell antigen. J Vet Intern Med 19:400, 2005.

13. Wardrop KJ, Reine N, Birkenheuer A, et al: Canine and feline blood donor screening for infectious disease. J Vet Intern Med 19:135-142, 2005.

14. Waddell LS, Holt D, Hughes D, et al: The effect of storage on ammonia concentration in canine packed red blood cells. J Vet Emerg Crit Care 11:23-26, 2001.

15. Abrams-Ogg AC, Kruth SA, Carter RF, et al: Preparation and transfusion of platelet concentrates. Am J Vet Res 54:635-642, 1993.

16. Abrams-Ogg AC: Triggers for prophylactic use of platelet transfusion and optimal platelet dosing in thrombocytopenic dogs and cats. Vet Clin North Am Small Anim Pract 33:1401-1418, 2003.

17. Jutkowitz LA, Rozanski EA, Moreau JA, Rush JE: Massive transfusion in dogs: 15 cases (1997-2001). J Am Vet Med Assoc 220:1664-1669, 2002.

18. Harrell KA, Kristensen AT: Canine transfusion reactions and their management. Vet Clin North Am Small Anim Pract. 25:1333-64. 1995.

19. Callan MB, Jones LT, Giger U: Hemolytic transfusion reactions in a dog with an alloantibody to a common antigen. J Vet Intern Med: 9:277-279, 1995.

20. Boshkov LK: Transfusion-related acute lung injury and the ICU. Crit Care Clin 21(3):479-495, 2005.

Chapter 4

Hemostasis and Disseminated Intravascular Coagulation

Daniel L. Chan

Overview of Hemostasis

Hemostasis is a complex but elegant process of forming blood clots to seal injured vessels and degrading such clots after they have served their purpose. The various reactions that comprise hemostasis are traditionally conceptionalized as having three distinct phases: primary hemostasis, secondary hemostasis, and fibrinolysis. Primary hemostasis involves the formation of a platelet plug. Secondary hemostasis begins with cross-linking of fibrin strands and stabilization of the platelet plug to form a mature clot. The degradation of the mature clot describes the process of fibrinolysis. While this over-simplified scheme is useful in the evaluation of coagulation, especially in relation to typical laboratory coagulation tests, it is important to realize that *in vivo*, coagulation likely proceeds in a different manner. More recently, a new "cell-based" model of coagulation has been proposed to better explain the process of coagulation that occurs in the body.[1,2] The purpose of this review is to outline the classical approach to coagulation, introduce newer concepts in coagulation, and describe perturbations in coagulation that may culminate in disseminated intravascular coagulation (DIC). A discussion of coagulation tests, their interpretation and rational therapy of coagulation disorders completes this overview of hemostasis.

Primary Hemostasis

The inciting events leading to activation of coagulation are endothelial damage and subsequent exposure of collagen on the subendothelial surface. One of the mechanisms by which platelets adhere to the subendothelium is mediated by von Willebrand factor (VWF). A key event is the bridging between exposed collagen and various platelet surface glycoprotein receptors via VWF. Following adhesion, platelets release substances including adenosine diphosphate (ADP), serotonin, and platelet activating factor (PAF), which serve to activate platelets. This is followed by aggregation forming the temporary hemostatic plug. The formation of this temporary plug is referred to as primary hemostasis and is degraded within minutes. Concomitant with platelet aggregation, platelets release a large number of procoagulants and clotting factors, providing an optimum environment for activating the coagulation cascade and, thereby, initiation of secondary hemostasis.

Secondary Hemostasis

Stabilization of the temporary platelet plug with cross-linked fibrin strands derived from serine proteases constitutes secondary hemostasis. Traditionally, this process was thought to be composed of intrinsic, extrinsic, and common pathways (Figure 4-1). Similarly to activation of primary hemostasis, an irregular vascular surface is the contact stimulus necessary for activating factor XII into factor XIIa, which initiates the intrinsic (factors XI, IX, VIII) pathway. The extrinsic pathway is initiated by the release of tissue factor (TF), a transmembrane glycoprotein present in most nonendothelial cell membranes (e.g., fibroblasts, vascular smooth muscle cells, monocytes). Tissue factor complexes with factor VII, and subsequently activates factors IX and X. Once factor X is activated, the common pathway of coagulation is initiated. Activated factors X and V culminate the conversion of prothrombin to thrombin, and finally thrombin converts fibrinogen into fibrin. Thrombin is also responsible for activating factor XIII which serves to cross-link fibrin strands and stabilize the clot, increasing its resistance to proteolytic degradation. Although the different pathways were once viewed as discrete events, it is now recognized that direct interactions occur between the pathways; the TF:factor VIIa complex (extrinsic pathway) also activates factors IX and X (intrinsic pathway). Nevertheless, the traditional scheme of secondary hemostasis offers a way to interpret common coagulation tests such as the prothrombin time (PT) and activated partial thromboplastin time (aPTT).

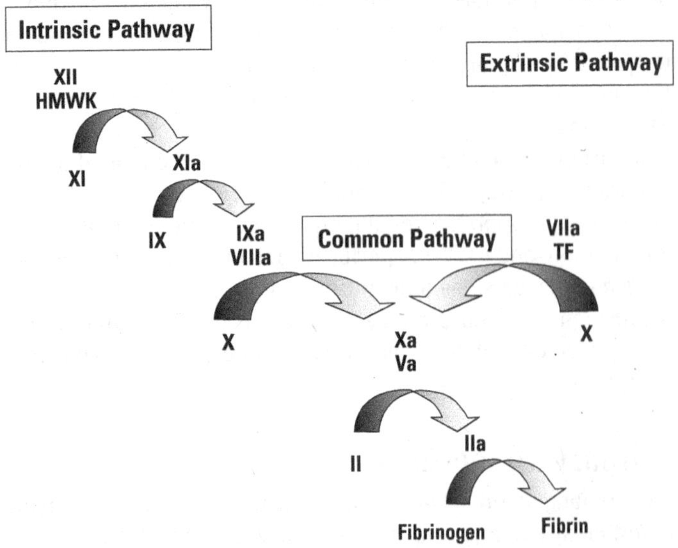

Figure 4-1. Classic coagulation cascade depicting reactions involved in the intrinsic, extrinsic, and common pathways, culminating in the production of the fibrin clot. HMWK = High molecular weight kalikrein, TF = tissue factor.

Fibrinolysis

Once the hemostatic plug has served its purpose it must be degraded and removed from the intravascular space. In addition to lysing fibrin and fibrinogen, plasmin biodegrades factors V, VIII, IX, and XI. Plasminogen, a proenzyme, is activated into plasmin by either factor XIIa or by a variety of poorly defined tissue factors. Several tissue activators of plasminogen have been recognized, including streptokinase, urokinase, and tissue plasminogen activator, and they may be used therapeutically in patients with thromboembolic disorders. The fibrinolytic system also has built-in inhibitory mechanisms that have a net procoagulant effect. Inhibitors of fibrinolysis include alpha-2 antiplasmin, alpha-2 macroglobulin and tissue plasminogen activator inhibitors 1 and 2. Plasmin biodegrades fibrinogen and fibrin-generating fibrin(ogen) degradation products (FDPs) that can be detected in plasma of dogs and cats. These FDPs also exert profound inhibitory effects on platelet function, contributing to the petechia and ecchymoses noted in patients with DIC.

New Model of Coagulation

Although the classic coagulation cascade is a convenient scheme that allows clinical assessment of coagulation status, it fails to explain why patients with severe congenital factor XII or XI deficiency do not exhibit significant bleeding disorders. In addition, it does not adequately explain why patients with deficiencies in factor VII but with intact intrinsic factors suffer from pronounced bleeding tendencies. It became apparent that coagulation in vivo must proceed differently from that demonstrated *in vitro*. A new model of coagulation emphasizes the role played by platelets and TF-bearing cells; hence it is referred to as the cell-based model of hemostasis (Figure 4-2).[1,2] This model is described as having three phases: initiation, amplification, and propagation (Figure 4-3).[1]

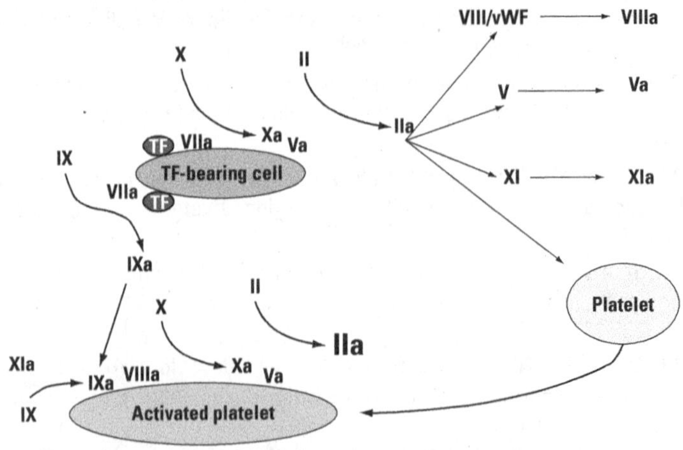

Figure 4-2. Cell-based model of coagulation. Tissue factor (TF)-bearing cells first activate factor VII into VIIa. The TF:VIIa complex converts X and IX into Xa and IXa, respectively. Xa combines with Va and generates a small amount of thrombin, which activates platelets and other coagulation factors. The surface of activated platelets then becomes the site of major thrombin generation necessary for fibrin formation. vWF = von Willebrand factor, TF = tissue factor.

During the *initiation phase*, vascular injury exposes TF expressed on TF-bearing cells such as fibroblasts, smooth muscle cells, and monocytes. Factor VII becomes activated when complexed with TF. This complex proceeds to activate small amounts of factors IX and X. Activated factor X combines and activates factor V on the surface of the TF-bearing cell to produce a prothrombinase complex that generates thrombin. The small amount of thrombin generated is insufficient to catalyze fibrin generation and is limited to the vicinity of the TF-bearing cell. However, this small amount of thrombin serves as a priming mechanism for subsequent hemostatic events (see Figure 4-2).

Platelet activation is central to the *amplification phase*, which sets the stage for subsequent large-scale generation of thrombin. The thrombin generated in the initiation phase stimulates release of factor V from circulating platelets, disengages factor VIII from VWF, and activates factors V, VIII, and XI on the platelet surface. Activated platelets also express receptors and binding sites for activated clotting factors. Uncoupled VWF can now mediate additional platelet adhesion and aggregation. The importance of the amplification phase is that platelets that were not directly stimulated by the inciting vessel-wall injury are recruited to participate in active coagulation.

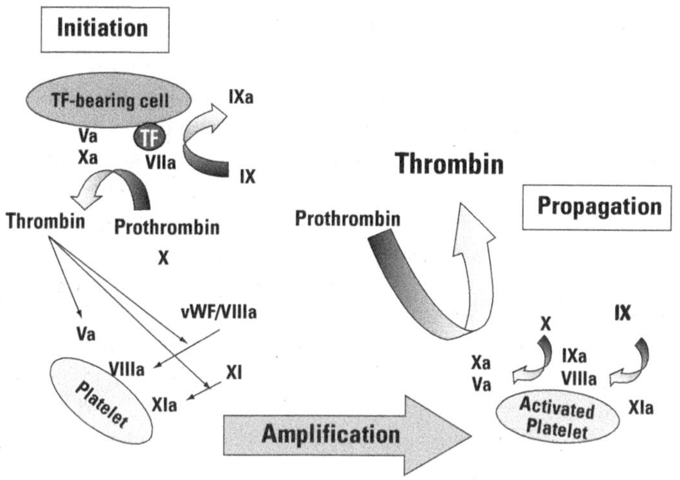

Figure 4-3. Stages of the cell-based model of coagulation. Initiation occurs on TF-bearing cells and results in the production of a small amount of thrombin. Thrombin produced by the initiation stage, activates platelets and other coagulation factors. Propagation occurs on the surface of activated platelets and results in the production of significant amounts of thrombin required for fibrin formation.

The *propagation phase* is typified by the production of thrombin and fibrin from their inactive precursors (see Figure 4-3). Activated factor XI produced in the amplification phase converts more factor IX into activated factor IX. Activated factor IX combines with its cofactor VIIIa to form the "tenase complex" (IXa/VIIIa). The tenase complex then recruits additional factor X from solution yielding more Xa on the surface of the platelet. Activated factor X, binds to activated factor V to form the "prothrombinase complex" that leads to a burst of thrombin generation of sufficient magnitude to clot fibrinogen and to the generation of the hemostatic plug.

Once the bleeding is abated, the clotting process must be limited to avoid thrombotic occlusion of adjacent normal areas of the vasculature. This may be thought of as a *termination phase*. The protein C/protein S/thrombomodulin system is an important mechanism confining coagulation to the site of injury.[3] Some of the thrombin generated during coagulation can diffuse away from the site of vascular injury. When thrombin reaches an intact endothelial cell, it binds to thrombomodulin (TM) expressed on the endothelial surface. The endothelial thrombin/TM complex then activates protein C, which binds to its cofactor protein S and inactivates any factors Va and VIIIa. This system illustrates the anticoagulant tendencies of the intact endothelium.

Disseminated Intravascular Coagulation

Rather than a disease, DIC is the pathologic consequence of many different disorders. It is characterized by an acute, generalized, widespread activation of coagulation, resulting in thromboembolic complications because of intravascular formation of fibrin, as well as diffuse hemorrhage, because of the consumption of platelets and coagulation factors.[4-6] Widespread fibrin deposition is associated with the genesis of multiple organ failure and poor outcome.[4-8] The clinical situation with simultaneous thrombosis and bleeding poses a difficult problem for the clinician in that replenishment of clotting factors with plasma does not attenuate the risk for thrombosis.

As DIC is always secondary to an underlying disorder, rational therapy should always be targeted at the primary disease. Common diseases associated with DIC are listed in Table 4-1. Disease processes characterized by capillary stasis, loss of vascular integrity, red cell hemolysis, inappropriate particulate matter in blood, or necrotic tissue release of tissue thromboplastin into the vasculature can produce this life-threatening complication.

Table 4-1. Common Disorders that may be Associated with DIC in Animals

Sepsis/severe infection
Severe trauma
Malignancy
Heat stroke
Severe burns
Severe hepatic failure
Pancreatitis
Hemolytic transfusion reactions
Adverse drug reactions
Immune-mediated hemolytic anemia

The pathogenesis of DIC in patients with severe infections may involve exposure to specific cell membrane components of microorganisms (e.g., lipopolysaccharides) or bacterial exotoxins. A generalized systemic inflammatory response ensues, characterized by the elevation of several cytokines. Cytokines, produced mainly by activated mononuclear cells and endothelial cells are partially responsible for the derangement of the coagulation system in DIC.[4-9] Neutrophil activation leads to platelet activation and decrease in antithrombin activity. Disturbances in the antithrombogenic functions of the endothelium induce adherence of platelets and granulocytes through the expression of cell adhesion molecules, such as P-, E-, and L-selectins, endothelial leukocyte-adhesion molecules (ELAM), such as ELAM-1, and intercellular adhesion molecule-1 (ICAM-1).[4-8] During this excessive intravascular coagulation, platelets are consumed in large quantities, causing thrombocytopenia. Tissue factor, which is exposed following injury to the endothelium and by activated monocytes, triggers the initiation of the coagulation cascade on the local endothelial surface.

Local generation of thrombin leads to the formation of thrombi. In this process of self-perpetuating coagulation, coagulation factors are consumed. Once the fibrinolytic system is activated, inactivation of clotting factors, and impaired platelet function follows. Fibrin degradation products, produced by clot lysis, are strong inhibitors of platelet function. Antithrombin, along with proteins C and S, are soon depleted in attempts to halt intravascular coagulation. The fibrinolytic system becomes inhibited by the release of plasminogen activator inhibitor 1 (PAI-1). PAI-1 release is chiefly mediated by TNF, endotoxin, IL-1, and IL-6. This imbalance between the systems fosters fibrin deposition. The formation of fibrin within the microcirculation leads to hemolytic anemia as the red blood cells are sheared by the fibrin strands. As a result, fragmented red blood cells or schistocytes are found in circulation.

Assessment of Coagulation

Prothrombin time (PT) is the primary laboratory test to evaluate the status of the extrinsic pathway. For this test, blood is collected into tubes containing citrate, which binds calcium and halts coagulation. A thromboplastin reagent (source of TF) and calcium are added to initiate coagulation. The time to fibrin formation is measured in seconds and prolongation greater than 25% as compared with normal is considered significant. The PT is prolonged by deficiencies in factors II, V, VII, and X. Typically, prolongation in PT indicates that factor activity must be depleted to less than 30%.

The activated partial thromboplastin time (APTT) primarily reflects the integrity of the intrinsic pathway. As with measurement of PT, coagulation is halted by collecting blood into citrated tubes. An activator (e.g., kaolin, celite, propyl gallate) is added, supplying negatively charged particles similar to basement membranes to activate the contact group (i.e., factors XII, XI). Partial thromboplastin (source of phospholipids surfaces) and calcium are then added and the time to fibrin formation is recorded in seconds. Prolongations in APTT occur if factor activity of factors VIII, IX, X, XI, and XII decrease below 30%. Severe depression in factor activity of factors II and V and depletion of fibrinogen will also prolonged the APTT.

Activated clotting time (ACT) is a coarse assessment of the intrinsic pathway. Tubes containing diatomaceous earth provide a contact activator. Platelets supplied by whole blood, provide phopholipid membranes needed to support coagulation reaction. While normal reference ranges for PT and APTT depend on the particular reagents used, it is generally accepted that the normal ACT for dogs is 60 to 110 seconds and for cats 50 to 75 seconds.

Plasmin-mediated degradation of fibrinogen and fibrin produces several fragments (fragments X, Y, D, and E) collectively referred to as FDPs. The measurement of FDPs can be semi-quantitatively evaluated via agglutination techniques and is used as an indicator of active fibrinolysis. It is important to note that FDPs are produced from lysis of both cross-linked and non-cross-linked fibrin. As such, elevation in FDP concentration is merely an indicator of increased generation of fibrin and increased fibrinolysis. Kits to evaluate dimers of D fragments (D-dimers) are commercially available and are becoming more commonly used.[10,11] D-dimers are more specific for fibrinolysis (particularly of cross-linked fibrin), however, it does not distinguish between physiologic or pathologic fibrinolysis.

Diagnosis of DIC

The association between the development of DIC and poor outcome is the impetus for early diagnosis; however, therapy should be directed at the primary disease rather than at coagulation abnormalities. Despite the desire to identify afflicted patients, currently no consensus exists in definitively diagnosing DIC. Several criteria have been proposed, and many include abnormalities in any three coagulation parameters (prolongation in PT, APTT, decrease in platelet count, elevated FDPs or D-dimers, depleted fibrinogen or AT).[12,13] In people, DIC scores and algorithms have also been proposed but are not widely recognized.[6,14] Various veterinary publications have each defined their criteria slightly differently, making development of similar schemes impossible.[10,12,13] Moreover, abnormalities in coagulation parameters are not specific enough for DIC and can be encountered in many disorders with vastly different prognoses.

In the CBC, schistocytes are indicative of mechanical damage to red cell membranes from microvascular fibrin strands. Whereas the presence of schistocytes is suggestive of DIC, they are only recognized in approximately 10% of patients with DIC.[12,13] Platelet counts can be variable in DIC because some inflammatory states can cause a reactive thrombocytosis and, therefore, it is more important to perform daily blood smears and manual platelet counts, as a drop in the platelet count often precedes other signs of DIC. In the future, increased platelet factor 4 and beta-thrombomodulin measurements could become pathognomonic for platelet destruction in DIC.[4-7] Dysfunctional platelets, resulting in thrombocytopathia, are caused by FDPs coating platelet membranes, which causes the release of platelet procoagulant materials.

Therapy for DIC

As DIC is a reflection of complete dysregulation of hemostasis, reversal can occur only if the primary stimulus is eliminated. However, as elimination of the initiating cause of DIC is almost never immediately possible, focus of therapy has traditionally been directed at halting further intravascular coagulation (administration of plasma, heparin, aspirin), promotion of capillary blood flow (aggressive fluid therapy), and supporting target organs at risk for hemorrhage, microthrombi, or ischemia (maintenance of perfusion and oxygenation, correction of acid-base status).[3-7] Despite these generic recommendations, no studies exist supporting the use of such therapies at ameliorating or reversing DIC.[7] The most commonly employed therapies include administration of plasma and heparin, yet improvement in outcome has not been demonstrated in either people or animals with these approaches.[2,15,16] There is even a suggestion that while heparin does improve AT activity, it does so at the expense of potent anti-inflammatory properties of AT, making recommendations for heparin therapy questionable in patients with DIC.[2,15,16] In the future, strategies directed at inhibiting TF-mediated activation of coagulation or restoration of physiologic anticoagulant systems may prove beneficial.[7]

Conclusions

As hemostatic disorders are commonly encountered in critically ill patients, many of which require surgical intervention, an understanding of coagulation, its assessment, and relationship to disease pathogenesis is crucial for the clinician. Since surgical removal of tumors may be the most effective way to treat DIC, the presence of coagulation abnormalities alone does not preclude surgical interventions. Interpretation of coagulation tests must be done in the context of clinical situations so as to guide the most appropriate course of action. Discordant results of coagulation tests with clinical assessment of clinical or surgical bleeding may reflect differences between the processes of coagulation *in vitro* and those encountered *in vivo.* In spite of the progress in the understanding of coagulation, therapeutic decisions are still controversial and should be individualized on the basis and severity of the coagulation abnormality.

References

1. Hoffman M: Remodeling the blood coagulation cascade. J Thromb Thrombolysis 16:17, 2003.
2. Hopper K, Bateman SW: An updated view of hemostasis: mechanism of hemostatic dysfunction associated with sepsis. J Vet Emerg Crit Care 15:83, 2005.
3. Hambleton J, Leung LL, Levi M: Coagulation: Consultative hemostasis. Hematology (Am Soc Hematol Educ Program): 335, 2002.
4. Levi M, de Jonge E, Van der Poll T, et al: Disseminated intravascular coagulation. Thromb Haemostasis 82:695, 1999.
5. Levi M, Cate H: Disseminated intravascular coagulation. N Engl J Med 341:586, 1999.
6. Taylor FB, Toh CH, Hoots WK, et al. Scientific subcommittee on disseminated intravascular coagulation (DIC) of the international society on thrombosis and haemostasis: Towards definition, clinical and laboratory criteria, and a scoring system for DIC: Thromb Haemost 86:1327, 2001.
7. Franchini M, Manzato F: Update on the treatment of disseminated intravascular coagulation. Hematology 9:81, 2004.
8. Johnson V, Gaynor A, Chan DL, et al: Multiple organ failure in humans and dogs. J Vet Emerg Crit Care 14:158, 2004.
9. Marshall JC: Inflammation, coagulopathy, and the pathogenesis of multiple organ dysfunction syndrome. Crit Care Med: 29(7 Suppl):S99, 2001.
10. Stokol T, Brooks MB, Erb HN, et al: D-dimer concentrations in healthy dogs and dogs with disseminated intravascular coagulation. Am J Vet Res 61:393, 2000.
11. Griffin A, Callan MB, Schofer, et al: Evaluation of a canine D-dimer point-of-care test kit for use in samples obtained from dogs with disseminated intravascular coagulation, thromboembolic disease, and hemorrhage. Am J Vet Res 64:1562, 2003.
12. Bateman SW, Mathews KA, Abrams-Ogg AC, et al: Evaluation of point-of-care tests for diagnosis of disseminated intravascular coagulation in dogs admitted to an intensive care unit. J Am Vet Med Assoc 215:805, 1999.
13. Bateman SW, Mathews KA, Abrams-Ogg AC, et al: Diagnosis of disseminated intravascular coagulation in dogs admitted to an intensive care unit. J Am Vet Med Assoc 215:798, 1999.
14. Levi M, de Jonge E, Meijers J: The diagnosis of disseminated intravascular coagulation. Blood Reviews 16:217, 2002.
15. Opal SM, Kessler CM, Roemisch J, et al: Antithrombin, heparin, and heparin sulphate. Crit Care Med: 30(5 Suppl):S325, 2002.
16. Hoffman JN, Vollmar B, Laschke MW, et al: Adverse effect of heparin on antithrombin action during endotoxemia: microhemodynamic and cellular mechanisms. Thromb Haemost: 88:242, 2002.

Chapter 5

Metabolism and Nutrition of the Surgical Patient

Elisa M. Mazzaferro

During states of health, the body's neuroendocrine system is in a constant state of flux in order to maintain homeostasis. Alterations in host substrate metabolism and endocrine pathways have been documented in both human and veterinary patients with critical illness and neoplasia.[1-6] In general, stressors such as injury, neoplasia, infection, anesthesia, and surgery can adversely influence the body's physiologic adaptive mechanisms and disturb homeostasis (Figure 5-1). The changes observed in metabolic pathways are intimately related to changes in the body's hormonal axes, including suppression of thyroid hormone activity and host release of glucocounterregulatory hormones, including cortisol and glucagon. Activation of the hypothalamic-pituitary-adrenal axis, thyroid axis, renin-angiotensin-aldosterone system, and release of proinflammatory cytokines during states of illness and injury can lead to protein and calorie depletion, negative nitrogen balance, organ dysfunction, suppressed immunity, delayed wound healing, changes in resting energy requirements, and increased morbidity and mortality.[7-8] Nutritional intervention is one modality that should be considered in all cases of critically ill and surgical patients to help restore homeostasis and aid in the healing and recovery process.

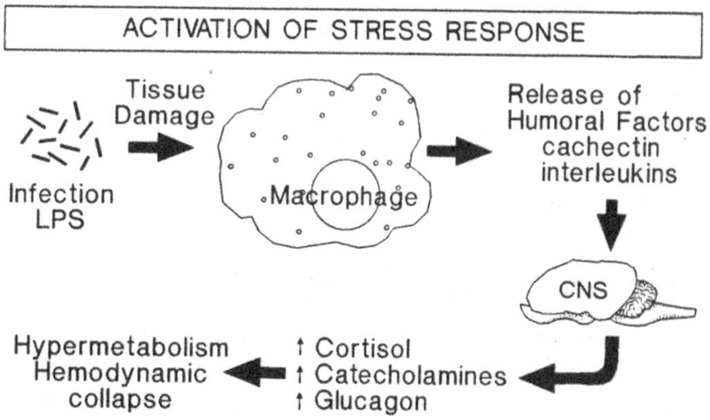

Figure 5-1. Activation of the stress response.

Stressed Versus Non-Stressed Starvation

In healthy patients, starvation occurs as a result of lack of available nutrients. This differs greatly from the "stressed starvation" that occurs in the face of illness and injury.

During non-stressed starvation, adaptations occur that favor utilization of fat for energy, sparing carbohydrate for glucose-dependent tissues and diverting host amino acids and protein to healing processes.[5,9] In healthy animals, hepatic glycogenolysis initially is utilized to maintain a state of euglycemia.[10] In dogs, hepatic glycogen becomes depleted within 48 to 72 hours,[11] and physiologic adaptations are utilized to break down muscle protein and provide gluconeogenic precursors such as alanine and glutamine for gluconeogenesis.[10,12] During non-stressed starvation, pyruvate becomes transaminated and is transported to the liver as alanine, where it becomes deaminated to pyruvate for gluconeogenesis. The kidney and the gastrointestinal tract also contribute alanine for gluconeogenesis, sparing muscle protein for other purposes. Skeletal muscle stores of alanine can become depleted during prolonged stressed starvation and can lead to dyshomeostasis and loss of function.[13] Obviously, continued proteolysis can result in lack of available amino acids for *de novo* protein synthesis and wound healing.

As starvation becomes more prolonged, down-regulation of the patient's metabolic rate and muscle proteolysis occurs, and the body adapts by reverting to lipolysis and fat oxidation for energy purposes. Muscle lactate, rather than muscle amino acids, are shuttled to the liver for gluconeogenesis by the Cori cycle (Figure 5-2) Although energy is formed in this process, it is largely an inefficient process by which the body maintains euglycemia.

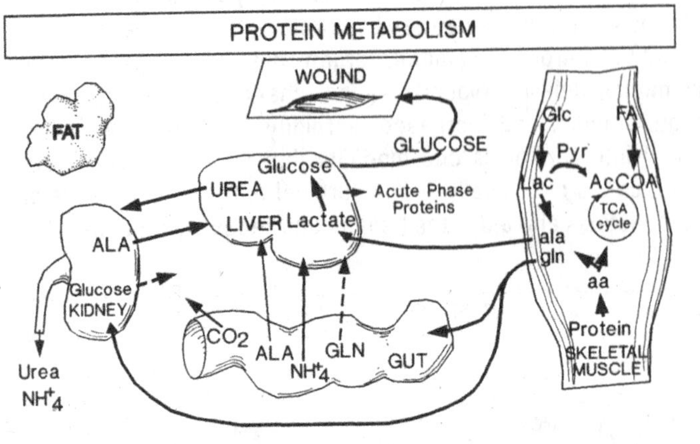

Figure 5-2. Protein metabolism.

Stressed Starvation

Lack of adequate nutrient intake is of particular importance in surgical patients and those with a variety of illnesses due to maladaptive responses that occur. Inadequate nutrient intake is common in veterinary patients during the pre- and post-operative periods. Many animals either cannot, or will not, voluntarily consume their nutritional requirements as a result of nausea, pain, facial masses or trauma, or anxiety. Food is often withheld in preparation for anesthesia and surgery. Sometimes, inadequate food orders can contribute to a decrease in nutrient intake, even in the realm of a hospital environment.[14] Suppression of resting energy expenditure occurs because of down–regulation of the hypothalamic-pituitary-adrenal axis. However, the release of proinflammatory cytokine mediators, including interleukin-1, interleukin-2, interleukin-10, and tumor necrosis factor (TNF), combined with the glucocounterregulatory hormones cortisol and glucagon has been implicated to play a role in the catabolic stress response.[15-17] Continued proteolysis in ongoing starvation leads to negative nitrogen balance.

During a variety of stressors, including anesthesia and surgery, activation of the sympathetic nervous system leads to the release of the catecholamine norepinephrine from peripheral nervous tissue and epinephrine from the adrenal medulla.[10] Activation of the hypothalamic-pituitary-adrenal axis leads to the release of cortisol from the adrenal cortex. Epinephrine indirectly stimulates hepatic glycogenolysis and gluconeogenesis. The actions of epinephrine also inhibit insulin release and promote the release of glucagon. An increase in glucagon relative to insulin helps to promote glycogenolysis, gluconeogenesis, and ureagenesis. Gluconeogenesis from muscle amino acids proceeds unchecked, and nitrogen utilization is increased relative to intake. Accelerated protein catabolism in stressed patients and urinary nitrogen loss contributes to protein-calorie malnutrition.[17] Negative nitrogen balance is characteristic of a catabolic state.

During stress, muscle protein appears to be the primary source of energy used for fuel, with approximately 25% of calories obtained from utilization of endogenous proteins.[15] In addition to endogenous nitrogen, amino acids are shuttled into the production of hepatic acute-phase protein synthesis during stress and illness. In canine surgical and critically ill patients, accelerated urinary nitrogen loss can occur even in the presence of enteral and parenteral nutritional supplementation.[16] As a result of diminished structure and functional protein synthesis, depressed immune function, impaired wound healing, and cardiorespiratory dysfunction can occur (Table 5-1).[18-20]

Table 5-1. Adverse Consequences of Malnutrition

Decreased protein synthesis
Delayed wound healing
Hypoalbuminemia
Increased risk of surgical site dehiscence
Enterocyte atrophy with increased bacterial translocation and nutrient malabsorption
Cardiac myocyte atrophy, decreased cardiac output, ventricular dysrhythmias
Respiratory muscle fatigue, hypercapnia, respiratory acidosis
Immune system suppression, increased risk of sepsis

Impaired carbohydrate utilization can also occur during critical illness. Any stressor, including surgery and anesthesia, that results in the release of glucocounterregulatory hormones, namely epinephrine, cortisol, and glucagon, can lead to impaired carbohydrate metabolism and inefficient glucose utilization. Glucocounterregulatory hormone release during illness can increase the synthesis of pyruvate carboxylase and phosphoenolpyruvate carboxylase, enzymes that favor the conversion of three-carbon intermediates to glucose.[21] As a result, glucose entry into the tricarboxylic acid (TCA) cycle is limited, and favors the shuttling of glucose through other pathways, including the Cori cycle or glucose-alanine shuttle (Figure 5-3).[21]

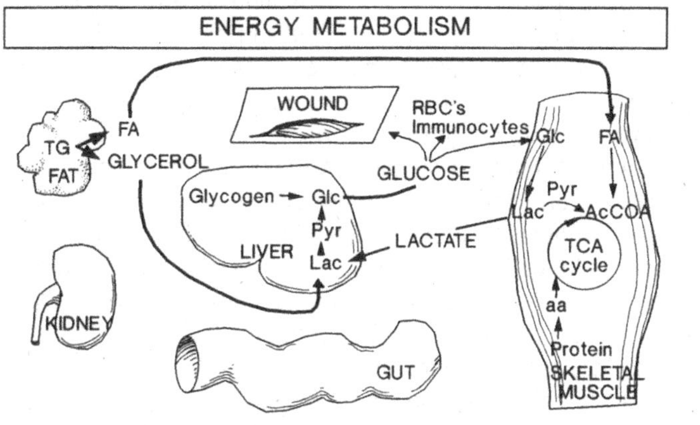

Figure 5-3. Energy metabolism.

Lipid Metabolism

Endogenous catecholamines released during stress promote lipolysis by increasing hormone-sensitive lipase in adipose tissue. Glycerol and free fatty acids are utilized as alternate energy sources, thus sparing endogenous amino acids for other purposes. Fatty acids are oxidized in the liver to the ketone bodies beta-hydroxybutyrate, acetone, and acetoacetate that can be utilized for energy purposes by some tissues, including the brain.[22] Glycerol released during lipolysis can also serve as a gluconeogenic precursor, further sparing muscle amino acids. In non-stressed starvation, lipolysis is a primary means by which euglycemia is achieved. However, during stress, peripheral insulin resistance can lead to catabolism in the face of lipolysis and hyperglycemia.

Resting Energy Expenditure

A patient's resting energy expenditure (REE) is the amount or number of calories (Kcal) expended by an animal in a post-absorptive state while resting in a thermoneutral environment.[8] Values used for REE and basal energy requirements (BER) in small animal patients have largely been obtained from healthy animals or extrapolated from those obtained from human subjects.[23-24] In human medicine, the precise measurement of resting energy expenditure has become fairly routine using bed-side indirect calorimetry units. In veterinary patients, relatively few studies have used similar methods to determine energy expenditure in small animal patients.[23-27] It was previously thought that all human and veterinary patients with illness and injury, including surgically induced trauma, were in a hypermetabolic state, and therefore required caloric intake in excess of their basal requirements.[25] This assumption led to the routine arbitrary use of an illness/injury/infection multiplication factor to apply to a patient's REE to determine the patient's actual daily caloric requirements. Indirect calorimetry analyses conducted in over 106 dogs with a variety of illnesses documented no significant increase in their resting energy expenditure compared with that of healthy controls.[23] Surgery and anesthesia, too, failed to increase a dog's REE.[25-27] In fact, research has demonstrated that an individual dog's REE can differ depending on the type, duration, and degree of illness; the REE may be increased, decreased, or normal.[28] Depending on the time that an individual patient's REE is measured, nutritional support may over- or underestimate caloric requirements throughout the course of illness and healing. Oversupplementation of calories, particularly in the form of carbohydrates, can lead to carbon dioxide retention and respiratory muscle fatigue. Oversupplementation of carbohydrates in human patients has been thought to contribute to impaired ability to wean from mechanical ventilation.[29] If, however, the patient's REE is measured at a time-point at which the patient is hypometabolic, nutritional support may underestimate the patient's changing caloric needs and may actually contribute to malnutrition. The most recent recommendations by veterinary nutritionists describe feeding veterinary patients at least 50% and no more than 100% of their calculated REE, in anticipation that the patient's actual energy needs will change over the course of disease and recovery.[30] In general, the formula: [(30 x Body weight in kg) + 70] = Kcal/day is used to calculate a patient's resting energy expenditure for nutritional support purposes.

The Hypothalamic-Pituitary-Thyroid Axis

The hypothalamic-pituitary-thyroid axis plays an important role in numerous cellular functions during states of health, including cellular oxygen consumption, basal energy metabolism, growth and development, regulation of cardiovascular indices, and regulation of carbohydrate and lipid metabolism.[31] During health, the hypothalamus secretes thyrotropin-releasing hormone (TRH) into the median eminence of the pituitary. The pituitary gland, in turn, releases thyroid-stimulating hormone (TSH), which stimulates the thyroid glands to produce and secrete the thyroid hormones thyroxine (T4) and triiodothyronine (T3). Triiodothyronine is the active form of thyroid hormone. Approximately 10 to 20% of T3 in circulation is released directly from the thyroid glands, and 80 to 90% is a result of conversion of T4 to T3 by enzymatic activity in the peripheral tissues. Both T4 and T3 feed back to the hypothalamus and pituitary gland to suppress further thyroid stimulation.

Down-regulation of the thyroid axis has been documented in a variety of systemic illnesses and injury in veterinary patients, including hyperadrenocorticism, pneumonia, sepsis, diabetes mellitus, renal and hepatic disease, and neoplasia.[32-33] During periods of stress and healing, down-regulation of thyroid hormone metabolism may be a teleological adaptive mechanism by which energy expenditure and protein loss decrease in order to allow healing to occur. During non-stressed starvation, T3 levels decline within 3 days of decreased nutrient intake.[34] Glucocorticoid release during stress is a primary mediator of inducing euthyroid sick syndrome in human and nonhuman animals. Euthyroid sick syndrome is characterized by impaired release of thyrotropin-releasing hormone from the hypothalamus, decreased pituitary responsiveness to TRH, decreased TSH release from the pituitary gland, and decreased level of thyroid-binding proteins in circulation. Complicating factors include decreased conversion of T4 to T3 owing to impaired monoiodinase enzyme activity, and decreased affinity of T3 for peripheral receptors. Euthyroid sick syndrome can be distinguished from true hypothyroidism by the presence of normal to low endogenous TSH in the presence of low T4. In true hypothyroidism, the lack of negative feedback of T4 to the pituitary gland results in elevated eTSH levels in the presence of low T4. Supplementation of thyroid hormone in euthyroid sick syndrome is ineffective at increasing patient survival.

In dogs, euthyroid sick syndrome has been documented in both acute[2] and chronic illnesses.[35-38] In one study, 67% of dogs admitted to a veterinary critical care unit displayed derangements of the thyroid axis, including decreased T3 and T4 concentrations.[2] Similarly, an increase in euthyroid sick syndrome was observed in surgical patients in the postoperative period compared with the same animals preoperatively.[32] In humans, severely decreased thyroid hormone function has been associated with an increase in morbidity and mortality.[1,39] Improvement of clinical condition was associated with similar improvements in thyroid axis function.

Nutritional Support and Glutamine

Nutritional support in surgical patients should be proactive, and ideally should aim to meet the patient's ongoing needs and prevent endogenous protein catabolism.[40] In every patient, a daily nutritional assessment should be considered. Is the patient able to eat? Is vomiting or diarrhea present that can increase nutrient loss or prevent nutrient absorption? Is there excessive loss of protein in the urine or from wound exudates? Is the animal third spacing fluid and protein? Based on the answers to these questions, the route and amount of nutritional support can be decided. In all cases, enteral nutrition is preferred, whenever possible. If enteral nutrition is impossible, parenteral nutrition should be implemented. Both enteral and parenteral nutritional support should provide not only a source of protein, carbohydrate, and lipids, but should also provide other nutrients that can become depleted during the course of illness. As a general rule, protein should compose 30 to 45% of a cat's diet and 15 to 30% of a dog's diet on an as fed dry matter basis.[41] Carbohydrates should be less than 50% of a cat's diet and approximately 50% of a dog's diet on an as fed dry matter basis.[41] Fat should constitute 10 to 30% of a cat's and 10 to 20% of a dog's diet on an as fed dry matter basis.[41] Enteral products formulated specifically for use in critically ill patients are available (Clinicare, Abbott Animal Health, North Chicago, IL; Maximum Calorie, The Iams Company, Dayton, OH; A/D, Hill's Pet Nutrition, Topeka, Kansas) and are an excellent source of calories, protein, and fat in ratios that are highly digestible for veterinary patients with critical illness or in the post-surgical period. A complete review of parenteral nutrition is located elsewhere in this text.

Glutamine

Glutamine is a nonessential amino acids that is required for numerous physiologic processes throughout the body, including normal enterocytes function, nucleic acid and protein synthesis, renal ammoniagenesis, carbohydrate metabolism and gluconeogenesis, and cellular immune function. Although glutamine is abundant in host tissues, demand quickly exceeds the body's synthetic capacity during states of illness, and the nutrient becomes "conditionally essential" in critically ill and surgical patients. Glutamine depletion has been associated with negative nitrogen balance, enterocyte atrophy, suppressed cellular immune function, and increased risk of bacterial translocation and sepsis. Glutamine supplementation in human enteral and parenteral formulations has been shown to increase muscle protein synthesis, peripheral leukocyte numbers, and overall nitrogen balance.[42] Although limited studies have been performed in veterinary patients, stable glutamine dipeptides are available in commercial enteral nutrition formulations (Clinicare, Abbott Animal Health, North Chicago, IL) and may help promote gastrointestinal health during the pre- and post-surgical periods.

Omega-3 Fatty Acids

The ratio of omega-3 to omega-6 polyunsaturated fatty acids has been implicated in playing a role in inflammatory conditions both in human and veterinary patients.[43] Omega-3 fatty acids are derived from alpha-linolenic acid, and omega-6 fatty acids are derived from linoleic acid. Both fatty acids are essential nutrients in cats and dogs. Breakdown of omega-3 and omega-6 fatty acids by cyclooxygenase and lipooxygenase ultimately results in the production of mediators of inflammation, namely, eicosanoids, prostaglandins, leukotrienes, and thromboxanes.[43] In general, proinflammatory mediators are the breakdown products of omega-6 fatty acids, whereas breakdown of omega-3 fatty acids, namely, eicosapentaenoic acid, produces anti-inflammatory mediators.[43] Fish oil supplementation, a potent source of omega-3 polyunsaturated fatty acids, may be beneficial in decreasing proinflammatory conditions in some species.

References

1. Kaptein EM, Weiner JM, Robinson WJ, et al: Relationship between altered thyroid hormone indices to survival in nonthyroidal illnesses. Clin Endocrinol 16:565-574, 1982.

2. Elliot DA, King LG, Zerbe CA: Thyroid hormone concentrations in critically ill canine intensive care patients. J Vet Emerg Crit Care 5(1):17-22, 1994.

3. Faber J, Kirkegaard C, Rasmussen B, et al: Pituitary-thyroid axis in critical illness. J Clin Endocrinol Metab 65:315-320, 1987.

4. Wartofsky L, Burman KD: Alterations in thyroid function in patients with systemic illnesses: the euthyroid sick syndrome. Endocrine Rev 3:164-217, 1982.

5. Mazzaferro EM, Hackett TB, Stein TP, et al: Metabolic alterations in dogs with osteosarcoma. Am J Vet Res 62:1234-1239, 2001.

6. Jackson NC, Carroll PV, Russell-Jones DL, et al: The metabolic consequences of critical illness: acute effects on glutamine and protein metabolism. Am J Physiol 276(Endocrinol Metab 39):E163-E170, 1999.

7. Remillard RL: Nutritional support in critical care patients. Vet Clin Small Anim 32:1145-1164, 2002.

8. Armstrong PJ, Lippert AC: Selected aspects of enteral and parenteral nutritional support. Semin Vet Med Surg (Small Anim) 3(3):216-226, 1988.

9. Webster NR, Galley HF: Nutrition in the critically ill patient. J R Coll Surg Edinb 5:373-379, 2000.

10. Chandler ML, Greco DS, Fettman MJ: Hypermetabolism in illness and injury. Compendium Cont Educ Pract Vet 14(10):1284-1290, 1992.

11. de Bruijne JJ: Ketone body metabolism in fasting dogs. PhD Thesis. University of Utrecht, 1982.

12. Bilbrey SA, Buffington CAT: Metabolism and nutrition in the surgical patient. *In* Disease Mechanisms in Small Animal Surgery, 2nd ed. Philadelphia: Williams & Wilkins, 1993, pp. 49-53.

13. Phillips GD, Odgers CL: Parenteral and Enteral Nutrition, 3rd ed. New York: Churchill Livingstone, 1986.

14. Remillard RL, Darden DE, Michel KE, et al: An investigation of the relationship between caloric intake and outcome in hospitalized dogs. Vet Therap 2(4):301-310, 2001.

17. Lunn JJ, Murray MJ: Nutritional support in critical illness. Yale J Biol Med 71:449-456, 1998.

15. Chang DW, DeSanti L, Demling RH: Anticatabolic and anabolic strategies in critical illness: a review of current treatment modalities. Shock 10(3):155-160, 1998.

16. Michel KE, King LG, Ostro E: Measurement of urinary nitrogen content as an estimate of the total amount of total urinary nitrogen loss in dogs in intensive care units. J Am Vet Med Assoc 210(3):356-359, 1997.

18. Falconer JS, Fearon KCH, Plester CE, et al: Cytokines, the acute-phase response, and resting energy expenditure in cachectic patients with pancreatic cancer. Ann Surg 219(4):325-331, 1994.

19. Barber MD, Fearon KCH, McMillan DC, et al: Liver export protein synthetic rates are increased by oral meal feeding in weight-losing cancer patients. Am J Physiol Endocrinol Metab 279:E707-E714, 2000.

20. Heyland DK: Enteral and parenteral nutrition of the seriously ill, hospitalized patient: a critical review of the evidence. J Nutr Health and Aging 4(1):31-41, 2000.

21. Wilmore DW: Hormonal responses and their effects on metabolism. Surg Clin North Am 56(5):999-1018, 1976.

22. Sacca L, et al: Insulin antagonistic effect of epinephrine and glucagon in the dog. Am J Physiol 237:E487, 1979.

23. Walton RS, Wingfield WE, Ogilvie GK, et al: Energy expenditure in 104 postoperative and traumatically injured dogs with indirect calorimetry. J Vet Emerg Crit Care 6:71-79, 1996.

24. O'Toole E, McDonnell WN, Wilson BA, et al: Evaluation and accuracy and reliability of indirect calorimetry for the measurement of resting energy expenditure in healthy dogs. Am J Vet Res 62(11):1761-1767, 2001.

25. Walters LM, Ogilvie GK, Salman MD, et al: Repeatability of energy expenditure measurements in clinically normal dogs by use of indirect calorimetry. Am J Vet Res 54(11):1881-1885, 1993.

26. Ogilvie GK, Walters LM, Salman MD, et al: Resting energy expenditure in dogs with nonhematopoietic malignancies before and after excision of tumors. Am J Vet Res 57(10):1463-1467, 1996.

27. Ogilvie GK, Salman MD, Kesel ML, et al: Effect of anesthesia and surgery on energy expenditure determined by indirect calorimetry in dogs with malignant and nonmalignant conditions. Am J Vet Res 57(9):1321-1326, 1996.

28. O'Toole EA, Miller CW, Wilson BA, et al: Comparison of the standard predictive equation for calculation of resting energy expenditure with indirect calorimetry in hospitalized and healthy dogs. J Am Vet Med Assoc 225(1):58-64, 2004.

29. Royall D, Fairholm L, Peters WJ, et al: Continuous measurement of energy expenditure in ventilated burn patients: an analysis. Crit Care Med 22(3):399-406, 1994.

30. Remillard RL, Armstrong PJ, Davenport DJ: Assisted feeding in hospitalized patients: enteral and parenteral nutrition. *In* Small Animal Clinical Nutrition, 4th ed. Marceline, MO: Walsworth Publishing Co, 2000, pp. 351-399.

31. Evinger JV, Nelson RW: The clinical pharmacology of thyroid hormones in the dog. J Am Vet Med Assoc 185:314-316, 1984.

32. Mazzaferro EM, Stein TP, Ogilvie GK, et al: The effect of glutamine on thyroid and adrenal axes in canine patients with critical illness. J Vet Emerg Crit Care13(3):164, 2003.

33. Prittie JE, Barton LJ, Peterson ME, et al: Pituitary ACTH and adrenocortical secretion in critically ill dogs. J Am Vet Med Assoc 220(5):615-619, 2002.

34. Vagenakis AG, Burger A, Portnay GI, et al: Diversion of peripheral thyroxine metabolism from activating to inactivating pathways during complete fasting. J Clin Endocrinol Metab 41:191-194, 1975.

35. Peterson ME, Ferguson DC, Kintzer PP, et al. Effects of spontaneous hyperadrenocorticism on serum thyroid hormone concentrations in the dog. Am J Vet Res 45(10):2034-2038, 1984.

36. Nelson RW, Ihle SL, Feldman EC, et al: Serum free thyroxine concentration in healthy dogs, dogs with hypothyroidism, and euthyroid dogs with concurrent illness. J Am Vet Med Assoc 138:1401-1407, 1991.

37. Vail DM, Panciera DL, Ogilvie GK. Thyroid hormone concentrations in dogs with chronic weight loss, with special reference to cancer cachexia. J Vet Int Med 8(2):122-127, 1994.

38. Scott-Moncrieff JCR, Nelson RW, Bruner JM, et al: Comparison of serum concentrations of thyroid-stimulating hormone in healthy dogs, hypothyroid dogs, and dogs with concurrent disease. J Am Vet Med Assoc 212:387-391, 1998.

39. Slag MF, Morley JE, Elson MK, et al: Hypothyroxinemia in critically ill patients as a predictor of high mortality. J Am Med Assoc 245(1):43-45, 1981.

40. Michel KE: Interventional nutrition for the critical care patient: optimal diets. Clin Tech Small Anim Pract 13(4):204-210, 1998.

41. Kerl ME, Johnson PA: Nutritional plan: matching diet to disease. Clin Tech Small Anim Pract 19(1):9-21, 2004.

42. Mazzaferro EM, Hackett TB, Wingfield WE, et al: The role of glutamine in health and disease. Comp Cont Educ Pract Vet 22:1094-1103, 2000.

43. Hickman MA: Interventional nutrition for gastrointestinal disease. Clin Tech Small Anim Pract 13(4):211-216, 1998.

Chapter 6

Enteral Nutrition

Elisa M. Mazzaferro

Nutritional support should be considered in any patient that is unable or unwilling to eat enough quantity to fulfill the caloric and nutrient requirements. Nutrient depletion is associated with increased patient morbidity and mortality.[1] Many veterinary patients have oral trauma, ulcers, or mass lesions that preclude them from prehending and swallowing food. In other cases, the patient may voluntarily eat, but has a disease process that causes severe vomiting or diarrhea and, therefore, the nutrients that are ingested do not have adequate time for digestion and absorption.[2] In one study, only 84% of dogs and 68% of hospitalized cats voluntarily consumed their resting energy requirements.[3] In another study, many patients were withheld from food prior to surgery, or had feeding orders during the postoperative period that led to inadequate offering and thus consumption of calories and other nutrients.[4]

Inappetance, whether voluntary or not in the situation of stress and illness, can lead to protein calorie malnutrition and negative nitrogen balance. Depending on the patient's overall condition, primary disease process, and anticipated length of time of inappetance, some form of nutritional support should be implemented as soon as possible. In general, if a patient has sustained a 10% decrease in body weight, has increased nutrient losses secondary to vomiting, diarrhea, renal disease, or wound exudates, or if oral intake has been or is anticipated to be diminished or ceased for more than 3 to 5 days, enteral support should be initiated.[5-6] The overall goals of nutritional support in any patient should be to replenish caloric intake and nutrients, reverse negative nitrogen balance, prevent tissue catabolism, decrease the incidence of complications, quicken recovery, and improve overall survival.[2] Enteral nutrition is preferred over parenteral nutrition for a variety of reasons including it being more cost-effective and physiologic, and for maintenance of gastrointestinal health and function, decreased incidence of bacterial translocation, and improved clinical outcome. Unless a specific contraindication exists to prevent some form of enteral nutrition, any portion of the gastrointestinal tract that is functioning should be utilized.[7]

Gastrointestinal Health

In addition to its important role in nutrient digestion and absorption, the gastrointestinal tract serves as a physical and immunologic barrier between the enteric bacteria and the relatively sterile environment of the rest of the body.[8] In critically ill and post-surgical patients, normal gastrointestinal protective defense mechanisms can be impaired by the use of glucocorticoids, immunosuppressive drugs, parenteral nutrition, and bowel rest.[8] The presence of luminal nutrients stimulates a complex cascade of events that serves to maintain enterocyte health, gastrointestinal barrier function, gastrointestinal immunity, and overall patient health. The cells lining the intestinal tract, enterocytes, derive approximately half their nutrient requirements from intraluminal substrates.[2] Research has documented that the presence of luminal nutrients is the single most important stimulus for intestinal mucosal growth and maintenance of barrier function.[9] Once ingested, the presence of substrates within the lumen of the gastrointestinal tract stimulates mesenteric blood flow and digestive enzyme and hormone secretion. Enteral nutrients stimulate the secretion of cholecystokinin and biliary flow.[10] Physical contact of fiber with mucosal cells directly stimulates mucosal cell proliferation. Fermentable fiber is metabolized to the short-chain fatty acid butyrate within the large intestine and provides a key substrate fuel for colonocyte health that exerts trophic effects on the gastrointestinal tract.[11-12]

As gastrointestinal nutrients are absorbed, mucin secretion is stimulated. Mucin functions to lubricate the ingesta and neutralize bacterial toxins and hydrogen ions.[8] Additionally, luminal nutrients stimulate the excretion of biliary secretory IgA, an important defense mechanism against bacterial adherence and endotoxin binding to the intestinal mucosa.[2,8,13] Without luminal nutrients, even patients receiving parenteral nutritional support undergo intestinal villous atrophy and mucosal atrophy. Luminal nutrition has been shown to maintain villous height and thus improve intestinal absorptive capacity and gastrointestinal barrier function.[10]

Benefits of Enteral Nutrition in the Critically Ill Surgical Patient

Within 24 hours of lack of enteral intake, enterocytes undergo atrophy and demonstrate decreased ability for digestion and absorption of nutrients.[14-15] The administration of enteral nutrition early after experimentally induced burn injury and abdominal surgeries has been shown to decrease bacterial translocation and improve clinical outcome.[16-17] In human patients undergoing small intestinal and colonic resection, early enteral nutrition maintained gastrointestinal mucosal integrity, improved wound healing, and had a lower incidence of complications.[18-21] Enteral administration of a liquid diet within 12 hours of admission caused a significant increase in weight gain and earlier return to function in canine patients with parvoviral enteritis.[22] Early enteral nutrition provided to canine and feline patients admitted to a university critical care unit was associated with a significantly increased rate of survival compared with patients that received parenteral nutrition alone.[23] The reported benefits of reduced complication rate, decreased length of hospital stay, and improved overall outcome have now led to the recommendation that enteral nutrition should be provided early in the course of illness, unless specific contraindications exist for using the gastrointestinal tract.[18]

Consequences of Inappetance and Parenteral Nutrition

The absence of luminal nutrients during courses of anorexia and administration of parenteral nutrition can result in intestinal villous atrophy, a decrease in enterocyte mass, impaired gastrointestinal barrier function, decreased biliary release of secretory IgA, and suppression of brush border enzyme activity necessary for nutrient breakdown and absorption.[24-25] The consequences of mucosal atrophy are increased gastrointestinal permeability and decreased mesenteric immunity. Bacterial translocation, with stimulation of mesenteric proinflammatory cytokine release, can lead to systemic inflammatory response syndrome, and contribute to multiple organ dysfunction (MODS) in critical patients.[26]

Nutritional Assessment

A patient's nutritional status should be documented ideally within 24 hours of admission to the hospital and then carefully evaluated on a regular basis in order to meet nutritional needs and monitor response to therapy. A variety of factors is typically used to determine a patient's nutritional status, and includes overall body condition, the presence or absence of muscle wasting, total protein and serum albumin concentrations, white blood cell count, and serum acute-phase protein concentrations.[7] Factors other than malnutrition such as fluid therapy, hepatic dysfunction, and increased protein loss can alter normal values; for this reason, the use of a specific indicator by itself when determining a patient's overall nutritional status is largely subjective.

Body condition score (BCS) is one method of evaluating a patient's general nutritional status. Various scales are used to determine overall BCS. This author uses a scale of 1 to 5, with 1 being cachexic and 5 being obese. A score of 3 is optimal. Negative nitrogen balance can occur in any patient with injury and illness. For this reason, even a morbidly obese patient should have caloric needs met based on their metabolic body size, not ideal body weight, while recovering from illness. To determine a patient's resting energy expenditure, use the formula: $(30 \times BW_{kg}) + 70$ = Kcal/day, where BWkg is the patient's body weight in kilograms and Kcal/day is the number of kilocalories per day required. In general, if caloric intake is optimal based on metabolic body size, a patient's protein and other nutrient requirements will be met, if veterinary formulas are administered. A more in depth description and discussion of metabolic nutrient requirements are discussed in, Chapter 5, Metabolism and Nutrition of the Surgical Patient.

Consideration of the individual patient's disease processes and ability to tolerate various forms of enteral feeding is necessary to determine a nutritional plan. First, optimal proportions of specific fuel sources in the form of carbohydrate, lipid, and protein should be determined.[27] Next, a specific diet and proposed means of nutrient delivery should be chosen.[27] Once nutritional support is initiated, the patient's response and tolerance to enteral feeding should be evaluated on a daily basis, at minimum. Changes to the nutritional plan should be made if complications occur or voluntary intake resumes. Once the patient's primary disease process has been treated, a plan should be formulated to transition the patient back to voluntary oral nutrient intake or to some form of indwelling feeding tube after discharge from the hospital.

Enteral Feeding Formulas

The type of enteral formula to administer should be considered based on the patient's clinical disease and ability to tolerate the type and route of feeding, the nutrient profile and specific disease or species requirements, and the individual patient's response to treatment, as well as on the cost and availability of the dietary formulation, its ease of storage and resistance to bacterial contamination and growth.[5-7,28] If a patient is going to require nutritional support for longer than 2 days, an indwelling feeding tube should be considered to minimize stress and potential trauma to the nasopharyngeal region.[2,6] The chosen diet should be balanced to provide the patient's carbohydrate, protein, lipid, and micronutrient requirements, and should be formulated to flow through an appropriately sized feeding tube without difficulty or risk of obstruction.[27] The ideal dietary formulation for tube feeding should be well tolerated, easily digested and absorbed, inexpensive, and have a long shelf life with minimal risk of bacterial contamination.[29] In general, if a feeding tube is less than 14 Fr in size, a liquid diet should be chosen. Blenderized soft food is appropriate for large (> 14 Fr) tubes, whenever possible.[30]

Blenderized Diets

Blenderized diets are an appropriate means of feeding through large-bore (esophagostomy and gastrostomy) feeding tubes. Soft food is usually higher in protein and fat, and lower in carbohydrate than liquid diets, and is generally well tolerated by the patient. Hill's P/D can be mixed with water (1/2 cup of P/D with 3/4 cup of water, blenderized then strained) to form a well balanced, calorie-dense diet that can be fed through esophagostomy and gastrostomy tubes. More recently, Hill's Pet Nutrition and the Iams Company have developed A/D and Maximum Calorie diets, respectively. Both diets are extremely palatable and do not require dilution with water or blending. An added benefit of the Maximum Calorie diet is its change in form by heating. The product can be warmed in the microwave, which changes its consistency to a liquid gruel that can be administered through feeding tubes without dilution.

Liquid Diets

A variety of liquid enteral products is available for use in veterinary and human patients (Table 6-1). Liquid enteral formulations are often associated with the development of diarrhea.[7] In some cases, the osmolality of the fluid causes osmotic diarrhea. In other cases, a lack of adequate fiber or fat in the diet results in diarrhea. Supplementing with fiber or fat can slow gastric emptying time and the rate of nutrient passage through the intestines and can improve fecal consistency.[7] In general, the nutrient density of most liquid formulations used for tube feeding approaches 1 Kcal/ml. Approximately 30% of the calories should be provided as protein, 34% of calories as carbohydrate, and

Table 6-1. Enteral Products Formulated for Human and Veterinary use.[14,31]

Veterinary Diets Liquid Diets	Manufacturer	Caloric Density	Osmolality mOsm/kg	% Content Carbohydrates % Kcal	Lipid % Kcal	Protein g/100 Kcal
Clinicare	Abbott	1	230	25	55	5.5
Moist Diets						
Eukanuba Maximum Calorie	Iams	2.1		5	66	7.4
Hill's A/D	Hill's	1.3		12	53	8.8
Hill's P/D	Hill's	0.9		7	56	9.3
Human Products*						
Monomeric Diets						
Vivonex HN	Sandoz Nutrition	1	630	83	2	2.1
Vital HN	(Ross Laboratories, Inc)	1	500	73	9	4.1
Polymeric Diets						
Osmolite HN	Ross Laboratories, Inc		300	54	29	4.2
Jevity	Ross Laboratories, Inc.		310	54	29	4.2

*** Suitable for short-term use in veterinary patients.**

36% of calories provided as lipid.[27] The addition of lipid and carbohydrates to a liquid diet improves feces consistency and decreases the incidence of diarrhea.[7] Many products developed for human use contain less than 20% of calories as protein and, therefore, are insufficient to meet canine and feline requirements.[5] Specific nutrients such as taurine are also not present in adequate quantities in human formulations. For these reasons, products developed specifically for veterinary use are preferred, whenever possible. While the caloric density is important in determining the volume of liquid to administer as continuous or bolus feeding, the type of diet can further contribute to a patient's ability to assimilate and absorb the nutrients provided. Two broad categories of enteral diets are currently available, and are classified based on the predigestion of carbohydrates and proteins present.

Monomeric Diets

Monomeric diets, or elemental diets, contain crystalline amino acids or dipeptides as a nitrogen source, dextrose or other simple sugars or oligosaccharides as a carbohydrate source, and are generally lower in fat. Fats are provided as long- or medium-chain triglycerides that require no digestion by pancreatic or brush border enzymes prior to absorption.[14] Hydrolysates of proteins provide amino acids as mono-, di- and oligopeptides.[14] It is thought that the digestion of di- and tripeptides and crystalline amino acids requires less fuel and energy than that of intact proteins and is thus more desirable in patients with impaired nutrient assimilation.[14,31] Because the nutrients are predigested, monomeric diets have a high osmolality (400 – 700 mOsm/kg) that often results in diarrhea.[5] Dilution of a monomeric diet with water sometimes can decrease the incidence of diarrhea by decreasing the solutions osmolality. However, dilution also decreases the caloric density of the diet, and requires administration of larger volumes to meet the patient's needs. It may not be physically possible to provide adequate caloric and nutrient intake when dilution is necessary to avoid diarrhea.

More recently, evidence suggests that administration of monomeric diets and elemental nutrition may influence gastrointestinal tract integrity. One study that investigated the use of a monomeric diet in cats with experimentally induced enterocolitis demonstrated that monomeric diets may contribute to gastrointestinal atrophy and increased morbidity even in the presence of gut-specific nutrients. Administration of intact nutrients, or a polymeric diet, helped retain gastrointestinal mucosal integrity.[5] For this reason, a polymeric diet is preferred over monomeric diets whenever possible. A monomeric diet should be offered only if a patient fails to tolerate the polymeric diets that are available.[31]

Polymeric Diets

Polymeric diets contain intact protein, intact carbohydrate, and lipids. In general, they contain a higher percent of calories as fat than do monomeric diets. Protein is provided as casein, soy, and egg albumin.[30] Proteins are provided primarily intact and require digestion by gastric hydrochloric acid and pancreatic enzymes prior to absorption and nutrient assimilation.[14] Intact lipids provided are usually of vegetable origin, such as corn oil, and are largely composed of long-chain triglycerides.[14] Lipids are digested into chylomicrons by pancreatic and enteric lipase prior to absorption.[29] Most polymeric diets are isoosmolar (300 – 450 mOsm/kg) and are better tolerated with fewer complications of diarrhea compared with monomeric diets.[31] Human products that have a caloric density greater than 1 Kcal/ml can be relatively hyperosmolar (600 – 700 mOsm/kg), and are often associated with diarrhea.[5]

Specific Nutrients

Glutamine

Glutamine is a nonessential amino acid that becomes "conditionally essential" during stress and critical illness. During nutrient depletion, intestinal glutaminase activity is upregulated, and glutamine utilization increases. Glutamine is extracted from luminal nutrients and from blood flow to the intestinal basement membrane to provide fuel for the gastrointestinal tract. Glutamine serves as an important substrate for the synthesis of protein and nucleic acids, glutathione, and gastrointestinal mucus.[32] Glutamine also is absolutely necessary for mesenteric immune function, glutathione synthesis, and nitrogen transport.[10,32] Glutamine depletion has been associated with gastrointestinal mucosal atrophy, increased permeability, depressed mesenteric immune function, and bacterial translocation. Enteral supplementation with glutamine-enriched formulas has been shown to ameliorate the negative consequences of depletion listed above.[32]

Arginine

Arginine is an essential amino acid for dogs and cats.[11] Arginine is known to stimulate the release of various anabolic hormones, including prolactin, insulin, and growth hormone. Arginine is also essential in mediating microvascular function and serving as a precursor for nitric oxide, and is an important vasodilatory substance.[10] Supplementation with arginine is thought to improve nitrogen balance by promoting nitrogen retention and to improve immune function and wound healing.[8] Veterinary nutritional supplements should contain arginine at a minimum of 146 mg arginine/100 Kcal for dogs and 250 mg arginine/100 Kcal for adult cats.[31] Most veterinary products contain arginine in sufficient quantities to meet the needs of critically ill patients, however, they do not meet the requirements necessary to promote improved immune function.[11]

Starch

A wide variety of carbohydrate sources is available in enteral formulations. In many products, carbohydrate is provided as corn starch or as mono- or disaccharides in elemental form. Mono- and disaccharides increase the relative osmolality of the preparation and may be associated with diarrhea.

Fiber

The addition of soluble and insoluble fiber to enteral diet formulations serves a dual purpose. Insoluble fiber such as lignin, cellulose, and hemicellulose is present in human formulations (Metamucil Regular or Psyllium fiber 10 – 13 g/100 Kcal) and stimulates enterocyte and goblet cell proliferation when in direct contact within the gut lumen.[31] Fiber can provide a barrier function and limit bacterial adherence and translocation. Additionally, soluble fiber such as pectin is fermented by enteric anaerobic bacteria to the short-chain fatty acid butyrate, acetate, and propionate.[14] Short-chain fatty acids enhance colonocyte health and decrease the incidence of diarrhea. Over-the-counter products that contain psyllium and pectin (1 gram/100 Kcal) can be administered in large-bore feeding tubes in combination with veterinary enteral formulations to decrease the incidence of diarrhea.[14] Oral fiber slows the rate of gastric emptying, and may help improve nutrient assimilation.

Fatty Acids

Enteral diets contain fats as medium- or long-chain triglycerides. Interest has been increased in providing varying proportions of the essential fatty acids linoleic (omega-3) and linolenic (omega-6) when dealing with inflammatory disease states. Omega-3 fatty acids are found in large quantities in flaxseed, canola, and fish oils. Omega-6 fatty acids are present in vegetable oils.[11] Essential long-chain fatty acids are precursors for arachidonic acid synthesis. Dogs can synthesize arachidonic acid from linoleic (omega-6) acid, and can synthesize eicosapentaenoic acid from α-linolenic (omega-3) acid. Cats are deficient in the enzymes necessary for arachidonic acid and eicosapentaenoic acid synthesis, and thus require both in their diets. Arachidonic acid is metabolized by cyclooxygenase enzymes to various pro- and anti-inflammatory mediators, including prostaglandins, thromboxanes, and leukotrienes. Collectively known as eicosanoids, these substances play an important role in mediating immune function, inflammation, platelet function and aggregation, and vascular tone.[11] Increasing the ratio of omega-3 to omega-6 fatty acids in the diet can promote the preferential substitution of linoleic acid into the phospholipid bilayer of cells and result in the production of less inflammatory cytokines. This can help decrease overall inflammation that is thought to contribute to the adverse consequences of systemic inflammatory response syndrome.

Protein

Protein in dietary supplements is typically provided as intact protein, crystalline amino acid, or as hydrolysates of protein. Di- and oligopeptide formulations have a higher osmolality than intact proteins and can cause diarrhea. Intact protein requires digestion by gastric hydrochloric acid and pancreatic enzyme activities. Crystalline amino acids can be absorbed in an energy-consuming active transport process. Di- and oligopeptides, in contrast, are absorbed in passive transport and do not consume energy in the process.[14]

Protein requirements for small animal patients differ across species and across disease states. In general, dogs require 3 to 4 grams of protein/100 Kcal, whereas cats require 4 to 6 grams protein/100 Kcal. Lower concentrations of protein are advisable if hepatic or renal dysfunction is present. Higher quantities of protein should be considered in cases of severe protein loss, including burns, excessive wound exudates, or protein-losing enteropathy or nephropathy. The concentration of protein in relation to caloric density should be considered when choosing an enteral formula appropriate for an individual patient. Protein concentration ranges from less than 5 g/100 Kcal to 15 g/100 Kcal.[14] The protein content of many human enteral nutrition products is deficient and should not be used for long-term nutritional support in small animal patients.[11] In general, if a patient's caloric requirements are met with a veterinary enteral product, its protein requirements will be met as well, unless excessive ongoing nitrogen loss occurs.[30]

Feeding Options and Considerations

Although enteral nutrition is preferred whenever possible, it is not a suitable mode of nutritional support for all small animal patients. Ideally, it is best to evaluate the patient's status at the time of presentation, or at the latest within 24 hours of admission. The nutritional status should be carefully assessed and the patient's individual needs determined prior to the onset of any complications. The anticipated time of enteral nutritional support and time to resume normal voluntary oral intake should be considered.[5] Animals that are poor anesthetic candidates, have coagulation defects, are recumbent or comatose, and cannot protect their airway will have increased risk of aspiration pneumonia, hemorrhage, or death if an indwelling tube is placed under general anesthesia.[5] Other contraindications to enteral feeding include gastrointestinal obstruction and severe malabsorptive syndromes.[8] Postoperatively, gastric ileus may be present for more than 5 days. In such cases, postgastric feeding in the form of duodenal or jejunal tubes should be considered.

Appetite Stimulation

If an animal is physically able to prehend food and does not have esophageal dysfunction or stricture or gastrointestinal obstruction, oral feeding may be possible if an animal is willing to eat and responds to appetite stimulants. Forcefeeding is extremely stressful for animal and caretaker alike and should be avoided. It is difficult to provide adequate calories to meet an animal's resting energy requirements. In some cases, the animal will associate the mere presence of a caregiver with the stress of forcefeeding and reactively and spontaneously vomit. This reverse Pavlovian response negates the goal of providing enteral nutrition and can lead to aspiration pneumonia, esophagitis, and further debilitation. Appetite stimulants that have been used with some success include benzodiazepene tranquilizers (Diazepam 0.05 – 0.5 mg/kg IV once daily to cats) and serotonin antagonists (2 mg/cat PO bid).[31,33] In some cases, warming a liquid diet or adding a small amount of spice to it can enhance odor and palatability.[33] Positive reinforcement and encouragement may entice a patient to eat. If voluntary feeding is not successful in meeting the patient's nutritional requirements, some form of involuntary feeding in the form of feeding tube or parenteral administration should be implemented.[3]

Nasoesophageal and Nasogastric Tubes

Nasogastric (NG) and nasoesophageal (NE) feeding tubes should be considered for short-term (< 1 week) administration of enteral nutrition.[5] Nasoesophageal and nasogastric tubes can be placed efficiently without anesthesia or sedation, in most cases.[2] Contraindications to nasoenteral feeding tube placement include facial or head trauma, impaired neurologic status (moribund or comatose patient without an intact gag reflex), or esophageal disorders including megaesophagus, masses, or stricture.[2]

The placement of nasoenteral feeding tubes has been discussed elsewhere.[5,34–37] Both silicone and polyvinylchloride tubes (Argyle Infant Feeding Tubes, Sherwood Medical, Inc; Sovereign Feeding Tube, Monoject,) are available for use. Because polyvinylchloride tubes can harden within days of exposure to hydrochloric acid, silicone tubes are preferable.[2] A 5 to 8 French tube can be placed in cats and small dogs that weigh less than 10 kg, while larger (8 to 10 Fr) tubes can be placed in larger dogs. Early studies documented that patients, in general, tolerated the NE or NG tube with mild to moderate coughing or sneezing as a common complaint. Gastroesophageal reflux can occur if the tip of the tube passes through the lower esophageal sphincter; however, gastric suctioning may be helpful in animals with severe ileus, to decrease gastric distention and vomiting.[22] In one study, 63% of patients demonstrated no complication with the nasogastric tube feeding, and 61% of patients maintained body weight while hospitalized.[7] Some animals were able to eat with the tube in place.[27,37] Administration of liquid enteral diets allowed maintenance of serum albumin, commonly used as a nutritional marker, in hospitalized small animal patients.[7] The most common complications observed were tube dislodgement, vomiting, and diarrhea, which may have been secondary to the patient's primary disease process(es), owing to the enteral feeding tube, or owing to dietary intolerance. In many patients, diarrhea was treated successfully by changing to a different dietary formulation.[7] More serious complications of nasoenteral feeding include epistaxis, rhinitis, vomiting, esophageal stricture, nasopleural intubation with pneumothorax, and aspiration pneumonitis.[5] Mechanical disruption of the tube by clogging is common, because of the small diameter necessary to bypass the nasal meatus. Sometimes, debris clogged within the tube can be dissolved with the use of pancreatic enzyme solutions or carbonated beverage products such as Coca Cola®.

Esophagostomy Tubes

Esophagostomy tubes are an excellent means of providing enteral nutritional support in a patient with full use and function of the gastrointestinal tract.[28,38] Several methods for esophagostomy tube placement have been described.[28,34,38,39–43] Advantages of esophagostomy tubes include their ease of placement, low risk of complication compared with other indwelling feeding tubes, low cost, lack of need for specialized equipment, immediate use, and positive owner and patient tolerance and use.[28] A recent study investigated the use of esophagostomy versus percutaneous endoscopic gastrostomy tubes, and found that 92% of clients with animals with E-tubes were comfortable and satisfied with their use, versus only 71% of clients whose animals had G-tubes placed.[28] Minor complications associated with E-tube use and placement included vomiting, inadvertent tube removal, patient scratching at the tube, and tube obstruction.[28] More serious complications that have been described, but are uncommon, include hemorrhage during tube placement, cellulitis, and mediastinal placement with pleuritis.

Gastrostomy Tubes

Percutaneous gastrostomy tubes can be placed with or without the assistance of an endoscope. Several techniques have been described.[33,44–46] Gastrostomy tubes are indicated in any patient that has a nonfunctional or injured esophagus, but still has normal gastric function. Gastric tubes are generally well tolerated by clients and animals alike.[34] Complications of gastric tubes include inadvertent tube removal, peritonitis, cellulitis, stoma site infection and pressure necrosis.[5,34] Disadvantages of a gastrostomy tube over esophagostomy tube include the need to wait a minimum of 12 to 24 hours prior to tube use to allow a seal to form, and the need to wait a minimum of 7 to 10 days prior to tube removal.

Jejunostomy Tubes

In general, jejunostomy tubes are well tolerated and provide an effective means of providing nutritional support if only a portion of the gastrointestinal tract is functional. Various methods for placement of jejunostomy tubes have been described.[47–50] Placement of a jejunostomy tube is indicated in patients with upper gastrointestinal obstruction or resection, gastroparesis, pancreatitis, and recurrent aspiration pneumonia.[5] Following placement of the jejunostomy tube, feeding should be initiated after 6 to 12 hours if peristalsis is present.[5] Without a reservoir to allow nutrients to slowly trickle into the gastrointestinal tract, intermittent bolus feeding through a jejunostomy tube is often associated with the development of diarrhea.[6] For this reason, continuous feeding is preferred. Providing a patient's nutrient requirements should be started slowly and then ramped up to full caloric intake over a period of 48 hours. A J-tube should ideally remain in place for a minimum of 7 to 10 days before removal, to decrease the risk of peritonitis. Complications associated with J-tube placement and feeding include orad migration of the tube, abdominal cramping with diarrhea, tube obstruction, focal cellulitis, and tube dislodgement with peritonitis.

Metabolic Complications Associated with Enteral Feeding

Enteral feeding has been associated with a variety of metabolic complications, including hypo- and hyperglycemia, uremia, vitamin and trace mineral deficiencies, and fluid and electrolyte imbalances.[5-10] Overfeeding with resultant vomiting and diarrhea is common. Whenever gastric function is marginal, it is best to aspirate and measure the residual volume in the stomach before the next feeding, to avoid gastric overdistention. If more than one third the volume of the previous feeding is still present, the scheduled feeding should be delayed to allow more time for the stomach to empty. Vomiting can increase the risk of aspiration pneumonia and should be prevented, whenever possible.[10]

Initiating Feeding

Enteral nutritional supplementation should be initiated gradually in the inappetant patient. Caution must be exercised when initiating enteral feeding support to a patient that has had inadequate fluid resuscitation. Research has indicated that administration of enteral nutrition to a patient with hypotension and intravascular fluid volume depletion can result in increased gastrointestinal work-load and oxygen consumption with impaired oxygen delivery, causing further compromise to the gut barrier.[11,51] If the stomach is functional, bolus meal feeding through an esophagostomy or gastrostomy tube can be administered as 6 small meals in a 24-hour period. Trickle feeding via constant-rate infusion is another method of administering liquid diets through nasoesophageal, nasogastric, and jejunostomy tubes. In some cases, a jejunostomy tube can be placed through a gastrostomy tube until the stomach and duodenum can tolerate feeding. Whether nutritional support is administered as a bolus or as a constant-rate infusion, approximately on quarter to on third of the patient's daily caloric requirements should be fed on the first day. Initially, nutrient boluses should equal 5 to 10 ml/kg until the patient is able to tolerate a larger volume.[31] The volume and caloric density should slowly be increased to full feeding over a period of 48 hours, to avoid oversupplementation and refeeding syndrome. Feeding should cease if clinical signs of salivation, retching, or vomiting occur.[31] The patient's acid-base and electrolyte status should be carefully monitored for hypokalemia, hypophosphatemia, and hyperglycemia during this time.

Refeeding Syndrome

Refeeding syndrome is an uncommon complication that occurs in dogs and cats when overzealous nutritional supplementation is administered to a patient that has been anorexic for a long period. Upon reintroduction of nutrients, insulin release drives potassium and phosphorus intracellularly with glucose.[52] A rapid decrease in serum potassium can result in cardiac dysrhythmias and muscle fasciculations. Hypophosphatemia (< 1 mg/dL) can result in severe red blood cell hemolysis.[53–54] Supplementation with phosphorus as potassium phosphate (0.03 – 0.12 mMol/kg/hour IV CRI or 100 mg/100 Kcal energy/day as oral supplement) and potassium chloride (not to exceed 0.5 mEq/kg/hour) or potassium gluconate (2 – 4 mEq/100 Kcal/day as oral supplement) may be necessary to alleviate clinical signs associated with hypophosphatemia and hypokalemia.[55] If clinical and metabolic signs of refeeding syndrome occur, enteral feeding should be decreased until electrolyte abnormalities have been normalized.

Gastric Atony

Gastric atony is a common complication observed in inappetant and post-surgical patients. Narcotic drugs administered to provide analgesia in the postoperative period often contribute to delayed gastric emptying, ileus, gastroesophageal reflux, and vomiting.[56] Empiric therapy with prokinetic agents can potentially decrease some of the complications associated with gastric atony in some patients.[56] Metoclopramide, a dopaminergic and 5-hydroxytryptamine (5-HT) receptor agonist-antagonist, functions as a central antiemetic and gastric promotility drug. Administration of metoclopramide (1 – 2 mg/kg/day IV CRI or 0.2 – 0.4 mg/kg SQ tid) has been shown to increase lower esophageal tone, increase the force of gastric contractions, and cause pyloric relaxation to promote gastric emptying.[56] The combined effects of metoclopramide serve to decrease vomiting and gastroesophageal reflux.

References

1. Webster NR, Galley HF: Nutrition in the critically ill patient. J R Coll Surg Edinb 45:373, 2000.

2. Armstrong PJ, Hand MS, Frederick GS: Enteral nutrition by tube. Vet Clin North Am Small Anim Pract 20(1):237, 1990.

3. Donoghue S: A quantitative summary of nutrition support services in a veterinary teaching hospital. Cornell Vet 81:109, 1991.

4. Remillard RL, Darden DE, Michel KE, et al: An investigation of the relationship between caloric intake and outcome in hospitalized dogs. Vet Therap 2(4):301, 2001.

5. Marks SL: The principles and practical application of enteral nutrition. Vet Clin North Am Small Anim 28(3):677, 1998.

6. Armstrong PJ, Lippert AC: Selected aspects of enteral and parenteral nutritional support. Semin Vet Med Surg (Small Anim) 3(3):216, 1988.

7. Abood SK, Buffington ACT: Enteral feeding of dogs and cats: 51 cases (1989 – 1991). J Am Vet Med Assoc 201(4):619, 1992.

8. Keithley JK, Eisenberg P: The significance of enteral nutrition in the intensive care unit patient. Crit Care Nursing Clin North Am 5(1):23, 1993.

9. Hadfield RJ, Sinclair DJ, Houldsworth, Evans TW: Effect of enteral and parenteral nutrition on gut mucosal permeability in the critically ill. Am J Resp Crit Care Med 152:1545, 1995.

10. Lunn JJ, Murray MJ: Nutritional support in critical illness. Yale J Biol Med 71:449, 1999.

11. Michel KE: Interventional nutrition for the critical care patient: optimal diets. Clin Tech Small Anim Pract 13(4):204, 1998.

12. Beaulieu AD, Drackley JK, Overton TR, et al: Isolated canine and murine intestinal cells exhibit a different pattern of fuel utilization for oxidative metabolism. J Anim Sci 80:1223, 2002.

13. Alverdy J, Chi HS, Sheldon G: The effect of parenteral nutrition on gastrointestinal immunity: the importance of enteral immunity. Ann Surg 202(6):681, 1985.

14. Proulx J: Nutrition in critically ill animals. *In* The Veterinary ICU Book. Wingfield WE, Raffe MR (eds). Jackson, WY: Teton Newmedia, 2002, p. 202.

15. Deitch EA, Winterton J, Li MA, et al: The gut as a portal of entry for bacteremia. Ann Surg 205:681, 1987.

16. Inoue S, Epstein MD, Alexander JW, et al: Prevention of yeast translocation across the gut by a single enteral feeding after burn injury. JPEN 13:565, 1989.

17. Zaloga GP, Bortenschlager L, Black KW, et al: Immediate postoperative enteral feeding decreases weight loss and improves healing after abdominal surgery in rats. Crit Care Med 20:115, 1992.

18. Heyland DK: Enteral and parenteral nutrition in the seriously ill, hospitalized patient: a critical review of the evidence. J Nutr Health Aging 1:31, 2000.

19. Carr CS, Ling E, Boulos P, et al: Randomised trial of safety and efficacy of immediate post-operative enteral feeding in patients undergoing gastrointestinal resection. Br J Med 312:869, 1996.

20. Schroeder D, Gillandes L, Mahr K, et al: Effect of immediate postoperative nutrition on body composition, muscle function and wound healing. JPEN 15:376, 1991.

21. Beier-Holgersen R, Boesby S: Influence of post-operative enteral nutrition on post-surgical infections. Gut 39:833, 1996.

22. Mohr AJ, Leisewitz AL, Jacobson LS, et al: Effect of early enteral nutrition on intestinal permeability, intestinal protein loss, and outcome in dogs with severe parvoviral enteritis. J Vet Intern Med 17:791, 2003.

23. Chan DL, Freeman LM, Labato MA, Rush JE: Retrospective evaluation of partial parenteral nutrition in dogs and cats. J Vet Intern Med 16:440, 2002.

24. Heel KA, Kong Se, McCauley RD, et al: The effect of minimal luminal nutrition on mucosal cellularity and immunity of the gut. J Gastroenterol Hepatol 13:1015, 1998.

25. Thatcher CD: Nutritional needs of critically ill patients. Comp Cont Educ Pract Vet 18:1303, 1996.

26. Moore EE, Moore FA: Immediate enteral nutrition following multisystemic trauma: a decade perspective. J Am Coll Nutr 10:633, 1991.

27. Donoghue S: Providing enteral nutritional support for hospitalized patients. Vet Med Sept: 910, 1992.

28. Ireland LM, Hohenhaus AE, Broussard JD, Weissman BL: A comparison of owner management and complications in 67 cats with esophagostomy and percutaneous endoscopic gastrostomy feeding tubes. J Am Anim Hosp Assoc 39:241, 2003.

29. Crowe DT: Tube feeding diets for nutritional support of the critically ill or injured patients. J Vet Emerg Crit Care 1:8, 1985.

30. Remillard RL: Nutritional support in critical care patients. Vet Clin North Am Small Anim 32:1145, 2002.

31. Remillard RL, Armstrong PJ, Davenport DJ: Assisted feeding in hospitalized patients: enteral and parenteral nutrition. *In* Small Animal Clinical Nutrition, 4th ed. Hand MS, Thatcher CD, Remillard RL, Roudebush P (eds). Marceline, MO: Walsworth Publishing Co, 2000.

32. Mazzaferro EM, Fettman MJ, Hackett TB, et al: Role of Glutamine in Health and Disease. Comp Contin Educ Pract Vet 22:1094, 2000.

33. Elliot DA, Riel DL, Rogers QR: Complications and outcomes associated with use of gastrostomy tubes for nutritional management of dogs with renal failure. J Am Vet Med Assoc 217:1337, 2000.

34. Han E: Esophageal and gastric feeding tubes in the ICU patients. Clin Tech Small Anim Pract 19(1):22, 2004.

35. Abood SK, Buffington CA: Improved nasogastric intubation techniques for administration of nutritional support in dogs. J Am Vet Med Assoc 199:577, 1991.

36. Ford RB: Nasogastric intubation in the cat. Comp Contin Educ Pract Vet 1:29, 1980.

37. Crowe DT: Clinical use of an indwelling nasogastric tube for enteral nutrition and fluid therapy in the dog and cat. J Am Anim Hosp Assoc 22:675, 1986.

38. Mazzaferro EM: Esophagostomy tubes: don't underutilize 'em! J Vet Emerg Crit Care 11:153, 2001.

39. Crowe DT, Devey JJ: Esophagostomy tubes for feeding and decompression: clinical experience in 29 small animal patients. J Am Anim Hosp Assoc 33:393, 1997.

40. Von Werthen CJ, Wess G: A new technique for insertion of esophagostomy tubes in cats. J Am Anim Hosp Assoc 37:140, 2001.

41. Devitt CM, Seim HB: Clinical evaluation of tube esophagostomy in small animals. J Am Anim Hosp Assoc 33:55, 2001.

42. Rawlings CA: Percutaneous placement of a midcervical esophageal tube: new technique and representative cases. J Am Anim Hosp Assoc 29:526, 1993.

43. Levine PB, Smallwood LJ, Buback JL: Esophagostomy tubes as a method of nutritional management in cats: a retrospective study. J Am Anim Hosp Assoc 33:405, 1997.

44. Fulton RB, Dennis JS: Blind percutaneous placement of a gastrostomy tube for nutritional support in dogs and cats. J Am Vet Med Assoc 201:607, 1992.

45. Mauterer JV: Endoscopic and nonendoscopic percutaneous gastrostomy tube placement. *In* Kirk's Veterinary Therapy Bonagura JD (ed). Philadelphia: WB Saunders, 1995, pp. 669 – 674.

46. Mauterer JV, Abood SK, Buffington CA, et al: New techniques and management guidelines for percutaneous and nonendoscopic tube gastrostomy. J Am Vet Med Assoc 207:574, 1994.

47. Heuter K: Placement of jejunal feeding tubes for post-gastric feeding. Clin Tech Small Anim Pract 19(1):32, 2004.

48. Crowe DT, Devey JJ: Clinical experience with jejunostomy feeding tubes in 47 small animal patients. J Vet Emerg Crit Care 7:7, 1997.

49. Swann HM, Sweet DC, Michel K: Complications associated with use of jejunostomy tubes in dogs and cats: 40 cases (1989 – 1994). J Am Vet Med Assoc 210:1764, 1997.

50. Hewitt SA, Brisson BA, Sinclair MD, et al: Evaluation of laparoscopic-assisted placement of jejunostomy feeding tubes in dogs. J Am Vet Med Assoc 225(1):65, 2004.

51. Tappenden KA: Provision of phosphorylatable substrate during hypoxia decreases jejunal barrier function. Nutrition 18:168, 2002.

52. Solomon SM, Kirby DF: The refeeding syndrome: a review. JPEN 14:90, 1990.

53. Adams LG, Hardy RM, Weiss DJ, et al: Hypophosphatemia and hemolytic anemia associated with diabetes mellitus and hepatic lipidosis in cats. J Vet Int Med 7:266, 1993.

54. Justin RB, Hoenhaus AE: Hypophosphatemia associated with enteral alimentation in cats. J Vet Int Med 7:52, 1993.

55. Michel KE: Preventing and managing complications of enteral nutritional support. Clin Tech Small Anim Pract 19(1):49, 2004.

56. Woosley KP: The problem of gastric atony. Clin Tech Small Anim Pract 19(1):43, 2004.

Chapter 7

Parenteral Nutrition

Elisa M. Mazzaferro

Too frequently, veterinary patients do not receive their daily nutritional requirements as a result of inadequate nutrient intake.[1] Advancements in veterinary nutrition and critical care have directed us to provide more aggressive nutritional support to critically ill small animal patients. A lack of essential nutrients and energy can contribute to increased patient morbidity, impaired wound healing, immunosuppression, and increased mortality. The goals of nutritional support are to treat and prevent malnutrition during times of critical illness until the patient is able to assimilate enteral nutrients alone.[2] Although the gold standard for administration of nutritional support is to utilize and feed whatever portion of the gastrointestinal tract is functional, some animals either cannot or will not voluntarily eat, or cannot digest or absorb nutrients provided enterally because of severe vomiting, ileus, inflammation, or surgical resection of the gastrointestinal tract.[2,3] The use of enteral nutrition may be contraindicated or impossible in such cases, and alternate forms of nutrition become absolutely necessary.

Parenteral nutrition is the provision of nutrients by any method other than the gastrointestinal tract.[4] Parenteral nutrition usually contains some form of carbohydrate in the form of dextrose, lipid, and a protein source in addition to vitamins and minerals (Table 7-1). Various phrases have been used to describe the type and method of parenteral nutrition. The term "total parenteral nutrition" (TPN) has frequently been used to indicate the provision of all of a patient's essential nutritional requirements via intravenous, intraperitoneal, or intraosseous route.[5,6] Because we rarely are able to provide every essential macro- and micronutrient to veterinary patients, the term TPN is actually a misnomer that should be abandoned.[4] Another recommendation was to simply use the terminology "Parenteral Nutrition (PN)" to be more accurate.[6]

Parenteral nutrition has also been named based on its route of administration. Solutions with an osmolality greater than 600 to 800 mOsm/L are typically infused via central venous catheters to prevent thrombophlebitis.[7] Such solutions have been called "central parenteral nutrition."[4] Interest has been renewed in the infusion of solutions with lower osmolalities into peripheral veins. This is termed "peripheral parenteral nutrition" or "partial parenteral nutrition" (PPN). Peripheral parenteral nutrition should be considered when short-term nutritional support is required, or as a bridge between parenteral and enteral nutrition as a patient becomes able to tolerate enteral feedings.

Table 7-1. Parenteral Nutrition Components

Name	Osmolality (mOsm/L)	pH	Manufacturer
10% Amino acid (Travasol)	998	6.0	Baxter Healthcare Corporation
Aminosyn	850	4.5-6.0	Abbott Pharmaceuticals
Procalamine	735	6.8	McGaw, Inc.
5% Dextrose	252-310	3.2-6.5	Abbott Pharmaceuticals
50% Dextrose	2530	4.2	Abbott Pharmaceuticals
20% Amino Acid (Aminosyn)	260	8.3	Abbott Pharmaceuticals

Parenteral Nutrients

In the past, the administration of parenteral nutrition in veterinary patients has been limited, largely because of the perceived increased expense, risk of potential complications including sepsis, and lack of technical expertise required for the placement and maintenance of central venous catheters.[7,8] Advancements in veterinary critical care have largely made parenteral nutrition a more viable option for critically ill small animal patients.[8] Parenteral nutrition can be formulated in-house or by commercial pharmacies by compounding a mixture of amino acids, dextrose, lipids, and vitamins.[7] "Three-in-One" mixtures can also be purchased from commercial sources. Ideally, parenteral nutrition solutions should be formulated and mixed under strict aseptic conditions, either in a compounding machine or in a laminar flow hood. In private practice, however, such techniques are often not possible. Mixing should occur, instead, in a surgical suite or low-traffic area, with the personnel wearing a surgical cap, mask, and sterile gloves.

Proteins

Essential and nonessential crystalline amino acid solutions (3.5%, 8.5%, and 15%) are available as a protein source for veterinary parenteral nutrition formulations. Most commonly, an 8.5% solution is used for small animal patients.[6] Amino acid solutions have a high osmolarity (300 – 1400 mOsm/L) and a relatively acidic pH (5.3 – 6.5).6,9,10 It has been recommended that amino acid solutions with concentrations greater than 3.5% should not be administered through a peripheral vein because of the high osmolality.[10] Commercial products containing varying amounts of glucose and electrolytes are also commercially available.[6] The amount of protein in parenteral formulations is usually calculated relative to the amount of nonprotein calories required by each patient. Protein requirements range from 1 to 6 grams of protein/100 Kcal nonprotein energy in small animal patients.6 In dogs, approximately 2 to 3 grams of protein/100 Kcal nonprotein calories should be administered on a daily basis. In cats, the value is slightly higher, at 4g protein/100 Kcal.[6] In patients with hepatic or renal insufficiency, smaller amounts of protein should be provided; in patients with large amounts of protein loss, larger portions should be considered. Because most amino acid solutions do not contain the amino acid taurine, taurine supplementation should be considered if parenteral nutrition is required for long-term management of feline patients.[2]

Lipids

Lipid emulsions are often a combination of soybean and safflower oil, and linoleic and linolenic acids.[6] Lipid sources for parenteral nutrition administration are available as 10 to 20% solutions, and are used to provide 40 to 60% of the patient's daily nonprotein calorie requirements.[11] Lipids traditionally supply essential fatty acids and provide a source of calories in an isotonic fluid. Because lipid emulsions typically have a lower osmolality (260 – 310 mOsm/L)[6,9,10] than amino acid solutions, lipids can be administered by peripheral catheters with minimal risk of causing thrombophlebitis.

Dextrose

Carbohydrate sources are typically provided as dextrose (2.5%-70%) in parenteral nutrition formulations. Most commonly, 50% dextrose is combined with lipid and amino acid solutions for a patient's daily nutritional needs. The exact ratio of dextrose to lipid to meet a patient's caloric requirements is a topic of debate. During states of stressed starvation, glucocounterregulatory hormones such as cortisol and epinephrine promote a state of insulin resistance. The body is unable to utilize carbohydrate sources for energy, and hyperglycemia develops. In humans, hyperglycemia secondary to oversupplementation of carbohydrates has been shown to increase patient morbidity, respiratory failure, and mortality. In small animal patients, dextrose as provided in parenteral nutrition formulations should not exceed 50% of total daily caloric requirements.

Electrolytes

Electrolyte abnormalities are a common complication of critical illness and parenteral nutrition administration. The most common electrolyte abnormalities observed are hypokalemia and hyperphosphatemia. Following a period of prolonged anorexia and malnutrition, infusion of supplemental dextrose alone or in combination with amino acids and lipids can stimulate insulin release, driving glucose, potassium, and phosphorus intracellularly. Provision of nutrients and the production of high-energy-containing compounds such as adenosine triphosphate (ATP) can deplete a patient's phosphorus stores, resulting in hypophosphatemia. Measuring a patient's levels of potassium and phosphorus is necessary in order to determine the appropriate amount of potassium and phosphorus supplementation. In most cases, adding 20 to 40 mEq/L of potassium chloride, or a mixture of potassium chloride with potassium phosphate (0.01 – 0.03 mmol/kg/hour) may be necessary to maintain normokalemia and normophosphatemia. Ten milliliters of 10% calcium gluconate solution can be administered in each liter of parenteral nutrition.[10]

Vitamins

Most patients do not require fat- and water-soluble vitamin supplementation unless the anorexia and weight loss have been prolonged or if nutrient absorption has been diminished because of excessive diarrhea or steatorrhea.[6] A weekly dose of Vitamin K1 (0.5 mg/kg) has been suggested at the onset of parenteral nutrition.[2,6] Other fat-soluble vitamins (A,D, and E) can be administered as a repository solution (1 ml IM, Schering-Plough Animal Healthcorp, Kenilworth, NJ) and will provide a sufficient store for approximately 3 months.[6] B-complex vitamins can be provided as a combination preparation in the parenteral solution (1 ml/100 Kcal or 3 ml/10 kg/day).[2] Because some B-vitamins degrade when exposed to light, the parenteral nutrition solution should be covered to prevent degradation of labile substances.

Formulating Parenteral Nutrition Solutions

Before actually formulating a patient's daily parenteral nutrition, one must first calculate the daily energy requirements (resting energy expenditure, REE), then determine what percent of the REE will be provided as carbohydrate (dextrose) and what percent will be provided as lipid. Veterinary studies have documented that critically ill small animal patients actually require basal energy requirements,[12] and are not "hypermetabolic" as previously suggested. A linear equation to calculate a patient's daily caloric requirements or resting energy expenditure (REE) is:

REE = (30 x Body weightkg) + 70 = Kcal/day

Once the REE is calculated, the amount of calories provided by fat as lipid emulsion and of carbohydrate as dextrose is then calculated. Finally, the REE is divided by 100, to provide a multiplication factor for the amount of protein to add to the mixture. In order to determine the amount of each solution to add to the total mixture, one must know the concentration of lipid, dextrose, and amino acid in each component solution. The volume of each component is added together and the sum divided by 24 hours, to yield a rate of ml/hour to administer the parenteral nutrition. An example of step-by-step calculation of parenteral nutrition formula for a canine and a feline patient is located in Table 7-2. Once a bag of parenteral nutrition has been formulated, it can be refrigerated for up to 48 hours. The parenteral nutrition should be administered at room temperature. Each bag should be administered over a period of 24 hours, then discarded.

Total Nutrient Admixture

A simple method of providing the patient's total daily nutritional and fluid requirements is to combine the parenteral nutrition within a Lactated Ringer's or other isotonic fluid (Normosol-R, Plasmalyte-A) bag. First, the volume of each parenteral nutrition component is determined. Next, the patient's total daily fluid requirement is determined. The volume of the parenteral nutrition is adjusted to meet the patient's daily fluid requirements by adding an isotonic fluid such as Lactated Ringer's, Plasmalyte-M, or Normosol-R into the bag of parenteral nutrition. The additions are made in a sterile manner, then the fluid is infused into a dedicated line. The advantages of administering a TNA solution are that the patient requires just one dedicated catheter, one fluid administration set, and one fluid pump.[4]

Central Catheter Placement

Infusion of a hyperosmolar substance into a peripheral vein is often associated with the development of thrombophlebitis. It is recommended, therefore, that parenteral nutrition solutions with an osmolality greater than 600 mOsm/L should be infused into a central venous catheter. In small animal patients, central venous catheters can be placed into the jugular, medial saphenous, and lateral saphenous veins with relative ease. Several single- and multiple-lumen catheter types are available. Polyurethane and silicone catheters are less irritating to the vessels and, therefore, are recommended over Teflon catheters.[6] A complete description of through-the needle and over-the-wire catheter placement is beyond the scope of this text. One of the most important concepts to remember when placing a central venous catheter is to maintain sterility at all times, to prevent catheter-related sepsis. First, the fur over the proposed site of catheter insertion should be clipped. Next, the clipped area should be aseptically scrubbed as with any surgical site. The area should be draped with sterile field towels to avoid contamination of the site. Wearing gloves, the practitioner can insert the catheter according to manufacturer's instructions, then secure it in place. The catheter entrance site should be covered with an antimicrobial ointment, then bandaged. The bandage should be labeled with the time and date of catheter placement, initials of the person who placed the catheter, and the date of bandaging. Once the catheter has been successfully placed and bandaged, the parenteral nutrition can be connected. The line should be labeled as a dedicated line and not be used for any purpose other than administration of the nutritional support. The line should not be disconnected for any reason except to change fluid/nutrition bags every 24 hours, even when taking the patient for a walk outside. The bandage should be changed and the catheter entrance site examined every 24 hours. Signs of phlebitis include erythema and pain at the catheter site, pain upon infusion into the vessel, and ropiness or hardening of the vessel on external palpation. In several retrospective studies regarding the use of central venous catheters for infusion of parenteral nutrition, catheter occlusion and kinking were among the most common complications observed.[13,14,15]

Partial Parenteral Nutrition

Partial parenteral nutrition is the provision of a portion of a patient's daily nutritional requirements. Partial parenteral nutrition should be used only in cases where nutritional support is anticipated for less than 5 days, or during a transition period when a patient is consuming only a portion of the daily nutritional requirements enterally. The osmolality of partial parenteral nutrition formulations is usually lower than 600 mOsm/L, and therefore, they can be administered through a peripheral vein. Because amino acid solutions are hyperosmolar, peripheral parenteral solutions typically contain small amounts of amino acid and provide a portion of the patient's caloric requirements as a mixture of dextrose and isoosmolar lipid solutions. Because of volume and osmolality constraints, peripheral parenteral nutrition only provides a portion of a patient's daily nutrient needs.[13,16]

Table 7-2. Step-wise Approach to Calculating Parenteral Nutrition Formulation

1. Calculate the patient's daily resting energy requirement (REE in Kcal/day)

   $REE = (30 \times BW_{kg}) + 70$

2. Calculate the patient's carbohydrate source, providing 20% of REE as dextrose.
3. Calculate the patient's lipid requirement, providing 80% of REE as lipid.
4. Calculate the patient's daily protein requirement (3 g/100 Kcal for dogs and 4 g/100 Kcal for cats)
5. Use the following guidelines to determine the volume of each parenteral nutrition component required.

   5% dextrose = 0.17 Kcal/ml

   50% dextrose = 1.7 Kcal/ml

   20% lipid = 2 Kcal/ml

   8.5% amino acid = 0.085 g/ml

   3% amino acid =0.03 g/ml

6. Add the volume of dextrose, lipid, and amino acid solution together to yield a daily volume to be administered.
7. Divide the volume obtained in Step 7 by 24 hours, to yield a ml/hour rate of infusion.

OR

8. Determine the patient's daily fluid requirement.
9. Subtract the volume obtained in Step 6 from the volume obtained in Step 8.
10. Add the volume obtained in Step 9 as an isotonic solution to the parenteral nutrition (components in Step 6) to obtain a daily fluid and nutrition solution.
11. Divide the total volume of Step 10 by 24 hours, to yield a fluid rate per hour.

Example of Calculating Parenteral Nutrition for a 30 kg dog:

1. Calculate the patient's daily REE.

   (30 x 30) + 70 = 970 Kcal/day

2. Calculate the daily carbohydrate source.

   20% = 0.2 x 970 Kcal/day = 194 Kcal/day carbohydrate (dextrose)

3. Calculate the daily lipid source.

   80% = 0.8 x 970 Kcal/day = 776 Kcal/day lipid

4. Calculate the daily protein requirement (4 g protein/100 Kcal in dogs)

   970 Kcal/day x 4 g protein/100 Kcal = 38.8 g protein/day

5. 50% dextrose = 1.7 Kcal/ml

   194 Kcal x 1 ml/1.7 Kcal = 114 ml of 50% dextrose/day

   20% lipid = 2 Kcal/ml

   776 Kcal x 1 ml/2 Kcal = 388 ml 20% lipid

   38.8 g protein/day x 1 ml/0.085 g protein = 456.5 ml/day 8.5% protein

6. Add the volume of dextrose, lipid, and protein required.

   114 ml 50% dextrose

   388 ml 20% lipid

   + 456.5 ml 8.5% amino acid = 958.5 ml/day

7. a. Divide the above volume by 24 to yield ml/hour rate of administration.

   958.5 ml/day ÷ 24 hours = 39.9 ≈ 40 ml/hour

OR

7. b. Determine the patient's daily fluid requirement (60 ml/kg/day)

   60 ml/kg/day x 30 kg = 1800 ml/day

8. Subtract the parenteral nutrition volume from daily fluid requirement.

   1800 ml/day – 985.5 ml/day = 814.5 ml

9. Add 814.5 ml of an isotonic fluid such as Normosol-R to the parenteral nutrition, to create a total nutrient admixture (TNA)
10. 1800 ml ÷ 24 hours = 75 ml/hour of total nutrient admixture.

Complications of Parenteral Nutrition

One of the most common reasons for not implementing parenteral nutritional support in critically ill veterinary patients is the perception of numerous complications. Several studies have been published investigating the use of parenteral nutrition in veterinary patients. Complications associated with parenteral nutrition administration can be categorized as mechanical, metabolic, or septic (Table 7-3).[3,13] Mechanical complications are most common and are typically associated with catheter dislodgement, kinks, and clogging.[3,13,14,15] Metabolic complications include transient hyperglycemia, hypokalemia, hyperlipidemia, hypophosphatemia, hyperbilirubinemia, hyponatremia, and hypochloremia.[3,13,14,15] In one study,[14] hyperglycemia at 24 hours after onset of PN infusion was associated with increased risk of mortality. In human patients, persistent hyperglycemia can contribute to respiratory fatigue and increased patient mortality. Administration of 10 units of regular insulin per liter of parenteral nutrition can decrease the hyperglycemia associated with PN administration.[3]

Lack of enteral nutrition can promote disuse atrophy of enterocytes and promote bacterial translocation and sepsis. In several veterinary studies, septic complications during administration of parenteral nutrition were few and were associated with the patient's primary disease process or to disruption of the patient's designated infusion line.[3,13,14,15]

Table 7-3. Mechanical and Metabolic Complications Associated with Parenteral Nutrition

Mechanical Complications
Catheter occlusion
Catheter malfunction
Line disconnection
Line or catheter breakage
Thrombus formation
Inability to re-catheterize patient
Metabolic Complications
Hyperammonemia
Hyperglycemia
Hyperkalemia
Hypokalemia
Hypomagnesemia
Hypochloremia
Hyponatremia
Hypophosphatemia
Elevated BUN

Conclusions

Parenteral nutrition should be considered in any patient that cannot tolerate enteral feeding. Nutritional plans should be formulated based on individual patient requirements, disease processes, anticipated length of required nutritional support, and risk of complications. The risks of increased patient morbidity and mortality and of delayed wound healing greatly exceed the perceived risks of increased patient expense and mechanical, metabolic, or septic complications. With increased use and technical proficiency, placement of dedicated central venous catheters and administration of parenteral nutrition can become commonplace in all veterinary hospitals, provided that aseptic techniques are strictly adhered to.

References

1. Remillard RL, Darden DE, Michel KE: An investigation of the relationship between caloric intake and outcome in hospitalized dogs. Vet Therap 2(4):301-310, 2001.
2. Lippert AC, Armstrong PJ: Parenteral Nutritional Support. *In* CVT X, pp. 25-30.
3. Lippert AC, Fulton RB, Parr AM: A retrospective study of the use of total parenteral nutrition in dogs and cats. JVIM 7:52-64, 1993.
4. Remillard RL: Nutritional support in critical care patients. Vet Clin Small Anim 32:1145-1164, 2002.
5. Reuter JD, Marks SL, Rogers QR, Farver TB: Use of total parenteral nutrition in dogs: 209 cases (1988 – 1995). J Vet Emerg Crit Care 8:201-213, 1998.
6. Remillard RL, Armstrong PJ, Davenport DJ: Assisted feeding in hospitalized patients: enteral and parenteral nutrition. *In* Small Animal Clinical Nutrition, 4th ed. Hand MS, Thatcher CD, Remillard RL, Roudebush P (eds). Marceline, MO: Walsworth Publishing Company, 2000.
7. Chandler ML, Guilford WG, Payne-James J: Use of peripheral parenteral nutritional support in dogs and cats. JAVMA 216(5):669-673, 2000.
8. Mauldin GE, Reynolds AJ, Mauldin GN, Kallfelz FA: Nitrogen balance in clinically normal dogs receiving parenteral nutrition solutions. AJVR 62:912-920, 2001.
9. Chan DL, Freeman LM, Rozanski EA, Rush JE: Colloid osmotic pressure of parenteral nutrition components and intravenous fluids. J Vet Emerg Crit Care 11(4):269-273, 2001.
10. Mathews KA: The various types of parenteral fluids and their indications. Vet Clin Small Anim 28(3):483-513, 1998.
11. Anorexia, inanition, and critical care nutrition. *In* Small Animal Clinical Nutrition, 3rd ed. Lewis LD, Morris ML, and Hand MS (eds). Topeka: Mark Morris Associates, 1993, pp.5-1–5-43.
12. Walton RS, Wingfield WE, Ogilvie GK, et al: Energy expenditure in 104 postoperative and traumatically injured dogs with indirect calorimetry. J Vet Emerg Crit Care 6:71-79, 1996.
13. Armstrong PJ, Lippert AC: Selected aspects of enteral and parenteral nutritional support. Semin Vet Med Surg (Small Anim) 3(3):216-226, 1988.
14. Freeman LM, Labato MA, Rush JE, Murtaugh RJ: Nutritional support in pancreatitis: a retrospective study. JVECCS 5(1):32-41, 1995.
15. Pyle SC, Marks SL, Kass PH: Evaluation of complications and prognostic factors

associated with administration of total parenteral nutrition in cats: 75 cases (1994-2001). JAVMA 225(2):242-250, 2004.
16. Chan DL, Freeman LM, Labato MA, Rush JE: Retrospective evaluation of partial parenteral nutrition in dogs and cats. JVIM 16:440-445, 2002.

Chapter 8

The Physiology of Pain and Principles for its Treatment

James S. Gaynor

Why is the Control of Pain Important?

The alleviation of pain is important for physiologic and ethical reasons.[1] Briefly, pain can induce a stress response in patients that is associated with elevations in ACTH, cortisol, antidiuretic hormone (ADH), catecholamines, aldosterone, renin, angiotensin II, and glucose, along with decreases in insulin and testosterone. These changes can result in a general catabolic state with muscle protein catabolism and lipolysis, in addition to retention of water and sodium and excretion of potassium.[2] A prolonged stress response can decrease the rate of healing. In addition, the stress response can have adverse effects on the cardiovascular and pulmonary systems, fluid homeostasis, and gastrointestinal tract function.[2,3]

Veterinarians have an ethical obligation to treat animal pain. Most under-treatment of animal pain is probably a result of lack of adequate knowledge and not a lack of concern. Outward show of concern for the pet and family is important to demonstrate a bond-centered approach to cancer therapy and pain management. Most owners who are willing to undergo the emotional stress and financial commitment to pet care have already shown they have a strong attachment to their pet. It is important for the veterinarian to foster good communication surrounding primary therapy and pain treatment and at the same time to demonstrate empathy for the owner. This fosters the doctor-client-patient relationship and will help build goodwill both within and outside of the practice.

Definitions

Having a working understanding of the terminology surrounding pain and analgesia is important. By knowing the terminology, practitioners can speak intelligently and accurately to one another when discussing their patients. Table 8-1 provides definitions, arranged alphabetically, that are commonly used when discussing pain.

Table 8-1. Definitions

- Acupuncture – The practice of inserting needles at certain points in the skin to achieve specific effects such as pain relief.
- Acute pain – Pain that follows some bodily injury, disappears with healing, and tends to be self limiting.
- Allodynia – Pain caused by a stimulus that does not normally cause pain.
- Analgesia –The loss of sensitivity to pain.
- Anesthesia – Total or partial loss of sensation.
- Breakthrough pain – A transient flare-up of pain in the chronic pain setting, which can occur even when chronic pain is under control.
- Chronic pain – Pain that lasts several weeks to months and persists beyond the expected healing time when nonmalignant in origin.
- Cancer pain – Pain that can be acute, chronic, or intermittent and is related to the disease itself or to the treatment.
- Epidural – The space above the dura mater.
- Hyperalgesia – An increased response to a stimulation that is normally painful (a heightened sense of pain) either at the site of injury or in surrounding undamaged tissue. Stimulated nociceptors respond to noxious stimuli more vigorously and at a lower threshold.
- Local anesthesia – The temporary loss of sensation in a defined part of the body without loss of consciousness.
- Multi-modal analgesia – The use of multiple drugs with different actions to produce optimal analgesia.
- Neuropathic pain – Pain that originates from injury or involvement of the peripheral or central nervous system and is described as burning or shooting, possibly associated with motor, sensory, or autonomic deficits.
- Opioid – A drug that is related naturally or synthetically to morphine.
- Pain – an unpleasant sensory and emotional experience associated with actual or potential tissue damage or described in terms of such damage.
- Preemptive analgesia – The administration of an analgesic drug prior to stimulation to prevent sensitization of neurons and wind-up (see below), thus improving postoperative analgesia.
- Regional anesthesia – The loss of sensation in part of the body by interrupting the sensory nerves conducting impulses from that region of the body.
- Somatic pain – Pain that originates from damage to bones, joints, muscle, or skin and is described in humans as localized, constant, sharp, aching, and throbbing.
- Wind-up – Sensitization of nociceptors, and peripheral and central pain pathways in response to a barrage of afferent nociceptive impulses resulting in expanded receptive fields and an increased rate of discharge.

Mechanisms of Pain

Textbook chapters and multiple review papers are dedicated to describing the mechanisms of nociception, transduction, modulations, and the perception of pain.[4-7] The following section provides an overview of what are considered the most important aspects of the mechanisms of pain. It is important to note that these concepts may change over time as we develop a better understanding on a basic science level and an improved interpretation of these aspects in the whole animal.

The detection of tissue damage by specialized receptors in the periphery is referred to as nociception. These peripheral receptors, nociceptors, can be found in the skin, mucosa, deep fascia, connective tissue of visceral organs, ligaments, muscles, tendons, articular capsules, periosteum, and arterial vessel walls. Nociceptors are the distal end of the axons of first order neurons in the pain pathway. They are responsible for detecting and transmitting the location, quality, and duration of the stimulus. Nociception occurs when the free nerve endings are activated on the distal terminals of A-delta and C nociceptors. The term nociception is used for the activity occurring from the periphery through the spinal cord to the brain. Pain, which is a conscious experience, requires integration with higher brain centers. Thermal, mechanical, chemical, and electrical stimuli may activate most nociceptors. Some, however, only respond to thermal or mechanical stimuli. The ability of a nociceptor to respond to a specific stimulus has been elucidated on a molecular basis. The cell bodies of the C fibers contain several unique molecules, which may be useful in the production of analgesic drugs in the future. These molecules include TTX-R, a tetrodotoxin-resistant Na^+ channel; VR-1, the vanilloid receptor that is targeted by capsaicin; P2X3, a subtype of purinergic receptor; and DRASIC, an acid-sensing ion channel.[8-18] Once activated via the nociceptors, the nerve signal is propagated to the central nervous system via C fibers or A-delta fibers.

A-delta are small (1-6 μm) diameter myelinated fibers. They conduct at relatively high speeds, 5 to 25 m/sec. C fibers are smaller (< 1 μm) diameter unmyelinated nerves with slower conduction velocity, typically less than 2 m/sec. The primary afferent nociceptors contain a variety of neurotransmitters, including glutamate, substance P, and calcitonin gene-related peptide. Glutamate is an excitatory amino acid, which acts upon several receptor subtypes to mediate rapid depolarization of dorsal horn neurons via an influx of Na^+ and an efflux of K^+. Substance P also activates subpopulations of dorsal horn neurons. Substance P can contribute to some of the long-term changes produced by persistent injury, as can the N_Methyl_D_Asparte (NMDA) receptor. The NMDA receptor gates Ca^{++} in addition to Na^+ and K^+ and can alter long-term dorsal horn processing.

The propagated stimulus from the periphery enters the spinal cord via the dorsal roots of the spinal nerves where the first synapse takes place. The spinal nerves then innervate the different laminae of the gray matter of the dorsal horn of the spinal cord. The laminae are distinct layers of cells that form columns extending the length of the spinal cord. Laminae I, II, V, and VI are locations where incoming A-delta and C fibers typically synapse.

Local inhibitory interneurons and descending inhibitory pathways with origins in the brain stem, both in the dorsal horn, help regulate dorsal horn nociception. Most inhibitory interneurons use glycine or gaba (gamma-aminobutyric acid) as their neurotransmitters. These inhibit the firing of dorsal horn neurons. Enkephalin and dynorphin also have inhibitory effects in some interneurons by causing hyperpolarization via increased K^+ conductance. Norepinephrine and serotonin have antinociceptive effects in the descending inhibitory pathways.

The second order neurons receive input from primary afferent fibers. These are located in the dorsal column nuclei and transmit signals to the higher centers of the brain via multiple parallel pathways including, but not restricted to, the spinothalamic, spinoreticular, spinocervicothalamic, neospinothalamic, and paleospinothalamic tracts. The importance of the various tracts is likely to have species-specific importance. The spinothalamic and spinocervicothalamic tracts seem to play an important role in conveying nociceptive input in domestic species.

The spinothalamic tract has neurons that originate in lamina I and ascend to the thalamus. The spinoreticular tract has origins deeper in the dorsal and ventral horns, with neurons coming from laminae VII and VIII. These axons project to reticular formations at all levels of the brainstem.

The sensation of pain is produced in the lateral thalamocortical system of the lateral thalamus and the primary and secondary somatosensory aspects of the cerebral cortex. Aversive reactions to noxious stimuli occur owing to projections to the medial thalamus, which sends projections to the limbic structures.

The gate control theory is a description of the physiologic mechanism of pain. Briefly, it states that sensory input is modulated by ascending and descending mechanisms in the central nervous system. In essence, the spinal cord acts like a gate, which increases or decreases the effect of the neural input before being processed by the brain, evoking pain perception and response.[19]

Traditional Chinese Medicine Aspects of Pain and Acupuncture Therapy

From a traditional Chinese medicine (TCM) perspective, pain can be a result of an excess condition leading to the obstruction of the circulation of Qi and blood. Examples of excess conditions contributing to pain include invasion of exterior pathogenic factors, interior cold or heat, stagnation of Qi or blood, obstruction by phlegm, and retention of food. Pain can also be caused by deficiency conditions such as deficiency of Qi and blood and consumption of body fluids from Yin deficiency. These conditions cause malnourishment of the channels, and hence, pain. Stagnation of Qi causes distention with distending pain and no fixed location. Stasis of blood causes a severe boring pain in a small defined area.[20]

The principles behind acupuncture therapy are the restoration of a balance in the body. Acupuncture needles placed in appropriate proximal, local, and distal locations can help resolve the underlying causes of pain. This ultimately restores Qi and blood circulation to normal. With no obstruction, there is no pain.

Acupuncture Pain Relief

Acupuncture can be used a pain relieving modality, often when conventional therapy does not work. It is also useful in conjunction with other therapy to allow lower doses of drugs that may have significant side effects. While some practitioners have difficulty accepting acupuncture because of traditional Chinese medical explanations, which may be scientifically untenable, it is important to remember that there exists well documented physiologic theory and evidence for its clinical effects.[21,22] In general acupuncture analgesia is extremely useful for pelvic, radius/ulna, and femoral bone pain as well as cutaneous discomfort secondary to radiation therapy. Acupuncture also helps alleviate nausea associated with chemotherapy and some analgesics, as well as promoting general well being.

Physiology of *Acupuncture* Pain Therapy

Placement of needles at specific acupuncture points can relieve pain through several different mechanisms. First, acupuncture may decrease muscle spasms when inserted into trigger points. Lack of spasms will increase comfort considerably. Acupuncture can also induce release of a variety of neurotransmitters, which can affect the processing of the pain impulse. This effect can be enhanced with specific types of electrical stimulation. Proper needle placement and low-frequency electrical stimulation (2-6 Hz) induces central release of endorphins and enkephalins, which may induce analgesia by inhibiting the transmission of nociceptive impulses from their origin to the brain and increasing the descending inhibition back to the periphery.[23] This type of stimulation usually produces analgesia in 10 to 20 minutes and is considered cumulative, meaning that subsequent treatments produce better and better analgesia. The analgesia produced by low-frequency stimulation can be abolished by the opioid antagonist naloxone.[24-26] High-frequency electrical stimulation (100-200 Hz) induces release of serotonin, epinephrine, and norepinephrine, inducing noncumulative analgesia.[27-28] As opposed to low-frequency-induced analgesia, analgesia from high-frequency stimulation is not affected by naloxone.[29] High-frequency-induced analgesia has its major effect by increasing descending inhibition of spinal tracts. For postoperative analgesia, low-frequency stimulation is most efficacious.

Approach to Pain Management in the Small Animal Patient

Drug treatment is the cornerstone of pain management. It is effective and affordable for most patients and owners. The general approach to pain management should follow the principles outlined further on. Individuals may suffer different side effects within the same category of drugs; therefore, if possible, it may be best to substitute drugs within a category before switching therapies. It is always best to try to keep dosage scheduling as simple as possible. The more complicated the regimen, the more likely that noncompliance will occur. Mild to moderate pain should be treated with a non-opioid such as a nonsteroidal anti-inflammatory drug (NSAID) or acetaminophen. As pain increases, some type of opioid should be added to the regimen. As pain becomes more severe, increase the dose of the opioid. Drugs should be given on a regular basis, not just as needed, as pain becomes moderate to severe. Continuous analgesia will facilitate maintaining patient comfort. Additional doses of analgesics may then be administered as pain is intermittently more severe. Adjuvant drugs may be administered to help with specific types of pain and anxiety.

Principles of Pain Management

Three simple principles may be followed to avoid acute and chronic pain. The first principle is that pain control is good medicine. This follows from the earlier description of the physiologic importance of avoiding pain. Once again, prevention and alleviation of pain keep normal patients reasonably healthy, prevent sick patients from developing unnecessary complications, and can preempt catastrophic events in critically ill patients. In the simplest sense, pain control helps patients heal more quickly and more effectively.

The second principle of pain management is the concept of preventative analgesia. This concept implies the provision of pain control before a potentially nociceptive or painful stimulus is induced. Problem pain is frequently associated with pathophysiologic changes that occur at the level of the spinal cord and brain. These changes frequently involve the activation of NMDA receptors, resulting in central neuronal hypersensitization, commonly referred to as wind-up. As wind-up develops, the central neurons begin to exaggerate the stimulus, which enters the spinal cord, making the stimulus that eventually makes it to the higher centers of the brain of greater intensity than its peripheral origination, thus resulting in worsening pain. This can result in any of the NSAIDs or other analgesics having a tapering effect over time, even though the origin of the pain has not worsened.

The third principle of pain control is to use drugs in a multimodal manner. This is simply the implementation of drugs or techniques that work at different levels of the nociceptive pathways and via different mechanisms. This means using some combination of opioids, nonsteroidal anti-inflammatory drugs, alpha-2 agonists, NMDA-antagonists, and local anesthetics.

Assessment of Pain

Assessment of pain in animals can be difficult and frustrating. Understanding types of pain and their causes can be helpful. Often veterinarians need to rely on the experience in humans to help define the pain in animals. Technicians and other staff members are usually the ones who experience the postoperative period more than the doctors. Pain assessment typically is delegated to these staff members. Recognition and assessment of pain is the first and probably the most difficult step in providing analgesia to dogs and cats. It is often easiest to assume an animal is in pain if a person undergoing similar trauma or surgery would be in pain.

A patient usually tolerates mild pain without a problem and does not exhibit any behavioral changes. Patients with mild pain often are not treated. Patients experiencing moderate pain usually exhibit changes in behavior, appetite, activity, positioning, or posture, at least in the absence of human interaction. These patients also tend to respond significantly to palpation of the painful area. Severe pain can be thought of as intolerable, and is often manifested as unprovoked crying, whimpering, or howling associated with violent thrashing. Nonspecific physiologic responses to pain include elevated heart rate and blood pressure, abnormal cardiac rhythm, panting, salivation, dilated pupils, and unhandleable behavior. It is important to remember that differences in variables will occur among individuals, breeds, and species.

Classification as to origin of pain is also important because some drugs have greater efficacy for different types of pain. Somatic pain originates from damage to bones, joints, muscles, or skin and is described in humans as localized, constant, sharp, aching, and throbbing. Visceral pain arises from stretching, distension, or inflammation of the viscera, and is described as deep, cramping, aching, or gnawing, without good localization. Neuropathic pain originates from injury or involvement of the peripheral or central nervous system and is described as burning or shooting, possibly associated with motor, sensory, or autonomic deficits.

Assessment of pain can be accomplished systematically with a pain scoring scale.[30-31] The objective of a pain scoring system is to place a quantitative value on a specific variable, add up the variables and compare the total to some predetermined assessment of pain. There are many different pain score scales and no one is perfect. Some investigators have also used a visual analog scale (VAS) in animals. A VAS would need to be validated for several people at each practice to assure consistent scoring.

Failure to assess pain initially and throughout the course of treatment is a leading factor of under-treatment. Pain should be assessed early with the goal of characterizing the pain as to location, intensity, and probable etiology. Client engagement in this process helps determine aggravating and relieving factors. After a good assessment is performed, goals for pain control can be set with the client.

Nonopioids

Nonopioid analgesics include drugs such as carprofen, meloxicam, tepoxalin, etodolac, deracoxib, firocoxib, acetaminophen, aspirin, ketoprofen, and etodolac (Table 8-2). All except acetaminophen are considered nonsteroidal anti-inflammatory drugs (NSAID). Despite the low anti-inflammatory activity of acetaminophen, it possesses beneficial analgesic effects, minimal risk of bleeding in thrombocytopenic patients, decreased gastrointestinal effects, and synergism with opioid analgesics, such as codeine. Acetaminophen should be avoided in cats because of their inadequate cytochrome P-450-dependent hydroxylation.[32]

Table 8-2. Commonly used Nonopioid Analgesics

Drug	Dog Dose	Cat Dose
Acetaminophen (Tylenol®)	10 mg/kg PO q 12 hrs	CI
Carprofen (Rimadyl®)	4 mg/kg PO q 24 hrs	Uknown oral dosing
Carprofen	4.0 mg/kg IV,IM,SQ q 24 hr	1-3 mg/kg SQ ONCE
Meloxicam (Metacam®)	0.2 mg/kg PO q 24 hrs ONCE then 0.1 mg/kg PO q 24 hrs	Variable#: 0.1 mg/kg PO q 24 hrs x 4 days, then 0.05 mg/kg PO x 4 days; then 0.05 mg/cat PO x 4 days, then 0.
Meloxicam (Metacam®)	0.2 mg/kg SQ	0.2-0.3 mg/kg SQ
Tepoxalin (Zubrin®)	10 mg/kg PO q 24 hrs	UK
Deracoxib (Deramax®)	1-2 mg/kg PO q 24 hrs	UK
Firocoxib (Previcox®)	5 mg/kg PO q 24 hrs	UK
Ketoprofen (Ketofen®)	2.0 mg/kg PO for 1st 24 hrs then 1.0 mg/kg PO q 24 hrs	2.0 mg/kg PO for 1st 24 hrs then 1.0 mg/kg PO q 24 hrs
Ketoprofen	2.0 mg/kg IV, SC, IM q 24 hr	2.0 mg/kg SC q 24 hr
Etodolac (Etogesic®)	10-15 mg/kg q 24 hrs	UK
Piroxicam (Feldene®)	0.3 mg/kg q 24 hrs for 2 days then 0.3 mg/kg q 48 hrs	0.3 mg/kg q 48 hrs
Misoprostal *(Cytotec®)	2-5 μg/kg PO q 8 hrs	UK

CI = Contraindicated for use in cats; UK = unknown dose

 # Oral dosing for meloxicam long term in cats has not been well established via pharmacokinetics, but clinical efficacy is based on variable dosing regimens

***Synthetic prostaglandin E used to increase the protective effects of endogenous prostaglandins ($PGE_{2\alpha}$) and nonselective cyclooxygenase inhibition to help prevent GI ulceration.**

Mild to moderate pain, especially that arising from intrathoracic masses, intraabdominal masses, minor fractures, mild soft tissue injuries, and bone metastases, can be relieved with NSAIDs. When pain increases, NSAIDs have an opioid-sparing effect so that better analgesia can be achieved with lower doses of opioids. NSAIDs have central analgesic and peripheral anti-inflammatory effects mediated via inhibition of cyclooxygenase. The choice of NSAID ultimately depends on available species information, clinical response, and tolerance of side effects. Most NSAIDs have been formally investigated only in dogs, leaving anecdotal information for use in cats. The most common side effect of NSAID administration in dogs is gastric irritation and bleeding owing to loss of gastric acid inhibition and of cytoprotective mucus production normally promoted by prostaglandins. Other side effects include renal failure and hepatic dysfunction that may lead to failure.[33] NSAIDs that are more selective for inhibition of cyclooxygenase-2 (COX-2) seem to have fewer gastrointestinal effects and potentially fewer renal effects.[34,35] Therefore, more selective COX-2 inhibitors, such as carprofen, meloxicam, deracoxib, tepoxalin, firocoxib, and etodolac, should be considered priority NSAIDs in pain patients. A blood chemistry panel should be performed prior to initiating NSAID therapy. If evidence exists of liver or renal disease, dehydration or hypotension, another approach to therapy should be considered. Therapy with NSAIDs, which are non-specific cyclooxygenase inhibitors, may also inhibit platelet function, leading to bleeding and oozing. Therapy with these NSAIDs should be stopped if this occurs. If clinical effectiveness is not achieved with one NSAID, it should be discontinued and another started 4 to 7 days later to avoid additive or synergistic cyclooxygenase inhibition effects. Aspirin should be avoided in dogs because of the increased possibility of gastrointestinal bleeding, even with buffered formulations.[36,37] Administering misoprostol can help provide gastrointestinal protection during the switchover period.

Opioids

Opioids are the major class of analgesics used in the management of moderate to severe pain. They are reasonably effective, predictable, and have low risk associated with them. The most common parenteral opioids used in small animals are morphine, oxymorphone, fentanyl, codeine, meperidine, buprenorphine, and butorphanol (Table 8-3). Parenteral opioids should be used in the perioperative period and should be discontinued when a patient can be switched to oral medication. Common oral opioids include morphine and codeine with or without acetaminophen. An opioid-like oral drug that is becoming more commonly administered is tramadol.

As a patient's pain increases, the required dose of opioid also increases. Veterinarians may be reluctant to administer high doses of opioids for fear of adverse side effects. It is important to remember that veterinarians have an ethical obligation to benefit the patient by alleviating pain. Opioids can be administered while managing side effects to maximally help the patient. Side effects of opioid administration include diarrhea and vomiting initially, constipation with long-term use, sedation, and dysphoria. The initial gastrointestinal effects occur most frequently with the first injection in the perioperative period and usually do not occur with subsequent dosing. These effects usually do not occur with oral dosing. When sending a patient home with oral medications, it is important to discuss with the owner that dosing is highly individual. It is possible that a given dose may be perfect, or it does not provide enough analgesia, induces sedation, or induces dysphoria or excitement. Adjusting of the dose requires excellent doctor-client interaction. Bradycardia is also possible after opioid administration, but is most common if opioids are administered parenterally. If bradycardia occurs, an anticholinergic, such as atropine or glycopyrrolate, should be administered, rather than discontinuing the opioid.

Opioids are classified as full mu-receptor agonists, partial agonists, and kappa agonist--mu antagonists. Examples of the full mu-receptor agonists include morphine, oxymorphone, fentanyl, codeine, and meperidine. In normal, healthy animals, opioids may produce sedation, which is usually acceptable, or dysphoria, an exaggerated unrest, which usually is undesirable. Full mu agonists induce the best analgesia in a dose-dependent manner and are not limited by a ceiling effect. As pain increases, larger doses may be administered. Morphine should be the most commonly used opioid for severe pain. It is available in multiple injectable and oral formulations, including short-duration tablets and liquids and sustained release tablets. Oral morphine may be the most effective method for providing longer term analgesia to dogs with moderate to severe pain. Patients receiving analgesics at set dosing intervals should also be provided with some short-duration opioid for breakthrough pain. While the pharmacokinetics of oral morphine in dogs are variable, the clinical efficacy seems to be highly reliable.[38,39]

Oxymorphone is only available as an injectable analgesic and may induce panting, by changing the temperature set point in the brain.[40] This usually is not an issue, except when attempting thoracic or abdominal radiography. Hydromorphone, like oxymorphone, is a pure mu-receptor agonist and can induce the same degree of analgesia as morphine. Meperidine is short acting in animals, limiting its use as an analgesic in patients with severe pain. Codeine is available alone or with acetaminophen, allowing some flexibility in choice of oral medications. Fentanyl is an injectable drug that is potent and equally effective as morphine. All of the previously mentioned parenteral opioids may be administered by intermittent intravenous, intramuscular, or subcutaneous routes. A problem with this type of intermittent dosing is that patients often develop pain before their subsequent dose, then are extremely sedate after dosing. An alternate dosing regimen would use continuous infusion of an opioid. Fentanyl, morphine, hydromorphone, and oxymorphone are appropriate drugs for continuous infusion. Fentanyl may be especially suited to continuous infusion therapy because it is short acting. This enables the practitioner to alter the dose as necessary from minute to minute to achieve good analgesia and potentially minimal sedation if desired.

Buprenorphine is an example of a partial mu agonist. It does not produce the same degree of analgesia as does morphine and has a ceiling effect. The advantage of buprenorphine is that it has a long duration of action, 6 to12 hours. It also has a long time to onset, approximately 40 minutes, even when given intravenously. Buprenorphine is a unique drug in that larger doses may actually produce less analgesia owing to a bell-shaped dose-response curve. Tapering the dose to the individual maybe difficult. If an animal does not have adequate analgesia after receiving buprenorphine, dosing with a morphine-like drug may not produce any results because of buprenorphine's strong affinity for mu-opioid receptors. Buprenorphine is not easily reversible. Experimentally, it takes 1000 times the normal dose of naloxone to reverse it in a normal dog.[41-43] Because of the inherent lack of maximal analgesia compared with morphine, buprenorphine should be used only for mild to moderate pain.

Buprenorphine can also be administered transmucosally in cats (Table 8-3). Owing to the pH of a cat's mouth, buccal buprenorphine has good uptake, resulting in pharmacokinetics that parallel intravenous administration.[44-46] Cats can usually tolerate 2 days of administration of buccal buprenorphine before developing unacceptable sedation.

Another group of opioids that are available are the kappa agonist--mu antagonists, of which butorphanol is an example. Butorphanol may reverse the effects of drugs like morphine, a pure mu agonist, but provides analgesia and sedation of its own. Butorphanol is also reversible with naloxone and nalmefene. Butorphanol cannot induce the same maximal analgesia as morphine, having a ceiling effect at moderate doses of pain. Even in large parenteral doses, butorphanol produces analgesia of short duration in dogs.[47] These last two properties may limit butorphanol's utility for treatment of severe pain.

Tramadol is an opioid-like drug that also inhibits serotonin reuptake.[48] Tramadol is a useful adjunct to NSAID therapy in patients with moderate pain. The pharmacokinetics seem to indicate the need for large doses administered frequently in dogs, although the clinical experience may indicate otherwise (Table 8-3).

Table 8-3. Commonly used Opioid Analgesics

Drug	Dog Dose (mg/kg) and Route	Duration in Dogs (hrs)	Cat Dose (mg/kg) and Route	Duration in Cats (hrs)
Morphine	0.5-2.2 SQ, IM	3-4	0.25-0.5 SQ, IM	3-4
Morphine	0.1-0.2 IV	1	0.05-0.1	1
Morphine: liquid; immediate release tablets	1.0-4.0 PO	4-6	0.5-1.0	4-6
Morphine: sustained release tablets* (MS Contin®)	1.0-4.0 PO	8-12	NA	NA
Morphine: preservative free (Astromorph®)	0.1 mg/kg epidural	6-24	0.1	6-24
Fentanyl	0.01 SQ	1-2	0.005 SQ	1-2
Fentanyl	0.002 IV	0.3-0.5	0.001-0.002 IV	0.3-0.5
Fentanyl	0.002-0.006 mg/kg/hr IV	**	0.001-0.004 mg/kg/hr IV	**
Fentanyl: transdermal patch (Duragesic®)	2-5 μg/kg/hr	72	2-5 μg/kg/hr	72-96
Codeine 60mg + acetaminophen 300 mg	1-2 based on codeine PO	3-4	CI	CI
Oxymorphone (Numorphan®)	0.1 SQ, IM	1.5-3	0.05 SQ, IM	1.5-3
Oxymorphone	0.06 IV	0.75	0.03 IV	0.75
Hydromorphone (Dilaudid®)	0.1-0.2 SQ, IM	1-3	0.05-0.1 SQ, IM	1-3
Hydromorphine	0.1 IV	0.75	0.05	0.75
Butorphanol (Torbugesic®)	0.4-0.8 SQ, IM	0.75-1.0	0.2-0.4	3-4
Butorphanol	0.2 IV	0.5	0.1	0.5
Buprenorphine (Buprenex® Carpuject®)	0.02-0.06 SQ, IM	4-12	0.005-0.01 SQ, IM	4-12
Buprenorphine	NAD	NAD	0.01-0.02 PO	8-12
Tramadol	2-6	6-12	1-3	6-12

***These tablets must not be cut. Dosing is appropriate for dogs weighing at least 15 kg**
NA: Not applicable to cats due to the size of the tablet
NAD: Not applicable to dogs due to oral pH
**** Duration is dependent upon infusion duration; CI= Contraindicated in cats**

An alternative to oral opioids for providing multiple-day analgesia is through transdermal fentanyl patches (Table 8-3). Fentanyl patches require 12 to 24 hours to take effect and last 2 to 4 days. Additional analgesia must be provided during the first 0.5 to 1 day after patch placement. One problem with transdermal fentanyl is related to unreliable plasma levels in dogs,[49-51] probably related to failure of patch application or inappropriate dosing. Fentanyl patches may not provide enough analgesia for severe pain,[52] but they allow lower doses of additional drugs. Fentanyl patches are expensive and should not be the first approach to chronic therapy. Transdermal fentanyl is most appropriate in those patients that do not tolerate oral medication.

Epidural opioids, especially morphine (Table 8-3), have been used as a method for perioperative analgesia. With placement of an epidural catheter, epidural opioids can be administered for days to weeks. Epidurals are discussed later in this chapter.

The appropriate dose of an opioid is that dose which produces analgesia with the fewest side effects. The need for increased doses often reflects progression of disease. Long-term use may produce opioid tolerance, increasing doses or frequency to achieve equivalent results. As previously mentioned, veterinarians should not be afraid of increasing doses in patients and should remember the need for analgesia. A distinct advantage of using opioids for pain control is that they are reversible with naloxone or nalmefene if unacceptable side effects occur. Prolonged use may produce constipation. Oral laxatives can help alleviate this problem.

Alpha-2 Agonists

Medetomidine and xylazine are two alpha-2 agonists approved for use in small animals in the United States (Table 8-4). They are non-controlled parenteral agents that provide excellent visceral analgesia, but only for 20 minutes to 2 hours.[53] Their effects can be nearly completely reversed with yohimbine or atipamezole, respectively. Xylazine and medetomidine should not be the first or sole choice in providing analgesia perioperatively to patients in moderate to severe pain because they greatly reduce cardiac function and, potentially, oxygenation.[54-56] Xylazine and medetomidine have synergistic effects with opioids. This effect,which can be achieved with microdoses, is useful postoperatively for inducing additional analgesia and alleviating dysphoria.

Ketamine

Ketamine has been used for many years as an induction agent to general anesthesia in normal and compromised patients (Table 8-4). It has been well established that ketamine provides reasonable somatic but poor visceral analgesia.[57] Recently, ketamine has been identified as a NMDA receptor antagonist. N-methyl-D-aspartate receptors are believed to play a role in the processes leading up to central sensitization and wind-up. As an NMDA receptor antagonist, ketamine reduces postoperative pain and cumulative opioid requirements for a variety of procedures in humans and dogs.[58-59] This is accomplished with doses that are much smaller than those for anesthesia. As such, it is uncommon for patients to develop behavioral or cardiovascular effects. Micro-dose ketamine appears to provide beneficial effects for a variety of surgical procedures, limb amputations, and major fracture repairs. When used in this manner, ketamine should be administered as a bolus (0.5 mg/kg IV) followed by an infusion (10 μg/kg/min) prior to and during surgical stimulation. A lower infusion rate (2 μg/kg/min) may be beneficial for the first 24 hours postoperatively and an even lower rate (1 μg/kg/min) for the next 24 hours. In the absence of an infusion pump, ketamine can be mixed in a bag of crystalloid solutions for administration during anesthesia. Using anesthesia fluid administration rates of 10 ml/kg/hr, 60 mg (0.6 ml) of ketamine should be added to a 1 liter bag of crystalloid fluids to deliver ketamine at 10 μg/kg/min.

Table 8-4. Adjunct Drugs to Management of Pain

Drug	Route	Dose
Acepromazine	IV	0.005-0.03 mg/kg
Acepromazine	SQ, IM	0.02-0.05 mg/kg
Diazepam /Midazolam (Versed®)	IV	0.1-0.2 mg/kg
Xylazine	IV	0.05-0.1 mg/kg
Xylazine	IM	0.2 mg/kg
Medetomidine (Domitor®)	IV	0.001 mg/kg
Medetomidine	IM	0.002 mg/kg
Amitriptyline (dog) (Elavil®)	PO	1-2 mg/kg q 12-24 hrs
Amitriptyline (cat)	PO	2.5-12.5 mg /cat q 24 hrs
Imipramine (dog) (Tofranil®)	PO	0.5-1.0 mg/kg q 8 hrs
Imipramine (cat)	PO	2.5-5 mg/kg q 12 hrs
Clomipramine (Comicalm®)	PO	2-4 mg/kg PO q 24 hrs
Ketamine	IV	0.5 mg/kg bolus followed by 0.6 mg/kg/hr during surgical stimulation followed by 0.12 mg/kg/hr for 24 hrs

Doses are the same for dogs and cats unless otherwise described

Tranquilizers

A concern that frequently arises with pain management is concurrent tranquilization and sedation. Most of the drugs used by veterinarians usually produce concurrent sedation. As mentioned previously, opioids have the greatest potential of producing dysphoria, instead of sedation. Dysphoria becomes more likely when cats are administered higher than necessary doses of opioids and when a patient is already experiencing high anxiety in the hospital. Dysphoric patients can sometimes be treated simply by petting and soothing, or by helping the patient change positions. Low-dose acepromazine, both IV and/or IM is reasonable drug therapy for dysphoria (Table 8-4). While acepromazine does not treat pain, it calms anxious patients very well and also makes them care less about their pain. For patients in which acepromazine is contraindicated, those with bleeding and seizure disorders, the benzodiazepines, diazepam and midazolam, often calm patients (Table 8-4). Benzodiazepines should not be used by themselves in most alert patients as they frequently cause excitement. Combined with opioids, sedation usually results. In patients that are hemodynamically stable, a microdose of medetomidine, IV, also can decrease dysphoria and increase analgesia.

Patients that develop dysphoria after oral analgesic medications often respond well to oral acepromazine or diazepam. It is important to discern whether the opioid dose is effective before changing the analgesia regimen.

Tricyclic Antidepressants

Tricyclic antidepressants, such as amitriptyline, imipramine, and clomipramine block the re-uptake of serotonin and norepinephrine in the central nervous system. They also have antihistamine effects. These drugs have been used in humans for the treatment of chronic and neuropathic pain at doses considerably lower than those used to treat depression.[60] Veterinarians have not used tricyclic antidepressants in this manner for long, but they appear to induce similar analgesic properties and enhance opioid analgesia as they do in humans (Table 8-4).

Local Anesthetics

The use of local and regional anesthetic techniques in small animals was common in the early 20th century. Interest has increased in these techniques, probably owing to their ability to provide preemptive analgesia and decrease wind-up. Local anesthetic techniques can be used instead of general anesthesia in selected cases or, more commonly, in combination.

The most commonly used local anesthetics include lidocaine and bupivacaine (Table 8-5). Lidocaine has a short onset (< 1 min) and lasts approximately 60 to 90 minutes. Doses of 1.5 to 2.0 mg/kg are safe in dogs and cats. Signs of toxicity are manifested as neurologic changes, including seizures. Bupivacaine takes approximately 20 minutes to take effect, but may last for 5 to 8 hours. Whereas lidocaine has antidysrhythmic effects at low to moderate intravenous doses, bupivacaine has cardiotoxic effects when administered intravascularly. Inadvertent IV administration can result in death.[61-64] Epinephrine may be added to bupivacaine in a 1:200,000 dilution to cause local vasoconstriction and prolonged duration. Epinephrine should not be used for peripheral blocks because collateral circulation may not be available to provide adequate perfusion to distal tissues. Combinations of lidocaine and bupivacaine are often used to achieve quick onset and long duration. This is especially necessary when using local anesthetics interpleurally. Because of its long onset, bupivacaine causes stinging and discomfort. Lidocaine administered concurrently limits the discomfort to a period of seconds.

Local anesthetics have numerous uses. They are often used epidurally to produce either better analgesia in low doses or anesthesia for caudal procedures in higher doses. They may be used interpleurally for thoracic and cranial abdominal pain. Intercostal nerve blocks are easily performed for lateral thoracotomy pain. Brachial plexus infiltration provides anesthesia for procedures distal to the elbow. Maxillary, infraorbital, mandibular, and mental nerve blocks are commonly used for procedures involving the face and mouth. Local infiltration is common for procedures involving the ear. Ring blocks have also been used for distal limb and digit amputations. Many of these techniques have been well described.[65]

Epidurals

Epidural administration of drugs requires additional skill and expertise that may not be available in all clinical settings. With epidural administration, a needle is placed on the dorsal midline and advanced at the lumbosacral junction through the ligamentum flavum until one encounters a loss of resistance. This technique has been well described.[65,66] Epidural morphine is commonly administered in the perioperative period to provide analgesia, but not anesthesia, for the abdomen or more caudally. In some instances, analgesia may be effective for the thorax and forelimb. This analgesia may last up to 24 hours.[67] Local anesthetics may also be administered epidurally as a low dose to augment epidural morphine-induce analgesia or at a higher dose to produce anesthesia.

Table 8-5. Doses of Local Anesthetic

Type of Block	Lidocaine (mg/kg)	Bupivacaine (mg/kg)
Epidural anesthesia to L2	2.0	1.5-2.0
Epidural anesthesia to T5	4.0-6.0	2.0
Epidural analgesia (administered with epidural morphine)	0.5-0.2	0.03-0.1
Interpleural	1.5 (given with bupivacaine)	1.5 (given with lidocaine)
Miscellaneous nerve blocks	1.5-2.0 maximum*	1.5-2.0 maximum*

***The maximum dose should be divided among all blocks to be performed**

A catheter can also be placed in the epidural space for severe pain that may be intractable in the caudal portion of the body. Maintenance of this catheter requires veterinarian and client vigilance to assure cleanliness and prevent infection migrating to the spinal cord. With proper care, an epidural catheter can remain in place for days to weeks.

Conclusion

The understanding of pain and its alleviation is a constantly evolving science. While we know more now than ever before, new information changes our approach to patients almost daily. Veterinarians have a physiologic and ethical obligation to treat pain to help assure optimal well being of their patients. The current understanding of pain medicine allows veterinarians to effectively treat the vast majority of patients with acute painand a large number of patients with chronic pain. While chronic pain may be more of a challenge, no patient should be euthanized because of pain if the owners have the means to explore multiple modalities.

References

1. Gaynor JS: Is postoperative pain management important in dogs and cats? Vet Med March Symposium:254-258, 1999.

2. Cousins MJ, Phillips GD: Acute Pain Management. New York: Churchill Livingstone, 1986, pp.19-48.

3. Hamill RJ: The physiologic and metabolic response to pain and stress. *In*. Handbook of Critical Care Pain Management, Hamill RJ,Rowlingson JC (eds). New York: McGraw-Hill, 1994.

4. Raja SN, Meyer RA, Ringkamp M, et al: Peripheral neural mechanisms of nociception. *In* Textbook of Pain, 4th ed. Wall PD, Melzack R (eds). Edinburgh: Churchill Livingstone, 1999, pp.11-58.

5. Doubell TP, Mannion RJ, Woolf CJ: The dorsal horn: state dependent sensory processing, plasticity, and the generation of pain. *In* Textbook of Pain, 4th ed. Wall PD, Melzack R (eds). Edinburgh: Churchill Livingstone, 1999, pp.165-182.

6. Muir WW: Physiology and pathophysiology of pain. *In* Handbook of Veterinary Pain Management. Gaynor JS, Muir WW (eds). St. Louis: Mosby, 2002, pp. 13-45.

7. Muir WW, Woolf CJ: Mechanisms of pain and their therapeutic implications. JAVMA 219:1346-1356, 2001;

8. Phelps PT, Anthes JC, Correll CC: Cloning and functional characterization of dog transient receptor potential vanilloid receptor-1 (TRPV1). Eur J Pharmacol 513:57-66, 2005.

9. Xie J, Price MP, Berger AL, et al: DRASIC contributes to pH-gated currents in large dorsal root ganglion sensory neurons by forming heteromultimeric channels. J Neurophysiol 87:2835-2843, 2002;.

10. Price MP, McIlwrath SL, Xie J, et al: The DRASIC cation channel contributes to the detection of cutaneous touch and acid stimuli in mice. Neuron 32:1071-1083, 2001.

11. Brauchi S, Orio P, Latorre R: Clues to understanding cold sensation: thermodynamics and electrophysiological analysis of the cold receptor TRPM8. Proc Natl Acad Sci USA 101:15494-15499, 2004.

12. Tominaga M, Caterina MJ: Thermosensation and pain. J Neurobiol 61:3-12, 2004.

13. Kobayashi K, Fukuoka T, Obata K, et al: Distinct expression of TRPM8, TRPA1, and TRPV1 mRNAs in rat primary afferent neurons with adelta/c-fibers and colocalization with trk receptors. J Comp Neurol 493:596-606, 2005.

14. Obata K, Katsura H, Mizushima T, et al: TRPA1 induced in sensory neurons contributes to cold hyperalgesia after inflammation and nerve injury. J Clin Invest 115:2393-2401, 2005.

15. Calixto JB, Kassuya CA, Andre E, et al: Contribution of natural products to the discovery of the transient receptor potential (TRP) channels family and their functions. Pharmacol Ther 106:179-208, 2005.

16. McKemy DD: How cold is it? TRPM8 and TRPA1 in the molecular logic of cold sensation. Mol Pain 1:16, 2005.

17. Harteneck C: Function and pharmacology of TRPM cation channels. Naunyn Schmiedebergs Arch Pharmacol 371:307-314, 2005.

18. Numazaki M, Tominaga M: Nociception and TRP Channels. Curr Drug Targets CNS Neurol Disord 3:479-485, 2004.

19. Melzack R: From the gate to the neuromatrix. [Review] [13 refs]. Pain Aug Suppl 6:S121-6, 1999.

20. Maciocia G: The Foundations of Chinese Medicine. Edinburgh: Churchill Livingstone, 1989.

21. Mittleman E: Acupuncture Analgesia: Mechanisms of Action and Nervous System Effects.

22. Skarda RT: Complementary and alternative (integrative) pain therapy. *In* Gaynor JS, Muir WW (eds). Handbook of Veterinary Pain Management. St. Louis: Mosby, 2002, pp. 281-328.

23. Vazquez J, Munoz M, Caceres JL: Modifications in the distribution of met-enkephalin in the limbic system of the cat brain after electroacupuncture. An immunocytochemical study. Histol Histopathol 10:577-582, 1995.

24. Lee DC, Lee MO: Endorphins, naloxone, and acupuncture. Calif Vet 24-33, 1979.

25. Lee DC, Ichiyanagi K, Lee MO, et al: Can naloxone inhibit the cardiovascular effect of acupuncture? Can Anaesth Soc J 26:410-414, 1979.

26. Mayer DJ: Antagonism of acupuncture analgesia in man by the narcotic antagonist naloxone. Brain Res 121:368-372, 1977.

27. Janssens LAA, Rogers PAM, Schoen AM: Acupuncture analgesia: a review. Vet Rec 122:355-358, 1988.

28. He L, Wang M, Gao M, et al: Expression of c-fos protein in serotonergic neurons of rat brainstem following electro-acupuncture. Acupunct Electro-Therap Res 17:243-248, 1992.

29. Chen SZ, Han JS: High frequency electroacupuncture induced changes of IP3 level in rat brain and spinal cord.

30. Holton LL, Scott EM, Nolan AM, et al: The development of a multidimensional scale to assess pain in dogs. Proceedings of the 6th ICVA 1997; 106.

31. Holton LL, Scott EM, Nolan AM, et al: Comparison on three methods used for assessment of pain in dogs. JAVMA 212:61-66, 1998.

32. Booth NH:. Nonnarcotic analgesics. *In* Veterinary Pharmacology and Therapeutics, 5th ed. Booth NH, McDonald LE, (eds). Ames: Iowa State University Press, 1982, pp. 297-320.

33. MacPhail CM, Lappin MR, Meyer DJ, et al: Hepatocellular toxicosis associated with administration of carprofen in 21 dogs. JAVMA 212 (12):1895-1901, 1998.

34. Golden BD, Abramson SB: Selective cyclooxygenase-2 inhibitors. Rheum Dis Clin Am 25:359-378, 1999.

35. Rubin BR: Specific cyclooxygenase-2 (COX-2) inhibitors. J Am Osteopath Assoc 99:300-301, 1999.

36. Shaw N, Burrows CF, King RR: Massive gastric hemorrhage induced by buffered aspirin in a greyhound. J Am Anim Hosp Assoc 33:215-219, 1997.

37. Bowersox TS, Lipowitz AJ, Hardy RM, et al; The use of a synthetic prostaglandin E1 analog as a gastric protectant against aspirin- induced hemmorhage in the dog. J Am Anim Hosp Assoc 32:401-407, 1996.

38. Dohoo S, Tasker RA, Donald A: Pharmacokinetics of parenteral and oral sustained-release morphine sulphate in dogs. J Vet Pharmacol Therap 17:426-433, 1994.

39. Machado C, Dyson D: Effects of oxymorphone and hydromorphone on isoflurane minimal alveolar concentration in dogs. Proceedings of the Annual Meeting of the American College of Veterinary Anesthesiologists

40. Booth NH: Neuroleptanalgesics, narcotic analgesics, and analgesic antagonists. *In* Veterinary Pharmacology and Therapeutics, 5th ed. Booth NH, McDonald LE (eds). Ames: The Iowa State University Press, 1982, pp. 267-296.

41. Heel RC, Brogden RN, Speight TM, et al: Buprenorphine: A review of its pharmacological properties and therapeutic efficacy. Drugs 17:81-110, 1990.

42. Rosland JH, Hole K: 1, 4-benzodiazepines antagonize opiate-induced actinociception in mice. Anesth Analg 71:242-248, 1990.

43. Hoskin PJ, Hanks GW: Opioid agonist - antagonist drugs in acute and chronic pain states. Drugs 41:326-344, 1991.

44. Robertson SA, Taylor PM, Sear JW: Systemic uptake of buprenorphine by cats after oral mucosal administration. Vet Rec 152:675-678, 2003.

45. Robertson S, Taylor P, Dixon M, et al: The effect of buprenophine, morphine and saline on thermal thresholds in cats. Proceedings of the Annual Meeting of the American College of Veterinary Anesthesiologists, San Francisco, 2001; 30.

46. Robertson SA, Taylor PM, Lascelles BD, et al: Changes in thermal threshold response in eight cats after administration of buprenorphine, butorphanol and morphine. Vet Rec 153:462-465, 2003.

47. Sawyer DC, Rech RC, Durham RA, et al: Dose response to butorphanol administered subcutaneously to increase viceral nociceptive threshold in dogs. Am J Vet Res 52:1826-1830, 1991.

48. Gaynor JS: Other drugs used to treat pain. *In* Gaynor JS, Muir WW (eds). Handbook of Veterinary Pain Management. St. Louis: Mosby, 2002, pp. 251-260.

49. Egger CM, Duke T, Archer J, et al: Comparison of plasma fentanyl concentrations by using three transdermal fentanyl patch sizes in dogs. Vet Surg 27:159-166, 1998.

50. Schultheiss PJ, Morse BC, Baker WH: Evaluation of a transdermal fentanyl system in the dog. Am Assoc Lab Anim Sci 34, No. 5:75-81, 1995.

51. Scherk-Nixon M: A study of the use of a transdermal fentanyl patch in cats. J Am Anim Hosp Assoc 32:19-24, 1996.

52. Robinson TM, Kruse-Elliot KT, Markel MD, et al: A comparison of transdermal fentanyl versus epidural morphine for analgesia in dogs undergoing major orthopedic surgery. J Am Anim Hosp Assoc 35:95-100, 1999.

53. Benson GJ, Grubb TL, Neff-Davis C, et al: Effect of medetomidine on surgically-induced endocrine responses. Proceedings of the 5th International Congress of Veterinary Anesthesia, August 1994; 165.

54. Tendillo FJ, Mascias A, Segura IAG, et al: Cardiopulmonary and analgesic effects of alpha-2 adrenergic receptor agonists, xylazine, detomidine and medetomidine and their antagonist atipamezole in the pig. ACVA85-82, 1992.

55. Savola JM: Cardiovascular actions of medetomidine and their reversal by atipamezole. Acta Vet Scand 85:39-47, 1989.

56. Serteyn D, Coppens P, Jones R, et al: Circulatory and respiratory effects of the combination medetomidine-ketamine in beagles. J Vet Pharmacol Therap 16:199-206, 1993.

57. Joubert K: Ketamine hydrochloride--an adjunct for analgesia in dogs with burn wounds. J South Afr Vet Assoc 69:95-97, 1998.

58. Felsby S, Nielsen J, Arendt-Nielsen L, et al: NMDA receptor blockade in chronic neuropathic pain: a comparison of ketamine and magnesium chloride. Pain 64:283-291, 1996.

59. Wagner AE, Walton JA, Hellyer PW, et al: Use of low doses of ketamine administrared by constant rate infusion as an adjunct for postoperative analgesia in dogs. JAVMA 221:72-74, 2002.

60. Merskey H: Pharmacologic approaches other than opioids in chronic non-cancer pain management. Acta Anaesthesiol Scand 41:187-190, 1997.

61. Lacombe P, Blaise G, Loulmet D, et al: Electrophysiologic effects of bupivacaine in the isolated rabbit heart. Anesth Analg 72:62-69, 1991.

62. Badgwell JM, Heavner JE, Kytta J: Bupivacaine toxicity in young pigs is age-dependent and is affected by volatile anesthetics. Anesth 73:297-303, 1990.

63. Moller R, Covino BG: Cardiac electrophysiologic properties of bupivacaine and lidocaine compared with those of ropivacaine. A new amide local anesthetic. Anesth 72:322-329, 1990.

64. Bader AM, Datta S, Flanagan H, et al: Comparison of bupivacaine- and ropivacaine-induced conduction blockade in the isolated rabbit vagus nerve. Anesth Analg 68:724-727, 1989.

65. Gaynor JSM, K.R. Local and regional anesthetic techniques for the alleviation of perioperative pain. *In* Gaynor JS, Muir WW (eds). Handbook of Veterinary Pain Management. St. Louis: Mosby, 2002.

66. Muir WW, Hubbell JAE, Skarda RT, et al: Handbook of Veterinary Anesthesia, 2 ed. St. Louis: Mosby, 1995.

67. Ravat F, Dorne R, Baichle JP, et al: Epidural ketamine or morphine for postoperative analgesia. Anesth 66:819-822, 1987.

Chapter 9

Principles of Metastasis

Susan E. Lana

In spite of the advances made in diagnostic approaches, surgical techniques, adjuvant chemotherapy, and radiation therapy, metastasis to distant sites remains the leading cause of cancer related death.[1-3] Unfortunately these metastatic foci can also be resistant to conventional therapies.[4] A significant amount of research has focused on the biologic and molecular events involved in this process, however much remains unknown. The purpose of this chapter is to provide an overview of the complex process of metastasis.

Metastatic Cascade

The process of metastasis is a series of sequential events or steps that must be completed for successful dissemination of a tumor to occur.[5] The metastatic cancer cell has often been referred to as the decathlete of cells for its ability to leave the primary tumor, enter the circulation, evade host defenses and physical stress, exit the vasculature and recognize an appropriate distant organ where it must interact in a sometimes hostile environment, divide, and continue to grow.[6] Because of theses multiple complex steps one can imagine that metastasis is a highly inefficient process. In fact, experimental models have shown that less than 0.01% of cells injected intravenously actually form viable tumor foci.[5] Additionally, the process of metastasis is not random and each step can be rate limiting, with failure to succeed at any point resulting in disruption of the process.

Several steps in this process, often referred to as the metastatic cascade, are discussed in the following.

Angiogenesis

As a tumor grows beyond a size that can be sustained by simple diffusion of nutrients from the immediate environment, hypoxic areas arise and the tumor initiates development of its own blood supply. This is usually the result of increased production of pro-angiogenic factors such as basic fibroblast growth factor (bFGF), vascular endothelial growth factor (VEGF), and platelet-derived growth factor (PDGF) either by the tumor or the surrounding host cells in response to tumor signals.[8,9] At the same time, suppression occurs of anti-angiogenic factors such as interferon alpha, thrombospondin, and endogenous protease inhibitors.[5] New vessel growth from existing vasculature has been believed to be the end result of this imbalance of factors; however, evidence is increasing to support the hypothesis that circulating endothelial progenitor cells (CEPs) derived from the bone marrow also play a significant role in tumor angiogenesis.[10] Regardless of the source, vascularization of tumor foci greatly increases the potential for metastasis.

Detachment

Cells must detach from the primary mass to start the journey to a distant location. To do this, down regulation occurs in cell-to-cell adhesion molecules such as E-cadherin as well as alterations in how the cell interacts with the extracellular matrix (ECM).[11] Change in cell mobility is also required and is associated with altered cytoskeletal elements in response to tumor-derived factors acting in an autocrine fashion, as well as host-secreted factors. Tumor cells may also secrete proteases that facilitate detachment.[5]

Invasion

Once a cell separates from the primary tumor and enters the ECM it must gain access to the vasculature. Degradative proteolytic enzymes are produced by the tumor or host support cells to facilitate this process. These include cathepsins, matrix metalloproteinases, and plasminogen activators. An increase in these enzymes has been associated with greater metastatic potential in several tumor types.[12] Tumor cells that bind to basement membrane components such as laminin or fibronectin also have a metastatic advantage.

Survival in the Circulation

At this point tumor cells must avoid host immune defenses and are susceptible to destruction by immune effector cells such as lymphocytes, monocytes, and natural killer cells. Other reasons for circulatory death include mechanical stresses associated with turbulent flow and high oxygen tension leading to toxicity. The host may also trigger apoptosis of tumor cells in the circulation through a variety of signals.[11]

Arrest and Extravasation

Cells or aggregates of cells (emboli) must stop at a distant vascular bed to begin the extravasation process. This arrest can be facilitated by the mechanical size of the emboli compared with the capillary or, more likely, is mediated by tumor cell attachment to specific cell surface markers such as E-selectin or CD-44. Arrest can also occur when endothelial cells are damaged and the basement membrane is exposed.[5] Cells can then attach to basement membrane components such as laminin, type IV collagen, and other proteoglycans similar to the process that occurs during invasion into the vascular space. These interactions are facilitated by cell surface adhesion molecules such as integrens.[11]

Organ Specificity

Clinical as well as experimental observations have shown that certain tumors tend to metastasize to certain locations preferentially. This is exemplified in Paget's "seed and soil" hypothesis, which was proposed to explain the apparent non-random pattern of tumor spread observed in visceral organs and bones.[4] This theory states that specific interactions between the metastasizing tumor cells and the target organ environment must occur and be favorable in order for tumor foci to survive and grow. Another theory of organ preference is based on hemodymanic factors such as the number of metastases that occur in an organ is related to the number of tumor cells delivered there by the flow of blood. In reality the theories are not mutually exclusive.[11] Rodent models demonstrating organ preference of metastatic cells are well documented in the literature. An example of this also exists in a clinical observation of ovarian cancer patients who have peritoneovenous shunts placed to palliate ascites build up. Ovarian cancer cells will readily grow in ascetic fluid and on peritoneal and organ surfaces. They rarely, however, spread beyond the abdominal cavity. When a shunt is placed, millions of tumor cells are dumped into the venous circulation, theoretically increasing the chance of hematogenous metastasis. Clinical observations at the time of patient death by Tarin and colleagues, however, did not show any increase in metastasis outside the abdominal cavity, supporting the need for the appropriate "soil" to ensure metastatic cell growth.[4,13] Our understanding of the tumor-host microenvironment has increased. Each organ likely has a unique set of growth factors, differentially expressed endothelial receptors and cell surface receptors that allow for unique cross talk with available metastasizing cells, encouraging or discouraging tumor growth.[4] One example of this cross talk is the finding that chemokine receptors may play a role in organ specificity. It has been shown in vitro that breast cancer cells have a high expression of CXCR4 and CCR7 and that the ligands for these receptors are highly expressed in organs where breast cancer preferentially spreads, including the lung and liver. Additionally, blocking the specific receptor ligand interaction can decrease metastasis experimentally.[14]

New Considerations

Disseminated Tumor Cells and Tumor Dormancy

The use of sensitive immunocytochemical stains and PCR strategies has allowed for the detection of disseminated tumor cells in sites such as the bone marrow where clinically evident macrometastases rarely occur. One example of this has been reported in 550 breast tumor patients where 30 to 40% of cells taken from the bone marrow had markers specific for epithelial tumors compared with 1% of the 200 non-cancer bearing individuals sampled. The presence of these cells also predicted a worse prognosis.[15] Additional studies have shown that 20 to 40% of patients with carcinomas from various primary sites have cells detectable in the bone marrow even with no evidence of lymph node or distant organ metastasis.[3] The implications of the discovery of these cells may indicate that the bone marrow may be a reservoir for malignant cells either to remain dormant or to adapt prior to establishing metastatic foci in other organs.

Genetic and phenotypic profiling of these cells compared with the primary tumor has shown significant differences, supporting the theory that these cells change and develop unique characteristics after leaving the primary tumor, perhaps even early in tumor development.[3] This theory proposes that cells neither proliferate or die, instead remain quiescent. These cells are probably resistant to traditional chemotherapeutics that typically target dividing cells.[1] The dormancy of cells can be reflected in the lag time that exists between the removal of a primary tumor and the development of detectable metastatic foci. Detection of disseminated cancer cells early in the course of disease might help guide therapy by predicting which patients actually need adjuvant therapy post-surgical excision of the primary tumor. For example 90% of breast cancer patients without lymph node metastasis will have adjuvant therapy recommended, whereas only 20 to 25% of those individuals will likely develop metastasis within the first 10 years, indicating that some patients may be overtreated.[16]

Therapeutic considerations also need to be given to these disseminated cells especially when targeted therapies become routinely incorporated into cancer treatment. If the primary tumor expresses one target and the disseminated cells another, one subpopulation may go untreated.

Gene Expression Profiling and the Metastatic Phenotype

In longstanding models of metastasis it has been believed that, within any given tumor, a small subpopulation of cells develop and are genetically altered to acquire the advantages needed to become metastatic.[2] This implies that the ability to metastasize happens late in tumor progression. Several studies have challenged this, including ones in breast cancer using microarray platforms to profile gene expression. These studies have shown that the differences in gene expression of the primary tumor can predict whether the tumor will spread or remain localized. In one study by Van De Vijver et al, tumors from 295 early-stage breast cancer patients were screened using a 70-gene prognosis profile dividing the population into poor and good gene signature groups. Patients with a poor signature (n = 180) had a 10-year survival of 55% compared with 94% for those in the good signature group (n = 115). Additionally the probability of remaining metastasis free was 51% in the poor prognosis group compared with 85% in the good prognosis group. Even in multivariate analysis, the gene profile status remained a strong independent factor at predicting disease outcome.[17] The authors of this study concluded that gene profiling was potentially a more powerful predictive tool than standard clinical and histopathologic criteria. The genetic background of the host may also influence the efficiency of the metastatic process, with certain individuals having the genetic profile that favorably supports tumor spread. If these individuals can be reliably identified, investigation of cancer preventative measures might be warranted.[18,19]

Conclusion

As more is learned about the process of metastasis, it is clear that many unanswered questions exist and that new technologies will help elucidate the intricacies of this complex process. From a therapeutic standpoint, it is also evident that not only must the metastatic tumor cell be targeted, but so must the host-produced factors that promote tumor cell growth, survival, invasion, and metastasis.

References

1. Tait CR, Dodwell D, Hrogan K: Do metastases metastasize? J Pathol 203:515, 2004.

2. Weigelt B, Peterse JL, van'tVer LJ: Breast cancer metastasis: markers and models. Nat Rev Cancer 5:591, 2005.

3. Pantel K, Brakenhoff RH: Dissecting the metastatic cascade. Nat Rev Cancer 4:448, 2004.

4. Fidler IJ: The pathogenesis of cancer metastasis: the seed and soil hypothesis revisited. Nat Rev Cancer 3:1, 2003.

5. Stetler-Stevenson WG, Kleiner DE: Molecular biology of cancer: Invasion and metastasis. *In* Cancer: Principles and Practice of Oncology, 7th ed. Devita VT, Hellman S, Rosenberg SA (eds). Philadelphia: Lippincott Williams & Wilkins, 2004.

6. Khanna C, Hunter K: Modeling metastasis in vivo. Carcinogenesis 26:513, 2005.

7. MacEwen EG, Khanna C, Radinsky R: Cancer biology and metastasis. *In* Small Animal Clinical Oncology, 3rd ed. Withrow SJ, MacEwen EG (eds). Philadelphia: WB Saunders Company, 2001, p 18.

8. Beckner ME: Factors promoting tumor angiogenesis. Cancer Invest 17:594-623,1999.

9. Fidler IJ, Kumar R, Bielenberg DR, et al: Molecular determinants of angiogenesis in cancer metastasis. Cancer J Sci Am 4:(1);S58-S66,1998.

10. Kerbel RS, Kamen BA: The anti angiogenic basis of metronomic chemotherapy. Nature Rev Cancer 4:423-436, 2004.

11. Khokha R, Voura E, Hill RP: Tumor progression and metastasis: cellular, molecular, and microenvironmental factors. *In* The Basic Science of Oncology, 4th ed. Tannock IF, Hill RP, Bristow RG, and Harrington L, (eds). New York: McGraw Hill, 2005, p 205.

12. Kumar R, Fidler IJ: Angiogenic molecules and cancer metastasis. In Vivo 18:27-34,1998.

13. Tarin D, et al: Mechanisms of human tumor metastasis studied in patients with peritoneovenous shunts. Cancer Res 44:3584-3592, 1984.

14. Muller A, Homey B, Soto H, et al: Involvement of chemokine receptors in breast cancer metastasis. Nature 410:50-56, 2001.

15. Braun S, et al: Cytokeratin positive bone marrow micrometastases and survival of breast cancer patients with stage 1-3 disease. N Engl J Med 342;525-533, 2000.

16. Goldhirsch A, et al: Meeting highlights: updated international expert consensus on the primary therapy of early breast cancer. J Clin Oncol 21:3357-3365, 2003.

17. Van De Vijver MJ, He YD, Van't Veer LJ, et al: A gene expression signature as a predictor of survival in breast cancer. N Engl J Med 347:1999-2009, 2002.

18. Hunter KW: Host genetics and tumour metastasis. Br J Cancer 90:752-755, 2004.

19. Cai Zhen, Chiu Jen-Fu, He Qing-Yu: Application of proteomics in the study of tumor metastasis. Geno Prot Bioinfo 4:152, 2004.

Chapter 10

Organ Transplantation – The Rejection Response

Clare R. Gregory
Andrew E. Kyles
Margo Mehl

In the late 1800s and early 1900s, surgeons gained the technical ability to transplant organs and tissues from one animal to another. It soon became evident that, following transplantation, the organ would rapidly become ischemic and necrotic. In 1923, Dr. Carl Williamson, at the Mayo Clinic, demonstrated that cells of the immune system were responsible for the death of transplanted tissues and organs. This discovery set the stage for the study of immune-mediated rejection and the development of effective immunosuppressive strategies.[1]

Transplantation of organs and tissues in veterinary medicine is becoming more common. Corneal transplantation is performed to replace diseased or scarred corneas. Corneoscleral transplantation is performed for the treatment of canine epibulbar melanomas. Allogeneic bone marrow transplantation has been performed in cats to aid in the treatment of lymphohematopoietic neoplasias, aplastic anemias, and feline retrovirus infections. In the dog and cat, for the treatment of acute and chronic renal failure, kidney transplantation is performed at university hospitals and private practices. Feline renal transplant patients have now survived for over 13 years with normal renal function.

Nomenclature

A graft is tissue or an organ used in a transplant procedure. An autograft is tissue or an organ that is removed from and then transplanted on or into the same individual. A common example is a cancellous bone graft used to speed fracture healing. Autografts do not incite a rejection response. An isograft is tissue or an organ transplanted between two genetically identical individuals; identical twins or closely inbred individuals. An allograft is tissue or an organ transplanted between genetically nonidentical members of the same species. Virtually all renal transplants performed in clinical veterinary medicine are allografts. A xenograft is tissue or an organ transplanted between members of different species.

Mechanism of the Immune Response to an Allograft[2-4]

Rejection of the transplanted tissue or organ is determined by T-cell (lymphocyte) recognition of differences in the composition of cell surface glycoproteins between graft and host tissues. These glycoproteins are termed histocompatibility antigens or histocompatibility molecules. The histocompatibility antigens that incite the most vigorous rejection response are encoded by genes of the major histocompatibility complex (MHC).

A MHC is found in all vertebrates. In dogs, this cluster of genes on a single chromosome is termed the dog leukocyte antigen (DLA); in cats it is termed the feline leukocyte antigen (FLA). Polymorphism, or the presence of many different variations of the same gene (alleles) at a single location, or locus, is characteristic of the MHC. Each individual will have two, one on each paired chromosome, of many possible alleles at each locus in his or her MHC. This variation in the genetic makeup of the MHC results in the production of a tremendous variety of cell surface histocompatibility antigens. This variety ensures that the host T-cells will recognize virtually all tissue and organ allografts as foreign, resulting in a rejection response.

The genes of the MHC are closely linked, and the genetic information inherited from each parent on a single chromosome is transferred as a block. This group of genes is termed the MHC haplotype; each offspring receives one haplotype from each parent. The genes of each haplotype are expressed codominantly; therefore, cell surface histocompatibility derived from each parent will be present in the offspring. This basic understanding of the genetics of the MHC is important clinically, particularly in a species like the dog, in which it is difficult to immunosuppress or control the rejection response. Because each offspring inherits one haplotype from each parent and each haplotype is expressed codominantly, 25% of littermates have the possibility of being MHC identical, 50% might share one haplotype, and 25% will not share a haplotype. Without the administration of immunosuppressive agents, renal allografts from MHC-nonmatched dogs survive approximately 10 days, renal allografts from dogs matched for one haplotype survive approximately 24 days, and MHC-matched allografts survive for 150 days or more. In the latter group, the rejection response can be more readily controlled using immunosuppressive agents; therefore, selection of MHC-identical littermates as donor/recipient pairs can greatly enhance the chance of long-term graft survival.

The fact that allograft survival is not indefinite when a dog receives a kidney from an MHC-identical donor demonstrates that the MHC is not the only genetic region coding for histocompatibility antigens. Minor histocompatibility genes have been isolated in mice and human beings and probably code for changes in peptide structure in endogenous proteins that allow recognition by host T-cells, but do not affect their physiologic function. Fortunately, the rejection response produced by minor histocompatibility differences is relatively easy to prevent using immunosuppressive agents.

It is important to understand that the MHC-encoded cell surface glycoproteins, or transplantation antigens, did not evolve to prevent the transplantation of genetically dissimilar tissue and organs, but rather to protect the host from invasion by viruses, fungi, nematodes, and other parasites. To do so effectively, the immune system must distinguish between antigens against which an immune response would be beneficial (pathogenic or allogeneic) or harmful (host or self). In the thymus, during fetal development, T-cells are propagated or destroyed based on their ability to recognize MHC glycoproteins as "self" or "nonself." The interaction between MHC glycoproteins and T-cells, in the presence of antigen, results in a series of transmembrane and cytosolic chemical reactions that result in T-cell cytotoxic activity and the production and/or release of cytokines. Cytokines (interleukins [ILs], tumor necrosis factor [TNF], and others) result in the further activation of T-cells, B-cells, macrophages, and other immunoreactive cells.

The cell surface glycoproteins of the MHC are divided into two major classifications: Class I and II. Class I glycoproteins or molecules are expressed on all nucleated cells. Class I molecules have a folded region that holds and presents antigens from virus-infected, tumor, and allogeneic cells to antigen-responsive cytotoxic ($CD8^+$) T-cells. The linkage of the T cell receptor – CD8 complex on the surface of cytotoxic T-cells with the class I molecule-antigen complex of allograft or antigen-presenting cells (monocytes, macrophages, Langerhans cells of the epidermis, and dendritic cells of lymphoid organs) results in the proliferation and differentiation of a clone of cytotoxic T cells specific for that class I-antigen combination. Thus, the cytotoxic activity of T-cells is both antigen specific and class I restricted.

Class II molecules are only constitutively expressed on the surface of cells that are essential for immune responses. These include B-cells (lymphocytes), thymic epithelial cells, and the cells listed above that present antigen to T-cells. T cells, vascular endothelial cells, smooth muscle cells, and others can express class II antigens when activated by cytokines such as interferon-γ (INF-γ). The function of class II molecules is similar to that of class I. Antigen-sensitive T helper cells ($CD4^+$) recognize the class II-antigen complexes on allogeneic or antigen-presenting cells. The linkage of the CD4-T-cell receptor complex with the class II-antigen complex results in the proliferation and differentiation of a clone of T helper cells specific for that class II-antigen complex. Activated T helper cells begin the cascade of events responsible for acute allograft rejection by the release of cytokines (IL-2, IL-3, IL-4, IL-5, IL-6, INF-γ, TNFs, granulocyte macrophage colony stimulating factor [GM-CSF], and others) that propagate an inflammatory response, activate cytotoxic cells, and promote antibody formation.

In addition to their role as antigen-presenting molecules, it is believed that foreign class I and class II molecules, in the absence of antigen, may stimulate alloreactive T cells and serve as the stimuli for rejection reactions. Also, rejection may be initiated following T-cell recognition of class I or II - minor histocompatibility antigen complexes.

The allograft rejection response begins with the migration of antigen-presenting cells of the host or donor organ to T-cell areas of secondary lymphoid organs. These T cells circulate between lymphoid tissues, regulated by chemokine and sphingosine-1 phosphate receptors. T-cell activation by allogeneic or antigen-presenting cells requires cell contact and cell surface molecule interaction. Cell surface molecules that interact are termed "ligand-receptor pairs." A ligand is any molecule that forms a complex with another molecule. Antigen presentation through class I or class II molecules can be split into four stages that produce three signals needed to stimulate the rejection reaction: adhesion, antigen-specific activation, co-stimulation, and cytokine signaling (Figure 10-1). Association of the antigen-presenting cells and T cells first involves nonspecific, reversible binding through adhesion molecules such as LFA-1and ICAM. When the T-cell receptor complex is presented with an alloantigen, a conformational change occurs in the adhesion molecules that results in tighter binding and prolonged cell to cell contact. The first signal of the rejection response is provided by the class I/antigen-CD8/T-cell receptor ligand-receptor pair and the class II/antigen-CD4/T-cell receptor ligand-receptor pair (CD3 complex) (Figure 10-2). The specific MHC/peptide – T-cell receptor interaction, although necessary, is not sufficient to fully activate the T cell. A second signal is required, otherwise the T cell becomes unresponsive. The second signal, also termed co-stimulation, is of critical importance (Figure 10-3). Two of the most potent co-stimulatory molecules expressed on antigen-presenting cells are B7-1 (CD80) and B7-2(CD86). They are ligands for the T-cell molecules CD 28 and CTLA-4. CD28 is the main co-stimulatory ligand expressed on naïve T cells. CD28 stimulation has been shown to prolong and augment the production of IL-2 and other cytokines and is probably important in preventing the induction of tolerance. CTLA-4, the alternative ligand for B-7 is an inhibitory receptor, limiting T-cell activation, and resulting in less IL-2 production. CD28, which is constitutively expressed, initially interacts with B7, producing signal 2 that leads to T-cell activation. The upregulation of CTLA-4, which has a higher affinity to B7 than CD28, limits the degree of activation. Signals 1 and 2 activate 3 signal transduction pathways: the calcium-calcineurin pathway, the RAS-mitogen-activated pathway (MAP), and the nuclear factor-κB pathway. These pathways activate transcription factors that bind to regulatory proteins in enhancer regions of specific genes involved in proliferation and differentiation, including cytokines such as IL-2, cytokine receptors such as IL-2R (CD25), and receptors involved in co-stimulation such as CD40L (CD154). Interleukin and other cytokines produce signal 3 via activation of the mammalian target of rapamycin (mTOR) pathway. This pathway is the trigger for cell proliferation (see Figure 10-2).

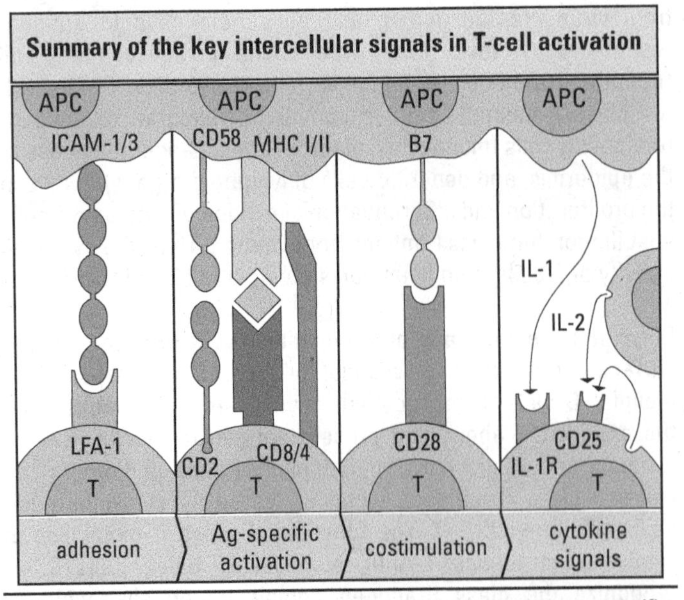

Figure 10-1. Association of APCs and T cells first involves non-specific, reversible binding through adhesion molecules, such as the LFA-1/ICAM interaction. Recognition of the peptide antigen in the MHC molecule by the TCR, which provides the specificity of the interaction, results in prolonged cell-cell contact. A second signal (co-stimulation) is necessary for the T cell to respond efficiently, otherwise tolerance may result. Activation results in upregulation of cytokines and their receptors, which boost the activatory signals and help to decide the cell fate.

Proliferation and differentiation lead to a large number of effector T cells. The primary mechanism of the destruction of an allograft is by generation of T cells that leave the lymph nodes, migrate to the allograft, and are cytotoxic for the cells of the graft. Graft-cell lysis is accomplished through the direct action of T cytotoxic cells, including release of secretory granules containing granzyme B and perforin and by the induction of apoptosis, and by the activation of cascading enzyme systems, including the complement, clotting, and the kinin pathways. Other cellular mediators such as plasma cells, macrophages, platelets, and

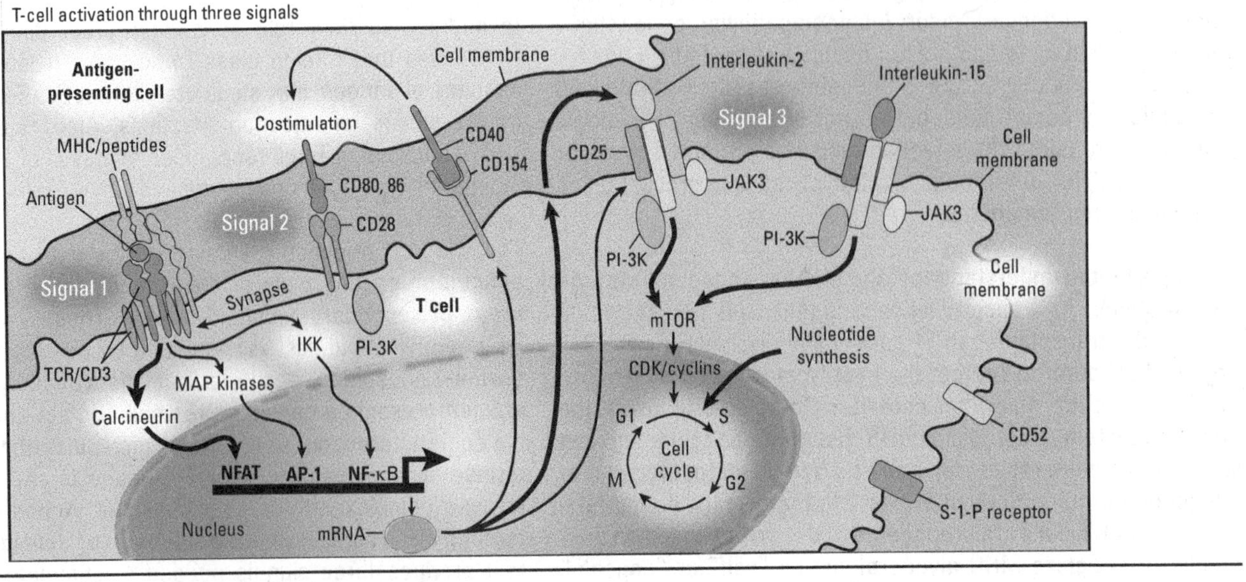

Figure 10-2. T-cell activation through three signals.

polymorphonuclear leukocytes also migrate into the allograft and have both a direct and indirect role in allograft rejection. B cells are activated when antigen engages their antigen receptors, usually in lymphoid follicles or in extrafollicular sites, such as the red pulp of the spleen or in the transplant, producing alloantibody against donor MHC antigens. Alloantibody targets capillary endothelium and fixes complement that results in cell lysis, thrombosis, and ischemia.

The severity of the immune response to allografts differs greatly between dogs and cats. Dogs mount a virulent rejection response, and without immunosuppression, a MHC-mismatched renal allograft is destroyed in 6 to 8 days. In cats, a MHC-mismatched renal allograft will function for approximately 23 days.

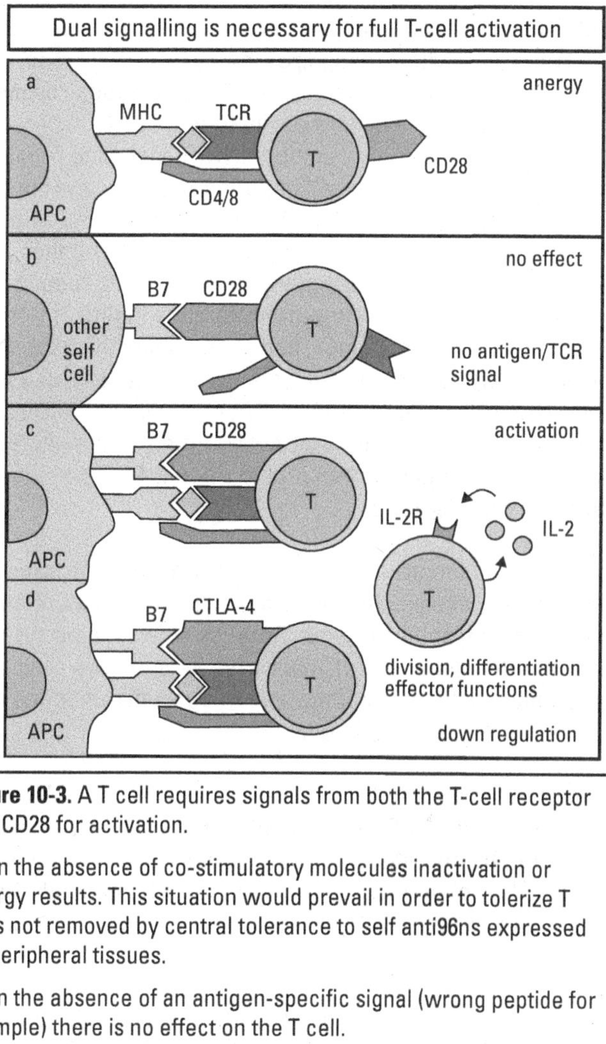

Figure 10-3. A T cell requires signals from both the T-cell receptor and CD28 for activation.

(a) In the absence of co-stimulatory molecules inactivation or anergy results. This situation would prevail in order to tolerize T cells not removed by central tolerance to self anti96ns expressed on peripheral tissues.

(b) In the absence of an antigen-specific signal (wrong peptide for example) there is no effect on the T cell.

(c) Co-reception of both signals, from the surface of a professional APC, activates the T cell to produce IL-2 and its receptor. The cell divides and differentiates into an effector T cell, which no longer requires signal 2 for its effector function.

(d) At the termination of the immune response, CTLA-4 replaces CD28 and downregulates T-cell function.

The Tempo of Rejection

Three overlapping types of organ rejection are recognized clinically. Hyperacute rejection is an accelerated form of rejection that is associated with naturally occurring or preformed circulating antibody in the serum of the recipient that reacts with donor cells, particularly the endothelium of blood vessel walls as described above. In hyperacute allograft rejection, the recipient has been sensitized to the allograft MHC antigens by previous blood transfusions, pregnancy, or transplantation. Preexisting antibody can be identified before transplantation by lymphocyte cross-match, which involves testing leukocytes of the potential donor with serum of the recipient in the presence of complement. If preexisting antibody is present in the serum, the host leukocytes will be lysed. In addition, antibodies against the donor's blood type (erythroid cell surface antigens) can cause hyperacute rejection. The donor and recipient should be tested for blood type compatibility and a blood cross match should be performed prior to transplantation.

Acute allograft rejection typically occurs 7 to 21 days after transplantation or when effective immunosuppression is terminated. Pathologic studies of the rejected organ reveal a predominant pattern of mononuclear leukocyte infiltration in the tissue.

Chronic rejection is characterized by gradual loss of organ function over months to years, often without any clinically recognized rejection episode. Chronic rejection is a major cause of death of all human organ transplant recipients and the primary cause of death for heart transplant recipients. Kidneys undergoing chronic rejection show severe narrowing of numerous arteries and thickening of the glomerular capillary basement membrane. Heart transplants show progressive thickening of the coronary arteries caused mainly by smooth muscle cell proliferation and migration. Occlusion of coronary artery blood flow results in diminished function of the cardiac muscle, and, eventually, in myocardial infarction. The factors causing chronic rejection are multiple and appear to produce chronic inflammation and injury via both immune and nonimmune mechanisms.[5] Factors that have been implicated in the development of chronic rejection in human beings include donor age, donor race, HLA mismatches, ischemia time, reperfusion injury to the allograft, viral infections, hyperlipidemia, hypertension, acute and subacute rejection, and drug toxicity. Many peptide growth factors, including transforming growth factor β, platelet-derived growth factor, and the fibroblast growth factors, have been shown to be upregulated in chronically rejecting organs. Growth factors have been shown *in vitro* and *in vivo* to promote fibroplasia, collagen synthesis, and smooth muscle cell proliferation and migration. Currently, growth factor inhibitors, coenzyme A reductase inhibitors, antiviral strategies, and changes in organ procurement and preparation are being investigated to reduce the incidence and severity of chronic rejection.

References

1. Gregory CR: Transplantation Immunology. *In* Kirk's Current Veterinary Therapy XIII. Bonagura JD (ed). Philadelphia: WB Sau nders, 1995, p 564.

2. Gregory CR, Bernsteen L: Organ Transplantation in Clinical Veterinary Practice. In Textbook of Small Animal Surgery, 3rd ed. Slatter D (ed). Philadelphia: WB Saunders, 2003, p 122.

3. Roitt I, Brostoff J, Male D: Immunology, 6th ed. New York: Mosby, 2001, p 105.

4. Halloran PF: Immunosuppressive drugs for kidney transplantation. N Engl J Med 351:2515, 2004.

5. Gregory CR, Morris RE: Strategies in the prevention of chronic rejection. Current Opinion Organ Transplant 3:19, 1998.

Chapter 11

Organ Transplantation – Immunosuppressive Agents

Clare R. Gregory
Andrew E. Kyles
Margo Mehl

Modification of the Rejection Response[1,2]

Transplanted organs are rejected by a process that occurs when the host's immune system recognizes the grafted tissue as foreign and mounts a response. Modification of this rejection response or altering the immune system's ability to respond to the grafted tissue can be produced in a number of ways including reducing the immune system's exposure to antigens, depleting the number of lymphocytes, suppressing antibody formation, and altering cellular function, such as blocking activation of lymphocytes. The most direct from of immunomodulation is to reduce the exposure of the host immune system to alloantigens. In organ transplantation, this is accomplished by matching the donor and recipient for MHC antigens. Transplantation antigens can also be hidden from allosensitive T cells. Prior to implantation into the peritoneal cavity, pancreatic islet cells can be encapsulated in fenestrated plastic spheres that prohibit T cells from coming into contact with the islet cells.

Lymphocyte populations can be depleted by the administration of cytotoxic drugs, antilymphocyte serum, lymphocytopheresis, or by irradiation of lymphoid organs. Organs of the immune system, in particular the spleen and thymus, can be surgically removed. Splenectomy results in impairment of phagocytic functions and a reduced production of antibodies.

Antibody formation may be suppressed by cytotoxic drugs or lymphoid irradiation of B cells and plasma cells. Destruction of T cells indirectly decreases antibody production by decreasing the effects of T-cell-derived cytokines on B cells. Antibodies and cytokines can be directly eliminated from the host by plasmapheresis.

Alteration of cellular function, directly or indirectly, without generalized cytotoxicity has been in the forefront of immunologic research for the past two decades. Cyclosporine was the first antirejection agent that specifically altered T-cell function. A number of antibodies have been developed that inhibit cell surface molecules involved in T-cell activation and/or T-cell-mediated cytotoxicity. OKT3 is a murine monoclonal antibody directed against the human CD3/T-cell receptor complex on the cell surface of T cells. Within minutes of administration, a marked decrease occurs in the number of circulating T cells. Gradually, these cells reappear but have internalized the CD3/T-cell receptor complex from the cell surface. Without this receptor complex, T cells cannot respond to the class I or class II antigen complex on the surface of allogeneic or antigen-presenting cells. Other antibodies have been directed against cytokines and cytokine receptors. Anti-IL-2 receptor antibodies are now available for human transplant patients and have been safely used to reduce the incidence and severity of acute rejection episodes. Anti-tumor necrosis factor, anti-INF-γ antibodies and others have been shown to increase allograft survival in animal models.

Antibodies have also been directed against the accessory cell-adhesion molecules, resulting in reduction of T cell binding and activation. Interference with the binding of LFA-1 on T cells and with ICAM-1 on allogeneic or antigen-presenting cells has prolonged allograft survival in rodent and primate models.

The antibodies used against T-cell receptors, cytokines, and adhesion molecules are usually murine in origin. Mice are challenged with the foreign glycoprotiens and produce antibody that is collected and administered to another animal or human being facing a rejection response. In most cases, the organ recipient will form antibodies against the murine antibody that eventually neutralize its effect. To reduce this problem in human transplantation, the new anti-IL-2 receptor antibodies have taken the active portion of the mouse antibody (antigen binding or Fab portion) and combined it in various ways to human antibody (Fc and variable regions) to produce antibodies of lower or nil antigenicity (Zenapax, Roche, Nutley, NJ; Simulect, Novartis, East Hanover, NJ).

Other schemes of specific immunosuppression are under investigation; for example, the generation of T-cell-specific antibody/toxin complexes. As T-cell activation and the factors involved in signal transduction are better understood, agents are being directed against the molecular events that occur in the cell membrane and in the cytosol following T-cell antigen recognition.

Immunosuppressive Agents[1,2]

Over the last half of the 20th century, immunosuppressive agents evolved from nonspecific cytotoxic drugs to agents that target specific enzyme pathways that catalyze reactions required for normal immune function. Much of our current knowledge of T-cell function was provided by research performed to understand the mechanism of action of cyclosporine. As each element of antigen recognition, T-cell activation, cytokine synthesis, and T-cell-dependent cytolysis are unraveled, investigators are devising more specific, less toxic and more efficacious agents for interrupting the immune response. This is termed rational drug development and replaces the selection of potential immunosuppressive agents based on their ability to lyse or inhibit the activation of T and B cells *in vitro*. Although specific immunosuppression using naturally induced and genetically engineered antibodies, soluble receptor fragments, and other biological methods are available for therapy of human diseases, most are not applicable or available for use in the treatment of animal diseases. For the foreseeable future, in clinical veterinary medicine, immunosuppression will continue to be accomplished using chemotherapies. As the new immunosuppressive agents become more readily available and clinicians become familiar with their indications, effects, and side effects, immunosuppression should become more specific, effective, and safe.

Myelotoxic Agents

The major effect of cyclophosphamide results from alkylation of deoxyribonucleic acid (DNA) during the S phase of the cell cycle. The alterations in DNA structure can be lethal to the cell or may produce miscoding errors that inhibit cell replication of DNA transcription. Cyclophosphamide produces T- and B-cell lymphopenia and suppresses both T-cell activity and antibody production. Cyclophosphamide is administered to dogs for the treatment of corticosteroid-resistant autoimmune hemolytic anemia, corticosteroid-resistant thrombocytopenia, rheumatoid arthritis, and polymyositis (in conjunction with corticosteroids). Cyclophosphamide is administered to cats for the treatment of autoimmune hemolytic anemia and rheumatoid arthritis. Myelosuppression, gastroenteritis, alopecia, and hemorrhagic cystitis are the major complications associated with cyclophosphamide therapy.

Azathioprine is a purine analog that is metabolized to ribonucleotide monophosphates. Poor conversion to diphosphates and triphosphates leads to an intracellular accumulation of monophosphates that produces a feed-back inhibition of enzymes required for the biosynthesis of purine nucleotides. The triphosphate analogs that do form become incorporated into DNA and result in ribonucleic acid (RNA) miscoding and faulty transcription. Azathioprine has a greater effect on humoral than on cell-mediated immunity. For the treatment of immune-mediated diseases in dogs, azathioprine is generally administered in conjunction with corticosteroids and/or cyclophosphamide. Azathioprine has been used for the treatment of autoimmune thrombocytopenia, autoimmune hemolytic anemia, autoimmune skin diseases, chronic hepatitis, myasthenia gravis, immune-mediated glomerulopathy, chronic atrophic gastritis, systemic lupus erythematosus, and inflammatory bowel disease. Although myelotoxic in cats, azathioprine has been used for the treatment of feline autoimmune skin diseases. Azathioprine and prednisolone, when administered at maximally tolerated levels, do not effectively suppress the rejection response against canine MHC-nonmatched renal allografts. However, when administered on an every other day schedule (1 to 5 mg/kg) with cyclosporine, azathioprine has been used to successfully maintain both canine MHC-matched and MHC-mismatched renal allografts. When administered at a dose of 0.3 mg/kg every third day, adjusting the dosage to maintain a white blood cell count of at least 3000 cells/μl, azathioprine has been used in combination with cyclosporine to reverse or control renal allograft rejection in cats. The primary complication encountered with the administration of azathioprine is bone marrow suppression that can result in leukopenia, anemia, and thrombocytopenia. Acute pancreatitis and hepatotoxicity may also occur.

Methotrexate competitively inhibits folic acid reductase necessary for the reduction of dihydrofolate to tetrahydrofolate and affects the production of both purines and pyrimidines. The effects of methotrexate occur during the S-phase of the cell cycle. Methotrexate is used primarily as an antineoplastic agent in dogs and cats for lymphomas, carcinomas, and sarcomas. In human medicine, methotrexate is administered for the treatment of rheumatoid arthritis and psoriasis. Gastrointestinal toxicity is the most common complication encountered with the administration of methotrexate.

Glucocorticoids

Glucocorticoids, and in particular, prednisolone, have both direct and indirect effects on the immune response. Glucocorticoids stabilize the cell membrane of endothelial cells and inhibit the production of local chemotactic factors, thus decreasing infiltration of neutrophils, monocytes, and lymphocytes. In allogeneic tissues, the secretion of destructive proteolytic enzymes such as collagenase, elastase, and plasminogen activator is inhibited. Glucocorticoids also inhibit the release of arachidonic acid from membrane phospholipids. This prevents the synthesis of prostaglandins, thromboxanes, and leukotrienes, which are major mediators of inflammation. Glucocorticoids redistribute monocytes and lymphocytes from the peripheral circulation to the lymphatics and bone marrow. This affects primarily T cells. T-cell activation and cytotoxicity are also reduced. Glucocorticoids suppress cytokine activity and alter macrophage function. Owing to their general efficacy and low cost, prednisolone or prednisone are considered to be the first line immunosuppressive agents for the treatment of immune-mediated and chronic inflammatory diseases in dogs and cats. Autoimmune hemolytic anemia and thrombocytopenia, autoimmune and allergic skin diseases, myasthenia gravis, allergic pneumonitis and bronchitis, immune-mediated arthritis, and systemic lupus erythematosus are just some of the indications for corticosteroid therapy in animals. Prednisolone at a dose of 0.25 to 2 mg/kg/day, has been used in both dogs and cats to slow allograft rejection; administered as a single agent, however, prednisolone is not capable of preventing allograft rejection. Although inexpensive and often effective, the chronic use of corticosteroids in both human beings and animals can result in severe complications, usually manifested as signs of hyperadrenocorticism. This complication, in addition to the fact that corticosteroids suppress multiple elements of the immune response, has led to the search for steroid-sparing immunosuppressive protocols.

Calcinurin Inhibitors

Cyclosporine is bound in the cytosol of lymphocytes by cyclophilins (cyclosporine-binding proteins). The cyclosporine-cyclophilin complexes associate with calcium-dependent calcineurin/calmodulin complexes to impede calcium-dependent signal transduction. Transcription factors that promote cytokine gene activation are either direct or indirect substrates of calcineurin's serine/threonine phosphatase activity. This enzymatic activity is reduced by association of the cyclosporine-cyclophilin bimolecular complex with calcineurin. Via this mechanism of action, cyclosporine inhibits early T-cell activation (Go phase of the cell cycle) and prevents synthesis of several cytokines, in particular, IL-2. Without stimulation by IL-2, further T-cell proliferation is inhibited, and T-cell cytotoxic activity is reduced. Cyclosporine may also exert an immunosuppressive effect as it stimulates mammalian cells to secrete transforming growth factor beta (TGF-β) protein. TGF-β is a potent inhibitor of IL-2-stimulated T-cell proliferation and generation of antigen-specific cytotoxic lymphocytes. Cyclosporine is not cytotoxic or myelotoxic, and is specific for lymphocytes. This specificity spares other rapidly dividing cells, and allows nonspecific host defense mechanisms to continue to function.

Cyclosporine is gaining wide use in veterinary medicine. Combination cyclosporine and prednisolone immunosuppression has maintained normal function of MHC-nonmatched feline renal allografts for over 13 years. Cyclosporine in combination with azathioprine and prednisolone, or with azathioprine, prednisolone, and antithymocyte serum has been used to maintain MHC-nonmatched canine renal allografts. Bone marrow transplantation has been successfully performed in cats using cyclosporine immunosuppression.

Cyclosporine has also been used to control corticosteroid-resistant autoimmune hemolytic anemia and thrombocytopenia in dogs. Cyclosporine is available in an ophthalmic preparation (Optimmune, Schering-Plough, Kenilworth, NJ) for the control of keratoconjunctivitis sicca in dogs. Recently, cyclosporine was found to significantly reduce the size and depth of perianal fistulas in dogs. Most dogs did not require further therapy, either medical or surgical, after 6 to 8 weeks of therapy.

Cyclosporine is available in two oral formulations: Sandimmune and Neoral (Sandoz, East Hanover, NJ). Both contain cyclosporine in a concentration of 100 mg/ml, but the two solutions are not biologically equivalent. Sandimmune consists of an olive oil base and absorption of cyclosporine requires emulsification of the agent by bile salts and digestion by pancreatic enzymes. Absorption percentage can be as little as 4% and tremendous variation exists in dose/trough whole blood concentrations among individuals of the same species. Neoral is a micro-emulsion preconcentrate of cyclosporine that becomes a microemulsion when in contact with gastrointestinal fluids. The microemulsion is directly absorbed through the gut epithelium, resulting in more sustained and consistent blood concentrations of the drug. When converting to Neoral from Sandimmune, most feline renal transplant recipients have had a reduction in dose level necessary to maintain the same trough whole blood concentrations. In addition, feline renal transplant patients were administered Sandimmune at 10 to 15 mg/kg/24 hours to initiate immunosuppression at the time of surgery. To achieve the same trough whole blood concentrations of cyclosporine (approximately 500 ng/ml), Neoral is administered at 4 to 6 mg/kg/24 hours. Owing to a more complete absorption that results in a more sustained and predictable blood concentration, Neoral appears be a more effective immunosuppressant than Sandimmune. In addition, it is more economical to use.

To achieve immunosuppression with cyclosporine in dogs, the authors recommend attaining a 12-hour whole blood trough (measured just before the next oral dose) concentration of at least 500 ng/ml. Using Sandimmune, this will require an oral dose of 10 to 25 mg/kg/24 hours divided into 2 doses. Neoral can be initiated at 6 to 10 mg/kg/24 hours divided into 2 doses. With either formulation, gastrointestinal inflammation will increase the dose requirements, and blood concentrations of the agent must be measured starting 24 to 48 hours after initiation of therapy to assure that adequate blood concentrations are achieved. Blood concentrations of cyclosporine should be measured at periodic intervals during the time of therapy.

To reduce the cost of cyclosporine necessary to treat medium- to large-size dogs, ketoconazole can be administered at 10 mg/kg/24 hours in addition to the cyclosporine. Ketoconazole interferes with the hepatic metabolism of cyclosporine, and will reduce the dose requirement of cyclosporine by as much as 60%. Possible toxic effects with the coadministration of these agents include hepatitis and cataract formation.

To achieve immunosuppression with cyclosporine in cats, the authors recommend attaining a 12-hour whole blood trough concentration of 250 to 500 ng/ml. Using Sandimmune, this will require an oral dose of 4 to 15 mg/kg/24 hours divided into 2 doses. Neoral can be initiated at 1 to 5 mg/kg/24 hours divided into 2 doses. Again, it is imperative to measure blood concentrations 24 to 48 hours after initiation of therapy to ensure that adequate blood concentrations have been achieved. Blood concentrations must also be measured periodically during the time of therapy.

Whole blood or plasma concentrations of cyclosporine can be determined by high-pressure liquid chromatography, fluorescence polarization immunoassay, and specific monoclonal antibody radioimmunoassay. Most medical centers that serve human patients perform cyclosporine assays and will serve veterinary needs.

Based on pharmacokinetic studies in the cat, trough whole blood concentrations of cyclosporine may not correlate well with drug exposure.[3] The whole blood concentration measured at 2 hours after administration of the drug may correlate better with drug exposure and give a better index for drug dosage and change in dose. The blood concentration of cyclosporine measured 2 hours after administration, or C_2, is recommended for therapeutic drug monitoring in human renal transplant patients.[3]

Unlike the situation in human beings, cyclosporine does not appear to be hepatotoxic in dogs and cats unless extremely high blood levels are maintained (> 3000 ng/ml). Although not as frequently encountered in human beings, cyclosporine can be nephrotoxic in the cat. Nephrotoxicity in the cat does not seem to be related to the concentration of the drug in the whole blood; it can occur at relatively low drug concentrations. Cats with extremely high concentrations in whole blood may show no nephrotoxicity at all. Whole blood concentrations of cyclosporine greater than 1000 ng/ml can cause inappetance in cats. If concentrations of 1000 ng/ml are maintained for several weeks or months, opportunistic bacterial and fungal infections can occur. As in human beings, cyclosporine can promote the development of neoplasia, particularly lymphomas, in cats and dogs. The administration of high levels (1 to 2 mg/kg/24 hours) of prednisolone with cyclosporine increases the likelihood of tumor formation. As in humans, cyclosporine has resulted in a marked increase in hair growth in several of our feline renal transplant recipients.

Cyclosporine has a distinctly unpleasant taste to both humans and animals. It is necessary to administer the drug in gelatin capsules. Novartis supplies capsules containing 25 mg or 100 mg of cyclosporine. For most cats, these capsules contain far too much drug. The authors place the oral solution in #0 or #1 gelatin capsules. Some cats require only a small dose of cyclosporine: 1 to 3 mg/dose. Measuring and administering this small amount (0.10 to 0.03 ml) of drug is difficult and imprecise. Sandimmune can be diluted and stored in olive oil. Neoral can be diluted in any oral solution, including tap water, but because it is a microemulsion concentrate, it must be administered immediately after it is diluted.

Cyclosporine is also available in an intravenous solution (Sandimmune IV) that must be diluted in 0.9% sodium chloride or 5% dextrose in water. The authors administer a dose of 6 mg/kg over 4 hours in the calculated maintenance fluid requirement. Intravenous cyclosporine is administered to control organ rejection episodes, an acute hemolytic crisis, or during periods when a patient cannot tolerate oral medications.

Tacrolimus (FK506, Prograf, Fujisawa USA, Dearfield, IL), although structurally different from cyclosporine, shares a similar mechanism of action. Tacrolimus binds in the cytosol of lymphocytes with an immunophilin, FK-binding protein (FKBP). As with the cyclosporine-cyclophilin complex, the tacrolimus-FKBP complex binds to calcineurin and inhibits its phosphatase activity. This directly and indirectly inhibits *de novo* expression of nuclear regulatory proteins and T-cell activation genes. The transcription of cytokines (IL-2, -3,-4, -5, IFN-γ, TNF-α, and GM-CSF) responsible for lymphocyte activation is suppressed as is the expression of IL-2 and IL-7 receptors. Tacrolimus, *in vitro*, is 50 to 100 times more potent an inhibitor of lymphocyte activation than cyclosporine. Tacrolimus also inhibits B-cell proliferation and production of antibody by unknown mechanisms. Tacrolimus decreases hepatic injury associated with ischemia/reperfusion injury, perhaps by inhibiting production of TNF and IL-6 by hepatocytes, and stimulates hepatic regeneration following liver injury.

Experimentally, allograft recipients from many species have been treated successfully with tacrolimus with doses several times less than for cyclosporine. Tacrolimus has prolonged the survival of renal, liver, pancreas, heart, lung, and vascularized limb grafts in rodents, dogs, and nonhuman primates. In human organ recipients, tacrolimus is superior to cyclosporine for the reversal of ongoing rejection. Tacrolimus also seems to have a greater steroid-sparing effect over Sandimmune but may not be superior to Neoral. The toxicity of tacrolimus is similar to that of cyclosporine in human beings.

Little, if any, use of tacrolimus has been applied clinically to veterinary patients. Experimentally, tacrolimus was shown to significantly prolong MHC-mismatched renal allograft survival in cats without serious side-effects.[4] Based on its effectiveness in other experimental animal trials, tacrolimus could be effective in controlling a wide range of immune-mediated conditions. Owing to its inhibition of antibody synthesis, in addition to T-cell proliferation, tacrolimus may be particularly effective in controlling immune-mediated anemia, thrombocytopenia, and arthritis.

Despite the potential benefits of tacrolimus for treating diseases in dogs, a major concern is the possible toxicity of the drug. A dose of 0.16 mg/kg/intramuscularly/day and 1.0 mg/kg/orally/day has been reported to be effective in prolonging renal allograft survival in beagle dogs. Side effects included anorexia, vasculitis, and intestinal intussusception. In a study using mongrel dogs, the same doses were not effective in prolonging renal allograft survival and most of the dogs developed severe vasculitis leading to fatal myocardial infarction, hepatic failure, and intussusception. Combination therapy with cyclosporine appears to have an additive effect with less toxicity. Blood concentrations of tacrolimus are assayed at human medical centers using monoclonal immunoassays. The effective serum trough concentration of tacrolimus in dogs is approximately 0.1 to 0.4 ng/ml; about 100 times lower than that of cyclosporine. Trough levels of 2.0 ng/ml or greater can result in death.

Inhibitors of Cytokine and Growth Factor Action

Sirolimus (rapamycin, Rapamune, Wyeth-Ayerst, Philadelphia, PA) is a macrocyclic antibiotic with a structure similar to tacrolimus that also binds in the cell cytosol to FKBP. However, sirolimus and tacrolimus affect different and distinct sites in the signal transduction pathway. The immunosuppressive activity of sirolimus appears to be a consequence in part of the sirolimus-FKBP complex blocking the activation of the mammalian target of rapamycin, (mTOR).[5] mTOR is a serine/threonine protein kinase and is involved in the regulation of cell proliferation through the initiation of gene translation in response to amino acids, growth factors, cytokines, and mitogens. The kinase activity of additional cell cycle regulatory proteins, cyclin-dependent kinase-2 and -4, is also inhibited by sirolimus. Sirolimus blocks IL-2 and other growth factor-mediated signal transduction (signal 3 of the allograft rejection response) and the calcium-independent CD28/B7 (CD80/CD86) costimulatory pathway. Whereas cyclosporine and tacrolimus block T-cell cycle progression at the G0 to G1 stage, sirolimus prevents cells from progressing from G1 to the S phase. Sirolimus blocks T-cell activation by IL-2, -4, and -6 and stimulation of B-cell proliferation by lipopolysaccaride. Sirolimus directly inhibits B cell immunoglobulin synthesis caused by interleukins. Sirolimus has been shown to prevent acute, accelerated, and chronic rejection of skin, heart, renal, islet, and small bowel allografts in rodent, rabbit, dog, pig, and nonhuman primate graft recipients. It has also been shown to be efficacious in models of autoimmunity; insulin-dependent diabetes, and systemic lupus erythematosus.

Sirolimus' antagonism of cytokine and growth factor action is not limited to cells of the immune system. Growth factor (PDGF, FGF)-induced proliferation of fibroblasts, endothelial cells, hepatocytes, and smooth muscle cells is inhibited by sirolimus. Sirolimus has been very effective in preventing intimal smooth muscle proliferation (arteriosclerosis) following mechanical or immune-mediated arterial injury. In human clinical trials, supplementation of cyclosporine-based protocols is associated with a reduction in acute renal allograft rejection; however, the combination of the two drugs increases the risk of nephrotoxicity, hemolytic-uremic syndrome, and hypertension.[5] Other reported side effects include hyperlipidemia, thrombocytopenia, delayed wound healing, delayed graft function, mouth ulcers, pneumonitis, and interstitial lung disease. Everolimus, another inhibitor of mTOR, is a derivative of sirolimus.

Mycophenolate mofetil (RS-61443, mycophenolic acid, Cellcept, Roche Laboratories, Palo Alto, CA) is a prodrug hydrolyzed by liver esterases to mycophenolic acid. Mycophenolic acid is cytostatic for lymphocytes owing to its inhibition of inosine monophosphate dehydrogenase (IMPDH), an enzyme necessary for *de novo* purine biosynthesis. Mycophenolic acid is a relatively selective inhibitor of T- and B-cell proliferation during the S phase of the cell cycle via its ability to prevent guanosine and deoxyguanosine biosynthesis. Mycophenolic acid has been shown to reduce allograft rejection in multiple animal models, being most effective when combined with cyclosporine, tacrolimus, and/or sirolimus. Mycophenolic acid was developed, in part, as a nonmyelotoxic replacement for azathioprine in human allograft patients. Early clinical trials in human renal allograft recipients showed a decrease in biopsy-proven acute rejection episodes in patients receiving mycophenolic acid in place of azathioprine. At therapeutic doses, mycophenolic acid can be toxic to animals. The primary dose-limiting effects are anemia and weight loss in rats; leukopenia, diarrhea, and anorexia in monkeys; and gastrointestinal hemorrhage, anorexia, and diarrhea in dogs. To reduce the toxic effects, the dose can be lowered or mycophenolic acid can be given in combination with other immunosuppressive agents. Mycophenolic acid can also inhibit growth factor-induced smooth muscle and fibroblast proliferation. Sirolimus and mycophenolic acid, in combination, are extremely effective in preventing arterial intimal smooth muscle proliferation following mechanical injury. This has marked implications for the control of chronic allograft rejection.

Leflunomide (Hoechst AG, Wiesbaden, Germany) is a synthetic organic isoxazole that the intestinal mucosa metabolizes to the active form, A77 1726. Leflunomide mediates at least part of its antiproliferative activity during the S phase of the cell cycle by inhibiting the *de novo* pathway of pyrimidine biosynthesis. The target of A77 1726 in this pathway is the enzyme dihydroorotate dehydrogenase. At higher concentrations, leflunomide is also an inhibitor of tyrosine kinases associated with growth factor receptors. In addition to T and B lymphocytes, leflunomide also has an antiproliferative effect on smooth muscle cells and fibroblasts, which is also owing to inhibition of the pyrimidine biosynthetic pathway in these cells. Leflunomide is currently approved for the treatment of rheumatoid arthritis in human beings. It has been shown to be an effective disease-modifying antirheumatic drug free from the side effects commonly associated with currently approved immunosuppressants. In addition to its efficacy in humans and animal models with autoimmune diseases, leflunomide has been found to control acute, ongoing, and chronic allograft rejection of the kidney, skin, heart, vessels, lung, and composite grafts in small and large animal models. Leflunomide has been used to successfully treat steroid-resistant autoimmune hemolytic anemia and systemic histiocytosis in dogs. In combination with cyclosporine, leflunomide has completely prevented the rejection of canine MHC-nonmatched renal allografts in both experimental and clinical studies.

At doses used in humans, leflunomide causes gastrointestinal toxicity in dogs because of the accumulation of a metabolite, trimethylfluoroanaline (TMFA). Fortunately, the canine lymphocyte is far more sensitive than the human lymphocyte to the effects of the active agent, A77 1726, and much lower oral doses are equally effective in achieving immunosuppression. The authors currently recommend a dose of 4 mg/kg/24 hours orally, and adjust the dose as needed to obtain a 24-hour serum trough concentration of 20 μg/ml. Early studies in the cat suggest that TMFA does not present the toxicity problem encountered in dogs; however, cats metabolize the drug much slower and require approximately half the oral dose to achieve effective blood concentrations. Both cats and dogs with diminished renal function may be subject to TMFA toxicity, as it is excreted by the kidneys. Leflunomide is marketed under the trade name, Arava. Owing to the short half-life of the drug in dogs, as compared with that in human beings, the use of leflunomide in dogs is very expensive.

Leflunomide analogs are currently being developed for transplantation applications. A combination of cyclosporine and FK778, a leflunomide analog, significantly prolonged MHC-mismatched canine renal allograft survival.[5]

Experimental Compounds

FTY 720 is derived from myriocin, a fungus-derived sphingosine analogue.6 After phosphorylation, FTY 720 engages lymphocyte sphingosine-1-phosphate receptors and profoundly alters lymphocyte traffic, acting as a functional sphingosine-1-phosphate antagonist. FTY 720 sequesters naïve and activated CD4+ and CD8+ T cells and B cells from the blood into lymph nodes and Peyer's patches, without affecting their functional properties. Importantly, FTY 720 does not impair cellular or humoral immunity to systemic viral infection, and it does not affect T- cell activation, expansion/proliferation, or immunologic memory.

FTY 720 synergizes effectively with inhibitors of T-cell activation and proliferation to prevent allograft rejection in a wide range of animal models. In combination with subtherapeutic concentrations of cyclosporine, FTY 720 has been shown to delay or prevent the rejection of skin, heart, small bowel, liver, and kidney allografts in rats, dogs, and nonhuman primates.[7] Similar results have been seen when FTY 720 is combined with rapamycin and tacrolimus. FTY 720 is extensively metabolized in the liver via cytochrome enzymes that are not involved in the metabolism of cyclosporine, rapamycin, or tacrolimus and, therefore, variations in drug concentrations when these agents are co-administered are unlikely to occur. In Phase I and II clinical trials in human renal transplant patients, FTY 720 was well tolerated and did not cause any significant toxicity, allograft loss, or increase in infection rates or other complications such as diabetes. The pharmacokinetic profile of FTY 720 was characterized by linear dose-proportional exposure over a wide range of doses, only moderate inter-patient variability, and a prolonged elimination half-life (89-150 hours). These factors suggest that FTY 720 will be administered once daily, without the need for monitoring blood concentrations or dose titration.[7] Human renal transplant patients experienced a significant reduction in peripheral blood lymphocyte counts by up to 85%. It is hoped that FTY 720 may be useful in the future design of more effective and less toxic immunosuppressive regimens for prevention of allograft rejection.

Combination Therapy

Most of the currently used or soon to be available immunosuppressant agents have differing mechanisms of action and are effective at different stages of the cell cycle. Experimentally and clinically, combining agents often results in more effective immunosuppression with fewer drug-induced side effects. In human transplant patients, cyclosporine and tacrolimus are currently considered to be the first line immunosuppressive agents. To increase their effectiveness and decrease toxicity, azathioprine, sirolimus, prednisolone, and/or mycophenolic acid are added to antirejection protocols. Few of the new non-myelotoxic agents have been used in veterinary patients, but many published experimental animal trials investigating autoimmune disease and organ transplantation provide indications and insight into their use. Based on experimental and clinical experience in canine MHC-nonmatched organ transplantation, the combination of cyclosporine and leflunomide or cyclosporine with azathioprine are extremely effective in preventing renal allograft rejection.

References

1. Gregory CR: Immunosuppressive agents. *In* Kirk's Current Veterinary Therapy XIII. Bonagura JD (ed). Philadelphia: WB Saunders Co, 1999, p. 509.

2. Gregory CR, Bernsteen L: Organ transplantation in clinical veterinary practice. *In* Textbook of Small Animal Surgery, 3rd ed. Slatter D (ed). Philadelphia: WB Saunders Co, 2003, p. 122.

3. Mehl ML, Kyles AE, Craigmill AL, et al: Disposition of cyclosporine after intravenous and multi-dose oral administration in cats. J Vet Pharmacol Ther 26:349, 2003

4. Kyles AE, Gregory CR, Craigmill AL, et al: Pharmacokinetics of tacrolimus after multidose oral administration and efficacy in the prevention of allograft rejection in cats with renal transplants. Am J Vet Res 64:926, 2003.

5. Kyles AE, Gregory CR, Griffey SM, et al: Immunosuppression with a combination of the leflunomide analog, FK778, and microemulsified cyclosporine for renal transplantation in mongrel dogs. Transplantation 75:1128, 2003.

6. Halloran PF: Immunosuppressive drugs for kidney transplantation. N Engl J Med 351:2515, 2004.

7. Dragun D, Fritsche L, Boehler T, et al: FTY720: early clinical experience. Transplant Proc 36:554S, 2004.

Chapter 12

Antimicrobial Prophylaxis

Dianne Dunning

Perioperative prophylactic antimicrobial therapy may be defined as the administration of antibiotics in the absence of infection, prior to surgery. The words antimicrobial and antibiotic are often used interchangeably; however, they are not equivalent. An antimicrobial is a general term that refers to a group of drugs that includes antibiotics, antifungals, antiprotozoals, and antivirals; whereas an antibiotic is a drug that is used to treat bacterial infections.[1] The general goal of this form of antimicrobial therapy is to reduce the number of viable bacteria present at the time of surgical incision to a level that normal host defenses can handle, thereby preventing postoperative surgical site infection (SSI).[2-9] Despite the widespread use and availability of antibiotics, however, postoperative wound infections or SSIs still continue to be a problem in people and animals.[9-17] Although the principles of antimicrobial prophylaxis in surgery have been clearly established, many reports continue to describe inappropriate drug selection and use.[2-4,10,18,19] Strict adherence to the recommended guidelines and avoidance of invalid indications or use of drugs with too broad a spectrum of activity should be eliminated to reduce risk of resistance and treatment failure.

Sources of Contamination

Even with appropriate hair removal, skin preparation, and aseptic technique, all surgical wounds are contaminated.[20] The skin and hair of animals provide the principal source of bacterial contamination entering the surgical wound and it is estimated that 20% of normal canine skin flora remains in situ, deep within the hair follicles, even after appropriate skin preparation.[1,9,11,13,16,20-22] Common bacteria residing on normal canine skin after preoperative preparation include (in order of descending prevalence): *Staphylococcus intermedius, coagulase-negative Staphylococcus spp, Bacillus spp., Acinetobacter spp., and Staphylococcus aureus.*[22] Clinical studies in the dog have revealed that the skin begins to reinstate its inherent bacteria colonies 90 minutes after aseptic preparation, turning a clean procedure into a clean contaminated surgery (Table 12-1).[1] It is also contraindicated to clip surgical sites any time before anesthetic induction, as they are 3 times as likely to develop infection owing to superficial skin infection resulting from superficial abrasions and cuts.[11] The risk of infection is the same whether or not the surgical site is clipped 4 hours or more before the induction of anesthesia.[11] Although the risk of SSI is not greater for most noninfected, properly performed gastrointestinal and urogenital procedures, the number and species of bacteria vary and must be considered when selecting an antimicrobial agent.[4,11,21] Each segment of normal bowel, beginning at the stomach, has an incrementally increasing load of bacterial colonies, culminating with the colon and rectum, and the most common pathogens encountered in the gastrointestinal tract are coliforms and anaerobes.

Although hematogenous sources of infection are uncommon, prolonged indwelling venous catheter sites should be inspected, as they pose a source of distant infection that may increase the risk of SSI if undetected. Multiple risk factors for the development of vascular catheter-related infection and bacteria have been identified, which include prolonged duration of catheterization (> 3 days), frequent manipulation of catheters and intravenous lines, improper aseptic insertion and maintenance, the use of transparent plastic dressing, contaminated skin-preparation solution, the location of the catheter, and the use of multilumen catheters.[16,21,23-25] Exogenous sources of bacteria are also infrequent, but they still should be considered when dealing with a SSI.[6,16,20] Commonly reported exogenous sources of bacteria in people and animals include: surgical equipment, the operating room, and personnel.[13,26,27]

A recent prospective study of postoperative SSIs in dogs and cats revealed "infection/inflammation" and "infected" rate of 5.8% and 3%, respectively.[13] In this particular study, a wound

Table 12-1. National Research Council Wound Classification Criteria

Classification	Criteria
Clean	Nontraumatic No inflammation encountered No break in technique Respiratory, gastrointestinal, genitourinary tracts not entered
Clean contaminated	Gastrointestinal or respiratory tracts entered with no significant spillage Oropharynx or vaginal vault entered Genitourinary or biliary tract entered in the absence of infection Minor error in aseptic technique
Contaminated	Major error(s) in aseptic technique Gross spillage from the gastrointestinal tract Traumatic wound < 4 hours after event Genitourinary or biliary tract entered in the presence of infection
Dirty	Acute bacterial inflammation encountered Penetration into necrotic or abscessed tissue Traumatic wound with gross fecal or foreign body contamination and devitalized tissue (> 4 hours after event)

was classified as "infected" if purulent drainage, an abscess, or a fistula was recorded, and a wound was classified as "infected/inflamed" when more than 3 of the following signs were present simultaneously: redness, swelling, pain, heat, serous discharge, and wound dehiscence.[13] These infection rates and definitions are in close agreement with previous studies in dogs and cats and also compare favorably to epidemiologic studies in people.[8,9,11,16,28]

Indications

SSIs usually develop within 30 days of a procedure and within 1 year of implant application.[21] To develop a SSI, two main conditions must be present: a bacterial inoculum (> 10^5 bacteria/gram of tissue) and an environment to support bacterial growth and nutrition. In most cases, the mere presence of bacteria is less important than the level of bacterial growth, as all contaminated wounds do not necessarily become infected.[20] A strong correlation exists, however, between wound contamination and SSI rates, with the rate of infection predictably increasing with increasing wound contamination.[8,9,13,17]

Classically, the four categories of wound contamination are the following: clean, clean contaminated, contaminated, and dirty (Table 12-1). Although the classification of wound type is important, it is insufficient by itself to accurately predict infection rates, because of the wide variety of presenting complaints and procedures it encompasses.[8,9,13,17] One prospective study revealed the three major risk factors for increasing the probability of surgical wounds becoming infected: the duration of surgery, increasing number of personnel in the operating room (particularly a problem in teaching hospitals), and a dirty surgical site classification.[13] Risk factors identified for a wound to become "infected/inflamed" include: a prolonged duration of anesthesia, admission to a postoperative intensive care unit, the presence of wound drainage, increasing patient weight, and a dirty surgical site classification.[13] For both "infected" and "infected/inflamed" wounds, antimicrobial prophylaxis was a protective factor, decreasing the rate of infection 6 to 7 times.[13] Additional risk factors from previously reported veterinary epidemiologic studies include: prior irradiation of the surgical site, chronologic age of the animal (dogs older than 8 years), sex (intact males), presence of a concurrent endocrinopathy, existence of distant sites of active infection, presence of abnormal body condition scores, administration of propofol as a part of the anesthetic protocol, the contamination of the surgical wound with more than 10^5 organisms/gram of tissue, excessive use of electrocautery, presence of foreign material and debris, use of braided or multifilament suture material, and presence of a contaminated surgical suction tip.[11,14,16,22,29-32]

In 1941, the American Society of Anesthetists, the forerunner of the American Society of Anesthesiologists (ASA), began to classify patients according to their preoperative physical status.[33] The ASA Physical Status Classification System was initially created with 6 classes, and then a seventh class was added. The modern ASA classification consists of 5 categories and was adopted in 1961 (Table 12-2).[34] Over the years, many clinical studies have utilized the ASA classification system to stratify patients for morbidity and mortality analysis associated with surgery and anesthesia. In people and in dogs, an ASA classification grade greater than 3 has been shown to be associated with an increased risk of SSI. However, this classification system was meant only to categorize physical status for the purpose of audit and statistical analysis. It was never intended to represent perioperative risk of morbidity for any individual patient, because, as with the surgical wound classification system, many other factors such as the surgical procedure, patient preparation, variability of surgeons and equipment used in different institutions can also affect outcome.[34]

Table 12-2. The ASA Physical Status Classification System.

Classification	Criteria
P1	A normal healthy patient
P2	A patient with mild systemic disease
P3	A patient with severe systemic disease
P4	A patient with severe systemic disease that is a constant threat to life
P5	A moribund patient who is not expected to survive without the operation
P6	A declared brain-dead patient whose organs are being removed for donor purposes

Pharmacologic Principles[1,35]

The key factors that determine a drug's delivery to the surgical site include: the absorption, distribution, and elimination characteristics of the selected antimicrobial agent (Figure 12-1). The disposition of most drugs is split between the central compartment of the vascular system and the tissue compartment, which are composed of less perfused areas, including the interstitial fluid which baths the surgical wound. The concentration of the antimicrobial agent in the interstitial fluid is critical to effective drug efficacy, as most antimicrobials penetrate tissues well but perform poorly in formed tissue exudates and clots.

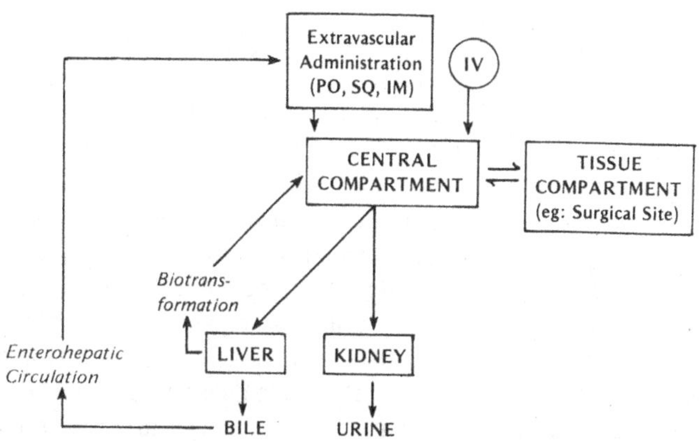

Figure 12-1. Schematic diagram of a drug's disposition in the body. PO, Per os; SQ, subcutaneous; IM, intramuscular; IV, intravenous.

Plotting the amount of intravenously administered drug in the central and tissue compartments as a function of time (Figure 12-2) clarifies the rationale for the general recommendations for perioperative antimicrobial prophylaxis. In the alpha phase, the drug is distributed from the central compartment to the peripheral or tissue compartment. When both compartments are at equilibrium, the beta phase ensues, with the onset of drug elimination. Peak tissue concentrations of the antimicrobials are only achieved once the distribution phase is complete. Therefore, for efficacious antimicrobial prophylaxis, antimicrobial administration should be initiated prior to the surgical incision at the start of the elimination phase, or within 30 minutes to an hour when using a cephalosporin or similar β-lactam antibiotic.

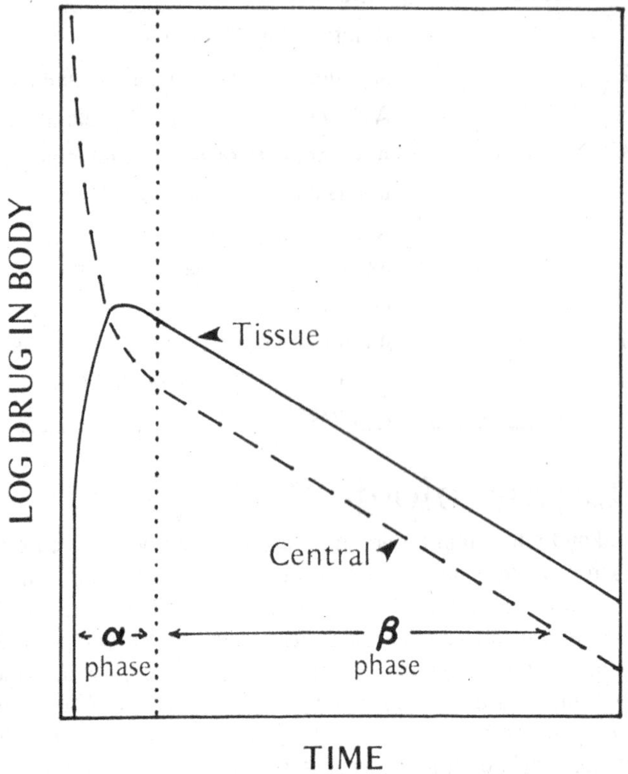

Figure 12-2. Plot of the amount of intravenously administered drug in the central and tissue compartments as a function of time. α, Distribution; β, elimination.

Following intravenous administration, an antimicrobial must reach a certain concentration to have an antimicrobial effect. The minimum inhibitory concentration (MIC) is defined as the lowest concentration that inhibits visible bacterial growth. Practically, the MIC represents the minimum concentration necessary for an antimicrobial to have an inhibitory effect in the plasma or tissues of the animal. The minimum bacteriocidal concentration (MBC) is defined as the lowest concentration that kills 99.9% of the bacteria and is sometimes also referred to as the minimal lethal concentration (MLC). If a drug has a low MBC to MIC ratio (< 4-6) it is referred to as a bacteriocidal drug, because it can be administered in safe doses to achieve high effect or bacterial kill. If a drug has a high MBC to MIC ratio (> 6) it is referred to as a bacteriostatic drug, because safe doses may not be possible to achieve a 99.9 % kill of the bacteria encountered. Depending on the dose administered, a drug may be both bacteriocidal and bacteriostatic. For purposes of perioperative prophylaxis, it is preferred that an antimicrobial be bacteriocidal rather than bacteriostatic to achieve greatest drug efficacy during the operative period.

The recommended dose of an antimicrobial is based on MIC studies performed in animal models of infection. Bacteriocidal antimicrobials are to be administered at 4 to 8 times the MIC for maximal drug efficiency; whereas bacteriostatic antimicrobials are administered at 1 time the MIC throughout the dosing period. Dosing recommendations are also based in part on efficacy studies where antimicrobials were classed as either a concentration or a time-dependent drug. Concentration-dependent drug efficacy (such as aminoglycosides or fluoroquinolones) relies upon achieving one peak concentration above the MIC for successful therapy. After achieving that peak, it is acceptable to allow the drug concentration to fall below the MIC for 8 to 12 hours over a 24-hour period. This is in contrast to time-dependent drug efficacy (such as β-lactams), which is reliant not only on achieving but on maintaining those peak concentrations above the MIC for successful drug therapy throughout the dosing interval.

General Recommendations

(Table 12-3)

Timing of Antimicrobial First Dose

The goal of perioperative antimicrobial prophylaxis is to achieve serum and tissue drug concentrations for the duration of the operation that exceed the MIC for organisms likely to be encountered during the operation. Landmark experimental studies in the early 1960s revealed that surgical incision contaminated with *Staphylococcus aureus* could not be distinguished from incisions that had not been contaminated when antimicrobial agents were administered before the incision.[36] Furthermore, in 1976, Stone et al demonstrated that the lowest SSI rates in patients undergoing gastrointestinal, biliary, and colon operations occurred when antimicrobial agents were administered within 1 hour before incision.[37] Administration of the first antimicrobial dose after surgery resulted in SSI rates almost identical to those in patients who did not receive prophylaxis.[370]

Ideally, based on numerous clinical and experimental studies in people and animals, the antimicrobial agent should be administered as near to the incision time as possible to achieve low SSI rates.[28,36-39] Although research in people has demonstrated that administration of the antimicrobial agent at the time of anesthetic induction is safe and results in adequate serum and tissue drug levels at the time of incision, in veterinary medicine we must take into account the time needed after induction for clipping and surgical preparation, which can be far more extensive and time consuming than in humans. If significant preoperative patient preparation is necessary, the initial dose of an antimicrobial should be delayed past anesthetic induction to more closely approximate 1 hour prior to the start of surgery to ensure appropriate drug concentrations in the peripheral compartments.[4,11,19,30,39] It is also advisable to deliver the entire antimicrobial dose 1 hour prior to applying a tourniquet to ensure local tissue concentrations distad to the vascular occlusion.[4]

Table 12-3. Summary of General Principals of Antimicrobial Selection

General Principal	Recommendation
Antibiotic timing	Infusion of the first antimicrobial dose should begin 60 minutes prior to the start of surgery
Duration of prophylaxis	Perioperative prophylactic antimicrobials should be discontinued after wound closure at the end of the surgical procedure
Antimicrobial dosing	The initial antimicrobial dose should be based on the animal's ideal weight. Administration should be repeated intraoperatively if the operation is continuing two half-lives after the first dose to ensure adequate antimicrobial levels until wound closure.
Screening for β-lactam allergy	Generally unnecessary, as sensitivity not widely documented in dogs and cats.[46] Clindamycin, vancomycin, or metronidazole are feasible options if β-lactam allergy suspected.

Duration of Antimicrobial Prophylaxis

The majority of published evidence demonstrates that antimicrobial prophylaxis after wound closure is unnecessary, and most studies comparing single- with multiple-dose prophylaxis have not shown benefit of additional doses.[3,5,8,31,40] The optimal duration of antimicrobial prophylaxis in veterinary surgery is unknown. In people, antimicrobial therapy is often continued for 24 hours beyond surgical wound closure, despite concerns regarding superinfection or selection for antimicrobial resistant pathogens.

Selection of an Antimicrobial Drug[1]

For most routine perioperative prophylaxis, the antimicrobial agents of choice are cephalosporins owing to their efficacy, safety, and cost effectiveness. Cephalosporins belong to the β-lactam family of antimicrobials, which also include the penicillins. Similar to other β-lactam antimicrobials, cephalosporins alter cell wall formation by interfering with bacterial peptidoglycan synthesis by inhibiting the final transpeptidation necessary for cross-links of the cell wall.

Cephalosporins are grouped into "generations" by their antimicrobial properties. The original cephalosporins were designated first generation with more extended-spectrum cephalosporin drugs being developed and sequentially classified as second, third, and fourth. In general, each new generation of cephalosporins has significantly greater gram-negative antimicrobial properties than its predecessor, however, the expense of the cephalosporin also usually increases with the generation bracket.

Specifically, most first generation cephalosporins have a spectrum of activity that includes penicillinase-producing, methicillin-susceptible staphylococci and streptococci. First generation cephalosporins also exhibit activity against *Staphylococci* spp., *Streptococci* spp., *Escherichia coli*, *Klebsiella* spp., and *Proteus mirabilis*, but they do not display effectiveness against anaerobic bacteria, *Pseudomonas*, *Enterococcus* spp., other *Proteus*, or *Serratia*. Second generation cephalosporins display a greater gram-negative spectrum while retaining some activity against gram-positive cocci and, therefore, are the antimicrobial of choice for most enteric and abdominal procedures. Second generation cephalosporins may also be active against some anaerobic bacteria as well as some strains of *Enterobacter*, *E. coli*, *Klebsiella*, *Proteus*, and *Serratia* that are resistant to first generation cephalosporins. Third generation cephalosporins exhibit a broad spectrum of activity against gram-negative bacteria but display less activity against *Staphylococci* and *Streptococci* species. The newest or fourth generation cephalosporins have a greater spectrum of activity against gram-positive organisms than the third generation cephalosporins. They also are useful and have a greater resistance to β-lactamases than the third generation cephalosporins.

In conclusion, SSIs in people and animals are the most common cause of postoperative morbidity and mortality because they often necessitate additional intervention and expense and prolong hospitalization.[7,9,10,12-17,28,30,41-45] Before considering whether antimicrobial agents are indicated, it is imperative that a surgeon consider the type of surgery to be performed, its expected duration, the potential pathogens that may be encountered, and the immunocompetence of the animal. While antimicrobial agents are an essential tool used to limit the incidence of SSIs and their associated complications, they do not replace good surgical technique, including gentle tissue handling, appropriate suture materials and patterns, and adequate preoperative planning.

References

1. Vaden SL, Riviere JE: Penicillins and related b-lactam antibiotics. *In* Veterinary Pharmacology and Therapeutics, 8th ed. Adams HR (ed). Ames: Iowa State University Press, 2001, pp. 818-827.

2. Antimicrobial prophylaxis in surgery. Med Lett Drugs Therap 43:92-97, 2001.

3. American Society of Health-System Pharmacists: ASHP therapeutic guidelines on antimicrobial prophylaxis in surgery. Am J Health Syst Pharm 56:1839-1888, 1999.

4. Bratzler DW, Houck PM: Antimicrobial prophylaxis for surgery: An advisory statement from the National Surgical Infection Prevention Project. Am J Surg 189:396-404, 2005.

5. Dellinger EP, Gross PA, Barrett TL, et al: Quality standard for antimicrobial prophylaxis in surgical procedures. Clin Infect Dis 18:422-427, 1994.

6. Fernandez AH, Monge V, Garcinuno MA: Surgical antibiotic prophylaxis: effect in postoperative infections. Eur J Epidemiol 17:369-374, 2001.

7. Malone DL, Genuit T, Tracy JK, et al: Surgical site infections: reanalysis of risk factors. J Surg Res 103:89-95, 2002.

8. Page CP, Bohnen JM, Fletcher JR, et al: Antimicrobial prophylaxis for surgical wounds. Guidelines for clinical care. Arch Surg 128:79-88, 1993.

9. Vasseur PB, Levy J, Dowd E, et al: Surgical wound infection rates in dogs and cats. Data from a teaching hospital. Vet Surg 17:60-64, 1988.

10. Barie PS, Eachempati SR: Surgical site infections. Surg Clin North Am 85:1115-1135, 2005.

11. Brown DC, Conzemius MG, Shofer F, et al: Epidemiologic evaluation of postoperative wound infections in dogs and cats. J Am Vet Med Assoc 210:1302-1306, 1997.

12. Delgado-Rodriguez M, Gomez-Ortega A, Sillero-Arenas M, et al: Epidemiology of surgical-site infections diagnosed after hospital discharge: a prospective cohort study. Infect Control Hosp Epidemiol 22:24-30, 2001.

13. Eugster S, Schawalder P, Gaschen F, et al. A prospective study of postoperative surgical site infections in dogs and cats. Vet Surg 33:542-550, 2004.

14. Heldmann E, Brown DC, Shofer F: The association of propofol usage with postoperative wound infection rate in clean wounds: a retrospective study. Vet Surg 28:256-259, 1999.

15. Lester S, Welsh E, Pratschke K: Complications of exploratory coeliotomy in 70 cats. J Small Anim Pract 45:351-356, 2004.

16. Nicholson M, Beal M, Shofer F, et al: Epidemiologic evaluation of postoperative wound infection in clean-contaminated wounds: A retrospective study of 239 dogs and cats. Vet Surg 31:577-581, 2002.

17. Pessaux P, Atallah D, Lermite E, et al: Risk factors for prediction of surgical site infections in "clean surgery." Am J Infect Control 33:292-298, 2005.

18. Gyssens I: Preventing postoperative infections: current treatment recommendations. Drugs 57:175-185, 1999.

19. Lallemand S, Thouverez M, Bailly P, et al: Non-observance of guidelines for surgical antimicrobial prophylaxis and surgical-site infections. Pharm World Sci 24:95-99, 2002.

20. Dunning D: Surgical wound infection and the use of antibiotics. *In* Textbook of Small Animal Surgery. Slatter D (ed). Philadelphia: WB Saunders, 2002, pp. 553-561.

21. Johnston JA, Murtauch RJ: Preventing and treating nosocomial infection: II. Wound, blood, and gastrointestinal infections. Compend Cont Educ Pract 19:693-703, 1997.

22. Whittem TL, Johnson AL, Smith CW, et al: Effect of perioperative prophylactic antimicrobial treatment in dogs undergoing elective orthopedic surgery. J Am Vet Med Assoc 215:212-216, 1999.

23. Blaiset M, Couto C, Evans K, et al: Complications of indwelling, silastic central venous access catheters in dogs and cats. J Am Anim Hosp Assoc 31:379-384, 1995.

24. Mathews K, Brooks M, Valliant A: A prospective study of intravenous catheter contamination. J Vet Emerg Crit Care 6:33-43, 1996.

25. Tan R, Dart A, Dowling B: Catheters: a review of the selection, utilisation and complications of catheters for peripheral venous access. Aust Vet J 81:136-139, 2003.

26. Emmerson M: A microbiologist's view of factors contributing to infection. New Horiz 6:S3-10, 1998.

27. Mangram A, Horan T, Pearson M, et al: Guideline for Prevention of Surgical Site Infection, 1999. Centers for Disease Control and Prevention (CDC) Hospital Infection Control Practices Advisory Committee. Am J Infect Control 27:97-132, 1999.

28. Polk HC Jr, Lopez-Mayor JF: Postoperative wound infection a prospective study of determinant factors and prevention. Surgery 66:97–103, 1969.

29. Sturgeon C, Lamport AI, Lloyd DH, et al: Bacterial contamination of suction tips used during surgical procedures performed on dogs and cats. Am J Vet Res 61:779-783, 2000.

30. Beal MW, Brown DC, Shofer FS: The effects of perioperative hypothermia and the duration of anesthesia on postoperative wound infection rate in clean wounds: a retrospective study. Vet Surg 29:123-127, 2000.

31. McDonald M, Grabsch E, Marshall C, et al: Single- versus multiple-dose antimicrobial prophylaxis for major surgery, A systematic review. Aust N Z J Surg 68:388-396, 1998.

32. Rosin E, Uphoff TS, Schultz-Darken NJ, et al: Cefazolin antibacterial activity and concentrations in serum and the surgical wound in dogs. Am J Vet Res 54:1317-1321, 1993.

33. Saklad M: Grading of patients for surgical procedures. Anesthesiol 2:281-284, 1941.

34. ASA grades. In: 2005.

35. Brown SA: Pharmacokinetics: Disposition and fate of drugs in the body. *In* Veterinary Pharmacology and Therapeutics, 8th ed. Adams HR (ed). Ames: Iowa State Press, 2001, pp. 15-56.

36. Burke JF: The effective period of preventive antibiotic action in experimental incisions and dermal lesions. Surgery 50:161-168, 1961.

37. Stone HH, Hooper CA, Kolb LD, et al: Antibiotic prophylaxis in gastric, biliary and colonic surgery Ann Surg 184:443-452, 1976.

38. Classen DC, Evans RS, Pestotnik SL, et al: The timing of prophylactic administration of antibiotics and the risk of surgical-wound infection N Engl J Med 326:281-286, 1992.

39. Polk HC Jr, Trachtenberg L, Finn MP: Antibiotic activity in surgical incisions. The basis for prophylaxis in selected operations. JAMA 244:1353-1354, 1980.

40. Meijer WS, Schmitz PIM, Jeekel J: Meta-analysis of randomized, controlled clinical trials of antibiotic prophylaxis in biliary tract surgery Br J Surg 77:293-290, 1990.

41. Basinger RR, Suber JT: Two techniques for supplementing interlocking nail repair of fractures of the humerus, femur, and tibia: results in 12 dogs and cats. Vet Surg 33:673-680, 2004.

42. Bass M, Howard J, Gerber B, et al: Retrospective study of indications for and outcome of perineal urethrostomy in cats. J Small Anim Pract 46:227-231, 2005.

43. Glickman LT: Veterinary nosocomial (hospital-acquired) Klebsiella infections. J Am Vet Med Assoc 179:1389-1392, 1981.

44. Kadar E, Sykes JE, Kass PH, et al: Evaluation of the prevalence of infections in cats after renal transplantation: 169 cases (1987-2003). J Am Vet Med Assoc 227:948-953, 2005.

45. Lizan-Garcia M, Garcia-Caballero J, Asensio-Vegas A: Risk factors for surgical-wound infection in general surgery: a prospective study. Infect Control Hosp Epidemiol 18:310-315, 1997.

46. Kunkle GA, Sundlof S, Keisling K: Adverse side effects of oral antibacterial therapy in dogs and cats: An epidemiologic study of pet owners' observations. J Am Anim Hosp Assoc 1995:46-55, 1995.

Part II

Soft Tissue Surgery

Chapter 13

Perineal Hernia

G. P. Dupré
H. N. Brissot

Perineal hernia (PH) results from weakness of muscles of the pelvic diaphragm. It occurs most likely in older male dogs, where its prevalence ranges from 0.1 to 0.4% from different hospital admisions.[1,2] It has also been described in cats, but one study describes only 40 cases in 12 years in three major American referral centers.[3] Some cases have also been mentioned in the female dog.

Clinical signs include straining to defecate and, less frequently, straining to urinate. Some other signs such as fecal incontinence, urinary incontinence, and flatulence have also been mentioned.[1-17]

The clinical diagnosis is based on appearance of a perineal swelling, most often right-sided or bilateral. A rectal examination demonstrates the presence of accumulated feces in an abnormally enlarged rectum. When the rectum is empty, the hernia may be difficult to diagnose. In these cases, the ability to push the finger through an enlarged rectum toward the sacrotuberous ligament demonstrates the loss of muscular support to the rectum wall and thus is diagnostic for perineal hernia.[1,4,5] Occasionally, an acute soft-tissue swelling increases the perineal deformation unilaterally. In these cases, a perineal cystocentesis usually confirms the diagnosis of an associated retroflexed bladder.[1,15] In most cases, besides the rectal wall deformity, periprostatic fat, omentum, digestive loops, or prostate may fill the perineal cavity.[1,2,18]

Causal Factors for Perineal Hernia

Predisposition

Breeds

Although breed over-representation has been mentioned for the Boston terrier, Pekingese, Boxer, Collies, and Old English sheepdogs,[1,2,12] this predisposition was not found in two other retrospective studies,[16,17] where Yorkshire terriers, Cotons, Bichons, German Shepherds, and Mixed-breeds have been the most common breeds encountered.

Male/Female

Perineal hernia occurs almost exclusively in male dogs. Some authors have shown that the levator ani muscle is larger and stronger in the female compared with the male dog to support parturition, thus explaining the low number of perineal hernias in the female.[19] However, when the weight of the pelvic diaphragm muscles was compared in some predisposed breeds (Corgie, Boxer)[1,2] to the weight of the same muscles in the Greyhound, no significant difference was found.[19] Therefore, based solely on the muscle weight, it is difficult to understand why perineal hernia occurs rarely in female dogs.[2]

Age

Perineal hernia occurs most commonly in dogs from 7 to 9 years of age.[1,5,12] Whether the age is associated with muscle weakness, prostatic disease, or any other underlying disease remains unknown.[15,20,21]

Side of the Hernias

Among different studies, 60% of perineal hernias were unilateral and 40% bilateral.[5,10-17] Among the unilateral hernias, almost 70% were right-sided. Studies have failed to demonstrate a relative weakness of the pelvic diaphragm muscles of the right side. On rectal examination of unilateral hernias, a contralateral weakness is often encountered. Failure to recognize this weakness and to reconstruct adequately this contralateral side makes it prone to future hernia.[17]

Increased Abdominal and Perineal Pressure

Chronic constipation resulting from bad feeding habits is usually associated with increased defecating efforts, which in turn, can increase abdominal and perineal pressure.[17,18,22,23] In cats, most cases were bilateral and associated with chronic constipation, megacolon, stranguria, or perineal urethrostomy surgery.[3] Increased abdominal pressure during coughing could be one predisposing factor in female dogs and in older male dogs prone to cardiac insufficiency.

Muscular Weakness and Atrophy

Perineal herniation commonly occurs between the external anal sphincter and the levator ani muscle and, more rarely, between the levator ani muscle and the coccygeal muscles. Frequently, the cranial remnants of the levator ani can be found close to the external anal sphincter or to the external coccygeal muscle. In severe cases, muscle atrophy will involve not only the levator ani muscle but also the external coccygeus, the internal obturator muscle, and the external anal sphincter.[1,2,18,24] Biopsy specimens of the levator ani muscle fibers of dogs suffering from perineal hernia have shown atrophy of neurologic origin,[24] but it remains unclear whether this atrophy is an expression of aging, neurologic disease, or excessive pressure.

Hormonal Imbalance

Androgen

Perineal hernias have frequently been associated with testicular tumors (2% of sertolinomas, 15% of interstitial tumors, 19% of seminomas, and 11% of mixed tumors),[25] which suggested an association between hormonal imbalance and pelvic diaphragm muscle atrophy. Currently, no influence of the androgen concentration has been demonstrated, although, in the rat, androgen receptors have been found in the levator ani muscle. Similar studies in the canine have failed to demonstrate any relation between testosterone levels and muscular fiber size.[19,26,27] In one study, the recurrence rate in castrated animals was 2.7 times less than in intact animals.[2] This is one of the reasons why castration is recommended as an adjunct therapy for perineal hernia.

Role of Prostate

The presence of relaxin in the canine prostate was evidenced and the hypothesis of relaxin being involved in perineal hernia formation in male dogs was tested. Based on preliminary results, relaxin of prostatic origin leaking from periprostatic cysts, usually seen in the perineum of affected dogs, is a possible factor in local connective tissue weakening and subsequently in perineal hernia formation.[28]

Different studies confirm that dogs with perineal hernia are prone to concurrent prostatic disease (range 10 to 51%)[12,14-17,29,30] In one study where ultrasonographic prostatic assessment was performed before any perineal hernia surgery, prostatic lesions were present in 17 dogs (41%); in 8 dogs (19.5%), prostatic disease had to be specifically treated surgically.[15] In another study on 41 bilateral or complicated hernias, 9 prostatic surgeries (omentalization or perineal cyst resection) were performed.[17] Given the high frequency of prostatic disease associated with perineal hernia, an ultrasound evaluation of the prostate is recommended prior to surgery. It remains unclear whether both diseases occur in the same type of patients (breed, age, and sex) or if a significant correlation does exist.[15-17,21]

Pathogenesis

Deterioration of the levator ani muscle results in a progressive loss of rectal wall support. The fissure between the external anal sphincter muscle and the pubocaudal part of the levator ani muscle progressively enlarges. Retroperitoneal fat naturally progresses through this fissure. The loss of muscular support and the progression of defecating efforts increase the chances of the rectum to progressively fill this new space into the perineal cavity. Then, because of lack of continuity of the rectum with the anus, feces cannot be expelled and defecating efforts even increase. Secondary rectal dilation occurs.[1,12,15,17,21] During this process, continual straining to defecate progressively enlarges the rectal dilatation and further weakens the pelvic diaphragm muscles.[17] Finally, persistent straining associated with a huge rectal dilatation and hernia can even promote secondary herniation of the prostate and retroflexion of the bladder into the perineal cavity.

Rectal Diseases

Rectal lesions associated with perineal hernia have previously been characterized as deviation (a change in rectal orientation from the midline), sacculation (enlargement not associated with tearing of the muscular wall), or diverticulum (protrusion of rectal mucosa through the muscular layers of the rectal wall).[12,14,17,21] Because differentiation between rectal deviation, sacculation, and diverticulum appears difficult clinically or radiographically,[12,13,21] a grading for the rectal dilatation was proposed.[17] In this study, a simple deviation with no dilatation was a grade 1, a mild rectal dilatation (asymmetric dilatation with fecal accumulation without visible perineal deformation) was a grade 2, and a severe rectal dilatation (asymmetric dilatation with a visible bulge of the perineum and a large amount of fecal accumulation and impaction) was a grade 3.

Bladder Retroflexion

Bladder retroflexion occurred in 12 to 29% of dogs.[8,6,10,12,15-17,29,31] In cases of retroflexion, the bladder rotates at least 180° around its neck. Although this finding was not statistically significant in all studies,[17] perineal hernias with bladder retroflexion carried a higher mortality rate (30%) and a worse prognosis than those without.[6,10,12] Following retroflexion, several complications can be encountered. Acute renal failure can occur secondary to complete urethral occlusion, bladder necrosis owing to occlusion of the urogenital arteries,[12] and overall, partial, total, temporary, or definitive loss of urinary continence can occur.[12,17]

Perineal Hernia Grading

In order to propose guidelines for surgical treatment, some authors have graded perineal hernias as unilateral, bilateral, and complicated. A perineal hernia was defined as complicated if it met the following criteria: recurrence of PH, unilateral PH with a severe (grade 3) rectal dilatation, PH with a concurrent surgical prostatic disease, and PH with retroflexed bladder.[15,16,17]

Considerations for Treatment

Closure of the Pelvic Diaphragm

Current approaches to treatment of perineal hernia rely on closure of the pelvic diaphragm. Because muscle appositional techniques resulted in excessive tension on the external anal sphincter, muscle transposition techniques were developed using the superficial gluteal muscle,[7,8] internal obturator muscle,[8-12] semitendinosus muscle flap,[32] or a combination of internal obturator muscle with superficial gluteal muscle flap.[13] Filling the defect with stainless steel, polypropylene mesh,[33,34] porcine intestinal submucosa,[35,36] and with fascia lata have been suggested.[37] Presently, the internal obturator flap with tenotomy is the most popular and seemingly the most appropriate technique for most cases of herniorraphy. In cases of severe muscle loss, we have successfully used the superficial gluteal muscle flap or the fascia lata free flaps.

Laparotomy in the Treatment of Perineal Hernia

Besides rupture of the pelvic diaphragm, rectal disease, bladder retroflexion, and prostatic disease often occur concurrently.[6,12,14-17,21,29-31] They contribute to the severity of perineal hernia, and may even discourage further treatment. After a report by Bilbrey et al in 1990,[29] some authors studied the incidence of rectal, prostatic, and bladder diseases associated with perineal hernia.[14-17,20] Since 1993 they have developed a "2-step protocol," where laparotomy was performed as the initial stage of repair in bilateral or complicated perineal hernia (recurrence of perineal hernia, unilateral perineal hernia with a grade 3 rectal dilatation, perineal hernia with a concurrent surgical prostatic disease, and perineal hernia with retroflexed bladder). During laparotomy, colopexy and cysto- or vas deferens-pexy and, if needed, prostatic surgery, are performed, and a perineal herniorraphy using an internal obturator muscle flap transposition[15-17] is performed 2 to 7 days later. Results compare favorably with those of previous studies.[6,9-13] Satisfactory results using colopexy and cysto- or vas deferens-pexy as sole or adjunctive treatment for perineal hernia have also been reported by others.[14,29,31]

Rationale For A Two-Step Protocol

Colopexy resolves rectal dilatation or deviation, vas deferens-pexy stabilizes the prostate, and cystopexy prevents abnormal motion of the bladder so that the perineal space becomes free of viscera after the abdominal surgery. At subsequent herniorraphy, perineal inflammation has resolved and the hernia is empty, which allows improved observation of important local anatomic structures such as the pelvic diaphragm muscles, pudendal and caudal rectal nerves and artery, internal obturator muscle and tendon, and rectal wall. This facilitates hernia repair (Figure 13-1).[15,17] Then guidelines for perineal repair can be proposed (Table 13-1).

Prognosis, Complication Rates and Causes

Prognosis and complication rates have been published. They depend on the severity of the hernia, associated disease, surgeon's experience, and surgical techniques (Table 13-2).

Colo-Recto-Anal Abnormalities

Preoperatively, external anal sphincter mechanism incompetence is rare. However, chronic distension of the rectal wall and chronic straining may weaken the external sphincter fibers. Whenever incompetence is suspected, electromyography of the external sphincter should be recommended prior to surgery. Although postoperative fecal incontinence and rectal prolapse have been described respectively in 3 to 15%[10,12,30] and 7 to 42%[10,12] of dogs with PH, none of the dogs sustaining a laparotomy as a first-step procedure experienced this complication.[17] When recorded, persistent postoperative tenesmus has been reported to occur in to 2 to 50% of dogs.[10,12,17] Causes of persistent postoperative tenesmus have not been determined, although rectal deformation associated with persistent rectocolitis has been suggested.[12] Colonic or rectal motility disorders can also be associated with long-term straining.[22,23] This could explain poor rectal emptying in some patients with good perineal reconstruction.[17]

Urinary Dribbling

Postoperative urinary incontinence has been described in 4 to 8% of dogs with perineal hernia.[6,10,12,14,17] Suggested mechanisms involve acute traction on the hypogastric and pelvic nerves or secondary deterioration of the detrusor muscle owing to retroflexion.[6,12,30] In one study,[17] 15 dogs (36%) presented with urine dribbling after surgery; 8 resolved within the first 6 months, but 7 (17%) had permanent dribbling. Possible associations between prostatic disease, bladder malposition as well as vas deferens- or cystopexy and urine dribbling remain to be determined.

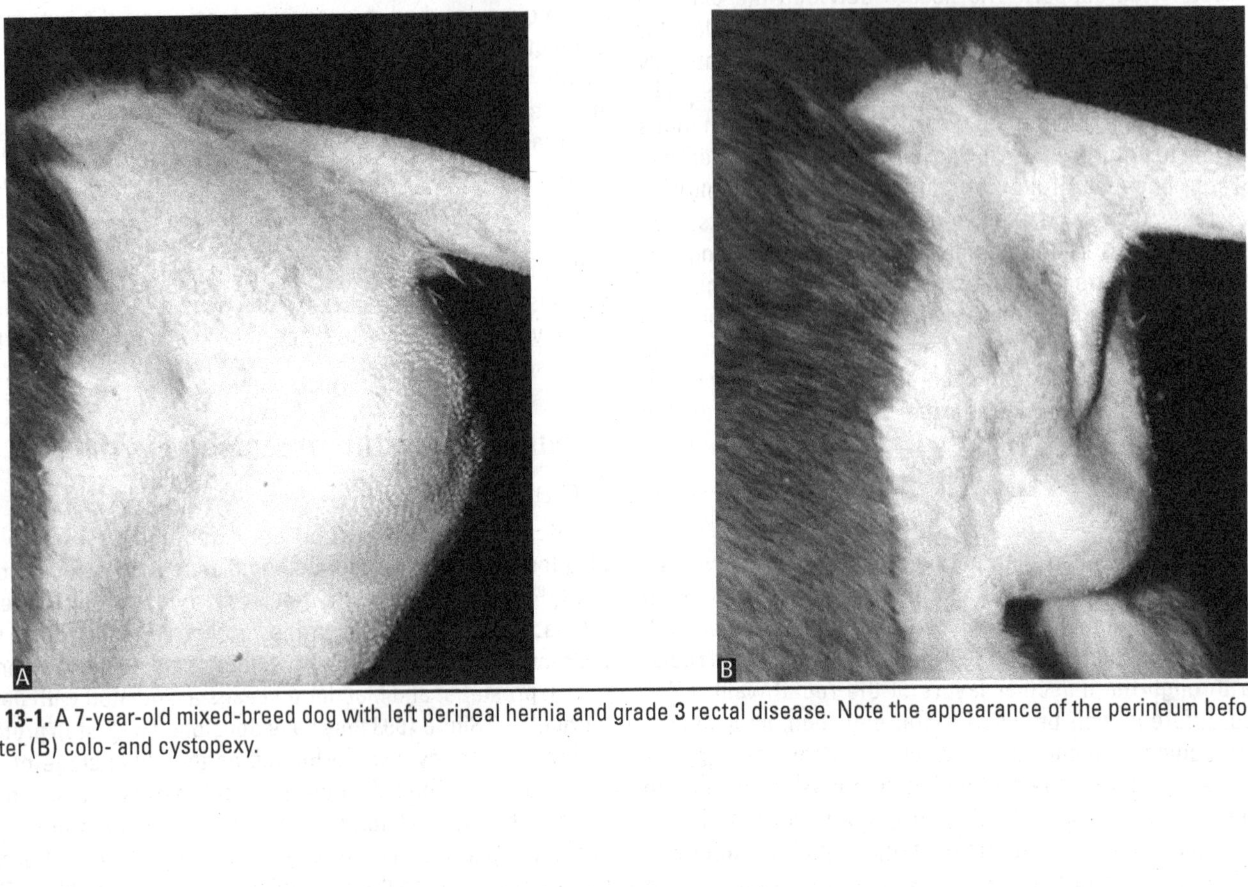

Figure 13-1. A 7-year-old mixed-breed dog with left perineal hernia and grade 3 rectal disease. Note the appearance of the perineum before (A) and after (B) colo- and cystopexy.

Perineal Wound Infection

Perineal wound infection is the most common complication described after perineal hernia repair, ranging from 5 to 45%.[9-13,17,30] Absorbable monofilament suture material, perioperative antibiotics, and anal closure are used to decrease the risks of postoperative infection.[10,12,30,38] Although laparoscopic colo- and vas deferens-pexy have been suggested,[39] these have been discouraged by some authors because of the high rate of septic complications at the colopexy site.[16,17]

Table 13-1. Current Guidelines for Perineal Hernia Repair[15-17]

1- Upon admission: Is the bladder in place?

If bladder retroflexion is suspected, catheterization is mandatory. In case of impossible catheterization, a perineal cystocentesis must be performed. Then the bladder can be manually reduced and catheterization becomes possible. Diuresis is monitored.

2- Complete physical exam and blood work

Given the age of the patients, concurrent diseases are not rare, particularly renal or cardiac diseases. In addition, some patients can be debilitated by tenesmus and anorexia. Preoperative enteral feeding may be necessary.

3- Diagnosis of associated lesions

After manual rectal emptying, grading of rectal disease is provided and prostatic ultrasonography is performed.

4- One- or two-step protocol

Candidates for a laparotomy before perineal herniorraphy include those with:

- retroflexion of the bladder
- surgical prostatic disease
- bilateral hernia
- recurrence
- unilateral hernia with grade 3 rectal disease

During laparotomy, only patients suffering from vesical retroflexion undergo a cystopexy, but colopexy, vas deferens-pexy, prostatic biopsies, and castration are done on all. In all other cases, a perineal herniorraphy and neutering are accomplished as the sole surgical treatment.

5- Medical care

When a laparotomy has been the first step, herniorraphy can be delayed for about 48 hours, during which rectal emptying and enteral feeding (no residue) can be accomplished. In some debilitated patients the herniorraphy can be delayed even further.

6- Perineal herniorraphy

Herniorraphy is the last step of this protocol. It usually involves an internal obturator flap, but a superficial gluteal muscle or fascia lata free flaps can also be added.

Table 13-2. Signalment, Description of Associated Lesions, Surgical procedures, Postoperative

Authors	Number of cases	Unilateral hernia	Bilateral hernia	Rectal disease	Prostatic disease
Hardie-1983	42	28	14	19/42	6 inside the hernia
Orsher-1986	31	14	17	11/31 postoperatively	Preoperative status not reported. Small prostate postoperatively in 30/31
Sjollema-1989	100	57	43	NR	Enlarged in 54 cases, displaced in 16 (clinical assesement and Xray survey)
Raffan-1993	44	27	17	24/44	Enlarged and/or cystic in 14 cases, inside hernia in 9 cases
Hosgood-1995	100 (2 females)	51	49	30/30 (Xray evaluation)	Prostatic disease in 5/43 (Xray evaluation) and 10/100 (clinical exam)
Maute-2001	32	19	9	NR	19/32 (clinical assesment, Xray and ultrasonography survey)
Brissot-2004	41	21	20	41/41 (clinical evaluation)	21/41 (clinical assesment and Xray survey, confirmed histologically in 17 cases)

NR: Non-Reported data
OIMT: Obturator Intern Muscle flap Transposition
SGMT: Superficial Gluteal Muscle flap Transposition

functional outcome and Recurrence rate published for Dogs suffering from Perineal Hernias.[9-12,14,17]

Bladder retroflexion	Surgery	Post-op ténesmus	Fecal incontinence	Urinary incontinence	Recurrence of herniation
7/42	IOMT	Reported but not calculated	Reported but not calculated	Reported but not calculated	1/42 (2%)
Reported but not calculated	IOMT	NR (+ 4 rectal prolaps)	NR	2	16/31 (50%) ventral and/or pelvic diaphgram defect
12/100 (clinical assesment and Xray survey)	IOMT and castration in case of prostatic enlargement	NR (+ 7 rectal prolaps)	15 (present in 7 cases preoperatively)	5	5/100 (5%)
6/44	IOMT + SGMT	4		3	3/44 (6.9%)
20/100	IOMT or standard herniorraphy. Castration in all but 17.	9 (8%) (+ 9 prolaps)	3	4	6/70 (8%)
9/32	Colopexy, cystopexy and castration	NR	NR	NR	7/32 (22%)
12	Colopexy, cystopexy, castration, treatment of prostatic disease, OIMT.	8 dog in short postop, 4 in long term (> 6months)	10	15 dog in short postop, 7 in long term (> 6 months)	4/41 (9%)

References

1. Bellenger CR: Perineal hernia in dogs. Aust Vet J 56:434-438,1980.

2. Hayes HM, Wilson GP, Tapone RE: The epidemiologic features of perineal hernia in 771 dogs. J Am Anim Hosp Assoc 14:703-707, 1978.

3. Welches CD, Scavelli TD, Aronsohn MG, et al: Perineal hernia in the cat: a retrospective study of 40 cases. J Am Anim Hosp Assoc 28:431-438, 1992.

4. Bojrab MJ, Toomey A: Perineal hernia in the dog. Comp Contin Educ Pract Vet : 3:8-15, 1981.

5. Burrows CF and Harvey CE: Perineal hernia in the dog. J Small Anim Pract. 14:315-332,1973.

6. White RAS, Herrtage ME: Bladder retroflexion in the dog. J Small Anim Pract 27:735-746,1986.

7. Spreull JSA, Frankland AL: Transplanting the superficial gluteal muscle in the treatment of perineal hernia and flexure of the rectum in dogs. J Small Anim Pract 21:265-278, 1980.

8. Weaver AD, Omamegbe JO: Surgical treatment of perineal hernia in the dog. J.Small Anim.Pract 22:149-158,1981.

9. Hardie E, Kolata R, Early T, et al: Evaluation of internal obturator muscle transposition in treatment of perineal hernia in dogs. Vet Surg 12:69-72, 1983.

10. Sjollema BE, Van Sluijs FJ: Perineal hernia repair in dog by transposition of the internal obturator muscle; I: Surgical technique; II: Complications and results in 100 patients. Vet Quart 11:12-23, 1989.

11. Orsher R: Clinical and surgical parameters in dogs with perineal hernia-analysis of results of internal obturator muscle transposition. Vet Surg 15:253-258, 1986.

12. Hosgood G, Hedlung SC, Pechman DR, et al: Perineal herniorrhaphy: perioperative data from 100 dogs. J Am Anim Hosp Assoc 31:331-342, 1995.

13. Raffan PJ: A new surgical technique for repair of perineal hernias in the dog. J Small Anim Pract 34:13-19, 1993.

14. Maute AM, Koch DA, Montavon PM: Perineal hernie beim hund-Colopexie, vasopexie, cystopexie und Kastration als therapie der wahl bei 32 hunden. Schweiz Arch Tierheilkd 143:360-367, 2001.

15. Dupré G, Bouvy B, Prat N: The nature and treatment of perineal hernia-related lesions. A retrospective study of 60 cases, and the definition of the protocol for treatment. Prat Med Chir Anim Comp 28:333-344, 1993.

16. Dupré G, Quéau E, Bouvy B: Use of laparoscopy and laparotomy in the treatment of perineal hernia. *In* Scientific proceedings WSAVA (World Small Animal Veterinary Association) - FECAVA (Federation of European Companion Animal Veterinary Association) World Congress, Amsterdam, 2000.

17. Brissot HN, Dupré GP, Bouvy BM: Use of laparotomy in a staged approach for resolution of bilateral or complicated perineal hernia in 41 dogs. Vet Surg 33:412-421, 2004.

18. Dorn AS, Cartee RE, Richardson DC: A preliminary comparison of perineal hernia in the dog and man. J Am Anim Hosp Assoc 18:624-632, 1982.

19. Desai R: An anatomical study of the canine male and female pelvic diaphragm and the effect of testosterone on the status of levator ani of male dogs. J Am Anim Hosp Assoc 18:195-202, 1982.

20. Dupré G, Dupuy-Dauby L, Bouvy B: The pathology and the surgical treatment of canine prostatic disease. Prat Med Chir Anim Comp 31: 503-514, 1996.

21. Krahwinkel DJ: Rectal diseases and their roles in perineal hernia. Vet Surg 12:160-165, 1983.

22. Guilford WG: Motility disorders of the bowel. *In* Strombeck's Small Animal Gastroenterology, 3rd ed. Guilford WG, Center SA, Strombeck DR, et al (eds). Philadelphia: WB Saunders, 1996, pp. 532-540.

23. Guilford WG: Approach to clinical problems in gastroenterology. In Strombeck's Small Animal Gastroenterology, 3rd ed. Guilford WG, Center SA, Strombeck DR, et al (eds). Philadelphia: WB Saunders, 1996, pp. 50-76

24. Sjollema BE, Venker-van Haagen AJ, Van Suijs FJ, et al: Electromyography of the pelvic diaphragm and anal sphincter in dogs with perineal hernia. Am J Vet Res 54:185, 1993.

25. Lipowitz AJ, et al: Testicular neoplasms and concomitant clinical change in the dog. J Am Vet Med Assoc 163:1364, 1973.

26. Mann FA, Boothe HW, Amoss MS, et al: Serum testosterone and estradiol 17-beta concentration in 15 dogs with perineal hernia. J Am Vet Med Assoc 194:1578-1580, 1989.

27. Mann FA, Nonnemand DJ, Pope ER, et al: Androgen receptors in the pelvic diaphragm muscles of dogs with or without perineal hernia. Am J Vet Res 56:134, 1995.

28. Niebauer GW, et al : Relaxin of prostatic origin might be linked to perineal hernia formation in dogs. Ann NY Acad Sci 1041:415-422, 2005.

29. Bilbrey SA, Smeak DD, DeHoff W: Fixation of the deferent ducts for retrodisplacement of the urinary bladder and prostate in canine perineal hernia. Vet Surg 19:24-27, 1990.

30. Matthiesen DT: Diagnosis and management of complications occurring after perineal herniorraphy in dogs. Comp Contin Educ Pract Vet 11:797-822, 1989.

31. Huber DJ, Seim HB, Goring RL: Cystopexy and colopexy for the management of large or recurrent perineal hernia in the dog: 9 cases (1994 to 1996). Vet.Surg (abstr) 26:253-254, 1997.

32. Chambers JN, Rawlings CA: Applications of semitendinosus muscle flap in two dogs. J Am Vet Med Assoc 199:84-86,1991.

33. Clarke RE: Perineal hernia in the dog: a modified technique of repair. Aust Vet Pract 13:173-174, 1983.

34. Clarke RE: Perineal herniorrhaphy in the dog using polypropylene mesh. Aust Vet Pract 19: 8-14, 1989.

35. Frankland AL: Use of porcine dermal collagen in the repair of perineal hernia in dogs- a preliminary report. Vet Rec 119:13-14, 1986.

36. Stoll MR, Cook JL, Pope ER, et al: The use of porcine small intestinal submucosa as a biomaterial for perineal herniorrhaphy in the dog. Vet Surg 31:379-390, 2002.

37. Bongartz A, Carofiglio F, et al: Use of autogenous fascia lata graft for perineal herniorrhaphy in dogs. ECVS Proceedings 2004; 293.

38. Lorinson D, Grösslinger K: The effect of preoperative anal closure on wound infection rate in perineal hernia surgery. Vet Surg (abstr) 31:301, 2002 .

39. Thompson SE, Hendrickson DA: Minimally invasive hernia repair: Ancillary procedures for perineal hernia. *In* Veterinary Endosurgery. Freeman LJ (ed). St Louis: Mosby, 1998, pp. 110-112.

Chapter 14

Abdominal Hernias

Daniel D. Smeak

An abdominal hernia is a defect or opening in the wall of the abdominal cavity (external abdominal hernia) or within a compartment of the peritoneal space (internal abdominal hernia). Under certain clinical conditions, the defect allows protrusion (herniation) of an abdominal structure. Organs or tissue located in the immediate vicinity are usually found within the defect. However, predicting the organ involved may be difficult because freely movable organs with long vascular pedicles may travel considerable distances to occupy the hernia. It is important to understand that the defect itself may not be the most important clinical problem presenting to the veterinarian for treatment. Instead, it is the cause and effect of vital structure entrapment within the confines of the defect (hernial ring) or concurrent organ damage from trauma, which often dictates whether prompt and aggressive medical or surgical treatment is needed. Frequency and types of complications, success of surgical repair, and ultimately, final outcome are often dependent on the initial condition of the patient and the organ involvement.[1-3] Whether an uncomplicated hernia defect requires surgery depends on the surgeon's estimate of the risk of future organ displacement. The causes of an abdominal hernia should also be determined so proper decisions can be made to help prevent perpetuation of the defect in offspring and to reduce the risk of incisional breakdown (dehiscence) or recurrence.

Hernia Classification and Terminology

Abdominal hernias are described in many ways depending on the nature of the herniation or defect, the location or anatomy of the hernia, the etiology, and most importantly, the condition of the structures protruding through the hernia and the functional alterations resulting from this protrusion.

The abdominal wall is composed of multilaminar arrangements of muscles, their aponeuroses, strong fascia, fat, and either skin or peritoneum. Generally speaking, the abdominal wall functions as a barrier to contain (limit movement) and offer protection for vital abdominal organs. Several normal anatomic openings lined with peritoneum penetrate the external abdominal wall, providing nourishment to the fetus (umbilical aperture), passageway and neurovascular supply for the testicles (inguinal canal), and neurovascular supply to the rear limbs (femoral canal).[4]

"True" hernias are generally formed from a **congenital** (present at birth) weakness or absence of tissues surrounding the normal abdominal apertures. More rarely, true hernias include midline abdominal wall fusion defects. This weakness or lack of a barrier leads to enlargement of the opening (hernial ring) and eventual organ protrusion. True hernias have a complete lining or sac of peritoneum (hernial sac) surrounding the contents. Congenital defects in the ventral midline of the abdominal wall, so called "ventral hernias or substernal hernias," often associated with internal hernias (diaphragmatic), are also considered true hernias because peritoneum usually covers the hernia contents. This slippery peritoneal lining helps reduce adhesion formation of herniated organs or tissue to periabdominal tissue so these hernias are frequently **reducible** (contents freely move from within the hernial sac to the abdomen) and often pose no immediate threat to the patient.

"False" hernias allow protrusion of organs outside the normal apertures of the abdominal wall. False hernias initially do not contain a complete peritoneal sac. Generally, these hernias are **acquired**, caused either by accidental trauma to the abdomen (traumatic hernias) or following breakdown of a surgical approach to the abdomen (incisional hernia). One recent report described a dog with a traumatic abdominal hernia caused by a fractured 12th rib penetrating through the paracostal musculature, resulting in liver herniation; this was termed an **"auto-penetrating hernia."**[5] Owing to the lack of a peritoneal covering, false hernias often lead to development of organ adhesion to surrounding periabdominal tissues causing complications such as **incarceration** (hernial contents become trapped or irreducible). In contrast to true hernias, contents of false hernias are exposed to local tissue inflammation and may sustain constriction of blood supply as the hernial rings contract during healing. When vascular supply to the contents within a true or false hernia is compromised it is said to be **strangulated**, and this is a surgical emergency.

Causes and Pathophysiology

The etiology of a hernia may be from a single obvious defect, such as trauma, or, more commonly, from multiple predisposing factors. Hernias may be the result of either congenital or acquired factors. Congenital defects result when injury or altered development of the fetus occurs as a result of various factors (developmental) or from genetic mechanisms that are transmissible from generation to generation (hereditary). Developmental hernias may be caused by lack or excess of some necessary substance (vitamin, protein) or by a toxin, resulting in abnormal fetal development. As investigation continues into causes of congenital hernias, more and more "developmental" hernias may be found, in some way to be caused by as yet unknown genetic influences. Therefore, until genetic causal factors have been eliminated for specific congenital abdominal hernias, it is prudent for the veterinarian to advise sterilization of affected patients.

Developmental Hernias

Congenital inguinal and umbilical hernias have well explained developmental causes. Male dogs develop congenital inguinal hernias more often than do females.[1] This is believed to be a result of delayed inguinal ring narrowing because of late testicular descent in dogs.[1,6,7] Congenital umbilical hernias result from failure or delayed fusion of the lateral folds (principally tissues forming the rectus abdominis muscle and fascia) at the umbilicus after normal return of the midgut (6th week of gestation) from the umbilical cord in the fetus.[8] Omphalocele congenitalis is a congenital defect formed when loops of intestine are delayed in their transit from the umbilical cord into the abdominal cavity. Gastroschisis is another congenital abnormality appearing similar to omphaloceles, except that the abdominal wall defect is paramedian.[9] Spontaneously occurring femoral and scrotal hernias seen in adult dogs are thought to be caused by an underlying congenital weakness of the musculofascial tissues surrounding the respective abdominal apertures. Factors such as trauma and increased intraabdominal pressure, from obesity or chronic straining from constipation for example, may then trigger hernia occurrence later in life.[3]

Hernias are often found in patients with other congenital defects. Cranioventral abdominal hernias, incomplete caudal sternal fusion, and umbilical defects with concomitant diaphragmatic hernias of various types have been described in puppies.[10] Successive breedings of a Laborador retriever and American foxhound with these defects created ratios of affected offspring suggesting an autosomal recessive mechanism.[11] Another investigation describing diaphragmatic, cardiac, and abdominal wall defects in a litter of cocker spaniel dogs, similar to thoracoabdominal ectopic cordis syndrome, however, suggested a developmental cause.[12] Cardiac malposition in humans may cause a mesodermal defect resulting in partial or complete failure of septum transversum development and subsequent supraumbilical fusion failure.[8,13] Congenital heart defects and portosystemic shunts may be associated with supraumbilical defects.[14] Defects associated with caudal ventral midline (infraumbilical) hernias include exstrophy of the bladder, hypospadius, and imperforate anus.[8,15] In addition, dogs with umbilical hernias often have cryptorchidism as well as other congenital defects.[16,17] These findings confirm the need to examine patients with congenital hernias closely for other important developmental problems before attempting surgical repair.[2]

Heritable Hernias

Many congenital umbilical and inguinal hernias are thought to be caused by hereditary influences. Heritable inguinal hernias have only been documented, however, in the golden retriever, cocker spaniel, and dachshund.[18] In man, persistence of the process vaginalis (opening into the evaginated peritoneum surrounding the testicle) and enlarged inguinal rings have a similar familial tendency. Although most umbilical hernias appear to be inherited, no definitive information has been presented regarding the mode or pattern of inheritance affecting the fibrosis and union of the abdominal aponeuroses. Results of one study indicated that this defect is probably the result of a polygenic threshold character, possibly involving a major gene whose expression is mediated by the breed background.[19,20] Umbilical hernias have also been associated with fucosidiosis, an inherited neurovisceral lysosomal storage disease. Of 31 English springer spaniels diagnosed with fucosidiosis, 10 had umbilical hernias and 1 had a scrotal hernia. This disease is believed to be inherited in an autosomal recessive manner.[21] Neutering should be recommended for all small animals with congenital inguinal or umbilical hernias until conclusive evidence is demonstrated regarding the heritable nature of this disease process.[6]

Hernias Caused by Metabolic and Hormonal Imbalance

Certain pathophysiologic conditions predispose to acquired abdominal herniation. Inguinal hernias are most commonly seen in older intact female dogs.[1] These hernias occur as a result of multiple factors including obesity, decreased connective tissue strength, and increased intraabdominal pressure. Obesity causes increased intraabdominal pressure, forcing fat through abdominal wall apertures and further dilating the hernial rings.[22] Onset of hernia occurrence is often associated with estrus or pregnancy, suggesting hormonal imbalance as a contributing cause.[23] Estrogen production is considered to have a close relationship with development of inguinal hernias. Sex hormones may change the strength or character of the connective tissue, weakening or enlarging the inguinal rings.[24] Experimentally, sex hormone imbalance has been directly linked to formation of inguinal hernia in male and female mice.[25] Ovariohysterectomy, therefore, is recommended to reduce the incidence of acquired inguinal hernias; this procedure may help to prevent recurrence following repair. Supporting structures of the abdominal wall may also become weak or stretch owing to nutritional or metabolic problems (for example, hyperadrenocortism or diabetes mellitus). Accumulation of fat around the round ligament may dilate the vaginal processes and inguinal canal, allowing herniation.[26] Maintenance of normal body weight and eliminating hormonal or metabolic disturbances should help reduce the incidence of acquired nontraumatic abdominal hernias.

Traumatic Hernias

It has been proposed that the contents of acute traumatic hernias may be more prone to adhesion formation to extra abdominal structures and to incarceration because such hernias lack a complete serosa lined hernial sac. Traumatic hernias may undergo organ strangulation owing to swelling caused by acute inflammation or from hernial ring contraction during healing.[22] However, adhesion formation, incarceration, and strangulation have not been found to be common sequelae of traumatic hernias in retrospective studies. The important cause of organ damage may be from the trauma itself, rather than from the hernia. None of the contents of 21 traumatic hernias in one retrospective study demonstrated any evidence of vascular obstruction from incarceration during abdominal exploration; although 2 dogs had evidence of traumatic intestinal devitalization.[27] One dog developed organ compromise as a result of mesenteric avulsion in a recent report of 36 traumatic body wall hernias in dogs and cats.[5]

Most abdominal hernias are caused by blunt trauma (automobile accidents, kicks, falls). Of 21 consecutively studied traumatic abdominal hernias, 17 were caused by blunt trauma (automobile accident) and 4 by penetrating trauma (dog fight).[27] Hernias can occur in a variety of locations, often dictated by the mode of trauma.[22,28] The most common areas of herniation caused by blunt trauma in one study were in the ventrolateral caudal abdominal (inguinal or prepubic areas) and paracostal regions.[27] In a more recent study, 28 of 36 dogs and cats with abdominal hernias were caused by bite wounds.[5] The lateral paralumbar site was the most common hernia location in dogs in Shaw's study,[5] whereas the ventral body wall and femoral sites were more common in cats. All pubic ligament ruptures in this study were caused by vehicular trauma.

Hernia location depends on various factors, including the local direction of the traumatic force and intraabdominal pressure changes. Blunt trauma, applied while abdominal muscles are contracted but the glottis is open, thus limiting increase in intraabdominal pressure, may result in traction or avulsion type injury to tissues with minimal elasticity (muscle attachments to bone).[22,27] Common hernias resulting from avulsion forces are the prepubic (ruptured cranial pubic ligament), inguinal, and dorsolateral hernias (muscle avulsion from transverse processes of lumbar vertebrae termed paralumbar or lateral hernias).[27,29] Rupture of the cranial pubic ligament is often associated with concurrent inguinal ligament damage (a traumatic femoral or inguinal hernia may result). A sudden increase in intraabdominal pressure may cause rupture in the weakest area of the abdominal wall. Paracostal hernias occur when the origin of the external oblique abdominal and transverse abdominal muscles avulse from their rib or costal cartilage origin, or they are caused by a broken rib lacerating adjacent musculature (autopenetrating hernia).[5] Abdominal viscera herniate laterally into the subcutaneous tissues in paracostal and paralumbar hernias. Paracostal hernias frequently occur with diaphragmatic rupture, presumably as a result of similar initiating forces. Direct local trauma caused by a blunt object (shoe, fence post) results in separation (tearing) of the wall at the location of impact.[30]

Blunt trauma may cause widespread crush, rupture, or avulsion damage to intraabdominal organs. Up to 75% of traumatized small animal patients with abdominal hernias have other significant injuries; most are orthopedic and usually involve the pelvis. In decreasing order of frequency, the respiratory, gastrointestinal, and genitourinary systems are also injured.[27] In a recent study, over 50% of patients with traumatic hernias suffered injury to other structures. One quarter had more than one associated injury. One third of the hernias had associated body cavity injuries including diaphragmatic hernia, kidney avulsion, bladder rupture, and mesenteric avulsion. In addition, 9 of 36 animals had concurrent orthopedic injuries.[5] A thorough examination of patients with traumatic hernias is imperative to assess for significant associated injuries.

Abdominal hernias may rarely occur through a fracture defect (sacroiliac luxation, pubic or symphyseal fracture).[31,32] In addition to the fracture, severe damage to underlying soft tissue structures, such as ligaments and mesenteric attachments, is required to allow organ herniation.[28] Traumatic body wall hernias may also result from shearing forces that are distributed over boney projections of the pelvis or caudal thorax rib cage. These forces result in the tearing of muscles or tendons from their boney attachments.[33]

Sharp trauma (bite wounds, gunshot, knife stabs) may cause herniation anywhere in the abdominal wall. Animal fight wounds are more apt to cause multiple hernias located in the dorsal or lateral abdominal wall.[5,27] Tears, perforation, and laceration of intraabdominal structures occur frequently with sharp trauma. Shaw reported that nearly 25% of animals with perforating abdominal wall trauma had evidence of intestinal damage requiring resection and anastomosis.[5] Therefore, patients with penetrating abdominal trauma and herniation should undergo emergency abdominal exploration after stabilization.[34,35]

Incisional Hernias

Incisional hernia incidence is reported to be between 1% and 11% in humans, and is as great as 16% in large animals, depending on the surgical approach to the abdomen, predisposing factors, and overall status of the patient.[36,37,38] Incisional hernia in small animals is less common. Sequelae to incisional hernia often are extremely serious and costly (e.g., total abdominal wound dehiscence in humans is associated with a 15 to 20% mortality rate).[24,39]

Predisposing causes of acute and chronic incisional hernia vary, appear interrelated, and occur at different times after surgery. Acute incisional hernias generally occur within the first 7 days after surgery, whereas chronic hernias are noted weeks to years postoperatively. Reported risk factors for acute incisional hernia include increased intraabdominal pressure because of pain, entrapped fat between hernia edges, inappropriate suture material use, infection, chronic steroid treatment, and poor postoperative care.[40] Technical error in surgery is the most common cause of **acute** wound disruption.[3,39] Factors associated with **chronic** incisional hernia in humans include obesity, hypoproteinemia, cardiopulmonary complications, abdominal distention, skin wound dehiscence, and deep fascial infection. Local wound complications, especially deep infection, are considered the most important predisposing causes of chronic incisional hernias.[37,41]

Incisional hernias result from either excessive forces acting on the abdominal incision or poor holding strength of the sutured wound.

Excessive Forces on the Incision

Forces disrupting the abdominal incision are mainly derived from excessive intraabdominal pressure or muscle tension. Experimentally created abdominal wounds healing under increased tension were less resistant to rupturing compared with wounds under normal tension, at 15 days.[42] Vigorous uncontrolled activity or violent coughing or straining postoperatively certainly predispose to wound breakdown. Increased intraabdominal pressure is observed in such conditions as obesity, abdominal effusions, pregnancy, or organ distention because of ileus or obstruction; all these problems increase incisional hernia risk.[39,42]

The gravity dependent ventral midline and paramedian approaches pose a greater risk for incisional herniation. Experimentally created transverse abdominal incisions in rabbits offer better security against dehiscence than ventral midline incisions because the suture/tissue interface is stronger in this area.[42] "Grid incisions" or those that involve muscle splitting, such as the flank approach, may be less susceptible to incisional hernia because wound edges are drawn together with muscle contraction.

Poor Holding Strength of the Wound

The choice of suture material for abdominal closure is rarely the sole cause of incisional hernia, provided the appropriate size is used.[39,42] Choice of suture type may be critical in patients that have prolonged wound healing or are severely catabolic and when wound infection is present, particularly when an unpredictable, rapidly absorbable suture such as chromic gut is used.[39]

A tied suture is only as strong as its knot. The nature of disruptive forces produced by normal physical activity applied to sutures and their knots remains unknown. An *in vitro* knot testing study found that suture materials placed in an interrupted pattern, except polydioxanone and monofilament nylon, were secure with three square throws. Square knots used to begin or end a continuous pattern require an additional one or two square throws, respectively, to be secure. Granny knots, loose asymmetrical square knots, and loosely tied square knots were not as secure as snug square knots for most suture materials tested.[43]

Whether suture is placed in an interrupted or continuous pattern or the abdomen is closed in a single or double layer has little significance in incisional hernia formation, provided the strength holding layer is incorporated.[42,43,44] Of 52 human patients with acute incisional hernia, 88% of the disruptions contained intact sutures that had pulled through tissue, whereas only 12% had broken sutures. The problem with most of the closures was inclusion of too little rather than too much tissue.[39] The holding power of abdominal wounds closed in a single layer was stronger than that of double layer closures in one experimental study involving rabbits.[42] Interrupted suture patterns are the more secure choice in situations where wound edges have questionable viability or strength or if other predisposing incisional hernia factors are present.

Successful, lasting abdominal wall closures must include the external rectus fascia. Identifying this layer before attempting closure is critical. Sutures should incorporate at least 5 mm of healthy fascia to ensure adequate anchorage.

Prevention of incisional dehiscence is best afforded by preventing excessive continual intraabdominal pressure (reducing coughing, straining) or abdominal distention, and preventing local wound complications (infection, seroma). Necrosis within a suture loop caused by excessive tightening should be prevented. Meticulous surgical technique placing sutures in strong tissue with adequate tissue bites using proper knot tying will reduce the incidence/occurrence/development of most acute wound dehiscences.

Causes of Hernia Recurrence

Overall, abdominal hernia recurrence appears to be much less frequent in small animals compared with humans. Abdominal hernia repair breakdown in humans ranges from less than 1% to 20%, depending on the cause and type of hernia and patient variables. Most hernia recurrences stem from infection, extreme tension on the repair, incorporating tissues with poor strength in the repair, poor anatomic reconstruction, or more obvious technical failure such as inappropriate suture type or size. Overall, it appears that the choice of suture material is less important than the technique and placement of sutures for prevention of hernia recurrence. The prime etiologic factor in late hernia recurrence is tension on the suture line, which is the cause of suture or tissue disruption. Increased intraabdominal pressure from vomiting, coughing, or straining to urinate or defecate greatly increases the risk of dehiscence. Severe obesity triples the risk of hernia recurrence in humans owing to increased intraabdominal pressure.[3]

High sac ligation to help reduce hernia recurrence, popularized by Marcy in some of the earliest reports of successful hernia repair, was until recently a universally accepted goal of hernia repair technique.[45] It is now known that the peritoneum lining the hernia sac is relatively weak and regenerates rapidly. Healing of large serosal defects is usually complete in less than one week.[46] Clinical and experimental studies have shown that the risk of incisional disruption is no greater if the peritoneum is not sutured at laparotomy or herniorrhaphy. Because of these findings, many surgeons now believe that high hernial sac ligation does not prevent recurrence, provided the other aspects of the repair are properly performed.[47] Suturing the peritoneum may cause deleterious effects such as local ischemia, delayed healing, increased postoperative pain, and adhesion formation.[48]

When a hernia recurs many times, it is unwise to always assume that the prior surgeon and surgical procedure were inadequate. Underlying tissue weakness may be responsible for the failure. In one recent experimental study, progressive fascial wound failure decreased the fidelity of subsequent incisional hernia repair, compared with identically sized acute abdominal wall defect repairs. The mechanism appears to include decreased fascial wound strength and decreased tissue compliance after herniorrhaphy.[49] Mesh reconstruction of these complicated recurrent hernias is now routinely recommended in humans because defects of any size can be repaired without tension. In addition, polypropylene mesh sets up a scaffolding that, in turn, induces the synthesis of collagen.[50] A biologic approach to combat acute wound failure is gaining more attention in human surgery. Treatment of experimentally created abdominal fascial incisions with growth factors in one study prevented development of incisional hernias in the rat model. TGF-beta stimulated fascial macrophage and fibroblast chemotaxis as well as collagen production.[51]

Sequelae to Organ Herniation and Trauma

Most abdominal wall defects can be reconstructed easily and successfully if the previously described surgical principles are observed. The overall success of a hernial repair (and often the prognosis for the patient), however, relies heavily on how the surgeon manages the sequelae to organ herniation or internal damage from trauma, which tend to impair normal body function. The severity of the functional alteration depends on the cause, location, and content of the hernia. Important, often life-threatening sequelae can be attributed to space-occupying effects or the condition termed "loss of domain," incarceration, or strangulation. The condition of the animal at presentation, concurrent injuries to distant structures, as well as organ compromise owing to the trauma must also be factored when attempting to predict patient outcome.[5]

Space-Occupying Effects

"Loss of domain" occurs when the abdominal cavity has become accustomed to a small intraabdominal volume so reduction of the hernia contents and primary closure of the defect are impossible. This is most commonly associated with closure of large chronic hernias. Repair of the abdominal wall and forcing the herniated contents back into the abdomen often result in excessive tension on the repair (increasing recurrence risk). Even more deleterious are acute pulmonary complications (caused by restriction of diaphragm function) and poor organ perfusion. High intraabdominal pressure has been documented in a series of client-owned dogs undergoing abdominal surgery, necessitating surgical decompression; one case was following hernia repair.[52]

Several techniques have been employed in human patients to reduce this "loss of domain" complication, using a tissue expansion principle.[53,54] Progressive pneumoperitoneum and tissue expansion using inflatable silastic expanders function to gradually expand the abdominal wall in much the same way that pregnancy does. Staged reduction of open congenital abdominal defects with a silastic sac has achieved excellent results with little mortality in infants. Most adult human patients with "loss of domain" are repaired using prosthetic materials to help span the defect to avoid tension and hernia recurrence, as well as postoperative complications.[54,55]

Other examples of space-occupying effects occur when organs herniate into the pleural or pericardial spaces. The negative pressure in the pleural space tends to draw abdominal organs into the chest. Organs herniating into the chest or pericardial sac reduce lung expansion and cardiac function, respectively, creating problems with patient management particularly at anesthetic induction. Severity of compromise depends on the volume and rate of expansion of the space-occupying herniated tissue. For example, a herniated liver lobe, spleen, or omentum rarely causes major problems for the patient unless strangulation occurs, so most are surgically repaired on an elective basis. A rapidly expanding herniated stomach, on the other hand, causes severe progressive respiratory distress and is a surgical emergency.

Incarceration

Incarceration of organs such as the intestine, uterus, or bladder most often alters normal function because of luminal obstruction. Incarcerated organs are irreducible and can become (within hours) lethal strangulated obstructions. The severity and onset of the clinical signs related to the incarcerated obstruction often depends on the contents of the hernia and size of the defect. Abdominal defects with small-sized, rather inelastic hernial rings, such as scrotal or femoral hernias, are at high risk for incarceration and strangulation.[1]

Incarceration of the uterus is often associated with inguinal hernias or large umbilical hernias. An irreducible viable, nongravid uterus within a hernia rarely causes clinical problems, however, incarceration of a pyometra or gravid uterus may lead to severe systemic alterations. Toxemia, resulting from obstructed drainage of an infected uterus or from uterine rupture, and dystocia are sequelae of uterine incarceration. Emergency surgical resection of the diseased uterus or caesarian section is given first priority following aggressive patient stabilization with appropriate fluid and antibiotic therapy. Surgical repair of the hernia is attempted only if the patient's vital parameters are stable following uterine surgery; otherwise repair is performed under more controlled conditions.

Small intestine may become incarcerated within any hernia, but it is my clinical impression that the risk is greatest when the hernial ring approximates the size of the bowel. Smaller hernias rarely allow intestinal protrusion. Larger hernias rarely trap or obstruct bowel unless they are caused by acute trauma or the entrapped intestines undergo torsion. Intermittent intestinal dysfunction may occur, however, even if intestines are reducible within the hernia. Once signs of intestinal obstruction occur (acute abdominal pain, vomiting, depression, anorexia) early intestinal decompression is warranted. Electrolyte, acid-base, and body fluid imbalances associated with the particular level of intestinal obstruction are corrected without delay before surgery. Adhesions, if present, are broken down and an incision is made in the hernial ring to help reduce the intestines and relieve the obstruction.

The urinary bladder may become obstructed in incarcerated perineal, ventral, inguinal, and traumatic pubic hernias. As urine flow becomes partially obstructed within the hernia, the bladder progressively distends, further obstructing outflow. Complete obstruction causes severe metabolic consequences such as azotemia, hyperkalemia, and metabolic acidosis, and eventually causes bladder-wall necrosis. Death results within 2 to 3 days if the obstruction is not relieved. Immediate bladder decompression and diversion of urine flow via needle cystocentesis, catheterization, or tube cystostomy are imperative. Diuresis is established with appropriate intravenous fluids following bladder decompression. If kidney function is not impaired, azotemia and electrolyte abnormalities usually normalize within 24 hours, after which surgical reduction of the bladder and hernia repair are attempted.

Strangulation

A strangulated hernia implies that the hernial contents are incarcerated and undergoing devitalization from arrested circulation. The arrested circulation may be from venous or arterial occlusion, or from a combination of the two. Early venous obstruction results in reversible organ engorgement, but eventually arterial stagnation occurs from back pressure at the capillary beds. Arterial stagnation or obstruction causes rapid organ necrosis if collateral blood supply is insufficient, resulting in organ rupture. Generally, venous obstruction occurs early in most strangulated hernias, but by the time surgical decompression is attempted, irreversible arterial stagnation has occurred.

Strangulation occurs from several mechanisms such as constriction of the blood supply at the hernial rings or from allowing organs more freedom of movement, resulting in torsion of a vascular pedicle. Organs with long, freely movable vascular pedicles (e.g., uterus, omentum, spleen, intestine, testicle) are more prone to torsion. Incarceration of a hollow viscus organ favors strangulation because increasing intraluminal pressure further obstructs venous outflow from the organ and opposes circulatory pressure. Traumatic hernias are more prone to incarceration and strangulation because organs are held within the hernia by adhesions, and the hernia ring eventually narrows from contraction during wound healing. Pleural effusions resulting from entrapped, compromised liver lobes in chronic diaphragmatic hernias are an example of this process. Decompression of ascites in humans with reducible umbilical hernias may result in rapid incarceration and strangulation. Decompression apparently reduces tension on the hernial margins, acutely narrowing the defect.

The threat of complication and death is 50% higher in human patients with incarcerated or strangulated hernias versus hernias containing reducible viable tissue. Early diagnosis and surgical correction of incarcerated hernias, therefore, is critical to prevent life-threatening sequelae relating to organ devitalization. Sequelae of hernia strangulation vary, depending on the organ involved and chronicity. Strangulated umbilical, inguinal, femoral, and prepubic hernia most often contain falciform ligament or omentum, uterus, prostatic fat, and urinary bladder, respectively.[12] The clinical course is affected by the degree of vascular compromise, volume of body fluids lost from obstruction or sequestration, and absorption of bacteria and toxins. Strangulated contaminated hollow viscus organs may result in significant blood, protein, and fluid loss, and often rupture, causing toxemia and septicemia. Bacteria migrate transmurally through devitalized intestine even before evidence of gross spillage occurs.[56] Before overt signs of infection or contamination occur, vasoactive substances such as arachadonic acid metabolites (cytokines, leukotrienes, kinins) from tissue and blood cell autolysis cause redistribution of body fluids and severe cardiopulmonary effects.[57]

Strangulated viscera within external abdominal hernias (when compared with intraabdominal strangulated viscera) are more isolated from the vascular system. Liberated vasoactive substances are not absorbed as quickly through the subcutanous tissue as the permeable peritoneal lining, and thus, external strangulated hernias may have a more delayed onset of clinical signs and shock. Initial management of patients with strangulated hernias include aggressive restoration of tissue perfusion, pain management, acid-base, and electrolyte balance, appropriate antimicrobial and shock therapy if infection and toxemia are present, and lastly, emergency surgical correction. Ventral midline celiotomy is the preferred approach to most strangulated hernias because it allows complete abdominal exploration, and the affected organ can be isolated with surgical towels to avoid further soilage of the peritoneum. Manual reduction of strangulated organs should not be attempted. Severely compromised patients often decompensate and die under anesthesia during attempts at surgical reduction and repair of strangulated hernias; this is thought to be caused by rapid release of vasoactive substances into the circulation from necrotic strangulated organs during surgical reduction. *En bloc* resection of the herniated devitalized tissue, releasing the constricting ring only after the vascular supply is occluded, may help reduce this fatal complication.[2]

Conclusion

Successful management of an abdominal hernia not only requires observation of sound surgical principles (anatomic closure of the defect without tension, incorporating strong tissue with meticulous technique) but a solid understanding of the disease mechanisms reviewed in this chapter. Attempts at hernia repair without searching and correcting for the underlying cause or the pathophysiologic consequences or effects associated with organ herniation often lead to hernia recurrence, severe postoperative complications, or death.[58]

References

1. Waters DJ, Roy RG, Stone EA: A retrospective study of inguinal hernia in 35 dogs. Vet Surg 22:44, 1993.

2. Smeak DD: Abdominal hernias. *In* Textbook of Small Animal Surgery. Slatter D (ed). Philadelphia: WB Saunders, 2003, p. 449.

3. Ponka JK: Herniation of the Abdominal Wall. Philadelphia: WB Saunders, 1980.

4. Evans HH: Millers Anatomy of the Dog. Philadelphia: WB Saunders, 1993.

5. Shaw SP, Rozanski EA, Rush JE: Traumatic body wall herniation in 36 dogs and cats. J Am Anim Hosp Assoc 39:35, 2003.

6. Fox MW: Inherited inguinal hernia and midline defects in the dog. J Am Vet Med Assoc 143:602, 1963.

7. Hobday FTG: Castration (Including Cryptorchidism and Caponing) and Ovariohysterectomy. London: Johnston, 1914.

8. Klein MD, Hertzler JH: Congenital defects of the abdominal wall. Surg Gynecol Obstet 152:805, 1981.

9. Nyberg DA, Mack LA: Abdominal wall defects. *In* Diagnostic Ultrasound of Fetal Anomalies. Nyberg DA, Mahony BS, Pretorias DH (eds). Chicago: Year Book Medical Publishers, 1990, pp. 395-432.

10. Nicholson C: Defective diaphragm associated with umbilical hernia. Vet Rec 98:433, 1976.

11. Feldman DB, Bree MM, Cohen BJ: Congenital diaphragmatic hernia in neonatal dogs. J Am Vet Med Assoc 153:942, 1968.

12. Bellah JR, Whitton DL, Ellison GW, Phillips L: Surgical correction of concomitant cranioventral abdominal wall, caudal sternal, diaphragmatic, and pericardial defects in young dogs. J Am Vet Med Assoc 195:1722, 1989.

13. Dobell AR, Williams HB, Long RW: Staged repair of ectopia cordis. J Ped Surg 17: 353, 1983.

14. Crowe DT, Archibald J: Abdominal wall and cavity. *In* Canine and Feline Surgery. Archibald J, Catcott EJ (eds).. Santa Barbara: American Veterinary Publishers, 1984, p. 23.

15. Sawyer SL: Defective diaphragm associated with umbilical hernia. Vet Rec 98: 490, 1976.

16. Bellenger CR: Inguinal and scrotal herniation in 61 dogs. Aust Vet Pract 26:58, 1996.

17. Pendergrass T W, Hayes HM: Cryptorchism and related defects in dogs: epidemiologic comparisons with man. Teratology 12:51, 1975.

18. Larsen RE, Dias E, Flores G, Selden JR: Breeding studies reveal segregation of a canine Robertsonian translocation along Mendelian proportions. Cytogenet Cell Genet 24:95, 1979.

19. Hayes HM: Congenital umbilical and inguinal hernias in cattle, horses, swine, dogs, and cats: Risk by breed and sex among hospital patients. Am J Vet Res 35:839, 1974.

20. Robinson R: Genetic aspects of umbilical hernia incidence in cats and dogs. Vet Rec 100:9, 1977.

21. Taylor RM: Canine fucosidosis: Clinical findings. J Small Anim Pract 28:291, 1987.

22. Parks J: Herniation. *In* Pathophysiology in Small Animal Surgery. Bojrab MJ (ed). Philadelphia: Lea & Febiger, p. 1981.

23. Strande A: Inguinal hernia in dogs. J Small Anim Pract 30:520, 1989.

24. Peacock EE, van Winkle W: Wound dehiscence. *In* Wound Repair. Peacock EE, van Winkle W (eds). Philadelphia: WB Saunders, 1976, p. 466.

25. Hazary S, Gardener WV: The influence of sex hormones on abdominal musculature and the formation of inguinal and scrotal hernias in mice. Anat Rec 136:437, 1960.

26. Ashdown RR: The anatomy of the inguinal canal in domestic mammals. Vet Rec 75:1345, 1963.

27. Waldron DR, Hedlund CS, Pechman R: Abdominal hernias in dogs and cats: A review of 24 cases. J Am Anim Hosp Assoc 22: 817, 1986.

28. Read R: Cranial abdominal hernias. *In* Textbook of Small Animal Surgery. Slatter D (ed). Philadelphia: WB Saunders, 1985, p. 853.

29. Greene JA: Lateral abdominal hernia repair in a cat. Feline Pract 8:23, 1978.

30. Dubois PM, Freeman JB: Traumatic abdominal wall hernia. J Trauma 21:72, 1981.

31. Dorn AS, Olmstead ML: Herniation of the urinary bladder through the public symphysis in a dog. J Am Vet Med Assoc 168:688, 1976.

32. Mann FA: Cranial pubic ligament rupture in dogs and cats. J Am Anim Hosp Assoc 22:519, 1986.

33. Damschen DD, Landercasper J, Thomas CH, Randall ST: Acute traumatic abdominal hernia: case reports. J Traum 36:273, 1994.

34. Bjorling DE, Crowe DT, Kolata RJ, Rawlings CA: Penetrating abdominal wounds in dogs and cats. J Am Anim Hosp Assoc 18:742, 1982.

35. Crowe DT: Dealing with visceral injuries of the cranial abdomen. Vet Med 83:682, 1988.

36. Akman PC: A study of five hundred incisional hernias. J Int Coll Surg 37:125, 1962.

37. George CD, Ellis H: The results of incisional hernia repair: A twelve year review. Ann R Coll Surg Engl 68:185, 1986.

38. Gibson KT, Curtis CR, Turner AS, et al: Incisional hernias in the horse. Incidence and predisposing factors. Vet Surg 18:360, 1989.

39. Alexander HC, Prudden JF: The causes of abdominal wound disruption. Surg Gynecol Obstet 122:1223, 1966.

40. Larson GM, Vandertoll DJ: Approaches to repair of ventral hernia and full-thickness losses to the abdominal wall. Symposium of hernias. Surg Clin North Am 64:335, 1984.

41. Fisher GD, Turner FW: Abdominal incisional hernias: a ten year review. Can J Surg 17:202, 1974.

42. Nilsson T: Abdominal wound repair: An experimental study of the wound healing mechanism in the rabbit. Dan Med Bull 30:394, 1983.

43. Rosin E, Robinson GM: Knot security of suture materials. Vet Surg 18:269, 1989.

44. Crowe DT: Closure of abdominal incisions using a continuous polypropylene suture: Clinical experience in 550 dogs and cats. Vet Surg 7:74, 1978.

45. Marcy HO: The Cure of Inguinal Hernia in the Male. Norwalk, Ohio, 1897.

46. Ellis H: Wound repair: Reaction of the peritoneum to injury. Ann R Coll Surg Engl 60:219, 1978.

47. Ellis H, Heddle R: Does the peritoneum need to be closed at laparotomy? Br J Surg 64:733, 1977.

48. Parulkar BG, Supe AN, Vora IM, Mathur SK: Effects of experimental non-closure of peritoneum on development of suture line adhesions and wound strength in dogs. Ind J Gastroenterol 5:251, 1986.

49. DuBay DA, Wang X, Adamson B, et al: Progressive fascial wound failure impairs subsequent abdominal wall repairs: a new animal model of incisional hernia formation. Surg 137:463, 2005.

50. Luijendijk RW, Hop WC, van den Tol MP, et al: A comparison of suture repair with mesh repair for incisional hernia. N Engl J Med 343:392, 2000.

51. Franz MG, Kuhn MA, Nguyen K, et al: Transforming growth factor beta(2) lowers incidence of incisional hernias. J Surg Res 97:109, 2001

52. Conzemius MG, Sammarco JL, Holt DE, Smith GK: Clinical determination of preoperative and postoperative intra-abdominal pressures in dogs. Vet Surg 24:195, 1995.

53. Boyd JB: Tissue expansion in reconstruction. South Med J, 80:430, 1987.

54. Carlson GW, Elwood E, Losken A, Galloway JR: The role of tissue expansion in abdominal wall reconstruction. Ann Plast Surg 44:147, 2000.

55. Kingsnorth AN, Sivarajasingham N, Wong S, Butler M: Open mesh repair of incisional hernias with significant loss of domain. Ann R Coll Surg Engl 86:363, 2004.

56. Bellhorn T, Macintire DK: Bacterial translocation. Comp Contin Educ Pract Vet 26:229, 2004.

57. Brady CA, Otto CM: Systemic inflammatory response syndrome, sepsis, and multiple organ dysfunction. Vet Clin North Am Small Anim Pract 31:1147, 2001.

58. Smeak DD: Management and prevention of surgical complications associated with small animal abdominal herniorrhaphy. Gastrointest Surg Complications. Probl Vet Med 1:254, 1989.

Chapter 15

Diaphragmatic Hernia

Geraldine B. Hunt

Anatomy

The diaphragm separates the abdominal and thoracic cavities and assists in ventilation. The muscular costal, sternal, and lumbar parts of the diaphragm surround a strong central tendon.[1] The costal and sternal muscles insert on the abaxial border of the central tendon, and the lumbar muscles insert on its axial border. The central tendon is approximately Y shaped, with each arm of the Y extending dorsally from the central region up to the 13th rib. The paired lumbar muscles form the diaphragmatic crura. The right crus is larger than the left. Each crus has a bifurcate tendon arising from the bodies of the third and fourth lumbar vertebrae, medial to the psoas minor muscles. The sternal muscle is unpaired and is continuous with the left and right costal muscles. It originates from the xiphoid cartilage, transverse fascia, and the eighth costal cartilages and extends forward to insert dorsally on the body of the central tendon.

The aorta, azygos and hemiazygos veins, and lumbar cistern of the thoracic duct pass through the aortic hiatus.

The thoracic surface of the diaphragm is adjacent to the lungs and is covered by endothelial fascia and pleura, the pleura being continuous with that of the mediastinum. The mediastinal attachment to the diaphragm is median dorsal to the esophagus. Ventral to the esophagus it deflects to the left in a wide semicircle across the left diaphragmatic costal muscles and returns to the midline at the sternum. A pleural reflection (plica vena cava), caudal to the heart around the caudal vena cava, is attached to the diaphragm on the right side. The plica vena cava and the mediastinum form a pouch cranial to the diaphragmatic central tendon that is occupied by the accessory lung lobe. Organs involved in diaphragmatic hernias may occasionally occupy this pouch, rather than the main part of the thoracic cavity. Motor innervation to the diaphragm is by the phrenic nerves.[1,2]

Embryology

Embryogenesis of the diaphragm is complex. The transverse septum is the initial incomplete partition between the pericardial and peritoneal cavities. This septum becomes the central tendon of the diaphragm. The dorsal mesentery of the esophagus develops simultaneously with the transverse septum and produces the median portion of the diaphragm. In adults, this mesentery forms the diaphragmatic crura, including the esophageal hiatus and aortic hiatus. The pleuroperitoneal folds develop along the lateral body walls and migrate medially, where they close the pleuroperitoneal canals by fusion with the esophageal mesentery and dorsal portion of the transverse septum, thereby completing the diaphragmatic partition. Finally, as the pleural cavities enlarge, myoblasts from the body wall invade the peripheral border of the diaphragm to form the costal muscles. Failure of development or fusion of any of the aforementioned structures may lead to formation of a pleuroperitoneal or peritoneopericardial hernia.[3]

Physiology

The diaphragm contracts during inspiration, pushing caudally on the viscera and displacing the abdominal wall outward.[4,5] At the same time, contraction of the diaphragmatic costal muscles expands the caudal thorax. The diaphragm plays a critical role in the maintenance of negative intrapleural pressure by resisting movement of abdominal viscera into the thorax during inspiration.

Types of Hernias

True diaphragmatic hernias are rare with the exception of hiatal hernias. Herniated viscera in false diaphragmatic hernias (traumatic or congenital) are not contained within a sac but lie free within the pleural cavity or pericardial sac. With peritoneopericardial hernias, the peritoneum is continuous with the visceral layer of the pericardium.

Traumatic Diaphragmatic Hernia

Following trauma, the diaphragmatic costal muscles are more often disrupted than the central tendon, whereas the stronger crural muscles are seldom damaged.[6] Despite early claims to the contrary, left to right distribution is probably uniform in dogs and cats, with sporadic cases having bilateral or multiple tears.[6-10] Tears are oriented circumferentially in about 40% of dogs, radially in 40%, or both in 20%. Cats had a preponderance of circumferential tears (59%) and fewer radial tears (18%) in one report.[9] In another series, tears were left-sided in 44% of cats, right-sided in 38%, ventral in 15%, and multiple in only 1 cat (23%).[8] In humans, the liver protects the right side of the diaphragm, and left-sided rupture of the tendon is 8 times more frequent than right-sided rupture.[11] In dogs and cats, the liver contacts both sides of the diaphragm and its protective effect is not as marked. The liver is found in the thoracic cavity in over 80% of cases with diaphragmatic hernia.[6] The small intestine, stomach, spleen, omentum, pancreas, colon, cecum, and uterus may be involved, in descending order of frequency. Herniation of a gravid uterus has been reported in a dog.[12] Herniation of a kidney, leading to urothorax has been reported in a cat.[13] Which organs occupy a hernia depend on various factors, including the site of the diaphragmatic tear, proximity of the organs, and range of movement of supporting ligaments or mesentery. The liver, small intestine, and pancreas tend to herniate through right-sided tears, whereas the stomach, spleen, and small intestine more commonly herniate through left-sided tears (Figures 15-1 and 15-2).

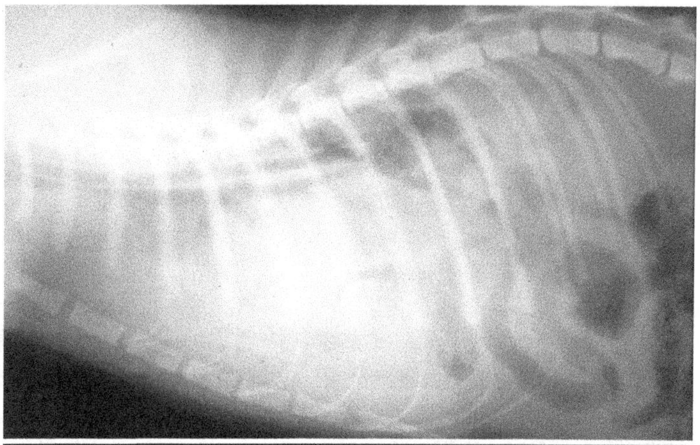

Figure 15-1. Lateral radiograph from a 9-year-old male neutered cat with a chronic diaphragmatic hernia.

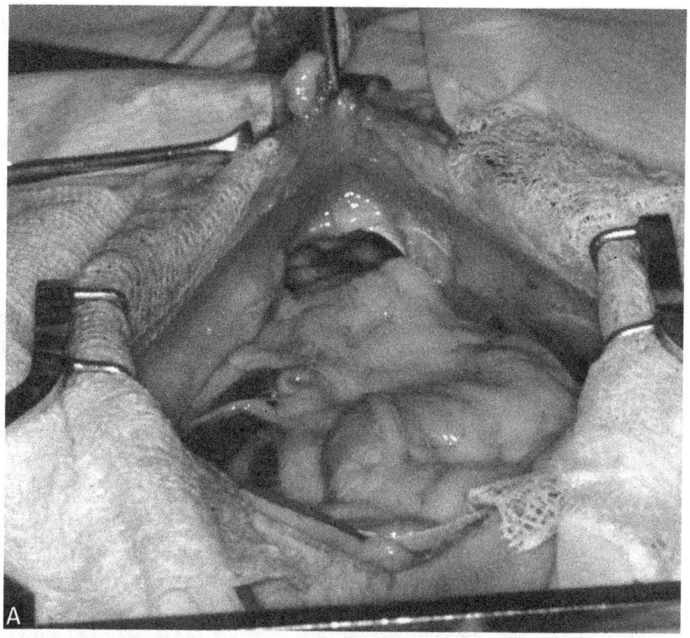

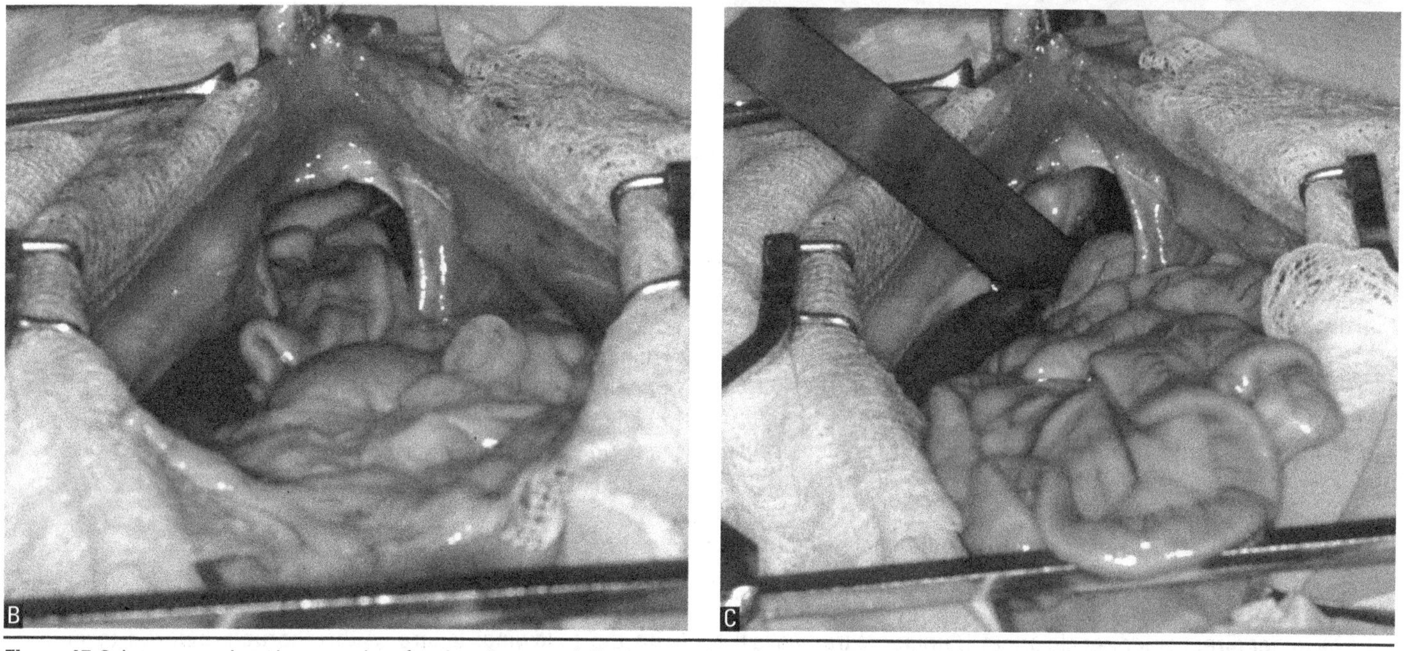

Figure 15-2. Intraoperative photographs of a chronic ventral diaphragmatic hernia in a cat. A: Herniated viscera is covered by omentum. B: Retraction of the omentum shows herniation of small intestine. C: Reduction of intestine reveals herniation of the quadrate lobe of the liver. The malleable retractor is indicating the gallbladder. Herniation and/or torsion of the liver lobes may lead to temporary or permanent signs of biliary and hepatocellular dysfunction such as obstructive jaundice, ascites, and hepatic encephalopathy.

Congenital Pleuroperitoneal Hernia

Canine congenital pleuroperitoneal hernias are rare, and usually take the form of a defect in the dorsolateral diaphragm, with or without central tendon involvement.[14] The intermediate part of the left lumbar muscle of the crus may be absent, leaving a defect of 1 to 2 cm in diameter, or the defect may be more extensive with both crura and parts of the central tendon absent. An autosomal recessive mode of inheritance of the defect was proposed in a series of related dogs.[14] Congenital pleuroperitoneal hernias have also been diagnosed in cats.[15]

Congenital Peritoneopericardial Hernia

Peritoneopericardial hernias commonly contain omentum, liver lobes, gallbladder, and small intestine, as a result of a simple communication between the peritoneal and pericardial cavities (Figure 15-3). Stomach, colon, falciform ligament, and spleen have also been reported. Cystic lesions in the pericardium have been reported in animals with small peritoneopericardial hernias and pathologic changes of the omentum or liver.[16,17]

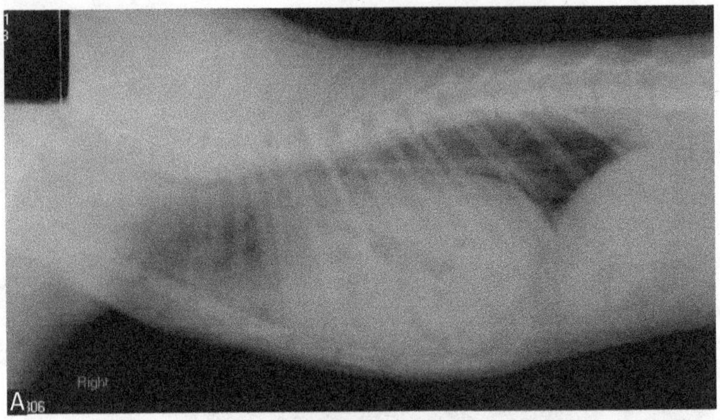

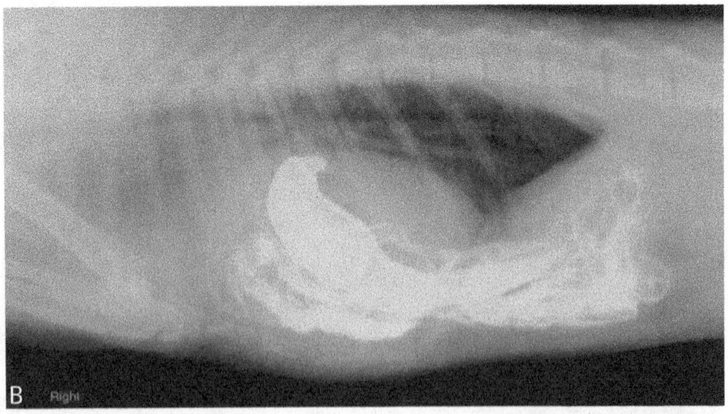

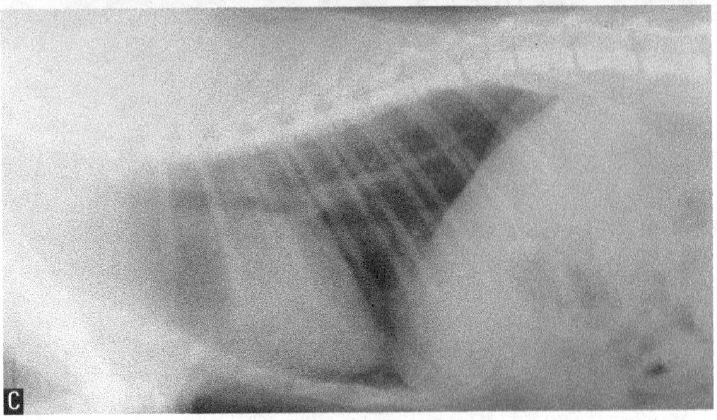

Figure15-3. Thoracic radiographs of a 5-month-old male cat with peritoneopericardial hernia. The cat presented with vomiting, decreased exercise tolerance, and hyperpnea. A: Plain radiographs (lateral and ventrodorsal views). Note the enlarged, rounded cardiac silhouette and the marked lung collapse. B: Contrast radiographs of the same cat after oral administration of barium sulfate. Small intestine and colon are present within the pericardial sac. Distention of gut with gas or ingesta, or effusion from herniated structures may lead to pericardial tamponade. C: Plain radiographs 2 months after surgical correction. The lungs were expanded gently over a period of 24 hours to avoid pulmonary reexpansion syndrome.

Causes of Hernias

Up to 85% of diaphragmatic hernias in small animals are traumatic in origin, 5 to 10% are congenital, and the rest are of unknown etiology.[6,7,18]

Pleuroperitoneal and peritoneopericardial hernias result from failure of development of the transverse septum and inappropriate patency of the pleuroperitoneal canals, with failure of ingrowth of myoblasts to form the muscular crura.[3] Breed predispositions for peritoneopericardial hernias have been reported for the Weimeraner,[19] domestic longhair, and Himalayan cat.[20]

Injury to the diaphragm, causing traumatic diaphragmatic hernia, can be either direct or indirect in origin. Blunt force trauma is the most common cause of diaphragmatic hernias in dogs and cats. Direct injuries from thoracoabdominal stab and gunshot wounds are a frequent cause of diaphragmatic injury in humans[21] but are rarely encountered in veterinary patients. Iatrogenic injury of the diaphragm has been reported with thoracocentesis, poorly positioned chest drains, or by extension of a midline celiotomy incision lateral to the xiphoid process.

Blunt force trauma likely to cause diaphragmatic hernia in animals includes motor vehicle trauma and falling from heights. Male dogs 1 to 3 years old are at significantly greater risk for traumatic diaphragmatic hernia, as a consequence of their increased risk of motor vehicle trauma. The mechanism of diaphragmatic rupture in these instances is probably the sudden increase in intraabdominal pressure at the same time as forced exhalation. Severe injuries of the thoracic cavity and organs have been reported in more than 39% of dogs and cats with musculoskeletal trauma.[22,23] Pulmonary contusions, pleural effusion, hemothorax, pneumothorax, and rib fractures are the most common of these injuries. Between 2% and 5% of animals with fractures have a diaphragmatic hernia.[22,24] Sudden exposure to elevated gravitational forces has been reported to cause diaphragmatic rupture in humans, but is unlikely to be a precipitating factor in veterinary patients. Diaphragmatic hernias have also been reported as a complication of parturition and excessive coughing in humans. Diaphragmatic hernias have been reported occasionally in animals with increased intraabdominal pressure but no obvious precipitating traumatic event.

Pathophysiology

Regardless of the etiology of the diaphragmatic defect, clinical signs related to diaphragmatic hernia are largely associated with the following: failure of the thoracic bellows to produce adequate negative inspiratory pressure, a mass effect from the abdominal organs present within the thorax or pericardium, and incarceration or strangulation of the herniated structures. Respiratory manifestations of diaphragmatic hernia may be further exacerbated by the presence of a pleuroperitoneal effusion or dilation of the gastrointestinal tract. Because of the nature of automobile trauma, multisystem injury and shock are potential complications in traumatic diaphragmatic hernia.

Respiratory Consequences of Diaphragmatic Hernia

Dyspnea and tachypnea are the most common clinical signs in diaphragmatic hernias. In addition to diaphragmatic dysfunction, rupture of the diaphragm causes loss of parietal pleural contact with the lungs and impairs the animal's ability to generate negative intrathoracic pressure. Pressures in the thoracic and abdominal cavities equalize and abdominal and thoracic wall muscles take over ventilation. Pain, rib fractures, and flail chest may limit thoracic expansion in patients with polytrauma. Pulmonary atelectasis following herniation of abdominal organs results in hypoventilation, ventilation/perfusion mismatch, and hypoxia. Dyspnea can also result from pleural effusion.[25] Effusions are commonly reported in association with diaphragmatic hernias, and result from obstruction to lymphatic drainage, inflammation of herniated or displaced organs, and leakage of bile, urine, and feces. Although in most cases the effusion is present in both the peritoneal and pleural cavity, in some instances abdominal organs seal the diaphragmatic defect and the effusion may be restricted to the pleural cavity.[13,26] Gastric tympany should be considered as a cause of respiratory compromise in cases where breathing deteriorates rapidly, particularly in animals known to have a diaphragmatic hernia.

Cardiovascular Consequences of Diaphragmatic Hernia

Cardiovascular abnormalities most commonly result from peritoneopericardial hernias. Pressure of herniated viscera within the pericardial sac may cause cardiac tamponade and right-sided congestive heart failure as a result of compression of the thin-walled right atrium and ventricle. Hypotension, tachycardia, venous distension, ascites, and pleural effusion (including chylothorax) may be seen. Concomitant cardiac defects in animals with congenital disease may produce a variety of hemodynamic effects.

Gastrointestinal Consequences of Diaphragmatic Hernia

The main effects of diaphragmatic hernias on the abdominal viscera are incarceration, obstruction, and strangulation. These effects result from pressure applied by the edge of the diaphragmatic tear as the organs pass over it, from formation of fibrous adhesions and strictures, or from malpositioning or torsion.

Incarceration of the stomach and intestine in a diaphragmatic hernia may result in partial or complete obstruction. Gastric tympany may cause rapid interference with cardiorespiratory function by compression of the caudal vena cava and lungs, and can be rapidly fatal. Recurrent vomiting, leading to dehydration, acid-base and electrolyte derangements, altered cardiac electrical conduction, and muscle weakness, was reported as a consequence of gastric outflow and duodenal obstruction in one dog.[27] Severe compromise of blood supply can also induce ischemic necrosis, intestinal perforation, and abscessation. In some instances, viscera may rupture, leading to bile peritonitis and pleuritis, fecal contamination of the body cavities, and uropleuritis.

Hepatic Consequences of Diaphragmatic Hernia

The liver may be injured at the time of diaphragmatic injury, or one or more lobes of the liver may herniate into the thoracic cavity. The latter may occur in both traumatic and congenital diaphragmatic hernia. Disease resulting from liver lobe herniation occurs as a result of hepatic congestion, hepatic necrosis, liver lobe torsion, or obstruction to biliary flow. A pressure gradient of up to 12 mm Hg normally exists across the hepatic sinusoids, between the portal vein and the hepatic vein. The caudal vena cava and hepatic veins are thin-walled, low-pressure vessels and are easily compressed. When the liver herniates or undergoes torsion, compression of these vessels results in occlusion to hepatic venous outflow. A rise in pressure in the hepatic veins or caudal vena cava relative to the intrahepatic sinusoidal pressure results in hepatic congestion, dilation of hepatic lymphatic vessels, and extravasation of copious quantities of high-protein hepatic lymph. Rapid accumulation of hydrothorax, ascites, or a combination may result. Hydrothorax and ascites develop in about 30% of animals with liver herniation.[6,7,10] The fluid typically is a modified serosanguineous transudate. In addition to fluid extravasation, the liver may undergo severe and sometimes irreversible changes (Figure 15-4). Hepatonodular myelolipomatosis has been reported in a cat with herniation of liver lobes into a peritoneopericardial hernia.[28] Diaphragmatic rupture with concomitant biliary tract injury, bile peritonitis, and bile pleuritis has been reported in dogs. Two cats with chronic diaphragmatic hernia were presented mainly for icterus resulting from extrahepatic biliary obstruction.[29] Although not yet reported in the setting of diaphragmatic hernias, bacterial proliferation (particularly of anaerobic organisms) is known to occur in devitalized liver, leading to sepsis and death.

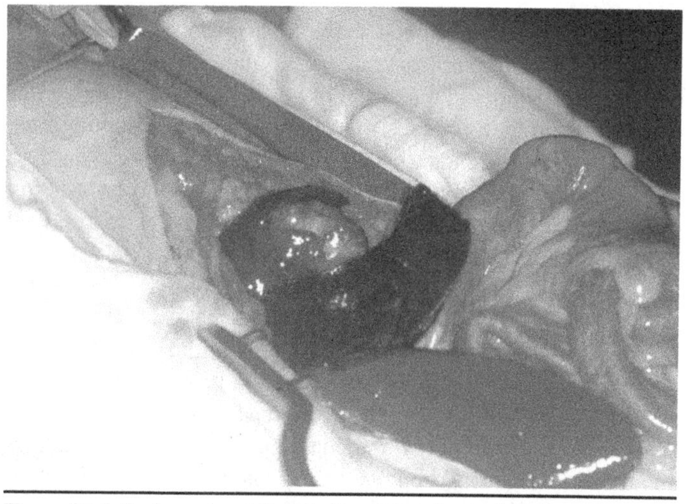

Figure 15-4. Darkened and fibrotic liver lobes (arrow) that have been reduced from a chronic diaphragmatic hernia in a cat. No clinical signs of hepatic dysfunction were present, but a preoperative biochemistry panel revealed markedly elevated activities of serum alanine aminotransferase and alkaline phosphatase. The nonherniated portion of the liver has undergone hyperplasia (open arrow). The discolored liver lobes were assessed as being viable despite the chronic changes and they were not resected. The cat made a complete recovery.

Pleural Effusion

Pleural effusion occasionally results from damage to viscera other than the liver. Hemothorax, chylothorax, urothorax, pneumothorax, and pyothorax have been reported. Pleural effusion may also occur as a result of right-sided congestive heart failure in animals with cardiac tamponade.

Mortality associated with Diaphragmatic Hernia

Prior studies have indicated that approximately 15% of animals die before presentation for anesthesia and surgical correction of traumatic diaphragmatic hernia. Preoperative deaths are due to hypoventilation, shock, multiorgan failure, and cardiac dysrhythmias. Restraint for examination, radiography, and pleural or peritoneal drainage may cause decompensation of critically compromised patients. Mortality may also result in animals with chronic hernias from sudden dilation of the stomach or intestine with ingesta or gas. The effect of acute gaseous distension of the stomach is equivalent to a tension pneumothorax. Emergency decompression of the stomach with a hypodermic needle or stomach tube may be required.

Anesthetic induction is a critical phase of management, and any undue delay in intubation and controlling ventilation can cause death. Induction of anesthesia and surgical intervention in patients that have not been adequately stabilized is likely to be the main reason for the poor outcomes observed previously in animals sent to surgery within 24 hours of injury.[9,36] More recent studies indicate that survival rate is between 80% and 94% and prognosis should be equally good for patients operated on within the first 24 hours, as long as appropriate adjunctive treatment is given.[8,37,38]

Postoperative complications that result in death fall into two groups and may result from the hernia, the surgical procedure, or the underlying traumatic event. In the first 24 hours after surgery, death is caused by hemothorax, pneumothorax, pulmonary edema, shock, pleural effusion, and sudden cardiac arrest. Deaths occurring later after surgery tend to be a result of rupture, obstruction, or strangulation of the gastrointestinal tract, secondary changes in herniated organs, or diseases unrelated to hernia.

Mortality may occur in up to 14% of dogs and cats undergoing surgery for peritoneopericardial hernia.[19,20,30] Mortality has resulted from cardiac arrest and persistence of preoperative signs such as chylothorax and vomiting. One animal developed ascites and signs of hepatic encephalopathy as a result of hepatic cirrhosis, presumably as a result of hepatic ischemia during herniation.[19] The author has also encountered this complication in an Australian cattle dog with a chronic diaphragmatic hernia.[15]

Complications of Diaphragmatic Hernia Repair

Complications reported after repair of diaphragmatic hernias result from changes to diaphragmatic function, physical impingement on structures passing through or near the diaphragm, changes in pleural and peritoneal pressure, and pulmonary reinflation.

Pulmonary dysfunction and edema are perhaps the most serious complications directly related to surgical repair of diaphragmatic hernias. Pulmonary reexpansion syndrome is a well described entity in humans and was first reported in a cat following diaphragmatic hernia repair in 1978.[39] Pulmonary reexpansion injury is commonly reported in humans following evacuation of pneumothorax, sometimes after just a few hours of lung collapse. It has since been identified as a major risk in many studies of small animal patients with diaphragmatic hernia. Pulmonary injury may result from barotrauma owing to overly zealous reinflation. Reexpansion pulmonary edema results from increased permeability of the pulmonary capillary bed. Experimental studies suggest that an inflammatory response follows mechanical injury to the alveolar-capillary membrane and is complicated by reperfusion injury. Reexpansion injury may be avoided by ensuring slow reexpansion by evacuation of air from the thorax using a negative pressure less than minus 10 mm Hg. Lungs should be reinflated slowly over a period of 12 to 24 hours.[40] Reexpansion injury is not just a complication of diaphragmatic hernia repair but may potentially occur in any animal undergoing pulmonary reexpansion after chronic lung collapse, for instance following drainage of pleural effusion or resection of a large space-occupying lesion of the thorax.

Hiatal hernia is a recognized complication of diaphragmatic hernia repair. Proposed mechanisms by which this occurs include physical damage to the esophageal hiatus, abnormal tension on the central tendon of the diaphragm and hence the hiatus, increases in intraabdominal pressure as a result of loss of abdominal domain following chronic diaphragmatic hernia, and alterations in vagal activity as a result of surgical trauma and organ repositioning.

Loss of abdominal domain is not, strictly speaking, a complication of diaphragmatic hernia repair, but it is a complicating factor that may impact the success of surgery. Loss of abdominal domain refers to reduction in the capacity of the abdominal cavity as a result of abdominal myofascial retraction in the presence of chronically reduced volume of abdominal contents. Muscles of the abdominal wall contract and lose the capacity to stretch immediately back to their original length. The fascial sheaths undergo remodeling. Muscles may also undergo fibrosis and retraction if they were damaged at the time of the original trauma. Therefore, following repositioning of herniated organs, direct closure of the celiotomy incision may be impossible, or may result in dangerously elevated intraabdominal pressures. Development of hiatal hernias subsequent to repair of chronic diaphragmatic hernias is likely to result, at least in part, from elevated intraabdominal pressure secondary to loss of domain. Strategies for overcoming the restrictions imposed by loss of domain include myofascial releasing incisions and mesh expansion.[41] The author has used relaxing incisions of the external rectus sheath parallel to the celiotomy incision to assist abdominal closure following repair of chronic diaphragmatic hernia in small animal patients.

Development of ascites immediately after surgery may signal an elevation in hepatic venous drainage pressure caused by repositioning the liver during herniorrhaphy or by chronic liver disease.

Gastric ulceration was a postoperative complication in two dogs that had chronic traumatic diaphragmatic hernia with intrathoracic adhesions to incarcerated liver.[42]

Hyperthermia was reported as a complication of peritoneopericardial hernia repair in 54% of cats in one study.[20] The authors speculated that this may be a result of hepatic manipulation and reperfusion. Hyperthermia has also been reported as a consequence of other major hepatic manipulations such as intrahepatic shunt attenuation in dogs and repair of hepatic injuries in humans.

Prognosis

Traumatic Diaphragmatic Hernia

The overall survival rate for animals diagnosed as having diaphragmatic hernias in the published literature is 52 to 94%. Two significant peaks in mortality were noted in a previous review. Survival rates for 40 dogs operated on within 24 hours was 67% and for 8 dogs operated on after 1 year was 37%.[18,36,43] Death in the early group was due entirely to shock and trauma and in the late group was largely unrelated to the hernia. By delaying surgery until 1 to 3 weeks after trauma, survival rates were greater than 90%. More recent reports, however, suggest that prognosis is equally good for animals operated on early, as long as the patient is stabilized appropriately prior to surgery, and following repair of chronic hernias.[8,37]

Recurrence rates of traumatic hernia, initially repaired with interrupted sutures of polyglactin 910 through an intercostal exposure, have been reported as 4% for dogs and 5% for cats.[44] Recurrence, in man and animals, is usually a result of a combination of tissue weakness and loss of abdominal domain, leading to elevated intraabdominal pressures.

Congenital Diaphragmatic Hernia

A surgical success rate of greater than 80% has been reported for repair of peritoneopericardial hernia in dogs and cats.[19,20,30]

References

1. Hermanson J, Evans HE: The muscular system. *In* Miller's Anatomy of the Dog, 3rd ed. Evans H (ed). Philadelphia: WBSaunders, 1993.

2. Hunt G, Johnson KA: Diaphragmatic, pericardial and hiatal hernia. *In* Slatter DH (ed). Textbook of Small Animal Surgery, 3rd ed. Philadelphia: WB Saunders, 2003, p. 473.

3. Noden D, deLahunta A: The Embryology of Domestic Animals. Developmental Mechanisms and Malformations. Baltimore: Williams & Wilkins, 1985.

4. De Troyer A, Sampson M, Sigrist S, PT: The diaphragm: two muscles. Science 213:237-238, 1981.

5. Macklem PT: Normal and abnormal function of the diaphragm. Thorax 36:161, 1981.

6. Wilson GP, Hayes HM Jr: Diaphragmatic hernia in the dog and cat: a 25-year overview. Semin Vet Med Surg (Small Anim) 1(4):318, 1986.

7. Wilson GP, Newton CD, Burt JK: A review of 116 diaphragmatic hernias in dogs and cats. J Am Vet Med Assoc 159:1142, 1971.

8. Schmiedt CW, Tobias K, McCrackin Stevenson MA: Traumatic diaphragmatic hernia in cats: 34 cases (1991-2001). J Am Vet Med Assoc 222:1237, 2003.

9. Garson HL, Dodman NH, Baker GJ: Diaphragmatic hernia. Analysis of fifty-six cases in dogs and cats. J Small Anim Pract 21:469, 1980.

10. Downs MC, Bjorling DE: Traumatic diaphragmatic hernias: a review of 1674 cases. Vet Surg 16:87, 1987.

11. Nursal TZ, Ugulu M, Kologlu M, et al: Traumatic diaphragmatic hernias: a report of 26 cases. Hernia 5:25, 2001.

12. Bellenger CR, Milstein M, McDonnell W: Herniation of gravid uterus into the thorax of a dog. Mod Vet Pract 56(8):553-555, 1975.

13. Stork C, Hamaide AJ, Schwedes C, et al: Hemiurothorax following diaphragmatic hernia and kidney prolapse in a cat. J Feline Med Surg 5:91, 2003.

14. Valentine BA, Cooper BJ, Dietze AE, et al: Canine congenital diaphragmatic hernia. J Vet Int Med 2: 109, 1988.

15. Voges A, Bertrand S, Hill RC, et al.: True diaphragmatic hernia in a cat. Vet Radiol Ultrasound 2:116, 1997.

16. Sisson D, Thomas, WP, Reed J, et al: Intrapericardial cysts in the dog. J Vet Intern Med 7:364, 1993.

17. Liptak J, Bissett SA, Allan GS, et al: Hepatic cysts incarcerated in a peritoneopericardial diaphragmatic hernia. J Feline Med Surg 4:123, 2002.

18. Boudrieau R: Pathophysiology of traumatic diaphragmatic hernia. *In* Mechanisms of Disease, 2nd ed. Bojrab MJ (ed). Philadelphia: Lea & Febiger, 1993, p. 103.

19. Evans S, Biery DN: Congenital peritoneopericardial diaphragmatic hernia in the dog and cat: A literature review and 17 additional case histories. Vet Radiol 21:108, 1980.

20. Reimer SB, Kyles AE, Filipowicz DE, Gregory CR: Long-term outcome of cats treated conservatively or surgically for peritoneopericardial diaphragmatic hernia: 66 cases (1987-2002). J Am Vet Med Assoc 224:728, 2004.

21. Degiannis E, Levy RD, Sofianois C, et al: Diaphragmatic herniation after penetrating trauma. Br J Surg 83:88, 1996.

22. Spackman CJA, Caywood DD, Feeney DA, et al: Thoracic wall and pulmonary trauma in dogs sustaining fractures as a result of motor vehicle accidents. J Am Vet Med Assoc 185:975, 1984.

23. Tamas PM, Paddleford RR, Krahwinkel DJ Jr: Thoracic trauma in dogs and cats presented for limb fractures. J Am Anim Hosp Assoc 21:161, 1985.

24. Kraje BJ, Kraje AC, Rohrbach BW, et al: Intrathoracic and concurrent orthopedic injury associated with traumatic rib fracture in cats: 75 cases (1980-1998). J Am Vet Med Assoc 216:51, 2000.

25. Roudebush P, Burns J: Pleural effusion as a sequela to traumatic diaphragmatic hernias: a review of four cases. J Am Anim Hosp Assoc 15:699, 1979.

26. Bellenger CR, Trim C, Summer-Smith G: Bile pleuritis in a dog. J Small Anim Pract 16:575, 1975.

27. Roe SC, Smith CW, Stowater JL: Diaphragmatic hernia producing gastric outflow obstruction, metabolic alkalosis, and hypokalemia in a dog. Comp Contin Edu Pract Vet 8:943, 1986.

28. Schuh JCL: Hepatic nodular myelolipomatosis (myelolipomas) associated with a peritoneo-pericardial diaphragmatic hernia in a cat. J Comp Pathol 97:231, 1987.

29. Cornell KK, Jakovljevic S, Waters DJ, Prostredny J, et al.: Extrahepatic biliary obstruction secondary to diaphragmatic hernia in two cats. J Am Anim Hosp Assoc 29:502-507, 1993.

30. Wallace J, Mullen HS, Lesser MB: A technique for surgical correction of peritoneal pericardial diaphragmatic hernia in dogs and cats. J Am Anim Hosp Assoc 28:503, 1992.

31. Sullivan M, Lee R: Radiological features of 80 cases of diaphragmatic rupture. J Small Anim Pract 30:561, 1989.

32. Williams J, Leveille R, Myer CW: Imaging modalities used to confirm diaphragmatic hernia in small animals. Comp Contin Educ Pract Vet 20:1199, 1998.

33. Berry C, Koblik PD, Ticer JW: Dorsal peritoneopericardial mesothelial remnant as an aid to the diagnosis of feline congenital peritoneopericardial diaphragmatic hernia. Vet Radiol 31:239, 1990.

34. White J, Tisdall PLC, Norris JM, et al: Diaphragmatic hernia mimicking a pulmonary mass. J Feline Med Surg 5:197, 2003.

35. Stowater JL, Lamb CR: Ultrasonography of noncardiac thoracic diseases in small animals. J Am Vet Med Assoc 195:514, 1989.

36. Sullivan M, Reid J: Management of 60 cases of diaphragmatic rupture. J Small Anim Pract 31:425,1990.

37. Gibson TWG, Brisson B, Sears W: Perioperative survival rates after surgery for diaphragmatic hernia in dogs and cats: 92 cases (1990-2002). J Am Vet Med Assoc 227:105, 2005.

38. Bellenger CR, Hunt GB, Goldsmid SE, et al: Outcomes of thoracic surgery in dogs and cats. Aust Vet J 74:25, 1996.

39. Stampley AR, Waldron DR: Reexpansion pulmonary edema after surgery to repair a diaphragmatic hernia in a cat. J Am Vet Med Assoc 203:1699,1993.

40. Sherman SC: Reexpansion pulmonary edema: a case report and review of the current literature. J Emerg Med 24:23, 2003.

41. Levine JP, Karp NS: Restoration of abdominal wall integrity as a salvage procedure in difficult recurrent abdominal wall hernias using a method of wide myofascial release. Plast Reconstr Surg 107:707, 2001.

42. Willard MD, Toal RL, Cawley A: Gastric complications associated with correction of chronic diaphragmatic hernia in two dogs. J Am Vet Med Assoc 184:1151, 1984.

43. Minihan A, Berg J, Evans KL: Chronic diaphragmatic hernia in 34 dogs and 16 cats. J Am Anim Hosp Assoc 40:51, 2004.

44. Stokhof AA: Diagnosis and treatment of acquired diaphragmatic hernia by thoracotomy in 49 dogs and 72 cats. Vet Q 8:177, 1986.

Chapter 16

Peritonitis

Jamie R. Bellah

Peritonitis is a clinical syndrome characterized by an inflammatory response to irritation of parietal serous membranes that line the abdominal cavity and the visceral membranes that cover the abdominal viscera, and it is a common initiator of the systemic inflammatory response syndrome.[1] It is most commonly secondary to diseases or trauma that result in bacterial contamination of the abdominal cavity in both dogs and cats. Introduction of microbes by any means can induce septic peritonitis, whereas nonseptic inflammation, or aseptic peritonitis, may be induced by neoplastic invasion, blood, urine extravasation, bile leakage, and irritating acid by-products of pancreatitis.[2-4] The latter nonseptic conditions may become septic (i.e., bowel obstruction) if damage to bowel allows transmural movement of bacteria.[3] Primary peritonitis is not common in small animals and is usually attributed to corona viral infection causing feline infectious peritonitis in cats, or to hematogenous infection if the source of peritonitis is not known in either dogs or cats.[5] The surface area of these inflamed membranes can be as much as 150% percent of the surface area of total body surface area,[6] so disorders that affect the abdominal cavity in either a generalized or local region can have a profound affect on the clinical health of the dog or cat.

Anatomy

The peritoneum is a serous membrane made up of mesenchymal cells supported by a stroma of collagenous and elastic fibers, called the transverse fascia.[6] Other cells and substances populate this stroma and include macrophages, lymphocytes, mast cells, adipose cells, and glycosaminoglycans. Special lymphatic collecting vessels and lacunae, especially common on the visceral surface of the diaphragm, are responsible for clearing fluid and particles from the peritoneal cavity,[6,7] but are also capable of increasing in diameter during peritonitis.[8] The peritoneal cavity normally has a small amount of serous fluid that serves a lubricating purpose. This fluid is produced by the mesenchymal cells.[6] The peritoneal membrane has been characterized as a semipermeable membrane that is capable of absorptive and exudative functions.[2] Circulation of normal peritoneal fluid occurs caudal to cranial (toward the diaphragm). Investigative dye studies show clearance times varying from 19 to 72 minutes, depending on a cranial or caudal location of the dye injection, respectively.[6,9] After absorption by diaphragmatic lymphatics, lymph is carried to mediastinal lymph nodes, to the thoracic duct, and finally to the systemic circulation. Omental lymphatics provide a route for drainage and aggregations of cells ("milky spots"), which include neutrophils, macrophages, and lymphocytes that are important to defense mechanisms. Peritoneal-associated lymphoid tissues are also capable of immunoglobulin production.[6]

The peritoneal cavity has a normal positive pressure, which varies from 1.5 to 5.5 mm Hg, which can be measured indirectly using a transurethral urinary bladder catheter. Increases in peritoneal pressure can result in decreased abdominal compartment compliance, which can cause cardiovascular, respiratory, and abdominal organ dysfunction. Peritoneal pressures greater than 15 mm Hg can be associated with tachycardia, hypertension, increased systemic vascular resistance, decreased cardiac output, decreased mesenteric blood flow, decreased intestinal mucosal blood flow, and increased bacterial translocation.[6] Intraabdominal pressures are increased after ovariohysterectomy and other causes of abdominal distention. Abdominal pressures greater than 22 mm Hg may require surgical decompression, especially in oliguric animals.[10]

Cytologic characteristics of normal peritoneal fluid include mostly macrophages, mesothelial cells and lymphocytes, and a protein content of less than 3 g/dl. Peritoneal fluid lacks fibrinogen, does not clot, and has antibacterial activity as a result of its complement and opsonizing fibronectin components.[6]

Etiology of Secondary Peritonitis

Gastrointestinal microorganisms gain access to the peritoneal cavity by leakage from perforation or other loss of bowel integrity and are the most common cause of secondary peritonitis.[6,11] Peritonitis may follow abdominal surgery and, when postoperative peritonitis occurs, the mortality rate is high.[11] Recently, preoperative peritonitis has been shown to be a risk factor for developing anastomotic leakage.[12] Bacteria and inflammatory cells produce collagenases, which decrease the collagen content of the intestinal wall and impair the strength of the anastomosis.[12] Gram-negative aerobes and anaerobes with an admixture of fluid and ingesta from the bowel result in initiation of inflammation from bacterial, chemical, and foreign materials. Leakage from bowel may occur from mechanical perforation, neoplastic invasion, foreign materials, sharp and blunt trauma, vascular disruption causing ischemia and necrosis, dehiscence of surgical incisions, and drug-induced lesions such as corticosteroid-induced ulceration or colonic perforation. Gastrointestinal perforation typically results in a plural population of bacteria within peritoneal fluids. A factor that determines the number and type of bacteria that escape into the peritoneal cavity is which region of gastrointestinal tract perforates. The more distally the site of perforation is located, the higher are the total bacteria count and the percentage of anaerobic microorganisms, as well as the incidence of mortality.[6] Two bacteria predominate with intestinal perforation: E. coli and *Bacteroides fragilus*. The aerobic and anaerobic characteristics of these organisms are thought to be synergistic. Endotoxin produced by E. coli is commonly integral in early mortality, and concomitant infection with *Bacteroides fragilis* is thought to enhance the lethal potential of E. coli.[13,14] Alpha-hemolysin, an exotoxin produced by E. coli, is thought to promote infection within the peritoneal cavity, as it is toxic to mammalian cells, and it alters the character of intraperitoneal fluid by lysing red blood cells and having detrimental effects on peritoneal leukocytes.[14,15] This exotoxin enhances the ability to recover E. coli and *Bacteroides fragilis* from peritoneal fluid, and it increases mortality.[14]

Rupture of a septic organ such as the pancreas, prostate, uterus, gallbladder, or urinary bladder, and rupture of intraabdominal abscesses (i.e., liver) usually result in single population of bacteria. The fluid content varies depending on the septic organ that ruptures. Peritoneal dialysis is commonly complicated by septic peritonitis, usually a result of tubing contamination during fluid exchanges or gastrointestinal perforation.[16] Peritonitis is rarely secondary to parasitic infections. *Toxoplasma gondii* infection in cats, *Porocephalus crotali*, and mesocetoides species in dogs have been identified.[17-19]

Secondary peritonitis that occurs in the absence of an infectious pathogen is termed aseptic peritonitis. Chemical agents (usually endogenous such as urine or bile), foreign materials such as starch or surgical sponges, mechanical irritation, and neoplasia may result in aseptic peritonitis. Surgical exposure and manipulation, including exposure to air during surgery or laparoscopic inflammation will cause peritoneal inflammation. Granulomatous peritonitis may result from glove powders, including starch, from talcum powder, and from silicone-based powders. Hypersensitivity to starch or corn is the proposed mechanism.[6] Sterile urine and bile within the peritoneal cavity does not result in significant inflammation of the peritoneum unless bacteria gain access to the fluid.[17,20,21] Sterile bile effusions have been reported for as long as 30 days.[21] Uroperitoneum usually has a more significant metabolic impact on the health of the animal; bacterial contamination from urine is not common. Sterile urine may remain in the peritoneal cavity for long periods without peritonitis if it is sterile.[22] If uroperitoneum is contaminated by bacteria, the need to correct the problem surgically is more urgent, whereas if the urine is sterile, urine diversion via peritoneal drainage can be performed until the patient is stable. Other chemicals that are iatrogenically placed into the abdominal cavity, such as antibiotics, barium, povidone-iodine solutions, and iodinated contrast agents cause varying degrees of peritoneal inflammation.[6]

Sclerosing encapsulating peritonitis, a chronic condition that results in the abdominal organs being encased in "cocoon-like" layers of collagenous connective tissue, has been reported in small animals.[6] This condition is nonseptic, with peritoneal fluid containing red blood cells, macrophages with phagocytized red cells, and fibroblasts. The etiology of this condition is uncertain.[23,24]

Inflammation of Peritonitis

The peritoneum utilizes immunologic mechanisms, absorptive function, and the ability to localize infectious processes to defend its surfaces. When peritoneal contamination or injury occurs, an immediate inflammatory response occurs beginning with activation of complement (C3a and C5a), and the influx of neutrophils. Mast cells and basophils degranulate, promoting vascular permeability and the elaboration of opsonins and complement. Opsonization of organisms, cell lysis and clearance of immune complexes is potentiated by complement. Phagocytosis is enhanced, and immunoglobulins are produced by peritoneum-associated lymphoid tissues.[25] Mast cells, neutrophils, macrophages, lymphocytes, and mesenchymal cells participate in release of cytokines, which results in further cell recruitments. Prostaglandin synthesis results from arachidonic acid metabolism stimulated by interleukin 1β and tumor necrosis factor-α. Such cytokines, with interleukin 8, enhance neutrophil emigration. The elevation of proinflammatory cytokines, such as tumor necrosis factor-α, and interleukins 8 and 6 are proportional to the severity of the clinical response.[6] Exudation of peritoneal fluid results from increased permeability of peritoneal capillary networks caused by mast cell histamines and prostaglandins. This peritoneal fluid exudation provides a large volume of fluid containing complement, immunoglobulins, clotting factors, and fibrin. Fibrin clearance is decreased because the fibrinolytic system is inactivated by inflammation, and clumps of fibrin can occlude peritoneal lacunae. Bacteria may be protected from the inflammatory response in regions of fibrin deposit; however, fibrin deposits are prerequisite to fibrous adhesion formation, which help localize regions of infection.[6,26]

The consequence of exudation of fluid from the vascular space into the peritoneal cavity is hypovolemia and hypoproteinemia. Hypovolemia and hypoproteinemia are exacerbated when ileus occurs secondary to sympathoadrenergic reflex inhibition[27] and fluid becomes sequestered in the bowel lumen. Translocation of bacteria is enhanced when intestinal motility is altered; therefore, in nonseptic types of peritonitis the associated ileus may allow transmural bacterial contamination of the peritoneal cavity.[6] Ileus may also occur from conditions such as ischemia or chronic distention from obstruction. As the volume of fluid in the peritoneal cavity continues to increase, loss of diaphragmatic compliance occurs and ventilation is compromised. When severe, hypoxemia and respiratory acidosis can result. Increasing volumes of peritoneal fluid eventually increase intraabdominal pressure, which may reduce venous return from abdominal capacitance vessels and negatively impact cardiac output. Acute renal failure will eventually result from decreased renal perfusion. Septic peritonitis has been associated with septic hepatopathy; intrahepatic cholestasis, icterus, and elevation of serum bile acids and liver enzymes.[28] Disseminated intravascular coagulation resulting in microembolization of parenchymal organ blood supply exacerbates insults to major organs from hypovolemia and hypoxia. Multiorgan dysfunction syndrome (MODS) may result from cell dysfunction and is mediated by cytokines.

Sepsis commonly occurs when peritonitis is secondary to bacterial contamination. Secondary effects of the bacterial pathogens and their by-products complicate the metabolic alterations already described. Experimentation has shown sepsis to be associated with a marked increase in peripheral oxygen demand, elevated levels of plasma insulin, glucagon, and catecholamines (the hyperdynamic state).[29,30] Endotoxin potentiates levels of proinflammatory cytokines, complement, and products of arachidonic acid metabolism, by stimulation of the innate immune response.[6] Anaerobic organisms produce exoenyzmes that make them particularly invasive to tissue, causing necrosis, suppuration, adhesion, and abscess formation.[6]

Substances that Potentiate Peritonitis

Substances that augment or potentiate local or systemic inflammatory responses in peritonitis or that worsen the prognosis for recovery in bacterial peritonitis are termed adjuvants of peritonitis.[29] Bile salts, gastric mucin, hemoglobin, and barium are recognized as adjuvants that enhance the virulence of contaminating bacteria.[6,31] Phagocytosis is inhibited by gastric mucin because of a heparin-like anticomplement effect and by hemoglobin, which disrupts phagocytic cell chemotaxis. Hemoglobin also interferes with phagocytosis, intracellular killing,[29] and lymphatic clearing mechanisms.[26,32] Bile salts lyse red blood cells and release hemoglobin and alter cellular adhesion mechanisms by lowering surface tension.[33] Another adjuvant effect is related to peritoneal fluid volume. Experimentally, incremental increases in volumes of fluid injected intraperitoneally while keeping the bacterial inoculums unchanged resulted in slowed bacterial clearance, increased bacterial proliferation, and increased mortality.[34] Barium and intestinal-content contamination resulted in a higher mortality rate than intestinal content contamination alone in an experimental study.[35] Despite this finding, barium is still used in upper gastrointestinal studies because it provides better radiographic detail. If leakage occurs, immediate exploratory surgery is performed to resolve the gastrointestinal perforation and to remove extravasated barium and foreign material by thorough lavage.

Clinical Signs of Peritonitis

It is common to think of clinical signs referable to peritonitis as acutely painful with vomiting, fever, and shock, but peritonitis in dogs and cats can present with a wide variation in clinical signs.[6] Anorexia, vomiting, malaise, depression, fever, weakness, and an abdominal pain response are common. Fever is not always present and rectal temperature can vary from hypothermic to hyperthermic. Fever may occur in either septic or aseptic peritonitis.[36] Dogs generally exhibit an abdominal pain response, however one third of cats with peritonitis do not exhibit an abdominal pain response.[37] Abdominal pain may be exhibited by a "praying position," which may provide pain relief in some dogs (also not a consistent observation). Varying degrees of abdominal fluid accumulation may or may not be detectable during physical examination. Large volumes of effusion may cause respiratory compromise. Sequestration of fluid in the peritoneal cavity and the intestinal lumen from ileus can quickly result in marked dehydration when accompanied by vomiting. In cats and dogs, peritoneal effusions have been associated with hyponatremia and hyperkalemia in the presence of normal adrenal gland function.[38] Auscultation of the abdomen may reveal the absence of borborygmi, consistent with ileus. Vital signs that may be suggestive of a hyperdynamic systemic inflammatory response syndrome include injected (brick red) mucous membranes, rapid capillary refill time, tachycardia, strong quick pulses, and pyrexia. As peritonitis progresses and hypovolemia worsens, tachycardia becomes severe with weak pulses, prolonged capillary refill time, pale membranes, and hypothermia (hypovolemic shock). In cats, bradycardia and hypothermia, pale mucous membranes, signs of diffuse abdominal pain, weak pulses, anemia, hypoalbuminemia, and icterus are indicative of severe sepsis.[39] Clinical signs may also reflect the organ system involved: icterus with septic cholecystitis and perforation; a vaginal discharge with ruptured pyometra; dysuria or pyuria with prostatic abscessation or septic prostatitis. Purulent drainage associated with abdominal pain after gastrointestinal surgery can be associated with dehiscence and leakage of bowel content.

Diagnosis

Many diagnostic tests contribute to and support the diagnosis of peritonitis, but cytologic examination of peritoneal fluid is the most important examination. The finding of degenerative neutrophils with intracellular bacteria is diagnostic for septic peritonitis. Culture (and susceptibility test) confirms bacterial infection.[40] A recent study recommended culturing nonseptic fluid, as lack of cytologic evidence for sepsis did not mean bacteria would not be cultured.[41] Often the volume of peritoneal fluid makes obtaining peritoneal fluid by abdominocentesis relatively simple, but ultrasound can guide aspiration when the fluid volume is low. In the absence of ultrasound guidance, a "four-quadrant" tap may be done. Diagnostic peritoneal lavage may also be used to "wash" peritoneal surfaces and collect fluid for examination; it is indicated when septic peritonitis is suspected despite low volumes or absence of abdominal fluid.[6] Exploration of the abdominal cavity is indicated if cytologic examination reveals degenerative or toxic neutrophils with phagocytized bacteria, free bacteria (be careful of stain contaminants), or plant material. Abdominal fluid obtained after uncomplicated gastrointestinal anastomosis surgery typically had nondegenerate neutrophils.[42] Neutrophil counts vary widely; cytologic characteristics are considered the most important criteria and should be used in conjunction with peripheral white blood cell counts. Peripheral blood WBC can vary from neutrophilia to neutropenia when neutrophilic consumption exceeds bone marrow production.[36] Culture of aerobic and anaerobic organisms and susceptibility testing is done.

Peritoneal fluid and serum in septic peritonitis have been compared, as bacterial isolation is not temporally realistic versus cytologic diagnosis. In this study, a presurgical white blood cell count of more than 2000 cells/dl and postsurgical white blood cell count of more than 9000 cells/dl was indicative of peritonitis in general. When blood and peritoneal fluid glucose were compared, a concentration difference of more than 20 mg/dl differentiated septic peritoneal effusions from nonseptic effusions in dogs and cats.[40] Lactate production occurs as a result of neutrophilic glycolysis and bacterial metabolites from an anaerobic microenvironment in peritoneal fluid with a resultant decrease in the pH of peritoneal fluid.[43] Septic effusions in cats were found to have a lower pH, but dogs did not show this trend.[40] Differences in blood to fluid pH were found to be insignificant in dogs and cats, blood to fluid glucose significant in dogs and cats, and blood to fluid lactate insignificant because of low numbers. Although not statistically significant, a blood to fluid lactate difference of less than -2.0 mmol/L was 100% sensitive and specific for septic peritoneal effusion in 7 dogs.[40] Blood to fluid glucose difference was more sensitive than glucose alone.[40] Another investigation in 19 dogs and 18 cats, showed dogs with septic peritoneal effusions to have peritoneal fluid lactate concentrations of more than 2.5 mmol/L and to have peritoneal fluid lactate concentrations that were higher than blood lactate concentrations (a negative blood to peritoneal fluid lactate difference); however, similar tests were not found to be accurate in cats.[43] It has been hypothesized that, because cats are deficient in glucokinase, they may have a tendency toward anaerobic metabolism with higher concentrations of lactate in peripheral blood.[43]

Suspicion of peritoneal fluid may occur during physical examination if a fluid wave is palpable and survey radiographs of the abdomen demonstrate loss of serosal detail (a ground glass appearance). In the absence of recent abdominal surgery, the appearance of free air in the abdominal cavity is indicative of gastrointestinal rupture.[41] Studies have shown gastrointestinal perforation to be the cause in 77% of 34 animals with pneumoperitoneum,[41] and in 74% of 54 animals with pneumoperitoneum but without history of penetrating trauma.[44] Residual free air can occur after abdominal surgery for as long as 30 days,[41] or from diagnostic procedures that utilize gas or air. Emphasematous change within abdominal organs may show air density as well, and be associated with peritonitis.[6] Ultrasonographic examination can reveal fluid and may be able to localize the potential source of leakage if a parenchymal organ is the source of septic purulent fluid. Corrugated small intestine was noted in 4 of 24 dogs with peritonitis, but was more commonly associated with pancreatitis (12 of 24 dogs).[45] Pleural effusion may occur concomitant with peritonitis and is considered a poor prognostic sign.[46] Imaging techniques such as CT and MRI may provide additional information prior to exploratory surgery, but ultrasonography provides a simple, practical, and widely available tool.

Complete blood count, serum chemistry evaluation, and coagulation profiles are preferentially done to assess the severity of disease. Biochemical analysis of peritoneal fluid can be helpful if uroperitoneum or bile leakage is suspected. Creatinine levels in peritoneal fluid greater than serum levels support a diagnosis of uroperitoneum; however, in icteric animals, reagent-based tests for bilirubin (i.e., urine reagent strips) are not accurate.[47] Determination of bilirubin concentration has been shown to be 100% effective in diagnosing bile leakage prior to exploratory surgery. It was consistently two and one-half times the serum concentration of bilirubin when bile leakage was occurring.[21] Hypoglycemia is often present during sepsis.[36] A glucose concentration in peritoneal fluid of less than 50 mg/dl was 100% specific for bacterial peritonitis when 55 cases of nonseptic abdominal effusion were compared with 16 cases of septic abdominal effusion.[48]

Management of Septic Peritonitis

When making a diagnosis of septic peritonitis supportive treatment is initiated typically with aggressive intravenous fluid resuscitation to restore hydration and to improve perfusion. Intravenous crystalloids are administered initially with the goal of achieving a urine output of 1 to 2 ml/kg/hour with a central venous pressure between 0 and 5 cm H_2O. Monitoring of central venous pressure can help tailor fluid therapy to achieve volume expansion and avoid fluid overload. Synthetic colloid administration or blood products may be appropriate, depending on the results of blood and serum evaluations. As fluid resuscitation progresses, serial testing of CVP, serum albumin, colloid osmotic pressure, acid base status, electroplytes, coagulation parameters, and blood pressure aid therapeutic decisions. Preoperative analysis can help to relate cardiovascular parameters to the effects of fluid administration. Fluid rates of 10 to 12 ml/kg/hour may be required to assure maintenance of blood pressure after surgery.[6] Antimicrobial therapy is initiated as soon as peritoneal fluid specimens are cultured and generally involves a combination of an aminoglycoside and a parenteral drug that is effective against anaerobes; however, this greatly depends on individual clinician's preference.[6] Administration of ntimicrobials, such as cefoxitin, that have broad spectrum and good activity against anaerobes, simplifies initial antimicrobial therapy. Antimicrobial therapy may be altered as soon as susceptibility tests are returned. Exploration and resolution of the source of bacterial contamination are required for successful treatment of septic peritonitis. Thorough lavage of the peritoneal cavity to dilute contaminants is believed to be important by most surgeons, but a recent investigation questions if evidence-based support exists for lavage.[49] Antimicrobials are not used in the lavage fluid during surgery as parenteral antimicrobials reach sufficient (therapeutic) levels in peritoneal fluid during peritonitis,[50] and adverse affects such as chemical irritation, adhesions, and delayed anastomotic healing are avoided.[51] In addition, use of antimicrobials in lavage fluids has not been shown to provide significant benefit over lavage alone. After correcting the source of bacterial contamination and thorough lavage, consideration is given to providing a gastric or enteral route of alimentation, so nutritional support can be provided in the early postoperative period. Corticosteroid and nonsteroidal use in septic peritonitis is controversial and is not routinely done, as there is no proven benefit.[36]

Drainage of the inflamed peritoneal cavity is the decision that seems most controversial. Closure of the abdominal cavity without drainage, sump drains for continued drainage (with or without intermittent lavage), open peritoneal drainage, and vacuum-assisted peritoneal drainage are used currently, although the latter technique is in its infancy in both human and veterinary medicine.[52-55] Open drainage allows the fluid to be removed from the abdomen in as little as 6 hours, whereas sump drainage requires 24 to 48 hours.[6] A retrospective investigation of 36 dogs and 6 cats, comparing open peritoneal drainage and primary closure techniques, found an overall survival rate of 71% with no significant difference in survival between groups. Iin the open drainage group, however, patients received more plasma and blood, more animals had jejunostomy tubes and longer intensive care unit hospitalization (a mean of 6 days versus 3.5 days for the primary closure group).[55] Prospective clinical trials comparing closed and open drainage techniques are not available in the veterinary literature.

Primary closure of the abdominal incision after exploration for septic peritonitis has been reported to have a mortality rate of 46%.[53] Although prospective comparison of open and closed methods of treating septic peritonitis has not been done, retrospective comparison of mortality rates in individual studies shows mortality rates to be similar, with gastrointestinal leakage being the most common cause and having the highest mortality.[52] A prospective randomized study that categorized septic peritonitis as gastrointestinal, biliary, and nonbiliary nongastrointestinal (i.e., uterus, prostate, renal) such that large numbers of animals managed by open and closed methods in each category would contribute to determination of when open peritoneal drainage is warranted and when primary closure is sufficient. In the author's opinion, septic peritonitis that originates from parenchymal organs such as the uterus, prostate, and kidney tends to have peritoneal contamination that is easily removed and diluted by large volume lavage. In situations of gastrointestinal content leakage, the decision for open peritoneal drainage is made based on judging the adequacy of lavage to dilute and remove foreign material and exudates and the extent of surface involvement (local or diffuse).

Septic peritonitis treated by primary closure and abdominal drains has not achieved strong support because drainage has been ineffective and because it benefits only a local region of the peritoneal cavity, undergoes premature partial occlusion by omentum, and can be complicated by ascending nosocomial infection. Bacterial contamination via an abdominal drain has been shown to occur in as little as 24 hours.[56] Sump drains allow better drainage than nonsump drains but also allow potential contamination because air is pulled into the peritoneal cavity if not filtered. Sump-Penrose drains were completely encased by omentum and omental adhesions in 96 hours in normal dogs.[54] Both the sump-Penrose drains and open peritoneal drainage in normal dogs caused a local inflammatory response.[54] Intermittent peritoneal lavage with a Parker peritoneal dialysis cannula has also been used, and an average of 91.4% of the infused lavage volume was recovered. Closed suction drains have also been used successfully to treat generalized peritonitis in dogs and cats without clinically important complications.[57,58]

Open peritoneal drainage has resulted in mortality rates varying from 22% to 48%.[52,54,55] Open peritoneal drainage provides the best and most complete drainage of the peritoneal cavity, essentially leaving it as an open wound or abscess would be treated and maintaining a microenvironment within the cavity less favorable to anaerobic bacteria. The efficacy of open peritoneal drainage is reported to be due to enhanced removal of bacteria, foreign material, and exudates (including inflammatory mediators).[59] Gross appearance of the wound, cytologic examination of the fluid, and the condition of the patient are factors that contribute to the optimum timing of abdominal closure. Reexploration of the abdomen may be performed if degenerative neutrophilic inflammation or bacterial contamination persists or returns. Bacterial culture is done prior to closing the abdomen; in previous studies, as high as 40% of cases had different bacteria isolated at closure than at initial exploration.[6] The most common complications of open peritoneal drainage include hypoproteinemia, hypoalbuminemia, anemia, and nosocomial infection.[6] Open peritoneal drainage in humans has been shown to have significantly more complications and no advantage over a primary closure technique when compared in a prospective clinical trial.[60] A study of 239 patients showed 31% mortality with closed technique and

44% mortality with open techniques.[61] The suggestion has been made that open peritoneal drainage is possibly enhanced by the animal's posture.[6]

Vacuum-assisted closure (VAC) is a new technique in both human and veterinary medicine and has application in acute and chronic wounds.[62,63] Vacuum-assisted peritoneal drainage is in its infancy, but is currently being evaluated in human patients and in a few veterinary centers. The technique has been shown to accelerate wound healing by increasing local blood flow, by reducing bacterial load, and by stimulating growth of granulation tissue.[64] In humans, use of temporary vacuum-assisted closure is being used for local and for generalized peritonitis. Techniques have been developed for using VAC to treat anastomotic leakage after rectal resection.[64] Vacuum-assisted wound closure has been reported to augment open abdominal wall repairs where human acellular dermal matrix is used to close open abdomens that cannot be closed by local tissue mobilization.[65] Use of VAC has also been successful in managing post-laparotomy wound dehiscence where compromised wound healing was thought to play a complicating role.[66] Technique modifications are being developed to allow treatment of local intraabdominal infections without dissemination of infection to other areas of the abdominal cavity.[67]

Supportive Care

Septic peritonitis results in massive protein and electrolyte losses in an animal that is unlikely to eat soon after surgery. Failure to provide nutritional support results in protein-energy malnutrition, which depletes energy stores, delays wound healing, impairs immunocompetance, and can result in weakness and eventually organ failure.[68] Early enteral nutrition is beneficial to enterocytes and also has been shown to decrease bacterial mural translocation, preserve or increase gastrointestinal blood flow, prevent ulceration, increase IgA concentration and stimulate other immune system defenses, and enhance wound repair;[68] therefore, a judgment as to what technique to use is important during surgery. Jejunostomy tubes allow direct infusion (as continuous rate infusion) of special diets into the small intestine; however, the complication rate with this technique is high, varying from 17.5% to 42%.[6] Esophagostomy tube placement and gastrostomy tube placement are alternatives to jejunostomy. Other noninvasive tube placement techniques include nasoesophageal and nasoenteric feeding tubes. Parenteral nutrition may be done in lieu of enteral feeding techniques and is capable of maintaining serum protein concentrations. Transfusion therapy is important to overall management as indicated by results of serial examination of hematocrit, albumin, and coagulation parameters, and management of pain with analgesics before and after surgery.

Prognosis

Survival rates for generalized peritonitis have varied from 52% to 79%. As has been noted,[6] more recent survival rates are improved and are likely related to improved diagnosis and preoperative and postoperative management. Septic bile peritonitis has been shown to be particularly lethal; only 27% of animals survived in one retrospective investigation.[21] In the same investigation, all six animals with sterile bile leakage survived.[21]

References

1. Swann H, Hughes D: Diagnosis and management of peritonitis. Vet Clin North Am Small Anim Pract 30:603, 2000.
2. Dulisch ML: Peritonitis. *In* Pathophysiology in Small Animal Surgery, 2nd ed. Bojrab MJ (ed). Philadelphia:WB Saunders, 2005, p. 109.
3. Ettinger SJ, Barrett KA: Peritonitis. *In* Textbook of Veterinary Internal Medicine, 4th ed. Ettinger SJ, Feldman EL (eds). Philadelphia: WB Saunders, 1995, p 68.
4. Wright KN, Gompf RE, DeNovo RC: Peritoneal effusions in cats: 65 cases (1981-1997). J Am Vet Med Assoc 214:375, 1999.
5. Birchard SJ: Peritonitis. *In* Birchard SJ, Sherding RG (eds). Saunders Manual of Small Animal Practice, 3rd ed. Philadelphia: WB Saunders, 2006, p. 853.
6. Kirby BM: Peritoneum and peritoneal cavity. *In* Slatter SL (ed). Textbook of Small Animal Surgery, 3rd ed. Philadelphia: WB Saunders, 2003, p. 414.
7. Heel KA, Hall JC: Peritoneal defenses and peritoneum-associated lymphoid tissue. Br J Surg 83:1031, 1996.
8. Maddus MA, et al: The biology of peritonitis and implications for treatment. Surg Clin North Am 68:431, 1988.
9. Hosgood GL, Salisbury SK: Pathophysiology and pathogenesis of generalized peritonitis. Prob Vet Med 1:159, 1989.
10. Conzemius MG, et al: Clinical determination of preoperative and postoperative intra-abdominal pressures in dogs. Vet Surg 24:195, 1995.
11. Hosgood G, Salisbury SK: Generalized peritonitis in dogs: 50 cases (1975-1986). J Am Vet Med Assoc 193:1448, 1988.
12. Ralphs SC, Jessen CR, Lipowitz AJ: Risk factors for leakage following intestinal anastomosis in dogs and cats: 115 cases (1991-2000) J Am Vet Med Assoc 223:73, 2003.
13. Johnson CC, et al: Peritonitis: Update on pathophysiology, clinical manifestations, and management. Clin Infect Dis 24:1035, 1997.
14. Hall JC, et al: The pathobiology of peritonitis. Gastroenterology 114:185, 1998.
15. May AK, et al: Contribution of Escherichia coli alpha-hemolysin to bacterial virulence and to intraperitoneal alterations in peritonitis. Infect Immunol 68:176, 2000.
16. Carter LJ, et al: Clinical experience with peritoneal dialysis in small animals. Comp Cont Educ Pract Vet 11:1335, 1989.
17. Reppas GP, et al: Anorexia and an abdominal mass in a cat. Aust Vet J 77:784, 1999.
18. Rogers KS, et al: Aberrant nymphal pentastomiasis in a dog. J Am Anim Hosp Assoc 21:417, 1985.
19. Crosbie PR, et al: Diagnostic procedures and treatment of eleven dogs with peritoneal infections caused by Mesocestoides spp. J Am Vet Med Assoc 213:1578, 1998.
20. Ackerman NB, et al: Consequences of intraperitoneal bile: Bile ascites versus bile peritonitis. Am J Surg 149:244, 1985.
21. Ludwig LL, McLoughlin MA, Graves TK, Crisp MS: Surgical treatment of bile peritonitis in 24 dogs and 2 cats: A retrospective study (1987-1994). Vet Surg 26;90, 1997.
22. Hardie EM: Peritonitis from urogenital conditions. Probl Vet Med 1:36, 1989.
23. Boothe HW, et al: Sclerosing encapsulating peritonitis in three dogs. J Am Vet Med Assoc 198:267, 1991.
24. Hardie EM, et al: Sclerosing encapsulating peritonitis in four dogs and a cat. Vet Surg 23:197, 1994.
25. Heel KA, Hall JC: Peritoneal defenses and peritoneum-associated lymphoid tissue. Br J Surg 83:1031, 1996.

26. Laroche M, Harding G: Primary and secondary peritonitis: An update. Eur J Clin Microbiol Infect Dis 17:542, 1998.

27. Glise H, et al: Reflex adrenergic inhibition of gastric motility by nociceptive intestinal stimulation and peritoneal irritation in the cat. Scand J Gastroenterol 15:673, 1980.

28. Taboada J, Meyer DJ: Cholestasis associated with extrahepatic bacterial infection in five dogs. J Vet Intern Med 3:216, 1989.

29. Heemken R, et al: Peritonitis: Pathophysiology and local defense mechanisms. Hepatogastroenterology 44:927, 1997.

30. Shaw JHF, Wolfe RR: A conscious septic dog model with hemodynamic and metabolic responses similar to responses of humans. Surgery 95:553, 1984.

31. Hosgood G, Salisbury SK: Pathophysiology and pathogenesis of generalized peritonitis. Probl Vet Med 1:159, 1989.

32. Hau T, et al: Mechanisms of the adjuvant effect of hemoglobin in experimental peritonitis. Surgery 83:223, 1978.

33. Walker EM, Ellis H: Relationship of the constituents of bile to biliary peritonitis in the rat. Gut 19:827, 1978.

34. Dunn DL, et al: The adjuvant effect of peritoneal fluid in experimental peritonitis: Mechanism and clinical implications. Ann Surg 37;199, 1984.

35. Cochran DQ, et al: An experimental study of the effects of barium and intestinal contents on the peritoneal cavity. Am J Roentgenol 89:883, 1963.

36. Macintire DK, Drobatz KJ, Haskins SC, Saxon WD: Peritonitis. *In* Manual of Small Animal Emergency and Critical Care Medicine. Philadelphia: Lippincott Williams & Wilkins, 2005, p. 219.

37. Costello MF, Drobatz KJ, Aronson LR, King LG: Underlying cause, pathopysiologic abnormalities, and response to treatment in cats with septic peritonitis: 51 cases (1990-2001). J Am Vet Med Assoc 225:897, 2004.

38. Bissett SA, Lamb M, Ward, CR: Hyponatremia and hyperkalemia associated with peritoneal effusion in four cats. J Am Vet Med Assoc 218:1590, 2001.

39. Brady CA, et al: Severe sepsis in cats: 29 cases (1986-1998) J Am Vet Med Assoc 217:531, 2000.

40. Bonczynski JJ, et al: Comparison of peritoneal fluid and peripheral blood pH, bicarbonate, glucose, and lactate concentration as a diagnostic tool for septic peritonitis in dogs and cats. Vet Surg 32:161, 2003.

41. Saunders WB, Tobias KM: Pneumoperitoneum in dogs and cats: 39 cases (1983-2002) J Am Vet Med Assoc 4:462, 2003.

42. Botte JR, Rosin E: Cytology of peritoneal effusion following intestinal anastomosis and experimental peritonitis. Vet Surg 12:20, 1983.

43. Levin GM, et al: Lactate as a diagnostic test for septic peritoneal effusions in dogs and cats. J Am Anim Hosp Assoc 40:364, 2004.

44. Smelstoys JA, et al: Outcome of and prognostic indicators for dogs and cats with pneumoperitoneum and no history of penetrating trauma: 54 cases (1988-2002). J Am Vet Med Assoc 225:251, 2004.

45. Moon ML, Biller DS, Armbrust LF: Ultrasonographic appearance and etiology of corrugated small intestine. Vet Radiol Ultrasound 44:199, 2003.

46. Steyn PF, Wittum TE: Radiographic, epidemiologic, and clinical aspects of simultaneous pleural and peritoneal effusions in dogs and cats: 48 cases (1982-1991). J Am Vet Med Assoc 202:307, 1993.

47. Crowe DT: Diagnostic abdominal paracentesis techniques: Clinical evaluation in 129 dogs and cats. J Am Anim Hosp Assoc 13:29, 1984.

48. Swann H, Hughes D: Diagnosis and management of peritonitis. Vet Clin North Am 30:603, 2000.

49. Whiteside OJ, et al: Intra-operative peritoneal lavage – who does it and why? Ann R Coll Surg Engl 87:255, 2005.

50. Gerding DN, et al: Antibiotic concentrations in ascitic fluid of patients with ascites and bacterial peritonitis. Ann Intern Med 86:708, 1977.

51. Withrow SJ, Black AP: Generalized peritonitis in small animals. Vet Clin North Am 9:363, 1979.

52. Greenfield CL, Walshaw R: Open peritoneal drainage for treatment of contaminated peritoneal cavity and septic peritonitis in dogs and cats: 24 cases (1980-1986). J Am Vet Med Assoc 191:100, 1987.

53. Lanz OL, et al: Surgical treatment of septic peritonitis without abdominal drainage in 28 dogs. J Am Anim Hosp Assoc 23:129, 2001.

54. Hosgood G, Salisbury SK, DeNicola DB: Open peritoneal drainage versus sump-penrose drainage: Clinicopathological effects in normal dogs. J Am Anim Hosp Assoc 27:115, 1991.

55. Staatz AJ, Monnet E, Seim HB: Open peritoneal drainage versus primary closure for the treatment of septic peritonitis in dogs and cats: 42 cases (1993-1999). Vet Surgery 31:174, 2002.

56. Casey BH: Bacterial spread in polyethylene tubing – a possible source of surgical wound contamination. Med J Aust 2:718, 1971.

57. Mueller MG, Ludwig LL, Barton LJ: Use of closed-suction drains to treat generalized peritonitis in dogs and cats: 40 cases (1997-1999). J Am Vet Med Assoc 15:789, 2001.

58. Chase JP, et al: Open peritoneal drainage in horses with experimentally induced peritonitis. Vet Surg 11:189, 1996.

59. Bosscha K, et al: Surgical management of severe secondary peritonitis. Br J Surg 86:1371, 1999.

60. Christon NV, et al: Surgical infection society intra-abdominal infection study: prospective evaluation of management techniques and outcome. Arch Surg 128:193, 1993.

61. Lanz OI: Vacuum assisted closure: A review and current veterinary applications. Abstract. American College of Veterinary Surgeons Annual Meeting, San Diego, CA October 27-29, 2005; 532.

62. Morykwas MJ, Argenta LC, Shelton-Brown, et al: Vacuum-assisted closure: a new method for wound control and treatment: animal studies and basic foundation. Ann Plast Surg 38:553, 1997.

63. Nagell CF, Holte K: Treatment of anastomotic leakage after rectal resection with transrectal vacuum-assisted drainage (VAC) A method for rapid control of pelvic sepsis and healing. Int J Colorectal Dis 31:1, 2006.

64. Scott BG, Welsh JF, Pham HQ, et al: Early aggressive closure of the open abdomen. J Trauma 60:17, 2006.

65. Heller L, Levin SL, Butler CE. Management of abdominal wound dehiscence using vacuum assisted closure in patients with compromised healing. Am J Surg 191:165, 2006.

66. Labler L, Keel M, Trentz O: New application of V.A.C. (vacuum assisted closure) in the abdominal cavity in case of open abdomen therapy. Zentralbl Chir 129:14, 2004.

67. Tennant B, Willoughby K: The use of enteral nutrition in small animal medicine. Comp Cont Educ Pract Vet 15:1054, 1993.

68. Devey JJ, Crowe DT: Microenteral nutrition. *In* Kirk's Current Veterinary Therapy XIII. Bonagura JD (ed). Philadelphia: WB Saunders, 2000, p. 136.

Part III

Cardiovascular

Chapter 17

Pericardial Disease

Eric Monnet

"The major function of most organs is readily apparent and requires no deep knowledge of biology or physiology. However, whether or not the pericardium serves an important function or not has been debated over the years and the debate continues."[1]

The pericardium is composed of two layers: the visceral pericardium and the parietal pericardium. The visceral pericardium is a serous membrane composed of mesothelial cells adherent to the epicardium. The parietal pericardium is fibrous and acellular. It contains collagen and elastin fibers. Collagen fibers are wavy when the pericardium is at low stretch. When the pericardium is stretched, the collagen fibers straighten, resulting in increased stiffness of the tissue.[2]

The parietal pericardium has ligamentous attachments to the diaphragm and the sternum. Therefore, the pericardium maintains the heart in its normal anatomic position in the chest by its attachment to the sternum. The pericardium provides a barrier against infection and provides lubrication between the parietal and visceral layers.[2] The pericardium is well innervated, including mechano- and chemoreceptors.[2] These nerve endings likely participate in reflexes resulting from irritation of the pericardium, epicardium, or both. An intact pericardium protects against atrial rupture in dogs with mitral insufficiency and myocardial hemorrhage induced by acute right-sided heart failure.

The pericardium also restrains cardiac filling and enhances diastolic ventricular coupling (Figure 17-1). The force exerted on the surface of the heart by the pericardium can significantly limit filling.[3-5] This effect is mostly important with high filling of the left and right ventricles. Under normal conditions, the contact pressure between the pericardium and the epicardium is 2 to 4 mm Hg.[3,4] With a left ventricular filling pressure of 25 mm Hg, the contact pressure has been estimated at 10 mm Hg.[3,4] By this mechanism, the pericardium prevents cardiac overdistention and helps balance the output of the right and left ventricles. The pericardium contributes to diastolic interaction (transmission of intracavitary filling pressure across the septum).[2,6] A portion of the right ventricular diastolic pressure is transmitted to the left ventricle across the interventricular septum and contributes to left ventricular end-diastolic pressure. If the cardiac volume increases, the pericardium contributes even more to the diastolic interaction.

The pericardium provides a gliding surface to accommodate heart motion. The pericardial cavity is filled with a variable amount of pericardial fluid. The volume of pericardial fluid present in normal dogs ranges from 1 to 15 ml (0.25 ml/kg). This fluid is an ultrafiltrate of serum containing between 1.7 and 3.5 g/dl of protein and having a colloid osmotic pressure approximately 25% that of serum. The pericardial fluid contains phospholipids that serve to lubricate the heart.[7,8] Because the pericardium is noncompliant and has a small reserve volume, intrapericardial pressure rises rapidly when the volume of its contents increases acutely (see Figure 17-1). Chronic stretching of the pericardium results in hypertrophy and augmentation of the pericardial volume.

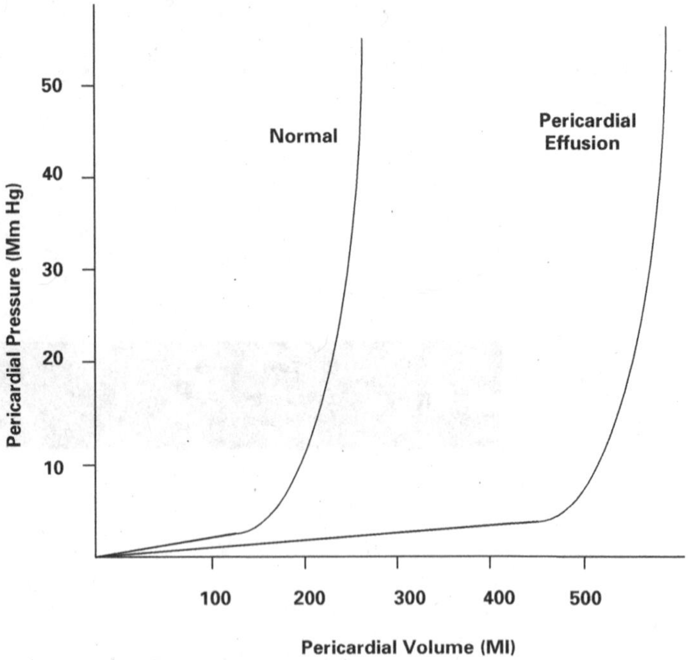

Figure 17-1. Pressure-volume relationship of the pericardium.

Congenital Pericardial Disease

Absence of Pericardium and Pericardial Defects

Absence of the pericardium is rare in dogs and cats. It does not precipitate clinical signs and is usually detected only at necropsy. Partial pericardial defects occur and represent a risk for cardiac herniation. Right atrial herniation through partial pericardial defects has been reported in dogs.[9,10]

Pericardial Cysts

Pericardial cysts have been described mostly in companion animals less than 3 years of age. Cysts are either unilocular or multilocular masses. On histologic analysis, they are thought to be cystic hematomas because they do not have an epithelial lining. In some cases, cysts were associated with a peritoneopericardial diaphramatic hernia. In other cases, cysts were on a stalk at the apex of the pericardium. This suggests that pericardial cysts result from entrapment of omentum, falciform ligament, or liver in the pericardium during development.[11-14] Dogs with pericardial cysts may show no clinical signs or may present with signs related to cardiac tamponade.

Acquired Pericardial Diseases

Pericardial Rupture

Traumatic rupture of the pericardium has been reported rarely in dogs.[10] Rupture of the pericardium after trauma (e.g., automobile accident or blunt thoracic trauma) likely occurs more frequently than it is diagnosed because it usually does not cause clinical signs. However, when the pericardium contracts around the herniated heart during healing, a stricture can develop that compresses the vena cava, causing a Budd Chiari syndrome with ascites and hepatomegaly, caval syndrome with swelling of the head and neck, or both.

Pericardial Effusion

Pericardial effusions are categorized by the clinical pathologic characteristics of the fluid. A transudate occurs secondary to congestive heart failure, peritoneopericardial diaphragmatic hernia, hypoalbuminemia, or increased vascular permeability.[15-22] An exudate results from infectious on noninfectious pericarditis.[17,23,24] Acute pericarditis is not associated with pericardial effusion.[2] Pericarditis has been associated with feline cardiomyopathy and feline infectious peritonitis.[17,25-28] Fungal pericarditis is unusual, with the exception of *Coccidioides immitis* in dogs living in the southwestern United States.[17,29] Renal failure can induce epicarditis and pericardial effusion in dogs.[30] Hemorrhagic pericardial effusion results from trauma, rupture of the left atrium secondary to mitral valve disease, intoxication with an anticoagulant, and neoplasia, or it may be idiopathic.[31-38] Idiopathic pericardial effusion is the most common cause of acute or chronic non-neoplastic hemorrhagic pericardial effusion in the dog.[15,16,20,29,37,38] Neoplasia of the heart, heart base, or pericardium is the second most common cause of hemorrhagic pericardial effusion in dogs. Hemangiosarcoma of the right atrium is the most common neoplasia. This tumor is often multicentric, involving the spleen or liver at the time of pericardial effusion. Chemodectoma is the second most common cardiac tumor and is most commonly seen in brachycephalic dogs. Mesothelioma of the pericardium is another cause of a hemorrhagic pericardial effusion.[15,18,20,22,23,27,37,39-43]

Cardiac Tamponade

The pericardium is fairly noncompliant, and pericardial pressure begins to rise after 5 to 60 ml of fluid accumulate within the pericardium (see Figure 17-1). The capacitance of the pericardium is influenced by the rate of fluid accumulation. Hypertrophy of the pericardium by slow stretching allows augmentation of pericardial volume and rightward shift of the pressure-volume curve of the pericardium. As a result, the pericardium can accumulate a larger volume of fluid before pressure begins to rise. However, beyond a certain point, pressure increases quickly with a small additional increase in volume. When the pericardium is thickened, as is the case with constrictive pericardial disease, a minor increase in volume causes a significant increase in pericardial pressure.[44-50]

The compensatory response to a pericardial effusion is an adrenergic stimulation and a parasympathetic withdrawal. It induces tachycardia and increased contractility.[2,51] Patients on beta-blocker therapy may not be able to show this response. Elevation in pericardial pressure increases diastolic pressure within the heart, which in turn reduces stroke volume. High pericardial pressure exerts its main effect on the right heart by impeding diastolic filling. The effect on the left side is secondary to decreased pulmonary venous return.[51-55] Because part of the vena cava is in the pericardial sac, increased pericardial pressure will directly affect blood flow in the vena cava. Pericardial pressure first equilibrates with right ventricular filling pressure (right-sided heart tamponade) and then with left ventricular filling pressure (left-sided heart tamponade). Right- and left-sided atrial and ventricular diastolic pressures raise and equilibrate at a pressure equivalent to the pressure in the pericardial sac (between 15 and 20 mm Hg). Cardiac output is significantly compromised and systemic venous pressure is elevated.[36,44-47,49,50] The small end-diastolic volume accounts for the small stroke volume. Compensatory mechanisms induce an augmentation in contractility, and a reduction of end-systolic volume, but not enough to normalize the stroke volume. Tachycardia is common as a reflex to maintain cardiac output. Also during cardiac tamponade, the flow of blood from the right atrium to the right ventricle is significantly reduced. Therefore, the y descent on the central venous pressure tracing is absent. Y descent is observed when the tricuspid valve opens. At this time no blood is leaving the heart, and because the right ventricle is fixed with a small volume, the y descent is lost. During cardiac tamponade, a transfer of blood volume occurs into the systemic circulation, resulting in a reduction of the pulmonary vascularity on thoracic radiographs.[56]

Decreased cardiac output results in activation of the renin-angiotensin-aldosterone system, causing retention of sodium and water. Activation of the sympathetic nervous system results in positive inotropic and chronotropic effects and vasoconstriction. Atrial natriuretic factor is not increased during cardiac tamponade to counteract the above effects because the atrium is still supported by the pericardium, which limits its dilation. As a result, cardiac tamponade is associated with increases in systemic venous and portal pressures, causing jugular distention and fluid transudation from systemic capillary beds to produce peripheral edema, liver congestion, and ascites.[36,44-47,49,50]

Arterial pressures may vary paradoxically with respiration during severe cardiac tamponade. During inspiration, pericardial pressure and right ventricular pressure decrease. Venous return to the right atrium and ventricle are increased. However, because the volume is limited by the pericardium, there is a leftward shift of the septum. Left ventricular end-diastolic volume is decreased, resulting in a reduction of cardiac output and arterial pressure during inspiration. This phenomenon, known as pulsus paradoxicus, is not a pathognomonic sign of cardiac tamponade. It can also occur with obstructive lung disease, restrictive cardiomyopathy, or hypovolemic shock.[36,44-47,49,50]

Constrictive Pericarditis

Constrictive pericarditis compromises cardiac filling by causing a non-distensible, thickened, and fibrotic pericardium. This condition has been reported in dogs aged from 3 to 10 years old.[57-59]

Chronic pericarditis resulting from any etiology can cause constrictive pericarditis. Chronic idiopathic pericardial effusion, neoplasia, foreign material (e.g., bullets), and infection (coccidiomycosis) are most commonly reported in cases with constrictive pericarditis.[58,59] In most cases, the parietal pericardium is more severely affected than the visceral pericardium. The parietal pericardium can be up to 8 mm thick. In some cases, the visceral and parietal pericardium are both affected, with severe adhesions between them. Pericardial fluid may be present, and if so, the condition is called effusive-constrictive pericarditis. Mesothelial proliferation, inflammation, and fibrosis are common findings on histopathology.[58-60]

Constrictive pericarditis affects late diastole. Early ventricular filling is normal and proceeds rapidly until the limit of pericardial distendibility is reached. The thickened, non-compliant pericardium abruptly limits ventricular filling in mid to late diastole. The atrial and ventricular pressure tracings classically show a rapid y descent followed by an abrupt rise to an elevated diastolic plateau. This is referred as the "square root sign" and is considered diagnostic for pericardial constriction (Figure 17-2). If a small amount of pericardial fluid is present, the rapid y descent is absent.

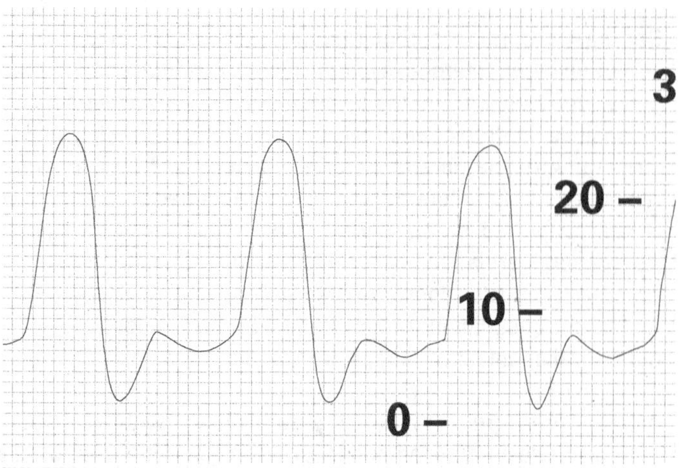

Figure 17-2. Constrictive pericarditis. Right ventricular pressure tracing showing the "square root sign" and an elevated end-diastolic pressure (8 mm Hg).

Pulmonary capillary wedge pressure, right ventricular diastolic pressures, right atrial, and left ventricular diastolic pressures are all elevated and equal with constrictive pericarditis. If localized fibrosis is affecting one cardiac chamber more than another, this hemodynamic occurrence may not be found. Also, if the patient is volume contracted from diuretics or other causes, volume loading with a crystalloid solution might be required to demonstrate these classic hemodynamic changes. As the condition worsens, cardiac output declines. Central venous pressure does not decrease during inspiration as normal because negative intrathoracic pressure during inspiration is not transmitted to the cardiac chambers. Changes of intrathoracic pressure are still transmitted to the pulmonary vasculature during respiration. During inspiration, the pressure gradient between the left atrium and the pulmonary circulation is reduced, resulting in less left atrial and ventricular filling. It results in an augmentation of right ventricular filling and deviation of the septum toward the left ventricle. The opposite occurs during expiration.[2,54] Augmentation of systemic venous pressure during inspiration with constrictive pericarditis is referred to as Kussmaul's sign.[2,60] High central venous pressure and reduced cardiac output result in compensatory retention of sodium and water by the kidney. Inhibition of the atrial natriuretic peptide (atrium cannot dilate) also contributes to the sodium retention. It further exacerbates increases in systemic, central venous, and left-sided filling pressures.

References

1. Shabetai R: The role of the pericardium in the pathophysiology of heart failure. *In* Congestive Heart Failure: Pathophysiology, Diagnosis, and Comprehensive Approach to Management. Hosenpud JD,Greenberg BH (eds). New York: Springer-Verlag, 1994, p. 95.

2. LeWinter MM, Kabbani S: Pericardial disease. *In* Braunwald's Heart Disease: A Textbook of Cardiovascular Medicine. Zipes DP, Libby P, Bonow RO, et al (eds). New York: Elsevier, 2005, p.1757.

3. Freeman GL, LeWinter MM: Determinants of intrapericardial pressure in dogs. J Appl Physiol 60:758, 1986.

4. deVries G, Hamilton DR, Ter Keurs HE, et al: A novel technique for measurement of pericardial pressure. Am J Physiol Heart Circ Physiol 280:H2815, 2001.

5. LeWinter MM, Pavelec R: Influence of the pericardium on left ventricular end-diastolic pressure-segment relations during early and later stages of experimental chronic volume overload in dogs. Circ Res 50:501, 1982.

6. Baker AE, Dani R, Smith ER, et al: Quantitative assessment of independent contributions of pericardium and septum to direct ventricular interaction. Am J Physiol 275:H476, 1998.

7. Santamore WP, Constantinescu MS, Bogen D, et al: Nonuniform distribution of normal pericardial fluid. Basic Res Cardiol 85:541, 1990.

8. Goto Y, LeWinter MM: Nonuniform regional deformation of the pericardium during the cardiac cycle in dogs. Circ Res 67:1107, 1990.

9. Gaag IV, Luer JT: Eight cases of pericardial defects in the dog. VetPathol 14:14, 1977.

10. Fine DM, Olivier NB, Walshaw R, et al: Surgical correction of late-onset Budd-Chiari-like syndrome in a dog. J Am Vet Med Assoc 212:835, 1998.

11. Less RD, Bright JM, Orton EC: Intrapericardial cyst causing cardiac tamponade in a cat. J Am Anim Hosp Assoc 36:115, 2000.

12. Marion J, Schwartz A, Ettinger S, et al: Pericardial effusion in a young dog. J Am Vet Med Assoc 157:1055, 1970.

13. Simpson DJ, Hunt GB, Church DB, et al: Benign masses in the pericardium of two dogs. Aust Vet J 77:225, 1999.

14. Sisson D, Thomas WP, Ruehl WW, et al: Diagnostic value of pericardial fluid analysis in the dog. J Am Vet Med Assoc 184:51, 1984.

15. Berg RJ, Wingfield W: Pericardial effusion in the dog: a review of 42 cases. J Am Anim Hosp Assoc 20:721, 1984.

16. Berg RJ, Wingfield WE, Hoopes PJ: Idiopathic hemorrhagic pericardial effusion in eight dogs. J Am Vet Med Assoc 185:988, 1984.

17. Bouvy BM, Bjorling DE: Pericardial effusion in dogs and cats. Part I. Normal pericardium and causes and pathyphysiology of pericardial effusion. Comp Cont Edu Pract Vet 13:417, 1991.

18. Brownlie SE, Clayton-Jones DG: Successful removal of a heart-base tumour in a dog with pericardial haemorrhagic effusion. J Small Anim Pract 26:191, 1985.

19. de Madron E, Prymak C, Hendricks J: Idiopathic hemorrhagic pericardial effusion with organized thrombi in a dog. J Am Vet Med Assoc 191:324, 1987.

20. Dunning D, Monnet E, Orton EC, et al: Analysis of prognostic indicators for dogs with pericardial effusion: 46 cases (1985-1996). J Am Vet Med Assoc 212:1276, 1998.

21. Lombard CW: Pericardial disease. Vet Clin North Am13:337, 1983.

22. De Madron E: Malignant pericardial effusion in dogs: seven cases clinical, electrocardiographic, radiographic, and echocardiographic aspects. Euro J Companion Anim Pract 1:52, 1991.

23. Aronson LR, Gregory CR: Infectious pericardial effusion in five dogs. Vet Surg 24:402, 1995.

24. Chastain CB, Greve JH, Riedesel DH: Pericardial effusion from granulomatous pleuritis and pericarditis in a dog. J Am Vet Med Assoc 164:1201, 1974.

25. Fossum TW, Miller MW, Rogers KS, et al: Chylothorax associated with right-sided heart failure in five cats. J Am Vet Med Assoc 204:84, 1994.

26. Owens JM: Pericardial effusion in the cat. Vet Clin North Am7:373, 1977.

27. Rush JE, Keene BW, Fox PR: Pericardial disease in the cat: a retrospective evaluation of 66 cases. J Am Anim Hosp Assoc 26:39. 1990.

28. Vacirca G, Mantelli F, Ferro E, et al: Pericardial effusion with feline infectious peritonitis. Companion Anim Pract 19:25, 1989.

29. Miller MW, Sisson DD: Pericardial disorders. *In* Textbook of Veterinary Internal Medicine, 5th ed. Ettinger SJ (ed). Philadelphia: WB Saunders, 2000, p. 923.

30. Madewell BR, Norrdin RW: Renal failure associated with pericardial effusion in a dog. J Am Vet Med Assoc 167:1091, 1975.

31. Berry CR, Lombard CW, Hager DA, et al: Pericardial effusion secondary to chronic endocardiosis and left atrial rupture in a dog. Comp Cont Edu Pract Vet 10:800, 1988.

32. Berry CR, Lombard CW, Hager DA et al: Echocardiographic evaluation of cardiac tamponade in dogs before and after pericardiocentesis: Four cases (1984-1986). J Am Vet Med Assoc 192:1597, 1988.

33. Buchanan JW, Botts RP: Clinical effects of repeated cardiac punctures in dogs. J Am Vet Med Assoc;161:814, 1972.

34. Kagan KG: Thoracic trauma. Vet Clin North Am 10:641, 1980.

35. Petrus DJ, Henik RA: Pericardial effusion and cardiac tamponade secondary to brodifacoum toxicosis in a dog. J Am Vet Med Assoc 215:647, 1999.

36. Price EK, Mullen PA: A case of haemopericardium in the dog. Vet Rec 78:480, 1966.

37. Vogtli T, Gaschen F, Vogtli-Burger R, et al: Hemorrhagic pericardial effusion in dogs. A retrospective study of 10 cases (1989-1994) with a review of the literature. Schweiz Arch Tierheilkd 139:217, 1997.

38. Weisse C, Soares N, Beal MW, et al: Survival times in dogs with right atrial hemangiosarcoma treated by means of surgical resection with or without adjuvant chemotherapy: 23 cases (1986-2000). J Am Vet Med Assoc 226:575, 2005.

39. Berg J: Pericardial disease and cardiac neoplasia. Semin Vet Med Surg (Small Anim) 9:185, 1994.

40. Bradley GA, Tye J, Lozano-Alarcon F, et al: Hemopericardium in a dog due to hemorrhage originating in a heart base thymic remnant. J Vet Diagn Invest4:211, 1992.

41. Closa JM, Font A, Mascort J: Pericardial mesothelioma in a dog: long-term survival after pericardiectomy in combination with chemotherapy. J Small Anim Pract 40:383, 1999.

42. Gonin-Jmaa D, Paulsen DB, Taboada J: Pericardial effusion in a dog with rhabdomyosarcoma in the right ventricular wall. J Small Anim Pract 37:193, 1996.

43. Madron E: Seven cases of pericardial effusion of cancerous origin in dogs. Clinical, electrocardiographic, radiographic and echocardiographic aspects. PMCAC 25:59, 1990.

44. Ameli S, Shah PK: Cardiac tamponade. Pathophysiology, diagnosis, and management. Cardiol Clin 9:665, 1991.

45. Fowler NO: Pulsus paradoxus. Heart Dis Stroke 3:68, 1994.

46. Hancock EW: Cardiac tamponade. Heart Dis Stroke 3:155, 1994.

47. Kirkland LL, Taylor RW: Pericardiocentesis. Crit Care Clin 8:699, 1992.

48. Reddy PS, Curtiss EI: Cardiac tamponade. Cardiol Clin 8:627, 1990.

49. Rodgers KG: Cardiovascular shock. Emerg Med Clin North Am 13:793, 1995.

50. Spodick DH: Pathophysiology of cardiac tamponade [published erratum appears in Chest 1998 Aug;114(2):662]. Chest 113:1372, 1998.

51. Spodick DH: Acute cardiac tamponade. N Engl J Med 349:684, 2003.

52. Fowler NO, Gabel M, Buncher CR: Cardiac tamponade: a comparison of right versus left heart compression. J Am Coll Cardiol 12:187, 1988.

53. Singh S, Wann LS, Schuchard GH, et al: Right ventricular and right atrial collapse in patients with cardiac tamponade--a combined echocardiographic and hemodynamic study. Circulation 70:966, 1984.

54. Oh JK, Hatle LK, Seward JB, et al: Diagnostic role of Doppler echocardiography in constrictive pericarditis. J Am Coll Cardiol 23:154, 1994.

55. Merce J, Sagrista-Sauleda J, Permanyer-Miralda G, et al: Correlation between clinical and Doppler echocardiographic findings in patients with moderate and large pericardial effusion: implications for the diagnosis of cardiac tamponade. Am Heart J 138:759, 1999.

56. Ditchey R, Engler R, LeWinter M, et al: The role of the right heart in acute cardiac tamponade in dogs. Circ Res 48:701, 1981.

57. Campbell SL, Forrester SD, Johnston SA, et al: Chylothorax associated with constrictive pericarditis in a dog. J Am Vet Med Assoc 206:1561, 1995.

58. Thomas WP, Reed JR, Bauer TG, et al: Constrictive pericardial disease in the dog. J Am Vet Med Assoc 184:546, 1984.

59. Wright KN, DeNovo RCJ, Patton CS, et al: Effusive-constrictive pericardial disease secondary to osseous metaplasia of the pericardium in a dog. J Am Vet Med Assoc209:2091, 1996.

60. Sisson D, Thomas WP: Pericardial disease and cardiac tumors. *In* Textbook of Canine and Feline Cardiology, 2nd ed. Fox PR, Sisson D, Moise NS (eds). Philadelphia: WB Saunders, 1999, p. 679.

Chapter 18

Perioperative Cardiac Arrhythmias

Janice McIntosh Bright

For every affection...that is attended with either pain or pleasure, hope or fear, is the cause of an agitation whose influence extends to the heart.
--- Sir William Harvey, 1628

That emotion and stress may affect the heart was recognized by William Harvey over three centuries ago. Stresses encountered by surgical patients predispose them to a variety of cardiac rhythm disturbances. Because these rhythm disturbances can contribute to morbidity and mortality, it is important to anticipate and avoid them when possible. When not possible, early recognition and intervention are usually advantageous. Monitoring heart rate and rhythm during and after surgery is, consequently, of utmost importance. Anesthesiologists and surgeons must be aware of normal variations of rate and rhythm in healthy anesthetized animals. In addition, they must be familiar with specific pathologic arrhythmias and appropriate treatment interventions for clinically significant rhythm perturbations. This chapter provides an overview of the identification and management of common perioperative arrhythmias. Other sources should be consulted for a discussion of arrhythmogenic properties of various preanesthetic and anesthetic agents.[1]

Risk Factors

Animals with a history of arrhythmia are at increased risk for recurrence or exacerbation of the arrhythmia during the perioperative period. Similarly, patients with preexisting structural heart disease are at risk of developing significant intraoperative and postoperative cardiac rate and rhythm abnormalities. The preoperative assessment of these animals should, therefore, include a complete cardiac evaluation, including Doppler/echocardiography, electrocardiography (ECG), thoracic radiographs, and blood pressure measurement. The data obtained from this evaluation is critical for choosing the safest anesthetic protocol and the most appropriate antiarrhythmic agents. A preoperative ECG in cats older than seven years of age is helpful for detecting the presence of left anterior fascicular block, which is a silent ECG abnormality often associated with myocardial disease in this species.

In people, risk factors identified for development of supraventricular tachyarrhythmias include advancing age, a previous history of supraventricular arrhythmia, type of surgery (intraabdominal, intrathoracic, or major vascular surgery), and preexisting congestive heart failure or chronic lung disease.[2] Risk factors for development of supraventricular arrhythmia in dogs during the perioperative period include atrial enlargement and a history of previous supraventricular ectopy. Furthermore, giant breeds and Labrador retrievers are predisposed.

Perioperative ventricular arrhythmias are strongly associated with underlying myocardial dysfunction or contusion, splenic surgeries, pheochromocytoma, hyperthyroidism, and surgery to correct gastric dilation/volvulus. Patients with preoperative ventricular tachyarrhythmias are also at high risk for intraoperative and postoperative ventricular ectopy. Animals receiving β-adrenergic antagonists preoperatively may develop either supraventricular or ventricular tachyarrhythmias associated with β-blocker withdrawal if these agents have been recently and abruptly discontinued.

An important bradyarrhythmia that must be anticipated preoperatively is the development of increasing severity of atrioventricular (AV) block in animals with conduction system disease. Bradyarrhythmias resulting from enhanced vagal tone occur frequently in animals with upper airway obstruction, those undergoing surgery of the cervical spine, and animals with increased intracranial pressure.

General Approach for Management of Perioperative Arrhythmias

Abnormalities of cardiac rate and rhythm that occur while the patient is anesthetized are often the result of alterations in depth of anesthesia. Arrhythmias may also occur under anesthesia as a result of autonomic imbalance and catecholamine release; direct effects of anesthetic agents including analgesics, muscle relaxants, and reversal agents; hypothermia (and rarely hyperthermia); and mechanical stimulation secondary to invasive procedures and surgical manipulation. All of these factors must be considered and specific interventions taken to alleviate the causative mechanism(s). Other factors involved in arrhythmogenesis during the intraoperative period include electrolyte abnormalities, acid-base disturbances, volume depletion, release of toxic metabolites, and myocardial ischemia. Again, these factors must be specifically treated to appropriately manage the resulting arrhythmias.

Although cardiac arrhythmias are common in the postoperative period, most are clinically benign, such as sinus bradycardia, sinus pauses, accelerated idioventricular rhythm, isorhythmic AV dissociation, and isolated ventricular premature contractions (VPCs). Tachycardia in the immediate postoperative period may reflect the sympathetic activation associated with recovery. However, in addition to anesthetic emergence, both supraventricular and ventricular tachyarrhythmias in the postoperative period may reflect hypoxemia, hypercarbia, acidosis, toxemia, hypovolemia, blood loss, electrolyte imbalances, fear, pain, or a combination of these factors. Residual effects of anesthetic agents such as ketamine may also play a role. Again, treatment should be directed at identification and reversal of underlying causative factors; however, antiarrhythmic therapy may be needed when the primary cause of a potentially fatal arrhythmia cannot be identified or quickly corrected. In summary, the following general approach for management of perioperative arrhythmias is proffered:

1) Have a precise ECG diagnosis for the arrhythmia, if possible.

2) Specifically treat noncardiac causes (e.g., electrolyte abnormalities, hypothermia, acidosis, hypovolemia, hypoxemia, pain, fear) before using an antiarrhythmic medication unless hemodynamic or electrical instability are present.
3) Consider discontinuing drugs that may be causing or contributing to the arrhythmia.

Identification and Management of Common Perioperative Tachyarrhythmias

Sinus Tachycardia

Post-anesthetic sinus tachycardia (canine > 180 beats/minute; feline > 240 beats/minute) may often result from the anesthetic agents used, including atropine, glycopyrrolate, ketamine, or adrenergic agonists. Sinus tachycardia in the perioperative period is rarely, if ever, a true cardiac arrhythmia, but, rather, a reflection of increased sympathetic tone, which may arise from a wide variety of pathologic and/or physiologic causes. Physiologic causes include excitement, stress, and fear. Pathologic causes include pain, hypovolemia, anemia, acidosis, hypoxemia, fever, hyperthermia, toxemia, cardiac failure, hypercapnia, hypotension, acute hemorrhage, and hyperthyroidism.

Treatment of sinus tachycardia should be directed at identification and correction of the underlying cause of the heightened adrenergic tone. Antiarrhythmic agents are rarely indicated and are often detrimental.

Atrial Fibrillation and Atrial Flutter

Atrial fibrillation and atrial flutter are common postoperative arrhythmias in human patients,[3] but development of either of these arrhythmias postoperatively is less common in dogs and extremely rare in cats. When atrial fibrillation and atrial flutter are noted in animals in the perioperative setting, these arrhythmias are usually present preoperatively. Nonetheless, both arrhythmias are clinically important because both may decrease cardiac output secondary to inappropriately fast heart rates that reduce stroke volume. Furthermore, atrial fibrillation abolishes the atrial contribution to ventricular filling and may, thereby, decrease cardiac output by as much as 39% while increasing left atrial pressure by as much as 9.5 mm Hg in otherwise healthy dogs.[4]

On ECG, atrial fibrillation is recognized by absence of P waves and completely irregular R-R intervals (Figure 18-1). Rapid, irregular fibrillatory waves that vary in size, shape, and timing are often visible. The QRS complexes are normal unless an intraventricular conduction abnormality is also present (e.g., right or left bundle branch block). The ventricular rate will depend on conduction velocity and refractoriness of the AV node and may be normal in dogs without structural heart disease. However, heart rate is typically very rapid in dogs and cats with heart failure as well as those with high circulating levels of catecholamines. In animals with atrial fibrillation that have been receiving oral medication for rate control, the heart rate often drops significantly following induction of anesthesia.

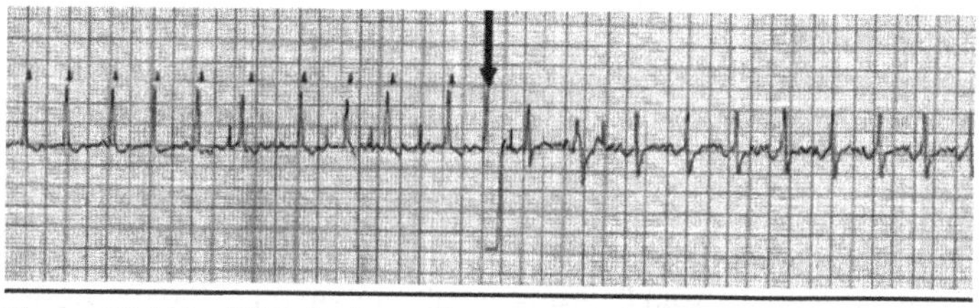

Figure 18-1. An ECG rhythm strip recorded during direct current (DC) cardioversion of atrial fibrillation in a dog with laryngeal paralysis. Atrial fibrillation is recognized as the underlying cardiac rhythm in the initial portion of the ECG by absence of P waves and completely irregular R-R intervals. Fibrillatory waves are present in the baseline. Prior to delivery of the synchronized electrical shock (at large arrow), the cardioversion device identifies QRS complexes with small arrows. As a result of the shock, normal sinus rhythm is restored. (lead II; 25 mm/s)

Management of atrial fibrillation is initially aimed at controlling heart rate. Intravenous calcium channel blockers or β-blockers are effective for slowing conduction through the AV node and can rapidly provide control of the ventricular response in patients with atrial fibrillation (Table 18-1). These drugs may be administered by bolus injection but require maintenance infusions or follow-up oral dosing to maintain adequate rate control. When continuous infusions are administered, blood pressure and heart rate should be closely monitored because these medications may cause hypotension and bradycardia. Because of the negative inotropic effects of β-blockers or calcium channel blockers, patients with myocardial systolic dysfunction may develop congestive heart failure or worsening of congestive heart failure after administration of these agents. Oral digoxin is used extensively for chronic heart rate control in dogs with atrial fibrillation because this drug will increase parasympathetic tone to the AV node with a resultant slowing of AV nodal conduction. However, in the postoperative period, sympathetic tone is often excessive, rendering this drug less effective in this setting. Furthermore, digoxin toxicity can cause nearly every known cardiac rhythm disturbance, and animals receiving digoxin may develop digoxin-induced arrhythmias in the perioperative setting if hypovolemia, hypoalbuminemia, or electrolyte depletion is induced by surgery or anesthesia.

Restoration of sinus rhythm with a synchronized direct current shock (DC cardioversion) has several advantages over heart rate control for management of atrial fibrillation in animals needing surgery. The cardioversion may be done immediately after induction of anesthesia, obviating the need to administer negative inotropic agents for rate control. Also, restoring sinus rhythm immediately after induction of anesthesia will improve cardiac performance and reduce ventricular filling pressures throughout the remainder of the anesthetic period and recovery.

Although similar to atrial fibrillation, atrial flutter is less common in veterinary patients. With atrial flutter the ECG recorded will show rapid, organized atrial activation with an abnormally rapid ventricular rate unless the patient is receiving medication to control heart rate or unless AV conduction block is also present. Unlike atrial fibrillation, the ventricular rate is usually regular. Although a "saw-toothed" pattern of flutter waves is typically described, this pattern of atrial activation may be difficult to appreciate when 2:1 AV conduction is present, and the arrhythmia may, therefore, be difficult to distinguish from other types of supraventricular arrhythmia. With administration of calcium channel blockers or β-blockers, or with induction of anesthesia, the flutter waves usually become easily visible. Management of atrial flutter is similar to management of atrial fibrillation, although rate control is often more difficult. DC cardioversion of atrial flutter is usually achieved at lower energy levels than those needed for cardioversion of atrial fibrillation.

Occasionally, atrial fibrillation and atrial flutter will develop in the postoperative period as a result of autonomic imbalance. This is recognized most frequently in patients that have had surgery on or trauma to the cervical spine. In this situation, the arrhythmias are often self-limiting with no treatment required (Figure 18-2).

Table 18-1. Drugs used for Acute Management of Tachyarrhythmias

Drug	Dose	Comments
Calcium channel blockers		
Diltiazem	Dog, Cat: 0.25 mg/kg IV bolus (may be repeated once after 3 minutes); then 2-6 μg/kg/min PRN	monitor for hypotension & bradycardia; may exacerbate congestive heart failure in animals with impaired myocardial function
Verapamil	Dog: 0.05 mg/kg IV (slow bolus) q 15-20 min PRN (up to 0.15 mg/kg total dose)	(Same as diltiazem)
Beta-blockers		
Esmolol	Dog, Cat: 50-100 μg/kg IV bolus q 5 min PRN (up to 500 μg/kg max); 50-200 μg/kg/min infusion	ultrashort acting; monitor for hypotension & bradycardia; may exacerbate congestive heart failure; reduced efficacy if β-agonists administered
Propranolol	Dog, Cat: 0.01-0.1 mg/kg IV (slow bolus)	monitor for hypotension & bradycardia; may exacerbate congestive heart failure; reduced efficacy if β-agonists administered; may induce bronchospasm
Digoxin	Dog: 0.0025 mg/kg IV bolus; repeat hourly 3-4 times up to 0.01 mg/kg	vagomimetic; toxicity enhanced by cachexia, renal dysfunction hypokalemia, hyponatremia, hypercalcemia, hyperthyroidism, hypoxemia, myocardial failure; many drug interactions
Lidocaine (without epinephrine)	Dog: 2-4 mg/kg IV bolus over 5 min (administer 2 mg/kg boluses slowly); then 40-80 μg/kg/min IV infusion Cat: 0.25-1.0 mg/kg IV bolus over 5 min (or 1 mg boluses, max of 4 mg, over 5 min); then 10-40 μg/kg/min IV infusion	serum [K^+] and serum [Mg^{++}] must be normal for max efficacy
Procainamide	Dog: 6-10 mg/kg slowly IV bolus to effect; then 25-50 μg/kg/min IV infusion Cat: (No data available for parenteral dosing)	serum [K^+] and serum [Mg^{++}] must be normal for max efficacy
Amiodarone	Dog: 2.5-5.0 mg/kg IV bolus over 2-5 min	Avoid preparations with polysorbate 80 and benzyl alcohol

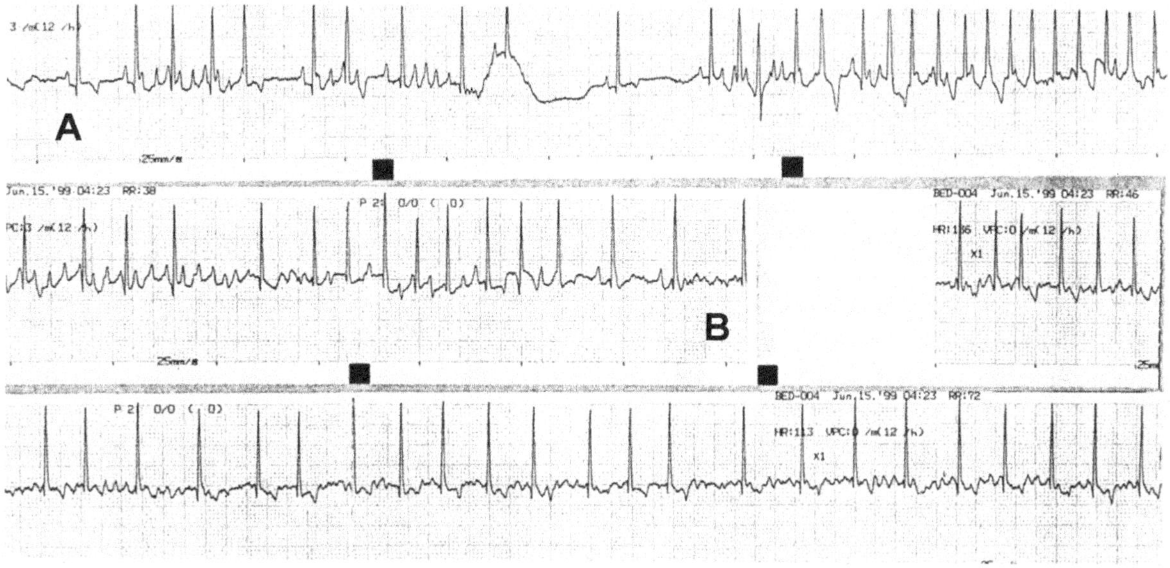

Figure 18-2. Continuous ECG rhythm strips obtained from a Labrador retriever during the early postoperative period following hemilaminectomy. Initially, the rhythm strip (A) shows sinus arrhythmia with brief paroxysms of atrial flutter. Ultimately (B), the rhythm degenerates to atrial fibrillation. This dog spontaneously converted to sinus rhythm within 24 hours, suggesting that the arrhythmias resulted from autonomic imbalance caused by surgical manipulation and stress. (lead II; 25 mm/s)

Paroxysmal Supraventricular Tachycardias

Although the term supraventricular tachycardia (SVT) in its broadest sense refers to any tachycardia originating above the ventricles, this term is generally reserved to describe supraventricular tachyarrhythmias other than sinus tachycardia, atrial fibrillation, or atrial flutter.

Paroxysmal SVT owing to impulse reentry in the AV node, impulse reentry within atrial tissue, or impulse reentry via an accessory atrioventricular conduction pathway has a similar ECG appearance, namely a rapid tachycardia with narrow (normal) QRS complexes (Figure 18-3). The QRS complexes will be abnormally wide, however, if there is intraventricular conduction delay such as right or left bundle branch block or when conduction from atria to ventricles occurs over an accessory conduction pathway. Regardless of the anatomic location of the reentry pathway, any of these SVTs may occur in the perioperative setting, causing a very rapid heart rate with hypotension. SVTs may occur in any age group and often are not associated with structural heart disease. These tachycardias are usually associated with enhanced adrenergic tone as well as with triggers such as premature atrial contractions or premature ventricular contractions. When paroxysmal, these SVTs begin and terminate abruptly (lack of gradual rate acceleration and deceleration).

The specific type of paroxysmal SVT can theoretically be identified from a multiple lead ECG (including chest leads) by evaluating P′ wave morphology and timing. However, P′ waves may be extremely difficult to identify with certainty during a rapid SVT. Furthermore, during anesthetic induction, surgery, or in the immediate recovery period, available ECG monitoring equipment is often not conducive to examination of multiple-lead ECG recordings. While vagal maneuvers may be helpful both diagnostically and therapeutically, many animals do not respond to them. Furthermore, aggressive vagal maneuvers may, on occasion, produce ventricular fibrillation. Therefore, administration of intravenous antiarrhythmic agents is generally a safer, more effective means of differentiating and treating SVTs. Ideally, blood pressure and ECG monitoring are done as antiarrhythmic agents are administered. Diltiazem is the drug of choice for initial treatment because of its ability to rapidly slow the ventricular response to atrial tachyarrhythmias, and for terminating most AV nodal and AV reciprocating tachycardias (see Table 18-1). Diltiazem has a negative inotropic effect and must be used cautiously in animals with myocardial failure; however, diltiazem has a less potent negative inotropic effect than verapamil or esmolol.[5] Although adenosine is used to terminate SVT in human patients, this agent does not appear to be effective for this purpose in dogs. Procainamide, a class IA antiarrhythmic, may also be administered intravenously for management for supraventricular tachyarrhythmias in dogs (see Table 18-1). This agent is most appropriately used after administering diltiazem and is useful for terminating atrial reentrant tachycardias and atrioventricular reentrant tachycardias.

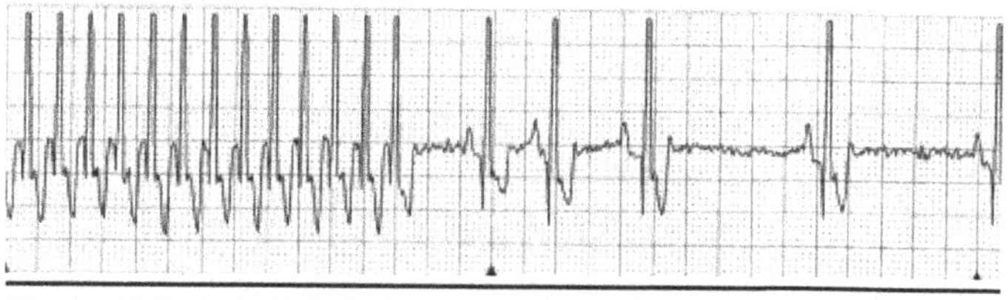

Figure 18-3. A lead II ECG rhythm strip obtained from a 1–year-old golden retriever. The ECG shows supraventricular tachycardia with a rate of 300 beats/minute. Abrupt conversion to sinus rhythm resulted from intravenous administration of diltiazem (0.25 mg/kg). Note that the QRS complexes during the arrhythmia are normal and identical to those during sinus rhythm. (lead II; 25 mm/s)

Ventricular Tachyarrhythmias

Perioperative ventricular ectopy may include relatively benign conditions such as ventricular premature contractions (VPCs) and accelerated idioventricular rhythm or potentially lethal arrhythmias such as sustained ventricular tachycardia (VT) and ventricular fibrillation (VF). The appearance of ventricular ectopy of any type should prompt measures to eliminate inciting factors such as hypoxemia, hypercarbia, electrolyte deficiencies, drug toxicities, and catecholamine excess. Antiarrhythmic therapy is indicated when the inciting cause cannot be identified or immediately reversed and the arrhythmia is responsible for hemodynamic compromise. Antiarrhythmic treatment is also indicated in animals at risk for sudden death triggered by fatal electrical instability.[6,7] In one postoperative study of 230 consecutive human patients with frequent VPCs or VT, adverse outcomes were not associated with the arrhythmias.[8] The adverse effects of ventricular arrhythmias in veterinary surgical patients has also been questioned, and the empiric use of antiarrhythmic agents has been challenged.[6,7] The decision that a ventricular arrhythmia is dangerous and should be suppressed with antiarrhythmic medication is based on the presence of weakness, syncope, hypotension, pallor, or exacerbation of heart failure directly attributable to the arrhythmia. Ventricular tachycardias vary in rate, morphology, and duration, and rate is generally the most important determinant of hemodynamic consequences. In general, the slower the rate of VT, the more benign the arrhythmia will be. In absence of clinical signs linked to the arrhythmia, the following characteristics of VT justify suppression with antiarrhythmic agents: rapid VT (rate appreciably greater than underlying sinus rate), sustained VT (> 30 seconds), VT with a short coupling interval to preceding sinus complex, and polymorphic VT. Furthermore, because of the known tendency for sudden death from ventricular ectopy, suppression of VPCs and VT is justified in boxers, Doberman pinschers, German shepherds, dogs with subaortic stenosis, and animals with significant myocardial dysfunction.

Ventricular premature contractions (VPCs) are identified on the ECG as wide QRS complexes that differ from the sinus complexes and occur prematurely (Figure 18-4). VPCs are frequently followed by a compensatory pause caused by retrograde conduction of the VPC into the His-Purkinje system with either block of the subsequent sinus beat or with retrograde conduction to the atrium resetting the sinus node. Ventricular ectopic complexes are classified as monomorphic or polymorphic according to whether the QRS complexes are uniform or variable. Ventricular tachycardia is defined as three or more consecutive ventricular premature beats (see Figure 18-4). VPCs may be difficult to distinguish from aberrantly conducted supraventricular beats; however, the presence of P waves that are not associated with QRS complexes or the presence of fusion beats indicates ventricular ectopy. It is also helpful to recall that ventricular tachycardia occurs much more frequently than supraventricular tachycardia with aberrancy. Ventricular tachycardia, particularly VT that is rapid, sustained, and polymorphic, may degenerate to ventricular fibrillation which is a rapid, chaotic, wide complex rhythm with absence of adequate cardiac output.

Ventricular tachycardia resulting in hemodynamic compromise (hypoperfusion or hypotension) should be treated immediately with DC cardioversion. Antiarrhythmic therapy can be administered to prevent a recurrence or as the initial therapy to terminate the VT in hemodynamically stable patients at risk for progression to hemodynamic instability. For veterinary patients, the antiarrhythmic agent of choice for immediate suppression of ventricular ectopy is lidocaine. This agent is highly effective with few side effects[3] (see Table 18-1). If lidocaine is not effective, substitution or addition of intravenous procainamide may provide arrhythmia suppression. Procainamide administration is particularly appealing when the ECG diagnosis of a wide complex tachycardia is uncertain. For refractory ventricular arrhythmias during the perioperative period, β-adrenergic blockers are often effective, particularly when combined with a class IA or IB antiarrhythmic agent, because the β-blockade antagonizes increased circulating catecholamines caused by stress. Regardless of the underlying mechanism of the ventricular arrhythmia, increased sympathetic tone can trigger the arrhythmia. Furthermore, adrenergic stimulation can render many antiarrhythmic drugs ineffective. Similarly, most antiarrhythmic agents are ineffective in the presence of hypokalemia or hypomagnesemia.

Amiodarone is now available for intravenous treatment of life-threatening VT and is recommended as a first line treatment for

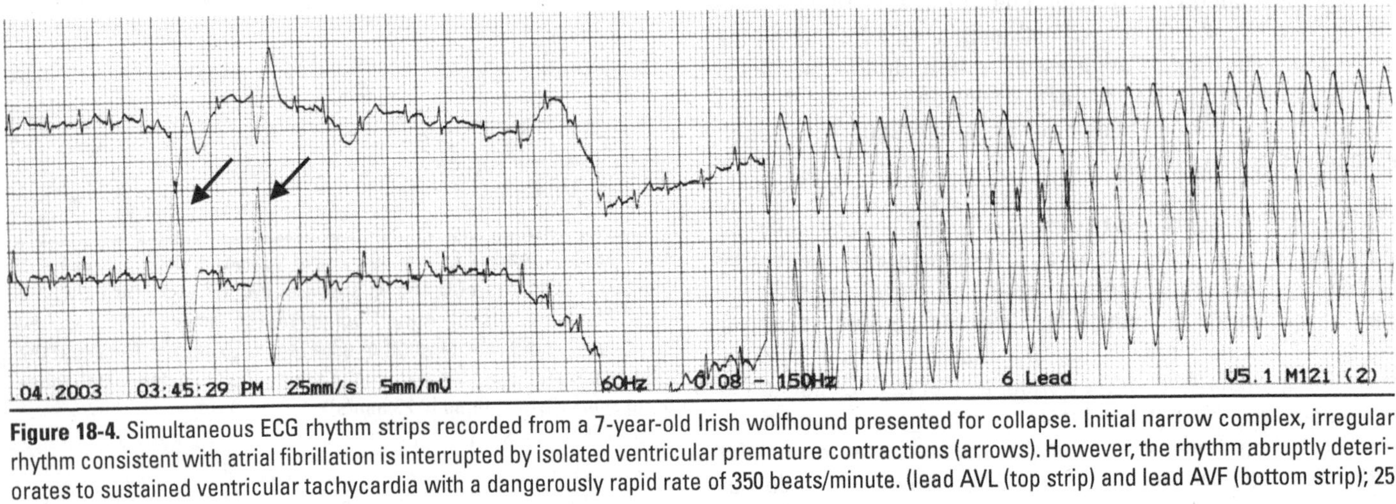

Figure 18-4. Simultaneous ECG rhythm strips recorded from a 7-year-old Irish wolfhound presented for collapse. Initial narrow complex, irregular rhythm consistent with atrial fibrillation is interrupted by isolated ventricular premature contractions (arrows). However, the rhythm abruptly deteriorates to sustained ventricular tachycardia with a dangerously rapid rate of 350 beats/minute. (lead AVL (top strip) and lead AVF (bottom strip); 25 mm/s; 5 mm/mV)

pulseless VT in people.[9] However, the most readily available intravenous preparation of amiodarone (Cordarone, Wyeth Laboratories Inc, Philadelphia, PA) contains polysorbate 80 and benzyl alcohol, both of which cause severe hypotension in dogs.[10,11] A newer aqueous formulation of amiodarone (Amio-Aqueous, Academic Pharmaceuticals Inc, Lake Bluff, IL) does not contain these agents and is better suited for dogs. Ventricular fibrillation should be managed by immediate DC defibrillation.

Accelerated Idioventricular Rhythm

Accelerated idioventricular rhythm develops frequently in dogs and cats during the intraoperative and postoperative periods. This arrhythmia is actually slow ventricular tachycardia, ventricular tachycardia at a rate slower than the sinus rate in a normal animal. Therefore, by heart rate criteria alone, this rhythm is not a tachycardia. Yet, because the ectopic ventricular focus responsible for the arrhythmia is depolarizing at a rate faster than a normal ventricular escape focus can depolarize, this rhythm is truly a ventricular tachycardia. Nonetheless, because the rate is slow, this form of VT is often referred to as accelerated idioventricular rhythm. The clinical importance of this terminology is that an accelerated idioventricular rhythm is usually benign whereas rapid VT is often malignant. The specific rates at which accelerated idioventricular rhythm becomes "true" ventricular tachycardia have not been precisely defined for dogs and cats. However, heart rates exceeding 180 beats/minute in dogs with VT and heart rates greater than 240 beats/minute in cats are most likely to be harmful.

Accelerated idioventricular rhythm often occurs in the perioperative setting in animals without underlying cardiac disease. This arrhythmia is frequent in dogs after gastric dilation/volvulus surgery, in dogs following splenic surgery, and in dogs with any type of abdominal disease (e.g., pancreatitis, prostatitis, enteritis, colitis). Accelerated idioventricular rhythm is also common in dogs with neurologic disease and with trauma.[12] Accelerated idioventricular rhythm in animals without underlying primary cardiac disease is nearly always benign, and antiarrhythmic treatment, in most cases, is unjustified.

On ECG, accelerated idioventricular rhythm is recognized as intermittent ventricular tachycardia that has a rate similar to or slightly greater than the sinus rate. The ventricular rhythm competes for the cardiac rhythm, meaning that the ventricular rhythm is apparent when the sinus rate slows or during sinus pauses (Figure 18-5). Although accelerated idioventricular rhythm usually has a uniform morphology, multiform ventricular complexes may occasionally be present.

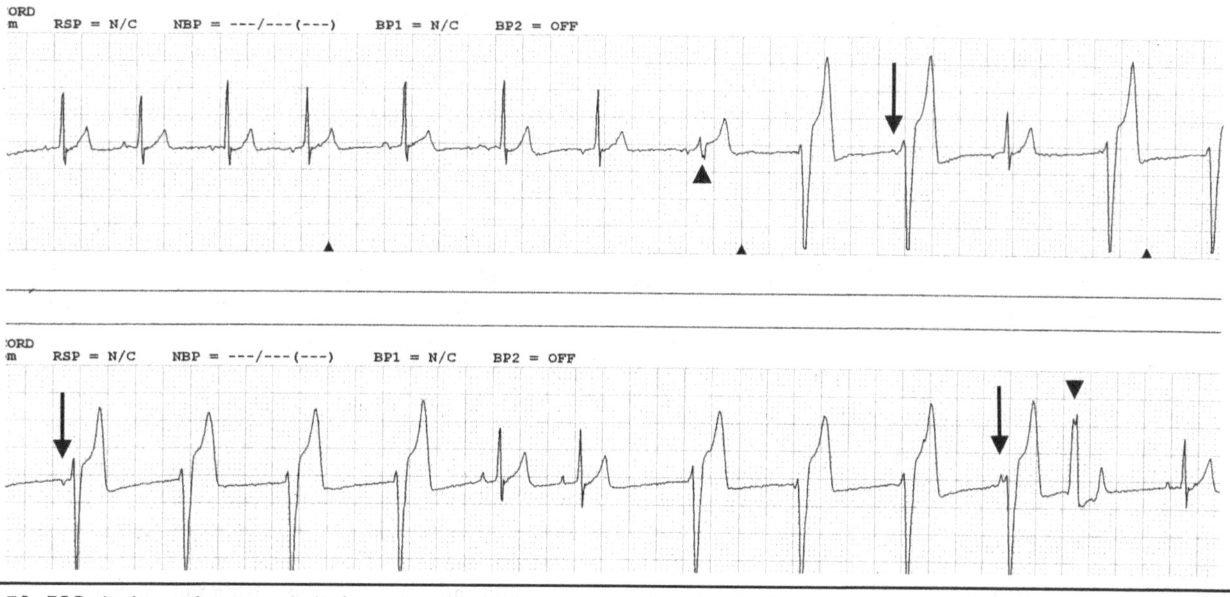

Figure 18-5A. ECG rhythm strips recorded after splenectomy from a canine patient. A sinus arrhythmia is present with wandering pacemaker during which the sinus rate varies from 83 to 107 beats/minute. The sinus arrhythmia is usurped intermittently by a wide QRS complex rhythm with a regular rate of 79 beats/minute. This wide complex rhythm is a slow ventricular tachycardia referred to as accelerated idioventricular rhythm. The idioventricular rhythm is evident only when the sinus rate drops below the ventricular ectopic rate. P waves unassociated with the QRS complexes are visible intermittently during the ventricular rhythm (arrows). Occasional fusion beats are present (arrow heads). (lead II; 25 mm/s)

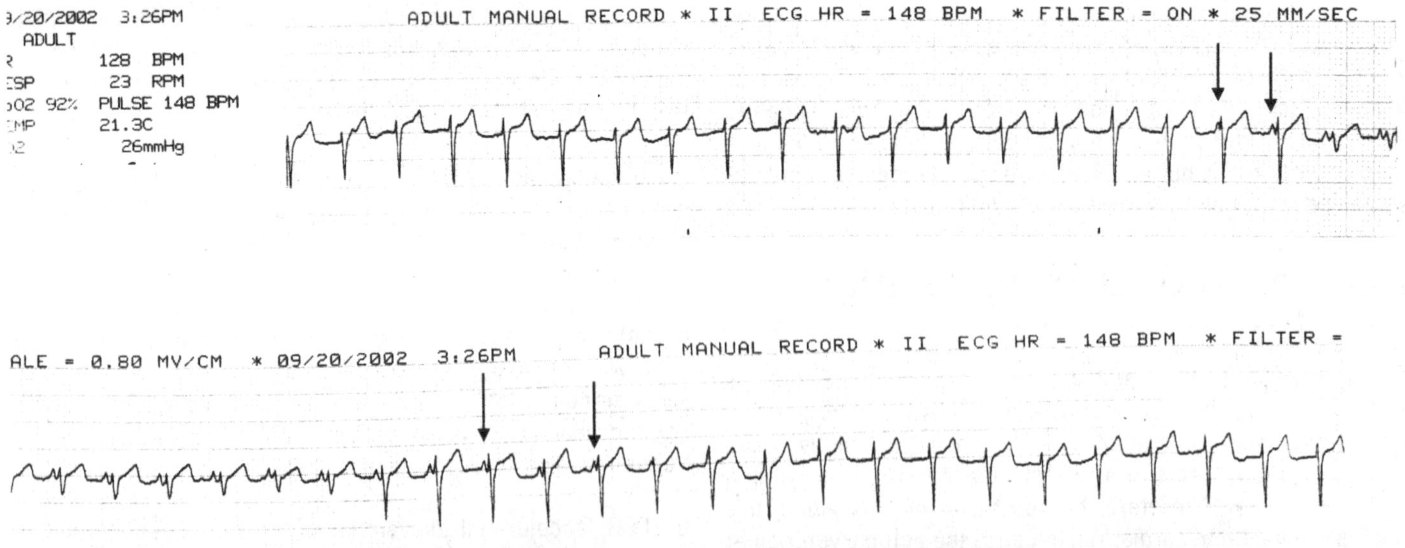

Figure 18-5B. ECG rhythm strip recorded from an anesthetized cat showing accelerated idioventricular rhythm. The cat was undergoing a subtotal colectomy. Initially a wide complex rhythm is seen with a regular rate of 142 beats/minute, during which P waves, unassociated with QRS complexes, are intermittently seen (arrows). Between the episodes of idioventricular rhythm is sinus rhythm with a similar rate (142 beats/minute). The accelerated idioventricular rhythm competes with the sinus rate as the dominant rhythm. (lead II; 25 mm/s)

Identification and Management of Perioperative Bradyarrhythmias

Bradyarrhythmias seldom cause significant problems in the perioperative period, and antiarrhythmic treatment is rarely indicated. Patients with symptomatic bradycardia resulting from disease of the cardiac pacing or conduction system should be evaluated for permanent pacemaker implantation prior to elective surgery. For patients with AV block or sinus node dysfunction without clinical signs or for those needing emergency surgery, temporary transvenous or transcutaneous pacing should be available. In the intraoperative and postoperative settings, bradycardia may signify a potentially serious underlying problem that requires specific intervention such as hypoxemia, hypothermia, surgical manipulation of the autonomic nervous system, excessive anesthetic depth, cardiac ischemia, hyperkalemia, increased intrathoracic pressure associated with pneumothorax, or drug toxicity (e.g., from opioids, α2-adrenergic agonists, digoxin, β-adrenergic antagonists, calcium channel blockers, halothane, or vagomimetic agents)[2,13,14] Profound sinus bradycardia and asystole have been described in association with spinal anesthesia in humans.[2]

Sinus bradycardia (sinus rhythm with rate < 60 beats/minute in dogs), sinus arrhythmia, and sinus pauses are common in healthy large and giant breed dogs with strong vagal tone. These physiologic, vagally mediated arrhythmias are often observed in dogs in the perioperative setting, particularly during sleep. Vagally mediated rate and rhythm alterations may also be associated with enhanced vagal tone caused by chronic airway diseases (particularly upper airway obstruction), chronic gastrointestinal diseases, increased intraocular pressure, increased intracranial pressure, and cervical spinal injuries or surgery.[14]

High-grade second-degree AV block and complete (third-degree) AV block often reflect intracardiac disease, and animals with these arrhythmias may require temporary or permanent heart rate support. Second-degree AV block is recognized on ECG by the presence of intermittent nonconducted P waves; whereas with complete AV block, the atrial and ventricular activity are completely dissociated, and the ventricular rate is slower than the atrial rate. Causes of high-grade AV conduction block in dogs and cats include degenerative disease of the conduction system, primary or secondary myocardial diseases, trauma, endocarditis, neoplasia, drug toxicity, and surgery or catheters within the heart. Transient third-degree AV block is occasionally due to vagal surges caused by pain, hypoxemia, or suctioning.[2]

Other than correcting reversible underlying causes, treatment of bradycardia is needed only if the rate is slow enough to cause hypoperfusion. Atropine may be administered intravenously at a dose of 0.02 to 0.04 mg/kg IV or IM. Intravenous infusion of isoproterenol (0.01-2.0 μg/kg/min) or dopamine (5-8 μg/kg/min) may also be considered. Temporary pacing for bradycardia may be performed transcutaneously in anesthetized patients; however, not all patients can be effectively paced in this manner because of high chest wall impedance. The discomfort induced by this pacing method limits its use to anesthetized or comatose patients. Transvenous pacing is more reliable and may be utilized as a bridge to permanent pacing in conscious or unconscious patients. However, temporary transvenous pacing is associated with risks including sepsis and sudden death from lead displacement. It should be recognized that any type of temporary pacing may produce pacemaker dependence.

Arrhythmias Associated with Specific Surgical Procedures

Instrumentation and Monitoring

Tracheal intubation may be associated with tachyarrhythmias caused by reflex sympathetic stimulation, and anxious patients with high adrenergic tone are particularly susceptible. Pretreatment with opioids, lidocaine, or β-blockers will reduce the cardiovascular responses to intubation.[1] Transient supraventricular or ventricular tachyarrhythmias have also been noted during placement of central venous pressure (CVP) monitoring catheters as the guidewire is passed into the right atrium or right ventricle.[1,15] Similar arrhythmias may occur from catheters passed through the right side of the heart into the pulmonary artery. Usually, these arrhythmias are transient and insignificant, but ventricular fibrillation has been reported.[16] Complete AV block has also occurred with guide-wire insertion during CVP cannulation.[17] To avoid these potential arrhythmias, it is recommended that guide-wire insertion be limited to the length necessary to reach the junction of the cranial vena cava with the right atrium. It is also important to monitor the patient's ECG or pulse and to have resuscitative drugs and equipment readily available during insertion of central venous or pulmonary artery catheters.

Acute Gastric Dilation and Gastric Dilation with Volvulus

A high incidence of ventricular arrhythmias (VT and VPCs) has been noted in dogs during and after surgery for acute gastric dilation (AGD) and gastric dilation with volvulus (GDV).[18] Continuous ECG monitoring is, therefore, recommended, and management of ventricular arrhythmias should be considered when formulating the anesthetic plan. The cause of ventricular ectopy associated with gastric dilation most likely is multifactorial. Ischemia almost certainly plays an important role.[19] Release of myocardial depressant factors from the pancreas has also been implicated.[20] Reperfusion injury is known to occur with GDV and will produce cardiac compromise and irritability.[21] Finally, the acid-base and electrolyte abnormalities in affected dogs undoubtedly play a contributing role. Ventricular ectopy in dogs with AGD and GDV rarely produces hemodynamic instability, and the value of antiarrhythmic treatment is unproven.[22] However, dogs with polymorphic VT, frequent pulse deficits, rapid VT, underlying heart disease, or hypotension associated with the arrhythmia should receive antiarrhythmic agents. Spontaneous resolution of the arrhythmia typically occurs within a few days with successful treatment of the underlying disease.

Splenectomy

Ventricular arrhythmias are also common in dogs undergoing splenectomy for neoplasia, torsion, or immune-mediated disease.[23,24] These arrhythmias may occur in the pre-, intra-, and postoperative periods, but arrhythmias most commonly develop 5 to 12 hours after surgery.[24] Therefore, continuous ECG monitoring throughout the perioperative period is advised. Proposed causes of the ventricular ectopy include release of emboli during manipulation of the spleen, arterial hypotension, anemia, free radical-induced myocardial damage, transient ischemia, and the effect of myocardial depressant factors.[23-25] Treatment should consist of restoring normal blood volume and red cell mass, treatment of hypotension, and correction of metabolic abnormalities. As with gastric dilation/volvulus, the ventricular arrhythmias associated with splenectomy are usually hemodynamically stable, and contribution of the ventricular ectopy to postoperative death is unlikely.[6] Monitoring cardiac rhythm and arterial blood pressure without administration of antiarrhythmic medication is a reasonable course of action in many patients. However, dogs with polymorphic VT, frequent pulse deficits, rapid VT, underlying heart disease, or hypotension associated with the arrhythmia should receive antiarrhythmic agents. In most dogs, ventricular arrhythmias associated with splenectomy resolve without antiarrhythmic treatment within 2 to 3 days following successful treatment of the underlying noncardiac abnormalities.

Thoracic Surgery

Cardiac surgical procedures frequently result in arrhythmias owing to direct stimulation of the myocardium. VPCs are a common manifestation of surgical manipulation or incision of the myocardium, and ventricular ectopy in this setting should be suppressed to prevent unstable VT or VF.[14] Preventive measures include discontinuing arrhythmogenic drugs (e.g., digoxin) in the preoperative period if possible; reversing electrolyte depletion caused by chronic diuretic administration; avoiding the use of halothane; and administration of lidocaine prior to and during manipulation, incision, or suturing of the myocardium.

Arrhythmias also occur frequently during thoracic surgeries that do not directly involve the heart. The etiology of these arrhythmias typically includes one or several factors including increased pulmonary vascular resistance, mediastinal shift, autonomic imbalance (vagal surges and release of catecholamines), hypoxemia, electrolyte and acid-base imbalance, and preexisting cardiac disease.[26]

Pheochromocytoma

Pheochromocytomas are functional tumors of the adrenal medulla that produce norepinephrine, epinephrine, and occasionally, dopamine. Large amounts of catecholamines may be released into the central circulation as a result of intraoperative tumor manipulation. This catecholamine release may cause or aggravate potentially fatal tachyarrhythmias. Direct monitoring of the ECG, arterial blood pressure, and central venous pressure throughout the perioperative period is advised. Supraventricular and ventricular tachycardias should be suppressed with intravenous administration of a β-adrenergic blocking agent such as esmolol or propranolol (Table 18-1). In addition, intravenous administration of phentolamine to control hypertension may indirectly mitigate ventricular tachyarrhythmias. Administration of lidocaine immediately prior to tracheal intubation has also been suggested.[27]

Thyroidectomy

Functional thyroid tumors (adenomatous thyroid hyperplasia) are common in older cats. In one series of 85 cats undergoing thyroidectomy, 10% had tachyarrhythmias during surgery.[28] When surgery on cats with this condition is necessary, intraoperative and postoperative cardiovascular complications, including supraventricular and ventricular tachyarrhythmias, can be minimized by medical induction of a euthyroid state prior to surgery. If this is not possible, recommendations for minimizing arrhythmia include administration of acepromazine prior to induction, avoidance of anticholinergic agents and α2-adrenergic agonists, and avoidance of halothane.[27]

References

1. Royster RL: Causes and consequences of arrhythmias *In* Anesthesia and Perioperative Complications, 2nd ed. Benumof JL, Saidman LJ (eds). St. Louis: Mosby, 1999, pp. 258-285.

2. Holshouser W, Hoyle J, Sackett M, Fitzgerald DM: Recognition and treatment of perioperative arrhythmias In Basic Science for Surgeons. Argenta LC (ed). Philadelphia: Saunders, 2004, pp. 741-759.

3. Rho RW, Bridges CR, Kocovic D: Management of postoperative arrhythmias. Semin Thorac Cardiovasc Surg 12:349, 2000.

4. Sisson D, Brown W, Riepe R: Hemodynamic effects of atrial fibrillation in dogs with experimentally induced mitral regurgitation. J Vet Intern Med (Abstr) 9:200, 1995.

5. Wright KN: Assessment and treatment of supraventricular tachyarrhythmias *In* Kirk's Current Veterinary Therapy XIII Small Animal Practice. Philadelphia: WB Saunders, 2000, pp. 726-730.

6. Knight DH: Reason must supersede dogma in the management of ventricular arrhythmias *In* Kirk's Current Veterinary Therapy XIII Small Animal Practice. Bonagura JD (ed). Philadelphia: WB Saunders, 2000, pp. 730-737.

7. Moise NS: Ventricular arrhythmias *In* Kirk's Current Veterinary Therapy XIII Small Animal Practice. Bonagura JD (ed). Philadelphia: WB Saunders, 2000, pp. 733-737.

8. Mahla E, Rotman B, Rehak P, et al: Perioperative ventricular arrhythmias in patients with structural heart disease undergoing noncardiac surgery. Anesth Analg 86:16, 1998.

9. AHA: 2000 Handbook of Emergency Cardiovascular Care for Healthcare Providers. Dallas:American Heart Association, 2000, p. 10.

10. Somberg JC, Cvetanovic I, Ranade V, et al: Comparative effects of rapid bolus administration of aqueous amiodarone versus 10-minute Cordarone IV infusion on mean arterial blood pressure in conscious dogs. Cardiovasc Drug Ther 18:345, 2004.

11. Platou ES, Refsum H: Acute electrophysiologic and blood pressure effects of amiodarone and its solvent in the dog. Acta Pharmacol Toxicol 58:163, 1986.

12. Kittleson MD, Kienle RD (eds): Small Animal Cardiovascular Medicine. St. Louis: Mosby, 1998, p. 481.

13. Muir WW, Hubbell JAE, Skarda RT, Bednarski RM: Cardiac emergencies *In* Handbook of Veterinary Anesthesia, 2nd ed. Muir WW, Hubbell JAE (eds). St. Louis: Mosby, 1995, pp. 408-417.

14. Raffe MR: Complications of anesthesia. *In* Complications in Small Animal Surgery. Lipowitz, AJ, Caywood DD, Newton, CD, Schwartz A (eds). Baltimore: Williams & Wilkins, 1996, pp. 73-97.

15. Reich DL, Moskowitz DM: Complications of cardiovascular monitoring *In* Anesthesia & Perioperative Complications, 2nd ed. Benumof JL, Saidman LJ (eds). St. Louis: Mosby, 1999, pp. 25-49.

16. Royster RL, Johnston WE, Gravlee GP, et al: Arrhythmias during venous cannulation prior to pulmonary artery catheter insertion. Anesth Analg 64:1214, 1970.

17. Eissa NT, Kvetan V: Guide wire as a cause of complete heart block in patients with preexisting left bundle branch block: Anesthesiol 73:772, 1990.

18. Rasmussen L: Stomach. *In* Textbook of Small Animal Surgery, 3rd ed. Slatter D (ed). Philadelphia: WB Saunders, 2003, pp. 592-640.

19. Muir WW, Weisbrode SE: Myocardial ischemia in dogs with gastric dilatation-volvulus. J Am Vet Med Assoc 181:363, 1982.

20. Wingfield WE, Betts CW, Rawlings CA: Pathophysiology associated with gastric dilatation-volvulus in the dog. J Am Anim Hosp Assoc 12:136, 1976.

21. Lantz GC, Badylak SF, Hiles MC, et al: Treatment of reperfusion injury in dogs with experimentally induced gastric dilation-volvulus. Am J Vet Res 53:1594, 1992.

22. Brockman DJ, Washabau RJ, Drobatz KJ: Canine gastric dilatation/volvulus syndrome in a veterinary critical care unit: 295 cases (1986-1992. J Am Vet Med Assoc 207:460, 1995.

23. Knapp DW, Aronsohn MG, Harpster NK: Cardiac arrhythmias associated with mass lesions of the canine spleen. J Am Anim Hosp 29:122, 1993.

24. Marino DJ, Matthiesen DT, Fox PR, et al: Ventricular arrhythmias in dogs undergoing splenectomy: A prospective study. Vet Surg 23:101, 1994.

25. Walshaw R: Hepato-biliary, pancreatic, and splenic surgery. *In* Complications in Small Animal Surgery. Lipowitz, AJ, Caywood DD, Newton, CD, Schwartz A (eds). Baltimore: Williams & Wilkins, 1996, pp. 399-453.

26. Caywood DD: Thoracic surgery. *In* Complications in Small Animal Surgery. Lipowitz, AJ, Caywood DD, Newton, CD, Schwartz A (eds). Baltimore: Williams & Wilkins, 1996, pp. 195-218.

27. Schwartz A: Endocrine surgery. *In* Complications in Small Animal Surgery. Lipowitz, AJ, Caywood DD, Newton, CD, Schwartz A (eds). Baltimore: Williams & Wilkins, 1996, pp. 287-331.

28. Birchard SJ, Peterson ME, Jacobson A: Surgical treatment of feline hyperthyroidism; results of 85 cases. J Am Anim Hosp Assoc 20:705, 1984.

Chapter 19

Pathophysiology of Congenital Heart Defects

E. Christopher Orton

Congenital heart defects are morphologic disorders of the heart and great vessels that are present at birth. Strong breed predilections for congenital heart defects suggest a genetic basis for most defects. Congenital heart defects result in a variety of pathophysiologic alterations that eventually can lead to progressive heart failure, cardiac arrhythmias, and sudden cardiac death, debilitating hypoxemia, or combinations of these adverse outcomes.

Patent Ductus Arteriosus

The ductus arteriosus is a vascular conduit between the pulmonary artery and descending aorta that diverts pulmonary flow away from the fetal lung circulation. Soon after birth, expansion of the fetal lung lowers pulmonary vascular resistance and reverses flow through the ductus. Oxygenated blood is detected by the vascular endothelium of the ductus arteriosus, and this, in turn, inhibits the release of the vasodilating prostaglandin that keeps the ductus patent. The vascular smooth muscle of the ductus arteriosus contracts and functionally closes the ductus within a few hours of birth.

Patent ductus arteriosus (PDA) results from a persistence of the ductus arteriosus after birth. Incomplete development of the medial layer of the ductus arteriosus wall has been implicated in the pathogenesis of PDA in dogs.[1] PDA allows a high-flow left-to-right shunt that overloads the volume in the left atrium and ventricle and overcirculates the lungs. The resultant chronic volume overload induces progressive dilation of the left ventricle with or without wall thickening. Secondary functional mitral regurgitation (MR) and overload-induced systolic dysfunction eventually contribute to the progression of heart failure as PDA becomes long standing. The overload is so overwhelming that most animals will succumb to progressive left-sided congestive heart failure within the first year of life. Closure of PDA is indicated for the vast majority of animals with this defect and is generally undertaken with curative intent unless secondary changes are advanced.

On occasion, increased pulmonary vascular resistance can elevate pulmonary artery pressures sufficiently to reverse flow through a PDA. Suprasystemic pulmonary hypertension results either from a failure of transition of the pulmonary circulation to extrauterine life or progressive pulmonary vascular remodeling caused by chronic pulmonary overcirculation. In the former case, right-to-left or "reverse" PDA is present from birth. In the latter, it typically develops in the first 8 months of life. Regardless of the inciting mechanism, the right-to-left shunt through a PDA causes selective hypoxemia to the caudal portions of the circulation and is responsible for the hallmark sign of differential cyanosis. Clinical consequences of the chronic hypoxemia include moderate to severe activity intolerance, pelvic limb weakness, and progressive polycythemia. Closure of right-to-left or "reverse" PDA causes severe acute cor pulmonale and is contraindicated.

Pulmonic Stenosis

Pulmonic stenosis (PS) in dogs is most often valvular, although supravalvular and subvalvular defects occur, either as isolated defects or in combination. Valvular PS represents a spectrum of abnormalities ranging from *simple commissural fusion*, consisting of incomplete separation of the valve leaflet commissurae, to valve *dysplasia*, characterized by varying degrees of narrowing of the valve annulus and/or thickening and immobility of the valve leaflets. In severe cases of PS, secondary hypertrophy of the right ventricular outflow tract (RVOT) can contribute to PS severity by causing dynamic obstruction to ventricular ejection of blood.

Chronic pressure overload caused by PS induces thickening of the right ventricular wall without chamber dilation (i.e., concentric hypertrophy). Right atrial dilation occurs as diastolic filling pressures increase in response to poor ventricular compliance and decreased cardiac output. If primary or secondary tricuspid regurgitation (TR) accompanies PS, then right ventricle dilation may accompany the ventricular wall thickening. Despite its relative importance as a congenital defect, the natural history of untreated PS in animals is not well documented. Dogs with mild to moderate PS may tolerate the defect relatively well for many years. Dogs with severe PS are likely at risk for both sudden cardiac death and progressive right-sided heart failure. Right-sided heart failure can manifest as either congestion behind the right heart (i.e., ascites) or low output failure, or both. Catheter-based or surgical procedures are generally recommended for dogs with moderate to severe PS to lessen the severity of RVOT obstruction, and decrease the risk for sudden death or heart failure.

Some dogs with PS, particularly English bulldogs and boxers, may have an accompanying anomalous left coronary artery. In dogs with this defect, the left coronary artery originates from the right coronary ostia and may course across the right ventricular outflow tract. As a result, the left circumflex coronary artery is at risk for injury during surgical or catheter-based treatments for PS.

Double-Chambered Right Ventricle

Double-chambered right ventricle (DCRV) is an uncommon congenital heart defect of dogs characterized by a fibromuscular diaphragm at the junction of the inflow and outflow portions of the right ventricle.[2] The defect obstructs flow through the mid-portion of the ventricle and causes hypertrophy of the proximal portion of the right ventricle, giving it a "double-chambered" appearance. The pathophysiology and natural history of DCRV are thought to be similar to those of PS.

Subvalvular Aortic Stenosis

Subvalvular aortic stenosis (SAS) is a common congenital defect in certain large and giant breed dogs. The typical defect consists of a discrete subvalvular fibrous membrane located millimeters below the aortic valve leaflets. The membrane traverses the ventricular septum and reflects onto the septal mitral valve leaflet. The defect can be associated with varying degrees of muscular septal hypertrophy and diffuse fibrosis of the left ventricular outflow tract (LVOT) that can contribute to outflow obstruction. The defect is often accompanied by varying degrees of aortic insufficiency. Mitral regurgitation may also be present if the fibrous membrane restricts motion of the septal mitral valve leaflet.

Subvalvular aortic stenosis causes a pressure gradient across the LVOT during left ventricular ejection that, in turn, increases left ventricular systolic pressure. The accompanying increase in ventricular systolic wall stress causes cardiomyocyte hypertrophy, leading to concentric thickening of the left ventricular wall and interventricular septum. Intramural coronary arterial pathology characterized by intimal hyperplasia and medial degeneration has been documented in dogs with SAS.[3] Myocardial oxygen demand is increased by the combination of high systolic wall stress (i.e., afterload) and cardiac hypertrophy. Myocardial oxygen delivery is impaired by abnormal coronary arteries. The resultant mismatch between oxygen demand and delivery causes myocardial ischemia that is exacerbated by activity or exercise. Myocardial ischemia is thought to be the cause of malignant ventricular tachycardia and sudden cardiac death. Median age at sudden death has been reported to be 18 months in dogs with untreated SAS.[4] Chronic β-adrenergic blockade therapy may reduce, but does not eliminate, the risk of sudden death.[5] Surgical intervention has not been shown to decrease the risk of sudden death in dogs with SAS.[5] Dogs that avoid early sudden death may develop left-sided congestive heart failure late in life.

Ventricular Septal Defect

Ventricular septal defect (VSD) is a congenital defect that occurs in dogs and cats. The defect allows left-to-right systolic shunt flow from the left to the right ventricle. The magnitude of the pathophysiologic change depends on the size of the defect. Small defects do not allow for equilibration of left and right ventricular systolic pressures and are termed "restrictive." Such defects are associated with low shunt flow. Large defects allow equilibration of ventricular systolic pressures and are associated with high shunt flow. Left-to-right shunt flow causes volume overload of the left heart and pulmonary circulation. The most common anatomic location for VSD in animals is high in the septum behind the septal leaflet of the tricuspid valve. Such defects, termed *perimembranous* VSD, typically spare the right ventricle from volume overload because shunt flow is ejected directly into the RVOT. Defects located low in the muscular septum may result in volume overload of both sides of the heart. On occasion, VSD occurs dorsal to the supraventricular crest (crista supraventricularis) in the RVOT. Such defects, termed *supracristal* VSD, are associated with a high incidence of aortic valve leaflet prolapse and concurrent aortic insufficiency. Surgical closure of VSD can be undertaken with the aid of cardiopulmonary bypass with curative intent. Pulmonary artery banding is a palliative surgical procedure intended to decrease shunt flow.

Restrictive VSD is generally well tolerated by both dogs and cats. Large hemodynamically significant defects cause progressive left-sided chamber dilation and congestive heart failure similar to PDA. High shunt flow also can trigger progressive pulmonary vascular remodeling, increased pulmonary vascular resistance, and increased pulmonary arterial pressures. If pulmonary artery pressures reach suprasystemic levels (i.e., exceed systemic arterial pressures), shunt flow reverses and becomes intermittently or continuously right-to-left. This condition, termed Eisenmenger's syndrome, is associated with varying degrees of hypoxemia and polycythemia.

Atrial Septal Defect

Various forms of atrial septal defect (ASD) or atrioventricular septal defect (AVSD) have been described in dogs and cats. Atrial septal defects (ASD) are classified as sinus venosus defects, coronary sinus ASD, ostium secundum (fossa ovalis type) ASD, or patent foramen ovale. Sinus venosus defects are situated cranial and dorsal in the atrial septum at the junction of the cranial vena cava and are frequently associated with anomalous pulmonary venous return. Coronary sinus ASD or unroofed coronary sinus results from an incomplete separation between the coronary sinus and the left atrium; this is often due to the persistence of the left cranial vena cava. Other types of ASD occur directly in the septum primum or the septum secundum, or both. Ostium secundum ASD (fossa ovalis type) occurs in the mid-dorsal portion of the atrial septum. Patent foramen ovale is usually an acquired defect secondary to pressure or volume overload of the right heart. Atrioventricular septal defects represent a spectrum of malformations that involve the septum primum, the inlet portion of ventricular septum, and the atrioventricular valves. Ostium primum ASD is currently classified as a partial AVSD. The defect is characterized by an ostium primum defect and a malformed mitral valve. The mitral valve defect consists of a cleft in the septal leaflet that changes the valve into a trileaflet structure. This malformation usually causes significant mitral regurgitation. Complete AVSD consists of an ostium primum defect above, a VSD below, and a single AV valve that is common to the right and left ventricle. The complete form of AV septal defect was formally termed an endocardial cushion defect.

Atrial septal defects share a common pathophysiology regardless of type. Left-to-right shunt through the defect causes volume overload of the right side of the heart. The right atrium and ventricle dilate in response to chronic volume overload. Increases in right ventricular diastolic pressure lead to progressive right-sided congestive heart failure. As right atrial pressures become elevated, bidirectional shunt and hypoxemia can complicate the clinical picture.

Tetralogy of Fallot

Tetralogy of Fallot (TF) is a complex congenital heart defect consisting of PS, VSD, an overriding aorta, and right ventricular hypertrophy. The defect occurs in both dogs and cats. The pathophysiology and natural history of TF depend on the magnitude of its two primary defects: PS and VSD. Animals with severe pulmonic stenosis and a large VSD will have significant right-to-left shunt resulting in severe hypoxemia. The clinical consequence is moderate to severe cyanosis at rest, profound activity intolerance, and progressive polycythemia. A shortened life span is expected owing to complications related to chronic hypoxemia, polycythemia, and sudden cardiac death. Animals with less severe pulmonic stenosis or restrictive VSD may tolerate the defect to varying degrees. Total correction of TF can be undertaken with the aid of cardiopulmonary bypass with curative intent.[5]

Tricuspid Valve Dysplasia

Tricuspid valve dysplasia (TVD) is a congenital malformation of the tricuspid valve that occurs in several large breeds of dog including Labrador retrievers, golden retrievers, and German shepherds. A spectrum of pathologic lesions has been associated with TVD, including shortening, thickening, or notching of leaflets; fusion, absence, or elongation of chordae tendineae; and malformation of papillary muscles. Tricuspid regurgitation (TR) is the most common hemodynamic manifestation, although tricuspid stenosis is possible. Tricuspid regurgitation results from restrictive motion of the valve leaflets and severe progressive dilation of the valve annulus. Severe TR causes volume overload of the right heart and eventual right-sided congestive heart failure. The age at onset of heart failure varies widely among individual dogs. Right-sided congestive heart failure is generally preceded by severe right atrial and ventricular dilation. Pulmonic stenosis or pulmonary hypertension will accelerate the course toward heart failure. Atrial fibrillation is a common late sequela that contributes to progression toward heart failure.

References

1. Patterson DF: Congenital defects of the cardiovascular system in dogs: Studies in comparative cardiology. Adv Vet Sci Comp Med 20:1, 1976.
2. Martin J, Orton EC, Boon J, et al: Surgical correction of double-chambered right ventricle in dogs. J Am Vet Med Assoc 220:770, 2002.
3. Flickenger GL, Patterson DF: Coronary lesions associated with congenital subaortic stenosis in the dog. J Pathol Bacteriol 93:133, 1967.
4. Kienle RD, Thomas WP, Pion PD: The natural clinical history of canine congenital subaortic stenosis. J Vet Intern Med 8:423, 1994.
5. Orton EC, Herndon GD, Boon J, et al: Intermediate-term outcome in dogs with subvalvular aortic stenosis: influence of open surgical correction. J Am Vet Med Assoc 216:364, 2000.
6. Orton EC, Mama K, Hellyer P, Hackett TB: Open surgical repair of tetralogy of Fallot in two dogs. J Am Vet Med Assoc 219:1089, 2001.

Chapter 20

Heart Failure

E. Christopher Orton

Heart failure is a clinical syndrome that represents a final common pathway of severe and progressive cardiac insufficiency. Heart failure is present when cardiac output is inadequate despite adequate diastolic filling pressures or when adequate cardiac output can only be maintained at the expense of elevated diastolic filling pressures. Heart failure results from the combined effects of acute or chronic cardiac insufficiency and compensatory neuroendocrine mechanisms. Heart failure manifests as either multiple organ dysfunction secondary to low cardiac output (termed *low output heart failure or forward heart failure*) or congestion of organs behind the heart (termed *congestive heart failure or backward heart failure*), or both. Congestion can occur behind the left heart, resulting in pulmonary edema or pleural effusion; or behind the right heart, resulting in ascites, peripheral edema, or pleural effusion; or both, resulting in any combination of the these.

Importance of the Frank-Starling Relationship

Cardiac output (ml/min) is the total effective flow coming from the heart and is the product of *stroke volume* and *heart rate*. Stroke volume is a function of the degree of myocardial fiber shortening in the ventricle. The stretch or load on myocardial fibers just prior to contraction profoundly influences the degree of myocardial fiber shortening. This load or stretch prior to contraction is termed *preload*. Within limits, an increase in preload increases myocardial fiber shortening and stroke volume. *Diastolic filling pressures* in the heart reflect the amount of stretch or preload on the ventricle prior to contraction and, in turn, are an important determinant of cardiac output. The *Frank-Starling curve* describes the direct relationship between cardiac output and diastolic filling pressures (i.e., preload) in the heart (Figure 20-1).

Cardiac output and diastolic filling pressures are not only functionally related, but are the physiologic parameters directly responsible for the two adverse manifestations of heart failure: namely, inadequate perfusion and congestion. The absolute amount of cardiac output is less important than the adequacy of tissue perfusion (i.e., how well cardiac output is meeting the metabolic needs of the patient). Initially, low cardiac output narrows the cardiac reserve, i.e., the ability to increase cardiac output during activity or exercise. The clinical manifestation is exercise or activity intolerance. Eventually, cardiac output can become low enough that it fails to meet the metabolic needs of organ systems and tissues even at rest. At this point, the patient is in low output heart failure. Multiple organ and tissue dysfunction are apparent. The patient is "cold" rather than "warm." While diastolic filling pressure exerts a positive influence on cardiac output, it also is the effective down stream pressure that resists venous return to the heart. Congestion occurs when diastolic filling pressure elevates capillary hydrostatic pressure to the point where a net efflux of water from capillaries to the interstitial space occurs. The result is edema of the organs and tissues behind the failing heart. The patient is "wet" rather than "dry."

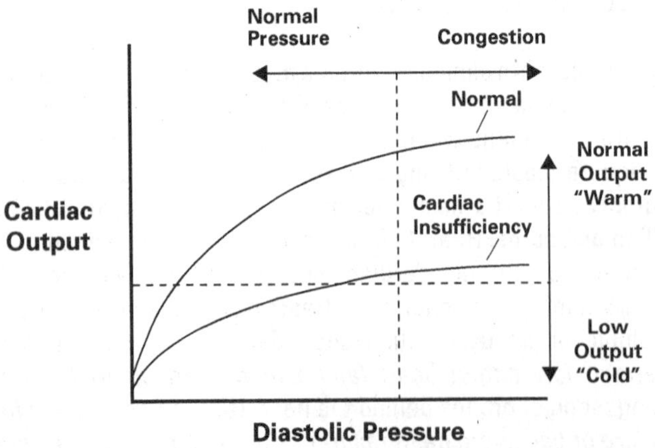

Figure 20-1. The Frank-Starling curve describes the direct relationship between cardiac output and diastolic filling pressures in the heart. When cardiac function is normal (upper curve), cardiac output will be adequate at normal diastolic pressures. The patient will remain "warm" and "dry" over a wide range of cardiac outputs. When cardiac insufficiency is present (lower curve), then cardiac output may be inadequate at normal diastolic pressures or cardiac output will only be adequate when diastolic filling pressures are high. In the former case, the patient is in *low output heart failure* or "cold." In the latter case, the patient is in *congestive heart failure* or "wet."

Causes of Cardiac Insufficiency

Most causes of cardiac insufficiency in small animals are chronic and insidiously progressive. Cardiac insufficiency is caused by one or a combination of four basic mechanisms: *primary myocardial failure, hemodynamic overload, diastolic dysfunction,* or *cardiac arrhythmias.* From a physiologic standpoint, primary myocardial failure is a loss of systolic function associated with a decrease in cardiac contractility or an inotropic state. The most common example of primary myocardial failure in dogs is heritable dilated cardiomyopathy. Myocardial infarction is a rare cause of primary myocardial failure in animals. Hemodynamic overload results when structural defects in the heart cause it to have to do excessive work. Excess cardiac work results from the heart having to pump a high volume of blood (i.e., *volume overload*) or against a high systolic pressure (i.e., *pressure overload*) in order to maintain an adequate cardiac output. Causes of volume overload include valve insufficiency (mitral regurgitation, tricuspid regurgitation, aortic insufficiency) and congenital left-to-right shunts (patent ductus arteriosus, ventricular septal defect, atrial septal defect). Causes of pressure overload include semilunar valve stenosis (subvalvular aortic stenosis, pulmonic stenosis) or hypertension (e.g., pulmonary hypertension). Diastolic dysfunction results from myocardial or pericardial disorders that decrease ventricular diastolic compliance (i.e., change in the pressure-volume relationship of the ventricle during diastole). Causes of diastolic dysfunction include hypertrophic cardiomyopathy, restrictive cardiomyopathy, pericardial effusion, and constrictive pericarditis. Cardiac arrhythmias can cause or contribute to heart failure by impairing cardiac output by either tachycardia or bradycardia. Tachyarrhythmias that cause or contribute to heart failure include chronic atrial fibrillation, atrial flutter, and sustained supraventricular tachycardias. Bradyarrhythmias that can cause or contribute to heart failure include third-degree atrioventricular block and persistent atrial standstill.

Response to Cardiac Insufficency

Progression of heart disease can be arbitrarily divided into three phases. The first phase of heart disease occurs when an initiating cardiac injury or insufficiency is present. If the initiating cardiac insufficiency is acute and overwhelming, then *low output heart failure* may immediately ensue. More often in veterinary patients, the cardiac insufficiency is not initially overwhelming or lethal, but rather slowly progressive. The presence of heart disease may be signaled only by the presence of physical findings such as abnormal heart sounds or murmurs and not associated with overt symptoms of heart failure other than possible activity or exercise intolerance.

The second phase of heart disease is hallmarked by activation of the *neuroendocrine response* to cardiac insufficiency (Table 20-1). This neuroendocrine response ensures that blood pressure and cardiac output are maintained principally through the retention of vascular blood volume and the constriction of arteries and veins. *Cardiac hypertrophy* generally begins during this phase, particularly when the initiating cardiac insufficiency results from hemodynamic overload. The type of cardiac hypertrophy depends on the nature of the cardiac insufficiency (Figure 20-2). During this phase, clinical evidence of cardiac insufficiency in the form of cardiomegaly occurs, although overt signs of heart failure are still not present. Symptoms would still be associated mostly with reduced activity or exercise capacity.

Although the neuroendocrine response is initially adaptive, ultimately this response becomes maladaptive. This is the third phase of heart failure. During this phase, the neuroendocrine response "overcompensates," producing high diastolic filling pressures and congestion in the form of tissue and organ edema. Inappropriate arterioconstriction is also present during this phase and may actually contribute to poor tissue perfusion. This state is termed *congestive heart failure.* It is possible in advanced cases of cardiac insufficiency for both congestive heart failure and low output heart failure to be present.

Table 20-1. Adaptive and Maladaptive Responses to Cardiac Insufficiency

Mechanism	Activating Stimuli	Physiologic Effects	Adaptive Consequences	Maladaptive Consequences
Epinephrine Norepinephrine	baroreceptors angiotensin II	vasoconstriction increase heart rate increase contractility	increase blood pressure increase cardiac output	decrease tissue perfusion tachyarrhythmias $beta_1$ down-regulation cardiomyocyte dysfunction cardiomyocyte apoptosis globoid ventricular dilation
Renin-Angiotensin	decreased RBF decreased [Na^+] sympathetic activation	vasoconstriction	increase blood pressure	decrease tissue perfusion cardiomyocyte dysfunction cardiac remodeling
Aldosterone	increased [K^+] angiotensin II	Na^+ retention (blood volume expansion)	increase cardiac output (preload)	venous congestion
Vasopressin	angiotensin II increased osmolality	water retention (blood volume expansion) vasoconstriction	increase cardiac output (preload) increase blood pressure	venous congestion dilutional hyponatremia decrease
Naturetic Peptides	angiotensin II atrial stretch increased [Na^+]	vasodilation naturesis	increase tissue perfusion decrease venous congestion	
Endothelin	vasopressin angiotensin II epinephrine, norepinephrine	intense vasoconstriction	increase blood pressure	decrease tissue perfusion cardiac remodeling
Cardiac Hypertrophy	systolic wall stress (pressure overload) diastolic wall stress (volume overload) angiotensin II epinephrine, norepinephrine endothelin	cardiac wall thickening cardiac chamber dilation	decrease afterload (wall thickening) increase cardiac mass (contractility)	increase afterload (chamber dilation) increase myocardial oxygen demand

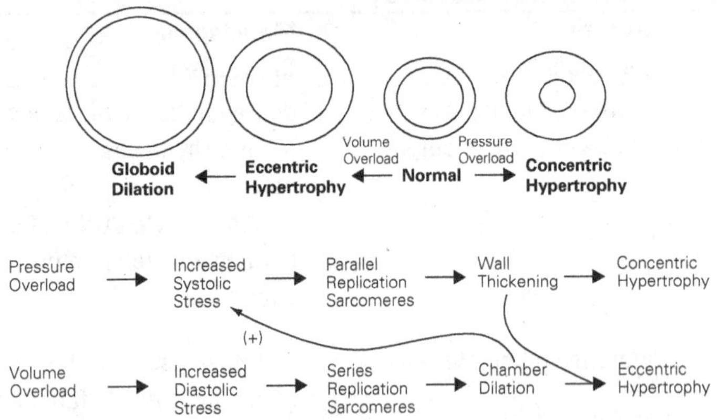

Figure 20-2. Cardiac hypertrophy is initially an adaptive response to hemodynamic overload in the heart. Pressure overload initiates a hypertrophic response that consists primarily of parallel replication of sarcomeres resulting in wall thickening. This pattern, termed *concentric hypertrophy*, normalizes afterload and thereby reduces the effect of pressure overload on the ventricle. Volume overload initiates a hypertrophic response that consists of both parallel and series replication of sarcomeres resulting in chamber dilation and wall thickening. This pattern, termed *eccentric hypertrophy*, increases the stroke volume capacity of the ventricle without increasing afterload. In advanced states of cardiac insufficiency, cardiac hypertrophy consists primarily of chamber dilation without wall thickening. This response, termed *globoid ventricular dilation*, is maladaptive because it places the ventricle at a mechanical disadvantage from the standpoint of afterload.

Neuroendocrine Theory of Heart Failure Progression

It has long been recognized that, regardless of the initiating cause of cardiac insufficiency, deleterious changes in the myocardium in the form of progressive systolic dysfunction will eventually contribute to the progression of heart failure. According to the neuroendocrine hypothesis, endogenous neuroendocrine systems activated by cardiac insufficiency are not only responsible for the deleterious hemodynamic derangements of heart failure, but also directly mediate progressive myocardial deterioration.[1-3] This myocardial deterioration takes the form of intrinsic loss of myocardial fiber contractility and, for many causes of heart failure, *globoid ventricular chamber dilation*. Several changes at the cellular and molecular level have been implicated in the loss of myocardial contractility, including down-regulation of beta-receptors, reversion of the cardiomyocyte to a less contractile fetal phenotype, and cardiomyocyte apoptosis. While some degree of ventricular dilation can be adaptive by increasing stroke volume capacity, particularly for volume overload, excessive ventricular chamber dilation places the ventricle at a substantial mechanical disadvantage from the standpoint of afterload, particularly when it is accompanied by thinning of the ventricular walls. In this regard, severe globoid dilation of the heart is considered a maladaptive response that contributes to heart failure progression. Evidence strongly implicates endocrine, paracrine, and autocrine mediators such as angiotensin II, aldosterone, catecholamines, endothelin, inflammatory cytokines, and peptide growth factors as mediators of or contributors to these deleterious myocardial effects. This understanding forms the current rationale for "cardioprotective" therapeutic strategies intended to slow progression toward heart failure. Drugs demonstrated to have a cardioprotective effect include angiotensin-converting enzyme inhibitors and beta-adrenergic antagonists.[2]

References

1. Packer M: The neurohormonal hypothesis: a theory to explain the mechanism of disease progression in heart failure. J Am Coll Cardiol 20:248, 1992.

2. Bristow MR: Pathophysiology and pharmacologic rationales for clinical management of chronic heart failure with beta-blocking agents. Am J Cardiol 21:12c, 1993.

3. Colucci WS, Braunwald E: Pathophysiology of heart failure. *In* HEART DISEASE: A Textbook of Cardiovascular Medicine, 5th ed. Braunwald E (ed). Philadelphia: WB Saunders, 1997.

Chapter 21

Thromboembolic Disease and Hypercoagulable States

Daniel L. Chan

Thromboembolic Disease

The formation of blood clots to seal injured vessels is an essential protective mechanism in animals and is referred to as coagulation. Once these clots have served their purpose, they are degraded by various enzymatic processes (fibrinolysis). The body also has in place several mechanisms to prevent the aberrant formation of blood clots (anticoagulation). Together, these processes form the complex but elegant system of hemostasis. Abnormalities in any of the components of hemostasis can result in thromboembolic disease with serious consequences. In fact, thromboembolic disease is one of the leading causes of death among critically ill people.[1,2]

As a point of clarification, the term "thrombus" refers to an aggregation of platelets and other blood components that causes partial or complete vascular obstruction. An "embolus" is a clot or other plug (e.g., fat or fibrocartilaginous material) that breaks off from an originating site and lodges in a distant vessel. Thromboembolic disease encompasses all types of thrombi and emboli.

Hypercoagulable or prothrombotic states are clinical conditions that predispose affected patients to blood clot emboli. The pathophysiology of thrombosis depends on three major factors: alterations in the vessel wall (endothelial injury), impairment of blood flow (blood stasis), and in abnormalities within the coagulation system (hypercoagulability). The interactions of these three processes culminating in thromboembolic disease are known as Virchow's triad.

Vascular injury leads to the exposure of subendothelial vessel wall components, such as collagen, resulting in platelet adhesion and activation of the contact phase of the coagulation system. Vascular integrity may be damaged with venipuncture, intravenous catheter placement, infectious and inflammatory vasculitis, and neoplastic invasion of vessels. Blood stasis favors thrombosis by retarding the removal of activated coagulation factors and by causing local hypoxia and vascular injury. Stasis can result from hypovolemia, shock, cardiac insufficiency, blood vessel compression, or immobility. Vascular obstruction by implants, foreign bodies, or neoplasms may induce local thrombosis as well. Cardiac chamber enlargement or vascular aneurysm leads to focal sludging of flow and thrombus formation. Hyperviscosity, as occurs with dehydration, polycythemia, leukemia, hyperglobulinemia, and hyperfibrinogenemia, also results in stasis.

Whereas vascular stasis and injury are prothrombotic, true hypercoagulability refers to a quantitative or qualitative change in the coagulation system. In the simplest sense, the coagulation system is composed of procoagulants (platelets and coagulation factors), anticoagulants (protein C, protein S, antithrombin, heparin cofactor II), and the fibrinolytic system. Any imbalance in these processes may result in excessive bleeding or hypercoagulation, depending on the nature of the imbalance. Hypercoagulation can result from platelet hyperaggregability, excessive activation or decreased removal of coagulation factors, deficiencies of natural anticoagulants, or defective fibrinolysis.

In regard to platelets, there appears to be no correlation between thrombocytosis and hypercoagulation. Hyperaggregability of platelets, however, can increase thromboembolic risk. Platelet aggregation is finely controlled by interactions between the platelets themselves and the vascular endothelium. Additionally, platelets produce and release various proaggregating substances, including thromboxane A_2, adenosine diphosphate (ADP), and prostaglandins G_2 and H_2. The endothelium in turn, releases several inhibitors of platelet aggregation, namely prostacyclin (PGI_2), ADPase, and nitric oxide. Disturbances in the balance between platelets and the endothelium can lead to thrombosis.

Increased activation of coagulation factors (by vascular injury or inflammatory mediators) or decreased removal of factors from areas of injury (owing to stasis or decreased activity of the reticuloendothelial system) may contribute to thrombosis. Whether increased levels of individual clotting factors alone heighten the trend toward a hypercoagulable state remains controversial, but elevated fibrinogen levels, and elevations of factors VIII and XII as seen with hyperadrenocorticism, have been incriminated in people.[3-5]

The mechanisms for triggering coagulation are offset by equally powerful mechanisms for controlling it. Three principal mechanisms are involved in this regulation: antithrombin (AT), protein C, and the fibrinolytic system. Protein C is a small (56,000 daltons) vitamin K-dependent serine protease that is synthesized in the liver. It circulates in plasma as an inactive protein, but is activated by thrombin complexed with thrombomodulin. Activated protein C (APC) then exerts its anticoagulant effect by inactivating membrane-bound factors Va and VIIIa (the amplifiers of coagulation). APC also encourages fibrinolysis by neutralizing plasminogen activator activity. Both actions of protein C are greatly enhanced by protein S.

Antithrombin is a serine protease inhibitor of low molecular weight (58,000 daltons) that is synthesized in the liver and endothelial cells. It is one of the most important inhibitors and effective modulators of hemostasis. AT functions as an inactivator of coagulation factors IIa, IXa, Xa, XIa, and XIIa. This effect occurs too slowly to be physiologically relevant unless heparin binds to AT, causing AT to undergo a conformational change that increases its anticoagulant activity by 1000-fold. Natural heparin-like substances (e.g., sulfated aminoglycans and heparin sulphates) are present on endothelial surfaces and are the major contributors to the anticoagulant properties of the endothelium. Heparin cofactor II (HC II) is a glycoprotein with a molecular mass of 64,000 daltons. It acts as an inhibitor of thrombin, with its action also accelerated by heparin.

AT deficiency is well described in dogs.[6,7] Acquired deficiencies occur because of decreased production, excessive losses, or consumption. Decreased hepatic production of AT occurs with hepatopathies, but thrombosis generally does not result because concomitant clotting factor deficiencies favor hemorrhage. A similar situation occurs with generalized protein loss, such as protein-losing enteropathies. However, there have been cases of thrombosis with protein-losing enteropathies.[8] In contrast, the increased glomerular permeability that accompanies protein-losing nephropathies (e.g., glomerulonephritis and amyloidosis) permits selective loss of lower molecular weight proteins, and consistently results in hypercoagulability.[6,7] AT is smaller than albumin (69,000 daltons) and procoagulant proteins, creating sufficient imbalance to favor a hypercoagulable state. Disseminated intravascular coagulation (DIC) is a situation of increased AT consumption. Measurement of AT activity has been helpful in detecting patients with DIC, and some authors have used it to guide therapy.[9]

The fibrinolytic system is extremely complex, and remains the least completely understood. Evidence is growing that fibrinolysis is exceedingly important in hypercoagulation.[10] Persistence of thrombi is abnormal and implies defective fibrinolysis. More recently, various degrees of hypofibrinolysis have been confirmed in many types of hypercoagulable states.[10,11]

In its simplest form, the fibrinolytic system consists of plasminogen and its activators, which convert plasminogen to plasmin. Plasmin is responsible for dissolution of the fibrin clot. The two physiologic plasminogen activators are tissue-type plasminogen activator (t-PA) and urokinase (UK). T-PA is released from intact endothelium in its active form, whereas UK is released as an inactive zymogen (pro-UK, which is converted to UK by kallikrein. Both t-PA and UK are inhibited by plasminogen activator inhibitor (PAI-1), the major inhibitor of the system. Other inhibitors include: histidine-rich glycoprotein, which interferes with the binding of plasminogen to fibrin; α2-antiplasmin, which inhibits plasmin; and C1-inhibitor, which inactivates kallikrein. Alpha2-macroglobulins are scavenging protease inhibitors that intervene in situations in which antiplasmin is markedly decreased (i.e., thrombolytic therapy). Hypofibrinolysis and resultant thrombosis can occur because of decreases in plasminogen, t-PA, or UK, or because of increases in circulating inhibitors. Increased levels of PAI-1 are by far the most frequent cause of ineffective fibrinolysis in people.[10]

Thrombosis associated with the development of antiphospholipid antibodies ("lupus-type anticoagulants") is common in people but has only been described in one dog with hemolytic anemia.[12] The exact mechanism by which lupus-type anticoagulants cause thrombosis is unclear, but these antibodies may develop secondarily to autoimmune disease, neoplasia, infectious or inflammatory diseases, or drug reactions. Defects of platelet function, dysfibrinolysis, plasminogen deficiency, dysfibrinogenemia, and t-PA deficiency may also lead to thrombosis in people, but have not yet been described in veterinary patients.

Specific Prothrombotic Disorders

Nephrotic Syndrome

Glomerular damage leads to leakage of small molecular weight proteins from blood. Because all of the major inhibitors of coagulation are proteins smaller than albumin, significant protein loss will result in acquired coagulation inhibitor deficiency. Antithrombin deficiency is well documented in protein-losing glomerulonephropathies.[6,7] The hypercoagulable state results from retention of high molecular weight hemostatic factors and selective loss of hemostatic regulators. Underlying inflammation also contributes to the hypercoagulable state by increasing production of acute-phase proteins that play a role in hemostatic reactions, e.g., fibrinogen, factor VIII, and α2-macroglobulin.[6,7] Hypoalbuminemia contributes to hypercoagulability owiing to the development of platelet hyperreactivity.[7] Pulmonary thromboembolism (PTE) is the most common manifestation of hypercoagulability in this disorder.[6]

Immune-Mediated Hemolytic Anemia (IMHA)

PTE is also a common complication of IMHA, occurring in up to 35% of IMHA patients.[13-19] The mechanism is incompletely understood but it has been suggested that endothelial exposure to anti-erythrocyte antibodies and the subsequent complement-mediated damage triggers thrombosis.[13-16] Other hypotheses include increased activity of clotting factors, decreased activity of anticoagulants, defective thrombolysis, increased platelet reactivity, and the presence of antiphospholipid antibodies.[16] In complement-mediated erythrolysis, a significant amount of thromboplastin may be released into the circulation. Other factors implicated in the development of PTE include the release of inflammatory cytokines, the use of corticosteroids, frequent venipuncture and catheterization, and patient inactivity, resulting in sluggish blood flow.[19]

Cardiac Disease

Arterial thromboembolism (ATE) occurs commonly in cats with cardiac disease, especially cats with hypertrophic cardiomyopathy.[20-24] ATE has also been reported in dogs, but the incidence is much lower.[25,26] Unlike other hypercoagulable states where the lesions center within veins, the thrombosis associated with cardiac disease affects arteries. Moderate to severe left atrial enlargement and swirling echocardiographic densities in the left atrium ("smoke") are considered risk factors for ATE.[22] The pathophysiology of ATE is thought to involve severe dilatation of the left atrium (resulting in stasis of blood flow), endothelial damage leading to platelet activation, increased platelet reactivity, and a number of as-of-yet unidentified factors.[21,22,24]

Hyperadrenocorticism

Patients with endogenous or exogenous glucocorticoid excess may develop venous, pulmonary, or arterial thrombosis. The mechanism of hypercoagulability associated with hyperadrenocorticism is incompletely understood. Contributing factors may include increased activity of coagulation factors (factors VIII, V, and prothrombin), which have been documented in dogs with hyperadrenocorticism, or the occurrence of secondary hypertension.[3] The presence of hyperadrenocorticism alone probably does not confer a high risk for thromboembolic complications necessitating prophylactic therapy. However, the presence of other concomitant risk factors may require anticoagulation.

Pancreatitis

The relationship between inflammatory conditions and the predisposition for developing thromboembolic events is well known. Proinflammatory cytokines such as TNF-α and IL-1 play a role in activating the coagulation system but are not the only contributors. In the case of severe pancreatitis, proteolytic enzymes that leak into the circulation are removed by the reticuloendothelial system once bound to α-macroglobulins.[27] Depletion of plasma α-macroglobulins or the inability of the reticuloendothelial system to remove bound proteases leads to activation of many plasma proteins, including those of the coagulation cascade and fibrinolytic system.[27] Athough the depletion of α-macroglobulins in patients with pancreatitis has been used to justify the use of fresh frozen plasma (FFP) transfusions, no veterinary trial has demonstrated an improvement in AT activity following transfusions.[15,28] A benefit to the course or outcome in human patients with severe pancreatitis by the administration of FFP has similarly not been demonstrated.[29,30]

Sepsis

In septic patients, several mechanisms exist by which thromboembolic events can occur. Generalized inflammation and circulation of cytokines are thought to activate the coagulation system. Furthermore, endotoxins and exotoxins released by microbes can contribute to thrombosis by causing direct endothelial damage, stimulating tissue factor (TF) expression, and activating clotting factors and platelets.[31] The progression of a hypercoagulable state to fulminant DIC occurs with concomitant dysfunction of the natural anticoagulant system. Depletion of AT, protein C, and protein S, and reduced plasmin activity, are key players in this progression. A more detailed discussion of DIC is found elsewhere. (See Chapter on Hemostasis and Disseminated Intravascular Coagulation). Necrotizing fasciitis is another important condition that exemplifies the relationship between infections and coagulation. Microorganisms can possess unique cell membrane components that elicit specific prothrombotic tendencies that result in the thrombosis of regional vessels and contribute to the extensive tissue necrosis and sloughing of muscle and skin seen with this condition.[32] In fact, the rapidity and extent of tissue destruction is more consistent with microvascular thrombosis and resultant ischemia than with direct microbial destruction of tissue.[31]

Orthopedic Surgery

The occurrence of PTE stemming from deep venous thrombosis in patients requiring orthopedic surgery is well documented in people, but this has not been described in the veterinary literature. However, the occurrence of thromboembolic events during or after total hip replacement in dogs has been described.[33-36] In the unique context of cemented total hip replacement, a marked increase occurs in proximal intramedullary pressure within the femur during femoral stem implantation. As cement intrudes into the cancellous bone, it dislodges particles of fat and bone, which enter the circulation and migrate to the right heart and pulmonary circulation.[35,36] This has been documented in studies using transesophageal echocardiography, capnography, pulmonary scintigraphy, and histologic evaluation.[33-36] Despite the fact that some form of thromboembolism occurs frequently in dogs undergoing total hip replacement, clinically significant abnormalities or fatalities remain rare. The pathophysiology of thromboembolism associated with total hip replacement differs from other diseases in that there is no direct perturbation of the coagulation system; therefore, preventative and therapeutic interventions should not involve the use of anticoagulants or antithrombotics. Nevertheless, a discussion of this phenomenon is important because the clinical manifestations (e.g., respiratory distress and sudden death) are identical to PTE caused by hypercoagulability. Techniques to reduce the risk of thromboembolic complications include controlling the rise in intramedullary pressure during implant insertion, use of vacuum drainage in the proximal femur, and meticulous, copious, pulsatile lavage of the bone-cement interface to remove embolic substrate.[35,36]

Laboratory Diagnosis of Hypercoagulation

The detection of hypercoagulability is extremely difficult in clinical practice. Little correlation exists between thrombocytosis, shortened coagulation times (decreased prothrombin time (PT), and activated partial thromboplastin time (aPTT)) and a prothrombotic tendency. Fibrin degradation products (FDP) are generated by the dissolution of fibrin by plasmin, and therefore, increased concentrations only indirectly imply thrombus formation.

Assessing risk for thromboembolic complications involves the recognition of predisposing conditions and populations rather than any single clinicopathologic abnormality. A list of predisposing conditions can be found in Table 21-1. Some authors have attempted to devise a predictive scheme based on the patient's plasma AT concentrations, but this algorithm has neither been validated nor is the AT assay widely available.[9] Such a scheme recommends AT supplementation and heparin therapy when AT activity levels fall below 60%. Other tests that have been developed include screening for elevations in the by-product of prothrombin activation (fragments F1 and F2) or fibrinogen cleavage (fibropeptides A and B), and increased concentrations of thrombin: AT complex.[36-39] Again, these markers indicate that thrombin has been generated rather than the likelihood of thromboembolism. Newer assays for D-dimers (a more specific indicator of cross-linked fibrin generation) are currently considered the best clinical test for diagnosing the presence of active coagulation.[40-42] Because of its high specificity, this semi-quantitative test may be best used to rule out cases of suspected PTE.[40] D-dimer concentrations > 2000 ng/dL had a 98.5% specificity in a heterogeneous population of dogs, and no dog with a confirmed embolus had a negative d-dimer test.[41] Thromboelastography, a global in vitro test of coagulation, is perhaps the best tool for assessing hypercoagulability, but remains a research tool optimally suited to characterize the degree of hypercoagulability seen with specific diseases.[43,44]

Table 21-1. Disorders that have been Associated with Thromboembolic Disease in Animals

Sepsis/severe infection
Severe trauma
Malignancy
Heat stroke
Severe burns
Pancreatitis
Immune-mediated hemolytic anemia
Protein-losing glomerulonephropathy
Protein-losing enteropathies
Hyperadrenocorticism
Exogenous glucocorticoid therapy
Vascular disease (heartworm infestation)

Anticoagulant and Antithrombotic Therapy

Unfractionated heparin is probably the most commonly employed form of anticoagulant therapy used in animals. The mechanism of action centers around the potentiation of AT, leading to the inactivation of factors IIa, Xa, IXa, XIa, and XIIa. Of these, the inactivation of IIa (thrombin) and Xa are considered the most important. Whereas heparin appears to increase tissue-type plasminogen activator (t-PA) activity, it does not appear to enhance fibrinolysis; however this subject remains highly controversial.[45] Various dosing schemes have been proposed and range from intermittent subcutaneous injections of 50 to 300 units/kg every 8 hours to continuous intravenous infusions of 5 to 20 units/kg/hour. It is important to realize that these dosing schemes are largely anecdotally derived, and studies to determine optimal dosing in patients with hypercoagulable tendencies have not been performed. Regardless of the dosing scheme, a common recommendation is to prolong the APTT by 1.5 to 2.5 times the baseline. Some limitations of monitoring heparin therapy via clotting times do exist, however, in that manipulation of the APTT does not necessarily decrease the risk of a thromboembolic event. Furthermore, considerable variation occurs in APTT sensitivity to heparin using different coagulometers.

One of the major concerns with heparin therapy is that it can lead to overt coagulopathy and major hemorrhage. Individual variation in the ability to metabolize heparin and changes in coagulation status in the course of many diseases explain the development of bleeding tendencies in previously hypercoagulable individuals. Although protamine sulfate is considered a reversal agent for heparin, few indications exist for its use given its side effects and the short half-life of heparin, particularly in hypercoagulable individuals. Another concern with the use of unfractionated heparin is that it can eliminate the important anti-inflammatory effects of AT, potentially limiting its use in critically ill patients.[46-49]

Given concerns over the possible complications of using unfractionated heparin, interest has been increased in the use of low molecular weight heparin (LMWH). Major advantages of LMWH include improved bioavailability, predictable renal clearance, predictable antithrombotic responses, more tempered effects on coagulation factors (mainly Xa), and supposedly prolonged half-life. However, several studies have shown that maintenance of a desirable anti-Xa activity level in both dogs and cats requires more frequent administration than the once daily dosing recommended for human patients.[50,51] A dose of 150 to 200 units/kg subcutaneously every 8 to 12 hours, in cats and dogs, respectively has been anecdotally reported with dalteparin.[20,50,51] Monitoring of APTT during LMWH therapy is not effective and may require assaying anti-Xa activity, which is not readily available. Because of the reduced risk of hemorrhage with LMWH, some authors have used it empirically without specific monitoring. However, further studies are needed to determine the optimal use of LMWH in dogs and cats, especially given the high cost of LMWH.

Coumarin-based anticoagulants (e.g., warfarin) block the g-carboxylation of several glutamate residues in factors II, VII, IX, and X, as well as the endogenous anticoagulant proteins C and S. The blockade results in incomplete molecules that are biologically inactive (unable to undergo calcium-mediated binding of prothrombin to platelet phospholipids), and are collectively known as PIVKA, or *proteins* induced by vitamin K antagonism or absence. The anticoagulant prevents the conversion of inactive vitamin K epoxide back to its active hydroquinone form that is required for proper clotting-factor synthesis. Therapy using coumadin should be carefully titrated against the PT, with the optimal goal of prolonging it to 1.5 to 2 times the patient's baseline PT. Recommended dose ranges are from 0.05 to 0.1 mg/kg PO SID for 3 days, then every other day to every third day, depending on individual response. Therapy should be recommended only in patients in which monitoring will be consistently and reliably performed.

Aspirin antagonizes thromboxane A_2, which is responsible for allowing platelets to alter their shape, release their granules, and aggregate. Aspirin is a mild platelet inhibitor that slightly attenuates aggregation responses to ADP and collagen but does not inhibit thrombin- or PAF-induced aggregation responses. Aspirin inhibits synthesis of thromboxane A_2 by irreversible acetylation of cyclooxygenase. Because the anuclear platelet cannot synthesize new proteins, it cannot manufacture any new enzyme during its 10-day lifetime. The typical dose of aspirin used as an anti-inflammatory agent may actually be procoagulant and, therefore, the use of an ultra-low dose has been recommended, which has been reported as 0.5 mg/kg/day PO.[52,53]

Fibrinolytic Agents

Although the practice is controversial, in the situation of a life-threatening thromboembolism, fibrinolytic drugs may be used to rapidly lyse thrombi and restore perfusion. This is accomplished by the ability of these agents to catalyze the formation of plasmin from its precursor plasminogen. These drugs create a generalized thrombolytic state when administered intravenously. Thus, both protective homeostatic thrombi and pathologic thromboemboli are broken down. In people, to reduce the nonselective systemic effects of fibrinolytic agents, intra-arterial administration has been used.[54] Given the high rate of complications, considerable cost, difficulty in obtaining these products, and high mortality of affected patients, experience with these treatment modalities is limited in veterinary medicine.

The use of streptokinase has been reported sporadically in the veterinary literature.[55-58] Streptokinase combines with a proactivator of inactive plasminogen, and this enzymatic complex catalyzes the conversion of inactive plasminogen to active plasmin, which degrades fibrin into fibrin degradation products. Since streptokinase does not have an affinity for fibrin-bound plasminogen, it can induce a state of systemic fibrinolysis and lead to significant hemorrhage. The dose in cats has been reported as a loading dose of 90,000 units per cat in 20 to 30 minutes, followed by a maintenance dose of 45,000 units per hour for 3 hours.[23] In dogs, dosage protocols include loading doses of 90,000 units intravenously administered slowly, followed by maintenance doses of 45,000 units per hour intravenous infusion over various periods of time, ranging from 30 minutes to 12 hours.[56,57] In one successfully treated case of arterial thromboembolism, a total of 8 streptokinase infusions were administered over a 50-hour period.[57]

Another potent thrombolytic agent is tissue-type plasminogen activator (t-PA), which is relatively clot-specific owing to its relative low affinity for circulating plasminogen and high affinity for cross-linked fibrin. In people, t-PA has been used for lysis of thrombi involved with acute myocardial infarction, PTE, and peripheral vascular thrombosis.[54] The clinical use of t-PA for the treatment of PTE in dogs and cats has not been reported. Only a few reports exist of successful thrombolysis in dogs using t-PA.[8,59] The cost and difficulty in obtaining this drug has precluded further evaluation of this treatment modality as a practical option. In cats, a total dose of 1 to 10 mg/kg administered as a 0.25 to 1 mg/kg/hour infusion has been reported, although the mortality rate associated with this therapy was 50%.[24]

The clinical use of urokinase in veterinary medicine is limited but has been reported in both cats and dogs with various types of thromboembolism.[26,60] The greatest experience is in cats with ATE, where the success rate was similar to that of other thrombolytic agents, but the complications were less severe and less common.[60] The one possible advantage suggested by the limited data available is that complications associated with UK therapy, as compared with other thrombolytics, may be less frequent and less severe; however, more studies are warranted to address this issue.

Conclusion

The occurrence of thromboembolic disease can have devastating consequences. Recognition of high-risk populations is important because timely intervention can be essential in the successful management of these cases, and preventative measures may be employed to decrease the likelihood of thromboembolic events. Knowledge of the pathophysiology involved in the development of thrombi in the context of different diseases can help in raising the index of suspicion in particular cases and in devising effective therapeutic strategies. Further research in the area of antithrombotics and anticoagulants is needed to determine optimal use of these agents in high-risk populations.

References

1. Spyropoulos AC: Emerging strategies in the prevention of venous thromboembolism in hospitalized medical patients. Chest 128:958, 2005.

2. Anderson FA Jr, Wheeler HB, Goldberg RJ, et al: A population-based perspective of the hospital incidence and case-fatality rates of deep vein thrombosis and pulmonary embolism: The Worcester DVT Study. Arch Intern Med 151:933, 1991.

3. Jacoby RC, Owings JT, Ortega T, et al: Biochemical basis for the hypercoagulable state seen in Cushing's syndrome. Arch Surg 136:1003, 2001.

4. Patrass GM, Dal Bo Zanon R, et al: Further studies on the hypercoagulable state of patients with Cushing's syndrome. Thromb Haemost 54:518, 1985.

5. Dal Bo Zanon R, Fomasiero L, Boscaro M, et al: Increased factor VIII associated activity in Cushing's syndrome: a probable hypercoagulable state. Thromb Haemostr 47:116, 1982.

6. Green RA: Pathophysiology of antithrombin III deficiency. Vet Clin North Am Small Anim Pract 18:95, 1988.

7. Abdullah R: Hemostatic abnormalities in nephrotic syndrome. Vet Clin North Am Small Anim Pract 18:105, 1988.

8. Clare AC, Kraje BJ: Use of recombinant tissue-plasminogen activator for aortic thrombolysis in a hypoproteinemic dog. J Am Vet Med Assoc 212:539, 1998.

9. Feldman BF, Kirby R, Caldin M: Recognition and treatment of disseminated intravascular coagulation. *In* Kirk's Current Veterinary Therapy XIII Small Animal Practice. Bonagura JD (ed). Philadelphia: WB Saunders, 2000, p. 190.

10. Booth NA: Fibrinolysis and thrombosis. Baillieres Best Pract Res Clin Haematol 12:42, 1999.

11. Good LI, Manning AM: Thromboembolic disease: Physiology of hemostasis and pathophysiology of thrombosis. Comp Contin Educ Pract Vet 25:650, 2003.

12. Stone SS, Johnstone IB, Brooks M, et al: Lupus-type "anticoagulant" in a dog with hemolysis and thrombosis. J Vet Intern Med 8:57, 1994.

13. Keyes ML, Rush JE, Knowles KE: Pulmonary thromboembolism in dogs. J Vet Emerg Crit Care 3:23, 1993.

14. Johnson LR, Lappin MR, Baker DC: Pulmonary thromboembolism in 29 dogs: 1985-1995. J Vet Intern Med 13:338, 1999.

15. Thompson MF, Scott-Moncrieff JC, Brooks MB: Effect of a single plasma transfusion on thromboembolism in 13 dogs with primary immune-mediated hemolytic anemia. J Am Anim Hosp Assoc 40:446, 2004.

16. Scott-Moncrieff JC, Treadwell NG, McCullough SM, Brooks MB: Hemostatic abnormalities in dogs with primary immune-mediated hemolytic anemia. J Am Anim Hosp Assoc 37:220, 2001.

17. Carr AP, Panciera DL, Kidd L: Prognostic factors for mortality and thromboembolism in canine immune-mediated hemolytic anemia: a retrospective study of 72 dogs. J Vet Intern Med 16:504, 2002.

18. Klag AR, Giger U, Shofer FS: Idiopathic immune-mediated hemolytic anemia in dogs: 42 cases (1986-1990). J Am Vet Med Assoc 202:783, 1993.

19. Klein MK, Dow SW, Rosychuk R, et al: Pulmonary thromboembolism associated with immune-mediated hemolytic anemia in dogs: ten cases (1982-1987). J Am Vet Med Assoc 246:246, 1989.

20. Smith CE, Rozanski EA, Freeman LM, et al: Use of low molecular weight heparin in cats: 57 cases (1999-2003) J Am Vet Med Assoc 225:1237, 2004.

21. Smith SA, Tobias AH, Jacob KA, et al: Arterial thromboembolism in cats: acute crisis in 127 cases (1992-2001) and long term management with low-dose aspirin in 24 cases. J Vet Intern Med 17:73, 2003.

22. Laste NJ, Harpster NK: A retrospective study of 100 cases of feline distal aortic thromboembolism: 1997-1993. J Am Anim Hosp Assoc 31:492, 1995.

23. Moore KE, Morris N, Dhupa N, et al: Retrospective study of streptokinase administration in 46 cats with arterial thromboembolism. J Vet Emerg Crit Care 19: 245, 2000.

24. Pion P, Kittleson M: Therapy for feline aortic thromboembolism. *In* Current Veterinary Therapy X. Kirk R (ed). Philadelphia: WB Saunders, 1989, p. 295.

25. Whelan MF, O'Toole TE, Lipitz L, et al: Aortic thromboembolism in dogs: 21 cases (1999-2004). Abstr J Vet Emerg Crit Care 15(Suppl): S8, 2005.

26.Whelan MF, O'Toole TE, Chan DL, Rush JE: Retrospective evaluation of urokinase use in dogs with thromboembolism (4 cases: 2003 – 2004). Abstr J Vet Emerg Crit Care 15(Suppl): S8, 2005.

27. Holm JL, Chan DL, Rozanski EA: Acute pancreatitis in dogs. J Vet Emerg Crit Care 13:201, 2003.

28. Rozanski EA, Hughes D, Scotti M, Giger U: The effect of fresh frozen plasma on plasma antithrombin III, prothrombin time and activated partial thromboplastin time in critically ill dogs. J Vet Emerg Crit Care 11:15, 2001.

29. Leese T, Holliday M, Watkins M, et al: A multicentre controlled clinical trial of high-volume fresh frozen plasma therapy in prognostically severe acute pancreatitis. Ann R Coll Surg Engl 73:207, 1991.

30. Leese T, Holloday M, Heath D, et al: A multicentre controlled clinical trial of low volume fresh frozen plasma therapy in acute pancreatitis. Br J Surg 74:907, 1987.

31. Bryant AE: Biology and pathogenesis of thrombosis and procoagulant activity in invasive infections caused by Group A Streptococci and Clostridium perfringes. Clin Microbiol Rev 16: 451, 2003.

32. Naido SL, Campbell DL, Miller LM, et al: Necrotizing fasciitis: a review. J Am Anim Hosp Assoc 41:104, 2005.

33. Reindl S, Matis U: Detection of embolic events by capnography and transesophageal echocardiography during total hip replacement. Vet Comp Orthop Traum 11:68, 1998.

34. Wheelwright EF, Byrick RJ, Kay JC, et al: Hypotension during cemented arthroplasty. J Bone Joint Surg Am 75:715, 1993.

35. Terrell SP, Chandra AMS, Pablo LS, Lewis DD: Fatal intraoperative pulmonary fat embolism during cemented total hip arthroplasty in a dog. J Am Anim Hosp Assoc 40:345, 2004.

36. Liska WD, Poteet BA: Pulmonary embolism associated with canine total hip replacement. Vet Surg 32:178, 2003.

37. Bateman SW, Mathews KA, Abrams-Ogg AC: Disseminated intravascular coagulation in dogs: Review of the literature. J Vet Emerg Crit Care 8:29, 1998.

38. Bateman SW, Mathews KA, Abrams-Ogg AC, et al: Evaluation of point-of-care tests for diagnosis of disseminated intravascular coagulation in dogs admitted to an intensive care unit. J Am Vet Med Assoc 215: 805, 1999.

39. Bateman SW, Mathews KA, Abrams-Ogg AC, et al: Diagnosis of disseminated intravascular coagulation in dogs admitted to an intensive care unit. J Am Vet Med Assoc 215:798, 1999.

40. Nelson OL, Andreasen C: The utility of plasma D-dimer to identify thromboembolic disease in the dog. J Vet Intern Med 17:830, 2003.

41. Nelson OL: Use of the D-dimer assay for diagnosing thromboembolic disease in the dog. J Am Anim Hosp Assoc 41:145, 2005.

42. Griffin A, Callan MB, Schofer, et al: Evaluation of a canine D-dimer point-of-care test kit for use in samples obtained from dogs with disseminated intravascular coagulation, thromboembolic disease, and hemorrhage. Am J Vet Res 64:1562, 2003.

43. Donahue SM, Otto CM: Thromboelastography: a tool for measuring hypercoagulability, hypocoagulability, and fibrinolysis. J Vet Emerg Crit Care 15:9, 2005.

44. Otto CM, Rieser TM, Brooks MB, et al: Evidence of hypercoagulability in dogs with parvoviral enteritis. J Am Vet Med Assoc 217:1500, 2000.

45. Minnema MC, ten Cate H, van Beck EJ, et al: Effects of heparin on fibrinolysis in patients with pulmonary embolism. Thromb Haemost 77:1164, 1997.

46. Opal SM, Kessler CM, Roemisch J, et al: Antithrombin, heparin, and heparin sulphate. Crit Care Med: 30(5 Suppl):S325, 2002.

47. Hopper K, Bateman SW: An updated view of hemostasis: mechanism of hemostatic dysfunction associated with sepsis. J Vet Emerg Crit Care 15:83, 2005.

48. Roemisch J, Gray E, Hoffman JN, et al: Antithrombin: a new look at the actions of a serine protease inhibitor. Blood Coag Fibrinolysis 13:657, 2002.

49. Hoffman JN, Vollmar B, Laschke MW, et al: Adverse effect of heparin on antithrombin action during endotoxemia: microhemodynamic and cellular mechanisms. Thromb Haemost 88:242, 2002.

50. Alwood AJ, Downend AD, Simpson SA, et al: Pharmacokinetics of dalteparin and enoxaparin in healthy cats. Abstr J Vet Emerg Crit Care 15(Suppl):S1, 2005.

51. Dunn M, Charland V, Thorneloe C: The use of low molecular weight heparin in 6 dogs. Abstr J Vet Intern Med 18(3):389, 2004.

52. Weinkle TK, Center SA, Randolph JF, et al: Evaluation of prognostic factors, survival rates, and treatment protocols for immune-mediated hemolytic anemia in dogs: 151 cases (1993-2002). J Am Vet Med Assoc 226:1869, 2005.

53. Brainard BM, Meredith CP, Callan MB, et al: Evidence of hypercoagulability in dogs treated with acetylsalicyclic acid (ASA). Abstr J Vet Emerg Crit Care 15(Suppl):S2, 2005.

54. Schneck MJ, Biller J: New treatments in acute ischemic stroke. Curr Treat Options Neurol 7:499, 2005.

55. Thompson MF, Scott-Moncrieff JC, Hogan DF: Thrombolytic therapy in dogs and cats. J Vet Emerg Crit Care 11:111, 2001.

56. Ramsey CC, Burney DP, Macintire DK, Finn-Bodner S: Use of streptokinase in four dogs with thrombosis. J Am Vet Med Assoc 209:780, 1996.

57. Tater KC, Drellich S, Beck K: Management of femoral artery thrombosis in an immature dog. J Vet Emerg Crit Care 15: 52, 2005.

58. Saoling L, HengLeng Y, HuiPi H, et al: Case report: management of canine pulmonary thromboembolism after adultcide administration in a heartworm-infected dog. Taiwan J Vet Med Anim Husb 66:225, 1996.

59. Bliss SP, Bliss Sk, Harvey HJ: Use of recombinant tissue-plasminogen activator in a dog with chylothorax secondary to catheter-associated thrombosis of the cranial vena cava. J Am Anim Hosp Assoc 38:431, 2002.

60. Whelan MF, O'Toole TE, Chan DL, Rush JE: Retrospective evaluation of urokinase use in cats with arterial thromboembolism. Abstr J Vet Emerg Crit Care 15(Suppl):S8, 2005.

Part IV

Gastrointestinal

Chapter 22

Periodontal and Endodontic Disease

Alexander M. Reiter
Colin E. Harvey

Periodontal and endodontic diseases are common in small animal practice and are similar in several ways:

- The basic pathology is inflammation resulting in bone resorption.
- The cause is most commonly contamination by oral flora.
- The end result of the pathologic process is loss of the tooth, permitting the adjacent tissues to recover from the chronic infection.

The major difference between periodontal and endodontic diseases is the location of the primary lesion.

Periodontal disease is centered in the periodontium (gingiva, periodontal ligament, alveolar bone, cementum), spreading along the periodontal space toward the root apex and causing loss of alveolar bone as it progresses. If allowed to continue to develop, it will eventually affect the periapical region of the tooth root, leading to retrograde pulpal infection. Thus, endodontic disease can occur as a result of severe periodontal disease.

Endodontic disease is centered in the pulp cavity, as a result of inflammation or necrosis of the pulp inside the tooth. The pathology spreads outward through foramina at the root apex or other areas of the root surface to involve the periodontal ligament and alveolar bone. If allowed to continue to develop, it will eventually affect more coronal areas of the periodontium. Thus, periodontal disease can occur as a result of severe endodontic disease.

Periodontal and endodontic disease may co-exist in the same tooth. It is often possible to recognize radiographically which condition was first to appear. When the condition starts as periodontal disease, subsequently spreading to involve the periapical region of the tooth root, it is referred to as *periodontal-endodontic lesion*. When the condition is primarily centered at the periapical region of the tooth root, secondarily affecting the mid- or coronal tooth-supporting alveolar bone and causing a fistula through the gingival attachment into the oral cavity, it is referred to as *endodontic-periodontal lesion*. Regardless of what came first, treatment must include both aspects of the disease (although many teeth with "perio-endo" or "endo-perio" lesions are so severely affected that extraction often is the only practical treatment option).

Periodontal Disease

Periodontal disease is the most common disease occurring in domestic dogs and cats and is defined as plaque-induced pathology of any part of the tissues that hold the tooth in the mouth - the gingiva, periodontal ligament, alveolar bone, and cementum. When accumulation of plaque is prevented by effective oral hygiene, periodontal disease does not develop.1 Local severity and systemic impact on the rest of the body are reasons that companion animals should receive an oral examination every time they are seen by a veterinarian. Periodontal disease is often separated into two clinical conditions.

Gingivitis is an inflammation of the gingiva, presenting clinically as reddening and edema initially at the gingival margin and progressing to visible ulceration and spontaneous bleeding. Gingivitis is reversible if dental plaque is removed by home or professional oral hygiene procedures.

Periodontitis is an inflammation and destruction of the non-gingival periodontal tissues and can be thought of as "alveolar bone osteomyelytis." It is diagnosed clinically as "loss of attachment" (i.e., the connective tissue attachment between the root and the alveolar bone no longer extends to the level of the cementoenamel junction [CEJ] of the tooth), which is recognized:

- Because gingival recession exposes part of the root.
- When a gently applied blunt-tipped probe can be passed between the tooth root and the gingiva into a periodontal pocket apical to the CEJ.
- Radiographically as horizontal or vertical alveolar bone loss.

Anatomy, Pathophysiology, and Oral Environment

The *gingiva* provides a thick protective cap to the alveolar margin (the tip of the alveolar bone closest to the crown). The marginal gingiva abuts the tooth crown and is not attached to bone but held in place by the hemidesmosomal attachment of the sulcular epithelium to the enamel surface. The *periodontal* ligament holds the tooth in the jaw by means of fibers and provides a shock-absorbing effect to prevent fracture of teeth during forceful occlusal action. The *alveolar bone* surrounding the roots has the most rapid turn-over of any bone in the body. The alveolar margin is the critical area in development of periodontitis.

Evaporation causes the salivary fluid to become deposited as a glycoprotein layer (the *pellicle*) on the tooth crowns, entrapping bacteria. *Plaque* is the developing biofilm on the surface of the teeth. The salivary fluid in which the teeth are bathed has antibacterial properties (lysozyme, lactoferrins, IgA with specific antibodies), and the combination of this antibacterial activity and daily occlusal scrubbing works well to keep the plaque from getting out of hand under "normal" conditions. Excellent long-term oral health is easy to achieve if daily oral hygiene is impeccable.[1] When oral hygiene is less than optimal and plaque is allowed to accumulate, it becomes thicker and more complex, and the protective components in oral fluids have less effect on the microbial inhabitants in the deeper layers. *Calculus* forms when calcium carbonate and other calcium salts in salivary fluid crystallize on the tooth surface, mineralizing the soft plaque into a hard material. Following dental scaling, it takes 2 to 3 days for plaque to become sufficiently mineralized to form calculus that resists being readily wiped off by dental abrasion. Calcium salts are more likely to be deposited on plaque in an alkaline environment. The mouths of dogs and cats are slightly alkaline (oral fluid in humans is usually slightly acidic). Thus, dogs and cats are more prone to deposition of calculus than are humans.[2]

Plaque Development and Periodontal Infection

When occlusal scrubbing is insufficient or infrequent, plaque thickens and matures. In the deeper part of plaque, the oxygen is strangled out of the fluid as a result of metabolism of aerobic organisms, and an anaerobic environment is established. This is unique to the plaque on teeth because of the lack of vascularity of the enamel surface on which plaque forms. Gingivitis and periodontitis are referred to as "bacterial infections," but several hundred bacterial species have been identified to date in normal and diseased mouths of dogs and cats.[3] Plaque development on a clean tooth surface following dental scaling follows a predictable pattern:

1. Colonization of the pellicle by aerobic cocci.
2. Adhesion of aerobic rods on the sticky and irregular surface provided by the growing coccal layer.
3. The aerobic cocci and rods multiply, and as they do so, the oxygen gradient in the thickening plaque changes so that at its deepest point oxygen is no longer available. The occasional obligate anaerobes caught deep in plaque can now grow. Plaque maturation to the point where it will support anaerobic organisms takes about 24 hours in the dog.
4. The biochemical environment changes, as plaque continues to mature, and is enriched by products of gingival inflammation. The mixture of microbial detritus and products of inflammation forms a physical and chemical environment that allows spirochetes and other organisms with complex growth requirements to thrive.
5. A "climax biofilm community" results - a semi-stable state in balance with available nutrients and oxygen, made more complex in the case of plaque by the presence of calculus, which provides protected spaces in an anoxic and nutrient-rich environment.

Periodontopathogens are bacteria that are the putative cause of gingivitis and periodontitis. They (a) are cultured more commonly from diseased individuals than from nondiseased individuals and from diseased areas of the mouth than from healthy areas in the same individual; (b) produce toxins or tissue-destructive enzymes such as matrix metalloproteinases; (c) show cytotoxic effects on tissue culture; and (d) reveal other "virulent factors." DNA probe technology has allowed recognition of a group referred to as *pathogen-related oral spirochetes* (PROS) in dogs as well as in humans.[4] Carnivore and human oral floras have many similarities, but also some important differences. The gram-negative anaerobic rod *Porphyromonas gingivalis* is considered to be the key human periodontopathogen. A catalase-positive form of *P. gingivalis* is found commonly in canine and feline periodontal specimens and is recognized as a distinct species - *Porphyromonas gulae.*[5] Other recognized canine and feline *Porphyromonas* organisms include *P. cangingivalis, P. canoris, P. cansulci, P. crevioricanis,* and *P. gingivicanis.*[6]

Progression of Periodontal Disease

As with bacterial infections in any other tissue, the initial effect is inflammation (gingivitis). Neutrophils are attracted to the site, move onto the epithelial surface through large intercellular spaces of the sulcular epithelium, and engulf, ingest, and digest the plaque bacteria. When a pathogenic plaque mixture is present, many neutrophils become over-full and burst, and some retire into the adjacent tissue before they burst; bursting neutrophils release bacterial toxins and destructive enzymes, including matrix metalloproteinases (e.g., collagenase) within tissue, causing breakdown of connective tissue integrity. The bursting neutrophils also release pro-inflammatory cytokines (e.g., IL-1β, IL-6, PGE2 and TNF-α) that propagate the inflammatory response. The sulcular epithelial layer ulcerates, exposing the more vulnerable connective tissue to direct bacterial invasion. As the destructive inflammatory-infective mixture descends deeper into the tissue, inflammation-induced resorption nibbles away the alveolar bone to produce periodontitis. Continuing bone loss causes instability of the attachment and mobility of the tooth, which is pushed against the remaining bone during chewing. This further enhances alveolar bone resorption by squeezing the blood vessels adjacent to the tooth. In an aging toy-breed dog with severe periodontitis, only a match-stick of mandibular bone may be present adjacent to the roots of the large first molar tooth, and pathologic fracture of the mandible is possible (Figure 22-1). If the process continues for long enough, the eventual result is loss of the tooth. This is actually a defense mechanism - finally, the remaining tissues can recover because the presence of the constant overwhelming plaque bacterial burden has been removed.

In the (usually long) period between the initial gingivitis and the final exfoliation of the tooth, bacteria adjacent to capillaries are squeezed into the vascular space, causing bacteremia. Bacteremia secondary to periodontal disease occurs daily in patients with gingivitis and active periodontitis, and it is normally rapidly cleared by the reticuloendothelial system in otherwise healthy patients.[7] Bacteremia is accompanied by chronic body-wide release of inflammatory mediators, immune complexes, and bacterial and cellular degradation by-products that may produce direct or immune-mediated distant organ pathology. The long-term consequences of these intravascular effects are the subject of ongoing investigations. It is known that an association exists between severity of periodontal disease and distant organ abnormalities in both humans (Table 22-1)[8] and dogs.[9,10] Circulatory markers of systemic inflammation are increased in dogs with more severe periodontal disease; they decrease following periodontal treatment.[11] Studies are underway to determine whether the cause (plaque $\rightarrow$ gingivitis/periodontitis $\rightarrow$ bacteremia/systemic inflammation) and effect (distant organ damage) hypothesis is correct.

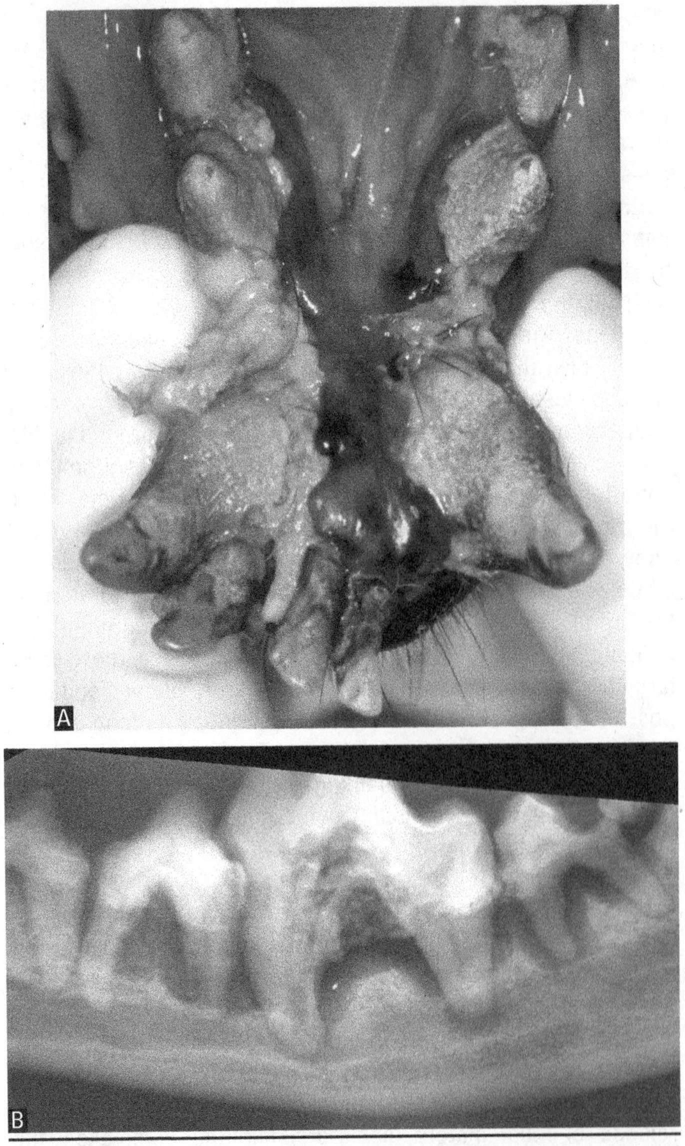

Figure 22-1. Dog with severe periodontitis. (A) Excessive plaque and calculus accumulation at mandibular incisor, canine, and premolar teeth. (B) Dental radiograph of left mandibular premolars and molars showing advanced loss of alveolar bone; the mandible is at risk of pathologic fracture.

Table 22-1. Confirmed or Suspected Interaction of Periodontitis with Systemic Diseases in Humans[21]

Cardiovascular diseases
Angina pectoris
Myocardial infarction
Endocarditis
Difficulties during pregnancy
Premature birth
Low birth weight
Increased infant mortality
Stroke, brain abscess
Pulmonary infections
Diabetes mellitus

Prevention and Therapy

Prevention is primarily directed at removing or reducing subsequent accumulation of plaque and calculus, or at suppressing the tissue-destructive effects of the inflammatory response. Professional supra- and subgingival scaling as needed, followed by daily tooth brushing, is the "gold standard" for prevention. Products that enhance dietary abrasion or chemically suppress plaque or calculus deposition are recognized by the Seal of Acceptance system of the Veterinary Oral Health Council (www.VOHC.org). Systemic antibiotic treatment is not indicated for periodontal patients except in very limited circumstances.[12] A trivalent *Porphyromonas* bacterin for use as a periodontal disease preventive in dogs is under development.[13] Treatment with anti-inflammatory drugs has been shown experimentally to have a protective effect on alveolar bone in dogs.[14] Anti-osteoclastic drugs such as bisphosphonates also retard alveolar bone loss experimentally in dogs.[15] Use of these pharmacologic agents long-term in veterinary patients has not been investigated and thus cannot be recommended at this time.

In some patients, several different types of procedures may be indicatedwith the patient under anesthesia. It is useful to differentiate between *preventive* and *treatment* procedures, both of which fit under the term periodontal *management*.[2] Frequent home oral hygiene and professional dental scaling are the primary preventive procedures. Professional scaling under anesthesia is necessary when accumulation of calculus is moderate. Gingivitis and mild or moderate periodontitis (periodontal pockets of up to 5 mm) can be managed effectively by scaling followed by frequent (daily) oral hygiene in an otherwise healthy dog or cat.

When periodontitis is extensive, or when complicating factors exist such as systemic illness, preventive procedures alone are insufficient. The most commonly indicated periodontal treatment in dogs and cats is extraction – it is also the most reliable means of preventing further local deep-seated periodontal infection and its systemic consequences. Some severely affected teeth can be successfully retained in the mouth by a combination of scaling, periodontal surgery, and conscientiously applied oral home hygiene.

Endodontic Disease

Endodontics refers to the branch of dentistry concerned with the anatomy, physiology, and pathology of the dentin, dental pulp, and periapical region and with the treatment of endodontic disease.[16] The periapical region of the tooth root becomes involved when bacteria invade the pulp, rendering it partially to totally necrotic. Exposed pulp in germ-free rats remains vital and relatively uninflamed, and the exposed site is repaired with reparative dentin. Thus, without bacteria and their by-products, periapical disease of endodontic origin does not occur.

Endodontic Anatomy

The pulp is a soft tissue with highly differentiated *odontoblasts* arranged peripherally in direct contact with the dentin. Because of the close relationship between odontoblasts and dentin, they are considered a functional entity and referred to as the *pulp-*

dentin complex.[17] The pulp also consists of loose connective tissue, intercellular substance, blood and lymph vessels, nerves, and fibers. The pulp connects with periapical tissues through the apex in each root. Root development in dogs and cats results in the formation of several *apical foramina*, in ground sections appearing as *apical delta. Secondary, accessory, lateral, and furcation canals* also may connect pulp tissue with periodontal ligament.[18,19] Endodontic success is influenced by obturation of all these canals. If bacteria from progressing periodontal disease reach and involve these canals, pulp involvement will result. Some epithelial cells persist within the periodontal ligament during tooth development, the *epithelial rests of Malassez*, forming a net-like structure around the tooth root.[20]

Arterioles enter through the apical foramina and pass centrally through the pulp, giving off lateral branches that divide further into capillaries. Minor vessels may enter through secondary, accessory, lateral, and furcation canals but do not provide sufficient collateral circulation. Venous return is collected by a network of capillaries that unite to form *venules* coursing down the central portion of the pulp. The blood supply diminishes with age, rendering a pulp more susceptible to irreversible damage. Inflammation in a localized coronal zone does not cause immediate strangulation of apical vessels and death of the pulp, as it is confined by a combination of ground substance and a unique blood supply. *Arteriovenous shunts* redistribute the blood and prevent buildup of unsustainable pressure in the rigid environment.[17,20] Autonomic and sensory nerve fibers enter the pulp with the vessels through the apical foramina. Individual axons branch into many terminal filaments, which may enter the dentinal tubules. The autonomic nerve supply consists of sympathetic fibers that control microcirculation. The two types of sensory fibers are *myelinated A fibers* and *unmyelinated C fibers.* The faster-conducting A fibers are responsible for sharp, localized pain owing to rapid movement of fluid in dentinal tubules, resulting in mechanical distortion of tissue in the pulp-dentin border and stimulation of A fibers. Stimulation of the slower-conducting C fibers gives rise to the duller, throbbing, less-localized pain.[17,20]

The primary role of the pulp is to produce dentin by mature odontoblasts, which are incapable of further division and, if damaged, may be replaced from undifferentiated mesenchymal cells. The odontoblast cell bodies are separated from mineralized dentin by an unmineralized *predentin* layer. *Primary dentin* is formed during tooth development. *Secondary dentin* is formed physiologically after the tooth is fully developed. Its formation continues throughout life, enabling the vital pulp to partially compensate for the loss of enamel or dentin caused by mechanical trauma or disease. Teeth of young adult animals have a fairly wide pulp cavity, whereas in old animals the pulp cavity is usually narrow. The narrower the pulp cavity, the thicker are the dentinal walls, and thus the stronger and more aged is the tooth. Comparing the radiographic appearance of the pulp cavity between ipsi- and contralateral teeth is an effective means of determining pulp vitality in teeth with suspected endodontic pathology. *Tertiary dentin (reparative dentin)* is formed in response to trauma or disease.[17,20]

Dentin consists of thousands of dentinal tubules radiating outward from the dental pulp to the enamel in the crown and cementum in the root. The tubules contain the long, narrow odontoblastic processes and are filled with *dentinal fluid.* A pressure gradient between the pulp and oral cavity accounts for the outward flow of fluid. Exposure of tubules from tooth fracture or cavity preparation results in outward movement of fluid to the exposed dentin surface. *Peritubular dentin* lines the tubules and is laid down by the odontoblastic process; *intertubular dentin* is found between tubules. Partial or complete occlusion of tubules may occur as a result of aging or in response to stimuli such as mechanical wear or caries. When tubules become filled with mineral deposits, the dentin becomes sclerotic and less permeable, shielding the pulp from irritation. *Dentinal sclerosis* gives aged teeth a characteristic translucency, and clinically the dentin appears glassy.[17,20]

Causes of Endodontic Disease

Rapid tooth wear removes enamel and dentin faster than odontoblasts can form dentin. The pulp may be exposed or eventually succumb to prolonged chronic inflammation. Causes of tooth wear include *abrasion* (tooth wear caused by contact of a tooth with a non-dental material), attrition (tooth wear caused by tooth-by-tooth contact in malocclusion), and *erosion* (demineralization of the tooth surface because of acids). *Caries* is the most common cause of endodontic disease in humans but is rather uncommon in dogs and has not yet been reported to occur in cats. It results from demineralization of the tooth surface by acids that are formed during fermentation of highly refined carbohydrates by cariogenic bacteria. Although the most common responses to caries are dentin sclerosis and formation of reparative dentin, the formation of a *dead tract* in dentin is not considered to be a defensive reaction. It is an area in dentin with tubules devoid of odontoblast processes, providing a channel for bacteria to reach the pulp.[20]

Crown infraction is an incomplete fracture of enamel without loss of tooth structure. Though these fractures are weak points through which bacteria and by-products can challenge the pulp, rarely do they result in permanent pulp damage. An *uncomplicated crown fracture* is a fracture of enamel only or enamel and dentin without pulp exposure. If enamel is involved only, the consequences are minimal; if dentin is exposed, a pathway exists for stimuli to pass through dentinal tubules to the pulp, resulting in formation of sclerotic and reparative dentin, chronic pulpitis, or pulp necrosis. A *complicated crown fracture* is a fracture of enamel and dentin with pulp exposure. If left untreated, this always results in pulp necrosis. This fracture is common in canine teeth of dogs and cats owing to motor-vehicle trauma, falls from great heights, kicks, and hits. Military, police, and prison dogs are more prone to fracture of canine teeth if their distal tooth surfaces are weakened by wear from chewing on cage bars (cage biter teeth). Fractures of carnassial teeth in dogs are frequently caused by chewing on hard objects (e.g., nylon bones, cow hooves, large ice cubes). Resorption initiating on external root surfaces and progressing into root and/or crown dentin are often the cause of crown fracture in cats, with root fragments remaining in the alveoli. A *crown-root fracture* is a fracture of enamel, dentin, and cementum. The pulp may or may not be involved. If a crown-root fracture cannot be made into an uncomplicated crown fracture by periodontal surgery and/or orthodontic extrusion, the tooth should be extracted. A *root fracture* is a fracture of cementum and dentin, usually with pulp exposure. The coronal segment is displaced and pulp necrosis may result, but generally the apical segment is not displaced and has an intact blood supply. Apical root and midroot fractures have a good to fair prognosis (root canal therapy and splinting of the coronal segment), while coronal root fractures have a poor prognosis.[20]

In *concussion* and *subluxation*, the tooth shows normal or slightly increased mobility and sensitivity to percussion, but no displacement. The tooth should be monitored radiographically to determine pulp vitality. *Luxation* refers to clinically or radiographically evident displacement of the tooth within its alveolus. Lateral and extrusive luxation occur most commonly and are often associated with fracture of the alveolus. Intrusive luxation is a rare complication associated with trauma that forced a tooth with periodontal disease into the nasal cavity, resulting in chronic rhinitis and nasal discharge. Surgical exposure through an intra-oral approach is required to remove the tooth. *Avulsion (exarticulation)* refers to complete extrusive luxation. The teeth most commonly avulsed in dogs are the incisors and canine teeth. The success of reimplantation of an avulsed tooth is greatly influenced by the length of time that the tooth is out of the alveolar socket. Luxated and avulsed teeth require repositioning, stabilization, and root canal therapy owing to the likely loss of blood supply to the pulp.[20]

Thermal injury causing pulp hyperemia, pulpitis, or pulp necrosis is caused by poor dental scaling and polishing techniques (insufficient cooling water, too much pressure on the working tip, prolonged scaling/polishing at the same location), restorative cavity and crown margin preparations; and careless use of thermocautery, diathermy, electrosurgery and laser units near teeth, and electric cord injuries. *Anachoresis* refers to infection of pulp tissue in a state of hyperemia by hematogenic invasion of bacteria through apical and non-apical ramifications. Progression of pulp hyperemia to pulpitis in the presence of bacteria ultimately results in pulp necrosis. Other causes of endodontic disease include *external tooth resorption*, progressive *internal tooth resorption*, severe *periodontitis*, *use of local anesthetics that contain a vasoconstrictor*, excessive *root planing*, unbased *restorations*, and rapid *orthodontic tooth movement*. Tooth resorption is common in cats, but infrequent in dogs. Periodontally diseased teeth have narrower root canal widths compared with healthy teeth owing to deposition of reparative dentin along the dentinal walls. Bacterial infection of the pulp is possible in areas devoid of cementum and through lateral, accessory, secondary, and furcation canals if exposed to oral fluids.[20]

Clinical Signs

Evaluation of the endodontic patient requires assessment of previous trauma and chewing history and inspection and palpation of intra- and extraoral tissues, focusing on tooth discoloration, crown defects, intra- and extraoral swellings, and sinus tract formation. Reduced biting pressure during play or aggression training and reluctance to eat hard or fibrous food may be noted. To relieve discomfort during late signs of abscess development, the animal may attempt to contact cool or cold surfaces and liquids. Regional lymphadenopathy and fever develop as the abscess reaches an acute stage. In cooperative patients, the occlusal surface of several healthy teeth and the suspect tooth can be percussed with a finger or the handle of a dental mirror. Hyperreaction indicates that the infection extended beyond the pulp into the periapical region. The pressure build-up in this small space from edema and inflammation will yield pain on percussion. Endodontic disease may result in crown discoloration (pink, red, purple, gray, or brown). Progressive tooth discoloration and/or radiographic changes can reasonably be interpreted as indicative of pulp necrosis. One study revealed that over 90% of teeth with crown discoloration are nonvital.[21] Transillumination of normal and suspect teeth reveals vital teeth to be rather translucent, whereas nonvital teeth tend to appear more opaque. Crown integrity is evaluated with a fine dental explorer. The tip of the explorer will find irregularities in the crown surface or catch in an open pulp chamber. Recent pulp exposures reveal bleeding pulp, whereas old pulp exposures show black debris and necrotic pulp tissue. Tooth mobility is directly proportional to the integrity of the attachment of the root. The degree of depressibility of the tooth within its alveolus should also be tested by pressing the tooth into its alveolus and watching for any vertical movement. The pressure exerted by purulent exudate in the periapical region may cause some transient tooth mobility. Crown-root and root fractures often result in mobility of a crown segment. Before incipient swelling becomes clinically evident, it may be detected by gentle palpation with the index finger. Swelling and sinus tracts originating from endodontically diseased maxillary fourth premolar teeth in dogs and cats often are located ventral to the medial canthus of the eye. Intraoral sinus tracts are commonly draining at the mucogingival junction. Swellings and sinus tracts owing to endodontic disease often have a history of responsiveness to antibiotics and recurrence when antibiotic therapy is discontinued. Sinus tracts can be traced with a gutta-percha cone, and a radiograph is obtained to locate their source.[16]

Pathophysiology and Radiographic Signs

A reversible pulpitis is pulp inflammation to the extent that thermal stimuli (usually cold) cause a quick, sharp, hypersensitive response that subsides as soon as the stimulus is removed. If the irritant is removed, the inflamed pulp will revert to an uninflamed state that is asymptomatic. An *irreversible pulpitis* may be acute, subacute, or chronic, partial or total, infected or sterile. The acutely inflamed pulp is symptomatic; the chronically inflamed pulp is usually asymptomatic. A symptomatic irreversible pulpitis elicits prolonged episodes of pain. A thickening of the apical periodontal ligament may become evident on radiographs in the advanced stage of disease. A reddish cauliflower-like growth of pulp tissue through an open pulp chamber is one variation of asymptomatic irreversible pulpitis and attributed to a low-grade chronic irritation of the pulp and the generous vascularity characteristically found in young animals. *Pulp necrosis* results from an untreated irreversible pulpitis, a traumatic injury, or any event that causes long-term interruption of the blood supply to the pulp, and may be partial or total. Total necrosis before it affects the periodontal ligament is asymptomatic. Protein breakdown products, bacteria and endotoxins will eventually spread beyond the apical foramina into the periapical region, leading to thickening of the periodontal ligament and manifesting as tenderness to percussion and chewing.[20]

Acute apical periodontitis is a painful inflammation around the apex before the bone begins to resorb and results from an extension of pulpal disease into the periapical tissue, an overextension of endodontic instruments or materials, or occlusal trauma such as bruxism. It may occur around vital and nonvital teeth. The apical periodontal ligament may be within normal limits or only slightly widened on dental radiographs because of edema. An *acute apical abscess* is a painful, purulent exudate around the apex. The periodontal ligament may be within normal limits or only slightly thickened on dental radiographs with a relatively normal (or slightly thickened) lamina dura because the fulminating infection has rapidly spread beyond the confines of the cortical plate before bone demineralization can be detected radiographically. Presenting signs include rapid onset of slight to severe swelling (cellulitis spreading into fascial planes), moderate to severe pain, and slight increase in tooth mobility; fever and general malaise are present in more advanced cases. *Chronic apical periodontitis (granuloma)* is generally asymptomatic and manifests radiographically. Bacteria and endotoxins, cascading out into the periapical region from a necrotic pulp, cause extensive demineralization of cancellous and cortical bone and large or small, diffuse or circumscribed, radiographically evident lesions. Slight tenderness may be evident on percussion and/or palpation testing. A sinus tract may yield frank suppuration. As pressure from pus is relieved by drainage, the sinus tract may close temporarily; if pressure from pus builds up again, the sinus tract returns. Epithelial rests of Malassez may respond to the stimulus in the apical periodontal ligament by proliferating to wall off the irritants coming through the apical foramina, creating a *periapical cyst.* A *phoenix abscess* is an acute exacerbation of chronic apical periodontitis, and symptoms identical to those present with an acute apical abscess will appear (Figure 22-2).[20]

Periapical osteosclerosis is excessive bone mineralization around the apex of a vital tooth caused by low-grade pulp irritation; this condition is asymptomatic and benign and does not require endodontic therapy. *Condensing osteitis (focal sclerosing osteomyelytis)* is excessive bone mineralization around the apex of a non-vital tooth caused by long-standing and low-toxic exudation from an infected pulp, resulting in mild irritation and circumscribed proliferation of the periapical bone. *Acute osteomyelytis* can arise directly from an endodontic infection. Live bacteria pass the apex and multiply in the marrow spaces and soft tissue of the bone, resulting in localized or widespread infection of the bone; if untreated, the acute form may progress to a chronic form, eventually leading to bone necrosis. *Calcification of pulp tissue* includes diffuse mineralization (often a pathologic process related to various forms of injury) or pulp stones *(denticles)* that form around epithelial cells remnants. Perhaps the greatest endodontic significance of pulp calcification is that it may hinder root canal shaping.[20]

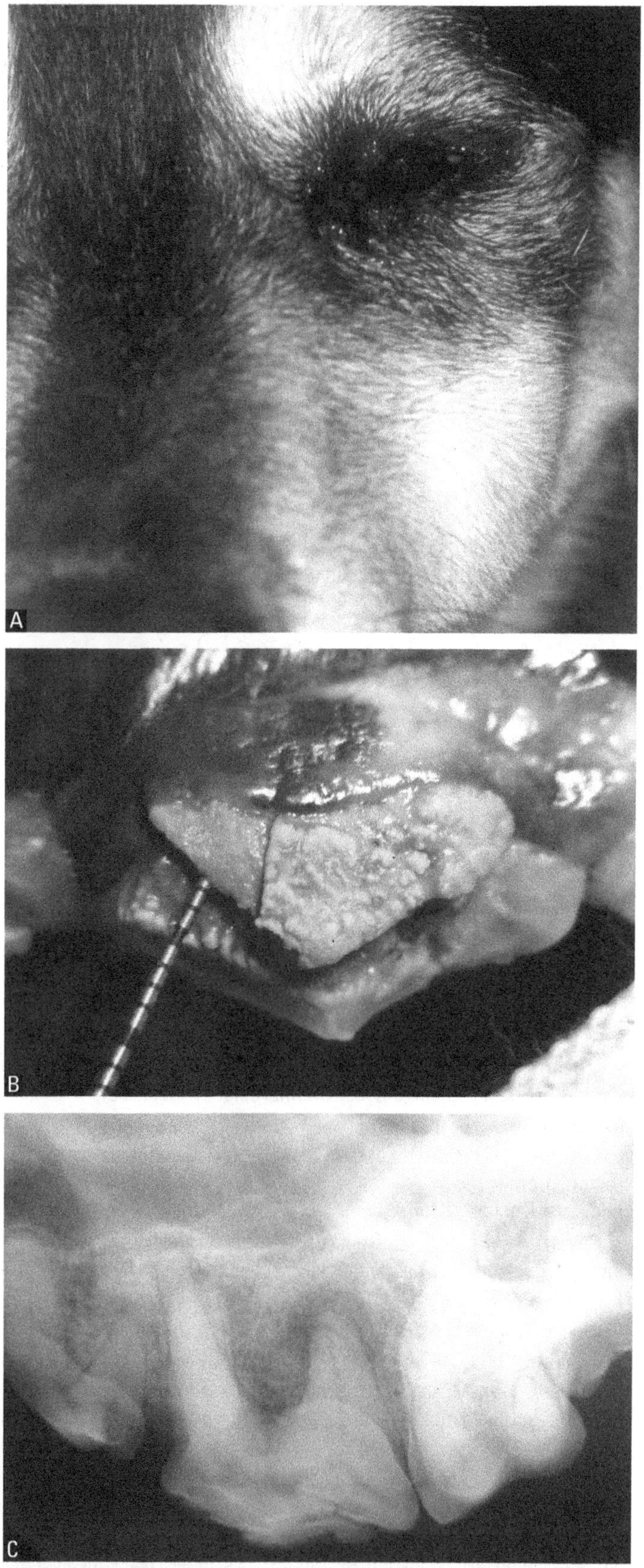

Figure 22-2. Dog with an apical abscess originating from the left maxillary fourth premolar tooth. (A) Left infraorbital swelling. (B) Crown-root slab fracture. (C) Dental radiograph showing a large radiolucent halo around apex of the distal root.

Endodontic Treatment

Vital pulp therapy is primarily utilized for "recent" tooth fractures or after intentional surgical crown reduction to preserve pulp vitality and increase strength of the tooth by allowing continued dentin formation. If the pulp is exposed for longer periods of time or has become necrotic, *standard root canal therapy* is performed and includes accessing the pulp cavity, debriding, shaping, disinfecting and obturating (filling) the root canal, and access restoration. An *apexification procedure* is a type of root canal therapy that is performed to stimulate the formation of a closed apex with hard tissue when a necrotic pulp is present in an incompletely developed permanent tooth in young animals or in teeth of adult animals that have "open" apices owing to apical root resorption. *Surgical root canal therapy* is performed when standard root canal therapy has failed or will likely fail in teeth with advanced periapical disease. This includes access through oral mucosa or skin, alveolectomy, apicoectomy and retrograde filling. Extraction is the treatment of choice for teeth fractured through the long axis of the tooth root(s) and teeth with advanced root resorption.

References

1. Lindhe J, Hamp S, Löe H: Plaque induced periodontal disease in beagle dogs. A 4-year clinical, roentgenographical and histometrical study. J Periodont Res 10:243, 1975.

2. Harvey CE: Management of periodontal disease: understanding the options. Vet Clin North Am Small Anim Pract 31:819, 2005.

3. Harvey CE, Thornsberry C, Miller BR: Subgingival bacteria - comparison of culture results in dogs and cats with gingivitis. J Vet Dent 12:147, 1995.

4. Riviere GR, Thompson AJ, Brannan RD, et al: Detection of pathogen-related oral spirochetes, Treponema denticola and Treponema socranskii, in dental plaque from dogs. J Vet Dent 13:135, 1996.

5. Fournier D, Mouton C, Lapierre P, et al: Porphyromonas gulae sp. nov., an anaerobic, gram-negative coccobacillus from the gingival sulcus of various animal hosts. Int J Syst Evol Microbiol 51:1179, 2001.

6. Collins MD, Love DN, Karjalainen J, et al: Phylogenetic analysis of members of the genus Porphyromonas and description of Porphyromonas cangingivalis sp. nov. and Porphyromonas cansulci sp. nov. Int J Syst Bacteriol 44:674, 1994.

7. Silver JG, Martin L, McBride BC: Recovery and clearance of oral micro-organisms following experimental bacteremia in dogs. Arch Oral Biol 20:675, 1975.

8. Wolf HF, Rateitschak EM, Rateitschak KH, et al: Color Atlas of Dental Medicine – Periodontology, 3rd ed. Stuttgart: Thieme, 2005, p. 64.

9. DeBowes LJ, Mosier D, Logan E, et al: Association of periodontal disease and histologic lesions in multiple organs from 45 dogs. J Vet Dent 13:57, 1996.

10. Pavlica Z, Petelin M: Systemic effects of chronically infected wounds in the oral cavity of dogs. Proceedings 12th European Congress of Veterinary Dentistry, 2003; 29.

11. Rawlinson JE, Goldstein RE, Reiter AM, et al: Tracking systemic parameters in dogs with periodontal disease. Proceedings 19th Annual Veterinary Dental Forum, 2005; 429.

12. Sarkiala E, Harvey C: Systemic antimicrobials in the treatment of periodontitis in dogs. Semin Vet Med Surg 8:197, 1993.

13. Hardham JM, Dreier K, Wong J, et al: Efficacy of companion animal Porphyromonas spp. vaccines in the mouse model of periodontal disease. Proceedings 18th Annual Veterinary Dental Forum, 2004; 267.

14. Jeffcoat MK, Willams RC, Wechter WJ, et al: Flurbiprofen treatment of periodontal disease in beagles. J Perio Res 21:624, 1986.

15. Ouchi N, Nishikawa H, Yoshino T, et al: Inhibitory effects of YM175, a bisphosphonate, on the progression of experimental periodontitis in beagle dogs. J Perio Res 33:196, 1998.

16. Lyon KF: Endodontic therapy in the veterinary patient. Vet Clin North Am Small Anim Pract 28:1203, 1998.

17. Nanci A: Ten Cate's Oral Histology, 6th ed. St. Louis: Mosby, 2003, p. 192.

18. Gioso MA, Knobl T, Venturini MA, et al: Non-apical root canal ramifications in the teeth of dogs. J Vet Dent 14:89, 1997.

19. Negro VB, Hernandez SZ, Maresca BM: Endodontic system of the carnassial teeth in cats. Proceedings 9th European Congress of Veterinary Dentistry, 2000; 25.

20. Cohen S, Burns RC: Pathways of the Pulp, 8th ed. Philadelphia: Mosby, 2002, pp. 411, 457, 603, 651.

21. Hale FA: Localized intrinsic staining of teeth due to pulpitis and pulp necrosis in dogs. J Vet Dent 18:14, 2001.

Chapter 23

Palate Defect

Alexander M. Reiter

Embryology

During embryogenesis the paired maxillary processes, the paired mandibular processes, and the median frontonasal process surround the primitive oral cavity. *Medial and lateral nasal processes* originate from the *frontonasal process* and extend on each side of the olfactory placodes. In contrast to humans, where the upper lip is formed by the maxillary and nasal processes, in dogs and cats the upper lip and the primary palate are both formed by the midline fusion of the maxillary processes.[1]

At this stage of the development, the choanae open at the caudal end of the primary palate. Later, the lateral palatine processes move toward the midline and fuse with the downwardly growing nasal septum that originates from the nasal process. This constitutes the secondary palate which will ossify *(hard palate)*, except in the caudal part where it will form the *soft palate*.[2]

Anatomy

The upper lip and most rostral hard palate supported by the palatine processes of the incisive bones constitute the *primary palate*. The hard palate that is supported by the palatine processes of the maxillary bones and the horizontal laminae of the palatine bones together with the soft palate constitute the *secondary palate*.[3] The junction of the hard and soft palate is at the level of the first maxillary molar teeth. The incisive bones carry the incisor teeth. The maxillary bones carry the canine, premolar, and molar teeth. The palatine bones do not contain teeth.

Cornified stratified squamous epithelium covers the oral surface of the hard and soft palates. The oral mucosa covering the hard palate is developed into 6 to 10 transverse ridges and depressions *(palatine rugae)*.[4] The mucosa ends abruptly laterally at its junction with the short palatal free gingiva and has a thick tough connective tissue support, the mucoperiosteum, which is continuous with the periodontal ligaments of the maxillary teeth.[5] The *incisive papilla* is located on the midline rostral to the first transverse ridge and just caudal to the maxillary first incisor teeth. On either side of this papilla are the *incisive ducts* that extend caudodorsally through the palatine fissures into the floor of the nasal fossae. This duct communicates with the *vomeronasal organ*.[3]

Unless stretched, the oral surface of the soft palate is thrown into many fine longitudinal folds and a few larger transverse ones, evidence of the mobility and slight elasticity of the soft palate. The oral mucosa of the soft palate is also richly endowed with palatine glands and lymphoid tissue. Dogs and cats possess several tonsil-like structures, but only the *palatine tonsils* are conspicuous as large, ovoid, discrete bodies, each partly concealed in its own tonsillar fossa by a tonsillar fold derived from the soft palate caudal to the palatoglossal folds.[3] Efferent lymphatics depart for the medial retropharyngeal lymph node.

The free edge of the soft palate curves laterally to form the left and right *palatopharyngeal arches*, which pass caudally and merge with the walls of the pharynx to create a large caudoventrally directed central hole – the intrapharyngeal ostium. The three parts of the pharynx (nasopharynx above, oropharynx below, and laryngopharynx behind) meet at this ostium, and a pair of palatopharyngeal muscles within the arches serves as its sphincter.[3] No uvula is present. There is no palatoglossal arch in the dog and cat comparable to that structure in humans, as they lack the palatoglossal muscle that forms the basis of the human arch. When the tongue is forcibly withdrawn from the mouth and moved to one side, a fold is developed on the opposite side, running from the body of the tongue to the initial part of the soft palate. Although this fold is not formed by muscle as in humans, is seems feasible to regard it as the *palatoglossal fold*, which distinguishes it from the palatoglossal arch of humans.[3] The minor palatine artery, infraorbital artery, and a common trunk that gives rise to the sphenopalatine and major palatine arteries are branches of the *maxillary artery* (Figure 23-1).[3,6] At its most caudal aspect the maxillary bone forms a small pointed spur, the pterygoid process. This process and the palatine bone form a notch or foramen, through which the *minor palatine artery* passes, which is the main blood supply to the soft palate.

The muscles of the soft palate consist of the paired *intrinsic palatine muscles* and the end ramifications of the paired *tensor and levator veli palatini muscles*.[3,7] The fibers of the palatine muscles are longitudinal and shorten the relatively long soft palate of the dog. Lateral radiographs in brachycephalic dogs reveal that their soft palate is thickened, suggesting that these animals have sustained contractions of their palatine muscles to maintain a patent airway. The tensor and levator veli palatini muscles stretch and lift the soft palate, respectively, with the aponeurosis of the tensor also serving as a structural support for the palate. The insertion of the tensor veli palatini muscle passes over the ventral edge of the hamular process of the pterygoid bone to reach rostrally in the soft palate. The main sensory supply to the soft palate is the minor palatine branch of the maxillary nerve (derived from the trigeminal nerve). The tensor veli palatini muscle is also supplied by a branch of the trigeminal nerve, while the levator veli palatini muscle is innervated by the facial nerve. Nerves from the pharyngeal plexus (derived from glossopharyngeal and vagus nerves) supply the palatopharyngeal muscles.[3]

The lateral surface of the palatine bone forms the medial wall of the *pterygopalatine fossa*. There is one large opening, the maxillary foramen for the infraorbital artery, and two smaller openings, the sphenopalatine foramen for the sphenopalatine artery and the caudal palatine foramen for the major palatine artery. The *infraorbital artery* runs in the infraorbital canal and emerges at the *infraorbital foramen*. The *sphenopalatine artery* extends to the nasal cavity. The *major palatine artery* passes through the palatine canal with a delicate vein and relatively large satellite nerve and emerges again at the *major palatine foramen*

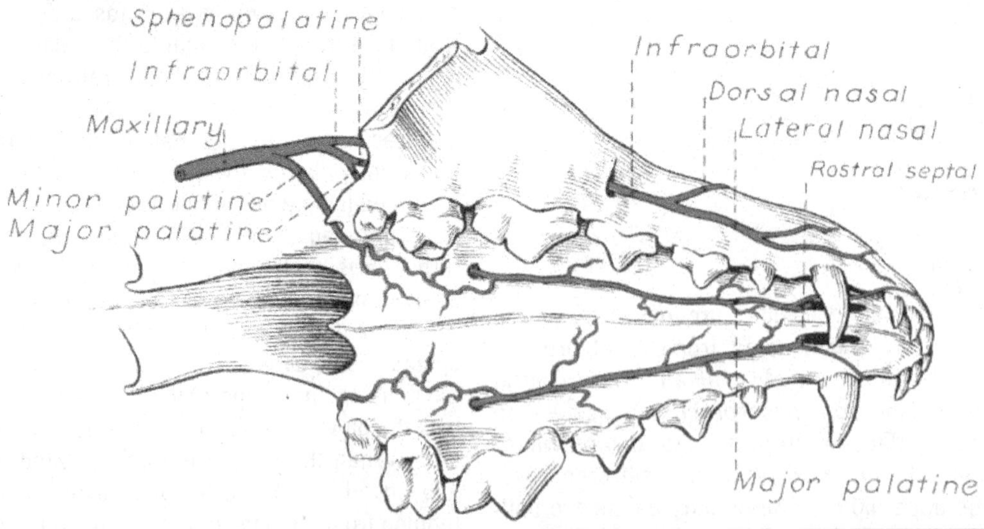

Figure 23-1. Terminal branches of the maxillary artery. (From Evans H (ed): Miller's Anatomy of the Dog, 3rd ed. Philadelphia: WB Saunders, 1993.)

that is located near the transverse palatine suture between the median palatine suture and the maxillary fourth premolar tooth, from where it runs rostrally in the *palatine sulcus* to the *palatine fissures.* This artery is the most important vascular structure of the palatal mucosa and needs to be preserved during surgical procedures. Within the palatine canal the nerve and artery divide so that one or more *accessory palatine arteries* and nerves emerge on the horizontal process of the palatine bone through *minor palatine foramina* situated caudal to the major palatine foramen.[3]

A small rostral septal branch of the major palatine artery passes through the palatine fissure dorsomedially and anastomoses with a branch of the sphenopalatine artery, which supplies the mucosa on the nasal side of the hard palate and the nasal septum. A small artery extends rostrolaterally and passes through the interdental space between the canine and third incisor teeth, anastomosing with the lateral nasal artery. The most rostral aspect of the major palatine artery branches profusely and anastomoses with its fellow. At the anastomosis a small vessel runs dorsally through the *incisive foramen* near the interincisive suture in the incisive canal, joining the right and left lateral nasal arteries. The main channel draining the area of the hard palate runs caudally in the soft tissue of the hard palate as a spongy, poorly developed venous plexus. The plexus continues in the soft palate, where it lies dorsal to the palatine glands and lateral to the palatine muscles. It empties into the maxillary vein caudal to the temporomandibular joint, ventrolateral to the tympanic bulla. The lymphatics go to the medial retropharyngeal lymph nodes.[3]

Etiology

Congenital defects of formation of the lip and palatal structures have been reported in both dogs and cats and may be inherited or result from an insult during fetal development.[5] A wide variety of dog and cat breeds have been affected. Brachycephalic dog breeds have been reported to be at higher risk. Growth of the palatine portions of facial bones must compete successfully with growth of the skull width to achieve midline closure of the palate. Broad-headed fetuses have a greater tendency to develop a cleft palate. The sporadic nature of these conditions and the wide range of dog and cat breeds that are affected suggest that in many cases the cause is an intrauterine insult rather than inheritance,[5] although all types of clefts, from partial unilateral to complete bilateral, have been produced in dogs in mating trials. As in children, unilateral harelips in dogs are almost always on the left side, and cleft lips may be associated with abnormalities of the secondary palate. According to the stage of development and the severity of the cause, other physical or neurologic abnormalities may be present. Clefts can occur if the intrauterine insult (trauma, stress, corticosteroids, antimitotic drugs, nutritional, hormonal, viral, and toxic factors) occurs at a specific time in fetal development (25th to 28th day in dogs).[2]

Acquired palate defects result from chronic infections (severe periodontal disease), trauma (e.g., high-rise syndrome, electric cord and gunshot injury, dog bites and foreign body penetration, and pressure wounds secondary to malocclusion), neoplasia, and surgical and radiation therapy (Table 23-1).[5] In all cases, the cause of the defect must be removed prior to repair. The most common cause of oronasal fistula is loss of incisive and/or maxillary bone associated with severe periodontal disease or tooth extraction. Traumatic cleft palate is commonly seen in cats after high-rise trauma. The defect that develops from electric cord injury is due to thermal necrosis of the soft and hard tissues of the palate.

Pathophysiology

Whereas the hard palate forms a rigid partition between the oral and nasal cavities, the soft palate forms a valve. When elevated during swallowing, it closes off the nasopharynx, and when depressed during nose breathing, it closes off the oropharynx.[3] During swallowing, it works with the epiglottis, which closes off the distal airway, to allow a bolus of ingesta to cross the respiratory tract. Thus, the palate allows independent functioning of the respiratory and digestive systems and is especially important during the neonatal period, when sucking requires an airtight oral cavity.[5]

Table 23-1. Causes of Palate Defects

- Inherited
  - Recessive or irregular dominant traits (congenital)
- Acquired
  - Intrauterine insult (congenital)
  - Periodontal disease
  - Traumatic
- High-rise syndrome
- Electric cord injury
- Gunshot injury
- Dog bites
- Foreign body penetration
- Pressure wounds secondary to malocclusion
  - Neoplasia
  - Previous surgery
  - Radiation therapy

Congenital palate defects manifest either as cleft lip or cleft palate. Defects of the primary palate are obvious at birth as an abnormal fissure in the upper lip *(harelip)* and/or a cleft of the most rostral hard palate (Figure 23-2A). Affected animals must be examined for coexisting clefts of the secondary palate. Except for being externally visible, clefts of the primary palate rarely result in clinical signs beyond local rhinitis, and repair may be performed for esthetic reasons. Clefts of the secondary palate *(cleft hard and/or soft palate)* are more common and more serious, although they are rarely visible externally. They are almost always along the midline and are usually associated with a midline soft palate abnormality (Figure 23-2B). Soft palate defects without hard palate defects may occur in the midline or may be unilateral.[8] The prognosis for congenital absence of the soft palate, as opposed to cleft soft palate, is poor because restoration of a palatopharyngeal sphincteric ring and normal swallowing function may not be achieved despite careful planning and meticulous surgical technique.[9,10] Clefts of the secondary palate frequently go unnoticed until a neonate demonstrates clinical signs, including failure to create negative pressure for nursing, nasal discharge (drainage of milk from the nares during or after nursing), coughing, gagging, sneezing, nasal reflux, tonsillitis, rhinitis, laryngotracheitis, aspiration pneumonia, poor weight gain, and general unthriftiness. Early diagnosis is important so that these secondary problems can be avoided. The prognosis without surgical repair is guarded because of the risk of aspiration.

An acute oronasal fistula following tooth extraction is diagnosed by direct visualization of the nasal cavity and hemorrhage at the nostril. Clinical signs of a chronic oronasal fistula include sneezing and ipsilateral nasal discharge. A defect in the area of a missing tooth that communicates with the nasal cavity may be noted on oral examination.[5] Patients with large acquired palate defects may show similar clinical signs as those with congenital defects of the secondary palate (Figure 23-3). The further caudal and the larger a defect, the more severe become the clinical signs.

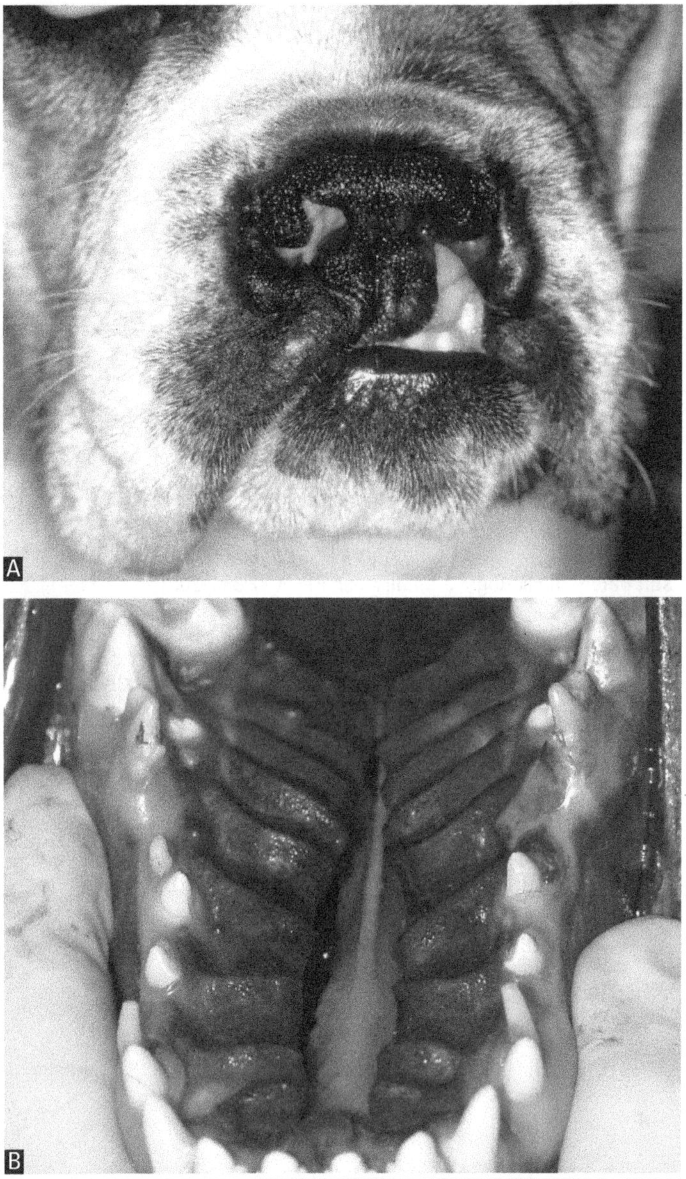

Figure 23-2. A. Defect of the primary palate presenting as harelip in a Bullterrier. B. Defect of the secondary palate presenting as cleft of the hard and soft palates in a German shepherd dog.

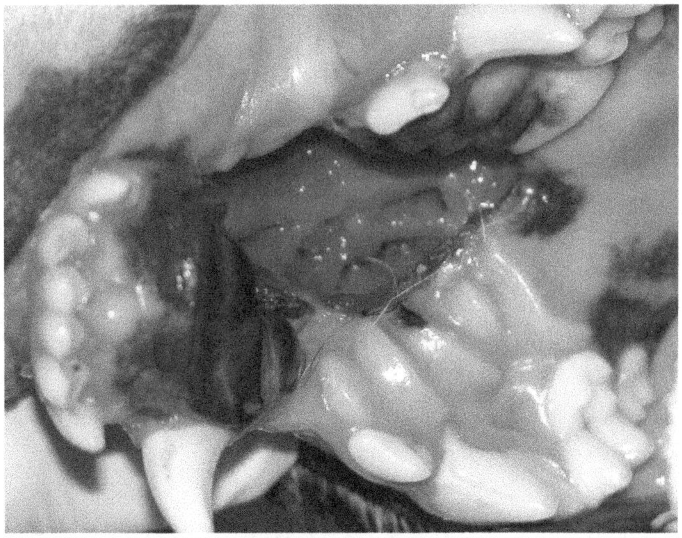

Figure 23-3. Acquired hard palate defect after gunshot trauma.

References

1. Senders CW, Eisele P, Freeman LE, et al: Observations about the normal and abnormal embryogenesis of the canine lip and palate. J Craniofac Genet Dev Biol 2:241, 1986.

2. Verstraete FJM: Self-Assessment Color Review of Veterinary Dentistry. Ames: Iowa State University Press, 1999, p. 18.

3. Evans HE: Miller's Anatomy of the Dog, 3rd ed. Philadelphia: WB Saunders, 1993, pp. 148, 387.

4. Orsini P, Hennet P: Anatomy of the mouth and teeth of the cat. Vet Clin North Am Small Anim Pract 22:1265, 1992.

5. Harvey CE: Palate defects in dogs and cats. Comp Cont Educ Pract Vet 9:404, 1987.

6. Gioso MA, Carvalho VGG: Oral anatomy of the dog and cat in veterinary dentistry practice. Vet Clin North Am Small Anim Pract 35:763, 2005.

7. Dyce KM: The muscles of the pharynx and palate of the dog. Anat Rec 127:497, 1957.

8. Warzee CC, Bellah TR, Richards D: Congenital unilateral cleft of the soft palate in six dogs. J Small Anim Pract 42:338, 2001.

9. Bauer MS, Levitt L, Pharr JW, et al: Unsuccessful surgical repair of a short soft palate in a dog. J Am Vet Med Assoc 193:1551, 1988.

10. Sylvestre AM, Sharma A: Management of a congenitally shortened soft palate in a dog. J Am Vet Med Assoc 211:875, 1997.

Chapter 24

Salivary Gland

Dianne Dunning

Diseases of the salivary glands and ducts are uncommon in the dog and cat, with a reported overall incidence of 0.17 to 0.3%.[1-3] Reported conditions involving the salivary glands include rupture, inflammation, dilation, necrosis, fistula, a foreign body, autoimmune disease, calculi, and neoplasia.[1,2,4-11] The onset of many of these conditions is frequently insidious, with vague findings on physical examination.[12] Definitive diagnosis often necessitates fine-needle aspiration and cytology, radiology, ancillary imaging, biopsy, and exploratory surgery. Complete knowledge of the anatomy of the head and neck, accurate dissection, removal of the affected glands and duct systems, and drainage may be necessary to successfully treat many of the conditions outlined in this chapter.

Anatomy and Function

The four major salivary glands in the dog and cat are the paired parotid, mandibular, sublingual, and zygomatic glands.[13] The parotid gland is a triangular bilobar gland located at the base of the horizontal ear canal. The parotid duct runs rostrally along the lateral surface of the masseter muscle between the dorsal and ventral buccal branches of the facial nerve and opens into the oral vestibule at the level of the 3rd-4th and 2nd cheek tooth in the dog and cat, respectively. Secretion from the gland is primarily thin and serous, with a mucous component also present in the dog. Sympathetic innervation is provided by the external carotid plexus of nerves, which travel in tandem with the parotid artery. Fibers of the auriculotemporal branch of the trigeminal nerve give parasympathetic input. The parotid artery is the main blood supply to this gland. Venous drainage is via the superficial temporal and great auricular veins.

Often mistaken as an enlarged lymph node on cervical palpation, the mandibular gland is located directly beneath the bifurcation of the external jugular vein, lying caudoventrally to the parotid gland, between the linguofacial and maxillary veins. It is an ovoid, capsulated gland that is fused to the monostomatic part of the sublingual gland. The mandibular duct travels rostrally, medial to the digastricus muscle to empty at the sublingual caruncle on the floor of the oral cavity. Secretion from this gland is mixed, both serous and mucous. Sympathetic never fibers reach the gland by means of a perivascular plexus around the glandular artery. Parasymphathetic innervation is provided by the chorda tympani of the facial nerve. The main artery supplying blood is the glandular branch of the facial artery, which enters the gland medially and in close association with the mandibular duct. Entering the dorsal part of the deep surface are one or two branches of the caudal auricular artery. The chief vein draining the gland terminates into the lingual vein. A second smaller vein drains the caudal portion of the gland and terminates in the facial, maxillary, or lingual veins.

The sublingual salivary gland is composed of both a monostomatic and a polystomatic component. The monostomatic portion is compact with a fibrous capsule that is contiguous with the rostral border of the mandibular gland. Its duct opens into the oral vestibule near the sublingual caruncle. The diffuse polystomatic part of the sublingual salivary gland spreads into tissues ventral to the floor of the oral cavity and drains via several ducts opening into the oral cavity on either side of the frenulum of the tongue. Similar to that of the mandibular gland, innervation is provided by perivascular plexus around the glandular artery and the corda tympani of the facial nerve. Blood supply to the monostomatic portion is provided by the facial artery; the sublingual artery supplies the small polystomatic part of the sublingual gland. Small satellite veins accompany the facial and sublingual arteries to drain the gland.

The zygomatic gland is seated deep to the zygomatic arch, on the dorsolateral surface of the medial pterygoid muscle, forming most of the orbital floor. It has both major and minor ducts that open into the vestibule opposite to the maxillary molar. The zygomatic gland is a mixed salivary gland, ovoid in shape, and is innervated by the glossopharyngeal nerve. Several ducts drain this small gland, but the major zygomatic duct opening is opposite the last maxillary molar. The minor duct openings are difficult to visualize with the naked eye, opening just caudal to the major duct. The first branch of the infraorbital artery provides blood supply to the gland. Venous drainage terminates into the deep facial vein on the lateral surface of the gland.

In addition to these primary glands, smaller, variable glands are present in the soft palate, lips, tongue, and cheeks and are collectively referred to as buccal glands. These glands drain into the oral cavity via numerous small ducts; the secretion is mixed serous and mucous in character.

Secretion of saliva is under control of the autonomic nervous system, which controls both the volume and type of saliva secreted.[14] Salivary secretions serve many functions in the dog and cat, some of which are to lubricate and bind masticated food into a consumable bolus, to solubilize dry food, to flush the oral cavity from debris, to prevent overgrowth of oral microbial population, to initiate starch digestion, and to provide evaporative cooling and maintain core body temperature homeostasis.[14]

Specific Disease Conditions

Salivary Mucocele (Sialocele)

Mucoceles are the most common salivary gland disorder of dogs, but are less frequent in the cat.[3,15,16] A mucocele, or sialocele, is defined as the accumulation of saliva in the subcutaneous tissue adjacent to the gland or duct. Unlike a cyst, a mucocele does not have an epithelial lining.[3,6,9,15,17-19] True brachial and zygomatic cysts have been reported in both the dog and cat, but these are rare.[18,19] The exact pathogenesis underlying mucolele formation is usually unknown, but trauma, foreign bodies, and infrequently, sialoliths have been implicated.[3,6,9,12,15,17] A case report of a mucocele associated with dirofilariasis has been reported in the dog.[17] Poodles, dachshunds, Australian silky terriers, and Siamese cats may be predisposed.[3,15]

Although a mucocele may arise from any one the salivary glands or their associated ducts, the sublingual and mandibular glands are most frequently implicated.[9,12,15,20] Clinical signs are dependent on the site of saliva accumulation. The most commonly reported clinical sign associated with mucocele formation is the appearance of a soft, fluctuant, painless mass that must be differentiated from abscesses, tumors, and other retention cysts of the neck.[9,12,15,20] Saliva will generally accumulate in a gravity-dependent site, within the cranial cervical or intermandibular region, but it can also appear within the oral cavity under the base of the tongue. The accumulations are referred to as ranulas.[9,12,15,20] A less common site is in the pharyngeal wall, which can obstruct airways and cause significant life-threatening dyspnea and heat stroke.[9,12,15,20]

In the initial phases of accumulation, the soft tissue surrounding saliva is inflamed and may be painful on palpation.[9,12,15,20] This stage is short-lived and usually not detected.[9,12,15,20] Once established, the slowly enlarging saliva-filled mass is non-painful; however, secondary infection should be suspected if the mass is persistently painful or a fever is noted.[9,12,15,20] Additional differentials for the swelling in this area include abscesses, neoplasia, and other retention cysts of the neck.[9,12,15,20] A complete oral exam should be performed in the event of a ranula, particularly if oral bleeding is noted.[12,18] Diagnosis of a mucocele is confirmed via paracentesis of a golden-brown or blood-tinged viscous fluid that typically does not need further analysis. If any question exists regarding the identity of the fluid, a mucus-specific stain, such as a periodic acid-Schiff will confirm the diagnosis.[12,15,20]

Definitive treatment requires surgical removal of the affected gland and duct.[15,20] Positioning the animal in dorsal recumbency usually delineates the affected side, as origin of the saliva is typically unilateral and most often originates from the mandibular sublingual gland complex. If the mucocele appears to be bilateral, exploration of the site of swelling will demarcate the side that is affected. The salivary glands may be removed bilaterally without any detrimental effects to saliva production, if any uncertainty remains as to the origin of the saliva acummulation.[12,15,20] Treatment limited to lancing and draining or periodic aspiration risks infection, does not address the primary problem, and is contraindicated. A retrospective review of mucoceles in the dog revealed a 42% recurrence rate when treatment was limited to surgical drainage.[15] Aspiration and drainage are indicated with pharyngeal mucoceles, but only as an emergency palliative procedure to relieve dyspnea until the animal can be anesthetized and the offending glands and the redundant tissue blocking the airway removed. If a ranula is present, marsupialization may be necessary in addition to glandular removal and drainage. Treated appropriately, mucocele recurrence is uncommon (less than 5%), unless the glandular tissue is not fully removed.[12,20]

Sialoadentitis

Inflammation of the salivary gland, or sialoadentitis, is an incidental finding frequently noted at necropsy in the dog that rarely manifests as a clinical problem. Blunt trauma, mucoceles, penetrating bite wounds, foreign body migration, invasive tumor infiltration, and systemic viral infection have been reported to cause inflammation of the salivary gland.[3,4,12,20,21] Sialodentitis has been reported with rabies, distemper, and paramyxovirus.[3,4,12] Clinical signs are characterized by pyrexia, lethargy, and painful, swollen salivary glands.[3,4,12] Severe inflammation can result in abscessation and rupture of the gland into the oral cavity or through the skin, with fistula formation.[3,4,12] Sialodentitis of the zygomatic gland frequently results in exopthalmos, retrobulbar swelling, divergent strabismus, and trismus.[3,4,12] Mild sialodentitis requires no treatment, and recovery is usually rapid and complete. A salivary abscess necessitates surgical drainage or removal of the gland and therapeutic antibiotics.[3,4,12]

Fistula

Salivary fistulas are typically the result of penetrating injury or abscessation of the salivary gland.[3,12] The transcutaneous flow of saliva prevents second intention healing. Definitive treatment entails dissection of the fistulous tract and salivary gland removal. In people, botulinum toxin A, injected into the involved gland with ultrasound guidance, has been successfully employed to abate the flow of saliva and allow wound healing via second intention, while preserving the gland in situ.[22,23]

Sialolithiasis

Salivary calculi or sialolithiasis is a rare condition; only two cases have been reported in the dog.[8,24] Clinically, these dogs present with a painful swelling and rupture of the affected parotid gland owing to obstruction of saliva outflow.[8,24] Diagnosis is made by palpation of the sialolith within the duct, skull radiographs, ultrasound and/or sialography.[8,24] Treatment entails removal of the calculi, with cannulation and lavage of the duct to remove any residual debris.[8,24] Healing is via second intention and closure of the duct in not necessary. Sialolith composition is usually calcium phosphate or calcium carbonate.[8,24]

Immune-Mediated Disease[25-28]

Immune-immediated disease localized to the salivary gland is rarely recognized in the dog and cat. Keratoconjunctivitis sicca and xerostoma (Sjögren syndrome) have been reported in the dog and are seen in association with other autoimmune diseases, such as rheumatoid arthritis, systemic lupus erythematosus, and polymyositis.

Necrotizing Sialometaplasia

In people, necrotizing sialometaplasia is a benign, mildly painful, self-limiting disease characterized by ischemic necrosis of the palatine gland with secondary proliferation (metaplasia) of the salivary duct.[5,29,30] Histologic changes in humans are difficult to differentiate from neoplasia and include: lobular necrosis of salivary tissue, squamous metaplasia conforming to duct and/or acinar outlines, preservation of salivary lobular morphology, variable inflammation, and granulation tissue.[5,29,30] In contrast, clinical signs in the dog and cat are characterized by severe acute retropharyngeal pain accompanied by enlarged, hard mandibular salivary glands, anorexia, gagging, and vomiting.[3,5,11,12,30] The underlying pathobiology is unclear; however, traumatic ischemia is suspected to be the cause of the vasculitis and thrombosis.[5,29,30] It has also been hypothesized that this syndrome may be an unusual form of limbic epilepsy.[31] Treatment consists of surgical excision of the affected gland and multimodal pain management or the short-term administration of anticonvulsants for their antiemetic properties.[5,29,30] The milder disease in humans is self-limiting; in some cases, facial or pharyngeal pain is more extensive.[5,29,30,32] The prognosis is guarded in the dog, as some animals continue to experience severe pain and vomiting, despite surgical excision and supportive care.[5,29,30] The prognosis in cats is more favorable for complete recovery.[5,29,30]

Neoplasia

Salivary gland neoplasia, like all other salivary gland disease, is rare, with an overall incidence of 0.17%.[1,2] Within the realm of salivary gland disease, however, neoplasia represents a relatively frequent condition, with 30% of all salivary gland biopsies being classified as neoplastic on histopathology.[2,3] Siamese cats are at higher risk than other breeds of cat, but there does not appear to be a breed predilection in the dog, as previously reported.[2,18] The glands most commonly affected are the parotid and mandibular salivary glands, accounting for approximately 80% of all the neoplastic cases reported (Table 24-1).[1,2,18] Clinical signs of salivary gland neoplasia include a mass affect in the region of the gland, dysphagia, weight loss, exophthalmos, and halitosis.[1,2] The most common histopathologic type of tumor was simple adenocarcinoma in both the dog and cat.[2] Other reported histopathologic tumor types include squamous cell carcinoma, mucoepidermoid carcinoma, anaplastic carcinoma, and complex carcinoma.[2] Adenomas are rarely reported and comprise only 5% of all salivary tumors. Fibrosarcomas, lipomas, mast cell tumors, and lymphomas may also incorporate salivary gland tissue by direct extension and invasion.[1,2]

In general, cats are diagnosed at a later stage of disease than dogs.[1,2] A retrospective study reviewing salivary gland neoplasia in the dog and cat revealed that early diagnosis significantly improved survival times in dogs but not in cats.[2] In this study, cats seemed to have a more aggressive disease, with over half the feline patients having nodal involvement, distant metastases, or both at the time of diagnosis.[2] Furthermore, clinical staging was prognostic in dogs, but not in cats.[2] The median survival times for dogs and cats reported in this multi-institutional study was 550 days and 516 days, respectively.[2] Local infiltration and metastasis to regional lymph nodes and lungs was common, as was local recurrence after surgical excision.[2] Radiotherapy, with or without surgery, offered the best prognosis.[2]

Table 24-1. Distribution of Salivary Gland Tumors in the Dog and Cat.

Gland	Dog	Cat
Mandibular	30%	59%
Parotid	50%	19%
Sublingual and minor glands	12%	6%
Zygomatic	4%	3%
Indeterminate	4%	13%

Reproduced with permission from: Hammer, A., Getzy, D., Ogilvie, G, et al. Salivary Gland Neoplasia in the Dog and Cat: Survival times and prognostic factors. J Am Anim Hosp Assoc 2001:37:478-482.

References

1. Carberry C, Flanders J, Harvey H, et al: Salivary gland tumors in dogs and cats: a literature and case review. J Am Anim Hosp Assoc 24:561-567, 1988.

2. Hammer A, Getzy D, Ogilvie G, et al: Salivary gland neoplasia in the dog and cat: survival times and prognostic factors. J Am Anim Hosp Assoc 37:478-482, 2001.

3. Spangler W, Culbertson M: Salivary gland disease in dogs and cats: 245 cases (1985-1988). J Am Vet Med Assoc 198:465-469, 1991.

4. Boydell P, Pike R, Crossley D: Presumptive sialadenosis in a cat. J Small Anim Pract 41:573-574, 2000.

5. Brown PJ, Bradshaw JM, Sozmen M, et al: Feline necrotising sialometaplasia: a report of two cases. J Feline Med Surg 6:279-281, 2004.

6. Durtnell RE: Salivary mucocoele in the dog. Vet Rec 101:273, 1977.

7. Glen JB: Canine salivary mucocoeles. Results of sialographic examination and surgical treatment of fifty cases. J Small Anim Pract 13:515-526, 1972.

8. Jeffreys DA, Stasiw A, Dennis R: Parotid sialolithiasis in a dog. J Small Anim Pract 37:296-297, 1996.

9. Mapes EL: Salivary mucocele in a dog. Mod Vet Pract 65:632-633, 1984.

10. Mazzullo G, Sfacteria A, Ianelli N, et al: Carcinoma of the submandibular salivary glands with multiple metastases in a cat. Vet Clin Pathol 34:61-64, 2005.

11. Schroeder H, Berry WL: Salivary gland necrosis in dogs: a retrospective study of 19 cases. J Small Anim Pract 39:121-125, 1998.

12. Brown NO: Salivary gland diseases. Problems in Veterinary Medicine: Gastrointestinal Surgical Complications 1:282-294, 1989.

13. Evans HE: The digestive apparatus and abdomen: The salivary gland. *In* Miller's Anatomy of the Dog, 3rd ed. Philadelphia: WB Saunders, 1993, pp. 415-419.

14. Harvey CE: Salivary gland disorders. In Mechanisms of Disease in Small Animal Surgery, 2nd ed. Smeak DD, Bojrab MJ, Bloomberg MS (eds). Philadelphia: Lippincott Williams & Wilkins, 1993, pp. 197-199.

15. Bellenger CR, Simpson DJ: Canine sialoceles - 60 clinical cases. J Small Anim Pract 33:376-380, 1992.

16. Rahal SC, Nunes AL, Teixeira CR, et al: Salivary mucocele in a wild cat. Can Vet J 44:933-934, 2003

17. Henry CJ: Salivary mucocele associated with dirofilariasis in a dog. J Am Vet Med Assoc 200:1965-1966, 1992.

18. Karbe E, Nielsen SW: Canine ranulas, salivary mucoceles and branchial cysts. J Small Anim Pract 7:625-630, 1966.

19. Speakman AJ, Baines SJ, Williams JM, et al: Zygomatic salivary cyst with mucocele formation in a cat. J Small Anim Pract 38:468-470, 1997.

20. Waldron DR, Smith MM: Salivary mucoceles. Probl Vet Med 3:270-276, 1991.

21. Stubbs WP, Voges AK, Shiroma JT, et al: What is your diagnosis? Infiltrative lipoma with chronic salivary duct obstruction. J Am Vet Med Assoc 209:55-56, 1996.

22. von Lindern JJ, Niederhagen B, Appel T, et al: New prospects in the treatment of traumatic and postoperative parotid fistulas with type A botulinum toxin. Plast Reconstr Surg 109:2443-2445, 2002.

23. Guntinas-Lichius O, Sittel C: Treatment of postparotidectomy salivary fistula with botulinum toxin. Ann Otol Rhinol Laryngol 110:1162-1164, 2001.

24. Mulkey C, Knecht CD: Parotid salivary cyst and calculus in a dog. J Am Vet Med Assoc 159:1774, 1971.

25. Monier JC, Fournel C, Lapras M, et al: Systemic lupus erythematosus in a colony of dogs. Am J Vet Res 49:46-51, 1988.

26. Halliwell RE: Autoimmune diseases in domestic animals. J Am Vet Med Assoc 181:1088-1096, 1982.

27. Quimby FW, Schwartz RS, Poskitt T, et al: A disorder of dogs resembling Sjogren's syndrome. Clin Immunol Immunopathol 12:471-476, 1979.

28. Quimby FW, Jensen C, Nawrocki D, et al: Selected autoimmune diseases in the dog. Vet Clin North Am 8:665-682, 1978.

29. Batsakis JG, Manning JT: Necrotising sialometaplasia of major salivary glands. J Laryn Otol 101:962-966, 1987.

30. Brooks DG, Hottinger HA, Dunstan RW: Canine necrozing sialometaplasia: A case report and review of the literature. J Am Anim Hosp Assoc 31:21-25, 1995.

31. Stonehewer J, Mackin AJ, Tasker S, et al: Idiopathic phenobarbital-responsive hypersialosis in the dog: an unusual form of limbic epilepsy? J Small Anim Pract 41:416-421, 2000.

32. Sneige N, Batsakis JG: Necrotising sialometaplasia. Ann Otol Rhinol Larnyngol 101:282-284, 1992.

Chapter 25

Swallowing Disorders

Andrew E. Kyles

Swallowing is a coordinated process consisting of three phases–oropharyngeal, esophageal, and gastroesophageal.[1] Swallowing disorders can be caused by a mechanical or anatomic lesion either intrinsic to the ailmentary tract or by compression from adjacent structures, by a functional or neurologic disturbance, or secondary to pain (Table 25-1).[2] The interruption to the normal coordinated sequence of swallowing may involve one or more of the contributing structures, including the muscles of the tongue, hyoid apparatus, soft palate, pharyngeal muscles, cranial esophageal sphincter, esophagus, and gastroesophageal junction.[2]

Table 25-1. Causes of Dysphagia

Mechanical or Anatomic Lesions

- Pharyngeal inflammation (abscess, inflammatory polyp, oral eosinophilic granuloma)
- Foreign body obstruction (oral, pharyngeal, nasopharyngeal, proximal esophagus)
- Acute oropharyngeal penetrating injuries
- Neoplasia
- Retropharyngeal lymphadenopathy
- Sialocele
- Necrotizing sialometaplasia
- Mandibular fracture
- Lingual frenulum disorder
- Cricopharyngeal achalasia
- TMJ disorder (luxation, fracture, ankalosis, malformation)
- Craniomandibular osteopathy
- Congenital (cleft palate, narrowed intrapharyngeal opening)
- Pharyngeal trauma

Functional or Neurologic Disorders

- Myasthenia gravis (focal or generalized)
- Acute polyradiculitis
- Masticatory myositis
- Tick paralysis
- Botulism
- Polymyositis
- Muscular dystrophy
- Sensory neuropathy
- Rabies
- Trigeminal paralysis or neuritis
- Neuropathies of cranial nerves VII, IX, X, or XII
- CNS disorders (brain stem lesion)
- Dysautonomia

Pain

- Stomatitis/glossitis/pharyngitis (FIV, FeLV, immune-mediated disease, uremic glossitis, ingestion of a caustic substance)
- Tooth-related problem (tooth root abscess, fracture, periodontitis)
- Trauma
- Electrical cord burns
- Retrobulbar abscess

Oropharyngeal Phase

The oropharyngeal phase of swallowing involves the prehension of food and formation of a bolus in the mouth and passage of the bolus into the cranial cervical esophagus. The oropharyngeal phase is subdivided into oral, pharyngeal, and cricopharyngeal stages.[1] These stages occur in rapid succession and can only be reliably differentiated by careful analysis of fluoroscopic studies. The oral stage is a voluntary process involving prehension and mastication of food, the formation of a bolus at the back of the tongue, and the delivery of the bolus into the pharynx. The pharyngeal stage is the first step of the involuntary phase of swallowing and is initiated by the delivery of a food bolus into the oropharynx. Pharyngeal constrictor muscles propel the bolus aborally to the cricopharynx. Contraction of the palatal and pharyngeal muscles closes the nasopharynx and prevents nasal reflux, while the epiglottis and adduction of the vocal folds close the larynx and prevent laryngotracheal aspiration. No obvious thickening occurs of the esophageal wall at the pharyngoesophageal junction to form a true cranial (or upper) esophageal sphincter. However, the cricopharyngeus and thyropharyngeus muscles and associated elastic tissue serve the function of a cranial esophageal sphincter. The cricopharyngeal stage of swallowing involves the relaxation of the cricopharyngeus and thyropharyngeus muscles and the delivery of the bolus into the cranial cervical esophagus. The oropharyngeal phase of swallowing is coordinated by cranial nerves V (trigeminal), VII (facial), IX (glossopharyngeal), X (vagus), and XII (hypoglossal).

Oral dysphagia is caused by abnormalities in prehension or interference in the voluntary process of bolus formation at the base of the tongue. The tongue plays the dominant role during the oral phase of swallowing, milking fluid aborally against the hard and soft palates. Food should be maintained in midline; oral dysphagia often results in lateral deviation of food into the buccal folds and loss of food from the mouth. The diagnosis can normally be made on the basis of the history, physical examination, and evaluation of swallowing. Fluoroscopy is not usually required for diagnosis. When performed, the dynamic study will show a reduced ability to form a bolus, with normal transport of the bolus after it reaches the oropharynx. Many animals with oral dysphagia learn to compensate by modifying their eating behavior.

Pharyngeal and cricopharyngeal dysphagia produce similar clinical signs. Affected animals are able to prehend and chew normally; these actions are followed by several, partially successful attempts to swallow. The animals then become anxious, gag, and expel the food from their mouth by forward motion of the tongue. The cycle is then repeated until the entire meal is swallowed. The animals may have an associated nasal discharge and coughing caused by aspiration of food material into the nasal cavities and trachea. Homogenized food is usually easier to swallow than chunks; although, oddly, water may be more difficult to swallow than food.[3]

Fluoroscopic examination of swallowing is needed to differentiate pharyngeal and cricopharyngeal dysphagias. In pharyngeal dysphagia, fluoroscopy demonstrates the absence of a strong aboral pharyngeal peristaltic contraction, resulting in incomplete bolus transport across the pharynx.[4] Associated reflux of contrast medium into the nasopharynx and laryngotracheal aspiration may occur. Cranial esophageal sphincter relaxation is proportionate to the size and consistency of the bolus delivered; therefore, pharyngeal dysphagia may result in a less pronounced relaxation of the sphincter compared with that in a normal animal. The deficient relaxation of the cricopharyngeal sphincter could result in an erroneous diagnosis of cricopharyngeal dysphagia. However, cricopharyngeal dysphagia is associated with vigorous contraction of the pharyngeal muscles, which causes distortion of the cricopharynx and/or transient pharyngeal outpouchings.[4]

Cricopharyngeal dysphagia is characterized by either cricopharyngeal asynchrony or achalasia. Cricopharyngeal asynchrony is caused by an incoordination between contraction in the dorsal cranial and middle pharyngeal constrictor muscles (hyopharyngeus, pteryopharyngeus and palatopharyngeus muscles) and relaxation of the cranial esophageal sphincter. In dogs with cricopharyngeal asynchrony, the time interval between onset of swallowing (closure of the epiglottis) and maximum pharyngeal contraction is normal, but the time to opening of the cranial esophageal sphincter is significantly prolonged.[5] Cricopharyngeal achalasia is a lack of relaxation of the cranial esophageal sphincter during the cricopharyngeal stage of swallowing. It is observed less commonly than asynchrony.[6] With both conditions, movement of the bolus into the caudal pharynx by movement of the tongue and pharyngeal constriction is normal. A thin stream of contrast medium may pass through the cranial esophageal sphincter. When the bolus of food in the cranial cervical esophagus is sufficient, primary esophageal peristalsis is initiated, and the food passes normally into the stomach. The food that does not pass through the cranial esophageal sphincter is expelled through the mouth, sometimes accompanied by nasal reflux and laryngotracheal aspiration.

Surgical management of cricopharyngeal dysphagia may be indicated. Surgery consists of a cricopharyngeal myotomy (incision of the cricopharyngeus muscle on dorsal midline of the larynx, sometimes accompanied by a partial or complete incision of the thyropharyngeus muscle) or myectomy. It is crucial to differentiate between pharyngeal and cricopharyngeal dysphagia as surgery can exacerbate signs of pharyngeal dysphagia.[2] Although it has been reported that surgery results in an immediate and continued resolution of all signs of dysphagia and nasal regurgitation in dogs with cricopharyngeal dysphagia,[7] one study reported poor long-term results.[8] In the latter study, complete, long-term resolution of signs occurred in one dog, transient complete resolution (with recurrence of dysphagia at 2 to 36 weeks after surgery) occurred in 3 dogs, a permanent, partial resolution occurred in 3 dogs, and no improvement was noted after surgery in 6 dogs. The reason for this disparity may reflect a lack of long-term follow-up in some earlier reports. In individual cases, there may be a failure to transect all the bands of the cricopharyngeus muscle, an incorrect initial diagnosis, or concurrent pharyngeal or esophageal dysfunction.[9] A poor outcome may be seen in older dogs, dogs with concurrent aspiration pneumonia or malnutrition that is not addressed prior to surgery, or where cricopharyngeal dysphagia is complicated by other anatomic or functional conditions, such as myasthenia gravis, laryngeal paralysis, or esophageal stricture.[8]

Esophageal Phase

Esophageal disorders are relatively common in the dog and cat. The entire length of the canine esophagus is composed of striated muscle, whereas the caudal one third to half of the feline esophagus is composed of smooth muscle. During normal swallowing, a food bolus is delivered to the cranial cervical esophagus through the relaxed cricopharynx. The bolus initiates a primary peristaltic wave in the esophagus, which propels the bolus aborally to the gastroesophageal junction. The transit time for the bolus from the cervical esophagus to the stomach is approximately 3 to 4 seconds.[3] Initiation of a primary peristaltic wave depends on the presence of a sufficiently large bolus distending the cervical esophagus; several swallows may be needed to produce a bolus that initiates a primary peristaltic wave. If the primary peristaltic wave fails to propel the bolus through the gastroesophageal junction, esophageal distention results in the generation of a secondary peristaltic wave. In normal animals, no significant amount of food should be retained in the esophagus at the end of eating.

The hallmark clinical sign of esophageal-phase dysfunction is regurgitation.[3] Regurgitation is the passive, retrograde expulsion of esophageal or gastric contents. Regurgitation, as distinct from vomiting, is characterized by minimal retching, minimal abdominal or thoracic muscle contraction, and the expulsion of a mucus-covered, sausage-shaped mass of food with a neutral or alkaline pH. Regurgitation may occur minutes to hours after eating. Other clinical signs may include weight loss accompanied by an increased appetite and signs of aspiration pneumonia.

Definitive diagnosis of esophageal-phase dysfunction is usually made by radiographic examination. Most esophageal-phase problems can be diagnosed by plain radiography or radiography following administration of a barium meal or liquid contrast medium.

The causes of esophageal-phase dysfunction can be broadly divided into mechanical or anatomic lesions, functional or neurologic disorders, and inflammatory conditions. Mechanical obstruction of the esophagus can result from the presence of a luminal or mural lesion or from compression from adjacent structures. Causes of mechanical obstruction include esophageal foreign bodies, strictures, neoplasms, vascular ring anomalies, hiatal hernias, and gastroesophageal intussusceptions. The presence of a mechanical obstruction results in a variable degree of obstruction of the esophagus. Esophageal obstruction results in the accumulation of food and secretions proximal to the obstruction and distention of the esophagus. Esophageal distention disrupts normal neuromuscular function and decreases peristalsis. The extent of distention of the esophagus proximal to the obstruction is the major determinant of long-term prognosis after successful relief of the obstruction.

Esophageal foreign bodies are a common problem in dogs and are occasionally diagnosed in cats. The most common foreign bodies in dogs are ingested bones. Esophageal foreign bodies most commonly lodge at the thoracic inlet, heart base, and caudal esophagus where extraesophageal structures restrict esophageal dilation.[9] Esophageal foreign bodies cause mechanical obstruction of the esophagus and can result in pressure necrosis and perforation of the esophageal wall.

Esophageal strictures are uncommon in dogs and cats. Acquired esophageal strictures are more common than congenital strictures. Acquired strictures result from severe, circumferential esophageal injury extending into the muscular layer of the esophageal wall. The damaged esophagus heals by fibrosis and wound contracture, resulting in a narrowed esophageal lumen and obstruction. The most common cause of acquired esophageal strictures in dogs and cats is esophageal reflux during anesthesia; other causes include chronic vomiting, ingestion of corrosive substances, thermal burns, radiation injury, foreign body ingestion, and surgery. The reader is referred to Chapter 26 for more information on vascular ring anomalies and to Chapter 27 for more information on hiatal hernias.

Causes of functional or neurologic disorders of the esophagus include congenital megaesophagus, acquired megaesophagus, and dysautonomia.

Esophagitis can be acute or chronic. Causes of esophagitis in dogs and cats include swallowing caustic substances, esophageal foreign bodies, and gastroesophageal reflux.

Gastroesophageal Phase

Dogs have an increase in thickness of the circumferential striated muscle layer at the gastroesophageal junction, which correlates with the accepted location of the high-pressure zone at the gastroeosphageal junction and may represent the anatomically ill-defined caudal (or lower or cardiac) esophageal sphincter.[10] Other proposed anatomic contributors to the lower esophageal high-pressure zone include the diaphragmatic crural muscles, the angle at which the esophagus and stomach meet and the folds of the gastroesophageal mucosa. It has also been suggested that the intraabdominal portion of the esophagus is subjected to higher pressure than the intrathoracic portion, although one anatomic study found that the intraabdominal portion of the esophagus in dogs could not be consistently demonstrated.[10]

The gastroesophageal phase is the final component of normal swallowing. As the peristaltic wave carries the bolus along the esophagus, the myenteric plexus mediates relaxation of the esophagus ahead of the bolus, permitting the passage of the bolus down the esophagus and through the gastroesophageal junction into the stomach. On fluoroscopic contrast examinations in normal dogs, the bolus of food will occasionally stop in front of the gastroesophageal junction and then enter the stomach with the following bolus. Reflux of food from the stomach into the distal esophagus also occurs occasionally; refluxed food is then carried by a secondary peristaltic wave through the gastroesophageal junction into the stomach.[3] In normal dogs, no food remains in the esophagus after completion of a meal.

Esophageal achalasia is a disease described in humans in whom a failure occurs of reflex relaxation of the gastroesophageal sphincter during swallowing. On thoracic radiographs in dogs with megaesophagus, the caudal thoracic esophagus narrows as it approaches the diaphragm and this "stenotic" appearance should not be misinterpreted as esophageal achalasia. Myotomy of the gastroesophageal sphincter is not recommended in cases of megaesophagus. In a single case report of a dog with apparent esophaghageal achalasia that responded to myotomy, the diagnosis was established by fluoroscopic contrast studies and was not confirmed by manometry.[11]

Gastroesophageal reflux is a disorder involving reflux of gastrointestinal contents into the esophagus. The severity of the resulting esophagitis depends on the frequency and composition of the refluxed material. The combination of gastric acid, pepsin, trypsin, and bile acids can produce severe esophagitis. Gastroesophageal reflux is poorly documented in dogs and cats, and is probably under-diagnosed.[12] It is associated with chronic vomiting, disorders of gastric emptying, hiatal hernia, and anesthesia-induced decreases in the pressure of the lower esophageal high-pressure zone.[12] The reader is referred to Chapter 27 for more information on hiatal hernias.

References

1. Watrous BJ, Suter PF: Normal swallowing in the dog: a cinefluorographic study. Vet Radiol 20:99, 1980.

2. Watrous BJ: Clinical presentation and diagnosis of dysphagia. Vet Clin North Am Small Anim Pract 13:437, 1983.

3. Rosin E: Swallowing disorders. Disease mechanisms 1993, p. 200.

4. Suter PF, Watrous BJ: Oropharyngeal dysphagias in the dog: a cinefluorographic analysis of experimentally induced and spontaneously occurring swallowing disorders I. Oral stage and pharyngeal stage dysphagias. Vet Radiol 21:24, 1980.

5. Pollard RE, Marks SL, Davidson A, Hornof WJ: Quantitative videofluoroscopic evaluation of pharyngeal function in the dog. Vet Radiol Ultrasound 41:409, 2000.

6. Watrous BJ, Suter PF: Oropharyngeal dysphagias in the dog: a

cinefluorographic analysis of experimentally induced and spontaneously occurring swallowing disorders II. Cricopharyngeal stage and mixed oropharyngeal dysphagias. Vet Radiol 24:24, 1983.

7. Niles JD, Williams JM, Sullivan M, Crowsley FE: Resolution of dysphagia following cricopharyngeal myectomy in six young dogs. J Small Anim Pract 42:32, 2001.

8. Warnock JJ, Marks SL, Pollard R, et al: Surgical management of cricopharyngeal dysphagia in dogs: 14 cases (1989-2001). J Am Vet Med Assoc 223:1462, 2003.

9. Kyles AE: Esophagus. *In* Textbook of Small Animal Surgery, 3rd ed Slatter D (ed). Philadelphia: WB Saunders, 2003, p. 573.

10. Pratschke KM, Fitzpatrick E, Campion D, et al: Topography of the gastro-oesophageal junction in the dog revisited: possible clinical implications. Res Vet Sci 76:171, 2004.

11. Boria PA, Webster CRL, Berg J: Esophageal achalasia and secondary megaesophagus in a dog. Can Vet J 44:232, 2003.

12. Washabau RJ, Holt DE: Pathophysiology of gastrointestinal disease. *In* Textbook of Small Animal Surgery 3rd ed. Slatter D (ed). Philadelphia: WB Saunders, 2003, p. 530.

Chapter 26

Vascular Ring Anomalies

Andrew E. Kyles

Vascular ring anomalies are developmental abnormalities of the great vessels that result in a complete or incomplete ring of vessels encircling the trachea and esophagus. Congenital anomalies of the great vessels have been reported in 20% of dogs, but most variants are not clinically significant.[1] The most common vascular ring anomaly in both human beings and dogs is aberrant right subclavian artery, although this is frequently not associated with clinical signs.[1] The most common clinical vascular ring anomaly is persistent right aortic arch (PRAA) with a left ligamentum arteriosum, an anomaly that accounts for 95% of canine clinical cases.[2] A patent ductus arteriosus is present in approximately 10% of dogs with a PRAA. Dogs with vascular ring anomalies may also have a persistent left cranial vena cava or left hemiazygous vein, which, although not clinically significant, may complicate the surgical approach.

Embryology of the Great Vessels

In the embryo, the paired dorsal and ventral aortas are separated by the foregut and pulmonary bud. The six pairs of aortic arches, corresponding to the six brachial arches, connect the dorsal and ventral aortas, and encircle the foregut. As the embryo develops, selective involution and reconnection of the vessels results in the formation of the definitive cardiovascular system and the release of the esophagus and trachea.

During normal embryonic development, the ventral aortas fuse caudally to form the heart and the dorsal aortas fuse caudally to form the descending aorta. The first, second and fifth aortic arches involute early in development. The paired ventral aortas between the third and fourth arches develop into the common carotid arteries and the corresponding sections of the dorsal aortas between the third and fourth arches disappear. The paired ventral aortas that served as the origin of the first two aortic arches develop into the external carotid arteries and the third aortic arches and the cranial dorsal aortas form the internal carotid arteries.

The left ventral aortic root of the fourth arch and the fourth left aortic arch develop into the adult aortic arch, which connects to the fused caudal dorsal aortas that form the adult descending aorta. The right ventral aortic root of the fourth arch becomes the brachiocephalic trunk and the right fourth aortic arch forms the right subclavian artery. The left subclavian artery arises from the left seventh intersegmental artery. The sixth aortic arches form the pulmonary arteries. The left aortic arch retains a connection to the fused dorsal aortas that serves as the left ductus arteriosus in the embryo and becomes the left ligamentum arteriosum after birth. The right ductus arteriosum involutes to release the esophagus and trachea.

Abnormal development of the third aortic arches will not produce a vascular ring anomaly, whereas abnormal development of the fourth and sixth aortic arches can produce a vascular ring anomaly. Complete vascular rings are formed when the right and left portions of the sixth aortic arches are retained, whereas abnormal development of the fourth aortic arches can result in an aberrant right or left subclavian artery and an incomplete vascular ring.

Types of Vascular Ring Anomalies

Several types of vascular ring anomalies have been described in dogs.

Persistent Right Aortic Arch

Persistent right aortic arch and left ligamentum arteriosum: The most common clinical vascular ring anomaly in which the aortic arch develops from the fourth right aortic arch and the ligamentum areteriosum connects the left pulmonary artery to the descending aorta, forming a complete ring around the esophagus.

Persistent right aortic arch, right ligamentum arteriosum, and aberrant left subclavian artery: The aberrant left subclavian artery courses over the esophagus and passes ventrally toward the ventral thoracic inlet.[3] The aberrant left subclavian artery can cause esophageal obstruction because it acts as a band, causing an incomplete vascular ring.

Persistent right aortic arch, left ligamentum arteriosum, and aberrant left subclavian artery: This anomaly forms two strictures, a complete vascular ring associated with the left ligamentum arteriosum and a more cranial incomplete vascular ring caused by the aberrant subclavian artery.[4]

Persistent right aortic arch and right ligamentum arteriosum: This is the mirror image of normal anatomy and does not result in the formation of a vascular ring. However, this anomaly has been associated with cranial thoracic esophageal dilation and regurgitation.[5] In dogs with a PRAA and left ligamentum arteriosum, fibrous, periesophageal bands are often present under the ligamanetum arteriosum; it was speculated that, although the left ligamentum arteriosum had involuted, similar bands may have been present.

Double Aortic Arch

Double aortic arch: This results from the persistence of both the right and left fourth aortic arches.[6] This anomaly can result in significant tracheal stenosis.

Left Aortic Arch

Left aortic arch and right ligamentum arteriosum: This is the mirror image of PRAA with a left ligamentum arteriosum.[7] Although it is uncommon, it is of particular significance because it cannot be corrected via a left lateral thoracotomy.

Left aortic arch, left ligamentum arteriosum, and aberrant right subclavian artery: This represents normal anatomy of the aortic arch and ligamentum arteriosum, with an aberrant right subclavian artery that passes dorsal to the esophagus, causing an incomplete vascular ring.[8]

Left aortic arch, right ligamentum arteriosum, and aberrant right subclavian artery: This anomaly forms two strictures, a complete vascular ring associated with the right ligamentum arteriosum and a more cranial incomplete vascular ring caused by the aberrant subclavian artery.[9]

Vascular ring anomalies are reported less frequently in cats. Vascular ring anaomalies that have been described in the cat include PRAA and left ligamentum arteriosum,[10] left aortic arch and right ligamentum arteriosum,[11] double aortic arch[12] and PRAA, right ligamentum arteriosum and aberrant left subclavian artery.[13]

Diagnosis

Vascular ring anomalies are reported in a variety of breeds; German shepherds and Irish setters have an increased risk compared with the general population.[14] The condition can affect multiple animals in the same litter; breeding of affected animals should be strongly discouraged. Most affected animals are considered normal until weaning, with the development of postprandial regurgitation after the introduction of solid food. In one study, 20% and 80% of dogs were diagnosed before 2 and 6 months of age, respectively,[14] though some animals are not diagnosed until later in life.

Clinical signs of vascular ring anomalies are caused primarily by a partial esophageal obstruction. The usual presenting complaint is regurgitation of undigested food. Affected animals are often smaller than their littermates and appear malnourished despite a ravenous appetite. Respiratory signs can develop secondary to aspiration pneumonia or tracheal compression in animals with a double aortic arch. Signs of cardiac disease are uncommon, except for an association between vascular ring anomalies and patent ductus arteriosus.

The diagnosis of a vascular ring anomaly can be confirmed by survey and positive-contrast radiography. On survey radiographs, the esophagus cranial to the heart may be dilated with air, fluid, or ingesta. On the ventrodorsal projection, it may be possible to identify the descending aorta on the right side of the esophagus in animals with a PRAA. Radiographic signs of aspiration pneumonia may be present. Positive-contrast radiography will confirm the presence of esophageal obstruction at the level of the base of the heart, with dilation of the esophagus cranial to the obstruction; the esophagus caudal to the obstruction is usually undilated. Angiography is rarely performed, but can be used to help determine the type of vascular malformation. Endoscopy can be used to rule out other causes of esophageal obstruction and may show a right-sided aortic pulse in animals with a PRAA.

Treatment

Long-term medical management is generally unrewarding as the degree of esophageal dilation usually increases with age. Preoperative medical management should be used in malnourished animals and patients with aspiration pneumonia. The aim of surgery is to divide the vascular ring by transecting the ligamentum arteriosum and the periesophageal fibrous bands that form under it. Aberrant subclavian arteries are ligated and divided. With double aortic arches, one branch is usually dominant, and the contralateral branch can be divided and oversewn.

Prognosis

The most common problem after surgery is persistent regurgitation. A loss of normal neuromuscular function occurs in the dilated section of the esophagus cranial to the vascular ring, and, although some reduction in esophageal dilation and improvement in motility can be expected following surgery, normal esophageal motility will not be regained. Factors that may affect prognosis include the degree of esophageal constriction and dilation, the severity of debilitation, the presence and severity of aspiration pneumonia before correction, and the medical management before and after surgery.[15]

The prognosis for surgical correction of vascular ring anomalies has improved. In 1981, Shires and Lui reported an excellent outcome (no regurgitation) in 9% of dogs, a good outcome (intermittent regurgitation) in 67%, and a poor outcome in 25%.[14] In 1997, Muldoon et al., using a similar classification scheme, reported the outcome as excellent in 92% and good in 8%.[16]

References

1. Smollich A: Abweichungen im bereich der aste des aortenbogens und ihre bedeutung. Arch Exp Veterinarmed 15:986, 1961.

2. van Grundy T: Vascular ring anomalies. Comp Cont Educ Pract Vet 11:36, 1989.

3. Buergelt CD, Wheaton LG: Dextroaort, atopic left subclavian artery and persistent left cephalic vena cava in a dog. J Am Vet Med Assoc 156:1026, 1970.

4. van der Ingh TS, van der Linde-Sipman JS: Vascular rings in dogs. J Am Vet Med Assoc 188:874, 1974.

5. Filipowicz DE, Kyles AE, Mehl ML, et al: Persistent right aortic arch without a vascular ring anomaly in two dogs with cranial thoracic esophageal dilation and regurgitation. J Am Anim Hosp Assoc (Submitted)

6. Aultman SH, Chambers JN, Verstre WA: Double aortic arch and persistent right aortic arch in two littermates: surgical treatment. J Am Anim Hosp Assoc 16:533, 1980.

7. Hurley K, Miller MW, Willard MD, Boothe HW: Left aortic arch and right ligamentum arteriosum causing esophageal obstruction in a dog. J Am Vet Med Assoc 203:410, 1993.

8. Tsukise A, Sugawa Y, Okano M: Two anomalous cases of the right subclavian artery arising from the aortic arch in dogs. Jpn J Vet 34:11, 1972.

9. Buchanan JW: Tracheal signs and associated vascular anomalies in dogs with persistent right aortic arch. J Vet Intern Med 18:510, 2004.

10. Douglas SW, Walker RG, Littlewort MCG: Persistent right aortic arch in the cat. Vet Rec 72:91, 1960.

11. McCandlish IA, Nash AS, Peggram A: Unusual vascular ring in a cat: left aortic arch with right ligamentum arteriosum. Vet Rec 114:338, 1984.

12. Yarim M, Gultiken ME, Ozturk S, et al: Double aortic arch in a Siamese cat. Vet Pathol 36:340, 1999.

13. White RN, Burton CA, Hale JSH: Vascular ring anomaly with coarctation of the aorta in a cat. J Small Anim Pract 44:330, 2003.

14. Shires PK, Lui W: Persistent right aortic arch in dogs: a long term follow-up after surgical correction. J Am Anim Hosp Assoc 17:773, 1981

15. Kyles AE: Esophagus. *In* Textbook of Small Animal Surgery 3rd ed. Slatter D (ed). Philadelphia: WB Saunders, 2003, p. 573.

16. Muldoon MM, Birchard SJ, Ellison GW: Long-term results of surgical correction of persistent right aortic arch in dogs: 25 cases (1980-1995). J Am Vet Med Assoc 210:1761, 1997.

Chapter 27

Hiatal Hernia

Geraldine B. Hunt

Hiatal hernias occur when abdominal contents protrude through the esophageal hiatus of the diaphragm into the thorax. Hiatal hernias are classified into two main types, sliding (or axial) and paraesophageal, according to the position of the gastroesophageal junction.[1,2] In dogs and cats, the most common type is the sliding hernia, in which the esophagus, esophagogastric junction, and part of the stomach move through the esophageal hiatus into the thoracic cavity.[3-5] This is also described as Type 1 (Figure 27-1). Paraesophageal (Type 2) hiatal hernia has been described infrequently and involves movement of the fundus of the stomach in a rolling fashion through a defect in the esophageal hiatus while the gastroesophageal junction remains fixed in its normal position. Type 2 hernias have been reported only sporadically in dogs, and never in cats.[3,6] In cases where a combination of the above two abnormalities occur, the hernia is classified as Type 3. In extreme cases, other abdominal organs may accompany the stomach in the thorax, in which case the hernia is classified as Type 4 (Figure 27-2).[7] Hiatal hernias may be fixed or dynamic, with herniated tissues moving in and out of the thorax according to changes in position and pleural pressure. Hence, clinical or radiographic signs may not always be present, and dynamic studies may be required to confirm a diagnosis.

Hiatal hernias may be diagnosed at any age. A distinction has been made between congenital and acquired sliding hiatal hernias in dogs, based on age of diagnosis.[2] However, reported case series demonstrate that acquired posttraumatic hiatal hernias can occur in animals as young as a few months.

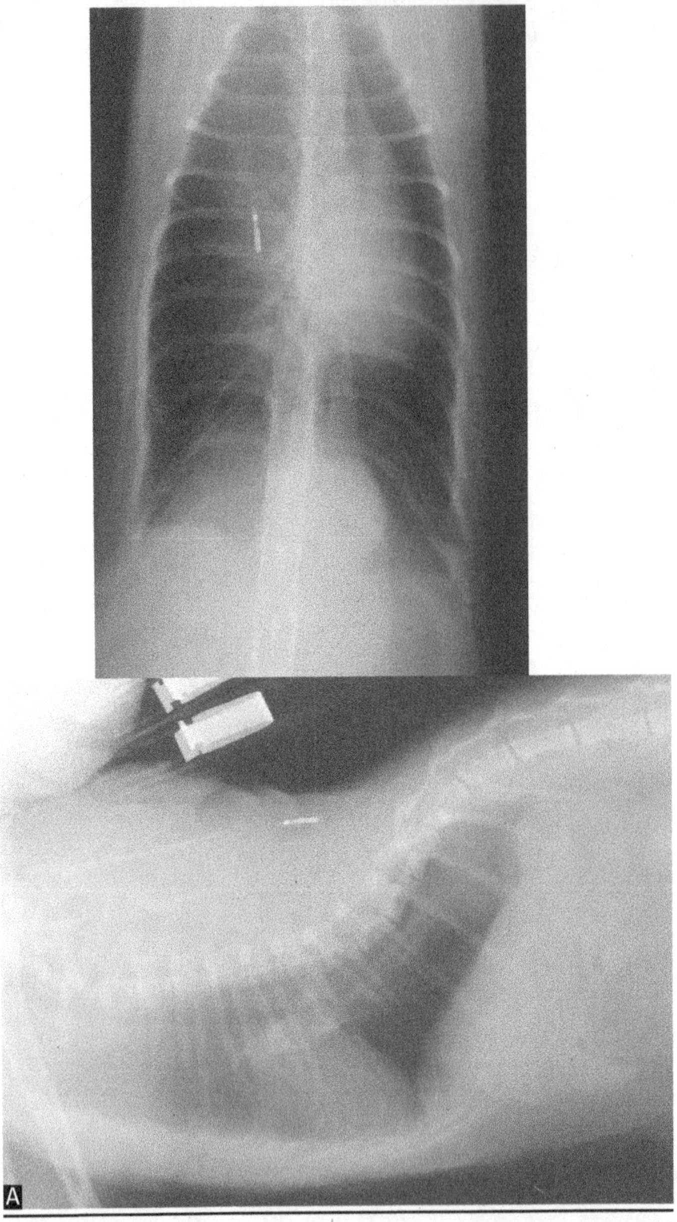

Figure 27-1A. Lateral and ventrodorsal radiographs of a 14-month-old Burmese cat with lordosis. A type 1 hiatal hernia was diagnosed coincidentally.

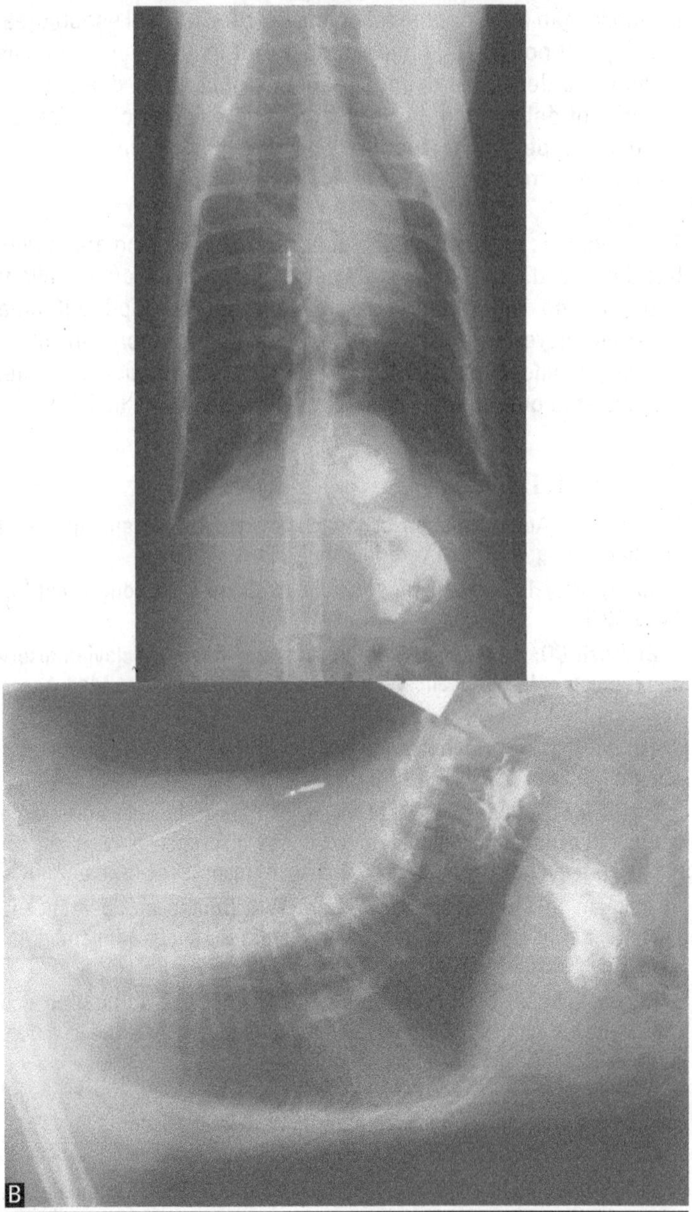

Figure 27-1B. Administration of barium paste reveals cranial malpositioning of the stomach through the diaphragmatic hiatus. This cat did show evidence of clinical signs associated with its hiatal hernia.

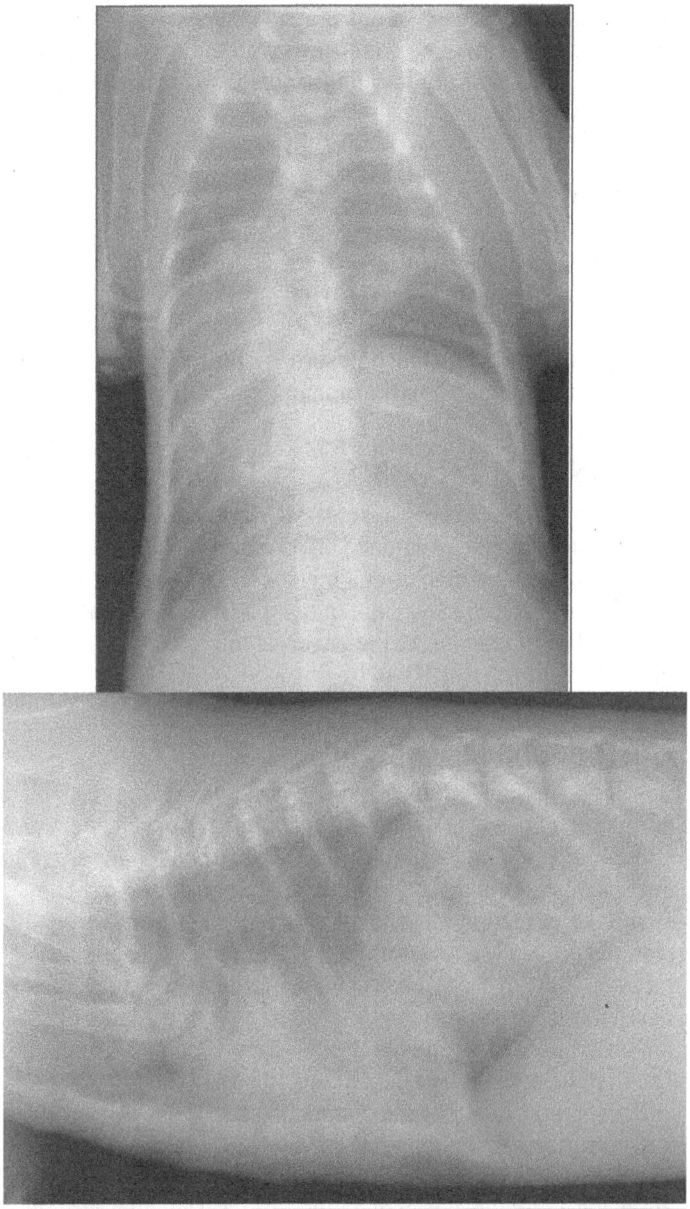

Figure 27-2. Lateral and ventrodorsal radiographs of a 10-week-old domestic shorthaired kitten with dyspnea. A large hiatal hernia is present, possibly incorporating other abdominal organs in addition to the stomach. A few days after these radiographs were taken, the kitten suffered a sudden deterioration in its respiratory function and died. Postmortem examination was not performed.

Anatomy and Physiology of the Diaphragmatic Hiatus and Gastroesophageal Junction

The diaphragm is a musculotendinous partition that separates the abdominal and thoracic organs, assists in ventilation, and has a role in the movement of lymphatic fluid. The diaphragm is composed of a strong central tendinous section and three separate muscles: the costal, sternal, and lumbar parts. The right crus is larger than the left. A tendon attaches each crus to the bodies of the third and fourth lumbar vertebrae, medial to the psoas minor muscles. Motor innervation of the diaphragm is from the phrenic nerves.[8]

Gastroesophageal reflux is normally controlled by a zone of increased pressure, the lower esophageal sphincter of the terminal esophagus.[9] At this point, the muscular layer is the thickest of the entire esophageal length. No anatomic or histologic differentiation exists between this zone and the rest of the esophagus. A complex arrangement of transverse, oblique, and longitudinal muscle fibers blends with the muscular layers of the stomach. A section of inner, transverse fibers blends with the inner muscular fibers of the stomach. Dorsal longitudinal fibers of the outer layer continue on the dorsal wall of the stomach. Oblique, inner fibers pass external to the transverse fibers to blend with longitudinal fibers of the stomach wall.[10] The lower esophageal sphincter (esophageal high-pressure zone) is traditionally considered to be part of the intraabdominal esophagus, situated between the diaphragmatic hiatus and the gastroesophageal junction. It has been contended that the intraabdominal esophagus is subjected to higher extraluminal pressures, increasing its resistance to gastroesophageal reflux. However, some anatomic studies challenge this concept by suggesting that in many canines there is little or no intraabdominal esophagus.[11] It has also been proposed that extrinsic influences imposed by diaphragmatic tone and the anatomic arrangement of the esophagus, hiatus, and stomach support the action of the increased pressure zone. Primary incompetence of the lower esophageal sphincter has not been demonstrated in dogs and cats.[28] Pratschke et al[12] demonstrated significant differences in the barrier pressure at the gastroesophageal junction in anesthetized dogs positioned in ventral versus lateral recumbency. Hence, the intrinsic muscular activity of the lower esophagus, exertion of extraluminal compression by surrounding structures such as the diaphragm, and geometric relationship of the cardia and esophagus seem most likely to work in concert to moderate gastroesophageal reflux.

Clinical Signs

In congenital hiatal hernias, clinical signs may be observed immediately after weaning onto solid food and are usually seen before the animal is 1 year of age. Acquired hiatal hernias can occur at any age and are most often associated with abdominal trauma. In some instances, animals with a congenital predisposition toward hiatal hernia may develop signs following development of an exacerbating problem such as upper respiratory tract obstruction or diaphragmatic dysfunction. In other individuals, such as the cat shown in Figure 27-1, hiatal hernias may be diagnosed incidentally during investigation for other problems. Clinical signs result from esophagitis, esophageal dysfunction, and the mass effect of herniated organs within the thorax. They include hypersalivation, regurgitation of frothy saliva and/or food, vomiting, dysphagia, dyspnea, and exercise intolerance.[2-4] The severity of disease may range from minor, with discomfort from mild esophagitis, to life-threatening, with cachexia, dehydration, and aspiration pneumonia. It is likely that, in contrast to humans in whom mild reflux esophagitis may be detected as a result of the patient's complaining of heartburn, most animals presenting for management of hiatal hernias will be diagnosed as a result of relatively severe clinical signs, such as hypersalivation, regurgitation, or dyspnea.

Predisposition to Hiatal Hernia

Breed

Multiple case reports and case series indicate that Chinese shar-peis appear to have a breed predisposition to the disease.[6,13,14] Hiatal hernias have also been described in a range of brachycephalic breeds. No breed predispositions have been reported in cats.

Upper Respiratory Obstruction

Evidence is growing that upper respiratory tract obstruction exacerbates the clinical signs associated with hiatal hernias.[15-19] A case-control study of bulldogs demonstrated that hiatal hernias were associated with the more severe manifestations of brachycephalic syndrome.[16] Single case reports have described complete remission of clinical signs associated with a sliding hiatal hernia in a Labrador-cross after surgical treatment of laryngeal paralysis,[15] and resolution of clinical signs and radiographic signs of a hiatal hernia following surgical correction of congenital stenosis of the soft palate in a dachshund.[17] A review of 30 dogs with brachycephalic obstructive airway syndrome revealed evidence of esophagitis in 25 and sliding hiatal hernias in 13.[18] Marked improvement in esophagitis and herniation followed surgical correction of the upper airway problems. Esophagitis (among other gastrointestinal tract lesions) was found in a substantial proportion of brachycephalic dogs with upper respiratory syndrome in another study.[19] Proposed mechanisms for exacerbation of hiatal hernias and gastroesophageal reflux by respiratory tract disease include increased force of ventilation, exaggerated negative pleural pressures, and aerophagia leading to gastric distention. Conversely, a strong association between gastroesophageal reflux and chronic respiratory and otolaryngeal disease has been identified in people, with speculation that gastroesophageal reflux may exacerbate airway disease by mechanisms including direct stimulation of the respiratory mucosa, aspiration pneumonia, and reflex bronchoconstriction.[20,21]

Other Disease Processes

Hiatal hernias may also occur as a result of other diseases that interfere with normal diaphragmatic function. Symptoms of hiatal hernias have been repeatedly observed following surgery for diaphragmatic hernias in cats and dogs.[3,4,22,23] Proposed mechanisms by which diaphragmatic hernia repair might predispose animals to clinical signs of hiatal hernias include physical damage to the diaphragmatic hiatus, abnormal tension on the central tendon of the diaphragm and hence the hiatus, increases in intraabdominal pressure as a result of loss of abdominal domain following chronic diaphragmatic hernia, and alterations in vagal activity as a result of surgical trauma and organ repositioning.

Four cases of hiatal hernias associated with generalized tetanus have been reported in dogs.[24-26] Proposed mechanisms relate to abnormal neuromuscular function of the diaphragm, distal esophagus, and abdominal musculature, causing diaphragmatic spasm or esophageal dysmotility with a subsequent tendency to herniation.

Regardless of the observations that clinical signs did not appear until after a precipitating event, it has not been possible to rule out the possibility of a preexisting predisposition to hiatal hernias in these patients.

Obesity

Excessive body weight has been reported as a significant factor predisposing both to hiatal hernia and esophagitis as a result of gastroesophageal reflux disease in humans. Obesity is considered to exacerbate the signs of hiatal hernias owing to an increase in intraabdominal pressure, increasing the likelihood of organ herniation and gastroesophageal reflux.[27]

Consequences of Hiatal Hernia

In humans, clinical signs associated with hiatal hernias do not result from the major anatomic abnormality (laxity of the esophageal hiatus of the diaphragm) but secondary to the events that occur as a result of movement of the gastroesophageal junction and axial displacement of the lower esophageal sphincter from the esophageal hiatus.[28]

Gastroesophageal Reflux

Gastroesophageal reflux is the major consequence of hiatal hernia,[29,30] causing esophagitis, esophageal dysmotility, airway contamination, and pneumonia.[3,4] Gastroesophageal reflux occurs as a normal event in humans when lower esophageal sphincter pressure falls below 4 mm Hg31, but regurgitated material is usually cleared promptly by esophageal peristalsis.[32,33] Increased exposure to gastric acid, increased acidity of gastric contents, reduced passage of saliva through the esophagus, and failure of normal esophageal clearance result in esophagitis. Esophagitis caused by reflux of acidic gastric contents induces vomiting, regurgitation, and hypersalivation. Severe esophagitis may progress to esophageal stricture.[34,35] In extreme cases, esophagitis may extend transmurally, resulting in fibrous adhesion between the esophagus and surrounding structures (such as the diaphragmatic hiatus), thereby reducing the elastic ability of the esophagus to stretch. This condition is termed "shortened esophagus syndrome" and carries a poor prognosis when addressed using normal surgical techniques.[3,36]

Regurgitation

Abnormal and decreased esophageal motility may be primary or secondary to hiatal hernia and reflux esophagitis. Up to 60% of patients with hiatal hernias have signs of megaesophagus on plain or contrast radiographs.[3,16,37]

Dysphagia in humans seems to result from obstruction to passage of a swallowed bolus by diaphragmatic impingement on the herniated stomach.[38]

Dyspnea

Dyspnea may occur in animals with hiatal hernias as a result of an intrathoracic mass effect (gastric distention in Types 1 to 4 or herniated organs in Type 4 hernia, Figure 27-2), failure of the thoracic bellows in animals with diaphragmatic dysfunction, or aspiration of gastric contents leading to bronchospasm or aspiration pneumonia.

Prognosis

Hiatal Hernia

Reflux esophagitis may be treated effectively with a variety of medical agents. However, surgery is indicated in animals with severe gastroesophageal reflux leading to chronic esophagitis, regurgitation, and airway disease. After surgical correction of hiatal hernia by use of an anatomic restoration technique, and with attention to exacerbating problems such as brachycephalic disease, uniformly good results may be expected.

References

1. Hunt GB, Johnson KE: Dipahragmatic, pericardial and hiatal hernia. *In* Textbook of Small Animal Surgery, 3rd ed. DH Slatter (ed)., Philadelphia: WB Saunders, 2003, p. 473.

2. Waldron DR, Leib MS. Hiatal hernia. *In* Disease Mechanisms in Small Animal Surgery, 2nd ed. Bojrab MJ (ed). Philadelphia: Lea & Febiger, 1993, p. 210.

3. Ellison GW, Lewis DD, Phillips L, et al: Esophageal hiatal hernia in small animals: Literature review and a modified surgical technique. J Am Anim Hosp Assoc 23:391, 1987.

4. Bright RM, Sackman JE, DeNovo C, et al: Hiatal hernia in the dog and cat: A retrospective study of 16 cases. J Small Anim Pract 31:244, 1990.

5. Lorinson D, Bright RM: Long term outcome of medical and surgical treatment of hiatal hernias in dogs and cats: 27 cases (1978-1996). J Am Vet Med Assoc 213:381, 1998.

6. Miles KG, Pope ER, Jergens AE: Paraesophageal hiatal hernia and pyloric obstruction in a dog. J Am Vet Med Assoc 193:1437, 1988.

7. Rahal SC, Mamprim MJ, Muniz LMR, et al: Type-4 esophageal hiatal hernia in a Chinese shar-pei dog. Vet Radiol Ultrasound 44:66, 2003.

8. Hermanson JW, Evans HE: The muscular system. *In* Miller's Anatomy of the Dog. Evans HE (ed). Philadelphia: WB Saunders, 1993,p. 304.

9. Patrikios J, et al: Relationship of transient lower esophageal sphincter relaxation to postprandial gastroesophageal reflux and belching in dogs. Gastroenterology 90:545, 1986.

10. Evans HE: The digestive apparatus and abdomen. *In* Miller's Anatomy of the Dog. Evans HE (ed). Philadelphia: WB Saunders, 1993, p. 424.

11. Pratschke KM, Fitzpatrick E, Campion D, et al: Topography of the gastro-oesophageal junction in the dog revisited: possible clinical implications. Res Vet Sci 76:171, 2004.

12. Pratschke KM, Bellenger CR, McAllister H, et al: Barrier pressure at the gastroesophageal junction in anesthetized dogs. Am J Vet Res 62:1068-1072, 2001.

13. Williams JM: Hiatal hernia in a shar-pei. J Small Anim Pract 31:251, 1990.

14. Callan MB, Washsabau RJ, Saunders HM, et al: Congenital esophageal hiatal hernia in the Chinese shar-pei dog. J Vet Intern Med 7: 210, 1993.

15. Burnie AG, Simpson JW, Corocoran BM: Gastro-oesophageal reflux and hiatus hernia associated with laryngeal paralysis in a dog. J Small Anim Pract 30:414, 1989.

16. Hardie EM, Ramirez O, Clary EM, et al: Abnormalities of the thoracic bellows: Stress fractures of the ribs and hiatal hernia. J Vet Intern Med 12:279, 1998.

17. Dvir E, Spotswood TC, Lambrechts NE, et al: Congenital narrowing of the intrapharyngeal opening in a dog with concurrent oesophageal hiatal hernia. J Small Anim Pract 44; 359-362, 2003.

18. Lecoindre P, Richard S: Digestive disorders associated with the chronic obstructive respiratory syndrome of brachycephalic dogs: 30 cases (1999-2001). Revue de Medicine Veterinaire 155:141, 2004.

19. Poncet CM, Dupre GP, Freiche VG, et al: Prevalence of gastrointestinal tract lesions in 73 brachcephalic dogs with upper respiratory syndrome. J Small Anim Pract 46:273, 2005.

20. Barbero GJ: Gastroesophageal reflux and upper airway disease. Otolaryngol Clin North Am 29:27, 1996.

21. Guill MF: Respiratory manifestations of gastroesophageal reflux in children. J Asthma 32:167, 1995.

22. Waldron DR, Moon M, Leib MS, et al: Oesophageal hiatal hernia in two cats. J Small Anim Pract 31:259, 1990.

23. Pratschke KM, Hughes JML, Skelly C, et al: Hiatal herniation as a complication of chronic diaphragmatic herniation. J Small Anim Pract 39:33, 1998.

24. Dieringer TM, Wolf AM: Esophageal hiatal hernia and megaesophagus complicating tetanus in two dogs. J Am Vet Med Assoc 199:87, 1991.

25. Van Ham L, van Bree H: Conservative treatment of tetanus associated with hiatus hernia and gastro-oesophageal reflux. J Small Anim Pract 33:289, 1992.

26. Acke E, Jones BR, Breathnach R, et al: Tetanus in the dog; a review and case-report of concurrent tetanus with hiatal hernia. Irish Vet J 57:593, 2004.

27. Wilson LJ, Wenzhou Ma MS, Hirschowitz BI: Association of obesity with hiatal hernia and oesophagitis. Am J Gastroenterol 94: 2841, 1999.

28. Sivacolundhu RK, Read RA, Marchevsky AM: Hiatal hernia controversies – a review of pathophysiology and treatment options. Aust Vet J 80:48, 2002.

29. Dhein CRM, Rawlings CA, Rosin E, et al: Esophageal hiatal hernia and eventration of the diaphragm with resultant gastroesophageal reflux. J Am Anim Hosp Assoc 16:517, 1980.

30. Marchand P: A study of the forces productive of gastrooesophageal regurgitation and herniation through the diaphragmatic hiatus. Thorax 12:189, 1957.

31. Dent J, Dodds WJ, Hogan WJ, et al: Factors that influence induction of gastroesophageal reflux in normal human subjects. Digest Dis Sci 33:270, 1988.

32. Baue AE, Hoffer RE: The effects of experimental hiatal hernia and histamine stimulation on the intrinsic esophageal sphincter. Surg Gynecol Obstet 125:791, 1967.

33. Helm JF, Dodds WJ, Riedel DR, et al: Determinants of esophageal acid clearance in normal subjects. Gastroenterol 85:607, 1983.

34. Pearson H, Darke PGG, Gibbs C, et al: Reflux oesophagitis and stricture formation after anaesthesia: a review of seven cases in dogs and cats. J Small Anim Pract 19:507, 1978.

35. Papazoglou LG, Patsikas M, Rallis, T, et al: Hiatal hernia with esophageal stricture in a cat. Feline Pract 28:3, 10, 2000.

36. Mattioli S, Lugaresi ML, Di Simone MP, et al: The surgical treatment of intrathoracic migration of the gastroesophageal junction and short esophagus in gastro-esophageal reflux disease. Eur J Cardiothorac Surg 25:1079, 2004.

37. Manderino D: Megaesophagus secondary to a hiatal hernia in a German shepherd puppy. Can Pract 14:5, 1987.

38. Kaul BK, DeMeester TR, Oka M, et al: The cause of dysphagia in uncomplicated sliding hiatal hernia and its relief by hiatal herniorrhaphy. A roentgenographic, manometric, and clinical study. Ann Surg 211:406, 1990.

Chapter 28

Pathopysiology Associated with Gastric Dilation-Volvulus Syndrome

Daniel J Brockman

Gastric dilatation – volvulus syndrome (GDVs) includes acute gastric dilation (GD), acute gastric dilation with gastric volvulus (GDV), and chronic gastric volvulus (cGV).[1] Although the overall prevalence of this disease in the population at risk is low, animals affected by GD and GDV are commonly presented as emergencies, so this remains an important syndrome for any clinician involved in emergency practice. Treatment protocols based on best current evidence regarding the pathophysiology resulting from GD and GDV, has resulted in good survival rates.[2-4] It is likely that any future improvements in the treatment of this condition will be as a direct result of a better understanding of the disease mechanisms involved. The most profound functional changes that occur are associated with GD and GDV and vary according to the extent of gastric dilation, the degree of gastric rotation, and the duration of each. Although it is often helpful to consider the pathophysiology on the basis of an organ or body system, the changes that occur are complex and interdependent. For the body as a whole, the consequences of GDVs are reduced oxygen delivery to tissues. These changes can be so mild that they are barely evident or they can be so severe that they result in irreversible "sepsis syndrome," either through uncontrolled infection (sepsis) or noninfectious systemic inflammatory response syndrome (SIRS).[5] The author will begin this review by describing the pathoanatomy of GDVs followed by a description of the effects this pathoanatomy has on body systems and organs based on data derived from experimental creation of GD or GDV. Data from clinical studies will be presented as confirmation, or otherwise, that each process is actually happening in dogs affected by GDVs. Again, however, it is important to remember that these processes are interdependent; no process or system can really be considered in isolation of other organs or systems. This is particularly germane to clinical treatment where a "global approach" to the patient aimed at optimizing oxygen delivery to tissues will yield the best clinical results in terms of overall outcome.

Pathoanatomy

Dilation of a normally positioned stomach, results in a 90- degree counter-clockwise gastric rotation around the gastroesophageal junction.[6] The majority of dogs affected with GDVs undergo simultaneous dilation and clockwise rotation (between 180 and 360 degrees) of the stomach about the gastroesophageal junction.[2-4] It has been suggested that gastric malposition must be present before gastric dilation results in classic GDV.[6] What conditions or factors trigger gastric rotation and whether it preceded gastric volvulus or vice versa, in an individual, are rarely clear at the time of diagnosis. From a pathophysiologic perspective, GD and GDV can create similar systemic effects, but evidence exists that the deleterious effects to the blood supply of local organs (stomach and spleen) are greater when volvulus has occurred.[6,7]

Splenic displacement has been documented in many patients with GDVs[2,6] and is considered inevitable because of its close anatomic association with the greater curvature of the stomach. The magnitude of displacement should, in theory, have a direct relationship with the degree of splenic vascular compromise.

Experimental Models of GDV

Attempts to precisely recreate the pathoanatomy of dogs with naturally occurring GDV have failed. In addition, all of the experimental models of this disease require general anesthesia, abolishing any conscious influence (such as release of endogenous catecholamines and cortisol) over events in these dogs. It seems that it is impossible to rotate the stomach of an otherwise normal dog and dilate it with air and have it remain in that state without additional "devices." Passi et al[8] ligated the thoracic esophagus around an orogastric tube, via thoracotomy, and ligated the pylorus through a right subcostal laparotomy. They inflated the stomach to a mean pressure of 25 +/- 11 mm Hg to create a model of GD. Merkley et al[9] used the experimental model of GD that was predominant at that time, using an intragastric balloon inflated to 80mm Hg. Orton and Muir[10] argued that such high intragastric pressures (80 mm Hg) should not be used because the intragastric pressure in dogs with naturally occurring disease varied from 9 to 62 mm Hg. They favored, therefore, using an intragastric balloon inflated to a pressure of 30 mm Hg.[10,11] In addition, these workers created a small celiotomy to allow concurrent rotation of the dilated stomach to create GDV. Subsequently, models of GDV have involved umbilical tape ligatures placed at the gastroesophageal junction and at the pylorus, in such a way that branches of the vagus nerve and the gastric vasculature are not compromised, to create an air-tight seal. The stomach is then inflated via a Foley catheter in the pyloric antrum, to a pressure of 30 mm Hg and the stomach is sutured in a rotated position to create GDV.[7,12-14] The length of time that these models of GD or GDV were maintained varied between 90 and 180 minutes. In addition to these models of GD and GDV, Lantz et al[7] studied the effect of gastric volvulus alone by suturing the nondistended stomach in position after rotating it 360 degrees. All models of GD or GDV that required celiotomy for their creation had the celiotomy closed before any measurements were made.

In summary, none of these models perfectly recreate the natural disease. In addition, anesthetic drug protocols have varied from model to model, which could have a significant effect on results. Because of the careful use of control animals, however, experiments using these models have provided a valuable insight into the events that follow GD and GDV.

Circulatory Pathophysiology

Passi et al[8] using their acute GD model, demonstrated that caudal vena cava flow rates fell rapidly from 51 ml $kg^{-1}min^{-1}$to between 0-9 ml $kg^{-1}min^{-1}$ within 31 minutes. Cranial caval flow rates fell from 28.9 ml $kg^{-1}min^{-1}$ to 24 ml kg-1min^{-1} during this time. Mean arterial pressure (MAP), during the same period, fell from 112 mm Hg to 90 mm Hg, and it took only a further 30 minutes for MAP to fall below 50 mm Hg. Pretreatment with lactated Ringer's solution (50 ml/kg), bilateral cervical vagotomy, and sympathectomy did not prevent the onset of these hemodynamic changes. Of 16 dogs, 12 required additional lactated Ringer's following gastric decompression to restore normal hemodynamics. These workers concluded that mechanical obstruction of the cava was responsible for an acute decrease in venous return, leading to systemic arterial hypotension, and that fluid administration was required to return these dogs to their predilation hemodynamic state. Orton and Muir[10,11] confirmed the earlier findings of Passi[8] and added further information regarding a fall in the maximum rate of left ventricular pressure change over time (dp/dt_{max}), increased heart rate, decreased cardiac output, and presumed neurohormonal reflex alterations in total peripheral resistance. Wingfield et al[15] provided angiographic evidence of caudal venous attenuation and obstruction in their model of acute gastric dilation. Barnes et al[16] provided indirect evidence of mechanical obstruction secondary to changes in intraabdominal pressure in an experiment that investigated the hemodynamic response to elevations in intraabdominal pressure (IAP). They documented hemodynamic changes similar to those that had been documented following experimental GD by increasing intraabdominal pressure to 40 mm Hg, alone. Together, the above experiments have demonstrated that acute gastric dilation, using intragastric pressures equivalent to those seen in dogs with natural disease, cause mechanical obstruction to the caudal vena cava with predictable consequences with respect to cardiac output. In addition, acute increases in IAP alone can be detrimental to blood flow through the low-pressure vascular systems (caudal cava and portal vein). Finally, because simply decompressing the stomach was not always enough to return hemodynamics to control levels, data from these experiments contained the clue that additional factors were mediating prolonged systemic hypotension in animals recovering from GD and GDV.

Impaired myocardial contractility has also been cited as a contributing factor in the poor circulatory status of dogs with GD and GDV. Such an influence could be secondary to an imbalance to the cardioinhibitory (e.g., myocardial depressant factor [MDF] or vagal mediated) and cardiostimulatory (circulating catecholamines) influences over myocardial function. In addition, myocardial ischemia could directly influence myocardial performance in these hypotensive patients. Orton and Muir[11] failed to detect cardioactive substances in their acute model of GDV, but they commented that, if MDF was being released by the pancreas, it could remain sequestered in the portal circulation until gastric decompression and mechanical release of the splanchnic circulation had occurred. Horne et al[17] investigated the direct effect of experimental GDV on myocardial blood flow and myocardial oxygen extraction in addition to more global changes in hemodynamic indices. They documented reduced myocardial blood flow (50% below control level) increased heart rate (similar to what has been previously described) and corresponding increase in myocardial oxygen extraction (30% above controls). Of the 8 experimental dogs, 6 developed subendocardial necrosis. Unfortunately, the long-term effects of MDF and the myocardial ischemia were not determined by either investigation.

Clinical evidence:
Good objective clinical data regarding the circulatory status of dogs with GDVs before fluid resuscitation is not contained in any of the large reports of this condition.[2-4] One small prospective study by Wagner et al[19] evaluated cardiopulmonary variables in 6 dogs that underwent gastropexy without partial gastrectomy for GDV. Unfortunately, 4 of these 6 dogs had intravenous fluid therapy before any measurements were made and all had intraoperative fluid therapy "according to the perceived needs of the patient, made by the attending clinician and anaesthetist." Wagner et al[19] concluded that not all dogs with naturally occurring GDVs have severe circulatory derangements. The study population did not include any dogs that required partial gastric resection -- creating study population bias -- and with so many uncontrolled variables, such as degree of gastric distention and fluid administration, and the small sample size, it is hard to interpret these data as being sound scientific evidence. Other evidence of the degree of systemic hypoperfusion was provided indirectly by De Papp et al[4] who retrospectively evaluated venous plasma lactate concentration as a predictor of gastric necrosis and survival in 102 dogs. In this study, the dogs with gastric necrosis were compared with dogs that did not have gastric necrosis, and mean venous plasma lactate concentrations were 6.6 mmol/L and 3.3 mmol/L, respectively. Originally, these workers hypothesized that the gastrointestinal tract was the source of the lactate; but ultimately they concluded that any ischemic tissue in the body could contribute to the venous plasma lactate concentration, especially if the sample was retrieved prior to gastric decompression and release of the splanchnic (portal venous) reservoir of gut-derived lactate. These authors suggested that high lactate was more likely to reflect systemic hypoperfusion than gut production alone and, as such, should be considered a marker of disease severity rather than a direct indicator of gastric-wall ischemia. In addition, dogs with naturally occurring GDVs frequently have rupture of the short gastric vessels and hemoperitoneum, both of which can affect regional organ blood flow (see later) and systemic hemodynamic parameters.

The prevalence of cardiac arrhythmias in dogs recovering from GDVs has been well documented.[2,3,19] Evidence of myocyte injury in the form of serum cardiac troponin I (cTI) and cardiac troponin T (cTT) has been demonstrated in dogs clinically affected with GDVs.[20] In the same study, 10 of 16 dogs that died had arrhythmias; all 16 had detectable cTI and CTT, but, it was not reported how many of the dogs that died did so as a direct result of a fatal arrhythmia.[20] In 4 of 5 dogs necropsied, myocardial necrosis was evident. In the absence of the identification of a direct myocardial depressant factor, another cardiotoxic element, or electrolyte derangements in the plasma of dogs affected with GDVs, reduced coronary blood flow and increased myocardial oxygen demand could be considered as a reflection of the systemic hypotension and hypoperfusion. Because coronary blood flow occurs predominantly during diastole, low diastolic pressures, in particular, would reduce coronary blood flow. Because diastolic pressure depends on systemic vascular resistance, perturbations of this in addition to total intravascular volume could have a detrimental effect on myocardial oxygen delivery.

In emergency practice, the clinician must rely on subjective indicators of perfusion such as mucous membrane color, capillary refill time, and pulse rate and quality. It would be an error to ignore these basic physiologic parameters when assessing the circulatory status of any patient.

Respiratory Pathophysiology

The effects of increasing gastric volume or increasing intraabdominal pressure on total thoracic volume and diaphragmatic excursions have been studied infrequently in an experimental setting.[15] These effects include a decrease in total thoracic volume, decreased diaphragmatic excursions, and partial lung lobe collapse (causing ventilation-perfusion mismatching), all resulting in hypoventilation and hypoxia. Compensatory mechanisms such a tachypnea and alterations in the lateral thoracic dimensions preserve lung function initially. Ultimately, the pulmonary blood flow falls secondary to systemic hypovolemia, magnifying the effect of ventilation-perfusion mismatching.

Clinical evidence:

No firm clinical evidence exists that these mechanisms occur in dogs clinically affected by GDVs, but anecdotal evidence of respiratory compromise abounds. It is understandable to anyone involved in emergency practice why objective documentation of this respiratory impairment has not been acquired. Improved pulmonary function, however, must remain one of the potential benefits of gastric decompression.

Dogs clinically affected by GDVs often make frequent attempts to vomit, and regurgitate any oral intake of fluid or food. This might place them at risk for aspiration pneumonia. Aspiration pneumonia is a finding that has been reported as a postoperative complication in several studies of this disease.[2,3] Aspiration of pharyngeal contents can have an acute and a longer term effect on pulmonary gas exchange and should be considered as one of the potential causes of poor lung performance in these animals.

Gastrointestinal, Hepatic, and Splenic Pathopysiology

The effect of 360-degree rotation of the blood supply of the nondistended dog stomach was investigated by Lantz et al.[7] These workers concluded that gastric venous obstruction contributed to mucosal and submucosal edema throughout the stomach, and that stretching of the short gastric arteries along the greater curvature of the stomach exacerbated the ischemic injury at that site. Davidson et al[13] demonstrated reduced blood flow to all tissues except liver and heart ventricles after experimental GDV lasting 270 minutes. In this experiment, pancreatic and jejunal blood flow were among those measured. The implication of the results of the two aforementioned experiments, is that gastric dilation causes reduced gastrointestinal blood flow either by direct compression of the portal vein or via reduced cardiac output. The compromise to gastric blood flow is worsened by gastric rotation and compression (or avulsion) of the short gastric and splenic arteries. It is important also to realize that the perfusion pressure in the gastric wall arterioles and capillaries must exceed the compressive force applied to these vessels by the tension in the gastric wall in order for blood to flow. The potential for gastric necrosis is, therefore, influenced by several factors: degree of gastric rotation, duration of rotation, intragastric pressure (gastric wall tension), systemic arterial pressure, and compression or injury to the short gastric branches of the splenic artery.

Increased levels of circulating endotoxin along with histologic evidence of intestinal villus injury were demonstrated by Davidson et al[13] in their experimental GDV group. The finding of high level of circulating endotoxin could indicate increased production of bacterial lipopolysaccharide (LPS) in the gut or increased permeability to LPS. Peycke et al[21] investigated the effect of experimental GDV on adenosine triphosphate (ATP) and conductance of the canine gastric and jejunal mucosa They concluded that the jejunal mucosa showed more profound changes and that the conductance values and ATP levels in jejunal mucosa were suggestive of cell-membrane dysfunction. These experiments could be taken as evidence for intestinal mucosal barrier compromise secondary to GDVs, resulting in systemic release of both bacterial products (e.g., LPS) and, potentially, whole bacteria.

Histologic evidence of hepatocellular damage following experimental GDV was provided by Davidson et al.[13] Several mechanisms could be responsible for this injury: ischemia-reperfusion injury, damage caused by endotoxin, and hypoxic damage. Alterations in hepatic function have not been assessed in experimental models of GDV but, in theory, acute diminution of hepatic function could have serious consequences. The effect of experimental GDV on the spleen has not been reported in detail.

Clinical evidence:

Gastric necrosis following naturally occurring GDVs has a predictable pattern, with the gastric fundus most commonly affected.[22] In clinical studies of this disease, rupture of the short gastric vessels and hemoperitoneum is often recorded, demonstrating that the natural disease causes changes that experimental models have not included, such as blood loss and irretrievable vascular compromise. In addition to necrosis of the fundus, necrosis at the cardia has been reported,[2] suggesting that twisting of the cardia can also directly affect local tissue integrity, probably by direct vascular occlusion. The reported prevalence of gastric necrosis in patients with naturally occurring GDV is between 10% and 30% in most studies.[2-4,22] This fact may give an indirect indication of the prevalence of "severe" disease among affected dogs, since the survival rate for dogs that do not require partial gastric resection as part of their treatment approached 100% in one study.[4] The intermediate-term effects of the gastric-wall insult are uncertain. Perhaps the abnormalities in gastric myoelectrical activity reported by Stampley et al14 and Hall et al[23] in dogs recovering from GDV and gastropexy represent these effects. Postoperative gastrointestinal ileus is an occasional complication in clinical patients recovering from GDVs, but the potential causes of this include anesthetic drug use, analgesic drugs, anxiety, and disease-related gastrointestinal compromise, so it is not possible to identify a single cause and effect relationship.

Splenic vascular compromise (vessel avulsion, intravascular thrombosis, infarction) occurs in approximately 16% of dogs that survive and 40% of dogs that die following acute GDVs.[2] Again, perhaps the presence of splenic complications implies more "severe" disease.

Although elevations in serum alkaline phosphatase and alanine aminotransferase have been documented in dogs recovering from GDVs, there is no clinical evidence of either acute or chronic hepatic dysfunction in these dogs.

Ischemia-Reperfusion Injury, Sepsis, Sirs, and Ards

(See Chapters 1 and 2)

Experimental evidence that ischemia-reperfusion injury occurs in dogs with acute GDVs was provided by Badylak et al[12] and Lantz et al.[25] Ischemia-reperfusion mediated production of reactive oxygen species directly through lipid peroxidation and indirectly through neutrophil activation will fuel the genesis of local and systemic inflammation. Endotoxin is a potent mediator of inflammation and has been demonstrated to be released in experimental models of GDVs.[13] Hypoperfusion and direct ischemic damage to many organs could also result in activation of neutrophils, monocytes, macrophages, and platelets, all of which contribute cytokines to the inflammatory cascade. In addition, inflammation associated with bacterial infection will feed local and systemic inflammation. Together these factors can trigger systemic inflammatory response syndrome (SIRS).

Clinical evidence:
High levels of circulating endotoxin have not been demonstrated in clinical patients with GDVs, nor have indicators of lipid peroxidation been measured from tissues of clinical patients. Large studies of GDVs do not frequently cite massive bacterial infections in dogs that die following treatment.[2-4] The most commonly cited causes of death are euthanasia because of massive gastric necrosis, and continued cardiovascular instability characterized by hypotension, despite appropriate resuscitation attempts, followed by multiple organ failure, notably pulmonary.[2,3] Such findings could be interpreted as circumstantial evidence, at least, that SIRS is a consequence for animals severely affected by GDVs.

Clinical Indicators of Disease Severity

Several preoperative clinical parameters that have been studied might best be considered indicators of the severity of disease in dogs suffering acute GDV rather than being a direct cause of morbidity or mortality. Such parameters include plasma lactate,[4] abnormal haemostatic profiles,[25] and the presence of cardiac arrhythmias.[3,19] Venous plasma lactate is considered an indicator of the degree of circulatory system compromise. Of course, other clinical data (pulse rate, capillary refill time, mucous membrane colour, packed cell volume, plasma protein levels) can also aid in the clinical evaluation of circulatory status. High lactate was associated with increased chance of having gastric necrosis in one study.[4] This study did not imply cause and effect, simply statistical association between a measure of perfusion status (plasma lactate) and the presence of gastric necrosis, an event influenced by many factors. It would seem, however, that high plasma lactate pre-resuscitation and, perhaps more importantly, elevated plasma lactate that is refractory to treatment, should be considered an indicator of severe disease.

The presence of abnormal laboratory hemostatic profiles in dogs clinically affected with GDV was associated with increased chance of gastric necrosis, in another study.[25] The authors of this study implied that microthrombi that either caused or resulted from the abnormal coagulation status in these dogs accelerated the demise of the gastric wall by local vessel occlusion.[25] Although it is difficult to determine whether stasis precedes thrombus formation in gastric-wall arterioles and capillaries or vice versa in dogs with GDV, abnormalities of hemostasis and evidence of disseminated intravascular coagulation (DIC) should be considered as clear evidence of severe disease.

The presence of cardiac arrhythmias was a negative prognostic indicator in one study[3] but was not thought to influence overall outcome in another.[2] Given that the majority of experimental and clinical evidence so far points to myocardial ischemia as a key factor in the development of cardiac arrhythmias, it would seem that dogs that have the most severely compromised circulation are going to be most likely to develop arrhythmias. Again, in this scenario, the presence of cardiac arrhythmias could be considered an indicator of disease severity.

The three parameters mentioned in this section are representative of many that could be considered in a similar way. Indeed, intraoperative findings such as gastric necrosis and splenic complications could also be considered markers of disease severity, as could postoperative findings such as intractable hypotension, intractable elevation in plasma lactate, fall in the partial pressure of oxygen in arterial blood, and intractable arrhythmias. The sensitivity of each with respect to the severity of disease is unknown and, given the potential complexity of the pathophysiologic events in these patients, the author would caution against using any single numberor event as a reason for withdrawing treatment from any patient. Rather, the patient should be considered as a whole in respect of clinical decision making.

References

1. Strombeck DR: Acute gastric dilation volvulus. *In* Strombeck's Small Animal Gastroenterology. Guilford WG, Center SA, Strombeck DR, et al (eds). Philadelphia: WB Saunders, 1996.

2. Brockman DJ, Washabau RJ, Drobatz KJ: Canine gastric dilatation/volvulus syndrome in a veterinary critical care unit: 295 cases (1986-1992) J Am Vet Med Assoc 207:460–464, 1995.

3. Brourman JD, Schertel ER, Allen DA, et al: Factors associated with perioperative mortality in dogs with surgically managed gastric dilatation-volvulus: 137 cases (1988-1993) J Am Vet Med Assoc, 208, 11:1855-1858, 1996.

4. de Papp E, Drobatz KJ, Hughes D: Plasma lactate concentration as a predictor of gastric necrosis and survival among dogs with gastric dilatation-volvulus: 102 cases (1995-1998). J Am Vet Med Assoc 215(1):49-52, 1999.

5. Brunn GJ, Platt JL: The etiology of sepsis: turned inside out. Trends Mol Med 12(1):10-16, 2006.

6. Blackburn PJ, McFarlane D: Acute fatal dilation of the stomach in the dog. J Comp Path Therap 54:189-199, 1944.

7. Lantz GC, Bottoms GD, Carlton WW, et al: The effect of 360° gastric volvulus on the blood supply of the nondistended normal dog stomach. Vet Surg; 13:189-196, 1984.

8. Passi RB, Kraft AR, Vasko JS: Pathophysiologic mechanisms of shock in acute gastric dilatation. Surgery 65(2) 298-303, 1969.

9. Merkley DF, Howard DR, Eyster GE:Experimentally induced acute gastric dilatation in the dog: Cardiopulmonary effects. J Am Anim Hosp Assoc 12:143-148, 1976

10. Orton EC, Muir WW: Hemodynamics during experimental gastric dilatation-volvulus in dogs. Am J Vet Res 44(8):1512-1515, 1983.

11. Orton EC, Muir WW: Isovolumetric indices and humoral cardioactive substance bioassay during clinical and experimentally induced gastric dilatation-volvulus in dogs. Am J Vet Res 44:1516-1520, 1983.

12. Badylak SF, Lantz GC, Jeffries M: Prevention of reperfusion injury in surgically induced gastric dilatation-volvulus in dogs. Am J Vet Res 51(2):294-9, 1990.

13. Davidson JR, Lantz GC, Salisbury SK, et al: Effects of flunixin meglumine on dogs with experimental gastric dilatation-volvulus. Vet Surg21(2):113-20, 1992.

14. Stampley AR, Burrows CF, Ellison GW, Tooker J: Gastric myoelectric activity after experimental gastric dilatation-volvulus and tube gastrostomy in dogs. Vet Surg 21(1):10-4, 1992.

15. Wingfield WE, Betts CW, Rawlings CA: Pathophysiology associated with gastric dilatation-volvulus in the dog. J Am Anim Hosp Assoc 12:136-141, 1976.

16. Barnes GE, Laine GA, Giam PY, et al: Cardiovascular responses to elevation of intra-abdominal hydrostatic pressure. Am J Physiol. 248(2 Pt 2):R208-13, 1985.

17. Horn WA, Gilmore DR, Dietz AE, Freden GO: Effects of gastric distention-volvulus on coronary blood flow and myocardial oxygen consumption in the dog. Am J Vet Res 46:(1) 98-104, 1985.

18. Wagner AE, Dunlop CI, Chapman PL: Cardiopulmonary measurements in dogs undergoing gastropexy without gastrectomy for correction of gastric dilatation-volvulus. J Am Vet Med Assoc 215(4):484-488, 1999.

19. Muir WW, Lipowitz AJ: Cardiac dysrhythmias associated with gastric dilation/volvulus in the dog. J Am Vet Med Assoc 172:683-689, 1978.

20. Schober KE, Cornand C, Kirbach B, et al: Serum cardiac troponin I and cardiac troponin T concentrations in dogs with gastric dilatation-volvulus. J Am Vet Med Assoc 221(3):381-8, 2002.

21. Peycke LE, Hosgood G, Davidson JR, et al: The effect of experimental gastric dilatation-volvulus on adenosine triphosphate content and conductance of the canine gastric and jejunal mucosa. Can J Vet Res 69(3):170-9, 2005.

22. Matthiesen DT: Partial gastrectomy as treatment of gastric volvulus: Results in 30 dogs. Vet Surg 14, 3:185-193, 1985.

23. Hall JA, Solie TN, Seim HB 3rd, Twedt DC: Gastric myoelectric and motor activity in dogs with gastric dilatation-volvulus. Am J Physiol 265(4 Pt 1):G646-53, 1993.

24. Lantz GC, Badylak SF, Hiles MC, Arkin TE: Treatment of reperfusion injury in dogs with experimentally induced gastric dilatation-volvulus. Am J Vet Res 53(9):1594-1598, 1992.

25. Millis DL, Hauptman JG, Fulton RB: Abnormal hemostatic profiles and gastric necrosis in canine gastric dilatation-volvulus. Vet Surg 22(2):93-97, 1993.

Chapter 29

The Gastric Mucosal Barrier: Why the Stomach does not Digest Itself

Colin F. Burrows

Ever since René Antoine Ferchault de Réamur, the 18th century man of many sciences, showed that juice secreted by the stomach could digest meat, philosophers, physiologists, and physicians alike have been puzzled by the question: why does the stomach not digest itself? One answer, of course, is that it sometimes does. Under certain circumstances, gastric juice can produce ulcers and even destroy most of the stomach lining. Normally, however, the stomach wall staunchly resists attack; as Claude Bernard observed, it behaves as if it were made of porcelain.[1,2]

Gastric juice contains hydrochloric acid, one of the most corrosive acids known. At the concentration secreted by the parietal cells in the gastric mucosa, gastric acid is capable of dissolving zinc and is deadly to cells. Yet in the stomach, hydrochloric acid ordinarily acts only to perform the useful functions of killing ingested bacteria, softening fibrous foods, and promoting pepsin production.[2] The corrosive juice is prevented from attacking the stomach wall by a complex physicochemical barrier termed the *gastric mucosal barrier* (GMB). The GMB was first defined by Davenport as "that property of the gastric mucosa which impedes diffusion of acid from the lumen into the mucosa and impedes diffusion of sodium ions from the mucosal space into the lumen."[3,4] The barrier cannot be defined on a strictly anatomic basis, but is rather a collection of interdependent physical and chemical processes that act in concert to protect the gastric mucosa against secreted acid and pepsin.[5,6] It is now generally agreed that the barrier has eight basic components: (1) epithelial cell tight junctions, (2) the ability of the gastric epithelial cells to change shape – a process called restitution, (3) mucosal bicarbonate (HCO_3^-) secretion, (4) the hydrophobic apical membrane of the gastric epithelial cells, (5) gastric mucosal blood flow and local acid-base balance, (6) gastric mucus production and secretion, (7) the protective and regulatory effect of mucosal prostaglandins, and (8) the basal lamina.[7-9]

In the normal stomach the gastric mucosa is under a continuous state of physical and chemical siege. It is exposed daily, not only to the potential ravages of acid and pepsin, but also to a wide variety of potentially damaging agents that include certain foods, a range of temperatures, hyperosmolar and abrasive substances, chemical damage from refluxed bile and pancreatic juice, as well as to bacterial toxins and a variety of potentially damaging drugs.[10] Some damage is inevitable under these circumstances, yet the gastric mucosa normally retains its integrity even under these attacks. The balance between normal gastric mucosal physiologic damage and repair is a dynamic process involving a variety of complex mechanisms. Clinically, however, when this process breaks down, acute gastric mucosal injury results, often with the accompanying signs of acute gastric disease. If the process is severe or ongoing, progression to chronic gastric disease is the almost inevitable sequel.

Although the mechanisms of disruption of the gastric mucosal barrier can vary widely, the end result is the same, namely erosion of the gastric mucosa, which allows acid to diffuse back into the submucosa and to initiate an inflammatory response. Mucosal epithelial erosion, hemorrhage, gastritis, and overt ulceration may develop if the process remains unchecked. Barrier disruption occurs to some extent in virtually every type of gastric disease as well as under a variety of sometimes less well appreciated circumstances such as neurologic disease, stress, hypotension, sepsis, and protein-calorie malnutrition. An appreciation of the mechanisms of acid secretion as well as barrier disruption and repair, therefore, are important for most clinicians, as is an understanding of approaches that enhance the repair process.

Gastric Acid Secretion

The mammalian stomach is a specialized organ of the digestive tract that serves to store and process food for subsequent intestinal absorption. One of its features, considered to be the hallmark of gastric function, is its ability to secrete acid. In most species this is a continuous process that varies in intensity in response to a variety of exogenous and endogenous stimuli. In the dog, however, and possibly in the cat, animals that ancestrally, at least, can go for days without eating, acid secretion is more variable, with the distinct possibility that little or no basal acid secretion occurs in these species.[11]

The gastric mucosa consists of a variety of cell types, predominantly mucus-filled tall columnar epithelial cells, which form a single protective layer. The secretory unit of the gastric mucosa is the gastric (or oxyntic) gland, of which the normal human stomach has been estimated to contain approximately one billion. These contain parietal (acid-producing and secreting) cells, chief (pepsinogen-producing and secreting) cells, mucous neck cells, and a variety of endocrine cells. Mucous neck cells are relatively few in number and are scattered among the parietal cells. Parietal cells are located mainly in the isthmus and neck region of the gland, whereas chief cells are located at its base (Figure 29-1).[12] Adjacent to the parietal cells are histamine-secreting enterochromaffin-like (ECL) cells and somatostatin-secreting "D cells." The surface epithelial cells have a life span of about three days and are replaced by division of cells just below the opening of the gastric glands. Immediately below the surface epithelial cell layer is a rich network of blood vessels, nerves, and lymphatics supported by a connective tissue matrix, which collectively form the submucosa.

The stomach secretes hydrogen ions, sodium, chloride, pepsinogen, lipase, and varying quantities of mucus into its lumen. Hydrogen ions are secreted into the lumen of the gastric gland in exchange for potassium by an energy-dependent exchange enzyme in the mucosal surface of the parietal cell called the hydrogen potassium-adenosine triphosphatase (H^+K^+ -ATPase) pump (Figure 29-2).[13] During acid secretion, the H^+K^+ -ATPase secretes H^+ ions into the lumen of the gland in exchange for K^+

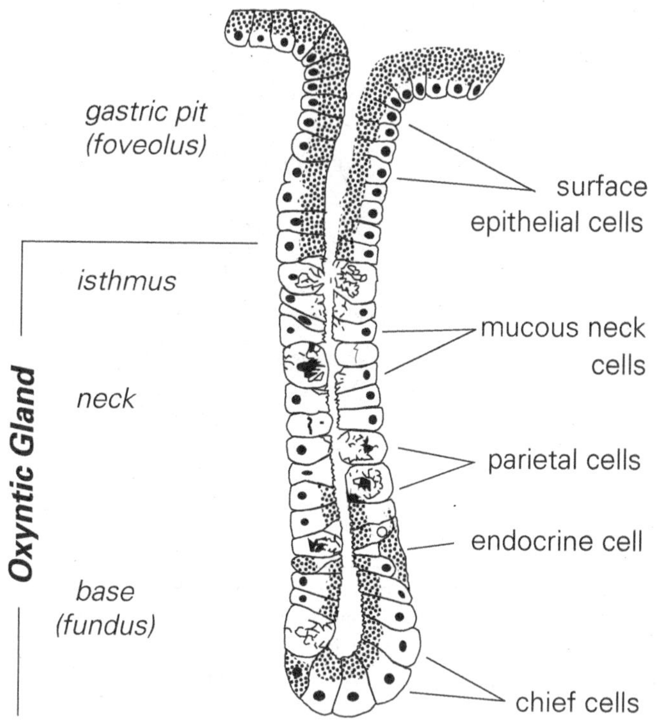

Figure 29-1. Diagram of tubular gastric (oxyntic) gland in the body of the mammalian stomach. (From I to S: Functional gastric morphology. *In* Physiology of the Gastrointestinal Tract, 2nd ed. Johnson LR (ed). Philadelphia: Lippincott Williams & Wilkins, 1987, with permission.)

ions, which have previously moved out of the cell down their concentration gradient. Simultaneously, chloride ions move from the cell into the lumen down an electrochemical gradient. Water moves out of the cell in response to the subsequent osmotic gradient, to form hydrochloric acid. This acid then flows from the glands through pores in the overlying mucus, which acts to prevent back-diffusion of acid from the lumen.[14]

Acid secretion can be stimulated by the binding of acetylcholine or histamine to specific receptors in the serosal membrane of the parietal cell. Gastrin, another important stimulus of acid secretion, is believed to bind to receptors on the ECL cells and to stimulate them to release histamine (Figure 29-3). It can, however, also stimulate the parietal cell directly via CCK-B(2) receptor. When gastrin, acetylcholine, or histamine bind with the cell, a variety of second messengers are stimulated that increase intracellular cyclic AMP (gastrin and histamine) or calcium (acetylcholine) concentration. These in turn stimulate acid secretion.

Gastric acid secretion is divided into four phases: basal, cephalic, gastric, and intestinal. The basal state, as has been mentioned, may be minimal in carnivores although it can be augmented by sepsis[15] and possibly by a variety of other stressful events. The cephalic phase of gastric secretion is activated by the thought (in man), sight, and smell of food via vagal impulses conducted from the brain to muscarinic receptors in the gastric mucosa. During the gastric phase of secretion, which accounts for 40 to 50% of the response to a meal, acid secretion is stimulated by both chemical and physical factors that include gastric distention and ingested protein. Amino acids in the duodenum are mainly responsible for initiation of the intestinal phase, primarily through stimulation of gastrin release.

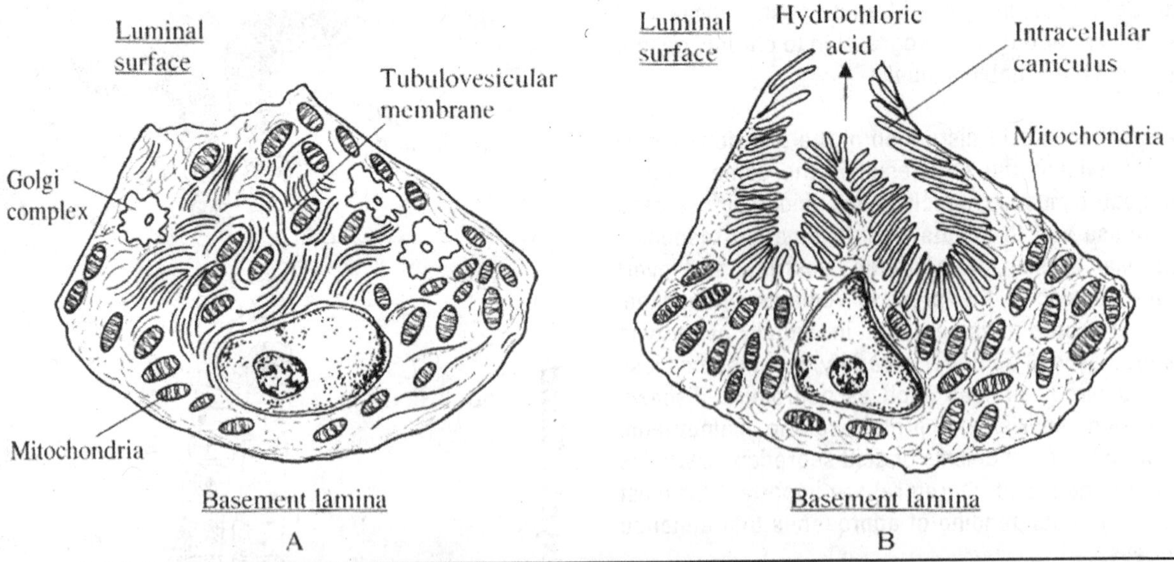

Figure 29-2. A. Non-secreting parietal cell. The cytoplasm is replete with tubulovesicular membranes, which contain H⁺K⁺-ATPase. B. Acid-secreting parietal cell. The tubulovesicular membrane has fused with the apical plasma membrane to form a secretory canalicular membrane with numerous microvilli. H⁺K⁺-ATPase is inserted into the membrane so that the cell can secrete acid. (From the BSAVA Manual of Canine and Feline Gastroenterology. Thomas DA, Simpson JW, Hall EJ (eds)., 1996, with permission.)

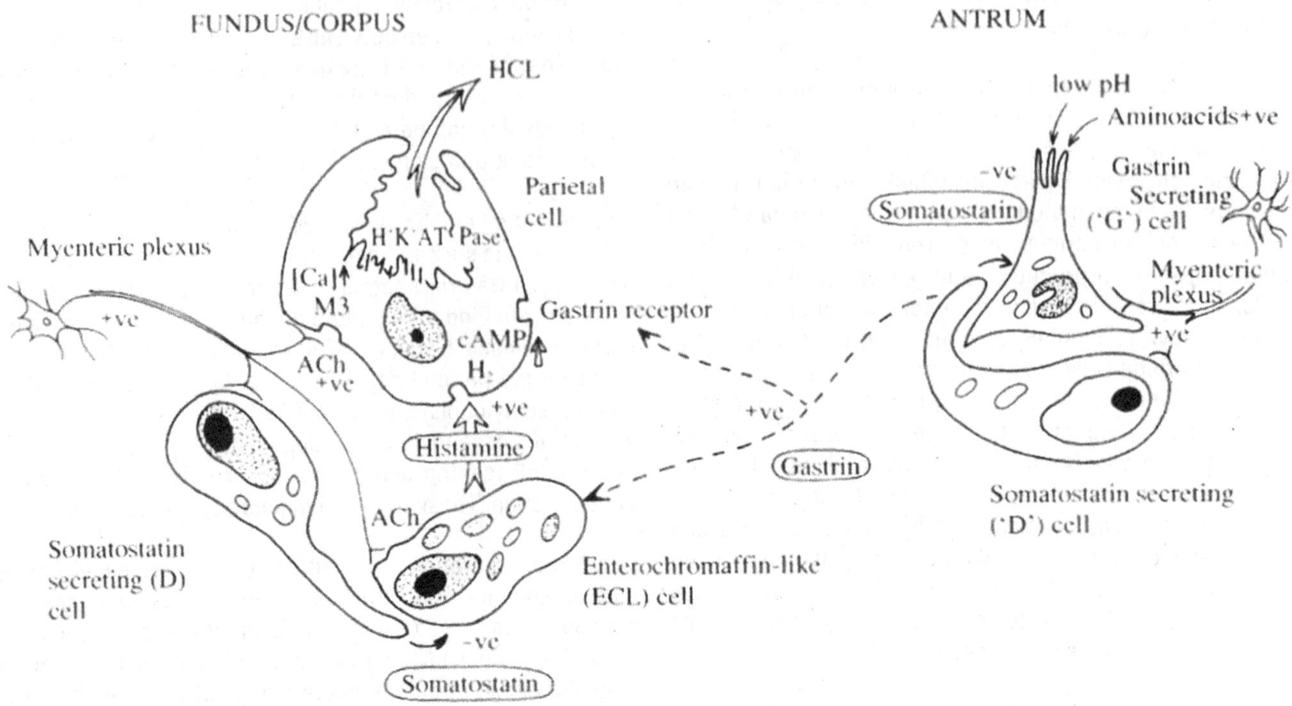

Figure 29-3. Current concept of the role of the enterochromaffin-like (ECL) cell, gastrin- (G) and somatostatin-secreting (D) cells in the peripheral regulation of acid secretion by parietal cells. Nervous stimulation from the CNS causes release of acetylcholine from the myenteric plexus. This binds with a muscarinic M3 receptor on the parietal cell, which results in an increase in intracellular calcium concentration. Calcium in turn stimulates insertion of H⁺K⁺-ATPase into the canaliculi membrane. Release of histamine is brought about by either gastrin or acetylcholine binding to receptors on the ECL cell. Histamine binds with H2 receptors on the parietal cell, which increases intracellular cAMP. This activates H⁺K⁺-ATPase in the membrane. Gastrin also probably reacts directly with the parietal cell in the dog. Somatostatin released from D cells in the gastric mucosa inhibits both histamine and gastrin release. (From the BSAVA Manual of Canine and Feline Gastroenterology. Thomas DA, Simpson JW, Hall EJ (eds)., 1996, with permission .)

After a meal, acid secretion is modulated by a negative feedback mechanism in which antral acidification inhibits further release of gastrin, possibly via the inhibitory effect of somatostatin.[12] The relative importance of and exact relationship between histamine, gastrin, and acetylcholine receptors in the stimulation of acid secretion is unclear. The two main activating receptors on the parietal cell are a histamine (H_2) receptor and a muscarinic (M_3) receptor. It is believed that the activity of the M_3 receptor is regulated by acetylcholine released from nerve fibers, whereas activity of the H_2 receptor depends on histamine released locally from the ECL cell. Release of histamine from the ECL cell results from the binding of either gastrin or acetylcholine to receptors in the ECL cell wall.[16]

Acetylcholine and histamine are also the major stimuli for pepsinogen secretion by chief cells, although secretin also stimulates its release. Pepsinogen is always secreted in parallel with acid and is converted to pepsin, its active form, by acid at a pH of about 1.5 as well as by previously converted pepsin. Stimulation of mucus secretion from the mucus neck cells also appears to be under the control of acetylcholine. This mucus is more viscid than mucus released by rupture of the surface epithelial cells. An acid-stable lipase is released from the chief cells and mucous-producing cells that is responsible for the digestion of up to 30% of dietary fat.[17,18]

Hydrogen ion secretion is accompanied by the passive secretion of chloride from the parietal cell and by the production of an equivalent amount of HCO_3^-. This is secreted from the base of the cell into the interstitium from where it is picked up by mucosal capillary vessels and carried to the systemic circulation.

Gastric secretion is inhibited by a low intraluminal pH, which inhibits gastrin secretion.[16] Secretion is also inhibited by hydrochloric acid, fatty acids, and hyperosmolar solutions contacting receptors in the duodenal mucosa. These negative feedback mechanisms ensure that acid secretion is proportional to need. Somatostatin secreted from D cells, adjacent to the parietal cells, is one of the principal inhibitors of acid secretion. D cells are also found in the gastric mucosa adjacent to the ECL cells where secreted somatostatin inhibits gastrin release (Figure 29-3). Prostaglandins, which are secreted by a variety of mucosal cells, also exert a tonic inhibitory effect on acid secretion by decreasing cyclic AMP production in the parietal cell.[16]

Components of the Barrier

Gastric Epithelial Cell Tight Junction

The stomach is lined by a layer of columnar epithelial cells, which form very tight junctions with each other and constitute the main anatomic portion of the gastric mucosal barrier.[19] These cells, however, are not completely impervious to luminal H^+ nor to diffusion of tissue Na^+. Small quantities of Na^+ and H^+ normally diffuse in both directions across the mucosa, with any H^+ that diffuses into the mucosa being neutralized by tissue buffers. Gastric mucosal cells are formed by division from mucus neck cells and have a life span of about 3 days, after which time they are sloughed into the lumen and replaced by lateral migration of younger cells from the neck of the oxyntic gland.[8] Mucus neck cells are located in the neck and isthmus region of gastric glands (Figure 29-1). Cells in the mucosal proliferative zone in the isthmus are responsible for the constant replacement of gastric epithelium in both health and disease.[20]

Restitution

Studies of the mechanisms of gastric repair after mucosal damage by such substances as alcohol, salicylates, and bile salts revealed that, in areas of relatively superficial cell disruption not extending deep into the mucosa, much of the damage is repaired within minutes. This is accomplished by a process called restitution, which occurs by migration of still viable epithelial cells from areas adjacent to or just beneath the injured surface cells.[13] After the necrotic surface cells exfoliate, the viable mucus cells in the upper gastric pits immediately flatten, extend finger-like projections called lamellipodia, and migrate across the exposed basal lamina to restore an intact cell layer over shallow defects (Figure 29-4). However, deeper lesions or ulcers require new cells to fill in the defect. The process of restitution occurs within minutes of injury and before the appearance of an extensive inflammatory response or cell proliferation.[9,19] The response is evoked, at lease in part, in response to hyperemia invoked by a capsaicin-sensitive emergency neural response system.[21] If gastric acid remains in contact with the mucosa, damage is ongoing, the basal lamina is destroyed along with the mucosa, and the substratum necessary for restitution is removed. This can result in persistent macroscopic lesions that may bleed, invoke a classic inflammatory response, and become clinically significant.

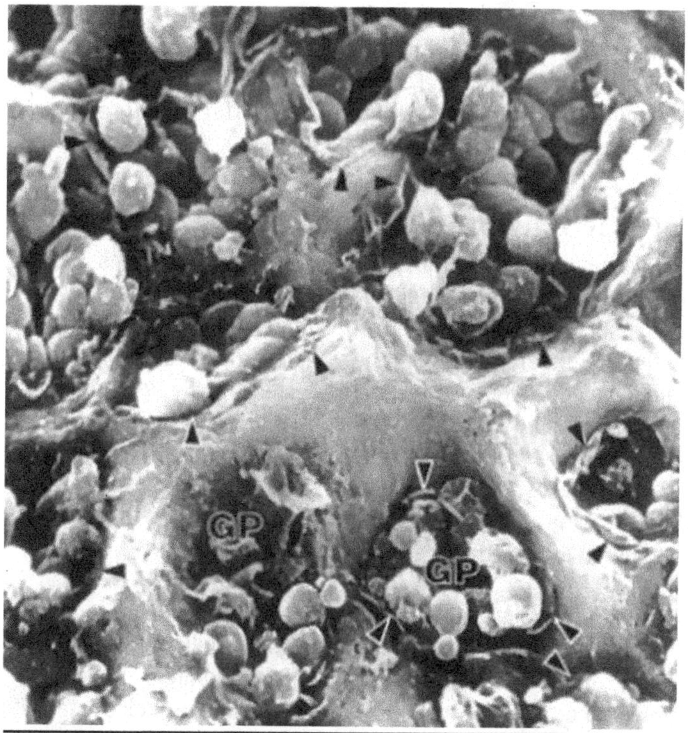

Figure 29-4. Low-power scanning electron micrograph of ethanol-disrupted rat gastric epithelium with much of the interpit basal lamina exposed. Many mucus cells from the gastric pits (GP) have lamellipodia (arrows) extending onto the basal lamina (x 1500). (From Lacy ER, Ito S: Rapid epithelial restitution of the rat gastric mucosa after ethanol injury. Lab Invest 51:573-583, 1984 with permission from Lippincott Williams & Wilkins.)

The shed surface cells are believed to play an important role in protecting the mucosa from further injury and to facilitate the process of re-epithelialization.[22] When traumatized, the apical plasma membrane of the shed cells ruptures, spilling mucoid contents and contributing to a gelatinous mass that contains mucus, cellular debris, necrotic tissue, and trapped alkaline exudate from damaged capillaries. It is believed that this layer may provide a protective microenvironment for reconstitution.[23] Each of these responses to superficial injury, namely formation of a protective mucoid layer, flow of alkaline mucosal fluid that may act to dilute luminal noxious agents, and rapid restitution of superficial epithelial cells appears to help prevent the formation of deeper hemorrhagic lesions and subsequent pathology.[23] Indeed, factors that facilitate or impair these early mucosal defense mechanisms are now believed to be of far greater importance in the development and repair of gastric damage than is the integrity of the classic gastric mucosal barrier itself.[23]

Bicarbonate Secretion

Under normal circumstances HCO_3^-, produced as a by-product of H^+ secretion, is present in abundance in the gastric mucosa. Some of this HCO_3^- is taken up by mucosal cells by means of a prostaglandin-dependent pump mechanism in exchange for chloride. The HCO_3^- is transported across the cell and secreted with mucus into the lumen. At one time it was believed that secreted HCO_3^- was trapped in the surface mucus where it neutralized H^+ back-diffusing from the lumen.[24-26] Until recently, epithelial HCO_3^- secretion was accepted as the most important defense mechanism against acid.[26] This theory has been called into question by more recent work that shows the surface pH is kept constant at a pH of about 4 by dual secretion of HCO_3^- and acid as needed into a surface unstirred layer.[27] In the mouse at least, pH control at the protective surface pH gradient is regulated by cyclooxygenase-1 (COX-1).[28]

Gastric Epithelial Cell Membrane

The luminal surface of gastric epithelial cells contains a layer of surface-active phospholipids that confers a degree of hydrophobicity to the cell surface.[29] Phosphatidyl-cholines are present in high concentrations in the luminal membrane of gastric mucosal cells and are oriented so that the hydrophobic end of the molecule is at the exterior surface. These hydrophobic molecules are believed to render the cell resistant to any acid that permeates the mucus layer. When the lipid layer is damaged however, the route is opened for acid to permeate into the cell and begin destruction.

A number of lipid-soluble nonionized substances can easily disrupt the membrane and penetrate the epithelial cells to initiate gastric mucosal damage. Bile salts, for example, have been shown to disrupt the mucosal barrier and initiate cell damage,[30] whereas lipid-soluble bile acids are taken up directly into the cell to cause mucosal injury from within the cell.[31] Reflux of bile into the stomach is a normal physiologic event in most species; however, it is usually quickly cleared so that no lasting damage is done to the gastric mucosa.[32] If normal clearance mechanisms fail, prolonged contact ensures membrane damage and development of gastritis.[33] Part of the damage caused by refluxed intestinal content is also caused by lysolecithin, a potent membrane-toxic phospholipid formed by the action of pancreatic phospholipase on biliary lecithin in the duodenal lumen.[34] Prolonged reflux of upper intestinal content causes extensive mucosal damage and chronic gastritis.[35] In endotoxemia, exposure of the stomach to bile causes macroscopic injury to the gastric mucosa.[36,37]

Aspirin has long been recognized as a substance that disrupts the mucosal barrier and causes extensive mucosal damage.[38] In humans, for example, ingestion of a single aspirin tablet results in the loss of between 0.5 and 2.0 ml of blood.[39] In some susceptible individuals much larger blood volumes may be lost and severe mucosal lesions may develop. The same situation can occur in the dog.[40] The mechanisms of aspirin damage are complex, but the most important is through a pH-dependent effect on mucosal hydrophobicity. At a pH of less than 3.5 to 4.0, acid is in its lipid-soluble form and disrupts the cell membrane. At a higher pH, aspirin is lipid-insoluble and little or no direct damage is done.[41] Another important effect is the inhibitory effect of aspirin and other NSAIDs on cyclooxygenase (see further on).

Gastric Mucosal Blood Flow and Local Acid-Base Balance

An adequate mucosal blood flow is critical for barrier integrity. If mucosal blood flow is decreased, gastric mucosal erosions and hemorrhage almost inevitably develop.[42] It was once thought that mucosal damage developed because of tissue hypoxia, but microanatomic and physiologic studies have shown that delivery of HCO_3^- to the mucosa and the prevention of local acidosis are much more important.

Anatomic studies have shown that the gastric arteries supply an arterial network in the submucosa from which arterioles penetrate the muscularis mucosae to supply the mucosal capillaries with blood (Figure 29-5). These capillaries run both in between and parallel to the oxyntic glands and are interconnected by short capillaries parallel with the mucosal surface. These capillaries form short loops around the mouth of the gastric gland before joining the collecting veins, which penetrate the muscularis mucosae vertically to form an extensive network of veins at the submucosal level.[7] Bicarbonate, produced as a by-product of H^+ synthesis in the parietal cells, escapes to be picked up by the vertically flowing capillaries, which are especially fenestrated at the mucosal surface to facilitate HCO_3^- flux. A small proportion of HCO_3^- escapes while the rest is carried to the systemic circulation (Figure 29-6).[43,44]

The epithelial cell membrane is not totally impervious to H^+ ions, which diffuse through the intact gastric mucosa in relatively small amounts. Mucosal HCO_3^-, however, normally neutralizes this acid to maintain a normal tissue acid-base balance. If the barrier is damaged, H^+ diffusion increases and HCO_3^- buffers are reduced.[9] When tissue buffers are exhausted, the tissues become acidotic and submucosal damage develops.

In that it carries HCO_3^- to the mucosa to maintain normal tissue acid-base balance, gastric mucosal blood flow is critical to the prevention of gastric lesions. Systemic acid-base balance is

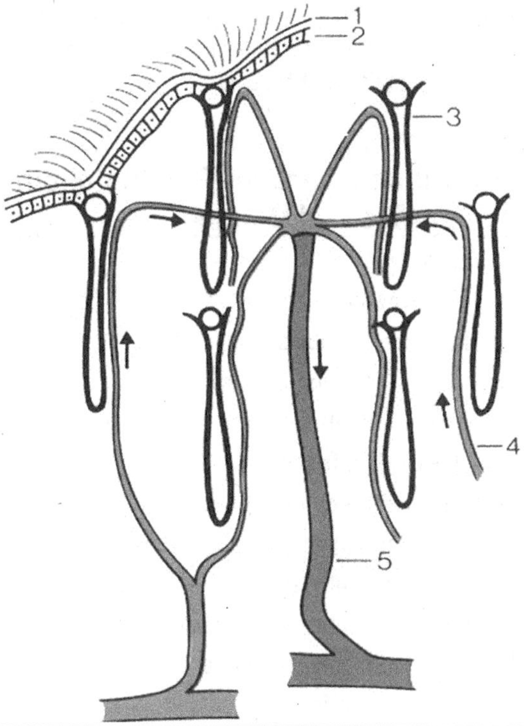

Figure 29-5. Three-dimensional view in the blood supply to the gastric mucosa. (From Miederer SE: The gastric mucosal barrier Hepatogastroenterology 33:88-91, 1986, with permission of IASG.)

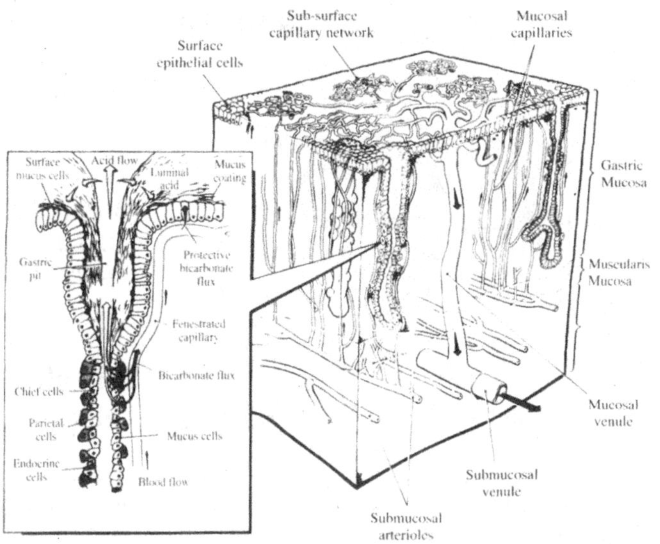

Figure 29-6. Schematic diagram of the vascular organization in oxyntic mucosa (right) and the proposed mechanism for vascular transport of bicarbonate toward the surface mucus cells from deeper within the mucosa (inset left). (From Gannon B, et al: Mucosal microvascular architecture of the fundus and body of the human stomach. Gastroenterology 86:866-875, 1984, with permis-sion of WB Saunders).

also important in that with acidosis less HCO_3^- is available for mucosal protection. This is one of the reasons advanced for the development of gastric lesions in critically ill or hypotensive individuals. It has been shown, for example, that intravenous sodium HCO_3^- not only prevents the decreases in gastric intramural pH induced by hemorrhagic shock but also prevents mucosal ulceration.[45] Plasma HCO_3^- concentration also plays a key role in mucosal resistance to ulceration in experimentally induced canine gastric dilatation.[46] It has also been observed that the absolute amount of H^+ that diffuses into the tissue from the luminal solution is less important in causing ulceration than the ability of the tissue to dispose of influxing H^+ by neutralization with mucosal HCO_3^-.[47]

Gastric mucosal blood flow is regulated by constriction and dilation of submucosal arterioles. Smooth muscle in these arterioles constricts to inhibit mucosal blood flow under a variety of conditions, including hypotension, stress, and sepsis as well as in response to a variety of vasoconstricting drugs.[48,49] Prostaglandins, beta-adrenergic agents, and gastrin all increase mucosal blood flow and, thereby, reduce gastric mucosal damage. This is one of the mechanisms by which prostaglandins are thought to exert cytoprotection (see further on).[50]

Gastric Mucus and Mucus Secretion

The gastric mucosa is covered by a variable layer of mucus between 5 and 200 μm thick that is believed to play a multifactorial role in mucosal defense. Composed of various mucopolysaccharides, glycoproteins, and water, mucus is secreted by the mucus neck cells in the parietal glands and by the gastric epithelial cells themselves. Mucus occurs in two physical forms: water soluble and water insoluble. The water insoluble form is produced by the mucus neck cells and consists of a thin layer of stable gel that firmly adheres to the gastric mucosal surface. Adherent mucus is impermeable to large proteins and thus protects the mucosa against peptic proteolysis. Water-soluble mucus comes from the surface epithelial cells, is less viscous, and acts as a lubricant to prevent mechanical damage to the mucosa. The adherent insoluble mucus provides a stable unstirred layer that traps secreted HCO_3^- to cause an alkaline interface between the surface and the lumen. Microelectrode studies showed a pH gradient within the mucus gel that varied somewhat among species and experimental conditions. The gradient peaks around 6.6 to 7.0 near the apical membrane.[9] More recent work has shown that this gradient may be only a part-time defender of the gastric epithelium, however, present only when the luminal pH is 3 or below.[51,52] The ability of mucus to form a pH gradient by trapping HCO_3^- at the epithelial cell surface (Figure 29-7) provides a mechanism that is believed to reduce acid diffusion into the mucosa by neutralization with concomitant production of carbon dioxide and water.[53]

The neural emergency response system enhances mucus production after gastric injury. Mucus flows copiously out of the gastric glands and spreads over the mucosal surface to form a protective cap over the damaged area and restituting cells beneath.[21] Much of the mucus cap, however, comes from mucus in the disintegrating damaged epithelial cells themselves. Viscous mucus produced by the mucus neck cells in the upper regions of the gastric glands forms strands of thicker mucus that hold the cap in place. This facilitation of repair, by holding a HCO_3^- -rich cap over damaged areas while epithelial integrity is reestablished, is believed to be one of the most important functions of gastric mucus.[54]

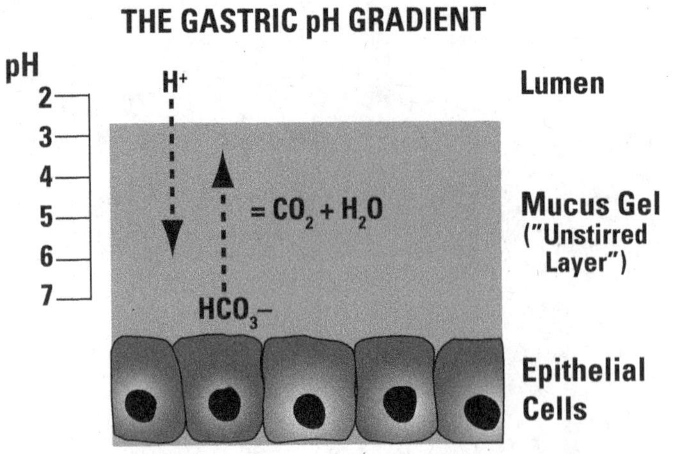

Figure 29-7. (still need full title and permission) Gastric mucus pH gradient. (From Turnberg LA: Gastric mucus, bicarbonate and pH gradients in mucosal protection. Clin Invest Med 10:178-180, 1987.

Various agents such as E-type prostaglandins, calcium, and glucagon stimulate both gastric mucus and HCO_3^- secretion, whereas compounds such as NSAIDs and bile salts decrease them.

Prostaglandins and Cytoprotection

Prostaglandins are found in high concentrations in the gastric mucosa and gastric juice and have been shown to protect the gastric and duodenal mucosa against injury, a function that has been termed cytoprotection.[54] Prostaglandins are found in a variety of cells in the gastric mucosa including mast cells, macrophages, and endothelial cells and are synthesized locally from arachidonic acid via the action of cyclooxygenase. Since Vane in 1971 showed that acetylsalicylic acid inhibits the cyclooxygenase system and thus the synthesis of prostaglandins, and hypothesized that this explained not only the therapeutic effects of acetylsalicylic acid but also its gastric side effects, there has been a tremendous amount of interest in the effect of prostaglandins on the stomach.[55] Prostaglandins promote mucosal defense through a variety of actions (Table 29-1), most important of which are the inhibition of acid output, augmentation of HCO_3^- and mucus secretion, and regulation of mucosal blood flow.[56,57] The wide range of effects of prostaglandins listed in Table 29-1 demonstrates their overall importance in gastric mucosal protection. Their synthesis can also be stimulated by a variety of mild irritants, with subsequent protection against more severe damage.[56] A deficiency of prostaglandins can result in a mucosa that looks and functions normally but that is more susceptible to injury.[56]

Given the wide range of beneficial effects of prostaglandins, it is no wonder that exogenous stimulation by the synthetic prostaglandin misoprostol offers some protection against NSAID-induced mucosal damage. Various other compounds have also been shown to exert a protective effect, at least in part, through stimulation of endogenous prostaglandin synthesis. These include sucralfate, arachidonic and linoleic acids, cimetidine, bismuth, and possibly, aluminum-containing antacids.[8,56] The hormone gastrin and salivary epidermal growth factor also have cytoprotective effects through a trophic effect on the gastric mucosa.[58] Even milk, the oldest ulcer remedy, has been shown to contain large quantities of PGE_2 and to protect against stress ulcers in rats.[59]

Table 29-1. Mechanisms for Prostaglandin Promotion of Mucosal Defense

Decreased acid secretion
Stimulation of bicarbonate secretion
Stimulation of mucus synthesis and release
Local control of gastric mucosal blood flow
Prevention of microvascular stasis
Prevention of H+ back diffusion
Promotion of cell restitution and renewal
Stimulation of surface active phospholipids
Stimulation of protein synthesis
Maintenance of cell membrane integrity
Stimulation of cell transport mechanisms
Inhibition of pepsin secretion
Maintenance of vascular endothelial permeability to bicarbonate

Basal Membrane

Destruction of the surface epithelial cells leaves the basement membrane exposed. This is permeable to alkaline proteinaceous tissue fluid, which exudes as part of the repair process. The basal membrane is the final barrier, however, and is essential as a surface for the spread of epithelial lamellipodia and associated reconstitution. Its destruction, which is heralded by the appearance of red blood cells on the mucosal surface, leaves the path open for erosion and ulcer formation and invokes the inflammatory process.[7]

The Response to Injury and Gastric Disease

One of the basic tenets of gastric pathophysiology has long been that a break in the gastric mucosal barrier results in increased gastric mucosal permeability to hydrogen ions and loss of sodium ions into the lumen. Back-diffusion of acid into the mucosa has a variety of consequences, including the stimulation of parietal and chief cells to secrete more acid and pepsinogen.[23] This acid diffuses across the broken barrier, repeating the cycle and exhausting intracellular and tissue buffers. Nerve endings are stimulated, invoking the neural emergency response system, which induces local smooth muscle contraction, and in humans at least, is associated with pain.[21] The decrease in mucosal pH also stimulates mucosal mast cells to release histamine and initiate an inflammatory response. This histamine stimulates the parietal cells to secrete even more acid and dilates precapillary sphincters, which increase mucosal blood flow through a prostaglandin-mediated response. Histamine is also believed to increase capillary permeability and to allow plasma protein and fluid to escape into the interstitium to cause local edema.

Rapid diffusion of acid into the mucosa can break down capillary walls and trigger hemorrhage (Figure 29-8). Events so far can be considered a virtually normal physiologic event because tiny superficial hemorrhages are sometimes seen during digestion of a meal. These, however, are transient and are quickly repaired. The same processes also occur in disease, but if the insult is non-physiologic, if it is widespread or ongoing, then the normal repair processes are inadequate, and gastritis, possibly with gastric hemorrhage and the signs of gastric disease, develops.

The gastric mucosal barrier is disrupted in virtually all types of gastric disease (Table 29-2) as well as in a variety of other and perhaps less well appreciated situations (Table 29-3). Of concern in the development of overt gastric disease in this latter group are factors that may delay or impair either epithelial cell restitution or the repair process. Corticosteroids have been shown to delay epithelial cell renewal and, in high doses, to cause mucosal damage.[60-62]

Gastric mucosal injury is well documented in a variety of clinical situations in humans. It occurs for example, during severe stress, hypotension, sepsis, and uremia, as well as with severe burns, intracranial lesions, and bile reflux. It also occurs after ingestion of certain agents such as alcohol, aspirin, or other NSAIDs.[8,48] Superficial erosions or ulcerations that develop in individuals who are victims of shock, trauma, burns, or sepsis, and especially, peritonitis are called stress ulcers (Table 29-4).[10] These are located primarily in the fundic mucosa and are superimposed on a background of erosive gastritis. It has been estimated that approximately 5% of patients who are the victims of shock, trauma, burns, and sepsis have major gastrointestinal hemorrhage during the course of their illness. Risk factors for gastric hemorrhage include hypotension, continued sepsis, jaundice, renal disease, and hypoxia.[63-65] Specific mechanisms for barrier disruption and inhibition of the normal restitution and repair processes in these patients are unclear, but it is believed that mucosal ischemia with subsequent local acidosis is most important.[10]

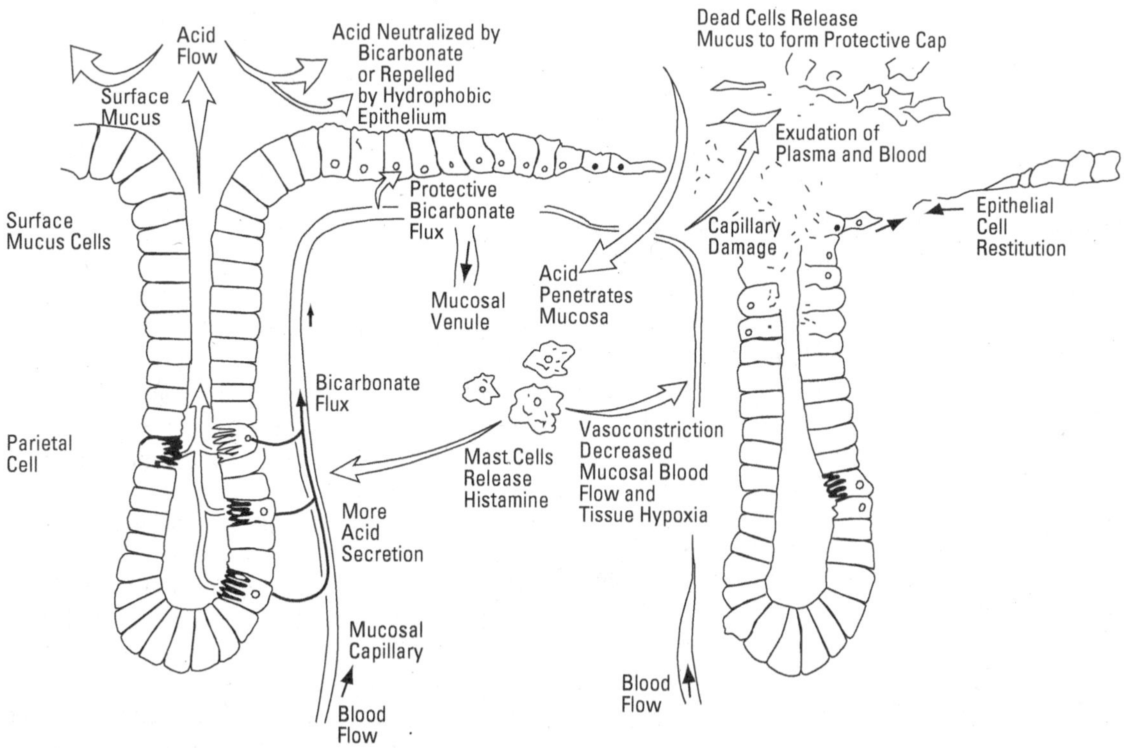

Figure 29-8. The normal gastric mucosal barrier (left) and the broken gastric mucosal barrier (right). The normal stomach is prevented from autodigestion by a variety of physical and chemi-cal defense mechanisms. Acid production in the parietal cells results in concomitant production of bicarbonate. The acid diffuses out of the cell into the mucosa where it is picked up by the uniquely arranged capillaries that flow beside each gastric gland and carry the acid to the surface. The acid then diffuses out of the vessels into the mucosa and the surface epithelial cells. It diffuses from the epithelial cells into the lumen where it is trapped in surface mucus secreted by mucus neck cells. Acid that diffuses back into the mucosa is thus neutralized by the bicarbonate. The biocarbonate maintains the surface of the cells at a pH of about 7 in contrast to the pH in the lumen, which can be as low as 2.5. The epithelial cells also contain a high proportion of hydro-phobic phospholipids in the apical surfaces that also acts to repel acid. The cells have tight junctions that prevent intracellular acid flow. The mucosal blood flow also maintains good tissue oxygenation and local acid-base balance. Mucosal blood flow is under the influence of prosta-glandins, particularly PGE2, which is produced by a variety of mucosal cell types. When the mucosa is damaged, mucosal cells rupture and release mucus that forms a protective cap. This cap protects undamaged cells at the periphery of the lesion that change shape and cover the lesion by growing over the basement membrane, a process called restitution. Acid in the mucosa over-whelms local buffering capacities and causes cell death and the release of histamine from mucosal mast cells. Histamine augments acid secretion from parietal cells and causes constriction of smooth muscles in blood vessel walls that diminishes mucosal blood flow and exacerbates tissue damage. Mucosal blood flow can also be disturbed by stress-induced submucosal vasoconstric-tion. This process also removes tissue buffer capacity and disrupts the barrier. (From Burrows CF: Vomiting and regurgitation in the dog. Viewpoints in Veterinary Medicine, 1990, with permis-sion of ALPO Pet Center, ALPO Petfoods Inc., Pennsylvania.)

Table 29-2. Diseases Associated with a Broken Gastric Mucosal Barrier

Acute gastritis
Chronic gastritis
Plasmacytic lymphocytic (idiopathic)
Hypertrophic
Eosinophilic
Atrophic
Reflux
Peptic ulceration
Gastric stasis
Gastric parasites
Gastric dilatation volvulus

Table 29-4. Risk Factors for Stress Ulceration

Shock
Sepsis, especially peritonitis
Respiratory failure
Renal failure
Hepatic failure

Table 29-3. Risk Factors for Barrier Disruption

Hypoadrenocorticism
Liver disease
Uremia
Sepsis (endotoxemia)
Shock (hypovolemic, sepsis, traumatic)
Reflux of intestinal contents
Acidosis
Hypoxia
Nonsteroidal anti-inflammatory drug therapy
Severe burns
Chronic or severe vomiting
Spinal trauma and surgery

Gastric mucosal injury and ulceration under such circumstances are less well documented in veterinary medicine, although clinical impression and anecdotal reports suggest that they may be much more widespread than is generally realized. Gastric hemorrhage occurred in 90% of dogs undergoing spinal surgery combined with administration of methylprednisolone sodium succinate.[66] In the dog, ulcers have been associated with peritonitis and liver disease,[67] with protein-calorie malnutrition,[68] and gastric erosions and hemorrhage with hypoadrenocorticism.[69] Gastroscopy in animals with such diverse conditions as peritonitis, hypoxia, pneumonia, chronic vomiting, systemic mastocytosis, liver disease, pyometra, feline infectious peritonitis, carcinomatosis, pancreatitis, and antral mucosal hypertrophy has revealed the presence of often severe and yet clinically unsuspected erosive gastritis with hemorrhage or frank ulceration (Burrows, unpublished observations).

Aspirin and other NSAIDs are notorious for the damage they cause to the mucosal barrier. This damage is achieved in a variety of ways, including damaging the mucosal cell membrane and enhancing mucosal cell permeability; inhibiting active mucosal ion transport; producing changes in mucosal blood flow; decreasing mucus production; and inhibiting prostaglandin synthesis.[70] Of all of these, the impact on prostaglandin synthesis through the inhibition of COX may be the most important. After Vane[55] showed that NSAIDs inhibited COX, the next great step in our understanding came in the early 1990s with the demonstration that COX had two isoforms: COX-1, which was constitutively expressed; and COX-2, which was inducible.[71] COX-2 is rapidly up-regulated at inflammatory sites and is responsible for the formation of pro-inflammatory prostanoids. COX-1 is responsible for the production of physiologically relevant prostanoids such as those in the stomach and platelets. Pharmacology defined the selectivity of existing NSAIDs on these COX enzymes and played a key role in producing a new generation of COX-2-selective drugs. These drugs would, it was hoped, have much reduced toxic side effects, particularly on the stomach.[71] COX-2, however, also has a physiologic role, being involved, for example, in the maintenance of fluid balance by the kidney. The COX-1 and -2 models, however, did not fully explain the antipyretic and analgesic effects and non-anti-inflammatory effects of acetaminophen. This might be explained by a variant of COX-2 now named COX-3.[72,73] The proposed pathways are shown in Figure 29-9. Different NSAIDs have different effects on the gastric mucosa but are most severe when the drugs are administered orally. Parenteral NSAIDs also have an effect, however. Much of the local effect perhaps can be attributed to the action of some NSAIDs, especially aspirin, in the acid milieu of the stomach to damage the hydrophobic lipid layer,[41] whereas the systemic effect is a result of the inhibition of COX.

Although all NSAIDs cause gastric mucosal damage, there is a wide interspecies susceptibility to specific drugs that may be associated with varying susceptibility of COX to different NSAIDs and to different metabolic pathways (Table 29-5). Aspirin, flunixine, and phenylbutazone for example, seem relatively well tolerated in the dog, although aspirin at a dose needed to obtain analgesic blood levels still causes gastric hemorrhage.[74] Wide individual susceptibility also exists. Flunixine, for example, appears to be relatively well tolerated over the short term in most dogs but caused severe ulceration after only 2 days of treatment in an apparently susceptible patient (Burrows, unpublished observations). These drugs, therefore, should always be used with caution because we currently have no means of identifying susceptible individuals. Other NSAIDs should never be used in veterinary medicine. Indomethacin and naproxen for example, cause severe, often fatal gastric and duodenal ulceration and hemorrhage in the dog.[75-78]

Facilitation of Barrier Repair

One of the basic tenets of medicine is that, in order to diagnose a disease, one has first to suspect it. The purpose of this chapter is to alert the reader to the possibility that gastric mucosal disease may be present not only in a variety of gastric diseases (Table

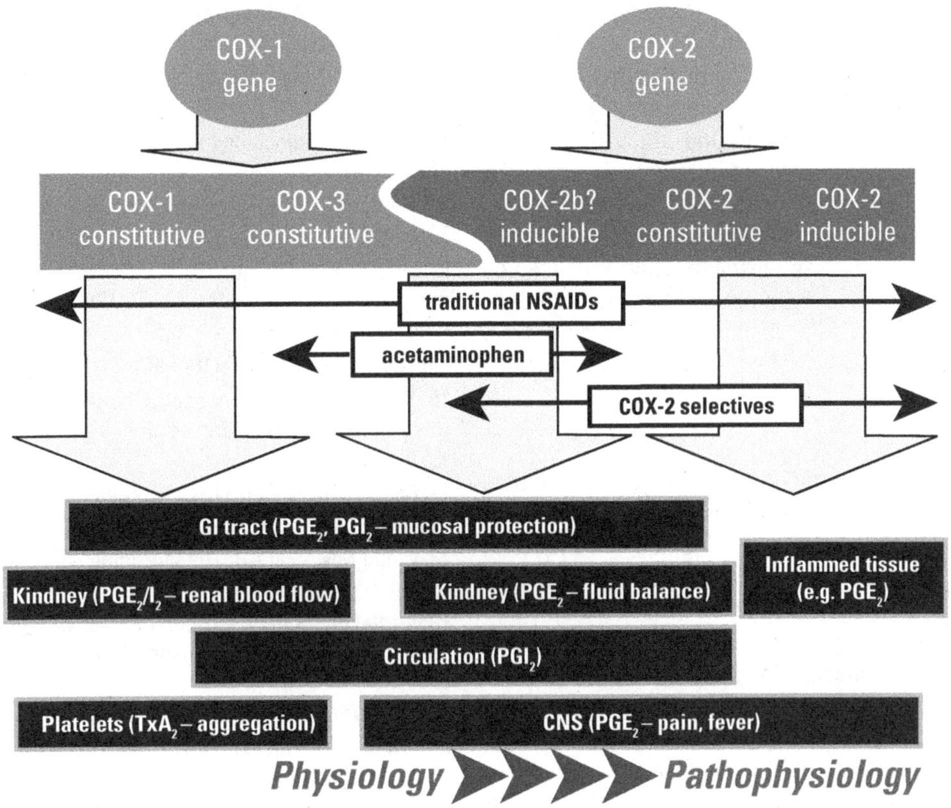

Figure 29-9. Current concept of the differing and overlapping roles of COX-1, COX-2, and proposed COX-3. Two distinct genes for COX-1 and -2 may give rise to a number of constitutive and inducible COX proteins with overlapping functions. Considering prostanoid production by a COX continuum may help us appreciate which enzymes underlie prostanoid production in different tissues as well as the actions of traditional NSAIDs, newer COX-2-selective drugs, and acetaminophen (COX-3 or COX-2b). (From Warner TD, Mitchell JA: Proc Natl Acad Sci 99(21):13371-13373, 2002, with permission. Copyright 2002 National Academy of Sciences, USA.)

Table 29-5. Drugs that Affect the Gastric Mucosal Barrier

Negatively	Positively
Corticosteroids	Misoprostol
Aspirin	Sucralfate
Naproxen	Cimetidine
Ibuprofen	Ranitidine
Indomethacin	Omeprazole
Flunixine	Bismuth sub-salts
Phenylbutazone	Aluminum salts
Alcohol	Linoleic and arachidonic acids

29-2) but also in a wide range of other disorders (Table 29-3). Recognition and appropriate treatment of barrier disruption may well reduce patient morbidity and mortality.

In dealing with the broken barrier, one first has to identify and, if possible, treat the underlying disease. All other actions are of secondary but nevertheless still considerable importance. Much of the mucosal damage comes from secreted acid, and one of the most important therapeutic approaches is to reduce acid output. This can be accomplished, at least to some extent, by dietary manipulation and, more importantly, by antisecretory drugs. Mucosal repair is also facilitated by a variety of cytoprotectants that protect the damaged mucosa from further acid damage.

As in most species, food is a potent stimulus to gastric secretion in the dog and cat. Since these species have little or no basal acid output, however, mucosal repair in many acute diseases may be facilitated by withholding food for 24 to 48 hours. Afterward, avoiding high-protein meals and providing frequent feedings in small quantities to reduce acid output may also be useful. This constitutes only supportive care, however, and most patients require additional antisecretory or cytoprotective drug therapy.

Antisecretory Drugs

The old maxim "no acid no ulcer"[79] is as true today as it ever was. A variety of substances can be used to reduce acid output but most widely used are the H_2 receptor antagonists and proton pump inhibitors (PPIs). Cimetidine, famotidine, and ranitidine are most widely used H_2 receptor antagonists in veterinary medicine. These drugs combine with the histamine receptors on parietal cells to inhibit histamine-stimulated secretion. They inhibit not only the acid secretory response to histamine, but also the response to cholinergic agents, gastrin, food, and vagal stimulation.[12] Their use should perhaps be routine as prophylaxis against mucosal injury in critically ill or stressed patients (Tables 29-3 and 29-4). Cimetidine is ineffective against aspirin-induced mucosal injury in the dog,[80] probably because in partly reducing acid synthesis, cimetidine also reduces HCO_3^- production and subsequent mucosal buffering.[70] Famotidine at a twice-daily dose appears to be the most effective drug in this class at reducing gastric acid secretion in the dog.[81]

The PPIs (e.g., omeprazole, pantoprazole, lansasoprole, esomeprazole) block the Na^+H^+-ATPase in the parietal cell in its secretory state. They are the most effective of the available drug classes in blocking acid secretion and are indicated in a spectrum of severe gastric diseases.[82] One study has shown that pantoprazole and omeprazole are effective in reducing acid secretion in dogs. Twice-daily dosing of omeprazole was the only regimen tested, however, that approached the potential therapeutic efficacy for acid-related disease when assessed by criteria used for human patients.[81] Omeprazole given once daily lessened aspirin-induced gastritis in the dog.[83] No data have been published for cats.

Cytoprotectants

Cytoprotection is defined as protection against gastric mucosal injury by a mechanism other than inhibition or neutralization of acid secretion.[84] Cytoprotective drugs include the synthetic prostaglandins, sucralfate, aluminum-containing antacids, bismuth compounds, and carbenoxolone (Table 29-5). It is possible that cimetidine also exerts some of its protective effect through this mechanism. In general, cytoprotective drugs promote the mechanisms responsible for maintaining a normal barrier, including increased mucus and HCO_3^- secretion, increased mucosal blood flow, promotion of apical cell restitution, phospholipid synthesis, and maintenance of vascular permeability to HCO_3^-.

Misoprostol and sucralfate are the most widely used cytoprotectants. Misoprostol, a synthetic prostaglandin that is effective when given orally, reduces the gastric mucosal side effects of NSAIDs. Sucralfate is a complex polymer of sucrose with multiple substitutions of aluminum sulfate. At a pH of less than 4.0 in the stomach, this compound undergoes a change in chemical configuration, develops a positive change, and binds electrochemically with negatively charged proteins leaking from the damaged mucosa.[85] In so doing, it forms a protective barrier over the damaged mucosa. The drug appears to be most useful in veterinary patients with gastric mucosal disease and was shown to be effective in lessening aspirin-induced gastritis.[83] It binds cimetidine, however, and the two drugs should not be given orally at the same time. Cimetidine, sucralfate, and misoprostol were ineffective in prophylaxis of gastrointestinal bleeding in dogs undergoing spinal surgery after having received methylprednisolone sodium succinate.[66] Omeprazole or pantoprazole may be more effective in these patients.

In conclusion, it should be appreciated that barrier disruption can occur under a wide variety of disease conditions. It should be considered as a complicating factor in most, if not all, critically ill patients. Mucosal protection therefore should be a routine part of therapy in such patients.

References

1. Bernard C: Leçons de physiologie expérimentale appliquée à la medicine. Paris Balliere, 1856, p. 408.

2. Davenport HW: Why the stomach does not digest itself. Sci Am 226(1):87, 1972.

3. Davenport HW: The gastric mucosal barrier. Digestion 5:162, 1972.

4. Davenport HW: The gastric mucosal barrier: past, present, and future. Mayo Clin Proc 50:507, 1975.

5. Allen A, Flemstron G, Gamer A, et al: Gastroduodenal mucosal protection. Physiol Rev 73:823, 1993.

6. Lamont TJ: Unlocking the secrets of the porcelain vase. Gastroenterol 119:1397, 2000.

7. Meiderer SE: The gastric mucosal barrier. Hepato-gastroenterol 33:88, 1986.

8. Holt KM and Hollander D: Acute gastric mucosal injury: pathogenesis and therapy. Ann Rev Med 37:107, 1986.

9. Fromm D: Mechanisms involved in gastric mucosal resistance to injury. Ann Rev Med 38:119, 1987.

10. Silen W: Gastric mucosal defense and repair. *In* Physiology of the Gastrointestinal Tract, 2nd ed. Johnson LR (ed). New York: Raven Press, 1987, p. 1055.

11. Emas S, Grossman MI: Comparison of gastric secretion in conscious dogs and cats. Gastroenterol 52(1):29, 1967.

12. Wolfe MM, Soll AH: The physiology of gastric acid secretion. N Engl J Med 319:1707, 1988.

13. Ito S: Functional gastric morphology. *In* Physiology of the Gastrointestinal Tract, 2nd ed. Johnson LR (ed). New York: Raven Press, 1987, p. 817.

14. Smith GW, Tasman-Jones C, Wiggins PM, et al: Pig gastric mucus: a one way barrier for H^+. Gastroenterol 89:1313, 1985.

15. Odonkor P, Mowat C, Hinal HS: Prevention of sepsis induced gastric lesions in dogs by cimetidine via inhibition of gastric secretion and by prostaglandin via cytoprotection. Gastroenterol 80:375, 1981.

16. Lloyd KCK, Debas HT: Peripheral regulation of gastric acid secretion. *In* Physiology of the Gastrointestinal Tract, 3rd ed. Johnson LR (ed). New York: Raven Press, 1994, p. 185.

17. Miled N, Canaan S, Depuis S, et al: Digestive lipases: from three dimensional structure to physiology. Biochem 82:973, 2000.

18. Steiner JM, Berridge BR, Wojcieszyn J, Williams D: Cellular immunologization of gastric and pancreatic lipase in various tissues obtained from dogs. Am J Vet Res 63:722, 2002.

19. Svanes K, Ito S, Takeuchi K, Silen W: Restitution of the surface epithelium of the in vitro frog gastric mucosa after damage with hyperosmolar sodium chloride. Gastroenterol 82:1409, 1982.

20. Eastwood GL: Epithelial cell renewal. *In* Gastric Cytoprotection: A Clinicians Guide. Hollander D, Tarnawski A (eds). New York: Plenum, 1989, p. 109.

21. Holzer P: Neural emergency system in the stomach. Gastroenterol 114:823, 1998.

22. Lacy ER, Ito S: Rapid epithelial restitution of the rat gastric mucosa after ethanol injury. Lab Investigation 51:573, 1984.

23. Lacy ER: Gastric mucosal defense after superficial injury. Clin Invest Med 10:189, 1987.

24. Flemstrom G, Turnberg LA: Gastroduodenal defense mechanism. *In* Clin Gastroenterol. Isenberg JI, Johansson C (eds). London: Saunders, 13:327, 1984.

25. Garner A, Flemston G, Allen A: Current concepts of gastroduodenal mucosal protection. Scand J Gastroenterol 19 (Suppl 92):78, 1984.

26. Flemstrom G, Isenberg JI: Gastroduodenal mucosal alkaline secretion and mucosal protection. News Physiol Sci 16:23, 2001.

27. Baumgartner HK, Montrose NH: Regulated alkali secretion acts in tandem with unstirred layers to regulate mouse gastric surface pH. Gastroenterol 126:774, 2004.

28. Baumgartner HK, Starodub OT, Joehl JS, et al: Cyclooxygenase 1 is required for pH control at the mouse gastric surface. Gut 53:1751, 2004.

29. Hills BA, Butler BD, Lichtenberger LM: Gastric mucosal barrier: hydrophobic lining to the lumen of the stomach. Am J Physiol 244:G561, 1983.

30. Duane WC, Wiegand DM: Mechanism by which bile salt disrupts the gastric mucosal barrier in the dog. J Clin Invest 66:1044, 1980.

31. Duane WC, Wiegand DM, Sievert CE: Bile acid and bile salt disrupt mucosal barrier in the dog by different mechanisms. Am J Physiol 242:G95, 1982.

32. Muller-Lissner SA, Sonnenberg A, Schattenmann G, et al: Gastric emptying and post prandial duodenogastric reflux in pylorectomized dogs. Am J Physiol 242:G9, 1982.

33. Twedt D: Bilious vomiting syndrome. *In* Five Minute Consult, 3rd ed. Tilley CP, Smith FWK (eds). Lippincott Williams & Wilkins, 2004, p. 155.

34. Duane WC, McHale AP, Sievert CP: Lysolecithin-lipid interactions in disruption of the canine gastric mucosal barrier. Am J Physiol 250:G275, 1986.

35. Ritchie WP: Other causes of GI mucosal injury: Upper intestinal content. Clin Invest Med 10:264, 1987.

36. Mercer DW, Casaneda AA, Denning JW, et al: Effects of endotoxin on gastric injury from luminal irritants in rats: potential role of nitric oxide. Am J Physiol 275:G449, 1998.

37. Helmer KS, West SD, Shipley GL, et al: Gastric nitric oxide synthetase expression during endotoxemia: implications in mucosal defense in rats. Gastroenterol 123:173, 2002.

38. Davenport HW: Damage to the gastric mucosa: effects of salicylates and stimulation. Gastroenterol 49:189, 1965.

39. Graham DY, Smith JL: Aspirin and the stomach. Ann Intern Med 104:390, 1986.

40. Shaw N, Burrows CF, King R: Massive gastric hemorrhage induced by buffered aspirin in a greyhound. J Am Anim Hosp Assoc 33:215, 1997.

41. Goddard PJ, Hills BA, Lichtenberger LM: Does aspirin damage canine gastric mucosa by reducing its surface hydrophobiticity? Am J Physiol 252:G421, 1987.

42. Cheung LY, Ashley SW: Gastric blood flow and mucosal defense mechanisms. Clin Invest Med 10:201, 1987.

43. Gannon B, Browning J, O'Brien P, et al: Mucosal microvascular architecture of the fundus and body of the human stomach. Gastroenterol 86:866, 1984.

44. Starlinger M, Schiessel R: Bicarbonate (HCO_3^-) delivery to the gastroduodenal mucosa by the blood: Its importance for mucosal integrity. Gut 29:647, 1988.

45. Starlinger M, Jakesz R, Mathews JB, et al: The relative importance of bicarbonate and blood flow in the protection of the rat gastric mucosa during shock. Gastroenterol 81:732, 1981.

46. Pfeiffer CJ, Keith JC, April M: Topographic localization of gastric lesions and key role of plasma bicarbonate concentration in dogs with experimentally induced gastric dilation. Am J Vet Res 48:262, 1987.

47. Silen W, Schiessel R, Kivilaakso E: The gastric mucosal barrier and ulceration. Brain Res Bull 5:3, 1980.

48. Yabana T, Yachi A: Stress-induced vascular damage and ulcer. Dig Dis Sci 33:751, 1988.

49. Helmer KS, West SD, Shipley GL, et al: Gastric nitric oxide synthesase expression during endotoxemia: implications in mucosal defense in rats. Gastroenterol 123:173, 2002.

50. Konturek SJ, Robert A: Cytoprotection of canine gastric mucosa by prostacyclin: Possible mediation by increased mucosal blood flow. Digestion 25:155, 1982.

51. Chu S, Tanaka S, Kauritz JD, et al: Dynamic regulation of gastric surface pH by luminal pH. J Clin Invest 103:605, 1999.

52. Baumgartner HK, Kirbiyuk U, Coskun T, et al: Endogenous-cyclooxygenase regulates mouse gastric surface pH. J Physiol (Lond) 544(3):871, 2002.

53. Turnberg LA: Gastric mucus, bicarbonate and pH gradients in mucosal protection. Clin Invest Med 10:178, 1987.

54. Silen W: The clinical problem of stress ulcers. Clin Invest Med 10:270, 1987.

55. Vane JR: Inhibition of prostaglandin synthesis as a mechanism of action of aspirin like drugs. Nature (New Biol) 231:232, 1971.

56. Cohen MM: Role of endogenous prostaglandins in gastric secretion and mucosal defense. Clin Invest Med 10:226, 1987.

57. Miller TA: Protective effects of prostaglandins against gastric mucosal damage: Current knowledge and proposed mechanisms. Am J Physiol 245:G601, 1983.

58. Kauffman GL: Mucosal damage to the stomach: How, when and why. Scand J Gastroenterol 19:19 (Suppl 101), 1984.

59. Materia A, Jatte B, Money S, et al: Prostaglandins in commercial milk preparations. Arch Surg 119:290, 1984.

60. Kuyama H, Eastwood GL: Effects of parenteral hydrocortisone sodium succinate on epithelial renewal in hamster gastric mucosa. Dig Dis Sci 33:1064, 1988.

61. Martin M, Menguy R: Influence of adrenocorticotropin, cortisone, aspirin and phenylbutazone on the rate of exfoliation and rate of renewal of gastric mucosal cells. Gastroenterol 58:329, 1970.

62. Rohrer CR, Hill RC, Fischer A, et al: Gastric hemorrhage in dogs given high doses of methylprednisolone sodium succinate. Am J Vet Res 60:977, 1999.

63. Cheung LY, Stephenson LW, Moody FG, et al: Direct effects of endotoxin on canine gastric mucosal permeability and morphology. J Surg Res 10:417, 1975.

64. Pollock TW, Goodwin CW, Schumate GR, et al: Effects of chronic hypoxia on canine gastric secretion. Am J Vet Surg 133:95, 1977.

65. Skillman JJ, Bushell LS, Goldman H, et al: Respiratory failure, hypotension, sepsis and jaundice. A clinical syndrome associated with lethal hemorrhage from acute stress ulceration of the stomach. Am J Surg 117:523, 1981.

66. Hanson SM, Bostwick DR, Twedt DC, et al: Clinical evaluation of cimetidine, sucralfate, and misoprostol for prevention of gastrointestinal tract bleeding in dogs undergoing spinal surgery. Am J Vet Res 58:1320, 1997.

67. Murray MM, Robinson PB, McKeating FJ, et al: Peptic ulceration in the dog: a clinico-pathologic study. Vet Rec 91:441, 1972.

68. Williams DA, Burrows CF: Short bowel syndrome – a case report in a dog and a discussion of the pathophysiology of bowel resection. J Small Anim Pract 22:263, 1981.

69. Burrows CF: Reversible megaesophagus in a dog with hypoadrenocorticism. J Small Anim Pract 22:1073, 1987.

70. Fromm D: How do non-steroidal anti-inflammatory drugs affect gastric mucosal defenses? Clin Invest Med 10:251, 1987.

71. Vane JR: The fight against rheumatism: from Willow Bark to COX-1 sparing drugs. J Physiol Pharmocol 51:573, 2000.

72. Chandresekaran NV, Dai H, Roos KL, et al: COX-3 a cyclooxygenase-1 variant inhibited by acetaminophen and other analgesic/antipyretic drugs: cloning, structure and expression. Proc Nat Acad Sci 99:13926, 2002.

73. Warner TD, Mitchell JA: Cyclooxygenase-3 (COX-3): filling the gaps towards a COX continum. Proc Nat Acad Sci 99:13371, 2002.

74. Lipowitz AJ, Boulay JP, Klausner JS: Serum salicylate concentrations and endoscopic evaluation of the gastric mucosa in dogs after oral administration of aspirin containing products. Am J Vet Res 47:1586, 1986.

75. Ewing GO: Indomethacin-associated gastrointestinal hemorrhage in a dog. J Am Vet Med Assoc 161:1665, 1972.

76. Daehler MH: Transmural pyloric perforation associated with naproxen administration in a dog. J Am Vet Med Assoc 189:694, 1986.

77. Gilmour MA, Walshaw R: Naproxen-induced toxicosis in a dog. J Am Vet Med Assoc 191:1431, 1987.

78. Pemberton RE, et al: A review of the upper GI side effects of the newer non-steroidal anti-inflammatory dugs. Dig Dis Sci 24:53, 1979.

79. Schwartz K: Über penetrierende magen und jejunalgeschwüre. Beit Klin Chir 67:96, 1910.

80. Boulay JP, Lipowitz AJ, Laupner JS: Effect of cimetidine on aspirin-induced gastric hemorrhage in dogs. Am J Vet Res 47:1744, 1986.

81. Besenas AME, Mathews KA, Allen DG, et al: Effect of ranitidine, famotidine, pantoprazole and omeprazole on intragastric pH in dogs. Am J Vet Res 66:425, 2005.

82. Jenkins CC, DeNovo RL: Omeprazole: a potent antiulcer drug. Comp Contin Educ 14:1578, 1992.

83. Jenkins CC, DeNovo RC, Patton CS, et al: Comparison of effects of cimetidine and omeprazole in mechanically created gastric ulceration and an aspirin-induced gastritis in dogs. Am J Vet Res 52:658, 1991.

84. Guth PH: Mucosal coating agents and other non-antisecretory agents. Are they cytoprotective? Dig Dis Sci 32:647, 1987.

85. McCarthy DM: Sucralfate. N Engl J Med 325:1017, 1991.

Chapter 30

Gastric Outflow Obstruction

Ronald M Bright

Anatomy and Physiology

The stomach is an unequal dilatation of the foregut, which extends as a J-shaped loop from below the esophagus and diaphragm in the upper left abdominal quadrant to the duodenum in the upper right quadrant.[1] The greater curvature of the stomach, facing caudally, is located mostly to the left of the midline. The lesser curvature faces cranially and is accentuated when the stomach is empty. The distal stomach is somewhat immobilized by the hepatogastric and hepatoduodenal ligaments. Within these structures are the common bile duct, the hepatic ducts, and the portal vein.

The stomach is divisible into four parts. The cardia is immediately distal to the gastroesophageal junction below the diaphragm. It blends into the fundus, which provides receptacle and storage functions and, along with the body, is the most expandable portion of the stomach. The cardia, body, and fundus comprise approximately two thirds of the proximal stomach. The fundus and body are histologically indistinguishable from each other. The pyloric antrum forms the remaining third of the stomach and leads into the pyloric sphincter. The mucosa of the body and fundus is rugose. The mucosa-submucosa are loosely attached to the underlying muscle, making it somewhat mobile. The antral mucosa contains fewer rugal folds and is flatter. The mucosa-submucosa are more firmly attached to the underlying muscle. When the stomach is empty, the rugal folds are most distinct.

The muscle layers of the stomach contain an outer layer of longitudinally arranged muscle fibers, an oblique layer, and deep to this are circularly arranged muscle fibers. The latter are plentiful in the antrum because of its important function of grinding, retropulsing, and emptying of gastric contents. The pylorus is a thickened continuation of the circular smooth muscle, which, along with its mucosal lining, forms an intraluminal bulge that can be palpated. The pylorus is considered a true antatomic sphincter owing to these abundant circular muscle fibers that encircle it.[2]

The blood supply to the stomach is by way of the celiac artery and some of its branches. The left and right gastroepiploic arteries primarily nourish the greater curvature, whereas the lesser curvature is supplied by the right and left gastric arteries, which eventually anastomose. Venous drainage is accomplished by the gastrosplenic and gastroduodenal veins emptying into the portal vein.

The proximal stomach serves a reservoir function and expands greatly in response to liquid and food. "Receptive relaxation" of the fundus and body of the stomach is induced when the animal swallows, resulting in decreased motor activity and pressure.[2] Gastric accommodation follows as pressure begins to increase within the fundus.

The primary role of the fundus is to empty liquids without allowing any modest change in the pressure within the fundus to raise intragastric pressure. Partial or complete removal of the fundus will raise the intragastric pressure more readily, however, resulting in an increased rate of emptying of liquids. This has no effect on the rate of emptying solids.[3]

The distal stomach is primarily responsible for grinding, filtering, and propelling solid food until it reaches a particle size of 1 to 2 mm in diameter. Even after antrectomy, up to 60% of emptied particles are smaller than 1 mm.[3]

In the fed state, peristaltic waves occur at a rate of 4 to 5 per minute, which helps propel the food toward the pylorus. The pylorus, as a "gate-keeper," is responsible for keeping material in the stomach until it reaches the appropriate particle size.[4] When the smaller particles begin to move aborally, the pylorus is partially relaxed and emptying occurs. Near the end of each antral contraction, the pylorus closes, forcing the larger particles to be retropulsed back into the antrum and body of the stomach so grinding can continue.

In the fasted state, the stomach and intestine alternate between quiescent time and short times of intense myoelectrical activity.[5] This results in vigorous aboral contractions and forms the migrating motor complexes, which extend through the entire intestinal tract. In the dog, this occurs every 2 to 3 hours. This is the period when nondigestable materials and cellular debris move out of the stomach. Antral contractions are stronger during the fed state and when relaxation of the pylorus is at its maximum.

The pylorus, besides regulating the size of particles that leave the stomach, is also responsible for limiting the amount of duodenogastric reflux.[4,6,7] It is known in dogs that bile, pancreatic juice, and intestinal contents have a deleterious effect on the gastric mucosa.[7] The amount of duodenal material inside the stomach depends on the rate and volume of duodenogastric reflux and the rate at which regurgitated material is removed from the stomach. Duodenogastric reflux is a common phenomenon and is not affected by the type of meal.[6] However, if gastric emptying is delayed, the reflux rate is stimulated, which may result in an erosive gastritis or ulcer formation.[6,7]

Similarly, when surgery of the pyloric sphincter or resection of the pylorus has occurred, the reflux of bile and pancreatic and intestinal secretions may increase. These secretions may be innocuous in some animals, but in others, reflux gastritis or bilious vomiting may occur. This is termed postoperative alkaline reflux gastritis.[8]

Gastric outflow obstruction is most often caused by mural, mucosal, and luminal abnormalities. Foreign bodies can produce either partial or complete obstruction as can inflammatory diseases caused by eosinophilic gastritis, fungal gastritis, chronic gastric ulcer disease, and neoplasia, most notably, adenocarcinoma. Suture-induced granuloma following pyloric surgery has also been reported.[9] Gastric volvulus, seen primarily in large or giant breeds, can result in outflow problems as well.

Vomiting is the most frequent sign seen with gastric outlet problems. The normal stomach is usually empty within 8 to 10 hours after eating. Vomiting after this time suggests a gastric retention disorder.[4]

The content of the vomitus may be bile and mucus when vomiting occurs on an empty stomach. This may suggest a duodenogastric reflux problem or gastric hypomotility. Conversely, in the absence of bile, the presence of nondigested material 12 to 24 hours after eating would suggest an outflow obstruction problem.[4]

Pyloric Stenosis (Congenital)

This condition is primarily seen in brachycephalic breeds and in the Siamese cat. This stenosis results from hypertrophy of the circular smooth muscle of the pylorus. Signs are usually not seen in the first 6 to 8 weeks of age. They appear when the animals are weaned and begin to take solid food. The difficulty of emptying solid food is the hallmark of this disease. Gastrin and its effects on the smooth muscle of the pylorus have been implicated but the mode of inheritance and exact pathogenesis are unknown.[5] Pentagastrin, a gastrin analogue, has been given to pregnant animals, resulting in pyloric stenosis in the neonate as a result of hypertrophy of the muscle. Surgery is necessary to correct this problem. Pyloromyotomy carries little risk and is accompanied by good results.[10,11]

Acquired Antral Pyloric Gastropathy

The acquired form of antral pyloric stenosis usually results from dramatic hypertrophic changes to the mucosa and, occasionally, to the circular smooth muscle as well. Type I hypertrophy involves the muscle; type II, the combination of muscle and mucosa; and type III, the mucosa.[7] Benign inflammatory infiltrates are commonly seen on biopsy samples. Grossly, these masses can resemble polyps. They can be smooth-surfaced or slightly lobulated. Some are somewhat sessile and can be single or multiple and confined to the antrum.

This acquired form of hypertrophy is typically seen in middle-aged small breeds, in which progressive vomiting is the most common clinical manifestation. The vomiting can be delayed up to 24 hours after eating, and it is not uncommon to see the absence of bile and undigested food in the vomitus. Melena and/or hematemesis would indicate erosive gastritis or ulcer disease that can also contribute to gastric emptying delays.

The treatment of choice is some type of pyloroplasty with resection of the hypertrophied polypoid-like masses (Figure 30-1).[10] The prognosis following surgery is good, with early return to normal gastric emptying. Any hypomotility that persists will usually respond to short-term use of a prokinetic agent.

Bilious vomiting following surgery may indicate an excessive amount of duodenogastric reflux caused by the pyloric operation. Sucralfate (Carafate, Hoechst Marion Roussel), systemic antacids and feeding a small meal before bedtime may be necessary on a short-term basis or indefinitely.

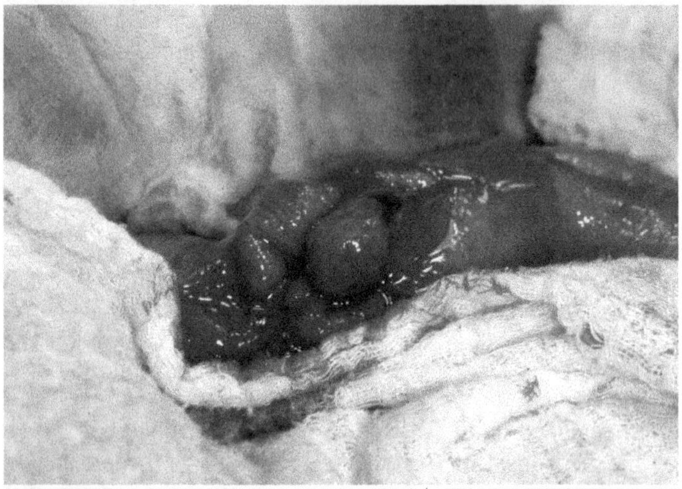

Figure 30-1. This intraoperative photo demonstrates the polypoid-type masses that are often seen in cases of antral mucosal hypertrophy.

Neoplasia

Gastric neoplasia is rare in the dog and no cause is known. Adenocarcinoma is the most common malignant tumor in dogs and it can manifest as an ulcerated mass, polypoid in appearance or scirrhous in nature.[12] Other gastric tumors include lymphosarcoma, (most common in cats), leiomyoma/sarcoma, and adenomatous polyps.[12]

Any of the gastric tumors can cause partial or complete gastric outflow obstruction (Figure 30-2). They can also result in gastric ulceration or altered gastric motility.

As is typical of any mass obstructing gastric outflow, progressive vomiting is the predominant sign. Hematemesis and melena are commonly seen with adenocarcinomas owing to their frequent ulceration.

Foreign Bodies

Foreign bodies are the most common cause of gastric outlet obstruction in dogs and cats. Vomiting is the sign most often

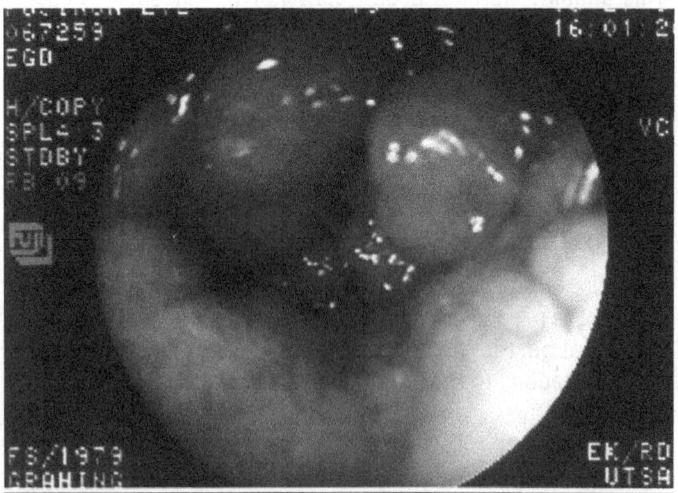

Figure 30-2. These multiple masses were diagnosed as adenocarcinoma based on biopsies taken endoscopically. Gastric outlet obstruction was almost complete in this case.

observed and, if the foreign body is sharp-edged, hematemesis may be seen. Many foreign bodies can pass through the pylorus during the interdigestive period owing to the migrating motor complexes. Ideally, foreign bodies can be retrieved by means of endoscopy, with surgery serving as a viable option if this is not possible.

Miscellaneous

Other causes of chronic intermittent vomiting include granulomatous conditions caused by Phythium and rarely, eosinophilic gastritis.[5] Fungal diseases are most commonly seen in the Gulf Coast states, affecting primarily male large-breed and younger dogs. The granulomas that form in the submucosa and muscularis mucosae are caused by the penetration of ingested spores that eventually enter the lymphatics.[5]

Eosinophilic gastritis can stimulate a large amount of granulation tissue to be formed anywhere in the stomach. If this lesion is large enough and present in the antrum, it can cause serious gastric emptying problems. This disease may be immune-stimulated.[13] These granulomas, when viewed grossly with endoscopy or during surgery, are indistinguishable from neoplastic lesions.

Extraluminal lesions can encroach on the antrum and, therefore, interfere with gastric emptying. Ultrasonography is usually helpful in distinguishing these lesions from intraluminal ones. Depending on the origin of the mass, systemic involvement may also occur.

Important causes of gastric emptying problems that can be confused with some type of mechanical obstruction are motility disorders. This is not well documented in dogs and cats and the diagnosis is usually made based on delayed gastric emptying in the absence of an obstructive lesion.[13]

Trichobezoars in cats may be caused by the lack of migrating motor complexes. Emptying of any type of foreign material in the stomach of a cat, therefore, may be impaired.[13]

Hypomotility disorder may occur in dogs that have survived an acute gastric-dilatation-volvulus episode. This may be associated with a large and flaccid stomach, which has been observed during acute gastric-dilatation-volvulus surgery. The vomiting associated with this is presumed to be related to delayed gastric emptying because response to a prokinetic agent is favorable. Long-term use of a prokinetic agent may be necessary in some instances.

Metabolic problems, although not as well documented in animals as in people, may delay gastric emptying. These include hypokalemia, diabetes mellitus, hypothyroidism, uremia, and hepatic encephalopathy.[13]

Perioperative Considerations

Regardless of the cause of gastric outflow obstruction, serious metabolic consequences can result from chronic and frequent vomiting that may accompany a gastric emptying disorder.

Dehydration and metabolic alkalosis with its accompanying electrolyte imbalances (hypochloremia, hypokalemia) should be corrected when possible before any surgical intervention.

A large, distended, fluid-filled stomach can present a serious risk to any animal undergoing anesthesia and/or surgery. These animals are at a greater risk of gastroesophageal reflux that could lead to an aspiration pneumonia or reflux esophagitis. Immediately after induction of anesthesia, an orogastric tube with a suction device attached should be passed into the stomach to remove it contents. In addition, a prokinetic agent and systemic antacid can be used during the perioperative period to decrease the risk of potential problems related to reflux of gastric contents.

References

1. Morson BC, Dawson IMP, Day DW, et al: Morson & Dawson's Gastrointestinal Pathology, 3rd ed. Oxford: Blackwell Scientific, 1990, p. 77.
2. Guilford WG, Strombeck DR: *In* Strombeck's Small Animal Gastroenterology, 3rd ed. Guilford WG, et al (ed). Philadelphia: WB Saunders, 1996, p. 239.
3. Rees WDW, Brown CM: Physiology of the stomach and duodenum. *In* Bockus Gastroenterology, 5th ed. Haubrich WS, Schaffner F, Berk JE (eds). Philadelphia: WB Saunders, 1995, p. 582.
4. Twedt DC, Magne ML: Diseases of the stomach. *In* Textbook of Veterinary Internal Medicine, 3rd ed. Ettinger SJ (ed). Philadelphia: WB Saunders, 1989, p. 1289.
5. Stanton MLE: Gastric outlet obstruction. *In* Disease Mechanisms in Small Animal Surgery, 2nd ed., Bojrab MJ, Smeak DD, Bloomberg MS (eds). Philadelphia: Lea & Febiger, 1993, p. 235.
6. Sonnenberg A, Muller-Lissner SA, Schattenmann G, et al: Duodenogastric reflux in the dog. Am J Physiol 242:G603, 1982.
7. Happe RP, Van Den Brom WE, Van Der Gaag I: Duodenogastric reflux in the dog, a clinicopathological study. Res Vet Sci 33:280, 1982.
8. Cooperman AM: Postoperative alkaline reflux gastritis. Surg Clin North Am 56:1445, 1976.
9. Bright RM, Jenkins C, DeNovo RC: Pyloric obstruction in a dog related to a gastrotomy incision closed with polypropylene. J Small Anim Pract 35:629, 1994.
10. Bright RM: Surgery of the stomach. *In* Saunders Manual of Small Animal Practice, 2nd ed. Birchard SJ, Sherding RG (eds). Philadelphia: WB Saunders, 2000, p. 777.
11. Dulisch ML. Pyloromyotomy, pyloroplasty, and pyloric resection. *In* Current Techniques in Small Animal Surgery, 4th ed. Bojrab MJ, Ellison GW, Slocum B (eds). Baltimore: Williams & Wilkins, 1997, p. 207.
12. Jenkins CC, DeNovo RC Jr: Diseases of the stomach. *In* Handbook of Small Animal Practice, 4th ed. Morgan RV, Bright RM, Swartout MS (eds). Philadelphia: WB Saunders, 2003, p. 335.
13. Johnson SE, Sherding, RG, Bright RM: Diseases of the stomach. *In* Saunders Manual of Small Animal Practice, 2nd ed. Birchard SJ, Sherding RG (eds). Philadelphia: W B Saunders, 2000, p. 753.

Chapter 31

Pancreatitis

Craig B. Webb
Jacqueline C. Whittemore

The diagnosis of severe acute pancreatitis carries with it a mortality rate of up to 50% in humans.[1] Although alcohol consumption and biliary disease (the two most common causes of pancreatitis in humans) are uncommon in veterinary patients, the underlying cellular pathophysiology is likely to be similar between species, and starts with premature activation of digestive enzymes within pancreatic acinar cells. Despite extensive research into the inflammatory mediators that promulgate the systemic effects of pancreatic inflammation, advances in treatment of the disease beyond pancreatic rest and nonspecific supportive care have been minimal. Pancreatitis in veterinary patients remains predominantly a medical disease unless a specific mass (e.g., a tumor, pseudocyst, or abscess) or structural defect (i.e., biliary obstruction) can be identified.

Physiology

The exocrine pancreas produces zymogens, pancreatic secretory trypsin inhibitor (PSTI), and active enzymes (lipase, amylase, and the pro-coenzyme, procolipase). The zymogens include trypsinogen, chymotrypsinogens, kallikreinogen, proelastases, procarboxypeptidases, and prophospholipase A_2. Zymogen granule secretion is the result of both neural and humoral mechanisms. Secretin and cholecystokinin (CCK) are believed to be the most important humoral mediators in stimulating zymogen secretion in dogs and cats. Trypsin is the only enzyme capable of activating itself and the other zymogens. This activation is largely controlled by the local calcium concentration. At a low calcium concentration, as is found within acinar cells, calcium binding protects the trypsinogen activation peptide from exposure. Increased calcium concentration, as is found in the pancreatic ducts and intestine, increases the sensitivity of trypsinogen to activation by trypsin. The lysosomal granules within exocrine pancreatic cells contain proteases, including cathepsin B, which can activate zymogens on contact.

Protective mechanisms that decrease the risk of premature zymogen activation include the inclusion of PSTI with zymogens, the segregation of zymogens within lipid structures, and the maintenance of high alkaline ductular flushing. Ductular PSTI protects the pancreas by binding to the active site on trypsin to prevent further zymogen activation.[2] Alkalinity is maintained by bicarbonate secretion through the cystic fibrosis transmembrane conductance regulator (CFTR).[3] The association of pancreatitis with CFTR mutations in humans emphasizes the importance of ductular bicarbonate secretion as a protective mechanism.[3] Duodenal brush border cells produce enterokinase, a strong protease that is responsible for zymogen activation within the intestinal lumen. This site-specific production of enterokinase helps ensure activation of zymogens within the intestinal lumen while limiting the risk of zymogen activation within the pancreas. Muscle sphincters in the pancreatic ducts help prevent reflux of enterokinase and duodenal contents into the pancreas, which is particularly important as enterokinase is not inactivated by PSTI and does not form complexes with anti-proteases.

Low levels of circulating exocrine pancreatic enzymes are commonly present in plasma and are cleared through the kidney. Circulating zymogens are bound by circulating enzyme inhibitors, α1-antitrypsin and α2-macroglobulin, which decrease their activity and increase monocyte-macrophage clearance, respectively.

Pathophysiology

Pancreatitis is a multifactorial process that eventually culminates in inappropriate activation of zymogens within the pancreatic parenchyma. In most patients, this is likely the result of abnormal fusion of lysosomal and zymogen granules within the acinar cells. A small subset of veterinary cases, like a large percentage of human cases, may be a result of inappropriate duodenal reflux into the pancreas.[4] The conversion of trypsinogen to trypsin starts a self-perpetuating cascade of zymogen activation with resulting auto-digestion of the pancreas and surrounding tissues. Endothelial membrane damage and increased capillary permeability lead to pancreatic edema, decreased microvascular circulation, increased free radical accumulation, and local ischemia.

As proteolytic enzymes propagate, they may overwhelm circulating anti-proteases and activate inflammatory cascades. The result may be refractory hypotensive and vasoactive shock, disseminated intravascular coagulation (DIC), multiple organ dysfunction syndrome (MODS), and death.[5] Pancreatic abscessation and pseudocysts may form in severe cases. Pancreatic pseudocysts are collections of pancreatic secretions that form secondary to fibrosis or inflammation.[6] Pancreatic abscessation may also occur and is usually sterile.[7] Both may require surgical intervention for successful outcomes.

In humans, defects in the trypsinogen, PSTI, and CFTR genes are associated with hereditary pancreatitis.[2] It is currently unknown whether there are specific hereditary causes of pancreatitis in dogs or cats, although terriers, miniature Schnauzers, and Siamese cats are over-represented.

Classification

Pancreatitis can be classified as either acute or chronic, and either form may be mild or severe. Acute pancreatitis is a completely reversible condition, despite the fact that this is often the more severe manifestation of the disease. In the cat, acute pancreatitis is further delineated as either acute necrotizing or acute suppurative disease.

Chronic pancreatitis entails irreversible histopathologic changes, including fibrosis and acinar atrophy with lymphoplasmacytic inflammation, although this form is often mild and subtle in its clinical presentation. Mild pancreatitis is associated with minimal systemic effects and low mortality. The pancreas may be edematous or show mild interstitial changes but the condition is rarely associated with necrosis of acinar cells. Severe pancreatitis is often associated with extensive pancreatic necrosis, hemorrhagic changes or suppurative inflammation, multiple organ involvement, and a poor prognosis.

Etiology and Examination Findings

Known or suspected risk factors for canine pancreatitis include breed (terriers, miniature Schnauzers), age (older than 5 years), concurrent endocrine disease (diabetes mellitus, hyperadrenocorticism, hypothyroidism, and hypertriglyceridemia), hypercalcemia, obesity, gastrointestinal disease, drugs (sulfonamides, azathioprine, L-asparaginase, estrogen, furosemide, potassium bromide, salicylates, tetracyclines, thiazide diuretics, and vinca alkaloids), toxins (cholinesterase inhibitor insecticides, cholinergic agonists, and zinc), epilepsy, infection, ischemia, and blunt abdominal trauma.[8] Glucocorticoids are no longer considered a risk factor for development of pancreatitis in humans; little support exists for an association between glucocorticoids and pancreatitis in either dogs or cats. Risk factors in cats include breed (Siamese), age (older than 7 years), trauma, and concurrent disease (hepatic lipidosis or diabetes mellitus).[4,9-11] Triaditis refers to concurrent inflammatory bowel disease (IBD), cholangiohepatitis, and pancreatitis. Feline cases may be caused by feline infectious peritonitis, toxoplasmosis, and liver or pancreatic flukes (*Erythremia procyonis, Amphimerus pseudofelineus,* or *Opisthorchis felineus*).[4,12]

Clinical signs in dogs include weakness, anorexia, vomiting, diarrhea, abdominal pain, fever, and collapse. Signs in cats include lethargy, anorexia, dehydration, and jaundice. Vomiting and diarrhea are uncommonly associated with feline pancreatitis; mild weight loss or atypical behavior may be the only clinical signs in this species. Findings on physical examination include dehydration, abdominal pain, icterus, tachycardia, tachypnea, fever or hypothermia, or the presence of an abdominal mass. In some animals, particularly cats, physical examination may be unremarkable.

Sequelae

The inappropriate activation and release of digestive enzymes have a number of systemic consequences. Direct injury to the pancreatic parenchyma results in cellular necrosis and the progression of the disease from edematous to hemorrhagic and/or necrotic pancreatitis. A variety of cascades are activated that cause systemic dissemination of the deleterious consequences of pancreatic inflammation. These include the kinin/coagulation cascades, the fibrinolytic, and the complement systems. A variety of inflammatory mediators are released that can quickly turn pancreatitis into a condition affecting multiple systems; free radicals released from neutrophils and macrophages also contribute to the adverse systemic consequences. Vascular injury leads to increased capillary permeability and activation of vasoactive amines. Effects can be significant fluid and protein loss, decreased blood flow to vital tissues, dehydration, hypovolemia, and shock. Plasma protease inhibitors are consumed; protease digestion of clotting factors may worsen shock and lead to DIC. In humans the cardiac system is particularly susceptible to the systemic signals set in motion by pancreatitis. Renal, pulmonary, and hepatic changes are the result of direct contact with digestive enzymes or secondary to altered blood flow and oxygen delivery. Hepatocellular necrosis, bile duct obstruction, pulmonary edema, acute renal failure and tubular degeneration, fibrosis, and clotting disorders are all recognized sequelae of pancreatitis in human patients.

References

1. Bhatia M, Wong FL, Cao Y, et al: Pathophysiology of acute pancreatitis. Pancreatology 5:132, 2005.

2. Rinderknecht H: Activation of pancreatic zymogens. Normal activation, premature intrapancreatic activation, protective mechanisms against inappropriate activation. Dig Dis Sci 31:314, 1986.

3. Whitcomb DC: Mechanisms of disease: Advances in understanding the mechanisms leading to chronic pancreatitis. Nat Clin Pract Gastroenterol Hepatol 1:46, 2004.

4. Weiss DJ, Gagne JM, Armstrong PJ: Relationship between inflammatory hepatic disease and inflammatory bowel disease, pancreatitis, and nephritis in cats. J Am Vet Med Assoc 209:1114, 1996.

5. Ruaux CG: Pathophysiology of organ failure in severe acute pancreatitis in dogs. Comp Contin Educ Pract Vet 22:531, 2000.

6. VanEnkewort BA, O'Brien RT, Young KM: Pancreatic pseudocysts in 4 dogs and 2 cats: Ultrasonographic and clinical pathologic findings. J Vet Intern Med 13:309, 1999.

7. Stimson EL, Espada Y, Moon M, et al: Pancreatic abscess in nine dogs. J Vet Intern Med 9:202, 1998.

8. Hess RS, Kass PH, Shofer FS, et al: Evaluation of risk factors for fatal acute pancreatitis in dogs. J Am Vet Med Assoc 214:46, 1999.

9. Hill RC, Van Winkle TJ: Acute necrotizing pancreatitis and acute suppurative pancreatitis in the cat. A retrospective study of 40 cases (1976-1989). J Vet Intern Med 7:25, 1993.

10. Akol KG, Washabau RJ, Saunders HM, et al: Acute pancreatitis in cats with hepatic lipidosis. J Vet Intern Med 7:205, 1993.

11. Ferreri JA, Hardam E, Kimmel SE, et al: Clinical differentiation of acute necrotizing from chronic nonsuppurative pancreatitis in cats: 63 cases (1996-2001). J Am Vet Med Assoc 223:469, 2003.

12. Dubey JP, Carpenter JL: Histologically confirmed clinical toxoplasmosis in cats: 100 cases (1952-1990). J Am Vet Med Assoc 203:1556, 1993.

Chapter 32

Pathophysiology of Hepatocellular Diseases

Pierre M. Amsellem
David C. Twedt

The liver is the largest solid organ and is involved in many critical metabolic functions of the body. It is important in metabolism, having a central role in synthesis, detoxification, excretion, and storage as well as host defensive mechanisms. The liver is also unique because of its dual blood supply derived from the portal vein and hepatic artery. The portal blood with its low oxygen tension provides approximately 70% to 75% of the hepatic blood flow to the liver. Disruption of liver function or circulation can have serious consequences to the patient. Lastly, the liver has the unique ability to regenerate. For example, following removal of one lobe, the liver will quickly regenerate to its original size. When dealing with the surgical patient, it is critical to understand basic liver function and to recognize conditions affecting the liver.

Identification of Liver Disease

The clinical history and physical examination may provide some insight to the presence of liver disease, but generally, the diagnosis of liver disease or circulatory disorders of the liver largely depends on combined information obtained from clinical findings, laboratory testing, ultrasonography, and histopathologic evaluation. Identification of abnormal liver enzymes or liver function tests such as bile acids, albumin, glucose, ammonia, and bilirubin indicate that the liver should be first investigated. It is important to point out, however, that the liver is also frequently a so-called "innocent by-stander," being affected by many non-hepatic metabolic or systemic disorders. Such hepatic changes are often referred to as reactive hepatopathies and rarely do they significantly alter hepatic function. Examples include certain drugs, endocrine disease, cardiovascular conditions, or intraabdominal disorders such as pancreatitis or inflammatory bowel disease.[1] Consequently, non-hepatic conditions and drug-associated liver dysfunction should be excluded first in the diagnostic work up before a primary investigation of the liver begins.

Radiographs will reveal liver size and shape and may aid in detecting other intraabdominal disorders. Ultrasonography is useful to detect parenchymal, biliary, and vascular abnormalities.[2] Hepatic cells for cytologic investigation are frequently obtained during ultrasonography using fine-needle aspiration; they may provide some useful information about the liver. Cytologic evaluation, however, is limited in the amount of information it can give. The best cytologic correlation with histopathologic findings is found with hepatic neoplasia and diffuse vacuolar disease.[3]

The definitive diagnosis of biliary or parenchymal disorders generally requires histopathologic evaluation. Histopathologic samples are obtained by needle biopsy, laparoscopy, or surgery. Each technique has certain advantages but also inherent limitations. For example, a needle biopsy is the least invasive but a core needle biopsy sample only represents one fifty-thousandth of the entire liver. It is recommended that at least 3 core biopsies of 16 g each be obtained from the liver to get an adequate quantity of tissue for interpretation.[4] The diagnostic accuracy of a needle biopsy is highest with diffuse hepatic disease. Laparoscopic or surgical wedge biopsies can be visually directed and provide larger pieces of tissue for examination. Laparoscopy is considered to be minimally invasive, but it is limited in that it is difficult to view the entire liver surface. The advantage over needle biopsies is that larger and more diagnostic samples are obtained when compared with the smaller needle biopsies.[5] Surgery, although more invasive, allows one to evaluate all liver lobes and obtain large samples with good hemostasis. In the appropriate clinical situations, liver culture and or hepatic copper analysis should be obtained on a liver biopsy sample.

Metabolic Considerations

Response to Injury

The liver can respond to an injury in only a limited number of ways. Reversible hepatocyte injury includes hepatocellular swelling, steroid-induced hepatopathy (in dogs only), and steatosis or lipidosis.[6] Hepatocellular swelling (hydropic degeneration) is the first manifestation of almost all forms of injury to cells and occurs when the cells are incapable of maintaining ionic and fluid homeostasis and accumulate water. Excessive corticosteroids will induce hepatocyte vacuolar changes owing to abnormal hepatic glycogen accumulation in dogs, but not cats. Lipidosis with hepatocyte accumulation of triglycerides occurs from abnormalities in fat metabolism or mobilization.

Nonreversible hepatocyte death occurs by either apoptosis or necrosis.[6] Hepatocytes may be killed by various insults, including hypoxia, toxins, drugs, microorganisms, immunologic events, and severe metabolic disturbances. The response following destruction of hepatic parenchyma results in inflammation, regeneration of parenchyma, fibrosis, and ductular proliferation.[6] The degree of clinical liver disease is dependent on the extent of hepatic damage and the ability of the liver to maintain normal functions. The liver has a great reserve capacity, and liver disease must be much advanced before clinical signs occur. Because the liver is involved in so many functions, no one test will determine the liver's overall function. When approximately 60% of the liver function is lost, function tests start to become abnormal, and when approximately 80% of liver function is lost, clinical evidence of liver failure usually becomes apparent.[7]

With persistent parenchymal damage (chronic hepatitis) or extensive loss of hepatocytes (massive hepatic necrosis) fibrosis can become extensive. In cirrhosis, collagen becomes deposited in the sinusoids, resulting in altered permeability, the formation of intrahepatic portovenous shunts, and regenerative parenchymal nodules. Impaired hepatic perfusion then results in portal hypertension.[8]

The liver has the special ability to regenerate when a loss of hepatocyte numbers occurs and as long as the reticulin framework remains intact. Following partial hepatectomy, hyperplasia and hypertrophy of the remaining cells occurs. This process is known as "liver regeneration."[9-11] However, regeneration may be a misnomer because the resected lobes never grow back. Potential stimuli for liver regeneration include cytokines and growth factors produced by the hepatocytes but also circulating substances (insulin, norepinephrin, or glucagon).[9-11] These stimuli induce changes in gene expression in hepatocytes, leading to mitotic proliferation of all cells composing the intact organ, including hepatocytes, biliary epithelial cells, and endothelial cells.[9,10]

In healthy dogs, 70% hepatectomy is well tolerated,[12] whereas 84% hepatectomy is usually fatal.[13] The cause of death remains unclear with extensive hepatectomies. It has been postulated that portal hypertension may occur because the reduced portal vasculature is insufficient to accommodate a constant volume of portal blood.[13] Secondary bacterial translocation and death may then ensue.[13] The decreased number of hepatic Küpffer cells after extensive hepatectomy may reduce clearance of bacteria by the liver and possibly lead to sepsis.[14] Changes in laboratory values following extensive hepatectomy have been studied in dogs. Following 70 % hepatectomy in healthy dogs, a small, transient increase in serum alkaline phosphatase, total bilirubin, and transaminases occurs.[12] Monitoring of blood glucose and supplementation of intravenous fluids with dextrose is recommended following extensive hepatectomy.[15] A small transient decrease in serum albumin occurs concurrently.[12] The result of ammonia-tolerance testing is normal following 40% hepatectomy but abnormal after 60% hepatectomy.[7] In one study in healthy dogs, 91% of the liver mass returned 6 weeks following 70 % hepatectomy.[12] Finally, the potential for regeneration after repeated sublethal partial hepatectomies has been studied in rats.[16] Twelve sequential partial hepatectomies were performed and complete regeneration occurred each time,[16] suggesting that the clonogenic potential of the liver may be endless.

Only when the normal hepatic stroma becomes disrupted from either collapse or from collagen deposition does hepatocyte regeneration become disorganized and regeneration result in nodular formation. Regenerative nodules in cirrhosis lose their ability to carry on normal hepatic function.[8]

Risk of Sepsis

The liver of healthy dogs may normally harbor various bacteria.[17] The portal vein of normal dogs often carries gastrointestinal bacteria, which are then normally cleared by the liver. Bacteria are phagocyted by reticuloendothelial cells referred to as Kupffer cells and then either killed or excreted into the bile. Immunoglobulin A production in the liver and bile also contributes to the protection against infectious agents. Impairment of these protective mechanisms may predispose to sepsis or resident bacterial colonization. Acute portal hypertension from loss of normal parenchymal function may allow for translocation of gastrointestinal organisms. Congenital or acquired portosystemic shunts allows gastrointestinal endotoxins or bacteria to bypass the liver, often leading to systemic enterotoxemia or bacteriemia.[18] Animals with intrahepatic or extrahepatic cholestasis,[19] hepatic ischemia, hepatic trauma, or portosystemic shunts may be at risk of sepsis and should be routinely treated with antibiotics perioperatively. The need for postoperative antibiotic is also based on the underlying disease and the condition of the animal.[15] Surgical resolution of biliary obstruction may result in release of bacteria into the biliary tract,[20] and postoperative antibiotic therapy has been recommended in those cases.[20] Antibiotics used should be non-hepatotoxic, have wide distribution in the hepatic tissue and biliary tract, and be bactericidal and effective against the gastrointestinal flora. Ideally, the antibiotic selection should be based on the results of bile or liver culture and sensitivity testing. Recommended empiric perioperative antibiotics include the use of second-generation cephalosporins or possibly a combination of penicillin and fluoroquinolone. In some cases, when anaerobic infections are suspected, metronidazole (Flagyl, Pharmacia) or clindamycin (Antirobe, Pfizer) may also be used.[21] Because metronidazole requires hepatic metabolism, it is recommended that lower doses be used with hepatic disease.

Risk of Hemorrhage

The liver plays a central role in hemostasis. The liver produces all coagulation factors except factor VIII, von Willebrand's factor, calcium, and tissue thromboplastin.[20] It also regulates anticoagulant and fibrinolytic mechanisms.[20] Studies in animals having liver disease found laboratory evidence of abnormal coagulation in 93% dogs and 82% of cats evaluated.[22,23] Mechanisms involved in coagulopathies occur from decreased factor synthesis, vitamin K deficiency,[24] excessive factor consumption, or inadequate clearance of activated factors. Thrombocytopenia and thrombocytopathies have also been reported in association with liver disease.[20] Disseminated intravascular coagulation (DIC) may also be initiated by liver disease because of release of thromboplastic substances by damaged hepatocytes, reduced clearance of intestinal bacterial endotoxins, decreased antithrombin III concentrations, stasis of mesenteric blood flow, and reduced clearance of activated clotting factors and fibrin degradation products.[25] As DIC progresses, fibrin degradation products (FDPs) accumulate, interfering with fibrin polymerization and platelet function.[20] Although mild coagulopathies are common in association with liver disease, clinical evidence of hemorrhage is uncommon.[20,26] In a large study in dogs, significant hemorrhage following ultrasound-guided liver biopsy occurred only when moderate thrombocytopenia was present.[27] Recommended testing in animals with liver disease should include a platelet count, prothrombin time (PT), and activated partial thromboplastin time (APTT). Buccal mucosal bleeding time should also be evaluated in animals with suspected platelet dysfunction. If DIC is suspected, fibrinogen, D-dimers, and FDP concentrations and antithrombin III activity are also measured. In cats with liver disease, measurement of protein invoked by vitamin K absence (PIVKA) is reported to be more sensitive than PT or APTT to detect coagulopathies.[24]

Risk of Gastrointestinal Ulcerations

Liver disease has been associated with ulcerations in both animals and humans. Blood loss from gastrointestinal ulceration not only results in anemia and protein loss but also precipitates hepatic encephalopathy in advanced liver disease or portosystemic shunting.[20] In one study, dogs with liver disease made up 28% of animals with identified gastroduodenal ulcerations.[28] Gastroduodenal ulcerations occur if the normal mucosal protective mechanisms are disrupted. Factors that reduce epithelial cell turnover, affect quality or quantity of gastric mucus production, or decrease gastrointestinal blood flow may induce gastrointestinal ulcerations. The duodenum is the most common site of ulceration in dogs with liver disease.[28] With severe liver disease, negative nitrogen balance and hypoalbuminemia also occur, resulting in decreased turnover of epithelial cells.[20] Portal hypertension also reduces gastrointestinal blood flow.[29-31] The role of gastrin in the pathogenesis of gastroduodenal ulceration secondary to liver disease remains unclear.[20] Because the gastric pH may actually be high in humans with cirrhosis, the prophylactic use of H-2 receptor antagonists in those patients is controversial.[20] Sucralfate (Carafate, Aventis) may be useful prophylactically because it provides cytoprotection and may increase gastric blood flow in cirrhotic animals.[32] Anti-inflammatories (steroidal and nonsteroidal) should be used cautiously in animals with severe liver disease because they may further disrupt mucosal defense mechanisms.[31] Some H-2 receptor antagonists drugs (i.e., cimetidine, Tagamet, SK-Beecham) and the proton pump inhibitors (i.e., omeprazole, Prilosec, Astrazeneca) require hepatic metabolism and are contraindicated in animals with liver disease. Ranitidine is a safe antacid in animals with liver disease because of its minimal involvement in hepatic metabolism.

Hepatic Encephalopathy and Portal Hypertension

These important complications of liver disease will be discussed in detail in the vascular anomalies chapter (Chapter 34).

Classification of Liver Disease

The basic classifications of liver disease in the dog and cat can be divided simply into one of four large categories: parenchymal, biliary, or circulatory disorders, and neoplasia.

Parenchymal Disorders

Damage involving hepatocytes is the hallmark of most of these disorders. The parenchymal disorders can be grouped into those causing reversible hepatocellular injury (cell swelling, steroid-induced hepatopathy, and steatosis), hepatic amyloidosis, hepatocellular death (apoptosis and necrosis), and acute and chronic hepatitis and cirrhosis. Hepatocellular death is a nonreversible injury most often associated with acute and chronic hepatitis, sometimes leading to cirrhosis.

Acute hepatitis is generally secondary to a hypoxic or toxic injury, infectious agents, or metabolic derangements.[33] Damage can be random, zonal, or diffuse throughout the liver. Diffuse or massive liver necrosis can lead to liver failure. Hepatic failure is complicated by the consequences of the loss of normal regulatory functions of synthesis, excretion, and metabolism. In these situations, recovery is possible if the patient can be maintained on life-support measures, if the reticulin framework remains intact, and if the liver retains it ability to regenerate. Metabolic consequences include hepatic encephalopathy, coagulopathies, cerebral edema, sepsis, and gastrointestinal ulceration.[34]

Chronic hepatitis may result secondary to infections, toxins, drugs, and immune mechanisms.[35-37] Many breeds of dogs also have primary metabolic defects in copper metabolism with hepatic copper accumulation causing hepatocyte death. In most clinical situations, the etiology is never determined. Hepatocellular necrosis results in production of cytokines that recruit inflammatory cells locally. In most cases, the inflammatory changes originate in the portal areas but expand into the parenchyma. Inflammation also becomes a stimulus for collagen deposition. If the reticulin framework is destroyed, regeneration becomes disorganized, sinusoidal circulation becomes permanently altered, and the hepatocyte regeneration develops as nodules. Cirrhosis is the end-stage of chronic hepatitis and is defined as a diffuse process characterized by fibrosis of the liver, the conversion of normal liver architecture into structurally abnormal nodules, and the presence of altered vascular circulation with portal-central vein anastomoses.[8]

In addition to the consequences listed with acute liver failure, portal hypertension results from the failure of the portal blood to adequately perfuse the sinusoids. The result of portal hypertension is the development of acquired portosystemic shunting and ascites. Portal collaterals become visible as multiple, tortuous vessels, particularly in the mediastinum along the esophagus, originating from the cardia of the stomach (cardioesophageal anastomoses), in the omentum between the spleen and the left dorsal abdominal wall cranial to the kidney (splenorenal anastomoses), and in the mesocolon and mesorectum (mesenteric anastomoses).[38,39]

Hepatic Biliary Disorders

The biliary disorders can be grouped into cystic disorders and cholangitis. Biliary cysts result from congenital defects in the development of the biliary tree.[40,41] They may be solitary or multiple, of variable size, and are characterized by dilatation of segments of the bile ducts. They are frequently associated with polycystic kidney disease especially in Persian cats. Cysts rarely have connection with the remaining biliary system and are often incidental findings on ultrasound, through palpation, or at surgery. Large cysts may be drained. Occasionally, they require surgical removal.

Cholangitis results from inflammation centered on the bile ducts within the liver. This condition is most commonly observed in cats. An acute neutrophilic (suppurative) cholangitis is thought to result secondary to enteric bacteria ascending the biliary system.[42] The extrahepatic biliary system can also be involved. Cholangitis can become chronic associated with mixed inflammatory infiltrates, bile duct proliferation, and variable fibrosis.[43] Chronic cholangitis is also reported to have an association with chronic pancreatitis and inflammatory bowel disease in cats. Liver flukes also produce bile ductal dilation and chronic cholangitis.

Hepatic Neoplasia

Liver tumors are divided into primary, metastatic, and hemolymphatic neoplasia.[44] In cats, hemolymphatic tumors are most common; whereas metastatic neoplasms are the most common form of liver tumors in dogs.[45] Primary liver tumors comprise less than 1% of findings in all canine and feline necropsies.[46,47] Malignant primary tumors are more common in dogs than in cats.[46,48] Primary liver neoplasms are categorized according to their histologic origin into hepatocellular, biliary, mesenchymal, and neuroectodermal.[46] They may also be divided into massive, nodular, and diffuse forms according to their distribution within the liver.[46] Biliary tumors are discussed in the biliary diseases chapter.

Most dogs and cats with primary liver tumors are 10-years old or older. The exception is in animals with carcinoids, which affect dogs at an average age of 8 years.[46,48] Clinical signs include anorexia, lethargy, vomiting, weight loss, polyuro-polydypsia, diarrhea, jaundice, and abdominal distension.[46,49] An abdominal mass may be palpated in 50% to 80% of cases.[44,49] Other reported findings include seizures associated with hypoglycemia or hepatic encephalopathy and, rarely, exercise-induced weakness owing to myasthenia gravis.[46,50] At the time of diagnosis of primary liver tumor, 28% of animals are asymptomatic.[49]

Laboratory findings are nonspecific and may include thrombocytosis, elevation of liver enzymes, and less commonly, hyperbilirubinemia or hypoglycemia.[45,46,48,51,52] In one study in cats, azotemia was the most common laboratory finding.[53] Thoracic radiographs should be performed to rule out lung metastasis, reported to occur in 14% of cases.[54,55] Abdominal ultrasonography allows confirmation of the hepatic origin of an abdominal mass and evaluation of other abdominal organs for metastasis (peritoneum, lymph nodes), and may help define the relation of the lesion to other abdominal structures such as the caudal vena cava and the gallbladder,[56,57] but it cannot differentiate neoplasia from benign nodular hyperplasia.[58] Fine-needle aspirate or core biopsies can be obtained with ultrasonographic guidance. Prior evaluation of hemostasis is advised as many large hepatic masses may be highly vascular and hemorrhage is a possible complication. MRI has also been proposed as a means to differentiate benign from malignant hepatic nodules in dogs.[59]

Hepatocellular tumors include hepatocellular adenoma, hepatocellular carcinoma, and hepatoblastoma. Hepatocellular adenoma is the most common hepatocellular tumor in cats and rarely has any clinical significance;[48] however, significant hemorrhage and hypoglycemia have been reported.[51] Prognosis is then based on tumor resectability. Hepatocellular carcinoma is the most common primary liver neoplasm in dogs.[44,46] The left liver lobes are most commonly involved.[46,56,60] Massive form is the most common HCC observed in dogs.[44,46,60] They are often resectable, rarely metastasize, and carry a good long-term prognosis after successful surgery.[56] Massive right-sided tumors may have a worse prognosis because of higher intraoperative mortality rate.[56] Nodular or diffuse forms of HCC are less common and carry a poor prognosis because they are rarely resectable and often metastasize.[56,60] Metastases to the lungs, peritoneum, and peritoneal lymph nodes are most common, but metastases to the kidneys, spleen, adrenal glands, gastrointestinal tract, and bone marrow have also been reported.[60] Prognosis is related to resectability and the presence of metastasis.56 Adjuvant therapies such as radiation or chemotherapy are uncommonly used because of poor efficacy.[56]

Carcinoid neoplasms are rare primary liver tumors in dogs and cats.[46,60,61] Carcinoids originate from neuroectodermal hepatic cells. These cells are also classified as enterochromaffin or APUD cells (they are capable of amine precursor uptake and decarboxylation). Prognosis is poor because of diffuse liver involvement and high rate of metastasis.[60]

Mesenchymal tumors or sarcomas are rare primary hepatic tumors in dogs and cats.[44,46,48,56,62] A poor prognosis has been suggested because of early metastasis.[44,46] A combination of surgical resection and adjuvant chemotherapy is recommended.[54,63]

Hepatic nodular hyperplasia (ENH) is a common necropsy finding in dogs.[64,65] It has been reported to occur in 70% of dogs older than 6 and 100% of dogs over 14 years.[64] The etiology of ENH is unknown. In dogs, ENH is not thought to be a preneoplastic lesion.[65] Macroscopically, superficial, multifocal, well-circumscribed, pinkish to pinkish-tan nodules may be seen;[64,65] however, deeper nodules, within the parenchyma are not visible.[64] In a postmortem study, nodule sizes ranged from 0.1 to 5 cm in diameter.[65] Microscopically, well differentiated hyperplastic hepatocytes with increased mitotic activity may be seen.[64,65] The lobular architecture is maintained.[64,65] In affected animals, clinical signs are often lacking.[66] Laboratory findings may include mild to severe increase in serum alkaline phosphatase (up to 14 times normal) and, less commonly, increase in serum alanine aminotransferase.[66] Ultrasonographic findings are nonspecific.[58,67] Hyperplastic nodules may be hyperechoic, isoechoic, or hypoechoic to the surrounding parenchyma.[58] ENH is clinically significant because it may easily be confused with primary or metastatic hepatic neoplasia on abdominal ultrasound or at surgery. Histopathologic study is required to differentiate ENH from neoplasia. However, even microscopically, it may be impossible to differentiate ENH from hepatocellular adenoma;[65] and large samples (wedge rather that needle biopsies) may be required to differentiate ENH from hepatocellular adenocarcinoma.[66]

Other Hepatic Conditions

Liver Torsion

Liver lobe torsion is a rare condition that has been reported in man, rabbits, pigs, horses, dogs, and in one cat.[68-80] The affected lobe rotates around its vascular pedicle causing congestion, cholestasis, and ischemic necrosis.[75-77] Clostridial proliferation may then occur,[73,77,81] occasionally leading to abscessation of the affected lobe.[69] As clostridial toxins and inflammatory mediators are liberated, septic shock and death may follow.[73,77] The left lateral liver lobe is most commonly affected in small animals, but torsion of the quadrate, caudate, and right medial lobes has also been reported.[69,73,75-77,80,82] Factors that cause stretching or rupture of the supporting ligaments of the liver may predispose to liver lobe torsion.[73,77] Congenital absence of the triangular ligaments, chronic gastric dilatation, traumatic diaphragmatic hernia, and tear of the hepatogastric ligament of the lesser omentum have been reported as possible causes.[73,76-78] Hepatic masses may also predispose to lobe torsion.[76] Liver lobe torsion has also been reported following routine ovariohysterectomy.[80] Clinical signs range from low-grade abdominal pain, anorexia, lethargy, vomiting, and ascites to acute abdominal crisis and death.[76] Occasionally a cranial abdominal mass can be palpated.[75] Intermittent clinical signs with intermittent lobe torsion have been described in a child.[83] Diagnostic findings may include an inflammatory leukogram, increased ALT, alkaline phosphatase (ALP), and total bilirubin.[69,76] Abdominal radiographs and ultrasound may reveal a cranial abdominal mass, but definitive diagnosis is often made at surgery or necropsy.[69,76] Preoperative management should include intravenous fluids and antibiotics directed against Clostridium sp. (e.g., ampicillin, Fort Dodge).[81] Immediate surgical intervention with liver lobectomy is indicated.[76] Derotation of the affected lobe is generally avoided because it may lead to systemic release of clostridial exotoxins.[69] The resected lobe should be submitted for cytologic and histopathologic studies and both anaerobic and aerobic bacterial cultures. Antibiotic therapy is continued postoperatively based on results of bacteriologic culture. Prognosis appears to be good if prompt surgical intervention is performed.[68,75,76]

Hepatic Abscesses

Hepatic abscesses are uncommonly reported in humans, dogs, and cats.[69,75,82,84-91] Abscesses may be single or multiple and are associated with high mortality rates in both humans and animals.[82,85] Underlying pathologies in humans include liver trauma, ascending infection from the biliary tract, malignant obstruction of the biliary tract, extension from an adjacent abdominal abscess, and hematogenous spread.[85] Hematogenous spread may be divided into systemic hematogenous (secondary for example to pneumonia, endocarditis, or otitis media) and portal spread from abdominal septic focus (e.g., inflammatory bowel disease, or pancreatitis).[85,88,89] Immunocompromised individuals are also predisposed.[85] In newborn puppies it may occur secondary to ascending omphalophlebitis.[87] In adult dogs and cats, hepatic abscess formation has been associated with diabetes mellitus,[86,90] liver lobe torsion,[69] ascending biliary tract infection,[91] and hepatic neoplasia.[90] In most cases, however, the underlying cause remains unknown.[82,90,91] Clinical signs often are nonspecific and include lethargy, anorexia, and fever.[82,85,90,91] Abdominal pain, jaundice, vomiting, and diarrhea are reported less frequently.[82,90,91] Laboratory findings may include an inflammatory leukogram, mild non-regenerative anemia, and increase in liver enzyme activities.[82,90,91] Hyperbilirubinemia may indicate sepsis or hepatic dysfunction. Hyperbilirubinemia may also be associated with primary biliary obstruction. Disseminated intravascular coagulation has been suspected in both dogs and cats.[82,91] Imaging modalities include abdominal radiographs, ultrasound, computed tomography, and scintigraphy.[85] In humans, the use of WBC-labeled scintigraphy may help differentiate an abscess from a metastatic lesion.[85] Ultrasound-guided or intraoperative aspiration and cytologic evaluation confirm the diagnosis.[82,85,90,91] If ultrasound-guided aspirate is chosen, a surgeon should be available if hemorrhage or contamination of the abdominal cavity occurs.[85] E. coli is the most common bacteria isolated but multiorganism infections are common and anaerobic infections have been reported.[82,85,90,91] Treatment consists of appropriate antibiotic therapy combined with drainage techniques or abscess resection.[85] However, antibiotic therapy alone may be adequate in selected cases, especially when multiple small abscesses are present.[92] Bactericidal antibiotics that are distributed in the liver should be used based on bacteriologic sensitivity results. While awaiting sensitivity results, a four-quadrant antibiotic therapy is recommended. Quinolones in combination with clindamycin have been recommended.[85] Drainage procedures may be surgical or ultrasound-guided. In humans, ultrasound-guided drainage for 11 to19 days with an in situ catheter is the modality of choice and has a high success rate (70-90%).[85] This technique fails in 10% to 30% of cases, and surgical intervention is then required.[85] Repeated ultrasound-guided drainage has also been successful in 10 of 14 dogs.[90] Resolution after ultrasound-guided drainage and alcohol injection has also been reported.[93] Surgical intervention may consist of drainage or abscess resection with partial or complete lobectomy.[82,90,91] Intraoperative identification of parenchymal abscesses may be difficult; however, the use of intraoperative ultrasound may help localize the abscess. Laparotomy allows thorough inspection of abdominal viscera and treatment of the primary disease. If the animal is stable, biopsies of the liver and intestinal tract are indicated to identify an underlying cause. Laparoscopic drainage has also been reported in humans.[94] Regardless of the modality of treatment, frequent ultrasonographic monitoring is indicated.[85] Antibiotic therapy should be continued for at least 2 weeks after ultrasonographic imaging indicates resolution of the abscess.[82] Prognosis is guarded, especially in debilitated animals with septic shock.[82,85,90,91] However, with early diagnosis and treatment, long-term successful outcomes are common in patients who survive the perioperative period.[82,85,90,91]

Hepatic Trauma

Following blunt or penetrating injury, disruption of hepatobiliary structures may occur. Isolated hepatic injuries are uncommonly recognized in small animals. In humans, capsular lacerations, parenchymal fractures, and subscapular hematomas are most common.[95,96] Trauma to the major vascular structures is uncommon.[95,96] In humans, peritoneal lavage, ultrasound, and computed tomography are used to identify and classify hepatic injuries and their severity.[95,96] Conservative management, with intravenous fluids and blood products is advocated in hemodynamically stable patients.[54,96] Heart rate, blood pressure, and packed cell volume (PCV) should be monitored to evaluate the need for surgical intervention. PCV should not be used as sole monitor during acute hemorrhage.[97] Indeed, acute hemorrhage results in splenic contraction and loss of both plasma and red cells.[97] Thus, PCV may remain normal in an animal that is bleeding heavily.[97] Abdominal exploration may be necessary to control severe hemorrhage.

References

1. Burt AD, Portmann BC, McSween RNM: Liver pathology associated with diseases of other organs or systems. *In* Pathology of the Liver, 4th ed. McSween MRN, Burt AD, Portmann BC, et al (eds). Edinburgh: Churchill Livingstone, 2002.

2. Biller DS, Kantrowitz B, Miyabayashi T: Ultrasonography of diffuse liver disease. A review. J Vet Intern Med 6:71, 1992.

3. Stockhaus C, Van Den Ingh T, Rothuizen J, et al: A multistep approach in the cytologic evaluation of liver biopsy samples of dogs with hepatic diseases. Vet Pathol 41:461, 2004.

4. de Rycke LM, van Bree HJ, Simoens PJ: Ultrasound-guided tissue-core biopsy of liver, spleen and kidney in normal dogs. Vet Radiol Ultrasound 40:294, 1999.

5. Cole TL, Center SA, Flood SN, et al: Diagnostic comparison of needle and wedge biopsy specimens of the liver in dogs and cats. J Am Vet Med Assoc 220:1483, 2002.

6. Meyer DJ: Hepatic pathology. *In* Strombeck's Small Animal Gastroenterology, 3rd ed. Guilford WG, Center SA, Strombeck DR, et al (eds). Philadelphia: WB Saunders, 1996, p. 633.

7. Prasse KW, Bjorling DE, Holmes RA, et al: Indocyanine green clearance and ammonia tolerance in partially hepatectomized and hepatic devascularized, anesthetized dogs. Am J Vet Res 44:2320, 1983.

8. Crawford JM: Liver cirrhosis. *In* Pathology of the Liver. McSween RNM, Burt AD, Portmann BC, et al (eds). Edinburgh: Churchill Livingstone, 2002, p. 575.

9. Michalopoulos GK, DeFrances MC: Liver regeneration. Science 276:60, 1997.

10. Fausto N, Riehle KJ: Mechanisms of liver regeneration and their clinical implications. J Hepatobiliary Pancreat Surg 12:181, 2005.

11. Francavilla A, Porter KA, Benichou J, et al: Liver regeneration in dogs: Morphologic and chemical changes. J Surg Res 25:409, 1978.

12. Mackenzie RJ, Furnival CM, O'Keane MA, et al: The effect of hepatic ischaemia on liver function and the restoration of liver mass after 70 per cent pàrtial hepatectomy in the dog. Br J Surg 62:431, 1975.

13. Ogata A, Miyazaki M, Ohtawa S, et al: Short-term effect of portal vein arterialization on hepatic protein synthesis and endotoxaemia after extended hepatectomy in dogs. J Gastroenterol Hepatol 12:633, 1997.

14. Arii S, Shibagaki M, Takahashi S, et al: Changes in the reticuloendothelial phagocytic function after partial hepatectomy. J Lab Clin Med 105:668, 1985.

15. Martin RA, Lanz OI, Tobias KM: Liver and biliary system. *In* Textbook of Small Animal Surgery, 2nd ed. Slatter D (ed). Philadelphia: WB Saunders, 2002, p.708.

16. Stocker E, Wullstein HK, Brau G: [Capacity of regeneration in liver epithelia of juvenile, repeated partially hepatectomized rats. Autoradiographic studies after continous infusion of 3h-thymidine (author's transl)]. Virchows Arch B Cell Pathol 14:93, 1973.

17. Niza MM, Ferreira AJ, Peleteiro MC, et al: Bacteriological study of the liver in dogs. J Small Anim Pract 45:401, 2004.

18. Howe LM, Boothe DM, Boothe HW: Endotoxemia associated with experimentally induced multiple portosystemic shunts in dogs. Am J Vet Res 58:83, 1997.

19. Cardoso V, Pimenta A, da Fonseca JC, et al: The effect of cholestasis on hepatic clearance of bacteria. World J Surg 6:330, 1982.

20. Center SA: Pathophysiology of liver disease: Normal and abnormal function. *In* Strombeck's Small Animal Gastroenterology, 3rd ed. Guilford WG, Center SA, Strombeck DR, et al (eds). Philadelphia: WB Saunders, 1996, p. 553.

21. Hirsh DC, Jang SS: Anaerobic infections. *In* Infectious Diseases of the Dog and Cat. Green CE (ed). Philadelphia: WB Saunders, 1998, p. 258.

22. Badylak SF, Dodds WJ, Van Vleet JF: Plasma coagulation factor abnormalities in dogs with naturally occurring hepatic disease. Am J Vet Res 44:2336. 1983.

23. Lisciandro SC, Hohenhaus A, Brooks M: Coagulation abnormalities in 22 cats with naturally occurring liver disease. J Vet Intern Med 12:71, 1998.

24. Center SA, Warner K, Corbett J, et al: Proteins invoked by vitamin k absence and clotting times in clinically ill cats. J Vet Intern Med 14:292, 2000.

25. Fiore LD, Brophy MT, Deykin D: Hemostasis. *In* Hepatology, A Textbook of Liver Disease, 4th ed. Zakim D, Boyer TD (eds). Philadelphia: WB Saunders, 2003, p. 549.

26. McVay PA, Toy PT: Lack of increased bleeding after liver biopsy in patients with mild hemostatic abnormalities. Am J Clin Pathol 94:747, 1990.

27. Bigge LA, Brown DJ, Penninck DG: Correlation between coagulation profile findings and bleeding complications after ultrasound-guided biopsies: 434 cases (1993-1996). J Am Anim Hosp Assoc 37:228, 2001.

28. Stanton ME, Bright RM: Gastroduodenal ulceration in dogs. Retrospective study of 43 cases and literature review. J Vet Intern Med3:238, 1989.

29. Albillos A, Colombato LA, Enriquez R, et al: Sequence of morphological and hemodynamic changes of gastric microvessels in portal hypertension. Gastroenterology 102:2066, 1992.

30. Sarfeh IJ, Tarnawski A, Malki A, et al: Portal hypertension and gastric mucosal injury in rats. Effects of alcohol. Gastroenterology 84:987, 1983.

31. Sarfeh IJ, Tarnawski A: Gastric mucosal vasculopathy in portal hypertension. Gastroenterology 93:1129, 1987.

32. Chen BW, Hiu WM, Lam SK, et al: Effect of sucralfate on gastric mucosal blood flow in rats. Gut 30:1544, 1989.

33. Hughes D, King LG: The diagnosis and management of acute liver failure in dogs and cats. Vet Clin North Am Small Anim Pract 25:437, 1995.

34. MacPhail CM, Lappin MR, Meyer DJ, et al: Hepatocellular toxicosis associated with administration of carprofen in 21 dogs. J Am Vet Med Assoc 212:1895, 1998.

35. Bunch SE, Castleman WL, Hornbuckle WE, et al: Hepatic cirrhosis associated with long-term anticonvulsant drug therapy in dogs. J Am Vet Med Assoc 181:357, 1982.

36. Rakich PM, Prasse KW, Lukert PD, et al: Immunohistochemical detection of canine adenovirus in paraffin sections of liver. Vet Pathol 23:478, 1986.

37. Twedt DC, Sternlieb I, Gilbertson SR: Clinical, morphologic, and chemical studies on copper toxicosis of Bedlington terriers. J Am Vet Med Assoc 175:269, 1979.

38. Kelly WR: The liver and biliary system. *In* Pathology of Domestic Animals, 4th ed. Jubb KVF, Kennedy PC, N (eds). San Diego: Academic Press, 1992, p. 319.

39. Szatmari V, van den Ingh TS, Fenyves B, et al: Portal hypertension in a dog due to circumscribed fibrosis of the wall of the extrahepatic portal vein. Vet Rec 150:602, 2002.

40. Bosje JT, van den Ingh TS, van der Linde-Sipman JS: Polycystic kidney and liver disease in cats. Vet Q 20:136, 1998.

41. Gorlinger S, Rothuizen J, Bunch S, et al: Congenital dilatation of the bile ducts (Caroli's disease) in young dogs. J Vet Intern Med 17:28, 2003.

42. Lucke VM, Davies JD: Progressive lymphocytic cholangitis in the cat. J Small Anim Pract 25:249, 1984.

43. van den Ingh TS, Rothuizen J, van Zinnicq Bergman HM: Destructive cholangiolitis in seven dogs. Vet Q 10:240, 1988.

44. Trigo FJ, Thompson H, Breeze RG, et al: The pathology of liver tumours in the dog. J Comp Pathol 92:21, 1982.

45. Hammer AS, Sikkema DA: Hepatic neoplasia in the dog and cat. Vet Clin North Am Small Anim Pract 25:419, 1995.

46. Patnaik AK, Hurvitz AI, Lieberman PH: Canine hepatic neoplasms: A clinicopathologic study. Vet Pathol 17:553, 1980.

47. Strombeck DR: Clinicopathologic features of primary and metastatic neoplastic disease of the liver in dogs. J Am Vet Med Assoc 173:267, 1978.

48. Lawrence HJ, Erb HN, Harvey HJ: Nonlymphomatous hepatobiliary masses in cats: 41 cases (1972 to 1991). Vet Surg 23:365, 1994.

49. Kosovsky JE, Manfra-Marretta S, Matthiesen DT, et al: Results of partial hepatectomy in 18 dogs with hepatocellular carcinoma. J Am Anim Hosp Assoc 25:203, 1989.

50. Krotje LJ, Fix AS, Potthoff AD: Acquired myasthenia gravis and cholangiocellular carcinoma in a dog. J Am Vet Med Assoc 197:488, 1990.

51. Strombeck DR, Krum S, Meyer D, et al: Hypoglycemia and hypoinsulinemia associated with hepatoma in a dog. J Am Vet Med Assoc 169:811, 1976.

52. Leifer CE, Peterson ME, Matus RE, et al: Hypoglycemia associated with nonislet cell tumor in 13 dogs. J Am Vet Med Assoc 186:53, 1985.

53. Post G, Patnaik AK: Nonhematopoietic hepatic neoplasms in cats: 21 cases (1983-1988). J Am Vet Med Assoc 201:1080, 1992.

54. Kudnig S, Monnet E: Liver. *In* Textbook of Small Animal Surgery, 2nd ed. Slatter D (ed). Philadelphia: WB Saunders, 2002, p.2378.

55. Evans SM: The radiographic appearance of primary liver neoplasia in dogs. Vet Radiol 28:192, 1987.

56. Liptak JM, Dernell WS, Monnet E, et al: Massive hepatocellular carcinoma in dogs: 48 cases (1992-2002). J Am Vet Med Assoc 225:1225, 2004.

57. Feeney DA, Johnston GR, Hardy RM: Two-dimensional, gray-scale ultrasonography for assessment of hepatic and splenic neoplasia in the dog and cat. J Am Vet Med Assoc 184:68, 1984.

58. Stowater JL, Lamb CR, Schelling SH: Ultrasonographic features of canine hepatic nodular hyperplasia. Vet Radiol 31. 1990.

59. Clifford CA, Pretorius ES, Weisse C, et al: Magnetic resonance imaging of focal splenic and hepatic lesions in the dog. J Vet Intern Med 18:330, 2004.

60. Patnaik AK, Hurvitz AI, Lieberman PH, et al: Canine hepatocellular carcinoma. Vet Pathol 18:427, 1981.

61. Alexander RW, Kock RA: Primary hepatic carcinoid (apud cell carcinoma) in the cat. J Small Anim Pract 23:767, 1982.

62. Minkus G, Hillemanns M: Botryoid-type embryonal rhabdomyosarcoma of liver in a young cat. Vet Pathol 34:618, 1997.

63. Hammer AS, Couto CG, Filppi J, et al: Efficacy and toxicity of vac chemotherapy (vincristine, doxorubicin, and cyclophosphamide) in dogs with hemangiosarcoma. J Vet Intern Med 5:160, 1991.

64. Bergman JR: Nodular hyperplasia in the liver of the dog: An association with changes in the ito cell population. Vet Pathol 22:427, 1985.

65. Fabry A, Benjamin SA, Angleton GM: Nodular hyperplasia of the liver in the beagle dog. Vet Pathol 19:109, 1982.

66. Prause LC, Twedt DC: Hepatic nodular hyperplasia. *In* Kirk's Current Veterinary Therapy 13. Bonagura JD (ed). Philadelphia: WB Saunders, 1999, p. 675.

67. Cuccovillo A, Lamb CR: Cellular features of sonographic target lesions of the liver and spleen in 21 dogs and a cat. Vet Radiol Ultrasound 43:275, 2002.

68. Bedda S, Bataille N, Montariol T, et al: Accessory liver lobe torsion mimicking a pancreatic tumor. Ann Chir 128:53, 2003.

69. Downs MO, Miller MA, Cross AR, et al: Liver lobe torsion and liver abscess in a dog. J Am Vet Med Assoc 212:678, 1998.

70. Grunz J, Luisiri A, Cradock T: Torsion of a hepatic lobe in the neonate--ultrasound findings. Pediatr Radiol 22:192, 1992.

71. Koplewitz BZ, Manson DE, Ein SH: Posttraumatic torsion of accessory lobe of the liver and the gallbladder. Pediatr Radiol 29:799, 1999.

72. Koumanidou C, Nasi E, Koutrouveli E, et al: Torsion of an accessory hepatic lobe in a child: Ultrasound, computed tomographic, and magnetic resonance imaging findings. Pediatr Surg Int 13:526, 1998.

73. McConkey S, Briggs C, Solano M, et al: Liver torsion and associated bacterial peritonitis in a dog. Can Vet J 38:438, 1997.

74. Sanguesa C, Esteban MJ, Gomez J, et al: Liver accessory lobe torsion in the infant. Pediatr Radiol 25:153, 1995.

75. Sonnenfield JM, Armbrust LJ, Radlinsky MA, et al: Radiographic and ultrasonographic findings of liver lobe torsion in a dog. Vet Radiol Ultrasound 42:344, 2001.

76. Swann HM, Brown DC: Hepatic lobe torsion in 3 dogs and a cat. Vet Surg 30:482, 2001.

77. Tomlinson J, Black A: Liver lobe torsion in a dog. J Am Vet Med Assoc 183:225, 1983.

78. Tate PS: Hepatic torsion and dislocation with hypotension and colonic obstruction. Am Surg 59:455, 1993.

79. Weisbroth SH: Torsion of the caudate lobe of the liver in the domestic rabbit (oryctolagus). Vet Pathol 12:13, 1975.

80. Woolfe DT, English B: Torsion of the left lateral and papillary lobes of the liver in a pup; a case report. J Am Vet Med Assoc 134:458, 1959.

81. Markowitz J, Rappaport A, Scott AC: The function of the hepatic artery in the dog. Am J Dig Dis 16:344, 1949.

82. Farrar ET, Washabau RJ, Saunders HM: Hepatic abscesses in dogs: 14 cases (1982-1994). J Am Vet Med Assoc 208:243, 1996.

83. Fogh J, Tromholt N, Jorgensen F: Persistent impairment of liver function caused by a pendulated accessory liver lobe. Eur J Nucl Med 15:326, 1989.

84. Berger H, Pratschke E, Berr F, Fink U: Percutaneous drainage treatment of primary liver abscesses. Rofo 150:167, 1989.

85. Frey CF, Zhu Y, Suzuki M, et al: Liver abscesses. Surg Clin North Am 69:259, 1989.

86. Grooters AM, Sherding RG, Biller DS, et al: Hepatic abscesses associated with diabetes mellitus in two dogs. J Vet Intern Med 8:203, 1994.

87. Hargis AM, Thomassen RW: Hepatic abscesses in beagle puppies. Lab Anim Sci 30:689, 1980.

88. Hazzan D, Fishman E, Heller E, et al. Liver abscess in Crohn's disease: A report of three cases. Mt Sinai J Med 71:351, 2004.

89. Margalit M, Elinav H, Ilan Y, et al: Liver abscess in inflammatory bowel disease: Report of two cases and review of the literature. J Gastroenterol Hepatol 19:1338, 2004.

90. Schwarz LA, Penninck DG, Leveille-Webster C: Hepatic abscesses in 13 dogs: A review of the ultrasonographic findings, clinical data and therapeutic options. Vet Radiol Ultrasound 39:357, 1998.

91. Sergeeff JS, Armstrong PJ, Bunch SE: Hepatic abscesses in cats: 14 cases (1985-2002). J Vet Intern Med 18:295, 2004.

92. Calvo-Romero JM, Lima-Rodriguez EM: Favourable outcome of multiple pyogenic liver abscesses with conservative treatment. Scand J Infect Dis 37:141, 2005.

93. Zatelli A, Bonfanti U, Zini E: Percutaneous drainage and alcoholization of hepatic abscesses in five dogs and a cat. JAm Anim Hosp Assoc 41:34, 2005.

94. Wang W, Lee WJ, Wei PL, et al: Laparoscopic drainage of pyogenic liver abscesses. Surg Today 34:323, 2004.

95. Feliciano DV: Surgery for liver trauma. Surgl Clin North Am 69:273, 1989.

96. Pachter HL, Spencer FC, Hofstetter SR, et al: Significant trends in the treatment of hepatic trauma. Experience with 411 injuries. Ann Surg 215:492, 1992.

97. Crane SW: Evaluation and management of abdominal trauma in the dog and cat. Vet Clin North Am 10:655, 1980.

Chapter 33

Extrahepatic Biliary Obstruction

Michael D. King
Robert A. Martin

Anatomy

The intrahepatic portion of the biliary system originates where bile, produced by sheets of liver cells surrounded by blood sinuses, is discharged into minute bile canaliculi that lie between these cells.[1] Interlobular ducts are formed from the unification of the canaliculi and lie between the lobules in the interstitial tissue. The interlobular ducts unite further to form lobar or bile ducts that exit the liver parenchyma as a variable number of hepatic ducts, beginning the extrahepatic portion of the biliary system. Usually there are four such ducts, two originating from the central division of the liver (quadrate and right medial lobes), and one each from the right (right lateral lobe and caudate process of the caudate lobe) and left (left lateral and medial lobes, papillary process of the caudate lobe) divisions.

The gallbladder is a pear-shaped structure, located within a fossa formed between the right medial and quadrate lobes of the liver. It is divided into a fundus, body, and neck and connects with the bile duct via the cystic duct. Its function is to store and concentrate bile and secrete a mucoid substance for lubrication and protection. The cystic duct extends from the neck of the gallbladder to the site of its junction with the first hepatic duct from the central liver division. From this level distally to the duodenum the main excretory channel that receives bile from the hepatic ducts from the left and right liver divisions is the bile duct.[1]

The free portion of the canine bile duct is approximately 5 cm long and 2.5 mm in diameter and courses through the lesser omentum to the duodenum within the hepatoduodenal ligament.[1] The intramural portion of the bile duct enters the mesenteric wall of the duodenum and courses obliquely for an additional 1.5 to 2 cm before terminating at the major duodenal papilla, separate from the ventral pancreatic duct. A double layer of smooth muscle (sphincter of Oddi) exists around the intramural portion of the bile duct, resulting in the discharge of bile being largely dependent on activity of the duodenum itself.[1]

An auxiliary retroportal network of bile ducts is reported to exist in dogs.[2] These additional ducts connect the intrahepatic lobar ducts of adjacent liver lobes to allow for continued drainage of bile when primary pathways are obstructed.

Specific features of note in the cat include the flexuosity of the feline cystic duct, and the existence of double or even triple gallbladders on occasion.[3,4] Additionally, the terminal intramural portion of the bile duct usually merges with the major pancreatic duct to empty into the duodenum through a common ampulla.[3-5]

Bile Formation, Flow, and Pathophysiologic Alterations

Bile is a slightly alkaline, isotonic solution that consists of water, inorganic electrolytes, and organic solutes such as bile acids, cholesterol, phospholipids, and bilirubin.[5,6] Primary bile is produced in the canaliculi as a result of several different active transport processes, with secretion of bile salts the most important factor in promoting bile flow.[7] This active transport of solutes by the hepatocytes is accompanied by passive water flow.[5]

Bile acids are produced from cholesterol, conjugated by hepatocytes, and secreted continuously into canaliculi. They are essential for the emulsification and absorption of fat from the small intestine.[6,8] The term bile acid refers to the molecular form in which the carboxylic acid side chain is nonionized; while the term bile salt refers to the ionized configuration. At physiologic pH the ionized bile salt form predominates.[5] More than 90% of the solutes within bile consist of bile acids and can represent a concentration 10^5-fold greater than serum bile acid concentrations.[5] They are maintained in solution in bile by formation of micelles, so an isosmotic balance is maintained with plasma. The rate of bile acid production is determined by the amount delivered to the liver for resecretion via enterohepatic circulation. With biliary obstruction, a decrease in bile acid production results from the increased plasma levels of bile acids.

Cholesterol is synthesized primarily in the liver, with the rate of synthesis related inversely to its level of dietary intake. Synthesis of bile acids from cholesterol with excretion through the gastrointestinal tract represents the major method of excretion of cholesterol from the body. Although not water-soluble, cholesterol exists in normal bile in the form of micelles. Because lipid solubility is the major determining factor for absorption of solutes by the gallbladder mucosa, cholesterol is present within bile in lower quantities than water-soluble compounds such as conjugated bile acids and bilirubin.[5]

Bilirubin, the major pigment in bile, is a product of hemoprotein degradation, two thirds of which is estimated to come from erythrocyte breakdown.[5] The unconjugated bilirubin is poorly water-soluble and binds to plasma proteins (predominantly albumin) for transport within the vascular space. Only a very small amount of unconjugated bilirubin remains unbound to plasma proteins because of albumin's high binding affinity for it, and this minimizes its renal filtration and excretion. Protein-bound unconjugated bilirubin is transported to liver for conversion by hepatocytes into a water-soluble form. The bilirubin is conjugated with glucuronic acid to diglucuronide in the smooth endoplasmic reticulum of the hepatocytes. Conjugated bilirubin is then either excreted into the bile canaliculi or removed from the body via renal filtration. More than two thirds of the bilirubin present within the liver at any time is unconjugated, yet less than 3% of bilirubin excreted within the bile is in this form.[5,9] This illustrates the importance of enzymatic presence and function as the rate-limiting steps in bilirubin conjugation.[5] Once excreted into the intestinal tract, the conjugated bilirubin undergoes bacterial deconjugation, with conversion to urobilinogen, some of which is resorbed through the enterohepatic circulation. The majority of this is returned to the liver, and a small portion is excreted in the urine. The remaining urobilinogen in the intestinal tract is further converted to stercobilin, which imparts normal fecal color.[9] Feces absent of normal color are termed acholic. This occurs from either a lack of bilirubin present within the intestinal tract (biliary obstruction) or a deficiency in intestinal bacterial activity.[5] Since only a small amount of bilirubin is needed for normal fecal pigmentation, complete cessation of bilirubin excretion is usually required for the formation of acholic feces. This is not seen until 7 to 10 days after complete blockage of the biliary system, when jaundice is also readily apparent.[5,9]

Biliary obstruction can occur in a variety of disease processes (Table 33-1). With biliary obstruction, bilirubin conjugation occurs normally but secretion in the bile is inhibited. Regurgitation of conjugated bile back into the plasma then occurs, causing hyperbilirubinemia. While the majority remains protein-bound in plasma, it has a less profound binding affinity when compared with unconjugated bilirubin. The liver maintains a high reserve capacity for bilirubin excretion, capable of increasing up to 30 to 60 times above normal.[5] Because of this reserve, dogs must regurgitate considerable amounts of bilirubin into the bloodstream before a significant increase in plasma levels occurs. The dog's renal threshold for bilirubin is low, with active excretion within the renal tubules possible. The renal threshold in cats is 9 times greater than that in the dog, and because of this, any bilirubin in the urine of cats should be considered abnormal.10 In cases of bile duct obstruction, renal filtration and excretion become essential.[5]

Table 33-1. Causes of Extrahepatic Biliary Obstruction

Congenital

- Biliary atresia
- Choledochal cysts

Acquired

- Luminal
  - Inspissated bile
  - Parasites (flukes)
  - Stones (choleliths, choledocholiths)
  - Blood clots
- Mural
  - Cholangitis (infectious, sclerosing)
  - Neoplasia (biliary carcinoma)
  - Cholecystitis
  - Stricture
  - Hematoma
- Extraluminal
  - Pancreatitis (chronic fibrosing, acute)
  - Neoplasia (pancreatic, lymph node, gastrointestinal)
  - Abscess
  - Duodenal foreign body
  - Diaphragmatic hernia
  - Perforating ulcer (gastric, duodenal)

Intra- or extrahepatic obstruction of the biliary system is the most common cause of conjugated hyperbilirubinemia (Table 33-1). However, nearly all hepatic diseases associated with hyperbilirubinemia consist of a mixture of conjugated and unconjugated bilirubinemia; differentiation is unlikely to be clinically useful.[9] Serum bilirubin levels over 0.3 mg/dl in the cat and 0.6 mg/dl in the dog are considered abnormal; at higher values, jaundice becomes visible clinically as yellow-stained tissues (serum levels > 2.0 mg/dl) or in serum (serum levels > 1.5 mg/dl).[9]

Flow of bile within the canine biliary system is dependent on pressure gradients because no valves are present. The increased pressure of the intramural component of the bile duct results in direction of the bile flow from the liver into the cystic duct and the gallbladder. The capacity of the gallbladder is about 1 ml per kg bodyweight; however, a much greater volume of bile can be accommodated by the gallbladder by mucosal absorption of water and electrolytes.[5] Active transport of sodium through the gallbladder epithelium is followed by passive transport of chloride, water, and other soluble constituents. Thus, bile is concentrated between 5- and 20-fold while in the gallbladder and this prevents a rise in pressure within the biliary system.[5,8]

The gallbladder does not simply fill continuously during fasting; rather, partial emptying occurs intermittently; approximately 75% of the bile excreted from the liver is released directly into the duodenum in this way.[5] The gallbladder has emptied 50% or more of its bile into the intestinal tract within 30 minutes following a meal.[4] The presence of chyme in the duodenum stimulates the release of cholecystokinin from duodenal mucosa as the primary regulator of gallbladder emptying. Cholecystokinin causes contraction of the gallbladder as well as relaxation of the terminal bile duct (sphincter of Oddi). In addition, vagal parasympathetic stimulation and, even more importantly, the presence of duodenal peristalsis itself contributes to relaxation of the smooth muscle surrounding the intramural bile duct, resulting in bile being expelled into the intestine with intermittent spurts[1,5,8] Obstruction of the bile duct increases intraductal pressure proximal to the obstruction, causing vascular dilatation. With increasing pressure bile flow decreases; at pressures of approximately 30 mm Hg it stops.[11] This increased hydrostatic pressure produces characteristic morphologic alterations to the liver.

Morphologic Alterations of the Liver

Soon after obstruction, intrahepatic cholestasis is followed by bile duct dilation and edema with inflammatory cell infiltration of portal areas. These changes occur from both initial increased hydrostatic pressure and toxic effects of bile leakage into periportal areas. In any disease process where cholestasis occurs there is the potential for hepatocellular damage. Bile acid retention causes injury to organelles, hydropic degeneration of hepatocellular tissue, and destruction of the cytochrome P-450 system.[5,7] In cases of chronic severe cholestasis, hepatocytes undergo degenerative necrosis and cirrhosis can occur.[5,7,12] An increase occurs in both fibroblast and hepatocyte collagen synthesis, with a concomitant reduction in hepatic collagenase activity, which results in fibrosis.[7,10]

Following bile duct obstruction, proliferation of both hepatocellular and preexisting biliary epithelial cells occurs, resulting in a new tortuous periportal ductal system. With prolonged duct obstruction, metaplasia of hepatocytes can occur and further contribute to the neo-duct network. Increased hydrostatic pressure in obstructed ducts is necessary for this proliferation, and once obstruction is relieved, additional bile ducts may regress.[5]

Physiologic Alterations of Digestion

Efficient digestion of fats in the intestinal tract largely depends on the presence and function of bile salts and the phospholipid lecithin.[5,8] Bile salts and lecithin act to first emulsify ingested lipids into smaller particles, and then to form micelles around monoglycerides and free fatty acids derived from pancreatic lipase activity. This allows for continued digestion of remaining fat globules and for efficient transport of the monoglycerides and free fatty acids to the intestinal epithelium. Bile salts and lecithin perform a similar transportation role in digestion of dietary cholesterol. Although intestinal absorption of free fatty acids can occur without bile salt micelles, absorption of cholesterol cannot, making the presence of bile even more critical.[8] The most important cause of clinically significant bile acid deficiency is extrahepatic biliary obstruction. Steatorrhea, weight loss, and acholic feces may result.

In situations of decreased intestinal absorption of fats, there is concurrent malabsorption of fat-soluble vitamins (A,D, E, and K), vitamin K being the most clinically significant.[7-9] The formation of functionally active forms of five important clotting factors (prothrombin, factors VII, IX, X, and protein C) is dependent on vitamin K, with its deficiency leading to potential blood dyscrasias. Because factor VII has the shortest half-life of these clotting factors, prothrombin time will usually be prolonged before partial thromboplastin time.[13] Vitamin K is continually produced by intestinal bacteria and clinical manifestation of deficiency is uncommon, except in cases of impaired fat absorption.[5,8,10,13]

Diversion of bile from the duodenum (extrahepatic biliary obstruction or surgical diversion via cholecystojejunostomy) not only affects fat digestion but also results in increased gastric acid secretion, with duodenal ulceration as a frequent sequela.[5,14] It is theorized that decreased absorption of fat in the duodenum results in a decrease in cholecystokinin activation (a competitive gastrin inhibitor), causing increased serum gastrin levels and subsequent peptic ulceration.[14] Also, hormonal inhibition of gastric acid secretion may be decreased in cases of biliary obstruction or surgical diversion of bile away from the duodenum.[14] Finally, neutralization of gastric acid is decreased in the absence of bile, which can lead to duodenal ulceration.

Cholelithiasis

Cholelithiasis is uncommon in animals and is often an asymptomatic incidental finding, usually at necropsy. Clinical signs are seen when biliary stones are associated with cholecystitis, biliary obstruction, or gallbladder rupture.[15] The incidence of cholelithiasis in dogs is reported at less than 1% of patients with biliary disease;[16] only a few cases have been reported in cats.[10,17] In animals, bile pigment stones predominate, in contrast to the cholesterol-based stones seen in people.[5] Choleliths seen in dogs and cats also tend to be lower in calcium than are human stones because of the efficiency of the gallbladder in resorbing free calcium from bile.[5]

Biliary stasis has been theorized as a potential cause of cholelith formation in animals because this is a common element seen in clinical disease. In contrast to humans, abnormal cholesterol metabolism does not seem to be a significant component of canine and feline choleliths.[5,15,18] Trauma, cholecystitis, dietary alterations, and parasitic or bacterial infections have also been proposed as predisposing factors.[10,15] Bile stasis results in pigment sludge formation with mucin-bilirubin particles present in the gallbladder. As the mucin component increases, sludge particles precipitate as stones.[5]

Both bile stasis and biliary infection are commonly seen in disease associated with cholelithiasis in animals; however, infection is not thought to be a necessary component of stone formation because choleliths occur frequently in the absence of infection. Also, the relatively high incidence of stones seen as an incidental finding at necropsy suggests clinical disease arises only when the biliary system containing stones becomes obstructed or infected. However, suppurative cholecystitis is inherently lithogenic because of prostaglandin-mediated inflammatory processes, increased mucin production, and the presence of bacterial enzymes.[5]

Although the gallbladder is the most common site of choledocholith formation, stones can form primarily within the bile duct.[11,19] This usually requires an abnormality that produces bile stasis such as partial obstruction and marked dilatation.[11]

Surgical Considerations

Preoperative Considerations

A vitamin K deficiency and subsequent coagulopathy can occur with complete bile duct obstruction over a period of weeks, but is unlikely in most clinical cases in the dog and cat.[5,9] Hemostasis testing is recommended, however, in patients with potentially chronic obstruction, most commonly by determination of prothrombin and partial thromboplastin times.[10,20] Prolonged partial thromboplastin time has been identified as a poor prognostic indicator in dogs undergoing extrahepatic biliary surgery.[21] The more specific test for potential vitamin K deficiency is that for "proteins induced by vitamin K absence or antagonists" (PIVKA).[5,22] This test evaluates the occurrence of both depleted vitamin K-dependent coagulation factors and build-up of PIVKA. PIVKA are circulating nonfunctional precursor forms of vitamin K-dependent proteins that are normally stored in the liver but accumulate and spill into the circulation when a vitamin K deficiency occurs. Results are expressed in seconds, with marked elevations in PIVKA time warranting treatment. Parenteral administration of vitamin K1 can correct the coagulopathy in these cases,[10,20] with an initial loading dose of 5 mg/kg bodyweight, followed by a 2.5 mg/kg bodyweight daily dose divided every 8 hours until the biliary obstruction has been relieved and coagulation times returned to normal.[22] Altough tests for PIVKA are sensitive and can detect early evidence of vitamin K deficiency, they are not as widely used clinically as other coagulation profile assessments.[22]

In addition to administration of vitamin K, patients with evidence of coagulopathies may require transfusion of whole fresh blood or fresh frozen plasma to replenish coagulation factors or packed red blood cells if they are anemic. It may take up to 12 hours for vitamin K administration to significantly decrease the prothrombin time and subsequently decrease bleeding.[22]

Antibiotics should be administered perioperatively when surgery is performed for biliary obstruction. Although normal bile is sterile, in situations of impaired bile flow, positive cultures have been frequently reported in people.[5] Hepatocellular damage secondary to biliary obstruction may decrease the effectiveness of the Kupffer cells in removing bacteria and bacterial endotoxins from the liver.[5] Empirical preoperative administration of broad spectrum intravenous antibiotics is recommended and should be active against enteric organisms commonly detected in biliary obstruction (Escherichia coli, Klebsiella, Proteus, Streptococcus, Pseudomonas, and Clostridium species). Examples include cephalosporins, or potentiated ampicillin, and fluoroquinolones plus metronidazole. These should be continued postoperatively depending on surgical findings, patient condition, and results of bacterial culture and antibiotic sensitivity testing of bile.

It has been well established that bilirubin is damaging to cells, with unconjugated bilirubin more toxic than the conjugated form because of its increased lipid affinity. However, the high binding affinity of unconjugated bilirubin with albumin reduces widespread tissue distribution and, therefore, limits its deleterious effects.[5] Free unconjugated bilirubin crosses the blood-brain barrier, causing neurotoxicity; this has been shown to result in hypotensive shock and death in dogs.[5] Additionally, hyperbilirubinemia is associated with renal failure in dogs and cats, theorized to be caused by direct cellular toxicity, hypotensive ischemia, or absorption of bacterial endotoxins.[5,21] Hypotension is commonly seen in cases of biliary obstruction and has been identified as a poor prognostic indicator. This is thought to be a result of a combination of the toxic effects of bilirubin and the development of systemic inflammatory response syndrome (SIRS).[21] Both preoperative and intraoperative efforts to monitor and maintain systemic blood pressure are essential in these patients.

Intraoperative Considerations

Liver biopsy should be performed routinely during surgery for extrahepatic biliary obstruction, including cases of cholelithiasis. Histopathologic evaluation of the liver provides information on the severity and progression of structural liver alterations and may prove beneficial in the diagnosis, prognosis, and long-term management of the patient postoperatively. A biopsy taken from the margin of a liver lobe (guillotine method) or from a more centrally located region of a lobe (biopsy punch technique) should be representative of the generalized parenchymal changes associated with extrahepatic biliary obstruction. Intraoperative culture of bile is essential to appropriately direct antimicrobial therapy in the postoperative period, as well as to provide prognostic information. The presence of septic bile peritonitis (traumatic rupture, cholecystitis, or extrahepatic biliary obstruction) is a negative prognostic indicator with 50% to 75% mortality in dogs, compared with less than 15% mortality for those patients with a nonseptic effusion.[21]

Cholecystectomy is preferred over cholecystotomy for stone removal. Secondary changes to the gallbladder that result from the presence of stones or concurrent infection include mucosal hyperplasia, inflammation, and necrosis. Removing the gallbladder eliminates a reservoir for subsequent stone formation and minimizes potential risks of dehiscence or increased morbidity that might occur with cholecystotomy.

Determination of patency of the remaining extrahepatic biliary tract is vital to surgical outcome. A duodenotomy created over the major duodenal papilla allows retrograde cannulation of the bile duct when patency cannot be determined from cannulation through the cystic duct. In cases of biliary obstruction or stricture unrelated to stones, a bile flow diversion procedure should be employed when the obstruction cannot be relieved. Furthermore, in extremely ill patients, temporary external biliary decompression using a cholecystostomy tube or intermittent percutaneous aspiration of the gallbladder should be considered until improved patient homeostasis can be achieved.[23] A definitive but more complicated diversion technique can be used when the patient's condition improves.

When bile diversion is required, cholecystoduodenostomy is the procedure of choice for the dog and cat. A wide anastomotic stoma (2.5 to 4 cm) can be created to reduce the possibility of postoperative stricture and secondary cholangitis. Bile that is redirected into the duodenum maintains normal digestion and intestinal homeostasis.

References

1. Evans HE: Miller's Anatomy of the Dog, 3rd ed. Philadelphia: WB Saunders, 1993.

2. Sleight DR, Thomford NR: Gross anatomy of the blood supply and biliary drainage of the canine liver. Anat Rec 166:153-160, 1970.

3. Bjorling DE: Surgical management of hepatic and biliary disease in cats. Comp Cont Educ Pract Vet 13:1419-1422, 1424-1425, 1991.

4. Hitt ME, Jones BD, Constantinescu G: The feline liver: what a practitioner needs to know. Vet Med 82:129-138, 1987.

5. Guilford WG, Center SA, Strombeck DR, et al: Strombeck's Small Animal Gastroenterology, 3rd ed. Philadelphia: WB Saunders, 1996.

6. Rogers WA: Disease of the Liver. *In:* Canine and Feline Gastroenterology. Jones BD (ed). Philadelphia: WB Saunders, 1986, pp. 345-379.

7. Twedt DC: Symposium on liver diseases. Vet Clin North Am Small Anim Pract 15:281, 1985.

8. Guyton AC, Hall JE: Textbook of Medical Physiology, 9th ed. Philadelphia: WB Saunders, 1996

9. Bunch SE: Hepatobiliary and exocrine pancreatic disorders. *In* Small Animal Internal Medicine, 3rd ed. Nelson RW, Couto CG (eds). St. Louis: Mosby, 2003, pp 472-567.

10. Zawie DA, Garvey MS: Feline hepatic disease. Vet Clin North Am Small Anim Pract 14:1201-1230, 1984.

11. Way LW, Sleisinger MH: Biliary obstruction, cholangitis, and choledocholithiasis. *In* Gastrointestinal and Liver Disease: Pathophysiology, Diagnosis, Management, 4th ed. Sleisinger MH, Fordtran JS (eds). Philadelphia: WB Saunders, 1989.

12. Center SA: Chronic liver disease: current concepts of disease mechanisms. J Small Anim Pract 40:106-114, 1999.

13. Neer TM, Hedlund CS: Vitamin K-dependent coagulopathy in a dog with bile and cystic duct obstructions. J Am Anim Hosp Assoc 25:461-464, 1989.

14. Fahie MA, Martin RA: Extrahepatic biliary tract obstruction: a retrospective study of 45 cases (1983-1993). J Am Anim Hosp Assoc 31:478-482, 1995.

15. Kirpensteijn J, Fingland RB, Ulrich T, et al: Cholelithiasis in dogs: 29 cases (1980-1990). J Am Vet Med Assoc 202:1137-1142, 1993.

16. Church EM, Matthiesen DT: Surgical treatment of 23 dogs with necrotizing cholecystitis. J Am Anim Hosp Assoc 24:305-310, 1988.

17. Heidner GL: Cholelithiasis in a cat. J Am Vet Med Assoc 186:176-177, 1985.

18. Eich CS, Ludwig LL: The surgical treatment of cholelithiasis in cats: a study of nine cases. J Am Anim Hosp Assoc 38:290-296, 2002.

19. Cantwell HD, Blevins WE, Hanika-Rebar C, et al: Radiopaque hepatic and lobar duct choleliths in a dog. J Am Anim Hosp Assoc 19:373-375, 1983.

20. Rothuizen J: Diseases of the biliary system. *In* BSAVA Manual of Canine and Feline Gastroenterology, 2005, pp. 269-278.

21. Mehler SJ, Mayhew PD, Drobatz KJ, et al: Variables associated with outcome in dogs undergoing extrahepatic biliary surgery: 60 cases (1988-2002). Vet Surg 33:644-649, 2004.

22. Couto CG: Hematology and immunology. *In* Small Animal Internal Medicine, 3rd ed. Nelson RW, Couto CG (eds). St. Louis: Mosby, 2003, pp. 1156-1228.

23. Herman BA, Brawer RS, Murtaugh RJ, et al: Therapeutic percutaneous ultrasound-guided cholecystocentesis in three dogs with extrahepatic biliary obstruction and pancreatitis. J Am Vet Med Assoc 227:1782-1786, 1753, 2005.

Chapter 34

Portosystemic Vascular Anomalies

Karen Tobias

Portosystemic shunts (PSS) are vascular anomalies that connect the portal system or its tributaries to the systemic circulation.[1-3] Portosystemic shunts may be congenital, in which case they are often singular, or they may be acquired secondary to portal hypertension. Blood shunting through the PSS bypasses the liver, circumventing extraction and detoxification processes normally performed by the hepatocytes. Clinical effects of shunts vary depending on the amount of blood shunted; in severe cases, PSS eventually results in death of the affected animal.[4] To understand the development and effects of PSS, a review of hepatic vascular anatomy and embryology is necessary.

Anatomy of the Hepatic Vasculature and Abdominal Venous Drainage

The portal vein provides up to 80% of blood flow and 50% of the oxygen content to the liver, with the remainder supplied by the hepatic artery. The portal vein is formed by the confluence of the cranial mesenteric vein, which drains the small intestines, and the caudal mesenteric vein, which drains the colon and proximal rectum. Cranially, the portal vein is joined by the splenic vein, which receives blood from the stomach (via the left gastric vein); the spleen; and, in dogs, the gastroduodenal vein, which drains portions of the pancreas, duodenum, and stomach.[2,3,5] The portal vein then bifurcates into the right and left portal veins. Branches of the right portal vein supply the right lateral liver lobe and the caudate process of the caudate lobe. The larger left portal vein gives off a central branch to the right medial liver lobe and a small papillary branch to the papillary process of the caudate lobe before dividing into quadrate, left medial, and left lateral branches.[5] In the cat, the portal vein divides into right, central, and left branches.[6] Within the liver lobes, blood flows through the portal venules and percolates through the hepatic sinusoids, mixing with blood from hepatic arterioles. It then collects within the central veins and is transported to the caudal vena cava via the hepatic veins.

Embryologic Development of the Portal System

The veins of the abdominal cavity are derived from the umbilical, vitelline, and caudal cardinal veins of the embryo.[7] The paired vitelline veins form the left hepatic vein, hepatic sinusoids, the hepatic portion of the caudal vena cava, and prehepatic portal vein and its tributaries. Portions of the vitelline and umbilical veins combine to form the ductus venosus and the left branch of the portal vein. The nonportal abdominal drainage, such as the renal and gonadal veins, is derived from the fetal cardinal venous system. The caudal cardinal veins also form the prehepatic caudal vena cava (caudal to the liver) and the azygos vein. In a normal animal, the only communication between the cardinal and vitelline systems is where the prehepatic and intrahepatic segments of the caudal vena cava join. Congenital extrahepatic portocaval and portoazygos shunts are developmental anomalies that result in abnormal, functional communication between these two systems.[7] Numerous nonfunctional portocaval and portoazygos communications are normally present in the fetus; these may become functional if chronic portal hypertension develops.[7] In rare instances, extrahepatic congenital PSS may result from persistence of the umbilical vein.[8]

Circulation through the ductus venosus permits at least 50% of the oxygenated blood from the placenta to reach the fetal heart without traversing hepatic sinusoids.[9-11] In most mammals it undergoes functional closure in the first 2 to 6 days after birth and structural closure within a few weeks.[9,10,12,13] The cause of functional closure of the ductus venosus is controversial.[13-15] Decreased portal blood flow and pressure and cessation of umbilical placental flow result in retraction and narrowing at the ductus origin.[10] In newborn puppies, no anatomic sphincter is evident, and the ductus appears to narrow uniformly after birth.[7,10,14,15] Ductus flow is not detectable by Doppler ultrasonography in 50% of Irish wolfhound puppies 4 days after birth and in 100% 9 days after birth.[13] Connective tissue proliferation at the junction of the ductus venosus and umbilical portal sinus in dogs expands to the termination of the ductus at the left hepatic vein, resulting in structural closure within 3 weeks after birth. Persistence of the fetal ductus venosus results in a left-sided intrahepatic PSS. If the ductus venosus remains patent in dogs, it may be secondary to underdevelopment or atresia of the hepatic portal system rather than a failure of primary closure mechanisms.[11] Etiology of central and right-sided shunts has not been determined and it is unknown whether these represent anomalous ductus venosus or other developmental errors.

Congenital Portosystemic Shunts

Etiology

Congenital PSS are reported in 0.18% of all dogs and 0.05% of mixed-breed dogs.

Because Yorkshire terriers, Irish wolfhounds, and a variety of other breeds are at increased risk for PSS, an underlying hereditary cause is suspected.[16,17] Familial relationships have been noted in Irish wolfhounds with PSS, and incidence of the disease has been reduced by breeding outside of these lines.[18] In Yorkshire and Cairn terriers, inheritance is not simple dominant, simple recessive, or sex-linked.[17,19] In humans, a recessive mode of inheritance is suspected for familial patent ductus venosus.[20] Inheritance of PSS in dogs is autosomal and most likely polygenic, or monogenic with variable expression or incomplete penetrance.[17,19] Genetic predispositions have also been noted in other portal vascular diseases, including muscular portal venular hypertrophy with secondary acquired portosystemic shunting in

Cocker spaniels and congenital portal hypoplasia (also known as hepatic microvascular dysplasia or HMD) in Cairn terriers.[21,22] Breeding of dogs with HMD can result in offspring with PSS, suggesting that the diseases may be related.

Clinical Signs

Neurologic, urinary, and gastrointestinal signs are reported in animals with congenital PSS. General clinical signs of animals with congenital shunts include small stature, poor hair coat, weight loss, fever, and anesthetic or tranquilizer intolerance.[2,3,23-26] Poor growth may be a result of decreased serum insulin-like growth factors (IGFs), which are anabolic and mitogenic polypeptide hormones that are responsible for prenatal tissue growth and postnatal development.[27]

Because of decreased urea production and increased ammonia excretion, animals can present with polyuria, pollakiuria, stranguria, and other clinical signs of urinary tract dysfunction and infection. Polydypsia and polyuria may also result from alterations in portal vein osmoreceptors, decreased renal medullary concentration gradient, potassium depletion, stimulation of thirst centers owing to hepatic encephalopathy, medullary solute washout, decreased responsiveness to ADH, shift in intrarenal blood flow from cortical to juxtaglomerular nephrons, and increased endogenous cortisol concentrations.[23] Animals with PSS may develop renomegaly secondary to increased glomerular filtration rate or changes in renal metabolic function or blood flow.[28]

Hepatic Encephalopathy

Pathophysiology

The most common clinical signs in dogs and cats with PSS are neurologic abnormalities associated with hepatic encephalopathy.[2,3,23,25,26] Clinical signs include depression, dementia, stupor, and coma. Muscle tremors, motor abnormalities, and focal and generalized seizures have also been reported.[2,29] The metabolic cause of hepatic encephalopathy is unknown, but is probably dependent on several factors, including alterations in amino acid neurotransmitters γ-amino butyric acid (GABA), glutamate, and glutamine; accumulation of cerebral toxins; and dysfunction of astrocytes.[29-46] Toxins that have been implicated in hepatic encephalopathy include ammonia, mercaptans, short-chain fatty acids, indoles, skatols, aromatic amino acids (AAA), and biogenic amines. None of these factors alone will consistently initiate an encephalopathic coma experimentally, but any may play a part in its development. Other metabolic alterations associated with portal blood shunting and impaired hepatic function include increases in blood levels of epinephrine, adrenocorticotropin, α-melanotropin, and cortisol.[46-49] Consequences of these increases on neurologic function of animals with PSS has not yet been thoroughly evaluated.

Ammonia

Ammonia is a side product of degradation of glutamine by glutaminase in the brain, small intestines, kidneys, and other tissues.[33] Ammonia produced by the small intestines is reabsorbed and transported through the portal system to the liver where 80 to 90% is transformed into urea via the Krebs-Hensleit urea cycle or used in the conversion of glutamate to glutamine.[29,32] Most urea is excreted by the kidneys into the urine; however, 20 to 25% is released into the intestinal lumen where urea and remaining amino acids, amines, and purines are degraded into ammonia by urease-producing coliforms and anaerobes within the colon. In the kidneys, a small portion of the ammonia produced during renal glutamine metabolism is reabsorbed and carried into the systemic circulation via the renal veins. Within skeletal muscle, ammonia is metabolized through glutamine synthesis; this process is coupled with the use of branched-chain amino acids for energy production.[32]

Because the brain lacks several enzymes of the urea cycle, ammonia must be removed by glutamine synthesis through amidation of glutamate in the astrocytes. Increased ammonia concentrations in the cerebrospinal fluid may cause neurotoxicity as a result of disturbances in cerebral energy metabolism, alteration in excitatory and inhibitory mechanisms, and interference with neuronal membrane transport and receptor function.[34-36] Structurally, hyperammonemia induces myelin splitting and brain vacuolation, preferentially within the white matter. Histologically, animals with hepatic encephalopathy develop Alzheimer type II cells and polymicrocavitation, particularly in the brainstem, cerebellar nuclei, and the border between grey and white matter.[34,39,50]

In people with acute liver failure, venous ammonia concentrations often increase with the severity of clinical signs, and arterial ammonia concentrations greater than 150 μmol/L predict a greater likelihood of dying from brain herniation.[35,51] In animals, the correlation between blood ammonia concentration and degree of encephalopathy is poor. Brain to blood concentration ratios in acute liver failure, however, may be 4 to 8 times normal because of increased ammonia uptake in the brain.[36] Mercaptans and short-chain fatty acids, products of bacterial activity in the intestines, may reduce ammonia metabolism or act synergistically with ammonia to increase inhibitory neurotransmission.[33]

Glutamine

In the brain, astrocytes are critical for ammonia metabolism, regulation of the extracellular environment, neuronal excitability, and neurotransmission. Accumulation of intracellular glutamine secondary to hyperammonemia causes osmotic stress and astrocyte swelling. This upregulates expression of peripheral benzodiazepine receptors, affects multiple ion channels and amino acid transport, alters receptor densities and neurotransmitter processing, induces deposition of glycogen and inhibition of glycogenolysis, and increases synthesis of neurosteroids that are potent modulators of neuronal GABA receptor activity.[35,36] Cerebrospinal fluid (CSF) concentrations of glutamine are significantly higher in dogs with PSS compared with healthy dogs fed a low-protein diet.[37]

Glutamate

The mammalian brain has four types of excitatory receptors that are defined by agonist selectivity, including N-methyl-D-aspartate

(NMDA), α-[3H]amino-3-hydroxy-5-methyl-4-isoxazoleproprionic acid (AMPA), kainite, and L-2-amino-4-phosphonobutyrate (L-AP4).[38] A fifth receptor subtype is linked to phophoinositol metabolism. L-Glutamate, the most important excitatory neurotransmitter, acts preferentially at AMPA and kainite sites. Effects of L-aspartate, another excitatory neurotransmitter, are thought to be mediated predominantly through the NMDA receptor. In dogs with congenital PSS and hepatic encephalopathy, glutamate concentrations are increased 65% in the CSF.[30,39] Kainate-receptor density and low-affinity AMPA sites are reduced, however, which may result in decreased excitatory neurotransmission and, therefore, a predominance of inhibitory neurotransmission.[38]

Gamma-Aminobutyric Acid (GABA)

Gamma-aminobutyric acid, the most important inhibitory neurotransmitter, is produced by enteric bacteria and is usually metabolized by the liver. Binding of GABA to its receptors increases chloride flow into the neuron, resulting in membrane hyperpolarization and inhibition of neurotransmission. The GABA receptor also has binding sites for barbiturates, benzodiazepines, and benzodiazepine-like substances called ligands. The majority of studies have found no significant alteration in brain GABA-receptor density or affinity in animal models of hepatic encephalopathy, and GABA concentrations are within normal range in dogs with congenital PSS.[30,38,39] Some researchers suggest, however, that ammonia may enhance selective binding of GABA to receptors, increase synaptic availability of GABA by inhibiting synaptic uptake, and upregulate peripheral-type benzodiazepine receptor release of neurosteroids that are potent agonists of GABA receptors, thus increasing inhibitory neurotransmission.[40]

Peripheral-type Benzodiazepine Receptors

Because GABA receptors contain binding sites for endogenous benzodiazepine receptor ligands, benzodiazepines were originally speculated to produce central nervous system (CNS) depression in animals with hepatic encephalopathy.[26] Although dogs with congenital PSS have increased concentrations of endogenous benzodiazepine receptor ligands in peripheral and portal blood, they do not have increased benzodiazepine binding activity in the CSF, and infusion of the benzodiazepine receptor antagonist flumazenil has little effect in reversing clinical and neurophysiologic dysfunction of dogs with chronic hepatic encephalopathy.[41,52] However, administration of sarmazenil, a drug that has both antagonistic and partial inverse-agonistic activity, results in significant improvement in electroencephalographic activity and clinical grade of dogs with hepatic encephalopathy.[41,42] Sarmazenil is thought to negatively modulate GABAergic tone by counteracting the actions of ammonia and neurosteroids on the GABA receptor, potentially balancing the effects of decreased excitatory glutamatergic neurotransmission.[42]

Unlike central receptors, peripheral-type benzodiazepine receptors have increased density and expression in hepatic encephalopathy models.[39] Ammonia is thought to upregulate these receptors, enhancing the production and release of neurosteroids that are potent agonists of the GABA receptor complex.[34,39,40] Manganese also increases expression of peripheral-type benzodiazepine receptors, resulting in increased inhibitory activity.[39]

Amino Acid Imbalances

Aromatic amino acids (phenylalanine, tyrosine, and tryptophan) are normally metabolized by the liver; whereas branched-chain amino acids (valine, leucine, and isoleucine) are used as energy sources in skeletal muscle and as substrates for CNS synthesis of the excitatory neurotransmitters norepinephrine and dopamine.[30,33,43,46] Dogs with PSS have significant increases in plasma concentrations of aromatic amino acids (AAA) owing to reduced hepatic clearance. Additionally, peripheral concentrations of branched-chain amino acids (BCAA) are significantly decreased in response to hyperammonemia, hyperinsulinemia, and hyperglucagonemia, resulting in a reduction of the peripheral BCAA:AAA ratio to 1.5 or less (normal is greater than 3.0).[30,33,43,46] Hyperinsulinemia decreases the rate of release of BCAA and stimulates the rate of utilization of BCAA by muscle and adipose tissue and incorporation of BCAA into proteins.[43] Because all amino acids compete for the same transport system into the brain, decrease in peripheral concentrations of BCAA means more AAA are transported into the CNS, resulting in reduction of CSF BCAA/AAA ratio to 0.5 (normal, 2.3).[30,43,46] Increased AAA may result in increased concentrations of inhibitory neurotransmitters and formation of weak or false neurotransmitters that disrupt normal synaptic impulse transmission.[37,46,53] Tryptophan hydroxylation is the rate-limiting step in CNS serotonin synthesis; therefore, increased CSF tryptophan could increase serotonin concentrations and thus inhibitory neurotransmission.[37] Increased tryptophan in the brain may result in increased amounts of its oxidative product quinolinic acid. Quinolinic acid is a known excitotoxin that acts at the NMDA receptor, causing irreversible damage to neurons.[44]

Precipitating Factors

Factors that may increase the chance of an encephalopathic episode include protein overload, zinc deficiency, arginine deficiency in cats, hypokalemia, alkalosis, hypovolemia, gastrointestinal hemorrhage, infection, azotemia, and constipation.[2-4,29,32,39,42,45,53] Blood that has been stored for 24 hours contains 170 μg of ammonia/dl; ammonia concentrations increase further with longer storage.[29] Diuretic agents promote hypokalemia, which increases renal ammonia production and alkalosis, increasing the availability of diffusible ammonia.[29]

Treatment

Medical management of animals with PSS-associated hepatic encephalopathy includes correction of fluid, electrolyte, and glucose imbalances and reduction of precipitating factors.[3,24,28,54] Reduction of total protein intake is more beneficial than altering the content of dietary amino acids; however, severe protein restriction may result in loss of skeletal muscle mass and subsequent reduction in ammonia metabolism.[46,55] Depletion of zinc can precipitate hepatic encephalopathy, and supplementation may improve psychomotor function in mildly affected patients.[56,57]

Lactulose is a poorly absorbed synthetic disaccharide that is hydrolyzed by colonic bacteria to short-chain fatty acids, lactic acid, and hydrogen. Proposed effects of lactulose include decreased colonic pH with subsequent entrapment of ammonium; inhibition of protein and amino acid metabolism, thereby reducing formation of ammonia and amino acid-derived short-chain fatty acids; decreased intestinal transit time; and increased fecal nitrogen excretion.[56] Nonabsorbable disaccharides have not consistently been shown to reduce or prevent signs of hepatic encephalopathy in human clinical trials, but are still used frequently in people and animals with hepatic encephalopathy.[58,59] Administration of nonpathogenic lactic acid bacteria may provide benefits similar to lactulose and may increase the proportion of non-urease-producing bacteria in the intestines.[60] Oral administration of antibiotics will also decrease colonic bacterial populations.

Other medications that improve clinical status of people with hepatic encephalopathy include arginine, sodium phenylacetate, sodium benzoate, L-ornithine L-aspartate, methionine sulfoximine, and sodium benzoate, which decrease ammonia production or increase ammonia metabolism.[35,36,44] L-ornithine L-aspartate (LOLA) may provide substrate to the liver for enhancing the residual urea cycle and serve as a substrate for ammonia detoxification in the muscles.[35,61] Administration of LOLA reduces brain edema in animals with acute liver failure.[32] Methionine sufloximine, an inhibitor of glutamine synthetase, prevents uptake of nonpolar amino acids, including tryptophan, by the CNS, ameliorating signs of hepatic encephalopathy in rats with surgically induced PSS.[37] Mild hypothermia may also be useful to reduce blood-brain ammonia transfer.[34]

Laboratory Abnormalities

Hemograms

Abnormalities on hemograms of animals with PSS include anemia, microcytosis, hypoproteinemia, and leukocytosis.[2,3,23] Other reported hemographic abnormalities include target cell formation, poikilocytosis, and hypochromasia. Potential causes of anemia include decreased red blood cell production because of poor nutritional status, low erythropoietin levels, decreased transferrin production and subsequent poor iron utilization, and abnormal cholesterol and lipid metabolism; decreased survival of red blood cells; dilution from increased extracellular fluid and plasma volume and total body water; or chronic loss from parasites or a coagulopathy.[2,3,23,28] Additionally, hematocrits may be considered low according to adult laboratory reference ranges but may be within normal limits for pediatric patients.[62] Microcytosis is thought to occur because of a problem with iron transport or utilization rather than an absolute iron deficiency. Dogs with congenital PSS have decreased serum iron concentrations and normal or decreased total iron binding capacity.[63,64] Some naturally affected animals and those with surgically created portocaval shunts may have accumulation of stainable iron in the liver.[63,64]

Presence of leukocytosis is variable and may occur in response to stress, hypercortisolemia, or infection. Inadequate clearance of bacteria and endotoxins from the portal system may play a role in development of leukocytosis; however, significant differences in concentration of endotoxins and in rates of positive portal blood cultures have not been found when comparing normal dogs with those with congenital PSS.[65,66] Recurrent bacterial infections, fever, leukocytosis, and hypergammaglobulinemia may occur with reticuloendothelial impairment, because 90% of reticuloendothelial function in dogs occurs within the liver.[67] Dogs with PSS have significantly impaired reticuloendothelial function secondary to a reduction in effective liver blood flow. Reticuloendothelial activity increases in the spleen and lung, but only partially compensates for the hepatic reductions.[67] Severity of preoperative leukocytosis is correlated with postoperative outcome.[68]

Serum Chemistry

In dogs with congenital PSS, decreased blood urea nitrogen and albumin and increased partial thromboplastin time are primarily the result of decreased hepatic production of proteins.[23,69] Hypoalbuminemia may also occur secondary to intestinal loss or fluid retention.[64] Decreased creatinine may occur with hepatic insufficiency or reduced muscle mass; the level of creatinine is also naturally lower in young patients.[28] Potential causes of hypoglycemia include decreased hepatic glycogen stores, increased insulin concentrations, decreased responsiveness to glucagon and insulin, and abnormal balance of counter-regulatory hormones (cortisol and epinephrine).[23,70] Dogs with congenital PSS have hyperinsulinemia and hyperglucagonemia secondary to insulin hypersecretion, insulin resistance, and decreased hepatic degradation of these hormones. Hypoglycemia is uncommon in cats with PSS, possibly because of their tendency to develop stress-induced hyperglycemia during sampling.[23]

Increases in alanine aminotransferase concentrations occur with hepatocellular necrosis and increased membrane permeability, possibly as a result of poor hepatic perfusion and cell hypoxia.[23,64] Because cholestasis is not a prominent feature of PSS, an elevation in serum alkaline phosphatase concentrations in young animals may actually be of osseous origin.[23]

Urinalysis

Low specific gravity may be secondary to polyuria/polydipsia or to alterations in the renal medullary concentration gradient from deficits in urea.[23] Chronic hypercortisolism induces inadequate osmoregulation of release of ADH and, thus, polyuria.[70] Animals with congenital PSS may have hematuria, pyuria, and proteinuria, and clinical signs of urinary tract infections secondary to urolithiasis or inflammation from urate crystal or calculus that form because of increased ammonia excretion.[2,23,24] Renal urate calculi may dissolve after shunt ligation.[71]

Bile Acids

Bile acids are synthesized in the liver from cholesterol. Within the liver they are conjugated to taurine (cats and dogs) or glycine (dogs) to increase their water solubility and enable micelle formation. Conjugated bile acids are excreted across the hepatocyte canalicular membrane into bile. Cholecystokinin, which is released in response to ingestion of a meal, stimulates gallbladder contraction and release of bile acids into the duodenum.[72] At least 95% of intestinal bile acids are actively reabsorbed in the ileum and are transported by portal blood back to the liver (the "enterohepatic cycle"), with the remainder lost in the feces.[72-74] At the sinusoidal surface of the hepatocyte, bile acid uptake relies on a sodium-coupled transporter. Serum bile acid concentrations increase in conditions that affect hepatocellular uptake, such as cholestasis or primary hepatic disease, or conditions that alter vascular flow to the liver, such as PSS. They are not significantly affected by dehydration, hypovolemia, or passive hepatic congestion. Effects of lipemia and hemolysis on spectrophotometric sample analysis of bile acids are unpredictable; theoretically they can overestimate bile acids by scattering light and increasing spectrophotometric absorption. However, lipemia may decrease bile acids by volume displacement of serum, and hemolysis can reduce bile acid recovery.[75] Falsely lowered results may occur with delayed absorption from prolonged intestinal transit time, lack of gallbladder contraction because of inadequate food intake or delayed gastric emptying, or malabsorption/maldigestion with subsequent decrease of enterohepatic recirculation. Postprandial bile acid concentrations are less than fasting in 20% of animals because of spontaneous interdigestive gallbladder contraction or with prolongation of gastric emptying or intestinal transit times.[4,23,76]

Increases in postprandial bile acids that were mild (> 31 μmol/L) or moderate to severe (> 80 μmol/L) were reported in 79% and 34% of Maltese dogs, respectively.[75] Most had normal ammonia tolerance tests, and bile acids were significantly lower when measured by high-performance liquid chromatography, indicating that bile acids measured spectrophotometrically in Maltese may be increased by some other cross-reacting substance.[75]

Plasma Ammonia Concentration

In dogs with PSS, sensitivity of postprandial ammonia is 91%[6] hours after feeding, compared with 81% before feeding; ammonia tolerance test is recommended to increase sensitivity.[77] Plasma ammonia levels may be normal in dogs with PSS after prolonged fasting or with effective medical treatment.[23] Because erythrocytes contain 2 to 3 times the amount of ammonia in plasma, improper sample cooling, hemolysis, incomplete plasma separation, or delays in sample analysis falsely increase ammonia values. Concentrations of ammonia measured with tabletop analyzers can be falsely increased if ammonia-based cleaners are used nearby or if ammonia-rich skin oils contaminate the apparatus.

Histology

Hepatic histologic changes in animals with PSS include generalized congestion of central veins and sinusoids, lobular collapse, bile duct proliferation, hypoplasia of intrahepatic portal tributaries, Kupffer cell hyperplasia, and proliferation of small vessels and lymphatics.[54] In dogs with surgically created PSS, direct infusion of insulin into the intrahepatic portal vein reduces atrophy, preserves hepatocyte ultrastructure, and increases cell renewal, indicating the first pass effect of insulin may be necessary for liver development.[70] Dogs with PSS have increased fragility of intracellular organelles, increased endoplasmic reticular and lysosomal enzymes, and increases in the biliary canalicular component of alkaline phosphatase activity.[78] Increased hepatic iron stores can be seen in some dogs with congenital PSS but this is not a consistent finding.[63,64] Histopathologic changes in the livers of dogs with congenital PSS are identical to those in dogs with primary hypoplasia of the intrahepatic portal venous system (HMD), reduced portal perfusion for any reason (e.g., portal vein thrombosis), and congenital arterioportal fistula; therefore, histopathology alone may not differentiate among these diseases.[22,54,79,80]

Surgery

Surgical options include acute ligation with suture; gradual occlusion with ameroid constrictors, cellophane banding, or hydraulic occluders; or embolization with coils.[2,3,81-86] When suture ligation is performed, portal and central venous pressures are measured to determine the acceptable degree of attenuation, because[32] 60% of animals cannot tolerate complete acute occlusion.[3,68,81-85,87,88]

Normal intraoperative portal pressures range from 6 to 15 cm H_2O (6-10 mm Hg); portal pressures in animals with PSS range from 0 to 12 cm H_2O.[2,3,87] Acute ligation of single PSS in animals with poorly developed or nonexpansile intrahepatic portal vasculature results in large increases in portal pressure and decreases in central venous pressure. Central venous pressure is an indirect measurement of right atrial pressure and cardiac preload. It is controlled by the tone of capacitance vessels and the intrathoracic pressure when right ventricular function is adequate and blood volume is stable. Because blood flow is proportional to the fourth power of vessel radius, small decreases in portal vessel size result in large decreases in venous return and central venous pressure.[87] Increases in portal pressure are caused by increased resistance to blood flow in the hepatic vascular bed. Mild increases in portal pressure accompanied by large decreases in central venous pressure and subjective evidence of portal hypertension during shunt occlusion suggest splanchnic venous compliance has increased and splanchnic pooling has occurred.[87,89] Portal pressure measurements can vary with depth of anesthesia, administration of inotropes, catheter position, abdominal viscera position, abdominal bandages, temperature, hydration status, phase of respiration, degree of splanchnic compliance, and other systemic factors.[89]

Multiple Acquired Portosystemic Shunts

Multiple acquired PSS are tortuous vessels that connect the portal system with tributaries of the caudal vena cava, most frequently the left renal or gonadal veins. They are thought to originate from pre-existing nonfunctional communications between the portal vein and the systemic circulation, secondary to portal hypertension from severe liver fibrosis, neoplasia, portal atresia, or congestion.[90,91] Animals with multiple acquired shunts often have neurologic and urinary tract signs similar to animals with congenital shunts.[90] Because of underlying portal hypertension and, in some cases, severe hypoalbuminemia, animals with multiple acquired shunts often develop ascites. Bleeding dyscrasias from decreased hepatic production of coagulation factors may also occur, resulting in prolonged bleeding of wounds and hematoma formation at venipuncture sites. Blood work results vary with the underlying cause but often include hypoalbuminemia, decreased blood urea nitrogen concentrations, increased liver enzymes, and increased bilirubin if cholestasis is present.

Hepatic Arteriovenous Fistulas

Hepatic arteriovenous (AV) fistulas are anomalous connections between the hepatic artery and the portal or hepatic vein. They are most often caused by congenital failure of embryologic vascular systems to differentiate into capillary, arterial, or venous structures; they may also occur as a result of trauma or surgery.[92-97] In animals with hepatic AV fistulas, high arterial pressure flow into the portal system results in retrograde portal flow, with subsequent intrahepatic portal hypoplasia, and portal hypertension with subsequent development of multiple acquired PSS. Clinical signs of hepatic arteriovenous fistula are associated with hepatic insufficiency (diarrhea, vomiting, neurologic abnormalities), portal hypertension (ascites), and decreased arterial blood volume (tachycardia, water-hammer pulses with decreased diastolic pressure, ventricular failure). On physical examination, a systolic cardiac murmur may be noted. Many dogs have water-hammer pulses and an auscultable continuous machinery-type murmur with the point of maximum intensity on the abdominal wall over or near the affected lobe.[96] Biochemical and hemogram abnormalities are similar to those of animals with PSS. Diagnosis of hepatic arteriovenous fistulas is made with Doppler ultrasonography. The presence of an extremely dilated and tortuous portal branch in a liver lobe is considered pathognomonic.[94,95,97] Ascites, hepatofugal blood flow in the portal vein, and multiple acquired shunts may also be noted. On exploratory laparotomy, affected liver lobes have multiple large, tortuous vessels; acquired extrahepatic shunts around the left renal and gonadal veins are also evident. Histologically, the fistulas consist of numerous thick-walled arteries and markedly dilated veins. The arteries and veins may contain smooth muscle hyperplasia, and hepatic lobules are atrophied, especially near the fistulas. Proliferation of bile ductules and thick-walled hepatic arterioles are found in the portal triads; portal veins in the triads may be reduced in size or absent.[98] Surgical ligation of the hepatic arteriovenous fistula or resection of the affected liver lobe will decrease clinical signs caused by arteriovenous shunting in 57% of dogs.[3,96] Animals are pretreated with glycopyrrolate or atropine to prevent reflex bradycardia (Branham reflex) with closure of the fistula.

References

1. Hickman J, Edwards JE, Mann FC: Venous anomalies in a dog. Anat Rec 104:137, 1949.

2. Swalec KM: Portosystemic shunts. *In* Disease Mechanisms in Small Animal Surgery. Bojrab MJ, Smeak DD, Bloomberg MS (eds). Philadelphia: Lea & Febiger, 1993, p. 298.

3. Tobias KM: Portosystemic shunts and other hepatic vascular anomalies. *In* Textbook of Small Animal Surgery, 3rd ed. Slatter DH (ed). Philadelphia: WB Saunders, 2003, p. 727.

4. Watson PJ, Herrtage ME: Medical management of congenital portosystemic shunts in 27 dogs–a retrospective study. J Small Anim Pract 39:62, 1998.

5. Tobias KMS, Rawlings CA: Surgical techniques for extravascular occlusion of intrahepatic shunts. Compend Contin Educ Pract Vet 18:745, 1996.

6. Breznock EM, Whiting PG: Portocaval shunts and anomalies. *In* Textbook of Small Animal Surgery. Slatter DH (ed). Philadelphia: WB Saunders, 1985, p. 1156.

7. Payne JT, Martin RA, Constantinescu GM: The anatomy and embryology of portosystemic shunts in dogs and cats. Semin Vet Med Surg (Small Anim) 5:75, 1990.

8. Brockman DJ, Brown DC, Holt DE: Unusual congenital portosystemic communication resulting from persistence of the extrahepatic umbilical vein. J Small Anim Pract 39:244, 1998.

9. Breznock EM, Berger P, Pendray D, et al: Surgical manipulation of intrahepatic portocaval shunts in dogs. J Am Vet Med Assoc 182:798, 1983.

10. Lohse CL, Suter PF: Comparative features relating to closure of the ductus venosus. Anat Rec 187:641, 1977.

11. White RN, Burton CA: Anatomy of the patent ductus venosus in dogs. Vet Rec 146:425, 2000.

12. Edelstone DI: Regulation of blood flow through the ductus venosus. J Develop Physiol 2:219, 1980.

13. Lamb CR, Burton CA: Doppler ultrasonographic assessment of closure of the ductus venosus in neonatal Irish wolfhounds. Vet Rec 155:699, 2004.

14. Burton CA, White RN: The angiographic anatomy of the portal venous systemic in the neonatal dog. Res Vet Sci 66:211, 1999.

15. Coceani F, Adeagbo ASO, Cutz E, Olley PM: Autonomic mechanisms in the ductus venosus of the lamb. Am J Physiol 247:H17, 1984.

16. Tobias KM, Rohrbach BW: Proportional diagnosis of congenital portosystemic shunts in dogs accessed by veterinary teaching hospitals: 1980-2002. J Am Vet Med Assoc 223:1636, 2003.

17. Tobias KM: Determination of heredity of single congenital portosystemic shunts in Yorkshire terriers. J Am Anim Hosp Assoc 39:385, 2003.

18. Ubbink GJ, van de Broek, J, Meyer HP, et al: Prediction of inherited portosystemic shunts in Irish Wolfhounds on the basis of pedigree analysis. Am J Vet Res 59:1553, 1998.

19. Van Straten G, Leegwater PAJ, de Vries M, et al: Inherited congenital extrahepatic portosystemic shunts in Cairn terriers. J Vet Intern Med 19:321, 2005.

20. Jacob S, Farr G, De Vun D, et al: Hepatic manifestations of familial patent ductus venosus in adults. Gut, 45:442, 1999.

21. Rand JS, Best SJ, Mathews KA: Portosystemic vascular shunts in a family of American Cocker Spaniels. J Am Anim Hosp Assoc 24:265, 1988.

22. Schermerhorn T, Center SA, Dykes NL, et al: Characterization of hepatoportal microvascular dysplasia in a kindred of Cairn Terriers. J Vet Intern Med 10:219, 1996.

23. Center SA, Magne ML: Historical, physical examination and clinicopathologic features of portosystemic vascular anomalies in the dog and cat. Semin Vet Med Surg (Small Anim) 5:23, 1990.

24. Winkler JT, Bohling MW, Tillson DM, et al: Portosystemic shunts: diagnosis, prognosis, and treatment of 64 cases (1993-2001). J Am Anim Hosp Assoc 39:169, 2003.

25. Havig M, Tobias KM: Outcome of ameroid constrictor occlusion of single congenital extrahepatic portosystemic shunts in cats: 12 cases (1993-2000). J Am Vet Med Assoc 220:337, 2002.

26. Kyles AE, Hardie EM, Mehl M, Gregory CR: Evaluation of ameroid ring constrictors for the management of single extrahepatic portosystemic shunts in cats: 23 cases (1996-2001). J Am Vet Med Assoc 220:1341, 2002.

27. Maxwell A, Hurley K, Burton C, et al: Reduced serum insulin-like growth factor (IGF) and IGF-binding protein-3 concentrations in two deerhounds with congenital portosystemic shunts. J Vet Intern Med 14:542, 2000.

28. Deppe TA, Center SA, Simpson KW, et al: Glomerular filtration rate and renal volume in dogs with congenital portosystemic vascular anomalies before and after surgical ligation. J Vet Intern Med 13:465, 1999.

29. Hardy RM: Pathophysiology of hepatic encephalopathy. Semin Vet Med Surg (Small Anim) 5:100, 1990.

30. Butterworth J, Gregory CR, Aronson LR: Selective alterations of cerebral spinal fluid amino acids in dogs with congenital portosystemic shunts. Met Brain Dis 12:299, 1997.

31. Roudebush P, Davenport DJ, Dimski DS: Hepatobiliary disease. *In* Small Animal Clinical Nutrition. Hand MS, Thatcher CD, Remillard RL, Roudebush P (eds). Marceline, MO: Walsworth Publishing, Mark Morris Institute, 2000, p. 811.

32. Shawcross D, Jalan R: Dispelling myths in the treatment of hepatic encephalopathy. Lancet 365:431, 2005.

33. Katayama K: Ammonia metabolism and hepatic encephalopathy. Hepatol Res 30S:73, 2004.

34. Butterworth RF: Pathogenesis of hepatic encephalopathy: new insights from neuroimaging and molecular studies. J Hepatol 39:278, 2003.

35. Jala R, Shawcross D, Davies N: The molecular pathogenesis of hepatic encephalopathy. Int J Biochem Cell Biol 35:1175, 2003.

36. Butterworth RF: Molecular neurobiology of acute liver failure. Semin Liver Dis 23:251, 2003.

37. Holt DE, Washabau RJ, Djali S, et al: Cerebrospinal fluid glutamine, tryptophan, and tryptophan metabolite concentrations in dogs with portosystemic shunts. Am J Vet Res 63:1167, 2002.

38. Maddison JE, Watson WEJ, Dodd PR, Johnston GAR: Alterations in cortical [^{3}H]kainate and alpha-[^{3}H]amino-3-hydroxy-5-methyl-4-isoxazoleproprionic acid binding in a spontaneous canine model of chronic hepatic encephalopathy. J Neurochem 56:1881, 1991.

39. Maddison JE: Newest insights into hepatic encephalopathy. Eur J Compar Gastroenterol 5:17, 2000.

40. Jones EA: Ammonia, the GABA neurotransmitter system, and hepatic encephalopathy. Metab Brain Dis 17:275, 2002.

41. Meyer HP, Rothuizen J: Modulation of the GABAergic tone by benzodiazepine receptor ligands in chronic hepatic encephalopathy in the dog. Vet Q 20:S100, 1998.

42. Meyer HP, Legemate DA, van den Brom W, Rothuizen J: Improvement of chronic hepatic encephalopathy in dogs by the benzodiazepine-receptor partial inverse agonist sarmazenil, but not by the antagonist flumazenil. Met Brain Dis 13:241, 1998.

43. Strombeck DR, Rogers Q: Plasma amino acid concentrations in dogs with hepatic disease. J Am Vet Med Assoc 173:93, 1978.

44. Barshaw ML, Robinson MB, Hyland K, et al: Quinolinic acid in children with congenital hyperammonemia. Ann Neurol 34:676, 1993.

45. Blei AT: Infection, inflammation and hepatic encephalopathy, synergism redefined. J Hepatol 40:327, 2004.

46. Meyer HP, Chamluleau RA, Legemate DA, et al: Effects of a branched-chain amino acid-enriched diet on chronic hepatic encephalopathy in dogs. Met Brain Dis 14:103, 1999.

47. Rothuizen J, de Kok Y, Slob A, Mol JA: GABAergic inhibition of the pituitary release of adrenocorticotropin and alpha-melanotropin is impaired in dogs with hepatic encephalopathy. Domestic Anim Endocrinol 13:59, 1996.

48. Sterczer A, Meyer HP, Van Sluijs FJ, Rothuizen J: Fast resolution of hypercortisolism in dogs with portosystemic encephalopathy after surgical shunt closure. Res Vet Sci 66:63, 1999.

49. Meyer HP, Rothuizen J: Increased free cortisol in plasma of dogs with portosystemic encephalopathy (PSE). Domest Anim Endocrinol 11:317, 1994.

50. Herden C, Beineke A, Hetzel U, et al: Unusual manifestation of hepatic encephalopathy in two Irish wolfhound siblings. Vet Rec 153:682, 2003.

51. Ong JJ, Aggarwal A, Krieger D, et al: Correlation between ammonia levels and the severity of hepatic encephalopathy. Am J Med 114:188, 2003.

52. Aronson LR, Gacad RC, Kaminsky-Russ K, et al: Endogenous benzodiazepine activity in the peripheral and portal blood of dogs with congenital portosystemic shunts. Vet Surg 26:189, 1997.

53. Holt D: Critical care management of the portosystemic shunt patient: Compend Contin Educ Pract Vet 16:879, 1994.

54. Allen L, Stobie D, Mauldin GN, Baer KE: Clinicopathologic features of dogs with hepatic microvascular dysplasia with and without portosystemic shunts; 42 cases (1991-1996). J Am Vet Med Assoc 214:218, 1999.

55. Cordoba J, Lopez-Hellin J, Planas M, et al: Normal protein diet for episodic hepatic encephalopathy: results of a randomized study. J Hepatol 41:38, 2004.

56. Marks SL: Nutritional support in hepatic disease. Part II. Dietary management of common liver disorders in dogs and cats. *In* Liver Disease: Nutritional Management in Dogs and Cats. Topeka: Hill's Pet Nutrition Inc, 1999, p. 37.

57. Grugreiff K: Zinc in liver disease. J Trace Elements Exper Med 15:67, 2002.

58. Als-Nielsen B, Gluud LL, Gluud C: Non-absorbable disaccharides for hepatic encephalopathy: systematic review of randomized trials. Br J Med 328:1046, 2004.

59. Rodes MAS, Sunyer L, Rodrigo L, et al: Comparison of rifaximin and lactilol in the treatment of acute hepatic encephalopathy: results of a randomized, double-blind, double-dummy, controlled clinical trial. J Hepatol 38:51, 2003.

60. Bongaerts G, Severijnen R, Timmerman H: Effect of antibiotics, prebiotics and probiotics in treatment for hepatic encephalopathy. Med Hypotheses 64:64, 2005.

61. Rose C, Michalak A, Pannunzio P, et al: Ornithine-L-Aspartate in experimental portal-systemic encephalopathy: Therapeutic efficacy and mechanism of action. Metab Brain Dis 13:147, 1998.

62. Clinkenbeard KD, Cowell RL, Meinkoth JH, et al: The hematopoietic and lymphoid systems. *In* Veterinary Pediatrics: Birth to Six Months. Hoskins JD (ed). Philadelphia: WB Saunders, 2001, p. 300.

63. Bunch SE, Jordan HL, Sellon RK, et al: Characterization of iron status in young dogs with portosystemic shunt. Am J Vet Res 56:853, 1995.

64. Simpson KW, Meyer DJ, Boswood A, et al: Iron status and erythrocyte volume in dogs with congenital portosystemic vascular anomalies. J Vet Intern Med 11:14, 1997.

65. Peterson SL, Koblik PD, Whiting PG, Breznock EM: Endotoxin concentrations measured by a chromogenic assay in portal and peripheral venous blood in ten dogs with portosystemic shunts. J Vet Intern Med 5:71, 1991.

66. Tobias KMS, Besser TE: Evaluation of leukocytosis, bacteremia, and portal vein partial oxygen tension in normal dogs and dogs with portosystemic shunts. J Am Vet Med Assoc 211:715, 1997.

67. Koblik PD, Hornof WJ: Technetium 99m sulfur colloid scintigraphy to evaluate reticuloendothelial system function in dogs with portosystemic shunts. J Vet Intern Med 9:374, 1995.

68. Mehl ML, Kyles AE, Hardie EM, et al: Evaluation of ameroid ring constrictors for treatment for single extrahepatic portosystemic shunts in dogs. J Am Vet Med Assoc 226:2020, 2005.

69. Niles JD, Williams JM, Cripps PJ, et al: Hemostatic profiles in 39 dogs with congenital portosystemic shunts. Vet Surg 30:97, 2001.

70. Starzl TE, Porter KA, Watanabe K, Putnam CW: Effects of insulin, glucagons, and insulin/glucagons infusions on liver morphology and cell division after complete portacaval shunt in dogs. Lancet I(7964):821, 1976.

71. Hardy RM, Klausner JS. Urate calculi associated with portal vascular anomalies. *In* Current Veterinary Therapy VIII. Kirk RW (ed). Philadelphia: WB Saunders, 1983, p. 1073.

72. Leveille-Webster C: Bile acids- what's new. Semin Vet Med Surg (Small Anim) 12:2, 1997.

73. Center SA: Serum bile acids in companion animal medicine. Vet Clin North Am Small Anim Pract 23:625, 1993.

74. Center SA: Diagnostic techniques and procedures for diseases of the liver and pancreas. Vet Int 9:13, 1997.

75. Tisdall PLC, Hunt GB, Tsoukalas G, and Malik R: Post-prandial serum bile acid concentration and ammonia tolerance in Maltese dogs with and without hepatic vascular anomalies. Austr Vet J 72:121, 1995.

76. Balkman CE, Center SA, Randolph JF, et al: Evaluation of urine sulfated and nonsulfated bile acids a s a diagnostic test for liver disease in dogs J Am Vet Med Assoc 222:1368, 2003.

77. Walker MC, Hill RC, Guilford WG, et al: Postprandial venous ammonia concentrations in the diagnosis of hepatobiliary disease in dogs. J Vet Intern Med 15:463, 2001.

78. Rutgers HC, Batt RM, Haywood S, Riley JE: Hepatic organelle pathology in dogs with congenital portosystemic shunts. J Vet Intern Med 5:351, 1991.

79. Van der Ingh TSGAM, Rothuizen J, Meyer HP: Circulatory disorders of the liver in dogs and cats. Vet Q 17:70, 1995.

80. Van der Ingh TSGAM, Rothuizen J, Meyer HP: Portal hypertension associated with primary hypoplasia of the hepatic portal vein in dogs. Vet Rec 137:424, 1995.

81. Sereda CW, Adin CA: Methods of gradual vascular occlusion and their applications in treatment of congenital portosystemic shunts in dogs: a review. Vet Surg 34:83, 2005.

82. Hunt GB, Kummeling A, Tisdall PLC, et al: Outcomes of cellophane banding for congenital portosystemic shunts in 106 dogs and 5 cats. Vet Surg 33:25, 2004.

83. Hurn SD, Edwards GA: Perioperative outcomes after three different single extrahepatic portosystemic shunt attenuation techniques in dogs: partial ligation, complete ligation, and ameroid constrictor placement. Austral Vet J 81:666, 2003.

84. Leveille R, Johnson SE, Birchard SJ: Transvenous coil embolization of portosystemic shunts in dogs. Vet Radiol Ultrasound 44:32, 2003.

85. Harvey J, Erb HN: Complete ligation of extrahepatic congenital portosystemic shunts in nonencephalopathic dogs. Vet Surg 27:413, 1998.

86. Hunt GB, Bellenger CR, Pearson MB: Transportal approach for attenuating intrahepatic portosystemic shunts in dogs. Vet Surg 25:300, 1996.

87. Swalec KM, Smeak DD: Partial versus complete attenuation of single portosystemic shunts. Vet Surg 19:406, 1990.

88. Papazoglous LG, Monnet E, Seim HB: Survival and prognostic indicators for dogs with intrahepatic portosystemic shunts: 32 cases (1990-2000). Vet Surg 31:561, 2002.

89. Swalec KM, Smeak DD, Brown J: Effect of mechanical and pharmacologic manipulations on portal pressure, central venous pressure, and heart rate. Am J Vet Res 52:1327, 1991.

90. Boothe HW, Howe LM, Edwards JF, Slater MR: Multiple extrahepatic shunts in dogs: 30 cases (1981-1993). J Am Vet Med Assoc 208:1849, 1996.

91. Langdon P, Cohn LA, Kreefer JM, Priddy NH: Acquired portosystemic shunting in two cats. J Am Anim Hosp Assoc 38:21, 2002.

92. Legendre AM, Krahwinkel DJ, Carrig CB, Michel RL: Ascites associated with intrahepatic arteriovenous fistula in a cat. J Am Vet Med Assoc 168:589, 1976.

93. Schaeffer IGF, Kirpensteijn J, Wolvekamp WTC, et al: Hepatic arteriovenous fistulae and portal vein hypoplasia in a Labrador retriever. J Small Anim Pract 42:146, 2001.

94. Szatmari V, Nemeth T, Kotair I, et al: Doppler ultrasonographic diagnosis and anatomy of congenital intrahepatic arterioportal fistula in a puppy. Vet Rad Ultrasound 41:284, 2000.

95. Bailey MQ, Willard MD, McLoughlin MA, et al: Ultrasonographic findings associated with congenital hepatic arteriovenous fistula in three dogs. J Am Vet Med Assoc 192:1099, 1988.

96. Whiting PG, Breznock EM, Moore P, et al: Partial hepatectomy with temporary hepatic vascular occlusion in dogs with hepatic arteriovenous fistulas. Vet Surg 15:171, 1986.

97. Szatmari V, Rothuizen J, van den Ingh TS, et al: Ultrasonographic findings in dogs with hyperammonemia: 90 cases (2000-2002). J Am Vet Med Assoc 224:717, 2004.

98. Moore PF, Whiting PG: Hepatic lesions associated with intrahepatic arterioportal fistulae in dogs. Vet Pathol 23:57, 1986.

Chapter 35

Intestinal Obstruction

Gary W. Ellison

By definition, intestinal obstruction implies the failure of ingesta or intestinal secretions to move in a normal aboral direction.[1] Obstructions are typically classified by their duration, their severity, and their location. Partial or incomplete obstruction is incomplete occlusion of the bowel lumen that allows limited passage of fluid or gas. Complete obstruction is total occlusion of the intestinal lumen, with failure of gas or fluid to pass the point of obstruction. Blockage in the duodenum or upper jejunum constitutes a high intestinal obstruction; blockage in the midjejunal area constitutes a midintestinal obstruction; and blockage in the distal jejunum, ileum, or ileocecal junction constitutes a low intestinal obstruction.

In terms of pathophysiologic changes, obstructions are usually best described as either simple mechanical or strangulating.[1] Simple mechanical obstruction is partial or complete obstruction of the bowel lumen, but the blood supply to the intestinal wall is usually not impaired. Conversely, with strangulation obstruction, the circulation to the involved segment of intestine is impaired, and usually complete obstruction is present.

Etiology of Simple Mechanical Obstruction

The causes of mechanical obstruction can be subdivided into three general categories: intraluminal mechanical obstruction, intramural mechanical obstruction, and extramural mechanical obstruction (Figure 35-1).[2]

Intraluminal mechanical obstruction is the most common type in small animals. The oropharyngeal opening is larger than any other orifice in the alimentary tract and foreign bodies such as bones, balls, or corncobs can traverse the esophagus and stomach and become lodged in the smaller-diameter intestine. Large intraluminal foreign bodies often cause signs consistent with complete luminal obstruction, although slow aboral passage of the foreign body may occur. Polypoid intestinal masses or linear foreign bodies such as string may cause partial or incomplete luminal obstruction. In cats, benign adenomatous polyps of the upper duodenum can cause intermittent hematotemesis.[3] The trailing end of linear foreign bodies often becomes anchored over the base of the tongue or in the pyloric antrum. Normal intestinal peristalsis moves the foreign body distally, but because it is fixed proximally the bowel plicates itself along the length of the foreign body.[4]

Intramural mechanical obstruction is most commonly caused by intestinal wall neoplasia or fungal granulomas. Intestinal neoplasms such as adenocarcinoma, leiomyoma, leiomyosarcoma, fibrosarcoma, and lymphosarcoma commonly invade the muscular layer of the intestinal wall. These tumors not only compromise lumen diameter, they also reduce the pliability of the intestinal wall at that point, reducing its distensibility and likening the occurrence of intussusception. In the Southeastern United States, intestinal granulomas caused by the algae Pythium species is a common cause of intestinal obstruction. This obligate organism creates mural thickening and fibrosis that interferes with normal intestinal absorption and also prevents normal intestinal distention. Both intestinal neoplasms and fungal granulomas tend to cause incomplete mechanical obstruction. Onset of clinical signs is often delayed or insidious.[4]

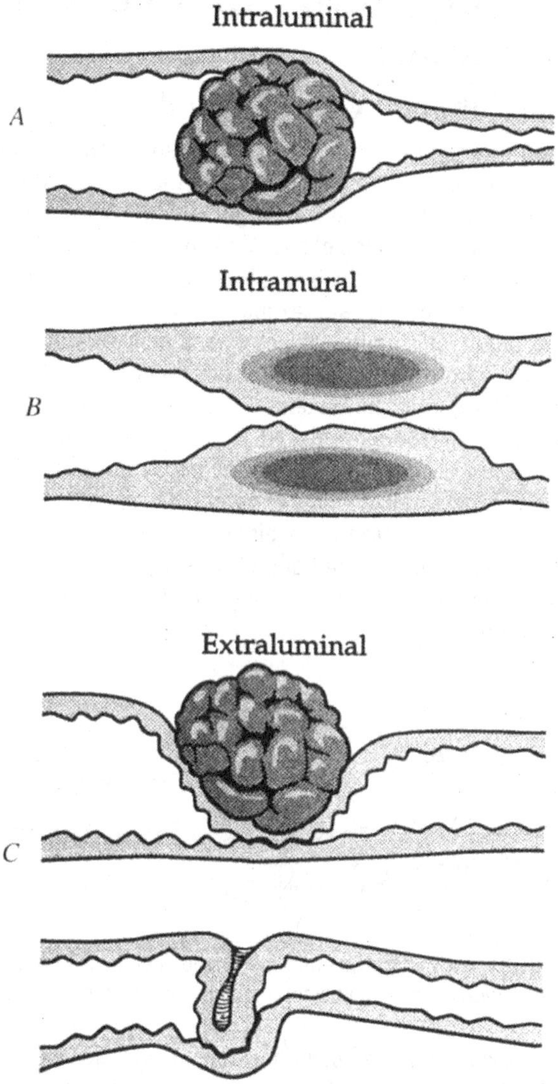

Figure 35-1. Types of mechanical obstruction. A. An intraluminal obstruction caused by a foreign body. B. An intramural obstruction created by neoplasia or granuloma. C. An extra-mural obstruction caused by an extramural mass (top) or kinking of the bowel wall to adhesions (below).

Extraluminal small intestinal obstruction resulting from adhesions is a potential sequela of elective abdominal surgery. Because of this, there is increasing emphasis on minimally invasive laparoscopy techniques in human and veterinary medicine. Most experimental and clinical studies in people found a reduction of adhesions with laparoscopy versus laparotomy.[5] Although adhesions do occur in the dog and cat abdomen following laparotomy, functional obstruction is less common. Studies of intestinal transit times after planned enteroplication techniques for intussusception in dogs have shown that no delay occurs in actual transit time when planned adhesions are created.[6] Clinical signs relating to extraluminal obstruction in small animals are more often a result of compression because of pancreatic abscess or neoplasia or translocation of the bowel through rents in the mesentery or through hernias in the diaphragm, umbilicus, or inguinal or femoral triangle region. These latter translocations usually lead to strangulation obstruction.

Pathophysiology of Mechanical Obstruction

Accumulation of Gas and Fluid

Complete intraluminal mechanical obstruction results in distention of the bowel proximal (oral) to the obstruction, owing to accumulation of gas and fluid (Figure 35-2). The gas accumulating proximal (oral) to the obstruction consists of swallowed air (72%) and gas formed in the body (28%).[1] Of the gas formed in the body, it is estimated that approximately 70% is gas that diffuses from the blood into the bowel lumen, and a smaller percentage (30%) results from intramural decomposition of food material by bacteria. The gas in the distended bowel is composed principally of nitrogen (70%), oxygen (10% to 12%), and hydrogen (1% to 3%), which mimics those percentages seen in atmospheric air. Additionally, small amounts of carbon dioxide (6% to 9%) can be formed from neutralization of bicarbonate in the bowel lumen. Organic gases such as methane (1%) or hydrogen sulfide (1% to 10%) when present are the result of low-level bacterial fermentation.[1]

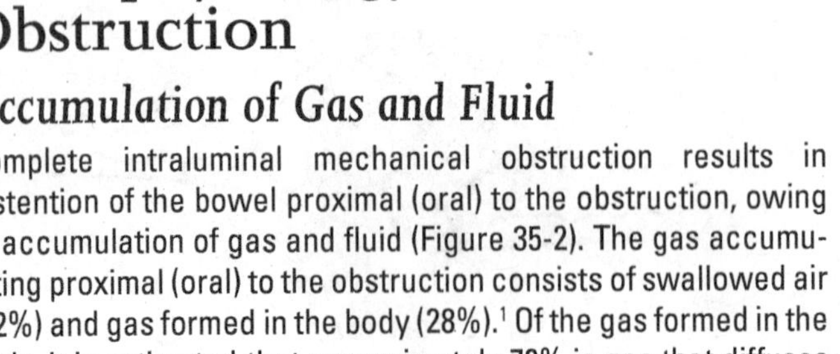

Figure 35-2. The pathophysiology of simple mechanical obstruction associated with an intraluminal foreign body. See text for details.

Fluid accumulation is a result not only of retention of ingested fluids but also of the significant production of secretions in the upper gastrointestinal tract. It is estimated that a 40 kg dog actually produces in excess of 2100 ml of secretions per day. Most of these secretions are reabsorbed in the lower jejunum and ileum; only an estimated 4% to 1% of the water volume reaches the colon.[7] Water transport in the gut is normally passively regulated, principally by hydrostatic pressure gradients that are created mainly by solute transfer. The intracellular solute pathway that allows passive diffusion between the pores and tight junctions of epithelial cells is controlled by electrochemical, osmotic, and hydrostatic pressure gradients.

During mechanical obstruction, the absorption of water from the gut lumen is reduced by several mechanisms. Transport of solutes through the epithelial cells is impaired, which normally occurs by active transport via sodium ion membrane pumps or brush border membrane carriers. Intraluminal osmolality is usually increased and additive factors such as lymphatic and venous congestion also reduce the absorption of solutes.[8] In addition, intestinal mucosal secretion is increased owing to the cyclic AMP mechanism. Factors believed to contribute to increased secretion and decreased absorption include increased concentration of intraluminal bacterial enterotoxins, increased levels of bile and fatty acids, or products of tissue ischemia.[9] The distended bowel may lose its ability to absorb fluids within 24 hours after onset of obstruction.

Normal intraluminal pressure in the canine small bowel is 2 to 4 mm Hg. It is estimated that normal peristalsis may produce pressures in the range of 15 to 25 mm Hg. Three days after creation of a total obstruction, intraluminal pressure in the small bowel of dogs can be as high as 44 mm Hg.[10] During vomiting it can rise as high as 95 mm Hg. Rapid lymphatic and capillary stasis occurs when intraluminal pressure reaches 30 mm Hg, and total occlusion of venous drainage occurs at 50 mm Hg.[9] Because the arterial supply is not affected, capillary congestion can occur at the microcirculatory level. The increased hydrostatic pressure at the capillary bed level produces a net shift of fluid into the interstitium, resulting in bowel wall edema. Eventually, fluid can shift not only from the bowel wall into the lumen but also through the serosal surface into the peritoneal cavity.

Increases in pressure also cause circulatory impairment of the submucosa and muscular layers of the bowel wall. Early impairment of the villous circulation within the mucosa is seen when the pressure reaches 20 mm Hg. Reductions in mesenteric and submucosal blood flow occur when the intraluminal pressures reach 30 mm Hg. Oxygenation of the intestinal mucosa decreases significantly when the intraluminal pressure exceeds 40 mm Hg. At 44 mm Hg arteriovenous shunting occurs at the mucosal villous base. Therefore, selective mucosal ischemia can follow simple mechanical obstruction if intraluminal pressure rises above 40 mm Hg. Because in naturally occurring mechanical obstruction physiologic pressure probably does not exceed 50 mm Hg, full-thickness devitalization of the wall usually does not occur in the dilated proximal segment.[10]

Reduced Motility and Bacterial Overgrowth

The bowel responds to gaseous and fluid distention with periodic bursts of neuromuscular activity, resulting in peristaltic rushes. These wave-like movements begin in the proximal bowel and traverse the entire length of intestine above the point of obstruction. Periods of hyperactivity are then followed by quiescent periods of varying duration. Experimental studies in dogs have shown increased myoelectric activity above the point of obstruction. The intestine distal to the obstruction simultaneously exhibits reduced peristaltic activity. With increased distention from prolonged obstruction, clusters of intense myoelectric activity are felt by the patient as intermittent cramps (colic). It is believed that this phenomenon is largely caused by stimulation of the proximal bowel through cholinergic pathways and by inhibition of the bowel distal to the obstruction through noncholinergic nonadrenergic pathways.[11]

Small intestinal stasis may lead to luminal bacterial over-growth. In normal intestinal mucosa, bacteria and their enterotoxins are not able to cross the mucosal barrier. In the impaired mucosal barrier, a potential exists for increased permeability and migration of bacteria and their toxic products into the systemic circulation or the peritoneal cavity.[1] Decompression of the distention usually allows reversal of the circulatory changes and provides for rapid mucosal regeneration.[10] However, if necrosis of the bowel wall occurs owing to prolonged severe distention or direct pressure from the obstructing object, the mucosal barrier may break down and transmural migration of bacteria and endotoxins beneath the obstructing foreign body may occur.

Level of Obstruction and Electrolyte Loss

The classic clinical signs associated with high (duodenal and proximal jejunal) obstruction are described as frequent vomiting that begins soon after the onset of obstruction. Yet experimental data support the observation that dogs and cats with high intestinal obstruction may not begin vomiting for 24 to 72 hours. Electrolyte loss is closely associated with the level of obstruction. With obstructions at the pylorus, gastric fluids that are rich in potassium, sodium, hydrogen, and chloride ions are vomited. Hypochloremic, hypokalemic, moderately hyponatremic metabolic alkalosis with dehydration may result in early stages.[4] Animals that vomit profusely do not survive as long as those that do not vomit at all.[8]

Severe vomiting associated with duodenal and proximal jejunal obstruction causes loss of gastric hydrochloric acid and bicarbonate-rich alkaline pancreatic secretions. Dehydration with mild metabolic acidosis usually results. With continued fluid depletion, progressive hypovolemic shock occurs. The major cause of mortality from upper small-intestinal obstruction is associated with this severe and rapid hypovolemia. Dogs with experimental complete upper intestinal occlusion usually died within 3 or 4 days without crystalloid fluid therapy.[8] Mortality was greatly reduced with parenteral infusion of physiologic saline or lactated Ringer's solution. Experimental reinfusion of vomitus into the dog's bowel below the obstruction was also life saving.[8]

With low small-intestinal obstruction, the onset of vomiting may not occur until 2 or 3 days after onset of obstruction and it is often intermittent. The distention usually is gaseous during the initial 24 hours, but thereafter is accompanied by loss of varying quantities of fluid into the bowel lumen. Fluid sequestered in low intestinal obstructions is usually mildly hyperosmotic and similar in composition to plasma. Analysis of intraluminal fluid after experimental low obstruction in dogs reveals a mean level of sodium of 140 mEq/L; of potassium, 16.8 mEq/L; and of albumin, 3.6 mg/dl.[8] The sequestration of these fluids from the upper gastrointestinal tract and the increase in secretion of new fluid electrolytes and protein cause a net loss of these compounds. The intraluminal fluid volume increases as the obstruction persists, although some sequestered fluid may move orally and eventually reach a nondistended loop of bowel, where normal reabsorption occurs. Lethargy and anorexia are often apparent in dogs with low intestinal obstruction. These animals exhibit steady weight loss and drink but do not eat. Dogs with experimentally created complete low intestinal obstructions may survive three weeks or longer if adequate water is provided.[9]

Evaluating Intestinal Viability

Intestinal viability is best evaluated after decompressing the dilated loops of bowel and removing the obstruction. In most cases of simple nonstrangulated obstruction, bowel viability is maintained and the appearance of dark distended loops of bowel improves rapidly after enterotomy and removal of the obstruction. Questionable areas of bowel viability are assessed with standard clinical criteria, including bowel-wall color, presence of arterial pulsations, and presence of intestinal peristalsis. The continued presence of intestinal myoelectric activity is the most important parameter of viability.[4] The *pinch test* should be performed on questionable areas of intestine, to determine whether smooth muscle contraction and peristalsis can be initiated.

Experimentally, bowel-wall viability has been assessed using temperature probes, pH monitors, Doppler devices, intravenous vital dyes, and surface oximetry. Fluorescein dye given intravenously through a peripheral vein at a dose of 20 mg/kg has been shown to be beneficial in determining intestinal wall (but not gastric wall) viability, particularly if the ischemia is mainly arterial versus venous in origin.[10] The tissues are subjected to 365-nm ultraviolet light (Wood's lamp). Normal bowel wall viability is represented by a bright green glow with smooth, uniform fluorescence. Areas of the bowel are considered viable if they have a normal or fine granular fluorescent pattern. Areas of bowel are considered nonviable if they have a patchy density where areas of nonfluorescence exceed 3 mm diameter or where only perivascular fluorescence is seen.[12] Pulse oximetry has also been utilized as a feasible technique to evaluate experimental intestinal ischemia in dogs. Dogs with bowel segment values exceeding PO_2 of 85% in general survived, whereas those with values lower than this had statistically higher incidence of ischemia and anastomotic breakdown. All anastomoses performed in segments with PO_2 values of 60 to 70% failed.[13]

Strangulation Obstruction

Causes and Classification

By definition, strangulation obstruction implies an obstructive process with loss of vascular integrity to the bowel wall. Common causes include intussusception, traumatic avulsion of the mesentery, mesenteric arteriothrombosis, mesenteric (intestinal) volvulus, and strangulated diaphragmatic, inguinal, or abdominal hernia. Foreign bodies can also create local small discrete areas of "pressure" strangulation necrosis. Strangulation obstruction may occur secondary to venous obstruction or thrombosis, arterial obstruction or thrombosis, or a combination of both. If the strangulating process incorporates the mesenteric vessels, devitalization of large segments of the intestinal tract may occur. Strangulation obstruction should be considered a medical and surgical emergency. Death is often rapid, the result of hypovolemia and septic shock secondary to devitalization of the intestinal wall.

Pathophysiology

Pathophysiologic changes as described under simple mechanical obstruction occur proximal to the strangulation obstruction in addition to the direct changes attributable to the strangulated bowel segment. Partial venous occlusion, such as that caused by partially strangulated hernia or intussusception, is a common type of intestinal strangulation in small animals. With venous occlusion alone, the arterial supply remains intact, allowing bowel-wall edema and sequestration of blood in the intestinal wall. Motility changes in the bowel wall are proportional to the duration of venous obstruction. Spike activity and motility of the affected bowel segment may be initially increased. As tissue hypoxia progresse, cyanosis becomes evident and motility gradually decreases until it ceases completely.

With complete venous occlusion or thrombosis, wall edema, hemorrhage, and mucosal epithelial sloughing can occur as early as 1 to 3 hours after the insult. The strangulated loop then gradually becomes more turgid, and whole blood begins accumulating in the bowel lumen and extravasating into the peritoneal cavity (Figure 35-3). The bowel wall becomes visibly thickened and dark red to blue. Eight to 12 hours after complete venous occlusion the bowel segment turns black and distends maximally. When complete arterial occlusion occurs, as with mesenteric volvulus, full-thickness ischemia of the bowel wall occurs and bacteria and red cells invade all layers of the wall within 20 hours of strangulation.

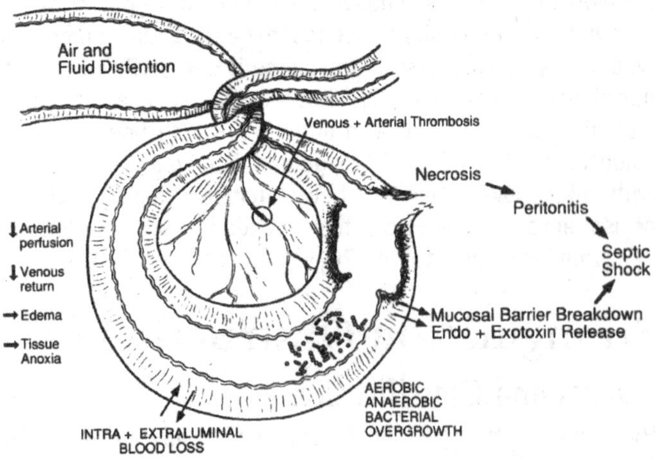

Figure 35-3. The pathophysiology of strangulation obstruction associated with intestinal volvulus. See text for details.

Translocation of Bacteria

The flora in the proximal small bowel consists primarily of gram-positive, facultative bacteria, whereas the distal small intestine contains primarily aerobic coliforms and anaerobic species. Organisms that are normally found in the terminal intestinemove to upper levels of the small intestine. Marked increases in aerobic coliform bacteria and Streptococcus species occur, in addition to large increases in anaerobic Clostridia and Bacillus species. Small intestinal bacterial concentrations that normally range from 10^2 to 10^4 per milliliter liquid secretion may increase to 10^8 to 10^{11} per milliliter within just 6 hours after the onset of strangulation.[14] A massive proliferation of resident bacteria also occurs within the strangulated section of bowel. Bacteria, particularly *Clostridium perfringens,* play a key role in the mortality of strangulation obstruction because germ-free animals live significantly longer than those with normal intestinal flora in experimental models.

Loss of mucosal function leads to passage of viable bacteria or endotoxins through the epithelial mucosa into the lamina propria and then to the intraabdominal cavity and systemic circulation. Bacterial translocation does occur in simple mechanical obstruction of the small bowel or colon. In strangulation obstruction, the loss of gut barrier function occurs more severely compared with simple obstruction because the ischemia promotes the rapid destruction of the intestinal epithelium. Three mechanisms that promote bacterial translocation have been identified: 1) intestinal bacterial overgrowth; 2) increased permeability of the intestinal mucosal barrier; and 3) deficiencies in host immune defenses.[14]

Clinical Presentation

Clinically, free peritoneal fluid begins to accumulate shortly after the development of strangulation obstruction. Initially, the fluid is a transudate resulting from effusion from serosal vessels secondary to venous congestion or obstruction. The initial fluid is pink, clear, and odorless, and relatively low in protein. As the length of time of strangulation obstruction increases, the appearance of the fluid changes: it becomes black and has a foul odor. This is thought to be caused by filtration of lumen contents through the devitalized bowel wall.[14] After prolonged strangulation obstruction, hypoxia in the intestinal wall results in complete breakdown of the mucosal barrier. With arterial thrombosis, full-thickness necrosis occurs, as does perforation and septic peritonitis, with resultant inflammatory cells, ingesta, and bacteria.

Many experimental and clinical studies have independantly proposed the hypothesis that the loss of gut barrier function and the consequent translocation of bacteria and their products may play an important role in the development of multiple organ failure (MOF) in strangulation obstruction. Evidence is growing that loss of gut barrier function to bacteria and or "endotoxins" might induce a local intestinal inflammatory response and lead to the subsequent release of cytokines (TNF, IL-1, 1L-6, IL-8, etc.).[15] Strangulation obstruction has been shown to cause increased release of IL-6 to intestinal venous blood in pigs.[16]

Plasma lactate has been shown to be of value in the diagnosis of gastrointestinal ischemia. In dogs with GDV, serum lactate values of more than 6 mm/L have been shown to be a positive predictor of gastric necrosis.[17] Likewise, peritoneal lactate levels in dogs with experimentally induced ischemia of the small intestine were found to be highly predictive for intestinal ischemia in these animals.[18]

Treatment

Treatment for strangulated intestinal obstruction involves not only fluid and electrolyte support but also aggressive antibiotic therapy, and possibly nonsteroidal anti-inflammatory drugs. If massive blood loss has taken place, blood transfusions may also be warranted. Early surgical removal of the devitalized section of bowel wall is essential. In experimental models of strangulated obstruction in dogs, death is delayed by the administration of broad-spectrum systemic antibiotics, particularly the aminoglycoside derivatives in combination with penicillins and metronidazole or third-generation cephalosporins.

Intestinal Pseudo-obstruction

Chronic intestinal pseudo-obstruction is a syndrome, originally described in humans, characterized by chronic or recurrent symptoms of intestinal obstruction. The obstruction occurs in the absence of both organic luminal obstruction and a recognized underlying disease. Although previously limited to the human literature, the disease syndrome has been described in two dogs and a cat.[19-21] Clinical manifestations result from delayed intestinal transit caused by disordered motility. Although all portions of the alimentary tract can be affected, the small bowel is most often involved. In some cases of pseudo-obstruction no pathologic abnormality can be found. In other cases, histologic examination has shown two distinct pathologic abnormalities. In humans, one pathologic subtype includes direct degeneration of intramural neurons, which are specifically associated with arrangement of the myenteric plexus, the celiac ganglion, the spinal cord, and even the brain. This type of chronic pseudo-obstruction has been labeled "visceral neuropathy." The second type of idiopathic intestinal pseudo-obstruction is caused by degeneration of intestinal smooth muscle cells -- so-called visceral myopathy. Histologic sections of bowel of this type have shown vacuolization of the smooth muscle and atrophy of muscle fibers in both the longitudinal and circular muscle layers of the bowel wall. All affected animals had chronic vomiting and weight loss with concurrent dilatation of the small intestine. In a mixed breed dog, atrophy of cecal smooth muscle fibers as well as infiltration of plasma cell lymphocytes and macrophages and mild lymphoplasmacytic enteritis were present.[19] In an English bulldog, both atrophy and fibrosis with monocellular infiltrate were noted from the duodenum to the colon.[20] In a cat, a regional jejunal area also displayed marked atrophy of the outer longitudinal muscular layer along with fibroplasia and vacuolar degeneration consistent with visceral myopathy in humans.[21] Clinical signs of idiopathic intestinal pseudo-obstruction in man include abdominal pain, constipation, diarrhea, and vomiting. In the acute stages, abdominal distention may occur. Surgery is usually avoided if possible; it is rarely beneficial. Stimulation of the gastrointestinal smooth muscle by prokinetic agents such as metoclopramide or cisapride might be helpful, as might nutritional support, in the form of enteral hyperalimentation. Results of surgery in animals have been similarly unsuccessful.

References

1. Lance GC: The pathophysiology of acute mechanical small bowel obstruction. Comp Contin Educ Small Anim Pract 3:910, 1981.

2. Holder WD: Intestinal obstruction. Gastroenterol Clin North Am 17:317, 1988.

3. MacDonald JM, Mullen HS, Moroff SD: Adenomatous polyps of the duodenum in cats: 18 cases (1985-1990). J Am Vet Med Assoc 202:647-651, 1993.

4. Ellison GW: Nontraumatic surgical emergencies of the abdomen. *In* Contemporary Issues in Small Animal Practice, Vol 2. Bright RM (ed). New York: Churchill Livingstone, 1986, p 127.

5. Gutt CN, Oniu T, Schemmer P, et al: Fewer adhesions induced by laparoscopic surgery? Surg Endoscop 18:898, 2004.

6. Lewis DD, Ellison GW: Intussusception in dogs and cats. Comp Contin Educ Small Anim Pract 9:523, 1987.

7. Strombeck D: Small Animal Gastroenterology. Davis, CA: Stonegate, 1979, pp. 165-166.

8. Mishra N, Appert HE, Howard JM, et al: The effects of distension and obstruction on the accumulation of fluid in the lumen of small bowel of dogs. Ann Surg 180:791, 1974.

9. Mirkovitch V, Cobo F, Robinson JW, et al: Morphology and function of the dog ileum after mechanical occlusion. Clin Sci Mol Med 50:123, 1976.

10. Shikata J, Shida T, Amino K, et al: Experimental studies on the hemodynamics of the small intestine following increased intraluminal pressure. Surg Gynecol Obstet 156:155, 1983.

11. Ishitani MB, Jones RS: Alterations in intestinal motility. *In* Surgery of the Stomach, Duodenum and Small Intestine. Scott HW, Sawyers JL (eds). Boston: Blackwell Scientific, 1987.

12. Ellison GW, Jokinen MC, Park RD: End-to-end intestinal anastomosis in the dog -- a comparative fluorescein dye, angiographic and histopathologic evaluation. J Am Anim Hosp Assoc 21:729, 1982.

13. Turkyilmaz Z, Sonmez K, Basaklar AC, et al: Assessment of anastomotic reliability with pulse oximetry in graded intestinal ischemia: an experimental study in dogs. J Pediatric Surg 32:1728, 1997.

14. O' Boyle CJ, MacFie J, Mitchell CJ, et al: Microbiology of bacterial translocation in humans. Gut 42:29-35, 1998.

15. Malnous MK, Ertel W, Chaudry IH, et al: The gut. A cytokine-generating organ in systemic inflammation? Shock 4:193-199, 1995.

16. Fevang J, Ovrebo K, Svanes K, et al: Endotoxin and cytokine release in strangulation obstruction and in partial occlusion of the mesenteric artery in pigs. Eur Surg Res 31:26, 1999.

17. de Papp E, Drobatz KJ, Hughes D: Plasma lactate concentration as a predictor of gastric necrosis and survival among dogs with gastric dilatation-volvulus: 102 cases (1995-1998). J Am Vet Med Assoc 215:49-52, 1999.

18. DeLaurier GA, Ivey RK, Johnson RH: Peritoneal fluid lactic acid and diagnostic dilemmas in acute abdominal disease. Am J Surg 167:302-305, 1994.

19. Eastwood JM, McInnes EF, White RN, et al: Caecal impaction and chronic intestinal pseudo-obstruction in a dog. J Vet Physiol Pathol Clin Med 52:43, 2005.

20. Duir E, Leisewitz AL, VanderLust JJ: Chronic idiopathic intestinal pseudo-obstruction in an English bulldog. J Small Anim Pract 42:243-247, 2001.

21. Harvey AM, Wall EJ, Day M.J, et al: Chronic intestinal pseudo-obstruction in a cat caused by visceral myopathy. J Vet Intern Med 19:111-114, 2005.

Chapter 36

Ileus

Gary W. Ellison

Ileus, also known as adynamic ileus, paralytic ileus, postoperative ileus, or intestinal dysmotility is a transient and usually reversible intestinal obstruction caused by delayed intestinal motility. Intestinal contents fail to progress aborally because of ineffective intestinal propulsion in the absence of mechanical occlusion of the lumen. Ileus is clinically manifested by abdominal distension, lack of bowel sounds, delayed passage of ingesta, and accumulation of gas and fluid in the bowel that may lead to nausea and vomiting. The exact pathophysiologic basis of ileus is unknown but is likely multifactorial with three major interrelated mechanisms -- neurogenic, inflammatory, and pharmacologic -- leading to its development.[1] It is among the most significant side effects of abdominal surgery in humans and horses, accounting for increased morbidity and prolonged hospitalization. The condition is less well understood in small animals. Whether it is less prevalent or whether the clinical signs are less severe than in other species is unclear.

Etiology

Ileus may be caused by a wide variety of intraabdominal, extra-abdominal, and systemic conditions, in addition to a host of chemical and pharmacologic agents (Table 36-1). Peritoneal inflammation, caused by infection, bile leakage, pancreatic enzymes, or surgery, can induce ileus in small animals. Systemic derangements owing to sepsis and electrolyte imbalances are also associated with ileus. In addition, ileus can be pharmacologically initiated via the administration of opioids, anticholinergic drugs, and the phenothiazine tranquilizers. Reported extra-abdominal causes may include systemic toxicity, uremia, spinal cord trauma, shock, and prolonged anesthesia.[2] Extra-abdominal thoracic lesions such as pneumonia, myocardial infarction, congestive heart failure, or rib fractures are reported causes of ileus in humans, but these remain undocumented in the dog and cat. Abrasion of the intestinal serosal surfaces with dry surgical sponges creates an ileus model in dogs that is used to study the human disease.[3] Postoperative ileus is inherent to any intraabdominal surgical procedure, but its severity and duration appear less with laparoscopic procedures.[1]

Table 36-1. Potential Causes of Ileus in Small Animals

Intraabdominal
Postsurgical
Septic peritonitis
Bile peritonitis
Inflammatory bowel disease
Pancreatitis
Uroperitoneum
Systemic
Shock
Septicemia
Electrolyte imbalance (potassium)
Metabolic acidosis
Uremia
Prolonged anesthesia
Spinal cord trauma
Pharmacologic
Anticholinergics
Phenothiazine tranquilizers
Opioids
Ganglionic blocking agents
Antihistamines
Vascular
Thrombophlebitis
Arteritis

Neurohormonal Mechanisms of Ileus

Parasympathetic (cholinergic) stimulation increases intestinal motility and secretion, whereas sympathetic (adrenergic) stimulation results in reduced motility and an increase in sphincter tone. Postoperative ileus may occur secondary to sympathetic hyperactivity and parasympathetic hypoactivity. Evidence of increased circulating levels of epinephrine and norepinephrine following abdominal surgery supports this theory. Stimulation of the sympathetic nervous system inhibits the interdigestive motor complexes that ordinarily propel the bowel contents aborally. Release of norepinephrine also appears to inhibit release of excitatory neurotransmitters such as acetylcholine, thereby allowing the inhibitory neurons to dominate.[2] The protective effect of alpha and beta sympathetic nerve blockers, splanchnic nerve division, or spinal anesthesia against the development of postoperative ileus in dogs and cats further supports this concept.[3]

The dog normally undergoes a period of reduced myoelectric activity after exploratory laparotomy. Studies in dogs have shown that normal small intestinal myoelectric activity usually resumes by 12 hours postoperatively, whereas gastric paresis persists for approximately 24 hours. Colonic motility is most affected; normal status does not return until approximately 48 hours after laparotomy.[4] Myoelectric slow waves still exist in the outer longitudinal muscles with ileus but do not initiate action potentials and associated contractile activity within the circular muscle layers. This electromechanical dissociation appears to result from a tonic discharge of inhibitory neurons and an absence of spike waves. Because the presence of ingesta may stimulate parasympathetic tone and resultant contractile activity, surgeons have noted that patients receiving enteral alimentation in the immediate postoperative period experience less postoperative ileus than do patients who are made to fast.[1]

Humoral intestinal peptides may also contribute to the pathophysiology of postoperative ileus. The hormone vasopressin disrupts jejunal motility and occurs in high levels in plasma following laparotomy, whereas the prokinetic hormones motilin and neurotensin stimulate small-intestinal activity and are suppressed for 24 hours following laparotomy.[4] Return of motilin to normal levels corresponds with return of motility. Release of endogenous opiates has also been proposed as a cause of ileus. Although naloxone does not relieve postoperative ileus in dogs, fedoztozine, a k-opioid agonist does restore intestinal motility in rats.[5]

Electrolyte imbalances have been associated with experimental ileus in dogs. A significant reduction in intestinal propulsion is associated with decreases in serum sodium and chloride values. Potassium deficits may play a more profound role than the sympathetic nervous system in the development of ileus. Hypokalemia may negatively effect the exchange of cellular potassium for plasma hydrogen ions when acidosis is present and greatly reduce smooth muscle contractility.[6]

Progression of Ileus

Ileus may affect the entire gastrointestinal tract or may be localized to one area. Obstruction in any one segment of the intestine may secondarily affect the rest of the intestinal tract via an intestinointestinal reflex whereby distention of bowel in one area inhibits motility in other areas. Therefore, segmental ileus can ultimately become diffuse. With prolonged ileus, pathophysiologic changes are similar to those seen in simple mechanical obstruction. Although there is no physical barrier to the passage of ingesta, the bowel becomes functionally obstructed owing to lack of effective intestinal motility. The lumen of the adynamic segment fills with swallowed air, gas from bacterial fermentation, ingested fluids, and secretions from the stomach, pancreas, intestine, and biliary tract. During ileus, these fluids are not resorbed and additional fluids are secreted from the distended gut wall. The net loss of circulating intravascular fluid results in dehydration and ensuing hypovolemic shock.[3]

Unresolved ileus perpetuates a vicious cycle, whereby distention promotes further ileus, which leads to greater distention. Prolonged ileus may also result in diffuse intestinal damage as a result of lymphatic and venous obstruction. Mucosal arteriovenous shunting, hypoxia, ischemia, and necrosis may all result. Early ischemia of the bowel wall initially results in hypermotility and spasms; complete cessation of motility occurs as the bowel-wall ischemia progresses toward necrosis. Similar to simple mechanical obstruction, bacterial over-growth occurs, and endotoxins may be produced in larger quantities than normal. In severe cases of long-standing ileus, transmural migration of bacteria and endotoxins may result in signs consistent with septic shock.

Pain-Induced Ileus

Animals that have post-laparotomy ileus characteristically do not show severe abdominal pain, although those that develop ileus secondary to septic peritonitis show abdominal splinting and clinical signs associated with abdominal pain. The mechanism of ileus secondary to peritonitis is a direct result of noxious stimuli of the abdominal viscera and parietal peritoneum. Visceral pain impulses stimulate sympathetic splanchnic nerves, which traverse the splenic ganglion and sympathetic chain to increase sympathetic tone. The inflammatory response must involve multiple nerve endings and be acute in order to create visceral abdominal pain (colic). This adrenergic stimulation of receptors in the gut wall is thought to inhibit intestinal motility.

Nerve endings of pain fibers are located in the submucosa of the bowel wall. Therefore, any process that causes fluid or gaseous distention, intestinal obstruction, forceful contraction, hypersegmentation, or traction (adhesions) may produce pain. Inflammation, whether it be secondary to peritonitis or due to tissue ischemia produces abdominal pain by creating a local intestinal inflammatory response, which leads to the subsequent release of cytokines (TNF, IL-1, IL-6, IL-8).[7] Nerve endings are also plentiful in the parietal peritoneum, and these are sensitive to the massive inflammatory response. This is why the splenic rigid abdominal posture and resistance to palpation are seen in most cases of ileus secondary to generalized peritonitis.[8]

Drug-Induced Ileus

Postoperative pain can cause bowel stasis, abdominal distention, discomfort, and vomiting. Analgesic intervention may alleviate these signs but may also have the potential to exacerbate ileus. Perioperative administration of drugs that inhibit intestinal motility may potentiate the severity of ileus in the postoperative period. In dogs, opioids such as morphine or hydromorphone act as gatrointestinal μ2 receptor agonists. They cause stasis by decreasing longitudinal muscle propulsive motility and increasing segmental contractions. Other opiates such as loperamide decrease pancreatic and biliary secretions and have antisecretory effects on the bowel that contribute to their antidiarrheal properties.[1] The effect on motility of other opioids such as butorphanol or pentazocine at recommended analgesic doses appears less inhibitory in dogs.[9]

The use of analgesics is particularly important with regard to intestinal motility in cats. The combination of ketamine (5 mg/kg) and midazolam (0.1 mg/kg) decreases gastrointestinal motility. Intramuscular acepromazine at 0.1 mg/kg combined with buprenorphine 0.01 mg/kg or medetomidine (50 μg/kg) does not affect orocecal transit time when used for short periods; however, oral buprenorphine used over several days may slow transit time.[10] Transdermal fentanyl patches do not seem to slow motility in dogs or cats. Anesthetic regime also will affect the incidence of postoperative ileus. In human medicine, the use of short-acting induction agents such as propofol, rapidly cleared inhalants such as sevoflurane, and minimally inhibitory opiates such as fentanyl is a preferred regime in the prevention of postoperative ileus.[9]

Clinical Signs

Clinical signs associated with ileus in dogs and cats are often obscure. Small-animal clinicians rarely auscultate the abdomens of their patients so reduction in intestinal sounds and borborygmi may be inconsistent findings. Gross abdominal distention may be present, and evidence of fluid and gas distention of the small intestine may be noted on radiographs or ultrasonography.

Distended loops of bowel also may be present on abdominal palpation. Loops of bowel distended by ileus are generally not as large, turgid, or painful as those distended by simple mechanical or strangulation obstruction. In long-standing cases of ileus, feces may be minimal or absent. In the absence of peritonitis, pain is not usually associated with ileus unless intestinal distention becomes severe. Gastric reflux on intubation is a hallmark of intestinal ileus in horses and humans, but its significance in small animals appears minimal.[2]

Treatment

Ileus that is uncomplicated and not associated with organic obstruction often resolves spontaneously without aggressive treatment. Early postoperative feeding is recommended to stimulate gastrointestinal motility and speed intestinal wound healing in patients recovering from gastrointestinal surgery. Failure of ileus to resolve spontaneously indicates that mechanical obstruction, strangulation obstruction, or septic peritonitis may be present. Abdominocentesis may be indicated to differentiate simple ileus from more severe strangulation obstruction.

Successful treatment of ileus involves the correction of concurrent electrolyte imbalances, elimination of underlying abdominal disease (including decompression of the distended bowel when possible), and possibly, promotililty drug therapy. Dehydration and serum electrolyte and acid-base status imbalances should be corrected. Serum potassium concentration is particularly important, because the concurrent movement of potassium from the extra-cellular to the intracellular space may result in hyperkalemia or hypokalemia. In the case of hypokalemia, supplementation with intravenous potassium is indicated. Bicarbonate supplementation may also be indicated to correct metabolic acidosis.

Because most cases of paralytic ileus in dogs and cats resolve spontaneously, the presence of continued, unaccounted for intestinal distention should warn the clinician of a residual problem that warrants exploratory laparotomy. Any areas of devitalized bowel must be removed at surgery. Gas and fluids should be removed from remaining distended loops of bowel, using a 22-gauge needle and continuous-suction apparatus. An indwelling nasogastric tube may also be placed, to decompress the stomach in the postoperative period. Continuous or intermittent suction can be applied to these tubes to facilitate continued gastric and intestinal decompression in the postoperative period.

Pharmacologic Therapy

Administration of drugs to stimulate intestinal motility and counteract the effects of ileus has not been consistently successful. Sympathetic blockade, parasympathetic stimulation, or both have been advocated. The anticholinesterase drug neostigmine does increase propulsive motility of the colon, although it decreases propulsive motility of the jejunum and delays gastric emptying. Pain may also occur secondary to intestinal spasm. In addition, neostigmine may increase the risk of anastomotic dehiscence and, therefore, is not recommended.[3]

Sympathetic nervous system blockade with phenothiazine derivatives such as chlorpromazine has been used to treat postoperative ileus in humans. This drug is a sympathetic alpha-blocker, which can potentiate shock. Therefore, animals should be well hydrated and their cardiovascular status stable before acetylpromazine or chlorpromazine is administered.[1] Sympathetic blockage with topical analgesics or opioids has been shown to counteract ileus in people, but is little used in dogs.

Metoclopramide is an anti-dopaminergic drug that appears to enhance coordination of gastroduodenal motor activity. Its gastrointestinal smooth muscle action is thought to result from antagonism of the inhibitory neurotransmitter dopamine; however, it now appears that metoclopramide acts to directly enhance gastrointestinal motility by augmenting release of acetylcholine, and perhaps by inhibiting serotonin release. Metoclopramide was shown to reverse decreased gastrointestinal myoelectric and contractile activity in surgically created adynamic ileus in dogs but its efficacy in humans is questionable.[1,11] Metoclopramide may decrease nausea and vomiting owing to its gastric effects rather than by correcting postoperative ileus.

Cisapride is a benzamide drug that stimulates gastrointestinal motility, most likely by facilitating acetylcholine release from myoenteric nerves. Unlike metoclopramide, cisapride possesses no antidopaminergic properties. In addition, it has no effect on gastrointestinal secretion. Experimentally it has been shown to increase lower esophageal sphincter tone, accelerate gastric emptying, and accelerate colonic transit. Experimental work in dogs indicates that cisapride increases the amplitude of intestinal peristaltic waves.[12] The drug was withdrawn from North American and Western European markets in 2000 owing to reported cardiac effects in people, but the drug is still available through compounding agencies in the United States. A new human prokinetic agent, tegaserod may prove useful in therapy of intestinal motility disorders of animals in the future. Tegaserod is a potent partial nonbenzamide agonist without the effect of prolonging cardiac QT intervals as does cisapride. Tegaserod at doses of 3 to 6 mg/kg has been shown to normalize intestinal transit time in opioid-induced bowel dysfunction in dogs.[13]

Nonsteroidal anti-inflammatory drugs may reduce the incidence of ileus by reducing postoperative pain and inflammation. The Cox-2 inhibitors in particular are thought to reduce the risk and duration of postoperative ileus in people, in part owing to reduction in the need for opiates by as much as 30%.[1] This, of course, must be balanced with the increased tendency toward gastrointestinal bleeding and nephrotoxicity.

Opioid antagonists such as naloxone and alvimopan have been used in human medicine in an attempt to reduce postoperative ileus. Naloxone has been unsuccessful but alvimopan was shown to reduce the incidence of postoperative ileus if given before surgery.[1]

Experimental work has demonstrated that electrical pacing can alter frequency and direction of propagation of the enteric myoelectric pacesetter in dogs. Potentially, antegrade pacing might be expected to enhance gastric or intestinal emptying or to play a positive role in disorders of intestinal atony or stasis.

Although these studies are experimental, clinical use may be feasible in the future.[3]

Summary

Motility of the intestinal tract depends on a highly integrated and coordinated response of the smooth muscle of the bowel wall. Motility of the small and large intestineis controlled by three basic mechanisms: myogenic, neural, and humoral. Present understanding of the control mechanisms and the physiologic and pathologic states that initiate ileus is not complete; however, it can be said that motor disorders usually affect the entire gastrointestinal tract. The disorders can be intrinsic to the gut wall itself, can be caused by an inflammatory process or myogenic dysfunction, or can result from inflammation of the bowel.

Surgical therapy is seldom indicated for the treatment of adynamic or postoperative ileus. Promotility agents, including metoclopramide, cisapride, and tegaserod may be useful in the supportive treatment of hypomotility disorders. Opiates prolong gastrointestinal transit time and may compound the problems seen with ileus. Opioid antagonists may show promise as potentiators of intestinal motility in the future. Laparoscopic procedures show promise of reducing the incidence and severity of postoperative ileus when compared with open laparotomy.

References

1. Bauer AJ, Boeckxstaens GE: Mechanisms of postoperative ileus. Neurogastroenterol Motil 16:54-60, 2004.

2. Guilford WG, Center SA, Strombeck DR, et al: Adynamic ileus. *In* Strombeck's Small Animal Gastroenterology, 3rd ed. Guilford WG, Center SA, Strombeck DR, et al (eds). Philadelphia: WB Saunders, 1996, pp. 535-537.

3. Brolin RE, Reddell MT, Thompson DA: Gastrointestinal myoelectric activity in fasting and nonfasting canine models of ileus. Arch Surg 120:417, 1985.

4. Summers RW, Yanda R, Prihoda, M, et al.: Acute intestinal obstruction: an electromyographic study in dogs. Gastroenterology 85:1301, 1983.

5. Livingston EH, Passaro EP: Postoperative ileus. Dig Dis Sci 35:121-132, 1990.

6. Streeton DHP, Vaughan-Williams EM: Loss of cellular potassium as a cause of intestinal paralysis in dogs. J Physiol 118:149, 1952.

7. Malnous MK, Ertel W, Chaudry IH, et al.: The gut. A cytokine-generating organ in systemic inflammation? Shock 4:193-199, 1995

8. Dillon AR, Spano JS: The acute abdomen. Vet Clin North Am 13:461, 1983.

9. Holzer P: Opioids and opioid receptors in the enteric nervous system: from a problem in opioid analgesia to a possible new prokinetic therapy in humans. Neurosci Lett 361:192-195, 2004.

10. Sparkes AH, Papasouliotis K, Kiner J, et al: Assessment of orocecal transit time in cats by the breath hydrogen method: the effects of sedation and a comparison of definitions. Res Vet Sci 60:243-246, 1996.

11. Graves GM, Becht JL, Rawlings CA: Metoclopramide reversal of decreased gastrointestinal myoelectric and contractile activity in a model of canine postoperative ileus. Vet Surg 18:27, 1989.

12. Fujii K, Oajima M, Kawahori K: Effect of cisapride on the cholinergic central mechanisms of gastrointestinal motility in dogs. Nippon Zashi 24:1, 1988.

13. Washabau RJ: Gastrointestinal motility disorders and gastrointestinal prokinetic therapy. Vet Clin North Am 33:1007-1028, 2003.

Chapter 37

Disorders of Visceral Healing

Gary W. Ellison

The small-animal surgeon routinely creates wounds in the gastrointestinal tract for biopsy, for foreign body or neoplasm removal, or for correction of strangulation obstruction. The urinary bladder wall is likewise wounded to remove calculi or to resect bladder wall tumors. The uterus is incised during cesarean section or removed in ovariohysterectomy, electively or when necessitated by infection. Although dehiscence of a skin wound is often easily remedied with appropriate local wound treatment, dehiscence of a hollow viscus is usually life threatening. Wound dehiscence of the digestive system often leads to generalized bacterial peritonitis and subsequent death. Wound dehiscence of the uterus can have the same outcome if pre-existing intrauterine sepsis is present. Leakage of cystotomy closure may also lead to uroperitoneum, uremia, hyperkalemia, and ultimate death as well. Therefore, factors that negatively affect visceral healing are potentially of great clinical significance to the surgeon.

Normal Wound Healing of the Viscera

The gastrointestinal, urinary, and reproductive tracts follow the same basic healing curve as the skin but have accelerated healing properties. The *lag* or *inflammatory* phase of healing lasts 3 to 4 days.[1] Immediately after wounding, blood vessels contract, platelets aggregate, the coagulation mechanism is activated, and fibrin clots are deposited to control hemorrhage. The fibrin clot offers some minimal wound strength on the first postoperative day, but the main wound support during the lag phase of healing comes from the sutures.[2] Enterocyte and uroepithelial regeneration begins almost immediately after wounding; however, the epithelium offers little biomechanical support.[2,3] The lag phase is the most critical period during visceral wound healing, because most dehiscences take place within 72 to 96 hours after the wound has been created.[2]

The *proliferative* or *logarithmic* phase of visceral wound healing lasts from day 3 or 4 through day 14.[1] Rapid proliferation of fibroblasts occurs logarithmically during this period. The fibroblasts produce large amounts of immature collagen, resulting in rapid gains in wound strength. The proliferative phase of wound healing is a dynamic process in which collagen synthesis takes place in the presence of collagenolysis. In the stomach, small intestine, and urinary tract, collagenase activity at the wound edge is minimal and rapid gains in tensile and bursting strength occur. At the end of 14 days, gastric and small-intestinal wound bursting strength is approximately 75% that of normal tissue. The urinary bladder heals even faster, regaining 100% of normal tissue strength at 14 to 21 days.[3] Conversely, the colon heals much more slowly owing to marked collagenase activity at the wound edge and regains only about 50% of its normal tensile strength 14 days after wounding.[1] Factors such as traumatic suturing, fecal material, bacterial contamination, and infection all increase the amount of local collagenase produced at the wound edge.[2]

The *maturation* phase of wound healing is characterized by reorganization and cross-linking of collagen fibers. This phase extends from day 14 through day 180 in the gastrointestinal tract of the dog,[1] and from day 14 through day 70 in the dog bladder.[3] As with skin wounds, the size and thickness of the scar decrease during this time without weakening the wound. The maturation phase is relatively unimportant clinically in visceral wound healing, because acceptable tensile and bursting strength have been established by the end of the proliferative phase of wound healing and leakage is virtually nonexistent at this point.[2]

Factors that Negatively affect Visceral Wound Healing

Nutritional Depletion

Tissue trauma, sepsis, burns, and major surgery induce major metabolic changes in small-animal patients. With each of these stresses, the animal's basic metabolic rate is accelerated and protein metabolism occurs, leading to a potential state of negative nitrogen balance. Protein-calorie malnutrition (PCM) occurs because of starvation, when a metabolic response to injury becomes prolonged, or when a hypermetabolic state occurs such as that caused by sepsis. It takes only 5 to 10 days of anorexia to compromise the immune system and deplete the body's muscular and hepatic glycogen stores.[4] When PCM is present, cell-mediated immunity is impaired, and there is a high risk of infection, anemia, and hypoproteinemia. Wound healing may also be impaired.

Caloric and protein depletion in experimental animals has been shown to inhibit dermal, muscular-fascial, and visceral healing, but only after a loss of 15% to 20% of body weight.[5] Decreases in wound breaking strength are directly proportional to the carcass weight loss. It is estimated that 75% of animals with elective surgical wounds attain functional wound union during the period of negative nitrogen balance;[6] however, extended PCM from muscle, visceral, or plasma tissue losses increases the risk for visceral wound disruption. Impaired visceral wound healing is due both to a prolonged lag phase of healing and to diminished capacity for fibroplasia within the logarithmic phase.[7]

Effect of Early Postoperative Enteral Feeding on Visceral Healing

Malnutrition induces intestinal mucosal atrophy, reduced motility, increased incidence of ileus, and the potential for bacterial translocation through the bowel wall, with resultant sepsis. Impaired wound healing owing to nutritional causes may be ameliorated by feeding an enteral or parenteral diet that supplies energy needs in the form of fatty acids and sugars and provides essential amino acids.[4,7] Feedings of high-protein meals after injury can optimize conditions for normal visceral wound healing. Amino acids provided through enteral nutrition are utilized for the synthesis of hexosamines, proteoglycan polymers, nucleic acids, and structural proteins such as actin, myosin, collagen, and elastin.[7]

Early, if not immediate, postoperative enteral feeding has been shown to have a positive influence on the healing rate of intestinal anastomosis in dogs. Bursting pressures and collagen levels of ileal and colorectal anastomosis were compared in Beagles fed elemental diets versus those fed only electrolyte and water for four days. The dogs fed elemental diets had nearly twice the bursting strengths of the control group and nearly double the amount of both immature and mature collagen at the wound site.[8] Total parenteral nutrition (TPN) does not appear to ameliorate the mucosal atrophy or increase collagen deposition as does enteral nutrition. In human studies, the incidence of septic complications was significantly lower in people fed between 8 to 24 hours after surgery versus those maintained on TPN. Additionally, those patients fed early had a reduced incidence of postoperative ileus and reduced hospital stay.[9]

Anemia

Small-animal patients with polytrauma, major burns, or malignancies are frequently anemic. Studies of experimental anemia in rats induced by phlebotomy or iron-deficient diet have shown suppression in wound healing only if the animals' blood volume remained deficient or significant malnutrition accompanied the iron-deficient diet.[5] With anemia resulting from phlebotomy, intravascular volume replacement results in normal wound healing.[10] Therefore, anemia in the absence of concurrent malnutrition or volume deficit does not appear to be a factor in suppressed visceral wound healing.

Leukopenia

Neutropenia caused by disease processes or induced by chemotherapy has been suspected of causing impaired wound healing. Contaminated wounds are more likely to become infected in the presence of neutropenia, but minimal problems are encountered with clean wounds. Neutropenic animals have been shown to have a reduced number of neutrophils at the wound site during the inflammatory phase of wound healing. However, normal progression of wound debridement occurs, owing to the presence of macrophages. When neutropenic rats are compared with controls, fibroplasia is unaffected, collagen deposition is unchanged, and wound strength is normal.[10]

Lymphopenia also fails to affect wound healing in rats. A normal inflammatory response is seen during the first 24 to 48 hours of the lag phase of healing, and normal wound strength and collagen content are found at 7 and 14 days.[10] Thus, leukopenia owing to either neutropenia or lymphopenia alone fails to suppress wound healing as assessed by histologic and biochemical techniques.

The macrophage plays a vital role in wound healing. Systemic hydrocortisone-induced monocytopenia can reduce tissue macrophage levels to approximately one third that of controls. Mild inhibition of wound debridement is observed, but collagen synthesis is unaffected. However, when antimacrophage serum and hydrocortisone are combined, clearance of wound debris is much decreased and fibroplasia and collagen synthesis are reduced. Macrophages are also important in enhancing neovascularization at the wound edge.[11] Activated macrophages are associated with a higher frequency of neovascularization.

Injection of activated peritoneal macrophages into dermis and subcutaneous tissues of rats immediately before wounding increases wound breaking strength at 8 days.[11]

Corticosteroids

The anti-inflammatory action of glucocorticoid hormones may prolong the inflammatory phase of wound healing. Specific mechanisms include the stabilization of lysosomal membranes, mobilization of neutrophils, decreased local phagocytosis, and inhibition of deoxyribonucleic acid (DNA) synthesis.[10] Hydrocortisone and methylprednisolone have a greater anti-inflammatory affect than does dexamethasone. Corticosteroids are also associated with increased risk of wound infection. They interfere with the logarithmic phase of healing by delaying fibroblast proliferation and collagen synthesis and crosslinking.

The negative effect on wound healing is critically dependent on the dose and timing of steroid administration. If glucocorticoids are started 3 days or more after creation of the wound, progression of cellular infiltration and resulting fibroplasia are histologically unchanged and produce no negative effect on wound tensile strength at 7 days.[10] Impairment of wound healing by corticosteroids is most obvious at 7 to 14 days, owing to their negative effect on fibroplasia during the logarithmic phase. However, by 3 to 4 weeks after injury the wound tensile strength in animals receiving corticosteroid treatment approaches that of control animals.

Dose is also an important factor. In rats, small doses (5 mg/kg) of hydrocortisone have no adverse effect on wound tensile strength, whereas larger doses significantly decrease it. The nutritional state of the animal is another important variable. Hydrocortisone at a dose of 5 mg/kg had no effect on the tensile strength of incised wounds in rabbits fed a regular diet but produced a marked inhibitory effect in rabbits that were 25% underweight. Along with the healing effects on the gastrointestinal tract, corticosteroid-induced gastric and colonic perforations are well documented in dogs being treated for concurrent spinal cord disease.[10]

It is possible that anabolic steroids may counteract the negative effects of glucocorticoids on wound healing. In one study, rats given 10 mg hydrocortisone for eight days had significantly weaker dermal wounds. However, rats supplemented with 5 mg testosterone propionate or nandrolone phenpropionate had similar wound strength to that in control animals.[12] In other studies, lower doses of testosterone did not reverse the detrimental effects of cortisone in rats five days after wounding.[12]

Nonsteroidal Anti-Inflammatory Drugs

Prostaglandins (PG) have been implicated as a major mediator in wound healing, particularly during the inflammatory phase. The PG-induced inflammatory response proceeds via lipid mediators metabolized from arachidonic acid through the cyclooxygenase pathway. Corticosteroids are thought to inhibit phospholipase A2 activity in cell membranes, resulting in reduced release of prostaglandin precursors (arachidonic acid). Nonsteroidal anti-inflammatory drugs (NSAID), on the other hand, inhibit the action of cyclooxygenase in the prostaglandin-formation cascade. Excessive doses of older NSAIDs such as aspirin, indomethacin, and phenylbutazone have been shown to significantly delay increases in skin wound strength in animals during the inflammatory phase. Flunixin meglumine was evaluated for its effects on dermal, fascial, gastric, and colonic wound healing in rats. Flunixin, 1.1 mg/kg b.i.d., significantly decreased the tensile strength of wounds in the skin and linea alba, but it did not affect visceral bursting strength at five days after surgery. At 14 days after surgery, no significant difference in wound strength was seen between the group given flunixin and control groups.[13] Other than liver toxicity, the newer Cox-2-inhibiting NSAIDs such as carprofen or deracoxib do not appear to negatively affect alimentary healing and may, in fact, reduce postoperative ileus by their analgesic and anti-inflammatory properties. The newer NSAIDs may work by reducing the release of cytokines (TNF, IL-1, IL-6, and IL-8) during the inflammatory stage of wound repair.[14] They probably do not effect the proliferative phase of visceral healing when fibroplasia is the factor influencing gain in visceral wound strength.[13]

Radiation

Radiation has a negative effect on wound healing for several reasons. Injury to the chromatin of dividing fibroblasts may decrease their accumulation in the wound. Collagen production is reduced in most irradiated wounds. Progressive fibrosis of blood vessels results in decreased blood flow and lower oxygen tension after radiation therapy. This delayed or impaired perfusion delays wound healing and also increases the risk of infection.[15]

Confusion exists about when to initiate radiation therapy in the perioperative period. Initiation of radiation therapy prior to or at the time of surgery may increase chances of dermal or visceral wound dehiscence. In one study of rats, a single dose of 2000 rad was given at seven days before, on the day of skin wounding, and at seven days thereafter. The wounds that were irradiated one week before surgery and at the time of surgery were significantly weaker than those irradiated one week after surgery. Because radiation interferes principally with the logarithmic proliferative phase of wound healing, it would be ideal to initiate radiation a minimum of 7 to 14 days after visceral wounding has occurred.[10] When suturing previously irradiated viscera, a nonabsorbable suture material or slowly absorbable synthetic monofilament absorbable suture should be chosen. Irradiated bladder wounds sutured with polyglycolic acid were stronger than those sutured with chromic catgut, but no difference was noted in nonirradiated bladders.[15]

Effects of Cancer on Wound Healing

Cancer has been incriminated in delayed wound healing, but impaired nutrition is probably the underlying cause. Except as a result of cancer cachexia, adverse wound healing owing to cancer is difficult to document. The presence of macroscopic tumor remote from the wound or microscopic tumor within the wound does not appear to impair healing.[10] Humans with esophageal cancer who have residual microscopic tumor at the surgical margins did not have a significantly higher rate of leakage at the anastomosis than did patients with no tumor present.[16] No evidence exists that the presence of tumor directly impedes healing; in selected cases, it may actually accelerate healing. In excisional biopsy for invasive cutaneous melanoma, those portions of the incision that contained residual tumor were stronger than those that did not. Further evidence indicates that presence of a tumor may have a positive effect on the wound strength of distant surgical wounds. Wounds were stronger in rats with hepatomas than in control rats. Increased wound strength in the presence of tumor may be due to the presence of growth factors that act as fibroblast mitogens. Other tumors such as mast cell tumors, which release vasoactive substances such as histamine, may retard wound healing.[17]

Effects of Chemotherapy

Chemotherapeutic agents affect wound healing in several ways. Neutropenia, a common side effect of chemotherapy, increases the risk of infection but does not interfere directly with wound healing. Interference with the inflammatory stage of wound healing is often not seen unless therapy is begun preoperatively.[10] Many chemotherapeutic agents exert their antineoplastic effect by interfering with DNA replication, RNA production, protein synthesis, or cell division.[12] Inhibition of fibroblast proliferation, reduced formation of collagen, and impaired neovascularization have been documented subsequent to chemotherapy in animals. Therefore, the greatest potential for impairment of wound healing would be during the proliferative or logarithmic phase, when fibroblasts are dividing and are metabolically active. In addition, anorexia and cachexia are common side effects of chemotherapy and may have an additive adverse effect with preexisting cancer cachexia. This can exacerbate negative nitrogen balance and PCM. Similar to corticosteroid therapy, the effects of chemotherapy are largely affected by time of administration and dose of the drug. The relative effects of various antineoplastic agents on wound healing are listed in Table 37-1.

Vincristine

Vincristine is commonly used to treat lymphosarcoma and other carcinomas in animals. The drug exerts its effect by binding with intracellular microtubular systems, causing mitotic arrest.[10,12] Impairment of dermal wound healing by this agent appears to be minimal. In mice treated with vincristine, mildly reduced dermal wound strength was seen 3 days after surgery, but not at 7 or 21 days thereafter.[18] Clinical trials in humans using preoperative vincristine do not indicate increased incidence of wound dehiscence or morbidity.

Vinblastine

Vinblastine is another plant alkyloid used to treat mast cell tumors and in some lymphoma protocols. This compound acts by binding to microtubules in the mitotic spindle, thereby preventing cell division. There is no direct association with disruption of wound healing, but gastroenterocolitis and myelosuppression are common.[19]

Table 37-1. Antineoplastic Agents and Wound Healing

Agents clearly detrimental to wound healing
Cisplatin
Cyclophosphamide (Cytoxan)
Methotrexate
Doxorubicin (Adriamycin)
5-Fluorouracil
Levamisole
Agents with variable or no effect on wound healing
Vincristine
Vinblastine
Azathioprine
Agents inadequately studied for effect on wound healing
Lomustine
Mitoxantrone
Mechlorethamine HCl

Doxorubicin

Doxorubicin (Adriamycin), an antitumor antibiotic, acts by inhibiting DNA and RNA synthesis. Doxorubicin inhibits cell division during the proliferative phase of wound healing. Doxorubicin given to rats reduced wound breaking strength at 5, 10, 15, 20, and 30 days after wounding when compared with controls.[20] In addition, doxorubicin impaired wound healing when it was given up to 5 weeks prior to wounding or as much as 4 weeks after wounding. The effects of doxorubicin on wound healing are dose dependent. Animals given high levels of the drug show significantly impaired wound healing, whereas those given normal therapeutic doses show little if any effect on wound healing.[17]

Cyclophosphamide

Cyclophosphamide is an alkylating agent that acts by cross-linking DNA strands and, thereby, preventing cell division. Cyclophosphamide interferes with fibroblast production and collagen production and also decreases neovascularization.[10] Experimental studies in animals indicate that cyclophosphamide significantly impedes healing at therapeutic doses. Rats given cyclophosphamide at the time of wounding had decreased strength of skin wounds at 1, 3, and 5 weeks after wounding. Larger doses of cyclophosphamide have also been shown to delay scar maturation in rats. However, in clinical studies of human patients, no adverse effect on visceral wound healing was observed, regardless of the time of administration of cyclophosphamide.[18]

Methotrexate

Methotrexate is an antimetabolite folic acid antagonist that prevents DNA maturation. High doses of methotrexate are associated with increased rates of wound infection in mice.[21] The effect is dose-dependent and is reversible with concurrent folic acid administration. Wound breaking strength is decreased and rate of wound healing was also retarded for as long as 21 days after wounding. However, these effects are not observed if methotrexate is given in therapeutic doses at the time of surgery.

Methotrexate given to humans at the time of surgery increases the rate of wound dehiscence. This complication is minimized by delaying chemotherapy 10 to 14 days or by concurrently administering folic acid. In mice, intraperitoneal methotrexate given in therapeutic doses causes decreased wound strength on day three but not on day 7 or 21.[10]

5-Fluorouracil

5-Fluorouracil (5-FU) has been used extensively in small animal patients with carcinomas and in humans with intestinal carcinomas. Because it is commonly given systemically or intraperitoneally after resection of carcinomas, its effect on intestinal wound healing has been studied directly but results have been conflicting. No impairment of healing of colon anastomoses occurred in rats when chemotherapy was given at operation and at 4, 7, and 11 days postoperatively.[22] However, rats given 5-FU alone or 5-FU in combination with levamisole were noted to have bursting strengths of healing colon anastomoses only 65% of that seen in the control group. In vitro studies showed that both of these agents significantly inhibit fibroblast proliferation. These effects were more pronounced in animals with weight loss or nutritional deficiencies;[23] however, the effect was dose related, and mice given therapeutic doses had minimal adverse effects. Although 5-FU is related to methotrexate in mode of action, the apparent risk for impaired visceral wound healing is much less with 5-FU than it is with methotrexate when given in therapeutic doses.[10]

Cisplatin and Carboplatin

Cisplatin, a heavy metal compound, has been used for various carcinomas including transitional cell carcinomas in dogs. Its effects on visceral wound healing have been evaluated in rats. Large- and small-bowel anastomoses were performed and compared at 4, 7, 14, and 28 days postoperatively.[24] Cisplatin was given in doses of 5 mg/kg 1 and 5 days preoperatively. At four days after surgery, wound breaking strength of both the large- and small-bowel anastomosis were too low to measure.[10,27] At all times during the study, wound breaking strength of treated animals was below that of controls. From these results and from studies in humans it appears that cisplatin is one of the most dangerous chemotherapeutic agents with regard to the potential for interfering with visceral wound healing. Carboplatin is a less toxic cousin to cisplatin that can be used in cats. Gastrointestinal irritation with this drug is reduced when compared with cisplatin, but the mechanism of action is the same and so caution should be exercised when using this drug concurrently with visceral surgery.[25]

Newer Chemotherapeutic Agents Requiring Further Study

Lomustine

This alkylating agent is used primarily in the treatment of canine mast cell tumor. No mention has been made of adverse wound healing, but vomiting, diarrhea, and stomatitis are common side effects.[25]

Mechlorethamine HCL

This alkylating agent is used as a rescue drug for lymphoma as well as for intracavitary administration of some neoplasms. It has significant gastrointestinal effects, which can lead to severe vomiting and diarrhea and may halt therapy.[25]

Mitoxantrone

This synthetic antitumor antibiotic has been used with some success in the treatment of lymphoma and transitional cell carcinoma, and as a radiation sensitizer against squamous cell carcinoma. Its side effects include myelosuppression, vomiting, and diarrhea.[25]

Conclusion

Healing of visceral wounds is negatively affected by a variety of factors. Chronic weight loss of 15% to 20% owing to cancer cachexia or other reasons has a negative effect on visceral wound healing. Correction of cachexia as well as early postoperative enteral feeding appears to increase collagen deposition and bursting wound strength. Glucocorticoids have a negative effect on wound healing when given in large doses prior to the third day after wounding. NSAIDs appear to affect the early inflammatory phase of wound healing, but do not appear to interfere with the proliferative phase of wound healing or have a significant negative effect on visceral healing strength. Radiation therapy interferes with fibroblast mobilization, replication, and collagen synthesis. It also causes sclerosis of the microvasculature, thereby reducing oxygenation at the wound site. Whenever possible, radiation therapy should be initiated after visceral wound healing is complete. The negative effects of cancer on wound healing appear to be secondary to nutritional deficiencies rather than direct tumor impairment of wound healing. Visceral wound healing may actually be mildly augmented owing to release of growth factors by the neoplasm. Effects of chemotherapeutic agents on visceral wound healing are variable. Drugs such as vincristine, vinblastine, and azathioprine seem to be safe when used in therapeutic doses. Drugs such as cyclophospha¬mide, methotrexate, 5-FU, and doxorubicin have been shown to delay wound healing in both experimental and clinical studies. Cisplatin appears to significantly impair intestinal wound healing in rats and should be used with caution after intestinal surgery. Newer antineoplastic drugs require further evaluation.

References

1. Peacock EE: The gastrointestinal tract. In Surgery and Biology of Wound Repair, 3rd ed. Peacock EE (ed). Philadelphia: WB Saunders, 1984.

2. Ellison GW: Wound healing in the gastrointestinal tract. Semin Vet Med Surg (Small Anim) 4:287, 1989.

3. Bellah JB: Wound healing in the urinary tract. Semin Vet Med Surg (Small Anim) 4:294, 1980.

4. Crowe DT: Enteral nutrition for critically ill or injured patients-Part III. Comp Pract Vet (Small Anim) 8:826, 1986.

5. Moore FD, Brennon MF: Surgical injury: Body composition, protein metabolism, and neuroendocrinology. *In* Manual of Surgical Nutrition. Ballinger WF (ed). Philadelphia: WB Saunders, 1975.

6. Haydock DA, Hill GL: Impaired wound healing in surgical patients with varying degrees of malnutrition. J Parent Ent Nutr 10:550, 1986.

7. Crane SW: Nutritional aspects of wound healing. Semin Vet Med Surg (Small Anim) 4:263, 1989.

8. Greenstein A: Double fourth-day colorectal anastomotic strength with complete retention of intestinal mature collagen following immediate full enteral nutrition. Surg Forum 29:78-81, 1978.

9. Braga M: Early postoperative enteral nutrition improves oxygenation and reduces costs compared with total parenteral nutrition. Clin Nutr 29:242-248, 2001.

10. McCaw DL: The effects of cancer and cancer therapies on wound healing. Semin Vet Med Surg 4:281, 1989.

11. Diegelman RF, Cohen IK, Kaplan AM: The role of macrophages in wound repair: a review. Plast Reconstr Surg 68:107, 1981.

12. Laing EJ: The effect of antineoplastic agents on wound healing. Comp Cont Educ Small Anim Pract 11:136, 1989.

13. Donner GS, Ellison GW, Peyton LC: Effect of flunixin meglumine on surgical wound strength and healing in the rat. Am J Vet Res 47:2247, 1986.

14. Mainous MR, Ertel W, Chaudry IH, et al: The gut: a cytokine-generating organ in systemic inflammation? Shock 4:193-199, 1995.

15. Shamberger R: Effect of chemotherapy and radiotherapy on wound healing: experimental studies. Recent Results Cancer Res 98:17, 1985.

16. Lin XS, Wu X, Chen BT, et al: Significance of residual tumor at the esophageal stump after resection for carcinoma. Semin Surg Oncol 2:257, 1986.

17. Dvorak HF: Tumors: wounds that do not heal. N Engl J Med 315:1650, 1986.

18. Bland KI, Palin WE, von Fraunhofer JA, et al: Experimental and clinical observa¬tions on the effects of cytotoxic chemotherapeutic drugs on wound healing. Ann Surg 199:782, 1984.

19. Plumb DC (ed): Veterinary Drug Handbook, 5th ed. Ames: Blackwell Publishing, 2005, pp 794-795.

20. Lawrence WT, Norton JA, Harvey AK, et al: Doxorubicin-induced impairment of wound healing in rats. J Natl Cancer Inst 76:119, 1986.

21. Cohen SC, Babelnick HL, Johnson RK, et al.: Effects of antineoplastic agents on wound healing in mice. Surgery 78:238, 1978.

22. Hillan K, Nordlinger B, Ballet F, et al: The healing of colonic anastomoses after early intraperitoneal chemotherapy: an experimental study in rats. J Surg Res 44:166, 1988.

23. de Waard JW, DeMan BM, Wobbes T, et al: Inhibition of fibroblast synthesis and proliferation by levamisole and 5-fluorouracil. Eur J Cancer 34(1):162-167, 1998.

24. Engelmann U, Grimm K, Gronniger J, et al: Influence of cisplatin on healing of enterostomies in the rat. Eur Urol 9:45, 1983.

25. Moore AS, Kitchell BE: New chemotherapy agents in veterinary medicine. Vet Clin Small Anim Pract 37:629-649, 2003.

Chapter 38

Short Bowel Syndrome

Michael Willard

Short bowel syndrome (SBS) has been described in people for over 30 years. Despite being a well recognized syndrome for decades, however, we do not yet have a universally accepted definition.[1] Occurring after major intestinal resection, the key features of SBS in people are generally acknowledged to include dehydration (caused by diarrhea), malabsorption, and subsequent malnutrition severe enough to cause morbidity and put the patient at risk for death. The best definitions of SBS generally describe the constellation of signs caused by resection of excessive amounts of intestine (i.e., dehydration, malabsorption) or their consequences, rather than the amount of intestine resected. For example, one definition of human SBS is based on intestinal failure following resection being so severe that the patient needs parenteral nutrition for more than 1 to 3 months post-surgery.[1]

Trying to define SBS based on how much bowel has been resected creates problems. Even though most surgeons agree that having less than 25% of the expected intestinal length left is almost always associated with SBS in people, one must also consider what portion of the bowel was resected (i.e., jejunum, ileum, colon), the functionality of the remaining bowel, and the body condition of the patient. For example, if one resects 65% of a person's intestines but leaves the ileum and colon intact, there is much less chance of SBS than if the ileum and colon were resected.[2] Furthermore, it has been stated that removal of the ileocolic valve is associated with a poorer prognosis; however, this seems to be based on a study in puppies[3] and may nor may not be true for people. In fact, although most papers describe how much intestine was removed, it would probably be more important to know how many centimeters of intestine remain in the patient, and which segments of bowel were left.

SBS in Veterinary Medicine

Defining SBS in veterinary medicine has principally consisted of taking the criteria used in people and applying them to dogs and cats. Part of the reason for this is that, while SBS is generally well recognized in people, only a handful of cases are reported in the veterinary literature.[4,6] This paucity of reports is probably because veterinary patients with such a guarded-to-poor prognosis and requiring intense therapy (total parenteral nutrition) for long periods of time are typically euthanatized instead of treated. Therefore, much of the discussion of SBS in dogs and cats must draw on experimental work done in dogs and rats, as well as on clinical reports in people. Obviously substantial species differences may exist, and one must be cautious about extrapolating from human beings to dogs and cats. For example, people are usually expected to develop SBS if more than 75% of the intestines are resected, but dogs have been reported to tolerate 80% to 85% resection and function well postoperatively.[3,5,7,8] Therefore, SBS in veterinary medicine should probably be defined by the inability of the patient to compensate adequately after massive intestinal resection as seen by the need for protracted nutritional/pharmacologic therapy to keep the patient alive until intestinal adaptation occurs.

Intestinal Adaptation

Adaptation refers to the functional and structural changes that occur in the intestines as they attempt to increase fluid and nutrient absorption to pre-resection levels. The primary goal of therapy of the patient with SBS is generally to maintain the patient until sufficient intestinal adaptation can occur so that parenteral nutrition may cease.

Shortly after massive intestinal resection, the remaining intestines begin to adapt by increasing in length and diameter. Hypertrophy and hyperplasia occur of all layers of the remaining intestines,[1] with epithelial hyperplasia in the intestinal crypts beginning within two to three days. Hyperplasia of the intestinal epithelium is one of the most important events.[2] The mechanisms for this adaptation are probably multifactorial and may include secretions from the remaining gastrointestinal tract (e.g., pancreatic) and various hormones, growth factors, and cytokines. However, the presence of enteral nutrition may in fact be the most important factor required for adaptation to occur. Studies in dogs[9] showed that enteral nutrition is associated with intestinal adaptation, whereas dogs feed strictly parenterally showed no evidence of intestinal adaptation. The composition of the enteral nutrition may be similarly critical. It is believed that complex nutrients are more trophic to the intestinal mucosa than are simple nutrients, and long-chain unsaturated fats may be the most important nutrients in this regard.

As intestinal adaptation takes place, usually some degree of dilatation of the diameter of the bowel lumen occurs,[9] which in turn, results in some degree of stasis of luminal contents.[10] Changes can also occur in intestinal myoelectrical activity that slow the velocity of duodenal and jejunal motor activity.[11] Whereas these changes are designed to aid in digestion and absorption of nutrients by prolonging the exposure of the intestinal mucosa to the nutrients, they also have some potential disadvantages. A dilated small intestine with slowed motility can promote bacterial overgrowth. Administering drugs designed to increase transit time (e.g., opioids such as loperamide) can make this situation even worse. In some patients, poor gut motility coupled with bacterial overgrowth can lead to bacterial translocation from the intestines to the blood, mesenteric lymph nodes, and spleen.[1]

Another problem that can be caused by an altered gut anatomy plus bacterial flora changes is d-lactic acidosis. When nutrients are malabsorbed in the small bowel, substantially increased amounts of carbohydrates may enter the colon. Colonic metabolism of these carbohydrates can result in acidification of the colon with subsequent overgrowth of bacteria that tolerate acidic environments, such as Lactobacilli. If overgrowth of Lactobacilli occurs, overproduction and subsequent absorption of d-lactate may follow as well.[12] The resulting acidosis can be so severe as to make patients weak and encephalopathic.

In people, intestinal adaptation may require months to years of support (i.e., parenteral nutrition to maintain the patient plus enteral nutrition to stimulate adaptation) before the intestines regain sufficient function and can maintain the patient without parenteral support.[1] No obvious, recognized relationship exists between the residual intestine length and the time required for adaptation. In general, about 75% of people with SBS ultimately adapt and are able to stop parenteral nutrition. In general, children seem to have more potential than adults to have successful intestinal adaptation, but this depends on many factors.[1]

Treatment

The most important aspect of treating SBS is trying to avoid massive resection in the first place. For example, when faced with a condition that seems to require massive intestinal resection, it may be better to leave questionable tissue instead of resecting it, even though a second operation will be required 1 to 3 days later to assess the viability of tissue left the first time. The risks involved with performing a second surgery may be less than the risks occurring if SBS develops.

If SBS occurs or seems highly likely to develop, then aggressive medical management is the first step. The first phase of therapy consists of stabilizing the patient; this generally requires up to 4 weeks in affected people.[13] Administration of intravenous fluids is generally required to maintain hydration as well as normal electrolyte and acid-base status. Oral rehydration solutions have been reported to be beneficial in some human patients,[14] but they have not replaced IV administration. Nutrition is best started sooner rather than later. If one anticipates SBS, then parenteral nutrition can begin two to three days after surgery. Partial parenteral nutrition is easier than total parenteral nutrition, but if long-term therapy is needed, and it usually is, then total parenteral nutrition may be preferable.[13]

The second phase of therapy consists of promoting intestinal adaptation by gradually increasing the amount of nutrients entering the intestines. Enteral nutrition should usually begin shortly after starting parenteral nutrition (during the first phase of therapy). Various studies have looked at the addition of glutamine and various other nutrients, hormones (e.g., growth hormone[15]), and/or enzymes (e.g., pancreatic enzymes[16]) to the enteral diet, but none has been shown to help unequivocally.[13,14] Use of hydrolyzed diets has not been shown to be beneficial in human infants with SBS.[17] People with SBS are generally expected to malabsorb 30% to 50% of ingested nutrients; therefore, these patients are often fed 50% more than their calculated caloric requirement.[10] Owing to the intestines' reduced ability to absorb water and nutrients, it is important to start administering relatively small amounts of more dilute enteral diets and gradually increase the volume, lest severe diarrhea occur with subsequent dehydration.[18] Therefore, a constant-rate infusion of enteral diet as opposed to bolus feeding is usually preferred. In people with SBS, the presence or absence of a colon affects the choice of diet.[19] For example, patients with colons can obtain energy from bacterial fermentation of carbohydrates within the colon. Whether the same occurs in dogs is unknown.

Initiating enteral nutrition is typically associated with severe diarrhea. Therefore, antidiarrheals (e.g., loperamide) have typically been used.[13] In people, loperamide has seemed more effective than other opioids.[10] However, the decreased intestinal absorption that characterizes SBS often means that higher than normal doses may be required. In some cases, IV administration is necessary. Occasionally, a combination of loperamide and another opioid (e.g., codeine) is necessary.

Gastric hypersecretion is commonly seen after massive intestinal resection[10,20] and seems to contribute substantially to the diarrhea. Therefore, inhibition of gastric secretion with H-2 receptor antagonists (e.g., famotidine) or proton pump inhibitors (e.g., omeprazole) is often necessary as well. Peptic ulcer disease and gastroesophageal reflux are recognized complications of SBS in people, ostensibly due, at least in part, to the gastric hypersecretion.[10] Rarely, somatostatin analogs (e.g., octreotide[10]) or other drugs (e.g., clonidine[21]) are required to control intestinal hypersecretion in people with SBS.

Bacterial overgrowth, for reasons stated earlier (intestinal dilatation, loss of ileocolic valve, altered motility), is a concern in human patients with SBS. In addition, pharmacologic suppression of gastric acid secretion necessary to minimize problems caused by gastric hypersecretion may help enable such overgrowth. The term "small bowel bacterial overgrowth" is controversial in dogs and cats, and the criteria used to diagnose small bowel bacterial overgrowth in people are not clearly appropriate for dogs and cats.[22,23] Nonetheless, dogs can have antibiotic-responsive enteropathies apparently caused, at least in part, by excessive numbers of bacteria in the small intestines.[23,24]

Bacterial overgrowth is usually suspected either when there is failure to respond to apparently appropriate therapy, or when unexpected weight loss occurs in a previously stable patient. Antibiotic therapy is often utilized in these patients. One cannot hope to eliminate all bacteria from the remaining small intestines; rather, one seeks to decrease the number of bacteria so that they no longer cause disease. Tetracycline, tylosin powder, metronidazole plus enrofloxacin, and cephalosporins are examples of therapy that have been used for this problem in veterinary medicine.[25] One must often experiment to see which antibiotic(s) will be most effective in a particular patient. Periodic rotation of antibiotics is sometimes practiced in people in an effort to prevent selection of resistant bacteria inhabiting the dilated section of intestine. Restriction of carbohydrates, use of probiotics (with or without concurrent prebiotics[26]), periodic small bowel irrigation with balanced hypertonic electrolyte solution,[27] and surgery (to reduce the lumen of the bowel[1]) have also been used to try to reduce bacterial overgrowth in affected people.

In people, the goal of therapy is eventually to wean the patient from parenteral nutrition (i.e., adequate intestinal adaptation occurs) and be able to maintain the patient on enteral nutrition. When this happens, one must consider whether supplementation of micronutrients (e.g., zinc, magnesium, cobalamin, fat-soluble vitamins) will be required. Some patients do not respond adequately to medical management alone.

Cases of SBS reported in Veterinary Medicine

To date, seven cases of canine SBS have been reported in the veterinary literature. The first case was a 12-month-old German shorthaired pointer that had an intussusception.[5] It was reported to have 1.5 meter of small bowel remaining and was euthanatized within eight weeks of surgery. The second case was an 8-year-old dog that had surgery 15 months prior to admission. It was euthanatized approximately six weeks after admission and had 66 cm of small and large intestines remaining.[4] Next there was a series of four dogs.[6] Three of these dogs (i.e., a 4-year-old pointer, a 4-month-old German shepherd, and an 8-year-old German shepherd) died within three months of surgery. One of these three dogs (i.e., the 4-year-old pointer) did well initially and declined only after it refused to eat the prescribed diet. It had received total parenteral nutrition promptly after surgery. The dog that did well was lost to follow up after 27 months. The last report is of a 10-year-old Doberman pinscher that had approximately 80% of its intestines, including the ileocolic valve resected. It did well and was primarily treated with enteral nutrition.[28]

Surgical Therapy of SBS

Surgery is considered in humans with SBS when it appears that medical/nutritional management will be inadequate. Intestinal transplantation seems to hold the most promise. It is unreported in clinical veterinary medicine but has been performed experimentally in dogs.[29] Surgical therapy of SBS has principally aimed at decreasing the diameter and/or increasing the length of the remaining intestines. Various techniques are reported in human SBS patients (e.g., intestinal tapering and plication, antiperistaltic segments, creation of intestinal valves, longitudinal lengthening, serial transverse enteroplasty, colonic interposition), and specific indications exist for each surgery.[1] For example, patients with a short, dilated bowel are candidates for serial transverse enteroplasty, whereas those with a dilated bowel that is sufficiently long might be managed by simple tapering enteroplasty. Because we have minimal experience with these techniques in clinical veterinary medicine, it appears that such surgeries should be reserved for those patients in which aggressive medical/nutritional management has failed or appears likely to fail.

References

1. Wales PW: Surgical therapy for short bowel syndrome. Pediatr Surg Int 20:647 657, 2004.

2. DiBaise JK, Young RJ, Vanderhoof JA: Intestinal rehabilitation and the short bowel syndrome: part I. Am J Gastroenterol 99:1386 1395, 2004.

3. Reid IS: The significance of the ileocecal valve in massive resection of the gut in puppies. J Pediat Surg 10:507 510, 1975.

4. Williams DA, Burrows CF: Short bowel syndrome a case report in a dog and discussion of the pathophysiology of bowel resection. J Small Anim Pract 22:263 275, 1981.

5. Joy CL, Patterson JM: Short bowel syndrome following surgical correction of a double intussusception in a dog. Can Vet J 19:254 259, 1978.

6. Yanoff SR, Willard MD, Boothe HW, Walker M: Short bowel syndrome in four dogs. Vet Surg 21:217 222, 1992.

7. Cuthbertson EM, Gilfillan RS, Burhenne HJ, Mackby MJ: Massive small bowel resection in the Beagle including laboratory data in severe under nutrition. Surgery 68(4):698 703, 1970.

8. Hutcher NE, Salzberg AM: Pre ileal transposition of colon to prevent the development of short bowel syndrome in puppies with 90 percent small intestinal resection. Surgery 70:189 197, 1971.

9. Feldman EJ, Dowling RH, McNaughton J, Peters TJ: Effects of oral versus intravenous nutrition on intestinal adaptation after small bowel resection in the dog. Gastroenterol 70:712 719, 1976.

10. DiBaise JK, Young RJ, Vanderhoof JA: Intestinal rehabilitation and the short bowel syndrome: part 2. Am J Gastroenterol 99:1823 1832, 2004.

11. Uchiyama M, Iwafuchi M, Matsuda Y, et al: Intestinal motility after massive small bowel resection in conscious canines: comparison of acute and chronic phases. J Pediatr Gastro Nutr 23:217 223, 1996.

12. Zhang DL, Jiang ZW, Jiang J, et al: D lactic acidosis secondary to short bowel syndrome. Postgrad Med J 79:110 112, 2003.

13. Keller J, Panter H, Layer P: Management of the short bowel syndrome after extensive small bowel resection. Best Pract Res Clin Gastroenterol 18:977 992, 2004.

14. Scolapio JS: Short bowel syndrome. J Parent Ent Nutr 26:S11 S16, 2002.

15. Weiming Z, Ling L, Jeishou L: Effect of recombinant human growth hormone and enteral nutrition on short bowel syndrome. J Parent Ent Nutr 28:377 381, 2004.

16. Layer P, Melle U: Indication for pancreatic enzyme substitution following small intestinal resection (short bowel syndrome). Pancreatol 1:49 54, 2001.

17. Ksiazyk J, Piena M, Kierkus J, Lyszkowska M: Hydrolyzed versus nonhydrolyzed protein diet in short bowel syndrome in children. J Pediatr Gastro Nutr 35:615 618, 2002.

18. Vanderhoof JA, Young RJ, Thompson JS: New and emerging therapies for short bowel syndrome in children. Pediatr Drugs 5:525 531, 2003.

19. Scolapio JS: Treatment of short bowel syndrome. Current Opinion Clin Nutr Metab Care 4:557 560, 2001.

20. Kato J, Sakamoto J, Teramukai S, et al: A prospective within patient comparison clinical trial on the effect of parenteral cimetidine for improvement of fluid secretion and electrolyte balance in patients with short bowel syndrome. Hepato Gastroenterol 51:1742 1746, 2004.

21. McDoniel K, Taylor B, Huey W, et al: Use of clonidine to decrease intestinal fluid losses in patients with high output short bowel syndrome. J Parent Ent Nutr 28:265 268, 2004.

22. Johnston KL: Small intestinal bacterial overgrowth. Vet Clin North Am 29:523 550, 1999.

23. German AJ, Day MJ, Ruaux CG, et al: Comparison of direct and indirect tests for small intestinal bacterial overgrowth and antibiotic responsive diarrhea in dogs. J Vet Intern Med 17:33 43, 2003.

24. Marks SL: Editorial: small intestinal bacterial overgrowth in dogs less common than you think? J Vet Intern Med 17:5 7, 2003.

25. Hall EJ, et al: Diseases of the small intestine. *In* Textbook of Veterinary Internal Medicine, 6th ed. Ettinger SJ, Feldman EC (eds). St. Louis: Elsevier, 2005, p. 1332.

26. Kanamori Y, Hashizume K, Sugiyama M, et al: Combination therapy with Bifidobacterium breve, Lactobacillus casei, and galactooligosaccharides dramatically improved the intestinal function in a girl with short bowel syndrome. Dig Dis Sci 46:2010 2016, 2001.

27. Vanderhoof JA, Young RJ, Murray N, Kaufmann SS: Treatment strategies for small bowel bacterial overgrowth in short bowel syndrome. J Pediat Gastro Nutr 27:155 160, 1998.

28. Pawlusiow JI, McCarthy RJ: Dietary management of short bowel syndrome in a dog. Vet Clin Nutr 1:163 170, 1999.

29. Zachariou Z, Daum R, Beiler HA, Gorgas K: Autogenic allotropic small bowel mucosa transplantation in beagles. A new perspective for treatment of small bowel syndrome? Eur J Pediatr Surg 8:230 233, 1998.

Chapter 39

Megacolon

Amy Zalcman
Ronald M. Bright

Megacolon describes the condition of prolonged dilation of the large bowel. It may contribute to or result from chronic constipation. In the absence of defining criteria, it is a diagnosis of radiographic and functional assessment with systematic elimination of potential underlying causes.

Only a small population presents with primary megacolon. The majority of patients who present with megacolon can be classified according to their primary disease: obstructive versus non-obstructive (colonic inertia). The various etiologies determine appropriate treatment (Table 39-1).

Table 39-1. Causes of Megacolon

Colonic Inertia
Idiopathic Megacolon*‡
Secondary to Neurologic Disease
Trauma to colonic innervation*‡
Associated with congenital abnormalities of caudal spine‡
Aganglionic (Hirschprung's disease) *
Autonomic neuritis
Multiple sclerosis*
Poliomyelitis*
Chagas' diease*
Secondary to medical conditions
Scleroderma*
Myxedema*
Pituitary insufficiency*
Toxic megacolon*
Secondary to prolonged colonic distention of any etiology (e.g., outlet obstruction)* ‡
Outlet obstruction
Pelvic fracture malunion‡
Colonic, rectal, or anal stricture or tumor*‡
Intrapelvic extraluminal mass*‡
Foreign body or improper diet‡
Anal or rectal atresia*‡
Aganglionic (Hirschprung's disease) *

*** Cited in the human literature**
‡ Cited in the veterinary literature

Adapted from Bertoy RW: Megacolon. In Mechanisms of Disease in Small Animal Surgery, 2nd ed. Philadelphia: Lea & Febiger, 1983.

Anatomy

The large intestine is that portion of the intestinal tract that is aboral to the ileum, is separated by the muscular ileocolic sphincter, and concludes at the rectum. At its proximal extent lies the cecum, a spiral diverticulum just wider in diameter than the ileum. From the ileocolic junction, the colon tracks cranially for a short distance and is relatively fixed in position by the mesocolon in the right caudal abdomen. The transverse colon travels the width of the abdomen to the descending colon; the large bowel joins the rectum at the pelvic inlet.[1] The junction between colon and rectum is ill defined and can be described as the abdomino-pelvic boundary, the 7th lumbar vertebra, or the point at which the cranial rectal artery dives below the seromuscular layer.[2]

The histologic anatomy of the colon consists of four layers: serosa, muscularis (longitudinal and circular), submucosa, and muscosa.[3] The serosa maintains no externally distinct property, whereas the mucosa is lined by a single layer of tall columnar epithelial cells.[3] In this portion of the gastrointestinal tract, the crypts of Lieberkühn maintain mature epithelial cells at the tip, while the proliferative epithelial cells are neighbored by the glandular cells at the base.[1] Goblet cells are abundant in the colon; their increased concentration allows space for a minimal amount of lamina propria and provides the histologic boundary from the ileum.[3] The submucosa houses the vascular supply and lymphatic system in loose connective tissue that also suspends the nervous supply.[1] As the rectum becomes a distinct structure, lymph nodules become more apparent.

The vascular supply to the large intestine is divided. The ileocolic junction to the midportion is supplied by branches of the cranial mesenteric artery as the ileocolic, midcolic, and right colic arteries. The caudal mesenteric artery, as the left colic artery, supplies the descending colon and cranial rectum. The venous system is established through the middle colic and ileocolic veins into the caudal mesenteric vein, leading to the portal vein.

All aspects of colonic innervation are maintained within the autonomic nervous system; this can be separated into intrinsic and extrinsic components. The intrinsic nervous supply coordinates global gastrointestinal movement. It is composed of the submucosal (Meissner's) and the myenteric (intramuscular, Auerbach's) plexuses that are linked in reflex circuits.[4] The intrinsic nervous system regulates secretion and absorption, vascular tone, and motility. Enteric primary afferent neurons transmit information about stretch or tension, although some communicate chemical or mechanical stimuli. These cells then stimulate others within their class to produce coordinated responses.[5] The arc is completed by effector nerve endings controlling secretory and smooth motor units.[4] Excitatory and inhibitory motor neurons produce coordinated events resulting in defecation. The interstitial cells of Cajal have been credited with controlling the rate of peristaltic waves.[5] Extrinsic innervation is supplied by parasympathetic (cholinergic) fibers, which stimulate muscle activity, whereas sympathetic (adrenergic) fibers inhibit.

Physiology

Motility

Motility is influenced by integrating cellular excitability, chemical control, and nervous input. The complex cellular events result in segmental and propulsive muscular contractions. In combination with interneuron stimulation of proximal contraction and distal relaxation, aboral movement ensues while mixing ingesta.[5] Evacuation of the colon by mass contractile movements originates in the distal segment of the colon. Colonic motility is also influenced by neurotransmitters, such as substance P, vasoactive intestinal polypeptide, somatostatin, and cholecystokinin.[6]

The ileocolonic junction permits a bolus of ingesta to enter the proximal segment of the colon; this ensures regulated filling and prevention of reflux.[1] Emptying of the proximal colon is controlled through the perception of tone in the presence of fatty acids as well as the volume and consistency of ingesta: both trigger waves of contraction.[5] Propagating waves are triggered more frequently in the proximal colon than in the distal, and they begin to dampen about midcolon.[5] This explains infrequent daily defecations when compared with the extensive movement of stool in the colon. Conversely, more frequent segmental contractions occur in the distal colon.

Defecation, as studied in humans, is a process that begins nearly an hour prior to the expulsion of feces.[5] Propagating waves increase in number in the distal colon, with a dramatic increase within 15 minutes, producing a conscious sensation. Sequentially, oral initiation of these waves results in a full distal colon and stimulation of the anorectal phase.[5] Stool and gas stretch the rectal wall and trigger the rectoanal inhibitory complex, allowing relaxation of the rectum and the involuntary internal anal sphincter. When the external anal sphincter is relaxed voluntarily, a coordinated muscle event assists the passage of feces.[5] Suppression of defecation results in storage of stool in the rectum (accommodation).

Chronic accommodation and retention of stool can result in megarectum and exacerbation of perineal hernia. Anal continence is the result of appropriate rectal capacity in the presence of sphincter coordination and reflexes. Normal reflexes and sphincter mechanism are insufficient, in the absence of an adequate reservoir, to maintain continence.

Absorption and Secretion

The majority of absorption occurs in the proximal half of the colon (absorbing colon); the distal portion serves to store feces prior to expulsion (storage colon). The majority of metabolite digestion and absorption for the body occurs in the small intestine; colonic bacteria complete this locally in the large intestine. Products of this metabolism, such as short-chain fatty acids, are rapidly absorbed by epithelial cells.[1] Short-chain fatty acids, specifically butyrate, provide energy to mucosal cells; deprivation leads to compromised colonic mucosal health.[1] Bacteria also digest dietary fiber; the remainder is fermented. Both processes allow the colon to take up carbohydrates inaccessible to the small intestine.

Water absorption is a passive process with the exchange of sodium. By means of Na^+/K^+ ATPase, sodium is actively pumped into the colonic epithelium. This action is preserved through the high sensitivity of tight junctions that prevent back-diffusion in this region of the bowel.[6] Because it has a higher electrical gradient than does the small intestine, the colonic epithelium permits diffusion across the apical membrane.[1] This activity is enhanced by glucocorticoids, mineralocorticoids, and catecholamines.

Bicarbonate is secreted in exchange for the absorption of chloride.[6] This assists in the neutralization of acidic bacterial byproducts. The gradient created by the exchange of sodium and chloride into the colonic epithelia allows water to follow passively.

Potassium exchange can occur in both directions.[6] Again, the potential difference generated is greater in the colon; a net secretion of potassium occurs, assisted by active conductance on the apical membrane.[1] Mucus is the predominant secretory product serving to lubricate formed feces, thereby facilitating defecation while protecting the mucosa.

Bacteria of the colon contribute to the production of nutrients in addition to aiding further digestion. Cellulose breakdown is of particular importance to herbivores. Vitamin K production by bacteria is essential to the support of the clotting cascade.[7]

Pathophysiology

Feces can be retained for several days in the normal dog and cat without permanent damage to the distal colon. Prolonged retention can derange the absorptive process such that the feces become more dehydrated and, therefore, firmer with time.[8] These concretions are painful to pass and can become impossible to eliminate (obstipation). When retention is severe and prolonged, irreversible changes in colonic motility can lead to colonic inertia. Significant distention in excess of three to four months is speculated to produce such effects.

Animals can demonstrate variable presenting signs. Central nervous system depression, anorexia, and weakness have been attributed to toxins absorbed by the compromised mucosa.[8] Abdominal pain and distention can result from the excessive amount of feces within the abdominal colon. Vomiting occurs secondary to the obstructive nature of colonic impaction, the effect of toxins on the chemoreceptor trigger zone, or vagal stimulation of intestinal distention.[8] Diarrhea may be observed as fluid bowel contents can pass about the solidified feces. Mucosal irritation by the mechanical obstruction results in increased mucus secretion by goblet cells and often exudation of blood. This produces a watery, mucoid, and potentially, bloody diarrhea. Common presenting complaints can include lethargy, anorexia, vomiting, tenesmus, weight loss, and diarrhea.[8]

Idiopathic Megacolon

Affecting middle-aged to older cats with few exceptions, idiopathic megacolon has an unknown etiology. Described as progressive intractable constipation, histologic evaluation does not identify abnormality in animals as it does in its human analog.

Hirschprung's disease (HD), described as aganglionosis of the distal large intestine, is often identified early in children owing to associated clinical features.[9] Important features of HD, characterized as a process of slow-transit constipation, are decreased ganglionic density and decreased concentration of Cajal cells.[10] These directly affect the motility of the distal large intestine and the production of a normal defecation reflex.

In the absence of histologic abnormalities, feline idiopathic megacolon (FIM) is attributed to inappropriate intrinsic or extrinsic innervation of the colon. Washabau and Stalis demonstrated the presence of myenteric neurons in colonic smooth muscle in cats with FIM as well as the neurons hyposensitivity to stimulation.[11] They postulated that the disorder is limited to the intrinsic nervous system in the absence of lower urinary tract signs.[11]

Many owners are not intimately aware of their animal's defecation habits and, so do not identify unusual behavior early in the disease. Most cats present with prolonged and, therefore, severe disease. FIM is an exclusionary diagnosis made through the elimination of other predisposing causes of constipation (i.e., renal insufficiency) by blood work, urinalysis, and imaging studies. The results of blood work can be consistent with pre-renal azotemia and electrolyte abnormalities compatible with metabolic acidemia in cases of severe, prolonged constipation. Abdominal radiographs demonstrate fecal distention in the colon with all causes of megacolon. Radiographs should be scrutinized for pelvic fracture malunions, distortions in the spine, and extramural compression. This can be supplemented by abdominal ultrasound and computed tomography for confirmation of soft tissue and bony obstructive etiologies, respectively. Rectal examination, colonoscopy, and contrast radiography can also assist in the systematic exclusion of causes.

Severity of dehydration and metabolic derangement must be addressed prior to intervention. Obstipation can then be the focus of treatment by the administration of stool softeners and enemas. Manual evacuation of stool should be performed gently in the anesthetized patient to minimize further mechanical trauma to already compromised mucosa. As the translocation of bacteria and toxins is a concern, administration of prophylactic antibiotics is recommended. Medical management includes high-fiber diet, stool softeners, bulk laxatives, prokinetic agents, and intermittent enemas. When aggressive medical therapy is unsuccessful, surgery can be considered.

Surgical management by subtotal colectomy is the treatment of choice. The surgeon must identify the objectives of colectomy when assessing the need to excise the ileocolic junction. Although removal of the ileocolic junction may produce looser stools, preservation may allow affected colonic tissue to remain. A survey of 22 cats undergoing subtotal or total colectomy demonstrated significantly looser stools in the group with total colectomy.[12] Recurrence of constipation occurred at comparable rates in the two populations, suggesting that the colonic tissue associated with the sphincter is insufficient to produce significant complications.[12] Removal of the ileocolic sphincter will likely allow some degree of recto-ileo reflux. Thus, preservation of the ileocolic junction has been recommended as surgical management of FIM. Initially, diarrhea is observed, but completely resolves or progresses to semi-formed stool in a period of weeks to months. The ileum and rectum are credited with the absorptive and reservoir capabilities that allow function to normalize with time.[13] Gregory et al evaluated the enteric functions of cats that had undergone colectomy; they found minimal differences between surgically-treated and untreated cats.[13] Serum concentrations of electrolytes remained within the normal limits. Trends in fecal concentrations of sodium and potassium were higher and lower, respectively, but not statistically significant; this was directly attributed to the removal of the proximal colon.[13]

Megacolon Secondary to Neurologic or Medical Disease

Disruption of the nervous supply of the large intestine can contribute to decreased or complete absence of colonic motility. Interruption of the appropriate signals can interfere with the normal defecation reflex and lead to constipation and megacolon. Removal of the affected colon may provide a satisfactory result when reflex mechanisms remain intact.

Manx cats have demonstrated abnormalities in their sacral spinal cord, producing urinary and fecal incontinence.[14] These abnormalities are manifested in bony structural deformities as well. Surgical intervention is not recommended owing to co-morbidities.

Megacolon secondary to autonomic ganglioneuritis was reported in a dog with a 6-week history of constipation and tenesmus.[15] Neurologic exam revealed only generalized muscle weakness. Histopathology demonstrated moderate lymphoplasmacytic infiltrates of the autonomic ganglia. The muscularis was normal, while the mucosa was edematous and mildly congested. The etiology of the neuritis was never identified.[15]

Constipation has been observed with poorly managed metabolic disease, potentiating the development of megacolon if the constipation is frequent and prolonged. Although not described in veterinary literature, toxic megacolon has been documented in humans.[16,17] Other neurologic and medical etiologies of megacolon have also been reported (Table 39-1).

Outlet Obstruction

Megacolon has been described secondary to a variety of processes physically obstructive to the outflow tract of the colon. Pelvic fracture malunion is one of the most common causes of secondary megacolon in the cat and the dog. Neoplasia, primary to the colon (intramural) or of adjacent tissue (extramural), can cause obstruction at a critical size. Altered anatomy, such as perineal hernia and anal or rectal atresia can result in constipation and then megacolon. In rare cases, foreign body or inappropriate nutrition can lead to obstruction of outflow.

Any disease process resulting in a prolonged, severe distention can result in permanent changes to colonic smooth muscle function.[18] Reduced motility or inertia can be particularly difficult to treat.

Clinical signs of outflow obstruction mimic those of idiopathic megacolon; therefore, diagnosis should place special importance on a thorough rectal examination. Following identification of the underlying obstruction, treatment is focused on surgical correction of the cause. Invasive procedures such as hemipelvectomy or pelvic reconstruction may be required to correct intrapelvic abnormalities. Schrader evaluated six animals with pelvic malunion and determined that surgical correction by pelvic osteotomy was successful in those animals whose clinical signs were less than six weeks in duration.[19] Clinical signs exceeding six weeks resulted in colonic inertia and, when obstipated, these animals were not managed successfully by pelvic reconstruction or ostectomy.[19] Removal of the ileocolic sphincter, in the subset of cats with megacolon secondary to pelvic malunion, is offered as a means to produce loose stools and minimize the intensity of continued medical management.[20] This population remains at risk of recurrent constipation despite total colectomy and may warrant continued medical management.

References

1. Strombeck DR: Small and large intestine: normal structure and function. *In* Strombeck's Small Animal Gastroenterology, 3rd ed. Guilford WG, Center SA, Strombeck DR, et al (eds). Philadelphia: WB Saunders, 1996, p. 318.

2. Evans HE: The digestive apparatus and abdomen. *In* Miller's Anatomy of the Dog, 3rd ed. Evans HE, ed.: Philadelphia: WB Saunders, 1993, p. 385.

3. Willenbueker RF, Snape WJ Jr: Pathophysiology of colonic motility disorders. *In* Bockus Gastroenterology, 5th ed. Haubrich, WS, Schaffner F, Berk JE (eds). Philadelphia: W.B. Saunders, 1995, p. 1592.

4. DeGeorgio R, Camilleri M: Human enteric neuropathies: morphology and molecular pathology (review). Neurogastroenterol Motil 16:515, 2004.

5. Cook IJ, Brookes SJ: Motility of the large intestine. *In* Sleisegner and Fordtran's Gastrointestinal and Liver Disease: Pathophysiology/ Diagnosis/Management, 7th ed. Feldman M, Friedman LS, Sleisenger MH (eds). Philadelphia: WB Saunders, 2002, p. 1679.

6. Chapter 65. Digestion and absorption in the gastrointestinal tract. *In* Textbook of Medical Physiology, 10th ed. Guyton AC, Hall JE (eds). Philadelphia: WB Saunders, 2000, p. 793.

7. Brooks M: Coagulopathies and thrombosis. *In* Ettinger SJ, Feldman EC (eds). Textbook of Veterinary Internal Medicine: Diseases of the Dog and Cat, 5th ed. Philadelphia: WB Saunders, 2000.

8. Bertoy RW: Megacolon in the cat. Vet Clin North Am 32: 901, 2002.

9. Chapter 35. Neuromuscular and mechanical disorders of the large intestine. *In* Morson BC, Dawson IMP, Day DW, et al (eds). Morson & Dawson's Gastrointestinal Pathology, 4th ed. Oxford: Blackwell Scientific, 2003, p. 452.

10. Wedel T, Spiegler J, Soellner S, et al: Enteric nerves and interstitial cells of Cajal are altered in patients with slow-transit constipation and megacolon. Gastroenterol 123:1459, 2002.

11. Washabau RJ, Stalis IH: Alterations in colonic smooth muscle function in cats with idiopathic megacolon. AJVR 57:580, 1996.

12. Sweet DC, Hardie EM, Stone EA: Preservation versus excision of the ileocolic junction during colectomy for megacolon: A study of 22 cats. JSAP 35:358, 1994.

13. Gregory CR, Guilford WG, Berry CR, et al: Enteric function in cats after subtotal colectomy for treatment of megacolon. Vet Surg 19: 216, 1990.

14. Deforest ME, Basrur PK: Malformations and the Manx syndrome in cats. Can Vet J 20:304, 1979.

15. Petrus DJ, Nicholls PK, Gregory SP: Megacolon secondary to autonomic ganglioneuritis in a dog. Vet Rec 148: 276, 2001.

16. Eyer F, Felgenhauer N, Zilker T: Toxic megacolon, an unusual complication of Amanita phalloides poisoning. Deutsche Medizinische Woechenschrift 129:137, 2004.

17. Lestin F, Pertschy A, Rimek D: Fungemia after oral treatment with Saccharomyces boulardii in a patient with multiple co-morbidities. Deutsche Medizinische Woechenschrift 128:2531, 2003.

18. Chapter 29. Congenital lesions. *In* Clinical Gastroenterology, 4th ed. Spiro HM (ed). New York: McGraw-Hill, 1993.

19. Schrader SC: Pelvic osteotomy as a treatment for obstipation in cats with acquired stenosis of the pelvic canal: Six cases (1978-1989). JAVMA 200:208, 1992.

20. Matthiesen DT, Scavelli TD, Whitney WO: Subtotal colectomy for the treatment of obstipation secondary to pelvic fracture malunion in cats. Vet Surg 20:113, 1991.

Part V

Neurology

Chapter 40

Injury to the Brain

Rodney S. Bagley
Chadwick R. West

Injury to the brain can occur from both endogenous and exogenous causes. Exogenous injury most commonly results from automobile-related trauma, although external blows to the head and face, penetrating wounds, gunshot injury, and impact from falling are also possible. At initial impact, primary mechanical disruption of intracranial tissues may occur. The force of impact can rupture axons, blood vessels, and other neural elements. Primary mechanical injury may then initiate numerous secondary pathophysiologic sequelae, such as metabolic alterations in neuronal or glial cells, impairment of vascular supply to normal tissue (ischemia), impairment of cerebrovascular autoregulation, hemorrhage (intraparenchymal, intraventricular, extradural, or subdural), irritation (seizure generation), obstruction of the ventricular system, edema formation, production of physiologically active products, and, most often, increased intracranial pressure (ICP). As ICP reaches life-threatening levels, shifts of brain parenchyma or brain herniation can occur. Differing types of brain herniation include subfalcial, rostral and caudal transtentorial, and foramen magnum herniation. Although some forms of herniation are treatable, brain herniation through the foramen magnum is often deadly.

The intracranial nervous system resides in a unique physiologic environment. Protected by, but also confined within, the bony limits of the cranium, nervous tissue exists with cerebrospinal fluid (CSF) and blood. Disease of the brain parenchyma or other intracranial tissues alters this physiologic equilibrium. As primary injury can be prevented but not treated per se, treatment of brain injury is directed toward treatment of secondary pathophysiologic events and basic life support. Important secondary pathophysiologic consequences of intracranial injury are discussed further so that a fundamental understanding of the intracranial environment following injury can be appreciated during the treatment process.

Cerebral Edema

Many intracranial diseases result in or are associated with brain edema. With acute injury, brain edema becomes maximal between 24 and 48 hours after injury, but may persist for a week or more.[1] Brain edema has been categorized as vasogenic, cytotoxic, or interstitial based on cause and anatomic areas of involvement.[2] Any or all of these types of edema may be present in an animal with brain disease.

Cytotoxic edema (intracellular edema) results from failure of cellular energy, with resultant failure to extrude sodium from within the cell. Intracellular water increases and cells swell. This edema most often results from disease processes such as toxicity, ischemia, or hypoxia.

Interstitial edema is defined as increased water content of the periventricular white matter owing to movement of CSF across the ventricular walls in instances of hydrocephalus. Periventricular white matter is reduced owing to the disappearance of myelin lipids secondary to increases in hydrostatic pressure or decreases in periventricular blood flow in the white matter.[3]

Vasogenic edema is the most common form of edema associated with CNS neoplasia. This type of edema results from vascular injury secondary to physical disruption of the vascular endothelium or functional alterations in endothelial tight junctions. Differences in transmural pressure gradients result in extravasation of fluid from cerebral vessels to the extracellular fluid (ECF) spaces of the brain.[4] These abnormalities allow for fluid to move from the vascular to perivascular spaces. Areas of the brain where ECF is normally enlarged provide a natural conduit for fluid movement. Increases in intravascular pressure owing to loss of autoregulation, vascular obstruction, or hypertension (e.g., Cushing's response and cerebral ischemic response) may perpetuate edema formation.

Vasogenic edema migrates away from areas of vascular disruption via bulk flow.[4] Fluid movement depends on a balance between the opposing forces of capillary hydrostatic pressure and tissue-resistance pressure. Vasogenic edema usually spreads readily through the white matter, possibly because of the orderly arrangement of nerve fibers found there. Also, the movement of this type of edema may be related to the low capillary density and blood flow in normal white matter. Deep white matter of the involved cerebral hemisphere is preferentially affected.

Hemorrhage

Hemorrhage, either within or around the brain may result in rapid cerebral dysfunction often by alterations in cerebral volume (mass effect). In comparison with humans, subdural hematomas are uncommon in dogs.[5] Systemic coagulation abnormalities (e.g., thrombocytopenia) and hypertension may potentiate hemorrhagic potentials. Vascular damage from therapeutic intervention (e.g., radiation therapy) may also influence the incidence of tumor-related hemorrhage. Also, loss of cerebral vascular autoregulation may predispose to hemorrhage or infarction.

Ventricular Obstruction

Space-occupying intracranial disease may impinge on the ventricular system, resulting in obstruction of CSF flow. Common areas of obstruction, owing to the inherently small diameter of the ventricular system, include the interventricular foramen (connection between the lateral and third ventricles) and the mesencephalic aqueduct. Knowledge of normal CSF flow allows for determination of the location of the obstruction. Sequestration of CSF in an obstructed component of the ventricular system may result in increases in intracranial pressure and interstitial brain edema.

Increases in Intracranial Pressure

Intracranial pressure is the pressure exerted between the skull and the intracranial tissues. As the skull is relatively inelastic compared with the other intracranial tissues, ICP is determined primarily by changes in intracranial tissue volume and the compensatory ability of these tissues to accommodate for volume changes.[1,6-8]

The three major components of volume residing within the intracranial space are the brain tissue (intracranial cellular elements), the cerebrospinal fluid, and blood.[7] Intracranial disease often increases the volume of one of these components. For ICP to remain normal, an increase in volume of one of these three intracranial components must be compensated for by a decrease in volume of one or both of the other components (intracranial compliance). Although compliance can initially aid in stabilizing ICP, it has finite limits. When compliance is exhausted, ICP will increase. This relationship may vary among individual patients and may be influenced by the extent and location of an intracranial mass as well as cerebral blood flow.[9] As ICP increases, the pressure within the intracranial space decreases cerebral blood flow. With decreased cerebral perfusion, neuronal ischemia, hypoxia, dysfunction, and death ultimately result.

Cerebral blood flow and CSF are in constant flux. ICP is dynamic and pulse-like, with a small pressure wave occurring almost simultaneously with each heart beat.[10,11] This wave form is referred to as the intracranial pulse pressure wave (ICPPW). Periodic fluctuations may occur in response to normal body functions, such as coughing or abdominal straining, via increases in intrathoracic pressure and venous pressure impairing venous return from the intracranial space. With intracranial disease, ICP may be elevated persistently or episodically, resulting in persistent or episodic clinical abnormalities, respectively. As exemplified by Lundberg, periodic elevations in ICP (plateau waves) with ensuing return of ICP to normal levels can occur in humans with intracranial disease.[12] These periodic elevations are thought to originate from cerebral vasodilation secondary to decreased cerebral perfusion in patients with intact cerebrovascular autoregulatory capacity.[13] In this situation, single-time measurements of ICP may not accurately reveal these episodic elevations, and critical periods of raised ICP will be overlooked.

Numerous physiologic and nonphysiologic variables influence ICP measurements. These include anesthetic agents[14-18] and body weight.[19] The effects of anesthetic agents on ICP are many and varied, and the need for anesthesia to measure ICP can potentially alter values obtained. Specific effects of anesthetic agents on ICP have been reviewed elsewhere.[14-18]

An absolute level wherein ICP is elevated has not been established. This may be the result of the inherent inaccuracies of the monitoring equipment and the normal variation in baseline ICPs. Most information from humans suggests that ICP higher than 15 to 20 mm Hg is elevated.[20] Cerebral blood flow may not be significantly decreased until ICP reaches about 30 mm Hg.[21] Experimentally, however, ICP was raised to very high levels (> 100 mm Hg) before brain death occurred.[22] We have seen ICPs as high as 30 to 40 mm Hg in dogs that subsequently have recovered from brain injury. Whereas some have suggested that the degree and persistence of ICP elevation is associated with outcome after head injury,[20] others have suggested that ICP monitoring does not influence overall prognosis.[23]

Clinical Effects of Intracranial Pressure Alterations

The major intracranial effect of increasing ICP is alteration of cerebral perfusion pressure (CPP) (Figure 40-1).[9,21,24,25] Cerebral perfusion is dependent on systemic blood flow and intracranial pressure expressed via the formula CPP = MABP - ICP (MABP = mean arterial blood pressure).[19] For CPP to remain constant, the effects of increased ICP on blood flow to the brain must be reciprocated by increases in systemic blood pressure. Cerebral perfusion pressure is a determinant of cerebral blood flow (CBF) but is not always equivalent; in many instances, however, as CPP decreases so does CBF. Intracranial pressure and CPP, however, have an inverse relationship (Figure 40-1). When CPP falls below 60 to 70 mm Hg, this creates physiologic abnormalities within the brain.

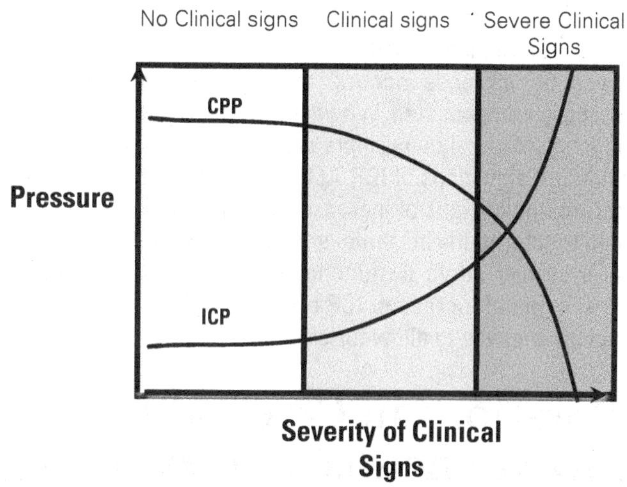

Figure 40-1. Schematic relationship between intracranial pressure (ICP) and cerebral perfusion pressure (CPP). As ICP increases, CPP ultimately decreases to result in clinical signs.

Blood flow to the brain is coupled to the cerebral metabolic rate. When CBF decreases, the brain recognizes the ischemia and evokes a spectrum of physiologic alterations known as the cerebral ischemic response.[26] These physiologic alterations are thought to emanate from vasomotor centers in the lower brain stem. Failure of adequate blood flow to remove CO_2 from receptors in these centers increases local CO_2 concentrations, which in turn, stimulates the sympathetic nervous system to increase systemic blood pressure. Systemic hypertension results as an attempt to maintain cerebral blood flow. Baroreceptors within the systemic vascular system recognize this hypertensive situation, and send this information to vagal centers also found in the lower brain stem. The resultant increase in systemic vagal tone reflexively causes bradycardia. The systemic hypertension and associated reflex bradycardia is commonly referred to as Cushing's reflex and may explain why many animals with intracranial disease have bradycardia.

As ICP increases and CPP subsequently decreases to a significantly low level, a large catecholamine release occurs.[22] This catecholamine release may result in myocardial ischemia known as brain-heart syndrome.[11,27] Clinically, arrhythmias are noted. Focal myocardial ischemia is the pathologic lesion, with focal white streaks seen grossly in the myocardium.[27] Histologically, myocardial degeneration is common. Brain-heart syndrome has been described with numerous intracranial and spinal pathologic lesions and in different species including dogs, sheep, cattle, horses, pigs, goats, and humans.

Intracranial pressure alterations are often responsible for clinical decline in many animals with brain disease. As stated previously, owing to the confining nature of the skull, changes in intracranial volume increase ICP when compensation is exhausted. With structural brain disease, the brain component usually enlarges as a result of neoplastic cell infiltration, edema, or inflammation. As the brain compartment volume increases, the CSF and blood compartments must decrease or ICP will increase. Compensation for increased brain tissue volume initially involves shifting of CSF out of the skull, decreased CSF production, and eventually decreased cerebral blood flow.

These compensatory mechanisms prevent increases in ICP for some undetermined period of time. In general, the more slowly the volume increase occurs, the more readily this volume increase is compensated. When compensatory mechanisms are exhausted, relatively small increases in intracranial volume result in dramatic elevations of ICP. At this time, clinical signs become apparent. Initial signs of increased ICP may be nonspecific and limited to alterations in mental status (progression to stupor and coma), cranial nerve dysfunction, and paresis. Unfortunately, clinical signs of increased ICP often become most obvious too late in the disease to allow for effective therapy.

Alterations in Cerebral Blood Flow (Ischemia and Hypoxia)

Because normal function of neurons depends on an adequate supply of oxygen, physical disruption of blood flow can significantly impair normal brain function. Cerebral vessels are directly responsive to $PaCO_2$ concentrations, with cerebral blood flow coupled to cerebral metabolic rate.[1] As $PaCO_2$ concentrations increase, cerebral vessels dilate to increase blood flow to the brain. The opposite effect is seen with decreased $PaCO_2$. This effect of $PaCO_2$ is a component of cerebral blood flow autoregulation. The cerebral vessels have the ability to change diameter in response to $PaCO_2$ (chemical autoregulation) as well as blood pressure (pressure autoregulation) in order to maintain a relatively constant cerebral blood flow. Cerebral vessels change diameter through perivascular changes in pH as a direct result of $PaCO_2$ concentrations similar to what occurs in the chemosensitive area of the medulla oblongata for stimulation of respiration.

If autoregulation is intact, hyperventilation to decrease $PaCO_2$ will cause cerebral vasoconstriction, decreased cerebral blood volume, and subsequently, decreased ICP. Cerebrovascular autoregulatory capability is affected by a variety of intracranial processes. For example, local acidosis, common in many hypoxic and ischemic events, will disrupt local autoregulatory functions.[28] If chemical autoregulation is absent in the diseased brain, hyperventilation will not alter the vascular diameter in the affected area. In this instance, two situations are possible, both dependent on the premise that cerebrovascular autoregulatory capacity is absent owing to local disease.

As $PaCO_2$ is decreased by hyperventilation, vessels in surrounding normal brain will constrict. Vessels in the damaged or abnormal area of the brain are already maximally dilated and, therefore, are unable to constrict. Because of the vasoconstriction in normal brain, vascular resistance increases in this area, shunting blood into the abnormal area (inverse steal or Robin Hood phenomenon).[28] This has the positive effect of increasing cerebral blood flow to the abnormal and potentially hypoxic areas of the brain. The negative effect, however, is potentiation of hemorrhage and cerebral edema in the abnormal area owing to the increased flow.

The opposite may occur as $PaCO_2$ increases. Vessels in normal brain surrounding the diseased area will dilate. Again, vessels in the abnormal area are already maximally dilated owing to loss of autoregulation. Vascular resistance will be decreased in surrounding normal brain, blood will be shunted away from abnormal areas, potentially decreasing hemorrhage and edema but resulting in further hypoxia (steal phenomenon).[28]

Autoregulation of cerebral blood flow can also occur in response to systemic changes in blood pressure in order to maintain relatively constant cerebral blood flow during times of both hypo- and hypertension.[1] This prevents underperfusion and resultant ischemia during times of hypotension and hemorrhage and edema at times of hypertension. In most instances, cerebral blood flow is maintained constant throughout shifts in systemic blood pressure of between 50 and 150 mm Hg.[1] Above and below these limits, cerebral blood flow depends directly on systemic blood pressure.

Whether autoregulation remains intact in brain disease is difficult to predict clinically. Global autoregulatory function of pressure has been assessed in human patients with head injury and found to be intact in about 69%.[29] It has been suggested that a crude clinical estimate of intact autoregulatory function is level of consciousness, with conscious patients thought to have intact autoregulatory capacity more often than do unconscious patients.[1] Local loss of autoregulation, however, is almost impossible to predict in the clinical setting without sophisticated testing that is not practically available.

Additionally, at least in the instance of exogenous head trauma, discrepancies can occur between the intact function of pressure versus chemical ($PaCO_2$-responsive) autoregulatory capacities.[29] With head trauma, pressure autoregulation is often abnormal; however, $PaCO_2$-responsive autoregulation remains intact. This is termed dissociative vasoparalysis and has important ramifications during treatment. As the cerebrovascular response to blood pressure changes are abnormal, a more intimate control of systemic blood pressure and central venous pressure is required to prevent large shifts of blood pressure and subsequent cerebral blood flow. While correction of hypotension is often necessary in the animal with concurrent head trauma and shock, hypervolemia should be avoided.[25] If pressure autoregulation is defective, significant increases in mean arterial blood pressure will increase cerebral blood flow and, ultimately, ICP.[29] If pressure autoregulation is intact, decreased blood pressure will cause cerebrovascular vasodilation, increasing cerebral blood flow, and ultimately, increasing ICP.

Pressure autoregulation may also falsely appear intact (false autoregulation) even when vasomotor paralysis is present.[28] In this situation, cerebral blood flow is found not to increase when systemic blood pressure is increased, suggesting intact pressure autoregulation. Because of associated cerebral swelling, however, further dilation of cerebral vessels is prevented. Therefore, no additional increase in cerebral blood flow is possible, regardless of blood pressure. All of these factors contribute to myriad intracranial blood flow alterations that can affect intracranial pressure.

Cerebral blood flow, therefore, is normally maintained through a combination of systemic blood flow (pressure) and cerebral vasculature autoregulation. Autoregulation is important to maintain a near constant cerebral blood flow over a range of systemic blood pressures. Brain injury may alter cerebral vascular autoregulatory mechanisms, thus making cerebral blood flow more dependent on systemic blood pressure. This results in inadequate perfusion of neurons during times of hypotension and overperfusion (possibly perpetuating edema formation) during times of hypertension (also referred to as luxury perfusion). Subsequent re-establishment of blood flow may also have possible detrimental effects (reperfusion injury) on spared brain through such processes as free radical formation and lactic acid accumulation.

Terminal Effects of Compartmentalized ICP Increases Brain Herniation

As intracranial volume continues to increase beyond the limits of compensation, ICP will increase so precipitously that shifts of brain parenchyma, termed brain herniation, will occur.[8] Coma and severe neurologic impairment are noted. Unfortunately, in many instances, brain herniation becomes a terminal event.

Five major types of brain herniation have been described; rostral or caudal transtentorial, subfalcial or cingulate gyrus, foramen magnum, and herniation through a craniotomy defect.[2,8] Of these, caudal transtentorial, subfalcial, and foramen magnum occur most commonly. Clinical signs of caudal transtentorial herniation are frequently the result of pressure distributed ventrally through the midbrain with subsequent compression of the oculomotor nerve. With unilateral herniations, an ipsilateral dilated pupil, unresponsive to light stimulation, may be seen. Monitoring for clinical signs of this type of herniation, therefore, should include periodic pupillary evaluations. If unilateral mydriasis is noted in this setting, immediate and aggressive attempts to decrease ICP should be instituted.

Foramen magnum herniation may occur quickly and results in respiratory arrest owing to associated pressure on the respiratory centers in the caudal brain stem. Foramen magnum herniation is invariably fatal, and surgical attempts at decompression after this type of herniation have not been helpful in affected dogs.

Treatment of Intracranial Pathophysiologic Sequelae

Effective treatment of the pathophysiologic sequelae of increased ICP depends on the determination and effective treatment of the primary disease. Unfortunately, in the situation of brain injury, the primary event has occurred prior to treatment. It is often necessary, therefore, to acutely treat the more immediately life-threatening secondary sequelae such as increased intracranial pressure to allow time for treatment of the primary disease. Treatment of secondary pathophysiologic events subsequent to intracranial injury is a more important determinant of acute survival than is treatment of the primary disease process. The following section provides an overview of treatment possibilities for these secondary pathophysiologic events. In-depth discussion of pros and cons of individual treatments have been discussed elsewhere.[30-33]

One of the most important aspects of treatment of intracranial injury is to maintain appropriate cerebral perfusion, primarily by maintaining effective intravascular volume. This is accomplished through the administration of intravenous crystalloids and/or colloids. Mannitol has been shown to decrease blood viscosity, which may contribute to increased cerebral perfusion and decreases in ICP.[34] Decreasing blood viscosity will increase cerebral perfusion at the same level of pressure. Vasoconstriction will result, lowering cerebral blood volume and concurrently lowering ICP. Other hypertonic solutions appear to be less effective at lowering ICP as compared with mannitol, however, hypertonic saline administration has shown some benefit.[35]

Treatment of intracranial hemorrhage varies depending on whether the hemorrhage has formed a discrete lesion that is increasing intracranial volume at the expense of the surrounding normal nervous tissue. In such an instance, surgical drainage may be necessary to bring about resolution. Although it is uncommon, traumatic subdural hematoma can be used as an example. As the lesion matures it becomes relatively hyperosmolar, resulting in imbibition of water and expansion of the lesion. The patient with traumatic subdural hematoma should, therefore, benefit from surgical drainage of the lesion.[5] It is also important to identify and treat any predisposing factors to hemorrhage such as hypertension or a bleeding disorder.

Craniotomy / Craniectomy

A major tenet of the Monro-Kellie doctrine is that intracranial contents are confined within the cranium. It would follow, therefore, that surgical removal of the skull would potentially decrease ICP. Unilateral or bilateral craniectomy has been used as a treatment for ICP elevations which cannot be decreased by the more conventional methods stated earlier.[36-40] Although skull removal alone may be beneficial, subsequent dural incision appears significantly more effective in lowering ICP. This has been shown clinically in humans and experimentally in dogs and cats.[41,42] Ultimate functional recovery, however, remains dependent on the underlying primary brain damage caused by the initial disease process. Postoperatively, the extent and magnitude of the decrease of ICP subsequent to surgery remains uncertain.

Craniectomy and durotomy have been shown to lower ICP by 15% and 65%, respectively, in dogs and cats, and humans.[41,38] Intracranial pressures in normal dogs approached atmospheric pressure when a bilateral or unilateral rostrotentorial craniectomy and durotomy were performed. Adequate decompression in animals with structural disease would be suggested if intraoperative ICP approached similar levels.

If large amounts of skull are removed, a cranioplasty may be necessary. Otherwise, postoperative scarring may result in brain compression similar to that which occurs because of the formation of laminectomy membrane after extensive laminectomy, resulting in spinal cord compression. Cranioplasty can be delayed until life-threatening elevations of ICP are stabilized. Some humans had improvement in persistent neurologic signs after delayed cranioplasty, suggesting that clinical signs after initial recovery may result from both the initial injury and surgical scarring.[52]

Other Treatments with Questionable Benefits

Much debate remains regarding the most appropriate head position for patients with head injury. Many current recommendations from human traumatologists suggest a horizontal or neutral position to maintain cerebral perfusion. Head elevation to 30° above heart level, however, has been shown to decrease ICP primarily by facilitating venous drainage.[43,44] Opponents suggest that head elevation may decrease cerebral perfusion and, therefore, be detrimental to brain functions. Reduction of ICP with this relatively simple treatment may be beneficial in combination with other ICP-decreasing measures.

If chemical autoregulation remains intact, hyperventilation can decrease ICP owing to the established effects of $PaCO_2$ concentrations on cerebral blood flow.[1,9] Hyperventilation is performed to maintain the $PaCO_2$ concentration between 25 and 35 mm Hg.

Cerebrospinal fluid aspiration may be used as the initial means to decrease ICP.[45] This is most helpful in humans if a ventriculostomy is present and if ICP elevations do not exceed 30 mm Hg.[9] The use of routine CSF collection alone for this purpose is not recommended in animals with suspected increased ICP owing to the increased risk of precipitating brain herniation.[46] In one study in animals, however, no increased risk of brain herniation was found in dogs and cats with intracranial disease after CSF collection.[47]

Corticosteroids have received much use in the treatment of spinal trauma, and have been recommended as a treatment for elevated ICP.[48,49] Although corticosteroids have shown to be beneficial by reducing cerebral edema in brain tumor patients, caution should be exercised when using corticosteroids for brain injury. One study in rats has suggested that corticosteroids may be advantageous in brain injury;[49] however, corticosteroids may not be efficacious in head trauma and are known to perpetuate neuronal damage if ischemia is operant.[50,51] Corticosteroid administration may increase blood glucose, a factor that may negatively influence outcome after head injury.[52] Also, the onset of beneficial effects of decreasing cerebral edema may be delayed too long to be helpful in acute elevations of ICP. Unfortunately, until further data are reported, the benefit of corticosteroid use in head injury and elevated ICP remains nebulous. Additionally, other treatments such as barbiturate-induced coma and hypothermia require further investigation.[24,53-55]

References

1. Shapiro HM: Intracranial hypertension: Therapeutic and anesthetic considerations. Anesthesiology 43:445-471, 1975.

2. Fishman RA: Brain edema. N Engl J Med 293:706-711, 1975.

3. Rosenberg GA, Saland L, Kyner WT: Pathophysiology of periventricular tissue changes with raised CSF pressure. J Neurosurg 59:606-611, 1983.

4. Reulen HJ: Vasogenic brain oedema, new aspects in its formation, resolution and therapy. Br J Anaesth 48:741-752, 1976.

5. Hopkins AL, Wheeler SJ: Subdural hematoma in a dog. Vet Surg 20:413, 1991.

6. Germon K: Interpretation of ICP pulse waves to determine intracerebral compliance. J Neurosci Nurs 20:344-349, 1988.

7. Kornegay JN: Pathogenesis of diseases of the central nervous system. *In* Textbook of Small Animal Surgery, 2nd ed. Slatter D (ed). Philadelphia: WB Saunders, 1993, pp. 1022-1037.

8. Kornegay JN, Oliver JE, Gorgacz EJ: Clinicopathologic features of brain herniation in animals. J Am Vet Med Assoc 182:1111-1116, 1983.

9. Lyons MK, Meyer FB: Cerebrospinal fluid physiology and the management of increased intracranial pressure. Mayo Clinic Proc 65:684-707, 1990.

10. Cardoso ER, Rowan JO, Galbraith S: Analysis of the cerebrospinal fluid pulse wave in intracranial pressure. J Neurosurg 59:817-821, 1983.

11. Graf CJ, Rossi NP: Catecholamine response to intracranial hypertension. J Neurosurg 49:862-868, 1978.

12. Lundberg N: Continuous recording and control of ventricular fluid pressure in neurosurgical practice. Acta Psychiatr Neurol Scand 36:1-193, 1960.

13. Rosner MJ, Becker DP: Origin and evolution of plateau waves. J Neurosurg 60:312-324, 1984.

14. Adams RW, Cucchiara RF, Gronet GA, et al:. Isoflurane and cerebrospinal fluid pressure in neurosurgical patients. Anesthesiology 54:97-99, 1981.

15. Cornick JL. Anesthetic management of patients with neurologic abnormalities. Comp Contin Educ Pract Vet 14:163-172, 1992.

16. Fenner WR: Neuroanesthesia. Proceedings 10th ACVIM Forum, San Diego, CA, May 1992; 722-724.

17. Grosslight K, Foster R, Colohan AR, Bedford RF: Isoflurane for neuroanesthesia: Risk factors for increases in intracranial pressure. Anesthesiology 63:533-536, 1985.

18. Shores A: Neuroanesthesia: A review of the effects of anesthetic agents on cerebral blood flow and intracranial pressure in the dog. Vet Surg 14:257-263, 1985.

19. Simpson ST, Reed RB: Manometric values for normal cerebrospinal fluid pressure in dogs. J Am Anim Hosp Assoc 23:629-632, 1987.

20. Obrist WD, Langfitt TW, Jaggi JL, et al: Cerebral blood flow and metabolism in comatose patients with acute head injury. J Neurosurg 61:241-253, 1984.

21. Hassler W, Steinmetz H, Gawlowski J: Transcranial doppler ultrasonography in raised intracranial pressure and in intracranial circulatory arrest. J Neurosurg 68:745-751, 1988.

22. van Loon J, Shivalkar B, Plets C, et al: Catecholamine response to a gradual increase of intracranial pressure. J Neurosurg 79:705-709, 1993.

23. Stuart GG, Merry GS, Smith JA, Yelland JDN: Severe head injury managed without intracranial pressure monitoring. J Neurosurg 59:601-605, 1983.

24. Marion DW, Obrist WD, Carlier PM, et al: The use of moderate therapeutic hypothermia for patients with severe head injuries: a preliminary report. J Neurosurg 79:354-362, 1993.

25. Rosner MJ, Daughton S: Cerebral perfusion pressure management in head injury. J Trauma 30:933-941, 1990.

26. Guyton AC: Arterial pressure regulation: I. Rapid pressure control. *In* Textbook of Medical Physiology, 7th ed. Philadelphia: WB Saunders, 1986, pp. 250-251.

27. King JM, Roth L, Haschek WM: Myocardial necrosis secondary to neural lesions in domestic animals. J Am Vet Med Assoc 180:144-148, 1982.

28. Enevoldsen EM, Jensen FT: Autoregulation and CO2 responses of cerebral blood flow in patients with acute severe head injury. J Neurosurg 48:689-703, 1979.

29. Bouma GJ, Muizelaar JP, Bandoh K, Marmarou A: Blood pressure and intracranial pressure-volume dynamics in severe head injury: relationship with cerebral blood flow. J Neurosurg 77:15-19, 1992.

30. Dewey CW: Emergency management of the head trauma patient: principles and practice. *In* Vet Clin North Am: Small Anim Pract. Vassallo, J (ed). Philadelphia: WB Saunders, 2000, pp. 207-225.

31. Dewey CW, Budsberg SC, Oliver JE Jr: Principles of head trauma management in dogs and cats -- part 1. Compend Contin Educ Pract Vet 14:199-206, 1992.

32. Platt SR, Radaelli ST, McDonnell JJ: The prognostic value of the modified Glasgow Coma Scale in head trauma in dogs. J Vet Intern Med 15:581-584, 2001.

33. Procaccio F, Stocchetti N, Citero G, et al: Guidelines for the treatment of adults with severe head trauma (part II). Criteria for medical treatment. J Neurosurg Sci 44:11-18, 2000.

34. Ravussin P, Archer DP, Meyer E, et al: The effects of rapid infusions of saline and mannitol on cerebral blood volume and intracranial pressure in dogs. Can Anaesth Soc J 32:506-515, 1985.

35. Qureshi AI, Wilson DA, Traystman RJ: Treatment of transtentorial herniation unresponsive to hyperventilation using hypertonic saline in dogs: effect on cerebral blood flow and metabolism. J Neurosurg Anesthesiol 14:22-30, 2002.

36. Fisher CM, Ojemann RG: Bilateral decompressive craniectomy for worsening coma in acute subarachnoid hemorrhage. Observations in support of the procedure. Surg Neurol 41:65-74, 1994.

37. Gaab MR, Rittierodt M, Lorenz M, Heissler HE: Traumatic brain swelling and operative decompression: a prospective investigation. Acta Neurochirurgica Suppl 51:326-328, 1990.

38. Jourdan C, Convert J, Mottolese C, et al:. Evaluation of the clinical benefit of decompression hemicraniectomy in intracranial hypertension not controlled by medical treatment. Neuro Chirurgie 39:304-310, 1993.

39. Rinaldi A, Mangiola A, Anile C, et al: Hemodynamic effects of decompressive craniectomy in cold induced brain oedema. Acta Neurochirurgica Suppl 51:394-396, 1990.

40. Venes JI, Collins WF: Bifrontal decompressive craniectomy in the management of head trauma. J Neurosurg 42:429-433, 1975.

41. Bagley RS, Harrington ML, Pluhar GE, et al: Effect of craniectomy/durotomy alone or in combination with hyperventilation, diuretics, and corticosteroids on intracranial pressure in normal dogs. Am J Vet Res 57:116-119, 1996.

42. Bagley RS, Keegan RD, Greene SA, et al: Intraoperative intracranial pressure monitoring in five dogs with structural brain disease. J Am Vet Med Assoc 5:588-591, 1995.

43. Feldman Z, Kanter MJ, Robertson CS, et al: Effect of head elevation on intracranial pressure, cerebral perfusion pressure, and cerebral blood flow in head-injured patients. J Neurosurg 76:207-211, 1992.

44. Schneider GH, von-Helden GH, Franke R, et al: Influence of body position on jugular venous oxygen saturation, intracranial pressure and cerebral perfusion pressure. Acta Neurochir Suppl Wien 59;107-12, 1993.

45. Caruselli G, Recchioni MA, Occhipinti C, et al: The role of CSF ventricular drainage in controlling intracranial hypertension in patients with brain lesions. Comparison of three methods. Preliminary results. J Neurosurg Sci 36:219-25, 1992.

46. Duffy GP: Lumbar puncture in the presence of raised intracranial pressure. Br Med J 1:407-409, 1969.

47. Speciale J, Steinberg SA, Van Winkle T: Morbidity and mortality related to cerebellomedullary spinal tap in dogs and cats. J Vet Intern Med 9:208, 1995.

48. Hall ED: The neuroprotective pharmacology of methylprednisolone. J Neurosurg 76:13-22, 1992.

49. Hall ED: High-dose glucocorticoid treatment improves neurological recovery in head-injured mice. J Neurosurg 62:882-887, 1985.

50. Braakman R, Schouten HJA, Dishoeck MB, Minderhound JM: Megadose steroid in severe head injury. J Neurosurg 58:326-330, 1983.

51. Sapolsky RM, Pulsinelli WA: Glucocorticoids potentiate ischemic injury to neurons: Therapeutic implications. Science 229:1397-1400, 1985.

52. Lam AM, Winn HR, Cullen BF, Sundling N: Hyperglycemia and neurological outcome in patients with head injury. J Neurosurg 75:545-551, 1991.

53. Lobato RD, Sarabia R, Cordobes F, et al: Posttraumatic cerebral hemispheric swelling. J Neurosurg 68:417-423, 1988.

54. Nordström CH, Messeter K, Sundbärg G, et al: Cerebral blood flow, vasoreactivity, and oxygen consumption during barbiturate therapy in severe traumatic brain lesions. J Neurosurg 64:231-237, 1986.

55. Pomeranz S, Safar P, Radovsky A, et al: The effect of resuscitative moderate hypothermia following epidural brain compression on cerebral damage in a canine outcome model. J Neurosurg 79:241-251, 1993.

Chapter 41

Surgical Diseases of the Brain

Rodney S. Bagley
Annie V. Chen

Intracranial surgery in animals is most commonly employed for removal of intracranial masses, biopsy of intracranial lesions, placement of ventricular cerebrospinal fluid (CSF) shunting devices, decompression and debridement of intracranial tissues, and short-term treatment of increased intracranial pressure (ICP). Surgery may include removal of sizable portions of the skull (craniotomy or craniectomy) or be limited to smaller burr holes for decompression and evacuation of hematoma or stereotactic biopsy. Additional indications for intracranial surgery in humans that may be employed in animals include treatment for seizures, chronic pain, and movement disorders.

Intracranial surgery used as treatment for intracranial disease is most appropriately considered following an appropriate diagnosis (both physical and anatomic) and with an understanding of the pathophyisology associated with the disease in question. Surgical approaches to intracranial lesions are chosen based on lesion location, extent, anticipated consistency, nature (inflammatory versus neoplastic versus hemorrhagic), and the goal of the surgery (tissue removal versus biopsy versus decompression).[1] Limited approaches are more often used for biopsy, hematoma decompression, and intraventricular shunt placement. The size and extent of bone removal are also limited by skull anatomy, surrounding soft tissues, and the associated vasculature. Surgical approaches to the brain have been reviewed elsewhere.[1-4] The more common disease processes in which intracranial surgery is currently utilized are discussed further.

Neoplasia

The most appropriate treatment for dogs with brain tumors has yet to be defined. Survival for dogs with brain tumors that are not treated, however, is reportedly dismal. In one study, median survival for dogs with varying tumor types that did not have treatment was 6 days.[5] Anecdotal reports exist, however, of dogs with brain tumors living for months to years without definitive treatment. The natural course and overall survival times of animals with brain tumors are not well established, making objective determination of treatment effects more difficult.

Surgical removal is most readily used for superficially located, encapsulated, relatively small, benign tumors of which meningiomas are the most common (Figure 41-1). Surgery also affords the possibility of cure that is uncommon with other treatment modalities for brain tumor. Depending on the type and location of the tumor, a surgical approach is made to the skull. The overlying skull is removed by performing a craniotomy or craniectomy. The mass is identified and, ideally, its borders are determined. The tumor can then be biopsied, debulked, or ideally, removed in total via a combination of sharp, blunt, and aspiration resection. Surgical equipment and techniques have been described elsewhere.[1] Tumor removal is performed with magnification or with the aid of an operating microscope to improve visualization of the microvascular anatomy and to provide a better view of the tissue. An ultrasonic aspirator unit may be useful in some instances to more safely remove softer tumor tissue or necrotic brain at the borders of the tumor.

Many brain tumors are removed in a piecemeal fashion to avoid compression of normal brain and further brain damage. The inner portions of the tumor are removed first to collapse the volume of the mass. Next, the capsule is identified and removed, if possible. The dura in contact with the lesion is incised with as large a margin as possible. In instances of meningioma, a biopsy of normal-appearing dura at the edge of the lesion is collected for histologic evaluation of tumor margins.

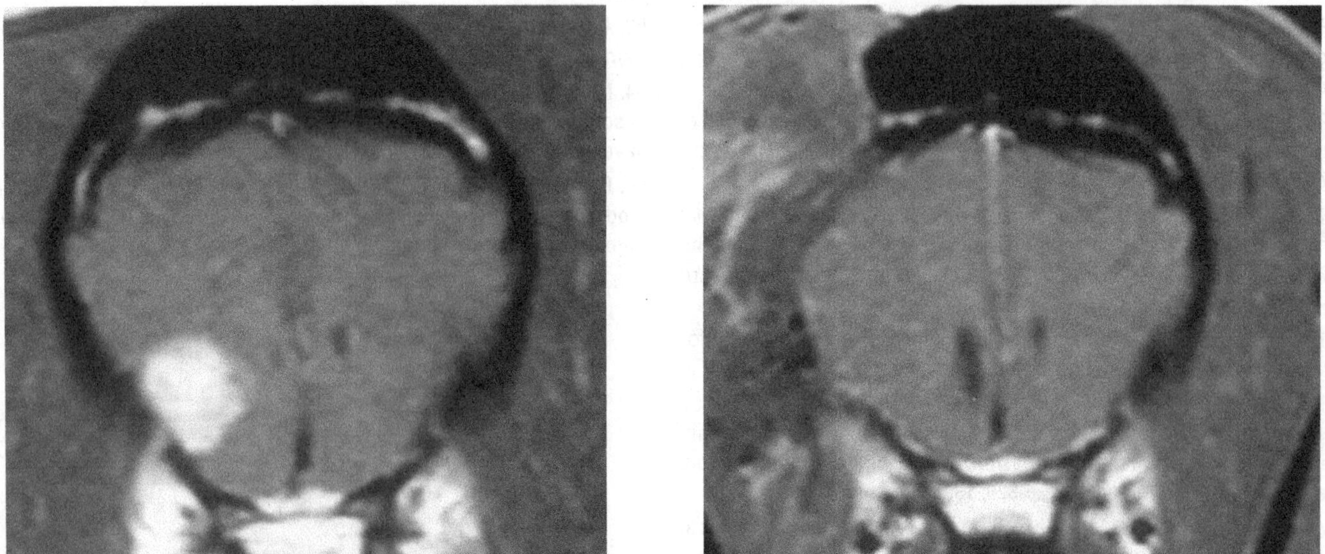

Figure 41-1 (A,B) Transverse, T1-weighted MR images following intravenous contrast administration of dogs with meningioma (left) before and (right) after surgical removal (From Bagley RS: Fundamentals of Veterinary Clinical Neurology, Ames, IA: Blackwell Publishing, 2005.)

In dogs, even when meningiomas are histologically benign, these tumors are often not well encapsulated and hence are difficult to differentiate from surrounding non-tumorous brain. Brain damage in areas adjacent to the tumor can make gross delineation of tumor borders difficult if not impossible. Tumor may be located in areas of the brain where access and exposure are limited, increasing the risk of surgical morbidity. Poor surgical access often leads to increased surgical mortality. If the tumor is within the parenchyma or within a ventricle, it is impossible to surgically access the lesion without damage to at least some surrounding or overlying brain. Many intracranial tumors have multiple vessels supplying them, leading to the risk of hemorrhage during resection. These factors may limit successful removal of brain tumors; in some instances, however, surgery is successful in bringing about cure or long-term remission of brain tumors.[1,2,5-12]

Surgical treatments for brain-stem tumors are often hindered by inadequate exposure of the lesion and infiltration or compression of vital brain structures. Cranial nerves are often entwined within these masses, making complete resection difficult. Tumors of the cranial nerves may also require surgical removal similar to other tumors of peripheral nerves.[7] Median survival times reported in dogs with all types of brain tumors after surgery vary but tend to cluster around 140 to 150 days.[1,2,5-12] For meningiomas, median survival times may be slightly longer (240 to 300+ days). Mortality is significant within the first 30 days of surgery for animals with infratentorial compared with supratentorial tumors.

Surgical excision is more readily accomplished in cats, as meningiomas in this species tend to be well encapsulated and easily delineated from normal brain. Studies have determined a median survival interval of cats after meningioma resection to be 22 and 27 months.[13,14]

Pituitary tumors may be treated surgically primarily through a transsphenoidal approach.[15-18] It can be difficult, however, to access larger tumors (> 1.0 cm) surgically, leading to incomplete removal and increased surgical morbidity.

Treatment of metastatic tumor to the brain is rarely performed in animals. With humans, however, surgical removal of metastases often improves survival. Tumors invading the skull, such as multilobular chondrosarcoma or osteosarcoma, may also be surgically removable depending primarily on size and anatomic location at the time of diagnosis.[19,20]

Many factors may affect survival following brain surgery, including neurologic and systemic abnormalities. In general, most dogs are probably diagnosed relatively late in the course of their disease and only when clinical signs become obvious. By this time, the tumors are relatively large, have caused significant associated brain injury, and are often infiltrative or tightly adherent to the nervous tissue. An overall deterioration of systemic health may have occurred prior to definitive treatment because of lack of adequate nutrition, chronic stress, pain, or deleterious effects of medications administered to control clinical signs, namely corticosteroids. Non-nervous system organ effects such as brain-heart syndrome may adversely compromise systemic health. In addition, as intracranial surgery in small animals has a relatively short history, the learning curve is still steep in regard to intracranial surgical techniques. All of these factors affect historical morbidity and mortality statistics of animals with brain tumors.

Unfortunately, primarily because of relatively small numbers of dogs with brain tumors that have been definitively treated, all dogs with tumors tend to be grouped for analysis. This means that all dogs with brain tumors, regardless of tumor location or tumor growth characteristics, are regarded as being equal, when the behavior and aggressiveness of the various tumor types and locations are ignored. Additionally, treatments given are variable even for animals with the same clinical characteristics. These factors introduce bias into the determination of overall survival. Finally, some lesions are diagnosed as brain tumors based primarily on imaging characteristics without a subsequent biopsy diagnosis. All of these potential influences make it difficult to communicate accurately with owners the prognosis of the many different types and locations of brain tumor. In an attempt to begin to determine whether certain characteristics influence overall survival, we have evaluated dogs with biopsy-diagnosed tumors regarding the influence of tumor type and location on survival after initial surgical treatment. Preliminary conclusions indicate that dogs with supratentorial tumors are more likely to survive longer than 30 days following surgery compared with dogs with infratentorial tumors. The mortality associated with supratentorial surgery is also lower than for infratentorial surgery in dogs with brain tumor. Overall, dogs have a 30-day survival rate of approximately 60% following intracranial surgery for brain tumor. Conversely, there is a 30-day mortality rate of approximately 40% for dogs with brain tumors. Survival for longer than six months depends on tumor type and location.

Surgical treatment of brain tumor should ideally not only cure the dog of the tumor but also improve or resolve the clinical signs associated with the tumor. Surgical resection of tumors, for example, may increase the likelihood of seizure control or help in the control of effects of increased ICP.

Syringomyelia and hydromyelia are increasingly diagnosed as a cause of spinal cord dysfunction in dogs and, rarely, in cats. Because several possible pathogenic mechanisms can result in or perpetuate syringomyelia and hydromyelia, an appropriate pathophysiologic diagnosis of the actual cause of these diseases is imperative for appropriate treatment planning. Commonly, syringomyelia and hydromyelia are associated with abnormal CSF dynamics at the level of the fourth ventricle/foramen magnum area. This may be the result of malformations of the foramen magnum or cranial cervical region, and may be associated with Chiari-like malformation of the infratentorial area.

If clinical signs are mild, non-surgical treatments with confinement, restricted activity, corticosteroids, or pain medication may provide symptomatic relief. Medical management of this condition may improve clinical signs in some dogs, and it is often attempted prior to, or concurrent with, surgical treatments. Corticosteroids (prednisone) are most often used at anti-inflammatory dosages (0.5-1 mg/kg every 12 to 24 hours). If medical treatment is the sole treatment to be used (i.e., because an owner does not wish to pursue surgical treatment), corticosteroid dosages are adjusted (increased) if clinical signs are not improved, and the animal is monitored closely for side effects. If improvement or resolution of clinical signs occurs within the first one to two weeks following corticosteroid therapy, this medication can be used in decreasing doses to achieve the lowest dose necessary to achieve remission of clinical signs.

If the clinical signs are the result of a Chiari-like malformation or other foramen magnum or infratentorial abnormality, surgical removal of any stenosis and decompression of the brain stem, cerebellum, and cranial spinal cord may alleviate clinical signs. Decompressive surgery of the foramen magnum usually includes a suboccipital craniectomy and durotomy.[21,22] After portions of the occipital bone and associated fibrous tissues are removed, a dura graft, such as a temporalis fascia graft, is placed over the foramen magnum area in an attempt to prevent further scaring of tissues in this area. In other situations where syringomyelia is associated with hydrocephalus, ventriculoperitoneal shunting may improve clinical signs (see further under hydrocephalus).

Primary cystic structures may also be present in the intracranial region, usually in or around the caudal and dorsal third ventricle. These cystic structures are often referred to as arachnoid or subarachnoid cysts. In some instances, surgical fenestration through a craniotomy or craniectomy can produce improvement in clinical signs. Similarly, epidermoid or dermoid cysts may be surgically resectable. Although there is no primary treatment for occipital dysplasia, the clinical consequences of Chiari-like malformation such as syringomyelia may be improved with a foramen magnum decompression via a suboccipital craniectomy with subsequent surgical reconstruction of this region.

Hydrocephalus

Several medical and surgical treatment options may be beneficial for animals with hydrocephalus. The choice of treatments is generally dictated by the degree of physical impairment, age of the animal, and cause of the hydrocephalus, if known. Medical treatment may include general supportive care and medications to limit CSF production and reduce intracranial pressure. Surgical treatment is designed to provide drainage of CSF from the brain to another site within the body for reabsorption.

Surgical treatment for hydrocephalus is generally required for those animals that do not improve within two weeks of the institution of medical therapy or for those animals whose clinical signs deteriorate during medical therapy. Surgical procedures are designed to provide controlled CSF flow from the ventricles of the brain to either the peritoneal cavity or the right atrium. Shunt systems designed for use in humans seem to be adaptable for animals. Ventriculoperitoneal (VP) shunts are technically easier to install and are most commonly used in human neurosurgery. Emergency placement of shorter-term CSF-removal devices may be used in the management of secondary hydrocephalus. Vascular access ports or similar subcutaneously implanted devices have been used for this purpose.

Ventriculoperitoneal shunt systems are used in the long-term management of hydrocephalus in humans and dogs. These shunt systems have three required components: a ventricular catheter, a siphon control mechanism, and a distal catheter. The three components can be obtained separately and fitted together at surgery, or purchased as a unit with the three parts permanently connected. The ventricular catheter is a fenestrated section of silicone tubing that is usually placed in a lateral ventricle via a small burr hole placed in the skull. This ventricular catheter is connected to a siphon control valve. The valve is designed to reduce the siphon effect of gravity-induced hydrostatic pressure in the distal catheter, thereby maintaining physiologic ventricular pressures. Hydrostatic pressure, which is greatest when the animal stands up, would cause overdrainage of CSF if not attenuated by the valve. There are low-, medium-, and high-pressure valves to maintain ventricular pressures within preset ranges. As normal ICP in dogs is thought to be between 8 and 12 mm Hg, a shunt that works at or above these pressures is usually used. The distal catheter carries CSF from the valve to the peritoneal cavity. Surgical placement of these shunts has been described elsewhere.

Regardless of the type of shunt used, strict aseptic technique and thorough hemostasis must be used to avoid shunt failure. The two most common complications of shunt placement in humans are infection and undershunting. Overshunting and seizures are less commonly encountered, but possible. Placement of VP shunts is contraindicated if systemic infections are present. All infections should be resolved prior to surgery.

Even if patients do not have a systemic infection at the time of surgery, they may develop an infection at a later time. Fever and deterioration of neurologic functions are the most common signs of shunt infection. If an infection is suspected, CSF can be collected from the subcutaneous shunt reservoir for culture and sensitivity examination. Prophylactic antibiotics are suggested for patients with VP shunts at times of potential for development of bacteremia or septicemia (e.g., dental procedures). Shunt nephritis has been reported in humans owing to chronic, low-level shunt infection causing immune complex deposition in renal glomeruli.

Undershunting (not removing enough CSF from the ventricle through the shunt) results from blockage, disconnection, or kinking of the catheter system. Possible causes of blockage include obstruction by choroid plexus and buildup of proteinaceous accretions, blood, or cellular debris (inflammatory or neoplastic). The blockage may occur in the ventricular catheter, siphon control valve, or distal catheter. Several methods, including shunt tapping and radiographic examinations, have been developed to evaluate shunt patency and locate the site of blockage.

Complications associated with overshunting have not been well described in animals, but they most likely do occur. In humans, overshunting results in formation of subdural hematomas and/or very small ventricular size (slit ventricle syndrome). Overshunting of CSF can cause collapse of the brain with tearing of vessels, which produces subdural hematoma formation. Animals with large dilated lateral ventricles and only a thin rim of cerebral cortex remaining have the highest risk for brain collapse and hemorrhage. The risk of brain collapse can be minimized by not allowing large amounts of CSF to escape during shunt placement. Additionally, a siphon control valve with the proper pressure range must be selected. Intracranial bleeding and brain collapse are most easily confirmed with advanced imaging studies such as MR or CT imaging following shunt placement.

Successful, long-term resolution of clinical signs of hydrocephalus has been achieved in dogs with these types of surgical shunting procedures. Experimental evidence suggests that reconstitution of the cerebral hemispheres after shunting occurs only in the white matter. Reconstituted white matter is characterized by myelin destruction, remyelination, and reactive astrocytosis. Because neuronal loss and cortical laminar destruction are irreversible, hydrocephalus should be treated aggressively as early as possible.

Inflammatory Diseases

Treatment of encephalitis and meningitis is ideally directed at a specific causative organism. In some instances, intracranial inflammation or infection will coalesce to form a discrete mass or abscess. As an abscess and its associated inflammation can rapidly increase intracranial pressure, surgical drainage and decompression of a focal abscess should occur as soon as possible after detection. Similarly, penetrating intracranial wounds may require debridement to avoid infectious complications.

Intracranial Hemorrhage and Vascular-Based Disease

Treatment for CNS bleeding includes treatment of any underlying bleeding disorder and stopping or resolving the local effects of any accumulated hemorrhage. Various treatments exist for individual coagulopathies and for thrombocytopenia. Current recommendations for treatment of these bleeding disorders should be reviewed.

Treatment for a localized hematoma within the CNS is focused on evacuation of the hematoma, usually via a craniotomy or craniectomy. If the underlying bleeding disorder is still active, a difficult choice exists between the need for surgical drainage of the hematoma and the risk of causing increasing amounts of hemorrhage. Short-term hemostatic support with blood products or platelets may provide a window of patient stability for a surgical procedure to be performed. Ultimately, if the accumulation of bleeding in the central nervous system is becoming life-threatening, surgical drainage is a necessity, which is undertaken in full recognition of the increased risk of hemorrhagic complications. While it is impossible to reverse all of the effects of the hemorrhage, decreasing the size of an expanding hematoma with the resultant decrease in nervous tissue pressure may improve clinical signs. Two caveats should be considered. One is that, by decreasing intraparenchymal pressure, blood flow to the area may be restored and a rebound hemorrhage may occur. Second, along the same lines, if the original cause of the bleeding was a ruptured vessel (aneurysm or arteriovenous malformation), hematoma removal may result in rebleeding. In both of these situations, however, hemostasis can be employed intraoperatively to decrease this possibility.

In chronic hematomas, especially if the initial bleeding tendency has subsided, surgical drainage is reasonably straightforward if the extent of the hematoma can be localized. Usually, a black, sometimes greenish, soft lesion consistent with an established hematoma is found. This can be removed with suction aspiration. The edges of the hematoma tend to be more organized and require blunt dissection for removal.

Intracranial Traumatic Injury

Surgical treatments for intracranial trauma are indicated primarily for decompression and debridement of abnormal tissue or blood. A major tenet of the Monro-Kellie doctrine is that intracranial contents are confined within the cranium. It would follow, therefore, that surgical removal of this structure would potentially relieve ICP elevations. Unilateral or bilateral craniectomy has been used as a treatment for ICP elevations that cannot be decreased by the more conventional methods stated earlier. Although skull removal alone may be beneficial, subsequent dural incision appears significantly more effective in lowering ICP.[23] This has been shown clinically in humans and experimentally in dogs as well as cats. Ultimate functional recovery remains dependent on the underlying primary brain damage inflicted by the disease process. Because ICP may increase during wound closure and anesthetic recovery, the magnitude of ICP decrease subsequent to surgery remains uncertain.

Craniectomy and durotomy have been shown to lower ICP by 15% and 65%, respectively, in dogs and cats, and humans. Intracranial pressures in normal dogs approached atmospheric pressure when a lateral rostrotentorial craniectomy and durotomy were performed. Adequate decompression of the brain in animals with structural disease would be suggested if intraoperative ICP approached similar levels.

Surgical Treatment for Diseases of Cranial Nerves

Cranial nerves can occasionally be affected with disease independent of the intracranial nervous structures.[24] Tumors, for example, often arise within or around the trigeminal nerve. Trigeminal nerve abnormalities can occur with infiltrating neoplasia (lymphosarcomas) that involve a branch or the entire nerve. Myelomonocytic leukemias and other hematocellular neoplasia may affect this nerve. Tumors of the coverings of the nerve (nerve sheath tumors) may arise on or around the trigeminal nerve. These tumors can infiltrate or compress the nerve, resulting in dysfunction. Unilateral muscle atrophy of the temporalis and masseter muscles is suggestive of an isolated disease of this cranial nerve. Surgical removal of these tumors has been performed, but can result in cosmetic consequences owing to complete trigeminal denervation of head muscles. Radiation therapy has been used in a limited number of cases with apparently encouraging results.

The vestibular nerve may be affected either peripherally (usually by disease of the middle or inner ear) or centrally at the brain stem level. Tumors of the ear more often occur in older animals. Squamous cell carcinoma and adenocarcinoma are most common. Treatment may include surgical resection or radiation therapy. Inflammatory polyps occur in cats. Surgical removal of these polyps is often helpful. Otitis media/interna may require systemic antibiotics (clavulanic acid), or surgical debridement (bulla osteotomy) may be necessary.

Future Directions-Surgical Treatments of Seizures

Surgical treatments for seizure control are used for selected human patients with seizures that are not controlled adequately with medical therapies. Similar surgical treatments are rare in animals, but we hope will increase with a better understanding of seizure generation and location.[25,26] This will occur through advances in intracranial imaging and electrophysiologic monitoring for animals.

References

1. Bagley RS: Surgical approaches to the central nervous system: Brain. *In* Textbook of Small Animal Surgery, 3rd ed. Slatter D (ed). Philadelphia: WB Saunders, 2003, pp. 1163-1173.

2. Bagley RS, Harrington ML, Pluhar GE, et al: Acute, unilateral transverse sinus occlusion during craniectomy in 7 dogs with space-occupying intracranial disease. Vet Surg 26:195-201, 1997.

3. Oliver JE Jr: Principles of Canine Brain Surgery. Anim Hosp 2:73-88, 1966.

4. Oliver JE Jr: Surgical approaches to the canine brain. Am J Vet Res 29:353-378, 1968.

5. Heidner GL, Kornegay JN, Page RL, et al: Analysis of survival in a retrospective study of 86 dogs with brain tumors. J Vet Intern Med 5:219-226, 1991.

6. Axlund TW, McGlasson ML, Smith AN: Surgery alone or in combination with radiation therapy for treatment of intracranial meningiomas in dogs: 31 cases (1989-2002). J Am Vet Med Assoc 221:1597-1600, 2002.

7. De Wet PD, Ali II, Peters DN: Surgical approach to the rostral cranial fossa by radical transfrontal craniotomy in the dog. J South Afr Vet Assoc 53:140-151, 1982.

8. Glass EN, Kapatkin A, Vite C, et al: A modified bilateral transfrontal sinus appraoch to the canine frontal lobe and olfactory bulb: Surgical technique and five cases. J Am Anim Hosp Assoc 36:43-50, 2000.

9. Jeffery N, Brearley MJ: Brain tumours in the dog. Treatment of 10 cases and review of recent literature. J Small Anim Pract 34:367-372, 1993.

10. Klopp LS, Simpson ST, Sorjonen DA, Lenz SD: Ventral surgical approach to the caudal brain stem in dogs. Vet Surg 29:533-542, 2000.

11. Kostolich M, Dulisch ML: A surgical approach to the canine olfactory bulb for meningioma removal. Vet Surg 16:273-277, 1987.

12. Niebauer GW, Dayrell-Hart BL, Speciale J: Evaluation of craniotomy in dogs and cats. J Am Vet Med Assoc 198:89-95, 1991.

13. Gallagher JG, Berg J, Knowles KE, et al: Prognosis after surgical excision of cerebral meningiomas in cats: 17 cases (1986-1992). J Am Vet Med Assoc 203:1437-1440, 1993.

14. Gordon LE, Thacher C, Matthiesen DT, et al: Results of craniotomy for treatment of cerebral meningioma in 42 cats. Vet Surg 23:94-100, 1994.

15. Meij BP, Voorhout G, van den Ingh TSGAM, et al: Transsphenoidal hypohysectomy in beagle dogs: evaluation of a microsurgical technique. Vet Surg 26:295-309, 1997.

16. Meij BP, Voorhout G, van den Ingh TS, et al: Results of transsphenoidal hypohysectomy in 52 dogs with pituitary-dependent hyperadrenocorticism. Vet Surg 27:246-261, 1998.

17. Niebauer GW, Eigenmann JE, Van Winkle TJ: Study of long-term survival after transsphenoidal hypophysectomy in clinical normal dogs. Am J Vet Res 51:677-681, 1990.

18. Niebauer GW, Evans SM: Transsphenoidal hypophysectomy in the dog. Vet Surg 17:296-303, 1988.

19. Dernell WS, Straw RC, Cooper MF, et al: Multilobular osteochondrosarcoma in 39 dogs: 1979-1993. JAAHA 34:11-18, 1998.

20. Straw RC, LeCouteur RA, Powers BA, et al: Multilobular osteochondrosarcoma of the canine skull: 16 cases (1978-1988). JAVMA 195:1764-1769, 1989.

21. Takagi S, Kadosawa T, Ohsaki T, et al: Hindbrain decompression in a dog with scoliosis associated with syringomyelia. J Am Vet Med Assoc 226:1359-1369, 2005.

22. Vemeersch K, Van Ham L, Caemaert J, et al: Suboccipital craniectomy, dorsal laminectomy of C1, durotomy and dural graft placement as a treatment for syringohydromyelia with cerebellar tonsil herniation in Cavalier King Charles spaniels. Vet Surg 33:355-360, 2004.

23. Bagley RS, Harrington ML, Pluhar GE, et al: Effect of craniectomy/durotomy alone or in combination with hyperventilation, diuretics, and corticosteroids on intracranial pressure in normal dogs. Am J Vet Res 57:116-119, 1996.

24. Bagley RS, Wheeler SJ, Klopp L, et al: Trigeminal nerve sheath tumor in 10 dogs. JAAHA 34:19-25, 1998.

25. Bagley RS, Baszler TV, Harrington ML, et al: Clinical effects of longitudinal division of the corpus callosum in dogs. Vet Surg 24:122-127, 1995.

26. Bagley RS, Harrington ML, Moore MP: Surgical treatment for seizures. Vet Clin North Am 26:827-842, 1996.

Chapter 42

Spinal Cord Compression

Lisa Klopp

Causes of Spinal Cord Compression

Diseases can affect the spinal cord by parenchymal disruption (intramedullary disease) or by compression of the tissue. Collectively, diseases that cause compression are probably the most common causes of spinal cord dysfunction. Compression can occur from pathology outside the dura (extradural compression) or within the dura (intradural-extramedullary compression). The mechanism of injury, rate of onset, force and kinetic energy of an injury, and the duration of compression all play a role in the severity and progression of clinical signs.[1-3] For example, an acute severe spinal cord compression is more likely to cause acute paraplegia in comparison with a spinal meningioma, which grows slowly and allows functional compensation to occur. However, once the limit of compensation is reached, deterioration of neurologic function can occur rapidly.[4] Clinical signs associated with spinal cord compression depend on the location of the lesion. Clinical signs of spinal cord dysfunction can be found in Chapter 46: Intervertebral Disk Disease. A list of the most common diseases that cause spinal cord compression can be found in Table 42-1. Images of various disease processes that cause spinal cord compression are shown in Figures 42-1 to 42-7.

Table 42-1. Diseases that Cause Spinal Cord Compression

Diseases that cause extradural spinal cord compression
Intervertebral Disk Disease
Type I
Type II
Articular facet joint synovial cysts
Cartilaginous exostosis
Vertebral canal stenosis
Caudal cervical vertebral malformation/malarticulation ("Wobbler's disease")
Congenital stenosis
Cervical bony stenosis
Stenosis associated with hemivertebra (usually thoracic in location)
Neoplasia
Sarcomas arising from the vertebra
Osteosarcoma
Chondrosarcoma
Fibrosarcoma
Hemangiosarcoma
Lymphosarcoma
Multiple myeloma
Epidural abscess
Fracture/luxation
Congenital
Atlantoaxial luxation
Traumatic
Hematoma (most commonly associated with intervertebral disk extrusion or trauma)
Diseases that cause intradural-extramedullary spinal cord compression
Arachnoid cyst
Arachnoid scarring/fibrosis
Hematoma
Neoplasia
Meningioma
Nerve root tumor
Metastatic neoplasia

Pathophysiology of Spinal Cord Compression

Morphologic and Histologic Changes

Spinal cord compression can occur relatively slowly over the course of time, with such disorders as developing neoplastic disease, arachnoid cyst, synovial cyst, or soft tissue hypertrophy/hyperplasia associated with caudal cervical vertebral malformation/malarticulation. In a chronic progressive process, the spinal cord tissue compensates for some period of time before clinical signs become evident.[5-7] Typically, this results in a large volume of pathology and severe compression prior to clinical dysfunction and diagnosis.

Acute spinal cord injuries occur as a result of rapid spinal cord compression, such as that seen with acute intervertebral disk extrusion and fracture/luxation. Acute spinal cord injuries involve both primary and secondary pathologic processes.[2,8-21] The primary injury is the inciting mechanical event itself, which then induces a complex series of vascular, biochemical, and cellular events that result in progressive secondary injury to the spinal cord parenchyma. Vascular events include ischemia, hemorrhage, impaired autoregulation of blood flow, microcirculatory disruption, vasospasm and thrombosis.[11,13,17,22,23] Secondary biochemical events ultimately result in edema, lipid peroxidation, and cytotoxic injury.[22-27] These include cellular ion derangement (increased intracellular sodium and calcium and extracellular potassium).[8-10,13] Extracellular release and accumulation of neurotransmitters (serotonin, catecholamines, and glutamate) occur and are injurious to the spinal cord cells in large quantities.[9,13,28] Induction of the arachidonic acid cascade, production of eicosanoids, and generation of free radicals result in progression of inflammation via cytokines and lipid peroxidation of cellular membranes of all spinal cord elements (endothelium,

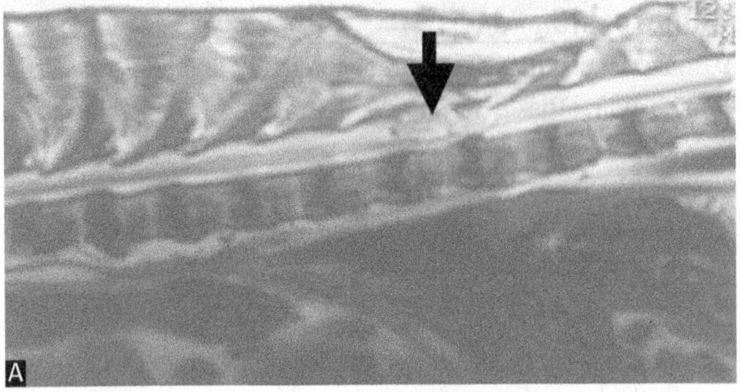

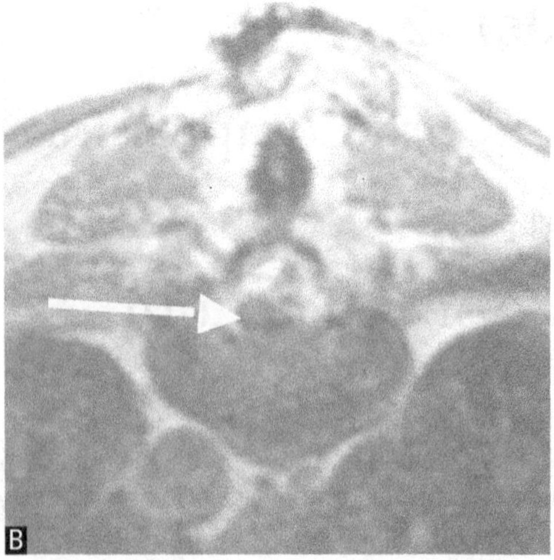

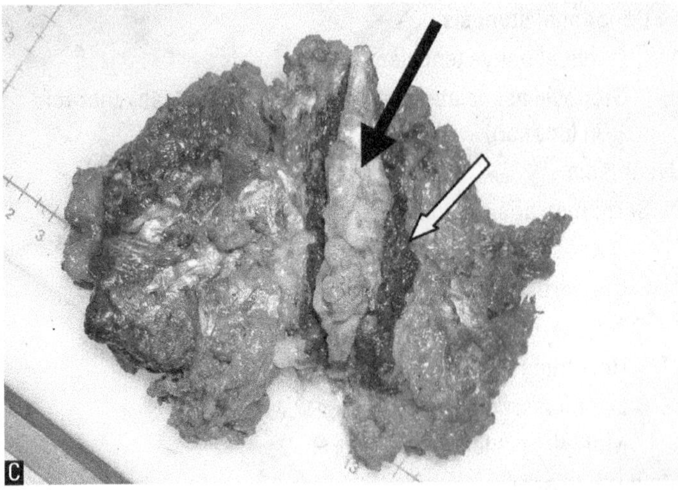

Figure 42-1. Extradural compression: T9 chondrosacroma in an 11-year-old MC bloodhound with acute deterioration of chronic paraparesis. The tumor was removed and the dog's neurologic function improved daily. A. T2-weighted, sagittal MRI. The tumor has severely and completely compressed the spinal cord. (arrow) B. T2-weighted, transverse MRI. The compressed spinal cord is indicated by the arrow. C. The tumor has been removed *en bloc* (ventral view of the dorsal lamina) and is surrounded by tumor capsule and normal muscle tissue. The dorsal lamina has been replaced by chrondoscarcoma (black arrow). The tumor margin has been outlined with paint (white arrow).

myelin, neurons, and glial cells).[15,29-32] Cellular energy failure via loss of adenosine-triphosphate pathways and cellular apoptosis also occurs.[13,30]

Most of what is known about the pathophysiology of spinal cord compression comes from acute spinal cord injury, cervical myelopathy, or animal models of spinal cord compression. In a clinical setting, histologic findings of spinal cord compression have been best described in human patients with cervical spondylitic myelopathy, which is a synonymous disease with canine caudal cervical vertebral malformation/malarticulation ("Wobbler's disease")[14,33-35] When the spinal cord is compressed, the central grey matter and medial portions of the white matter are usually the most severely affected with cystic cavitation (syrinx), gliosis, edema, and demyelination.[3,33,36-42] Wallerian degeneration is observed cranial to the compression site in the posterior and posteriolateral columns.[3,39,43] Lower motor neuron dropout occurs at the site of compression, and demyelination and axonal degeneration occur in the corticospinal tracts caudal to the compression site.[14,33,39,44] Studies have shown that clinical signs typically appear after the spinal cord has been compressed by 30%.[8,33,45,46] In addition, because of the relative tolerance of the cervical spinal cord to encroachment, the development of clinical myelopathy was found to be highly correlated to pre-existing congenitally narrow spinal canal.[33,47]

Ogino et al.[48] followed nine patients with cervical myelopathy throughout their clinical course and postmortem. He found that the severity of compression was correlative to the pathologic changes. Minor compression was most associated with degeneration of the posteriolateral white matter (including the corticospinal tracts). Advancing severity of compression resulted in infarction and loss the α-motor neurons in the anterior horn grey matter. As compression became more severe, extensive grey matter infarction ensued. The dorsal horn columns and lateral white matter tracts were also affected only in cases of severe compression. However, anterior white matter appeared remarkably resistant to degeneration, a finding supported by other studies.[49] The severity of histologic findings correlated well to the clinical neurologic findings in all patients.

In a study by Yamaura et al.,[35] twy/twy mice, which spontaneously develop dorsolateral calcified deposits at C1 and C2 vertebrae by four months of age, were used to study chronic spinal cord compression. At six months of age, the spinal cords in these mice were already significantly compressed. Grey matter degeneration was observed as small, flattened neurons that were decreased in number, especially in the dorsal horns where the compression was most significant. Loss of axonal and glial elements and myelin destruction were observed in the white matter at the site of the compression as well as in descending tracts caudally and ascending tracts cranially.

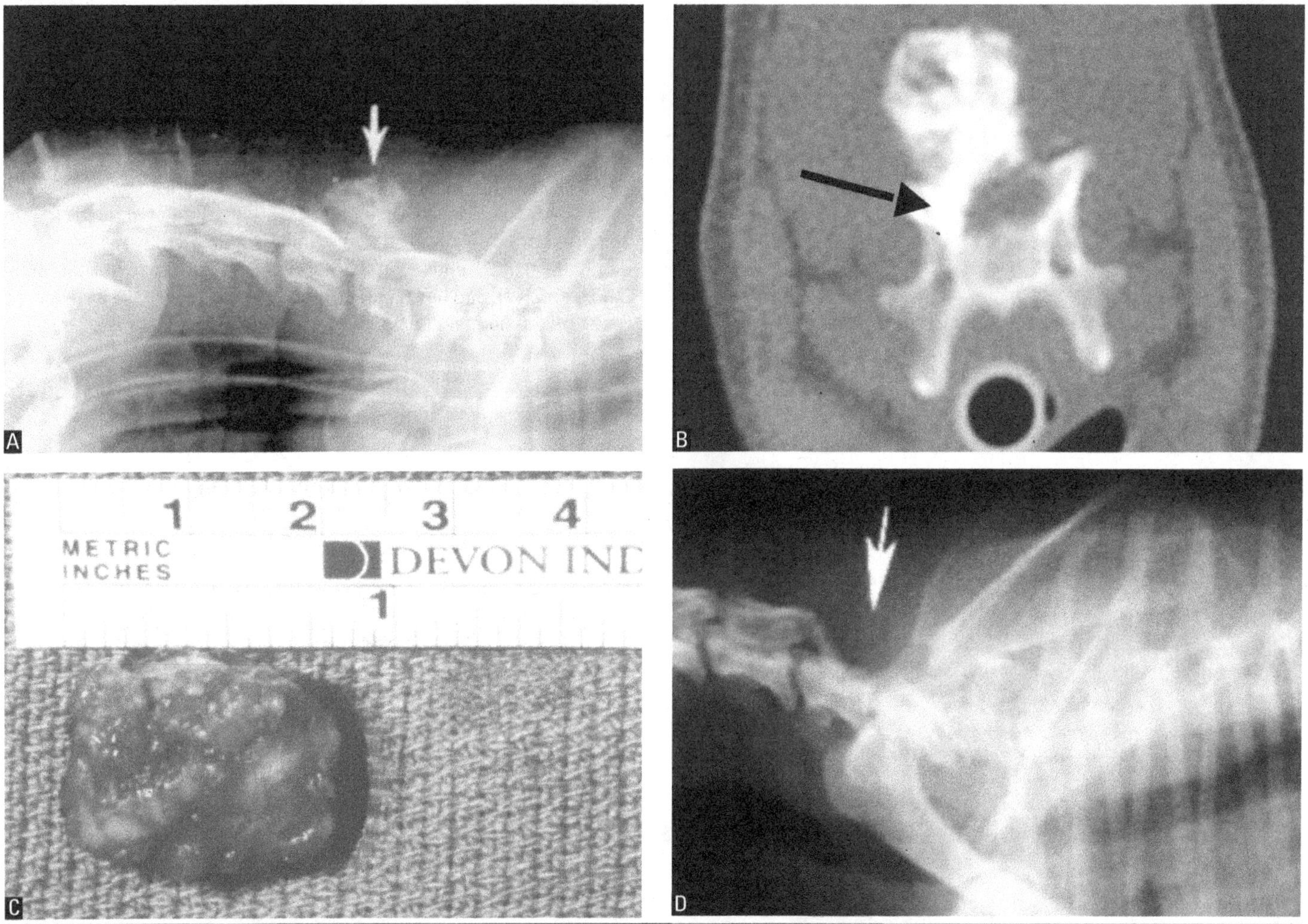

Figure 42-2. Extradural compression: Low-grade osteosarcoma of the lamina and pedicles of C6 in a 6-year-old, FS Yorkshire terrier. The tumor was removed *en bloc* and there was no recurrence until the animal was lost to follow-up 2 years later. A. Lateral image of a myelogram. Note the significant dorsal compression of the spinal cord (arrow). B. Computed tomographic scan following myelogram. The tumor has extended into the pedicle on one side (arrow). C. The tumor has been removed *en bloc*. D. A radiograph taken 1 year postoperatively.

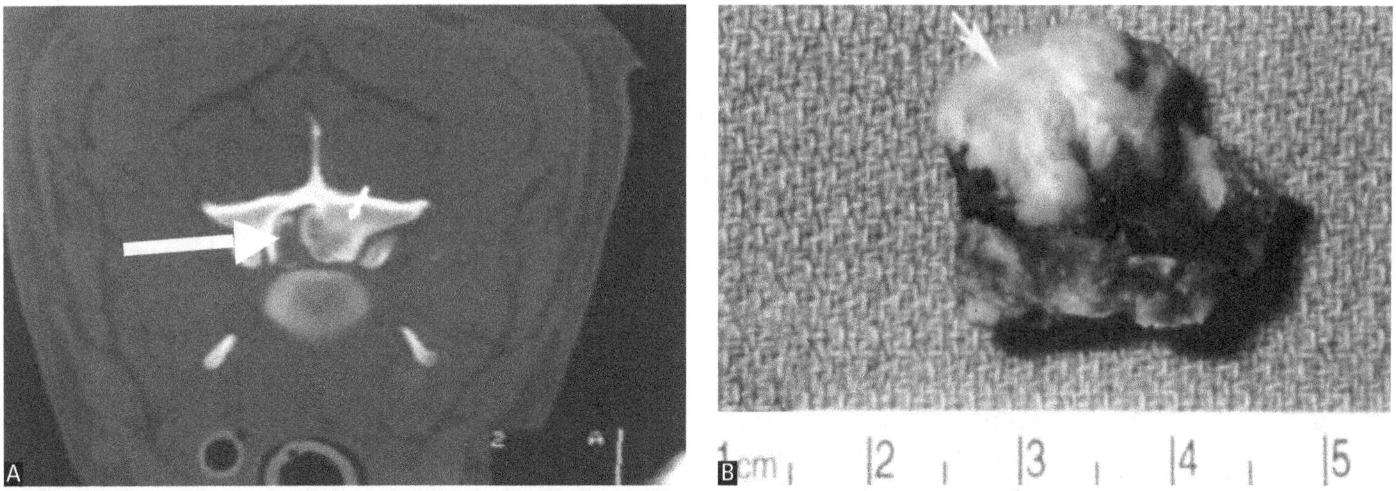

Figure 42-3. Extradural compression: Cartilaginous exostosis of the C4 caudal articular process in an 11-month-old, MC Airedale terrier mix with a 6-month history of progressive tetraparesis. A. Postmyelogram transverse computed tomographic scan. The spinal cord (large arrow) has been compressed to about 25% of its normal diameter by the mass (small arrow). B. The benign tumor was removed, the dog recovered to normal neurologic status and was still normal at 5 years postoperative.

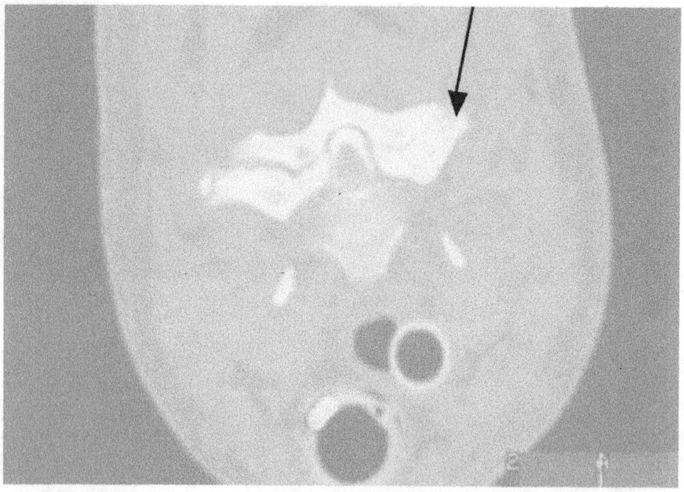

Figure 42-4. Extradural compression: severe stenosis at the level of the C4-5 facet joint in a 7-year-old, FS Basenji with unremitting cervical pain and mild neurologic dysfunction. A computed tomographic scan of the C4-5 spinal level. The spinal cord is triangular-shaped from the compression. A hyperplastic facet joint is indicated by the arrow. This dog had similar stenoses at 3 other levels in her cervical spine (C3-4, C5-6, and C6-7). She had modified medial facetectomies at all levels and recovered to normal function and her pain resolved.

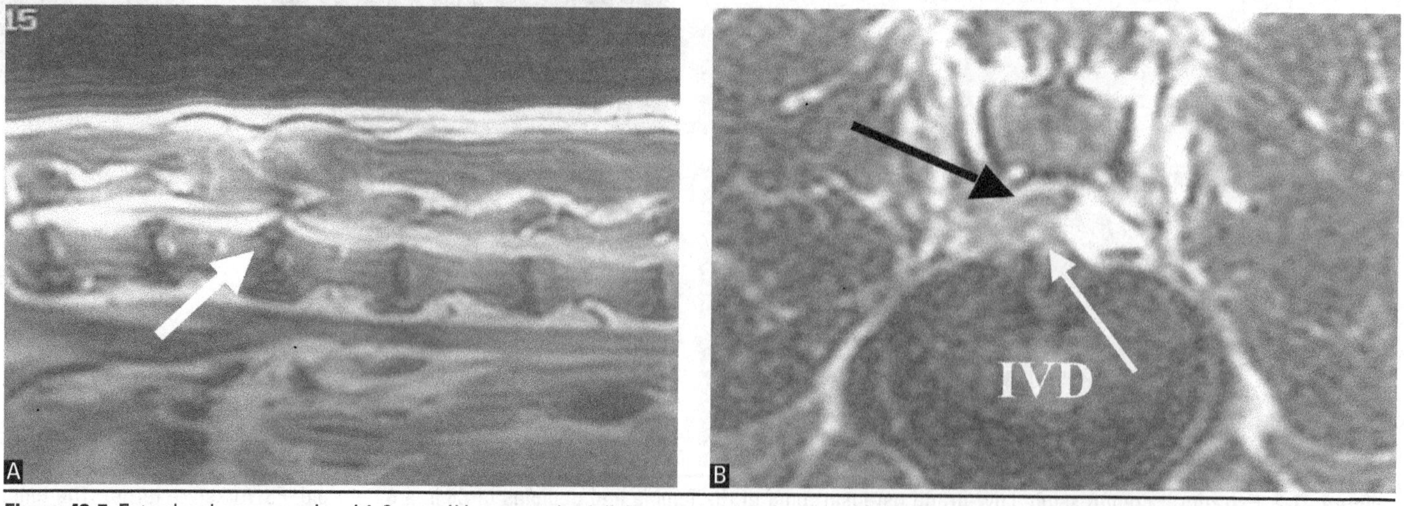

Figure 42-5. Extradural compression: L1-2, type II intervertebral disk extrusion in a 4-year-old, MC German shepherd dog that displayed mild paraparesis and significant thoracolumbar pain. A. T2-weighted, sagittal MRI. The spinal cord is severely compressed by the disk extrusion (arrow). B. T2-weighted, transverse MRI. The spinal cord is compressed to the right and dorsally (black arrow) by the protruding intervertebral disk (white arrow). (IVD = intervertebral disk)

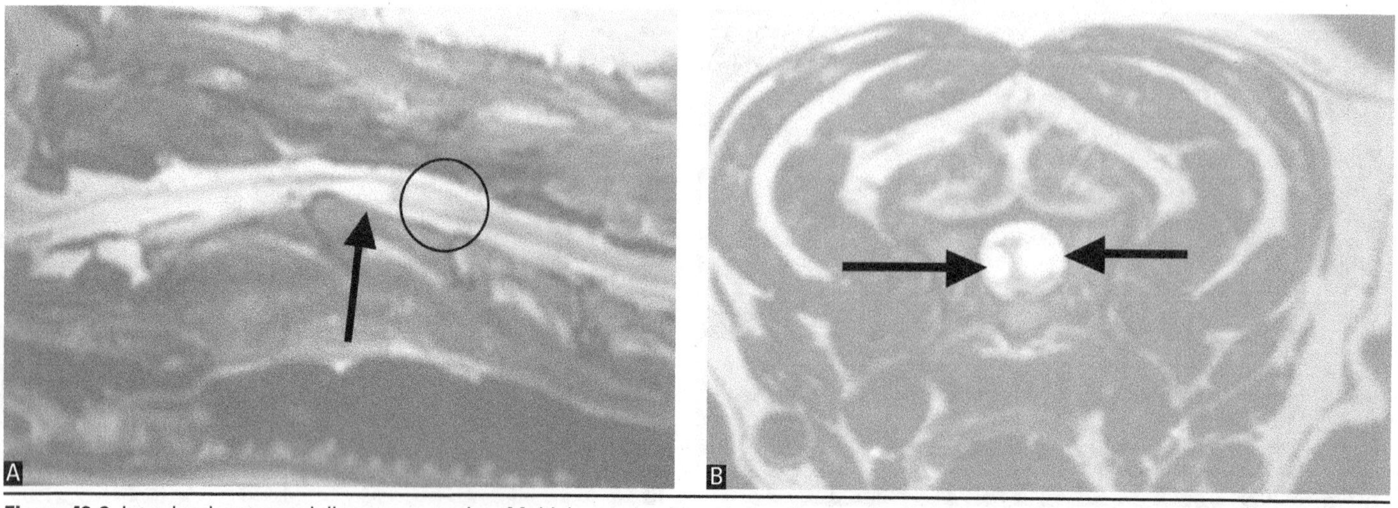

Figure 42-6. Intradural, extramedullary compression: Multiple arachnoid cysts in a 7-year-old, Springer spaniel that had a history of cervical pain and mild tetraparesis after being hit by a car 2 years earlier. At the time of the MRI the dog was poorly ambulatory. The arachnoid cysts were believed to have formed secondary to arachnoiditis from hemorrhage and inflammation. The arachnoid cysts were addressed surgically and she recovered to ambulatory tetraparesis but began to slowly deteriorate over time. Repeat MRI revealed that the cysts were resolved, but that there were progressive parenchymal changes in the spinal cord. A. Preoperative T2-weighted, sagittal MRI. The arrow indicates one arachnoid cyst. Signal hyperintensity within the parenchyma is seen within the circle. This was likely an area of malacia, edema, or early syrinx formation. B. T2-weighted, transverse MRI. The cysts are indicated by the arrows. The spinal cord has taken on an "apple-core" shape due to the intradural compression.

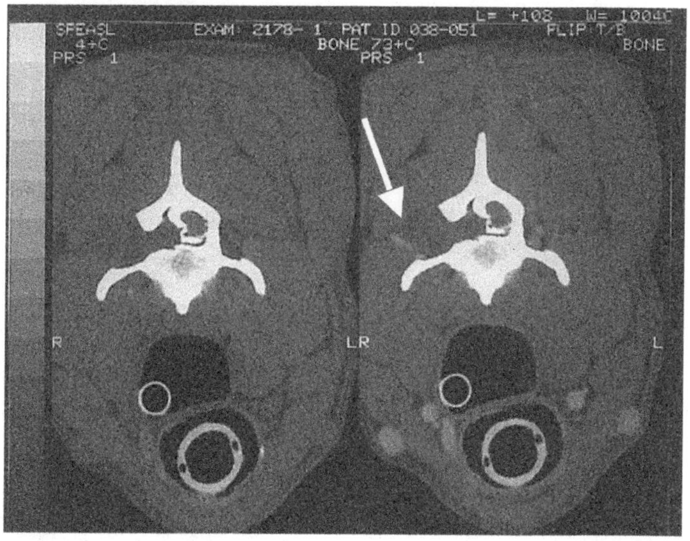

Figure 42-7. Intradural-extramedullary compression: C3 nerve root tumor in a 7-year-old, FS Doberman pinscher that presented with ataxia and cervical pain. Post-myelogram computed tomographic scan with the precontrast image on the left and the postcontrast image on the right. The tumor has caused pressure necrosis of the pedicle and the foramen is widened. (Note the presence of pedicle bone on the left side.) The tumor did not contrast-enhance with the exception of a small blush at the periphery (arrow).

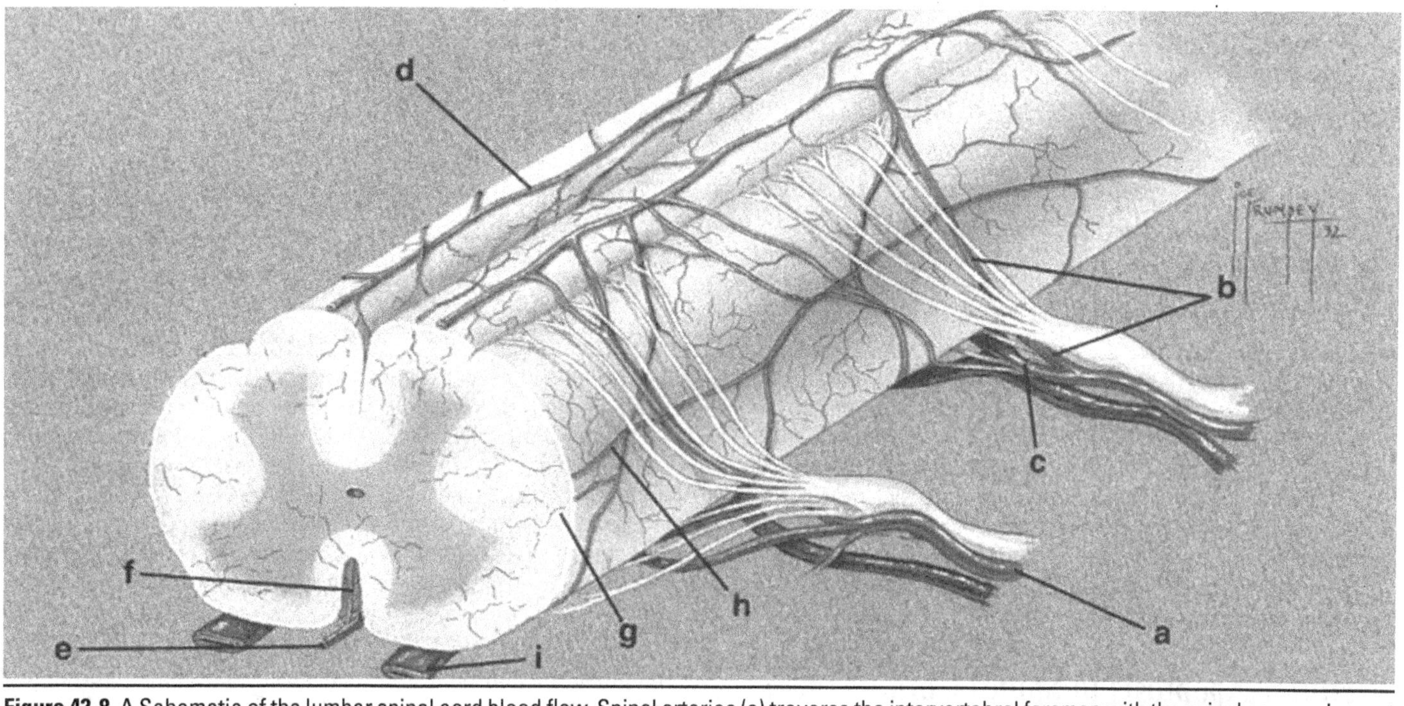

Figure 42-8. A Schematic of the lumbar spinal cord blood flow. Spinal arteries (a) traverse the intervertebral foramen with the spinal nerves. In most cases these arteries are bilateral and present at every level. The spinal artery branches into the dorsal radicular artery (b) and the ventral radicular artery (c). The dorsal spinal arteries (d) that arise from the dorsal radicular arteries are paired and take a more tortuous course than depicted in the drawing. The unpaired ventral spinal artery (e) arises from branches of the ventral radicular arteries and perforates the ventral fissure of the spinal cord, giving rise to the vertical arteries (f) that supply much of the spinal cord grey matter and ventral white matter. (g) Radial arteries arise from the superficial surface arteries to supply much of the white matter and some peripheral grey matter. Venous blood from the capillaries goes to the surface veins (h) that drain into the venous sinuses (i) that are found on the floor of the spinal canal. (With permission from Wheeler SJ, Sharp NJH. Functional anatomy. In Small Animal Spinal Disorders: Diagnosis and Surgery. Wheeler SJ, Sharp NJH (eds). London: Mosby-Wolfe, 1994. Illustration by Joseph E. Trumpey, North Carolina State University.)

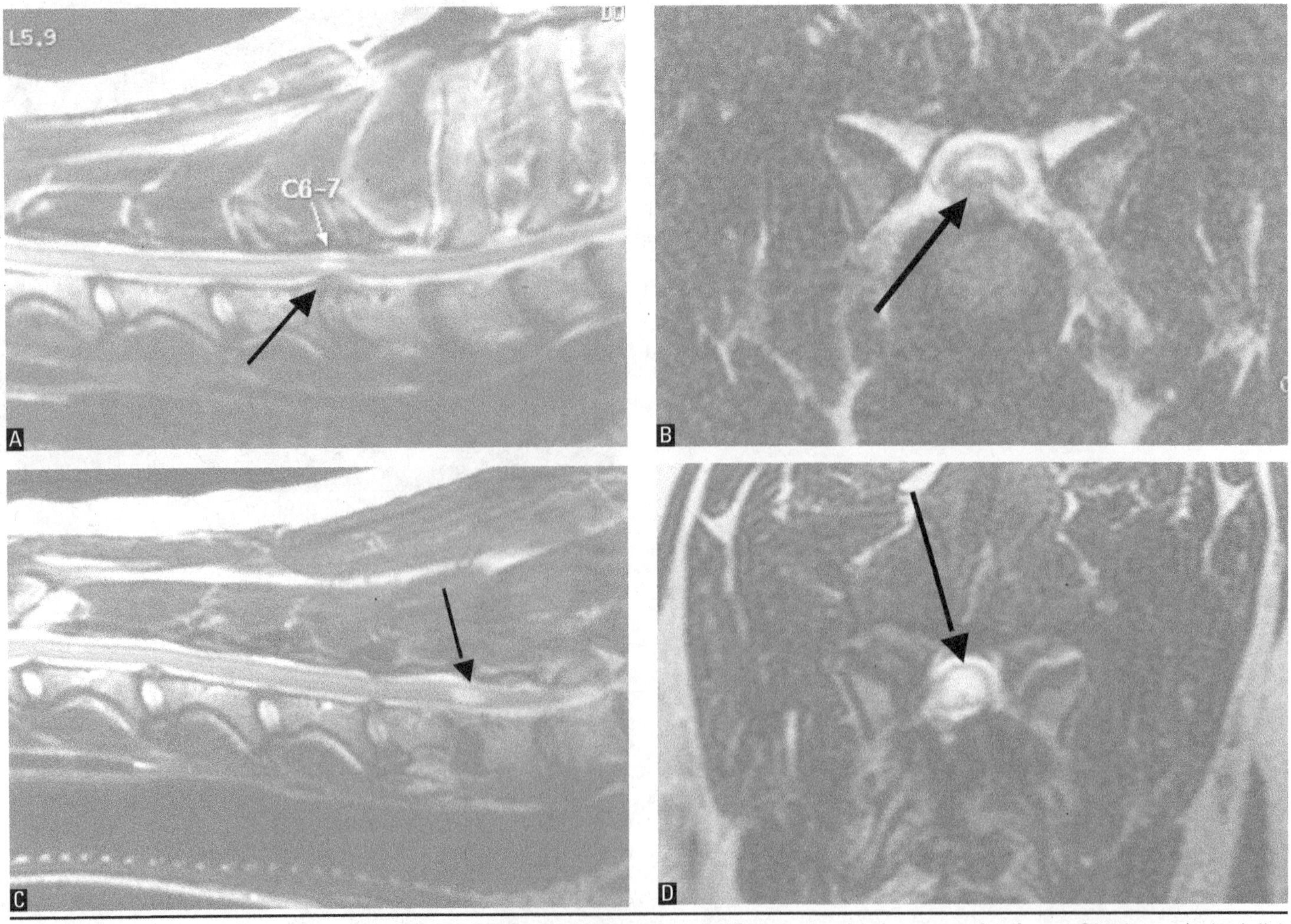

Figure 42-9. Syrinx progression in an 11-year-old, MC Dalmatian that was treated for an extradural compression from a C6-7 intervertebral disk extrusion. He initially presented with mild neurologic deficits and mild spinal discomfort. He recovered well from surgery but at 1 year postoperative, developed progressive tetraparesis and severe, unremitting pain. A. Preoperative T2-weighted, sagittal MRI. The C6-7 intervertebral disk (black arrow) has protruded and is compressing the spinal cord. There is signal hyperintensity in the spinal cord, which may have indicated edema, malacia, or syrinx formation. B. T2-weighted, transverse MRI. Note the signal hyperintensity in the middle of the parenchyma. The disk extrusion is indicated by the arrow. C. T2-weighted, sagittal MRI taken 18 months postoperative. The spinal cord has been decompressed at C6-7 but the signal hyperintensity in the parenchyma has progressed. D. The severity of progression in the parenchyma is best observed on the T2-weighted, transverse MRI. This was believed to be a large syrinx at the time. Because the dog was in a great deal of pain and surgery was unlikely to result in resolution of pain, the dog was euthanized.

Cellular Apoptosis in Spinal Cord Compression

Apoptosis, or programmed cell death, is a natural process of self-destruction in certain cells that are genetically programmed to have a limited life span or are damaged. Apoptosis plays an important role in development and homeostasis by controlling cellular density and deletion of abnormal cells.[33,50] Apoptosis is differentiated from necrosis by the lack of inflammation, karyorhhexis, and karyolysis. In apoptosis, the cells disintegrate into membrane-bound particles that are then eliminated by phagocytosis.[23,33,51,52] Apoptosis can be induced either by a stimulus, such as trauma, compression, irradiation, or toxic drugs or by the removal of a repressor agent. Necrosis can be induced by similar injuries to the spinal cord, and which cellular pathway is taken may depend on the severity of cellular damage.[23]

Apoptosis in the central nervous system has been shown to be controlled by several promoting and blocking genes.[33,53-55] Apoptosis of neuronal and glial cells has been reported with pathologic processes in the spinal cord, including injury, ischemia, and neurodegenerative conditions such as amyotrophic lateral sclerosis and spinal muscular atrophy.[33,40,56-66] Apoptosis in acute spinal injury has been proposed as a mechanism of degeneration of neuronal elements at the site of the injury and as a cause of chronic demyelination some distance away from the injury.[40,56,59-61,66] In the previously mentioned twy/twy mouse chronic compression model,[35] apoptosis was identified in both the white and grey matter at the most severely compressed location. Oligodendrocytes displayed markers of apoptosis, suggesting that programmed loss of these cells may be a cause of demyelination and of poorly myelinated cells some distance from the lesion.

Derangements in Neuronal Conduction

Alterations in myelin (demyelination and remyelination) and axonal integrity and caliber occur soon after spinal cord injury and impact the conduction capabilities of axons at both the site of injury and for some distance from the site of injury.[3,67-71] Changes in axonal conduction and spinal cord morphology following spinal cord injury have been studied in several different animal models[69,71-84] and in postmortem evaluation of human patients.[85,86] Morphologically, significant reduction in axonal numbers, axonal degeneration, and reactive astrocytosis has been reported. In addition, myelin sheaths are thinner, and remyelination of axons by invading Schwann cells (peripheral nervous system myelinating cells) as well as by oligodendrocytes (central nervous system myelinating cell) has been observed.[71,74,75,77-80,87-89] In a study by Wrathall et al.,[90] mRNA levels of important myelin structural proteins (myelin basic protein and proteolipid protein) were decreased in the chronically injured spinal cord of rats, suggesting either aberrant metabolism of or a decrease in the number of functional oligodendrocytes. Changes in axonal diameter, observed as either reduced median diameter in a spinal tract or enlarged axonal swellings, are dependent on the white matter tract evaluated and possibly the species as well.[3,71,72,74,75,77-80,87,91-94] Swollen axons are likely terminal bulbs, which are the accumulation of organelles that occurs when axonal transport is disrupted.[71,85]

Electrophysiologic testing has revealed that the injured spinal cord axons display decreased compound action potential (CAP) amplitude, reduced conduction velocity, prolonged refractory periods, and inability to respond to high-frequency stimulation. These axons were considerably less excitable and required a much higher stimulus intensity to elicit even half the maximal response of that seen in the spinal cords of the non-injured control group.[71,76] Reduction in the amplitude of the CAP is a function of many factors including axonal density, axonal diameter, and axonal input resistance and channel activation.[71] Reduction in the CAP in spinal cord injury can be explained by the altered spinal cord morphology (reduced axonal numbers, reduced axonal diameter) as well as by the changes in conduction (increased stimulus intensity required to cause an action potential and prolonged refractory period) that would result in lower than normal number of axons conducting during testing.[71] Conduction velocity depends on the fastest conducting fibers, thus the large caliber, heavily myelinated fibers. Alterations in the axonal size, myelin loss, reduced myelin thickness, and disrupted axonal integrity observed in these studies would all result in reduced conduction velocity.[71] Myelin reduces capacitance and limits the exchange of ions to the nodes of Ranvier and, allows more rapid repolarization of the axonal membrane. The faster membrane repolarization occurs, the faster action potentials can be propagated. Therefore, the alterations of myelin in injured spinal cord axons previously described would also explain the prolongation of the refractory period and inability to respond to high frequency stimulation.[71]

Derangements in Spinal Cord Blood Flow and Cerebrospinal Fluid Flow

Considerable evidence exists that interruption to the vascular supply of the spinal cord plays a role in the pathophysiology of spinal cord compression.[33,34,36,37,39,48,95-103] The spinal cord is relatively protected from circulatory insufficiency owing to segmental blood flow and a rich vascular plexus. The arterial supply to the spinal cord arises from the usually paired segmental spinal arteries adjacent to the spinal nerve roots within the intervertebral foramen.[104] These arteries bifurcate into ventral and dorsal radicular arteries that supply rich anastamotic networks on the ventral and dorsal pial surfaces of the spinal cord.[104] The dorsal spinal arteries are paired and tortuous on the dorsal pial surface, whereas the ventral spinal artery is a distinct single artery located in the ventral spinal fissure.[104] These arteries are connected by several anastomotic connections. The ventral spinal artery gives rise to the vertical arteries, which penetrate the ventral fissure of the spinal cord and supply most of the grey matter and some white matter of the spinal cord.[104] Radial arteries arise from the superficial surface arteries to supply much of the white matter and some peripheral grey matter (Figure 42-8).[104-111] The capillary network within the spinal cord and nerve roots are continuous and lined with vascular endothelial cells bound by tight cellular junctions that form the blood-spinal cord or blood-nerve barrier.[112] In one study, an intravenous injection of a protein tracer did not leak through the blood-nerve barrier; but when it was injected into the cerebrospinal fluid, it was taken up by capillary pinocytotic vesicles and excreted in to the veins, suggesting that there is no blood/spinal fluid barrier.[113]

The venous drainage occurs via radial veins that drain into a network of surface veins that ultimately drain into the vertebral venous plexus located on the floor of the vertebral canal. The venous plexus also receives venous drainage from the vertebral bodies. The venous plexus drains via the intervertebral veins that are also associated with the spinal nerve root at the intervertebral foramen (Figure 42-8).[104,109-111]

In cervical spondylotic myelopathy in people, the relative sparing of the anterior columns and subpial posterior columns is believed to be related to the architecture of the blood supply.[33,97] For example, the dorsal spinal arteries are paired and tortuous and are, thereby, resistant to tension when the cord elongates in flexion.[33,97] The anterior spinal artery travels in a longitudinal direction, and forces that compress the spinal cord tend not to disrupt the flow. In contrast, the transversely oriented perforating vessels that arise from the vertical artery in the ventral sulcus supply and the grey and medial white matter may be more susceptible to compression.[33,97]

Ligation of a single radicular artery in animal models was not shown to induce spinal cord dysfunction.[112,114-116] In one study in dogs, ligation of five pairs of thoracic spinal nerve roots and associated radicular arteries and veins resulted in only a 20% to 30% reduction in blood flow and oxygen tension and did not result in clinical loss of neurologic function.[112] The findings of this study suggest that collateral circulation from the pial vascular plexus and intact segmental arteries were adequate to maintain spinal cord metabolism. It was also hypothesized that the cerebrospinal fluid flow system plays a supplementary role in supplying nutrients to the spinal cord.[117]

Vascular derangements in spinal cord compression may actually be associated with impairment in venous blood flow rather than with impairment in arterial flow.[4,112,118-120] In one dog model, chronic compression as a result of chronic arachnoid scarring was induced by applying a circumferential silicone tube for three months. Histologic evaluation at termination revealed a patent superficial medullary artery, whereas the superficial medullary vein was compressed and thrombosed. In addition to these findings, syrinx formation was identified in the dorsal column.[121] A study using kaolin injection in the subarachnoid space in rabbits resulted in total circumferential occlusion of the arachnoid space in 86% of the animals and partial occlusion in 14%. In the animals in which total occlusion occurred, intramedullary edema secondary to increased vascular permeability was also present. In addition, syringomyelia and/or hydromyelia were found histologically in this group.[122] The findings from both studies suggest that total circumferential ablation of the subarachnoid space results in loss of nutrient supply and lack of removal of cellular waste products via the cerebrospinal fluid as well as disturbing venous blood flow, resulting in spinal cord edema, necrosis, syrinx formation, and neurologic dysfunction.[24,26,27,41,121,122] A comparison of the effects in the spinal cord from arterial obstruction (thoracic aorta) versus venous obstruction (caudal vena cava) was studied in a dog model. The blood-nerve (spinal cord) barrier remained intact when the thoracic aorta was obstructed. However, the blood-spinal cord barrier was disrupted as revealed by leakage of an Evans Blue albumin protein tracer and edema in the parenchyma of the spinal cord and nerve roots.[123] The results of these laboratory models may correlate with the findings of parenchymal edema and formation of syringomyelia and/or hydromyelia seen on T2-weighted magnetic resonance imaging and histologically in chronic myelopathy (Figure 42-9).[3,24,26,27,41,124,125]

Role of Duration of Spinal Cord Compression

Much debate has occurred in human as well as veterinary medicine on the timing of decompression. Compression is considered to play a role in initiation and progression of secondary spinal cord injury.[126] Whereas several studies and clinical experience have shown the importance of decompression in mitigating secondary spinal cord injury, poor consensus exists on the appropriate timing for surgical intervention.[126-136] Several animal studies have been done on the time-dependent pathologic effects of spinal cord compression. Many of these studies have established a relationship between increased duration of compression and neurologic recovery.[126,134-138] In a dog study by Carslon et al,[2] thoracic spinal cord compression was induced by a loading device precalibrated to indent the spinal cord at a constant of 0.17 mm/min and maintained for either 30 or 180 minutes. The loading pressure of the spinal cord was maintained at a constant once the somatosensory evoked potentials were decreased by 50% of baseline values. The peak loading spinal cord interface pressures were highest at the end of dynamic loading and actually decreased by more than 50% once sustained compression was maintained for five minutes. After 30 minutes of sustained pressure, the interface pressures decreased to 25% of the peak pressure. Dogs were allowed to recover and were evaluated for 28 days by parameters that included spinal cord somatosensory evoked potentials (intraoperative and preterminally), functional neurologic assessment, magnetic resonance imaging, and histologic study. Amplitude of somatosensory evoked potentials (SSEP) decreased to about 90% of baseline values at the time of peak loading pressures. SSEP amplitudes improved to 63% of baseline within 90 minutes after decompression in the 30-minute compression model. Recovery of SSEP did not occur in the 180-minute compression model. All dogs in the 30-minute compression model had functional recovery and were walking normally or with mild deficits within 21 days of the surgery. Only 50% of the dogs in the 180-minute compression model developed the ability to bear weight, but none were ever able to walk with, at best, minimal deficit. T2-weighted MRI imaging at 28 days postoperatively revealed increased signal intensity in the central area of the spinal cord; these lesions were significantly larger in volume in the 180-minute compression model. Both groups of dogs developed central cavitation in the spinal cord (syrinx formation), but the 180-minute compression group had significantly larger lesions, correlating to the finding on magnetic resonance imaging. These findings agreed with an earlier model of compression by Delmarter et al,[137] using circumferential ligature and decompression at time zero, 1, 6, and 24 hours, and 6 weeks after compression.

One important difference between this and many other studies evaluating the effects of spinal cord compression was that, in most of the other studies, spinal cord compression was applied with an unremitting interface force utilizing weights, balloon, or dynamic clips in which interface forces did not rapidly decline. It is hypothesized that the clinical causes of spinal cord compression were associated with interface pressures that were greatest at the time of impact with relaxation of interface pressures ensuing. This phenomenon is known as a visoelastic relaxation response to dynamic spinal cord loading.[1,139] There appears to be a range of maximum pressures that occur prior to declines in SSEP amplitudes; pressures above this limit may cause aberrations in regional blood flow.[1,140,141] This was determined in a previous dog study by Carlson et al.[1] The spinal cord was compressed until SSEP amplitudes were diminished to 50% of baseline. The spinal cord was then either decompressed at 5 minutes or subjected to sustained compression for 3 hours without decompression. Regional spinal cord blood flow was evaluated using a fluorescent microsphere extraction technique. Spinal cord blood flow decreased by about 33% at the time of maximum interface pressures. Within 5 minutes of sustained compression, interface pressure dissipated by 51%; however, the SSEP amplitudes continued to decrease to 16% of baseline values. In the group that underwent decompression, regional blood flow and SSEP amplitudes recovered to baseline within 30 minutes. This initial hyperemic response was followed by a mild decline in regional spinal cord blood flow. In the 3-hour sustained compression group, interface pressures relaxed to 13% of the maximum values within 90 minutes, but there was no recovery of SSEP values. Regional spinal cord blood flow remained significantly lower than baseline values at 30 minutes, but was similar to the decompression group at 180 minutes. Results of both of these studies imply that, in spite of visoelastic relaxation, sustained compression was associated with regional hypoperfusion and ischemia, poorer SSEP recovery, poorer functional outcome, and lesions visible on magnetic resonance imaging and histologic evaluation.[1,2]

Dynamic movement of the spine in addition to static spinal cord compression also plays a role in spinal cord injury.[142-144] This phenomenon is most commonly observed in the condition of cervical myelopathy associated with vertebral malformation/malarticulation. In a cat study by Wolfa et al,[144] a C3 corpectomy was performed and the vertebra was replaced with a hinged anterior compression device with and without C3 dorsal laminectomy to evaluate the impact of spinal movement on the pathologic processes of static compression. The results of this study revealed several findings. First, in the cats that did not undergo laminectomy, as the degree of compromise of the spinal canal rose above 20%, the epidural pressure began to rise as well, suggesting that some compensatory mechanism exists in the spinal cord and dura until that point. At spinal canal compromise greater than 20%, the compensatory mechanisms are overwhelmed, and it is at this point that clinical dysfunction and electrophysiologic (somatosensory evoked potential) changes occur.[1,144] Epidural pressures were higher in cervical extension than in a neutral position, whereas pressures were not affected in flexion. This finding supports the hypothesis that the dorsal structures (ligamentum flavum and joint capsule) contribute to compression when the neck is in extension.[144] Another important finding in this study was that the mean epidural pressure was significantly higher during passive neck movement than was the mean pressure in neutral positioning. It appears that during repeated flexion and extension visoelastic relaxation does not have time to occur, resulting in increases of both mean and maximum epidural pressures. In the laminectomized animals with spinal canal compromise of less than 75%, mean epidural pressure was remarkably lower in neutral positioning, in all degrees of spinal compromise associated with flexion and extension, and during spinal neck movement, supporting the benefit of dorsal decompression on mitigating progressive spinal cord injury.

Spasticity and Spinal Cord Compression

Spasticity is an inevitable consequence of chronic spinal cord injury or disease[145,146] and contributes to clinical complications such as limb contractures and decubital ulcers.[145,146] Spasticity is defined as an abnormal increase in tone (hypertonicity), which is observed as a resistance to passive limb movement that is proportional to the velocity of the movement.[145,146] The velocity-dependent stiffness of the affected limbs is associated with increased stretch-evoked reflexes.[147-151] However, decreased compliance of the surrounding soft tissue structures of the limb (muscles, tendons and ligaments) may also contribute to spacticity.[152,153]

Although spasticity has been studied in numerous experimental models, the exact mechanisms that induce spasticity are not completely understood. Spasticity is most often associated with chronic spinal cord disease in which spasticity develops in a time-dependent fashion with lasting neuroanatomic, neurophysiologic, and neuropharmocologic changes in the spinal cord.[145,146,154-156] Once established chronically it is unlikely to improve without pharmacologic and/or surgical intervention.[145,146,154-156] It is proposed that the changes in the spinal cord are related to increased excitability of the monosynaptic reflexes that originate in the muscle-stretch receptor and synapse on the α-motoneuron that directly innervates the same muscle (e.g., the patellar reflex).[145,147,151,157-161] Studies in cats and rats (as well as observations from clinical cases) have demonstrated increased magnitude of the lumbar monosynaptic reflexes (hyper-reflexia) caudal to severe thoracic transverse myelopathy (i.e., hemisection of the spinal cord).[155,156,162-164] The changes in reflex responses have been shown to be associated with fundamental processes that control reflex excitability, namely reduction in rate modulation of synaptic activity during repetitive stimulation.[145,146,156] In normal rat monosynaptic reflex neurons, the amplitude of recorded CAPs declines as the frequency of afferent stimulation is increased.[146] In animals with midthoracic spinal cord contusion injuries, the influence of rate-depression on the reflex CAP magnitude is attenuated and decreases in a time-dependent manner following injury.[146,165-167] Rate-depression of reflex magnitude is just one of three processes, including facilitation and potentiation, that compete to control the expression of the monosynaptic reflex.[146,168-172] The change in the magnitude of the reflex is not related to decreased action potential or to excitability of the α-motoneuron directly, but rather is associated with long-acting presynaptic inhibition in the spinal cord afferent neurons mediated by γ-aminobutyric acid (GABA) and the $GABA_B$ receptor.[145,173-177] GABA is one of the most important inhibitory neurotransmitters in the central nervous system and the $GABA_B$ receptor modulates voltage-gated calcium channels.[145,173-177] Calcium entry into the terminal axon is necessary for neurotransmitter release; therefore, activation of voltage-gated calcium channels on the presynaptic afferent neuron in the reflex arc leads to decreased amplitude of the postsynaptic excitatory potentials without altering the conductive properties of the α-motoneuron itself.[145,173]

In addition to altered $GABA_B$ receptor function, loss of spinal cord interneurons has also been implicated in alterations in rate depression.[145] Loss of interneurons at the site of injury does not explain changes in rate depression in segments caudal to the lesion. It is recognized that the interneurons that mediate presynaptic inhibition are influenced by descending input from other spinal cord regions, the brain stem, and the cerebral cortex.[178-186] It has been postulated that the time-dependent development of spasticity is associated with secondary pathology that occurs in the descending pathways.[145,154-156] One descending pathway believed to be involved in modulation of sensory input and rate depression is the midbrain nucleus locus coeruleus which has been shown to send axons to all levels of the spinal cord.[146,187] Norepinephrine is the primary neurotransmitter in this pathway. The influence of this system on spinal cord spasticity has been studied by using an immunotoxin for dopamine β-hydroxylase, an enzyme in the cellular pathway that produces norepinerphine.[156,188-190] Results of these studies have suggested that loss of input from descending noradrenergic fibers that contribute to $GABA_B$-mediated rate depression in the monosynaptic reflex contributes to the development of spasticity in the chronically injured spinal cord.[145,146] The development of spasticity and altered rate depression serving as an adaptive recovery process rather than a maladaptive process has been proposed an alternative theory.[191-194]

Pain and Spinal Cord Compression/Injury

Pain that originates from the spinal cord or nervous tissue (also referred to as central pain syndrome) is reported primarily in human patients following severe spinal cord injury.[170,195,196] Following initial injury, the patient usually manifests acute pain, which is the result of injury to the spinal column and adjacent soft tissue. This nociceptive type of pain is most often described as dull, aching, and movement-related. It tends to resolve well with appropriate treatment such as rest, opioids, and anti-inflammatory medications, as well as time.[4] Pain associated with spinal cord injury tends to occur months to years after the initial injury and is difficult to manage and treat.[195-201] This type of pain should be considered a disease in and of itself, rather than a clinical manifestation of some other problem. The incidence is reported to be between 10% and 90% of all spinal cord injured patients and is often more of a concern to the patient than the residual functional disabilities.[202-204] This is not a commonly recognized phenomenon in veterinary patients that are managed long-term following spinal cord injury, but is reported in rodent models of spinal cord injury.[195,200,205-209]

Pain associated with spinal cord injury may be spasticity related or may arise from the nervous system or both. The types of pain sensations reported are variable among patients.[145,196] In people, pain of spinal cord injury can be divided into transitional-zone pain and central dysesthesia syndrome. Transitional-zone pain occurs at the level of the spinal cord injury and is often associated with nerve root injury. This type of pain seems to arise most commonly with injuries at the thoracic level. It is often present at a few contiguous spinal segments and is often asymmetrical. Transitional-zone pain often "mimics" pain sensations that have been felt in the past. The pain occurs early as allodynia or hyperalgesia and may improve spontaneously.[196] This type of pain is often addressed early in the course of the disease, therefore decreasing the chances of it's becoming a long-standing illness. Severe, persistent cases are often treated with nerve blocks or dorsal root entry zone (DREZ) procedures.[196]

Central dysesthesia syndrome is associated with a "burning" sensation below the level of the spinal cord injury.[196] In contrast to transitional-zone pain, it is often diffuse and symmetrical. The pathophysiology behind this syndrome has been studied but remains somewhat of an enigma. Multiple hypotheses have been generated, but it is not known if the same mechanisms underlie all central pain syndromes, because there appears to be no one lesion type or location that is associated with a higher relative risk. This type of pain has been attributed to abnormal associations of the spinothalamic and dorsal column pathways that transmit pain information.[145,210] The functional spinothalamic tracts, which normally transmit protopathic sensations such as temperature and pain, are severely impaired. The dorsal column pathways, which normally transmit epicritic information about light touch, discrimination of touch, and vibratory sensations, are spared. In central pain, it is believed that the dorsal column pathways begin to transmit pain sensations normally transmitted by the spinothalamic pathways. Patients with central pain often have abnormal pain and temperature sensibilities. Of interest is that lesions within the spinothalamic pathways are not required to induce this phenomenon, but rather tend to influence the character of the abnormal sensations. It appears that the critical disinhibition occurs in the ventroposterior, medial, and intralaminar thalamic nuclei that receive and integrate information from the spinothalamic pathways.[211-213] These thalamic regions in general tend to have an inhibitory influence on pain sensation. Abnormal functioning in this pathway results in abnormally high levels of pain and hypersensitivity. How these cells ultimately become disinhibited after spinal cord injury is not truly known;[145,214] however, on a cellular level excitatory amino acids, glutaminergic N-methyl-D-aspartate (NMDA), and serotonergic receptors have been implicated.[17,214-216] The excitatoxic amino acids may influence cytokine production, breakdown of structural proteins, second messengers, and transcriptional proteins in ways that result in abnormal signaling in the pain processing pathways.[145,170,200,217,218] In experimental models of spinal cord injury, abnormal electrical activity has been identified in segments surrounding the injury site on electrophysiologic testing.[206,219,220] The abnormal activities reported include increased stimulus response, increased spontaneous background activity, and increased after-discharge responses. In a rat spinal cord clip-compression study by Bruce et al,[214] the influence of serotonin in development of central pain of spinal cord injury was investigated. Serotonin immunoreactivity in the dorsal horn was found to be decreased caudal to the thoracic injury site (T9-11) and increased three-fold in regions rostral to it. The decrease caudal to the injury was believed to be consistent with loss of descending serotonergic antinociceptive pathways. The presence of increased serotonin activity in dorsal horns rostral to the injury was an unexpected finding. Because serotonin is also known to possess pronociceptive properties, it was postulated that this observation may be involved in the disruption of inhibition of pain pathways.

Central pain may remain stable, escalate in severity, or decrease over time and it can be very difficult to treat.[145,210,221,222] Autonomic dysnergia, such as distended bladder or constipation, can result in increased pain transmission, raising baseline pain levels in these patients.[223]

Another complication of spinal cord injury is the development of syrinx within the parenchyma of the spinal cord (syringomyelia).[196,198] This injury most commonly occurs years after the injury and is associated with ascension of the sensory and motor level dysfunction owing to the expansion as well as to the development of new pain sensations. Typically, this pain is located in the region of the syrinx but may cause a burning-type pain above the level of the injury or syrinx. The natural course of syringomyelia is continued escalation of the pain that is often not responsive to medications or surgical intervention with syringopleural shunting. Post-injury or post-compression syrinx formation appears to be a more common source of pain in dogs than is the enigmatic central pain syndrome (Figure 42-9).

References

1. Carlson GD, Warden KE, Barbeau JM, et al: Viscoelastic relaxation and regional blood flow response to spinal cord compression and decompression. Spine 22(12):1285-1291, 1997

2. Carlson GD, Gorden CD, Oliff HS, et al: Sustained spinal cord compression: part I: time-dependent effect on long-term pathophysiology. J Bone Joint Surg Am 85A(1):86-94, 2003.

3. Harrison BM, McDonald WI: Remyelination after transient experimental compression of the spinal cord. Ann Neurol 1(6):542-551, 1977.

4. Kim P, Haisa T, Kawamoto T, et al: Delayed myelopathy induced by chronic compression in the rat spinal cord. Ann Neurol 55(4):503-511, 2004.

5. Baba H, Maezawa Y, Imura S, et al: Quantitative analysis of the spinal cord motoneuron under chronic compression: an experimental observation in the mouse. J Neurol 243(2):109-116, 1996.

6. Baba H, Maezawa Y, Uchida K, et al: Three-dimensional topographic analysis of spinal accessory motoneurons under chronic mechanical compression: an experimental study in the mouse. J Neurol 244(4):222-229, 1997.

7. Baba H, Maezawa Y, Uchida K, et al: Plasticity of the spinal cord contributes to neurological improvement after treatment by cervical decompression. A magnetic resonance imaging study. J Neurol 244(7):455-460, 1997.

8. Agrawal SK, Fehlings MG: Mechanisms of secondary injury to spinal cord axons in vitro: role of Na^+, Na(+)-K(+)-ATPase, the Na(+)-H^+ exchanger, and the Na(+)-$Ca2^+$ exchanger. J Neurosci 16(2):545-552, 1996.

9. Agrawal SK, Fehlings MG: Role of NMDA and non-NMDA ionotropic glutamate receptors in traumatic spinal cord axonal injury. J Neurosci 17(3):1055-1063, 1997.

10. Agrawal SK, Nashmi R, Fehlings MG: Role of L- and N-type calcium channels in the pathophysiology of traumatic spinal cord white matter injury. Neuroscience 99(1):179-188, 2000.

11. Aki T, Toya S: Experimental study on changes of the spinal-evoked potential and circulatory dynamics following spinal cord compression and decompression. Spine 9(8):800-809, 1984.

12. Allen AR: Surgery for experimental lesions of spinal cord equivalent to crush injury of fracture dislocation of spinal column: a preliminary report. J Am Med Assoc 57:878-880, 1911.

13. Fehlings MG, Sekhon LH: Cellular, ionic and biomolecular mechanisms of the injury process. *In* Contemporary Management of Spinal Cord Injury: From Impact to Rehabilitation. Benzel E, Tator CH (eds). Chicago: AANS, 2000, pp. 33-50.

14. Fehlings MG, Sekhon LH, Tator C: The role and timing of decompression in acute spinal cord injury: what do we know? What should we do? Spine 26(24 Suppl):S101-S110, 2001.

15. Hung TK, Albin MS, Brown TD, et al: Biomechanical responses to open experimental spinal cord injury. Surg Neurol 4(2):271-276, 1975.

16. Morino T, Ogata T, Horiuchi H, et al: Delayed neuronal damage related to microglia proliferation after mild spinal cord compression injury. Neurosci Res 46(3):309-318, 2003.

17. Tator CH, Fehlings MG: Review of the secondary injury theory of acute spinal cord trauma with emphasis on vascular mechanisms. J Neurosurg 75(1):15-26, 1991.

18. Thienprasit P, Bantli H, Bloedel JR, et al: Effect of delayed local cooling on experimental spinal cord injury. J Neurosurg 42(2):150-154, 1975.

19. Wagner FC Jr, Stewart WB: Effect of trauma dose on spinal cord edema. J Neurosurg 54(6):802-806, 1981.

20. Young W, Koreh I: Potassium and calcium changes in injured spinal cords. Brain Res 365(1):42-53, 1986.

21. Zhang Y, Hillered L, Olsson Y, et al: Time course of energy perturbation after compression trauma to the spinal cord: an experimental study in the rat using microdialysis. Surg Neurol 39(4):297-304, 1993.

22. Lu J, Waite P: Advances in spinal cord regeneration. Spine 24(9):926-930, 1999.

23. Lu J, Ashwell KW, Waite P: Advances in secondary spinal cord injury: role of apoptosis. Spine 25(14):1859-1866, 2000.

24. al-Mefty O, Harkey LH, Middleton TH, et al: Myelopathic cervical spondylotic lesions demonstrated by magnetic resonance imaging. J Neurosurg 68(2):217-222, 1988.

25. Matsumoto M, Toyama Y, Ishikawa M, et al: Increased signal intensity of the spinal cord on magnetic resonance images in cervical compressive myelopathy. Does it predict the outcome of conservative treatment? Spine 25(6):677-682, 2000.

26. Ohshio I, Hatayama A, Kaneda K, et al: Correlation between histopathologic features and magnetic resonance images of spinal cord lesions. Spine 18(9):1140-1149, 1993.

27. Takahashi M, Yamashita Y, Sakamoto Y, et al: Chronic cervical cord compression: clinical significance of increased signal intensity on MR images. Radiology 173(1):219-224, 1989.

28. Osterholm JL, Mathews GJ: Altered norepinephrine metabolism, following experimental spinal cord injury. 2. Protection against traumatic spinal cord hemorrhagic necrosis by norepinephrine synthesis blockade with alpha methyl tyrosine. J Neurosurg 36(4):395-401, 1972.

29. Anderson DK, Means ED, Waters TR, et al: Spinal cord energy metabolism following compression trauma to the feline spinal cord. J Neurosurg 53(3):375-380, 1980.

30. Anderson DK, Hall ED: Pathophysiology of spinal cord trauma. Ann Emerg Med 22(6):987-992, 1993.

31. Demopoulos HB, Flamm ES, Pietronigro DD, et al: The free radical pathology and the microcirculation in the major central nervous system disorders. Acta Physiol Scand Suppl 492:91-119, 1980.

32. Hall ED, Yonkers PA, Horan KL, et al: Correlation between attenuation of posttraumatic spinal cord ischemia and preservation of tissue vitamin E by the 21-aminosteroid U74006F: evidence for an in vivo antioxidant mechanism. J Neurotrauma 6(3):169-176, 1989.

33. Fehlings MG, Skaf G: A review of the pathophysiology of cervical spondylotic myelopathy with insights for potential novel mechanisms drawn from traumatic spinal cord injury. Spine 23(24):2730-2737, 1998.

34. Ito T, Oyanagi K, Takahashi H, et al: Cervical spondylotic myelopathy. Clinicopathologic study on the progression pattern and thin myelinated fibers of the lesions of seven patients examined during complete autopsy. Spine 21(7):827-833, 1996.

35. Yamaura I, Yone K, Nakahara S, et al: Mechanism of destructive pathologic changes in the spinal cord under chronic mechanical compression. Spine 27(1):21-26, 2002.

36. Hoff J, Nishimura M, Pitts L, et al: The role of ischemia in the pathogenesis of cervical spondylotic myelopathy: a review and new microangiographic evidence. Spine;2:100-108, 1972.

37. Hughes JT: Disorders of the spine. *In* Pathology of the Spinal Cord. (Anonymous.) London: WB Saunders, 166-176, 1978.

38. Kameyama T, Hashizume Y, Ando T, et al: Spinal cord morphology and pathology in ossification of the posterior longitudinal ligament. Brain 118 (Pt 1):263-278, 1995.

39. Mair WG, Druckman R: The pathology of spinal cord lesions and their relation to the clinical features in protrusion of cervical intervertebral discs; a report of four cases. Brain 76(1):70-91, 1953.

40. Nakahara S, Yone K, Sakou T, et al: Induction of apoptosis signal regulating kinase 1 (ASK1) after spinal cord injury in rats: possible involvement of ASK1-JNK and -p38 pathways in neuronal apoptosis. J Neuropathol Exp Neurol 58(5):442-450, 1999.

41. Takahashi T, Suto Y, Kato S, et al: Experimental acute dorsal compression of cat spinal cord: correlation of magnetic resonance signal intensity with spinal cord evoked potentials and morphology. Spine 21(2):166-173, 1996.

42. von Euler M, Seiger A, Sundstrom E: Clip compression injury in the spinal cord: a correlative study of neurological and morphological alterations. Exp Neurol 145(2 Pt1):502-510, 1997.

43. Wilkinson M: The morbid anatomy of cervical spondylosis and myelopathy. Brain 83:589-617, 1960.

44. Bunge MB, Puckett WR, Becerra JL, et al: Observations on the pathology of human spinal cord injury. A review and classification of 22 new cases with details from a case of chronic cord compression with extensive focal demyelination. Adv Neurol 59:75-89, 1993.

45. Fujiwara K, Yonenobu K, Ebara S, et al: The prognosis of surgery for cervical compression myelopathy. An analysis of the factors involved. J Bone Joint Surg Br 71(3):393-398, 1989.

46. Penning L, Wilmink JT, van Woerden HH, et al: CT myelographic findings in degenerative disorders of the cervical spine: clinical significance. Am J Roentgenol 146(4):793-801, 1986.

47. Arnold JG Jr: The clinical manifestations of spondylochondrosis (spondylosis) of the cervical spine. Ann Surg 141(6):872-889, 1955.

48. Ogino H, Tada K, Okada K, et al: Canal diameter, anteroposterior compression ratio, and spondylotic myelopathy of the cervical spine. Spine 8(1):1-15, 1983.

49. Bohlman HH, Emery SE: The pathophysiology of cervical spondylosis and myelopathy. Spine 13(7):843-846, 1988.

50. Burek MJ, Oppenheim RW: Programmed cell death in the developing nervous system. Brain Pathol6(4):427-446, 1996.

51. Cohen JJ: Apoptosis. Immunol Today 14(3):126-130, 1993.

52. Raff M: Cell suicide for beginners. Nature 396(6707):119-122, 1998.

53. Gillardon F, Klimaschewski L, Wickert H, et al: Expression pattern of candidate cell death effector proteins Bax, Bcl-2, Bcl-X, and c-Jun in sensory and motor neurons following sciatic nerve transection in the rat. Brain Res 739(1-2):244-250, 1996.

54. Macaya A: Apoptosis in the nervous system. Rev Neurol 24(135):1356-1360, 1996.

55. White FA, Keller-Peck CR, Knudson CM, et al: Widespread elimination of naturally occurring neuronal death in Bax-deficient mice. J Neurosci 18(4):1428-1439, 1998.

56. Crowe MJ, Bresnahan JC, Shuman SL, et al: Apoptosis and delayed degeneration after spinal cord injury in rats and monkeys. Nat Med 3(1):73-76, 1997.

57. Kato H, Kanellopoulos GK, Matsuo S, et al: Neuronal apoptosis and necrosis following spinal cord ischemia in the rat. Exp Neurol 148(2):464-474, 1997.

58. Katoh K, Ikata T, Katoh S, et al: Induction and its spread of apoptosis in rat spinal cord after mechanical trauma. Neurosci Lett 216(1):9-12, 1996.

59. Li GL, Brodin G, Farooque M, et al: Apoptosis and expression of Bcl-2 after compression trauma to rat spinal cord LI1996. J Neuropathol Exp Neurol 55(3):280-289, 1996.

60. Li GL, Farooque M, Holtz A, et al: Apoptosis of oligodendrocytes occurs for long distances away from the primary injury after compression trauma to rat spinal cord. Acta Neuropathologica 98(5):473-480, 1999.

61. Liu XZ, Xu XM, Hu R, et al: Neuronal and glial apoptosis after traumatic spinal cord injury. J Neurosci 17(14):5395-5406, 1997.

62. Mackey ME, Wu Y, Hu R, et al: Cell death suggestive of apoptosis after spinal cord ischemia in rabbits. Stroke 28(10):2012-2017, 1997.

63. Mu X, He J, Anderson DW, et al: Altered expression of bcl-2 and bax mRNA in amyotrophic lateral sclerosis spinal cord motor neurons. Ann Neurol 40(3):379-386, 1996.

64. Schrank B, Gotz R, Gunnersen JM, et al: Inactivation of the survival motor neuron gene, a candidate gene for human spinal muscular atrophy, leads to massive cell death in early mouse embryos. Proc Natl Acad Sci U S A 94(18):9920-9925, 1997.

65. Shuman SL, Bresnahan JC, Beattie MS: Apoptosis of microglia and oligodendrocytes after spinal cord contusion in rats. J Neurosci Res 50(5):798-808, 1997.

66. Wada S, Yone K, Ishidou Y, et al: Apoptosis following spinal cord injury in rats and preventative effect of N-methyl-D-aspartate receptor antagonist. J Neurosurg 91(1 Suppl):98-104, 1999.

67. Anthes DL, Theriault E, Tator CH: Characterization of axonal ultrastructural pathology following experimental spinal cord compression injury. Brain Res 702(1-2):1-16, 1995.

68. Eidelberg E, Straehley D, Erspamer R, et al. Relationship between residual hindlimb-assisted locomotion and surviving axons after incomplete spinal cord injuries. Exp Neurol 56(2):312-322, 1977.

69. Fehlings MG, Nashmi R: Assessment of axonal dysfunction in an in vitro model of acute compressive injury to adult rat spinal cord axons. Brain Res 677(2):291-299, 1995.

70. Fehlings MG, Nashmi R: A new model of acute compressive spinal cord injury in vitro. J Neurosci Meth 71(2):215-224, 1997.

71. Nashmi R, Fehlings MG: Changes in axonal physiology and morphology after chronic compressive injury of the rat thoracic spinal cord. Neuroscience 104(1):235-251, 2001.

72. Balentine JD: Pathology of experimental spinal cord trauma. I. The necrotic lesion as a function of vascular injury. Lab Invest;39(3):236-253, 1978.

73. Blight AR: Axonal physiology of chronic spinal cord injury in the cat: intracellular recording in vitro. Neuroscience 10(4):1471-1486, 1983.

74. Blight AR: Cellular morphology of chronic spinal cord injury in the cat: analysis of myelinated axons by line-sampling. Neuroscience 10(2):521-543, 1983.

75. Blight AR, DeCrescito V: Morphometric analysis of experimental spinal cord injury in the cat: the relation of injury intensity to survival of myelinated axons. Neuroscience 19(1):321-341, 1986.

76. Bostock H, Grafe P: Activity-dependent excitability changes in normal and demyelinated rat spinal root axons. J Physiol365:239-257, 1985.

77. Bresnahan JC, King JS, Martin GF, et al: A neuroanatomical analysis of spinal cord injury in the rhesus monkey (Macaca mulatta). J Neurol Sci 28(4):521-542, 1976.

78. Bresnahan JC: An electron-microscopic analysis of axonal alterations following blunt contusion of the spinal cord of the rhesus monkey (Macaca mulatta). J Neurol Sci 37(1-2):59-82, 1978.

79. Fehlings MG, Tator CH: The relationships among the severity of spinal cord injury, residual neurological function, axon counts, and counts of retrogradely labeled neurons after experimental spinal cord injury. Exp Neurol 132(2):220-228, 1995.

80. Griffiths IR, McCulloch MC: Nerve fibres in spinal cord impact injuries. Part 1. Changes in the myelin sheath during the initial 5 weeks. J Neurol Sci 58(3):335-349, 1983.

81. Honmou O, Felts PA, Waxman SG, et al: Restoration of normal conduction properties in demyelinated spinal cord axons in the adult rat by transplantation of exogenous Schwann cells. J Neurosci 16(10):3199-3208, 1996.

82. Kaji R, Sumner AJ: Ouabain reverses conduction disturbances in single demyelinated nerve fibers. Neurology 39(10):1364-1368, 1989.

83. Sakatani K, Ohta T, Shimo-Oku M: Conductivity of dorsal column fibers during experimental spinal cord compression and after decompression at various stimulus frequencies. Cent Nerv Syst Trauma 4(3):161-179, 1987.

84. Sakatani K, Iizuka H, Young W: Randomized double pulse stimulation for assessing stimulus frequency-dependent conduction in injured spinal and peripheral axons. Electroencephalogr Clin Neurophysiol 81(2):108-117, 1991.

85. Povlishock JT, Christman CW: The pathobiology of traumatically induced axonal injury in animals and humans: a review of current thoughts. J Neurotrauma 12(4):555-564, 1995.

86. Puckett WR, Hiester ED, Norenberg MD, et al: The astroglial response to Wallerian degeneration after spinal cord injury in humans. Exp Neurol 148(2):424-432, 1997.

87. Balentine JD: Pathology of experimental spinal cord trauma. II. Ultrastructure of axons and myelin. Lab Invest 39(3):254-266, 1978.

88. Brook GA, Plate D, Franzen R, et al: Spontaneous longitudinally orientated axonal regeneration is associated with the Schwann cell framework within the lesion site following spinal cord compression injury of the rat. J Neurosci Res 53(1):51-65, 1998.

89. Koenig H, Bunge MB, Bunge RP: Nucleic acid and protein metabolism in white matter. Observations during experimental demyelination and remyelination; a histochemical and autoradiographic study of spinal cord of the adult cat. Arch Neurol 6:177-193, 1962.

90. Wrathall JR, Li W, Hudson LD: Myelin gene expression after experimental contusive spinal cord injury. J Neurosci 18(21):8780-8793, 1998.

91. Bunge MB, Holets VR, Bates ML, et al: Characterization of photochemically induced spinal cord injury in the rat by light and electron microscopy. Exp Neurol 127(1):76-93, 1994.

92. Martin D, Schoenen J, Delree P, et al: Experimental acute traumatic injury of the adult rat spinal cord by a subdural inflatable balloon: methodology, behavioral analysis, and histopathology. J Neurosci Res 32(4):539-550, 1992.

93. Ramon y Cajal S: Degeneration and Regeneration of the Nervous System. London: Oxford University Press, 1928.

94. von Euler M, Seiger A, Sundstrom E: Clip compression injury in the spinal cord: a correlative study of neurological and morphological alterations. Exp Neurol 145(2 Pt 1):502-510, 1997.

95. Bittigau P, Ikonomidou C: Glutamate in neurologic diseases. J Child Neurol 12(8):471-485, 1997.

96. Brain WR: Discussion on rupture of the intervertebral disc in the cervical region. Proc R Soc Med 41:509-511, 1948.

97. Breig A, Turnbull I, Hassler O: Effects of mechanical stresses on the spinal cord in cervical spondylosis. A study on fresh cadaver material. J Neurosurg 25(1):45-56, 1966.

98. Choi DW: Excitotoxic cell death. J Neurobiol 23(9):1261-1276, 1992.

99. Gooding MR, Wilson CB, Hoff JT: Experimental cervical myelopathy. Effects of ischemia and compression of the canine cervical spinal cord. J Neurosurg 43(1):9-17, 1975.

100. Gooding MR, Wilson CB, Hoff JT: Experimental cervical myelopathy: autoradiographic studies of spinal cord blood flow patterns. Surg Neurol 5(4):233-239, 1976.

101. Nurick S: The pathogenesis of the spinal cord disorder associated with cervical spondylosis. Brain 95(1):87-100, 1972.

102. Shimomura Y, Hukuda S, Mizuno S: Experimental study of ischemic damage to the cervical spinal cord. J Neurosurg 28(6):565-581, 1968.

103. Taylor AR: Mechanism and treatment of spinal-cord disorders associated with cervical spondylosis. Lancet 1(15):717-720, 1953.

104. Wheeler SJ, Sharp NJH: Functional anatomy. *In* Wheeler SJ, Sharp NJH (eds). Small Animal Spinal Disorders: Diagnosis and Surgery. London: Mosby-Wolfe, 1994, pp. 8-20.

105. Caulkins SE, Purinton PT, Oliver JE Jr: Arterial supply to the spinal cord of dogs and cats. Am J Vet Res 50(3):425-430, 1989.

106. Parker AJ: Clinical significance of traumatic occlusion of segmental spinal arteries. J Am Vet Med Assoc 162(12):1041-1042, 1973.

107. Parker AJ: Distribution of spinal branches of the thoracolumbar segmental arteries in dogs. Am J Vet Res 34(10):1351-1353, 1973.

108. Parker AJ, Park RD, Stowater JL: Traumatic occlusion of lumbar segmental arteries. J Trauma 14(4):330-333, 1974.

109. Parker AJ. Traumatic occlusion of segmental spinal veins. J Trauma 14(10):868-872, 1974.

110. Worthman RP: The longitudinal vertebral venous sinuses of the dog. II. Functional aspects. Am J Vet Res 17(64):349-363, 1956.

111. Worthman RP: The longitudinal vertebral venous sinuses of the dog. I. Anatomy. Am J Vet Res 17(64):341-348, 1956.

112. Yoshizawa H. Presidential address: pathomechanism of myelopathy and radiculopathy from the viewpoint of blood flow and cerebrospinal fluid flow including a short historical review. Spine27(12):1255-1263, 2002.

113. Wagner HJ, Pilgrim C, Brandl J: Penetration and removal of horseradish peroxidase injected into the cerebrospinal fluid: role of cerebral perivascular spaces, endothelium and microglia. Acta Neuropathol (Berl) 27(4):299-315, 1974.

114. Bradshaw P: Arteries of the spinal cord in the cat. J Neurol Neurosurg Psychiatry 21(4):284-289, 1958.

115. Fried LC, Di CG, Doppman JL: Ligation of major thoraco-lumbar spinal cord arteries in monkeys. J Neurosurg;31(6):608-614, 1969.

116. Toribatake Y: The effect of total en bloc spondylectomy on spinal cord circulation. Nippon Seikeigeka Gakkai Zasshi 67(11):1070-1080, 1993.

117. Ukai T: Effect of stagnant cerebro-spinal fluid on spinal cord. 10:155-176, 1991.

118. Gooding MR: Pathogenesis of myelopathy in cervical spondylosis. Lancet 2(7890):1180-1181, 1974.

119. Taylor AR: Vascular factors in the myelopathy associated with cervical spondylosis. Neurology 14:62-68, 1964.

120. Wilson CB, Bertan V, Norrell HA Jr, et al: Experimental cervical myelopathy. II. Acute ischemic myelopathy. Arch Neurol;21(6):571-589, 1969.

121. Nishimoto S: Experimental study on chronic spinal cord compression: the effect of chronic dural strangulation on spinal cord. 13:1325-1352, 1995.

122. Kato K: Experimental study of syringomyelia. 15:1321-1353, 1996.

123. Nakagawa M: Pathophysiology of lumbo-sacral spinal nerve root compression. 12:227-251, 1994.

124. Mehalic TF, Pezzuti RT, Applebaum BI: Magnetic resonance imaging and cervical spondylotic myelopathy. Neurosurgery 26(2):217-226, 1990.

125. Ramanauskas WL, Wilner HI, Metes JJ, et al: MR imaging of compressive myelomalacia. J Comput Assist Tomogr 13(3):399-404, 1989.

126. Carlson GD, Minato Y, Okada A, et al: Early time-dependent decompression for spinal cord injury: vascular mechanisms of recovery. J Neurotrauma 14(12):951-962, 1997.

127. Benzel EC, Larson SJ: Functional recovery after decompressive operation for thoracic and lumbar spine fractures. Neurosurgery 19(5):772-778, 1986.

128. Bohlman HH, Freehafer A, Dejak J: The results of treatment of acute injuries of the upper thoracic spine with paralysis. J Bone Joint Surg Am 67(3):360-369, 1985.

129. Brodkey JS, Richards DE, Blasingame JP, et al: Reversible spinal cord trauma in cats. Additive effects of direct pressure and ischemia. J Neurosurg 37(5):591-593, 1972.

130. Brodkey JS, Miller CF Jr, Harmody RM: The syndrome of acute central cervical spinal cord injury revisited. Surg Neurol 14(4):251-257, 1980.

131. Dolan EJ, Tator CH, Endrenyi L: The value of decompression for acute experimental spinal cord compression injury. J Neurosurg 53(6):749-755, 1980.

132. Levi L, Wolf A, Rigamonti D, et al: Anterior decompression in cervical spine trauma: does the timing of surgery affect the outcome? Neurosurgery 29(2):216-222, 1991.

133. Maiman DJ, Larson SJ, Benzel EC: Neurological improvement associated with late decompression of the thoracolumbar spinal cord. Neurosurgery 14(3):302-307, 1984.

134. Nystrom B, Berglund JE: Spinal cord restitution following compression injuries in rats. 78(6):467-472, 1988.

135. Rivlin AS, Tator CH: Effect of duration of acute spinal cord compression in a new acute cord injury model in the rat. 10(1):38-43, 1978.

136. Tarlov IM: Spinal cord compression studies. III. Time limits for recovery after gradual compression in dogs. AMA Arch Neurol Psychiatry 71(5):588-597, 1954.

137. Delamarter RB, Sherman J, Carr JB: Pathophysiology of spinal cord injury. Recovery after immediate and delayed decompression. J Bone Joint Surg Am 77(7):1042-1049, 1995.

138. Guha A, Tator CH, Endrenyi L, et al: Decompression of the spinal cord improves recovery after acute experimental spinal cord compression injury. Paraplegia 25(4):324-339, 1987.

139. Ichihara K, Taguchi T, Sakuramoto I, et al: Mechanism of the spinal cord injury and the cervical spondylotic myelopathy: new approach based on the mechanical features of the spinal cord white and gray matter. J Neurosurg 99(3 Suppl):278-285, 2003.

140. Guha A, Tator CH, Smith CR, et al: Improvement in post-traumatic spinal cord blood flow with a combination of a calcium channel blocker and a vasopressor. J Trauma 29(10):1440-1447, 1989.

141. Kearney PA, Ridella SA, Viano DC, et al: Interaction of contact velocity and cord compression in determining the severity of spinal cord injury. J Neurotrauma 5(3):187-208, 1988.

142. Robinson R, Afeiche N, Dunn E: Cervical spondylotic myelopathy: etiology and treatment concepts. Spine 2:89-99, 1987.

143. White AA III, Panjabi MM: Biomechanical considerations in the surgical management of cervical spondylotic myelopathy. Spine 13(7):856-860, 1988.

144. Wolfla CE, Snell BE, Honeycutt JH: Cervical ventral epidural pressure response to graded spinal canal compromise and spinal motion. Spine 29(14):1524-1529, 2004.

145. Burchiel KJ, Hsu FP: Pain and spasticity after spinal cord injury: mechanisms and treatment. Spine 26(24 Suppl):S146-S160, 2001.

146. Thompson FJ, Parmer R, Reier PJ, et al: Scientific basis of spasticity: insights from a laboratory model. 16(1):2-9, 2001.

147. Herman R: The myotatic reflex. Clinico-physiological aspects of spasticity and contracture. Brain 93(2):273-312, 1970.

148. Ju MS, Chen JJ, Lee HM, et al: Time-course analysis of stretch reflexes in hemiparetic subjects using an on-line spasticity measurement system. J Electromyogr Kinesiol 10(1):1-14, 2000.

149. Kamper DG, Rymer WZ: Quantitative features of the stretch response of extrinsic finger muscles in hemiparetic stroke. Muscle Nerve 23(6):954-961, 2000.

150. Kuhn RA: Functional capacity of the isolated human spinal cord. Brain 73(1):1-51, 1950.

151. Powers RK, Rymer WZ: Effects of acute dorsal spinal hemisection on motoneuron discharge in the medial gastrocnemius of the decerebrate cat. J Neurophysiol 59(5):1540-1556, 1988.

152. Sinkjaer T, Toft E, Larsen K, et al: Non-reflex and reflex mediated ankle joint stiffness in multiple sclerosis patients with spasticity. Muscle Nerve 16(1):69-76, 1993.

153. Dietz V, Quintern J, Berger W: Electrophysiological studies of gait in spasticity and rigidity. Evidence that altered mechanical properties of muscle contribute to hypertonia. Brain 104(3):431-449, 1981.

154. Thompson FJ, Reier PJ, Lucas CC, et al: Altered patterns of reflex excitability subsequent to contusion injury of the rat spinal cord. J Neurophysiol 68(5):1473-1486, 1992.

155. Thompson FJ, Reier PJ, Parmer R, et al: Inhibitory control of reflex excitability following contusion injury and neural tissue transplantation. Adv Neurol 59:175-184, 1993.

156. Thompson FJ, Parmer R, Reier PJ: Alteration in rate modulation of reflexes to lumbar motoneurons after midthoracic spinal cord injury in the rat. I. Contusion injury. J Neurotrauma 15(7):495-508, 1998.

157. Calancie B, Broton JG, Klose KJ, et al: Evidence that alterations in presynaptic inhibition contribute to segmental hypo- and hyperexcitability after spinal cord injury in man. Electroencephalogr Clin Neurophysiol 89(3):177-186, 1993.

158. Diamantopoulos E, Zander Olsen P: Excitability of spinal motor neurons in normal subjects and patients with spasticity, Parkinson rigidity and cerebellar hypotonia. J Neurol Neurosurg Psychiatry 30:325-331, 1967.

159. Ishikawa K, Ott K, Porter RW, et al: Low frequency depression of the H wave in normal and spinal man. Exp Neurol 15(1):140-156, 1966.

160. Little JW, Halar EM: H-reflex changes following spinal cord injury. Arch Phys Med Rehabil 66(1):19-22, 1985.

161. Nielsen J, Petersen N, Ballegaard M, et al: H-reflexes are less depressed following muscle stretch in spastic spinal cord injured patients than in healthy subjects. Exp Brain Res 97(1):173-176, 1993.

162. Hultborn H, Malmsten J: Changes in segmental reflexes following chronic spinal cord hemisection in the cat. I. Increased monosynaptic and polysynaptic ventral root discharges. Acta Physiol Scand 119(4):405-422, 1983.

163. Malmsten J: Time course of segmental reflex changes after chronic spinal cord hemisection in the rat. Acta Physiol Scand 119(4):435-443, 1983.

164. McCouch GP, Austin GM, Liu CN, et al: Sprouting as a cause of spasticity. J Neurophysiol 21(3):205-216, 1958.

165. Brodal P: The Central Nervous System: Structure and Function. New York: Oxford University Press, 1998.

166. Shefner JM, Berman SA, Sarkarati M, et al: Recurrent inhibition is increased in patients with spinal cord injury. Neurology 42(11):2162-2168, 1992.

167. Young RR: Spasticity: A review. Neurology 44(11 Suppl 9):S12-S20, 1994.

168. Dusart I, Schwab ME: Secondary cell death and the inflammatory reaction after dorsal hemisection of the rat spinal cord. Eur J Neurosci 6(5):712-724, 1994.

169. Edgar RE, Best LG, Quail PA, et al: Computer-assisted DREZ microcoagulation: posttraumatic spinal deafferentation pain. J Spinal Disord 6(1):48-56, 1993.

170. Eide PK, Stubhaug A, Stenehjem AE: Central dysesthesia pain after traumatic spinal cord injury is dependent on N-methyl-D-aspartate receptor activation. Neurosurgery 37(6):1080-1087, 1995.

171. Eriksson MB, Sjolund BH, Nielzen S: Long term results of peripheral conditioning stimulation as an analgesic measure in chronic pain. Pain 6(3):335-347, 1979.

172. Eyssette M, Rohmer F, Serratrice G, et al: Multi-centre, double-blind trial of a novel antispastic agent, tizanidine, in spasticity associated with multiple sclerosis. Curr Med Res Opin 10(10):699-708, 1988.

173. Glynn CJ, Jamous MA, Teddy PJ, et al: Role of spinal noradrenergic system in transmission of pain in patients with spinal cord injury. Lancet 2(8518):1249-1250, 1986.

174. Hachen HJ: Psychological, neurophysiological and therapeutic aspects of chronic pain: preliminary results with transcutaneous electrical stimulation [proceeedings]. Paraplegia 15(4):353-367, 1978.

175. Hansebout RR, Blight AR, Fawcett S, et al: 4-Aminopyridine in chronic spinal cord injury: a controlled, double-blind, crossover study in eight patients. J Neurotrauma 10(1):1-18, 1993.

176. Hao JX, Xu XJ, Aldskogius H, et al: Allodynia-like effects in rat after ischaemic spinal cord injury photochemically induced by laser irradiation. Pain 45(2):175-185, 1991.

177. Hao JX, Xu XJ, Urban L, et al: Repeated administration of systemic gabapentin alleviates allodynia-like behaviors in spinally injured rats. Neurosci Lett 280(3):211-214, 2000.

178. Andersen P, Eccles JC, Sears TA: Presynaptic inhibitory action of cerebral cortex on the spinal cord. Nature 194:740-741, 1962.

179. Carpenter D, Engberg I, Lundberg A: Primary afferent depolarization evoked from the brain stem and the cerebellum. Arch Ital Biol 104(1):73-85, 1966.

180. Lundberg A, Vyklicky L: Inhibition of transmission to primary afferents by electrical stimulation of the brain stem. Arch Ital Biol 104(1):86-97, 1966.

181. Martin RF, Haber LH, Willis WD: Primary afferent depolarization of identified cutaneous fibers following stimulation in medial brain stem. J Neurophysiol 42(3):779-790, 1979.

182. Proudfit HK, Larson AA, Anderson EG: The role of GABA and serotonin in the mediation of raphe-evoked spinal cord dorsal root potentials. Brain Res 195(1):149-165, 1980.

183. Rudomin P, Engberg I, Jankowska E, et al: Evidence of two different mechanisms involved in the generation of presynaptic depolarization of afferent and rubrospinal fibers in the cat spinal cord. Brain Res 189(1):256-261, 1980.

184. Rudomin P, Engberg I, Jimenez I: Mechanisms involved in presynaptic depolarization of group I and rubrospinal fibers in cat spinal cord. J Neurophysiol 46(3):532-548, 1981.

185. Rudomin P, Jimenez I, Solodkin M, et al: Sites of action of segmental and descending control of transmission on pathways mediating PAD of Ia- and Ib-afferent fibers in cat spinal cord. J Neurophysiol 50(4):743-769, 1983.

186. Sastry BS, Sinclair JG: Tonic inhibitory influence of a supraspinal monoaminergic system on presynaptic inhibition of an extensor monosynaptic reflex. Brain Res 124(1):109-120, 1977.

187. Remy-Neris O, Denys P, Daniel O, et al: Effect of intrathecal clonidine on group I and group II oligosynaptic excitation in paraplegics. Exp Brain Res 148(4):509-514, 2003.

188. Bose P, Parmer R, Thompson FJ: Velocity-dependent ankle torque in rats after contusion injury of the midthoracic spinal cord: time course. J Neurotrauma 19(10):1231-1249, 2002.

189. Harkema SJ, Hurley SL, Patel UK, et al: Human lumbosacral spinal cord interprets loading during stepping. J Neurophysiol 77(2):797-811, 1997.

190. Wrenn CC, Picklo MJ, Lappi DA, et al: Central noradrenergic lesioning using anti-DBH-saporin: anatomical findings. Brain Res 740(1-2):175-184, 1996.

191. Goldberger ME, Murray M: Patterns of sprouting and implications for recovery of function. Adv Neurol 47:361-385, 1988.

192. Goldberger ME, Murray M: Lack of sprouting and its presence after lesions of the cat spinal cord. Brain Res 241(2):227-239, 1982.

193. Murray M, Goldberger ME: Restitution of function and collateral sprouting in the cat spinal cord: the partially hemisected animal. J Comp Neurol 158(1):19-36, 1974.

194. Goldberger ME, Murray M: Restitution of function and collateral sprouting in the cat spinal cord: the deafferented animal. J Comp Neurol 158(1):37-53, 1974.

195. Tasker RR: Central pain states. *In* Bonica's Management of Pain, 3rd ed. Loeser JD, Butler SH, Chapman CR, et al (eds). Philadelphia: Lippincott Williams & Wilkins, 2001, pp. 433-457.

196. Loeser JD: Pain in spinal cord injury patients. *In* Bonica's Management of Pain, 3rd ed. Loeser JD, Butler SH, Chapman CR, et al (eds). Philadelphia: Lippincott Williams & Wilkins, 2001, pp. 613-619.

197. Loeser JD, Ward AA, Jr., White LE Jr: Chronic deafferentation of human spinal cord neurons. J Neurosurg 29(1):48-50, 1968.

198. Yezierski RP: Pain following spinal cord injury: the clinical problem and experimental studies. Pain 68(2-3):185-194, 1996.

199. Yezierski RP, Liu S, Ruenes GL, et al: Excitotoxic spinal cord injury: behavioral and morphological characteristics of a central pain model. Pain 75(1):141-155, 1998.

200. Yezierski RP: Pain following spinal cord injury: pathophysiology and central mechanisms. *In* Progress in Brain Research. Sandkuhler J, Bromm B, Gebhart GF (eds). Amsterdam: Elsevier, 2000, pp. 429-449.

201. Yezierski RP: Spinal cord injury: a model of central neuropathic pain. Neurosignals 14(4):182-193, 2005.

202. Defrin R, Ohry A, Blumen N, et al: Characterization of chronic pain and somatosensory function in spinal cord injury subjects. Pain 89(2-3):253-263, 2001.

203. Rintala DH, Loubser PG, Castro J, et al: Chronic pain in a community-based sample of men with spinal cord injury: prevalence, severity, and relationship with impairment, disability, handicap, and subjective well-being. Arch Phys Med Rehabil 79(6):604-614, 1998.

204. Stormer S, Gerner HJ, Gruninger W, et al: Chronic pain/dysaesthesiae in spinal cord injury patients: results of a multicentre study. Spinal Cord 35(7):446-455, 1997.

205. Hubscher CH, Johnson RD: Changes in neuronal receptive field characteristics in caudal brain stem following chronic spinal cord injury. J Neurotrauma 16(6):533-541, 1999.

206. Hulsebosch CE, Xu GY, Perez-Polo JR, et al: Rodent model of chronic central pain after spinal cord contusion injury and effects of gabapentin. J Neurotrauma 17(12):1205-1217, 2000.

207. Siddall P, Xu CL, Cousins M: Allodynia following traumatic spinal cord injury in the rat. Neuroreport 6(9):1241-1244, 1995.

208. Siddall PJ, Taylor DA, McClelland JM, et al: Pain report and the relationship of pain to physical factors in the first 6 months following spinal cord injury. Pain 81(1-2):187-197, 1999.

209. Vierck CJ Jr, Siddall P, Yezierski RP: Pain following spinal cord injury: animal models and mechanistic studies. Pain 89(1):1-5, 2000.

210. Bowsher D: Central pain: clinical and physiological characteristics. J Neurol Neurosurg Psychiatry 61(1):62-69, 1996.

211. Milhorat TH, Kotzen RM, Mu HT, et al: Dysesthetic pain in patients with syringomyelia. Neurosurgery 38(5):940-946, 1996.

212. Nathan PW, Smith MC, Cook AW: Sensory effects in man of lesions of the posterior columns and of some other afferent pathways. Brain 109 (Pt 5):1003-1041, 1986.

213. Weng HR, Lee JI, Lenz FA, et al: Functional plasticity in primate somatosensory thalamus following chronic lesion of the ventral lateral spinal cord. Neuroscience 101(2):393-401, 2000.

214. Bruce JC, Oatway MA, Weaver LC: Chronic pain after clip-compression injury of the rat spinal cord. 178(1):33-48, 2002.

215. Eide PK: Pathophysiological mechanisms of central neuropathic pain after spinal cord injury. 36(9):601-612, 1998.

216. Cui MY, Feng DJ, McAdoo DJ, et al: Periaqueductal gray stimulation-induced inhibition of nociceptive dorsal horn neurons in rats is associated with the release of norepinephrine, serotonin, and amino acids. 289:868-876, 1999.

217. Bethea JR, Castro M, Keane RW, et al: Traumatic spinal cord injury induces nuclear factor-kappaB activation. J Neurosci 18(9):3251-3260, 1998.

218. Willis WD: Central sensitization and plasticity following noxious stimulation. *In* Basic and Clinical Aspects of Chronic Abdominal Pain. Raybound HE (ed). Amsterdam: Elsevier, 1993, pp. 212-217.

219. Hao JX, Yu W, Wiesenfeld-Hallin Z, et al: Treatment of chronic allodynia in spinally injured rats: effects of intrathecal selective opioid receptor agonists. Pain 75(2-3):209-217, 1998.

220. Yezierski RP, Park SH: The mechanosensitivity of spinal sensory neurons following intraspinal injections of quisqualic acid in the rat. Neurosci Lett 157(1):115-119, 1993.

221. Beric A: Altered sensation and pain in spinal cord injury. *In* Recent Achievements in Restorative Neurology. Dimitrijevic MR, Wall PD (eds). Basel: Karger, 1990, pp. 27-36.

222. Levitt M, Levitt JH: The deafferentation syndrome in monkeys: dysesthesias of spinal origin. Pain 10(2):129-147, 1981.

223. Davis L, Martin J: Studies upon spinal cord injuries: II. The nature and treatment of pain. J Neurosurg 483-491, 1947.

Chapter 43

Peripheral Neuropathy

Joan R. Coates
G. Diane Shelton

Neuropathies comprise a group of disorders that affect the neuron of the motor unit. It is important for the veterinary surgeon to understand the pathophysiology of peripheral neuropathy in order to recognize clinical signs and make appropriate decisions for surgical intervention. Clinical presentation of orthopedic, spinal and muscle disorders often will mimic peripheral neuropathy and pose a diagnostic dilemma for the clinician. Conversely, polyneuropathy can cause paraparesis or tetraparesis that must be differentiated from orthopedic or spinal cord disease or other components of the motor unit (neuromuscular junction or muscle). In this chapter we review basic anatomy and physiology of the peripheral nervous system and associated clinical features of peripheral neuropathy. Other excellent resources to consider for more in-depth knowledge relevant to specific neuromuscular diseases and their categorical descriptions are provided by Shelton[1,2] and Braund.[3]

Anatomy and Physiology

The peripheral nervous system (PNS) consists of those structures (including cranial nerves and spinal nerves) containing motor, sensory, and autonomic nerve fibers or axons that connect the central nervous system (CNS) with somatic and visceral end organs. Anatomic structures that comprise the peripheral nervous system are derived from the neural crest from which several cranial nerves also receive contributions from ectodermal placodes.[4] Nerve fibers that terminate either in striated muscles or viscera are termed somatic or visceral, respectively. There are 12 pairs of cranial nerves with afferent and efferent fibers that traverse to and from the brainstem.[5] The spinal nerves usually number in 36 pairs for the dog and cat.[6] Of the spinal nerves, 8 are in the cervical (C1-8) region, 13 in the thoracic (T1-13) region, 7 in the lumbar (L1-L7) region, 3 in the sacral (S1-3) region, and 5 or more in the caudal region. Each pair of spinal nerves communicates with the spinal cord segment of the same number. The somatic peripheral nervous system (PNS) consists of ventral and dorsal rootlets, spinal nerve roots, spinal nerves, dorsal and ventral rami, plexuses, and individual peripheral nerves and their branches.[6] The C6-T2 spinal cord segments comprise the cervical intumescence from where the nerve roots of the brachial plexus originate.[7,8] The L4-S3 spinal cord segments comprise the lumbosacral intumescence which contributes to the cauda equina and the lumbosacral plexus.[9,10] Nerve roots are minimally myelinated and traverse within the subarachnoid space containing cerebrospinal fluid (CSF). Thus, nerve roots are more susceptible to traction injury, and exposure to toxic and infectious agents. The nerve roots exit as spinal nerves through intervertebral foramina as myelinated fibers. Similarly, cranial nerves exit from foramina of the skull.

The visceral nervous system includes components of the central and peripheral nervous system that are involved in the homeostatic control of body functions.[11] The autonomic nervous system is subdivided into parasympathetic and sympathetic and includes only the general visceral efferent or motor components.[12] The neural pathway consists of two neurons; the first neuron (preganglionic neuron) is located in the CNS and terminates in ganglia in the PNS. The second neuron (postganglionic neuron) is located outside the CNS in the ganglion and terminates on an effector organ. The parasympathetic division is known as the craniosacral division of the autonomic nervous system because preganglionic neurons are located in the brainstem and the sacral spinal cord. Preganglionic neurons are located in the parasympathetic nuclei of cranial nerves III, VII, IX, X, and XI and in the intermedial lateral gray matter of the sacral spinal cord. The sympathetic division is known as the thoracolumbar division of the autonomic nervous system. The preganglion neurons are located in the intermedial lateral gray matter of the thoracic and first four to five lumbar spinal cord segments. Preganglionic neurotransmission in both systems is cholinergic, by which acetylcholine binds to the nicotinic receptors on the postganglionic neuron. In the parasympathetic system, postganglionic neurotransmission occurs with the binding of acetylcholine to a muscarinic receptor of the effector organ; in the sympathetic system, the postganglionic neurons synapse on noradrenergic receptors via the neurotransmitter norepinephrine.[11]

An individual peripheral nerve contains a variable mix of nerve fibers, myelinated and unmyelinated.[6] Most peripheral nerves contain both motor and sensory axons. Motor axons of spinal nerves and cranial nerves originate from neurons that lie within the gray matter of the spinal cord (ventral horn) and brainstem, respectively. Cell bodies for sensory axons are contained within the dorsal root ganglia or ganglia of cranial nerves. One nerve fiber consists of an axon surrounded by a myelin sheath which is composed of neurolemma (sheath of Schwann). Afferent fibers (sensory) can be myelinated or unmyelinated. Efferent fibers (motor) to striated muscle are always myelinated. Unmyelinated efferent fibers are postganglionic sympathetic fibers supplying smooth muscles.

The peripheral nerve in cross-section is composed of many nerve fibers arranged into fascicles (Figure 43-1). The nerves have three separate connective tissue sheaths: endoneurium, peineurium, and epineurium.[13] The loosely arranged endoneurium immediately surrounds myelinated and unmyelinated fibers. Bundles of fibers are gathered into fascicles surrounded by a perineurium. The epineurial epineurium encases the nerve trunk, containing fascicles that are separated by mesoneurium (epifascicular epineurium). The epineurium contains connective tissue, small lymphatics, and blood vessels that supply the nerve. The number and size of fascicles within a nerve can vary from one nerve to another but also within the same nerve along its course.[14]

Neuron

A neuron consists of three parts: cell body (perikaryon or soma), dendrite, and axon. The cell body contains the nucleus. Dendrites are extensions of the cell body and function to transmit excitatory or inhibitory impulses toward the cell body. Axons are usually single, straight structures that project further away from the cell body than dendrites and branch near their synaptic terminus. Axons often acquire a myelin sheath. Communication of an electrical signal (action potential) between an axon terminal and the dendrite or somatic membrane of another neuron is called electrical transmission. The electrical impulse occupying the axonal terminal (presynapse) leads to release of a transmitter (chemical transmission) which interacts with receptor molecules in the postsynaptic membrane of the receiving cell.[15]

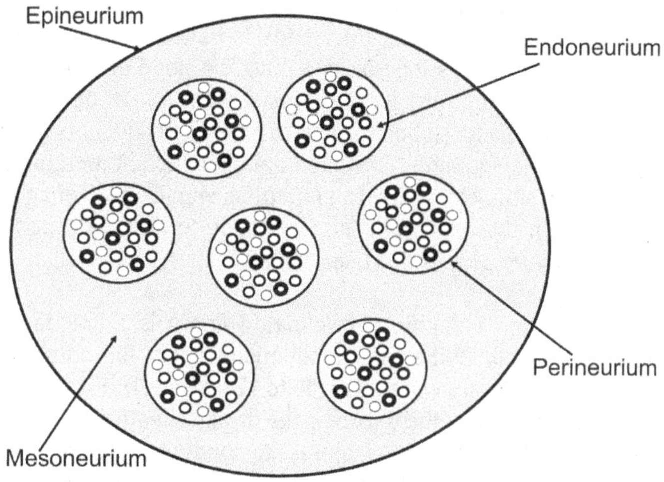

Figure 43-1. Peripheral nerve in cross section of 7 fascicles surrounded by perineurium that is ensheathed by epineurium and mesonerium. Nerve fibers of varying myelin thicknesses are separated by endoneurium.

Axon

The origin of the axon from the cell body is the axon hillock and initial segment, which are unmyelinated.[13] The axon hillock and initial segment are considered the trigger zone, which contains a high concentration of voltage-gated sodium channels.[15] This area is considered to have a low threshold and be the site for generation of an action potential. Conduction of an action potential is considered polarized relative to the cell body; it propagates in an orthodromic direction toward the terminus. An action potential that is artificially induced on the axon also can conduct toward the cell body (antidromic propagation).

The axoplasm contains neurofilaments, mitochondria, and agranular endoplasmic reticulum.[13] Axoplasmic flow is bidirectional along the axon. Longitudinally oriented neurofilaments and microtubules interconnected by cross-bridges transport substances away from the cell body to the axon terminal (anterograde transport) and from the distal axon to the cell body (retrograde transport). Anterograde and retrograde transport play an important pathophysiologic role in the transmission of neurotoxins (i.e., tetanus toxin) and neurotropic pathogens (i.e., rabies and pseudorabies viruses).[16] Flow rates differ as slow (1 mm/day) and fast (10 mm to 2 m/day).[13] Slow flow consists of soluble proteins and of particulate matter for growth and maintenance of the neuron. Fast flow consists of organelles, mitochondria, and materials for enzymatic reactions to facilitate synaptic transmission. Microtubules are organelles that facilitate fast axonal flow.

Myelin

Myelin is formed by Schwann cells in the PNS and oligodendrocytes in the CNS. Processes from these cells wrap around an axon in a unique multilamellar structure analogized as a "Swiss roll" to fuse with the inner axonal membrane. Myelin provides a role in axonal support and maintenance.[17] The correct thickness of the myelin sheath is regulated by a transmembrane protein expressed by the axon.[18] The myelin sheath is not continuous over the length of the axon but is interrupted at regular intervals (1 μm) at the ***nodes of Ranvier***, so that the axon membrane is in direct contact with the extracellular fluid.[13] The cylindrical sheath of myelin between the nodes is called the ***internode***. Internodes can be as long as one mm. The node of Ranvier is considered an electrotonic sink consisting of a high density of sodium channels for depolarization to occur.[19] Myelin acts as an insulator by having high resistance and low capacitance to the internode region. This allows an electrical impulse to propagate rapidly down the axon, jumping from node to node, a process called ***saltatory conduction*** (Figure 43-2).

The conduction velocity in myelinated fibers is much faster than in nonmyelinated axons. Conduction velocity for motor and sensory nerve fibers varies from 50 to 120 m/sec. The larger the diameter of the axon, the thicker is the myelin sheath. The longer the internodal distance, the faster is the conduction of the action potential. Small myelinated fibers (fast, sharp pain) conduct at rates of 12 to 30 m/sec; unmyelinated C fibers (slow, dull pain) conduct at much slower rates of 0.5 to 2 m/sec.

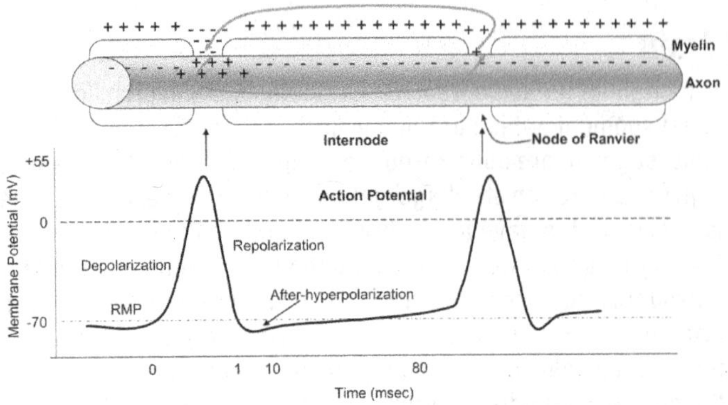

Figure 43-2. Saltatory conduction of an action potential along a myelinated axon. Transmembrane action potential currents (inward sodium movement and outward potassium movement) occur only at the nodes of Ranvier that contain a high density of voltage-gated sodium changes. The internodal region of the axon facilitates very rapid movement of currents down the axon. (Modified with permission from Blankenship JE: Neurophysiology. St. Louis, Mosby Inc. – Elsevier Science, 2003)[19]

Action Potential

The basis of electrical transmission within the nervous system is the action potential.[19] The action potential, "nerve impulse," is a brief electrical signal within nerve and muscle cells (Figure 43-2). The change in membrane potential represents a transient change from the resting state, in which the internal potential of the neuron moves from an equilibrium resting state (resting membrane potential -70 mV) to a positive value and then back to the resting state. At the resting potential (-60 mV), the electrical and concentration gradients act on sodium and potassium ions across the membrane. The gradients at rest are nearly equal for potassium, but for sodium both the concentration and electrical gradients are directed inward. The action potential is caused by the membrane's becoming suddenly permeable to sodium ions (depolarization) until the membrane potential reaches the sodium equilibrium potential (+55 mV). As the electrical gradient of sodium and potassium become equal, the electrical gradient for potassium is directed outward. If the neuron is made highly permeable to potassium and impermeable to sodium, the potassium ions readily move out of the cell in response to the outwardly directed concentration and electrical gradients. The efflux of potassium ions causes the neuron to become increasingly negative (repolarization) until the membrane reaches a potassium equilibrium potential (-75 mV; hyperpolarization).

Motor Unit

A motor unit is composed of a neuron cell body, its axon, the neuromuscular junction, and associated muscle fibers. A group of myofibers innervated by one neuron is considered a motor unit. An abnormality in any portion of the motor unit can result in clinical signs of neuromuscular disease – lower motor neuron. The functional component of the motor unit involves the ***reflex arc***. The arc consists of a sense organ, an afferent neuron (cell body in dorsal root ganglion), one or more synapses centrally, an efferent neuron, and an effector organ. An all-or-none action potential is generated in the afferent nerve and modulated centrally to be generated again as an all-or-none potential in the efferent nerve. A reflex with a single central synapse is a monosynaptic reflex (i.e., patellar reflex); a reflex with more than one central synapse (interneurons) is a polysynaptic reflex (i.e., flexor withdrawal reflex).

The LMN system consists of three functional divisions: general somatic efferent, special visceral efferent, and general visceral efferent systems.[20] The general somatic efferent system consists of spinal motor neurons and cranial nerves III, IV, VI, and XII, which innervate voluntary striated muscles. The special visceral efferent system consists of cranial nerves V, VII, IX, X, and XI, which innervate voluntary striated muscle associated with respiratory and gastrointestinal functions. The general visceral efferent system consists of the parasympathetic and sympathetic nervous systems that innervate involuntary smooth muscle.

Pathophysiology of Neuropathy

Peripheral neuropathies consist of disorders that affect the axon -- axonopathies; the Schwann cells or myelin directly -- myelinopathies (demyelinating diseases); or both the axons and Schwann cells -- mixed axonal and demyelinating diseases. Underlying pathologic processes of the peripheral nerve include Wallerian degeneration, axonal degeneration, and segmental and diffuse myelin degeneration (Figure 43-3).[21] In most cases, these pathologic reactions are not disease-specific but occur in various combinations with peripheral nerve disease. Axonal degeneration and demyelination specify the underlying pathologic process and location to the peripheral nerve, but rarely occur as separate disease entities. Central neuropathies that affect the neuronal cell bodies are termed motor neuron disease.

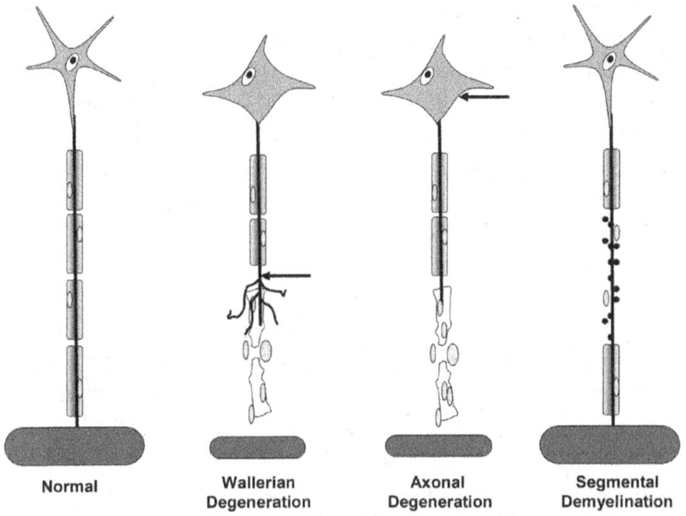

Figure 43-3. Basic pathologic processes affecting peripheral nerves. Wallerian degeneration shows degeneration of the axon and myelin distal to the site of axonal damage (arrow). In axonal degeneration, primary neuronal disease causes distal degeneration of the axon and myelin (arrow). Note the eccentric displacement of the nucleus and swelling of the neuron cell body with Wallerian degeneration and axonal degeneration. Both Wallerian and axonal degeneration cause neurogenic muscle atrophy. With segmental demyelination the axon is spared, thus no muscle atrophy occurs.

Wallerian Degeneration

Original classifications of peripheral nerve disorders were based on anatomic and clinical observations following focal nerve damage. Waller demonstrated predictable degeneration of nerve fibers in the distal stump of a transected nerve, describing alterations of the axolemma with subsequent dissolution of axons and myelin.[22] Seddon followed with a clinical classification of nerve injury, using morphologic and electrophysiologic studies.[23] ***Neurapraxia*** is a transient interruption of the nerve function and conduction without associated axonal degeneration. Pathology involves myelin injury or an ischemic process. Recovery can occur within hours to weeks. ***Axonotmesis*** describes focal destruction of axons and myelin sheaths from the neuronal cell body. The endoneurium and Schwann cell sheath remain intact. Axonal and myelin degeneration (***Wallerian degeneration***) occurs distal to the lesion site. Wallerian degeneration consists of degeneration of both the axon cylinder and myelin sheath distal to the site of axonal damage. Severance of the axon prevents transport of organelles to the distal axon for replenishing membrane reconstruction and neurotransmitter processes. The motor neuron undergoes chromatolysis with rounding of the cell body, eccentrically displaced nucleus, and dispersion of chromatin. Recovery is prolonged (1 mm per day), occurring first in nerve segments closest to the site of damage. Completeness and length of recovery depend on the degree of nerve disruption and the distance to the end organ. ***Neurotmesis*** describes complete transection of the nerve from its cell body. Regenerating axons often take an aberrant course with fibroblastic formation to form a neuroma. Both axonotmesis and neurotmesis are followed by Wallerian degeneration.

Axonal Degeneration

Axonal degeneration results from disease within the neuronal cell body or of the axon itself. Often the degeneration of the axon and its myelin sheath begins distally and extends proximally. The neuron undergoes chromatolysis. This process has been termed as "dying-back" neuropathy, distal axonopathy, or distal sensorimotor neuropathy. These processes preferentially affect long, large-caliber, myelinated nerve fibers. Clinical signs usually are recognized first in the distal limbs as a consequence of the distance of the nerve from the cell body. Both axonal degeneration and Wallerian degeneration cause neurogenic muscle atrophy. The time of onset usually is considered chronic, with a progressive time-course. These disorders often are inherited, idiopathic, or toxic in origin.

Demyelination

Demyelination is caused by disease of the Schwann cell or myelin sheath. Demyelination is loss of the myelin sheath along the length of the internode (segmental demyelination) or near the paranodal area (paranodal demyelination). Disease can occur continuously (diffuse demyelination) or randomly along the nerve path. Diffuse myelinopathies occur with inherited, metabolic, and toxic disorders. In immune-mediated neuropathies, nerves are damaged by cellular or humoral mechanisms on various components of myelin. Repeated processes of demyelination and remyelination also occur with some disease processes, i.e., inflammatory demyelinating polyneuropathies. Remyelination restores function. Disruption of the myelin sheath causes the electrical current to dissipate through the internode as a result of increased capacitance and decreased resistance. This results in a longer time to charge the next internode, thus prolonging the conduction time. Conduction failure occurs with severe demyelination.

Diagnostic Approach

Establishing an accurate diagnosis is based on following a logical sequence of diagnostic tests. History provides the signalment, presenting clinical signs, background, and time of onset and temporal progression of clinical signs. Specifically, disorders of the motor unit with acute onset include polyradiculoneuritis, tick paralysis, botulism, and fulminant myasthenia gravis. Myopathic and neuromuscular junction (i.e., myasthenia gravis) diseases often are episodic in onset. Signalment is especially important in young animals with a predilection for breed-specific neuropathies. A physical examination is performed to localize the clinical signs and detect other systemic abnormalities. The neurologic examination will establish the existence of peripheral nervous system disease and further assist with determining disease symmetry and distribution (focal, multifocal, or diffuse). The neurologic examination should include sensory testing. Proper neuroanatomic localization is crucial to the direction of the diagnostic approach. A complete blood count, serum chemistry (including creatine kinase concentration and electrolytes), and a urinalysis serve to establish a baseline health profile and further identify other systemic abnormalities. Thoracic radiography may show evidence of concurrent megaesophagus and aspiration pneumonia, which can be a sequela of peripheral neuropathy.

Additionally, thoracic radiography and abdominal ultrasonography are used to screen for underlying metastatic disease and evidence of paraneoplastic neuropathy. CSF analysis will show abnormalities in cellularity and protein concentration with some peripheral neuropathies. Serology is useful to evaluate for infectious and immune-mediated diseases. Endocrine function testing, especially thyroid hormone, will further delineate any underlying cause of the neuropathy.

Diagnostic Electrophysiology

Electrophysiology is useful for determining disease localization within the motor unit and the extent of the disease process.[24] Temporal development of neuropathies has important implications for diagnostic yield of the electrophysiologic examination. Neuropathic disease must be present for 3 to 7 days before evidence can be detected by electrodiagnostic examination.[25] Diagnostic electrophysiology is thoroughly reviewed in Chapter: Electrodiagnosis

Briefly, ***electromyography*** (EMG) will assess electrical activity within a discrete region of an accessible muscle. The activity is recorded by inserting a needle electrode into the muscle. The pattern of electrical activity in muscle has been characterized and abnormalities have been correlated with some disorders at different levels of the motor unit. Relaxed muscle normally shows no spontaneous electrical activity except in the end-plate region, but various types of abnormal activity occur spontaneously in diseased muscle. Typically, abnormalities caused by denervation occur on EMG with axonal disease but not with pure demyelinating disorders.

Nerve conduction studies provide a technique of confirming the presence and extent of peripheral nerve damage. Studies of several types of acquired and hereditary axonal and demyelinating neuropathies have shown different patterns of distribution, which further assist with differential diagnosis. ***Motor nerve conduction studies*** are performed by recording the electrical response of a muscle to stimulation of its motor nerve at two or more points along its course. This permits the conduction velocity, amplitude, and duration of action potentials to be determined in the fastest-conducting motor fibers between the points of stimulation. Results may give an indication of altered function of axons and myelin. ***Sensory nerve conduction studies*** are performed by determining the conduction velocity and amplitude of action potentials in sensory fibers when these fibers are stimulated and responses recorded at another point along the course of the nerve. Conduction studies do not provide information regarding smaller fiber function; thus autonomic nerve abnormalities go undetected. ***F wave- response studies*** evaluate the latter motor response; F waves may be abnormal when lesions of the proximal portions (nerve roots) of the peripheral nervous system are present.

Muscle and Nerve Biopsy

Histopathologic examination of a muscle biopsy specimen is a critical part of the evaluation of a motor unit disease and can indicate whether the underlying weakness is neurogenic or myopathic in origin.[26] With neuropathic disease, myofibers can show angular atrophy, small and large grouped atrophy, fiber-type grouping if denervation has been followed by reinnervation, replacement of muscle fibers by fatty tissue, and pyknotic nuclear clumps in end-stage disease (Figure 43-4). In myopathic disease, pathologic changes can include variability in fiber size, necrosis and phagocytosis, cellular infiltrations, connective tissue expansion, cytoarchitectural abnormalities, and inclusions and vacuoles (Figure 43-5).

A properly processed peripheral nerve biopsy often provides insight into the pathologic process of peripheral nerve disease. Techniques for collection of nerve biopsies have been described in detail, but often consist of a fascicular biopsy.[26,27] Evaluation of resin-embedded semi-thin sections provides the most information regarding axonal degeneration and regeneration, demyelination and remyelination, and abnormalities of supporting structures (Figure 43-6). In selected cases, electron microscopy, teased nerve fibers, and nerve fiber morphometry can provide additional information. Processing of peripheral nerve biopsies for only paraffin or frozen sectioning provides only limited information.

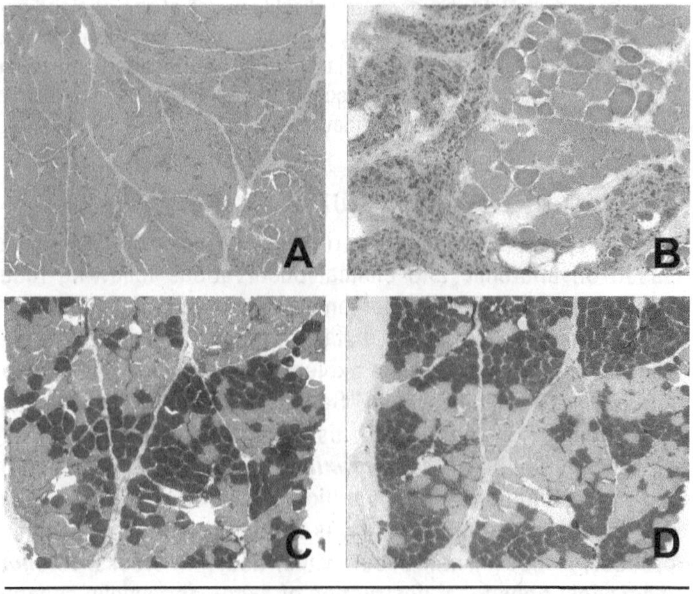

Figure 43-4. Specific patterns of muscle fiber atrophy are present in denervation. Angular atrophied fibers may be scattered among fibers of normal size or be present in small and large groups (A: H&E stain). With end-stage denervation, pynotic nuclear clumps are obvious (B: H&E stain), and muscle fibers are replaced with fatty or connective tissue. Fiber type grouping is an indicator of chronicity and reinnervation (C: ATPase reaction at pH 9.8; type 1 fibers are light and type 2 fibers are dark; D: acid reversal of ATPase reaction at pH 4.3 with type 1 fibers dark and type 2 fibers light). Note loss of the normal mosaic pattern of muscle fiber types. Magnification X 100 for all images.

Clinical Features and Differentials

Pattern recognition of clinical signs assists with ascertaining an underlying cause and formulating a diagnostic plan and possibilities of treatment. Specifically, establishing a time course of the disease process is informative. Most acute polyneuropathies develop over 2 to 3 days and include inflammatory, immunologic, toxic, or vascular causes. Some toxic, nutritional, and systemic

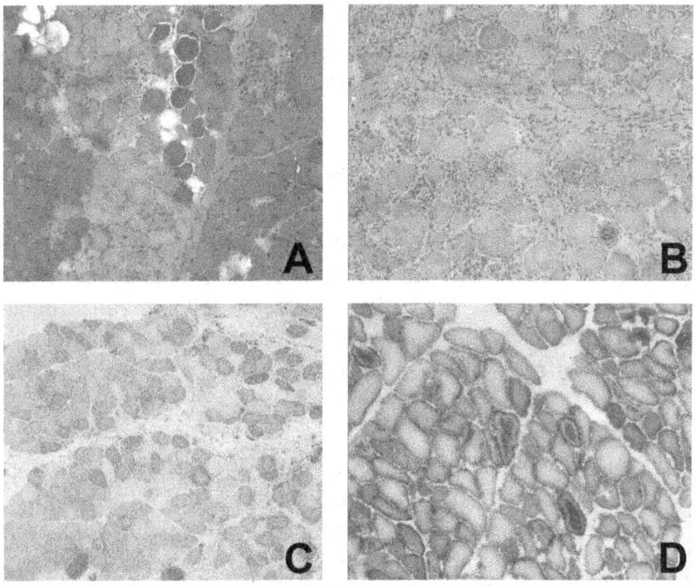

Figure 43-5. Pathologic changes typical of muscle disease include degeneration and regeneration as in muscular dystrophy (A: H&E), multifocal areas of mononuclear cell infiltration in inflammatory myopathy (B: H&E), excessive accumulation of storage products such as neutral triglycerides in lipid-storage myopathy (C: oil red O stain), and cytoarchitectural changes such as the central accumulations of mitochondria in inherited myopathy of Great Danes, previously called central core myopathy (D: succinic dehydrogenase reaction). Magnification X 100 for all images.

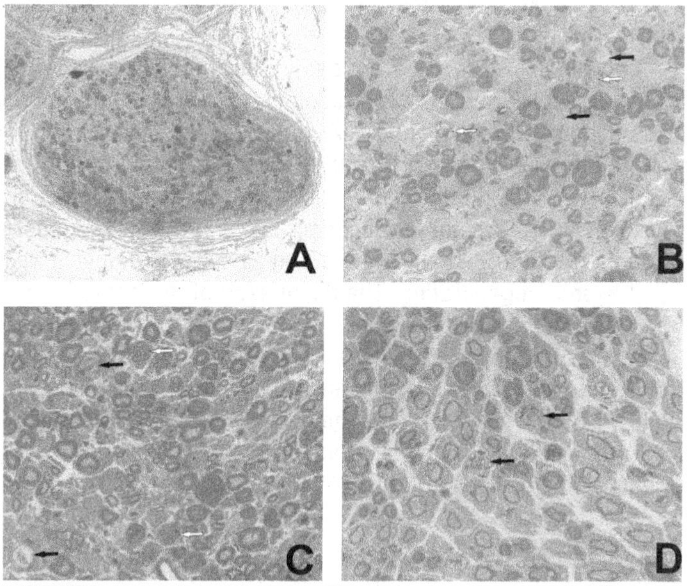

Figure 43-6. Pathologic changes in resin-embedded nerve-biopsy sections typical of peripheral nerve disease. Nerve fiber loss and endoneurial fibrosis (A) are common findings in dogs with chronic peripheral neuropathy and may also be found in cats. Nerve fiber loss is usually a sequelae of chronic axonal degeneration (B). Myelin ovoids (black arrows) and foamy macrophages (white arrows) may be seen. Active axonal degeneration (C; black arrows) and regenerating clusters (white arrows) are commonly found. In chronic demyelinating disorders (D), onion bulbs (arrows) and inappropriately thinly myelinated fibers are typical of recurrent episodes of demyelination and remyelination. Toluidine blue-basic fucshin, magnification X 40 for A and X 100 for B-D.

diseases of the nerve will develop over weeks. Chronic neuropathies that develop over weeks to months include inherited and/or degenerative, metabolic, paraneoplastic, and idiopathic diseases. Chronic neuropathy also may have a time course with intermittent periods of improvement.

Patterns of peripheral neuropathy are described based on distribution: neuronopathy, polyneuropathy, polyradiculopathy, mononeuropathy, and plexopathies. Neuronopathies are selective for loss of sensory or motor neurons. Polyneuropathies are diffuse lesions of the peripheral nerves that produce weakness, sensory disturbance, and/or reflex abnormalities. In general, polyneuropathies involve several nerves and are bilateral and symmetrical. Differential diagnoses for symmetric neuropathies include degenerative, metabolic, idiopathic, and toxic diseases. Idiopathic polyneuropathy is the most common diagnosis. Polyradiculopathies imply nerve root involvement and present with asymmetric signs, weakness, and multifocal sensory disturbance. Asymmetric and multifocal neuropathies often are associated with inflammatory, immune–mediated, or ischemic disease.

Mononeuropathy is a disorder of a single peripheral or cranial nerve, often owing to trauma or entrapment and, less commonly, from tumor infiltration, inflammation, and ischemic infarction. Mononeuropathies of cranial nerves also occur as idiopathic disease. Plexopathies involve multiple nerves within the brachial or lumbar plexus and usually affect one limb. Disorders of the brachial plexus and other mononeuropathies (Table 43-1) are covered in more detail in Chapter 44: Traumatic and Neoplastic Diseases of the Brachial Plexus.

Table 43-1. Differentials for Mononeuropathies in Dogs and Cats

Disease Category	Specific Diseases
Neoplasia	Nerve sheath tumor, lymphosarcoma, metastasis
Inflammation	Brachial plexus neuritis
Trauma	Brachial plexus avulsion, injection injury, iatrogenic surgical trauma, lumbosacral injury, pelvic fractures, humeral and femoral fractures
Toxic	Tetanus
Vascular	Thromboembolic disease, fibrocartilagenous embolism

Peripheral Nerve Disease

Peripheral neuropathies are broadly classified as motor neuron disease, motor neuropathy/radiculopathy, sensory neuropathy, autonomic neuropathy, and mixed neuropathy. Most peripheral neuropathies or polyneuropathies involving spinal nerves are considered mixed neuropathies that affect motor, sensory, and autonomic nerves in varying degrees. Pathologic studies of peripheral neuropathies show a combination of demyelination and axonal degeneration. The distal axon of the nerve is more sensitive to disease as a result of its distance from the cell body and interruption of axonal transport. Some peripheral nerve diseases affecting the axons and myelin involve both the CNS and PNS, but clinical signs manifest as disease of the PNS. Differential diagnoses for polyneuropathy consist of a wide spectrum of diseases (Table 43-2).

Motor Neuron Disease

Motor neuronopathies are disorders of the ventral horn cells that cause generalized weakness. Loss of motor neurons results in progressive weakness with muscle atrophy. A characteristic feature of motor neuron disease that differs from peripheral neuropathy is muscular weakness and fasciculations with muscle atrophy, but preservation of reflexes until the disease is advanced.[28] Motor neuron diseases are rare, usually occur in young growing animals, and have an insidious and progressive clinical disease course. Inherited forms have been described in the Brittany spaniel,[29] English pointer,[30] Swedish Lapland dogs,[31] and the Maine coon cat,[32] and are suspected for other breeds.[28] An adult form has been reported in cats.[33]

Motor Neuropathy/Radiculopathy (Polyneuropathies and Mononeuropathies)

Peripheral neuropathies that involve the motor nerve and nerves roots often manifest as hallmark signs of lower motor neuron disease with impairment of motor function. Motor neuropathies are characterized by a flaccid paresis or paralysis, postural reaction deficits, neurogenic muscle atrophy, and reduced to absent spinal reflexes.[22] Muscle fasciculations, spasms, and cramps also can occur. Tremors can be a clinical feature with some pure demyelinating diseases.[34,35] Neurogenic muscle atrophy is rapid and severe, occurring within 1 to 2 weeks from onset of clinical signs and progressing to joint contracture in chronic cases.[3] Muscle atrophy is a clinical feature for Wallerian degeneration and axonal degeneration, but not for pure myelinopathies (axons still remain intact).

Gait evaluation commonly reveals moderate to severe sensory ataxia with loss of proprioceptive fibers. Animals with lower motor neuron dysfunction often have a shortened stride and an inability to support weight associated with the appendicular and axial musculature. Limb tone is reduced, and flaccidity often becomes more apparent in the distal limbs.[36] Limb posture will be crouched with tendency for joints to be flexed. Ventroflexion of the neck also signifies generalized weakness. Dogs with only distal polyneuropathy often show a high-steppage or pseudohypermetric pelvic limb gait.[37] This represents a compensatory response to allow the carpi or tarsi to flip forward for limb placement. It is not uncommon for polyneuropathy to manifest as paraparesis before tetraparesis because the longer (sciatic nerve) and more myelinated proprioceptive fibers usually are affected first.

Loss of tendon and flexor withdrawal reflexes is a sign of peripheral nerve disease. Early in acute polyneuropathy, the reflexes may be diminished although not absent, but they become more reduced from day to day. In disease of small fibers, tendon reflexes still may be retained.[38] Conversely, reflexes can be diminished out of proportion to weakness because of involvement of the large afferent fibers of muscle spindles.

Disease of spinal nerves (mixed nerves) often causes sensory loss along with motor deficits distal to the lesion.[39] Hypesthesia or anesthesia may be evident with involvement of the sensory component of the nerve. Hypesthesia denotes decreased sensation or partial lesion; anesthesia refers to a complete lesion. Sensory function may be normal or decreased with polyneuropathy. A hallmark feature of mononeuropathy associated with complete nerve transection is anesthesia of a specific dermatome. A dermatome refers to a cutaneous region innervated by afferent nerve fibers from a single spinal nerve.[6] Cutaneous sensory testing uses the ***two-step pinch technique*** to assess nociception (superficial and deep pain) with the autonomous zone of the dermatome being tested.[40] A conscious response or withdrawal reflex indicates function of the peripheral nerve being tested. Loss of deep nociception indicates a poor prognosis.

Sensory disturbance also may reflect increased sensitivity to stimuli. Pain associated with disease of the peripheral nerve is termed *neuropathic* pain.[38] In humans, types of neuropathic pain manifest as symptoms (i.e., tingling, burning, prickling, etc.) that we are unable to recognize in animals. Sensory disturbances in animals may manifest as clinical signs of dysesthesia (paresthesia) and hyperesthesia.[39] Hyperesthesia is a general term for increased cutaneous sensitivity from a non-noxious stimulus. Dysesthesia denotes an abnormal sensation without application of an external stimulus. Animals with peripheral nerve regeneration are predisposed to mutilation of the anatomic area undergoing reinnervation as a result of axonal sprouting and excessive excitation causing dysesthesia.[39] Dysesthesia also may result from irritation of the nerve sheath itself. Tactile stimuli may cause a perversion of sensation or allodynia, which refers to a type of stimulus that evokes another type of sensation (i.e., touch as pain). This may be related to the type of pain observed with polyradiculopathies and diabetes mellitus.

Sensory Neuropathy

An animal with a *pure* sensory neuropathy may show gait and postural reaction deficits (sensory ataxia), decreased nociception, paresthesia, evidence of self-mutilation, and reduced to absent spinal reflexes *without* muscle atrophy.[36] Pure sensory neuropathies are rare and often have an inherited cause.[41] Some acquired diseases also may show sensory disturbances.[42] Unlike in humans, clinical signs of sensory loss (numbness, pain, temperature alterations) associated with polyneuropathy in animals often are impossible to recognize or go undetected.

Table 43-2. Differentials for Polyneuropathies in Dogs and Cats

Disease Categories		Specific Disorders in Dogs	Specific Disorders in Cats
Motor Neuronopathy			
Inherited		Brittany spaniels, English pointer, German shepherd, Rottweiler, Doberman pinscher, Griffon Briquet Vendeen dog, saluki, collie, giant breed dogs, Swedish Lapland dog	Maine coon cat, domestic short-haired
Idiopathic		Dysautonomia	Dysautonomia
Motor Neuropathy/Radiculopathy			
Inherited	Storage diseases	Fucosidosis, globoid cell leukodystrophy	Globoid cell leukodystrophy, glycogenosis type IV, mannosidosis, Niemann–Pick disease type A
	Distal sensorimotor polyneuropathies	Alaskan malamute, German shepherd, Great Dane, Leonberger dog, Rottweiler, Doberman pinscher (dancing Doberman disease), laryngeal paralysis polyneuropathy complex (Dalmatian, Rottweiler, Pyrenean mountain dog)	
	Myelin-associated polyneuropathies	Congenital hypomyelination (Golden retriever), hypertrophic neuropathy (Tibetan mastiff)	Laminin alpha2-deficient muscular dystrophy (domestic short-haired cat, Siamese cat), hypertrophic polyneuropathy (domestic long-and short-haired cats)
	Central-peripheral distal axonopathy	Progressive axonopathy in Boxers, giant axonal neuropathy in German shepherd	Birman cat distal polyneuropathy
Metabolic		Hypothyroidism, hypoglycemia, insulinoma, diabetes mellitus	Diabetes mellitus, hyperchylomicronemia in cats, hyperoxaluria in cats
Paraneoplastic		Multiple myeloma, bronchogenic carcinoma, leiomyosarcoma, hemangiosarcoma, anaplastic sarcoma, synovial sarcoma, adenocarcinomas, mammary gland neoplasms, lymphosarcoma	Rare in cats, lymphosarcoma
Nutritional			Phenylalanine and tyrosine deficiency
Idiopathic		Chronic relapsing demyelinating polyradiculoneuritis, canine chronic axonal degeneration, chronic polyneuritis, distal sensorimotor polyneuropathy	Acute idiopathic polyneuropathy, chronic inflammatory demyelinating polyneuropathy, chronic relapsing polyneuropathy, vaccine-induced polyneuropathy
Inflammatory/Immune		Protozoal polyradiculoneuritis, acute canine polyradiculoneuropathy (Coonhound paralysis)	Feline leukemia virus, feline immunodeficiency virus
Toxic		Drugs – vincristine, cisplatin, aminoglycosides; heavy metals (lead, mercury, thallium, zinc); insecticides – organophosphate compounds	Insecticides – organophosphate delayed neuropathy, pyrethrins; drugs – vincristine, salinomycin; heavy metals – thallium, mercury
Vascular		Vasculitis, multifocal thromboses	Vasculitis
Sensory Neuropathy			
Inherited		Long-haired Dachshund, English pointer, Short-haired pointer, Jack Russell terrier	
Metabolic		Diabetic neuropathy	Diabetic neuropathy
Idiopathic		Sensory ganglioneuritis	
Traumatic		Reinnervation	Reinnervation
Autonomic Neuropathy			
Idiopathic		Dysautonomia	Dysautonomia
Toxic		Strychnine, tetanus, botulism, organophosphate compounds	Strychnine, tetanus, organophosphate compounds

Autonomic Neuropathy

Autonomic nerve dysfunctions arise coincident with a variety of diseases. Autonomic neuropathy can occur as a single disease entity (dysautonomia) or in conjunction with other polyneuropathies. In veterinary medicine, the term ***dysautonomia*** refers to acute or subacute idiopathic panautonomic failure in animals.[43] Common clinical signs of autonomic nerve dysfunction include pupillary impairment, altered tear production and salivation, micturition dysfunction, gastrointestinal stasis, and decreased heart rate variability. These signs can be isolated to a single nerve (i.e., Horner's syndrome) or be multiple as with panautonomic nerve dysfunction. Horner's syndrome (miosis, enophthalmos, ptosis, and third-eyelid protrusion) can occur with disease of the first, second, or third order neuron system. Differential diagnoses include trauma, inflammation, neoplasia, or idiopathic causes.[44] Lower motor neuron injuries (trauma, iatrogenic) are the most common cause of Horner's syndrome in animals.[45]

Cranial Nerve Disease

Peripheral neuropathy of cranial nerves can occur with focal, multifocal, or diffuse (polyneuropathy) disease. Mentation, gait, postural reactions, and spinal reflexes are normal with focal neuropathy of a cranial nerve. Typically, only one cranial nerve is affected. If disease is in the brainstem, mentation, postural reactions, gait, and multiple cranial nerves will show abnormalities. Neurologic deficits are more severe on the ipsilateral side. Myopathic and neuromuscular junction diseases also can mimic neuropathy of cranial nerves, i.e,. myasthenia gravis will manifest clinical signs of megaesophagus (regurgitation). Some neuropathies are specific for a particular cranial nerve (Table 43-3, page 242).[46-48] These disorders usually are congenital or idiopathic in origin. Idiopathic neuropathies more commonly affect cranial nerves V and VII.[47] Multifocal disease processes include some hematogenous neoplasms and inflammatory diseases that may cause asymmetric multiple cranial nerve deficits.[49] Neoplastic disease can affect multiple cranial nerves by mass effect or direct extension. Many cranial nerves are located within the superficial structures of the head and are more susceptible to trauma.[47]

Multiple cranial nerve deficits with generalized LMN signs should suggest polyneuropathy. Cranial nerves V, VII, VIII, IX, X, and XI usually are involved. Animals with polyneuropathy may also have clinical signs of dysphagia, dysphonia, and dyspnea.[47] Dyspnea associated with upper respiratory tract signs suggests laryngeal paralysis.[50] The laryngeal abductor muscles are innervated by the recurrent laryngeal nerve, which is one of the longest peripheral nerves and thus susceptible to distal neuropathy. Polyneuropathy must be considered as an underlying cause of laryngeal paralysis.[51] Diffuse motor neuropathies also cause respiratory compromise if the intercostal and phrenic nerves are involved.

References

1. Shelton GD: The Veterinary Clinics of North America: Small Animal Practice Neuromuscular Diseases I. Philadelphia:WB Saunders, 2002.

2. Shelton GD: Veterinary Clinics of North America: Small Animal Practice Neuromuscular Diseases II. Philadelphia:WB Saunders, 2004.

3. Braund KG: Neuropathic disorders. *In* Clinical Neurology in Small Animals - Localization, Diagnosis and Treatment. Braund KG (ed). Ithaca: International Veterinary Information Service (www.ivis.org), 2003.

4. Noden DM, de Lahunta A: Peripheral nervous system and ear. *In* The Embryology of Domestic Animals: Developmental Mechanisms and Malformations. Noden DM, de Lahunta A (eds)., Baltimore: Williams & Wilkins, 1985, pp. 120-139.

5. Evans HE, Kitchell RL: Cranial nerves and cutaneous innervation of the head. *In* Miller's Anatomy of the Dog. Evans HE, de Lahunta A (eds).. Philadelphia:WB Saunders, 1993, pp. 953-987.

6. Kitchell RL, Evans HE: The spinal nerves. *In* Miller's Anatomy of the Dog. Evans HE, de Lahunta A (eds). Philadelphia:WB Saunders, 1993, pp. 829-893.

7. Bailey CS, Kitchell RL, Johnson RD: Spinal nerve root origins of the cutaneous nerves arising from the canine brachial plexus. Am J Vet Res 43:820-825, 1982.

8. Bailey CS: Patterns of cutaneous anesthesia associated with brachial plexus avulsions in the dog. J Am Vet Med Assoc 185:889-899, 1984.

9. Bailey CS, Kitchell RL, Haghighi SS, Johnson RD: Spinal nerve root origins of the cutaneous nerves of the canine pelvic limb. Am J Vet Res 49:115-119, 1988.

10. Haghighi SS, Kitchell RL, Johnson RD, et al: Electrophysiologic studies of the cutaneous innervation of the pelvic limb of male dogs. Am J Vet Res 52:352-362, 1991.

11. Hasser EM, Schadt JC: Autonomic physiology. Semin Vet Med Surg (Small Anim) 5:12-16, 1990.

12. Amann JF, Constantinescu GM: The anatomy of the visceral and autonomic nervous systems. Semin Vet Med Surg (Small Anim) 5:4-11, 1990.

13. Peters A, Palay SL, Webster H: The Fine Structure of the Nervous System: Neurons and Their Supporting Cells. New York:Oxford University Press, 2001.

14. Stewart JD: Peripheral nerve fascicles: Anatomy and clinical relevance. Muscle Nerve 28:525-541, 2003.

15. Kandel ER, Schwartz JH, Jessell TM: Principles of Neural Science. New York: McGraw-Hill, 2000.

16. Von Bartheld CS: Axonal transport and neuronal transcytosis of trophic factors, tracers, and pathogens. J Neurobiol 58:295-314, 2003.

17. Edgar JM, Garbern J: The myelinated axon is dependent on the myelinating cell for support and maintenance: molecules involved. J Neurosci Res 76:593-598, 2004.

18. French-Constant C, Colognato H, Franklin RJM: The mysteries of myelin unwrapped. Science 304:688-689, 2004.

19. Blankenship JE: Neurophysiology. Philadelphia:Mosby, 2003.

20. de Lahunta A: Veterinary Neuroanatomy and Clinical Neurology. Philadelphia:WB Saunders, 1983.

21. Duncan ID: Peripheral neuropathy in the dog and cat. Prog Vet Neurol 2:111-128, 1991.

22. de Lahunta A: Lower motor neuron-general somatic efferent system. *In* de Lahunta A (ed). Veterinary Neuroantaomy and Clinical Neurology. Philadelphia:WB Saunders, 1983, pp. 53-94.

23. Seddon HJ: Three types of nerve injury. Brain 66:237-288, 1943.

24. Cuddon PA: Electrophysiology in neuromuscular disease. Vet Clin North Am Small Anim Pract 32:31-62, 2002.

25. Griffiths IR, Duncan ID: Some studies of the clinical neurophysiology of denervation in the dog. Res Vet Sci 17:377-383, 1974.

26. Dickinson PJ, LeCouteur RA: Muscle and nerve biopsy. Vet Clin North Am Small Anim Pract 32:63-102, 2002.

27. Braund KG, Walker TL, Vandevelde M: Fascicular nerve biopsy in the dog. Am J Vet Res 40:1025-1030, 1979.

28. Olby N: Motor neuron disease: inherited and acquired. Vet Clin North Am Small Anim Pract 34: 1403-1418, 2004.

29. Lorenz MD, Cork LC, Griffin JW, et al: Hereditary spinal muscular atrophy in Brittany Spaniels: clinical manifestations. J Am Vet Med Assoc 175:833-839, 1979.

30. Inada S, Sakamoto H, Haruta K, et al: A clinical study on hereditary progressive neurogenic muscular atrophy in Pointer dogs. Nippon Juigaku Zasshi 40:539-547, 1978.

31. Sandefeldt E, Cummings JF, de Lahunta A: Animal model of human disease. Infantile spinal muscular atrophy, Werdnig-Hoffman diease. Animal model: hereditary neuronal abiotrophy in Swedish Lapland dogs. Am J Pathol 82:649-652, 1976.

32. He Q, Lowrie C, Shelton GD, et al: Inherited motor neuron disease in domestic cats: a model of spinal muscular atrophy. Pediatr Res 57:324-330, 2005.

33. Shelton GD, Hopkins AL, Ginn PE, et al: Adult-onset motor neuron disease in three cats. J Am Vet Med Assoc 212:1271-1275, 1998.

34. Bagley RS: Tremor syndromes in dogs: diagnosis and treatment. J Small Anim Pract 33:485-490, 1991.

35. Cuddon PA: Tremor syndromes. Prog Vet Neurol 1:285-299, 1990.

36. Glass EN, Kent M: The clinical examination for neuromuscular disease. Vet Clin North Am Small Anim Pract 32: 1-29, 2002.

37. Shelton GD, Podell M, Poncelet L, et al: Inherited polyneuropathy in Leonberger dogs: a mixed or intermediate form of Charcot-Marie-Tooth disease. Muscle Nerve 27:471-477, 2003.

38. Victor M, Ropper AH: Diseases of the peripheral nerves *In* Adams and Victor's Principles of Neurology. Victor M, Ropper AH (eds). New York: McGraw-Hill, 2001, pp. 1370-1445.

39. Lorenz MD, Kornegay JN: Paresis of one limb. *In* Handbook of Veterinary Neurology. Lorenz MD, Kornegay JN (eds). St. Louis: Elsevier, 2004, pp. 113-129.

40. Bailey CS, Kitchell RL: Cutaneous sensory testing in the dog. J Vet Intern Med 1:128-135, 1987.

41. Coates JR, O'Brien DP: Inherited peripheral neuropathies in dogs and cats. Vet Clin North Am Small Anim Pract 34:1361-1401, 2004.

42. Cuddon PA: Acquired canine peripheral neuropathies. Vet Clin North Am Small Anim Pract 32:207-249, 2002.

43. O'Brien DP, Johnson GC: Dysautonomia and autonomic neuropathies. Vet Clin North Am Small Anim Pract 32:251-265, 2002.

44. Boydell P: Idiopathic Horner's's syndrome in the golden retriever. J Small Anim Pract 36:382-384, 1995.

45. Morgan RV, Zanotti SW: Horner's syndrome in dogs and cats: 49 cases (1980-1986). J Am Vet Med Assoc 194:1096-1099, 1989.

46. Shell LG: The cranial nerves of the brain stem. Prog Vet Neurol 1:233-245, 1990.

47. Jeffery N: Neurological abnormalities of the head and face. In BSAVA Manual of Canine and Feline Neurology. Platt SR, Olby NJ (eds). Gloucester: Woodrow House, 2004, pp. 172-188.

48. Penderis J: Common cranial nerve disorders in dogs and cats. *In* Practice April:178-189, 2003. Auth: Volume number?

49. Dewey CW: Encephalopathies: Disorders of the brain. *In* A Practical Guide to Canine and Feline Neurology. Dewey CW (ed). Ames: Iowa State Press, 2003, pp. 99-178.

50. Monnet E: Laryngeal paralysis and devocalization. *In* Textbook of Small Animal Surgery. Slatter DH (ed). Philadelphia: Elsevier Science, 2003, pp. 837-845.

51. Braund KG, Steinberg HS, Shores A, et al: Laryngeal paralysis in immature and mature dogs as one sign of a more diffuse polyneuropathy. J Am Vet Med Assoc 194:1735-1740, 1989.

Table 43-3. Common Differentials for Cranial Neuropathies in Dogs and Cats

Cranial Nerve	Clinical Signs	Specific Focal Cranial Neuropathies	Acquired Neuropathies
Olfactory nerve (CN I)	Anosomia, behavior change, depressed appetite	Idiopathic	Neoplasia, inflammation (encephalitis)
Optic nerve (CN II)	Blindness, absent menace response, absent pupillary light reflex	Sudden acquired retinal degeneration, optic hypoplasia, optic disc atrophy	Neoplasia or space-occupying masses, inflammation (infectious, noninfectious), trauma, vascular
Oculomotor nerve (CN III)	Decreased to absent PLRs, external ophthalmoplegia, lateral strabismus, ptosis	Resting anisocoria (CNIII, sympathetic n.), dysautonomia	Spastic pupil syndrome (FeLV, inflammation, lymphosarcoma), neoplasia, inflammation (encephalitis), increased ICP
Trochlear nerve (CN IV)	Dorsal lateral rotation of pupil (cats); lateral deviation of dorsal retinal vessels	Rare as solely affected	Neoplasia, inflammation (encephalitis)
Trigeminal nerve (CN V)	Sensory and motor deficits, dropped jaw, masticatory muscle atrophy, loss of palpebral and corneal reflexes, loss of facial sensation, neurogenic keratopathy	Idiopathic trigeminal neuritis – dropped jaw	Neoplasia (nerve sheath tumor), inflammation (encephalitis)
Abducens nerve (CN VI)	Medial strabismus, absence of retractor bulbi reflex	Rare as solely affected	Neoplasia, inflammation (encephalitis)
Facial nerve (CN VII)	Lip/ear droop, loss of palpebral reflex, deviation of nasal philtrum, decreased tear production – exposure keratopathy, neurogenic KCS	Idiopathic facial nerve paralysis, hemifacial spasm	Neoplasia, inflammation (otitis media/interna, encephalitis), iatrogenic surgical trauma, hypothyroidism
Vestibular/cochlear nerve (CN VIII)	Deafness Vestibular signs – head tilt, spontaneous nystagmus, deficits of physiologic nystagmus, strabismus	Congenital deafness Idiopathic vestibular disease, congenital vestibular disease	Neoplasia, inflammation (encephalitis, nasopharyngeal polyp, otitis media/interna), toxicity, hypothyroidism
Glossopharyngeal nerve (CN IX), Vagus nerve (CN X), Accessory nerve (CN XI)	Dysphagia, regurgitation, megaesophagus, dysphonia, upper respiratory tract signs	Idiopathic/congenital megaesophagus, dysautonomia, idiopathic/congenital laryngeal paralysis, laryngeal paralysis polyneuropathy complex	Neoplasia, inflammation (encephalitis), iatrogenic surgical trauma, polyneuropathy, myasthenia gravis
Hypoglossal nerve (CN XII)	Ipsilateral paresis	None	Trauma, neoplasia, inflammation (encephalitis)
Sympathetic nerve	Miosis, enophthalmos, third eyelid protrusion, ptosis	Idiopathic Horner's syndrome	Iatrogenic surgical trauma, brachial plexus avulsion, neoplasia, inflammation (otitis media/interna)

Chapter 44

Traumatic and Neoplastic Diseases of the Brachial Plexus

Andy Shores
Laurie Pearce

The brachial plexus is the collective name for the lower motor neuron (LMN) components of the lower cervical and upper thoracic spinal cord segments (C6 toT2), which innervate the shoulders and forelimbs.[1] Injuries to the brachial plexus, either by trauma or neoplasia, result in dysfunction of muscle groups innervated by the involved nerves. In this chapter we present an overview of the anatomy and function of the brachial plexus and a review of the incidence, mechanisms of injury, diagnostic methods, prognosis, and treatment options for traumatic and neoplastic diseases of the brachial plexus.

Anatomy and Function

Figure 44-1 depicts the location of the spinal cord segments, peripheral nerves, and forelimb muscles associated with the brachial plexus' general somatic efferent (GSE) function. Each LMN consists of a cell body located in the ventral gray matter of the spinal cord, the ventral root, the spinal nerve, the peripheral nerve, and the myoneural junction.[2] Motor nerves of the forelimb are formed by ventral branches of spinal cord segments C6, C7, C8, and T2.[3] The fifth cervical segment occasionally contributes to the plexus, but when it does, the second thoracic segment usually contributes nothing. When both C5 and T2 contribute to the brachial plexus, the ventral branches of each are small. The ulnar, median, radial, axillary, musculocutaneous, subscapular, suprascapular, thoracodorsal, and lateral thoracic branches are the motor nerves formed by the brachial plexus, and they innervate intrinsic and extrinsic muscles of the shoulder, brachium, and antebrachium.[1]

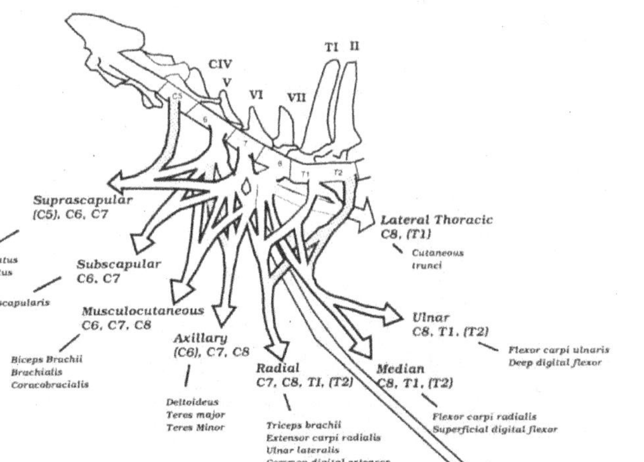

Figure 44-1. Anatomy of the brachial plexus: cervical vertebrae (Roman numerals), spinal cord segments, distribution of the spinal cord segments to the peripheral nerves of the brachial plexus, and muscles innervated by the peripheral nerves of the brachial plexus.

Injuries to the Brachial Plexus

Causes

Automobile accidents are the most frequent cause of injuries to the brachial plexus. Additional causes include projectiles, falling or jumping from moving vehicles, and foreign bodies that enter the axillary region.[4]

Mechanism

Avulsion of the brachial plexus follows extreme abduction of the shoulder or traction of the forelimb caudally, placing traction and longitudinal forces on the nerves.[3] Spinal nerve roots, the ventral nerve root branches, and the brachial plexus are subject to injury. Spinal nerve root avulsion probably occurs more frequently because these structures contain less connective tissue and, so, are less elastic than the extravertebral components of the LMN. Peripheral nerve dysfunction resulting from an avulsion injury is usually severe and permanent, although one study showed a 28% (8/29) rate of return to acceptable limb function 4 months after injury. Loss of radial nerve function is most critical because adequate limb function cannot be achieved without at least partial triceps muscle function.[5]

Classification

Neuropraxia is a temporary loss of nerve function without structural damage. *Axonotmesis* is loss of function from separation of the axons when the endoneurium remains intact. Complete severance of the nerve trunk defines *neurotmesis* (Figure 44-2). Return of function following neuropraxia may take 1 to 3 weeks. With axonotmesis or neurotmesis, the nerve undergoes Wallerian (axonal and myelin) degeneration distal to the site of injury. Regeneration of the axon fibers can occur, albeit slowly, if unimpeded by organized blood clots in the neural sheath (which occurs with axonotmesis) or by separation of the neural sheath (neurotmesis).[6]

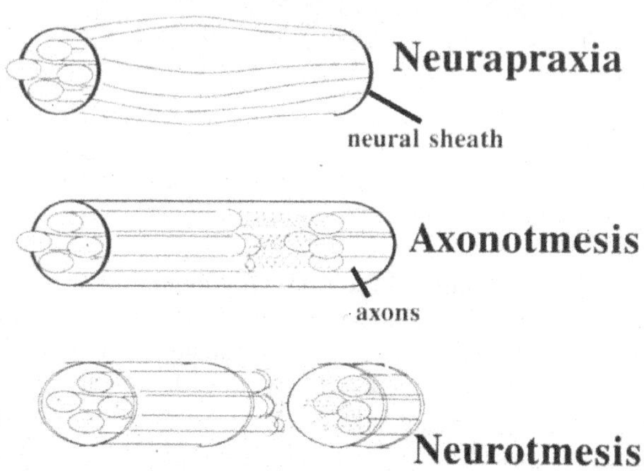

Figure 44-2. Classification of nerve injuries and associated structural changes.

Clinical Signs

Animals with brachial plexus injuries frequently have a history of loss of function in one forelimb noted immediately following trauma. Bilateral brachial plexus injuries are rare. Readily apparent clinical signs may include inability to fully extend the elbow or bear weight on the limb, and knuckling of the forepaw. Ipsilateral miosis, protruding third eyelid, enophthalmos, and ptosis (Horner's syndrome, Figure 44-3) may be evident, and the cutaneous trunci (panniculus) reflex may be absent on the affected side. Animals presented 10 to 14 days after brachial plexus injury exhibit neurogenic atrophy of the affected muscles (Figure 44-4).[3]

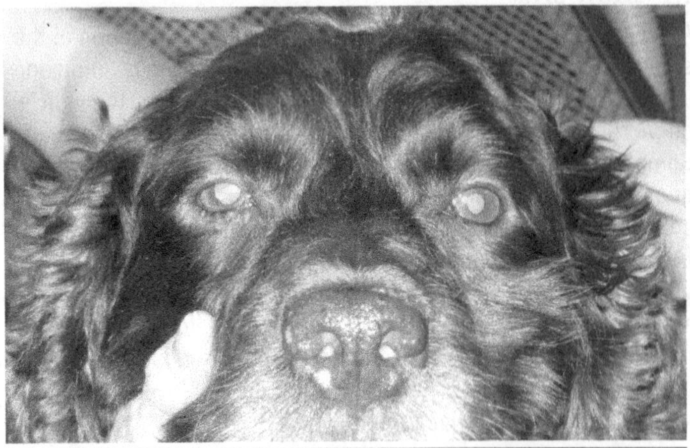

Figure 44-3. Anisochoria/partial Horner's syndrome in a dog with a left brachial plexus avulsion. The miotic left pupil results from a reduced or absent sympathetic nerve supply.

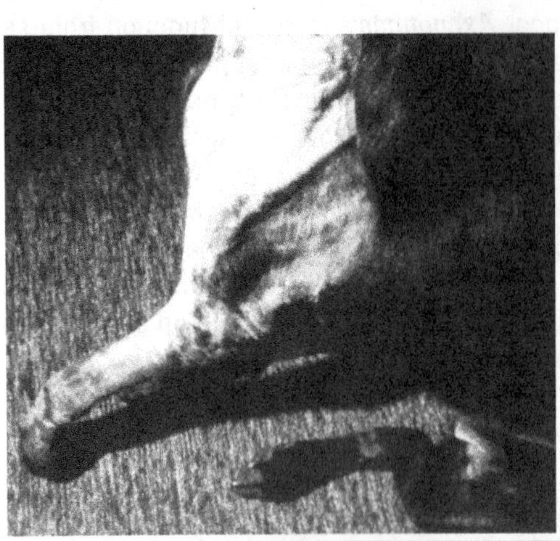

Figure 44-4. Right forelimb of a dog 2 weeks after a partial brachial plexus avulsion. Complete loss of ulnar, median, radial, and axillary nerves was noted; minimal musculotaneous and suprascapular nerve function was preserved. Notice the extreme neurogenic atrophy.

Injury to any component of the LMN, whether temporary or permanent, results in dysfunction of the entire unit. The *neuropathic syndrome* characterizes the clinical signs accompanying LMN dysfunction: decreased or absent muscle tone (hypotonia, atonia), reduced or absent segmental reflex responses (hyporeflexia, areflexia), and neurogenic muscle atrophy.[7]

Complete avulsion of the brachial plexus spinal nerve roots (C6 toT2) results in a flaccid, fully extended limb that is incapable of bearing weight. Avulsion of only the caudal plexus roots (C8 to T2) causes the animal to carry the limb with the elbow and shoulder flexed as a function of the remaining musculocutaneous, axillary, and suprascapular nerves.[8] Injury to the T1 nerve root may also damage sympathetic innervation to the eye, causing ipsilateral Horner's syndrome. Avulsion of the C8 nerve root results in ipsilateral loss of the cutaneous trunci reflex.[3]

Radial, axillary, and thoracodorsal nerve dysfunction caused by direct nerve damage or injury to the C7, C8, and T1 roots results in more ventral carriage of the elbow from loss of a majority of the shoulder flexors. The limb is unable to support weight. Cutaneous analgesia includes the caudal scapular region, a small area of the lateral brachium, the dorsum of the paw, and portions of the cranial and lateral antebrachium.[3,8]

Peripheral nerve injuries not caused by traumatic avulsions of the brachial plexus can involve specific nerves, and the level of injury dictates the type of dysfunction. Radial nerve injury distal to the triceps muscle branches causes knuckling of the forepaw and loss of carpal and digital extensor function. Most animals compensate by learning to flip the carpus forward when walking or running. Distal radial nerve damage causes analgesia of the dorsal surface of the paw and of portions of the cranial and lateral antebrachium. More proximal radial nerve damage creates similar cutaneous sensory loss but more severe motor dysfunction. The elbow is carried more ventrally because the shoulder flexor function of the long head of the triceps muscle is lost. Intact elbow and shoulder extensor function causes the limb to be carried upward (flexed). Attempts to use the limb result in knuckling of the forepaw and collapse of the limb. An animal with radial nerve injuries that cause loss of triceps function is unable to bear weight on the limb.[3]

Selective involvement of specific nerves of the brachial plexus other than the radial nerve does not produce substantial disability.[3] Sensory loss is evident in areas associated with the injured nerve (Figure 44-5). Loss of ulnar nerve function, which provides sensory innervation to the lateral aspect of the foot, predisposes animals to abnormal wear and abrasions of the lateral aspect of the footpads as the foot is allowed to slide laterally when bearing weight.[9]

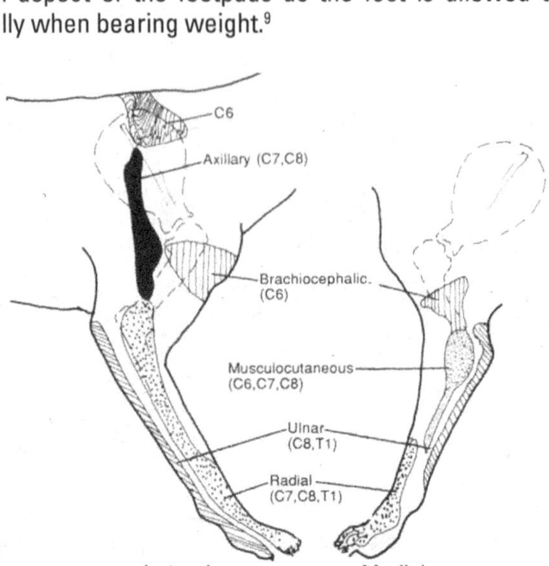

Figure 44-5. Autogenous zones on the lateral and medial aspects of the canine forelimb.

Tumors of the Brachial Plexus

Nerve sheath tumors are infrequent in dogs, rare in cats, and most often involve peripheral nerves derived from the brachial plexus. A survey of all entries from 21 veterinary colleges to the Veterinary Medical Data Program records for a 10-year period revealed the incidence was less than 1 per 32,000 dogs (0.003%) and less than 1 per 160,000 cats (0.0006%). These neoplasms have been described as schwannomas, neurilemmomas, neurinomas, and neurofibrosarcomas. Collagen content, encapsulation characteristics, and structures from which the tumors arise have been used to differentiate the tumor types; however, even with special staining and electron microscopy, differentiation is frequently a difficult and speculative process in veterinary pathology. Nerve sheath tumor is perhaps the best accepted term for these neoplasms in dogs and cats.[10]

Lymphosarcomas occasionally involve peripheral nerves or spinal nerve roots.[7,11] Other primary neoplasms such as meningiomas, which are extramedullary and intradural, can produce signs referable to the brachial plexus. Metastatic neoplasms, especially those involving the vertebrae, can also cause signs referable to the brachial plexus.[7]

Nerve sheath tumors of the brachial plexus are usually slow growing, rarely metastasize, and are classified as extramedullary and intradural when growth of the mass extends into the spinal canal.[10] The most caudal cervical (C7, C8) and the first thoracic spinal roots were more frequently involved in two clinical reports, but any of brachial plexus spinal nerve roots, ventral branches, or peripheral nerves can be primary sites of origin.[10,12] Clinical signs are slowly progressive and usually manifest as pain followed by muscle atrophy, limb dysfunction, and finally, spinal cord compression with continued growth of the tumor. Occasionally, the first sign noted is the animal's licking or chewing of the foot or carpus of the affected limb. Involvement of the T1 spinal nerve root may result in ipsilateral Homer's syndrome; with C8 spinal nerve root neoplasms, the cutaneous trunci reflex may be decreased or absent on the involved side.[3,10]

Diagnosis is based on typical history and clinical signs, palpation of a mass in the axillary region, electrodiagnostic tests, myelographic changes consistent with an extramedullary or intradural structure, and surgical biopsy findings. Early diagnosis is crucial to successful long-term management of animals with nerve sheath tumors, but it is frequently delayed by incomplete diagnostic evaluations and symptomatic treatment for suspected musculoskeletal or intervertebral disk disease.[7,10] One study reported an interval of more than 6 months from onset of signs to diagnosis in a survey of 18 dogs with nerve sheath tumors.[10]

Diagnostic Methods

History and Signalment

Brachial plexus injuries are usually associated with a history of trauma, although injuries from foreign bodies that penetrate the axillary region may be the exception. Owners of animals with brachial plexus tumors often relate a history of obscure lameness, resistance to palpation of the limb, possibly licking and chewing of the foot or carpus, and finally a reluctance to bear weight on the limb. The course of this history may be a few days to several weeks.[10,13]

A survey of brachial plexus nerve sheath tumors reported from 21 veterinary colleges to the Veterinary Medical Data Program during a 10-year period did not reveal a breed predisposition for brachial plexus nerve sheath tumors. Large-breed dogs (i.e., Labrador retrievers) appear to be over-represented in the literature, but this likely represents breed popularity rather than increased incidence rate.

Physical and Neurologic Examinations

Thorough examination is important when brachial plexus injury or neoplasia is suspected. Animals presented following motor vehicle trauma should be assessed for thoracic and abdominal injuries as well as fractures or nervous system injuries remote to or associated with the brachial plexus. In addition to a thorough physical examination, animals with suspected brachial plexus tumors are carefully assessed for the presence of other tumors.

Neurologic deficits found with brachial plexus injuries or tumors reflect the location and extent of brachial plexus and spinal cord involvement. Early signs of a nerve sheath tumor may not include neurologic deficits, but advanced signs may include hyporeflexia, muscle flaccidity, cervical spinal cord compression, and involvement of the contralateral limb. Brachial plexus trauma produces lower motor neuron dysfunction of the injured spinal nerve roots, ventral branches, or peripheral nerves. Complete brachial plexus involvement abolishes triceps, biceps, and forelimb flexor reflexes.[3]

Sensory innervation mapping is used to locate areas of cutaneous anesthesia on the limb. This examination requires a patient examiner, a cooperative patient, and a quiet, uninterrupted environment. Beginning on the dorsum of the paw, small, curved Halsted forceps are used to pinch the skin in a two-step procedure (Figure 44-6). An assistant gently restrains the animal while distracting its attention from the examiner. First, a small amount of skin is grasped lightly and lifted slightly with the forceps. Next, the hemostats are used to pinch the skin. Intact sensation is determined by vocalization of the animal, looking at the site of stimulation, or attempts to discourage the examiner from pinching the skin. Only consistent and repeatable results

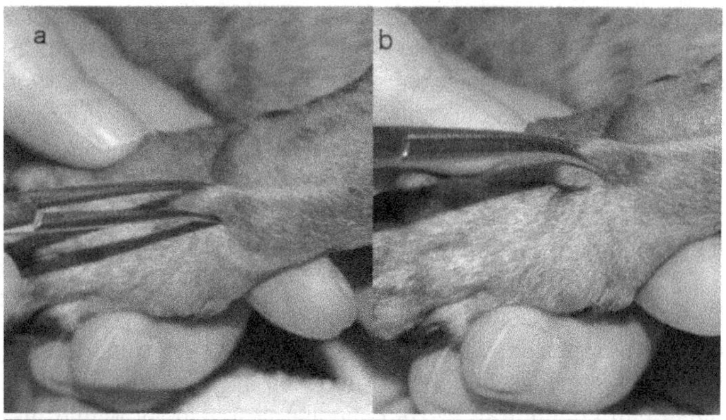

Figure 44-6. A and B. Two-step method for cutaneous sensory evaluation of the forelimb, a modification of the technique described by Bailey.

are considered valid. The examination is continued, proceeding up the antebrachium on the medial, lateral, cranial, and caudal sides. A cutaneous zone is the total cutaneous area supplied by a peripheral nerve. Some peripheral nerves have cutaneous zones that overlap. Autogenous zones are cutaneous regions that receive sensory innervation from only one peripheral nerve. Analgesia in an autogenous zone implies a loss of sensory function for the nerve represented by that zone.[3,4] Figure 44-5 illustrates the autogenous and cutaneous zones of the forelimb in the dog; the distribution is similar in cats. Certain dorsal spinal nerve branches in the brachial plexus region also have cutaneous and autogenous zones. The distribution of the cutaneous analgesia is used to determine which spinal and peripheral nerves are impaired.

Electrodiagnostic Tests

Several electrodiagnostic tests can be used to confirm and further characterize suspected nerve dysfunction. The electromyogram (EMG) is a graphic and auditory analysis of muscle function. Certain waveforms and sounds recorded from muscles may reflect denervation, reinnervation, or normal function.

Spontaneous activity consisting of fibrillation potentials and positive sharp waves are patterns associated with denervation and can be recorded 5 to 14 days after denervation. Low-amplitude monophasic or polyphasic motor unit action potentials (MUAP) or giant MUAP may be demonstrated from muscle undergoing reinnervation. Early stages of reinnervation can result in small MUAP when the number of regenerated axons is few, and polyphasic waves indicate a disparity in the degree of remyelination among the regenerating fibers. Giant MUAP occur when denervated muscles are reinnervated by adjacent functional nerves, resulting in a low muscle nerve branch to muscle fiber ratio.

Early evidence of reinnervation is not predictive of full recovery of function. Serial EMG evaluations that produce consistent physical and electrophysiologic evidence of active muscle reinnervation are more reliable indicators of a reinnervation process sufficient to produce some return of function. Serial microscopic examination of muscle biopsy specimens from the most proximal affected muscles (e.g., supraspinatus, deltoid) may be used to further confirm the regenerative process. Normal muscle exhibits insertional activity as the EMG electrode is passed through it; in anesthetized animals, however, electrical silence is evident after the electrode is stationary. A thorough EMG examination 2 to 3 weeks after a brachial plexus injury documents the extent of muscle denervation and confirms the distribution of nerve root injury. The EMG may be helpful in early diagnosis of brachial plexus tumors, especially when limb dysfunction is minimal or absent and a pattern of scattered spontaneous activity indicative of denervation (fibrillation potentials, positive sharp waves) is found in the distribution of one nerve.

Nerve conduction studies are of limited value in the assessment of brachial plexus dysfunction. Soon after avulsion, before Wallerian degeneration has proceeded far distally, a motor nerve can conduct an evoked impulse at a velocity within the normal range. After Wallerian degeneration, impulses cannot be conducted. This information adds little to the findings of physical and electromyographic examination. Sensory nerve conduction studies may be useful in determining the location of the nerve injury. When sensory nerve fibers are avulsed proximal to the dorsal root ganglia, however, the sensory fibers of the peripheral nerve do not degenerate and are capable of conducting an evoked impulse, even with complete analgesia in the autogenous zone.[14]

Spinal evoked potentials (cord dorsum potentials) may be more valuable for determining the integrity of the sensory nerve function. Stimulation of the nerve in the distal portion of the limb and recording an evoked response from an electrode over vertebra C6 or C7 indicate that a portion of the sensory tracts is functional for that nerve. The value of this test for predicting return of function is unknown.

Other motor evoked responses that might be useful but have not been sufficiently evaluated in veterinary medicine are the H wave and F wave. The H wave is produced by a submaximal stimulation and is equivalent to a monosynaptic reflex. The H wave can be recorded only if the dorsal and ventral roots are intact. The F wave is produced by a supra¬maximal stimulus, represents antidromal and orthodromal transmission of the electrical impulse, and requires an intact peripheral nerve, ventral root, and ventral horn cell. Presence of an F wave indicates a functional motor nerve.[15]

Radiography and Advanced Imaging

Radiography and advanced imaging techniques (myelography, ultrasonography, computed tomography, magnetic resonance imaging) are used to evaluate the vertebrae and spinal cord of the caudal cervical region.[16-20] Brachial plexus nerve sheath tumors that invade the spinal canal often create bony lysis at the intervertebral foramen. The widened foramen may be demonstrated on lateral views of the spine. Myelography usually depicts spinal cord compression and an extramedullary intradural pattern.[19] With brachial plexus avulsions of the spinal roots, the contrast material may be seen outside the subarachnoid space, at the site of the avulsion. The expanded availability of ultrasonography, computed tomography, and magnetic resonance imaging in veterinary medicine has proven useful in determining avulsion sites and the extent of nerve sheath tumors in the caudal cervical region (Figure 44-7).[16-18]

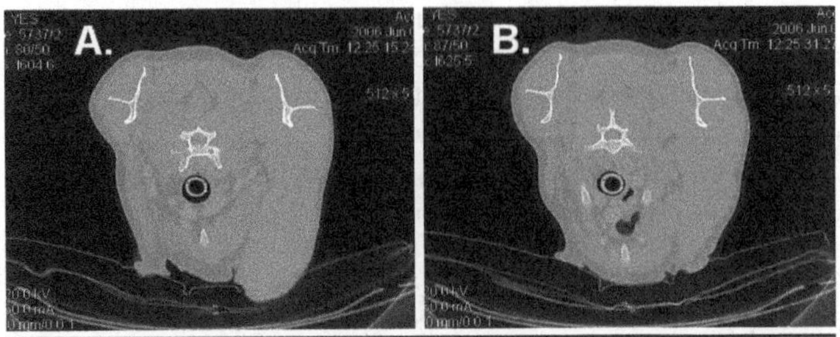

Figure 44-7. Computed tomographic images of a patient with brachial plexus avulsion. Note the extreme atrophy of the right appendicular muscles, but relatively mild atrophy of the scapular muscles. Electrodiagnostics in this patient indicated avulsion of the caudal cervical nerve roots (C7 through T2) and, therefore, some sparing of the suprascapular and subscapular nerves. A. Level of the C6 vertebra; B. Level of the C7 vertebra.

Therapeutic Options and Guidelines

Injuries to the Brachial Plexus

Most brachial plexus injuries unfortunately result in permanent dysfunction of the affected nerves and associated muscles of the forelimb. Most plexus avulsions occur at or within the spinal cord, and surgical repair would require extraordinary effort, expertise, and expensive equipment (e.g., operating microscope, microsurgical instruments).[9] More distal injuries, involving peripheral nerves, warrant surgical exploration and, when indicated, primary surgical repair. Caution and prudence should guide the decision for primary nerve root repair. Low-frequency laser technology for nerve anastomosis may warrant consideration in the future.

Definitive therapy for brachial plexus injury is delayed until the full extent of injury is known. Figure 44-8 is an algorithm that outlines a schedule for serial evaluation of brachial plexus injuries and the various treatment options available. The initial concern is protection of the limb from further injury and prevention of flexor tendon contracture. If elbow flexion is not sufficient to prevent the carpus from dragging on the ground, the carpus is bandaged. Limb carriage and sensory mapping are documented in the medical record for future reference. In 7 to 14 days the limb is re evaluated: sensory mapping is repeated, muscle atrophy is noted, and EMG evaluation is performed if available. Evidence of self-mutilation, skin abrasions on the dorsal surface of the carpus, and flexor tendon contracture are addressed at this time. Amputation is considered if there is total analgesia distal to the elbow and evidence of self-mutilation and if improvement is not noted within three weeks. To prevent flexor tendon contracture, a coaptation splint can be applied or the owners can perform hyperextension exercises on the limb for 10 minutes four times a day. The latter approach requires cooperation from the animal and strict compliance from the owner. Weekly reevaluations are scheduled for three weeks. If improvement is noted, conservative therapy is continued. Axon regeneration does not begin until 7 to 14 days after injury, and neuropraxia may take three to six weeks to fully resolve.[6] Muscle biopsy and EMG are needed to confirm evidence of reinnervation. If no improvement is noted during the three weekly visits, therapeutic options are these: conservative (no further treatment) and surgical (amputation, tendon transposition, nerve-muscle transposition).

When no improvement is noted, if the limb is not constantly subjected to trauma (dorsal carpal skin abrasions, self-mutilation) and limb appearance is acceptable to the client, no additional care is needed or indicated.

Tendon transpositions have been reported by several authors as therapeutic options when musculocutaneous function is intact;[9,21-23] however, most reports are of experimental and not clinical data. In most spontaneous brachial plexus injuries, any musculocutaneous nerve function remaining is partial, and neither the brachialis nor the biceps brachii muscles have sufficient functional muscle fibers to both flex and extend the elbow.[5] The transposition procedure is intended to supply function to the triceps muscle, allowing extension of the elbow. Even if sufficient triceps function can be supplied, sensory deficits remain and self-mutilation can begin any time after the injury. If the tendon transposition is successful, carpal arthrodesis should be considered as an adjunct to triceps function. Arthrodesis should align the carpus in slight hyperextension (8° to 12°) and 5° to 8° outward rotation.[9] With each step of the tendon transposition or carpal arthrodesis therapy, owners are again counseled about the ever present threat of self-mutilation.

Nerve-muscle transpositions have shown limited success in experimental radial nerve transection. The efficacy of nerve allografts has varied, with failure usually related to immune-mediated reactions.[9] Intact neurovascular muscle pedicle grafts have been considered; this requires microvascular technique and may have future clinical applications.

Tumors of the Brachial Plexus

Early diagnosis is the single most important factor in successful treatment of brachial plexus tumors. Any well founded suspicion of a brachial plexus tumor is an indication for surgical exploration, although the more common items in the differential diagnosis must first be ruled out. Brachial plexus neuritis, trauma, and vascular thrombus are all characterized by acute onset of substantial lower motor neuron dysfunction of one or both pelvic limbs.[5] Radicular and spinal cord compression may have a slower, more insidious onset, although clinical signs and radiographic studies should differentiate these conditions from brachial plexus tumors. Radicular compression from an intervertebral disk extrusion involves only one cervical segment, even when progressive, and should be demonstrable on plain film radiography or myelography. Caudal cervical spinal cord compression from an intervertebral disk extrusion or spinal cord neoplasm usually produces clinical signs, which are more evident in the hind limbs than the forelimbs, although neck pain can be the only sign. Again, radiographic studies should demonstrate the lesion.

When brachial plexus tumors are diagnosed or when other more common causes of forelimb LMN dysfunction are ruled out, exploration of the brachial plexus to determine the extent and distribution of the suspected neoplasm is the best method of definitively diagnosing the problem. All too often, the decision to explore is delayed unnecessarily.[5]

The surgeon tailors the surgical approach to the location of the suspected mass. Careful palpation, before and after induction of anesthesia, is helpful, as is a through knowledge of brachial plexus anatomy, EMG changes in the limb, and results of the neurologic examination. If the tumor is palpable and located distal to the mid-humerus, a linear incision is made from the proximal third of the humerus to the middle of the antebrachium. The tumor is identified and resected, along with a margin of normal-looking nerve proximal and distal to the mass.[5]

Exploration of the region from the brachial plexus to the spinal canal is accomplished through an incision over the scapula followed by muscle dissection on the cranial, caudal, and dorsal

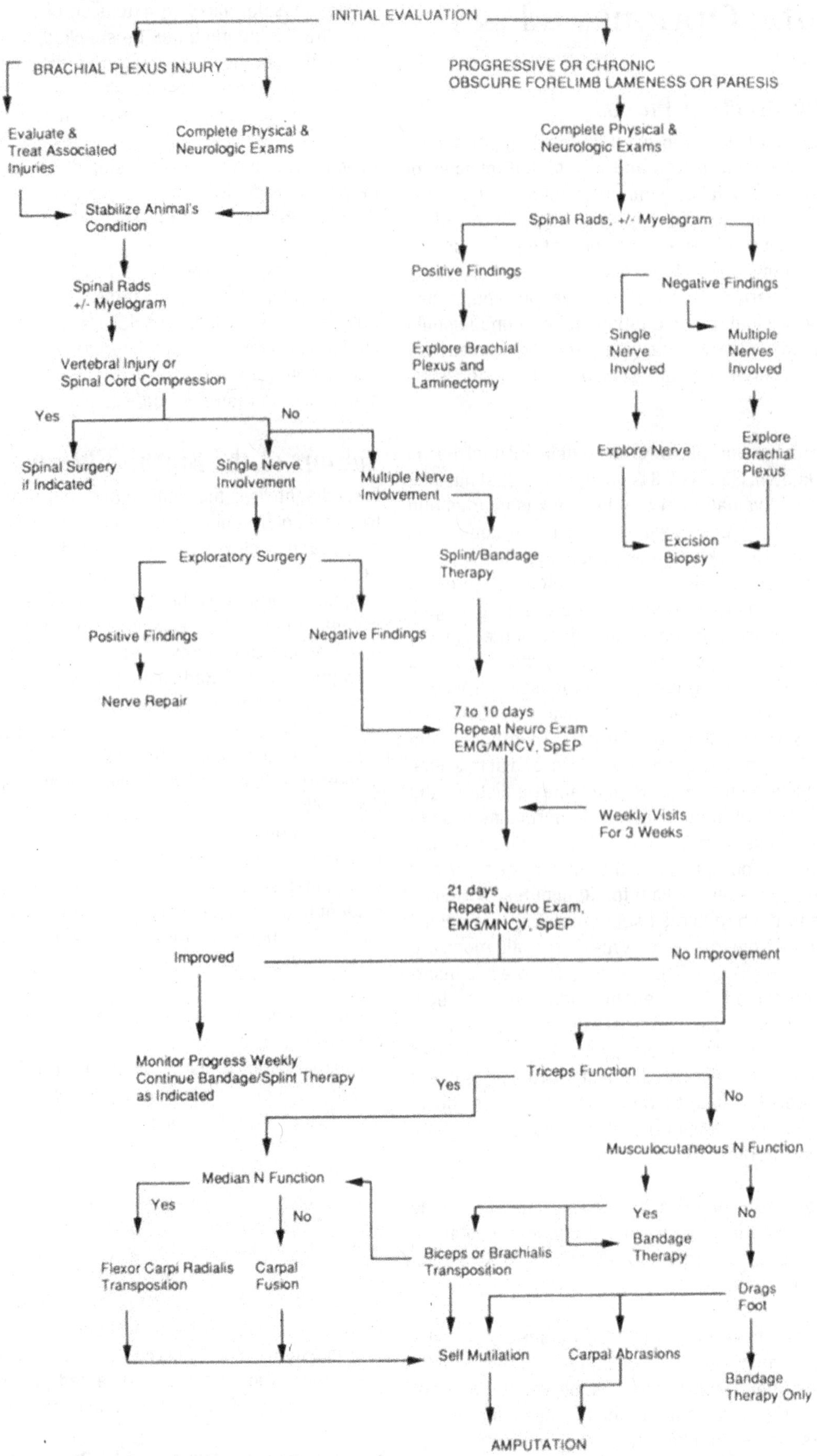

Figure 44-8. Algorithm of serial evaluation and treatment options for brachial plexus injuries. EMG, electromyography; MNCV, motor nerve conduction velocity; SpEP, spinal evoked potential. (Adapted from Knecht CD, Raffe MR: Diseases of the brachial plexus. *In* Textbook of Small Animal Orthopaedics. Newton CD, Nunamaker DM (eds). Philadelphia: JB Lippincott, 1985.

aspects of the scapula and reflecting the scapula toward the surgeon (Figure 44-9). Neural structures from the spinal canal to the mid-humerus can be explored with this exposure. The axillary lymph node can be biopsied with this approach. Prior knowledge of the precise location of the mass, through palpation or advanced imaging techniques, allows some modification of this approach. If the mass is in the cranial-most brachial plexus area, transection of the omotransversarius muscle and retraction plus blunt dissection allow exposure of this region. For the caudal brachial plexus, the rhomboideus muscle is transected and retraction plus blunt dissection are adequate for exposure of this area.[5]

An alternative surgical approach is the craniolateral approach. The reported advantage is improved exposure of the proximal brachial plexus; whereas the craniomedial approach described above offers a better exposure of the peripheral nerves.[24]

If the mass extends into the spinal canal, the tumor is resected to the point of the intervertebral foramen and the spinal canal is explored later (preferably within a week). Nerve sheath tumors that invade the spinal canal may also extend to the opposite side, necessitating extensive exposure of the canal for resection.

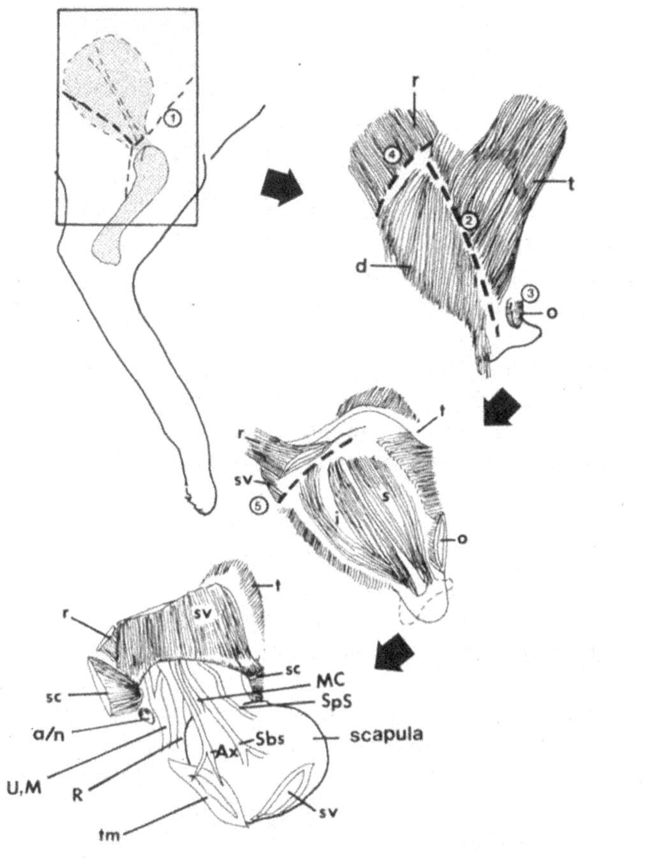

Figure 44-9. Exploration of the brachial plexus. 1, Initial skin and subcutaneous tissue incision; 2, incision through tendinous attachments to the spine of the scapula; 3, incision through omotransversarius (O) muscle attachment to the scapula; 4, incision through rhomboideus (r) muscle attachment to the scapula (t, trapezius; d, deltoideus); 5, incision through serratus ventralis (sv) muscle (s, supraspinatus; i, infraspinatus); abduction of the scapula follows, to expose the brachial plexus nerves (aln, axillary lymph node; sc, scalenus; U, ulnar nerve; M, median nerve; R, radial nerve; tm, teres major; Ax, axillary nerve; MC, musculocutaneous nerve; Sbs, subscapular nerve; SpS, suprascapular nerve).

Limb amputation is a practical consideration if the mass extensively involves the brachial plexus or if resection will cause permanent triceps muscle dysfunction. If the mass extends into the spinal canal and has extensive brachial plexus involvement, euthanasia is a rational decision for the owners to make, since a cure is unlikely, long-term prognosis is poor, and the postoperative discomfort, physical rehabilitation, and dysfunction may be considerable. Palliative therapy is reserved for animals that cannot or should not undergo surgery for any reason (including recurrence of the tumor) and whose pain or discomfort can be controlled well enough to allow quality life in the time remaining.

Estimating Prognosis

Estimating prognosis is difficult early in the course of brachial plexus injuries and when proof exists of complete removal of a nerve sheath tumor on microscopic examination of tissue margins. Most avulsions cause permanent damage. Most nerve sheath tumors recur. It is the responsibility of the veterinarian to give clients accurate information so that they may make an informed decision.

Postoperative Rehabilitation

Care of the animal with brachial plexus injury that has undergone surgery for tendon transposition or nerve repair includes immobilization of the limb for at least 2 weeks. When arthrodesis of the carpus is performed, 6 to 8 weeks' immobilization is needed to allow fusion. Amputees seldom require major care after the immediate postoperative period. Animals recovering from surgery for brachial plexus neoplasms require physical therapy and much the same care as animals with traumatic brachial plexus injuries: protection of the carpus and hyperextension exercises to prevent flexor tendon contraction. Because the involved nerves are usually severed and return of function is not a consideration, the owners are made aware of the need for life-long commitment to this care. Any changes in the animal's ability to use the limb, signs of pain, or other factors that might herald recurrence of the mass should be reported immediately.

References

1. Miller ME, Christensen GC, Evans HE (eds): Anatomy of the Dog. Philadelphia: WB Saunders, 1964.

2. Redding RW: Anatomy and physiology. *In* Canine Neurology, 3rd ed. Hoerlein B (ed). Philadelphia: WB Saunders, 1978.

3. deLahunta A: Veterinary Neuroanatomy and Clinical Neurology, 2nd ed. Philadelphia: WB Saunders, 1983.

4. Bailey CS: Patterns of cutaneous anesthesia associated with brachial plexus avulsions in the dog. J Am Vet Med Assoc 185:889, 1984.

5. Steinberg HS: Brachial plexus injuries and dysfunctions. Vet Clin North Am Small Anim Pract 18:565,1988.

6. Shores A: Peripheral nerve surgery. *In* Current Techniques in Veterinary Surgery, 4th ed. Bojrab MJ (ed). Baltimore: Williams & Wilkins, 1998.

7. Braund, KG: Clinical Syndromes in Veterinary Neurology. Baltimore: Williams & Wilkins, 1986.

8. deLahunta A., Habel RE: Applied Veterinary Anatomy. Philadelphia: WB Saunders, 1986.

9. Knecht CD, Raffe MR: Diseases of the brachial plexus. *In* Textbook of Small Animal Orthopaedics. Newton CD, Nunamaker DM (eds). Philadelphia: JB Lip¬pincott, 1985.

10. Bradley RL, Withrow SJ, Snyder SP: Nerve sheath tumors in the dog. J Am Anim Hosp Assoc 18:915, 1982.

11. Spodnick GJ, et al: Spinal lymphoma in cats: 21 cases (1976-1989). J Am Vet Med Assoc 200[3]:373-376 1992.

12. Wheeler S, Jones DGC, Wright JA: The diagnosis of brachial plexus disorders in dogs: a review of twenty-two cases. 1. Small Anim Pract 27:147,1986.

13. Braund KG: Neoplasia. *In* Veterinary Neurology. Oliver JE Jr, Mayhew IG, Hoerlein BF (eds). Philadelphia: WB Saunders, 1987.

14. Kline DG, Hackett ER, Happel LB: Surgery for lesions of the brachial plexus. Arch Neurol 43:170, 1986.

15. Knecht CD, Redding RW: Monosynaptic reflex (H wave) in clinically normal and abnormal dogs. Am J Vet Res 42:1586, 1981.

16. Rudich SR, et al: Computed tomography of masses of the brachial plexus and contributing nerve roots in dogs.Vet Radiol Ultrasound 45[1]:46-50 2004.

17. Mellanby RJ, et al: Magnetic resonance imaging in the diagnosis of lymphoma involving the brachial plexus in a cat. Vet Radiol Ultrasound 44[5]:522-5 2003.

18. Platt SR, et al: Magnetic resonance imaging and ultrasonography in the diagnosis of a malignant peripheral nerve sheath tumor in a dog.Vet Radiol Ultrasound 40[4]:367-71 1999.

19. Forterre F, et al: CT myelography for diagnosis of brachial plexus avulsion in small animals. Tierarztl Prax Ausg K Klientiere Heimtiere 26[5]:322-9 1998.

20. McCarthy RJ, et al: Preoperative diagnosis of tumors of the brachial plexus by use of computed tomography in three dogs. J Am Vet Med Assoc 202[2]:291-4 1993.

21. Sterner W, Moller AW: Tendon transplantation--a surgical approach to radial paralysis in the dog. J Am Vet Med Assoc 137:71,1960.

22. Bennett D, Vaughn L: The use of muscle relocation techniques in the treatment of peripheral nerve injuries in dogs and cats. J Small Anim Pract 17:99,1976.

23. Simpson ST, Kornegay JN, Raffe MR: Surgical diseases of peripheral nerves. *In* Textbook of Small Animal Surgery. Slatter DH (ed). Philadelphia: WB Saunders, 1985.

24. Sharp NJH: Craniolateral approach to the canine brachial plexus. Vet Surg 17[1]:18-21, 1988.

Chapter 45

Atlantoaxial Subluxation in the Dog

Daniel P. Beaver

Atlantoaxial subluxation is typically a congenital or developmental disease affecting immature toy breed dogs.[1,2] Atlantoaxial subluxation has also been reported in other mammals including cats, horses, and cattle. In people, both the ligamentous laxity associated with Down's syndrome and the bony destruction of erosive rheumatoid arthritis can cause atlantoaxial subluxation.[2,3,4,5] In dogs with atlantoaxial subluxation, instability of the atlantoaxial joint results from a loss of ligamentous support of the axis, often with concurrent aplasia, hypoplasia or dysplasia of the dens. Acute or chronic spinal cord compression causing clinical signs consistent with an upper cervical myelopathy can result from this instability.[2]

Anatomy

The occipitus, atlas, and axis are the three bones that comprise the craniovertebral junction. Through their specialized shapes and interrelationships of movement, they allow a wide range of motion of the head.[6] The atlanto-occipital joint is the cranial part of the overall occipito-atlanto-axial complex. It allows for dorsoventral motion of the head on the neck. The more caudal atlantoaxial joint allows for rotational movement of the head about the longitudinal axis of the vertebral column. At the center of this rotation is the dens, a bony protuberance that extends cranially from the axis and lies along the floor of the vertebral foramen of the atlas. The dens is the major point of attachment for ligaments that stabilize the atlantoaxial joint. The synovial joint cavities of the occipito-atlanto-axial complex are interconnected to form a single composite joint cavity.[7]

Interosseous ligaments provide stability to the occipito-atlas-axis complex (Figure 45-1).[8] The apical ligament attaches the cranial aspect of the dens to the ventral aspect of the foramen magnum. The paired alar ligaments attach the dens to each of the occipital condyles. The transverse ligament is a tough fibrous band that acts as a restraint, keeping the dens against the body of the atlas. The transverse ligament allows rotational movement, but prevents the dens from tipping up into the vertebral canal. The dorsal atlantoaxial ligament and membrane extending between the vertebral arches of the atlas and axis also contribute to atlantoaxial stability.[8]

Pathophysiology

Dogs with atlantoaxial subluxation usually have congenital abnormalities that predisposed them to injury. Although various congenital malformations of the entire occipito-atlanto-axial complex have been described in association with atlantoaxial subluxation, most commonly only aplasia or hypoplasia of the dens is present in dogs.[2,9] Dorsal deviation and so-called "nonunion" or separation of the dens have also been reported in the dog.[2,10,11,12]

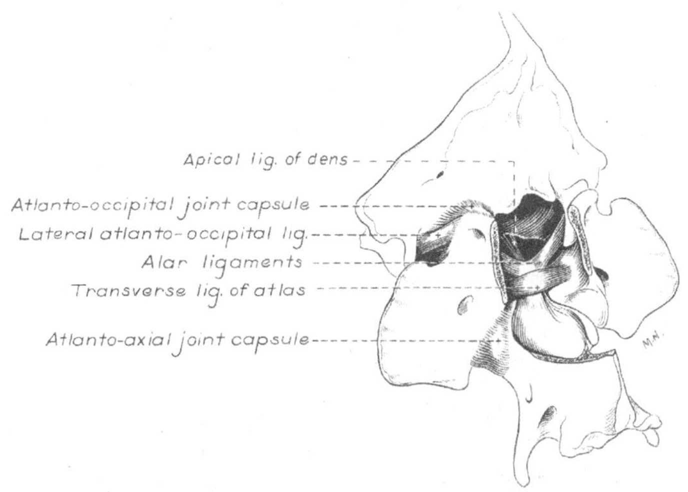

Figure 45-1. The ligaments of the occiput, atlas, and axis in a normal dog. (Reprinted with permission from: Evans HE, Christensen GC: Millers Anatomy of the Dog, 3rd ed. Philadelphia: WB Saunders, 1993, p. 227.

The cause of aplasia, hypoplasia, or dysplasia of the dens is unknown. At birth, the axis is composed of four separate ossification centers: the right and left neural arches, centrum 1 and centrum 2. Three additional ossification centers develop in the axis in postnatal life: intercentrum 2, the epiphysis, and the centrum of the proatlas (Figure 45-2.) An early hypothesis was that an assumed single ossification center for the dens fails to develop prenatally.[11] Subsequent investigation of the postnatal

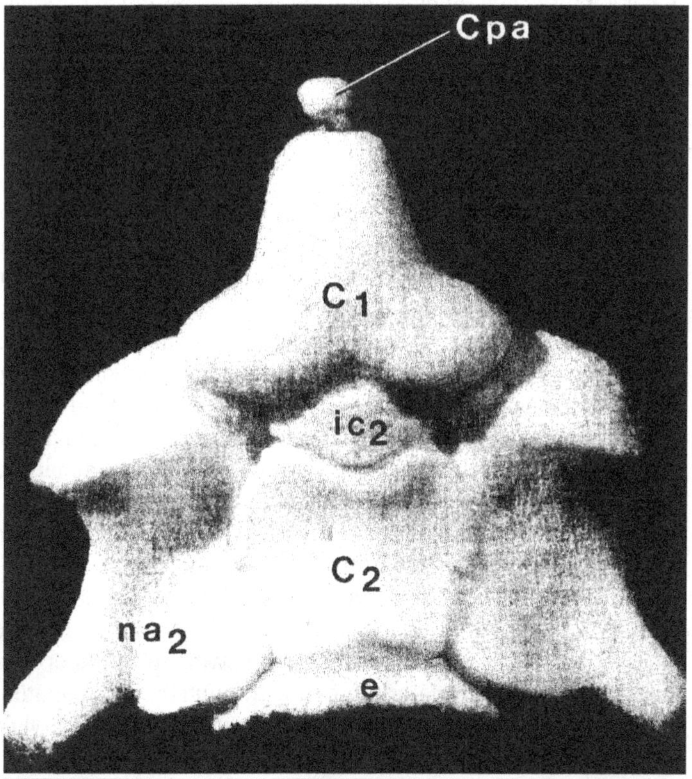

Figure 45-2. Ventral aspect of the axis from a 10-week-old Miniature Schnauzer, revealing 7 ossification centers: Cpa = centrum of the proatlas; C_1, C_2 = centrum 1 and centrum 2, respectively; ic_2 = intercentrum 2; na_2 = right neural arch center of the axis; e = epiphysis; x 5. (Photo courtesy of Dr. Alastair Watson. Reprinted from: Watson AG, Stewart JS: Postnatal ossification centers of the atlas and axis in Minature Schnauzers. Am J Vet Res 51:264, 1990.

ossification centers of the atlas and axis in Miniature Schnauzers and other breeds revealed that the dens originates from two ossification centers.[6,13] The cranial one quarter originates from the centrum of the proatlas, and the caudal three quarters of the dens as well as the cranial part of the axis body originate from centrum 1 of the axis. The authors of this study thus contended that dens hypoplasia or aplasia is unlikely owing to congenital absence of an ossification center. They proposed that a vascular-related ischemia may lead to postnatal resorption of at least the middle part of the dens, resulting in dens dysplasia.[13]

As the dens is a major attachment point for ligaments that stabilize the atlantoaxial joint, dogs with absent or hypoplastic dens are susceptible to trauma causing subluxation of the joint. Tearing of the dorsal atlantoaxial ligament and membrane often occurs with subluxation of the joint. With flexion of the head on the neck, ventral compression of the spinal cord occurs. Trauma to the spinal cord can come in the form of an apparently single acute episode or from more chronic progressive damage.

Atlantoaxial subluxation can occur in dogs with normal dens conformation as well. These cases usually result from traumatic rupture of the transverse ligament or fracture of the dens. A case of a dog with normal dens conformation with instability secondary to absence of the transverse ligament has been reported.[14] Such soft tissue abnormalities may be present in other cases of atlantoaxial subluxation in dogs with normal dens conformation. Dogs with atlantoaxial subluxation and a normal dens conformation may be at greater risk of severe spinal cord compression as the intact dens tilts dorsally into the vertebral canal. In one study, however, the conformation of the dens, whether it was normal, hypoplastic, or aplastic, did not affect the odds of a successful surgical outcome.[9]

Clinical Findings

Atlantoaxial subluxation is a disease that most often affects immature, toy breed dogs of both sexes. Breeds most commonly affected include the Yorkshire terrier, toy and miniature poodle, Pomeranian, Pekingese, Chihuahua, and Maltese. However, atlantoaxial subluxation may occur in any size and breed of dog and at any age if significant trauma to the neck occurs.

Toy breed dogs with atlantoaxial subluxation often do present with a history of trauma, although this is often a mild incident such as jumping off a chair or being dropped by a child. Clinical signs of atlantoaxial subluxation may be mild to severe depending on the degree of compression and the chronicity of the disease. Most, but not all, dogs with atlantoaxial subluxation have neck pain, exhibited by rigid guarding of the neck, reluctance to move, or pain on cervical palpation. Mild cases of atlantoaxial subluxation may have ataxia or a spastic gait. Front and hind limb reflexes may be normal or increased, and postural reaction deficits may be present. More severe cases exhibit tetraparesis or tetraplegia. True paralysis from atlantoaxial subluxation is also associated with respiratory arrest and death owing to injury to the respiratory centers in the cervical spinal cord.

Occasionally, dogs with atlantoaxial subluxation have neurologic signs that may be localized to the caudal brainstem.[9,15,16,17,18]

These may be seen more often in more neurologically compromised patients or following surgical manipulation. The cause of these signs often goes undiagnosed. They may be a result of concurrent congenital brain abnormalities, iatrogenic cervical spinal cord and brainstem trauma , or hypothetically, ischemia in the brainstem owing to compression of the basilar artery.[18]

Diagnosis

The diagnosis of atlantoaxial subluxation is usually confirmed with radiography. Lateral radiographic views will show dorsal displacement of the axis in relation to the atlas, with an abnormally increased distance between the dorsal arch of the atlas and the dorsal spine of the axis, and dorsal displacement of the body of the axis (Figure 45-3). On occasion, there may not appear to be enough distance between the dorsal aspects of the atlas and axis to be able to confirm atlantoaxial subluxation. General anesthesia may aid in getting diagnostic radiographs. Stressed views may be made by slightly flexing the neck; however, this maneuver can be very dangerous especially in the anesthetized unguarding animal. Fluoroscopy can aid in visualization of instability during flexion and extension. Myelography may also demonstrate spinal cord compression. Ventrodorsal radiographs of the atlantoaxial joint that demonstrate an absent or hypoplastic dens support a diagnosis of atlantoaxial subluxation (Figure 45-4). An open-mouth radiographic view demonstrates the conformation of the dens; however, because flexion of the neck is required for this view, it is usually not recommended. Computed tomography and magnetic resonance imaging modalities are also useful in diagnosing atlantoaxial subluxation.

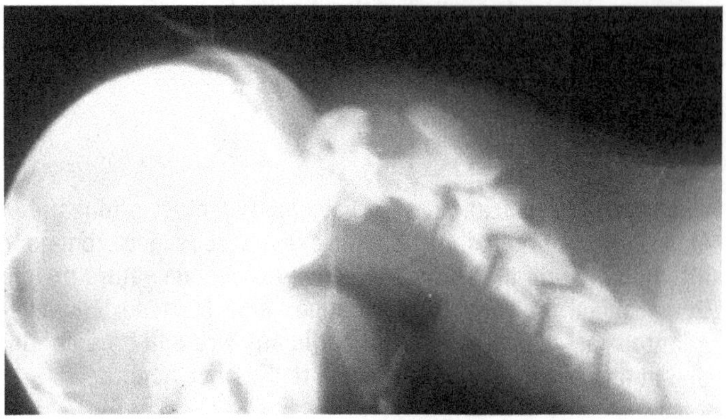

Figure 45-3. Lateral radiograph of caudal head and neck of an immature dog with atlantoaxial subluxation. Note the increased distance between arch of atlas and spine of axis.

Differential diagnosis for cranial cervical spinal cord lesions in toy breed dogs includes focal myelitis associated with canine distemper, toxoplasmosis, or granulomatous myelitis and meningitis (most often immune-mediated in the young dog). Cervical disc disease is common in the middle-aged to older small breed dog. Neoplasia is also a rare possibility.

Treatment

Treatment of atlantoaxial subluxation consists of relieving spinal cord compression by reduction and permanent stabilization of the atlantoaxial joint. This has been achieved through both surgical and conservative methods.

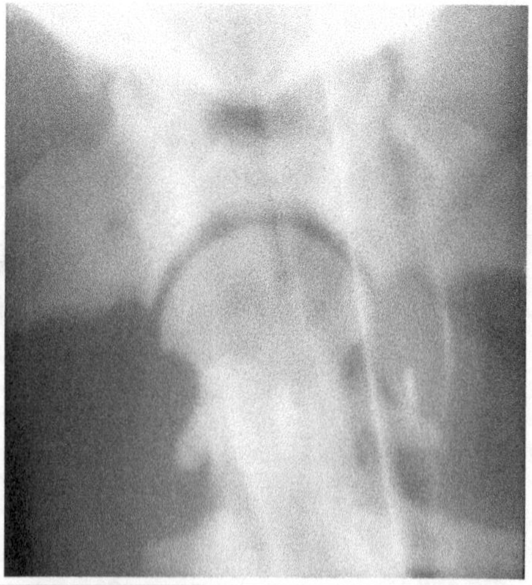

Figure 45-4. Ventrodorsal radiograph of caudal head and the neck of an immature dog with atlantoaxial subluxation. Note the absence of the dens on the axis.

Surgical Management

Surgical stabilization of the atlantoaxial joint is technically demanding. The vertebrae in toy breeds are extremely small and little margin for error exists when placing implants. The bone in immature dogs is soft. Implants can break the bone, migrate out of position, or cause impingement on the spinal cord. Manipulation of the atlantoaxial joint during surgery can also cause significant spinal cord trauma with subsequent death. However, most authors have recommended surgical stabilization for atlantoaxial subluxation. In dogs, both dorsal and ventral approaches to the atlantoaxial joint have been successfully used, with the goal of permanent fixation.

Dorsal Techniques

The first surgical stabilizations of the atlantoaxial joint in dogs were performed dorsally.[1,15,16,19] They consisted of orthopedic wire or suture material (even the nuchal ligament[19]) placed through the epidural space, then over the arch of the atlas, and finally, attached to the dorsal spine of the axis. A dorsal technique using a metal retractor[20] and a dorsal technique using a combination of pins and polymethylmethacrylate[21] have subsequently been described. Surgical implants applied on the dorsal surfaces of the atlas and axis have a theoretical biomechanical advantage as they are placed on the tension side of the joint subluxation; therefore, less implant strength is required to hold the joint reduced. Another advantage of the dorsal approach is the ease of surgical approach and the good exposure of the dorsal aspects of the atlas and axis. Complications of the dorsal techniques include resubluxation owing to suture or wire breakage or to these materials tearing through the soft immature bone. Also, life-threatening spinal cord damage may occur while attempting to pass material through the dorsal epidural space to the atlas. Dorsal surgical techniques do not allow access to the ventral articular surfaces of the atlantoaxial joint to attempt an arthrodesis. Long-term stability after dorsal procedures presumably is attributable to fibrosis across the dorsal aspects of the atlas and axis.

Ventral Techniques

Ventral stabilization techniques are advocated by most authors. The first ventral stabilizations involved placement of two transarticular Kirschner wires from the ventral aspect of the axis bilaterally through the joint to just medial to the alar notches on the wings of the axis.[10,16] This technique allowed for curettage of the articular surfaces of the atlantoaxial joint and the placement of bone graft to promote a permanent bony fusion. The ventral technique also allowed access to the dens for odontoidectomy procedures if necessary. More recently described ventral atlantoaxial stabilization techniques are modifications of the two-Kirschner-wire technique that often use additional Kirschner wires or bone screws in the atlas and axis.[17,22,23] The exposed ends of the Kirschner wires or bone screws are usually incorporated within a mass of polymethylmethacrylate bone cement. Other surgical methods that have been described to stabilize the atlantoaxial joint from a ventral approach include bone plating[16] and lag screw techniques.[15,16]

Postoperatively, dogs should be managed in a cervical splint (as described in the following section) to protect the surgical fixation. Cage rest should be enforced for six to eight weeks. Radiographs may be made 8 weeks after surgery to confirm atlantoaxial alignment and progression of arthrodesis.

Conservative Management

Although most authors have recommended surgical stabilization, conservative management of atlantoaxial subluxation by use of a cervical splint has been reported,[24] and more recently advocated.[25] If a cervical splint is used, the neck must be positioned in extension to allow for healing with the atlantoaxial joint reduced. Cervical splints must be light weight so that they are well tolerated by the pet. They may be circumferential or ventral only and should incorporate fiberglass, x-ray film, formable plastic splint material, or aluminum bars for stiffness. Cervical splints should be maintained for six to eight weeks. Radiographic evaluation should be performed prior to splint removal to confirm atlantoaxial alignment.

Restriction of activity is important to maintain atlantoaxial joint reduction and to keep the cervical splint from causing sores or loosening prematurely. Controlled, limited activity may have therapeutic value in the rehabilitation of dogs with neurologic compromise.

The success of conservative management relies on scar tissue formation across the atlantoaxial joint. As these dogs may be at risk of resubluxation later in life, long-term exercise restriction (e.g., preventing them from jumping off furniture) should be considered.

Corticosteroids such as oral prednisone have often been used in conjunction with both conservative management and surgical management. No scientific information is currently available showing that they improve the prognosis of these patients.

Prognosis

Nonsurgical management of atlantoaxial subluxation with a cervical splint was evaluated in a retrospective study.[25] Of 16 dogs, 10 (62%) were considered to have a good outcome 12 months after removal of the cervical splint. The authors of this study suggested that dogs with an acute onset of clinical signs and no prior history of neurologic disease, young dogs with immature bone in which surgical fixation may not provide adequate stability, or dogs for which there are financial constraints, should be considered for nonsurgical management. The authors of this study did not find that severity of deficits at admission was a reason to opt for a surgical approach.

Most authors consider surgical management the preferred treatment for atlantoaxial subluxation, especially in dogs with neurologic compromise. A 1995 review of the literature on surgical management of atlantoaxial subluxation revealed a 61% (32/52 dogs) success rate for dorsal procedures and a 62% (21/34 dogs) success rate for ventral procedures. Success was defined as improvement in clinical signs with no reported recurrence or necessity of reoperation.[2] These modest success rates have caused surgeons to strive to develop more reliable techniques to provide permanent rigid immobilization of the atlantoaxial joint. Three more recent studies reported modified surgical techniques with a combined 87.5% (35/40) of dogs having a good or excellent outcome.

A retrospective review of 46 cases of atlantoaxial subluxation in dogs identified risk factors affecting the outcome of surgical treatmenet.[9] Age of onset of clinical abnormalities of less than 24 months was significantly associated with greater odds of a successful first surgery and outcome. Duration of clinical abnormalities of less than 10 months was significantly associated with greater odds of a successful first surgery. Preoperative neurologic status was only marginally sensitive and specific in predicting a successful first surgery. Potential risk factors that did not affect the odds of a successful outcome include the type of surgery performed (the dorsal wire or suture technique vs. the ventral two-Kirschner-wire technique), grade of atlantoaxial joint reduction, conformation of the dens, and the need for a second surgical procedure. The long-term prognosis for dogs with atlantoaxial subluxation managed with surgery appears to be good provided the animal survives the perioperative period.[9]

References

1. Geary JC, Oliver JE, Hoerlein BF: Atlantoaxial subluxation in the canine. J Small Anim Pract 8:577, 1967.

2. McCarthy RJ, Lewis DD, Hosgood G: Atlantoaxial subluxation in dogs. Comp Contin Educ Pract Vet 17:215, 1995.

3. Menezes AH, Ryken TC: Craniovertebral abnormalities in Down's syndrome. Pediatr Neurosurg 18:24, 1992.

4. McRorie ER, McLoughlin P, Russell T, et al: Cervical spine surgery in patients with rheumatoid arthritis: an appraisal. Ann Rheum Dis 55:99, 1996.

5. Shelton SB, Bellah J, Chrisman C, et al: Hypoplasia of the odontoid process and secondary atlantoaxial subluxation in a Siamese cat. Prog Vet Neurol 2:209, 1991.

6. Watson AG, Evans HE, de Lahunta A: Ossification of the atlas-axis complex in the dog. Anat Histol Embryol 15:122, 1986.

7. Watson AG, de Lahunta A, Evans HE: Prenatal development of the composite occipito-atlanto-axial synovial joint cavity in the dog. Anat Rec 216:423, 1986.

8. Evans HE, Christensen GC: Millers Anatomy of the Dog, 3rd ed. Philadelphia: WB Saunders, 1993, p. 227.

9. Beaver DP, Ellison GW, Lewis DD, et al: Risk factors affecting the outcome of surgery for atlantoaxial subluxation in dogs: 46 cases (1978-1998). J Am Vet Med Assoc 216:1105, 2000.

10. Johnson SG, Hulse DA: Odontoid dysplasia with atlantoaxial instability in a dog. J Am Hosp Assoc 25:400, 1989.

11. Ladds P, Guffy M, Blauch B, Splitter G: Congenital odontoid process separation in two dogs. J Small Anim Pract 12:463, 1970.

12. Zaki FA: Odontoid process dysplasia in a dog. J Small Anim Pract 21:227, 1980.

13. Watson AG, Stewart JS: Postnatal ossification centers of the atlas and axis in Minature Schnauzers. Am J Vet Res 51:264, 1990.

14. Watson AG, de Lahunta A: Atlantoaxial subluxation and absence of transverse ligament of the atlas in a dog. J Am Vet Med Assoc 195:235, 1989.

15. Denny HR, Gibbs C, Waterman A: Atlanto-axial subluxation in the dog: a review of thirty cases and evaluation of treatment by lag screw fixation. J Small Anim Pract 29:37, 1988.

16. Thomas WB, Sorjonen DC, Simpson ST: Surgical management of atlantoaxial subluxation in 23 dogs. Vet Surg 20:409, 1991.

17. Platt SR, Chambers JN, Cross A: A modified ventral fixation for surgical management of atlantoaxial subluxation in 19 dogs. Vet Surg 33:349, 2004.

18. Jaggy A, Hutto VL, Roberts RE, Oliver JE: Occipitoatlantoaxial malformation with atlantoaxial subluxation in a cat. J Small Anim Pract 32:366, 1991.

19. LeCouteur RA, McKeown D, Johnson J, Eger CE: Stabilization of atlantoaxial subluxation in the dog, using the nuchal ligament. J Am Vet Med Assoc 177:1011, 1980.

20. Kishigami M: Application of an atlantoaxial retractor for atlantoaxial subluxation in the cat and the dog. J Am Anim Hosp Assoc 20:413, 1984.

21. Jeffery ND: Dorsal cross pinning of the atlantoaxial joint: New surgical technique for atlantoaxial subluxation. J Small Anim Pract 37:26, 1996.

22. Schulz KS, Waldron DR, Fahie M: Application of ventral pins and polymethylmethacrylate for the management of atlantoaxial instability: results in nine dogs. Vet Surg 26:317, 1997.

23. Sanders SG, Bagley RS, Silver GM, et al: Outcomes and complications associated with ventral screws, pins and polymethyl methacrylate for atlantoaxial instability in 12 dogs. J Am Anim Hosp Assoc 40:204, 2004.

24. Gilmore DR: Nonsurgical management of four cases of atlantoaxial subluxation in the dog. Vet Med Small Anim Clin 65:583, 1984

25. Havig ME, Cornell KK, Hawthorne JC, et al: Evaluation of nonsurgical treatment of atlantoaxial subluxation in dogs: 19 cases (1992-2001). J Am Vet Med Assoc 227:257, 2005.

Chapter 46

Intervertebral Disk Disease

Lisa S. Klopp

Anatomy of the Intervertebral Disk and Supporting Structures

Related Anatomic Structures of the Spine

The joining of two adjacent vertebrae is facilitated by several types of articulations (syndesmoses, arthroses, and amphiarthroses). The supporting structures of the spine include the various ligamentous structures (syndesmoses), the articular facets (arthroses), and the intervertebral disks (amphiarthoses). The ligaments of the spinal column include the interspinous and supraspinous ligaments, the intertranversarious ligaments, ligamentum flava, transverse intercapital ligaments, and the longitudinal ligaments (ventral and dorsal) (Figure 46-1).[1] The intertranversarious ligaments unite the adjacent transverse processes of the lumbar spine. The supraspinous ligament is a thick ligament extending along the apices of the dorsal spinous processes from the first thoracic vertebra to the third sacral vertebra.[1] This ligament plays an important role in preventing excessive separation of the dorsal spinous processes during spinal flexion. The interspinous ligaments blend with the interspinous muscles and connect adjacent dorsal spinous processes of the thoracic and lumbar vertebrae on midline. Some fibers from this ligament blend with the supraspinous ligament. These ligaments play a role in maintaining the relationship between the dorsal spinous processes when the spine is in flexion; however, they are not as strong as the supraspinous ligament.[1]

The transverse intercapital ligaments attach to the rib heads bilaterally by crossing the spinal canal perpendicularly to its long axis at each intervertebral disk beneath the dorsal longitudinal ligament. These ligaments are associated with the second through the tenth thoracic vertebrae in the dog. Although present between the eleventh rib heads, the transverse intercapital ligament is much less developed there. These ligaments aid in maintaining tight opposing rib head attachments to the vertebrae at the costovertebral joints, resulting in minimal cranial to caudal movement of the rib head.[1] The presence of this additional stabilizing ligamentous structure, in addition to the rigidity of the rib cage, is believed to play a role in the small numbers of clinically significant intervertebral disk extrusions observed in the thoracic region.

The dorsal longitudinal ligament courses along the entire length of the floor of the vertebral canal (dorsal to the vertebral body and dorsal annulus fibrosus). It is arranged as a parallel bundle of fibers that is approximately 2 millimeters or less in thickness when healthy. It is firmly attached to the dorsum of the vertebral body at its midline and fans out to blend fibers with the dorsal annulus fibrosus of the intervertebral disk.[2] Its anatomic location and relationship to the intervertebral disk allow it to help contain

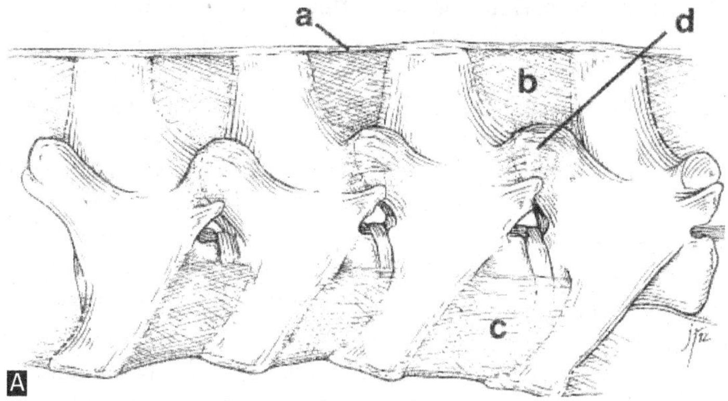

Figure 46-1A. Extrinsic spinal ligaments. a. dorsal spinous ligament; b. interspinous ligament; c. intertransverse ligament; d. joint capsule of the articular facet. (With permission from Wheeler SJ, Sharp NJH: Functional anatomy. In Small Animal Spinal Disorders: Diagnosis and Surgery. Wheeler SJ, Sharp NJH (eds). London: Mosby-Wolfe, 1994. Illustration by Joseph E. Trumpey, North Carolina State University.)

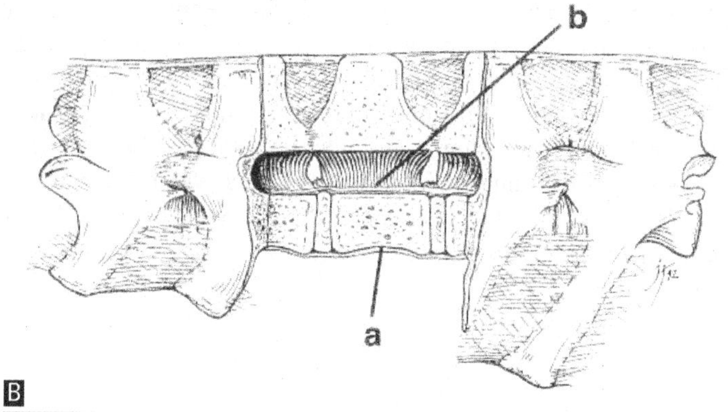

Figure 46-1B. The longitudinal ligaments of the spinal column. a. dorsal longitudinal ligament; b. ventral longitudinal ligament. (With permission from Wheeler SJ, Sharp NJH: Functional anatomy. In Small Animal Spinal Disorders: Diagnosis and Surgery. Wheeler SJ, Sharp NJH (eds). London: Mosby-Wolfe, 1994. Illustration by Joseph E. Trumpey, North Carolina State University.)

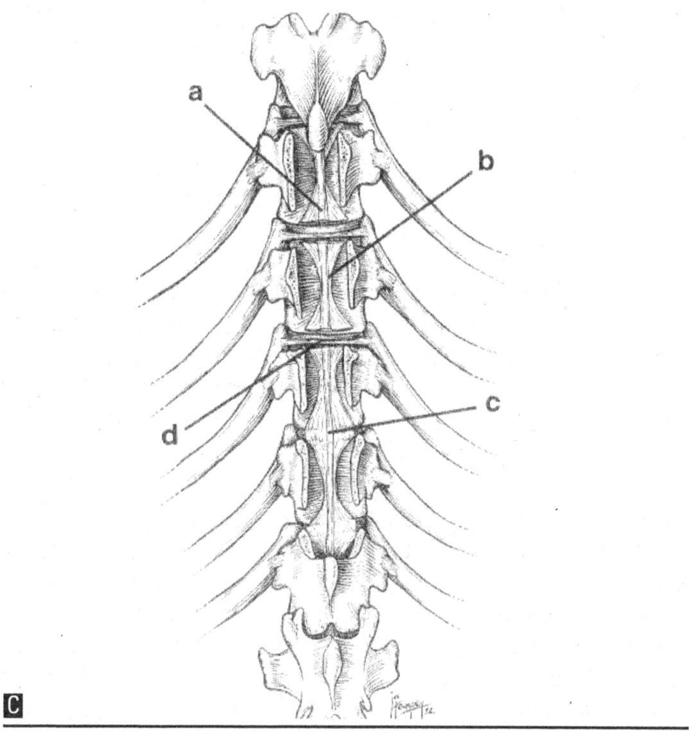

Figure 46-1C. The intrinsic ligaments of the spinal column. a., b, and c. course of the dorsal longitudinal ligament over the vertebral body and intervertebral disk; d. transverse intercapital ligament. (With permission from Wheeler SJ, Sharp NJH: Functional anatomy. In Small Animal Spinal Disorders: Diagnosis and Surgery. Wheeler SJ, Sharp NJH (eds). London: Mosby-Wolfe, 1994. Illustration by Joseph E. Trumpey, North Carolina State University.)

centrally extruded intervertebral disk material between it and the spinal cord.[2] The ventral longitudinal ligament is a similar type of ligament that traverses the ventral aspect of the vertebral bodies. In the dog, it is thinner than the dorsal longitudinal ligament and is probably of limited significance in support of the spine.[1]

The articular facets are true arthrodial joints that posses a typical synovial joint capsule and articular cartilage on the opposing surfaces.[3] The cranial articular process of the caudal vertebra and caudal articular process of the cranial vertebra forms this joint between two adjacent vertebrae. In the cervical region, the joint is in a nearly horizontal plane and the caudal articular process lies dorsally over the cranial articular process. In the cranial thoracic region, these joints become more perpendicular in their orientation to the longitudinal spinal axis, whereas in the lower thoracic and lumbar regions the cranial articular process is lateral to the medially situated caudal articular process. The facet joints play an important role in the stability of the spine in rotation and flexion. In extremes of spinal motion, it is not uncommon for these joints to fracture.

The Intervertebral Disk

The dog has 26 intervertebral disks excluding those found between coccygeal vertebrae. There are no intervertebral disks between the first two cervical vertebrae or, in a normal situation, between the sacral segments. The intervertebral disk is an amphiarthrodial joint (an articulation between bony surfaces that provides limited movement and is connected by ligaments or elastic cartilage) that binds adjacent vertebral bodies.[2,3] The intervertebral disk is mechanically and structurally required to be extremely strong as it provides for protective alignment of the spinal column and withstands the various physiologic forces imparted to it. In spite of the minimal movement of this type of joint, the multiple vertebral segments impart an overall flexibility to the spine. The disks differ somewhat in size and detail between spinal regions but are essentially identical in structural organization. The disks are widest in the cervical and lumbar area; the caudal cervical intervertebral disks are the widest disks in the dog. The intervertebral disk can be divided anatomically, histologically, and functionally into two sections: the nucleus pulposus (an internal semi-fluid mass) and the annulus fibrosus (an external layer of fibrous connective tissue) (Figure 46-2).

The nucleus pulposus develops from the embryonic notochord.[1] In neonates, it is large and contains a large number of cells of notochordal origin.[4] These cells tend to disappear with age, and chondrocyte-like cells then predominate.[4-6] The nucleus pulposus is positioned eccentrically within the confines of the fibrous annulus pulposus. The ventral aspect of the annulus fibrosus is approximately two times the height of the dorsal annulus, thus leaving the nucleus pulposus closer in position to the spinal canal (Figure 46-2). The nucleus pulposus is composed of loose, delicate fibrous strands in a gelatinous matrix that suspends fibrocyte- and chondrocyte-like cells in an avascular environment.[7] Most of the fibers within the nucleus are not arranged in any fashion, but those closest to the vertebral endplate embed into it at an angle.

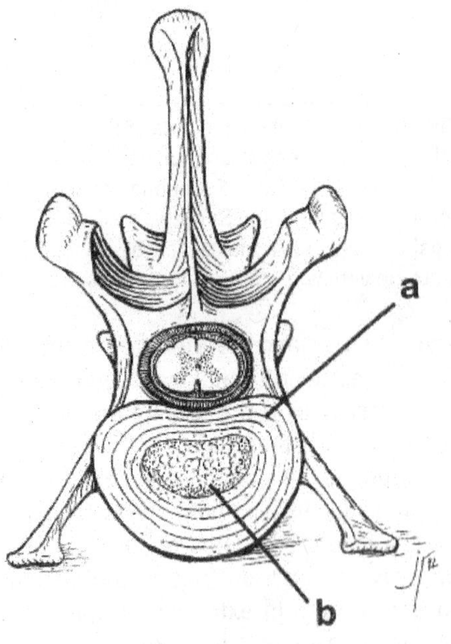

Figure 46-2. Schematic transverse drawing of a lumbar vertebra at the level of the intervertebral disk. a.annulus fibrosus; b.nucleus pulposus. (With permission from Wheeler SJ, Sharp NJH: Functional anatomy. In Small Animal Spinal Disorders: Diagnosis and Surgery. Wheeler SJ, Sharp NJH (eds). London: Mosby-Wolfe, 1994. Illustration by Joseph E. Trumpey, North Carolina State University.)

The annulus fibrosus forms the confinement of the nucleus pulposus and strongly attaches to the adjacent intervertebral bodies. The primary cell type in this portion of the intervertebral disk has fibrocyte characteristics.[8] The cells are located between bundles of fibrocartilage that is arranged in parallel fiber bundles (lamellae) that course in oblique orientation, crossing at angles of 100 to 120 degrees to each other.[7,9,10] When cut transversely, these fibers have an appearance of concentric rings surrounding the nucleus pulposus.[7,9,10] The lamellae are thinner and more densely packed in the dorsal aspect (closer to the spinal canal) of the annulus fibrosus. By comparison, the lamellar bands are thicker and more distinct in the ventral aspect of the annulus.[2] No definable structural interface exists between the nucleus pulposus and annulus fibrosus; their fibers blend imperceptibly in a transitional zone. In this region, the lamellae of fibrocartilage become less organized and the collagenous and cellular composition begins to change.[7] Cells in the outer annulus fibrosus are similar to fibroblasts but the cells in the transitional zone are more chondrocytic in nature.[2] This region is involved in the postnatal development of the intervertebral disk and has been observed to be broader in immature disks from chondrodystrophic breeds of dogs.[11]

The articular surface of the vertebral body, or the vertebral endplate, is concave in its center and covered with cribriform cartilage that renders this region porous.[12] Unlike typical arthrodial joints, the surface of the endplate does not possess compact cartilage tissue between the medullary cavity of the vertebral body and the nucleus pulposus of the intervertebral disk. In this region, the bony trabelculae blend with the chondrous endplate and the fibers of the nucleus pulposus and inner lamellae of the annulus fibrosus.[13-17] Adjacent to the central depression of the endplate, dense compact bone forms the edges of the vertebral body. This region of the endplate serves as an apophysis for attachment of the fibers of the annulus fibrosus and dorsal and ventral longitudinal ligaments.[18] The osseous outer ring provides the firmest attachment of the disk to the vertebral body where the outer lamellar bands of the annulus fibrosus (also referred to as Sharpey's fibers) penetrate it.[18-20] The outermost lamellar fibers of the annulus extend beyond the confines of the disk to blend with the vertebral periosteum and longitudinal ligaments.[1,2]

Physiology of the Intervertebral Disk

Macromolecular Composition

The major macromolecular components of the intervertebral disk are collagenous and noncollagenous proteins, proteoglycans, and glycoproteins.[7,17,21-24] Collagen forms the strong structural fibrocartilage network of the disk and anchors it to the vertebral endplates, allowing containment of the cells and extracellular matrix.[5,7,25] It is found in the highest concentration in the annulus fibrosus. The annulus fibrosus possesses mostly type I and some type II collagen; the nucleus pulposus only possesses type II collagen.[22,26,27] In transition from the inner lamellae of the annulus fibrosus to the nucleus pulposus, the concentration of type II collagen increases and type I decreases.[27,28] The type of collagen present in each region is related to its mechanical function. Type II collagen is most suited to load-bearing functions, whereas type I collagen is better at withstanding tensile loads.[25,29-31] Other collagen types are found in much lesser concentrations within the disk.[5,28,32] Elastic fibers are also present within the disk and are oriented parallel to the collagen fibers.[5] They are found in dense concentration between the lamellae of collagen fibers and likely play a role in sliding and recoil of the lamellar fibers during deformation.[5,33]

The proteoglycans found in the extracellular matrix are composed of glycosaminoglycans or GAGs (long chains of monosaccharides) covalently bound to a central protein core (Figure 46-3).[34-39] Aggrecan is the most abundant of these proteoglycans in the intervertebral disk.[4,27,40] The GAGs present in the intervertebral disk are primarily chondroitin sulfate and keratan sulfate.[12,24] The highest concentration of proteoglycans is found in the nucleus pulposus, which is associated with type II collagen,[41] but these proteins are also present in the intercellular matrix of the annulus fibrosus. Proteoglycans are negatively charged macromolecular complexes. Those concentrated in the nucleus pulposus and transitional zones possess polar groups (carboxyl and sulfonyl) that convey a high degree of hydrophilicity. Binding of water to the hydrophilic groups, up to 9 times the volume of the proteins,[5,12,26,27,34,40,42,43] is responsible for the gelatinous consistency of the nucleus pulposus.[24,27] The normal intervertebral disk is highly hydrated; the water content of a young intervertebral disk is approximately 80 to 85% in the nucleus pulposus and 60 to 78% in the annulus fibrosus.[24,27] The nucleus pulposus of a young disk has seven to eight times more proteoglycan than the annulus fibrosus, and half as much collagen.[44-46] Proteoglycan turnover varies with age, but in people, the average turnover rate is two to three years.[12,40] With age, the nucleus pulposus becomes more collagenous in structure.

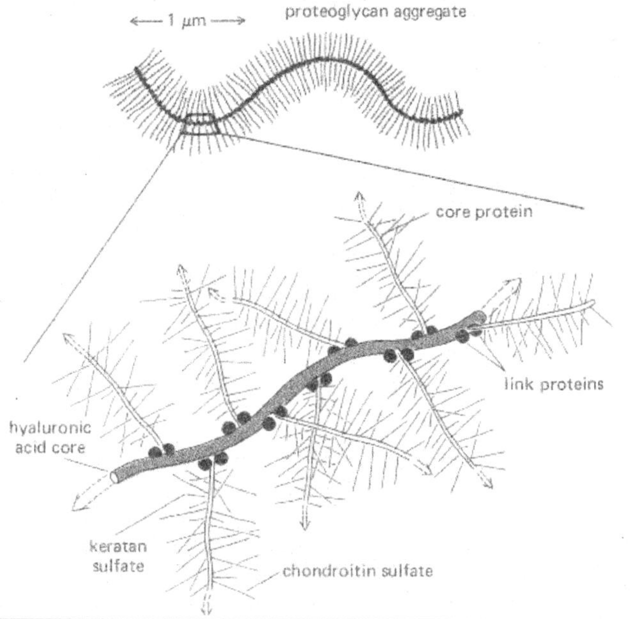

Figure 46-3. Schematic of the glycosaminoglycan aggregate and its associated molecular components. (With permission from Alberts B, Bray D, Lewis J, et al: Molecular Biology of the Cell, 2nd ed. New York: Garland Press, 1989.)

Blood Supply and Nutrition of the Intervertebral Disk

The intervertebral disk is the largest avascular structure in the body, but it is biochemically vital. It is characterized by a high rate of metabolic activity[4,47,48] and, unlike arthrodial joints that receive nutrition through synovial fluid, it receives its nutrition and disposes of metabolic waste via diffusion. Nutrition and metabolic waste product removal are brought to and from the disk, respectively, by diffusion from two sources: the bone-disk interface vasculature of the vertebral endplate, which supplies the majority of the disk, and an adjacent peripheral vascular plexus, which supplies the outermost one to two mm of the annulus fibrosus and surrounding soft tissues.[5,16,48-52] In some instances the nutrients may need to diffuse several millimeters to parts of the disk farthest from the endplate capillary system.[5,50] The endplate arterial supply to the disk arises from the same supply as the vertebral body and drains into either a venous network or into bone marrow veins.[53] The endplate capillary system forms terminal loops that penetrate the subchondral endplate,[13,54-58] and diffusion of materials to and from the disk occur at this interface. The concentration of capillaries is highest at the center and decreases toward the periphery of the disk.[17] This vasculature, like the systemic vasculature, is regulated by the autonomic nervous system (muscarinic receptors) and is responsive to external stimuli.[59]

Like most systems that are dependent on diffusion for equilibrium of solutes, two properties affect this diffusion: the partition coefficient and diffusion coefficient.[12] The partition coefficient defines the equilibrium of solutes between that found in the plasma and the intervertebral disk.[12] It depends on both the size and charge of the particle of interest.[12,17,60] Small uncharged solutes will be near equilibrium between the plasma and the intervertebral disk, whereas large molecules such as albumin and lysozyme are excluded.[12,50,60,61] In regard to ionic solutes, the intervertebral disk matrix possesses a high content of proteoglycans, which behave as fixed, negatively charged aggregates.[26,34,42,43,45,60,62] The concentration of these molecules is much higher in the nucleus pulposus and inner annular lamellae compared with that in the outer annulus fibrosus.[17] Particles or solutes with positive charge diffuse easily into this region, allowing for a higher concentration of cationic particles in the disk compared with that in the plasma.[12,17,60] Negatively charged particles are repulsed by the existing overall negative charge of the disk and tend to be in higher concentration in the plasma.[12,14,17] This differential in ionic permeability has been supported by studies on antibiotic concentrations in the intervertebral disk; negatively charged antibiotics (penicillin and cefuroxime) penetrate much less effectively than positively charged antibiotics (aminoglycosides).[61,63,64] Because of differential concentrations of proteoglycans, and thus, fixed negative charges throughout the disk, some difference may exist between the sources of diffused solutes based on the partition coefficient. Cationic solutes may diffuse more easily from the endplate interface vasculature and anions from the peripheral vasculature, whereas small uncharged particles are equally distributed from both vascular capillary systems (Figure 46-4).[12,60]

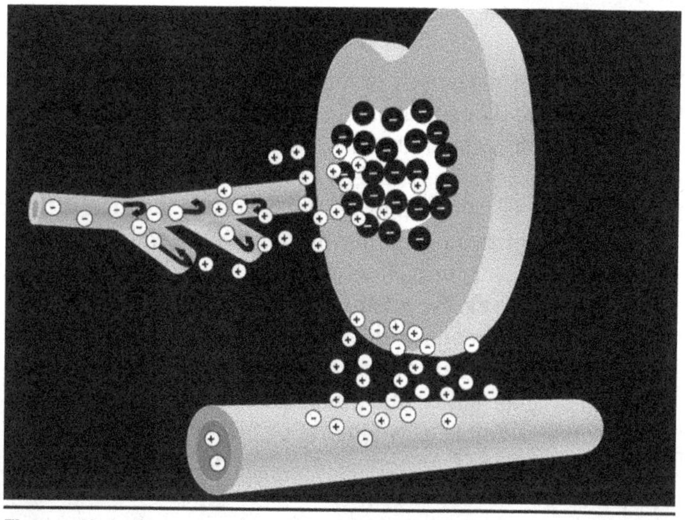

Figure 46-4. The central portion of the intervertebral disk (nucleus pulposus and inner lamellae of the annulus fibrosus) possesses a predominately negative charge owing to higher concentrations of proteoglycans. Because of the differential charge in the inner and outer regions of the disk, the partition coefficient for charged particles differs between the peripheral vascular plexus and interface vasculature at the vertebral endplate. Cationic solutes more readily diffuse from the interface vasculature than do anionic solutes. Anionic solutes are more likely to diffuse from the peripheral vascular plexus.

The diffusion coefficient characterizes solute mobility.[12] Solute mobility is slower in the intervertebral disk compared with that in the plasma because of the presence of large compact molecules such as collagen and proteoglycans.[12] Without considering solute charge, the diffusion coefficient is 40 to 60% of that in water.[12,14] Mobility is greatest where the water content is higher, as seen in the nucleus pulposus and inner annular lamellae.[12]

Movement along the spine may provide a "pumping" action, and likely aids in diffusion of the larger molecules into the disk.[12] This "pumping action" may induce some degree of convective transport by which negatively charged and larger molecules with lower diffusion coefficients may move into the disk.[65-68] Convective transport may also aid in the movement of molecules synthesized by the disk cells.[17]

Like any organ, the intervertebral disk requires an adequate supply of nutrients and biochemical building blocks to maintain its integrity. Glucose is consumed at a high rate as the primary energy source of the intervertebral disk.[69] Because of low oxygen concentration in the disk, anaerobic glycolysis with production of lactic acid is the primary metabolic pathway.[17,27] The intervertebral disk develops mechanisms by which to survive in an acidic environment.[27] When glucose demands are not met, disk cell vitality is adversely affected.[70-75] In addition, when lactic acid production is decreased, the increasing pH of the intervertebral disk results in reduced production of extracellular matrix components. The production and activation of proteases that breakdown the extracellular matrix is not likewise impaired.[76] Thus, the overall net effect of inadequate energy supply is impaired cellular viability and loss of extracellular matrix components. The disk is not as dependent on oxygen supply as it is on glucose. Under hypoxic conditions, the cells become dormant and synthesis of extracellular matrix is impaired.[5,72,76,77] Long-term, however, this would result in a net loss of extracellular matrix as well.

The diffusion of molecules is regulated by the rate of metabolism leading to diffusional gradients. Gradients for oxygen and glucose exist throughout the disk, especially toward the center of the disk where concentrations are lowest.[71,72,77] For example, glucose consumption is up to 100 times greater than the rate of incorporation of sulfate during proteoglycan synthesis.[16] The diffusional gradient for sulfate is low because it is consumed and replenished easily, whereas the diffusional gradient for glucose is steep because the concentration is low.[16] Accordingly, high cellular density in certain regions of the disk also results in steeper diffusional gradients simply by the nature of higher demand. Cell density tends to be highest where the diffusional distances are the shortest; thus, cell density is dictated by nutrient diffusional constraints.[78]

Function of the Intervertebral Disk

The primary function of the intervertebral disk is both to contribute to protective structural alignment and to resist and redistribute stresses along the spine.[29] It must be strong enough to withstand normal physiologic loads (torsion, shear, bending, and compression)[7,10,56,79-85] and yet deformable enough to allow flexibility and mobility.[12,23,86-89] Whereas the spinous ligaments and articular facets tend to withstand torsional, bending, and shear forces, the intervertebral disk is biomechanically best constructed to withstand compressive forces.[12,23,86,88,89] The mechanical properties of the intervertebral disk are conferred upon it by its biochemical nature related to the quantity and quality of its matrix glycosaminoglycans.[5,10,40] Altered biochemistry of the intervertebral disk alters its mechanical properties and ability to withstand axial stresses. The nucleus pulposus is anatomically situated within the intervertebral disk along the center of the axis of movement, which is the equilibrium between tension generated on the convex side and compression on the concave side when the spine is bent.[31,90-93] Because of its gelatinous make up, the nucleus pulposus behaves as a viscous fluid under applied pressure (compression) with considerable elastic rebound and return to its original position on release of the pressure. The nucleus pulposus essentially serves as a "hydraulic shock absorber" allowing disk deformity and dissipation of forces equally over the annulus fibrosus and vertebral end plates.[23,29,31,94,95] Fluid is essentially incompressible; therefore, the internal pressure achieved during compression of the nucleus pulposus pushes the annulus out radially in a horizontal plane of distortion (Figure 46-5).[12,31,84,94-96] The annulus fibrosus itself is normally highly elastic and readily absorbs axial stresses, but it is constructed to best resist the high tensile forces generated during compression by sliding of the lamellar fibers across one another.[12,29,31,40,87,94,95] The lamellae of the annulus fibrosus are strongest when forces are generated along the direction of its fibers and these forces, therefore, are best counterbalanced by the alternating, oblique arrangement of these lamellae.[31,84,97,98] The tensile forces are the highest in the outer lamellar layers and this is where the majority of injuries to the intervertebral disk occur.[31] Initially, the intervertebral disk is easily deformed, but as compressive force increases, it becomes "stiffer" to prevent structural collapse.[90,96,99,100] With increasing sustained compression, gradual efflux of interstitial fluid out of the disk will result in additional microscopic movement of the disk known as "creep."[96,101] This is particularly noted as a diurnal effect in people, in whom 25% of the fluid is expressed during the day with loading and reimbibed when they sleep at night when the axial stresses are relieved.[5]

The spine is loaded both by external forces and internal forces generated by muscles (preload).[5,102] Regular movement and normal physiologic loads are necessary for extracellular matrix composition; metabolic activity of the disk cells is regulated in response to these loads.[103-109] Nucleus pulposus cells primarily respond to changes in hydrostatic and osmotic pressure, whereas the annulus fibrosus responds to tensile strains that originate from flexion or extension.[5] Dynamic compression of the spine has been shown to result in alterations of gene expression and histochemisty within 2 hours to 1 week of loading.[110,111] Biomechanical stresses modulate the maintenance and remodeling of the connective tissue and extracellular matrix of the disk. In turn, the quality and quantity of these components are responsible for the effectiveness of these tissues to withstand these loads.[109]

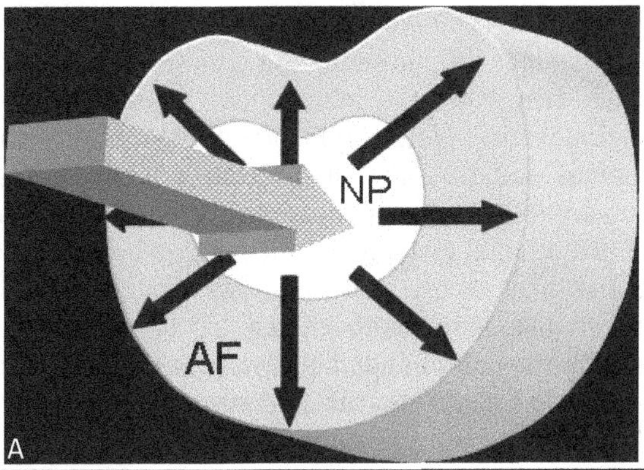

Figure 46-5A. The nucleus pulposus (NP) absorbs axial compressive forces along the spine. The nucleus is fluid by its nature and, thus, incompressible.

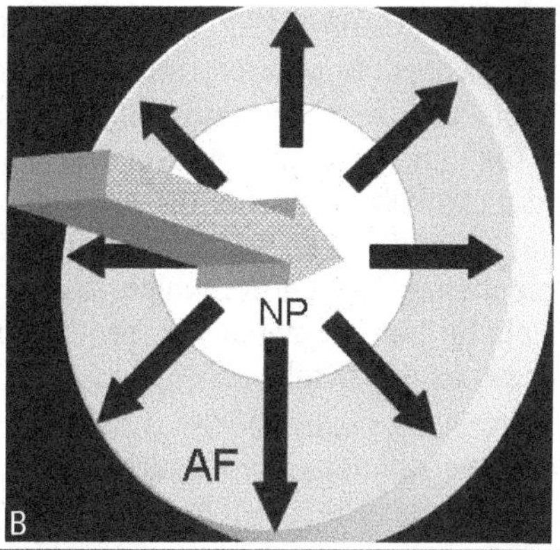

Figure 46-5B. The nucleus (NP) transmits the forces radially across the disk to the annulus fibrosus (AF) which is elastic and can expand to accommodate the tensile forces.

Aging and Pathology of the Intervertebral Disk

Degeneration is a deterioration of the physical properties of a tissue with changes in cellular function and tissue content that result in destruction or inhibition of function. Degeneration is an ultimate consequence of aging. Although aging is the most common cause of tissue degeneration, genetics, nutrition, and external factors (i.e., lifestyle) also play a role.[50,59,112-123] Aging and degeneration of the intervertebral disk usually occur in parallel and may be a continuum of the same process.[17,27,124] Distinguishing aging from degeneration is difficult; separating these two processes may be the key to understanding degenerative changes that are not age-related.[17,25,27,124] With degeneration, alteration of the intrinsic structure, biochemical characteristics, and cellular function and apoptosis ensues.[27] The biochemical and biomechanical alterations that occur lead to further progression of degeneration of the intervertebral disk.[38,125-130]

Although the cellular component is only about 1% of the disk composition,[5] these cells are responsible for the production and maintenance of all the macromolecules. Not only do they produce the extracellular matrix, but they also produce enzymes that break it down. In the healthy disk, the rates of synthesis and catabolism are in equilibrium.[5] Matrix degradation occurs when the rate of production decreases and/or rate of breakdown increases.[5] With a limited cell density, it is not surprising that the cells cannot maintain the health of the disk indefinitely. Degeneration is associated with both an alteration in cellular activity and celluar density.[124,131] The chondrocytic cells change the characteristics and decrease the synthesis of new extracellular matrix components.[132,133] Initially, clusters of cells involved in a reparative process may be present within the disk, but cells undergo limited cell division.[17] As degeneration progresses, cells undergo both apoptosis and necrosis.[17,134,135]

Several cytokines have been implicated in intervertebral disk degeneration. The role of cytokines in health and in the cause or effect of degeneration of intervertebral disks is not yet understood. Implicated cytokines include tumor necrosis factor (TNF), interleukin-1a and 1b (IL-1), vascular endothelial growth factor (VEGF), nerve growth factor (NGF), and matrix metalloproteinases (MMPs). Ingrowth and proliferation of nerve fibers,[136] endothelial cells,[137,138] and fibroblasts have been observed in relation to the degenerative disk, suggesting that biochemical events are occurring that have autocrine and paracrine effects.[25] Expression of VEGF has been demonstrated in the intervertebral disk.[139] Synthesis of NGF by vessels growing into the disk has been demonstrated,[25] suggesting that the neovasculature is influencing the ingrowth of nerve fibers. IL-1 has been shown to be involved in cartilage homeostasis[140] and is associated with a switch from anabolic to catabolic metabolism in the chondrocyte.[141,142] IL-1 has been shown to regulate angiogenesis, potentially by activating VEGF.[143,144] It has also been implicated in both the initiation of extracellular matrix degeneration and pain associated with disk disease.[145] The release of prostaglandins involved with the mediation of pain, such as prostaglandin $E2_{\alpha}$ ($PgE2_{\alpha}$), and production of degradative enzymes, such as matrix metalloproteinases (MMPs), have been shown to be increased under the influence of IL-1b.[145] Concentrations of interleukin-6 (IL-6) and $PgE2_{\alpha}$ were shown to be higher than normal in culture of herniated disks.[145] The stimulus for production of these cytokines has not been identified. In cartilage, these molecules may be intermediaries in the suppression of proteoglycan synthesis by interleukin-1 (IL-1),[146] promoting a net loss of proteoglycans. Conversely, IL6 is a tissue inhibitor of MMP (TIMMP) in articular cartilage and may actually serve a protective role by inhibiting matrix degeneration.[147]

Interest has been intense over the last 10 years in the role of matrix metalloproteinases (MMPs) in degenerative joint disease. Less is known about their role in intervertebral disk metabolism and degeneration; however, herniated disks cultured in vitro have been shown to produce relatively high levels of MMPs, primarily gelatinase and stromelysin (which degrade gelatin and the core proteins of proteoglycans, respectively).[145,148-153] Matrix metalloproteinase expression is highly regulated by cytokines and proinflammatory mediators such as TNF, IL1, IL8, and prostaglandins.[151,154-156] The exact role of MMPs is not known, but they have been shown to be involved in the inflammatory cascade and may play a role in radiculopathy and disk matrix degeneration. This is especially true of disk matrix proteoglycans.[151] Because the production of these enzymes in normal intervertebral disks is low, MMPs may also play a role in disk maintenance by acting as a stimulus to remodel and by partially resorbing herniated disk.[151] One problem with previous studies evaluating MMPs is that healthy "control" disk material was not compared with degenerative herniated material.[149,157] Two possibilities exist for the production of MMPs during intervertebral disk degeneration: 1. degenerating disks make more matrix degenerative enzymes and cytokines, resulting in breakdown of the disk matrix; or 2. the herniated disk itself stimulates the production. However, it is possible that both events are concurrent. The degenerative cells may be biochemically altered, which is followed by disk herniation, which further promotes the production of matrix degenerative enzymes and cytokines.[151]

Many macromolecular changes occur with normal aging and with degeneration of the intervertebral disk. Some of these changes are likely "preprogrammed" events during development such as loss of notochordal cells, mesenchymal apoptosis, and loss of the congenital vasculature.[27] With these events, the characteristics of homeostasis within the disk change dramatically.[27] The most significant of these in aging and degeneration of the disk are alterations in the structure and function of the proteoglycans and collagens. Alterations in these macromolecules subsequently lead to loss of hydration and impairment of biomechanical function of the disk. As the disk ages, aggrecan is proteolyzed by matrix metalloproteinases and cleaved by free radicals,[23] and its concentration decreases within the disk.[23,158] This is particularly prominent in the nucleus pulposus.[159] In addition to proteolysis of aggrecan, the chain length of chondroitin sulfate is shortened on the proteoglycan, and a shift occurs from chondroitin sulfate to keratan sulfate as the predominant glycosaminoglycan.[127] The synthesis of chondroitin sulfate, but not keratan sulfate, requires oxidation of glucuronic acid. The alteration in chain length and ratio of these GAGs may reflect decreased supply of oxygen as the disk grows in size and the nuclear cells move farther away from the vasculature.[160] With degeneration, loss of nutrient and oxygen supply to the disk results from altered diffusion through the endplate, further contributing to the altered GAG ratio. It is the aggregate negative charge of the proteoglycans and their GAGs that maintains adequate hydrostatic pressure within the disk. Proteolysis results in a high concentration of nonaggregating proteoglycans that are too large to diffuse from the disk.[7,27] These retained nonaggregating proteoglycans may still contribute to the hydrostatic pressure of the disk, but are not as functional.[5,7,27] Therefore, the disk, losing as much as 20% of its water content, becomes dehydrated and the disk height decreases.[7] In addition, there is an increase in collagen type II production in the nucleus pulposus,[161,162] with more relative decreases in water and proteoglycan content.[132] The nucleus begins to become more fibrocartilaginous in structure and less distinct grossly from the annulus fibrosus. The fluid-like behavior of the nucleus pulposus transforms into more solid-like properties,[163] and the function of the nucleus pulposus in dissipating compressive forces fails.

Collagenous tissues change structure with age, wear, and time.[25] As the disk collagen ages, collagenase damages the fibrillar collagen.[132,164] Damage to the collagen increases with age and becomes more extensive. Accumulation of these damaged fibers reflects the slow metabolic rate and repair of collagen in the intervertebral disk.[27,132,164] Damaged collagen fibers fray and fibrillate,[114] resulting in loss of lamellar organization.[124] In addition to collagen damage, the fibril diameter tends to increase over time by cross-linking via glycation.[23] Thickening of the fibrils results in impaired sliding of the lamellae and adversely affects the biomechanical properties of the disk.[165] As these injuries accumulate over time, the mechanical strength of the disk eventually weakens.[27] With the concurrent degenerative changes in the nucleus pulposus, the annulus bears higher percentage of the compressive forces than normal, further contributing to injury.[25,166] Both radial and concentric fissures begin to develop, and the disk may bulge. With progressive degeneration and injury, the annulus may eventually fail and collapse.[7,167] Microfractures in the vertebral endplate also occur and may actually precede the disk pathology as a consequence of increased intradiskal pressure and altered nutrition.[20,167-169]

Alterations in normal motion and mechanical loading of the intervertebral disk may also play a role in accelerating degeneration.[40,102] The cells can exhibit both catabolic and anabolic responses depending on type, magnitude, duration, and localization of the forces exerted on the intervertebral disk. With low to moderate magnitude of static compression, anabolic activity increases in the inner AF and NP. For example, normal tensile forces have been shown to induce type I collagen synthesis,[10,162] promoting maintenance of disk function. Abnormal intradiskal pressures, either too high or low, have a catabolic effect, inhibiting prostaglandin synthesis and increasing synthesis nitrous oxide and matrix metalloproteinases.[10170] Most likely, magnitudes and frequencies of forces exist that are physiologically healthy for each cell type within the intervertebral disk to promote maximal biosynthesis and repair.[102,171]

The effects of both overload and immobilization have been studied by Stokes et al.[102] In vitro motion segment testing revealed that annular tears can occur with both excessive static or repetitive loading.[172,173] The annulus fibrosus is damaged by both fiber disruption and separation of lamellar layers. Multiple fissures and microfailure occur before complete failure. Periods of static compression induced changes in the cell synthesis and gene expression for collagen, PGs, and proteases as well as increased cellular apoptosis[161,174-181] Overload to the spine results in "wear and tear," with localized trauma to the intervertebral disk, which is difficult to heal because of slow metabolic turnover.[7] Accumulation of injury continues to weaken the disk until its ability to repair is overcome by recurrent injury.[182] Conversely, hypomobility may not necessarily be beneficial for the intervertebral disk. Most of what is known about hypomobility of joints has been studied in articular cartilage and is not yet proven for the spine.[102,183-188] Stokes et al[102] postulated that hypomobility will also lead to degeneration of the intervertebral disk. In a state of hypomobility, the stimulus to cellular activity is altered as is transport of nutrient metabolites, which alters the viability of the disk.

Both hypermobility and hypomobility may occur in the early and late stages of disk degeneration, respectively. Degeneration initially results from increased movement and excessive loading, which ultimately leads to pain, resulting in tissue stiffening owing to limitation of motion. People with low back pain develop altered muscle activation patterns that change the physiologic loading of the spine, which ultimately results in even more axial compression and shear loading.[189] Altered muscle activation patterns with resultant change in forces generated on the intervertebral disk likely occur in animals as well, as evidenced by abnormal postures (e.g., kyphosis).

Adequate blood supply is necessary for continued health of the intervertebral disk; derangements in nutrient supply are associated with disk degeneration.[17,50] The integrity of the vasculature is affected by both aging[115,190] and injury.[115,21190] Blood and nutrient supply to the disk may be affected in several ways. Diseases that may block blood flow through the vasculature, such as atherosclerosis[118,120] and thrombotic disorders,[113,117] have been associated with degenerative disk disease. Other factors observed in people such as smoking[50] and chronic exposure to vibration[59] (such as long-haul trucking) may impair the vasculature by affecting muscarinic receptors[191] and are shown to have an association with higher incidence of disk degeneration. OIn addition, the thickness of the vertebral endplate diminishes with age and becomes calcified.[25,27,94,192,193] Sclerosis of the subchondral bone and vertebral endplate calcification alters the permeability of the endplate and has been associated with degenerative disk disease.[73,192] It is not known, however, if these endplate changes precede or are a part of the degenerative process.[17] As the intervertebral disk becomes dessicated, the relative content of proteoglycan increases and the movement of solutes becomes even more restricted, setting up a vicious cycle of loss of nutrition.[17]

Degenerative Disk Disease of the Dog

In the dog, morphologic and physiologic changes in the intervertebral disk have been divided into two categories: Hansen's type I and type II. Hansen's type I disk degeneration is associated with chondroid metaplasia, which is characterized by extracellular matrix degeneration, peripheral and central mineralization of the nucleus pulposus, and cellular death.[11] These changes are biochemically associated with a 40 to 50% decrease of proteoglycan and reversal of the chondroitin sulfate: keratan sulfate ratio. Decreased GAG content results in decreased water imbibition by the disk and loss of properties of "shock absorption" and deformability.[2,22,46,194,195] The annulus is then subject to increased loading by axial pressures. Failure of the mechanical properties of the nucleus pulposus results in dysfunction of the annulus fibrosus, causing fissures and displacement of the nucleus pulposus.[2] Alternatively, it is possible that the changes in the annulus pulposus are primary rather than secondary. It is theorized that an increased proteolysis of type I collagen and elastin leads to the weakening of the annulus pulposus.[2] Hansen's type I disk degeneration is associated frequently with massive extrusion of nucleus pulposus material and dorsal annulus pulposus (Figure 46-6). Hansen's type I disk material consistency ranges from soft and cheesy to firm with a granular appearance (mineralization). Historically, the period of time over which the disk extrusion occurs in the clinical setting varies from acute to slowly progressive.

Hansen type I intervertebral disk disease is primarily seen in chondrodystrophic breeds of dogs.[2] The breed most commonly affected with this form of disk degeneration by far is the dachshund, with a relative risk[12] six times greater than any other breed.[196] Other affected breeds include the Shih tzu, Lhasa apso, Pomeranian, beagle, poodle, Basset hound, Cocker spaniel, and the Welsh corgi. However, other less commonly considered breeds appear to have similar changes. For example, the author has seen many Dalmatians with this form of disk pathology, particularly in the cervical disks. In these breeds, the aging pattern of the interverteberal disk is different from that found in Hansen's type II disk degeneration. Degeneration of the disk may start as early as four months of age and is usually complete by 12 to18 months.[2] Mechanical properties of the disk are usually decreased by two to three years of age, about the time when clinical signs first occur.[2] Although disk degeneration is seen in dachshunds as old as 13 to15 years of age, most animals are between two and eight years of age when clinical signs first occur. Although the older dog probably has disk degeneration, the change in the disk may reach a stage where the intradiskal pressure is so low that the annulus is no longer affected.[2] Genetics have been shown to play a role in the disease in the beagle and dachshund.[2] In dachshunds, intervertebral disk disease is thought to be governed by polygenetic, nondominant, factors that are not sex-linked.[197] Environmental factors such as life-style and nutrition probably play a role.

Hansen's type II IVDDz is most commonly seen in nonchondrodystrophic dogs and is an aging change that results in fibroid metaplasia of the intervertebral disk, particularly the nucleus pulposus.[2] This type of degeneration is more similar to the aging and degenerative changes in the intervertebral disk commonly observed in people. The disease is usually seen in middle-aged-to-older large breed dogs but any nonchondrodystrophic breed is susceptible to type II disk disease.[2] Even chondrodystrophic breeds may develop this type of disk degeneration with advancing age. As the intervertebral disk ages, the nucleus pulposus is gradually replaced by more mature fibrocartilage (fibroid metaplasia), and eventually the difference between the nucleus pulposus and the annulus fibrosus is difficult to determine grossly. The disk eventually changes in its biochemistry to possess lower GAG levels.[2,47,124] Mineralization of the disk is uncommon in this type of degeneration. Typically, type II disk disease is associated with a partial rupture (fissures) in the dorsal annulus. This is observed as a herniation (or bulging) of the dorsal annulus.[2] Although massive ejection of the nucleus pulposus is not considered to be part of the disease process, acute rupture with concussive spinal cord injury is possible. Typically, when this occurs and surgery is performed, the material removed from the spinal canal is more ligamentous and similar to the annulus fibrosus in appearance.

The pathogenesis of spinal cord injury with intervertebral disk extrusion is associated with both concussive and compressive forces. Although compression secondary to extrusion is associated with some degree of concussion, concussive injury does not always result in compression of the spinal cord. In the author's experience, concussive disk extrusions without significant compression are seen most commonly in poodles and Cocker spaniels. Paucity or complete absence of disk material has been observed by many surgeons during surgical intervention.

The velocity and force of the intervertebral disk extrusion is the single most important factor responsible for irreversible paraplegia. In experimental spinal cord injury, it is the magnitude of the force of the injury (=/> 400 g/cm) that produces irreversible changes.[198] The the sequelae of the concussive event are hemorrhage, ischemia, and vascular spasm.[198] This results in release of potent inflammatory mediators, as well as iron and propagation of ischemia with a final common pathway to the production of oxygen free radicals.[198] These biochemical events induce an inherent, progressive autodestruction of the spinal cord.[198] These autodestructive processes may continue for 24 to 48 hours[198] and are probably responsible for those animals that are presented for surgery within a few hours of onset with good deep-pain response and wake from anesthesia without a deep-pain response. When these autodestructive processes are not limited to a focal area of injury, they may continue in both directions from the injury and result in ascending/descending myelomalacia. Impacts of lesser magnitude and rate often produce more transient dysfunction and are associated with reversible changes.[198] Improvement in these cases is probably secondary to resolution of edema, hemorrhage, demyelination, and ischemia.

Compression of the spinal cord may result in a grossly swollen, indented, flattened, or atrophied spinal cord, depending on the duration of the compression. Adherence of disk material to the dura is sometimes observed with chronic lesions. Extensive epidural and/or subdural hemorrhage may be present with highly concussive disk extrusions. The disk material may migrate over one to two vertebral bodies. Microscopic changes in the spinal cord depend on the force of disk extrusion and duration of compression. Severe concussion of the cord will result in edema, inflammation, and focal and multifocal hemorrhage and malacia in the gray and white matter.[199-221] Astrocytosis and skeletonized trabeculae of blood vessels are observed in old malacic lesions.[200,206-227] Chronic compression is associated with demyelination, remyelination, Wallerian degeneration, and focal areas of ischemia.[200,206-227] The pathomechanisms of spinal cord compression are discussed in depth in Chapter 42.

Clinical Signs of Intervertebral Disk Disease

Clinical signs associated with intervertebral disk disease depend on both the location (lesion localization) and the degree and severity of disk extrusion. One of the earliest clinical signs of intervertebral disk disease is pain. The origins of pain associated with disk disease are presented in the following section. Neurologic abnormalities occur either concurrently or may follow pain when intervertebral disk extrusion results in compression and concussion of the spinal cord. Determining the localization of a neurologic lesion is important for choosing the appropriate clinical diagnostic tests, list of differential diagnoses, and occasionally, prognosis. Lesion localization can be divided into four anatomic spinal cord syndromes: C1-C5 (cervical), C6-T2 (cervicothoracic), T3-L3 (thoracolumbar), and L4-S3 (lumbosacral). Clinical signs of spinal cord disease can be divided into anatomic syndromes because, in general, the clinical signs are similar for lesions inclusive in these spinal cord segments. This is because of the location of the lower motor neurons supplying the thoracic (C6-T2) and pelvic limbs (L4-S3). Not all of the clinical signs (neurologic deficits) will be present in each case. The signs associated with each syndrome can be found in Tables 46-1 through 46-4.

No evidence exists that trauma plays a role in the pathogenesis of intervertebral disk extrusion; however, clinical signs may be precipitated by a seemingly minor trauma or normal activity. Many dogs that become acutely paralyzed with Hansen's type I thoracolumbar intervertebral disk extrusions have a recent history of jumping off a piece of furniture. Trauma is not necessary, however, for clinical signs to occur. Significant trauma is usually required to cause extrusion (rupture) of a healthy disk. This has been most commonly observed by the author in animals that have been hit by motor vehicles or have run head first into a solid immovable object (i.e., tree or wall).

Approximately 70% of intervertebral disk extrusions are between T11-12 and L2-3. C2-3 is reported to be the most common location of cervical intervertebral disk extrusions,[2] but extrusion is seen commonly in all cervical disks up to C6-7. C7-T1 extrusions do occur but are rare. Dogs are less likely to be neurologically affected with cervical disk extrusions compared with thoracolumbar intervertebral disk extrusions unless they are severe and/or acute. Advanced imaging, such as computed tomography or magnetic resonance imaging, has helped to identify severe compression of the spinal cord (e.g., disk material filling 75% of the canal) when the only clinical sign the dog displays is unremitting cervical pain (Figure 46-6). Dogs with thoracolumbar disk extrusions are more likely to show neurologic deficits than are those with cervical disk extrusion, but dogs may have significant compression of the spinal cord and show only spinal pain clinically.[228] Cervical and lumbar disk extrusions in the intervertebral foramen can result in radiculopathy and nerve root signature as the only clinical sign.

Pathogenesis of Pain Associated with Intervertebral Disk Disease

Animals with acute intervertebral disk extrusion are almost always in pain. This differentiates disk extrusion from fibrocartilagenous emboli, which are almost never associated with persistent pain. Pain associated with disk disease in the thoracolumbar region is usually manifested by a kyphotic posture. A dog with pain from cervical disk disease will often keep its neck flexed with the nose pointed to the ground and roll the eyes upward when spoken to or encouraged to move. Because of the low head carriage, these animals may also appear to have a kyphotic posture. Pain may be elicited by palpation of the neck and cervical spine manipulation, such as lifting the head or turning the neck laterally. Pain often decreases in intensity over time and with the use of analgesics or anti-inflammatory medications. Animals with Hansen's type II disk extrusions are often not in overt pain or may not be experience pain on spinal palpation if the lesion is chronic.

Table 46-1. Clinical Signs of C1-C5 (Cervical) Syndrome

Signs	Comments
Mentation	Normal
Gait	May be ataxic in all 4 limbs, or just in pelvic limbs if compressive lesion is very mild
	May be weak or paralyzed in all 4 limbs (tetraparesis/tetraplegia) or in the ipsilateral limbs on one side (hemiparesis/plegia) if a lesion is affecting only one side of the spinal cord (uncommon)
Postural reactions	Hopping may be decreased to absent in all 4 limbs or in the limbs on the side that is ipsilateral to the lesion (uncommon)
	Conscious proprioception may be decreased to absent in all 4 limbs or any of the limbs
Spinal reflexes	Limb tone is normal to exaggerated (spastic)
	Myotatic reflexes are normal to exaggerated (hyperreflexic) in all 4 limbs
	Crossed extensor reflexes may be elicited in all or any of the limbs
Pain	Painful diseases include: intervertebral disk disease, vertebral neoplasia, diskospondylitis, osteomyelitis, meningomyelitis, trauma/fracture, spinal cord neoplasia (+/-), and vertebral anomalies (+/-)
	Nonpainful diseases include: vascular injuries (i.e., FCE), spinal cord degenerative diseases, neoplasis, and vertebral anomalies
Urinary incontinence as seen in table 46-2	Spinal cord neoplasia, and vertebral anomalies
Horner's syndrome	If present, usually partial*
Respiratory difficulties	May occur with severe lesions (breathing maintained by diaphragmatic muscles; the chest wall muscles are weak or paralyzed from injury to descending motor axons from the respiratory center in the medulla)**
	Loss of diaphragm function may occur with lesions in the mid-cervical region (C4)

***Partial Horner's signs are usually anisocoria and occasionally mild enophthalmos. These signs are attributed to injury of the lateral tectotegmental spinal tracts that carry information from the posterior hypothalamus (which exerts excitatory activity on the sympathetic nervous system) through the brain and cervical cord to the preganglionic nerve cell bodies in the thoracic spinal cord. Usually these signs are observed in only severe cases of C1-5 syndrome (e.g., acute tetraparesis/plegia).**

**** Usually these signs are observed in only severe cases of C1-5 syndrome (e.g., acute tetraparesis/plegia).**

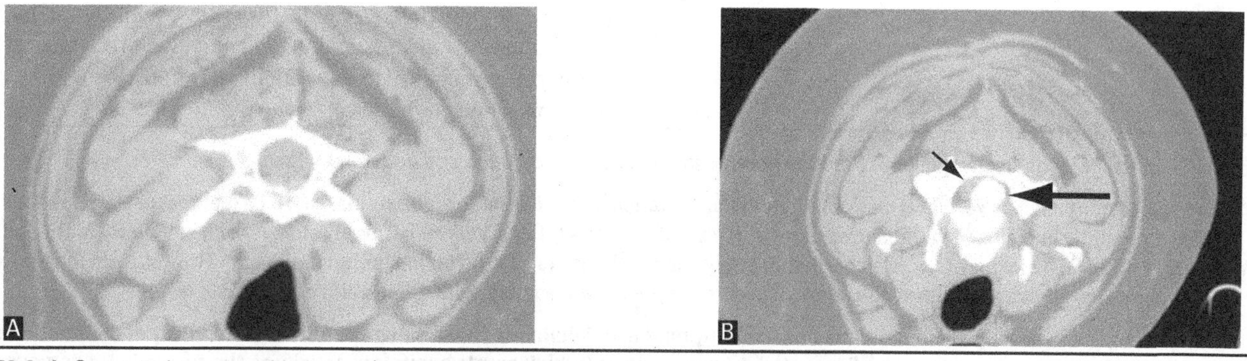

Figure 46-6. A. Computed tomographic image (uncontrasted) of a normal vertebral canal and spinal cord; B. massive Type I disk extrusion (large arrow) has severely compressed the spinal cord to about 20% of its normal diameter to the left of the disk (small arrow).

Table 46-2. Clinical Signs of C6-T2 (Cervicothoracic) Syndrome

Signs	Comments
Mentation	Normal
Gait	May be ataxic in all 4 limbs, or only in pelvic limbs if compressive lesion is very mild May be weak or paralyzed in all 4 limbs (tetraparesis/tetraplegia) or in the ipsilateral limbs on one side (hemiparesis/plegia) if a lesion is affecting only one side of the spinal cord (uncommon)*
Postural reactions	Hopping may be decreased to absent in all 4 limbs or in the limbs on the side that is ipsilateral to the lesion (uncommon) Conscious proprioception may be decreased to absent in all 4 limbs or in any of the limbs
Spinal reflexes	Thoracic limbs Muscle tone is decreased (hypotonic) to absent (flaccidity)** Myotatic reflexes are decreased (hyporeflexic) to absent (areflexic) in the thoracic limbs (some or all reflexes) May have neurogenic muscle atrophy (chronic) Pelvic limbs Muscle tone is normal to exaggerated (hyperreflexic) Myotatic reflexes are normal to exaggerated (hyperreflexic) Muscle atrophy is not present unless the animal is paralyzed and has disuse atrophy Panniculus reflex may be decreased to absent on the ipsilateral side or on both sides from a lesion in the T1-2 area (the motor component of this reflex) with normal sensation along the back Crossed extensor reflexes may be elicited in the pelvic but not thoracic limbs May have decreased to absent deep pain response in all 4 limbs
Pain	Painful diseases include: intervertebral disk disease, vertebral neoplasia, diskospondylitis, osteomyelitis, meningitis, trauma/fracture, spinal cord neoplasia (+/-) and vertebral anomalies (+/-) Nonpainful diseases include: vascular injuries (i.e., FCE), spinal cord degenerative diseases (degenerative myelopathy), spinal cord neoplasia, and vertebral anomalies
Urinary incontinence	Upper motor neuron bladder (uncommon unless the signs are severe, i.e., tetraplegia)
Horner's syndrome	If present, usually partial if the lesion is cranial to T1*** May have a complete ipsilateral Horner's syndrome if the lesion is in the T1-2 region
Respiratory difficulties	May occur with severe lesions (breathing maintained by diaphragmatic muscles; chest wall muscles are weak or paralyzed from injury to descending upper motor neuron axons from the respiratory center in the medulla)

*** Occasionally an animal will display postural reaction deficits in just one thoracic limb and both pelvic limbs.**

****Caudal cervical lesions such as vertebral malformation/malarticulation may have some signs similar to C1-C5 lesion (spasticity in the thoracic limbs), but when carefully examined significant weakness in myotatic biceps brachii and withdrawal reflexes with spasticity in triceps muscle tone are observed. Mild C6-T2 lesions (e.g., disk herniation) may appear similar to a C1-C5 lesion (normal reflexes). The ability to localize a lesion to the cervical region vs. other areas is probably more important; signalment may help with differential diagnoses.**

****Partial Horner's signs are usually anisocoria and occasionally mild enophthalmos. These signs are attributed to injury of the lateral tectotegmental spinal tracts that carry information from the posterior hypothalamus (which exerts excitatory activity on the sympathetic nervous system) through the brain and cervical spinal cord to the preganglionic sympathetic nerve cell bodies in the thoracic spinal cord. Usually these signs are observed in only severe cases of C1-5 syndrome (e.g., acute tetraparesis/plegia).**

Table 46-3. Clinical Signs of T3-L3 (Thoracolumbar) Syndrome

Signs	Comments
Mentation	Normal
Gait	Normal thoracic limbs
	May be ataxic in the pelvic limbs
	May be weak or paralyzed in the pelvic limbs (paraparesis/ plegia)
Postural reactions	Normal in thoracic limbs
	May be decreased to absent in the pelvic limbs
Spinal reflexes	Normal in thoracic limbs
	Muscle tone is normal to hypertonic in pelvic limbs
	Myotatic reflexes are normal to hyperreflexic in the pelvic limbs
	Crossed extensor reflexes may be elicited in one or both pelvic limbs
	Deep pain response may be decreased to absent caudal to the lesion
	May have Schiff-Sherrington syndrome (usually a severe injury)
Pain	Painful diseases include:
	intervertebral disk disease, vertebral neoplasia, diskospondylitis, osteomyelitis, meningitis, trauma/fracture, spinal cord neoplasia (+/-), and vertebral anomalies (+/-)
	Nonpainful diseases include:
	vascular injuries (i.e., FCE), spinal cord
	degenerative diseases (degenerative myelopathy), spinal cord neoplasia, and vertebral anomalies
Urinary incontinence	May have upper motor neuron bladder with severe lesions (about the time the animal can no longer walk)

Table 46-4. Clinical Signs of L4-S3 (Lumbosacral) Syndrome

Signs	Comments
Mentation	Normal
Gait	Normal thoracic limbs May be ataxic in the pelvic limbs May be weak or paralyzed in the pelvic limbs (paraparesis/plegia)
Postural reactions	Normal in thoracic limbs May be decreased to absent in the pelvic limbs
Spinal reflexes	Normal in thoracic limbs Muscle tone is decreased (hypotonic) to absent (flaccidity) in pelvic limbs Myotatic reflexes are decreased to absent (hyporeflexia) in the pelvic limbs* Deep pain response may be decreased to absent caudal to the lesion
Pain	Painful diseases include: intervertebral disk disease, vertebral neoplasia, diskospondylitis, osteomyelitis, meningitis, trauma/fracture, spinal cord neoplasia (+/), and vertebral anomalies (+/-) Nonpainful diseases include: vascular injuries (i.e., FCE), spinal cord degenerative diseases (degenerative myelopathy), spinal cord neoplasia and vertebral anomalies
Urinary incontinence	May have lower motor neuron bladder dysfunction May dribble urine
Other	May have fecal incontinence and/or dilated anal sphincter Nerve root signature (less common than C6-T2 lesions) May have tail weakness/paralysis/hypoesthesia

***An increased patellar reflex may be observed when a lesion affects the nerve cell bodies and spinal roots that form the sciatic nerve (L6, L7, S1) but not those that form the femoral nerve (L4-6). This arises because there is a loss of function in the antagnostic muscles innervated by the sciatic nerve. This is not truly hyperreflexia and is, therefore, termed "pseudohyperreflexia."**

The spinal cord itself does not possess pain receptors. Pain associated with intervertebral disk degeneration has been shown to be secondary to both biochemical mediators and nervous tissue impingement. The ligaments, joint capsule and bone of the spinal column are highly innervated.[7] The external periosteum, articular facet joint capsule, and longitudinal ligaments receive sensory innervation by way of the medial branches of the dorsal rami of the spinal nerves. These rami form the recurrent sinuvertebral nerve.[12] The dorsal longitudinal ligament and the ventral meningeal surface are highly innervated by complex encapsulated nerve endings as well as poorly myelinated free nerve endings.[12] These fibers also innervate the outer lamellae of the dorsal annulus fibrosus,[12,136,229] and direct stimulation of the intervertebral disk has been shown to induce pain.[7] Although the innervation to these structures is diverse and includes postganglionic efferent fibers from the thoracolumbar autonomic ganglia (which mediate smooth muscle function of the vasculature of the spinal canal) and proprioceptive fibers (which modulate postural reactions), the majority of these fibers are nociceptive in function.[12,136] In fact, it has been shown experimentally that stimulation of tissues innervated by the sinuvertebral nerve elicits back pain.[12] In the clinical setting, mechanical impingement of the nerve roots (radiculopathy) and meninges by extruded disk material and hypertrophy of supporting structures play a role in generation of pain.[36,230] For example, as the intervertebral disk space narrows, concomitant settling of the facet joint and narrowing of the cross-sectional area of the intervertebral foramen occur, which may result in nerve root compression.[231,232] The production of osteophytes may also play a role by contributing to pre-existing narrowing of the intervertebral foramen.[231] In addition, arthritic changes often occur in the facet joint synovium and joint capsule.

Disruption of the intervertebral disk and its ligaments and compression of nervous tissue lead to production of neuropeptides. Algesic molecules can activate nociceptors in the dorsal longitudinal ligament and dorsal annulus.[40,230] The somata of the dorsal root ganglia make various algesic neuropeptides that are transported to central and peripheral terminals.[230] Implicated neurogenically derived cytokines include substance P and calcitonin gene-related protein (CRGP). Substance P has been shown be a part of the inflammatory cascade and of the generation of pain in radiculopathy. CGRP found in primary sensory neurons has been shown to mediate nociception and mechanoreception.[230] Non-neurogenic-derived chemicals released during tissue damage (e.g., bradykinin, serotonin, histamine, and Pgs) also sensitize pain fibers.[230] Extruded intervertebral disk material itself has been implicated as a source of biochemical mediators in the pathophysiology of radicular pain.[157,233-235] In an in vitro study of human herniated disk material removed during decompressive surgery, nitric oxide, prostaglandin E2a, and interleukin 6 concentrations were elevated compared with nonherniated control disks from patients undergoing spinal surgery for other reasons (e.g., scoliosis correction).[151] Nitric oxide is a novel mediator of inflammation and immune regulation.[235] This biochemical has been shown to have both proinflammatory and anti-inflammatory functions. As a proinflammatory agent, it exerts strong vasodilatory effects, promoting vascular leakiness resulting in edema. As an anti-inflammatory agent, it has been shown to inhibit production of IL-6, PgE_2, and thromboxane. The exact function of nitric oxide in the disk and disk degeneration is not known at this time, however.

References

1. Evans HE, Christensen GC: Joints and ligaments. *In* Miller's Anatomy of the Dog, 2nd ed. Evans HE, Christensen GC (eds). Philadelphia: WB Saunders, 2007, pp. 225-268.

2. Braund KG: Intervertebral disk disease. *In* Disease Mechanisms in Small Animal Surgery, 2nd ed. Bojrab MJ, Smeak DD, Bloomberg MS (eds). Philadelphia: Lea & Febiger, 1993, pp. 960-970.

3. Hoerlein BF: Intervertebral disk disease. *In* Veterinary Neurology. Oliver JE, Hoerlein BF, Mayhew IG (eds). Philadelphia: WB Saunders, 1987.

4. Urban JPG, Roberts S, Ralphs J: The nucleus of the intervertebral disk from development to degeneration. Am Zool 40:53-61, 2007.

5. Bibby SR, Jones DA, Lee RB, et al: The pathophysiology of the intervertebral disc. Joint Bone Spine 68(6):537-542, 2001.

6. Taylor JR, Twomey LT: Development of the human intervertebral disc. *In* The Biology of the Intervertebral Disc, vol. 1. Ghosh P (ed). Boca Raton: CRC Press, 1988, pp. 40-82.

7. Urban JP, Roberts S: Development and degeneration of the intervertebral discs. Mol Med Today 1(7):329-335, 1995.

8. Errington RJ, Puustjarvi K, White IR, et al: Characterisation of cytoplasm-filled processes in cells of the intervertebral disc. J Anat 192 (Pt 3):369-378, 1998.

9. Roberts S: Disc morphology in health and disease. Biochem Soc Trans 30:864-869, 2002.

10. Setton LA, Chen J: Cell mechanics and mechanobiology in the intervertebral disc. Spine 29(23):2710-2723, 2004.

11. Hansen HJ: A pathologic-anatomical study on disc degeneration in dog, with special reference to the so-called enchondrosis intervertebralis. Acta Orthop Scand Suppl 11:1-117, 1952.

12. Parke WW: Applied anatomy of the spine. *In Rothman-Simeone* The Spine, 4th ed. Herkowitz HN, Garfin SR, Balderston RA, et al (eds). Philadelphia: WB Saunders, 1992, pp. 29-73.

13. Crock HV, Goldwasser M: Anatomic studies of the circulation in the region of the vertebral end-plate in adult Greyhound dogs. Spine 9(7):702-706, 1984.

14. Gibson MJ, Karpinski MR, Slack RC, et al: The penetration of antibiotics into the normal intervertebral disc. J Bone Joint Surg Br 69(5):784-786, 1987.

15. Hirano N, Tsuji H, Ohshima H, et al: Analysis of rabbit intervertebral disc physiology based on water metabolism. I. Factors influencing metabolism of the normal intervertebral discs. Spine 13(11):1291-1296, 1988.

16. Maroudas A, Stockwell RA, Nachemson A, et al: Factors involved in the nutrition of the human lumbar intervertebral disc: cellularity and diffusion of glucose in vitro. J Anat 120(Pt 1):113-130, 1975.

17. Urban JP, Smith S, Fairbank JC: Nutrition of the intervertebral disc. Spine 29(23):2700-2709, 2004.

18. Bick EM: The osteohistology of the normal human vertebra; its relation to scoliosis and certain lesions incident to growth and senescence. J Mt Sinai Hosp NY 19(3):490-527, 1952.

19. Inoue H: Three-dimensional architecture of lumbar intervertebral discs. Spine 6(2):139-146, 1981.

20. Marchand F, Ahmed AM: Investigation of the laminate structure of lumbar disc anulus fibrosus. Spine 15(5):402-410, 1990.

21. Bayliss MT, Johnstone B: Biochemistry of the intervertebral disc. *In* The Lumbar Spine and Back Pain. Jayson MI (ed). New York: Churchill-Livingstone, 1992, pp. 111-131.

22. Ghosh P, Bushell GR, Taylor TF, et al: Collagens, elastin and noncollagenous protein of the intervertebral disk. Clin Orthop Relat Res (129):124-132, 1977.

23. Oegema TR Jr: Biochemistry of the intervertebral disc. Clin Sports Med 12(3):419-439, 1993.

24. Puschel J: Der Wassergehalt normaler and degenerierter Zwischenwirbelscheiben. Beitr Path Anat 84:123-130, 1930.

25. Freemont AJ, Watkins A, Le MC, et al: Current understanding of cellular and molecular events in intervertebral disc degeneration: implications for therapy. J Pathol 196(4):374-379, 2002.

26. Eyring EJ: The biochemistry and physiology of the intervertebral disk. Clin Orthop 67:16-28, 1969.

27. Roughley PJ: Biology of intervertebral disc aging and degeneration: involvement of the extracellular matrix. Spine 29(23):2691-2699, 2004.

28. Eyre DR, Muir H: Quantitative analysis of types I and II collagens in human intervertebral discs at various ages. Biochim Biophys Acta 492(1):29-42, 1977.

29. Adams MA: Biomechanics of the lumbar motion segment. *In* Modern Manual Therapy. Boyling JD, Palastanga N, Jull GA, et al (eds). NY: Churchill Livingstone, 1995, pp.109-129.

30. Evans JM, Barbenel JC: Structural and mechanical properties of tendon in relation to function. Eq Vet J 7:1-8, 1975.

31. White AA, Panjabi MM: Clinical Biomechanics of the Spine. Philadelphia: JB Lippincott, 1978.

32. Roberts S, Ayad S, Menage PJ: Immunolocalisation of type VI collagen in the intervertebral disc. Ann Rheum Dis 50(11):787-791, 1991.

33. Yu J, Winlove PC, Roberts S, et al: Elastic fibre organization in the intervertebral discs of the bovine tail. J Anat 201(6):465-475, 2002.

34. Bernardi G, Happey F, Naylor A: Mucopolysaccharides from cartilage and nucleus pulposus. Nature 180(4598):1341-1342, 1957.

35. Buckwalter JA, Pedrini-Mille A, Pedrini V, et al: Proteoglycans of human infant intervertebral disc. Electron microscopic and biochemical studies. J Bone Joint Surg Am 67(2):284-294, 1985.

36. Burke MJ, Banks WJ, Nelson AW, et al: Histochemical study of the anulus fibrosus in normal canine caudal cervical intervertebral discs. Res Vet Sci 40(1):18-23, 1986.

37. Emes JH, Pearce RH: The proteoglycans of the human intervertebral disc. Biochem J 145(3):549-556, 1975.

38. Stevens RL, Ewins RJ, Revell PA, et al: Proteoglycans of the intervertebral disc. Homology of structure with laryngeal proteoglycans. Biochem J 179(3):561-572, 1979.

39. Sylven G, Paulson S, Hirsch C, et al: Biophysical and physiological investigations on cartilage and other mesenchymal tissues. II. The ultrastructure of bovine and human nuclei pulposi. J Bone Joint Surg Am 33-A(2):333-340, 1951.

40. Kuiper JI, Verbeek JH, Frings-Dresen MH, et al: Keratan sulfate as a potential biomarker of loading of the intervertebral disc. Spine 23(6):657-663, 1998.

41. Scott JE, Haigh M: Proteoglycan-collagen interactions in intervertebral disc. A chondroitin sulphate proteoglycan associated with collagen fibrils in rabbit annulus fibrosus at the d-e bands. Biosci Rep 6(10):879-888, 1986.

42. Hendry NG: The hydration of the nucleus pulposus and its relation to intervertebral disc derangement. J Bone Joint Surg Br40-B(1):132-144, 1958.

43. Naylor A, Horton WG: The hydrophilic properties of the nucleus pulposus of the intervertebral disc. Rheumatism 11(2):32-35, 1955.

44. Ghosh P, Taylor TK, Braund KG, et al: The collagenous and non-collagenous protein of the canine intervertebral disc and their variation with age, spinal level and breed. Gerontology 22(3):124-134, 1976.

45. Ghosh P, Taylor TK, Braund KG, et al: A comparative chemical and histochemical study of the chondrodystrophoid and nonchondrodystrophoid canine intervertebral disc. Vet Pathol 13(6):414-427, 1976.

46. Ghosh P, Taylor TK, Braund KG: Variation of the glycosaminoglycans of the intervertebral disc with ageing. II. Non-chondrodystrophoid breed. Gerontology 23(2):99-109, 1977.

47. Brown MD: The Pathophysiology of Intervertebral Disc: Anatomical, Physiological and Biomedical Considerations. Philadelphia: Jefferson Medical College, 1969.

48. Maroudas A: Nutrition and metabolism of the intervertebral disk. *In* The Biology of the Intervertebral Disc. Ghosh P (ed). Boca Raton: CRC Press, 1988.

49. Hassler O: The human intervertebral disc. A micro-angiographical study on its vascular supply at various ages. Acta Orthop Scand 40(6):765-772, 1969.

50. Holm S, Maroudas A, Urban JP, et al: Nutrition of the intervertebral disc: solute transport and metabolism. Connect Tissue Res 8(2):101-119, 1981. START

51. Ogata K, Whiteside LA: 1980 Volvo award winner in basic science. Nutritional pathways of the intervertebral disc. An experimental study using hydrogen washout technique. Spine 6(3):211-216, 1981.

52. Rudert M, Tillmann B: Detection of lymph and blood vessels in the human intervertebral disc by histochemical and immunohistochemical methods. Ann Anat 175(3):237-242, 1993.

53. Crock HV, Yoshizawa H, Kame SK: Observations on the venous drainage of the human vertebral body. J Bone Joint Surg Br 55(3):528-533, 1973.

54. Crock HV, Goldwasser M, Yoshizawa H: Vascular anatomy related to the intervertebral disc. *In* Biology of the Intervertebral Disc. Ghosh P (ed). Boca Raton: CRC Press, 1995, pp. 109-133.

55. Oki S, Matsuda Y, Shibata T, et al: Morphologic differences of the vascular buds in the vertebral endplate: scanning electron microscopic study. Spine 21(2):174-177, 1996.

56. Selard E, Shirazi-Adl A, Urban JP: Finite element study of nutrient diffusion in the human intervertebral disc. Spine 28(17):1945-1953, 2003.

57. Urban JP, Holm S, Maroudas A. Diffusion of small solutes into the intervertebral disc: an in vivo study. Biorheology 15(3-4):203-221, 1978.

58. Whalen JL, Parke WW, Mazur JM, et al: The intrinsic vasculature of developing vertebral end plates and its nutritive significance to the intervertebral discs. J Pediatr Orthop 5(4):403-410, 1985.

59. Hirano N, Tsuji H, Ohshima H, et al: Analysis of rabbit intervertebral disc physiology based on water metabolism. II. Changes in normal intervertebral discs under axial vibratory load. Spine 13(11):1297-1302, 1988.

60. Urban JPG, Maroudas A: Measurement of fixed charge density and partition coefficients in the intervertebral disc. Biochim Biophys Acta 586:166-178, 1979.

61. Shibuya K: Experimental and clinical studies on metabolism with the intervertebral disc. J Jpn Orthop Assoc 44:1-24, 1970.

62. Oegema TR Jr, Bradford DS, Cooper KM: Aggregated proteoglycan synthesis in organ cultures of human nucleus pulposus. J Biol Chem 254(21):10579-10581, 1979.

63. Tai CC, Want S, Quraishi NA, et al: Antibiotic prophylaxis in surgery of the intervertebral disc. A comparison between gentamicin and cefuroxime. J Bone Joint Surg Br 84(7):1036-1039, 2002.

64. Thomas RW, Batten JJ, Want S, et al: A new in-vitro model to investigate antibiotic penetration of the intervertebral disc. J Bone Joint Surg Br 77:967-970, 1995.

65. Boubriak OA: Nutrient supply to the cells of the intervertebral disk. Trans Am Orthop Res Soc 28:1127, 2003.

66. Ferguson SJ, Ito K, Nolte LP: Fluid flow and convective transport of solutes within the intervertebral disc. J Biomech 37(2):213-221, 2004.

67. Mauck RL, Hung CT, Ateshian GA: Modeling of neutral solute transport in a dynamically loaded porous permeable gel: implications for articular cartilage biosynthesis and tissue engineering. J Biomech Eng 125(5):602-614, 2003.

68. O'Hara BP, Urban JP, Maroudas A: Influence of cyclic loading on the nutrition of articular cartilage. Ann Rheum Dis 49(7):536-539, 1990.

69. Nimer E, Schneiderman R, Maroudas A: Diffusion and partition of solutes in cartilage under static load. Biophys Chem 106(2):125-146, 2003.

70. Bibby SR, Fairbank JC, Urban MR, et al: Cell viability in scoliotic discs in relation to disc deformity and nutrient levels. Spine 27(20):2220-2228, 2002.

71. Bibby SR, Jones DA, Ripley RM, et al: Metabolism of the intervertebral disc: effects of low levels of oxygen, glucose, and pH on rates of energy metabolism of bovine nucleus pulposus cells. Spine 30(5):487-496, 2005.

72. Horner HA, Urban JP: 2001 Volvo Award Winner in Basic Science Studies: Effect of nutrient supply on the viability of cells from the nucleus pulposus of the intervertebral disc. Spine 26(23):2543-2549, 2001.

73. Roberts S, Urban JP, Evans H, et al: Transport properties of the human cartilage endplate in relation to its composition and calcification. Spine 21(4):415-420, 1996.

74. Urban MR, Fairbank JC, Bibby SR, et al: Intervertebral disc composition in neuromuscular scoliosis: changes in cell density and glycosaminoglycan concentration at the curve apex. Spine 26(6):610-617, 2001.

75. Urban MR, Fairbank JC, Etherington PJ, et al: Electrochemical measurement of transport into scoliotic intervertebral discs in vivo using nitrous oxide as a tracer. Spine 26(8):984-990, 2001.

76. Razaq S, Wilkins RJ, Urban JP: The effect of extracellular pH on matrix turnover by cells of the bovine nucleus pulposus. Eur Spine J 12(4):341-349, 2003.

77. Ishihara H, Urban JP: Effects of low oxygen concentrations and metabolic inhibitors on proteoglycan and protein synthesis rates in the intervertebral disc. J Orthop Res 17(6):829-835, 1999.

78. Holm S, Nachemson A: Cellularity in the intervertebral disc and its relevance to nutrition. ISSLS (Conf Proc), 1983.

79. Acaroglu ER, Iatridis JC, Setton LA, et al: Degeneration and aging affect the tensile behavior of human lumbar anulus fibrosus. Spine 20(24):2690-2701, 1995.

80. Adams MA, Green TP: Tensile properties of the annulus fibrosus. Eur Spine J 2(4):203-208, 1993.

81. Ebara S, Iatridis JC, Setton LA, et al: Tensile properties of nondegenerate human lumbar anulus fibrosus. Spine 21(4):452-461, 1996.

82. Fujita Y, Duncan NA, Lotz JC: Radial tensile properties of the lumbar annulus fibrosus are site and degeneration dependent. J Orthop Res 15(6):814-819, 1997.

83. Galante JO: Tensile properties of the human lumbar annulus fibrosus. Acta Orthop Scand Suppl:91 1967.

84. Nachemson A: Lumbar intradiscal pressure. Experimental studies on post-mortem material. Acta Orthop Scand Suppl 43:1-104, 1960.

85. Wu HC, Yao RF: Mechanical behavior of the human annulus fibrosus. J Biomech 9(1):1-7, 1976.

86. Brown T, Hansen RJ, Yorra AJ: Some mechanical tests on the lumbosacral spine. J Bone Joint Surg Am (39):1135-1164, 1957.

87. Hoerlein BF: Intervertebral disc protrusions in the dog. I. Incidence and pathological lesions. Am J Vet Res 14(51):260-269, 1953.

88. Panjabi MM, Goel VK, Takata K: Physiologic strains in the lumbar spinal ligaments. An in vitro biomechanical study. 1981 Volvo Award in Biomechanics. Spine 7(3):192-203, 1982.

89. Shah JS, Hampson WG, Jayson MI: The distribution of surface strain in the cadaveric lumbar spine. J Bone Joint Surg Br 60-B(2):246-251, 1978.

90. Farfan HF, Cossette JW, Robertson GH, et al: The effects of torsion on the lumbar intervertebral joints: the role of torsion in the production of disc degeneration. J Bone Joint Surg Am 52(3):468-497, 1970.

91. Nachemson A, Morris JM: In vivo measurements of intradiscal pressure. Diskometry, a method for the determination of pressure in the lower lumbar disks. J Bone Joint Surg Am 46:1077-1092, 1964.

92. Townshend HGG, Leach DH: Relationship between intervertebral joint morphology and mobility in the equine lumbar spine. Eq Vet J 16:461-465, 1984.

93. Virgin WJ: Experimental investigations into the physical properties of the intervertebral disc. J Bone Joint Surg Br 33-B(4):607-611, 1951.

94. Nachemson A, Elfstrom G: Intravital dynamic pressure measurements in lumbar discs. A study of common movements, maneuvers and exercises. Scand J Rehabil Med Suppl 1:1-40, 1970.

95. Szirmai JA: Structure of the intervertebral disc. *In* Chemistry and Molecular Biology of the Intercellular Matrix. Balazs EA (ed). Philadelphia: Academic Press, 1970, pp. 1279-1308.

96. Horton WG: Further observations on the elastic mechanism of the intervertebral disc. J Bone Joint Surg Br 40-B(3):552-557, 1958.

97. Gertzbein SD, Holtby R, Tile M, et al: Determination of a locus of instantaneous centers of rotation of the lumbar disc by moire fringes. A new technique. Spine 9(4):409-413, 1984.

98. Hirsch C, Nachemson A: New observations on the mechanical behavior of lumbar discs. Acta Orthop Scand 23(4):254-283, 1954.

99. Keller TS, Spengler DM, Hansson TH: Mechanical behavior of the human lumbar spine. I. Creep analysis during static compressive loading. J Orthop Res 5(4):467-478, 1987.

100. Koreska J, Robertson D, Mills RH, et al: Biomechanics of the lumbar spine and its clinical significance. Orthop Clin North Am 8(1):121-133, 1977.

101. Pattison ST, Melrose J, Ghosh P, et al: Regulation of gelatinase-A (MMP-2) production by ovine intervertebral disc nucleus pulposus cells grown in alginate bead culture by Transforming Growth Factor-beta(1) and insulin like growth factor-I. Cell Biol Int 25(7):679-689, 2001.

102. Stokes IA, Iatridis JC: Mechanical conditions that accelerate intervertebral disc degeneration: overload versus immobilization. Spine 29(23):2724-2732, 2004.

103. Caterson B: Immunological aspects of markers of joint disease. J Rheumatol Suppl 27:19-23, 1991.

104. Fujisawa T, Hattori T, Takahashi K, et al: Cyclic mechanical stress induces extracellular matrix degradation in cultured chondrocytes via gene expression of matrix metalloproteinases and interleukin-1. J Biochem (Tokyo) 125(5):966-975, 1999.

105. Handa T, Ishihara H, Ohshima H, et al: Effects of hydrostatic pressure on matrix synthesis and matrix metalloproteinase production in the human lumbar intervertebral disc. Spine 22(10):1085-1091, 1997.

106. Hascall VC, Glant TT: Proteoglycan epitopes as potential markers of normal and pathologic cartilage metabolism. Arthritis Rheum 30(5):586-588, 1987.

107. Lane NE, Buckwalter JA: Exercise: a cause of osteoarthritis? Rheum Dis Clin North Am 19(3):617-633, 1993.

108. Thonar EJ, Masuda K, Hauselmann HJ, et al: Keratan sulfate in body fluids in joint disease. Acta Orthop Scand Suppl 266:103-106, 1995.

109. Urban JP: The chondrocyte: A cell under pressure. Br J Rheumatol 33:901-908, 1994.

110. MacLean JJ, Lee CR, Alini M, et al: Anabolic and catabolic mRNA levels of the intervertebral disc vary with the magnitude and frequency of in vivo dynamic compression. J Orthop Res 22(6):1193-1200, 2004.

111. Walsh AJ, Lotz JC: Biological response of the intervertebral disc to dynamic loading. J Biomech 37(3):329-337, 2004.

112. Andersson GBJ: Intervertebral disk herniation: epidemiology and natural history. *In* Low Back Pain: A Scientific and Clinical Overview. Weinstein JN, Gordon SL, (eds). Rosemont, IL: American Academy of Orthopaedic Surgeons, 1996, pp. 7-21.

113. Babhulkar S, Babhulkar S: Osteonecrosis in Sickle Cell hemoglobinopathy. *In* Osteonecrosis- Etiology, Diagnosis and Treatment. Urbaniak JR, Jones JPJ (eds). Am Orthop Assoc 131-133, 1997.

114. Bernick S, Cailliet R: Vertebral end-plate changes with aging of human vertebrae. Spine 7(2):97-102, 1982.

115. Donisch EW, Trapp W: The cartilage endplates of the human vertebral column (some considerations of postnatal development). Anat Rec 169(4):705-716, 1971.

116. Hansson TH, Holm S: Clinical implications of vibration-induced changes in the lumbar spine. Orthop Clin North Am 22:247-253, 1991.

117. Jones JPJ: Subcondral osteonecrosis can conceivably cause disk degeneration and primary osteoarthritis. *In* Osteonecrosis-Etiology, Diagnosis and Treatment. Am Orthop Assoc 1997, pp.135-142.

118. Kauppila LI: Prevalence of stenotic changes in arteries supplying the lumbar spine. A postmortem angiographic study on 140 subjects. Ann Rheum Dis 56(10):591-595, 1997.

119. Kelsey JL, Golden AL, Mundt DJ: Low back pain/prolapsed lumbar intervertebral disc. Rheum Dis Clin North Am 16(3):699-716, 1990.

120. Kurunlahti M, Tervonen O, Vanharanta H, et al: Association of atherosclerosis with low back pain and the degree of disc degeneration. Spine 24(20):2080-2084, 1999.

121. Moore RJ, Osti OL, Vernon-Roberts B, et al: Changes in endplate vascularity after an outer anulus tear in the sheep. Spine 17(8):874-878, 1992.

122. Mundt DJ, Kelsey JL, Golden AL, et al: An epidemiologic study of non-occupational lifting as a risk factor for herniated lumbar intervertebral disc. The Northeast Collaborative Group on Low Back Pain. Spine 18(5):595-602, 1993.

123. Wilder DG, Pope MH, Frymoyer JW: The biomechanics of lumbar disc herniation and the effect of overload and instability. J Spinal Disord 1(1):16-32, 1988.

124. Urban JP, Roberts S: Degeneration of the intervertebral disc. Arthritis Res Ther 5(3):120-130, 2003.

125. Buckwalter JA: Aging and degeneration of the human intervertebral disc. Spine 20(11):1307-1314, 1995.

126. Kitano T, Zerwekh JE, Usui Y, et al: Biochemical changes associated with the symptomatic human intervertebral disk. Clin Orthop Relat Res (293):372-377, 1993.

127. Lyons G, Eisenstein SM, Sweet MB: Biochemical changes in intervertebral disc degeneration. Biochim Biophys Acta 673(4):443-453, 1981.

128. Pearce RH, Grimmer BJ: Target tissue models: the proteoglycans and degeneration of the human intervertebral disc. J Rheumatol Suppl 11:108-110, 1983.

129. Pearce RH, Grimmer BJ, Adams ME: Degeneration and the chemical composition of the human lumbar intervertebral disc. J Orthop Res 5(2):198-205, 1987.

130. Yoganandan N, Larson SJ, Pintar FA, et al: Intravertebral pressure changes caused by spinal microtrauma. Neurosurgery 35(3):415-421, 1994.

131. Boos N, Weissbach S, Rohrbach H, et al: Classification of age-related changes in lumbar intervertebral discs: 2002 Volvo Award in basic science. Spine 27(23):2631-2644, 2002.

132. Antoniou J, Steffen T, Nelson F, et al: The human lumbar intervertebral disc: evidence for changes in the biosynthesis and denaturation of the extracellular matrix with growth, maturation, ageing, and degeneration. J Clin Invest 98(4):996-1003, 1996.

133. Ishihara H, Warensjo K, Roberts S, et al: Proteoglycan synthesis in the intervertebral disk nucleus: the role of extracellular osmolality. Am J Physiol 272(5 Pt 1):C1499-C1506, 1997.

134. Gruber HE, Hanley EN Jr: Analysis of aging and degeneration of the human intervertebral disc. Comparison of surgical specimens with normal controls. Spine 23(7):751-757, 1998.

135. Gruber HE, Hanley EN Jr: Ultrastructure of the human intervertebral disc during aging and degeneration: comparison of surgical and control specimens. Spine 27(8):798-805, 2002.

136. Freemont AJ, Peacock TE, Goupille P, et al: Nerve ingrowth into diseased intervertebral disc in chronic back pain. Lancet 350(9072):178-181, 1997.

137. Kauppila LI: Ingrowth of blood vessels in disc degeneration. Angiographic and histological studies of cadaveric spines. J Bone Joint Surg Am 77(1):26-31, 1995.

138. Yasuma T, Arai K, Yamauchi Y: The histology of lumbar intervertebral disc herniation. The significance of small blood vessels in the extruded tissue. Spine 18(13):1761-1765, 1993.

139. Tolonen J, Gronblad M, Virri J, et al: Platelet-derived growth factor and vascular endothelial growth factor expression in disc herniation tissue: and immunohistochemical study. Eur Spine J 6(1):63-69, 1997.

140. Cawston T, Billington C, Cleaver C, et al: The regulation of MMPs and TIMPs in cartilage turnover. Ann NY Acad Sci 878:120-129, 1999.

141. Nishida Y, D'Souza AL, et al: Stimulation of hyaluronan metabolism by interleukin-1alpha in human articular cartilage. Arthritis Rheum 43:1315-1326, 2000.

142. van den Berg WB: The role of cytokines and growth factors in cartilage destruction in osteoarthritis and rheumatoid arthritis. Z Rheumatol 58(3):136-141, 1999.

143. Jackson JR, Minton JA, Ho ML, et al: Expression of vascular endothelial growth factor in synovial fibroblasts is induced by hypoxia and interleukin 1beta. J Rheumatol 24(7):1253-1259, 1997.

144. Lindholm D, Heumann R, Meyer M, et al: Interleukin-1 regulates synthesis of nerve growth factor in non-neuronal cells of rat sciatic nerve. Nature 330(6149):658-659, 1987.

145. Kang JD, Stefanovic-Racic M, McIntyre LA, et al: Toward a biochemical understanding of human intervertebral disc degeneration and herniation. Contributions of nitric oxide, interleukins, prostaglandin E2, and matrix metalloproteinases. Spine 22(10):1065-1073, 1997.

146. Nietfeld JJ, Wilbrink B, Den OW, et al: The effect of human interleukin 1 on proteoglycan metabolism in human and porcine cartilage explants. J Rheumatol 17(6):818-826, 1990.

147. Lotz JC: Animal models of intervertebral disc degeneration: lessons learned. Spine 29(23):2742-2750, 2004.

148. Crean JK, Roberts S, Jaffray DC, et al: Matrix metalloproteinases in the human intervertebral disc: role in disc degeneration and scoliosis. Spine 22(24):2877-2884, 1997.

149. Fujita K, Nakagawa T, Hirabayashi K, et al: Neutral proteinases in human intervertebral disc. Role in degeneration and probable origin. Spine 18(13):1766-1773, 1993.

150. Goupille P, Jayson MI, Valat JP, et al: Matrix metalloproteinases: the clue to intervertebral disc degeneration? Spine 23(14):1612-1626, 1998.

151. Kang JD, Georgescu HI, Intyre-Larkin L, et al: Herniated lumbar intervertebral discs spontaneously produce matrix metalloproteinases, nitric oxide, interleukin-6, and prostaglandin E2. Spine 21(3):271-277, 1996.

152. Roberts S, Caterson B, Menage J, et al: Matrix metalloproteinases and aggrecanase: their role in disorders of the human intervertebral disc. Spine 25(23):3005-3013, 2000.

153. Weiler C, Nerlich AG, Zipperer J, et al: 2002 SSE Award Competition in Basic Science: expression of major matrix metalloproteinases is associated with intervertebral disc degradation and resorption. Eur Spine J 11(4):308-320, 2002.

154. Burke JG, Watson RW, McCormack D, et al: Intervertebral discs which cause low back pain secrete high levels of proinflammatory mediators. J Bone Joint Surg Br 84(2):196-201, 2002.

155. Burke JG, Watson RW, McCormack D, et al: Spontaneous production of monocyte chemoattractant protein-1 and interleukin-8 by the human lumbar intervertebral disc. Spine 27(13):1402-1407, 2002.

156. Olmarker K, Blomquist J, Stromberg J, et al: Inflammatogenic properties of nucleus pulposus. Spine 20(6):665-669, 1995.

157. Smyth MJ, Wright V: Sciatica and the intervertebral disc; an experimental study. J Bone Joint Surg Am 40-A(6):1401-1418, 1958.

158. Hickey DS, Hukins DW: X-ray diffraction studies of the arrangement of collagenous fibres in human fetal intervertebral disc. J Anat 131(Pt 1):81-90, 1980.

159. Setton LA, Zhu W, Weidenbaum M, et al: Compressive properties of the cartilaginous end-plate of the baboon lumbar spine. J Orthop Res 11(2):228-239, 1993.

160. Taylor JR, Scott JE, Cribb AM, et al: Human intervertebral disc acid glycosaminoglycans. J Anat 180 (Pt 1):137-141, 1992.

161. Hutton WC, Toribatake Y, Elmer WA, et al: The effect of compressive force applied to the intervertebral disc in vivo. A study of proteoglycans and collagen. Spine 23(23):2524-2537, 1998.

162. Terahata N, Ishihara H, Ohshima H, et al: Effects of axial traction stress on solute transport and proteoglycan synthesis in the porcine intervertebral disc in vitro. Eur Spine J 3(6):325-330, 1994.

163. Iatridis JC, Setton LA, Weidenbaum M, et al: Alterations in the mechanical behavior of the human lumbar nucleus pulposus with degeneration and aging. J Orthop Res 15(2):318-322, 1997.

164. Hollander AP, Heathfield TF, Liu JJ, et al: Enhanced denaturation of the alpha (II) chains of type-II collagen in normal adult human intervertebral discs compared with femoral articular cartilage. J Orthop Res 14(1):61-66, 1996.

165. Vernon-Roberts B: Age-related and degenerative pathology of the intervertebral discs and apophyseal joints. *In* Jayson MIV (ed). The Lumbar Spine and Back Pain. NY: Churchill Livingstone, 1992, pp. 17-41.

166. Nachemson AL: Disc pressure measurements. Spine 6(1):93-97, 1981.

167. Osti OL, Vernon-Roberts B, Moore R, et al: Annular tears and disc degeneration in the lumbar spine. A post-mortem study of 135 discs. J Bone Joint Surg Br 74(5):678-682, 1992.

168. Cassidy JJ, Hiltner A, Baer E: Hierarchical structure of the intervertebral disc. Connect Tissue Res 23(1):75-88, 1989.

169. Tsuji H, Hirano N, Ohshima H, et al: Structural variation of the anterior and posterior anulus fibrosus in the development of human lumbar intervertebral disc. A risk factor for intervertebral disc rupture. Spine 18(2):204-210, 1993.

170. Liu GZ, Ishihara H, Osada R, et al: Nitric oxide mediates the change of proteoglycan synthesis in the human lumbar intervertebral disc in response to hydrostatic pressure. Spine 26(2):134-141, 2001.

171. Hutton WC, Elmer WA, Boden SD, et al: The effect of hydrostatic pressure on intervertebral disc metabolism. Spine 24(15):1507-1515, 1999.

172. Adams MA, Hutton WC: The effect of fatigue on the lumbar intervertebral disc. J Bone Joint Surg Br 65(2):199-203, 1983.

173. Adams MA, McMillan DW, Green TP, et al: Sustained loading generates stress concentrations in lumbar intervertebral discs. Spine 21(4):434-438, 1996.

174. Ariga K, Yonenobu K, Nakase T, et al: Mechanical stress-induced apoptosis of endplate chondrocytes in organ-cultured mouse intervertebral discs: an ex vivo study. Spine 28(14):1528-1533, 2003.

175. Chin JR, Lotz JC: Cell death and matrix gene expression are upregulated in intervertebral discs during recovery from short durations of moderate static compression. Trans Orthop Res Soc 26:874, 2001.

176. Hsieh AH, Lotz JC: Prolonged spinal loading induces matrix metalloproteinase-2 activation in intervertebral discs. Spine 28(16):1781-1788, 2003.

177. Iatridis JC, Mente PL, Stokes IA, et al: Compression-induced changes in intervertebral disc properties in a rat tail model. Spine 24(10):996-1002, 1999.

178. Lee CR, Proveda L, Iatridis JC, et al: Intervertebral disc organ culture system: application for mechanobiology. Trans Orthop Res Soc 29:838, 2004.

179. Lotz JC, Colliou OK, Chin JR, et al: Compression-induced degeneration of the intervertebral disc: an in vivo mouse model and finite-element study. Spine 23(23):2493-2506, 1998.

180. Lotz JC, Chin JR: Intervertebral disc cell death is dependent on the magnitude and duration of spinal loading. Spine 25(12):1477-1483, 2000.

181. Ohshima H, Urban JP, Bergel DH: Effect of static load on matrix synthesis rates in the intervertebral disc measured in vitro by a new perfusion technique. J Orthop Res 13(1):22-29, 1995.

182. Adams MA, Freeman BJ, Morrison HP, et al: Mechanical initiation of intervertebral disc degeneration. Spine 25(13):1625-1636, 2000.

183. Hong SP, Henderson CN: Articular cartilage surface changes following immobilization of the rat knee joint. A semiquantitative scanning electron-microscopic study. Acta Anat (Basel) 157(1):27-40, 1996.

184. Leroux MA, Cheung HS, Bau JL, et al: Altered mechanics and histomorphometry of canine tibial cartilage following joint immobilization. Osteoarthritis Cartilage 9(7):633-640, 2001.

185. Muller FJ, Setton LA, Manicourt DH, et al: Centrifugal and biochemical comparison of proteoglycan aggregates from articular cartilage in experimental joint disuse and joint instability. J Orthop Res 12(4):498-508, 1994.

186. Narmoneva DA, Cheung HS, Wang JY, et al: Altered swelling behavior of femoral cartilage following joint immobilization in a canine model. J Orthop Res 20(1):83-91, 2002.

187. Saamanen AM, Tammi M, Jurvelin J, et al: Proteoglycan alterations following immobilization and remobilization in the articular cartilage of young canine knee (stifle) joint. J Orthop Res 8(6):863-873, 1990.

188. Setton LA, Mow VC, Muller FJ, et al: Mechanical behavior and biochemical composition of canine knee cartilage following periods of joint disuse and disuse with remobilization. Osteoarthritis Cartilage 5(1):1-16, 1997.

189. Marras WS, Davis KG, Ferguson SA, et al: Spine loading characteristics of patients with low back pain compared with asymptomatic individuals. Spine 26(23):2566-2574, 2001.

190. Bernick S, Walker JM, Paule WJ: Age changes to the anulus fibrosus in human intervertebral discs. Spine 16(5):520-524, 1991.

191. Wallace AL, Wyatt BC, McCarthy ID, et al: Humoral regulation of blood flow in the vertebral endplate. Spine 19(12):1324-1328, 1994.

192. Nachemson A, Lewin T, Maroudas A, et al: In vitro diffusion of dye through the end-plates and the annulus fibrosus of human lumbar intervertebral discs. Acta Orthop Scand 41(6):589-607, 1970.

193. Roberts S, Menage J, Eisenstein SM: The cartilage end-plate and intervertebral disc in scoliosis: calcification and other sequelae. J Orthop Res 11(5):747-757, 1993.

194. Braund KG, Ghosh P, Taylor TK, et al: The qualitative assessment of glycosaminoglycans in the canine intervertebral disc using a critical electrolyte concentration staining technique. Res Vet Sci 21(3):314-317, 1976.

195. Yasuma T, Makino E, Saito S, et al: Histological development of intervertebral disc herniation. J Bone Joint Surg Am 68(7):1066-1072, 1986.

196. Goggin JE, Li AS, Franti CE: Canine intervertebral disk disease: characterization by age, sex, breed, and anatomic site of involvement. Am J Vet Res 31(9):1687-1692, 1970.

197. Ball MU, McGuire JA, Swaim SF, et al: Patterns of occurrence of disk disease among registered dachshunds. J Am Vet Med Assoc 180(5):519-522, 1982.

198. Das GD: Perspectives in anatomy and pathology of paraplegia in experimental animals. Brain Res Bull 22:7-32, 1989.

199. al-Mefty O, Harkey HL, Marawi I, et al: Experimental chronic compressive cervical myelopathy. J Neurosurg 79(4):550-561, 1993.

200. Allen AR: Remarks on the histopathological changes in the spinal cord due to impact: An experimental study. J Nerve Ment Dis 41:141-147, 1914.

201. Anthes DL, Theriault E, Tator CH: Characterization of axonal ultrastructural pathology following experimental spinal cord compression injury. Brain Res 702(1-2):1-16, 1995.

202. Arbit E, Galicich W, Galicich JH, et al: An animal model of epidural compression of the spinal cord. Neurosurg 24(6):860-863, 1989.

203. Bedford PD, Bosanquet FD, Russell WR: Degeneration of the spinal cord associated with cervical spondylosis. Lancet 2(2):55-59, 1952.

204. Blight AR: Cellular morphology of chronic spinal cord injury in the cat: analysis of myelinated axons by line-sampling. Neuroscience 10(2):521-543, 1983.

205. Bohlman HH, Emery SE: The pathophysiology of cervical spondylosis and myelopathy. Spine 13(7):843-846, 1988.

206. Bunge MB, Puckett WR, Becerra JL, et al: Observations on the pathology of human spinal cord injury. A review and classification of 22 new cases with details from a case of chronic cord compression with extensive focal demyelination. Adv Neurol 59:75-89, 1993.

207. Carlson GD, Gorden CD, Nakazowa S, et al: Perfusion-limited recovery of evoked potential function after spinal cord injury. Spine 25(10):1218-1226, 2000.

208. Carlson GD, Gorden CD, Oliff HS, et al: Sustained spinal cord compression: part I: Time-dependent effect on long-term pathophysiology. J Bone Joint Surg Am 85-A(1):86-94, 2003.

209. Delamarter RB, Sherman J, Carr JB: Pathophysiology of spinal cord injury. Recovery after immediate and delayed decompression. J Bone Joint Surg Am 77(7):1042-1049, 1995.

210. Fehlings MG, Skaf G: A review of the pathophysiology of cervical spondylotic myelopathy with insights for potential novel mechanisms drawn from traumatic spinal cord injury. Spine 23(24):2730-2737, 1998.

211. Fujiwara K, Yonenobu K, Hiroshima K, et al: Morphometry of the cervical spinal cord and its relation to pathology in cases with compression myelopathy. Spine 13(11):1212-1216, 1988.

212. Fukui K, Kataoka O, Sho T, et al: Pathomechanism, pathogenesis, and results of treatment in cervical spondylotic myelopathy caused by dynamic canal stenosis. Spine 15(11):1148-1152, 1990.

213. Gambardella G, Staropoli C, Toscano S, et al: Clinical, morphometric and ultrastructural aspects in a new model of spinal cord compression. J Neurol Sci 35(3):131-138, 1991.

214. Gledhill RF, Harrison BM, McDonald WI: Demyelination and remyelination after acute spinal cord compression. Exp Neurol 38(3):472-487, 1973.

215. Gledhill RF, Harrison BM, McDonald WI: Pattern of remyelination in the CNS. Nature 244(5416):443-444, 1973.

216. Gledhill RF, McDonald WI: The pattern of demyelination and remyelination following transient experimental spinal cord compression. Ann Neurol 1:552, 1977.

217. Gooding MR: Pathogenesis of myelopathy in cervical spondylosis. Lancet 2(7890):1180-1181, 1974.

218. Gooding MR, Wilson CB, Hoff JT: Experimental cervical myelopathy. Effects of ischemia and compression of the canine cervical spinal cord. J Neurosurg 43(1):9-17, 1975.

219. Griffiths IR: Vasogenic edema following acute and chronic spinal cord compression in the dog. J Neurosurg 42(2):155-165, 1975.

220. Griffiths IR, Pitts LH, Crawford RA, Trench JG: Spinal cord compression and blood flow. I. The effect of raised cerebrospinal fluid pressure on spinal cord blood flow. Neurol 28(11):1145-1151, 1978.

221. Holtz A: Spinal cord compression injury. Acta Univ Ups 209:1-43, 1989.

222. al-Mefty O, Harkey HL, Marawi I, et al: Experimental chronic compressive cervical myelopathy. J Neurosurg 79(4):550-561, 1993.

223. Anthes DL, Theriault E, Tator CH: Characterization of axonal ultrastructural pathology following experimental spinal cord compression injury. Brain Res 702(1-2):1-16, 1995.

224. Arbit E, Galicich W, Galicich JH, et al: An animal model of epidural compression of the spinal cord. Neurosurg 24(6):860-863, 1989.

225. Bedford PE, Bosanquet FD, Russell WR: Degeneration of the spinal cord associated with cervical spondylosis. Lancet 2(2):55-59, 1952.

226. Blight AR: Cellular morphology of chronic spinal cord injury in the cat: analysis of myelinated axons by line-sampling. Neuroscience 10(2):521-543, 1983.

227. Bohlman HH, Emery SE: The pathophysiology of cervical spondylosis and myelopathy. Spine 13(7):843-846.,1988.

228. Penning V, Platt SR, Dennis R, et al: Association of spinal cord compression seen on magnetic resonance imaging with clinical outcome in 67 dogs with thoracolumbar intervertebral disc extrusion. J Small Anim Pract 47(11):644-650, 2006.

229. Mayer TG: Lumbar musculature: anatomy and function. *In Rothman-Simeone* The Spine, 4th ed. Herkowitz HN, Garfin SR, Balderston RA, et al (eds). Philadelphia: WB Saunders, 1992, pp.75-82.

230. Brower RS: Cervical disk disease. *In Rothman-Simeone* The Spine, 4th ed. Herkowitz HN, Garfin SR, Balderston RA, et al (eds). Philadelphia: WB Saunders, 1992, pp. 455-474.

231. Garfin SR, Rydevik BL, Lipson SJ, et al: Spinal stenosis. *In Rothman-Simeone* The Spine, 4th ed. Herkowitz HN, Garfin SR, Balderston RA, et al (eds). Philadelphia: WB Saunders, 1992, pp. 779-796.

232. Revel M, Mayoux-Benhamou MA, Aaron C, et al: [Morphological variations of the lumbar foramina during flexion-extension and disk collapse]. Rev Rhum Mal Osteoartic 55(5):361-366, 1988.

233. McCarron RF, Wimpee MW, Hudkins PG, et al: The inflammatory effect of nucleus pulposus. A possible element in the pathogenesis of low-back pain. Spine 12(8):760-764, 1987.

234. Saal JS, Franson RC, Dobrow R, et al: High levels of inflammatory phospholipase A2 activity in lumbar disc herniations. Spine 15(7):674-678, 1990.

235. Wehling P, Molsberger A, Schulitz KP: [Pain and the spine. A review. 1. On the pathophysiology of radicular pain syndromes. Current concepts explaining pain in nerve entrapment syndromes]. Z Orthop Ihre Grenzgeb 127(2):197-201, 1989.

Chapter 47

Discospondylitis: Diagnostic and Therapeutic Aspects

Laurent Cauzinille

Discospondylitis is a bacterial or fungal infection of the intervertebral disc space and contiguous vertebral endplates. When the lesion involves only the vertebral body, the terminology is spondylitis. Nestel provided the first description of discospondylitis in a dog secondary to tuberculosis in 1957.[1] Since then, this disease has been reviewed multiple times.[2] The avascular nucleus pulposus is nourished by the dense capillary bed of the adjacent vertebral end plates. Commonly, the infectious agent migrates hematogenously toward the slowly flowing venous channels of the vertebral end plates, proliferates, and spreads to the disk by local diffusion. Remote infected sites, vegetal material migration, extension of paravertebral abscess, penetrating wounds, or vertebral surgeries are often implicated in bacterial or fungal discospondylitis. It is a painful condition that, later in the course of the disease, may induce neurologicl deficits because of extradural spinal cord or nerve root compression.

Diagnosis

The diagnosis of discospondylitis is based on clinical findings and complementary examination results.

Clinical Findings

Discospondylitis has been more often described in young adult to middle-aged dogs of large or giant breeds; males are twice more often affected than females.[3,4] Although rare, discospondylitis has also been described in cats.[5,6] The clinician should look for a history of interdigital wound or inhaled grass awn, recent use of immunomodulating drugs to treat immune-mediated diseases of young dogs (e.g., suppurative aseptic meningomyelitis, polyarthritis), or recent viral infection with immunosuppressive capacity (e.g., parvovirus). Any chronic skin, ear, bladder, prostatic, uterine, or oral infection may also be a source of bacteria.

Hyperesthesia and lameness are the most common initial clinical signs that the owner describes. The pain may stay unlocalized, and the owner will report only decreased spontaneous physical activity. Pain and lameness often decrease with administration of anti-inflammatory drugs but recur as soon as the drugs are discontinued. Depending on the immune status of the patient and the nature of the infectious agent, the disease evolves in a subacute or chronic manner. Later, pain may become so severe that the animal is reluctant to move and becomes aggressive if manipulated. Excruciating pain is usually associated with severe cord or nerve root compression, subluxation, or pathologic vertebral fracture. Systemic signs of infection are often not present initially; hyperthermia may be the only sign but it is not a constant finding. Later in the course of the disease, weight loss, anorexia, and localized pain become more obvious. Reactive inflammatory osseous or discal tissues protrude in the vertebral canal and induce spinal cord or nerve root compression, which explains signs of ataxia and paresis. The localization of the affected vertebrae along the vertebral column determines the clinical presentation. With a C1-C5 or T3-L3 compressive lesion, the clinical findings are decreased conscious proprioception and upper motor neuron signs on the four limbs or rear limbs only, respectively. With a C6-T2 compressive lesion, decreased conscious proprioception in all four limbs, lower motor neuron signs in the front, and upper motor neuron signs in the rear limbs are present. The vertebral segment most commonly involved is L4-S1, especially the lumbosacral junction. With this lesion, the patient will manifest a more or less complete *"cauda equina syndrome"*: rear end pain, short-strided pelvic limb gait, pelvic limb lameness or root signature, and later, lower motor neuron signs, i.e., rear limb weakness, tail paralysis, and urinary and fecal incontinence. In lesions of the cervical spine, which is rarely involved, pain precedes paresis or paralysis usually weeks before the lesion protrudes enough to cause spinal cord or spinal root compression. When the diagnosis is made late in the course of the disease, lesions may be multiple with adjacent or nonadjacent vertebrae involved.

Complementary Exam Findings

Early in the course of the disease, the differential diagnosis may include many conditions. Systemic disease inducing hyperthermia and generalized weakness, orthopedic conditions such as polyarthritis or panosteitis, other neurologic diseases such as polymyositis or juvenile meningitis have the same clinical presentation as discospondylitis. When pain is localized to the vertebral column or when neurologic deficits are more obvious, plain radiographs under general anesthesia are the first diagnostic tools of choice. It is essential to radiograph the entire vertebral column because more than one space may be involved, pain may not be localized above the involved vertebrae, or the major radiographic changes may not be localized at the most painful sites. Radiographic characteristics of discospondylitis are decreased size of the intervertebral space (Figure 47-1), lysis of the vertebral endplates, sclerosis of the adjacent vertebral bodies, and sometimes, spondylosis. The time interval between the onset of clinical signs and the first radiographic signs (i.e., irregularity or lysis of the middle endplates area) may be two to four weeks.[7] This is why radiographs must be repeated in a few weeks when initial radiographs are not diagnostic but the suspicion of discospondylitis is high. More advanced lesions may show shortening of the vertebral bodies or subluxation or collapse of the vertebral bodies. Once discospondylitis has been diagnosed, a thorough physical examination is essential to look for a primary site of infection (urinary or genital tract, ear canals, teeth, etc.).

Myelographic findings indicate extradural compression because of a protruding infected disc, swollen and displaced ligaments, or periosteal reaction. However, a myelographic study is rarely necessary unless multiple affected sites are present and the clinician wants to evaluate which one is the most compressive for surgical decompression and culture.

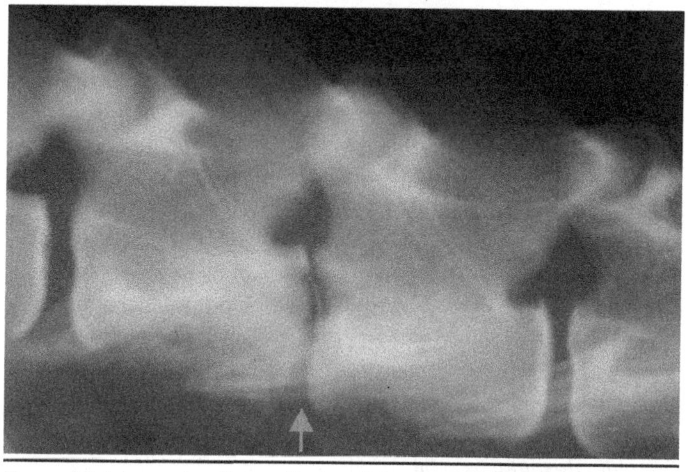

Figure 47-1. Lateral radiograph of a midlumbar discospondylitis; notice the early signs of end plate lysis and intervertebral space collapsus.

Computed tomography and magnetic resonance imaging are also useful tools for the diagnosis of discospondylitis (Figures. 47-2 and 47-3).[8] Magnetic resonance imaging, especially, may detect subtle nucleus and annulus changes earlier than radiographic identification.9 Increased T2 and decreased T1 signal intensity of intervertebral discs, end plates, and subvertebral soft tissues, as well as interface contrast enhancement are classically described.[10,11] These advanced imaging techniques do not eliminate the need for culture of the causative organism for definitive diagnosis and treatment (see below).

Bone scintigraphy with gallium-67 or technetium-99m may also detect a disc inflammation sooner than radiographs, especially if spondylosis is misleading; a hot spot will be found in the first case, not in the second. However, the sensitivity of this test is poor; on an aged dog, it does not rule out neoplasia. Discospondylitis and spondylitis may be difficult to distinguish initially from a primary vertebral neoplasm in adult dogs; except for osteoblastic sarcoma, a primary vertebral neoplasm should not cross the intervertebral space.

White blood cell count and urine analysis usually do not show a neutrophilic leukocytosis unless there is a concurrent systemic infection. Cerebrospinal fluid collection and culture are not necessary. A moderate proteinorachia and, more rarely, a mild pleocytosis may be found. Diffuse suppurative meningitis associated with an extension of an abscess to the subarachnoid space is uncommon; when it does occur, prognosis is extremely poor and generalized sepsis is highly probable.

In order to isolate the causative organism, aerobic and anaerobic bacterial culture (and fungal culture depending on the geographic region the patient has visited) should be done prior to treatment. Urinary culture may help to detect the causative agent up to 50% of the time. Blood culture is positive in up to 75% of cases.[12] When a draining tract of the paravertebral region is present, it should be cultured during the surgical exploration for a foreign body. The infectious agent may also be cultured from a spinal needle-aspiration guided by fluoroscopy. An ultrasound-guided aspirate is also technically possible on lumbar or lumbosacral sites. Finally, a surgical biopsy must be considered if the previous cultures are negative and treatment is ineffective.

The most commonly encountered agents are *Staphylococcus sp* coagulase positive, *Streptococcus sp*, *Aspergillus sp*, and *Mycobacterium sp.* More recently, discospondylitis caused by *Pseudomonas earuginosa*, *Enterococcus faecalis*, *Staphylococcus epidermidis*, and *Bordetella sp* have been published.[9,13,14] Before breeding dogs, an agglutination test must always be performed to confirm the absence of *Brucella canis*; this test has an excellent predictive value.[15,16] Infection with this organism is considered an important public health consideration in many countries, as the disease is transmissible to humans, especially those handling aborted puppy fetuses. Results of blood culture are less likely to be positive for *Brucella canis* than for discospondylitis caused by other organisms.[17] The fungal agents able to induce discospondylitis are *Aspergillus sp*, *Paecilomyces sp*, *Coccidioides immitis*, and *Actinomyces sp.*[18-20]

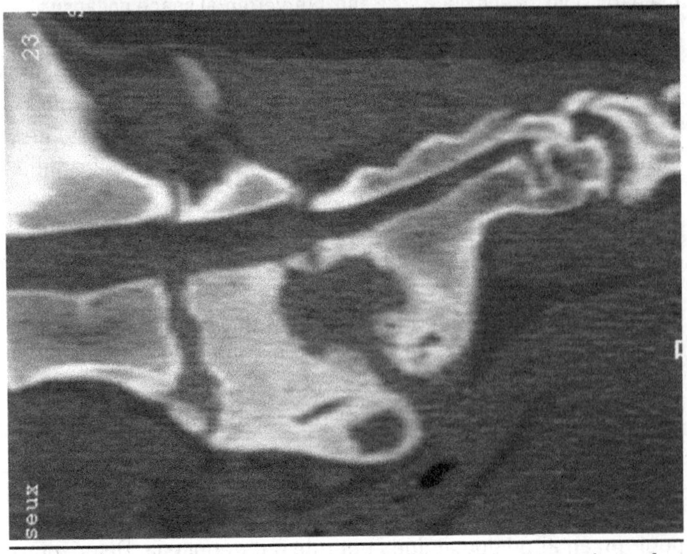

Figure 47-2. Sagittal computed tomographic reconstruction of a lumbosacral discospondylitis in a dog; notice the bone window setting that enlightens the lesion.

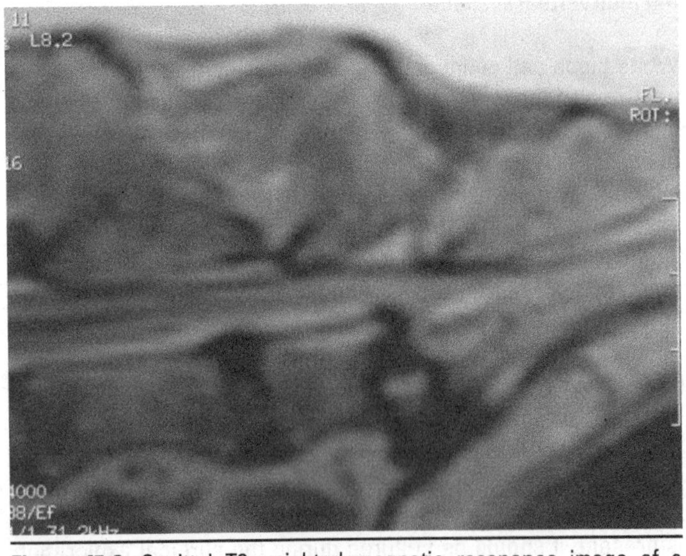

Figure 47-3. Sagittal T2-weighted magnetic resonance image of a lumbosacral discospondylitis in a dog; notice the contrast enhancement of the intervertebral space.

Therapeutic Aspects

Ideally, identification of the causative organism and sensitivity results help to select the antimicrobial of choice. Bactericidal antibiotics are recommended for patients that may be immunocompromized. A treatment lasting a minimum of 6 weeks is necessary. Without identification of the organism or pending the results, assuming that *Staphylococcus* sp coagulase positive is the most common agent, the following are appropriate first choice antibiotics: cephalosporins (cephalexin: Rilexine, Virbac, 20-30 mg/kg b.i.d., IV, IM, or PO), beta lactamase-resistant penicillins (amoxicillin and clavulanic acid: Clavamox, Pfizer, 12.5 mg/kg b.i.d., PO), and clindamycin (Antirobe, Pharmacia, 11 mg/kg b.i.d., PO). Intravenous treatment is preferred initially if the disease is long standing. Nonsteroidal anti-inflammatory drugs or narcotic agents may be necessary for pain control. The author regularly uses steroids at an anti-inflammatory dosage (prednisolone: Megasolone, Merial, 0.2-0.3 mg/kg b.i.d., PO) to alleviate the pain when nonsteroidal drugs are not effective. They must be tapered and discontinued within a week or two. Clinical improvement must be noticed within one week; by that time, steroids, when used, are tapered. When the lysis is extensive, because pathologic fractures are possible, the patient must have only minimal physical activity for the first weeks. If the patient is responsive to therapy, radiographs should be repeated no more than every 4 weeks to assess the progression or regression of the lytic lesions. In adult dogs, the radiographic deterioration continued, despite a successful clinical response, for 3 to 9 weeks.[7] Radiographic evidence of healing may take 4 to 6 months.

In a patient that fails to improve, the clinician should consider reassessment and culture of the disc space by aspiration or open biopsy, especially if the neurologic deficit progresses. Fluoroscopy-guided percutaneous discectomy or surgical exploration must then be considered in order to fenestrate and decompress the infected site.[21] Biopsies for histopathologic analysis and culture are submitted along with urine and blood. Internal stabilization (plates, pins, screws, and methylmetacrylate) may be necessary if stability is compromised, although the risk of implant superinfection is high. A surgical technique involving distraction and stabilization of the lumbosacral vertebral segment using external skeletal fixation associated with or without cancellous bone graft has been described.[22]

Dogs infected with Brucella canis should not be treated. In the countries where this disease is considered a zoonosis, the infected dogs are euthanized.

Fungal infection must be treated with ketoconazole (Nizoral, Janssen, 10 mg/kg, PO, q 24 h) or itraconazole (Sporanox, Janssen, 5 mg/kg, PO, q 24 h). Temporary remission is more common that definitive cure.[13,20,23]

Prognosis

Patients with severe neurologic deficit have a poorer prognosis than those with pain only. However, in a multicenter retrospective study, neither significant correlation between the degree of compression in the affected site and the clinical outcome, nor between ambulatory status and the final outcome was found.[24]

References

1. Nestel BL, Nestel HM: Spinal tuberculosis in the dog. J Am Vet Med Assoc 131:234-236, 1957.

2. Thomas WB: Diskospondylitis and other vertebral infections. Vet Clin North Am Small Anim Pract 30:169-182, vii, 2000.

3. Kornegay JN, Barber DL: Diskospondylitis in dogs. J Am Vet Med Assoc 177:337-341, 1980.

4. Hurov L, Troy G, Turnwald G: Diskospondylitis in the dog: 27 cases. J Am Vet Med Assoc 173:275-281, 1978.

5. Northworthy GD: Discospondylitis as a cause of posterior paresis. Feline practice 9:39, 1957.

6. Kornegay JN: Diskospondylitis. *In* Kornegay JN (ed). Problems in Veterinary Medicine: Feline Neurology. Philadelphia: JB Lippincott, 1991, pp. 369-370.

7. Shamir MH, Tavor N, Aizenberg T: Radiographic findings during recovery from discospondylitis. Vet Radiol Ultrasound 42:496-503, 2001.

8. Oakley R: Computed tomography as an aid to diagnosing vertebral osteomyelitis. Prog Vet Neurol 6:95, 1995.

9. Cherubini GB, Cappello R, Lu D, et al: MRI findings in a dog with discospondylitis caused by Bordetella species. J Small Anim Pract 45:417-420, 2004.

10. Gonzalo-Orden JM, Altonaga JR, Orden MA, et al: Magnetic resonance, computed tomographic and radiologic findings in a dog with discospondylitis. Vet Radiol Ultrasound 41:142-144, 2000.

11. Kraft SL, Mussman JM, Smith T, et al: Magnetic resonance imaging of presumptive lumbosacral discospondylitis in a dog. Vet Radiol Ultrasound 39:9-13, 1998.

12. Kornegay JN: Diskospondylitis. In Kirk RW (ed). Current Veterinary Therapy. Philadelphia: WB Saunders, 1986, p. 810.

13. Dallman MJ, Dew TL, Tobias L, et al: Disseminated aspergillosis in a dog with diskospondylitis and neurologic deficits. J Am Vet Med Assoc 200:511-513, 1992.

14. Adamo PF, Cherubini GB: Discospondylitis associated with three unreported bacteria in the dog. J Small Anim Pract 42:352-355, 2001.

15. Wanke MM: Canine brucellosis. Anim Reprod Sci 82-83:195-207, 2004.

16. Henderson RA, Hoerlein BF, Kramer TT, et al: Discospondylitis in three dogs infected with Brucella canis. J Am Vet Med Assoc 165:451-455, 1974.

17. Kerwin SC, Lewis DD, Hribernik TN, et al: Diskospondylitis associated with Brucella canis infection in dogs: 14 cases (1980-1991). J Am Vet Med Assoc 201:1253-1257, 1992.

18. Moore MP: Discospondylitis. Vet Clin North Am Small Anim Pract 22:1027, 1992.

19. Butterworth SJ, Barr FJ, Pearson GR, et al: Multiple discospondylitis associated with Aspergillus species infection in a dog. Vet Rec 136:38-41, 1995.

20. Booth MJ, van der Lugt JJ, van Heerden A, et al: Temporary remission of disseminated paecilomycosis in a German shepherd dog treated with ketoconazole. J SAfr Vet Assoc 72:99-104, 2001.

21. Kinzel S, Koch J, Buecker A, et al: Treatment of 10 dogs with discospondylitis by fluoroscopy-guided percutaneous discectomy. Vet Rec 156:78-81, 2005.

22. Auger J, Dupuis J, Quesnel A, et al: Surgical treatment of lumbosacral instability caused by discospondylitis in four dogs. Vet Surg 29:70-80, 2000.

23. Berry WL, Leisewitz AL: Multifocal Aspergillus terreus discospondylitis in two German shepherd dogs. J S Afr Vet Assoc 67:222-228, 1996.

24. Davis MJ, Dewey CW, Walker MA, et al: Contrast radiographic findings in canine bacterial discospondylitis: a multicenter, retrospective study of 27 cases. J Am Anim Hosp Assoc 36:81-85, 2000.

Chapter 48

Caudal Cervical Vertebral Malformation/Malarticulation

Lisa S. Klopp

Anatomy and Pathophysiology

Caudal cervical malarticulation/malformation (CCVMM), also known in lay terms as "Wobbler's syndrome," is referred to by many names in the literature including: cervical vertebral instability, cervical vertebral spondylopathy, caudal cervical spondylomyelopathy and cervical spondylolithesis.[1-19] The plethora of terminology indicates the confusion and lack of understanding about the underlying pathogenesis of this disease. This is a fairly common spinal column disease of mature Doberman pinschers that appear to have instability-related pathology and young Great Danes and Mastiffs that appear to have congenital stenosis of the spinal canal.[2,5,6,9,11-14,16,17,19] The Boerboel, an African relative of the Mastiff, which is becoming a more popular breed in the United States, appears to have similar pathology to the Mastiff breed. These syndromes have been observed much less frequently in other large breed dogs such as the Weimaraner, Dalmatian, German shepherd, Borzoi, and Samoyed. The Borzoi may have a recessive mode of inheritance for this disease.[20] A similar syndrome of vertebral malformation/malarticulation has been recorded in many breeds, but the changes are often recognized in the cranial part of the cervical spine.[1-3,5-7,8-12,14,16-22] The author has recognized similar severe changes in the caudal cervical vertebrae of middle-aged-to-older Yorkshire terriers as well. Whether this finding is related to a similar underlying pathogenesis is not known.

The cervical spinal column possesses the greatest range of motion of all the vertebrae. In addition to the paracervical musculature, several soft tissue structures play a role in the anatomy and stability of the cervical spine.[13,21,23] A more complete description of this anatomy is found in the first section of Chapter 46: Intervertebral Disk Disease. The dorsal longitudinal ligament, the articular facet joint capsules, the intervertebral disk, and ligamentum flavum bind the vertebral elements together and help prevent excessive motion that could damage the spinal cord and nerve roots. Motion induced by physiologic loads should not cause spinal cord damage in an anatomically stable spine. Malformation and malalignment of the cervical spine may result in spinal cord injury when the intervertebral movement is within normal or less than normal ranges.

The true underlying cause of CCVMM is not known; the pathogenesis is highly complex and may include genetic, nutritional and growth rate factors. The pathologic changes that account for clinical signs are well described.[2,3,5,8-12,14,16,17,19,20] For purposes of understanding the pathophysiology, the disease can be subdivided into instability and congenital/developmental stenosis. In the Doberman pinscher, the most likely basis for the degenerative changes is a malformation and malarticulation of the caudal vertebrae, which result in abnormal stressors on the soft tissues (ligaments, intervertebral disks, joint capsule of the articular facet, and paraspinal musculature).[2,3,5,9,13,14,16,17,19] With this micro-instability, the ligamentous elements that confer stability, hypertrophy and osteophytes (spondylosis, articular facet osteophytes) form at joint spaces. These degenerative changes result in static and dynamic compression of the spinal cord (Figures 48-1 and 48-2). The early events that lead to these changes are not completely known but likely include genetic and nutritional factors as is suspected for most diseases of abnormal bone development; evidence of these changes has been shown in very young Doberman pinscher puppies.[2] The three chronic degenerative changes of the spinal column that are associated with this type of CCVMM are chronic degenerative disk disease (Hansen's type II), osteoarthritic changes, and hypertrophy of the ligamentum flavum and dorsal longitudinal ligament. A dog with this disease may have one, multiple, or all of the changes described.[2,3,5,9,11,12,14,16,17,19]

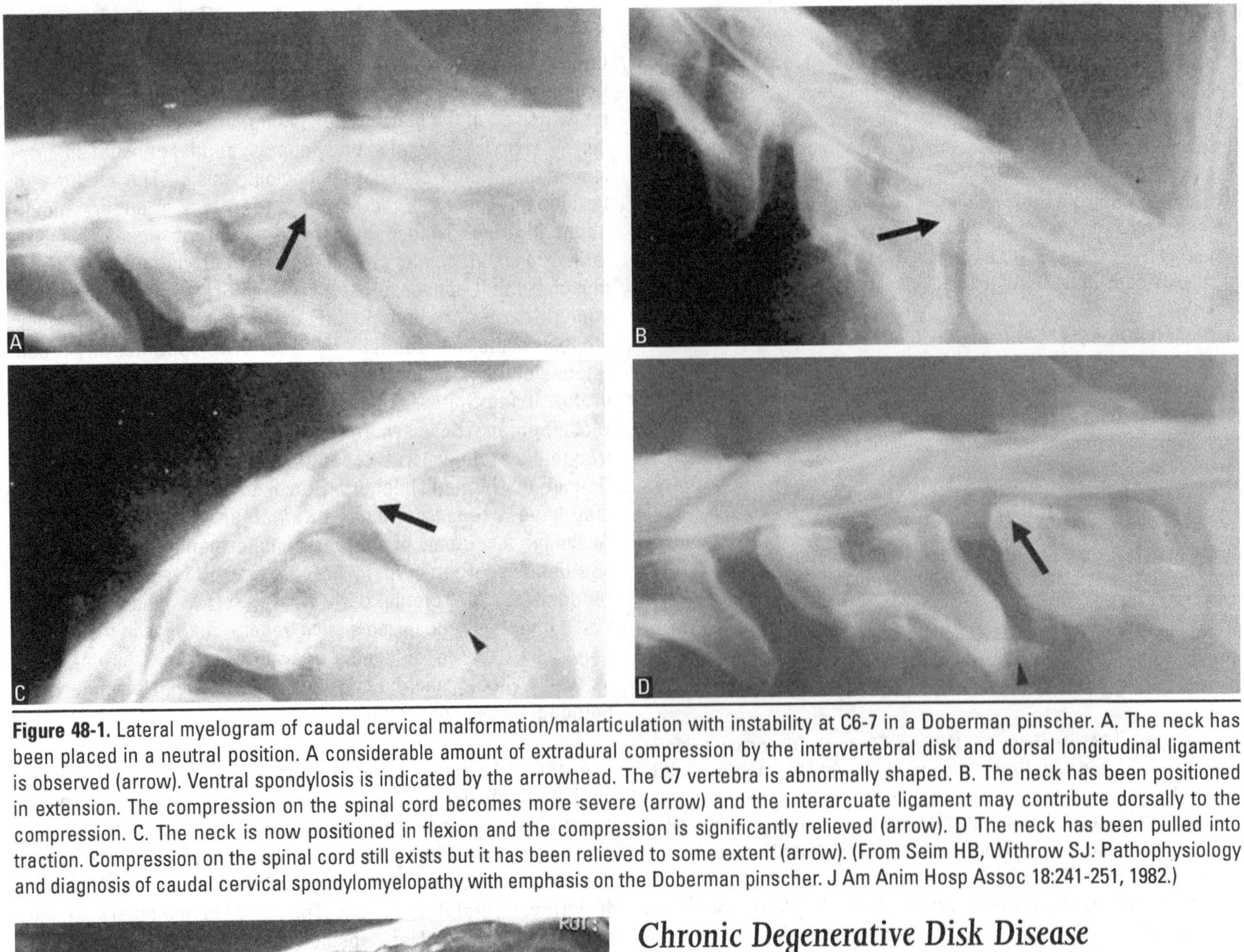

Figure 48-1. Lateral myelogram of caudal cervical malformation/malarticulation with instability at C6-7 in a Doberman pinscher. A. The neck has been placed in a neutral position. A considerable amount of extradural compression by the intervertebral disk and dorsal longitudinal ligament is observed (arrow). Ventral spondylosis is indicated by the arrowhead. The C7 vertebra is abnormally shaped. B. The neck has been positioned in extension. The compression on the spinal cord becomes more severe (arrow) and the interarcuate ligament may contribute dorsally to the compression. C. The neck is now positioned in flexion and the compression is significantly relieved (arrow). D The neck has been pulled into traction. Compression on the spinal cord still exists but it has been relieved to some extent (arrow). (From Seim HB, Withrow SJ: Pathophysiology and diagnosis of caudal cervical spondylomyelopathy with emphasis on the Doberman pinscher. J Am Anim Hosp Assoc 18:241-251, 1982.)

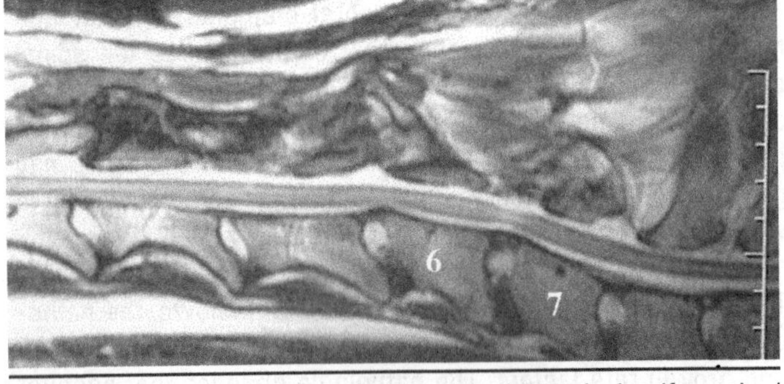

Figure 48-2. A T2-weighted lateral MRI of caudal cervical malformation/malarticulation. The C6 and C7 vertebrae are malformed. The C5-6, C6-7, and C7-T1 intervertebral disks are mildly degenerative as indicated by loss of signal intensity. Mild spinal cord compressions are at C5-6 and C6-7. Mild hydromyelia is observed in the spinal cord over the C6-7 disk space.

Chronic Degenerative Disk Disease (Hansen's type II)

This change is observed mostly as a proliferative (hypertrophied, hyperplastic, or both) dorsal aspect of the annulus fibrosus and hypertrophied dorsal longitudinal ligament causing compression of the spinal cord from the ventral aspect. Although fibrous metaplasia and degeneration of the IVD is seen, extrusion of the nucleus pulposus is uncommon. It is not known if the type II disk degeneration is a cause or effect of the pathology. One source claims it is the underlying disease; however, from the chronicity of the anatomic changes, it would appear that the disk degeneration is an effect of chronic abnormal anatomy and instability.

Osteoarthritic Changes

Articular facet joint capsule hypertrophy, spondylosis, and

rounding of the cranial ventral aspect of involved vertebrae may be observed. Articular facet osteophytes and capsule hypertrophy may contribute to spinal cord compression from a dorsal or dorsolateral direction. Osteochondrotic changes (cores of retained cartilage, subchondral cysts, and osteoporosis) have been observed in the articulations of dogs with CCVMM.

Hypertrophy of the Ligamentum Flavum and Dorsal Longitudinal Ligament

Hypertrophy of the ligamentum flavum is probably an attempt at stabilization and can be a source of significant dynamic compression on the spinal cord from the dorsal direction. The dorsal longitudinal ligament also hypertrophies (although some sources disagree). The dorsal longitudinal ligament and type II disk herniation cause compression of the spinal cord from the ventral direction.

Congenital or developmental osseous anomalies are the more common changes seen in young Great Dane, Mastiff, Boerboel, and other large breed dogs.[1,3,5,9,11,14,16,19] A component of cervical stenosis often exists. The most common change seen is enlarged articular facets resulting in a dorsolateral stenosis at the level of the joint (Figure 48-3). Multilevel stenosis is a common finding. In other cases, the neural canal may be flattened in the dorsoventral direction, but lateral stenosis from the laminae/pedicle is also observed. Instability may also be involved in the development in some of these dogs, because spondylosis and articular facet osteoarthrosis are not unusual findings.

In both types of this disease, the primary pathophysiology is a reduction in the diameter of the spinal canal, which results in spinal cord compression and traction injury, causing neurologic deficits.[1-3,5,7-10,14-16,19,20,22,24] An extensive description of the pathology of spinal cord compression is found in Chapter 42.

Clinical Presentation

The disease is usually chronic and progressive over many months to years. Clinical signs may be present from two days to two years. The average age of Doberman pinschers with clinical signs of disease is six to eight years (range 1-11 years),

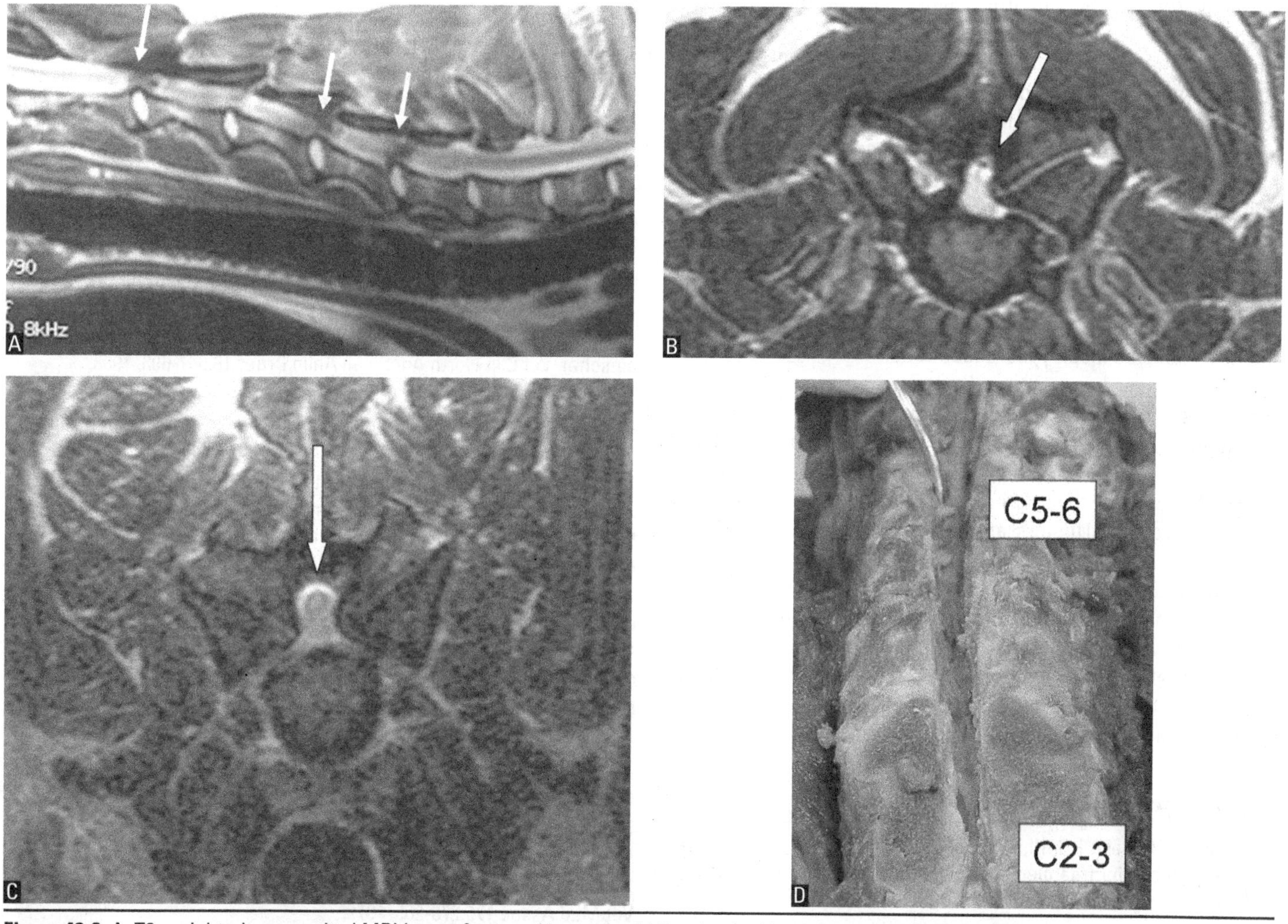

Figure 48-3. A. T2-weighted parasagittal MRI image from an 11-month-old Boerboel with severe ataxia and mild tetraparesis. The arrows indicate the location of the multiple enlarged facet joints that are compressing the cord laterally. B. T2-weighted axial MRI image at the level of C2-3. The stenotic change at the facets has resulted in severe spinal cord compression and changes in spinal cord signal intensity (increased signal) that may indicate edema or malacia. C. T2-weighted axial MRI image at the level of C5-6. Less severe stenosis has occurred with severe spinal cord compression. D. Postmortem evaluation of the spinal canal reveals severe stenosis of the canal at C2-3 and a sharp indentation (hemostats) of the canal at C5-6.

whereas the average age for Mastiffs and Great Danes is 11 to 24 months.[2-5,7-11,14-20,22,23,24] Animals may present with acute exacerbation with neurologic deterioration. The underlying malformation and instability occur during development. The chronic changes probably occur over many years.[2-5,7-10,14-20,22-24] By the time dogs show clinical signs with CCVMM, permanent damage to the spinal cord may be significant. Although some animals may present with an apparently acute onset of severe clinical signs, the pathology suggests chronicity. The degree of neurologic dysfunction is highly variable. Initial signs are wide-based stance and abnormal gait in the pelvic limbs. Clients may not recognize these signs early in the course of the disease. Dogs usually begin with pelvic limb ataxia and conscious proprioceptive deficits followed by or concurrent with a short, stilted thoracic limb gait if the lesion occurs at C6-7. Signs usually progress over time to mild-to-moderate tetraparesis and dysmetria. Some dogs become nonambulatory. Signs progress at variable rates; some dogs deteriorate acutely from mild trauma or massive intervertebral disk extrusion.

The most common lesions are at C6-7, with the next most common changes at C5-6.[2-5,7,24,8-10,13,14,16-19,21-24] This is particularly true for the instability seen in the Doberman pinscher. The gray matter in this area contributes to brachial plexus nerves responsible for supplying innervation to the shoulder and flexors of the elbow (suprascapularis and musculocutaneus nerves). When closely examined, these dogs often have some degree of atrophy in the scapular and biceps brachii muscles. When severely affected, these dogs may not be able to flex their limbs to withdrawal of their limbs or to lie in sternal recumbency. Thus, the lesion may result in lower motor neuron signs to the flexors and upper motor neuron signs to the extensor muscles. The extensor muscles are the most dominant muscle group in the thoracic limb of the dog. When opposing tone and function to flexor groups are lost, the extensor muscles display increased tone.

CCVMM is not typically considered a painful disease. Dogs may carry their head in ventroflexion. Although dogs may sometimes display discomfort when the head and neck are extended, they do not often display the degree of pain that is seen in type I disk extrusions, vertebral tumors, and meningitis. Mild discomfort may be representative of meningeal compression, arthritis, or nerve root pain. Dogs that display significant pain may have a massive disk extrusion or radiculopathy from nerve root impingement. Discussions of the pathogenesis of pain associated with intervertebral disk disease and nerve root compression are found in Chapter 46: Intervertebral Disk Disease, and Chapter 50: Lumbosacral Disease, respectively.

References

1. Bruecker KA, Seim HB, III, Withrow SJ: Clinical evaluation of three surgical methods for treatment of caudal cervical spondylomyelopathy of dogs. Vet Surg 18:197-203, 1989.

2. Burbidge HM, Pfeiffer DU, Guilford WG: Presence of cervical vertebral malformation in Doberman puppies and the effects of diet and growth rate. Aust Vet J 77:814-818, 1999.

3. Denny HR, Gibbs C, Gaskell CJ: Cervical spondylopathy in the dog--a review of thirty-five cases. J Small Anim Pract 18:117-132, 1977.

4. Dixon BC, Tomlinson JL, Kraus KH: Modified distraction-stabilization technique using an interbody polymethyl methacrylate plug in dogs with caudal cervical spondylomyelopathy. J Am Vet Med Assoc 208:61-68, 1996.

5. Drost WT, Lehenbauer TW, Reeves J: Mensuration of cervical vertebral ratios in Doberman pinschers and Great Danes. Vet Radiol Ultrasound 43:124-131, 2002.

6. Ellison GW, Seim HB III, Clemmons RM: Distracted cervical spinal fusion for management of caudal cervical spondylomyelopathy in large-breed dogs. J Am Vet Med Assoc 193:447-453, 1988.

7. Gage ED, Hall CL: Surgical repair of caudal cervical subluxation in a dog. J Am Vet Med Assoc 160:424-426, 1972.

8. Parker AJ, Park RD, Cusick PK, et al: Cervical vertebral instability in the dog. J Am Vet Med Assoc 163:71-74, 1973.

9. Parker AJ, Park RD, Gendreau C: Cervical disk prolapse in a Doberman Pinscher. J Am Vet Med Assoc 163:75-76, 1973.

10. Parker AJ, Park RD, Henry JD Jr: Cervical vertebral instability associated with cervical disk disease in two dogs. J Am Vet Med Assoc 163:1369-1371, 1973.

11. Raffe MR: Cervical vertebral malformation in Bull Mastiffs. J Am Anim Hosp Assoc 14:593-594, 1978.

12. Raffe MR, Knecht CD: Cervical vertebral malformation: A review of 36 cases. J Am Anim Hosp Assoc 16:881-883, 1980.

13. Read RA, Robins GM, Carlisle CH: Caudal cervical spondylomyelopathy (Wobbler syndrome) in the dog: a review of thirty cases. J Small Anim Pract 24:605-621, 1983.

14. Seim HB, Withrow SJ: Pathophysiology and diagnosis of caudal cervical spondylomyelopathy with emphasis on the Doberman pinscher. J Am Anim Hosp Assoc 18:241-251, 1982.

15. Swaim SF: Evaluation of four techniques of cervical spinal fixation in dogs. J Am Vet Med Assoc 166:1080-1086, 1975.

16. Trotter EJ, deLahunta A, Geary JC, et al:Caudal cervical vertebral malformation-malarticulation in Great Danes and Doberman Pinschers. J Am Vet Med Assoc. 168:917-930, 1976.

17. VanGundy TE: Disc-associated Wobbler syndrome in the Doberman pinscher. Vet Clin North Am Small Anim Pract 18:667-696, 1988.

18. Wilson ER, Aron DN, Roberts RE: Observation of a secondary compressive lesion after treatment of caudal cervical spondylomyelopathy in a dog. J Am Vet Med Assoc 205:1297-1299, 1994.

19. Wright F, Rest JR, Palmer AC: Ataxia of the Great Dane caused by stenosis of the cervical vertebral canal: comparison with similar conditions in the Basset Hound, Doberman Pinscher, Ridgeback and the thoroughbred horse. Vet Rec 92:1-6, 1973.

20. Jaggy A, Gaillard C, Lang J, et al: Hereditary cervical spondylopathy (Wobbler syndrome) in the Borzoi dog. J Am Anim Hosp Assoc 24:454-460, 1988.

21. Vasseur PB, Saunders G, Steinback C: Anatomy and function of the ligaments of the lower cervical spine in the dog. Am J Vet Res 42:1002-1006, 1981.

22. Wright JA: The use of sagittal diameter measurement in the diagnosis of cervical spinal stenosis. J Small Anim Pract 20:331-344, 1979.

23. Wright JA: A study of the radiographic anatomy of the cervical spine in the dog. J Small Anim Pract 18:341-357, 1977.

24. Hurov LI: Treatment of cervical vertebral instability in the dog. J Am Vet Med Assoc 175:278-285, 1979.

Chapter 49

Degenerative Myelopathy

Laurent Cauzinille

Many, if not all, disease processes will eventually terminate in degenerative changes of the involved organ. In neurology, the terminology "degenerative myelopathy" may be used as a broad descriptive term, for example in association with any compressive spinal cord process (chronic disc disease, vertebral instability, spinal meningioma, etc.). Based on clinical signs and neuropathologic features, the terminology "degenerative myelopathy," used in its strictest sense, is a chronic, progressive leukomyelopathy that may represent an abiotrophic type of degenerative disease.[1] Several forms of degenerative myelopathy (DM), although clinically similar, may exist. One of these clinical and pathologic conditions is most often observed in 5- to 14-year-old German shepherd dogs.[2,3] However, a similar condition has been described in other breeds of different size, as well as in mongrels and even in a cat.[4,5,6] Corgi and Boxer breeds, for instance, have a high incidence of late onset, non-painful, non-compressive degenerative myelopathy. Research into these conditions is being supported by breed clubs and other foundations. Until more information becomes available, the etiology of these degenerative conditions remains idiopathic.

History and Clinical Presentation

The time course of the disease prior to presentation is usually long (i.e., months) and is progressive in nature. The owner often describes an insidious gait abnormality of the hind limb with dysmetria and crossing of the feet of the pelvic limbs, especially when making a sudden turn. Knuckling of the toes is another common complaint. Deficits may initially be more pronounced on one side. Later, paresis will appear along with difficulty rising, dragging of the toes, and wearing of the nails of digits III and IV.[7] Over the next 6 to 36 months, these signs progress slowly in the pelvic limbs to obvious truncal ataxia and severe paresis without apparent bladder dysfunction.[7] On neurologic examination, one finds proprioceptive deficits in the hind limbs, normal to exaggerated patellar reflexes, and crossed extensor reflexes. Nociception is unimpaired. This upper motor neuron presentation is reflective of a partial loss of spinal cord function between the brachial and lumbar medullary intumescences (T3-L3). The patellar reflexes may be depressed and the withdrawal reflex may be increased, uni- or bilaterally.[3] This type of presentation is more consistent with an L4-L6 spinal cord or nerve root involvement, although neurologically normal dogs may have an age-dependent decline in patellar reflex.[8] However, sciatic, caudal, and sphincter functions remain normal, which reflects sparing of the caudal lumbosacral intumescence or nerve roots. Such lower motor neuron clinical findings may be more common in Boxer dogs with signs of progressive DM (unpublished data).

Diagnosis

Diagnosis is based on signalment, clinical signs, and complementary tests, which rule out any of the other common causes of myelopathy. The T3-L3 clinical presentation associated with this degenerative syndrome is identical to numerous other chronic spinal cord or vertebral diseases. The differential diagnosis should include, at least initially when neurologic deficits are subtle, any orthopedic disease (hip dysplasia, cruciate ligament rupture, degenerative joint disease) or caudal abdominal disease (prostatic disease, perineal hernia). When neurologic deficits are more obvious, *cauda equina* signs, common in large breeds and especially in German shepherd dogs, should be ruled out by neurologic examination and diagnostic imaging. Lumbosacral diseases that induce rear limb and tail weakness or paralysis, and fecal or urinary incontinence, do not belong on the list of differential diagnoses for DM, which has generally a T3-L3 clinical presentation. A misleading finding may be the weak patellar reflex when the degenerative lesion involves the cranial lumbar intumescence or its nerve roots. Overall, pain is a common clinical sign in lumbosacral compressive or infiltrative diseases; pain is not found in DM.

A slowly protruding disc herniation of the T3-L3 spinal segment is probably the most common disease that the clinician has to rule out. It cannot be done solely based on clinical signs or plain vertebral radiographs and will require advanced imaging. Other diseases such as dorsal spinal cord compression by articular facet spondylosis, synovial cyst formation, slow growing vertebral or meningeal tumors, or a low-grade myelitis must also be ruled out. Results of hematologic studies, blood chemistries, and urinalysis are normal in dogs with DM.

It is not uncommon to find a mild to moderate increase in protein content (proteinorachia) of the lumbar cerebrospinal fluid without pleocytosis.[9] This albumino-cytologic dissociation is neither sensitive nor specific for DM.

Spinal radiographs may show spondylosis; this finding, often multifocal in older large breed dogs, does not rule out DM. Compressive medullary consequences of spondylosis cannot be assessed without spinal cord imaging unless foraminal calcification of a protruding disc is visible above the degenerative site. A myelographic study, high-quality computerized tomography or magnetic resonance imaging are necessary to rule out any compressive or infiltrative vertebral or medullary disease. Myelography should not demonstrate the presence of a compromised subarachnoid space in cases of DM, ruling out compressive lesions. High-quality magnetic resonance imaging is very sensitive; interpretation of the images requires a considerable expertise if the reader does not want to under- or over-appreciate the significance of any abnormality.

To the author's knowledge, high-field magnetic resonance imaging does not reveal intraparenchymal lesions throughout the spinal cord in DM cases.

Electrodiagnostic findings are unremarkable unless clinical presentation belongs to the rare lower motor neuron form.

Spinal cord evoked potentials may confirm an intramedullary conduction defect. Stimulation is applied at the level of the sciatic nerve and the compound evoked potentials are recorded at the cisterna magna. Diminished amplitude and prolonged or separated N1 wave changes are not sensitive at detecting a peculiar form of myelopathy; however, they tend to worsen as the signs of DM progress.[3]

Dogs with signs of progressive DM have a depressed response to mitogens associated with the presence of peripheral blood suppressor cells, especially if they are severely affected.[10] A mitogen response assay performed twice failed to confirm the diagnosis of DM, although histopathology did, in one reported case.[11]

A change in the dog leucocyte antigen gene region has been found at the University of Florida in German shepherd dogs that have a high suspicion for DM based on standard diagnostic testing. Sensitivity and specificity of this DNA marker is being evaluated as a test for DM.

In a patient with chronic spinal cord disease, especially a German shepherd, the diagnosis of DM based on clinical signs alone is no more likely to be accurate than a diagnosis of chronic protruding disc. Vertebral and spinal cord imaging and cerebrospinal fluid analysis can increase the degree of suspicion to "most probable." Definitive diagnosis still requires histopathologic confirmation.

Histopathologic Findings

Several forms of degenerative myelopathies may be distinguished histopathologically, even if they are clinically similar. Ideally, no obvious macroscopic changes should be found once the spinal cord has been removed from the vertebral canal. However, any compressive lesion of discal, vertebral (chronic disc disease, major spondylosis, or vertebral degenerative changes) or meningeal origin (major dural ossification or masses) should be evaluated. Once the meninges are removed, dorsal and ventral roots and rootlets should appear normal.

At a microscopic level, DM is a disease of white matter although in some cases the central gray matter may also be involved; this may account for signs related to specific peripheral nerve involvement.[2,7] All white matter funiculi, especially dorsolateral and ventromedial, appear affected throughout the length of the spinal cord in a diffuse manner. Both motor and sensory tracts are involved. On longitudinal sections, the lesions are not continuous.[12] The myelopathy is more obvious in the thoracic segments; this explains the classic T3-L3 clinical presentation. Macrophages invade the degenerative areas; myelin sheaths appear swollen, and dystrophic axons tend to disappear. Astrocytosis and gliosis may be present. The cases presenting with lower motor neuron signs tend to have similar changes in the low lumbar spinal nerve roots. In early publications, lesions were not found extending into the brainstem.[2] More recently, chromatolysis, gliosis, and neuronal loss were observed in the red, lateral vestibular, and occasionally, in the dentate nuclei.[13] In some dogs, if ventral roots are unaffected, dorsal roots, dorsal root ganglions, and dorsal gray horns may show degenerative changes.[2,7]

Pathogenesis

The pathogenesis of DM is unknown. The theory of a "dying back" motor and sensory neuropathy is not supported by morphologic and morphometric data.[7,12,13]

As a similar disorder has been described in young German shepherds and Siberian huskies, it may be that this disease has a genetic origin.[5,12] Based on the theory that DM may be a late-onset neurodegenerative disease that has a heritable basis, a search for candidate genes is in progress.[7,13]

A depressed response to mitogens has been described in dogs affected with DM. This may be related to the release of prostaglandins, reflecting an attempt by the host to control an immune event.[10] Immunoglobulin G and the third component of complement have been found in spinal nerve tracts of affected German shepherds.[14] Depression of cell-mediated immune responses, increased circulating immune complexes, plasma cell infiltrates in kidneys and intestinal tracts suggest that DM may be an immune-mediated neurodegenerative disease.[9]

An associated enteropathy, bacterial overgrowth, and decreased serum levels of cobalamin (vitamin B12) have also been described in dogs with DM.[15,16] However, parenteral administration of cobalamin has not reversed the clinical evolution of developing DM in dogs.[13]

Indications exist that vitamin E transport may be involved, resulting from an impaired function of the hepatic alpha-tocopherol transfer protein.[17] The alpha tocopherol transfer protein gene could then be used for pre mortem diagnosis of DM in comparison with human patients with familial ataxia associated with vitamin E deficiency. Recent research to determine whether a deficiency or a defect of the canine alpha-tocopherol transfer protein could be a primary factor in DM suggests that this is unlikely.[18]

Treatment

Because dogs with various types of compressive myelopathy may also have concomitant DM, treatable diseases should be addressed first. However, in the case of a strong suspicion of DM in a dog that also has other mild chronic disease (hip dysplasia, chronic disc protrusion), it is essential to avoid any unnecessary surgical procedure that might be useless or that might accelerate clinical deterioration.

No treatment is known to be effective in either reversing or slowing of the progression of clinical signs of DM. Although no controlled experiments have been published, each pathogenesis theory may support a therapy. Recommended treatments involve a combination of different protocols: exercise, massive corticosteroid therapy, multiple vitamin and mineral supplementation, dietary manipulation, acupuncture, and aminocaproic acid.

Nonsteroidal anti-inflammatory drugs are recommended to alleviate other inflammatory conditions (degenerative joint disease, spondylosis, nerve root signature, etc.) that may aggravate the clinical signs. Prednisolone, (Megasolone, Merial,) 1 mg/kg/day for a few days, then reduced to maintenance levels of 0.5 mg/kg every other day, is indicated if clinical deterioration is acute.[19] However, long-term use of corticosteroids favors muscle atrophy and other side effects. No other immunosuppressive trials have been published.

Although not proven, tocopherol (vitamin E) supplementation at high dosage (2000 IU /day) along with B complex vitamins are recommended.

Aminocaproic acid (Amicar, Immunex), a blocker of the final common pathway of tissue inflammation, given at 500 mg PO t.i.d., has been reported to alter the course of the disease.[3,19] Improvement is usually seen within 2 months. No recent retrospective or prospective study has been published for this drug protocol or for others addressing the same mechanism.

Exercise should be sustained or even increased when possible to maintain muscle mass and joint elasticity.

Prognosis is poor; the time course for progression may take from weeks to months for signs to reach the level of a complete disuse of the pelvic limbs. When the dog's neurologic deficits reach the point that it is no longer ambulatory, decubitus care, passive physiotherapy, bladder control, and the use of a cart may still preserve a reasonable quality of life.

References

1. de Lahunta A: Abiotrophy in domestic animals: a review. Can J Vet Res;54:65-76, 199.

2. Averill DR Jr: Degenerative myelopathy in the aging German Shepherd dog: clinical and pathologic findings. J Am Vet Med Assoc 162:1045-1051, 1973.

3. Clemmons RM: Degenerative Myelopathy. *In* Current Veterinary Therapy. Kirk RW (ed). Philadelphia: WB Saunders, 1989, pp. 830-833.

4. Matthews NS, de Lahunta A: Degenerative myelopathy in an adult miniature poodle. J Am Vet Med Assoc 186:1213-1215, 1985.

5. Bichsel P, Vandevelde M, Lang J, et al: Degenerative myelopathy in a family of Siberian Husky dogs. J Am Vet Med Assoc 183:998-1000, 1965, 1983.

6. Mesfin GM, Kusewitt D, Parker A: Degenerative myelopathy in a cat. J Am Vet Med Assoc 176:62-64, 1980.

7. Griffiths IR, Duncan ID: Chronic degenerative radiculomyelopathy in the dog. J Small Anim Pract 16:461-471, 1975.

8. Levine JM, Hillman RB, Erb HN, et al: The influence of age on patellar reflex response in the dog. J Vet Intern Med 16:244-246, 2002.

9. Clemmons RM: Degenerative myelopathy. Vet Clin North Am Small Anim Pract 22:965-971, 1992.

10. Waxman FJ, Clemmons RM, Hinrichs DJ: Progressive myelopathy in older German shepherd dogs. II. Presence of circulating suppressor cells. J Immunol124:1216-1222, 1980.

11. Romatowski J: Degenerative myelopathy in a German shepherd. Mod Vet Pract 65:535-537, 1984.

12. Braund KG, Vandevelde M: German Shepherd dog myelopathy--a morphologic and morphometric study. Am J Vet Res 39:1309-1315, 1978.

13. Johnston PE, Barrie JA, McCulloch MC, et al: Central nervous system pathology in 25 dogs with chronic degenerative radiculomyelopathy. Vet Rec 146:629-633, 2000.

14. Barclay KB, Haines DM: Immunohistochemical evidence for immunoglobulin and complement deposition in spinal cord lesions in degenerative myelopathy in German shepherd dogs. Can J Vet Res 58:20-24, 1994.

15. Sheahan BJ, Caffrey JF, Gunn HM, et al: Structural and biochemical changes in a spinal myelinopathy in twelve English foxhounds and two harriers. Vet Pathol 28:117-124, 1991.

16. Williams D, Batt R, Sharp N: Degenerative myelopathy in German Shepherd dogs: an association with mucosal biochemical changes and bacterial overgrowth in the small intestine. Clin Sci 66:24, 1984.

17. Traber MG, Pillai SR, Kayden HJ, et al: Vitamin E deficiency in dogs does not alter preferential incorporation of RRR-alpha-tocopherol compared with all rac-alpha-tocopherol into plasma. Lipids 28:1107-1112, 1993.

18. Fechner H, Johnston PE, Sharp NJ, et al: Molecular genetic and expression analysis of alpha-tocopherol transfer protein mRNA in German shepherd dogs with degenerative myelopathy. Berl Munch Tierarztl Wochenschr 116:31-36, 2003.

19. Clemmons RM, Wheeler S, LeCouteur RA: How do I treat degenerative myelopathy. Prog Vet Neurol 6:71-72, 1995.

Chapter 50

Lumbosacral Disease

Lisa Klopp

Anatomy of the Lumbosacral Spine

The structural anatomy of the lumbosacral spine includes the intervertebral disk, the articular facet joints, and spinal ligaments. Detailed descriptions of these structures are discussed in Chapter 46: Intervertebral Disk Disease. The last lumbar vertebra (L7) attaches to the fused three-segment (S1-3) sacrum rather than to another individual vertebra (Figure 50-1). The range of motion of the sacrum is limited by its attachment to the pelvis.

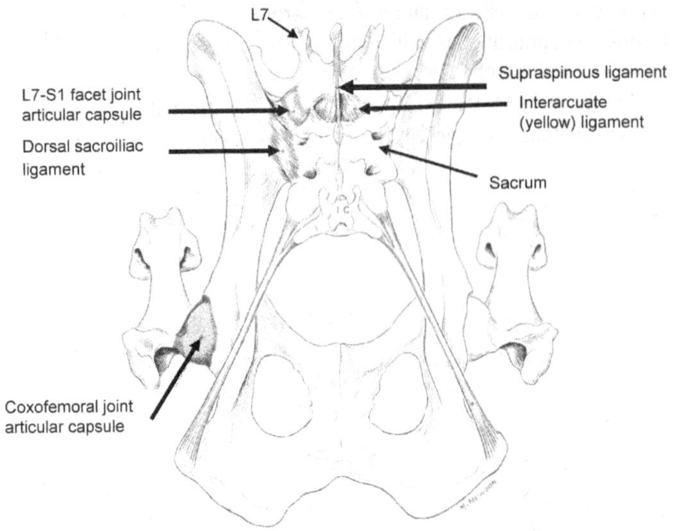

Figure 50-1. A schematic drawing of the anatomy of the lumbosacral junction. (From Miller ME, Christensen GC, and Evans HE: Anatomy of the Dog. Philadelphia: WB Saunders, 1964. Drawn by M. Newsom)

This anatomic difference leads to different biomechanical loading forces at this level in comparison with the other lumbar vertebra.[1,2] The characteristic that renders the lumbosacral joint unique clinically is that, in most instances in the dog and cat, the spinal cord itself does not extend into this region. At birth the spinal cord extends through the vertebral canal of the sacrum.[3] Differential growth rates between the vertebral column and spinal cord result in termination of the spinal cord around the L6 vertebra in medium-to-large breed dogs and at L7 cats (Figure 50-2).[3] Small-breed dogs (< 7 kg) may have longer spinal cords in which case the spinal cord may terminate as far caudally as the lumbosacral junction.[3] Caudal to the lumbar intumescence, the spinal cord tapers to an elongated cone, or the conus medullaris, which contains the sacral and caudal spinal cord segments.[3] The spinal cord itself terminates as the filum terminale, which is a band composed of glial and ependymal cells.[3] The filum terminale unites with the dura and arachnoid layers to form the caudal ligament around the S1 vertebra. The caudal ligament anchors the spinal cord by fusing with the periosteum and dorsal

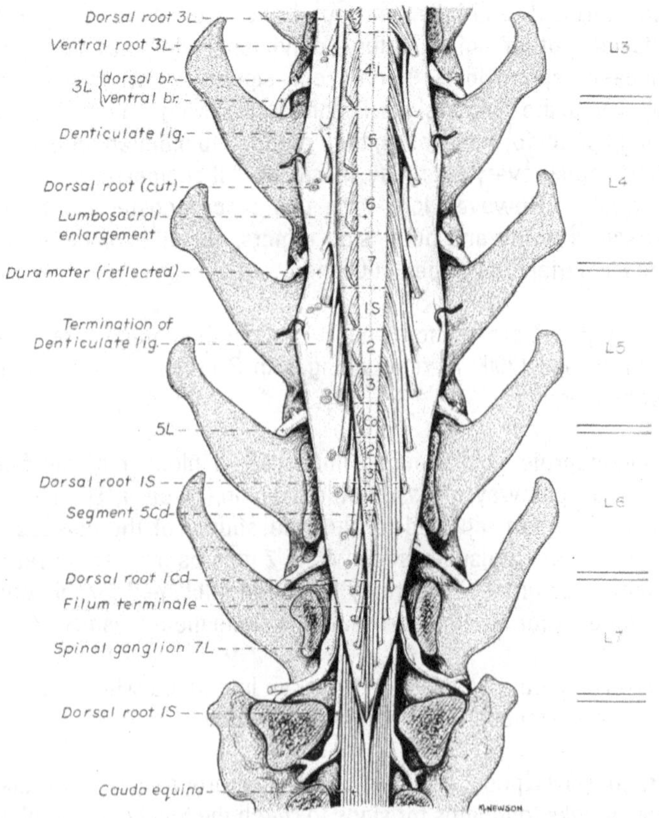

Figure 50-2. Spinal cord segmental relationship to the vertebral bodies. From T11 through the caudal segments the spinal cord, roots, ganglia, and nerves have been exposed by removal of the vertebral arches. The dura mater has been removed except on the right side. The numbers on the right represent the levels of the vertebral bodies. (From Miller ME, Christensen GC, and Evans HE: Anatomy of the Dog. Philadelphia: WB Saunders, 1964. Drawn by M. Newsom)

longitudinal ligament in the caudal vertebrae. The thecal sac and arachnoid space, which contain cerebrospinal fluid, extend beyond the filum terminale up to 2 cm and may extend as far as the S1 vertebra.[2] Because the spinal cord terminates before the lumbosacral junction, the caudal lumbar, sacral, and caudal nerve roots travel the remaining distance to exit the spinal canal at the appropriate intervertebral foramen. This collection of the nerve roots is referred to as the cauda equina.[3] The dorsal and ventral nerve roots fuse distal to the dorsal root ganglion near the intervertebral foramen to form the spinal nerves. The spinal nerves carry the axonal fibers that form the sciatic, pudendal, parasympathetic, and caudal nerves (Figure 50-3).[3] Throughout the thoracic and lumbar spinal cord, spinal nerves exit caudally to the vertebra of the same number (e.g., L7 nerve root exits at the L7-S1 intervertebral foramen) just cranially to the intervertebral disk. Therefore, with lumbosacral disease, typically the last lumbar and sacral roots are most clinically affected. However, degenerative disease at L6-7 can occur independently or in conjunction with lumbosacral disease. The nerve roots, like the spinal cord, are covered by epidural fat which acts as a protective layer against injury. Paired venous sinuses, present the length of the spinal canal, diverge laterally over the disk spaces and converge toward the midline as they reach the mid-body of the vertebrae.

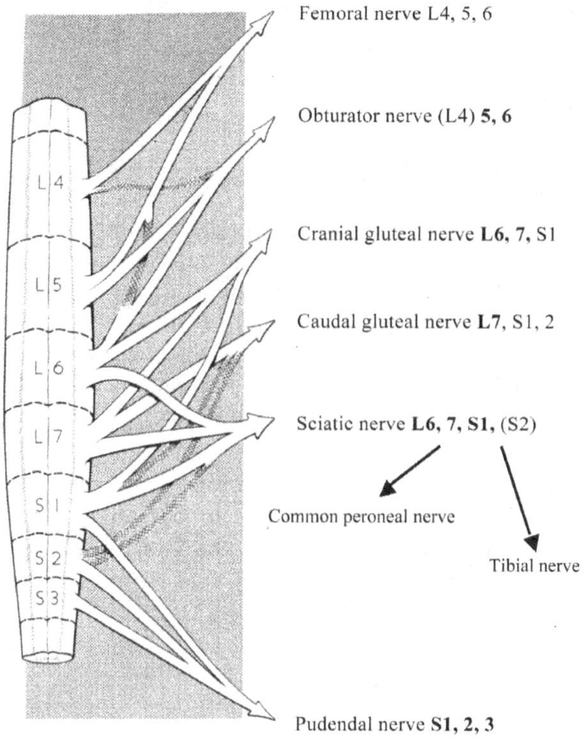

Figure 50-3. Peripheral nerve formation from the spinal cord segments of the lumbar intumescence in the dog. (Modified from De Lahunta A: Veterinary Neuroanatomy and Clinical Neurology, 2nd ed. Philadelphia: WB Saunders, 1983.)

Two adjacent vertebral bodies and the intervening intervertebral disk constitute a motion segment. In the vertebral motion segment are three joints: two articular facets and the intervertebral disk. Motion is constrained by associated joint capsules and ligaments.[4] As these structures reach the limits of their elasticity and tensile forces are encountered, flexibility is reduced.[1] Movement in the joint is primarily flexion with more restricted degrees of rotation, lateral bending, and extension.[1,5] Flexion in the sagittal plane is limited by the supraspinous, intraspinous, interarcuate, and dorsal longitudinal ligaments and the articular facet joint capsules.[1,5] Extension is restricted by the ventral longitudinal ligament and articular facet joint capsules.[1,5] Lateral bending is controlled by the articular facet joint capsules, the intertranverse ligaments, the annulus fibrosus of the intervertebral disk, and to some degree, by the pelvis.[1,5] Finally, axial rotation is controlled by the articular facets and annulus fibrosus of the intervertebral disk.[1,4]

Gross Pathology of Lumbosacral Disease

The most common cause of cauda equina pathology is stenosis, or narrowing of the spinal canal, resulting in compression of the cauda equina (Figure 50-4).[2,4-8] Although stenosis can be congenital in nature, it is often secondary to degenerative lumbosacral disease, which encompasses multiple changes in the structural anatomy at this location. Most often, these changes affect the intervertebral disk, the articular facets, and the ligaments of the spine. Congenital abnormalities, such as instability, transitional vertebrae, and osteochondrosis of the sacral or L7 endplate,[8,9] as well as trauma are also associated with lumbosacral disease. These abnormalities usually result in acquired secondary degenerative changes, which ultimately contribute to clinical signs at a later time.[2,4,5,7,8,10] True congenital lumbosacral spinal stenosis may present early with clinical signs prior to development of degenerative changes if the canal diameter is narrowed severely enough. However, congenital abnormalities and prior trauma are not required for degenerative changes to occur at this level and are certainly not as common as aging and degenerative changes. Other diseases that affect the lumbosacral spine and cauda equina are neoplasia, trauma (fracture), inflammation, infection, and vascular injuries. In this chapter, the focus is on degenerative lumbosacral disease. The anatomic pathology associated with degenerative lumbosacral disease is found in Table 50-1.

Table 50-1. Anatomic Pathology Associated with Degenerative Lumbosacral Disease

Acquired disease
- Degenerative disk disease
  - Type II *
- Degenerative changes of other spinal structures
  - Ligamentum flavum (interarcuate ligament) hypertrophy/inflammation
  - Dorsal longitudinal ligament hypertrophy/inflammation
  - Articular facet joint capsule hypertrophy/inflammation
  - Articular facet osteophytes
  - Thickening and induration of epidural fat
  - Fibrous adhesions to nerve roots
  - Spondylosis

Congenital diseases that may cause lumbosacral disease and contribute to degenerative changes
- Congenital stenosis
- Malarticulation or malformation of the lumbosacral joint (e.g., instability)
- Transitional vertebrae
- Osteochondrosis of the L7 or S1 vertebral endplate

*** Type I disk extrusion can occur in this region but is relatively uncommon even in chondrodystrophic breeds.**

The lumbosacral joint is one that transitions between a more freely flexible region of the spine (lumbar segments) and one that is static in position (sacrum) because of the attachment to the pelvis. The range of motion is higher at this location than at any of the other lower lumbar motion segments.[11] It is not surprising that this joint can undergo excessive biomechanical stresses. It is postulated that the disease is most prevalent in large breed dogs owing to an imbalance between body weight and dimension of the lumbosacral contact area not seen in smaller breeds and resulting in higher loading forces around the joint.[12] Spondylosis and osteophyte production around the articular facet joints commonly observed with degenerative lumbosacral disease may be one way of reducing the loading forces.[12,13] German shepherds, which have a high reported incidence of the disease, have been shown to have hypermobility and increased longitudinal extension.[8,12]

One of the earliest changes occurs in the intervertebral disk and is related to type II degeneration. An extensive review of type II intervertebral disk disease can be found in Chapter 46. As the disk degenerates at the lumbosacral joint, derangements occur in the normal load-bearing functions. As the disk begins to herniate or collapse, the normal disk height is lost, the facet joints begin to share more than their normal biomechanical load,[8,14] and subluxate to some extent.[15] Although collapse of the disk results in foramen narrowing,[5,16] the significance of this is not known. The clinical significance of foraminal narrowing without spinal canal stenosis has been challenged in the human literature.[17] As in other diarthrodial joints, development of periarticular osteophytes occurs in response to excessive biomechanical stressors.[18] Osteophytes often form on the ventromedial side of the facet and the dorsolateral endplate of L7.[18-20] They may severely restrict the foramen and L7 root, especially if the joint is extended.[14] In addition, changes in the function of the motion segment may cause interarcuate ligament hypertrophy and infolding into the spinal canal, which may contribute to stenosis and compression of the nerve roots dorsally.[4,5,21,22] Ventral spondylosis is a typical finding; however, it is most often an indicator of degenerative changes rather than a true cause of clinical signs.

Congenital anomalies tend to accentuate the effects of excessive biomechanical loads and contribute to lumbosacral degenerative changes. Congenital instability is typically related to malformation and malarticulation of the facets and abnormal vertebral alignment. The response to instability at this joint can be likened to that seen with caudal cervical malformation/malarticulation ("Wobbler's disease"). Osteochondrosis is the most recently reported congenital anomaly that contributes to degenerative changes at the lumbosacral joint. The cartilaginous endplate defect is more commonly seen in the cranial sacral endplate than the caudal lumbar endplate.[9] Not surprisingly, this anomaly has been most commonly observed in German shepherd dogs, with a higher male: female ratio.[9] It is often seen clinically in dogs younger (as early as 18 months) than the typical patient

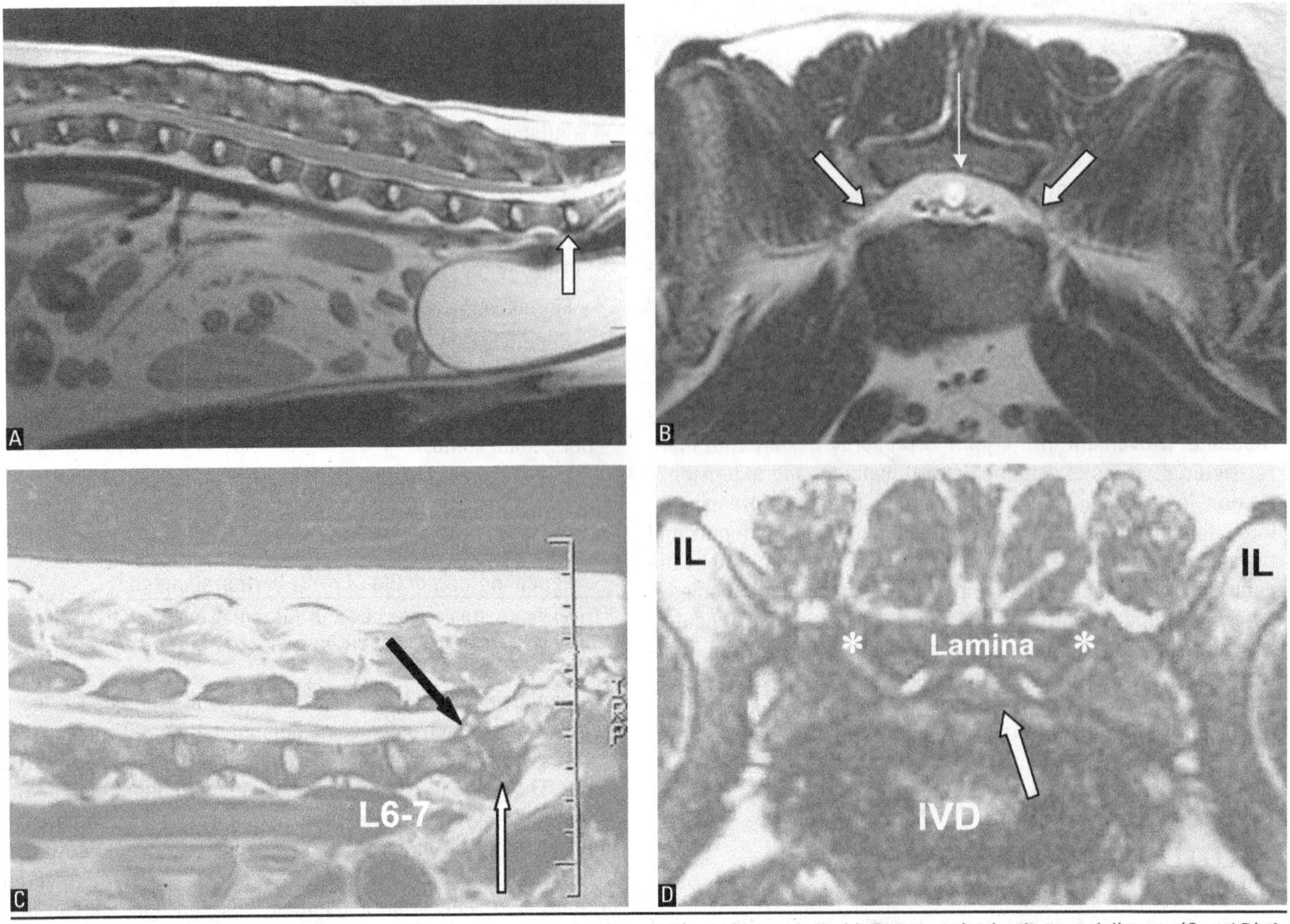

Figure 50-4. MRI images of a dog with a normal lumbosacral junction (A and B) and from a dog with degenerative lumbosacral disease (C and D). A. T2-weighted sagittal plane MRI. All of the intervertebral disks are well hydrated. The neural tissue and fat are easily identified in the lower lumbar and sacral spinal canal. White arrow = L7-S1 disk B. T2-weighted transverse plane MRI through the L7-S1 joint. Thin arrow = spinal canal containing the dural tube, nerve roots and epidural fat. Block arrows = L7 nerve roots exiting the L7-S1 intervertebral foramen. C. T2-weighted, sagittal plane MRI. There is a large disk extrusion at the L7-S1 disk and the canal is severely stenotic. (black arrow) Multiple degenerative intervertebral disks (noted by loss of signal owing to dehydration) are at L3-4, L4-5, and L7-S1. Ventral spondylosis is noted at the lumbosacral joint (white arrow) and other disk spaces as well. D. T2-weighted, transverse plane MRI through the L7-S1 disk space. The spinal canal is obliterated with extruded disk material (white arrow), and the neural anatomy is difficult to appreciate. IL = wing of the ilium; IVD = intervertebral disk; * = L7-S1 facet joint.

presenting with lumbosacral disease.[9] Degenerative changes at the lumbosacral joint may be attributable to an increase in abnormal stresses and possibly impairment of intervertebral disk nutrition at an age earlier than that of typical type II intervertebral disk degeneration.

The term transitional vertebrae encompasses a variety of congenital osseous abnormalities seen in vertebrae between the spinal segments. Most commonly, these changes have been seen in the lumbosacral motion segment.[23] This abnormality displays morphologic characteristics of both lumbar and sacral vertebrae.[24-26] Normally, the development and alignment of the last lumbar vertebrae are such that the transverse processes are not in contact with the ilia.[23] Abnormal development arises through abnormal mechanisms during growth in the ossification centers of the sacrum and/or L7 vertebrae.[23] The most distinct abnormalities usually occur in the transverse processes, which may or may not be attached to the ilium or sacrum.[23,24,26] Variations in the morphology of the vertebral body are less common.[23,26] These abnormalities may result in abnormal sacroiliac attachments (usually shortening of the attachment on the affected side) and abnormal rotation of the pelvis.[23] The abnormal anatomic alignment likely results in altered biomechanics and excessive loading on the intervertebral disk and facet joints. Transitional vertebrae may, therefore, be clinically relevant to degenerative lumbosacral disease, especially in German shepherd dogs, which have a high reported incidence of degenerative lumbosacral disease.[23,24,26-28]

Transitional vertebrae in people are more likely to be associated with degenerative disk disease and facet joint degeneration at the joint above the transitional vertebra, and this malformation is somewhat protective against degenerative changes to the disk below.[29] The joint between the transverse process of the transitional vertebra and the sacrum may be restrictive to rotation and bending, thus protecting the lumbosacral disk (L5-S1 disk in people) from excessive biomechanical forces.[29,30] The disk height below the transitional vertebra is found to be shorter than disc heights of the upper levels in young men, but the disk height is similar in people with this condition in comparison with that in normal men in the middle-aged population.[29] The shortened disk height in the unaffected older population is presumably a result of degeneration.[29,31] The protective effect of the transitional vertebra on the disk below is stronger for the annulus fibrosus than the endplate and nucleus pulposus but it is postulated that the degenerative changes seen in these structures may be induced by another mechanism, i.e., natural aging of the disk.[29]

Clinical Signs of Lumbosacral Disease

Clinical signs of lumbosacral spinal disease are differentiated from injury to the lumbosacral spinal cord segments. Because of the neurologic anatomy at the lumbosacral joint, the L7 and the sacral and caudal nerve roots are typically affected rather than the spinal cord by pathology at the lumbosacral junction. Compression of the cauda equina is most often associated with pain, gait changes, and mild-to-moderate degrees of neurologic dysfunction compared with injury to the lumbosacral spinal cord segments that may be more complete or severe. Table 50-2 is a list of the possible findings during the neurologic examination in animals with cauda equina syndrome. It is important to note that not all of the deficits listed in the table are necessarily present in any one patient.

The most common disease entity affecting the cauda equina is stenosis, or narrowing of the spinal canal, which results in compression of the nerve roots.[2,4-7] Dogs often display signs of lumbosacral pain observed on deep lumbosacral palpation with or without hip extension, dorsal elevation of the tail base, rectal palpation (pressing dorsally), and pelvic limb wheelbarrowing. Clients often comment on lower tail carriage or lack of tail wagging. Pain associated with lumbosacral disease may originate from the disk (diskogenic pain), nerve root and inflamed articular facet capsules, and spinal ligaments. Radicular, or nerve root, pain may be manifested as allodynia, dysesthesia, hyperesthesia, orparesthesia.[32] Definitions of these pain syndromes are shown in Table 50-3. The pathogenesis of pain associated with lumbosacral disease will be discussed further.

It is critical to rule out the presence of coxofemoral osteoarthritis as a source of lumbar area pain, which can also be present concurrently. Lumbosacral pain often leads to lameness, which is either intermittent or persistent, and a bunny hopping gait. These gait changes are also seen with coxofemoral disease. Difficulty rising, exercise intolerance, and inability to perform tasks that were once normal activities may be attributed to both pain and/or weakness.

Neurologic examination may be normal in an animal with only lumbosacral pain, or, if the results are abnormal, the examination may reveal pain and mild deficits in postural reactions and spinal reflexes. Earlier recognition of signs, improved health care for pets, and finally, improvements in diagnostic modalities and therapies may contribute to the lower incidence of significant neurologic deficits seen by the author. However, the disease may result in variable degrees of dysfunction in the postural reactions and reflexes innervated by the sciatic, sacral, and caudal nerves. These include deficits in conscious proprioception, hopping reactions, decreased-to-absent spinal reflexes, urinary and/or fecal incontinence, and abnormal tail and perineal function or sensation.

The patellar reflex is spared because the nerve roots that supply the femoral nerve (L4-L6) have exited the spine rostral to the lumbosacral joint. Paraplegia is rare because when femoral nerve function is intact, the pelvic limb can extend and bear weight. In cases of severe sciatic nerve dysfunction, the animal may be very weak, but not usually nonambulatory. When the sciatic nerve is extremely dysfunctional, the patellar reflex may appear to be exaggerated. This is called "pseudohyperreflexia" because it is not a true "upper motor neuron" sign, but occurs secondary to loss of antagonist muscle action in the biceps femoris, semitendinosus, semimembranosus, and gatrocnemius muscles. Typically, this "false" reflex is observed as a brisk extension of the limb with a poor rebound of flexion of the hock. True hyperreflexia is associated with clonus of the limb.

Table 50-2. Neurological Examination Findings with Lumbosacral Disease

Signs	Comments
Mentation	Normal
Gait	Normal thoracic limbs
	May be ataxic in the pelvic limbs
	May be weak (paraparesis or monoparesis) in the pelvic limbs, primarily in the muscles innervated by the sciatic nerve (weakness is usually mild and paralysis is rare)
	Lameness (intermittent or persistent)
	Bunny-hopping gait
	Difficulty rising
	Decreased exercise tolerance
Postural reactions	Normal in thoracic limbs
	Conscious proprioception may be normal or decreased-to-absent in the pelvic limbs, depending on the severity of the nerve root injury
	Hopping reactions may be normal-to-decreased; rarely absent unless injury to nerve roots is severe (spinal fracture with root avulsion)
Spinal reflexes	Normal in thoracic limbs
	Muscle tone in pelvic limbs and anal sphincter may be normal, or decreased (hypotonic)-to-absent (flaccid) depending on the severity of the nerve root injury
	Myotatic femoral (patellar) reflex is normal*
	Myotatic reflexes are normal or decreased-to-absent (hyporeflexia to areflexia) in the distribution of reflexes innervated by the sciatic and sacral nerves, depending on severity of the nerve root injury
	Deep pain response is often intact but may be decreased-to-absent in the lateral toes, tail, and perineal region, depending on severity of the nerve root injury
Pain	Most diseases in this region cause pain: intervertebral disk disease/degenerative acquired disease vertebral neoplasia diskospondylitis osteomyelitis trauma/fracture vertebral anomalies (+/-)
	Non-painful diseases Nerve root avulsion without spinal fracture
Urinary incontinence	May have lower motor neuron bladder dysfunction
	May dribble urine
Other	May have fecal incontinence and/or dilated anal sphincter
	Nerve root signature (less common than C6-T2 lesions)
	May have tail weakness/paralysis
	Paresthesia may lead to self-mutilation (tail, pelvic limbs)
	Dysesthesia

Table 50-3. Definitions of Pain Syndromes that May Occur with Nerve Root Injury[32]

Allodynia	Pain caused by a stimulus that does not normally induce pain
Dysesthesia	An unpleasant abnormal sensation, whether spontaneous or evoked
Hyperalgesia	Increased response to a stimulus that is normally considered painful
Paresthesia	An abnormal sensation, whether spontaneous or evoked

Occasionally, the single or most severe clinical sign of lumbosacral disease is loss of autonomic function, such as urinary and/or fecal incontinence. The function of the bladder is impaired by disruption of the S1-3 parasympathetic nerve fibers that form the pelvic nerve and control function of the detrusor muscle of the urinary bladder. The somatic fibers that are present in the S1-3 spinal nerves control the external urinary sphincter, or urethralis muscle. In addition, the sensory afferent fibers are also affected. The sensory afferent fibers send information to the sacral spinal cord that facilitates local reflex activity. Ascending information from these fibers also converges on the sympathetic preganglionic nerve cell bodies in the thoracolumbar spinal cord (around L1-4) which form the hypogastric nerve that innervates the internal urinary sphincter. The varying degree of loss of ascending information to these cell bodies may result in inefficient internal urinary sphincter tone as well. However, this sphincter may be somewhat more functional than the urethralis muscle and may contribute to any retention of urine present. Presence of significant autonomic dysfunction typically results in a guarded prognosis even with therapy.[5,33]

An animal sometimes displays nerve root signature with compression of the cauda equina. This is characterized by lifting the pelvic limb on ceasing movement. It is probably related to an attempt to improve comfort by decreasing stretch of the nerve root that has been compressed. Nerve root signature appears to be much more common with cervical radiculopathy in which the animal will hold up a thoracic limb.

Pathophysiology of Pain in Lumbosacral Disease

Pain is one of the key clinical features of lumbosacral stenosis and degenerative disease. Although the causes of pain might seem some what obvious, the variable nature of the degree of pain and the lack of resolution of pain following decompressive surgery among individual human and animal patients remain an enigma.[34] Direct mechanical compression of the nerve roots plays a role in the pathogenesis of pain, but it is not the sole cause. A tremendous amount of research has been conducted in both experimental and clinical settings to elucidate the underlying causes of low back pain with lumbosacral degenerative disease. Pain results from compression and inflammation of sensory nerve roots (radicular pain) and from degenerative and inflammatory changes in the articular facet joints, other supporting structures, and the intervertebral disk (diskogenic pain).[35]

Many of the neuropathic pain models that have been developed experimentally involve the manipulation of the sciatic nerve, the cauda equina, or an isolated nerve root. Injury to the nerve, nerve root(s), or cauda equina has been induced by many mechanisms: manipulation, transaction, ligation, cryoneurolysis, crush, and chronic constriction.[36-39] Local pathophysiology at the site of nerve injury has implicated a plethora of potential mediators of pain. Compression of the nerve or nerve roots results in mechanical deformation with spontaneous (ectopic) depolarization of the nerve, vasogenic edema, infiltration of immune cells with subsequent up-regulation of immune mediators in both the nerve roots and spinal cord, and central sensitization of the spinal cord to up-regulate pain perception.[35,40] These factors are not independent entities and are interrelated in a complex pathway (Figure 50-5).

Nociception in the Anatomic Structures of the Spine

On a basic nociceptive level, sensory innervation is present to all of the structures of the spine.[41] Innervation to these structures primarily arises from the primary dorsal nerve root distal to the dorsal root ganglion.[42,43] Recurrent articular nerves innervate the vertebral periosteum, articular facet joint capsules, and ligamentous tissues of the dorsal neural arch (e.g., interarcuate ligament).[42] Another branch forms the sinuvertebral nerve, which enters back into the intervertebral foramen and gives rise to cranial and caudal branches that supply rich innervation to the dorsal longitudinal ligament and dorsal annulus fibrosus of the intervertebral disk.[42] These fibers were recently shown to possess sensory-specific sodium-gated pain channels (SNS/PN3 and NaN/SNS2), which may provide a new therapeutic mechanism for analgesia.[41] The extension of these fibers over one to two vertebral segments may limit precise localization of pain to a specific intervertebral joint.[41] These two sensory nerves also have an intimate association with the autonomic plexus.[41] Painful or pathologic conditions of these nerves or of structures innervated by them may result in autonomic manifestations.

Because the articular facet is a true arthrodial joint, facet-associated pain can be attributed to mechanical stresses, osteoarthritis, and synovial inflammation.[44-47] Similar to other load bearing joints, degenerative changes in the articular facet include hyaline cartilage degradation, remodeling and osteosclerosis of subchondral bone, and osteophyte formation.[47] Although inflammatory processes in typical joints (i.e., knee and hip) have been well documented, studies evaluating the facet joint are few.[47] Pain secondary to osteoarthritis and joint degeneration is associated with cytokines produced by the arachidonic acid cascade. In one study, multiple prostaglandins and leukotrienes, both products of the arachidonic acid cascade, were produced in the facet joint, disk tissues, and subchondral bone of human patients with degenerative lumbosacral spinal disorders. The cytokines produced were similar to those obtained from cartilage and subchondral bone tissues of other osteoarthritic joints.[48] In another human clinical study,[47] the synovium and joint cartilage of 40 patients undergoing lumbar spinal surgery were harvested for evaluation of cytokine production. Although the focus of the study was to identify the presence of interleukin-Iβ

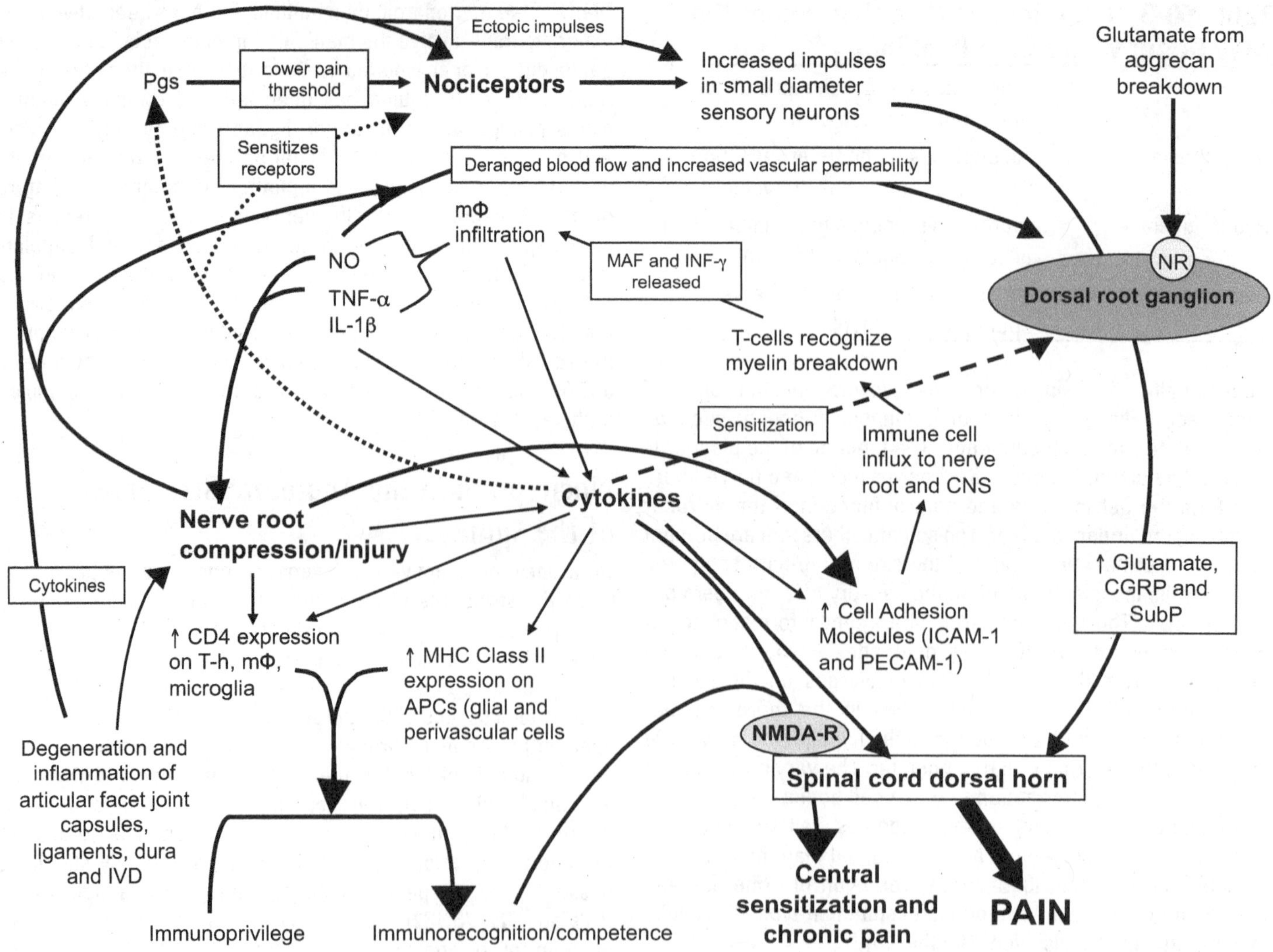

Figure 50-5. A schematic overview of the interplay of factors in acute and chronic radicular pain with nerve root compression. Abbreviations: Pgs = prostaglandins; NO = nitric oxide; mΦ = macrophages; TNF-α = Tumor Necrosis Factor-α; IL-1β = Interleukin-1β; MAF = Macrophage Activating Factor; INF-γ = Gamma-interferon; NR = nociceptive receptor; T-h = T-helper cells; APCs = antigen presenting cells; ICAM-1 = Intercellular Adhesion Molecule 1; PECAM = Platelet Endothelial Cell Adhesion Molecule-1; CGRP = Calcitonin Gene Related Peptide; SubP = Substance P; NMDA-R = N-Methyl-D-Aspartate Receptor; IVD = intervertebral disk.

(IL- Iβ) and tumor necrosis factor-α (TNF-α), the authors were surprised to find that these cytokines were not found in a high concentration in patients with either lumbar disk disease or spinal canal stenosis. However, interleukin 6 (IL-6) concentration was elevated in both groups of patients. IL-6 production has been found to be induced by both IL-Iβ and TNF-α. Both of these cytokines are believed to be present early in acute inflammation and subsequent production of IL-6, further contributing to the inflammatory cascade.[49-54] The presence of elevated IL-6 without increased IL-Iβ and TNF-α may be attributed to the chronic nature of degenerative lumbar disease.

Less attention has been given to pain generated from compression and inflammation of the dura mater. Sensory innervation of the dura mater is provided by the sinuvertebral nerve which carries both sensory and sympathetic fibers.[55] Many peptidergic (pain-associated) nerve fibers are distributed throughout the dura mater[55] and likely play a role in generation of pain.

Mechanical Deformation of the Nerve Roots and Cauda Equina

In the normal state, the nerves of the cauda equina are somewhat moveable within the spinal canal and intervertebral foramen to accommodate changes in spinal extension and flexion and movement of the pelvic limbs. When the nerve roots become compressed or entrapped by extruded intervertebral disk, hypertrophied tissues, or canal stenosis, the movement of the nerve root becomes limited and traction and compression of the nerve root induce pain mechanisms and morphologic changes in the nerve. Chronic compression can be thought of as repeated episodes or persistence of acute compression.[40] The basic underlying pathophysiology of pain in degenerative lumbar spinal disease has been extensively studied. It begins with nerve root compression within the entire cauda equina or with compression of select nerve roots. Direct mechanical, chemical injury or mechanical injury to lumbar roots in the rat produces mechanical allodynia and thermal hyperalgesia.[56] Pain, allodynia, and numbness are subjective symptoms of lumbar radiculopathy that may be induced by ectopic or spontaneous firing of nociceptive sensory neurons.[43,57] Excitability and spontaneous firing in the dorsal root ganglion have been shown to be linked to sensory nerve sodium-gated channels (SNS/PN3 and NaN/SNS2) recently implicated in neuropathic pain.[41] Mechanical compression has additionally been shown to lead to intraneurial tissue reaction, including edema, demyelination, and fibrosis.[40,58,59] Various morphologic and physiologic changes occur with separate phases (acute, subacute, and chronic) of nerve root compression.[37,40,59-62] A study by Kobayashi et al[40] evaluated the morphologic derangements induced by clip compression of the L7 nerve root in a dog model. The clip was retained postoperatively and the nerve roots were evaluated at 1 and 3 weeks postoperatively. Three characteristic processes were observed: Wallerian degeneration, influx of macrophages, and radiculitis. Wallerian degeneration was observed in the nerve root proximal and ventral to the dorsal root ganglion. In the regions of Wallerian degeneration, macrophages were observed metabolizing necrotic debris. Macrophages are involved in the inflammatory cascade by enhancement of vascular permeability, production of chemotactic signals for other inflammatory cells, and modulation of these cells' activity the exact origin of the macrophages is unknown.[63,65] Nervous tissue does not possess a lymphatic system; however, the cerebrospinal fluid may play a role similar to the lymphatic system because the flow of the fluid can remove metabolites and waste products from the spinal cord and nerve roots.[63-65]

Many studies have been performed elucidating the pathogenesis of radiculitis associated with nerve root compression. Chemically induced inflammation of the nerve root by the presence of ruptured disk tissue disseminated along the root sheath has been proposed.[35,63,66] Disk substances thought to play a role in inducing chemical radiculitis include glycoproteins, immunoglobulin G, phospholipase A_2, cytokines, and hydrogen ions.[35,63,64,66-69] Although these findings do not explain the production of inflammation with lumbar canal stenosis, compression of a nerve root results in intraneurial edema and macrophage influx, which is associated with production of inflammatory cytokines, such as IL-1β, IL-6, and TNF-α, nitric oxide, and proteases.[49-54,67]

In a study paralleling the dog nerve-clipping model,[63] changes in the dorsal root ganglia were evaluated at 24 hours, 1 week, or 3 weeks after clipping. Compression of the dorsal roots proximal to the dorsal root ganglion resulted in an impairment to axonal flow in the root and morphologic changes including central chromatolysis in cell bodies of the dorsal root ganglion. Axonal transport plays a role in both the retrograde and anterograde movement of neurotransmitters, nutrients, and neurotrophic factors that are synthesized by dorsal root ganglion cells. Disturbance of axonal flow would be expected, then, to cause neurologic dysfunction. Central chromatolysis and other morphologic changes seen in the ganglion were considered a reflection of decreased synthesis of neurotransmitters and other neuronal homeostatic factors in favor of structural proteins such as the cytoskeleton and neurotrophic factors required for repair.[63,70;71] Nerve growth factors and other neurotrophic factors are thought to be involved in the maintenance of sensory neurons and may actually inhibit cell death after nerve transecton.[63,72-76] When compression results in mild central chromatolysis, the neuron can usually recover fully once the compression is relieved. However, sustained compression could result in irreversible damage to the dorsal root ganglion, which may, in part, explain those patients that do not recover neurologic function after decompressive surgery.

Intraneurial Blood Flow and Edema

Decreased blood flow within nerve roots or the cauda equina may play a role in the symptoms seen in patients with degenerative or stenotic lumbosacral disease.[77] Blood flow is shown to be negatively affected by experimental nerve root constriction,[61,78-81] and hypoxic stress was shown to induce ectopic firing in the dorsal root ganglion and increased sensitivity to mechanical stimuli.[78,82] A large number of sensory roots pass through the dorsal root ganglion, which has an abundant vascular network and no blood-nerve barrier.[80,83] Compression likely occurs first in thin-walled venules, which results in impaired perfusion of the capillary system that feeds the nerve roots, producing ischemia and augmenting radicular edema.[58,62,82,84,85] Increased vascular permeability and subsequent edema in the remainder of the root are attributable to a break down in the blood-nerve barrier.[40,63,84,86] Endoneurial edema, which has been shown experimentally to be temporally associated with the onset of nerve root pain and neurologic dysfunction, is observed in the dorsal root ganglion during compression.[57,80] Edema results in high pressures being exerted on the ganglion cells because the perineurium prevents leakage into the epineurium and the fluid is retained[87,88] (Figure 50-6). The edema may then increase the functional compression in addition to the mechanical stress and contribute to the impaired cell function.[80] In the aforementioned study of canine L7 clipping by Kobayashi et al,[40] increases in vascular permeability were most marked at 1 week postoperatively and began to resolve by 3 weeks. The early marked edema was attributed to loss of vasomotor control induced by vasoactive amines and neuropeptides produced in response to injury at this site. The persistence of increased vascular permeability beyond the acute injury phase was attributed to a greater demand for blood flow to provide nutrients and metabolic building blocks during regeneration.[40,89] Support of the contribution of vascular compromise in nerve root compression was offered by Hida,[90] who showed that nerve-root blood flow measured intraoperatively during spinal lumbar decompressive surgery was increased in those patients whose neurologic deficits or pain resolved shortly after operation compared with those patients whose neurologic deficits or pain did not resolve after surgery.

Neuroimmune Responses, Inflammatory Mediators, and Central Sensitization

The process of nociception involves the generation of nerve impulses in small-diameter sensory neurons and propagation of those impulses to the spinal cord. A complex interplay exists between the nociceptors and the inflammatory cascade. Inflammatory mediators cause sensitization or enhanced responsiveness to stimuli, which are also accentuated by neuropeptides released in the inflammatory cascade.[34] Leukocyte trafficking into spinal cord has been observed in nerve root compression.[91]

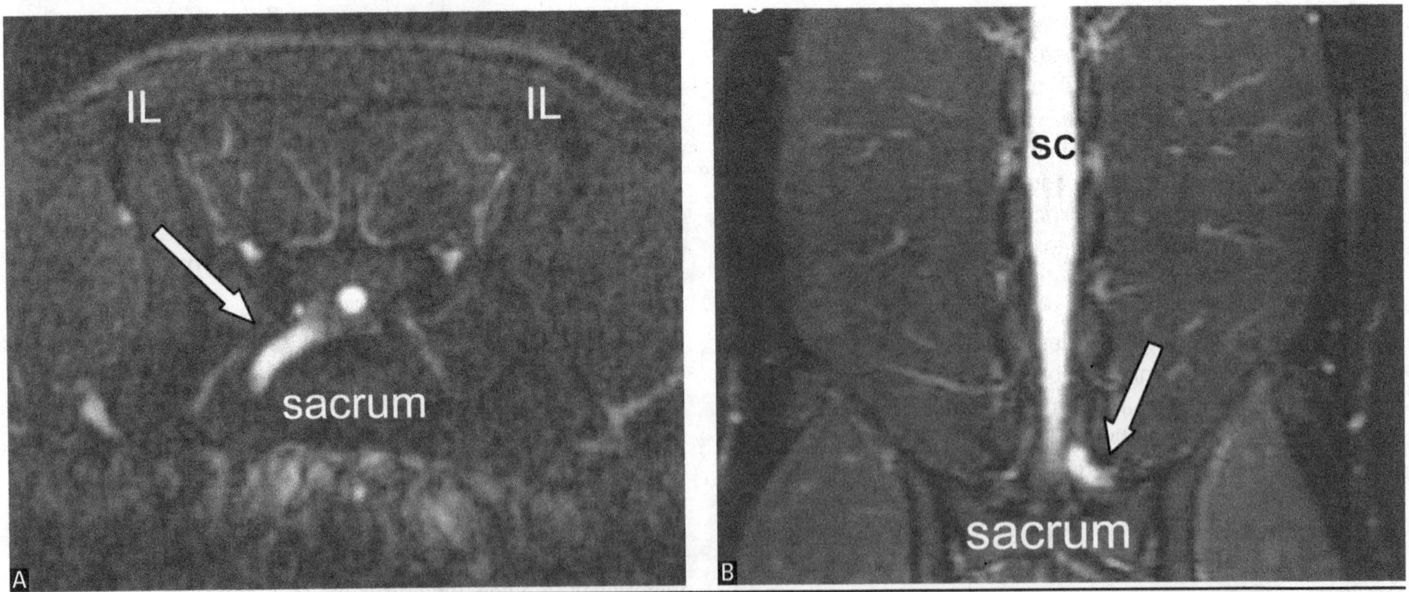

Figure 50-6. A. T2-weighted, transverse plane MRI image at the level of the lumbosacral joint of a dog with left pelvic limb muscle atrophy and lumbar and limb pain. The dog had mild conscious proprioceptive deficits and weakness in the left pelvic limb. Severe swelling of the nerve root was identified (white arrow) intraoperatively and confirmed by biopsy. A foraminotomy was performed; the dog improved and was normal at 6 months postoperative. IL = wing of the ilium B. T2-weighted, coronal plane MRI image of the same dog. White arrow = edematous nerve root. SC = spinal cord.

The nervous system is considered immunologically privileged, meaning that it is not typically surveyed by circulating lymphocytes as are other organs. Immune-membrane glycoproteins (CD4 and major histocompatibility complex, or MHC class II) and cell adhesion molecules (intracellular adhesion molecule-1, or ICAM-1, and platelet endothelial cellular adhesion molecule-1, or PECAM-1), which are integral to immunologic activation, and influx of immune cells were found to increase in response to nerve root injury.[91] MCH class II molecules are usually expressed on antigen-presenting cells (APCs) for interaction with T-cells in immune recognition. The antigen-presenting cells in the nervous system are perivascular cells and microglia.[92,93] Glial cells do not usually express MHC class II molecules, but expression can be induced by cytokines.[94] CD4 membrane glycoprotein, expressed on T-helper cells, macrophages, and microglia,[95] plays the role of antigen recognition by APCs in association with MHC class II molecules. Lumbar nerve root injury resulted in enhanced CD4 expression in the grey matter of the spinal cord compared with sham operated and normal rats.[91] The role of the CD4 molecules is not completely known, but contribution to immunocompetence and response in the CNS after nerve root injury is likely. The nervous system constitutively expresses very low levels of these membrane proteins, which contribute to the nervous system's immunoprivileged status.[91]

Nerve root injury may produce a cascade of events that upregulates ICAM-1, which enables entry of the hematogenous cells into the CNS, contributing to neuroinflammation and the development of central sensitization.[91,91,96-98] The upregulation of these molecules has been temporally associated with the onset of mechanical allodynia after nerve root injury.[91] Additionally, these changes are associated with the dorsal horn laminae in which nociceptive sensory fibers terminate.[91] Increased expression of cell adhesion molecules and membrane glycoproteins has been demonstrated with various disease processes of the CNS and PNS, including infection, autoimmune inflammation, and nerve root compression.

Experimental models have produced evidence for central neuroinflammation from nerve root compression, which includes astrocyte and glial activation and increased expression of proinflammatory cytokines.[98-100] Local production of proinflammatory cytokines via immune-cell activation has been implicated in enhanced nociceptor activity.[101] The CNS becomes infiltrated by immune cells from the peripheral circulation.[91,02] Microglia and astroctyes also become activated in response to peripheral nerve or nerve root injury[37] and release pro- and anti-inflammatory molecules, chemokines, and cellular adhesion molecules.[96,97,102]

T cells recognize myelin sheath breakdown products and release macrophage-activating factors such as γ-interferon.[103] Activated macrophages begin to infiltrate locally to remove cellular debris and release inflammatory cytokines such as IL1-β, nitric oxide, and TNF-α. When applied epineurially, TNF-α was shown to produce hypersensitivity that was blocked when antibodies against TNF-α were co-administered.[101] TNF-α and nitric oxide may potentiate demyelination by Schwann cell injury. Nitric oxide also contributes to increased vascular permeability[104,105] and pain.[106-108] Prostaglandins, which also play an important role in inflammation, have not been shown to have a direct nociceptive effect but may lower the pain threshold at sensory nerve endings.[109] In addition, algesic spinal neuropeptide expression (calcitonin gene-related peptide, or CGRP and substance P, or SP) was shown in models of nerve root compression.[110] Mechanical compression of the dorsal root ganglion in rats resulted in an increase of substance P concentration in the ipsilateral dorsal root ganglion and spinal dorsal horn cells, which was linked to the onset of pain.[111] Accumulation of SP inside the axons of the central branches increased distal to the dorsal root ganglion as the strength and duration of compression increased, suggesting neurotransmitter dynamics are involved in the appearance of radicular pain.[112]

The amino acid glutamate is one of the most ubiquitous neurotransmitters and has been shown to be associated with pain processing throughout the nervous system.[113-117] Glutamate antagonists that work at NMDA, AMPA, and kainite receptors have been shown to attenuate pain responses in rat models.[113-120] Although the actions of glutamate in the dorsal root ganglion are not completely known, the cell bodies have been shown to possess a high density of glutamate receptors[121-124] colocalized with nociceptive neurons,[114,125,126] and mechanisms for reuptake of glutamate from the neuromuscular junction have been identified.[122,123,127-129] Consequently, glutamate is also found in high concentrations in aggrecan, the most prevalent proteoglycan in the extracellular matrix of the intervertebral disk.[117,130-133] Harrington et al[134] hypothesized that glutamate released by proteoglycan degradation during disk degeneration may be a potential source of biologically active neurotransmitter by diffusing across the extradural space to affect glutamate receptors in the dorsal root ganglion.[117,133,135,136] Human herniated and non-herniated intervertebral disks were evaluated using both high-performance liquid gas chromatography and immunohistochemistry to test for the presence of glutamate. Glutamate was found to be abundant in the extracellular matrix of the intervertebral disk with concentrations significantly higher in the herniated disk material, suggesting release of glutamate from the proteoglycan structure. In addition to identification and semi-quantification of glutamate from the intervertebral disk, they evaluated the ability of tritiated-glutamate to diffuse across the epidural space and bind with glutamate receptors on dorsal root ganglion cells in a rat model. Tritiated glutamate was found to be bound to dorsal root ganglion receptors when infused into the epidural space at levels two magnitudes lower than that measured in the herniated disk material. These results suggested that the dorsal root ganglion cells were capable of glutamate uptake from the epidural space and that the concentration of glutamate normally present in the epidural space was relatively low, resulting in a steep concentration gradient diffusing from the herniated intervertebral disk material into the dorsal root ganglion. Further studies are required to understand how free glutamate affects nociceptive pathways in the dorsal root ganglion.

Pain from lumbosacral disease is characteristically chronic in its nature. Nerve injury may lead to potentiation of central sensitization and the development of chronic lumbar radiculopathy.[34] It has been shown that long-term potentiation occurs in the spinal cord in response to noxious stimulation or injury to peripheral nerves.[137] Repeated nerve root injury in a rat model produced significant increases in the magnitude and duration of mechanical allodynia in the paw of the rat.[34] Studies have shown the involvement of chemical factors (cytokines) around the nerve root associated with radicular pain.[138-141] Moreover, early on, pronounced spinal neuroimmune activation and inflammation induce central sensitization by directly or indirectly inhibiting interneuron inhibitory activity at the dorsal horn in the spinal cord.[37] Glial and neuronal proinflammatory cytokines can sensitize the peripheral nociceptive fields and dorsal root ganglia.[142,143] Glial cells synthesize proinflammatory cytokines, proteases, inducible-NO, excess glutamate, oxygen free radicals, eicosanoids, and other toxins that act at the NMDA (N-methyl-D-aspartate) receptors that are implicated in central nervous system sensitization.[56,144-149] Finally, supporting the concept of central sensitization, nerve root compression exhibits the features of mirror pain.[34] Mirror pain is the presence of pain sensation in the opposite limb when only unilateral nerve root compression is present.

References

1. Evans JH: Biomechanics of lumbar fusion. Clin Orthop 193:38-46, 1985.

2. Wheeler SJ. Lumbosacral disease. Vet Clin North Am Small Anim Pract 22(4):937-950, 1992.

3. Evans HE, Christensen GC: Miller's Anatomy of the Dog, 2nd ed. Philadelphia: WB Saunders, 1979, pp. 945-947.

4. Chambers JN. Degenerative lumbosacral stenosis in dogs. Vet Med Report 1:166-180, 1989.

5. Palmer RH, Chambers JN: Canine lumbosacral diseases. Part 1:Anatomy, pathophysiology, and clinic presentation. Cont Ed Pract Vet 13(1):61-69, 1991.

6. De Risio L, Thomas WB, Sharp NJ: Degenerative lumbosacral stenosis. Vet Clin North Am Small Anim Pract 30(1):111-32, 2000.

7. Indrieri RJ: Lumbosacral stenosis and injury of the cauda equina. Vet Clin North Am Small Anim Pract 18(3):697-710, 1988.

8. Oliver JE Jr, Selcer RR, Simpson S: Cauda equina compression from lumbosacral malarticulation and malformation in the dog. J Am Vet Med Assoc 173(2):207-214, 1978.

9. Hanna FY: Lumbosacral osteochondrosis: radiological features and surgical management in 34 dogs. J Small Anim Pract 43(6):272-278 2001.

10. Natarajan M, Prabhakaran T, Surendranathan R: An analysis of lumbar intervertebral disc prolapse. Int Surg 64(6):27-30, 1979.

11. Burger R, Lang J: [Kinetic studies of the lumbar vertebrae and the lumbosacral transition in the German shepherd dog. 2. Our personal investigations]. Schweiz Arch Tierheilkd 135(2):35-43, 1993.

12. Breit S: Functional adaptations of facet geometry in the canine thoracolumbar and lumbar spine (Th10-L6). Ann Anat 184(4):379-385, 2002.

13. Wright JA: Spondylosis deformans of the lumbosacral joint in dogs. J Small Anim Pract 21:45-58, 1980.

14. Weinstein PR: The application of anatomy and pathophysiology in the management of lumbar spine disease. Clin Neurosurg 27:517-540, 1980.

15. Macnab I: The surgery of lumbar disc degeneration. Surg Annu 8:447-480, 1976.

16. Crock HV: Isolated lumbar disk resorption as a cause of nerve root canal stenosis. Clin Orthop Relat Res (115):109-115, 1976.

17. Cinotti G, De SP, Nofroni I, et al: Stenosis of lumbar intervertebral foramen: anatomic study on predisposing factors. Spine 27(3):223-229, 2002.

18. Atarvin GB, Prata RG: Cauda equina compression syndrome. In Bojrab MJ (ed). Current Techniques in Small Animal Surgery, 2nd ed. Philadelphia: Lea & Febiger, 1983, pp. 594-598.

19. Schneck CD: The anatomy of lumbar spondylosis. Clin Orthop Relat Res (193):20-37, 1985.

20. Burton CV, Heithoff KB, Kirkaldy-Willis W, et al: Computed tomographic scanning and the lumbar spine. Part II: Clinical considerations. Spine 4(4):356-368, 1979.

21. Burton CV, Heithoff KB, Kirkaldy-Willis W, et al: Computed tomographic scanning and the lumbar spine. Part II: Clinical considerations. Spine 4(4):356-368, 1979.

22. McIvor GW, Kirkaldy-Willis WH: Pathological and myelographic changes in the major types of lumbar spinal stenosis. Clin Orthop Relat Res (115):72-76, 1976.

23. Damur-Djuric N, Steffen F, Hassig M, et al: Lumbosacral transitional vertebrae in dogs: classification, prevalence, and association with sacroiliac morphology. Vet Radiol Ultrasound 47(1):32-38, 2006.

24. Morgan JP: Transitional lumbosacral vertebral anomaly in the dog: a radiographic study. J Small Anim Pract 40:167-172, 1999.

25. Simoens P, De Vos NR, Lauwers H, Nicaise M: Numerical vertebral variations and transitional vertebrae in the goat. Vet Med J Anat Histol Embryol 12:97-103, 1983.

26. Morgan JP: Congenital anomalies of the vertebral column of the dog: a study of the incidence and significance based on radiographic and morphologic study. J Am Vet Radiol Soc 9:21-29, 1968.

27. Breit S, Knaus I, Kunzel W: Differentiation between lumbosacral transitional vertebrae, pseudolumbarisation, and lumbosacral osteophyte formation in ventrodorsal radiographs of the canine pelvis. Vet J 165(1):36-42, 2003.

28. Winkler W, Loeffler K: [Lumbosacral transitional vertebrae in the dog]. Berl Munch Tierarztl Wochenschr 99(10):343-346, 1986.

29. Luoma K, Vehmas T, Raininko R, et al: Lumbosacral transitional vertebra: relation to disc degeneration and low back pain. Spine 29(2):200-205, 2004.

30. MacGibbon B, Farfan HF: A radiologic survey of various configurations of the lumbar spine. Spine 4(3):258-266, 1979.

31. Hsieh CY, Vanderford JD, Moreau SR, et al: Lumbosacral transitional segments: classification, prevalence, and effect on disk height. J Manipulative Physiol Ther 23(7):483-489, 2000.

32. Turk DC, Okifuji A: Pain terms and taxonomies of pain. *In* Loeser JD, Butler SH, Chapman RC, and Turk DC (eds). Bonica's Management of Pain, 3rd ed. Philaderphia: Lippincott Williams & Wilkins, 2001, p. 18.

33. De RL, Sharp NJ, Olby NJ, et al: Predictors of outcome after dorsal decompressive laminectomy for degenerative lumbosacral stenosis in dogs: 69 cases (1987-1997). J Am Vet Med Assoc 219(5):624-628, 2001.

34. Hunt JL, Winkelstein BA, Rutkowski MD, et al: Repeated injury to the lumbar nerve roots produces enhanced mechanical allodynia and persistent spinal neuroinflammation. Spine 26(19):2073-2079, 2001.

35. Kang JD, Georgescu HI, Intyre-Larkin L, et al: Herniated lumbar intervertebral discs spontaneously produce matrix metalloproteinases, nitric oxide, interleukin-6, and prostaglandin E2. Spine 21(3):271-277, 1996.

36. DeLeo JA, Coombs DW, Willenbring S, et al: Characterization of a neuropathic pain model: sciatic cryoneurolysis in the rat. Pain 56(1):9-16, 1994.

37. DeLeo JA, Winkelstein BA: Physiology of chronic spinal pain syndromes: from animal models to biomechanics. Spine 27(22):2526-2537, 2002.

38. Przewlocka B, Mika J, Labuz D, et al: Spinal analgesic action of endomorphins in acute, inflammatory and neuropathic pain in rats. Eur J Pharmacol 367(2-3):189-196, 1999.

39. Seltzer Z, Dubner R, Shir Y: A novel behavioral model of neuropathic pain disorders produced in rats by partial sciatic nerve injury. Pain 43(2):205-218, 1990.

40. Kobayashi S, Yoshizawa H, Yamada S: Pathology of lumbar nerve root compression. Part 1: Intraradicular inflammatory changes induced by mechanical compression. J Orthop Res 22(1):170-179, 2004.

41. Bucknill AT, Coward K, Plumpton C, et al: Nerve fibers in lumbar spine structures and injured spinal roots express the sensory neuron-specific sodium channels SNS/PN3 and NaN/SNS2. Spine 27(2):135-140, 2002.

42. Branch CL Jr: Anatomic principles guiding surgery of degenerative lumbar spine disease. Clin Neurosurg 41:258-269, 1994.

43. Howe JF, Loeser JD, Calvin WH: Mechanosensitivity of dorsal root ganglia and chronically injured axons: a physiological basis for the radicular pain of nerve root compression. Pain 3(1):25-41, 1977.

44. Evans HE, Christensen GC: Miller's Anatomy of the Dog, 2nd ed. Philadelphia: WB Saunders, 1979, p. 161.

45. Lawrence JS, Bremner JM, Bier F: Osteo-arthrosis. Prevalence in the population and relationship between symptoms and x-ray changes. Ann Rheum Dis 25 (1):1-24, 1966.

46. Adams MA, Hutton WC: The mechanical function of the lumbar apophyseal joints. Spine 8(3):327-330, 1983.

47. Igarashi A, Kikuchi S, Konno S, et al: Inflammatory cytokines released from the facet joint tissue in degenerative lumbar spinal disorders. Spine 29(19):2091-2095 2004.

48. Willburger RE, Wittenberg RH: Prostaglandin release from lumbar disc and facet joint tissue. Spine 19(18):2068-2070, 1994.

49. Akira S, Taga T, Kishimoto T: Interleukin-6 in biology and medicine. Adv Immunol 54:1-78, 1993.

50. Guerne PA, Zuraw BL, Vaughan JH, et al: Synovium as a source of interleukin 6 in vitro. Contribution to local and systemic manifestations of arthritis. J Clin Invest 83(2):585-592, 1989.

51. Houssiau FA, Devogelaer JP, Van DJ, et al: Interleukin-6 in synovial fluid and serum of patients with rheumatoid arthritis and other inflammatory arthritides. Arthritis Rheum 31(6):784-788, 1988.

52. Miyasaka N, Sato K, Hashimoto J, et al: Constitutive production of interleukin 6/B cell stimulatory factor-2 from inflammatory synovium. Clin Immunol Immunopathol 52(2):238-247, 1989.

53. Rosenbaum JT, Cugnini R, Tara DC, et al: Production and modulation of interleukin 6 synthesis by synoviocytes derived from patients with arthritic disease. Ann Rheum Dis 51(2):198-202, 1992.

54. Yoshizaki K, Nakagawa T, Kaieda T, et al: Induction of proliferation and Ig production in human B leukemic cells by anti-immunoglobulins and T cell factors. J Immunol 128(3):1296-1301, 1982.

55. Konnai Y, Honda T, Sekiguchi Y, et al: Sensory innervation of the lumbar dura mater passing through the sympathetic trunk in rats. Spine 25(7):776-782, 2000.

56. Hashizume H, DeLeo JA, Colburn RW, et al: Spinal glial activation and cytokine expression after lumbar root injury in the rat. Spine 25(10):1206-1217, 2000.

57. Winkelstein BA, Weinstein JN, DeLeo JA: The role of mechanical deformation in lumbar radiculopathy: an in vivo model. Spine 27(1):27-33, 2002.

58. Rydevik B, Brown MD, Lundborg G: Pathoanatomy and pathophysiology of nerve root compression. Spine 9(1):7-15, 1984.

59. Yoshizawa H, Kobayashi S, Morita T: Chronic nerve root compression. Pathophysiologic mechanism of nerve root dysfunction. Spine 20(4):397-407, 1995.

60. Gelfan S, Tarlove IM: Physiology of spinal cord, nerve root and peripheral nerve compression. Am J Physiol 185(1):217-229, 1956.

61. Yoshizawa H, Kobayashi S, Kubota K: Effects of compression on intraradicular blood flow in dogs. Spine 14(11):1220-1225, 1989.

62. Yoshizawa H, Kobayashi S, Hachiya Y: Blood supply of nerve roots and dorsal root ganglia. Orthop Clin North Am 22(2):195-211, 1991.

63. Kobayashi S, Yoshizawa H, Yamada S: Pathology of lumbar nerve root compression. Part 2: morphological and immunohistochemical changes of dorsal root ganglion. J Orthop Res 22(1):180-188, 2004.

64. Nathaniel EJ, Nathaniel DR: Electron microscopic studies of spinal ganglion cells following crushing of dorsal roots in adult rat. J Ultrastruct Res 45(3):168-182, 1973.

65. Nielsch U, Bisby MA, Keen P: Effect of cutting or crushing the rat sciatic nerve on synthesis of substance P by isolated L5 dorsal root ganglia. Neuropeptides 10(2):137-145, 1987.

66. Iwamoto H, Kuwahara H, Matsuda H, et al: Production of chronic compression of the cauda equina in rats for use in studies of lumbar spinal canal stenosis. Spine 20(24):2750-2757, 1995.

67. Cornefjord M, Olmarker K, Farley DB, et al: Neuropeptide changes in compressed spinal nerve roots. Spine20(6):670-673, 1995.

68. Kuraishi Y, Hirota N, Sato Y, et al: Evidence that substance P and somatostatin transmit separate information related to pain in the spinal dorsal horn. Brain Res 325(1-2):294-298, 1985.

69. Morton CR, Hutchison WD: Release of sensory neuropeptides in the spinal cord: studies with calcitonin gene-related peptide and galanin. Neuroscience 31(3):807-815, 1989.

70. Bisby MA: Dependence of GAP43 (B50, F1) transport on axonal regeneration in rat dorsal root ganglion neurons. Brain Res 458(1):157-161, 1988.

71. Oblinger MM, Szumlas RA, Wong J, et al: Changes in cytoskeletal gene expression affect the composition of regenerating axonal sprouts elaborated by dorsal root ganglion neurons in vivo. J Neurosci 9(8):2645-2653, 1989.

72. Acheson A, Conover JC, Fandl JP, et al: A BDNF autocrine loop in adult sensory neurons prevents cell death. Nature 374(6521):450-453, 1995.

73. Edwards SN, Tolkovsky AM: Characterization of apoptosis in cultured rat sympathetic neurons after nerve growth factor withdrawal. J Cell Biol 124(4):537-546, 1994.

74. Lieberman AR: The axon reaction: a review of the principal features of perikaryal responses to axon injury. Int Rev Neurobiol 14:49-124, 1971.

75. Persson H, Ibanez CF: Role and expression of neurotrophins and the trk family of tyrosine kinase receptors in neural growth and rescue after injury. Curr Opinion Neurol Neurosurg 6(1):11-18, 1993.

76. Tong JX, Eichler ME, Rich KM: Intracellular calcium levels influence apoptosis in mature sensory neurons after trophic factor deprivation. Exp Neurol 138(1):45-52, 1996.

77. Olmarker K, Holm S, Rosenqvist AL, et al: Experimental nerve root compression. A model of acute, graded compression of the porcine cauda equina and an analysis of neural and vascular anatomy. Spine 16(1):61-69, 1991.

78. Garfin SR, Rydevik B, Lind B, et al: Spinal nerve root compression. Spine 20(16):1810-1820, 1995.

79. Kobayashi S, Yoshizawa H, Nakai S: Experimental study on the dynamics of lumbosacral nerve root circulation. Spine 25(3):298-305, 2000.

80. Kobayashi S, Yoshizawa H: Effect of mechanical compression on the vascular permeability of the dorsal root ganglion. J Orthop Res 20(4):730-739, 2002.

81. Naito M, Owen JH, Bridwell KH, et al: Blood flow direction in the lumbar nerve root. Spine 15(9):966-968, 1990.

82. Sugawara O, Atsuta Y, Iwahara T, et al: The effects of mechanical compression and hypoxia on nerve root and dorsal root ganglia. An analysis of ectopic firing using an in vitro model. Spine 21(18):2089-2094, 1996.

83. Bergmann L, Alexander L: Vascular supply of the spinal ganglia. Arch Neurol Psychiat 46:761-82, 1941.

84. Kobayashi S, Yoshizawa H, Hachiya Y, et al: Vasogenic edema induced by compression injury to the spinal nerve root. Distribution of intravenously injected protein tracers and gadolinium-enhanced magnetic resonance imaging. Spine 18(11):1410-1424, 1993.

85. Parke WW: The significance of venous return impairment in ischemic radiculopathy and myelopathy. Orthop Clin North Am 22(2):213-221, 1991.

86. Kobayashi S, Baba H, Uchida K, et al: Effect of mechanical compression on the lumbar nerve root: localization and changes of intraradicular inflammatory cytokines, nitric oxide, and cyclooxygenase. Spine 30(15):1699-1705, 2005.

87. Arvidson B: Distribution of intravenously injected protein tracers in peripheral ganglia of adult mice. Exp Neurol 63(2):388-410, 1979.

88. Shanthaveerappa TR, Bourne GH: Perineural epithelium: a new concept of its role in the integrity of the peripheral nervous system. Science 154(755):1464-1467, 1966.

89. Hara H, Kobayashi S: Adrenergic innervation of the vasa nervorum in the cranial nerves and spinal roots in the subarachnoid space. Exp Neurol 98(3):673-676, 1987.

90. Hida S, Naito M, Kubo M: Intraoperative measurements of nerve root blood flow during discectomy for lumbar disc herniation. Spine 28(1):85-90, 2003.

91. Rutkowski MD, Winkelstein BA, Hickey WF, et al: Lumbar nerve root injury induces central nervous system neuroimmune activation and neuroinflammation in the rat: relationship to painful radiculopathy. Spine 27(15):1604-1613, 2002.

92. Ford AL, Goodsall AL, Hickey WF, et al: Normal adult ramified microglia separated from other central nervous system macrophages by flow cytometric sorting. Phenotypic differences defined and direct ex vivo antigen presentation to myelin basic protein-reactive CD4+ T cells compared. J Immunol 154(9):4309-4321, 1995.

93. Wekerle H: T-cell autoimmunity in the central nervous system. Intervirology35(1-4):95-100, 1993.

94. Kreutzberg GW: Microglia: a sensor for pathological events in the CNS. Trends Neurosci 19(8):312-318, 1996.

95. Buttini M, Westland CE, Masliah E, et al: Novel role of human CD4 molecule identified in neurodegeneration. Nat Med 4(4):441-446, 1998.

96. DeLeo JA, Yezierski RP: The role of neuroinflammation and neuroimmune activation in persistent pain. Pain 90(1-2):1-6, 2001.

97. Nottet HS, Jett M, Flanagan CR, et al: A regulatory role for astrocytes in HIV-1 encephalitis. An overexpression of eicosanoids, platelet-activating factor, and tumor necrosis factor-alpha by activated HIV-1-infected monocytes is attenuated by primary human astrocytes. J Immunol 154(7):3567-3581, 1995.

98. Sweitzer SM, Colburn RW, Rutkowski M, et al: Acute peripheral inflammation induces moderate glial activation and spinal IL-1beta expression that correlates with pain behavior in the rat. Brain Res 829(1-2):209-221, 1999.

99. DeLeo JA, Colburn RW, Rickman AJ: Cytokine and growth factor immunohistochemical spinal profiles in two animal models of mononeuropathy. Brain Res 759(1):50-57, 1997.

100. DeLeo JA, Colburn RW, Rickman AJ, et al: Intrathecal catheterization alone induces neuroimmune activation in the rat. Eur J Pain 1(2):115-122, 1997.

101. Sorkin LS, Doom CM: Epineurial application of TNF elicits an acute mechanical hyperalgesia in the awake rat. J Peripher Nerv Syst 5(2):96-100, 2000.

102. Sweitzer SM, White KA, Dutta C, et al: The differential role of spinal MHC class II and cellular adhesion molecules in peripheral inflammatory versus neuropathic pain in rodents. J Neuroimmunol 125(1-2):82-93, 2002.

103. Misko TP, Trotter JL, Cross AH: Mediation of inflammation by encephalitogenic cells: interferon gamma induction of nitric oxide synthase and cyclooxygenase 2. J Neuroimmunol 61(2):195-204, 1995.

104. Ialenti A, Ianaro A, Moncada S, et al: Modulation of acute inflammation by endogenous nitric oxide. Eur J Pharmacol 211(2):177-182, 1992.

105. Lacroix S, Rivest S: Effect of acute systemic inflammatory response and cytokines on the transcription of the genes encoding cyclooxygenase enzymes (COX-1 and COX-2) in the rat brain. J Neurochem 70(2):452-466, 1998.

106. Choi Y, Raja SN, Moore LC, et al: Neuropathic pain in rats is associated with altered nitric oxide synthase activity in neural tissue. J Neurol Sci 138(1-2):14-20, 1996.

107. Duarte ID, dos Santos IR, Lorenzetti BB, et al: Analgesia by direct antagonism of nociceptor sensitization involves the arginine-nitric oxide-cGMP pathway. Eur J Pharmacol 217(2-3):225-227, 1992.

108. Khalil Z, Helme RD: The quantitative contribution of nitric oxide and sensory nerves to bradykinin-induced inflammation in rat skin microvasculature. Brain Res 589(1):102-108, 1992.

109. Seibert K, Zhang Y, Leahy K, et al: Pharmacological and biochemical demonstration of the role of cyclooxygenase 2 in inflammation and pain. Proc Natl Acad Sci USA 91(25):12013-12017, 1994.

110. Rothman SM, Kreider RA, Winkelstein BA: Spinal neuropeptide responses in persistent and transient pain following cervical nerve root injury. Spine 30(22):2491-2496, 2005.

111. Badalamente MA, Dee R, Ghillani R, et al: Mechanical stimulation of dorsal root ganglia induces increased production of substance P: a mechanism for pain following nerve root compromise? Spine 12(6):552-555, 1987.

112. Kobayashi S, Kokubo Y, Uchida K, et al: Effect of lumbar nerve root compression on primary sensory neurons and their central branches: changes in the nociceptive neuropeptides substance P and somatostatin. Spine 30(3):276-282, 2005.

113. Corderre TJ: The role of excitatory amino acid receptors and intracellular messengers in persistent nociception after tissue injury in rats. Mol Neurobiol 7:229-246, 1994.

114. Heuttner JE: Glutamate receptor channels in rat DRG neuron: activation by kainate and quisqualate and blockade of desensitization by Con A. Neuron 5:255-266, 1990;

115. Gronblad M, Virri J, Tolonen J, et al: A controlled immunohistochemical study of inflammatory cells in disc herniation tissue. Spine 19(24):2744-2751, 1994.

116. Jensen TS, Yaksh TL: Brainstem excitatory amino acid receptors in nociception: microinjection mapping and pharmacological characterization of glutamate-sensitive sites in the brainstem associated with algogenic behavior. Neuroscience 46(3):535-547, 1992.

117. Upholt WB, Chandrasekaran L, Tanzer ML: Molecular cloning and analysis of the protein modules of aggrecans. Experientia 49(5):384-392, 1993.

118. Kitao Y, Robertson B, Kudo M, et al: Neurogenesis of subpopulations of rat lumbar dorsal root ganglion neurons including neurons projecting to the dorsal column nuclei. J Comp Neurol 371(2):249-257, 1996.

119. Maeshima T, Ito R, Hamada S, et al: The cellular localization of 5-HT2A receptors in the spinal cord and spinal ganglia of the adult rat. Brain Res 797(1):118-124, 1998.

120. Zhou S, Bonasera L, Carlton SM: Peripheral administration of NMDA, AMPA or KA results in pain behaviors in rats. Neuroreport 7(4):895-900, 1996.

121. Herrero I, Miras-Portugal MT, Sanchez-Prieto J: Functional switch from facilitation to inhibition in the control of glutamate release by metabotropic glutamate receptors. J Biol Chem 273(4):1951-1958, 1998.

122. Kuslich SD, Ulstrom CL, Michael CJ: The tissue origin of low back pain and sciatica: a report of pain response to tissue stimulation during operations on the lumbar spine using local anesthesia. Orthop Clin North Am 22(2):181-187, 1991.

123. Li JL, Ohishi H, Kaneko T, et al: Immunohistochemical localization of a metabotropic glutamate receptor, mGluR7, in ganglion neurons of the rat; with special reference to the presence in glutamatergic ganglion neurons. Neurosci Lett 204(1-2):9-12, 1996.

124. Partin KM, Patneau DK, Winters CA, et al: Selective modulation of desensitization at AMPA versus kainate receptors by cyclothiazide and concanavalin A. Neuron 11(6):1069-1082, 1993.

125. Lee CJ, Bardoni R, Tong CK, et al: Functional expression of AMPA receptors on central terminals of rat dorsal root ganglion neurons and presynaptic inhibition of glutamate release. Neuron 35(1):135-146, 2002.

126. Small B, Thomas J, Kemp M, et al: LY339434, a GluR5 kainate receptor agonist. Neuropharmacol 37(10-11):1261-1267, 1998.

127. Cangro CB, Sweetnam PM, Wrathall JR, et al: Localization of elevated glutaminase immunoreactivity in small DRG neurons. Brain Res 336(1):158-161, 1985.

128. Duce IR, Keen P: Selective uptake of [3H]glutamine and [3H] glutamate into neurons and satellite cells of dorsal root ganglia in vitro. Neurosci 8(4):861-866, 1983.

129. Kai-Kai MA, Howe R: Glutamate-immunoreactivity in the trigeminal and dorsal root ganglia, and intraspinal neurons and fibres in the dorsal horn of the rat. Histochem J 23(4):171-179, 1991.

130. Barry FP, Gaw JU, Young CN, et al: Hyaluronan-binding region of aggrecan from pig laryngeal cartilage. Amino acid sequence, analysis of N-linked oligosaccharides and location of the keratan sulphate. Biochem J 286 (Pt 3):761-769, 1992.

131. Lohmander LS, Neame PJ, Sandy JD: The structure of aggrecan fragments in human synovial fluid. Evidence that aggrecanase mediates cartilage degradation in inflammatory joint disease, joint injury, and osteoarthritis. Arthritis Rheum 36(9):1214-1222, 1993.

132. Neame PJ, Barry FP: The link proteins. Experientia 49(5):393-402, 1993.

133. Vilim V, Fosang AJ: Proteoglycans isolated from dissociative extracts of differently aged human articular cartilage: characterization of naturally occurring hyaluronan-binding fragments of aggrecan. Biochem J 304 (Pt 3):887-894, 1994.

134. Harrington JF, Messier AA, Bereiter D, et al: Herniated lumbar disc material as a source of free glutamate available to affect pain signals through the dorsal root ganglion. Spine 25(8):929-936, 2000.

135. Inkinen RI, Lammi MJ, Lehmonen S, et al: Relative increase of biglycan and decorin and altered chondroitin sulfate epitopes in the degenerating human intervertebral disc. J Rheumatol 25(3):506-514, 1998.

136. Nguyen Q, Liu J, Roughley PJ, et al: Link protein as a monitor in situ of endogenous proteolysis in adult human articular cartilage. Biochem J 278 (Pt 1):143-147, 1991.

137. Sandkuhler J, Liu X: Induction of long-term potentiation at spinal synapses by noxious stimulation or nerve injury. Eur J Neurosci 10(7):2476-2480, 1998.

138. Gertzbein SD, Tait JH, Devlin SR: The stimulation of lymphocytes by nucleus pulposus in patients with degenerative disk disease of the lumbar spine. Clin Orthop Relat Res (123):149-154, 1977.

139. Gronblad M, Weinstein JN, Santavirta S: Immunohistochemical observations on spinal tissue innervation. A review of hypothetical mechanisms of back pain. Acta Orthop Scand 62(6):614-622, 1991.

140. Nachemson A. Intradiscal measurements of pH in patients with lumbar rhizopathies. Acta Orthop Scand 40(1):23-42, 1969.

141. Urban L, Somjen GG: Reversible effects of hypoxia on neurons in mouse dorsal root ganglia in vitro. Brain Res 520(1-2):36-42, 1990.

142. Junger H, Sorkin LS: Nociceptive and inflammatory effects of subcutaneous TNFalpha. Pain 85(1-2):145-151, 2000.

143. Ozaktay AC, Kallakuri S, Takebayashi T, et al: Effects of interleukin-1 beta, interleukin-6, and tumor necrosis factor on sensitivity of dorsal root ganglion and peripheral receptive fields in rats. Eur Spine J15:1-9, 2006.

144. Chao CC, Hu S: Tumor necrosis factor-alpha potentiates glutamate neurotoxicity in human fetal brain cell cultures. Dev Neurosci 16(3-4):172-179, 1994.

145. Huang ZF, Massey JB, Via DP: Differential regulation of cyclooxygenase-2 (COX-2) mRNA stability by interleukin-1 beta (IL-1 beta) and tumor necrosis factor-alpha (TNF-alpha) in human in vitro differentiated macrophages. Biochem Pharmacol 59(2):187-194, 2000.

146. Kalaria RN, Cohen DL, Premkumar DR: Cellular aspects of the inflammatory response in Alzheimer's disease. Neurodegeneration 5(4):497-503, 1996.

147. Morioka N, Takeda K, Kumagai K, et al: Interleukin-1beta-induced substance P release from rat cultured primary afferent neurons driven by two phospholipase A2 enzymes: secretory type IIA and cytosolic type IV. J Neurochem 80(6):989-997, 2002.

148. Nicol GD, Lopshire JC, Pafford CM: Tumor necrosis factor enhances the capsaicin sensitivity of rat sensory neurons. J Neurosci 17(3):975-982, 1997.

149. Serou MJ, DeCoster MA, Bazan NG: Interleukin-1 beta activates expression of cyclooxygenase-2 and inducible nitric oxide synthase in primary hippocampal neuronal culture: platelet-activating factor as a preferential mediator of cyclooxygenase-2 expression. J Neurosci Res 58(4):593-598, 1999.

Part VI

Respiratory System

Chapter 51

Brachycephalic Upper Airways Syndrome

Gilles P. Dupré
Cyrill Poncet

Brachycephalic breeds are usually distinguished from mesocephalic and doliocephalic breeds by their shortened skull, which is a result of early ankylosis of the skull cartilages. Brachycephalic breeds have been defined by different measurements:[1,2] A skull width to length ratio greater than 0.81, a face to skull ratio of 1.6 to 3.44, or a craniofacial angle less than 14° (angle between the base of the skull and the facial skull). Breeds usually recognized as brachycephalic by these definitions include: Boston terrier, English and French bulldog, pug, Pekinese, Shi-tzu, and Cavalier King Charles. Some miniature breeds as Yorkshire terriers and miniature pinschers are also often included in this list.

Upper respiratory syndrome has been described in brachycephalic dogs (BD). Clinical signs usually include snoring, inspiratory dyspnea, exercise intolerance, stridor, cyanosis, or even syncopal episodes in more severe cases. These problems are usually aggravated with stress, exercise, or heat. Labored breathing is accompanied by over dilatation of the chest, because a higher intrathoracic negative pressure tends to suck the abdomen into the thoracic cavity. The upper respiratory syndrome usually becomes more severe with increasing age. Vomiting or regurgitation of saliva is also frequently encountered in association with this syndrome.

Anatomy of the Upper Airways in Brachycephalic Dogs

Several anatomic abnormalities can be found in the brachycephalic dog.[1,2,3] The cartilaginous skeleton of the external nares is usually shorter, thicker, and medially displaced compared with non-brachycephalic breeds, causing secondary obstruction of the nostrils. Owing to shortening of the skull, the size and shape of the conchae are modified, leading to potential intranasal stenosis. The transition from hard to soft palate is usually caudal to the last molar in dolichocephalic and mesocephalic breeds, whereas it is more caudally located in BD. The soft palate, which normally extends to the top of the epiglottis, can extend up to 1 to 2 cm beyond the epiglottis and can be readily aspirated into the rima glottidis during inspiration. On radiographic examination (Figures 51-1 and 51-2) one can readily see that, in BD, the soft palate is not only overlong but also over-thick.[4] In many BD, especially French and English bulldogs, the base of the tongue is also hyperplastic; the term macroglossia has usually been used to define this abnormality. Besides these findings, other tissue redundancies can be found, especially in the oro- and nasopharynx region.

The rima glottidis, the narrowest airflow passage of the upper airways, is formed by the paired arytenoid cartilages and the vocal folds. The laryngeal saccules, or ventricles, are located cranial to the vocal folds and cannot be seen in a normal dog. In many BD, the laryngeal ventricles can be seen protruding into the laryngeal lumen.[5] Owing to an abnormal embryogenesis, the trachea of some brachycephalic dogs (mainly English bulldogs) is hypoplastic, which further decreases the upper respiratory air flow.[6]

These anatomic anomalies are responsible for a multifocal obstruction of the upper-airways. The nostrils are narrowed by medially displaced nares, the nasopharynx and the oropharynx are "blocked" between a hyperplastic tongue and an overthick soft palate, and the rima glottidis is obstructed by the overlong soft palate. These anatomic abnormalities have secondary adverse functional consequences on laryngeal function.

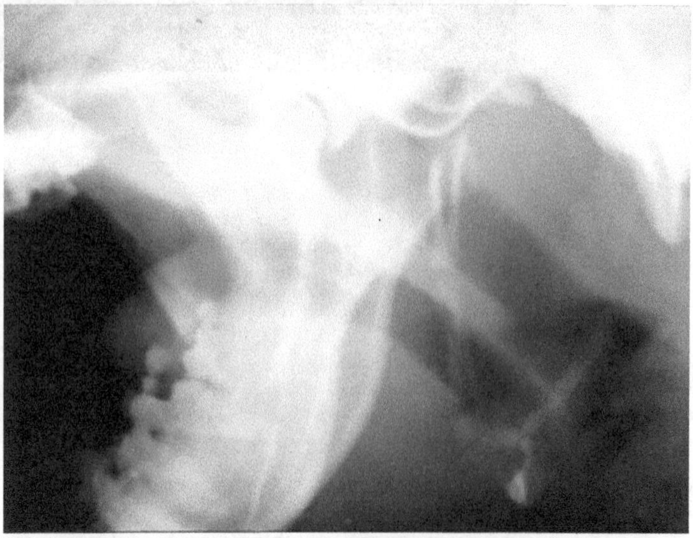

Figure 51-1. Lateral radiograph of pharyngeal region of a mesocephalic dog. The oro- and nasopharynx can be readily seen as two broad stripes of aeric density.

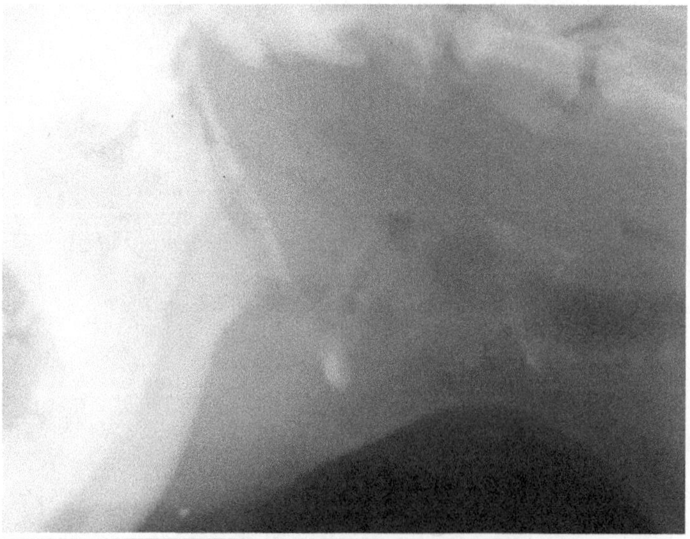

Figure 51-2. Lateral radiograph of pharyngeal region of a brachycephalic dog. The two broad stripes of aeric density have disappeared and the soft palate appears both elongated and thickened.

Pathophysiologic Consequences

Brachycephalic dogs must produce higher negative pressure to breathe properly given their narrowed nostrils and nasal passages. During inspiration, the soft palate flutters into the rima glottidis and can even obstruct it. In some instances when negative pressure is high enough, it may exceed the natural resistance of the tissues, causing their collapse. This can be observed clinically in the nostrils and also in the larynx. The cuneiform and corniculate cartilages are drawn into the glottal opening following increased inspiratory efforts, causing laryngeal collapse. In these cases, an inspiratory stridor and even suffocation can be observed. In such patients the laryngeal ventricles are usually everted into the laryngeal lumen. Everted laryngeal ventricles and laryngeal collapse are secondary events that lead to even more severe respiratory compromise.[2,5,7]

Other Findings in Brachycephalic Dogs Suffering from Upper Airway Compromise

Many owners describe signs of regurgitation or vomiting when their BD becomes excited or suffers respiratory distress.[7,8,9] In these instances, signs of respiratory distress are usually relieved when the dog vomits or regurgitates large packs of "foam." In one study on 73 brachycephalic dogs suffering from upper airway syndrome,[9] respiratory and digestive signs were graded as minimal (grade 1), moderate (grade 2), or severe (grade 3), according to their frequency and severity. Respiratory signs were moderate in 20 dogs (27.4%) and severe in 51 (69.9%). Nineteen dogs (26%) were presented with grade 1 digestive disorders, 19 (26%) with grade 2, and 35 (48%) with grade 3. Among the 35 dogs with grade 3 digestive signs, 28 (80%) suffered from grade 3 respiratory disorders, 5 (14.3%) from grade 2, and 1 (5.7%) from grade 1. A correlation between the severity of gastric and respiratory signs was demonstrated ($p=0.059$).

Diagnosis

Several steps should be undertaken in order to make an accurate diagnosis of brachycephalic syndrome.

History And Clinical Signs

The history usually describes snoring and progressive exercise intolerance aggravated by warm temperature when the dog is 1 to 2 years old.[5,9,10] Therefore, most owners become aware of the problem during the second summer of the dog's life.[7,9,11] Unfortunately, because snoring is considered a normal respiratory feature of BD by most owners, breeders, and even practitioners, no further diagnostic or therapeutic steps are usually undertaken. With time, the condition worsens until signs of laryngeal collapse occur (inspiratory stridor). In these cases, most owners spontaneously find a way to open their pets' upper airways by opening the mouth and pulling the tongue forward. Concomitantly, vomiting or regurgitating food or saliva usually happens and this is also considered to be a normal feature of BD in most owners' and breeders' minds.

Radiographic Examination

Radiographic examination of the head can be used to assess the length and thickness of the soft palate. It can often be observed that both oropharynx and nasopharynx are equally compressed by mucosal hyperplasia (Figures 51-1 and 51-2). Thoracic radiographs are recommended in order to diagnose hypoplastic trachea, aspiration pneumonia, and/or secondary right-sided heart failure.[2,11]

Endoscopy

Given the common involvement of upper airways and the upper gastrointestinal tract, endoscopy should be conducted as part of a basic diagnostic work-up.

Length and thickness of the soft palate are assessed and, after removal of the endotracheal tube, the motion of the arytenoid cartilages and position of the ventricles are evaluated. In some cases, especially in very small brachycephalic dogs (e.g., pugs or Pekinese) the arytenoid cartilages are flaccid and have a tendency to rotate inward into the laryngeal lumen.[7] During the same procedure, upper gastrointestinal endoscopy is done. The esophagus, cardia, stomach, pylorus, and duodenum are evaluated. Gastric and duodenal biopsies are recommended.[7,8,9]

Macroscopic and Endoscopic Findings

Stenotic nares and soft-palate hyperplasia are the two most common anomalies (present in 50 to 85% and 96 to 100% of cases, respectively.[5,8,10,11] Everted ventricles are usually found in 54 to 60% of cases,[10,11] and although more rarely mentioned in the past,[5,11] a moderate to severe laryngeal collapse was present in 64% (39/61) of the patients in a retrospective study.[9]

Although many anatomic malformations of the gastrointestinal tract have been described in BD,[12-15] some authors specifically studied digestive disorders in BD affected by upper airway compromise.[7,8,9] In one such study,[9] 71 of 73 dogs (97.2%) were presented with esophageal, gastric, or duodenal anomalies. Forty-four dogs suffered esophageal anomalies; 12 presented with an esophageal deviation, 28 had cardial atony, 23 had gastro,esophageal reflux, 3 had axial hiatal hernia and 27 had distal esophagitis. Chronic vomiting, slow gastric emptying, and hiatal hernias have been classically described to explain gastroesophageal reflux.[16] In brachycephalic breeds, a possible explanation is the high positive abdominal pressure generated by recurrent vomiting as well as the negative intrathoracic pressures generated by increased inspiratory work.[17-21] In the same study,[9] among the 71 dogs suffering gastric anomalies, 65 presented with diffuse inflammation of the body or antrum and a punctiform inflammation was seen in 28 dogs; 23 presented with gastric stasis, 63 with pyloric mucosal hyperplasia, 22 with pyloric stenosis, 4 with pyloric atony, and 6 with duodenogastric reflux. A chronic diffuse or follicular gastritis was found in 50 of 51 specimens (98%). Gastritis was histologically graded as minimal in 13 cases (26%), moderate in 25 cases (50%), and severe in 10 cases (24%).

Gastrointestinal and Respiratory Signs: A Common Pathophysiologic Pathway

Gastroesophageal reflux associated with regurgitation and vomiting can contribute to upper esophageal, pharyngeal, and laryngeal inflammation. These phenomena have been documented experimentally in animals[22] and clinically in infants.[23] They can further contribute to upper respiratory problems. In turn, respiratory distress could stimulate the autonomous sympathetic nervous system, which would slow gastric motility and increase the gastric emptying time. Furthermore, the dilated antrum would stimulate gastrin-producing cells responsible for muscular hyperplasia.[13,24] In a study in exercising race horses, the pressure over the lower esophageal sphincter was shown to be related to the obstruction of upper respiratory tract.[25] In humans, a high prevalence of hiatal hernia and gastroesophageal reflux has been demonstrated in asthma patients.[26] Finally, in the dog several cases of gastroesophageal diseases or hiatal hernia have been described associated with upper airway obstruction.[7-9,26,27] The correlation between respiratory and digestive disorders suggests the influence of upper respiratory tract diseases on gastroesophageal diseases, and vice versa. The gastroesophageal disorders, ptyalism, regurgitation, vomiting, and reflux, can aggravate the respiratory signs by encumbering the pharyngeal region and stimulating persistent inflammation. Conversely, chronic respiratory depression promotes gastroesophageal reflux. The close relation between respiratory and digestive problems is sustained by the fact that most of these animals "vomit" large packs of saliva when excited or stressed or during respiratory distress.

Treatment

Early Relief of Respiratory Compromise

According to the pathophysiology of the syndrome, early relief of the proximally located obstruction should be attempted because it is postulated that early correction could prevent or even reverse ventricular eversion or laryngeal collapse.[5] Therefore, as soon as snoring is observed, rhinoplasty and palatoplasty are recommended. This has been done as early as at six months of age but the value of an earlier rhinoplasty is still debated.

Medical Treatment of Gastroesophageal Disease

The influence of surgical treatment of the upper airway on improvement in gastrointestinal signs has also been studied.[28] In this study, when an inflammatory gastrointestinal disease was observed endoscopically, a medical treatment, based on inhibition of hydrogen ion secretion (omeprazole 0.7 mg/kg per os every 24 hours) and prokinetic medication (cisapride 0.2 mg/kg per os every 8 hours), was recommended immediately after surgery. If distal esophagitis was noted, an antacid was prescribed for 15 days (magnesium hydroxide, 1 ml/kg per os after meals). Following histologic results, medical treatment was adjusted for each case. For moderate to severe gastritis, a 2-month course of treatment was recommended, including an inhibitor of hydrogen ion secretion (omeprazole, 0.7 mg/kg per os every 24 hours), a prokinetic (cisapride, 0.2 mg/kg per os every 8 hours), a surface protector (sucralfate, 1g per os every 12 hours apart from the meals). For severe gastritis and/or duodenitis with parietal fibrosis, the same treatment was advised for 3 months and corticosteroids were added (prednisolone starting at 0.5 mg/kg per os every 12 hours).

This study also suggested that, after surgical treatment of the upper airways and despite discontinuation of medical treatment in more than 80% of the cases, a clear improvement of upper gastrointestinal tract disease was observed. In the cases where a control gastroesophageal endoscopy could be obtained six months after upper airway surgery, it always showed a complete resolution of the gastroesophageal endoscopic and histopathologic signs. These findings support the previous hypothesis of a common pathophysiologic pathway for upper respiratory and upper gatroesophageal disease in brachycephalic dogs.

Surgical Treatment

Nostrils

Several techniques of rhinoplasty have been developed.[2,5] They all aim at opening the lateral wings of the nostrils. Removing this part increases the diameter and contributes to improvement of the nasal air flow.

Elongated and Hyperplastic Soft Palate

Current techniques for treatment of elongated soft palate involve excision of the elongated part.[2,5] Although the level of excision has been recommended to be somewhere between the midpoint and the end of the tonsils, it is also considered wise to cut the soft palate at a level where it just comes into contact with the tip of the epiglottis. A new technique of palatoplasty, the so-called "Folded flap palatoplasty," has been developed to address both the pharyngeal and the laryngeal obstruction.[4] This technique achieves a marked reduction of the thickness of the soft palate, thereby relieving the nasopharynx and oropharynx from obstruction. As with the conventional techniques, the soft palate is shortened and the laryngeal obstruction is also relieved.

Laryngeal Collapse

In one study,[9] 64% (39/61) of the patients were presented with moderate to severe laryngeal collapse and 54% (33/61) with everted ventricles. Because it is postulated that laryngeal collapse and ventricular eversion are secondary events most likely a result of increased respiratory depression, relief of proximal obstruction should alleviate signs of laryngeal collapse. This has been observed clinically. In this study, only 1 dog out of 61 had laryngeal surgery (arytenoid lateralization) and 1 had an oral ventriculectomy. Although ventriculectomy has been recommended as a treatment for ventricular eversion, it increases local inflammation and can result in laryngeal webbing. Its benefit in improving clinical signs has not yet been proven. To the contrary, in a retrospective study looking at dogs with ventricular eversion, the overall prognosis was better in those that did not have a ventriculectomy.[10]

Treating laryngeal collapse remains challenging. In cases where clinical signs are not improved after rhinoplasty and palatoplasty, lateralization of one of the arytenoid cartilages can be attempted. This usually provides an adequate laryngeal opening in cases where the cartilage is stiff enough. In some cases, the arytenoid cartilages are flaccid and have a tendency to invert into the laryngeal lumen. In our experience, these dogs do not respond favourably to lateralization and a permanent tracheostomy should be recommended.

Prognosis

Following this overall medicosurgical protocol, the prognosis 6 months after surgical treatment was graded as good in 22% and excellent in 67% of the cases.[29] Results with this protocol compare favorably with previous studies conducted at the same institution not accounting for gastroesophageal treatment.[10]

Conclusion

In brachycephalic breeds, anatomic anomalies of the upper respiratory tract, (i.e., stenotic nares and over-long and over-thick soft palate) progressively lead to further impairment of breathing owing to progressive laryngeal compromise (i.e., laryngeal collapse and ventricular eversion). In addition, gastroesophageal disease can be found clinically, endoscopically, and histologically in many brachycephalic dogs suffering from upper airway impairment. To relieve the upper airway obstruction, an early surgical treatment of the stenotic nares and of the over-long and over-thick soft palate is recommended. A concurrent medical treatment of gastroesophageal signs has also been shown to improve the overall prognosis.

References

1. Chaudieu G, Denis B: Génétique des races canines dites brachycéphales. PMCAC 5:571-576, 1999.

2. Koch D, Arnold S, Hubler M, Montavon P: Brachycephalic syndrome in dogs. Compendium 25:48-55, 2003.

3.Evans HE: Miller's Anatomy of the Dog, 3rd ed. Philadelphia: WB Saunders, 1993.

4. Dupre G, Findji L, Poncet C: The folded flap palatoplasty: a new technique for the treatment of elongated soft palate in dogs. ECVS Proceedings, 14th Annual Meeting, Lyon France.

5. Harvey C: Upper airway obstruction surgery. J Am Anim Hosp Assoc 18:535-569, 1982.

6. Harvey CE, Fink EA: Tracheal diameter, analysis of radiographic measurements in brachycephalic and non brachycephalic breeds. J Am Anim Hosp Assoc 18:570, 1982.

7. Dupre G, Freiche V: Ronflements et vomissements chez les bouledogues: traitement médical ou chirurgical? AFVAC-CNVSPA Annual Congress Proceeding, Paris. France. 2002; 235-236.

8. Lecoindre P, Richard S: Digestive disorders associated with the chronic obstructive syndrome of brachycephalic dogs: 30 cases. Revue Méd Vét 155(3):141-146, 2004.

9. Poncet C, Dupre G, Freiche V, et al: Prevalence of gastro-intestinal tract lesions in brachycephalic dogs with upper respiratory syndrome. J Small Anim Pract 46(6):273-279, 2004.

10. Ducarouge B : Le syndrome obstructif des voies respiratoires supérieures chez les chiens brachycéphales. Etude clinique à propos de 27 cas. University Thesis, Lyon, France, 2002 ; 142.

11. Lorinson D, Bright RM, White RAS: Brachycephalic airway obstruction syndrome - A Review of 118 Cases. Canine Pract 22:18-21, 1997.

12. Callan MB, Washabau RJ, Saunders HM, et al: Congenital esophageal hiatal hernia in the chinese shar-pei dog. J Vet Intern Med 7 :210-215, 1993.

13. Peeters ME: Pyloric stenosis in the dog: developments in its surgical treatment and retrospective study in 47 patients. Tijdschr Diergeneeskd 116:137-141, 1991.

14. Walter MC, Goldschmidt MH, Stone EA, Chronic hypertrophic pyloric gastropathy as a cause of pyloric obstruction in the dog. J Am Vet Med Assoc 186:157-161, 1985.

15. Woods C, Rawlings C, Barber D: Esophageal deviation in four english bulldogs. J Am Vet Med Assoc 172:934-938, 1978.

16. Washabau RJ: Diseases of the esophagus. *In* Textbook of Veterinary Internal Medicine, 5th ed. Ettinger SJ (ed). Philadelphia:WB Saunders, 2000, pp. 1142-1154.

17. Burnie A, Simpson J, Corcoran B: Gastro-oesophageal reflux and hiatus hernia associated with laryngeal paralysis in a dog. J Small Anim Pract 30:414-416, 1989.

18. Hall JA: 2000 Diseases of the Stomach. *In* Textbook of Veterinary Internal Medicine, 5th ed. Ettinger SJ (ed). Philadelphia:WB Saunders, 2000, pp. 1154-1182.

19. Hardie EM, Ramirez O, Clary EM, et al: Abnormalities of the thoracic bellows: stress fractures of the ribs and hiatal hernia. J Vet Intern Med 12:279-287, 1998.

20. Hunt GB, O'Brien C, Kolenc G, Malik R: Hiatal hernia in a puppy. Austral Vet J 80:685-686, 2002.

21. Miles KG, Pope ER, Jergens AE: Paraesophageal hiatal hernia and pyloric obstruction in a dog. J Am Vet Med Assoc 193:1437-1439, 1988.

22. White D, Heavner S, Hardy S, Prazma J: Gastroesophageal reflux and eustachian tube dysfunction in an animal model. Laryngoscope 112:995-961, 2002.

23. Halstead LA: Role of gastroesophageal reflux in pediatric upper airway disorders. Otolaryngol Head Neck Surg 120:208-214, 1999.

24. Guilford W, Strombeck D: Chronic gastric disease. *In* Strombeck's Small Animal Gastroenterology, 3rd ed. Guilford W, Center S, Strombeck. D (eds). Philadelphia: WB Saunders,1996, pp. 275-302.

25. Hackett R, Ducharme N, Ainsworth D, et al: Effects of extrathoracic airway obstruction on intrathoracic pressure and pulmonary artery pressure in exercising horses. Am J Vet Res 60:485-49, 1999.

26. Bright R, Sackman J, Denevo C, Toal C: Hiatal hernia in the dog and cat: a retrospective study of 16 cases. J Small Anim Pract 31:244-250, 1990.

27. Carmona-Sanchez C, Valdovinos-Diaz M, Facha M: Hiatal hernia in asthmatic patients: prevalence of and its association to gastroesopahgeal reflux. Revista de Investigacion Clinica 54(4):214-220, 1999.

28. Poncet C, Dupre G, Freiche V, et al: Long term results of upper respiratory syndrome surgery and gastrointestinal tract medical treatment in 51 brachycephalic dogs (2000-2003). J Small Anim Pract 46:1-6, 2004.

Chapter 52

Laryngeal Paralysis

Catriona MacPhail

The function of the larynx is to regulate airflow, protect the lower airway from aspiration during swallowing, and control phonation. Laryngeal paralysis is the failure of the arytenoid cartilages to properly abduct secondary to muscle or nerve damage. This results in upper airway obstruction because of interference with airflow, particularly during inspiration. Although laryngeal paralysis can occur in cats, this condition is far more common in dogs and should be considered as a possible differential diagnosis for animals presenting with respiratory distress and stridor.

Functional Anatomy

The larynx is a term used to describe the cartilages that surround the rima glottidis and that are responsible for control of airflow during respiration. The four cartilages that make up the larynx are the paired arytenoids, and the unpaired epiglottis, cricoid, and thyroid cartilages. The base of the epiglottis attaches to the cranial trough of the thyroid cartilage. Laterally the epiglottis is connected to the cuneiform processes of the arytenoid by mucosa that makes up the aryepiglottic fold. The apex of the epiglottis extends into the oropharynx just beyond the caudal edge of the soft palate. The thyroid cartilage is a U-shaped structure with dorsal horn-shaped projections on each end known as the rostral and caudal cornu. The rostral cornu articulate with the thyrohyoid bones of the hyoid apparatus, whereas the caudal cornu connect with the cricoid cartilage. The cricoid cartilage is a ring-shaped structure that is wider dorsally than it is ventrally. The caudal aspect of the cricoid cartilage connects with the trachea. The paired arytenoid cartilages are irregular structures with four sets of processes: the corniculate process dorsally, the cuneiform process rostrally, the muscular process caudally, and the vocal process ventrally. The rima glottidis is the elongated opening between the arytenoid cartilages, and it is the narrowest part of the larynx. The glottis consists of the rima glottidis dorsally and the vocal folds ventrally, which are created by vocal ligaments extending from the vocal processes of the arytenoid cartilage.

The cricoarytenoideus dorsalis muscle is solely responsible for enlarging the glottis. The muscle originates on the dorsolateral surface of the cricoid and inserts on the muscular process of the arytenoids. Contraction of the muscle results in external rotation and abduction of the arytenoids that then pulls the vocal processes laterally. The recurrent laryngeal nerve innervates all of the intrinsic muscles of the larynx except the cricothyroid muscle, which is supplied by the cranial laryngeal nerve. The right side branches from the vagus nerve at the level of the middle cervical ganglion in the thoracic inlet, curves dorsocranially around the right subclavian artery, and then courses cranially along the dorsolateral surface of the trachea. The left side leaves the vagus nerve at about the level of the middle cervical ganglion, but travels caudally and then medially around the aortic arch before coursing cranially along the ventrolateral aspect of the trachea.

Etiology

Laryngeal paralysis is a common unilateral or bilateral respiratory disorder that primarily affects older large breed dogs. However, a congenital form does occur in certain breeds. Laryngeal paralysis is caused by damage to the recurrent laryngeal nerve or cricoarytenoideus dorsalis muscle resulting in failure of arytenoid abduction during inspiration.

Congenital Laryngeal Paralysis

Congenital laryngeal paralysis has been reported in a variety of canine breeds. An autosomal dominant trait has been documented in the Bouvier des Flandres, resulting in Wallerian degeneration of the recurrent laryngeal nerves and abnormalities of the nucleus ambiguous.[1,2] Although a precise mode of inheritance has not been established, a hereditary predisposition has also been identified in Siberian husky dogs, Alaskan malamutes, and crosses of those two breeds.[3-5] Laryngeal paralysis-polyneuropathy complexes have been described in Dalmatians, Rottweilers, and Leonberger dogs.[6-8] Other reported breeds with congenital laryngeal paralysis include bull terriers and white-coated German shepherd dogs.[9,10] Respiratory signs are often apparent within the first few months of life, but most dogs are diagnosed at less than a year of age. The prognosis for dogs with congenital laryngeal paralysis is poor, especially in those with concurrent polyneuropathy.

Acquired

Acquired laryngeal paralysis is a common condition of older large and giant breed dogs. The Labrador retriever is by far the most common breed reported, but Golden retrievers, Saint Bernards, Newfoundlands, and Irish setters are also overrepresented.[11-16] Average age of onset ranges from 9 to 11 years. In most studies, male dogs appear to be more commonly affected.[12,14,15] Laryngeal paralysis has also been described in cats.[17] Proposed causes of laryngeal paralysis include accidental trauma, intrathoracic masses, cervical masses, and neuromuscular disease (Table 52-1). There is an association between acquired laryngeal paralysis and hypothyroidism, but a direct link has not been determined.[18] For dogs that are diagnosed with concurrent hypothyroidism, thyroid supplementation should be instituted, but this typically does not improve the clinical signs of laryngeal paralysis. An underlying cause of laryngeal paralysis often cannot be determined, and these cases are then deemed idiopathic.

Diagnosis

Suspicion of laryngeal paralysis arises from the history of the dog as well as from consistent clinical signs. A routine work-up for a dog suspected to have bilateral laryngeal paralysis includes physical examination, neurologic examination, complete blood count, biochemical profile, urinalysis, thoracic radiographs, thyroid function screening, and laryngeal examination. Definitive

Table 52-1. Proposed Etiologies of Laryngeal Paralysis

Congenital
Accidental trauma
Cervical penetrating wounds
Strangulating trauma
Iatrogenic surgical trauma
Ventral slot
Thyroidectomy / parathyroidectomy
Tracheal surgery
Cervical / Intrathoracic masses
Thyroid carcinoma
Thymoma
Lymphoma
Abscess
Granuloma
Neuromuscular Disease
Immune-mediated disease
Endocrinopathy
Idiopathic

diagnosis of laryngeal paralysis requires visual examination of the larynx. However, laryngoscopy is a poorly specific diagnostic test, as false positives are common owing to the influence of anesthetic agents on laryngeal function. By definition, laryngeal paralysis is the absence of arytenoid abduction on inspiration. In particular, the corniculate process of the arytenoid cartilages that frame the rima glottidis dorsally are observed for purposeful motion (Figure 52-1). However, an absolute diagnosis should not be made based solely on the lack of arytenoid movement. Laryngeal paralysis is a fixed upper airway obstruction that results in inflammation and swelling of the laryngeal cartilages. Diagnosis may also be confused by the presence of paradoxical movement of the arytenoids, which can lead to a false negative result. In this situation, the arytenoid cartilages move inward during inspiration owing to negative intraglottic pressure that is created by breathing against an obstruction. The cartilages then return to their original position during the expiratory phase, giving the impression of abduction. An assistant can state the stage of respiration during laryngoscopy to help distinguish normal from abnormal motion.

Treatment

Dogs often do not have severe clinical signs until they have bilateral laryngeal paresis or paralysis. For dogs with bilateral laryngeal paralysis, the decision to institute surgical treatment is based on the quality of life of the dog, the severity of clinical signs, and the time of the year. Surgical treatment of laryngeal paralysis is primarily directed at increasing the functional area of the rima glottidis. This is most commonly performed by unilateral arytenoid lateralization, but other methods include variations of partial laryngectomy and castellated laryngofissure. Permanent tracheostomy is also described as a surgical treatment as a means of bypassing the upper airway obstruction entirely. Bilateral arytenoid lateralization is no longer considered a reasonable option for this disease because of the number of postoperative complications; also, it is not necessary to enlarge the area of the rima glottidis to that degree to alleviate clinical signs.[15,19] According to Poiseuille's law, air flow through the glottis is directly proportional to the radius of glottis to the fourth power (Figure 52-2). For example, if the radius of the rima glottidis is doubled, resistance to air flow through the glottis is reduced by a factor of 16. However, this equation is used most appropriately to describe laminar low velocity flow through a straight tube, generally the small peripheral airways. Movement of air through the trachea, rima glottidis, nose, and mouth is high velocity turbulent flow with heavy resistance. Yet, different methods of unilateral arytenoid lateralization have resulted in varying degrees of increase in rima glottidis area without any difference in short-term clinical outcome or complication rate.[20] Cricoarytenoid laryngoplasty, in which the suture is passed from the muscular process of the arytenoid cartilage to the dorsocaudal aspect of the cricoid cartilage, results in a 207% increase in the area of the rima glottidis. This is compared with a 140% increase in rima glottidis area for dogs with thyroarytenoid lateralization, in which the suture travels from the muscular process of the arytenoid cartilage to the caudodorsal aspect of the thyroid catilage.

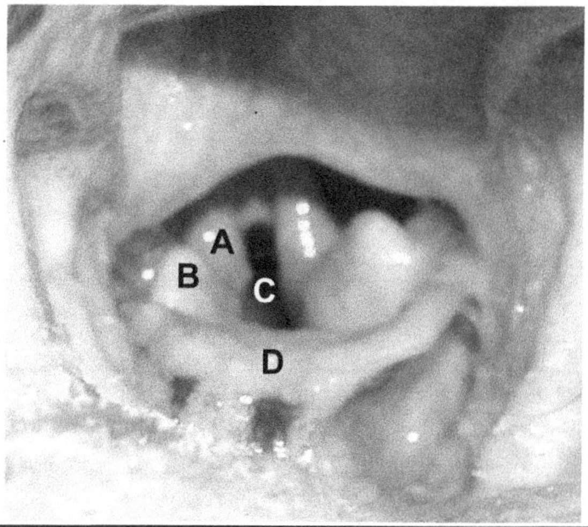

Figure 52-1. Laryngeal anatomy as visualized during laryngeal examination: A = Right corniculate process of the arytenoid cartilage; B = Right cuneiform process of the arytenoid cartilage; C = Rima glottidis; D = Epiglottis.

The effect of the degree of suture tension on the area of the rima glottidis has also been evaluated in canine cadavers.[21] It was found that a low-tension suture (the suture was tied until resistance was felt from the cranial part of the cricoarytenoid articulation joint capsule) increased the area of the rima glottidis when the epiglottis was open without an increase in the area of the rima glottidis not covered when the epiglottis is closed. A high-tension suture (the suture was tied as tight as possible) resulted in a significant increase in the area not covered by the epiglottis in a closed position (467% larger than the low-tension suture). It was suggested that the use of a low-tension suture in clinical cases may reduce the potential risk of postoperative aspiration pneumonia.

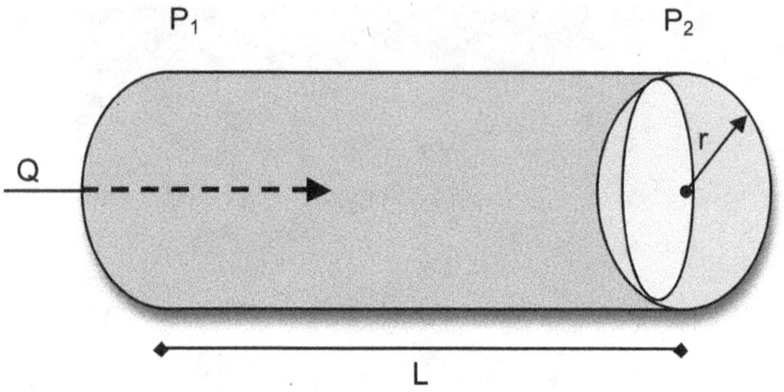

Figure 52-2. Schematic representation of Poiseuille's ($Q = \pi r^4 P/8\eta L$) law where Q = flow rate, r = radius of the tube, L = Length of the tube, P = pressure within the tube, and η = viscosity.

Surgical Complications

Following surgical treatment of laryngeal paralysis, postoperative aspiration pneumonia has been reported to occur in 8 to 19% of dogs following unilateral arytenoid lateralization.[15,22] Although aspiration pneumonia is most likely to occur in the first few weeks following surgery, it has been recognized that these dogs are at risk for aspiration pneumonia for the rest of their lives.[15] Factors that have been significantly associated with a higher risk of developing complications include preoperative aspiration pneumonia, postoperative megaesophagus, temporary tracheostomy placement, and concurrent neoplastic disease.[15]

The use of a temporary tracheostomy tube before surgery has been found to be a significant negative risk factor in dogs with laryngeal paralysis. Of dogs that had a temporary tracheostomy preoperatively, 50% developed complications postoperatively. The increased risk was not related to whether the dog was presented as an emergency. The presence of a tracheostomy tube results in loss of cilia, epithelial ulceration, submucosal inflammation, and retained secretions. The trachea becomes colonized with bacteria from oropharyngeal flora within 24 hours after tracheostomy tube placement. It is theorized that tracheostomy tubes significantly interfere with the normal function of the mucociliary apparatus such that these dogs are then unable to effectively clear aspirated substances.[23]

Prognosis

Without surgical complications, unilateral arytenoid lateralization for treatment of canine laryngeal paralysis results in less respiratory distress and stridor and improved exercise tolerance. Owner satisfaction with this procedure has been reported as excellent, with the majority of owners believing the quality of their dog's life was dramatically improved.[14,22,24]

Laryngeal Paralysis in Cats

Laryngeal paralysis is an uncommon condition in the cat. Clinical presentation is similar to that of the dog and both unilateral and bilateral laryngeal paralysis have been reported. Cats with unilateral laryngeal paralysis can present with significant clinical signs, unlike dogs, which are rarely symptomatic. There also appears to be a prevalence of left-sided unilateral laryngeal paralysis in cats, which is similar to what is reported in humans and horses. The specific etiology of laryngeal paralysis in cats is unknown, but several cases have been associated with trauma, neoplastic invasion, and iatrogenic damage. Successful surgical treatment primarily utilizing unilateral arytenoid lateralization has been reported.[17]

References

1. Venker-van Haagen AJ, Hartman W, Goedege SA: Spontaneous laryngeal paralysis in young Bouviers. J Am Anim Hosp Assoc 1914:714, 1978.

2. Venker-van Haagen AJ, Bouw J, Hartman W: Hereditary transmission of laryngeal paralysis in bouviers. J Am Anim Hosp Assoc 18:75, 1981.

3. O'Brien JA: Hereditary laryngeal paralysis in the racing sled dog (husky). Vookjaarsdagen International Congress, Amsterdam, The Netherlands, 1985.

4. O'Brien JA, Hendriks J: Inherited laryngeal paralysis. Analysis in the husky cross. Vet Q 8:301, 1986.

5. Polizopoulou ZS, Koutinas AF, Papadopoulos GC, et al.: Juvenile laryngeal paralysis in three Siberian husky x Alaskan malamute puppies. Vet Rec 153:624, 2003.

6. Braund KG, Shores A, Cochrane S, et al: Laryngeal paralysis-polyneuropathy complex in young Dalmatians. Am J Vet Res 55:534, 1994.

7. Mahony OM, Knowles KE, Braund KG, et al: Laryngeal paralysis-polyneuropathy complex in young Rottweilers. J Vet Intern Med 12:330, 1998.

8. Shelton GD, Podell M, Poncelet L, et al: Inherited polyneuropathy in Leonberger dogs: a mixed or intermediate form of Charcot-Marie-Tooth disease? Muscle Nerve 27:471, 2003.

9. Baker GJ: Surgery of the canine larynx and pharynx. J Small Anim Pract 13:505, 1972.

10. Ridyard AE, Corcoran BM, Taker S, et al: Spontaneous laryngeal paralysis in four white-coated German shepherd dogs. J Small Anim Pract 41:558, 2000.

11. Burbridge HM: A review of laryngeal paralysis in dogs. Br Vet J 151:71, 1995.

12. Gaber CE, Amis TC, LeCouteur RA: Laryngeal paralysis in dogs: A review of 23 cases. J Am Vet Med Assoc 186:377, 1985.

13. Greenfield CL: Canine laryngeal paralysis. Comp Cont Educ Pract Vet 9:1011, 1987.

14. LaHue TR: Treatment of laryngeal paralysis in dogs by unilateral cricoarytenoid laryngoplasty. J Am Anim Hosp Assoc 25:317, 1989.

15. MacPhail CM, Monnet E: Outcome of and postoperative complications in dogs undergoing surgical treatment of laryngeal paralysis: 140 cases (1985-1998). J Am Vet Med Assoc 218:1949, 2001.

16. Ross JT, Matthuesen DT, Noone KE, et al: Complications and long-term results after partial laryngectomy for the treatment of idiopathic laryngeal paralysis. Vet Surg 20:169, 1991.

17. Schachter S, Norris CR: Laryngeal paralysis in cats: 16 cases (1990-1999). J Am Vet Med Assoc 216:1100, 2000.

18. Jaggy A, Oliver JE, Ferguson DC, et al: Neurological manifestations of hypothyroidism: a retrospective study of 29 dogs. J Vet Intern Med 8:328, 1994.

19. Burbridge HM: Laryngeal paralysis in dogs: An evaluation of the bilateral arytenoid lateralization procedure. J Small Anim Pract 34:515, 1993.

20. Griffiths LG, Sullivan M, Reid SW: A comparison of the effects of unilateral thyroarytenoid lateralization versus cricoarytenoid laryngoplasty on the area of the rima glottidis and clinical outcome in dogs with laryngeal paralysis. Vet Surg 30:359, 2001.

21. Bureau S, Monnet E: Effects of suture tension and surgical approach during unilateral arytenoids lateralization on the rima glottidis in the canine larynx. Vet Surg 31;589, 2002.

22. Snelling SR, Edwards GA: A retrospective study of unilateral arytenoids lateralization in the treatment of laryngeal paralysis in 100 dogs (1992-2000). Aust Vet J 81:464, 2003

23. Colley P, Huber M, Henderson R: Tracheostomy techniques and management. Comp Cont Educ Pract Vet 21:44, 1999.

24. White RAS: Unilateral arytenoid lateralization: An assessment of technique and long term results in 62 dogs with laryngeal paralysis. J Sm Anim Pract 30:543, 1995.

Chapter 53

Tracheal Collapse

Catriona MacPhail

The primary function of the trachea is to serve as a conduit for air into and away from the bronchial tree. Tracheal collapse occurs when there is malacia of the tracheal cartilages leading to varying degrees of dorsoventral flattening, impeding airflow. Controversy exists over management of tracheal collapse as medical management is directed only at symptomatic therapy, and surgical treatment is burdened by complications.

Functional Anatomy

The trachea of the dog or cat is composed of 35 to 45 incomplete C-shaped cartilage rings, although variations may exist between breeds and individual animals.[1,2] The ends of the cartilages are connected by the dorsal tracheal membrane, which is the thin, strap-like muscle on the dorsal surface of the trachea. The first tracheal ring is complete and partially covered by the cricoid cartilage. The remaining tracheal rings are linked together by elastic annular ligaments that result in the rigid, yet flexible tube.

The blood supply to the trachea is from the cranial thyroid artery, caudal thyroid artery, and bronchoesophageal arteries. Branches of the thyroid arteries penetrate the tracheal rings on either side and then arborize in the submucosa to create a rich subepithelial plexus in the cervical and proximal thoracic trachea. Branches of the bronchoesophageal arteries supply the terminal trachea, carina, and mainstem bronchi. The trachea is innervated by the autonomic nervous system; stimulation results in muscle contraction and glandular secretion.

The trachea is composed of four distinct layers: mucosa, submucosa, musculocartilaginous layer, and adventitia.[3] The mucosa is made up of pseudostratified, ciliated, columnar epithelium and goblet cells, and is oriented in longitudinal folds. Tracheal glands within the submucosa contribute mucus to respiratory secretions. The musculocartilaginous layer is composed of hyaline cartilage, fibroelastic tissue, and smooth muscle that blend with the connective tissue of the adventitia.

The main function of the trachea is to channel air through the phases of respiration. The lumen diameter of the trachea is capable of changing in size by contraction of the dorsal tracheal membrane. Muscle contraction brings the ends of the incomplete cartilage rings closer together, narrowing the diameter, and thus reducing ventilatory dead space and increasing airflow velocity. The tracheal diameter can also enlarge to accommodate increases in airflow volume and reduce airway resistance. Insult to the tracheal wall can affect how the trachea adapts to changes in airflow and external pressures. Airflow velocity increases as diameter decreases and, according to the Bernoulli effect, internal pressure decreases. A normal trachea is rigid enough to withstand external pressure, but weakened tracheal cartilages are subject to collapse.

Another important role of the trachea is to trap aspirated debris and transport this material back up the tracheobronchial tree. The mucociliary apparatus is responsible for clearance of small particles (1 to 5 μm) that are able to pass through the nasopharynx.[4] These particles adhere to the mucus lining of the large airways; cilia of the epithelial cells beat in the mucus layer, pushing material back toward the pharynx. Normal cilia beat at a rate of 15 to 20 times per second, resulting in a clearance time in the normal dog of 5 to 26 mm per minute.[5] The mucociliary apparatus and clearance rate can be markedly affected by airway disease and mucosal trauma.

Pathophysiology

Tracheal collapse results from structural abnormalities of the cartilage rings and secondary changes in the dorsal tracheal membrane. Histopathology and ultrastructural analysis of tracheal cartilage in dogs with tracheal collapse found hypocellularity leading to decreased chondroitin sulfate and glycosaminoglycans and transformation of normal hyaline cartilage to fibrous cartilage.[6] This chondromalacia makes the trachea less rigid and less able to withstand external pressures, resulting in dorsoventral flattening. The specific etiology of tracheal collapse is unknown but is thought to be multifactorial with a congenital or inheritable component.[7]

Tracheal collapse may be confined to an isolated segment or may involve the entire trachea and bronchial tree. The thoracic inlet is the most commonly involved area (Figure 53-1). Collapse typically occurs in a dorsoventral direction as the cartilages weaken and the dorsal tracheal membrane thins and lengthens; however, lateral collapse of the tracheal walls has been reported.[8]

Collapse in the cervical tracheal and thoracic inlet classically occurs on inspiration as pressure within the lumen drops and the walls are susceptible to atmospheric pressure; intrathoracic trachea collapses on expiration. Although pressure within the trachea decreases on inspiration, luminal pressure still exceeds intrapleural pressure, which keeps airways open. On expiration, intrapleural pressure becomes less negative and exceeds intraluminal pressure. Dogs with weakened cartilages lack sufficient strength to withstand the increased intrapleural pressure. The thoracic inlet is most susceptible to tracheal collapse as this is the site of the equal-pressure point: where intrapleural pressure equals intraluminal airway pressure and where the transition from intrapleural to atmospheric pressure occurs.[7] One study, however, found occasional evidence of dogs that had intrathoracic collapse on inspiration and extrathoracic collapse on expiration, although no explanation could be offered.[9]

Dogs with tracheal collapse have varying degrees of secondary injury owing to chronic coughing. Coughing causes further increase in intrapleural pressure and worse tracheal collapse. In cases of moderate to severe collapse, opposing epithelial linings come into contact causing mucosal lesions and irritation. This chronic irritation leads to inflammation, mucus gland hyperplasia, epithelial desquamation, and disruption of the mucociliary clearance.[7]

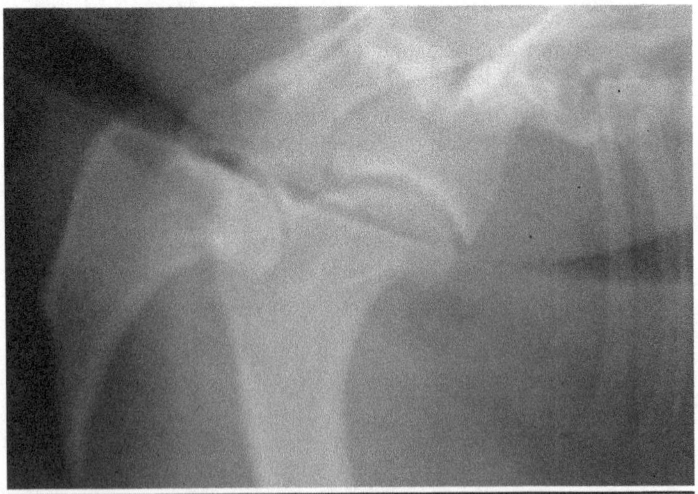

Figure 53-1. Lateral thoracic radiograph showing severe tracheal collapse at the thoracic inlet.

Signalment/Presentation

Tracheal collapse is typically associated with middle-aged toy and miniature breed dogs. Classic breeds include Yorkshire terriers, toy poodles, miniature poodles, Pomeranians, Chihuahuas, and pugs. This condition has also occasionally been described in young large breed dogs[10,11] and in cats.[12-14] In cats, tracheal collapse has been associated with intraluminal, extraluminal, or nasal masses.

Most dogs are diagnosed around 6 to 7 years of age; however, it has been reported that 25% of affected dogs are symptomatic by 6 months of age.[15] Dogs present with an easily solicited cough that is most often described as a "goose-honk." Severely affected dogs may have exercise intolerance, respiratory distress, and syncope. Clinical signs are exacerbated by stress or excitement.

Dogs with tracheal collapse may suffer from a variety of concurrent problems. Almost 50% of dogs suffer from a degree of obesity that worsens clinical signs.[7] Laryngeal paresis or paralysis has been reported in 20 to 30% of dogs, while one third of dogs have concurrent systolic heart murmurs consistent with mitral valve insufficiency.[7,15,16] Upper respiratory signs may be aggravated by an enlarged left atrium, putting pressure on the carina and mainstem bronchi.

At least 40% of dogs are believed to have a degree of dental or periodontal disease.[7] Aspiration of oral bacteria into diseased airways is hypothesized to contribute to exacerbation of clinical signs owing to increased airway inflammation or increased coughing. In a study of 37 dogs with tracheal collapse, 83% had a positive large-airway culture, with 59% growing greater than one species of bacteria.[17] This is of interest as oropharyngeal flora have been found in the trachea of normal dogs, but only 17% had multiple, mixed colonization.[18] Concurrent cytologic inflammation however, was not consistently found in a population of dogs with tracheal collapse; therefore, an association between bacterial colonization of large airways and clinical signs has not yet been proven.[17]

Concurrent hepatomegaly and hepatopathy are also common in dogs with tracheal collapse. In a study of 26 dogs, 46% had increased serum activity of two or more liver enzymes, with 92% having elevated serum basal bile acid concentrations.[19] The reason for this association is still unclear, although speculative theories include passive hepatic congestion or centrilobular liver cell necrosis secondary to chronic hypoxia.

Diagnosis

The diagnosis of tracheal collapse is often suspected based on signalment, history, and physical examination findings. Lateral survey thoracic radiographs of the neck and thorax can confirm this diagnosis. Views should be taken of the cervical and thoracic trachea on both inspiration and expiration. Cervical trachea narrows during inspiration owing to negative pressure within the trachea, whereas intrathoracic trachea collapse occurs during expiration owing to increased intrapleural pressure. Static radiographs may only detect collapse in 59 to 92% of cases,[9,15,16] yet radiographs should be closely evaluated for signs of concurrent airway pathology or cardiac disease.[7,20] Dynamic evaluation of the trachea can be performed using fluoroscopy and is particularly helpful for identification of intrathoracic collapse. When comparing fluoroscopy and standard radiographic evaluation, radiography has been found to underestimate the frequency and degree of tracheal collapse.[9] Detection of tracheal collapse using ultrasonography has also been described.[21]

Bronchoscopy allows direct visualization and evaluation of the entire tracheobronchial tree (Figure 53-2A). In particular, bronchoscopy allows evaluation of the main stem bronchi (Figure 53-2B). Airway samples for cytology and bacterial culture can be obtained by tracheal brushing or bronchoalveolar lavage, as tracheobronchitis or bronchopneumonia may play a role in the severity of clinical signs. The disadvantage of bronchoscopy is that general anesthesia is required. However, this provides an opportunity to assess laryngeal anatomy and function.

Tracheal collapse can been graded by its appearance on fluoroscopy or bronchoscopy (Table 53-1; Figure 53-3). This grading scheme allows for the determination of the severity of the collapse, establishes a baseline from which to assess disease progression, and identifies or eliminates the potential for surgical intervention.

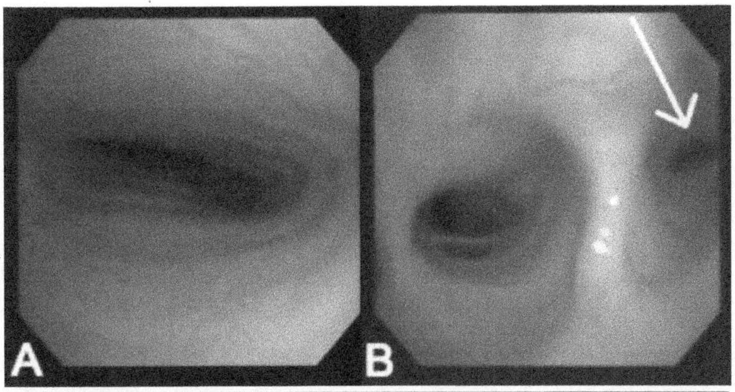

Figure 53-2A and 53-2B. Bronchoscopic view of cervical trachea collapse and left mainstem bronchi (arrow) of the same dog.

Table 53-1. Grades of Tracheal Collapse

Grade	Reduction in airway diameter (%)	Characteristics
1	25	Mild protrusion of dorsal tracheal membrane into lumen
2	50	Mild to moderate elongation and flattening of tracheal rings
3	75	Marked flattening of tracheal rings
4	> 90	Dorsal deviation of ventral tracheal surface

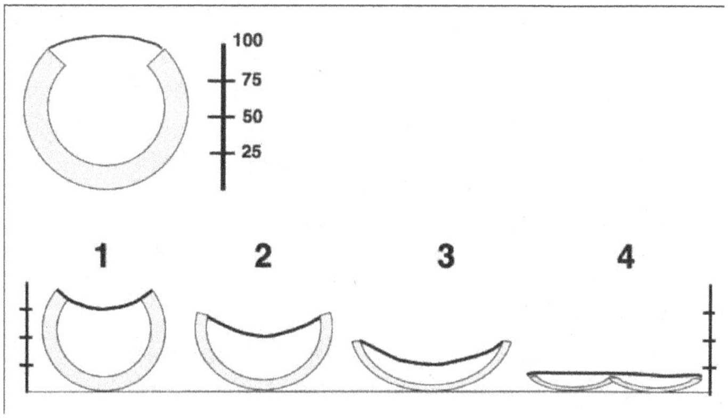

Figure 53-3. Graphic representation of tracheal collapse grading scheme.

Treatment

Medical management of tracheal collapse results in improvement in most dogs.[15] Weight loss is critical to the success of other medical therapies. Environmental modifications, such as the use of a harness instead of a collar and creation of a nonsmoking environment, may help some dogs, as will management of concurrent underlying conditions. It has also been advocated to perform dental prophylaxis in affected dogs to decrease the bacterial load that can be aspirated into the trachea.[7] Frequently used medications include cough suppressants, bronchodilators, anti-inflammatories, and antibiotics.

Surgical intervention is suggested in patients with moderate to severe tracheal collapse that are refractory to medical management. Surgery is not recommended in patients with mainstem bronchi collapse, underlying laryngeal disease, and concurrent cardiopulmonary disease. Although other techniques have been described, surgical treatment of tracheal collapse is currently achieved by either extraluminal ring prostheses or endoluminal stenting.

Extraluminal tracheal ring prostheses can be implanted in dogs with cervical tracheal collapse or proximal intrathoracic tracheal collapse. Good to excellent outcomes have been reported in 75 to 85% of patients, however, this technique is limited by candidate selection and surgical complications.[16,22] Following surgery, laryngeal paralysis, laryngeal necrosis, and postoperative distress requiring permanent tracheostomy have been reported.[22] Dogs older than 6 years appear to have worse outcomes than younger dogs regardless of the degree of collapse.[22]

Endoluminal stenting has been reported in a variety of settings and using a large array of materials.[23-25] Endoluminal stenting can be used in dogs with intrathoracic tracheal collapse or diffuse tracheal collapse to provide rapid relief of clinical signs, and has been used in dogs with coexisting bronchial collapse. Complications reported with endoluminal stent implantation include stent migration, stent fracture, granuloma formation, pneumonia, and chronic coughing.[26,27]

Conclusion

Tracheal collapse is a challenging condition to diagnose and treat. Diagnosis is complicated by concurrent illnesses that exacerbate clinical signs, and treatment standards of care have not been established. Appropriate medical management may alleviate clinical signs in a large percentage of dogs affected, however dogs refractory to pharmacologic intervention may benefit from extraluminal or endoluminal support.

References

1. Evans HE: The respiratory system. *In* Miller's Anatomy of the Dog, 3rd ed. Evans HE (ed). Philadelphia: WB Saunders, 1993, pp. 463-493.

2. Grandage J: Functional anatomy of the respiratory system. *In* Textbook of Small Animal Surgery, 3rd ed. Slatter DH (ed). Philadelphia: WB Saunders, 2000, pp. 763-780.

3. Fingland RB: Trachea and bronchi. *In* Disease Mechanisms In Small Animal Surgery, 2nd ed Bojrab MJ (ed). Philadelphia: Lea & Febiger, 1993, pp. 376-385.

4. Tucker A: Respiratory pathophysiology. *In* Textbook of Small Animal Surgery, 3rd ed. Slatter DH (ed). Philadelphia: WB Saunders, 2000, pp. 781-797.

5. Bridger GP, Proctor DF: Mucociliary function in the dog's larynx and trachea. Laryngoscope 52:218, 1972.

6. Dallman MJ, McClure RC, Brown EM: Histochemical study of normal and collapsed tracheas in dogs. Am J Vet Res 49:2117, 1988.

7. Johnson LR: Tracheal collapse. Diagnosis and medical and surgical treatment. Vet Clin North Am Small Anim Pract 30:1253, 2000.

8. Johnson LR, Krahwinkel DJ, McKiernan BC: Surgical management of atypical lateral tracheal collapse in a dog. J Am Vet Med Assoc 203:1693, 1993.

9. Macready DM, Johnson LR, Pollard RE: Fluoroscopic and radiographic evaluation of tracheal collapse in dogs: 62 cases (2001-2006). J Am Vet Med Assoc 230:1870, 2007.

10. Spodnick GJ, Nwadike BS: Surgical management of extrathoracic tracheal collapse in two large-breed dogs. J Am Vet Med Assoc 211:1545, 1997.

11. Radlinsky MA, Fossum TW: Tracheal collapse in a young boxer. J Am Anim Hosp Assoc 36:313, 2000

12. Hendricks JC, O'Brien JA: Tracheal collapse in two cats. J Am Vet Med Assoc 187:418, 1985.

13. Fujita M, Miura H, Yasuda D, et al: Tracheal narrowing secondary to airway obstruction in two cats. J Small Anim Pract 45:29, 2004.

14. Bell R, Philbey AW, Marineau H, et al: Dynamic tracheal collapse associated with disseminated histiocytic sarcoma in a cat. J Small Anim Pract 47:461. 2006.

15. White RAS, Williams JM: Tracheal collapse in the dogs: Is there really a role for surgery? A survey of 100 cases. J Small Anim Pract 35:191, 1994.

16. Tangner CH, Hobson HP: A retrospective study of 20 surgically managed cases of collapsed trachea. Vet Surg 11:146, 1982.

17. Johnson LR, Fales WH: Clinical and microbiologic findings in dogs with bronchoscopically diagnosed tracheal collapse: 37 cases (1990-1995). J Am Vet Med Assoc 219:1247, 2001.

18. McKiernan BC, Smith AR, Kissil M: Bacterial isolates from the lower trachea of clinically healthy dogs. J Am Anim Hosp Assoc 20:139, 1982.

19. Bauer NB, Schneider MA, Neiger R, et al: Liver disease in dogs with tracheal collapse. J Vet Intern Med 20:845, 2006.

20. Marolf A, Blaik M, Specht A: A retrospective study of the relationship between tracheal collapse and bronchiectasis in dogs. Vet Radiol Ultrasound 48:199, 2007

21. Rudorf H, Herrtage ME, White RAS: Use of ultrasonography in the diagnosis of tracheal collapse. J Small Anim Pract 38:513, 1997

22. Buback JL, Boothe HW, Hobson HP: Surgical treatment of tracheal collapse in dogs: 90 cases. J Am Vet Med Assoc 208:380, 1996.

23. Radlinsky MG, Fossum TW, Walker MA, et al: Evaluation of the Palmaz stent in the trachea and mainstem bronchi of normal dogs. Vet Surg 26:99, 1997.

24. Gellasch KL, Gomez TD, McAnulty JF, et al: Use of intraluminal nitinol stents in the treatment of tracheal collapse in a dog. J Am Vet Med Assoc 221:1719, 2002.

25. Moritz A, Schneider M, Bauer N: Management of advanced tracheal collapse in dogs using intraluminal self-expanding biliary wallstents. J Vet Intern Med 18:31, 2004.

26. Mittleman E, Weisse C, Mehler SJ, et al: Fracture of an endoluminal nitinol stent used in the treatment of tracheal collapse in a dog. J Am Vet Med Assoc 225:1217, 2004.

27. Ouellet M, Dunn ME, Lussier B, et al: Noninvasive correction of a fractured endoluminal nitinol tracheal stent in a dog. J Am Anim Hosp Assoc 42:467, 2006.

Chapter 54

Lung Lobe Torsion

Prudence J. Neath

Anatomy and Etiology

The lungs of the dog and cat are divided into specific lobes by deep fissures, which allow the lungs to alter position in response to movement of the diaphragm or spine.[1] The extent of movement of each lung lobe is usually limited by the presence of adjacent lobes, as well as the surrounding structures such as the heart, mediastinum, diaphragm, and thoracic wall. Pulmonary ligaments are thin sheets of pleura that extend from the caudal lobe of each lung to the mediastinum and provide further stabilization of these lobes.[2] The accessory lobe is isolated between the mediastinum and the plica vena cavae, providing significant support for this lobe. The space between the parietal and visceral pleura contains only a thin film of pleural fluid, which eases a sliding movement of the lung lobes, but the normal negative pressure within this pleural space helps to minimize excessive movement of the lobes.[3]

Development of a lung lobe torsion requires the lobe to overcome the stabilizing forces of these anatomic features in order to twist around its longitudinal axis. Various theories have been considered, and any condition that may increase the mobility of a lung lobe might predispose it to developing a torsion. Review of the human literature indicates lung lobe torsion to have occurred in association with pleural effusion, pneumothorax, and accidental or surgical trauma. The most common predisposing cause in humans appears to be surgical manipulation of the lung lobes. It is thought that the division of pulmonary ligaments during a thoracic procedure, in combination with deflated lung lobes, may predispose a consolidated lobe to twist about its axis.[4] Similarly, reports of lung lobe torsion in the dog have proposed that suspension of a consolidated or atelectatic lung in fluid (pleural effusion) or air (pneumothorax) could predispose the lobe to rotational movement.[5,6] Lung atelectasis can result from a variety of causes such as trauma, pneumonia, pleural effusion, pneumothorax, or surgical manipulation, although surgical trauma is rarely the predisposing cause of lung lobe torsion in dogs or cats. There have also been reports of lung lobe torsion occurring without any history of predisposing factors; therefore,spontaneous torsion may occur.[7-9] Reports of lung lobe torsion in cats are rare, and have all been associated with underlying disease such as chylothorax, pyothorax, or chronic asthma.[10,11]

As a lung lobe rotates about its axis, the pulmonary vessels and bronchus become occluded by the rotation at the hilus, leading initially to obstruction of the thin-walled pulmonary vein. Because some blood continues to flow through the pulmonary artery, the lobe becomes congested. Fluid leaks from the blood vessels into the interstitial tissues and airways, leading to consolidation of the lobe. The parietal pleura is eventually breached, leading to the accumulation of pleural effusion in the majority of cases.[6,9]

The thin, narrow right middle lobe of the lung is affected most commonly in dogs and cats, although the left cranial lobe is affected almost as often in the dog. Torsion of each lung lobe has been reported, as have occasional episodes of multiple lobe torsions. The right middle and left cranial lobes may be predisposed to torsion because they have less extensive attachments and, therefore, increased mobility compared with the other lobes.[5-11]

Clinical reports of lung lobe torsion are dominated by descriptions of large, deep-chested dogs, and it is thought that this thoracic shape might predispose to rotation of a lung lobe. The Afghan hound was found to be 133 times as likely to develop lung lobe torsion as other breeds in one study.[6] More recent reports have noted a trend for lung lobe torsion to occur in the pug, and the barrel-shape of the chest has been suggested as a predisposing factor in these dogs.[7-9]

Clinical Signs and Investigations

Clinical history commonly includes dyspnea or tachypnea, coughing, and lethargy, often accompanied by anorexia and vomiting. Physical examination usually reveals varying degrees of respiratory distress, often accompanied by dull cardiopulmonary sounds on thoracic auscultation. Absence of breath sounds may be extensive if significant pleural effusion is present, or there may be a focal absence over the affected lung lobe. Other signs such as pyrexia, cardiovascular instability, vomiting, and depression have also been reported.[5-11]

Analysis of a complete blood count and serum biochemistry panel usually reveals mild non-specific results in these patients, but may be influenced by the presence of an underlying thoracic disease process.[6,9]

Imaging of the thorax will reveal pleural effusion in the majority of patients, and thoracocentesis may be required before radiographic details of the lungs can be revealed.[5-11] Lung lobe consolidation is typically seen, and occasionally more than one lobe is consolidated.[6,9] One severely consolidated lung lobe with minimal abnormalities of the other lung lobes is highly suggestive of lung lobe torsion, especially if accompanied by abnormal bronchial positioning. Air bronchograms or air alveolograms may been seen if the lobe has twisted recently, but as fluid or blood moves into the airways, the lobe will become opacified.[5-11] The differential diagnosis for the opacified lung lobe includes atelectasis, neoplasia, pneumonia, edema, and pulmonary contusions.

Thoracic ultrasonography may confirm the presence of pleural effusion and can provide further details of the underlying reasons for opacification of the affected lung lobe, as well as revealing any fluid accumulation in the bronchi.[6,9] Ultrasound-guided biopsy may be performed to determine whether any underlying disease process is present.[7] Confirmation of bronchial occlusion using fiberoptic bronchoscopy has been reported.[9,12] Thoracoscopy would allow confirmation of lung lobe torsion, but has not been reported in any clinical case reports to date in the author's knowledge.

Pleural fluid collected from these patients is usually serosanguinous or hemorrhagic, although chylous effusion has been reported in many cases.[5-11] Cytologic findings often indicate an inflammatory cell population with high levels of neutrophils, lymphocytes, and some erythrocytes.[6] Underlying disease processes may complicate interpretation of the pleural fluid. Reactive mesothelial cells may be seen as a result of pleural inflammation: these should not be over-interpreted because mediastinal mesothelioma is rare.[6] Bacterial culture may yield growth in some cases, although pyothorax is rarely reported to accompany lung lobe torsion.[5,6,9] Identified bacteria have included *Escherichia coli*, *Staphylococcus* spp., *Proteus* spp., and *Pseudomonas* spp.[6,9] Chylous effusion is suspected when a milky-white opaque fluid is obtained, and confirmed by demonstration of a triglyceride concentration greater than that of the serum.

Treatment

Medical stabilization is required before surgical intervention. Provision of oxygen via a mask, nasal catheter, or oxygen cage may be necessary. Removal of all pleural effusion by thoracocentesis will improve ventilation of the unaffected lung lobes, relieving signs of respiratory distress. Many patients require fluid resuscitation prior to induction of general anaesthesia. Administration of intravenous antibiotics is recommended as intraoperative contamination from the respiratory tract is likely to occur.

Exploratory thoracotomy is performed via a lateral intercostal approach at the appropriate intercostal space. The affected lung lobe usually appears dark and consolidated and may be friable. Necrosis may have already begun, increasing the fragility of the lobe. Lung lobectomy without untwisting of the pedicle is recommended to minimize the risk of cytokine release into the circulation and potential reperfusion injury. The bronchus should be clamped prior to lobectomy, and the pedicle can then be ligated by hand or with an appropriate stapling device. A portion of the lung lobe should be submitted for bacterial culture, and the rest of the lobe for histologic examination. Evaluation of the other lung lobes and the rest of the thoracic structures should be performed. Any abnormal tissue is biopsied to allow submission for histologic study and bacterial culture. If chylothorax is present, thoracic duct ligation and pericardectomy might be performed. This treatment decision may be influenced by the breed of the patient. Although chylothorax has been reported to resolve following lung lobectomy in many patients, Afghan hounds appear to be predisposed to development of chylothorax and are likely to require further surgical treatment of the condition following the initial lung lobectomy.[5,6] Prior to closure of the thorax, a chest tube should be placed and adequate inflation and correct orientation of the other lung lobes should be confirmed.

Postoperative care involves analgesia, antibiotics, and intravenous fluid therapy as indicated by regular assessment of the patient. Oxygen supplementation is sometimes required. Drainage of the chest tube takes place at regular intervals until fluid production is less than 5 ml/kg/day and the chest tube can be safely removed.

Histopathologic examination of the excised lung lobe usually reveals bronchi filled with hemorrhagic fluid, thrombosis of blood vessels, plasma cell and lymphocyte infiltration of the tissues, and necrosis.[6,9] Occasionally, an underlying disease is revealed such as pneumonia or neoplasia that may have predisposed the lobe to twisting.[6,11]

Prognosis

The majority of patients treated for spontaneous lung lobe torsion without an underlying disease process will recover quickly without significant complications.[5-9] If neoplasia is responsible for the development of pleural effusion and subsequent lung lobe torsion, the prognosis is likely to be poor.[6,9] Some patients will develop systemic inflammatory response syndrome pre- or postoperatively, leading to death or euthanasia. This is believed to result from cytokine release by necrotic lung tissue and may be complicated by cardiovascular compromise, disseminated intravascular coagulation, or acute respiratory distress syndrome.[6,9]

Persistent pleural effusion may occur in these patients, and persistent chylothorax is reported most often.[5,6,9] It is thought that disruption or impedance of the thoracic duct or thoracic lymphatic vessels leads to lymphangiectasia, resulting in chylous effusion into the pleural cavity.[13] Although chylothorax has been detected at the time of diagnosis of lung lobe torsion, it is usually reported to develop following surgical correction of lung lobe torsion.[5,6,9,10] Resolution of the chylothorax will occur within 7 days in most patients, but persistent chylothorax has been reported in Afghan hounds and a cat.[5,6,9,10] It has been suggested that Afghan hounds may have a thoracic lymphatic system that has a lower tolerance for any degree of trauma, predisposing them to development of chylothorax.[6] The prognosis for Afghan hounds who developed chylothorax in association with lung lobe torsion has been reported to be poor,[6,9] but reports of surgical treatment for chylothorax have revealed a more favorable outcome for dogs and cats than has been reported in the past.[13-15]

References

1. Diaconescu N, Veleanu C: Die Rolle der brunstwirbelsaulendynamik bei der lobierung des lungenparenchyms (The role of thoracic spine dynamics in lobation of the lung parenchyma). Anat Anz 117(2):96, 1965.

2. Evans HE: Miller's Anatomy of the Dog, 3rd ed. Philadelphia: WB Saunders, 1993.

3. Miserocchi G, Nakamura T, Mariani E, et al: Pleural fluid pressure over the interlobar mediastinal and diaphragmatic surfaces of the lung. Respir Physiol 46:61, 1981.

4. Schamaun M: Postoperative pulmonary torsion: report of a case and survey of the literature including a spontaneous and posttraumatic torsion. Thorac Cardiovasc Surgeon 42:116, 1994.

5. Johnston GR, Feeney DA, O'Brien TD, et al: Recurring lung lobe torsion in three Afghan hounds. J Am Vet Med Assoc 184:842, 1984.

6. Neath PJ, Brockman DJ, King LG: Lung lobe torsion in dogs: 22 cases (1981-1999). J Am Vet Med Assoc 217:1041, 2000.

7. Rooney MB, Lanz O, Monnet E: Spontaneous lung lobe torsion in two pugs. J Am Anim Hosp Assoc 37:128, 2001.

8. Hofeling AD, Jackson AH, Alsup JC. et al: Spontaneous midlobar lung lobe torsion in a 2-year-old Newfoundland. J Am Anim Hosp Assoc 40:220, 2004.

9. Murphy KA, Brisson BA: Evaluation of lung lobe torsion in Pugs: 7 cases (1991-2004). J Am Vet Med Assoc 228:86, 2006.

10. Kerpsack SJ, McLoughlin MA, Graves TK, et al: Chylothorax associated with lung lobe torsion and a peritoneopericardial diaphragmatic hernia in a cat. J Am Anim Hosp Assoc 30:351, 1994.

11. Dye TL, Teague HD, Poundstone ML: Lung lobe torsion in a cat with chronic feline asthma. J Am Anim Hosp Assoc 34:493, 1998.

12. Moses BL: Fiberoptic bronchoscopy for diagnosis of lung lobe torsion in a dog. J Am Vet Med Assoc 176:44, 1980.

13. Fossum TW, Birchard SJ, Jacobs RM: Chylothorax in 34 dogs. J Am Vet Med Assoc 32:263, 1986.

14. Fossum TW, Mertens MM, Peacock JT, et al: Thoracic duct ligation and pericardectomy for treatment of idiopathic chylothorax. J Vet Intern Med 18:307, 2004.

15. Hayashi K, Sicard G, Gellasch K, et al: Cisterna chyli ablation with thoracic duct ligation for chylothorax: results in eight dogs. Vet Surg 34:519, 2005.

Chapter 55

Pneumothorax

David A. Puerto
Susan W. Volk

Pneumothorax is defined as the accumulation of free air or gas in the pleural space. This accumulation of air may come from three general sources but rupture of the visceral pleura with secondary leakage from the lung via a pleuropulmonary leak is the most common cause. Alternatively, atmospheric air may enter from disruptions to the esophageal, tracheal, bronchial, or chest walls. Gas may also be formed within the pleural space from infection with gas-forming organisms, although this is a rare occurrence.

Pneumothorax may be categorized into four broad categories: traumatic, iatrogenic, spontaneous, and infectious. Traumatic pneumothorax is the most common form and develops when disruption of the integrity of the lung, esophagus, or thoracic wall allows air to leak into the pleural space. Traumatic pneumothorax can be further subdivided according to whether there has been loss of integrity to the chest wall (open pneumothorax) or no discernible disruption (closed pneumothorax). Iatrogenic pneumothorax is a consequence of thoracotomy, but also can occur as a result of inadvertent trauma to the lungs during diagnostic or therapeutic procedures. Spontaneous pneumothorax is defined as a pneumothorax that occurs with no history of prior trauma and results from a pleuropulmonary leak, which is usually found at a site of pulmonary tissue damage secondary to a variety of underlying causes. Pneumothorax may also occur secondary to infection of the pleural space with a gas-producing organism.

Regardless of underlying etiology, the progression of the pneumothorax depends on the defect size, ability to seal itself, and whether it acts as a one-way valve or allows air to enter and exit the pleural space. The patient's respiratory pattern may also influence progression of the pneumothorax.

Physiology and Pathophysiology

The visceral (pulmonary) pleura is the serous membrane tightly adhered to the lungs, following all irregularities of their surfaces.[1] The parietal pleura covers the walls of the thoracic cavity and diaphragm, as well as the inner surface of the mediastinum. The pleurae of dogs and cats are approximately 20 microns thick.[2] The pleurae form two complete sacs on either side of the chest and are referred to as the pleural cavities. The right pleural cavity is larger than the left owing to the displacement of the mediastinum to the left caudal to the heart. Except for a thin film of capillary fluid moistening the flat mesothelial cells of the pleurae, the visceral pleura lies in contact with the parietal pleura. This fluid effectively couples the lungs to the thoracic wall while allowing the lungs to move within the thoracic cavity during the phases of respiration. Owing to the fluid coupling of the two pleural surfaces and negative intrathoracic pressure, changes in thoracic volume confer changes in lung volume.

Only during pathologic conditions in which fluid or air accumulate between these two layers does the pleural cavity exist as a true cavity. The opposing elastic recoil of the lung and thorax creates negative interpleural pressure relative to both atmospheric and alveolar pressure.[3] For optimal function, the pleural space must be devoid of both air and fluid. Fluid secreted into the pleural cavity normally is reabsorbed by lymphatics underlying the parietal pleura. The relative negative total gas pressure of the surrounding tissue favors absorption of gas from the pleural space.

With introduction of air into the pleural space, as occurs with pneumothorax, the pressure of gas in the space approaches or eventually reaches atmospheric pressure. By comparison, the pressure within the surrounding tissues remains subatmospheric. This pressure difference favors reabsorbtion of the pneumothorax, with each gas being reabsorbed independently. Pleural oxygen diffuses down its concentration gradient (from approximately 149 mm Hg to 40 mm Hg), out of the pleural cavity and into the interstitial fluid. With the loss of oxygen from the pleural space, the volume of gas decreases and the relative concentration of nitrogen increases. The residual oxygen and nitrogen within the pleural space, followed by carbon dioxide and water vapor, continue to be absorbed until all gases are evacuated from the cavity. The rate of resorption depends on several factors, including: the quality of the pleural surface (pathologic conditions leading to increased pleural thickness will decrease the resorptive rate), the total surface area of the thoracic cavity, and the initial volume of air to be resorbed. Oxygen therapy has been shown to hasten the resolution of pneumothorax by decreasing the alveolar nitrogen partial pressure and, therefore, venous nitrogen pressure.[4,5] The increased gradient between pleural and alveolar space nitrogen facilitates its diffusion from the pleural to the alveolar space, thus speeding the absorption of the pleural air.

The cardiopulmonary effects of progressive pneumothorax have been investigated in both anesthetized and conscious dogs.[6-11] As the pleural surfaces separate, and elastic recoil is abolished, the thoracic cavity expands with simultaneous collapse of the lungs, although degree of lung collapse is disproportionately greater than that of thoracic cavity expansion.[10] In addition to a decrease in tidal volume, the collapse of the lung creates a ventilation/perfusion mismatch, leading to diminished arterial partial pressures of oxygen.[10,12] This fall in PaO_2 leads to a concomitant increase in respiratory rate via a vagally mediated elimination of the abdominal expiratory muscle activity.[7] As pneumothorax progresses, hypoxemia induces resistance vessels of the lungs to undergo vasoconstriction (hypoxic vasoconstriction), in an effort to reduce ventilation-perfusion mismatch by diverting blood from hypoxic regions and to maintain PaO_2. Initially, early compensatory mechanisms are capable of maintaining alveolar ventilation despite reductions in tidal volume, but as the degree of pneumothorax increases, they are overcome and additional cardiopulmonary derangements become evident.[10,11] It is also of clinical significance that many compensatory mechanisms are abolished during anesthesia, augmenting the cardiorespiratory depression in anesthetized patients with pneumothorax.[13] Respiratory rate, central venous pressure, and alveolar-to-arterial O_2 tension difference increase in a linear relationship proportional to the degree of pneumothorax, while tidal volume, and arterial and mixed-venous pH and PaO_2 decrease in a linear relationship and a manner inversely proportional to the degree of pneumothorax. Heart rate and mean arterial pressure are not significantly affected by mild to moderate pneumothorax.[10,11] As the pneumothorax progresses, cardiovascular effects become more evident. Increased intrathoracic pressure may impair venous return directly by compression of the great vessels and indirectly by eliminating the thoracic pump. Additionally, pulmonary artery pressure elevation and myocardial ischemia may diminish cardiac output.

Tension pneumothorax occurs when the torn edge of lung or thoracic wall forms a flap and acts as a one-way valve allowing air to enter but not to exit the pleural space. Air accumulation may be rapid and initial pathophysiologic changes described above can rapidly progress to cardiopulmonary collapse if not promptly detected and treated. As supra-atmospheric pressure develops in the pleural space, severe compression atelectasis of the lung, flattening of the diaphragm, and compression of the major vessels occur. These events lead to ventilatory impairment, profound hypoxemia, and dramatically reduced venous return, which are ultimately fatal if not aggressively treated.

Although it is clear that increasing volume of air within the pleural space correlates with the degree of cardiorespiratory dysfunction, underlying lung pathology has a substantial impact on clinical presentation. In normal experimental subjects, pneumothorax equivalent to 150% of the calculated lung volume were well tolerated;[11] however, patients with concurrent pulmonary disease and ventilatory compromise may exhibit pathophysiologic derangements with much smaller volumes of pneumothorax. Furthermore, concurrent head trauma, fractures, large airway disruptions, diaphragmatic hernias, myocardial contusions, and intraabdominal disease seen in trauma patients with pneumothorax may further compromise these patients.

Syndromes and Pathogenesis

The categorical designation of a patient with regard to underlying etiology is an important step in logical diagnostic and therapeutic decision-making.

Traumatic Pneumothorax

Pneumothorax attributable to a traumatic event has been estimated to occur in up to 87% (92/105) of pneumothorax cases and is most often the result of an automobile accident.[14] Less commonly, a bite or stab wound, gunshot or shearing injury may cause a penetrating injury and disruption of the integrity of the thoracic wall (open pneumothorax). In the absence of a pleurocutaneous defect (closed pneumothorax), air may gain access to the pleural space through a pleuropulmonary leak or disruption of the conducting airways or esophagus. This may occur from barotrauma secondary to massive, sudden increase in intrathoracic pressure, which occurs with blunt-force chest compression against a closed glottis or from shearing or tensile forces generated from impact.

Rib fractures and penetrating foreign bodies may also directly lacerate pulmonary parenchyma. Concurrent pneumothorax has been shown to occur in 56% of cats with traumatic rib fractures and 58% of dogs and cats with flail segments.[15,16] In a study that included 92 cases of traumatic pneumothorax, the most common nonrespiratory-associated injury was to the musculoskeletal system, with an incidence of approximately 50% of these cases.[14] Similarly, over one half (6/11) of dogs and cats treated for thoracic bite wounds in one study were diagnosed with pneumothorax.[17] Pneumothorax associated with high-rise syndrome has been reported to occur in 32% of dogs and in 63% of cats.[18,19] Owing to the chance of concurrent injuries, animals may be less likely to tolerate smaller volumes of pneumothorax. In addition, more aggressive treatment for the pneumothorax may be necessary in the event that the concurrent disease necessitates emergency surgical management, because anesthesia may abolish compensatory cardiorespiratory mechanisms. Interestingly, in one study, survival rate was not significantly affected by the presence of concurrent injury in treated animals.[14]

Open pneumothorax results when the thoracic wall is disrupted and air is able to enter the pleural space via the wound: penetrating foreign bodies (i.e., gunshots, sticks, etc), and combined blunt/sharp trauma secondary to bite wounds or vehicular trauma. An open chest wound results in significant compromise of pulmonary function because it allows rapid equilibration of intrathoracic pressure with atmospheric pressure with an inability to expand the lung.

Iatrogenic Pneumothorax

Iatrogenic traumas associated with diagnostic and therapeutic veterinary procedures are reported causes of pneumothorax in the dog and the cat. Pneumothorax is an accepted risk of thoracocentesis, thoracostomy tube placement, fine-needle lung aspiration biopsy, or biopsy of other intrathoracic structures.[20,21] Pneumothorax was reported to occur in 31% of dogs undergoing transthoracic needle biopsy.[21] Animals undergoing general anesthetic procedures are at risk for barotrauma to conducting airways and alveoli.[22,23] Of dogs and cats undergoing prolonged periods of therapeutic mechanically-assisted ventilation, the incidence of pneumothorax was 29% and 28%, respectively.[24,25] The combination of pulmonary pathology and positive end-expiratory pressures makes these patients particularly susceptible to the development of pneumothorax. Furthermore, the use of positive pressure ventilation may convert a simple pneumothorax into a tension pneumothorax. Pneumothorax is a reported complication of thoracolumbar disk fenestration.[26] Physical restraint during venipuncture was theorized to be the cause of pneumothorax in a kitten.[27] Other procedures in which pneumothorax has been induced include closed-chest cardiopulmonary resuscitation, central venous cannula placement, pacemaker implantation, and inadvertent diaphragmatic incision during celiotomy.

Spontaneous Pneumothorax

In the absence of a preceding traumatic event, a pneumothorax is categorized as spontaneous (with the rare exception of those caused by gas-forming bacteria). In comparison with cases of trauma-induced pneumothorax, spontaneous pneumothorax occurs much less frequently and has an estimated prevalence of 0.11%. Underlying pulmonary parenchymal pathology may be the site of the leak. Alternatively, rupture of the air-containing space within or immediately beneath the visceral pleura may lead to the pleuropulmonary communication and are referred to as blebs or bullae, depending on location.

Blebs are contained entirely within the pleura between the two layers of the lamina elastica (interna and externa), but they communicate directly with adjacent alveolar spaces.[28,29] They are most frequently found at the apices and appear as small "bubbles" or "blisters" on the surface of the lung. Bullae are lined by a combination of thickened pulmonary tissue and by emphysematous lung (Figure 55-1). In the largest study of canine spontaneous pneumothorax cases to date, 68% of cases in which a definitive diagnosis was reached were attributable to bullous emphysema,[30] supporting reports from smaller studies that blebs and bullae were the most frequent cause of spontaneous pneumothorax in the dog.[31-34] Interestingly, Siberian huskies were over-represented in the case population studied at the University of Pennsylvania.[30] In a study of 12 dogs with spontaneous pneumothorax attributable to bullae or blebs, all 12 had lesions in one or both cranial lung lobes, with 10 of the dogs having multiple lesions. Bilateral lesions were seen in 36 to 58% of dogs and multiple lung lobes were affected by bullae in 37% of dogs.[3,30] By comparison, this condition appears to be much less prevalent in cats, with only seven cats reported in the literature.[35,36]

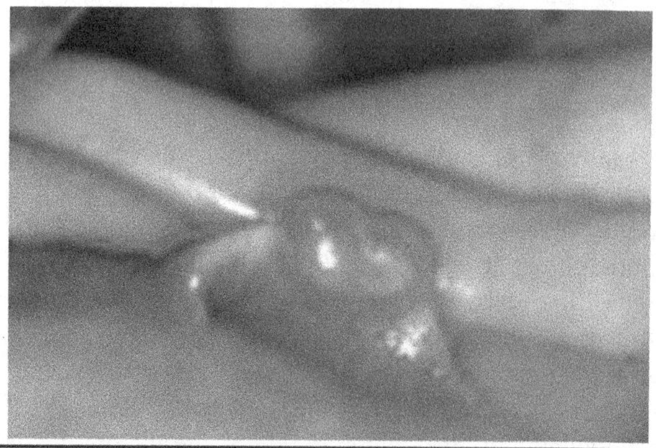

Figure 55-1. Intraoperative view of a pulmonary bleb/bulla in a dog with spontaneous pneumothorax. (Courtesy of David Holt, University of Pennsylvania)

The pathogenesis of pulmonary blebs and bullae in dogs and humans is poorly defined. Exposure to cigarette smoke has been shown to be a significant risk factor for the development of these lesions in humans.[37] In addition, increased distensile forces associated with conformation, changes in atmospheric pressure, and certain inflammatory conditions have all been theorized to predispose to their development.[38-42] Although no studies have specifically examined pathogenesis of blebs and bullae in dogs, histologic similarities between these human and canine lesions suggest that similar mechanisms in their development may exist.

Less commonly, spontaneous pneumothorax develops secondary to a specific pulmonary pathology, which has caused weakening of the alveolar walls and visceral pleura with subsequent formation of a pleuropulmonary leak. Bullae may be grossly visible in the pathologic tissue. In dogs, spontaneous pneumothorax has been associated with a variety of infectious and inflammatory conditions, including pulmonary abscesses, pneumonia, parasitic granulomas and associated pulmonary arterial thromboembolism, and heartworm disease, as well as pleuritis.[30,43-47] Neoplasia, primary or metastatic, has also been implicated in the development of pneumothorax.[30,48,49]

Infectious Pneumothorax

Pneumothorax that occurs secondary to an infection with gas-producing organisms is a rare condition in dogs and cats.

Pneumomediastinum with Pneumothorax

Pneumomediastinum is defined as the presence of free air within the tissues of the mediastinum. Pneumomediastinum can be seen radiographically in some animals with pneumothorax. Additionally, air may be seen dissecting in fascial planes of the neck, the pericardium, and the retroperitoneal space. This can occur with disruption of the lower airways, esophagus, and marginal aleveoli of the lung.[22,50-56] Mediastinal pleura may commonly rupture with over-distention and lead to pneumothorax, but pneumothorax cannot cause a pneumomediastinum.[55,56] When pneumomediastinum occurs, it is rarely of clinical significance, but clinicians should be aware that it may lead to pneumothorax.

Treatment for patients with minimal respiratory compromise is conservative. Placing the patient in lateral recumbency with the affected side down may be of benefit, even in patients that are mechanically ventilated. Thoracocentesis or placement of thoracostomy tubes with intermittent or continuous suction may be needed. If the leakage is secondary to positive pressure ventilation, positive end-expiratory pressure (PEEP) should be discontinued if possible. Surgery is rarely necessary and is reserved for patients that do not respond to conservative treatment. The recommended treatment of spontaneous pneumothorax involves stabilization of the patient by thoracocentesis or tube thoracostomy followed by early surgical exploration with median sternotomy for patients that do not have identifiable non-surgical disease or diffuse pulmonary disease. Cases of spontaneous pneumothorax treated surgically had a lower recurrence, 3%, and mortality, 12%, versus 50% recurrence and 53% mortality for non-surgically managed cases.[30]

References

1. Evans HE: The respiratory system. *In* Miller's Anatomy of the Dog. Evans HE (ed). Philadelphia: WB Saunders, 1993, p. 463.
2. Lai-Fook SJ, Kaplowitz MR: Pleural space thickness in situ by light microscopy in five mammalian species. J Appl Physiol 59:603, 1985.
3. Lipscomb V, Hardie RJ, Dubielzig RR: Spontaneous pneumothorax caused by pulmonary blebs and bullae in 12 dogs. J Am Anim Hosp Assoc 39:435, 2003.
4. England GJ, Hill RC, Timberlake GA, Harrah JD, et al: Resolution of experimental pneumothorax in rabbits by graded oxygen therapy. J Trauma Injury Infection Crit Care 45:333, 1998.
5. Zierold D, Lee SL, Subramanian S, DuBois JJ: Supplemental oxygen improves resolution of injury-induced pneumothorax. J Pediatr Surg 35:998, 2005.
6. Lee BP, Lin YC, Chiang ST: Role of vagal reflex in maintaining alveolar ventilation during pneumothorax in anaesthetized dogs. J Formosan Med Assoc 86:1133, 1987.
7. Hollstein SB, Carl ML, Schelegle ES, Green JF: Role of vagal afferents in the control of abdominal expiratory muscle activity in the dog. J Appl Physiol 71:1795, 1991.
8. De Troyer A, Sampson M, Sigrist S, Macklem PT: Action of costal and crural parts of the diaphragm on the rib cage in dogs. J Appl Physiol 54:465, 1983.
9. Shannon R: Respiratory pattern changes during costovertebral joint movement. J Appl Physiol 48:862, 1980.
10. Walker M, Hartsfield S, Matthews N, et al: Computed tomography and blood gas analysis of anesthetized bloodhounds with induced pneumothorax. Vet Rad Ultrasound 34:93, 1993.
11. Bennet RA, Orton EC, Tucker A, Heiller CL: Cardiopulmonary changes in conscious dogs with induced progressive pneumothorax. Am J Vet Res 50:280, 1989.
12. Moran JF, Jones RH, Wolfe WG: Regional pulmonary function during experimental unilateral pneumothorax in the awake state. J Thorac Cardiovasc Surg 74:396, 1977.
13. Kilburn KH: Cardiorespiratory effects of large pneumothorax in conscious and anesthetized dogs. J Appl Physiol 18:279, 1962.
14. Krahwinkel DJ, Rorhbach BW, Hollis BA: Factors associated with survival in dogs and cats with pneumothorax. J Vet Emerg Crit Care 9:7, 1999.
15. Kraje BJ, Kraje AC, Rorhbach BW, et al: Intrathoracic and concurrent orthopedic injury associated with traumatic rib fracture in cats: 75 cases, J Am Vet Med Assoc 216:51, 2000.
16. Olsen D, Renberg W, Perrett J, et al: Clinical management of flail chest in dogs and cats: A retrospective study of 24 cases (1989-1999). J Am Anim Hosp Assoc 38:315, 2002.
17. Shahar R, Shamir M, Johnston DE: A technique for management of bite wounds of the thoracic wall in small dogs. Vet Surg 26:45, 1997.
18. Whitney WO, Melhaff CJ: High-rise syndrome in cats. J Am Vet Med Assoc 191:1399, 1987.
19. Gordon LE, Thacher C, Kapatkin AS: High-rise syndrome in dogs: 81 cases (1985-1991). J Am Vet Med Assoc 202:118, 1993.
20. Tillson DM: Thoracostomy tubes, part II, placement and maintenance. Comp Cont Educ Pract Vet 19:1331, 1997.
21. Teske E, Stokhof AA, van den Ingh TS, et al: Transthoracic needle aspiration biospy of the lung in dogs with pulmonic diseases. J Am Anim Hosp Assoc 27:289, 1991.
22. Cimino Brown D, Holt D: Subcutaneous emphysema, pneumothorax, pneumomediastinum and pneumopericardium associated with positive pressure ventilation in a cat. J Am Vet Med Assoc 206:997, 1995.

23. Evans HE: Pneumothorax, pneumomediastinum, and subcutaneous emphysema in a cat due to barotrauma after equipment failure during anesthesia. J Am Vet Med Assoc 164:1107, 1998.

24. King LG, Hendricks JC: Use of positive-pressure ventilation in dogs and cats: 41 cases (1990-1992). J Am Vet Med Assoc 204:1045, 1994.

25. Lee JA, Drobatz KJ, Koch MW, King LG: Indications for and outcome of positive-pressure ventilation in cats: 53 cases (1993-2002). J Am Vet Med Assoc 226:924, 2005.

26. Bartels KE, Creed JE, Ytrurraspe DJ: Complications associated with the dorsolateral muscle-separating approach for thoracolumbar disk fenestration in the dog. J Small Anim Pract 38:237, 1997.

27. Godfrey DR: Bronchial rupture and fatal tension pneumothorax following routine venipuncture in a kitten. J Am Anim Hosp Assoc 33:260, 1997.

28. Ohata M, Suzuki H: Pathogenesis of spontaneous pneumothorax. Chest 77:771, 1980.

29. Murphy DM, Fishman AP: Bullous disease of the lung. *In* Pulmonary Diseases and Disorders. New York: McGraw-Hill, 1988, p. 1219.

30. Puerto DA, Brockman DJ, Lindquist C, Drobatz K: Surgical and nonsurgical management of and selected risk factors for spontaneous pneumothorax in dogs: 64 cases (1986-1999). J Am Vet Med Assoc 220:1670, 2002.

31. Valentine A, Smeak D, Allen D, et al: Spontaneous pneumothorax in dogs. Comp Cont Educ Pract Vet 18:53, 1996.

32. Yoshioka MM: Management of spontaneous pneumothorax in 12 dogs. J Am Anim Hosp Assoc 18:57, 1982.

33. Kramek BA, Caywood DD, O'Brien TD: Bullous emphysema and recurrent pneumothorax in the dog. J Am Vet Med Assoc 186:971, 1985.

34. Holtsinger RH, Beale BS, Bellah JR, King RR: Spontaneous pneumothorax in the dog: A retrospective analysis of 21 cases. J Am Anim Hosp Assoc 29:195, 1993.

35. White HL, Rozanski EA, Tidwell AS, et al: Spontaneous pneumothorax in two cats with small airway disease. J Am Vet Med Assoc 222:1573, 2003.

36. Cooper ES, Syring RS, King LG: Pneumothorax in cats with a clinical diagnosis of feline asthma: 5 cases (1990-2000). J Vet Emerg Crit Care 13:95, 2003.

37. Bense L, Eklaund G, Odont D, Wiman LG: Smoking and the increased risk of contracting spontaneous pneumothorax. Chest 92:1009, 1987.

38. Vawter DL, Matthews FL, West JB: Effect of shape and size of lung and chest wall on stresses in the lung. J Applied Phys 39:9, 1975.

39. Dermksian G, Lamb LE: Spontaneous pneumothorax in apparently healthy flying personnel. Ann Intern Med 51:39, 1959.

40. Bense L: Spontaneous pneumothorax related to falls in atmospheric pressure. Eur J Respir Dis 65:544, 1984.

41. Scott GC, Berger R, McKean HE: The role of atmospheric pressure variation in the development of spontaneous pneumothoraces. Am Rev Respir Dis 139:659, 1989.

42. Schramel FM, Postmus PE, Vanderschueren RG: Current aspects of spontaneous pneumothorax. Eur Resp J 10:1379, 1997.

43. Saheki Y, Ishitani R, Miyamoto Y: Acute fatal pneumothorax in canine dirofilariasis. Jpn J Vet Sci 43:315, 1981.

44. Burrows CF, O'Brien JA, Biery DN: Pneumothorax due to Filaroides osleri infestation in the dog. J Small Anim Pract 3:613, 1982.

45. Schaer M, Gamble D, Spencer C: Spontaneous pneumothorax associated with bacterial pneumonia in the dog--two case reports. J Am Anim Hosp Assoc 17:783, 1981.

46. Forrester SD, Fossum TW, Miller MW: Pneumothorax in a dog with a pulmonary abscess and suspected infective endocarditis. J Am Vet Med Assoc 200: 351, 1992.

47. Busch DS, Noxon JO: Pneumothorax in a dog infected with Dirofilaria immitis. J Am Vet Med Assoc 201:1893, 1992.

48. Pechman RD Jr: Pulmonary paragonimiasis in dogs and cats: a review. J Small Anim Pract 21:87, 1980.

49. Dallman MJ, Martin RA, Roth L: Pneumothorax as the primary problem in two cases of bronchioloalveolar carcinoma in the dog. J Am Anim Hosp Assoc 24:710, 1988.

50. Manning MM, Brunson DB: Barotrauma in a cat. J Am Vet Med Assoc 205:62, 1994.

51. White RN, Burton CA: Surgical management of intrathoracic tracheal avulsion in cats: long-term results in 9 consecutive cases. Vet Surg 29:430, 2000.

52. White RN, Milner HR: Intrathoracic tracheal avulsion in three cats. J Small Anim Pract 36:343, 1995.

53. Hardie EM, Spodnick GJ, Gilson SD, et al: Tracheal rupture in cats: 16 cases (1983-1998). J Am Vet Med Assoc 214:508, 1999.

54. Kellagher REB, White RN: Tracheal rupture in a dog. J Small Anim Pract 28:29, 1987.

55. Van den Broek A: Pneumomediastinum in 17 dogs: aetiology and radiographic signs. J Small Anim Pract 27:747, 1986.

56. Rogers K, Walker MA: Disorders of the mediastinum. Comp Cont Educ Pract Vet 19:69, 1997.

Chapter 56

Pyothorax

Trent Gall
Matthew Rooney

"In cases of empyema treated by the cautery or incision, when the matter is pure, white, and not fetid, the patient recovers; but if of a bloody and dirty character, he dies."..

Hippocrates (470-410 BC) in his original works on empyema.[1]

Pyothorax or thoracic empyema is a disease that affects dogs and cats. This disease has been recognized in humans for over 2000 years, with Hippocrates being one of the first people to document it.[1] Pyothorax is characterized by a septic thoracic effusion and infection of the pleural space. This rare but life-threatening disease has many proposed etiologies and often the cause is not found antemortem.

Etiology

The many proposed mechanisms for pyothorax include: inhaled or ingested plant material (plant awns), migrating foreign bodies, esophageal perforation, parasitic migration, penetrating thoracic wounds, hematogenous or direct extension of infection (systemic sepsis), secondary to bronchopneumonia, parapnuemonic spread, mediastinitis, iatrogenic causes, and subphrenic infection.[2-4] The majority of the time the inciting cause of pyothorax is never determined antemortem.

In cats, one of the widely believed mechanisms for pyothorax is penetrating thoracic bite wounds. Although bite wounds account for a small percentage of documented cases of pyothorax, this cause is rarely identified antemortem.[2,3,5] The mechanism of development of pyothorax from a bite wound is contamination from normal oral flora.[3,6,7] This has been popularized because there is an overrepresentation of cats from multi-cat households, but interestingly enough, intact male outdoor cats are not overrepresented in some studies.[3,5] Also no statistical difference exists in the number of indoor cats versus outdoor cats in these studies.[3,5] The most commonly held description for the overrepresentation of cats from multi-cat households is that these bite wounds are small and go unnoticed, and the wounds go on to abscess and rupture intrathoracically.[3,5] The authors of one paper contest this belief and subscribe to the thought that parapneumonic spread of infection after colonization and invasion of lung tissue by oropharyngeal anaerobes is the most frequent cause of feline pyothorax.[3] The overrepresentation of cats from multi-cat households can be attributed to the fact that cats from this population are more predisposed to upper airway infections, thus leading to pneumonia and then parapneumonic spread of bacteria, leading to pyothorax.[3] Because of the controversy surrounding the cause of pyothorax in cats a complete physical exam (including dermatologic examination for bite wounds) and a thorough history (inquiring about recent upper airway infections) should be performed on all cats.

In dogs, the most commonly accepted etiology is the migration of plant awn material via inhalation, ingestion, or trandsdermal migration from the awn penetrating elsewhere in the body. Common species of plants that have been identified have been grasses of the *Poaceae* family, *Hordeum jubatum* (in the majority of the United States), *Stipa* and *Setaria* (in the southern United States), and *Hordeum murinum* in France and Australia.[8] This etiology has gained support because of the predominace of sporting breeds in the reported literature.[2,8-13] The inhaled or ingested plant material is thought to carry oral flora into the lungs with the awn as well as environmental contaminants such as *Actinomyces* spp. and *Nocardia* spp. The plant awns that migrate through the skin are thought to carry environmental bacterial species as well as skin contaminants. This idea is supported by the fact that in most cases the pyothorax is composed of polymicrobial populations that contain these oral and environmental microorganisms.[2,3,9,10,12,14,15] Adding further confusion to the problem, some dogs that have pyothorax have not had exposure to plant awn material. With any case of pyothorax, a complete physical and thorough history should be performed, although it is uncommon to find the inciting cause in many cases of pyothorax.[2,10,11,14]

Microbes

Pleural fluid that is suspicious for pyothorax (exudative fluid) should be submitted to a labratory for cultures and antimicrobial sensitivity analysis for aerobic, Mycoplasma, and anaerobic microbes. Pyothorax has a high prevalence of polymicrobic infections.[2,3,9,10,12,14,15] Both *Actinomyces* spp. and *Nocardia* spp. are common environmental microorganisms that are thought to be introduced into the animal through plant material foreign bodies. *Actinomyces* spp. can also be found as part of the normal oropharynx flora in both dogs and cats.[4] *Actinomyces* spp. are opportunistic pathogens that rely on mechanical disruption of normal mucosal barriers, such as what happens with plant awn migration.[4] Infections with *Nocardia* spp. are thought to be similar in nature because Nocardia spp. are ubiquitous soil saprophytes that degrade organic matter and are found in soil, water, and on plants.[4] The most common isolated microorganisms from dogs and cats are *Bacteroides, Clostridium, Peptostretococcus,* and *Pasteurella multocida.*[7,15] These bacteria are considered normal flora of the oropharynx and upper respiratory system of dogs and cats. (Table 56-1).[16]

History, Signalment, and Physical Examination Findings

Pyothorax has been recognized in dogs with a mean age of 3 to 4 years (range: 1-11 years) with one case report of a neonate boxer puppy.[2,9,11-14,17] Cats range in age from 1 to 11 years with a mean of 3.83 to 5.8 years with one report of a 4-month-old lion cub and a report of 1-month-old kitten.[3,5,11,18-22] Sex predilection for pyothorax is still somewhat disputed. Several studies report that canine males are more predisposed than females: 2:1 in one study and 1.25:1 in another;[2,9,11,14] but other studies suggest that no sex predilection exists.[12,13,15] Some discrepancy in sex predilection seems to exist in cats as well. One study suggested a male to female ratio of 2 to 2.5:1,[5,11] and other studies showed no

Table 56-1. Reported Microbes Associated with Canine and Feline Pyothorax[2,7,10,11,15,17]

Anaerobic bacteria	Aerobic bacteria	Fungus
Bacteroides species	*Actinomyces* species	*Candida albicans*
Clostridium species	*Escherichia coli*	
Eubacterium species	*Enterobacter* species	
Fusobacterium species	*Klebsiella* species	
Peptostreptococcus species	*Mycoplasma* species	
Porphyromonas species	*Nocardia* species	
Prevotella species	*Pasteurella* species	
Propionibacterium species	*Proteus* species	
	Pseudomonas species	
	Staphylococcus species	
	Streptococcus species	

difference between the sexes.[3,15,21] The majority of affected dogs are medium- to large-breed dogs, with hunting/working dogs being overrepresented in certain geographies.[12] No specific breed predilection is apparent, with most cases occurring during fall and winter months, which corresponds with typical hunting seasons.[10]

Dogs and cats often present with clinical signs consistent with pleural effusion but this can vary depending on the severity of the effusion. The signs include: exercise intolerance, poor athletic performance, shortness of breath, tachypnea, lethargy, and weight loss. Other signs are open-mouth breathing with dyspnea on the inspiratory phase, abducted elbows, extended head and neck, labored breathing, muffled heart sounds, decreased lung sounds, dull percussive sounds of the ventral thorax, thoracic and/or abdominal wall swellings, penetrating wounds or other trauma.[2,3,9-11,13,14,17,23] The majority of cats present with a history of partial or complete anorexia as the most common historical finding,[3] with other signs similar to that of dogs. Owners often miss the subtle signs in cats with pleural effusion. Less common signs such as lethargy, reluctance to lie down, and anorexia can be initial complaints for dogs.[2,3,9-11,13,14,17] Less common presenting complaints include cough, diarrhea, polyuria, and polydipsia. The most severe cases present with acute respiratory distress, shock, dehydration, pale mucous membranes, and hypothermia.[10,19]

Complete Blood Count and Biochemical Analysis

Biochemical analysis is not specific for pyothorax; the most common abnormality is hypoalbuminemia. Other abnormalities include hyponatremia, hypochloremia, hyperglobulinemia, elevations in alanine aminotransferase or alkaline phosphatase, hyperglycemia, hypoglycemia, increase in blood urea, increase in creatinine, and increased bile acids.[2,3,5,11,14,19]

It is recommended that all cats with pleural effusion be tested for feline leukemia virus (FeLV), feline immunodeficiency virus (FIV), and heartworm disease.[24]

Results of hematology studies vary and are typically indicative of bacterial infections. These abnormalities include neutrophilic leukocytosis with or without a left shift, monocytosis, and eosinophilia. Anemia may or may not be present.[2,3,5,11,14,19]

Diagnostic Imaging

Right and/or left lateral and either ventrodorsal or dorsoventral views can be taken in patients that are stable. Findings include blurring of the cardiac silhouette, presence of interlobar fissure lines, rounding of the lung margins at the costrophrenic angles, separation of the lung borders away from the thoracic wall, scalloping of the lung margins dorsal to the sternum, lung lobe collapse or suspected pulmonary mass, elevation of the trachea, widened mediastinum, thickening of visceral pleura, enlarged sternal lymph nodes, diffuse and focal alveolar infiltrates, air bronchograms within consolidated lung lobes, bronchointerstitial disease, and diffuse interstitial disease.[2,3,10,11,25] Atelectasis can be documented in some cases. It is not always possible to distinguish among recoil atelectasis, lobar consolidation, and encapsulated pleural fluid.[3] It is advantageous to remove as much of the pleural effusion as possible before attempting radiographs. This will improve visualization of thoracic anatomy and often makes the patient more comfortable while positioning for the radiographs. If the patient is in respiratory distress, horizontal-beam radiographs can be taken.[21] These views are often useful because they help the clinician to differentiate pyopneumothorax from gas-producing bacteria. Radiographs can detect as little as 50 to 100 ml of fluid; the recumbent ventrodorsal position appears to be the most sensitive for detecting the smaller amounts of fluid.[26] It has been reported that animals with radiodense lesions in the mediastinum or pulmonary fields have a poorer prognosis if they are treated medically rather than surgically.[2]

The majority of affected dogs and cats present with bilateral effusion.[2,3,5,11,21] One study reported 82% (of total animals) presenting with bilateral effusion; 29% of cats had unilateral effusion, and 14% of dogs had unilateral effusion.[11] Another study in cats reported a similar finding of 76% bilateral and 24% unilateral effusion.[3] In this study, 40% of cats had radiographic evidence of concurrent pneumonia.

Thoracic ultrasonography can be helpful in the diagnosis of

pyothorax and may be used to find small volumes of pleural fluid not detected radiographically, to quantitate or further characterize an effusion, or to guide thoracocentesis.[27] Abnormal findings include free pleural fluid, consolidated or collapsed lung lobes, and/or fibrinous or fibrous tags that can extend between the parietal and visceral pleura.[5,11] Occasionally, effusions have been accompanied by septations and parietal pleural thickening.[27] Cranial mediastinal masses, pulmonary abscesses, pericardial effusion, and restrictive pleuritis can be detected using ultrasonography.[11,27] It is also feasible to conclude that foreign bodies could be detected with ultrasound; however, to our knowledge, this has not been documented in published reports. It is advantageous to have pleural effusion present when performing ultrasound in the thorax as the fluid provides an "acoustic window" that allows the ultrasonographer to visualize more of the thoracic anatomy.[27]

Computed tomography (CT) and MRI are commonly used in human medicine to diagnose thoracic disease and with these modalities becoming more and more common in veterinary medicine, it is a resource that can be used depending on whether the patient is stable enough for general anesthesia or heavy sedation. These modalities are especially helpful for diagnosing certain disease processes such as neoplasia28 and pulmonary abscesses.

Pleural Fluid Analysis

Thoracocentesis is a procedure that is simple, diagnostic, and therapeutic. The complications of thoracocentesis are minimal if proper technique is used. These complications can include laceration of underlying lung tissue, causing pneumothorax, hemothorax, or pulmonary hemorrhage.[10] If the pleural effusion is "pocketed," radiographs or ultrasound can help guide the clinician to draw from these "pockets." Approximately 5 to 10 ml of aspirated fluid should be saved for bacterial culture and antimicrobial sensitivity testing as well as analysis. Ideally these samples would be taken at the time of therapeutic thoracocentesis and before antibiotic therapy is initiated. A portion of the fluid should be placed in an EDTA tube for total nucleated cell count, total protein count, specific gravity, and cytologic examination.[10,25,29] The remainder of the sample fluid should be placed in a glass serum tube (red top without clot activator) for biochemical analysis as well as into culture-transport media for aerobic, *Mycoplasma*, and anaerobic cultures, and antimicrobial sensitivity analysis.[10,29] Samples that are going to be submitted for culture and sensitivity must be handled properly to maximize identification. Refrigeration of the samples must be avoided, and they must be submitted to the laboratory within 24 hours.[10,30] At the time of fluid collection for analysis 4 to 6 direct smears of fluid onto a microscope slide should be made, especially if the samples are to be sent out to a laboratory.[25,31] If these slides are to be sent to an outside laboratory, several should be unstained. If the clinician is going to examine the slides, they should be Gram stained and/or Diff Quick stained for examination.[3,25]

Pleural effusion samples should be analyzed for physical, chemical, and cytologic characteristics. Physical parameters include volume, color, turbidity, viscosity, presence of sulfur granules, and odor.[10,25,29,31,32] Increased turbidity, high viscosity, bad odor, and varying color (e.g., sanguineous, brown, tan, white/greenish, or "creamy" red) are characteristics of septic effusions.[10,25] Degenerating leukocytes and bacteria can compose flocculent debris in the form of yellow flecks or sulfur granules.[10,25] If possible, this debris should be included in the direct smears and in the samples that are submitted for culture and sensitivity.[10]

Normal pleural fluid contains less than 1.5 g/dl of protein and less than 500 cells/μl. Exudative fluids typically contain more than 3 g/dl of protein and more than 7,000 cells/μl with variable cell types and have a specific gravity greater than 1.025.[10,29] Some chemical properties have been shown to be useful in evaluating pleural fluid in humans and cats. To the authors' knowledge these have not been determined to be accurate in canine fluid analysis.[10,32] These parameters include lactate dehydrogenase (LDH), pH, and glucose levels. LDH levels greater than 200 IU/L, acidic fluid, and glucose measurements less than 30 mg/dl have been shown to be consistent with exudative fluids in cats.[10,33] In humans, increased levels of LDH are consistent with cell damage or inflammation.[10,32,34]

When evaluating pleural effusion, the lack of microorganisms and/or degenerative neutrophils seen on cytologic analysis does not rule out an infectious cause.[10,29] Some bacteria may not produce enough toxins to cause toxic changes to neutrophils, and the absence of microorganisms may be a result of antibiotic administration prior to sampling or owing to the presence of microorganisms without cell walls (e.g., *Mycoplasma*).[10]

Prognosis

Pyothorax carries a fair to good prognosis in both dogs and cats treated with aggressive medical or surgical management. Reports of survival rates range from approximately 60% to 90%, depending on early diagnosis, underlying etiology, and aggressiveness of treatment.[2,10] In one retrospective study, dogs that had confirmed infection with *Actinomyces* spp. had a significant difference in disease-free intervals between those that were treated medically versus those treated surgically (1.56 to 15.78).[2] In dogs that had evidence of mediastinal or pulmonary lesions, the difference in disease-free intervals was also significant between medically versus surgically treated animals (2.16 to 22.46).[2] This evidence suggests that animals with confirmed *Actinomyces* spp. and/or mediastinal or pulmonary lesions have a better prognosis when they are treated surgically versus medically.[2] Cats with pyothorax were more likely to come from multi-cat households than single-cat households.[5] Hypersalivation and bradycardia were more common in non-surviving cats with pyothorax than in survivors.[5]

Conclusion

Pyothorax carries a fair to good prognosis with the appropriate management. Often the inciting cause cannot be identified during antemortem examinations. Successful resolution of pyothorax depends on early detection, appropriate antimicrobial selection, and aggressive management. Aggressive management includes early surgical intervention when surgery is warranted.

References

1. Hippocrates: The Genuine Works of Hippocrates. New York: Dover, 1868.

2. Rooney MB, Monnet E: Medical and surgical treatment of pyothorax in dogs: 26 cases (1991-2001). J Am Vet Med Assoc 221:86-92, 2002.

3. Barrs VR, Allan GS, Martin P, et al: Feline pyothorax: a retrospective study of 27 cases in Australia. J Feline Med Surg 7:211-222, 2005.

4. Greene CE: Infectious Diseases of the Dog and Cat, 2nd ed. Philadelphia: WB Saunders, 1998.

5. Waddell LS, Brady CA, Drobatz KJ: Risk factors, prognostic indicators, and outcome of pyothorax in cats: 80 cases (1986-1999). J Am Vet Med Assoc 221:819-824, 2002.

6. Love DN, Johnson JL, Moore LV: Bacteroides species from the oral cavity and oral-associated diseases of cats. Vet Microbiol 19:275-281, 1989.

7. Love DN, Jones RF, Bailey M, et a:. Isolation and characterisation of bacteria from pyothorax (empyaemia) in cats. Vet Microbiol 7:455-461, 1982.

8. Brennan KE, Ihrke PJ: Grass awn migration in dogs and cats: A retrospective study of 182 cases. J Am Vet Med Assoc 182:1201-1204, 1983.

9. Robertson SA, Stoddart ME, Evans RJ, et al: Thoracic empyema in the dog; a report of twenty-two cases. J Small Anim Pract 24:103-119, 1983.

10. Scott JA, Macintire DK: Canine pyothorax: clinical presentation, diagnosis, and treatment. Comp Cont Educ Pract Vet 25:180-193, 2003.

11. Demetriou JL, Foale RD, Ladlow J, et al: Canine and feline pyothorax: a retrospective study of 50 cases in the UK and Ireland. J Small Anim Pract 43:388-394, 2002.

12. Piek CJ, Robben JH: Pyothorax in nine dogs. Vet Q 22:107-111, 2000.

13. Frendin J: Pyogranulomatous pleuritis with empyema in hunting dogs. Zentralbl Veterinarmed A 44:167-178, 1997.

14. Turner WD, Breznock EM: Continuous suction drainage for management of canine pyothorax - A retrospective study. J Am Anim Hosp Assoc 24:485-494, 1988.

15. Walker AL, Jang SS, Hirsh DC: Bacteria associated with pyothorax of dogs and cats: 98 cases (1989-1998). J Am Vet Med Assoc 216:359-363, 2000.

16. Love DN, Vekselstein R, Collings S: The obligate and facultatively anaerobic bacterial flora of the normal feline gingival margin. Vet Microbiol 22:267-275, 1990.

17. Schoeffler GL, Rozanski EA, Rush JE: Pyothorax in a neonatal boxer. J Vet Emerg Crit Care 11:147-152, 2001.

18. Dickie CW: Feline pyothorax caused by a Borrelia-like organism and Corynebacterium pyogenes. J Am Vet Med Assoc 174:516-517, 1979.

19. Brady CA, Otto CM, Van Winkle TJ, et al: Severe sepsis in cats: 29 cases (1986-1998). J Am Vet Med Assoc 217:531-535, 2000.

20. Buergelt CD: Pleural effusion in cats. Vet Med 97:812-818, 2002.

21. Davies C, Forrester SD: Pleural effusion in cats: 82 cases (1987 to 1995). J Small Anim Pract 37:217-224, 1996.

22. Cannon JE, Higgins WY: Pyothorax in a lion cub. Mod Vet Pract 53:40, 1972.

23. Frendin J: Thoracic and abdominal wall swellings in dogs caused by foreign bodies. J Small Anim Pract 35:499-508, 1994.

24. Forrester SD: The categories and causes of pleural effusion in cats. Vet Med 894-906, 1988.

25. Forrester SD, Troy GC, Fossum TW: Pleural effusions: Pathophysiology and diagnostic considerations. Comp Cont Educ Pract Vet 10:121-136, 1988.

26. Lord PF, Suter PF, Chan KF, et al: Pleural, extrapleural and pulmonary lesions in small animals: a radiographic approach to differential diagnosis. J Am Vet Radiol Soc 13:4-17, 1972.

27. Tidwell AS: Ultrasonography of the thorax (excluding the heart). Vet Clin North Am Small Anim Pract 28:993-1015, 1998.

28. Henninger W: Use of computed tomography in the diseased feline thorax. J Small Anim Pract 44:56-64, 2003.

29. Cowell RL, Tyler RD, Meinkoth JH: Abdominal and thoracic fluid. In Cowell RL, Tyler RD, Meinkoth JH (eds). Diagnostic Cytology and Hematology of the Dog and Cat. St Louis: Mosby, 1999, pp.142-158.

30. Hirsh DC, Jang SS: Anaerobic infections. *In* Infectious Diseases of the Dog and Cat. Greene CE (ed). Philadelphia: WB Saunders, 1998, pp. 258-263.

31. Perman V, Osborne CA, Stevens JB: Laboratory evaluation of abnormal body fluids. Vet Clin North Am 4:255-268, 1974.

32. Christopher MM. Pleural effusions. Vet Clin North Am 17:255-270, 1987.

33. Stewart A, Padrid P, Lobinger R: Diagnostic utility of differential cell counts and measurement of LDH, total protein, glucose and Ph in the analysis of feline pleural fluid [abstract]. Proc ACVIM 1990;1121.

34. Light RW: Pleural effusions. Med Clin North Am 61:1339-1352, 1977.

Chapter 57

Pleural Effusion

MaryAnn G. Radlinsky

Pleural effusion results in ventilatory compromise by preventing pulmonary expansion in response to diaphragmatic and thoracic movements. With large amounts of effusion, diaphragmatic and thoracic movement may be severely limited. The etiology of the effusion, volume, and rate of accumulation determine clinical signs and severity of the ventilatory compromise. The impairment of pulmonary expansion results in decreased vital capacity and maximum tidal volume, inspiratory reserve volume, and functional residual capacity, or pulmonary volume at the end of exhalation.[1] Atelectasis results, which may further exacerbate ventilation and perfusion abnormalities. Supportive treatment for cases of pleural effusion often includes thoracocentesis, fluid therapy, nutritional support, and other treatments depending on the type and etiology of the effusion. Repeated drainage of pleural fluid may result in significant loss of fluid, protein, electrolytes, and perhaps lipid, vitamins, and white blood cells, which underscores the need for supportive and specific therapeutic measures.

An understanding of the etiologies and pathophysiologies of pleural effusion is therefore vital to the management of clinical cases. In this chapter we provide insight into the diagnosis and pathophysiology of the different types and causes of pleural effusion.

Normal Anatomy

The normal pleural space is lined by a single layer of mesothelial cells with an adjacent layer of elastic connective tissue containing vascular and lymphatic channels. The parietal pleura lines the thoracic wall, diaphragm, and mediastinum, and the visceral pleura lines the pulmonary surfaces including the interlobar fissures. The normal pleural space is occupied by a small amount (2-3 ml) of fluid that is low in both cell numbers (< 500 cells/ml) and protein (< 1.5 g/dl).[2] The pleural fluid lubricates the surfaces of the lungs and surrounding structures as they move throughout the ventilatory cycle. The parietal pleura is supplied by the systemic circulation (intercostal, diaphragmatic, and pericardial arteries), and venous drainage is via the azygous and internal mammary veins. The visceral pleura is supplied by the lower pressure pulmonary circulation (pulmonary and bronchial arteries) and drains via the bronchial veins. Stomas between mesothelial cells of the parietal pleura increase in numbers ventrally along the thoracic wall and diaphragm, increasing the drainage of lymph from the parietal pleura.[3] The parietal pleural lymphatic drainage proceeds into the intercostal lymphatics and eventually into the thoracic duct.[4]

The visceral pleural lymphatic drainage enters the peribronchial and interlobar lymphatics and into the thoracic and right lymphatic duct, which receives lymph from the lungs, heart, abdomen, mediastinum, and diaphragm. The diaphragmatic lymphatics allow some communication between the peritoneal and pleural cavities. The thoracic duct is the continuation of the cisterna chyli, located ventral to the first through fourth lumbar vertebrae, and carries lymph from the abdominal viscera and caudal half of the body. The duct travels dorsolaterally to the aorta on the right in the dog and on the left in the cat. The duct crosses to the left in the dog at the fifth or sixth thoracic vertebra and terminates in the left external jugular or jugulosubclavian angle in most members of both species.

Normal Physiology

Fluid production in the pleural space is based on Starling's law, primarily on hydrostatic and colloid osmotic pressure differences between the capillary and lymphatic beds of the parietal and visceral pleura. The following equation provides the determinants of pleural fluid dynamics, including vascular permeability:[1]

Movement of fluid =
K x ([HPc parietal – HPc visceral) – HPif] – [COPc – COPif])
Adjust the equation – there are an unequal number of open- and closed-paretheses

K = filtration coefficient (ml/sec/cm^2/cm H_2O)
HP = hydrostatic pressure (cm H_2O)
c = capillary
if = interstitial fluid
COP = colloid osmotic pressure (cm H_2O)

General pressure gradients for fluid production and absorption are shown in Figure 57-1. Because the systemic and pulmonary capillary hydrostatic pressures are greater than that of the pleural space, hydrostatic pressure favors fluid production. The gradient between the systemic circulation, or parietal pleura, and the pleural space is greater than that formed on the pulmonary side, or from the visceral pleura. Osmotic pressure of both the systemic and pulmonary vascular beds is greater than that of the fluid in the pleural space, favoring absorption of fluid across the parietal and visceral pleura. When the net hydrostatic and osmotic pressure gradients are added together, fluid tends to enter the pleural space from the parietal pleura and be absorbed by the visceral pleural lymphatics and capillaries. However, the parietal pleura contains many stomas, and parietal lymphatics may absorb fluid.[5] Absorption via parietal lymphatics is encouraged by the movement of the intercostal and diaphragmatic musculature and the lungs. Parietal lymphatics may play an important role in cases of pleural effusion in which pulmonary capillary absorption decreases or cannot maintain absorption in the face of high-volume effusion.

Pathophysiology

Abnormal fluid accumulation occurs upon alterations in hydrostatic pressure, osmotic pressure, vascular permeability, or with lymphatic dysfunction. Increased systemic hydrostatic pressure, as with right-sided congestive heart failure, may lead to increased fluid production. Decreased osmotic pressure, as in hypoalbuminemia, will affect fluid reabsorption in that the osmotic pressure of the vascular system is decreased, which decreases the gradient favoring fluid resorption by the parietal

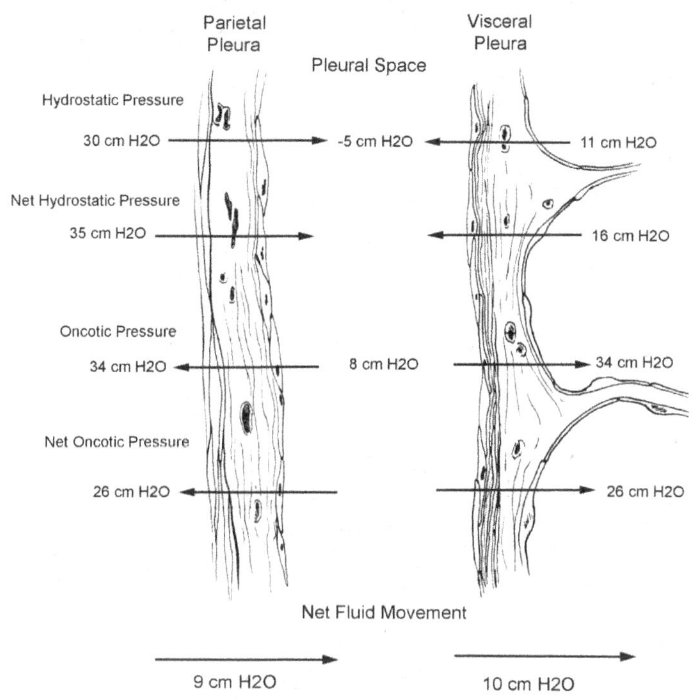

Figure 57-1. Forces and resultant gradients responsible for pleural fluid production and absorption. (Adapted from Pathophysiology in Small Animal Surgery, MJ Bojrab (ed). Philadelphia: Lea & Febiger, 1981.)

and visceral pleura. Inflammatory conditions of the pleural space lead to increased vascular permeability, increasing pleural fluid production. Concurrent vascular or lymphatic obstruction may alter hydrostatic pressures and lymphatic reabsorption of fluid. Lymphatic obstruction owing to reduction of flow or obstruction at the lymphaticovenous junction also decreases pleural fluid resorption and may lead to the leakage of fluid from the thoracic duct(s).

Other factors, such as trauma, neoplasia, or focal conditions may cause fluid accumulation by different forces. Generalized increases in hydrostatic pressure are not present, for example, in cases of lung lobe torsion, but a localized severe increase in hydrostatic pressure will cause fluid accumulation. Trauma to blood vessels or hemorrhage from abnormal blood vessels (e.g., neoplasia) leads to the accumulation of blood within the pleural space. Alterations in coagulation may also result in hemothorax from minimal trauma.

Types of Pleural Effusion

Pleural fluid is generally classified into three categories based on the protein concentration, cell count, and potentially the types of cells present and specific gravity of the fluid. Classification of the fluid is usually the first step in developing the definitive diagnosis of the condition. When the signalment, history, physical findings, and fluid type are combined with the laboratory classification of the fluid, the differential list is narrowed dramatically, and the etiology becomes apparent.

Laboratory classification of fluid includes transudate, modified transudate, and exudate. The protein content and cell count increase along the classification scheme. Some variation exists in the literature, but general divisions in protein content and cell numbers are listed in Table 57-1. The etiology of fluid accumulation is not included in this classification scheme. Further diagnostic testing may elucidate the cause of effusion and ultimately its diagnosis. Clinically useful classification of pleural fluid includes pure transudate, serosanguineous, sanguineous (or hemorrhagic), inflammatory, chylous, and neoplastic. Differentials for each type of effusion are listed in Table 57-2.

Pure Transudate

Pure transudates most often develop secondary to hypoproteinemia. Lack of serum protein, mainly albumin, results in decreased oncotic pressure of the vascular system. Lack of oncotic pressure results in increased fluid leakage (increased production) and decreased reabsorption, which causes fluid accumulation in the pleural space. Decreased protein production may be due to hepatic dysfunction, starvation, or severe nutritional deficiency. Significant protein loss may occur with conditions such as protein-losing enteropathy or nephropathy. Congestive heart failure may also result in production of a pure pleural transudate via increased hydrostatic pressure, but more often heart failure is associated with a modified transudate. Any chronic pure transudate may become modified over time; therefore, transudative etiologies must be considered in the diagnostic plan for a modified transudate.

Table 57-1. Laboratory Classification of types of Pleural Fluid

Type	Protein (g/dl)	Specific Gravity	Cell Ct. (x10^9/L)	Cytology
Transudate	< 3	< 1.018	< 3	Mesothelial, macrophages, lymphocytes
Modified Transudate	3-5		< 5	RBCs, lymphocytes, mesothelial cells
Exudate	> 3	> 1.018	> 7 Septic 30-200 Non-septic 5-15	Neutrophils (degenerate if septic)

Table 57-2. Clinical Classification and Etiologies of Pleural Effusion

Type	Etiology	Type	Etiology
Transudate	Congestive heart failure	Inflammatory	Idiopathic
	Hypoproteinemia		Foreign body
	Ascites associated effusion		Trauma
	Hyperthyroidism		Esophageal or tracheal disruption
Serosanguineous	Lung lobe torsion		Surgery
	Diaphragmatic hernia		Thoracocentesis
	Pericardial effusion		Systemic infection
	Neoplasia		Mediastinitis
	Thromboembolism		Extension of cervical infection
Sanguineous	Trauma		Pulmonary abscess
	Surgery		Pancreatitis
	Neoplasia		Feline infectious peritonitis
	Coagulopathy	Neoplastic	Mesothelioma
Chylous	Idiopathic		Primary or secondary pulmonary tumor
	Congestive heart failure		Heart-base tumor
	Neoplasia		Carcinomatosis
	Trauma		Lymphosarcoma
	Cranial vena caval compression or obstruction		Other neoplasia
	Fungal infection		
	Dirofilariasis		
	Congenital anomaly		

Serosanguineous Effusion

Serosanguineous effusion most often is concurrently categorized as a modified transudate. Red blood cell numbers, and thus the hematocrit, of the fluid are far below that of the peripheral blood. Many conditions can result in serosanguineous effusion via different pathologic routes. Lung lobe torsion causes venous and lymphatic occlusion in the presence of intact arterial blood flow. This results in significant increased hydrostatic pressure and increased production of pleural fluid. Lymphatic absorption is concurrently decreased. The initial effusion associated with lung lobe torsion may be sanguineous; however, lung lobe torsion may be primary or secondary.[5] Suspension of pulmonary parenchyma in a pre-existing pleural effusion may predispose more mobile lung lobes, such as the right middle lobe or caudal lung lobes, to twist around their long axis.[5] Primary effusion, such as chylothorax, must be ruled out, as pneumolobectomy will not result in resolution of the effusion. Diaphragmatic hernia with hepatic entrapment may similarly cause venous and lymphatic obstruction. Fluid leaks from the congested hepatic parenchyma. Pericardial effusion resulting in cardiac tamponade and right-sided heart failure cause increased fluid production owing to increased vascular hydrostatic pressure. Neoplasia can result in a variety of effusions via lymphatic or vascular obstruction, decreasing serum protein concentrations, or by inciting inflammation. Diffuse neoplasia such as mesothelioma or carcinomatosis commonly results in serosanguineous effusion. Lastly, idiopathic pleuritis and pleural effusion has been diagnosed in both dogs and cats. It is most often associated with a modified transudate.[6]

Sanguineous Effusion

Hemorrhage into the pleural space is commonly associated with trauma, which may be blunt, penetrating, or surgical. The packed cell volume of the blood in the effusion is similar to that of the periphery, but owing to rapid defibrination, it may not clot. The source of iatrogenic hemorrhage depends on the approach taken and the procedures performed. Intercostal, internal thoracic, pulmonary, pericardial, mediastinal, and cardiac vasculature are all possible sources. Intercostal vessels are at risk during lateral thoracotomy, which may also traumatize the internal thoracic vessels if extended ventrally on the thorax. The other vessels may be traumatized depending on the procedure done and the condition of the structures. Mediastinal vessels may be increased in size and number with inflammatory conditions of the thorax. Tumors within the chest can erode into vessels or adjacent tissue, leading to significant hemorrhage. Common tumors include chemodectoma, which may invade adjacent great vessels, and hemangiosarcoma of the right atrial appendage. Certain tumors (e.g., hemangiosarcoma) or diffuse neoplasia can be associated with disseminated intravascular coagulopathy and hemothorax.

Life-threatening hemorrhage of any etiology requires aggressive stabilization and potentially surgical intervention. Blood loss and atelectasis must both be considered prior to surgical intervention. Supportive care and stabilization are appropriate and may preclude surgery, allowing for reabsorption of blood from the pleural space. Autotransfusion may be considered as well, as contamination of the effusion with bacteria is rare. Neoplastic cells may be present in the transfusate, and the long-term prognosis should be considered in light of the need for autotransfusion. It is unlikely that the neoplastic cells in the transfusate will significantly decrease prognosis in a case of neoplasia-induced hemothrax.[3]

Chylous Effusion

Chylothorax is usually grossly apparent, as the fluid is milky white or white with a pink hue. Chyle is classified as a modified transudate with protein values usually less than 4 g/dl, cell counts less than 7000/ml, and specific gravity less than 1.032.[2] The cells may be predominantly lymphocytes, but with time nondegenerate neutrophils may be more numerous. A definitive diagnosis is made by comparing serum triglyceride and cholesterol levels with those of the effusion. Triglyceride is higher and cholesterol lower in the fluid compared with serum levels. Pseudochylous effusion in which the cholesterol level is elevated compared with serum, triglyceride content is low, and chylomicrons are not present has been described in people but not in dogs or cats. Other diagnostic tests include staining chylomicrons in the fluid with Sudan black or performing an ether clearance test. Pleural fluid is placed into two tubes and both are alkalinized with potassium hydroxide. Ether is added to one tube and tap water to the other. The ether will cause clearance of the opacity, water will not.

Chylous effusion can result from any condition that increases hydrostatic pressure in the cranial vena cava; obstruction or relative obstruction of the lymphaticovenous junction leads to dilation and leakage from the thoracic lymphatics. Pulmonary lymphatics may also be a source of chylous effusion.[7] Blunt or penetrating trauma can cause chylothorax, but the thoracic duct is expected to heal spontaneously.[8] Other conditions associated with chylothorax are listed in Table 57-1. Specific conditions include cardiomyopathy, mediastinal masses (e.g., lymphosarcoma and thymoma), dirofilariasis, blastomycosis, jugular venous thrombosis, diaphragmatic hernia, pericardial effusion, congenital anomalies (e.g., tetrology of Fallot, tricuspid dysplasia, cor triatriatum dexter, or a thoracic duct anomaly), and heart-based tumors. Despite the numerous conditions associated with chylothorax, the most common cause is idiopathic and is associated with thoracic lymphangiectasia. Afghan hounds and Siamese cats may be affected more often than other breeds, and lung lobe torsion may be associated with long-standing chylous effusion.

The etiology of the effusion is determined by performing thoracic radiographs after removal of the effusion to rule out mass lesions. Failure of the lungs to expand after therapeutic thoracocentesis suggests fibrosing pleuritis. Fibrin deposition on the visceral pleura occurs secondary to chronic inflammation, which causes mesothelial cell changes. Cellular changes include altered permeability, increased desquamation, and coagulation cascade activation.[9] Increased collagen production and subsequent fibrosis with decreased fibrinolysis leads to constriction of the pulmonary parenchyma.[9] Decreased fibrinolysis may be a dilutional effect of the pleural fluid on plasminogen activator or may be due to alterations in mesothelial cell function.[9]

Ultrasound of the chest requires some fluid to obtain an acoustic window to evaluate structures in the mediastinum; the heart and its function should also be examined. Routine blood work may show lymphopenia and hypoproteinemia secondary to loss into the effusion. Diagnostic testing should be complete before backing into the most frequently diagnosed etiology – idiopathic chylothorax. Cases of idiopathic chylothorax usually also undergo further imaging with lymphangiography, which is traditionally performed by catheterizing an intestinal lymphatic vessel. Water-soluble contrast is injected at a dose of 1 ml/kg diluted 1:1 in sterile saline. Thoracic radiographs are taken to identify the number and location of thoracic duct branches to be ligated. Post-ligation lymphangiography is used to confirm complete occlusion of all duct branches.[10]

Inflammatory Effusion

Inflammation of the pleural space may or may not be associated with infection. Nonseptic effusions are usually associated with a much lower nucleated cell count than is septic inflammation (Table 57-1). Lymphocytes, macrophages, and neutrophils may be present; degenerative changes of the neutrophils occur with septic inflammation. Septic exudate filling the pleural space is referred to as "pyothorax" or "thoracic empyema." Fluid accumulation secondary to inflammation is a result of increased production owing to vasodilation and increased vascular permeability. Decreased fluid reabsorption may also occur owing to increased oncotic pressure of the pleural space and thickening of the pleura as the condition becomes more chronic.

Nonseptic inflammation may be caused by infectious diseases (e.g., feline infectious peritonitis), chronic chylous effusion, diaphragmatic herniation of abdominal organs, neoplasia, or abdominal conditions such as pancreatitis. The inflammatory effusion associated with pancreatitis may be a result of the localized inflammation associated with the diaphragm and release of pancreatic enzymes known to cause localized fat necrosis and inflammation.[3] The exudate associated with feline infectious peritonitis is high in protein (5-12 g/dl) and specific gravity (> 1.017); the nucleated cells are usually nondegenerate neutrophils, but with chronicity, macrophages, plasma cells, and lymphocytes appear.[1] Chronic diaphragmatic hernia, chronic chylothorax, and chronic lung lobe torsion may also cause nonseptic inflammation. Fungal and bacterial cultures should be pursued in any case of pleural exudation to rule out the possibility of an infectious process, even if organisms are not apparent on cytologic examination. Idiopathic pleural effusion has also been associated with exudative effusion.[6]

Septic inflammation is primarily traumatic in origin. The route of bacterial access to the pleural space may be extension from any of the following: penetrating thoracic wall trauma, esophageal trauma or foreign body, tracheal trauma, foreign body inhalation and migration through the small airways or lung, caudal cervical trauma or infection leading to mediastinitis, repeated thoracocentesis, or cervical or thoracic surgery. Extension from a systemic infection, pneumonia, or rupture of a pulmonary abscess less commonly results in a septic pleural exudate. Both aerobic and anaerobic cultures should be performed on any pleural exudate.

Exudates are most often polymicrobial, and anaerobes are common in polymicrobial pleural infection.[11] Special care should be taken to evaluate and culture for *Actinomyces* and *Nocardia*, which are frequently present in chronic septic exudates.[12]

Neoplastic Effusion

Obstruction of vessels and lymphatics, inflammation, decreased serum albumin, and increased oncotic pressure within the pleural space may all contribute to fluid accumulation associated with a neoplastic condition within the pleural space. Specific tumor types erode vessels (e.g., hemangiosarcoma) to cause hemorrhagic effusion or may obstruct or erode into the thoracic duct (e.g., mediastinal neoplasia) to cause chylous effusion. Diffuse neoplasia may be primary, as with mesothelioma, or secondary, as in cases of carcinomatosis. Diffuse neoplasia usually results in the accumulation of a modified transudate; however, neoplastic cells are rarely identified within the fluid. Cytologic evaluation rarely provides the diagnosis of neoplasia, because reactive mesothelial cells display many characteristics of neoplasia, making the two cell types difficult to differentiate. The diagnosis may require more invasive techniques with tissue sampling for histopathologic examination.

Clinical Signs

Pleural fluid accumulation usually results in tachypnea owing to the lack of pulmonary expansion. The ventilatory pattern is referred to as "restrictive," and is characterized by rapid and shallow ventilation in an effort to maintain minute ventilation. The duration and rapidity of fluid accumulation will determine the severity of clinical signs. Animals with a small amount of effusion may be asymptomatic. Likewise, a slow accumulation of fluid allows the animal to compensate and adapt to the change in residual capacity until stressed by activity, increased ambient temperature, or anxiety. The rapid accumulation of a large volume of pleural fluid results in more severe signs such as an acute onset of tachypnea, dyspnea, and/or collapse. Cyanosis, orthopnea, and a distended thoracic cage may also occur with large volumes of pleural fluid. Other clinical signs accompanying pleural effusion include exercise intolerance, cough, lethargy, inappetance, reluctance to lie down, and weight loss. Additional clinical signs may depend on the etiology of the effusion.

Physical examination findings consistent with pleural effusion include a restrictive ventilatory pattern and diminished heart and lung sounds, especially ventrally. Bronchovesicular sounds may be increased dorsally. The chest may sound dull on percussion, or percussion may demonstrate a fluid line. Cats may exhibit apparent "breath holding" in which inspiration seems forced and exhalation is somewhat delayed. Fever may accompany exudative effusions, a heart murmur, jugular venous distention, hepatomegaly, ascites, or lymphadenopathy may be present depending on the primary disease process.

Conclusion

Noncardiogenic pleural effusions should be approached based on their type (transudate, modified transudate, etc.) and etiology. The forces resulting in the accumulation of fluid include decreased oncotic pressure, increased hydrostatic pressure, increased vascular permeability, abnormal lymphatic function or permeability, and relative lymphatic volume overload. These forces should be understood, as they are vital in the diagnosis of pleural effusion. Sampling of the pleural fluid provides the type of effusion, prompts further specific testing, and narrows the list of possible causes. Definitive diagnosis then allows for the development of therapeutic options and provides a prognosis for the patient.

References

1. Silverstein DC: Pleural space disease. *In* Textbook of Respiratory Disease in Dogs and Cats. King LG (ed). Philadelphia: Saunders, 2004, p. 49.

2. Fossum TW: Small Animal Surgery. St. Louis: Mosby, 2004, pp. 788-820.

3. Birchard SJ: Noncardiogenic pleural effusion. *In* Disease Mechanisms in Small Animal Surgery. Borjab MJ (ed). Philadelphia: Lea & Febiger, 1993, p. 404.

4. Bezuidenhout AJ: The lymphatic system. *In* Miller's Anatomy of the Dog. Evans HE (ed). Philadelphia: WB Saunders, 1993, p. 717.

5. Neath PJ, Brockman DJ, King LG: Lung lobe torsion in dogs: 22 cases (1981-1999). J Am Vet Med Assoc 217:1041, 2000.

6. Kovak JR, Ludwig LL, Bergman PJ, et al: Use of thoracoscopy to determine the etiology of pleural effusion in dogs and cats: 18 cases (1998-2001). J Am Vet Med Assoc 221:990, 2002.

7. Bilbrey SA, Birchard SJ: Pulmonary lymphatics in dogs with experimentally induced chylothorax. J Am Anim Hosp Assoc 30:86, 1994.

8. Hodges CC, Fossum TW, Evering W: Evaluation of thoracic duct healing after experimental laceration and transection. Vet Surg 22:431-5, 1993.

9. Fossum TW: Feline chylothorax. Comp Cont Educ Pract Vet 15:549, 1993.

10. Fossum TW, Mertens MM, Miller MW, et al: Thoracic duct ligation and pericardectomy for treatment of idiopathic chylothorax. J Vet Intern Med 18:307, 2004.

11. Walker AL, Jang SS, Hirsh DC: Bacteria associated with pyothorax of dogs and cats: 98 cases (1989-1998). J Am Vet Med Assoc 216:359-63, 2000.

12. Rooney MB, Monnet E: Medical and surgical treatment of pyothorax in dogs: 26 cases (1991-2001). J Am Vet Med Assoc 221:86, 2002.

Chapter 58

Thoracic Wall and Sternum

Dennis Olsen

The thoracic wall and sternum play an integral role in various normal physiologic processes that are essential in maintaining homeostasis. The physiologic roles of the thoracic wall and sternum include housing and protecting the thoracic viscera as well as providing the semirigid framework that supports respiratory effort and function. When the functions of the wall and sternum are altered through malformation (congenital or acquired) or trauma, homeostasis can be disrupted with results ranging from inconsequential to catastrophic. Therefore, it is incumbent on the veterinarian to understand the normal functions of the thoracic wall and sternum as well as to recognize potential consequences when these functions are disrupted. Unfortunately, clinical signs that indicate the presence of thoracic wall pathology may be either overshadowed by concurrent, more obvious, clinical signs from separate problems or be insidious in presentation and relatively difficult to detect.

Thoracic wall trauma is considered to be more common than congenital and acquired deformities,[1] and traumatic injuries to the thoracic wall can be categorized as blunt or penetrating.[1-4] Blunt injuries to the thoracic wall result from vehicle accidents, adverse interactions with other animals or humans, falling from heights, and crushing injuries. The pliant nature of the thoracic wall in small animals has been suggested as a primary reason that blunt trauma may not always be manifest by visible pathology to the thoracic wall.[5-10] However, owing to the enclosure of vital thoracic organs, absence of visibly obvious pathology does not preclude the possibility of damage to these organs. Many reports have indicated that injury to pulmonary and cardiac tissues are common sequelae to blunt injury despite the lack of visible damage to the thoracic wall.[2,11-13] When injuries to the thoracic wall are apparent, it should be assumed that damage to the underlying organs has also occurred, and therapy addressing this damage may take priority over other less threatening injuries. Pulmonary damage, alterations of the pleural space, disruption of tracheobronchial structures, damage to the heart and great vessels, and diaphragm rupture are common potential sequelae to blunt thoracic trauma.

Penetrating injuries to the thoracic wall are not as common as blunt injury and result from high- and low-velocity projectiles, animal bites, and impalement (accidental or purpose driven). The integrity of the pleural space and underlying organs becomes a primary concern in that loss of the integrity and function can be rapidly fatal. Penetrating wounds must also be considered contaminated and the potential for infection realized.[3] The degree of trauma resulting from penetration is dependent on several factors. Among these are the type of tissue, the mass, shape, size, and velocity of the penetrating object, and the behavior of the object on penetration.[14,15] Generally speaking, the more kinetic energy transmitted to the tissues, the greater the tissue damage will be. This generalization, however, does not take into account that vital functions may be completely disrupted by even relatively little tissue damage, depending on the organ involved. Penetrating wounds to the thoracic wall alone would rarely be a cause of major concern if not for the role the thoracic wall plays in respiration and in protecting vital organs.

Deformities of the thoracic wall and sternum, as previously mentioned, are much less common than is traumatic injury.[1] The pathologic results of deformities can alter normal physiologic function of the chest wall and major organ systems housed within the thoracic cavity.[1,3,6,16] However, such disruption of function is not common and is relative to the severity of the deformity. Congenital deformities include pectus excavatum, pectus carinatum, and various rib and spinal deformities. Finding a significant congenital deformity of the thoracic wall and/or sternum is not an automatic indication for surgical or medical intervention because in many cases those affected are asymptomatic.[16,17] Acquired deformities of the thoracic wall may be a result of neoplasia or infection. Neoplastic disorders may arise from soft tissue or skeletal structures of the thorax or be a metastatic extension from a distant site.[17] Infections can result from bacterial or fungal invasion secondary to chest wall trauma or migrating foreign bodies. These infections can present as mass lesions or can disrupt the integrity of the thoracic wall, leading to pleural space and possibly pulmonary disease.

In this chapter, I focus on the basics of anatomy and physiology to provide sufficient information for the reader to recognize pathophysiology of selected disorders of the thoracic wall and sternum.

Anatomy

The thoracic cage provides the dorsal, lateral, and ventral peripheral boundaries of the thoracic cavity, which contains all or part of the heart and great vessels, lungs, pleurae and pleural space, trachea, esophagus, thymus, lymph nodes, and nerves of the somatic and autonomic systems. Also protected by the thoracic cage are the diaphragm, liver, gall bladder, stomach, and all or part of the spleen, right kidney and adrenal gland, intestines, and abdominal extensions of the great vessels and autonomic nerves.[18] The morphology of the thoracic wall can generally be described as a laterally compressed cone with the base as the caudal extent and the apex cranial. The lateral compression results in a greater dimension in the dorsoventral direction.[16,18] The skeletal components include the sternum, thoracic vertebral bodies, and ribs. The sternum is composed of 8 individual bones called sternebrae, which make up the floor of the thoracic cage. The cranial- and caudal-most sternebrae are specifically designated as the manubrium and xiphoid process, respectively. Interposed between the sternebrae are cartilaginous plates, and extending caudally from the xiphoid process is the flattened xiphoid cartilage. The dorsal aspect of the thoracic cage is formed by the 13 thoracic vertebral bodies and the vertebral extremities of the ribs. Thirteen pairs of ribs constitute the lateral walls of the thoracic cage, each with osseous dorsal and cartilaginous ventral components. Each rib has synovial articulations dorsally with the vertebrae in two locations, the head with the vertebral bodies (or body) at or near the intervertebral disc and the tubercle with the transverse process. Ventrally the first 9 pairs of ribs have synovial articulations with the sternum. The first pair with the manubrium, pairs 2 to 7 with the corresponding intersternebral cartilage plates, and pairs 8 and 9 share an articulation site at the last intersternebral cartilage. Pairs 10 to 12 attach to the preceding rib through the ventral costal cartilages and form the costal arch. The 13th pair are commonly known as floating ribs because they do not articulate with the sternum and the ventral cartilaginous portions are enclosed in the surrounding abdominal muscles.[6,16,18] The diverging nature of the sternum and vertebral bodies and the increasing arch of the ribs from cranial to caudal account for the aforementioned cone shape.[18]

The soft tissue components of the thoracic wall include the costal parietal pleura, the endothoracic and external thoracic fasciae, and various muscles that are important structurally as well as functionally for respiration. The parietal pleura is a serous membrane that has a layer of mesothelial cells supported by a layer of delicate elastic fibers. The parietal pleura also lines the surface of the diaphragm.[18,19] The parietal pleura is supported by the endothoracic fascia which is deep to the thoracic musculature. The external thoracic fascia covers the external surfaces of the muscles and the chest wall.[18]

The intercostal muscles are confined within the space between each rib. Closest to the parietal pleura are the internal intercostals. These muscles extend from the cranial borders of ribs 2 to 13 and course in a cranioventral direction to insert on the caudal border of the preceding rib.[16,18] In the interosseous area of the thoracic cage, this arrangement results in the ribs being pulled in a caudal direction. Other muscles of the thoracic wall also function to pull the ribs caudally. These include the external intercostals of the caudal-most interspaces, rectus abdominus muscles on the ventral aspect, the costal portions of the external abdominal oblique muscle at the ventrolateral aspect of the chest wall, the caudal portion of the serratus dorsalis located caudodorsally, and the transverses thoracis on the internal surface of the ventral thorax.[16,18,20,21] The external intercostals, as the name implies, lie lateral or external to the internal intercostals. These muscles arise from the caudal border of ribs 1 to 12 and course caudoventrally to insert on the cranial border of the succeeding rib.[16,18] The fibers run at a right angle to the fibers of the internal intercostals and in the craniodorsal interspaces have essentially the opposite action, that of pulling the ribs cranially. The other muscles of the thoracic wall that pull ribs cranially include the interchondral portion of the internal intercostals, rectus thoracis located cranioventrally, the scalenus on the ventrolateral aspect, and the cranial portion of the serratus dorsalis on the dorsolateral aspect of the chest wall.[16,18,20,21] The other muscles that cover the thoracic wall and function in mobility of the spine and thoracic limb include the epaxial muscles over the dorsal thoracic region, the serratus ventralis on the craniolateral surface, the rhomboideus and trapezius muscles over the craniodorsal walls, the pectoral muscles on the ventral surface, and the latissimus dorsi along the lateral wall.[16,18] Finally, loose subcutaneous tissues, the cutaneous trunci muscle and the skin form the outer layers and covering of the thoracic wall.

Vascular supply to the thoracic wall is generally through the intercostal arteries and veins. The arteries originate either from the costocervical trunk or the dorsal intercostals from the thoracic aorta and course along the caudal border of the ribs to anastomose with the ventral intercostal arteries arising from the internal thoracic arteries that lie on the internal surface of the ventral thoracic wall. Branches of the ventral intercostals can be found on the cranial and caudal aspect of the ribs. The intercostal veins course with the arteries along the caudal border of the ribs and drain into the azygous vein between the vertebral bodies and thoracic aorta.[18]

Innervation to the thoracic wall is primarily from branches of the thoracic spinal nerves. The intercostals nerves arise from the ventral branches and course with the arteries and veins along the caudal border of the ribs.[18]

Physiology

Respiration can be divided into four major functions: pulmonary ventilation, diffusion of O_2 and CO_2 between alveoli and the blood, transport of O_2 and CO_2 within the blood to the cells of the body, and regulation of ventilation.[22] The anatomic morphology of the thoracic wall contributes primarily to pulmonary ventilation. The cone-like shape of the thoracic cage and the muscle attachments allow for expansion and contraction of the thoracic cavity. Because the diaphragm is located near the base of the "cone," as it contracts the craniocaudal dimension of the thoracic cavity is increased. The combination of rib morphology, rib articulation with the spine and sternum, and thoracic wall musculature lead to a "bucket-handle" type of motion to the ribs.[6,23] As the ribs are pulled in a cranial direction by thoracic wall muscles, the sternum moves further away from the spine and the arches of the ribs become more abaxially positioned. This results in an increase in both the dorsoventral and lateral dimensions of the thoracic cavity. Those muscles that function to pull the ribs cranially are called muscles of inspiration while those that pull the ribs caudally are muscles of expiration.

By convention it has been thought that the external and internal intercostal muscles have distinctly inspiratory and expiratory functions, respectively. This convention has changed and the individual effects of these muscles on respiration are determined more by topography and nervous input.[20,21] It is now thought that the external intercostals in the craniodorsal interspaces and the interchondral portion of the internal intercostals (a.k.a. parasternal intercostals) are inspiratory and pull the ribs in a cranial direction.[20,21]

The parasternal intercostal contribution to the cranial movement of the ribs is estimated at approximately 80%.[24] The interosseous portion of the internal intercostals and the external intercostals of the caudal-most interspaces are expiratory and pull the ribs caudally.[20,21]

The pleural space contained within the thoracic cavity is, in actuality, only a potential space. This is because the subatmospheric or negative pressure within the space keeps the pulmonary pleura held in contact with the parietal pleura of the thoracic wall. This negative pressure is created by fluid movement into and out of the pleural space.[22] Starling's forces and pleural membranes that are porous allow protein-containing interstitial fluid to transude into and out of the pleural space. The net effect of capillary hydrostatic pressures and colloid osmotic pressures between systemic capillaries and pulmonary capillaries favors flow from the systemic capillaries through the pleural space and absorption into the pulmonary capillaries. As the volume of fluid increases above that which is necessary for lubrication of the pleural surfaces, the lymphatic vessels pump excess fluid away. The pumping action of the lymphatic system helps to produce the negative intrapleural pressure. Fluid flow dynamics and the lymphatic actions produce a "liquid coupling" between the pulmonary and parietal pleural surfaces. This coupling allows complete transmission of changes in the thoracic cavity volume to the lungs.[19] So, as thoracic cavity dimensions are increased in response to respiratory muscle action, the lungs are able to expand.

The thoracic wall and lungs have an elastic nature that is independent of each other. Without fluid coupling, the thoracic wall would expand to a point where, when relaxed, a specific thoracic volume (V_0) would exist.[6] When muscles of inspiration increase the thoracic volume above V_0, the thoracic wall has a tendency to recoil inward until V_0 is reached. If thoracic volume is less than V_0, the thoracic wall has a tendency to spring outward, again until Vo is reached.[6] The elastic nature of the lungs, without fluid coupling, would result in an inward collapse to a point where only a residual volume of air remained. The opposing elastic recoil of the thoracic wall and lungs, with fluid coupling, has a point where balance is achieved. That is, the inherent tendency of the lungs to collapse is prevented by the inherent tendency of the thoracic wall to spring outward and vice versa. At this point of balance, the thoracic volume is less than V_0 and the volume within the lungs is the functional residual capacity (FRC).[6,23] When the muscles of inspiration cause expansion of the thoracic volume, the lungs also expand owing to fluid coupling. This results in an increase in the negative pleural pressure, which generates negative pressure within the airways and alveoli relative to the atmosphere (transpulmonary pressure) and allows air to flow into the lungs. Because the thoracic volume is held to less than V_0, the inherent tendency of the thoracic wall to spring outward actually assists in the inspiratory effort until V_0 is reached or exceeded. Then, when inspiratory muscle contraction ceases, the thorax passively returns to the point of balance.

The change in volume of the lungs and thoracic cavity in response to changes in pressure is called compliance.[6,22,23] The compliance of the lungs and the thoracic wall together make up the total compliance of the pulmonary system. When the ability of either the thoracic wall or the lungs to change volume in response to change in pressure occurs, the total compliance will change. The effort required to generate sufficient negative transpulmonary pressure to overcome the compliance of the pulmonary system and the resistance to airflow within the airways for inspiratory flow or to overcome resistance to expiratory flow is the work of respiration. The work of respiration will be altered if compliance is altered.[1,6] If thoracic wall compliance is decreased because of trauma or disease, the work of respiration will increase.

Trauma

Blunt Trauma

Blunt trauma to the thorax induces tissue injury by transference of the kinetic energy of the impacting object to the chest wall without creating an opening between the pleural space and thoracic organs and the external environment. The greater the kinetic energy transmitted the greater potential for damage to the thorax. Additionally, the energy is also transferred to the thoracic organs with potential damage to those organs. Direct trauma produces crush and shear injury to the soft tissues and skeletal structures. Low-speed trauma produces a localized crushing injury to the tissues.[1] With this type of trauma the skin may appear relatively undamaged owing to the resilience of the cutaneous epithelium. Underlying tissues such as muscle and bone however, may exhibit a greater degree of damage. Muscle tissue is extremely sensitive to pressure.[25] This sensitivity can result in muscle damage with localized rhabdomyolysis, and myoglobin, potassium, phosphorus, and creatinine phosphokinase are released into the surrounding tissues. When more than 200 grams of muscle are injured, the serum myoglobin levels can be increased and myoglobin may be detected in the urine.[26] Despite the fact that myoglobinemia is rapidly cleared, it must be remembered that the products of myoglobin breakdown are nephrotoxic.[27,28] Skeletal muscle contains more potassium than any other body structure.[29] Extensive damage to muscle tissue with muscle necrosis can lead to hyperkalemia.[30] Phosphorus can leak from damaged muscle tissue and contribute to hyperphosphatemia.[31] Creatinine phosphokinase is an enzyme released from damaged muscle; an increase in levels of creatinine phosphokinase is a sensitive indicator of muscle injury from any cause, and the increase will parallel the degree of damage. Muscle that has been injured in this manner becomes edematous and swollen and looses its elasticity and ability to contract efficiently. This decreases the compliance of the thoracic wall and, therefore, increases the work of respiration. However, the resulting pain may contribute to a decreased respiratory effort, which may contribute to hypoventilation.

Higher speed trauma produces shearing injury in addition to crushing.[1] Shearing injury results when two adjacent tissues with different specific gravities are suddenly accelerated or decelerated.[1,32] Because of the specific gravity variation, the momentum of the tissues during the abrupt change is also different. This generates shear forces at the junction of the two tissues. If the shear forces exceed the inherent elasticity of the tissue junction, the result will be a separation between the tissues. Although soft tissue damage of the thoracic wall is rarely a major cause of morbidity or mortality,[1] it is critical to remember that the kinetic energy of the impact is also transmitted to the thoracic organs, and crush and shear injuries may occur to these structures.

The resistance of skeletal structures of the thoracic cage to injury through blunt trauma is attributed to inherent resilience.[2,4,6,9] Despite this resilience, the lack of obvious skeletal damage does not preclude the possibility of severe, even life-threatening soft tissue or thoracic organ damage because considerable force is required to induce fracture and that force is also transmitted to the thoracic organs. Blunt trauma that results in fractures of the thoracic cage most commonly is from a direct force applied to the lateral body wall resulting in rib fractures.[4] Ventral-dorsal compression of the thorax from bite wounds or falls from heights can result in sternal and rib fractures, but these are considered rare.[4,33] Research has shown that local bending and shear are some of the primary loading modes during impact trauma.[34] When the force or load applied to skeletal components exceeds the ultimate strength, the failure point is reached and a fracture is produced. Interestingly, the rate at which a force is applied to the cortical bone of ribs will affect the material characteristics of the bone. The ultimate strength of the bone is lower if the load is applied slowly. Conversely, high-speed application results in a higher ultimate strength. This property is known as viscoelasticity.[35] This property can affect the amount of kinetic energy absorbed by the bone when a force is applied. Slow application of load to failure results in less kinetic energy absorbed and the resulting fracture will likely be a simple two-piece fracture with minimal energy released and subsequently minimal damage to the surrounding tissues. High-speed load to failure will result in an increase in absorbed kinetic energy and a more complex fracture with more surrounding tissue damage.[35] The proximity of the pleural space and lungs to the thoracic cage puts them at risk when a fracture occurs; the more complex the fracture, the higher the risk to these vital structures. Rib and sternal fractures alter the function of the thoracic cage by decreasing compliance. However, in simple nondisplaced fractures and displaced fractures that will not damage the underlying pleural space and lung, therapy should be directed at the underlying pulmonary damage and pain rather than at the fractures. If the fracture fragments endanger these vital organs, then therapy is directed at stabilization of the fragments.

Flail Chest

When the trauma to the thoracic wall is severe enough to fracture adjacent ribs (at least two) in two locations, the result is flail chest. This complex fracture eliminates the costal arch support of the section of thoracic wall between the fractures. The section "flails" asynchronously with normal thoracic motion and is characterized by inward displacement during inspiration and outward displacement during expiration. The degree of paradoxical motion is determined by the pleural pressure becoming more negative during inspiration and the action of the parasternal intercostal (interchondral internal intercostal) muscles which pulls the flail segment inward.[36,37] This paradoxical motion can be a dramatic clinical finding, which may overshadow the less apparent but clinically more significant damage to the thoracic organs. It has been shown in a nontraumatic model of flail chest in the canine that arterial blood gases and the respiratory pattern did not change while the flail segment existed. This suggests that the severe effects of traumatic flail chest are a result of pulmonary damage, pleural space disruption, and the accompanying pain from the trauma rather than the paradoxic motion of the flail segment.[5,38] Disruption of the thoracic wall from fractured ribs will decrease the compliance of the thoracic cage and the work of respiration will increase; however, the accompanying pain causes a restriction in the ventilatory efforts. Understanding the pathophysiology of flail chest has refocused primary therapy from flail segment stabilization to improving respiratory function and pain control.[1,5] If the trauma or fracture fragments have resulted in pleural space disruption or if they endanger the pulmonary parenchyma, it is important that therapy also include restoration of the pleural integrity and stabilization of the fractures.

Penetrating Trauma

Penetrating injury usually results when a mechanical force is abruptly applied to a focal area and the integrity of the thoracic wall and pleural space is breached. The resulting damage is from severe stretching and crushing of tissues in the direct path of penetration. Penetration of the thoracic wall itself would not be a primary cause of concern except that the pleural space and thoracic organs may be damaged. The severity of penetration injury depends on the resulting degree of dysfunction and the degree of damage to vital organs.

Low-velocity penetration injury is essentially limited to the confined area because relatively little energy is transferred from the penetrating object to the tissues. Simple bite wounds, stabs, arrows, and some pneumatically propelled projectiles are examples of low-velocity penetration. Cutaneous and subcutaneous tissue, muscle, fascia, and possibly bone are damaged in the path of penetration. When the parietal pleural layer is penetrated and direct communication with the external atmosphere occurs, the negative pressure within the pleural space is lost and air now fills the pleural space. Fluid coupling of the thoracic wall and parietal pleura with the visceral pleura and lung is disrupted and the inherent elasticity of the lung causes an inward collapse while the thoracic wall expands. The individual compliance of the lungs and thoracic wall decreases and the work of respiration necessarily increases. Without the assistance of the thoracic wall, the lungs are unable to expand adequately and the degree of negative transpulmonary pressure needed to allow efficient airflow into the airways is not generated. The result is an expanded thoracic cage and a compensatory rapid shallow respiratory pattern.[6]

Impalement injury is another type of low-velocity penetration in which a foreign object traverses and remains transfixed within the thoracic wall. This uncommon injury is generally the result of collision or impact between the body and an immovable object.[39] Even though this injury is classified as penetrating, it can be argued that there are characteristics of blunt trauma as well.[40,41] The distance and trajectory of the penetration dictate which (if any) thoracic organs or other body areas may also be involved. In impalement injury, the foreign object may fill the wound sufficiently such that the pleural space is effectively closed and also provide a tamponade effect to the surrounding organs or vessels.[4,42,43] It is recommended for this reason that the impaling object not be blindly removed from the body but left in place and stabilized for transport to a hospital for removal under direct visualization and controlled surgical conditions.[40-43] It may be necessary to cut and shorten the object for patient extrication and this should be done with extreme care so as not to cause further disruption or accidental dislodgement. Impaled wounds may be contaminated with unusual pathogens from the environment as well as with resident microorganisms from cutaneous tissues and potential hollow viscus disruption.[43]

Bites are a relatively common source of low-velocity penetrating thoracic wounds. Bite wounds, like impalement, also have characteristics of blunt trauma but they also introduce the potential of severe tearing injury away from the point of penetration owing to the scissor action of teeth and the shaking that may accompany a bite wound. The blunt trauma aspect of bite wounds to the thoracic wall is a relatively common source of fractures.[4,5,8] Tearing of the intercostal muscles and potential fracture can severely disrupt the thoracic wall and pleural space such that pulmonary herniation may occur.[6] Occasionally, the cutaneous epithelium may remain intact despite complete disruption of muscular and skeletal structures. When this occurs, the skin may move in a paradoxic manner and mimic flail chest.[6] As with other penetrating thoracic wounds, microorganism contamination is inevitable, with the possibility of subsequent infection. The spectrum of contaminating organisms includes normal cutaneous flora and numerous intraoral microorganisms.

Penetrating injury through high-velocity projectiles most commonly results from either accident or malicious intent. As mentioned previously, the amount of kinetic energy a penetrating object transfers to the tissues dictates the amount of damage. Several formulas calculate the amount of kinetic energy. The simplest of these is:

$$KE = 1/2\, mv^2$$

Where KE is the kinetic energy, m is the mass of the projectile and V is velocity.[44] As is readily seen from the equation, velocity is the most important factor when it comes to kinetic energy transfer and therefore tissue damage. The transfer of energy to the tissues produces injury in various ways. Lower velocity projectiles, such as those from air guns, damage tissues primarily through crushing and laceration. Higher velocity projectiles also have crushing and laceration components in the path of penetration, but they also produce a temporary cavity that is formed by forward acceleration of the tissues in the wake of the projectile, which causes radial stretch of the wound cavity. Cavitation can lacerate tissues, create contusions, damage vascular lining, and rupture large vessels. The greater the energy transferred to the tissue, the further from the bullet track these injuries will extend. Another method of injury is through shock waves that travel ahead of and to the sides of the projectile. At lower velocities these shock waves produce little damage, but at high velocity the pressure created can be significant.[14]

Another factor includes the type of tissue penetrated. The major characteristics of body tissues that influence the degree of damage are specific gravity (density) and elasticity.[14] These characteristics have differing influences on the degree of tissue damage when penetrated by a high-velocity projectile. Tissues that have a high specific gravity will incur greater damage whereas tissues that are highly elastic will have less damage. Muscle has a relatively high density and some elasticity and, therefore, is severely damaged. The variable density of bone may divert the trajectory of the projectile. If the bone is fractured by the projectile, the created fragments can in turn become projectiles.[45]

Structural Deformities

Pectus Excavatum

Pectus excavatum (PE) is a morphologic deformity of the thoracic wall characterized by sternal and costal cartilage abnormalities that can result in dorsoventral flattening of the thorax to concave deformation of the ventral thoracic wall.[1,3,6,16] Although the condition is generally considered congenital in small animals, the etiology is largely unknown. Various theories exist as to the cause, including defective development of cartilage and bone such that the sternum and costal cartilages are readily deformed by respiratory pressure gradients; anatomic variations in soft tissue attachments to the sternum; excessive costal cartilage growth; and abnormal intrauterine pressures.[1,3,46] Because PE is seen most commonly in brachycephalic dogs and Burmese cats and has been reported in cases of mucopolysaccharidosis, it is feasible that a genetic basis for the condition exists.[1,6,46-48] It is also possible that there is an acquired aspect of PE as can be seen in humans with upper airway obstruction.[1,46,49,50] In brachycephalic dogs the upper airway obstruction that results from brachycephalic airway syndrome may lead to an increase in the negative pleural pressure, which deforms the immature cartilage and bone of the thorax. Generally, the condition is localized in the caudal sternal area but cranial sternal deformities have also been reported.[51]

Patients with PE may show an increased work of respiration, and this suggests a decrease in the compliance of the pulmonary system. Abnormal anatomy of the sternum and costal cartilage will decrease compliance of the thoracic wall, and pulmonary compression will decrease pulmonary compliance. Clinically, this can be seen as varying degrees of tachypnea, exercise intolerance, dyspnea, and cyanosis. Other signs may include recurrent respiratory infection, cardiac murmurs, vomiting, weight loss, and decreased growth.[1,46] Deviation of the heart owing to PE can lead to heart murmurs, conduction abnormalities, and apparent enlargement.[1,6,16,46,52] It is important to differentiate potential congenital cardiac defects from the secondary effects of cardiac compression and malposition. Many of the clinical abnormalities associated with PE can be alleviated or eliminated by repair of the defect.

Diagnosis of PE is usually made by thoracic palpation. However, in some, the flattening of the chest is not as apparent as evidenced by diagnosis later in life when clinical signs indicate a potential cardiovascular or respiratory problem. Radiographs of the thorax can provide a means of objective measurement of the relative degree of PE. The frontosagital index is a ratio between the width of the chest at the 10th vertebral body and the dorsoventral measurement from the ventral surface of the 10th vertebra to the sternum. The range of normal ratios for nonbrachycephalic dogs is 0.8 to 1.4, for brachycephalic dogs is 1.0 to 1.5, and for cats is 0.7 to 1.3. The vertebral index has also been used and is calculated as the dorsoventral measurement from the dorsal surface of the vertebral body selected to the sternum and the dorsoventral measurement of the vertebral body itself. Nonbrachycephalic dogs have a vertebral index range of 11.8 to 19.6, brachycephalic dogs from 12.5 to 16.5, and cats from 12.6 to 18.8.[52] Although these measurements and ratios can help classify the degree of PE and help to determine anatomic improvement after repair procedures, they do not necessarily correlate to the severity of clinical presentation or physiologic abnormalities.[1]

Other Congenital Deformities

Pectus carinatum is essentially the reverse of pectus excavatum and is described as a protrusion deformity of the sternum.[16,53] Because the thoracic cage of small animals is laterally compressed, this condition would be inherently difficult to detect. In fact, to the author's knowledge, no cases have been reported in small animals. Other chest-wall deformities include missing ribs, extra ribs, and rib malformations. Toxin exposure in utero may lead to these types of abnormal skeletal formations.[54] Although there are scattered reports of such anomalies in the veterinary literature, they are often incidental findings. Severe spinal malformations such as scoliosis and kyphosis may lead to thoracic cage malformation and decreased compliance.[46] The abnormality may also lead to pulmonary restriction with decreased compliance and abnormal respiratory function.[55] These abnormalities are also rare, and reports in the veterinary literature are uncommon.

Acquired Deformities

Acquired deformities of the thoracic wall that lead to dysfunction are uncommon. Such deformities can present as mass lesions readily visible externally or as a mild chest-wall thickening with significant intrathoracic extension that leads to respiratory or cardiovascular dysfunction.[3,6,17] These deformities include primary chest-wall tumors, metastatic tumors, and pyogranulomatous or purulent infection.

Infection

The contaminating nature of penetrating wounds raises the potential of clinical infection at or near the site of the wound. The infectious process may produce cellulitis, abscesses, or granulomas. Various aerobic and anaerobic bacteria and fungal organisms have been isolated from thoracic-wall lesions. Migrating foreign bodies such as grass awns ("fox tails") may be the source of the infection, and the degree of tissue involvement can be extensive. Lesions from infectious microorganisms can adversely affect the function of localized areas of the thoracic wall through alteration of muscle action and destruction of musculoskeletal tissues. However, extension of the infection into the pleural space and organs of the thoracic cavity can produce more serious conditions such as pyothorax, lymphadenopathy, and pulmonary infiltration.[17] Therapy for infectious conditions may be simple drainage and appropriate antimicrobial medications, but it may require extensive debridement or excision of diseased tissue to facilitate resolution. In this case, therapy may also contribute to altered thoracic function.

Neoplasia

Tumors of the thoracic wall can originate from skeletal structures or soft tissues; the type of tumor will determine the biologic behavior. Although tumors of the thoracic wall are considered uncommon, it is important to differentiate between benign and malignant tumors in order to plan the appropriate therapy. Benign tumors can often be removed without wide or radical types of excision, and a cure can be expected. Malignant tumors should be removed with a variable margin of normal tissue, depending on the tumor type and the tissues involved. Those that have a high probability of recurrence should have large borders of normal tissue removed three dimensionally around the tumor.[56] The extent of the surgical excision may not only affect the function of the thoracic wall but will dictate the type of closure or thoracic wall reconstruction required.

Primary tumors affecting the supporting skeletal structures of the thoracic wall are malignant more often than they are benign.[1,3,6,16,46,57] Most authors report that osteosarcoma is the most common type of malignant rib tumor, with chondrosarcoma being second;[1,3,6,16,46,57] however, some authors have this order reversed.[17] The common site of occurrence in dogs for both types of tumor is the costochondral junction; rarely the sternum is the site.[1,3,16,57] These tumors are often firmly attached to other tissues of the thorax, making them relatively immobile. This characteristic may be an indication of malignancy.[46] Younger to middle-aged dogs seem to be affected more often with these tumors.[1,16,57,58] The occurrence of these tumors in this location in the cat is rare.[57]

The most common bone tumor in dogs is osteosarcoma; approximately 25% occur in the axial skeleton, with 10% of those occurring in the ribs.[59] Clinically, dogs with osteosarcoma of the thorax present with a palpable mass of the ribs or sternum that may be painful,[59] although many authors describe them as nonpainful.[16,17,57] Dyspnea has been reported as a clinical sign by various authors with suggestions that pulmonary impingement owing to intrathoracic extension, pleural effusion, and pulmonary metastasis may be the cause.[1,16,57,58] Others state that respiratory signs owing to these conditions are not commonly seen.[59] One characteristic that is generally agreed on is that the biologic behavior of osteosarcoma in the rib is similar to that in other locations. Locally, osteosarcoma is aggressive, with lysis and production of bone and replacement with neoplastic tissue.[59] Early metastasis is a hallmark of osteosarcoma with the lungs as the primary location for tumor spread.[6,57,58] This predilection for metastasis is responsible for the poor prognosis for osteosarcoma. The median survival times for patients treated by en bloc excision and excision plus adjunctive chemotherapy are 3 and 8 months, respectively.[59,60,61] The poor prognosis emphasizes the need for accurate diagnosis.

Chondrosarcoma seems to have a predilection for flat bones; it occurs in these 61% of the time.[59] In dogs, the range of occurrence on the ribs is from 6% to as high as 33%, according to various sources.[17,57] In cats, common locations near the thorax are the scapula and vertebrae; rarely, if ever, the ribs or sternum. Ostensibly not as aggressive as osteosarcoma, this tumor may attain large dimensions before diagnosis. It is locally invasive, invades the pleural space, and may cause pleural effusion.17 Metastasis is reported to be slower than with osteosarcoma and the prognosis is somewhat better.[17,59] A wide variation exists in reported median survival times for dogs with chondrosarcoma of the ribs, but they are considerably longer than with osteosarcoma, with sources reporting survival up to 1080 days.[59,61] As with osteosarcoma, therapy for chondrosarcoma is en bloc resection of the tumor with reconstruction of the thoracic wall if needed.

Metastatic neoplasms of the thoracic wall have been described and the ribs are considered a common site, whereas the sternum is rarely reported.[1,59] When metastasis to the ribs (and other bones) occurs, it seems to be localized near the diaphyseal area near the nutrient foramen rather than the costochondral junction.[17,59] The incidence of metastasis of osteosarcoma to other bones such as the ribs may be increased following chemotherapy regimens.[59]

Primary tumors of thoracic soft tissues include various sarcomas (e.g., fibrosarcoma, hemangiosarcoma, hemangiopericytoma, and malignant fibrous histiocytoma) and occasional discrete cell tumors (i.e., mast cell tumor).[3,46,62] Wide three-dimensional surgical excision is recommended for these tumors. If removal requires en bloc excision of the thoracic wall, reconstruction may be required.

References

1. Fossum TW: Thoracic Wall and Sternum: Diseases, Disruptions, and Deformities *In* Disease Mechanisms in Small Animal Surgery, 2nd ed. Bojrab MJ (ed). Philadelphia: Lea & Febiger, 1993, p. 411.

2. Cockshutt JR: Management of fracture-associated thoracic trauma. Vet Clin North Am Small Anim Pract 25:1031, 1995.

3. Sweet DC, Waters DJ: Role of surgery in the management of dogs with pathologic conditions of the thorax – part II. Comp Cont Educ Pract Vet 13:1671, 1991.

4. Spackman CJA, Caywood DD: Management of thoracic trauma and chest wall reconstruction. Vet Clin North Am Small Anim Pract 17:431, 1987.

5. Olsen D, Renberg W, Perrett J, et al: Clinical management of flail chest in dogs and cats: a retrospective study of 24 cases (1989-1999). J Am Anim Hosp Assoc 38:315, 2002.

6. Orton EC: Small Animal Thoracic Surgery. Philadelphia: Williams & Wilkins, 1995, p. 73.

7. Anderson M, Payne JT, Mann FA, et al: Flail chest: pathophysiology, treatment, and prognosis. Comp Cont Educ Pract Vet 15:65, 1993.

8. Kolata RJ: Management of thoracic trauma. Vet Clin North Am Small Anim Pract 11:103, 1981.

9. Tamas PM, Paddleford RR, Krahwinkel DJ: Thoracic trauma in dogs and cats presented for limb fractures. J Am Anim Hosp Assoc 21:161, 1985.

10. Crowe DT: Traumatic pulmonary contusions, hematomas, pseudocysts, and acute respiratory distress syndrome: an update – part I. Comp Cont Educ Pract Vet 5:396, 1983.

11. Hackner SG: Emergency management of traumatic pulmonary contusions. Comp Cont Educ Pract Vet 17:677, 1995.

12. Griffon DJ, Walter PA, Wallace LJ: Thoracic injuries in cats with traumatic fractures. Vet Comp Orthop Trauma 7:98, 1994.

13. Kraje BJ, Kraje AC, Rohrbach BW, et al: Intrathoracic and concurrent orthopedic injury associated with traumatic rib fractures in cats: 75 cases (1980-1998). J Am Vet Med Assoc 216:51, 2000.

14. Adams DB: Wound ballistics: a review. Mil Med 147:831, 1982.

15. Bartlett CS: Clinical update: gunshot wound ballistics. Clin Orthop Relat Res 408:28, 2003.

16. Fossum TW: Surgery of the lower respiratory system: lungs and thoracic wall *In* Small Animal Surgery, 2nd ed.Fossum TW (ed). St. Louis: Mosby, 2002, p. 780.

17. Bauer T, Woodfield JA: Mediastinal, pleural and extrapleural diseases. *In* Textbook of Veterinary Internal Medicine, 4th ed. Ettinger SJ, Feldman EC (eds). Philadelphia: WB Saunders, 1995, p. 815.

18. Smith BJ: Canine Anatomy. Philadelphia: Lippincott Williams & Wilkins, 1999, p. 333.

19. Monnet E: Pleura and pleural space *In* Textbook of Small Animal Surgery, 3rd ed. Slatter D (ed). Philadelphia: Elsevier Science, 2003, p. 387.

20. DeTroyer A, Legrand A, Wilson TA: Respiratory mechanical advantage of the canine external and internal intercostals muscles. J Physiol 518:283, 1999.

21. DeTroyer A, Kirkwood PA, Wilson TA: Respiratory actions of the intercostal muscles. Physiol Rev 85:717, 2005.

22. Guyton AC, Hall JE: Textbook of Medical Physiology, 11th ed. Philadelphia: Elsevier Science, 2005, p. 471.

23. West JB: Respiratory Physiology – the Essentials, 4th ed. Williams & Wilkins 1990, p. 99.

24. DeTroyer A: Inspiratory elevation of the ribs in the dog: primary role of the parasternals. J Appl Physiol 70:1447, 1991.

25. Bettor OS, Abassi Z, Rubenstein I, et al: The mechanism of muscle injury in the crush syndrome: Ischemic versus pressure stretch myopathy. Minor Electrolyte Metab 16:181, 1990.

26. Kagan LJ: Myoglobinemia and myoglobinuria in myositis syndrome. Arthritis Rheum 14:457, 1971.

27. Better OS: Traumatic rhabdomyolysis ("crush syndrome"). Israel J Med Sciences 25:69, 1989.

28. Monroe WE, Waldron DR: Renal failure: Surgical considerations *In* Disease Mechanisms in Small Animal Surgery, 2nd ed. Bojrab MJ (ed). Philadelphia: Lea & Febiger, 1993, p. 411.

29. Better OS, Rubenstein I, Winaver J: Recent insights into the pathogenesis and early management of the crush syndrome. Semin Nephrol 12:217, 1992.

30. Gabow PA, Kaehny WD, Kelleher SP: The spectrum of rhabdomyolysis. Medicine 61:141, 1982.

31. Pettifer G: Fluids, electrolytes, and acid-base therapy *In* Textbook of Small Animal Surgery, 3rd ed. Slatter D (ed). Philadelphia: Elsevier Science, 2003, p. 17.

32. Berkwitt L, Berzon JL: Thoracic trauma, newer concepts. Vet Clin North Am Small Anim Pract 15:1031, 1985.

33. Mitten RW: Radiographic examination of the ribs and sternum in the dog and cat. Comp Cont Educ Pract Vet 2:738, 1980.

34. Shen W, Nin Y, Stuhmiller JH: Biomechanically based criteria for rib fractures induced by high speed impact. J Trauma 58:538, 2005.

35. Schwarz PD: Fractures biomechanics of the appendicular skeleton: Causes and assessment *In* Disease Mechanisms in Small Animal Surgery, 2nd ed. Bojrab MJ, (ed). Philadelphia: Lea & Febiger, 1993, p. 1009.

36. Cappello M, Legrand A, DeTroyer A: Determinants of rib motion in flail chest. Am J Respir Crit Care Med 159:886, 1999.

37. Cappello M, DeTroyer A: Actions of the inspiratory intercostals muscles in flail chest. Am J Respir Crit Care Med 155:1085, 1997.

38. Cappello M, Yuehua C, DeTroyer A: Rib cage distortion in a canine model of flail chest. Am J Respir Crit Care Med 151:1481, 1995.

39. Ketterhagan JP, Wassermann DH: Impalement injuries: the preferred approach. J Trauma 23: 258, 1983.

40. Eachempati SR: Impalement injuries. Duke Trauma Center Newsletter 6:6, 1998.

41. Asch MJ, Lippman J, Nelson RJ, et al: Truck aerial impalement injury of the thorax: report of a case in an 8-year old boy. J Pediatric Surg 9:251, 1974.

42. Horowitz MD, Dove DB, Eismont FJ: Impalement injuries. J Trauma 25:914, 1985.

43. Santanello SA: Impalement injuries: the "ins and outs" of management. Life Link Log 5: 2, 2001.

44. Mendelson JA: The relationship between mechanisms of wounding and principles of treatment of missile wounds. J Trauma 31:1181, 1991.

45. Bartlett CS, Helfet DL, Hausman MR, et al: Ballistics and gunshot wounds: effects on musculoskeletal tissues. J Am Acad Orthop Surg 8: 21, 2000.

46. Orton EC: Thoracic wall. *In* Textbook of Small Animal Surgery, 3rd ed. Slatter D (ed). Philadelphia: Elsevier Science, 2003, p. 373.

47. Sturgess CP, Waters L, Gruffydd-Jones TJ, et al.: Investigation of the association between whole blood and tissue taurine levels and the development of thoracic deformities in neonatal Burmese kittens. Vet Rec 141:566, 1997.

48. Schultheiss PC, Gardner SA, Owens JM, et al: Mucopolysaccharidosis VII in a cat. Vet Pathol 37:502, 2000.

49. Fan L, Murphy S: Pectus excavatum from chronic upper airway obstruction. Am J Dis Child 135:550,1981.

50. Olsen KD, Kern EB, O'Connell EJ: Pectus excavatum: resolution after surgical removal of upper airway obstruction. Laryngoscope 90:832, 1980.

51. Ellison G, Halling KB: Atypical pectus excavatum in two Welsh terrier littermates. J Small Anim Pract 45:311, 2004.

52. Fossum TW, Boudrieau RJ, Hobson HP: Pectus excavatum in 8 dogs and 6 cats. J Am Anim Hosp Assoc 25:595, 1989.

53. Fonkalsrud EW: Pectus carinatum: the under treated chest malformation. Asian J Surg 26:189, 2003.

54. Panter KE, Keeler RF, Bunch TD, et al: Congenital skeletal malformations and cleft palate induced in goats by ingestion of Lupinus, Conium and Nicotiana species. Toxicon 28:1377, 1990.

55. West JB: Pulmonary pathophysiology – the Essentials, 4th ed. Williams & Wilkins 1990, p. 89.

56. Withrow SJ: Surgical Oncology. *In* Small Animal Clinical Oncology, 3rd ed. Withrow SJ, MacEwen EG (eds). Philadelphia: WB Saunders, 2001, p. 70.

57. Bell FW: Neoplastic diseases of the thorax. Vet Clin North Am Small Anim Pract 17:387, 1987.

58. Feeney DA, Johnston GR, Grindem, et al: Malignant neoplasia of canine ribs: clinical, radiographic and pathologic findings. J Am Vet Med Assoc 180:927, 1982.

59. Dernell WS, Straw RC, Withrow SJ: Tumors of the skeletal system *In* Small Animal Clinical Oncology, 3rd ed. Withrow SJ, MacEwen EG (eds). Philadelphia: WB Saunders, 2001, p. 378.

60. Matthiesen DT, Clark GN, Orsher RJ, et al: En bloc resection of primary rib tumors in 40 dogs. Vet Surg 21:201, 1992.

61. Pirkey-Ehrhart N, Withrow SJ, Straw RC, et al: Primary rib tumors in 54 dogs. J Am Anim Hosp Assoc 31:65, 1995.

62. MacEwen EG, Powers BE, Macy D, et al: Soft tissue sarcoma *In* Small Animal Clinical Oncology, 3rd ed. Withrow SJ, MacEwen EG (eds). Philadelphia: WB Saunders, 2001, p. 283.

Part VII

Special Senses

Chapter 59

Ear

Jamie R. Bellah

Surgical procedures of the ear fit into two basic categories. They are adjunctive to medical therapy of ear disease, or they attempt to provide complete resolution of local neoplastic or inflammatory disease. Occasionally, traumatic injuries to the ear are resolved surgically. Ear disease is most commonly inflammatory and complicated by secondary infection with bacteria and/or yeast. The ear canal, as an extension of the skin is affected by generalized skin disorders such as atopy, food allergy, and generalized seborrhea. The warmer, more humid microclimate is a predisposing factor to secondary infection. Neoplastic processes, whether benign or malignant, obstruct ear canal drainage, alter defense mechanisms, and often result in secondary local infection. Congenital stenosis, stenosis from wound healing processes, and vascular disorders also may affect the ear canal and pinna. Whereas the middle ear is most commonly affected because it is the near neighbor of the external ear canal, disease that begins within the middle ear can secondarily affect the external ear canal and nasopharyngeal passages. The proximity of the temporomandibular joint and facial and sympathetic nerve branches may result in clinical signs being referred to more distant structures. The ear may also be affected by vascular disorders that in some instances require surgery. My mission in this chapter is to focus on pathophysiologic processes that affect the ear and how surgery may be used to support treatment efforts or to resolve the disease process.

External Ear Canal

The pinna of the external ear is a breed characteristic, but more importantly, it has specific functions. As a funnel, its cartilaginous plate and shape receive vibrations and transmit or direct them down the ear canal to the tympanic membrane. The ear canal provides protection for the tympanic membrane from direct injury, and provides or maintains an open conduit for conduction of sound to the eardrum.[1] The shape of the pinna is altered by 19 auricular muscles attached to each ear that control movement independently.[2] The convex surface of the pinna is the medial and caudal surface of the ear, whereas the concave surface is the rostral and lateral surface and directs sound down the ear canal. The blood supply to the pinna is provided by the medial, intermediate, and lateral branches of the caudal auricular arteries, which arise at the base of the ear in subcutaneous tissue at the base of the convex side of the ear.[2]

Auricular Cartilage

The auricular cartilage includes the helix, anthelix, tragus, and antitragus. The helix is the free edge of the auricular cartilage, which has medial and lateral parts that meet at the apex. The anthelix is located on the medial wall of the ear canal, forms a low horizontal ridge, and has a prominent tubercle that is seen near the entrance. The tragus is the lateral wall of the entrance to the ear canal. The intertragic notch separates the thicker dense tragus from the more caudal and thinner antitragus. The aforementioned structures and the medial and lateral crura of the helix encircle the ear canal (Figure 59-1). The auricular cartilage of the ear canal attaches to the skull at the dorsolateral-facing external acoustic meatus. The vertical ear canal extends to the transversely oriented horizontal canal, which terminates at the end (most medial aspect) of the ear canal, formed by the tympanic membrane. The tympanic membrane is also the lateral wall of the middle ear (Figure 59-2). The annular cartilage is located medial to, and in part telescopes into, the rolled portion of the auricular cartilage and then has ligamentous attachment to the temporal bone.

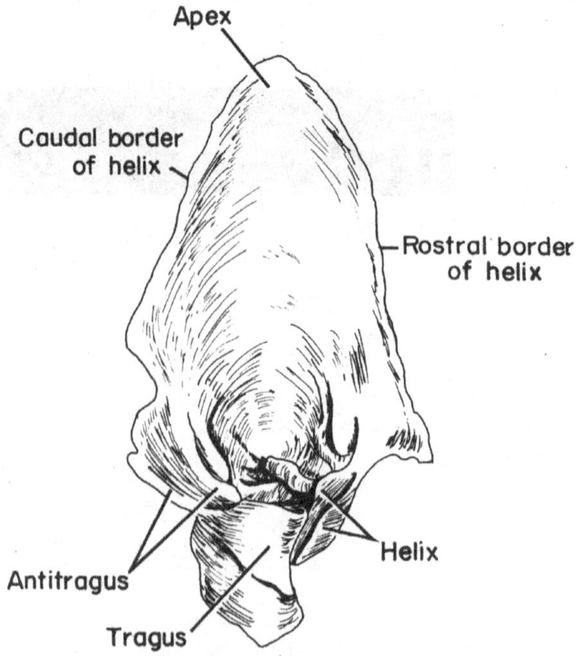

Figure 59-1. Diagram of pinna and auricular cartilages. (Redrawn from Miller's Anatomy of the Dog, 2nd ed. Evans HE, Christensen GD, (eds). Philadelphia: WB Saunders, 1979.)

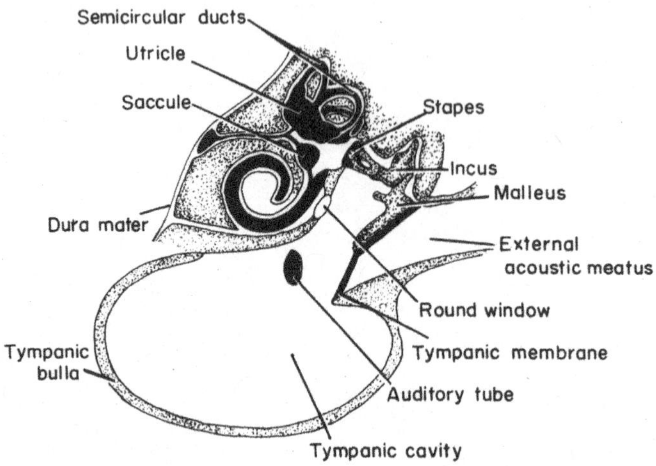

Figure 59-2. Diagram of the middle ear and inner ear. (Redrawn from Miller's Anatomy of the Dog, 2nd ed. Evans HE, Christensen GD, (eds). Philadelphia: WB Saunders, 1979.)

External Acoustic Meatus

The external acoustic meatus is lined by a continuation of stratified squamous epithelium from the ear canal and the adnexa, which include the more superficial sebaceous glands, tubular apocrine (ceruminous) glands located in the deeper connective tissue layer, and hair follicles. Both apocrine and sebaceous glands are responsible for the production of the cerumen. Although there is breed variation, hair follicles are located on the pinna and within the ear canal. The density of follicles, sebaceous glands, and tubular glands decreases in the depth of the canal and is least within the osseous meatus. Dogs with heavy hair coats have more compound hair follicles and have a consistent follicle density throughout the horizontal canal. Short-coated breeds tend to have fewer follicles and simple follicles near the eardrum.[1,3] Cats have little hair in the ear canal, and have more adnexa in the proximal third of the horizontal canal. Hair tends to point outward and, therefore, facilitates cerumen and debris moving out of the ear canal and resists movement toward the eardrum.

The skin of the entire ear canal is supported by a dense layer of connective tissue and gradually becomes thinner as it extends into the external acoustic meatus (Figure 59-3). Coiled apocrine glands are noted in the deeper dermal layers of the peripheral ear canal. Normal canine ear canals contain actively secreting sebaceous follicles, which produce a holocrine substance that is secreted through ducts near the surface of the skin and occasionally directly to the skin surface.[2] Cerumen is a combination of desquamated corneocytes, apocrine secretions and sebaceous secretions, which contain protein, lipids, amino acids, and mineral ions. Cerumen tends to be sticky, and this adhesive character is considered a local protective mechanism, helping to prevent debris from moving toward the tympanum. Small coiled tubular apocrine glands are not common in healthy ears and are located below the sebaceous glands. In long-standing otitis externa, secretions from both sebaceous and apocrine glands become copious and accumulate within the external auditory meatus. The increased activity of the cerumen glands results in excessive cerumen accumulation, which is a good growth medium for bacteria, especially for pathologic microorganisms.[2,3]

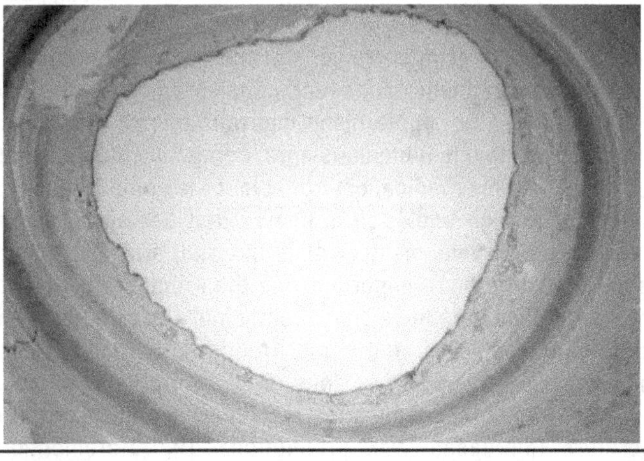

Figure 59-3. Histopathologic photomicrograph of a transverse section of a normal canine ear canal (H & E). Photomicrograph courtesy of Dr. Pam Ginn, University of Florida. (Reprinted with permission from Bellah JR: When should you recommend total ear canal ablation and lateral bulla osteotomy? Vet Med June:544-550, 1997.)

Peripheral Nerves

Peripheral nerves that supply the ear canal are the vagus nerve, which provides sensory innervation to the external auditory meatus, and the facial nerve, which is responsible for motor innervation but also provides two branches that enter the caudal and caudolateral aspect of the vertical canal. These branches provide sensory innervation to a portion of the pinna.[4] These small sensory branches of the facial nerve are transected during ear canal ablation.[4]

Epithelial Migration

The ear is hypothesized to have a self-cleaning function that is thought to be a mechanism that keeps the external auditory meatus clean.[5] Investigative work has suggested that epithelial migration occurs from the tympanic membrane outward toward the opening of the ear canal. The tympanic membrane has a generation center (a region where epithelial cell mitosis is increased) that is thought to replace cells that migrate actively off the tympanum and outwardly or distally along the ear canal wall. Cells in the stratum basale and stratum spinosum are implicated as being important in this process because of their asymmetrical shape and their long-axis orientation in the direction of epithelial movement. These cells also have a high concentration of contractile proteins when compared with other cells.[2] In this way, the debris is passively transported toward the canal opening. The hypothesized lateral epithelial migration may explain, in part, the rapid wound healing potential within the ear canal and the general lack of debris within the canal.

Tympanic Membrane

The eardrum or tympanum is a thin, transparent barrier between the external ear canal and the middle ear. It is made up of the pars flaccida, the small triangular region that is located between the lateral process of the malleus and the margins of the tympanic incisure, and the pars tensa, the larger region of the membrane. The umbo membranae tympani is a depressed point opposite to the distal end of the manubrium. Otoscopically, the stria malleolaris is seen running dorsocaudally from the umbo membranae tympani toward the pars flaccida. The pars tensa is attached firmly to the surrounding bone by a fibrocartilaginous ring, known as the annulus fibrocartilaginous, and the latter is attached by fibrous tissue to the external acoustic meatus.[1]

The Middle Ear

The middle ear is located just medial to the ear drum in the tympanic cavity, which is an oval-shaped cavity in the petrous temporal bone. The middle ear includes the auditory (Eustachian) tube, the larger bulbous or pear-shaped cavity known also as the osseous bulla, and the epitympanic recess, which houses the three auditory ossicles. In the cat, the tympanic cavity is bisected into a dorsolateral compartment and a ventromedial compartment by a boney septum. Structures of importance in the middle ear are the auditory ossicles (malleus, incus, and stapes), the vestibular (oval) window, the cochlear (round) window, and the auditory tube (Eustachian tube). The vestibular window is occupied by the base of the stapes (Figure 59-4). The auditory tube ostia is located rostrodorsally near the cochlear window. The chorda tympani nerve, a branch of the facial nerve, passes through the dorsal aspect of the tympanic bulla, crossing the manubrium of the malleus, and eventually joins the lingual nerve. The vital structures within the tympanic bulla are located dorsomedial in the cranial-most region. The tympanic bulla is bordered externally by the digastricus muscle laterally and by the styloglossus and hyoglossus muscles medially. The hypoglossal nerve is located medial to the bulla. The tympanohyoid cartilage of the hyoid apparatus attaches to the mastoid process of the skull, which is caudal to the external acoustic meatus and caudolateral to the tympanic bulla. The air-filled tympanic cavity is lined by columnar ciliated epithelium, which forms an essentially translucent membrane lining which continues into the Eustachian tube. Simple squamous epithelium lines the ventral aspect of the tympanic cavity and also invests the auditory ossicles, the inner surface of the tympanic membrane, and the membranes over the vestibular (oval) and cochlear (round) foramina.

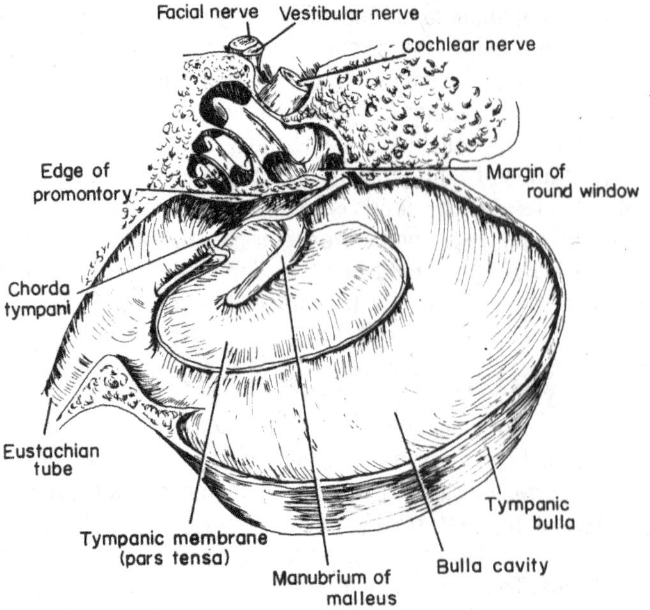

Figure 59-4. Sculptured medial view of the right middle ear and cochlea. (Redrawn from Miller's Anatomy of the Dog, 2nd ed. Evans HE, Christensen GD, (eds). Philadelphia: WB Saunders, 1979.)

The Inner Ear

The osseous labyrinth within the petrous temporal bone contains the cochlea, vestibule, and the semicircular canals. Within the osseous labyrinth are membranes that form a closed system that contains endolymph and is termed the membranous labyrinth. The membranous labyrinth is made up of three parts -- the vestibule (saccule and utricle), the cochlea, and three semicircular canals -- and is the sensory end organ for the vestibulo-cochlear nerve and the vestibular mechanism. Changes in the position of the head are detected by this proprioceptive apparatus, which then directs tenseness of postural muscles. It is this mechanism of the ear that when damaged results in vestibular signs, including a head tilt toward the affected side and horizontal nystagmus. The fast phase of horizontal nystagmus is away from the affected side when the injury or disease is peripheral. Small animals that are severely affected often cannot walk and will roll toward the affected side. The median longitudinal fasciculusand accompanying cranial nerves III, IV, and VI allow communication from the vestibular nuclei to the ocular muscles and, therefore, are the neurologic pathway that results in nystagmus.

Developmental Anomalies

Congenital problems within the ear canal are rare in dogs and cats. Anotia, the absence of an ear canal, usually occurs in conjunction with anophthalmia and other deformities, and affected animals often die or are euthanized prior to weaning. In puppies the external ear canal membrane occludes the ear canal until 14 to 17 days of age, when the canal opens. Complete failure of this membrane to disintegrate usually results in deafness, whereas a partially retained ear canal membrane will predispose to otitis externa secondary to poor aeration and drainage. Suspected atresia of the distal acoustic meatus has been reported in a Bouvier des Flandres, and associated otalgia was resolved by total ear canal ablation and lateral bulla osteotomy.[6]

Dentigerous cysts and temporal odontomas may occur from ectopic tooth development. The incompletely developed tooth is usually found near the mastoid process of the petrous temporal bone and causes a sinus tract to form and drain near the base of the ear canal. Surgical removal of the sinus tract and the cyst resolves the condition.

Congenital deafness occurs as a result of a defect of the inner ear or because of a lesion of the auditory center and is either perceptive or central, respectively. These defects are associated with a lack of cilia in the organ of Corti, improper development of the cochlear nerve, or agenesis of the cochlea.

Acquired Disease of the Ear Canal

Otitis Externa

Inflammation of the ear canal may be caused by predisposing, primary, and perpetuating factors, and the degree of involvement may include one or more regions of the ear. Factors that alter the microenvironment of the ear canal predispose the canal to pathogenic and opportunistic microorganisms. Examples of such factors include pendulous ears, congenital stenosis of the ear canal, and mechanical obstruction of the canal by ear canal tumors or foreign bodies. It is known that ear anatomy plays a role in the development of otitis externa, and otic humidity seems to play a more important role than temperature.[3,7] Dogs with pendulous ears have significantly more otitis externa than dogs with erect ears, and some breeds (Labrador retrievers, American cocker spaniels, and English Springer spaniels) have greater numbers of apocrine (ceruminous) glands and, therefore, increased wax production.[3] The aforementioned breeds also had a higher density of hair follicles throughout the horizontal canal when compared with greyhounds and mongrel dogs.[3] Poodle and Lhasa apso breeds have a higher density of compound hair follicles, which promotes accumulation of ear wax and debris and interferes with migration of material out of the canal. Beagles and setters are breeds that are the exception to the above and are less frequently affected by otitis than are other pendulous-eared breeds. Alternatively, German shepherd dogs, as an erect-eared breed, are over-represented. The Chinese Sharpei breed tends to have a narrow, long vertical ear canal, which is essentially a stenosis in comparison with other breeds. Ear canal stenosis can be coincidental in other breeds; Chow-chows and their crosses also tend to have narrow canals. Acquired canal stenosis occurs from periaural masses such as neoplasia. Microflora that normally occur in the ear may be more apt to cause otitis externa when the microenvironment of the ear canal better supports organism growth. The stratum corneum can be broken down by increased moisture content in the ears, as maceration of the epidermis occurs, allowing microorganisms to colonize the ear canal resulting in otitis. Excessive moisture in the ear from swimming, excessive bathing, and environmental humidity and temperature (characteristic of the southeast region of the United States) can cause maceration of the surface of the ear canal and can influence the incidence of otitis externa. An investigation of first-time otitis externa cases over five geographic regions in North America found that monthly variations in ambient temperature, rainfall, and relative humidity correlated positively with the incidence of initial ear infection. The investigation found a 2-month delay between a climatic change and an increased incidence of otitis externa.[3]

Mechanical trauma to the ear canal from excessive cleaning or from the excessive use of cleaning agents or drying agents may damage the ear canal. Systemic diseases may predispose to otitis externa as they may impair cell-mediated immunity. Ulcerative otitis externa has been reported to respond to immunosuppressive therapy in dogs.[8] Examples of diseases that may result in such immune impairment include feline leukemia virus, feline immunodeficiency virus, canine distemper, and canine parvovirus. Endocrine disease such as hyperadrenocorticism, hypoadrenocorticism, hypothyroidism, and diabetes mellitus may also be associated with otitis externa.[3]

Parasites such as Otodectes cyanotis and Demodex canis are commonly responsible for otitis externa in young animals,[9] especially in cats in which approximately 50% of cases are secondary to mite infestation. Ear mites cause mechanical irritation but the dog or cat can also become sensitive to antigens in mite saliva. When hypersensitization is present, it takes very few mites to cause severe inflammation. Demodex mite infestation generally causes a severe ceruminous otitis in dogs and in cats, and the presence of otitis may be the only sign of infestation. Other mites and Otobius megnini, the spinous ear tick may also be found in the canal, but these are less common than those previously mentioned. Grass awns, foxtails, and other foreign material including impacted wax may initiate otitis. The most common cause for bilateral otitis externa in the dog is hypersensitivity. Allergic conditions that commonly produce secondary otitis externa include atopy, food allergy, and contact allergy. Atopy, for example, affects as many as 50% of dogs at a given time, and is commonly associated with secondary infection. When atopy and other hypersensitivities that affect the ear are uncomplicated, the pinna and the vertical ear canal are reddened and pruritic, and the horizontal canal can be normal.[2] Otitis externa is present in 88% of dogs with food allergy.[10] Contact allergies are most commonly due to topical therapy; the indication of this is a worsening of the otitis and lack of improvement with the initiation of therapy.[3,5]

Seborrhea is a disorder of keratinization that can result in ceruminous otitis. Other endocrine disorders that may be associated with otitis externa include hypothyroidism, male feminizing syndrome (Sertoli or interstitial cell tumors), and ovarian imbalance.[3]

Tumors within the ear canal cause mechanical interference with normal movement of the cerumen from the ear canal and with drainage of exudates once otitis externa has occurred. Ceruminous gland adenoma and adenocarcinoma, sebaceous adenocarcinoma, mast cell tumor, squamous cell carcinoma, and benign conditions such as polyps can obstruct the ear canal.

Perpetuating factors that prevent resolution of otitis externa or that worsen preexisting otitis are usually microorganisms. The normal ear canal has microflora in low numbers that include both commensal and pathogenic bacteria. *Staphylococcus intermedius* is a common bacterium involved in otitis externa, and other species frequently encountered include Pseudomonas spp, Proteus spp, *Escherichia coli*, enterococcus spp, and Corynebacterium spp. Pseudomonas is cultured from 12 to 35% of ears with otitis externa.[11] Multiple organisms can occur in otitis externa. In 20% of cultures another organism may be missed, and this is one criteria that should be considered in treatment failure.[12] These organisms benefit by alteration of the microenvironment within the ear canal and impaired drainage from the canal, which results in their proliferation and potentiation of the inflammatory response. Malassezia spp is the most common fungal organism found in the ear canal, and it can be present in both normal and inflamed ears, but is highly opportunistic in macerated and inflamed ears, and is common as a secondary complication in atopic skin disease or food allergy. Other fungi, such as Candida, Aspergillus, and Microsporum may cause otitis externa.[3]

Otitis externa results in progressive injury to the ear canal if medical therapy is not able to control the cause and the inflammatory response. Initially, when otitis is acute, canal erythema and swelling occur as many inflammatory cells infiltrate the dermis and epidermis. Apocrine glands hypertrophy and dilate, with an accompanying increase in the production of cerumen. The cerumen that is produced differs in composition as well. Normally, epidermal migration occurs toward the opening of the ear canal, but if the inflammatory response is progressive the epidermis begins to fold (Figure 59-5) and epidermal migration is inhibited. Eventually, the increased glandular activity, epidermal thickness, and decreased epidermal migration lead to excessive wax production with a buildup of keratinaceous debris, and proliferation and overgrowth of bacteria occurs. Persisting inflammation results in dermal fibrosis within the horizontal canal and calcification of annular and auricular cartilages, usually from deeper regions to the exterior, and ossification can occur late. The end-stage result is permanent stenosis of the ear canal lumen.[3,5] Complete obstruction of the ear canal lumen can result, and the inflammatory process can "break-out" of the ear canal and result in development of periaural fistulae (Figures 59-6 and 59-7)

Clinical signs of ear canal disease do not necessarily differentiate the varying causes of otitis. Pruritus, pain, erythema, swelling, and drainage are common. Depending on the severity and amount of drainage from the ear and whether the middle ear is involved, a head tilt may be noted to the affected side. Excessive head shaking may lead to aural hematoma. A discharge or foul order is often present. Periauricular excoriations and alopecia may be noted. In uncomplicated allergic otitis externa, erythema of the pinna and the vertical canal may occur and the horizontal canal may be relatively unaffected. Proliferative disease may be limited to the vertical canal. Ulcerations and erosions of the ear canal may occur with contact dermatitis or gram-negative bacterial infections. As the otitis externa becomes more chronic, the compliance of the cartilage support of the ear canal is lost as it becomes mineralized. Acute otitis externa is painful to dogs and cats; but as the condition becomes more chronic, less dramatic pain responses are elicited during examination. However, calcified ear canals are associated with intense pain. Hearing loss is often detected by the owners as otitis becomes end-stage.

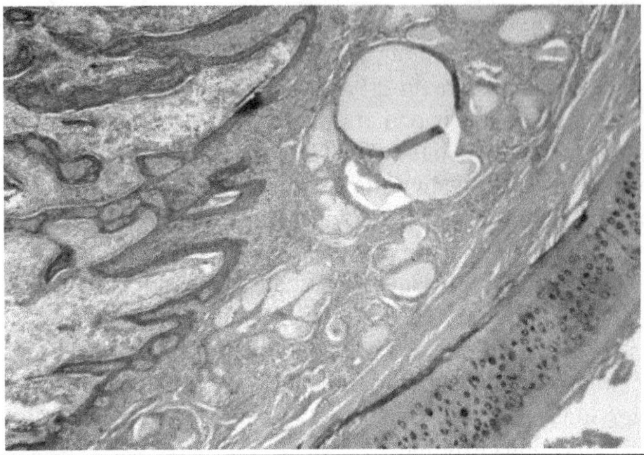

Figure 59-5. Histopathologic photomicrograph of a transverse section of an ear canal in a dog with otitis externa (H & E). Note hyperplasia of apocrine tubular glands, thickening of the epidermis, and a buildup of keratinaceous debris. (Photomicrograph courtesy of Dr. Pam Ginn, University of Florida.)

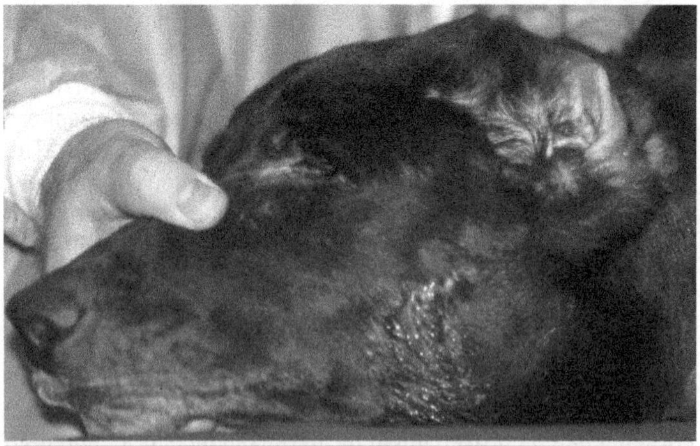

Figure 59-6. Labrador retriever with end-stage otitis externa and break-out abscessation with the draining fistulae. The ear canal was ablated (see Figure 59-7). (Reprinted with permission from Bellah JR: When should you recommend total ear canal ablation and lateral bulla osteotomy? Vet Med June:544-550, 1997.)

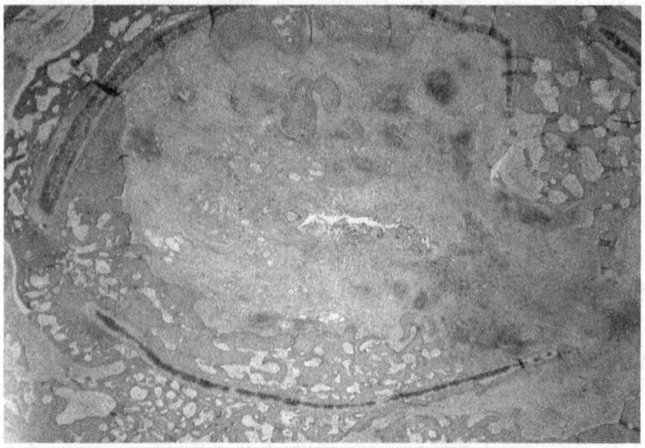

Figure 59-7. Histopathologic photomicrograph of a transverse section of an ear canal in a dog with severe end-stage otitis externa (the dog in Figure 59-6). Note the obstruction of the ear canal owing to cartilage mineralization and the severe hyperplasia and microabscessation within the canal lumen (H & E). Photomicrograph courtesy of Dr. Pam Ginn, University of Florida. (Reprinted with permission from: Bellah JR: When should you recommend total ear canal ablation and lateral bulla osteotomy? Vet Med June:544-550, 1997.)

Tympanic Injury

Tympanic injury is most commonly secondary to otitis externa in small animals.[13] Proteolytic enzymes that accumulate from bacterial release and from the degradation of inflammatory cells have destructive effects on the epithelial surface of the tympanic membrane. Once a perforation occurs, the bacteria, enzymes, and debris have access to the respiratory epithelium of the middle ear.[13] Traumatic perforations occur from direct trauma (i.e., cotton-tipped applicator or excessive fluid pressures against a weakened membrane) during ear canal cleansing. Masses, such as nasopharyngeal polyps in cats, may cause pressure necrosis as they push against the tympanic membrane, and secondary infection and its by-products cause additional injury.

The tympanum is capable of healing, and will attempt to do so if remnants of the eardrum remain. Two factors are required to accomplish tympanic membrane healing: a satisfactory blood supply and an intact germinal epithelium. The blood supply to the germinal epithelium arises from vessels within the pars flaccida; therefore, this region of the eardrum must be intact for healing to occur. The germinal epithelium that produces the epidermal layer of the tympanum is located near the manubrium of the malleus. From that location, the tympanic epithelium grows radially toward the annulus of the tympanic membrane, and healing can be complete in a period of 3 weeks to 4 months.[13]

Tympanic membrane wound healing has been investigated. Keratinocytes proliferate on the external surface of the eardrum simultaneously with proliferation of fibrous connective tissue cells in the middle layer. The inner layer of epithelium differentiates into ciliated and secretory cells at the border of the perforation. Early healing and closure of the tympanic wound is by the migration of the superficial epithelial layers of the eardrum, and permanent apposition and closure of the defect is by the slower-migrating basal epithelium.[13] In naturally occurring eardrum perforations, pathologic changes tend to be progressive, such that inflammation, fibrosis, tympanosclerosis, and hyperkeratosis are found to impair wound healing progress. Keratinized epithelial proliferation may localize to the medial side of the tympanum and protrude into the middle ear cavity. Otitis media, because of the production of mucous and purulent exudates, including proteolytic enzymes, impairs eardrum healing. If lysis of the malleus occurs and the germinal epithelium is destroyed, or if fibrous scar devitalizes the pars flaccida, perforation will be permanent.[13] A ring of hyperkeratotic epithelium in the region of the perforated tympanum is an indication of chronic permanent perforation. Persistent drainage with relapsing otitis media occurs in this condition.

Surgery of the External Ear Canal

Surgical treatment of the external ear canal is done to treat relapsing or persisting otitis externa, stenosis of the vertical or horizontal ear canal, neoplasia, vascular disease of the pinna, and traumatic injuries to the ear canal. Specific techniques for specific conditions of the ear are not the objective of this chapter, but commentary on specific areas of the ear and the surgery appropriate for those areas follows.

Pinna

The pinna of dogs and cats is important functionally to pets but also cosmetically to pet owners. Traumatic lacerations and injuries to the pinna are common and result from skirmishes between cats, between dogs, between cats and dogs, and from gunshot and other missiles. Many partial-thickness lacerations do not require suturing, but apposition using fine sutures (3-0 to 5-0) often improves the cosmetic result. Full-thickness lacerations benefit by including the cartilage of the ear canal in the suture loop (i.e., vertical mattress), so careful apposition of the cartilage edges is done, followed by suturing the skin on the opposite side. Lacerations on the haired (convex) side of the ear canal may be more easily apposed and sutured because subcutaneous tissue separates the dermis and cartilage on that side of the pinna.[2,14]

When it is necessary to remove a mass, from the pinna,the haired surface of the convex surface of the ear canal has sufficient skin that may be undermined and closed after tumor excision. Depending on the location of the mass, it is possible to remove masses up to 2 cm in size 14 with the expectation of achieving primary closure without creating a flap from the head or neck. Moveable skin is more readily available near the base of the pinna. On the concave surface, the skin and cartilage are in close contact, so undermining is difficult. Small non-malignant masses may be excised with narrow margins, and the small minor wound may heal by second intention. Small malignant masses may be excised by removing skin, mass, and underlying perichondrium and cartilage, whereas larger masses with known malignant character are best aggressively removed by excision of the entire pinna. This results in cosmetic asymmetry but is preferable to leaving microscopic tumor at the excision site.

Large defects of the lateral non-haired skin of the pinna are difficult to correct because of the inability to undermine skin extensively and because the auricular cartilage is inelastic. Various reconstructive techniques are available including the creation of local skin flaps from the skin of the cheek or neck. Flaps of varying shapes may be designed to repair the ear cosmetically using staged techniques. The different hair color or direction and the thickness of the skin are disadvantages to consider. Defects of the central portion of the pinna may also be resolved with similar techniques.

Amputation of a portion of the pinna is simplest when neoplastic involvement or traumatic devitalization of a portion of the pinna is located at the periphery of the ear. Full-thickness incisions, using a scalpel blade, can be done by obtaining a margin of normal pinna to be removed with the tumor. A scalpel is the instrument of choice as it is the least traumatic instrument for incision versus traumatically crushing the auricular tissues with scissors. Occasionally, curvilinear incisions at the edge of the pinna may be made with very sharp scissors as it is sometimes easier to make a more cosmetic (rounded) incision. The concave and convex skin margins are sutured over the cartilage, using fine suture. Excisions of masses along the anterior or posterior margins of the ear canal may done by removing a triangular portion of the edge of the canal (a wedge), and apposing the full-thickness margins in two layers. Sometimes this will narrow the pinna of pendulous ears or make the pinna slightly more convex in erect ears, but once the hair grows back, a good cosmetic result is often attained.

Lateral Ear Resection (LER)

Lateral ear resection, the Zepp procedure, has been done to aid management of otitis externa in dogs since 1949.[15] Over the years, veterinary surgeons have altered their approach to otitis externa, from recommending lateral ear resection frequently in dogs that have relapsing otitis externa, to rarely recommending this surgery. The advent of better ear care in general and the knowledge that the results of lateral ear resection surgery are not the panacea for resolution of otitis that might have been anticipated. The potential for adjunctive surgical therapy to be efficacious was a sincere goal, as approximately 4% of veterinary hospital admissions involve some form of otitis externa.[16] Lateral ear resection does result in a significant change in the microclimate of the ear, and in one study relative humidity was reduced by 10% in operated external ear canals.[17] In a study of 281 dogs with otitis externa, Tufvesson found LER to resolve approximately 50% of otitis externa in dogs, with another 15% of the dogs showing improvement, and the remaining 35% showing minimal or lack of improvement.[18] In this study, age or breed did not affect the outcome; however spaniels, poodles, and Airedale terriers were predisposed.[18] A similar outcome was reported by Gregory and Vasseur in a small number of dogs (N=26), where 41% had good outcomes, 12% improved, and 47%

had a poor outcome.[19] They concluded that a technically correct LER does not ensure a successful outcome, but also noted that clinical signs improved in some instances where the surgery was a technical failure.[19] A post-surgical investigation by Lane and Little, of 135 dogs with persistent aural drainage after ear surgery found concurrent otitis media, irreversible disease of the medial vertical ear canal, and unsatisfactory drainage from the horizontal canal to be the most common factors recognized with surgical failure.[20] Surgical outcome in another study showed LER to achieve acceptable results in 45% of the dogs treated and 55% to be unacceptable. Acceptable outcomes were rated excellent (the ears no longer required regular cleaning and the dog had no more than 2 bouts of otitis externa since the surgery) or good (the ears had occasional flare-ups of otitis externa, no more that 2 per year that readily responded to topical medical management. Unacceptable outcomes were rated fair (the ears required regular cleaning in order to prevent a relapse of the otitis and the dog experienced an average of 3 or more bouts of otitis annually) or poor (the ears progressed to an end-stage with an occluded canal as determined by follow-up physical examination). The Cocker spaniel breed had poorer results than other breeds, showing a failure rate of 86.5%. Non-Cocker spaniel breeds had an LER acceptable result percentage of 63%. The Shar pei breed was found to have narrower vertical ear canals.[21] Other studies have shown varied acceptable results from LER surgery.[19] Johnston found disappointing results when LER was performed in 41 dogs, after otitis media was present and severe changes developed in the ear canal with ruptured tympanums. Aggressive middle ear flushing and appropriate antimicrobial use based on culture and susceptibility testing in addition to LER found in these dogs clinical improvement, but head shaking and drainage from the horizontal canal persisted.[22] A lesser affected group in this study, 70 dogs with a history of 1 to 2 years of otitis externa and minimal canal changes were treated by LER. In this group, 50 had severe eardrum perforations and the other 20 had diseased and likely ruptured eardrums; LER resulted in slight to moderate discharge with reduced discomfort and head shaking.[22] The third group of 33 dogs in this study were dogs that had been affected by lifelong otitis externa at 12 to 18 months of age (based on breed, a minimum of 3 episodes of otitis externa after treatment and evidence of atopy or other allergic skin disease). Dogs in this group did not have tympanic rupture. In this latter group of 33 dogs, all dogs had resolution of ear discharge and discomfort at 6 months after surgery, and no dogs had eardrum perforation.[22] The conclusion was made that LER (Zepp) was definitively indicated once a predisposition to otitis externa was diagnosed and before irreversible changes are present within the ear canal, tympanum, and the middle ear.[22] If surgical intervention is considered a last resort after proliferative disease and canal obstruction is in progress, the procedure is doomed to fail.

Indications for recommending surgical resection of the lateral wall of the vertical ear canal or creating a lateral ear canal flap that is positioned ventrally (Zepp) may be when masses involve the lateral aspect of the vertical ear canal or when opening the vertical canal to change the microclimate of the ear canalis judged beneficial to the individual dog with otitis externa.[23] The latter indication presents a more difficult decision as lateral ear resection is an adjunctive measure and not considered a curative procedure for otitis externa. The procedure does change the microclimate of the ear canal and can have a positive impact on aiding treatment of otitis externa. In addition to altering the microclimate of the ear canal, LER improves drainage of fluid and exudates from the horizontal canal by eliminating the vertical canal "reservoir" that must be overcome by head shaking. The region aerates better and is more easily cleaned, and in some dogs at the least this is palliative. A horizontal ear canal with minimal chronic proliferative changes is necessary for this surgery to be considered.[24]

Lateral ear resection does not require special equipment and it is not a difficult procedure to complete. The most common error made is an inaccurate incision of the vertical canal. This can happen if the lateral canal flap is made too thin on the lateral aspect, making the base of the flap too narrow, or on the medial side, resulting in a narrow strip of vertical ear canal remaining and a lateral canal flap that is difficult to bend to a ventral location. The goal is to incise the flap so the ventral aspect of the horizontal canal is wide open and the lateral flap makes a smooth cranioventral bend. The flap created is trimmed to a length of approximately 2 cm and sutured such that it remains ventral. The method of suturing is up to the individual surgeon's preference. The most difficult area to suture is the deep corner of the lateral ear canal flap where it bends away from the vertical ear canal. A figure-of-eight mucocutaneous suture pattern (similar to that used for mucocutaneous apposition) may be used to make the sutures more accessible at suture removal.[23,25]

Vertical Ear Resection (VER)

A slightly more aggressive ear canal excision is the vertical canal resection. It is less commonly used for otitis externa.[26] Complete resection of the vertical ear canal is more commonly done when trauma has lacerated and injured the vertical canal badly or when neoplasia involves the vertical segment of the ear canal. Atopic dogs and dogs with food allergy, in which inflammation and swelling are more focally located within the vertical canal, benefit by having the proliferative changes in the vertical ear canal removed.[27] The horizontal canal is commonly spared severe inflammatory effects in these two allergic conditions; the most pruritic region seems to be the vertical canal and extending upward toward the pinna.[3] When vertical ear canal excision is considered for aural tumor excision, the most important factor is determining the presence of sufficient horizontal canal for wound closure after resection. Imaging the ear canal and skull by computed tomography (CT) prior to surgery aids preoperative decisions. In the absence of CT, local inspection to explore the canal during surgery by means of a lateral ear resection approach may be necessary. If the horizontal canal is insufficient, a total ear canal ablation is done to achieve the best surgical margin possible beyond the tumor. The surgical approach for vertical canal resection requires conservation of periaural skin for wound closure and, therefor, differs from lateral ear canal resection. A T-shaped incision is commonly used, and the incision correlating to the top of the "T" can meander along the margin of the tragus cartilage if the skin is normal. to preserve all available skin for closure under the pinna. Conserving skin facilitates apposition of wound edges between the horizontal ear canal stoma and the pinna.

The vertical canal is isolated around its entire circumference by dissection next to the cartilage of the ear canal and pushing or making a minor incision in the parotid salivary gland to aid exposure. Remaining directly adjacent to the ear canal is especially important on the concave surface of the canal so the auricular vessels that supply the pinna of the ear are not damaged. The level of the incision at the dorsal aspect of the ear canal is dependent on the position of the tumor being excised or the level of proliferative disease if done for atopy. Once the resection is completed and hemostasis obtained, the horizontal canal remaining may be divided into dorsal and ventral baffle plates if enough canal is present. If not, the skin is sutured directly to the circular remnant of the horizontal canal. The figure-of-eight mucocutaneous suture pattern is useful when little horizontal canal remains. The apposition of skin around the horizontal canal is done first, followed by apposing the skin to the pinna from the anterior and posterior edges.

Total Ear Canal Ablation and Lateral Bulla Osteotomy (TECA-LBO)

End-stage otitis externa results in obstruction of the ear canal to the extent that normal lateral epidermal migration of debris and keratinized epithelium does not occur, and in most canals the eardrum is ruptured, and otitis media is present as well. Removing the entire ear canal is a common procedure in dogs, and less common in cats.[28-30] In cats, the most common indication for TECA-LBO in one investigation was neoplasia,[29] with 86% of the neoplasms being ceruminous gland adenocarcinoma.[29] Total ear canal ablation is indicated to resolve the discomfort and chronic infection and drainage from end-stage otitis externa and calcified canals, from neoplastic disease located deep within the ear canal with or without secondary infection, and to resolve para-aural abscessation that results from traumatic avulsion and secondary stricture of the ear canal.[31,32] Traumatic avulsion of the annular cartilage from the external auditory meatus in a cat has also been reported and was treated by ablation of the ear canal.[33] Traumatic ear canal separations may be managed by isolating the distal end of the horizontal ear canal (annular cartilage) and suturing the open end to the skin to allow cleaning and maintenance of patency.[34]

Many references and texts contain reviews of the surgical technique for ablation of the ear, and each surgeon has specific methods to facilitate exposure and completion.[28-30,35,36] Many surgeons use a "T-shaped" incision similar to that used for vertical canal resection; however, the author's preference is to make an incision from the cranial aspect of the opening of the ear canal in a caudoventral direction but following the edge of the ear canal to the caudal aspect of the ear canal opening, and then extending ventrally parallel to the vertical ear canal to a level below the horizontal canal. The purpose of this incision is to conserve as much skin as possible to aid closure after resection of the ear canal, essentially in the manner of a single pedicle advancement toward the concave surface of the pinna. Once the incision is made, dissection is carried to the level of the cartilage and soft tissues are removed by sharp and blunt dissection around the entire circumference of the vertical ear canal. The level of the incision made to release the dorsal aspect of the vertical canal depends on where the proliferative disease extends. All proliferative disease should be removed, but the higher the level of the vertical canal resected the more important it is to carefully remain intimate with the cartilage of the ear canal so auricular vessels supplying the pinna are protected. Dissection down to the horizontal ear canal and continuing down to the external acoustic meatus is carefully continued. Note that branches of the facial nerve, the caudal internal auricular nerve and the lateral internal auricular nerve penetrate the caudal and lateral aspects of the horizontal canal, respectively.[4] Each is associated with an artery that is ligated. The facial nerve is located just caudal and ventral to a boey protuberance about 5 o'clock or 7 o'clock, depending on whether the left or right ear canal is being ablated. The facial nerve need not be identified at surgery as its trunk is located just caudal to the external acoustic meatus and just ventral to the mastoid process, a protuberance that can be palpated during surgery. These landmarks allow the location of the facial nerve to be kept in mind so careful retraction of neighboring soft tissues may be done and care is taken not to compress this region as the nerves movement is restricted by the close proximity to the stylomastoid foramen where the nerve exits the skull. Rarely, facial nerve is incorporated in an inflammatory response that extends from the ear canal, but more often is simply pushed away by the expansion of the canal tissues.

The dorsal-most aspect of the circumference of the horizontal canal is the location that allows the most convenient entry into the tympanic cavity. The ear canal can usually be pushed away from the meatus using a Freer elevator. The remainder of the circumference is then released by gradually extending the separation around the entire circumference. The caudo-ventral aspects of the canal attachment are the most difficult and this is also where bony proliferation is the most extensive. The retroarticular foramen should be avoided so hemorrhage from the retroglenoid vein does not occur. Tissues or debris are collected for culture and histopathologic examination once the canal is released. Bacteria cultured from TECA-LBO sites commonly include *Streptococcus canis* and *E. coli*.[37] One investigation showed bacteria to remain after debridement and lavage of the tympanic cavity, and in this study, only 26% of isolates showed susceptibility to cefazolin.[38]

Access to the tympanic bulla is accomplished by lateral bulla osteotomy and is done to allow thorough removal of debris and tissue extending into the middle ear. An air drill is the most efficacious method for removing the thick cortical bone of the external acoustic meatus. Ronguers can be used effectively. Care must be taken to avoid wrapping up soft tissues around the canal if a drill is used and also to carefully inspect the tissues just ventral to the external meatus so no secretory epithelium remains. Branches of the carotid artery are located deep to the tympanic bulla and severe hemorrhage may result if these vessels are torn during dissection. Thorough lavage is done and closure of the surgical wound is performed.

Drains are not necessary to maintain drainage after TECA-LBO.[35] Primary closure is most commonly done after TECA-LBO but passive drains may be used at the discretion of the surgeon. Drains may be used in some instances where "breakout" abscessation has occurred and fistulae are apparent prior to ablation, as the extent of wound infection can be well beyond the region of the ear canal. Soft tissues are apposed, being careful to avoid deep suture bites that may penetrate vessels. Subcutaneous tissues are apposed and cartilage may be included in the suture pattern if necessary for wound strength. The apposition of the wound margin of the pinna (remainder of the auricular cartilage) to the skin flap is done from a cranial to caudal direction, as "dog-ear" correction is simple to do at the caudoventral aspect of the incision.

Facial paralysis is the most common complication and likely results from ischemia caused by compression or traction of the facial nerve near the mastoid process. Incidences vary from 5% to 58%.[30] Ischemia, if sustained long enough, will cause fiber degeneration within the nerve and result in loss of function. As long as the facial nerve is intact, function should return, as the fibers regenerate at a rate of approximately 1mm per day. Although the incidence of facial nerve paralysis is high, careful technique in the region of the mastoid process and ventral to the external acoustic meatus will protect nerve function. In cats, facial nerve paralysis occurred in 56% of cats that underwent TECA-LBO, and 42% had Horner's syndrome.[29] Nerve fragility was suggested to be greater in cats in comparison with dogs.[29]

Persistent otitis media and development of periaural sinus have been reported to be as high as 30% in dogs undergoing total ear canal ablation;[30,39] however, most veterinary surgeons would estimate that less than 10% are affected.[40,41] The source of the fistulae may be tissue or material within or outside the tympanic cavity.[40] Plain radiographs and sinography may be used to demonstrate the source of drainage.[42] It is uncommon for persisting otitis media with sinus tract development to be successfully treated with drainage and antimicrobial therapy; only 1 of 17 and 1 of 8 dogs in 2 reports were successfully treated in that way.[41,43] In the author's opinion, lateral bulla osteotomy is the procedure of choice to attempt resolution of draining sinuses and persisting otitis media. Although a ventral bulla osteotomy may be used and will accomplish good exposure of the tympanic cavity, it is difficult with this procedure to access the region of the acoustic meatus, especially laterally where remnants of secretory epithelium may be found. Retraction of the external carotid artery and at least partial transaction of the digastricus muscle is required to obtain exposure to the lateral aspect of the external acoustic meatus if a ventral approach is used.[40] Facial nerve location is difficult with the lateral approach after TECA-LBO as the canal landmark is not present. The mastoid process is still palpable, however, and careful dissection along the deeper portions of the sinus will help protect the facial nerve. A lateral approach allows the sinus tract to be followed (inserting a red rubber catheter into the tract is an effective method for following the tract during surgery) to the remnant of the external acoustic meatus and for the tympanic cavity to be reopened to a wide enough dimension and be debrided of debris and any adnexal structure that may be causative.

Vestibular signs, including nystagmus, head tilt, and postural abnormalities may occur when trauma to the promontory and the oval and round windows occurs during curettage of the tympanic cavity.[30] This is a rare complication but is probably the most disconcerting to an owner because the dog shows such anxiety as it tries to walk. Usually, vestibular signs abate over a period of weeks, but residual signs such as a persisting head tilt may remain.[40]

Necrosis of the pinna from careless dissection, hemorrhage, and airway obstruction have been reported to occur after ear canal ablation. The latter complication has been noted when severe hemorrhage occurs, and when bilateral ear canal ablations are done during one anesthetic episode. Airway structures are in close proximity to the tympanic bullae such that severe hemorrhage or edema may result in airflow resistance when dogs are extubated. Cervical bandages that are too tight may also restrict good air flow.

Multiple regimens exist to provide analgesia for aural surgery. Opioids and combinations of systemic administration and local nerve blocks are used commonly.[44] Bupivicane splash blocks and bupivicane administration by analgesia catheter placement have also been used.[45] A comparison of systemic opioids with systemic opioids and preoperative nerve blocks found no advantage to the latter protocol.[44] The great auricular and auriculotemporal nerves may be blocked.[36] Extended release morphine tablets and transdermal patches may be used as well.[36] Tranquilization may be necessary, not for analgesia, but to provide restraint from head shaking and pawing at the incision in some animals. Physical restraint with E-collars to prevent the dog or cat from traumatizing the surgical site is also used.

Perioperative antimicrobial use is recommended for ear canal surgery, especially for TECA-LBO, and therapeutic use beyond the post-operative period should be based on the results of culture and susceptibility testing.[38]

Auditory Function after Ear Canal Ablation

Pet owners are commonly worried about the effect of ear canal ablation on their pet's hearing. Dogs with bilateral end-stage otitis externa have been evaluated before and after surgery by auditory evoked response.[46] Prior to surgery, all dogs could hear a loud voice or noise, 3 dogs could hear a voice at a normal volume level, and 13 of 14 ears of the 7 dogs had a positive brainstem auditory-evoked response (air-conducted or bone conducted). After surgery, 2 dogs responded to a normal voice and all 7 dogs responded to a loud voice or noise. There were 3 of 13 ears that did not respond to an air-conducted stimulus that did prior to surgery, but all 13 ears in the dogs responded to a bone-conducted stimulus.[46] Experimentally, normal dogs that underwent ventral bulla osteotomy had reduced auditory evoked potentials after wound healing.[47] Proliferation of scar and bone in a subperiosteal location in some dogs impaired function of the auditory ossicles and tympanum. Although most dogs in the study reformed a tympanic cavity without bearing impairment, the internal surfaces were found to easily produce new bone, which if extensive, can affect hearing function in dogs.[47]

Conductive hearing loss was evaluated in dogs experimentally using brain stem auditory evoked response threshold and latency-intensity. Dogs had their ears canals obstructed by an ear plug rated at 26 decibels, had mechanical irritation to induce transient stenosis of the external ear canal, a needle puncture of the tympanum, and extensive destruction of the tympanum with electrocautery.[48] The investigators found that only the mechanical plug and the destruction of a major portion of the eardrum produced pronounced hearing loss.[48] The size and location of the perforation and especially the loss of integrity of the auditory ossicles were factors that affected the severity of auditory-evoked response.[48]

Otoacoustic emission (termed tinnitus in humans), an audible ringing from the ear canal, has been reported in a dog. Otoacoustic emission is the term used in animals because it cannot be determined if the animal consciously perceives the sound.[49] The dog was reported to have a normal brain-stem auditory evoked-response test, indicating the intitial phases of sound processing in the affected ear were normal.[49]

Otitis Media

Otitis media is defined as inflammation of the middle ear, and is usually caused by bacterial infection that has extended directly from the external ear canal.[50,51] In most situations the tympanum has ruptured, but the tympanum may appear intact at examination, as small defects may have healed.[52] Positive cultures of the middle ear cavity may often be obtained by myringotomy in the presence of an intact eardrum. In one investigation of 46 ears in dogs with otitis media, 71% of the ears had intact eardrums.[52] Bacteria are the most common cause of otitis media but yeast may be the causative agent as well.[52] Hematogenous route and the Eustachian tube are also sources of infection for otitis media.[53] Bacterial infection of the middle ear is usually secondary, from extension of otitis externa or cholesteatoma. Primary otitis media may occur owing to neoplasia, inflammatory polyps, and rarely, primary infections. Middle ear disease has been associated with congenital palatine defects in both dogs and a cat, without evidence of external ear disease.[54]

The initial clinical sign of primary otitis media is pain, causing the dog to hold the affected ear down.[2] Clinical signs of disease involving the middle ear can be similar to those in other types of ear disease, but the routine head shaking, pawing at the ear, and drainage from the ear canal are more common in otitis media. Drainage may occur if the eardrum should perforate. Otoscopic or videoscopic examination of the eardrum, which often requires anesthesia, may reveal it to be discolored or possibly bulging into the external ear canal, and to have congested blood vessels.[2] A bulging discolored tympanum (dull, and grey to yellow) in the presence of a normal external ear canal suggests an origin of disease to be hematogenous or via the Eustachian tube. A myringotomy is done to obtain specimens for cytologic examination and for culture and susceptibility testing.

Disease of the middle ear can be expansile and result in an enlargement of the volume of the tympanic cavity ventrally, or the disease process can break through the boundaries of the tympanum. This can result in a mass that is sometimes palpable ventral to the bulla. Because of the proximity of the osseous bulla to the nasopharynx, if the expansile mass becomes large enough that it extends down toward the soft palate and compresses against these structures, oral examination may reveal the region of the dorsal tonsillar pillar and soft palate to bulge into the oropharynx. Noisy respiration may be noted if the nasopharynx is compromised. In addition, the osseous bulla is in close proximity to the temporomandibular joint so disease processes that cause inflammation and pain in this region may cause irritation when the mandible moves, resulting in dysphagia.

Diagnostic evaluation includes basic otoscopic examination, radiographs of the tympanic bulla, and cytologic evaluation of drainage from the ear. Computerized tomography is an ideal imaging technique for the middle ear, and use of contrast can provide valuable diagnostic information.[22,55] One report showed that CT was more accurate than skull radiographs for diagnosing middle ear disease when the degree of disease was moderate to high; however, when the severity of involvement of the middle ear was low, skull radiographs and CT were more variable in their ability to detect abnormalities.[56] Findings of proliferation of bone, lysis of bone, and in particular, extension of invasive processes toward or into the calvarium allow judgments to be made to avoid surgery as well as to help plan exploratory surgery. Once the diagnostic imaging is done, specimens from the middle ear can be obtained if the ear canal is not obstructed. Soft catheters may be placed by myringotomy if the tympanum is intact, or through a perforated tympanum, to obtain specimens for cytologic examination and for culture and susceptibility testing.

In dogs, aural cholesteatoma can be a sequela to ear canal occlusion and chronic otitis externa.[3] A cholesteatoma is an epidermal cyst that is found within the middle ear cavity and originates from a pocket of tympanic membrane that bulges into the tympanic cavity. This prolapse of epidermis adheres to the inflamed mucosa of the middle ear cavity and fills with keratin lamellae (Figure 59-8) which is produced by the tympanic membrane epidermis.[3,57] This process can result in expansion of the osseous tympani bulla with remodeling of the bone that normally borders the dimensions of the normal tympanic cavity (Figure 59-9). Cholesteatomas are most commonly secondary to otitis externa in dogs, but can be congenital or acquired.[57] Cholesteatomas that expand within the middle ear can cause oropharyngeal compression and partial obstruction of the nasopharyngeal tube.[57,58] Cholesteatomas that are secondary to chronic otitis externa can be managed successfully by total ear canal ablation and lateral bulla osteotomy. The large epidermal-lined cystic structure can be gently removed from the middle ear cavity. A ventral bulla osteotomy can be done and the epidermal cyst removed; however, if the cholesteatoma is secondary to chronic otitis externa, the tympanum and residual epidermis may remain.

Surgical Approaches to the Middle Ear

The three methods of access to the middle ear include myringotomy, ventral bulla osteotomy, and lateral bulla osteotomy.

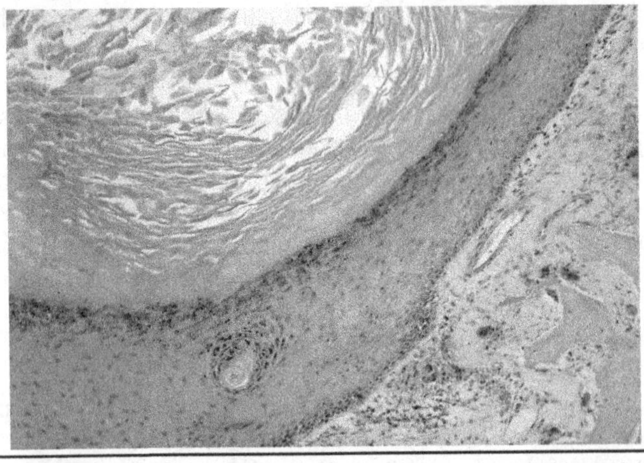

Figure 59-8. Histopathologic photomicrograph of a section of the tympanic bulla in a dog with cholesteatoma. Note the epithelium and keratin flakes. (Photomicrograph courtesy of Dr. Pam Ginn, University of Florida.)

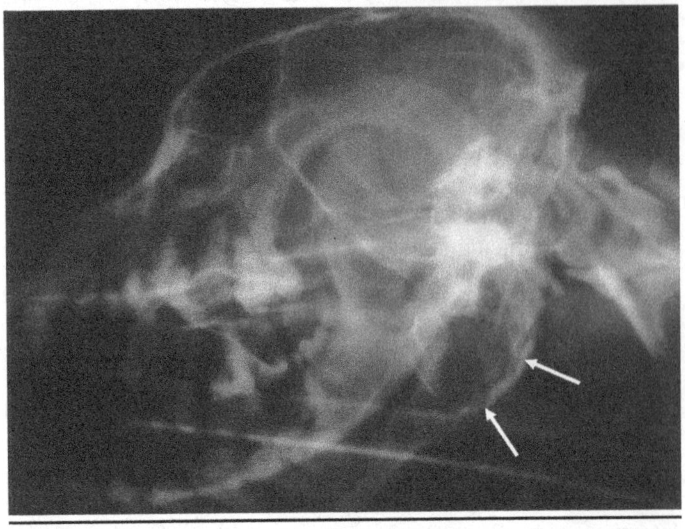

Figure 59-9. Lateral radiograph of the affected tympanic bulla (Figure 59-8) in a dog with cholesteatoma. Note the lacy expanded margin of the tympanic bulla (open arrows).

The most conservative approach is myringotomy, which is most commonly done to obtain specimens for culture and susceptibility testing and cytology when otitis media is suspected. Lateral bulla osteotomy is the more common surgical approach but is done in conjunction with total ear canal ablation for the purpose of debriding tissue and debris from the tympanic bulla. Ventral bulla osteotomy is done to explore the tympanic bulla,to remove tissue, tumors, and debris for histopathology and for culture and susceptibility testing. It is also done for removal of cholesteatomas and to promote ventral drainage. The ventral approach to the tympanic bulla is usually done when diagnostic evaluation reveals focal disease within the bulla, or if otitis media is not responsive to myringotomy and medical therapy, and if all efforts done to salvage hearing function are desired by the owner.

Surgical judgment is required when deciding which approach to perform for middle ear disease. Lateral bulla osteotomy is most appropriate for treatment of otitis media secondary to end-stage otitis externa. A ventral approach can be done but provides poor access to the lateral aspects of the external acoustic meatus. Ventral bulla osteotomy provides the most complete exposure to the tympanic cavity and is used when primary otitis media and other middle ear diseases are present. In dogs, breed differences cause ventral bulla osteotomy to vary in difficulty. For example, dissection is deep in stocky breeds such as the English bulldog and Boxer, whereas in dolicocephalic breeds the dissection seems easier. In cats, the osseous bullae are palpable prior to incision; however the tympanic bulla is partitioned into dorsolateral and ventromedial compartments. The surgical anatomy is basically the same, but the degree of difficulty of getting to the bulla may vary greatly. Vital structures encountered during the approach include the hypoglossal nerve, the external carotid artery, the lingual artery, and the sublingual salivary gland. Remember, the vital structures within the tympanic bulla are located dorsally and cranially; thus, the initial osteotomy approach must be made ventrally and caudally. The bulla is located between the angle of the mandible and the jugular process of the skull, but a convenient landmark that aids in finding the bulla is the hyoid apparatus. The tympanohyoid cartilage (attached at the stylohyoid bone) attaches caudal to the external auditory meatus, which is caudolateral to the tympanic bulla. It is also important to remember that, in addition to the vital structures in the periphery of the approach to the ventral aspect of the tympanic bulla, the oropharynx is just a few millimeters away and cavalier medial dissection can result in exposure of the oral cavity.

Inflammatory Polyps in Cats and Dogs

Inflammatory polyps are common in young cats and have been rarely reported in dogs.[59-61] These polyps are non-neoplastic and the exact etiology is not known, as neither a congenital origin or a secondary result of middle ear infection has been confirmed.[62] Polyps in cats do not appear to be associated with feline leukemia virus or feline immunodeficiency virus infections.[62] Attempts to find viral evidence by polymerase chain reaction (PCR) have been unsuccessful.[63] Chronic irritation to the mucosal surface of the middle ear may lead to the production of the inflammatory polyp, which is typically composed of well vascularized fibrous tissue stroma covered with respiratory epithelium. The ulcerated epithelium has an underlying stroma that contains both acute and inflammatory cells. Although the polyps can occur in cats of any age, the average age at diagnosis is 1.5 years.[62] Inflammatory polyps in cats are thought to originate most commonly in the middle ear near the junction of the auditory tube and the tympanic bulla, and from this location migrate into the horizontal ear canal by protrusion through the tympanum or into the nasopharynx via the auditory tube. Because the respiratory epithelium is continuous within the tympanic cavity, the Eustachian tube, and the nasopharynx, it is difficult to know the exact location of origin.[62] In the pharynx, polyps may attain a large enough size to cause stertorus respiration. Rarely, dysphagia may result. Surgical removal is accomplished by avulsing the polyp from the horizontal ear canal, or by ventral bulla osteotomy, or by an oral approach that may or may not require incision of the soft palate. Ventral bulla osteotomy to allow removal of the septum of the middle ear and curretage of the polyp base decreases recurrence of the polyps.[64,65] The polyp usually originates from the dorsolateral compartment. Curettage of both areas must be complete or recurrence of the polyp is likely. Horner's syndrome is usually transient after bulla curettage in cats (as many as 48% can have this complication).[62]

Traction or avulsion of the inflammatory polyp can be done from either canal or nasopharyngeal locations. A lateral ear resection can improve exposure.[62] Regrowth of the polyp may occur if the polyp stalk remains. In 22 cats that had inflammatory polyps treated by traction alone, 41% had recurrence.[66] Prednisolone was also used in cats reported in this investigation and was believed to aid suppression of recurrence, as 8 cats that received the corticosteroid did not have recurrence and 9 of 14 cats that did not receive the drug had recurrence of the polyps.[66] It has also been reported that nasopharygeal polyps are 4 times more likely to be successfully treated by traction alone than those that occur in the ear canal.[62,66] Perendoscopic trans-tympanic excision (PTTE) has been described and utilizes endoscopic view and endoscopic forceps to pinch away the polyp. In one report, 8 of 10 cats had complete resolution for 24 months, 2 cats required repeating PTTE, and 2 cats had temporary Horner's syndrome.[67]

Laser ablation of inflammatory polyps can be done using videoscopic exposure and a CO_2 laser.[62] Small polyps may be vaporized and gradually removed until the polyp stalk can no longer be seen. Larger polyps are removed by initially vaporizing a portion of the polyp stalk, avulsing the polyp, and then going back to finish vaporization of the polyp stalk.[62] Corticosteroid and azithromycin therapy are also recommended.[62] Antimicrobial therapy should be based ultimately on antimicrobial culture and susceptibility testing.

The tympanum is commonly destroyed when inflammatory polyps extend out into the horizontal canal. Although remnants of the tympanum and proliferation of scar tissue may result in reformation of the tympanum and partitioning of the middle ear from the external ear, persistence of this communication may result in relapse of otitis externa and media with persisting drainage from otitis media. In some cats, TECA-LBO may be necessary to resolve chronic otitis externa and media that may result.

In dogs, nasopharyngeal polyps and aural polyps rarely develop.[62] Polyps can enter the nasopharyngeal tube and affect the airway. In one dog, a polyp was removed by a staphylotomy approach, which allowed the polyp to be grasped and removed.[59] Polypoid masses are often large ceruminous-gland adenomas, rather than inflammatory polyps.[62]

Complications of bulla osteotomy include injury to vital structures such as the hypoglossal or glossopharyngeal nerves, creation or exacerbation of otitis interna (vestibular signs), Horner's syndrome when sympathetic fibers are damaged, facial nerve paralysis, and hemorrhage. Head tilts present prior to surgery, especially if chronic, may persist despite resolution of disease.

Aural Hematomas

Aural hematomas are most commonly diagnosed in dogs but are occasionally seen in cats. They occur within the cartilaginous plate (intrachondral) of the auricle (pinna) of the ear. The hematoma, which consists of blood, serum, or both, has classically been thought to result from self-inflicted trauma to the ear. Pruritus, owing to allergy or ectoparasites or secondary to otitis externa, results in head shaking or scratching. The trauma is believed to cause a shearing force that causes separation of the cartilage of the pinna. The hematoma is painful and irritating to the dog or cat and causes more head shaking and pawing at the ear with subsequent extension of the region of involvement. In cats, aural hematomas are most commonly diagnosed when ear mite infestation and otitis externa are concurrent.[2] Aural hematomas show trauma to be a precipitating rather than an underlying factor. They are uncommonly associated with chronic skin diseases, and commonly occur when there is no other evidence of ear disease in the affected dog.[68]

The aforementioned pathogenesis of aural hematomas in dogs was challenged in the late 1980s. Most veterinary surgeons have made the diagnosis of aural hematoma in the presence of a pristine ear canal; therefore, understanding the association of otitis externa and trauma is sometimes in question. An immune-mediated pathogenesis had been hypothesized on the basis of one study where 30% of affected dogs were LE cell positive, 100% of affected dogs were Coomb's test positive, and 52% of affected dogs had positive antinuclear antibody titers.[69] It was suggested that the inflammatory disease in the ears might serve as a triggering mechanism for an autoimmune reaction that could be responsible for cartilage degeneration, cartilage clefts, and subsequent development of the aural hematoma. Local treatment of aural hematoma remains unchanged, but judgment as to whether systemic therapy is appropriate is warranted. Dexamethasone has been recommended, based on these papers, to control the immune-mediated component thought to be responsible. This treatment remains controversial, and what works for some veterinarians may not work for others. Reported causes (or associations) include fungi, bacteria, parasites, atopy, aural foreign bodies, and aural neoplasia. An autoimmune pathogenesis posited in the literature in the past, has not been substantiated by more recent investigation.[68] The latter investigation did find cartilage degeneration associated with fibrovascular granulation tissue that may have been the end result of a macrophage-mediated process.[62,68]

It is important to treat aural hematomas, because if left untreated, the result is usally a thickened fibrous scar that causes the ear to fold. The auricular cartilage perichondrium is highly chondrogenic, and chondroblast invasion into an organizing aural hematoma results in a firm hard cartilaginous mass of scar, and distortion of the pinna occurs. The end result of a conservatively treated aural hematoma is an abnormal shape that is most noticeable in breeds with erect ears. Various methods of treatment exist but all must be combined with careful otoscopic examination to discern whether self-inflicted trauma or head shaking is evident, as medical management of a concurrent problem is important for complete treatment.

Conservative techniques to drain aural hematomas are effective, and because a large incision is not made, minimal scarring of the pinna occurs. Active drainage technique or pressure can be an aid to evaluation of fluid from the aural cavity.[70] Each type of drain is placed into the cavity encompassing the hematoma after a small stab incision is made. The teat cannula is placed in the dependent portion of the hematoma. The drain must be cleansed daily to assure patency, and it may be necessary to leave it in place 14 to-21 days. If the drain becomes clogged by exudate, or if it is removed prematurely, recurrence of the hematoma is likely. Bandaging protects the ear from further trauma related to head shaking and also prevents soiling of areas in the home when drainage occurs.

More invasive techniques usually involve making incisions parallel to the pinna, evacuating the fluid, and suturing to appose the tissue layers with the hope of resolving and preventing recurrence of the aural hematoma. Various incision and suture patterns can be used to accomplish this; the choice depends on the individual surgeon. Too much tension on sutures may cause secondary contracture and deformation of the ear so care should be taken when placing sutures. Some surgeons feel a large curvilinear incision does not allow contraction to deform the pinna of the ear. A narrow gap is desired to aid maintenance of drainage from the concave surface of the ear. Nonadherent contact dressings are used. Bandaging techniques also vary but are used to protect the ear from head shaking and to absorb drainage. Sutures are often left in place for 14 or more days.

More chronic aural hematomas may be firm and organized, as after 7 to 10 days fibroblastic infiltration of the hematoma occurs, and eventually cartilage forms. It is helpful to remove this material surgically and obliterate the space using sutures. In this state, drainage by the aforementioned techniques is not feasible. Organized hematomas must be removed by incision on the concave surface of the ear. The hematoma is removed and bleeding vessels are cauterized or ligated. The incisional margins are excised such that the edges do not meet and drainage is promoted. The dead space in the cavity is obliterated with through-and-through mattress sutures placed parallel to and on each side of the incision, with the knots on the external surface of the ear. An alternative technique is to place the mattress sutures from inside the ear through the cartilage without penetrating the opposing skin surface. A better cosmetic result is obtained as the development of stitch abscesses on the haired side of the pinna is prevented. Noncapillary suture material should be used (i.e., monofilament nylon or polypropylene), and mattress sutures should be placed parallel to the long axis of the pinna to preserve blood vessels that are oriented in that direction. The carbon dioxide laser can also be used to treat aural hematomas.[71] Regardless of technique, a protective bandage and head wrap are applied and changed every 2 to 3 days, and sutures are removed in 10 to 14 days.

Antibiotic therapy is not indicated unless infection is suspected or confirmed by culture and sensitivity testing, but corticosteroids are used by those who feel an immune-mediated component contributes to the development of aural hematomas. Corticosteroids are also important to lessen head shaking and for patient comfort. Use of corticosteroids may also be therapeutic if the inflammatory response is in part responsible for cartilage separation and development of the aural hematoma.

Marginal Auricular Dermatosis and Ear Margin Fissures

Short-haired dogs with pendulous ears occasionally develop thickened areas at the apical edges of the pinna. These areas eventually become scab-like, which when removed reveal a raw bleeding surface. As these wounds heal, exposed cartilage disappears but the edge of the flap remains eroded and thickened.[2] Pinnal necrosis, often idiopathic, can affect toy breeds and requires surgical excision of the edge or apex of the pinna. (Figures 59-10A and 59-10B) Biopsy of lesions of the pinna, especially on the concave surface, may be done using a 3 mm skin punch. Hemorrhage can be controlled by digital pressure, needle-tip cautery, or a cauterizing agent. It is important to obtain dermal tissue in the specimen. A small hypodermic needle can be used to tease the fibrous tissue off the cartilage base.

Ear margin fissures occur as a result of scratching or flapping the ears. This lesion appears as small wounds at the margin of the distal aspect of the pinna, and with continued trauma may become several centimeters long.[2] Treatment of the primary

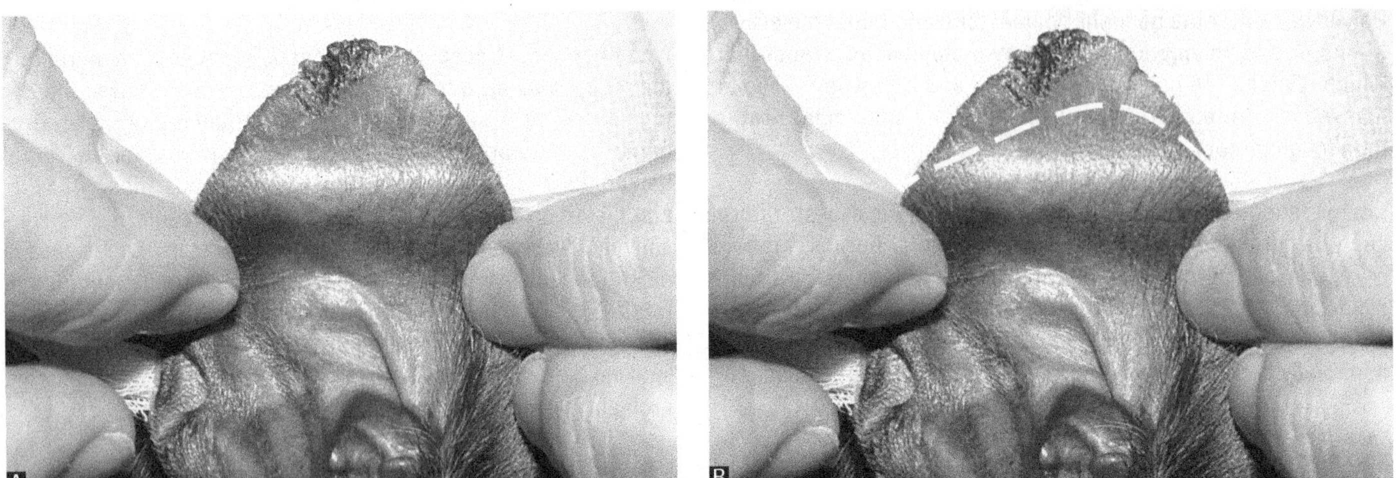

Figure 59-10A. Photograph of the ear of a Chihuahua with idiopathic pinnal necrosis. Surgical biopsy of this lesion is indicated and (B) cosmetic distal pinna excision, depicted by the dashed line, may be curative. (Photograph courtesy of Dr. Robert Kennis, Auburn University.)

reason for the discomfort and head shaking (flapping) is important to break the cycle that results in recurrent injury. Treatment of long fissures requires debridement and suturing. Multiple small fissures are usually treated by excision of the most superficial edge of the pinna. A scalpel or sharp scissors (depending on the thickness of the edge of the pinna) can be used to excise the affected edge just proximal to the fissure. Sutures are not always required, but the ear must be bandaged across the head to prevent trauma to the wound margin from head shaking. Alternatively, the medial and lateral edges of the skin can be apposed gently over the cartilage edge with fine interrupted sutures of non-absorbable material, taking care to avoid penetrating the cartilage where possible. While the ear margin is healing primarily or by secondary wound healing, the primary cause for the irritation and trauma must be treated, so that once the ears are left unbandaged, ear flapping is minimized.

Auricular chondritis, resulting in bilateral thickening of the pinnae was reported in a cat. Slight curling of the pinna, intense erythema, and pain were evident. The cat responded to treatment with prednisolone.[72]

Otolithiasis

Rarely, mineralized opacities may occur in the tympanic bullae. Mineralized necrotic material from previous otitis media may be the source of otolithiasis. Otolithiasis has been reported in three dogs and was detected by skull radiographs and CT.[73] Otoliths may be identified in active cases of otitis media, or in some dogs, maybe an incidental finding.

Aural Neoplasia

In dogs and cats, tumors of the ear canal are relatively rare, comprising between 2% and 6% of dog ear surgery admissions and 1% to 2% of cat ear surgery admissions, respectively.[74] Malignant aural tumors in dogs and cats include ceruminous gland adenocarcinoma, squamous cell carcinoma, and carcinoma of undetermined origin.[74] It has been stated that malignant tumors in dogs are less aggressive than those in cats.[75] It is expected that dogs generally live longer than 2 years after surgical excision of an aural tumor, whereas cats' median survival is about 1 year.[75] The median survival rates for dogs and cats with malignant tumors in a 1996 study were longer than 58 months and 11.7 months, respectively.[74] A more recent study in cats showed a median survival time of 50.3 months for those with ceruminous gland adenocarcinoma.[29] Negative prognostic factors were extensive tumor involvement, neurologic signs at the time of diagnosis, diagnosis of squamous cell carcinoma or of carcinoma of undetermined origin, and lymphatic or blood vessel invasion.[74] Squamous cell carcinoma is known to arise from the middle ear in cats, and may cause Horner's syndrome, vestibular dysfunction, and facial paraylsis.[29,76] In the more recent study in cats, a mitotic index of greater or equal than 3 found cats living significantly less than cats with a mitotic index of less than or equal to 2.29 Approximately 25% of malignant aural tumors will have tympanic bulla involvement; therefore, imaging studies such as CT are helpful to plan surgical removal.[75] Metastasis to the thorax or to regional lymph nodes is present in about 10% of dogs and cats at the time of diagnosis.[75] For both dogs and cats, aggressive surgical resection of malignant tumors (i.e., total ear canal ablation with lateral bulla osteotomy), results in the longest survival times. Benign ear canal tumors can be managed with more conservative surgical resection, depending on the location of the tumor and the condition of the ear canal. Radiation may be used adjunctively where resection is incomplete, but little is known about the efficacy of chemotherapy.[75]

References

1. Cole LK: Diseases of the ear. *In* Morgan RV, Bright RM, Swartout MS (eds). Handbook of Small Animal Practice, 4th ed. Philadelphia: Saunders, 2003, p. 1047.

2. Bojrab MJ, Griffin CE, Renegar WR: The ear. *In* Bojrab MJ (ed). Mechanisms of Disease in Small Animal Surgery. Philadelphia: WB Saunders, 1998, p. 120.

3. Logas DB, Bellah JR: Otitis externa. *In* Handbook of Small Animal Practice, 4th. Morgan RV, Bright RM, Swartout MS (eds). ed. Philadelphia: WB Saunders, 2003, p. 1049.

4. McClure RC: The cranial nerves. *In* Evans HE, Christensen GC (eds). Miller's Anatomy of the Dog. Philadelphia: WB Saunders,: 1979, p. 924.

5. Logas D: Otitis externa etiology and pathogenesis. Course Notes, Two Day Intense Otitis Seminar, North American Veterinary Conference, January 2002.

6. House A: Atresia of the distal external acoustic meatus in a Bouvier des Flandres. J Small Anim Pract 42:88, 2001.

7. Huang HP, Huang HM: Effects of ear type, sex, age, body weight, and climate on temperatures in the external acoustic meatus of dogs. Am J Vet Res 60:1173, 1999.

8. Hendricks A, Brooks H, Pocknell A, Bond R: Ulcerative otitis externa responsive to immunosuppressive therapy in two dogs. J Small Anim Pract 43:350, 2002.

9. Griffen CE: Otitis externa and otitis media. *In* Current Veterinary Dermatology. Griffin CE, Kwochka KW, MacDonald JM (eds). Philadelphia: Mosby Year Book, 1993, p. 245.

10. Rosser EJ: Diagnosis of food allergy in dogs. J Am Vet Med Assoc 203:259, 1993.

11. Nuttall TJ: Use of ticarcillin in the management of canine otitis externa complicated by Pseudomonas aeruginosa. J Small Anim Pract 39:165, 1998.

12. Graham-Mize CA, Rosser EJ: Comparison of microbial isolates and susceptibility patterns from the external ear canal of dogs with otitis externa. J Am Anim Hosp Assoc 40:102,2004.

13. Gotthelf, LN: Healing of the ruptured eardrum. *In* Small Animal Ear Diseases, an Illustrated Guide. Gotthelf LN (ed). St. Louis: Elsevier Saunders, 2005, p. 305.

14. Swaim SF, Henderson RA:. Small Animal Wound Management, 2nd ed. Philadelphia: Williams & Wilkins, 1997, p. 212.

15. Zepp CP: Surgical technique to establish drainage of the external ear canal and corrections of hematoma of the dog and cat. J Am Vet Med Assoc 115:91, 1949.

16. Griffin CE: Otitis externa. Comp Cont Educ Pract Vet 3:741, 1981.

17. Grono LR: Studies of the microclimate of the external auditory canal in the dog. Res Vet Sci 11:316, 1970.

18. Tufvesson G: Operation for otitis externa in dogs according to Zepp's method. Am J Vet Res 16:565, 1955.

19. Gregory CR, Vasseur PB: Clinical results of lateral ear resection in dogs. J Am Vet Med Assoc 182:1087, 1983.

20. Lane JG, Little CJL: Surgery of the canine external auditory meatus: A review of failures. J Small Anim Pract 27:247, 1986.

21. Sylvestre AM: Potential factors affecting the outcome of dogs with a resection of the lateral wall of the vertical ear canal. Can Vet J 39:157, 1998.

22. Johnston DE: Early lateral drainage procedure for chronic otitis externa in dogs. Abstract, the 4th Annual Scientific Meeting of the ECVS, Constance, Germany, 1995; 38.

23. Blakely CL: Otorrhea and surgical drainage. *In* Canine Surgery, 4th edd., Mayer K, et al (eds). Santa Barbara: American Veterinary Publications, 1957, p. 309.

24. Bellah JR: How and when to perform lateral and vertical ear canal resection. Vet Med June:535, 1997.

25. Layton CE: The role of lateral ear resection in managing chronic otitis externa. Semin Vet Med Surg (Small Anim) 8:24, 1993.

26. Fraser G, Withers AR, Spreull JA: Otitis externa in the dog. J Small Anim Pract 2:32, 1961.

21. McCarthy RJ, Caywood DD: Vertical ear canal resection for end-stage otitis externa in dogs. J Am Anim Hosp Assoc 28:545, 1992.

28. Bellah JR: When should you recommend total ear canal ablation and lateral bulla osteotomy? Vet Med June:544, 1997.

29. Bacon NJ, Gilbert RL, Bostock DE, White RAS: Total ear canal ablation in the cat: indication, morbidity and long-term survival. J Small Anim Pract 44:430, 2003.

30. Henderson JT, Radasch RM: Total ear canal ablation with lateral bulla osteotomy for the management of end-stage otitis in dogs. Comp Pract Vet (Small Animal) 17:157, 1995.

31. McCarthy PE, Hosgood G, Pechman: Traumatic ear canal separations and para-aural abscessation in three dogs. J Am Anim Hosp Assoc 31:419, 1995.

32. Connery NA, McAllister H, Hay CW: Para-aural abscessation following traumatic ear canal separation in a dog. J Small Anim Pract 42:253, 2001.

33. Smeak DD: Traumatic separation of the annular cartilage from the external auditory meatus in a cat. J Am Vet Med Assoc 211:448, 1997.

34. Boothe HW, Hobson HP, McDonald DE: Treatment of traumatic separation of the auricular and annular cartilages without ablation: Results in five dogs. Vet Surg 25:376, 1996.

35. Devitt DM, Seim HB, Willer R, et al: Passive drainage versus primary closure after total ear canal ablation – lateral bulla osteotomy in dogs: 59 dogs (1985-1995) 26:210, 1997.

36. Waldron DR: Ear canal surgery: Palliation vs. cure. Vet Forum January:24, 2006.

37. Vogel PL, Komtebedde J, Hirsh DC, Kass PH: Wound contamination and antimicrobial susceptibility of bacteria cultured during total ear canal ablation and lateral bulla osteotomy in dogs. J Am Vet Med Assoc 214:1641, 1999.

38. Hettlich BF, Boothe HW, Simpson, et al: Effect of tympanic cavity evaluation and flushing on microbial isolates during total ear canal ablation with lateral bulla osteotomy in dogs. J Am Vet Med Assoc 227:748, 2005.

39. Grono LR: The surgical treatment of canine otitis externa. Aust Vet J 38:235, 1962.

40. Holt D, Brockman DJ, Sylvestre AM, Sadanaga KK: Lateral exploration of fistulas developing after total ear canal ablations: 10 cases (1989-1993). J Am Anim Hosp Assoc 32:527, 1996.

41. Smeak DD, Crocker CB, Birchard SJ: Treatment of recurrent otitis media that developed after total ear canal ablation and lateral bulla osteotomy in dogs: nine cases (1986-1994). J Am Vet Med Assoc 209:937, 1996.

42. Lamb CR, White RN, McEvoy FJ: Sinography in the investigation of draining tracts in small animals: Retrospective review of 25 cases. Vet Surg 23:129, 1994.

43. Matthieson DT, Scavelli T: Total ear canal ablation and lateral bulla osteotomy in 38 dogs. J Am Anim Hosp Assoc 26:257, 1990.

44. Buback JL, Boothe HW, Carroll GL, Green RW: Comparison of three methods for relief of pain after ear canal ablation in dogs. Vet Surg 25:380, 1996.

45. Radlinsky M, Mann D, Roush J, et al: Continuous infusion of bupivicane for analgesia following total ear canal ablation in dogs (abstract). Presented at the 12th Annual Veterinary Symposium of the American College of Veterinary Surgeons, San Diego, October, 2002.

46. Krahwinkel DJ, Pardo AD, Sims MH, Bubb WJ: Effect of total ablation of the external acoustic meatus and bulla osteotomy on auditory function in dogs. J Am Vet Med Assoc 202:949, 1993.

47. McAnulty JF, Hattle A, Harvery CE: Wound healing and brain stem auditory evoked potentials after experimental ventral tympanic bulla osteotomy in dogs. Vet Surg 24:9, 1995.

48. Steiss JE, Wright JC, Storrs DP: Alterations in the brain stem auditory evoked response threshold and latency-intensity curve associated with conductive hearing loss in dogs. Prob Vet Neurol 1:205, 1991.

49. Sims MH, Brace JJ, Arthur DA, Harvey RC: Otoacoustic emission in a dog. J Am Vet Med Assoc 198:1017, 1991.

50. Logas DB: Diseases of the ear canal. Vet Clinic North Am (Small Anim Pract) 24:905, 1994.

51. Neer TM, Howard PE: Otitis media. Comp Cont Educ Pract Vet 4:410, 1982.

52. Cole LK, Kwochka KW, Kowalski JJ, Hillier A: Microbial flora and antimicrobial susceptibility patterns of isolated pathogens from the horizontal ear canal and middle ear in dogs with otitis media J Am Vet Med Assoc 212:534, 1998.

53. Bruette DS, Lorena MD: Otitis externa and otitis media: diagnostic and medical aspects. Semin Vet Med Surg (Small Anim) 8:3, 1993.

54. Gregory SP: Middle ear disease associated with congenital palatine defects in seven dogs and one cat. J Small Anim Pract 41:398, 2000.

55. Bischoff MG, Kneller SK: Diagnostic imaging of the canine and feline ear. Vet Clin North Am (Small Anim) 34:437, 2004.

56. Rohleder JJ, Jones JC, Duncan RB, et al: Comparative performance of radiography and computed tomography in the diagnosis of middle ear disease in 31 dogs. Vet Radiol Ultrasound 47:45, 2006.

57. Ellison GW, Donnell RL, Daniel GB: Nasopharyngeal epidermal cyst in a dog. J Am Vet Med Assoc 207:1590, 1995.

58. Little CJL, Lane JG, Gibbs C, et al: Inflammatory middle ear disease of the dog: the clinical and pathological features of cholesteatoama, a complication of otitis media. Vet Rec 128:319, 1991.

59. Fingland RB, Gratzek A, Vorhies MW, et al: Nasopharyngeal polyp in a dog. J Am Anim Hosp Assoc 29:311, 1993.

60. Kapatkin AS, Matthiesen DT, Noone KE, et al: Results of surgery and long-term follow-up in 31 cats with nasopharyngeal polyps. J Am Anim Hosp Assoc 26:387, 1990.

61. Pratschke KM: Inflammatory polyps in the middle ear in 5 dogs. Vet Surg 32:292, 2003.

62. Gotthelf LN: Inflammatory polyps. *In* Small Animal Ear Diseases, An Illustrated Guide. Gotthelf LN (ed). St. Louis: Elsevier Saunders, 2005, p. 318.

63. Veir JK, Lappin MR, Foley JE, et al: Feline inflammatory polyps: historical, clinical, and PCR findings for feline calicivirus and feline herpesvirus-1 in 28 cases. J Feline Med Surg 4:195, 2002.

64. Trevor PB, Martin RA: Tympanic bulla osteotomy for the treatment of middle ear disease in cats; 19 cases (1984-1991). J Am Vet Med Assoc 202:123, 1993.

65. Boothe HW: Surgery of the tympanic bull (otitis media and nasopharyngeal polyps). Prob Vet Med 3:254, 1991.

66. Anderson DM, White RAS, Robinson RK: Management of inflammatory polyps in 37 cats. Vet Rec 147:684, 2000.

67. Mortenello CM, Alfieri C, DeFrancesco I, et al: Perendoscopic transtympanic excision (PTTE) of ear canal polyps in cats: 10 case reports. World Small Animal Veterinary Association Proceedings, 2001.

68. Joyce J, Day M: Immunopathogenesis of canine aural haematoma. J Sm Anim Pract 38:152, 1997.

69. Kuwahara J: Canine and feline aural hematoma: Clinical, experimental and clinicopathologic observations. Am J Vet Res 47:2300, 1986.

70. Swaim SF, Bradley DM: Evaluation of closed-suction drainage for treating auricular hematomas. J Am Anim Hosp Assoc 32:36, 1996.

71. Dye TL, Teague HD, Ostwald DA, Ferreira SD: Evaluation of a technique using the carbon dioxide laser for the treatment of aural hematomas. J Am Anim Hosp Assoc 38:385, 2002.

72. Delmage DA, Kelly DF: Auricular chondritis in a cat. J Small Anim Pract 42:499, 2001.

73. Ziemer LS, Schwarz T, Sullivan M: Otolithiasis in 3 dogs. Vet Radiol Ultrasound 44:28, 2003.

74. London CA, Dubilzeig RR, Vail DM, et al: Evaluation of dogs and cats with tumors of the ear canal: 145 cases (1978-1992). J Am Vet Med Assoc 208:1413, 1996.

75. Vail DM, Withrow SJ: Tumors of the skin and subcutaneous tissues. In Small Animal Clinical Oncology. Withrow SJ, MacEwen EG (eds). Philadelphia: Saunders, 2001, p. 252.

76. Indrieri RJ, Taylor RF: Vestibular dysfunction caused by squamous cell carcinoma involving the middle ear and inner ear in two cats. J Am Vet Med Assoc 184:471, 1984.

Chapter 60

Feline Aural and Nasopharyngeal Polyps

Rod A.W. Rosychuk

Feline aural-nasopharyngeal polyps are non-neoplastic growths that originate from the middle ear and/or the adjacent entrance to the auditory canal. Aural polyps are those that extend from the middle ear, through the tympanum into the horizontal canal of the ear. Nasopharyngeal polyps are those that extend through the auditory canal into the posterior pharynx. Aural-nasopharyngeal polyps are the most common nasopharyngeal disease of young cats and the most common non-neoplastic mass of the feline ear.[1,2]

Polyps are seen in young to middle-aged cats, with the mean age at presentation variably reported as 18 months 3-5 or 6.0 years.[6,7] The range is 3 months to 18 years.[3-7] There does not appear to be any breed or sex predisposition.[3-7]

Etiopathogenesis

Polyps appear to be inflammatory or post inflammatory lesions. Histologically, the growths are characterized by loosely arranged fibrous tissue throughout which are scattered plasma cells, lymphocytes, neutrophils, lymphoid aggregates or follicles, and variable numbers of mucus-secreting glands.[4,8,9] Often, just beneath the epithelium, are focal areas of increased vascularity and, at times, heavy infiltrations of both acute and chronic inflammatory cells.[8,9] Polyps are covered by a stratified squamous to ciliated columnar epithelium that may be ulcerated.[3,8,9] The ciliated columnar epithelium cannot be differentiated from that covering the nasopharynx, auditory canal, or lining of the middle ear.[10] Grossly, polyps may be smooth or lobulated and pale pink or grey.[9] Nasopharyngeal polyps and many aural polyps are usually firm or rubbery on cut section.[9] This firmness facilitates grasping with forceps for purposes of removal by traction or avulsion. Some aural polyps tend to be more myxomatous, and friable, suggesting a shorter duration of growth.[8]

The etiology of polyps remains unclear. Because the lesions have an inflammatory component, the most likely initiating cause would be irritant in nature.[10] Both viral[2,7,11] and bacterial infections[9] have been hypothesized. Support for an infectious etiology is suggested by the occasional observation of multiple, unrelated cats all developing polyps at about the same time.[11]

Although reports exist of calicivirus isolation from polyp material,[11,12] the incidence is low and is likely an incidental finding. In a study of 41 polyps, feline *herpesvirus*-1 and feline *calicivirus* were not found by RT-PCR and PCR.[7] The fact that the samples in this study were formalized may have contributed to some false negative results. Although this data suggests that viral persistence is not a likely cause of the problem, it does not rule out the possibility that viruses may initiate the syndrome, but are eventually cleared.

It is also possible that bacterial infection that has ascended the auditory tube may be responsible for initiating and perpetuating polyp growth.[9] Cats are prone to viral upper respiratory infections that may be complicated by secondary bacterial infection. However, most cats do not have a history of upper respiratory infections antedating polyp development,[7] and the middle ear of cats with nasopharyngeal polyps are usually sterile.[4] This again does not preclude the possibility that bacterial infection may have initiated the problem.

A role for other infectious organisms such as *Bartonella, Mycoplasma,* and/or *Chlamydia* has not been evaluated to date.

Because polyps have been noted in very young individuals, it has also been hypothesized that they may be congenital defects arising from remnants of brachial arches.[13] However, no data exist to support this conjecture.

The initiating cause of polyp growth is likely no longer present at the time of clinical presentation. This is supported by the fact that relatively complete removal utilizing ventral bulla osteotomy (VBO) results in a lack of regrowth in the vast majority of cases of both aural and nasopharyngeal polyps.[3,4,6,7]

Site of Origin

The middle ear of the cat is divided into a smaller dorsolateral and a larger ventromedial chamber by a thin bony plate. The dorsolateral chamber is bordered medially by the bony cochlear promontory and petrous temporal bone and laterally by the tympanum. It contains the auditory ossicles and a postganglionic sympathetic nerve plexus that fan out over its medial wall.[14,15] The communication between these chambers is limited to a narrow fissure between the bony plate and cochlear promontory on the caudomedial aspect of the compartment. Toward its caudal extremity, the fissure enlarges into a triangular foramen.[14,15] The round window of the cochlea makes up part of the medial wall of this opening. The auditory canal, which is 5 to 8 mm long,[15] arises from the anterior-most aspect of the dorsolateral chamber and extends into the posterior pharynx.

Only rare reports exist of post-mortem dissection to document the site of origin of polyps. In one young cat with nasopharyngeal and middle ear polyps, the only site of attachment for both was in the region of the opening of the middle ear into the auditory canal.[16] Site of origin correlations are otherwise presumptive and based on radiographs and observations made during surgical therapy.

A middle ear site of origin for both aural and nasopharyngeal polyps is supported in the vast majority of cases by the observation that a middle ear mass is seen radiographically and by surgical exploration via ventral bulla osteotomy.[4,5] A dorsomedial chamber site of origin is supported by the observation that, during ventral bulla osteotomy in affected cats, polyps are attached to the walls of the dorsolateral compartment but not to the walls of the ventromedial chamber. Polyp growth likely extends from the dorsolateral chamber through the communicating fissure and foramen to fill the ventromedial chamber. Its growth may produce pressure necrosis of the thin bony plate that separates the chambers. This would explain the observed absence of the bony plate at the time of ventral bulla osteotomy in many patients. Nasopharyngeal polyps are occasionally seen without radiographic middle ear involvement. In these individuals, polyp growth appears to occur from around the opening to the auditory canal.[4] After traction for removal of nasophyaryngeal polyps, a stalk is seen attached to the polyp that corresponds to the approximate length of the feline auditory canal.[4]

The attachment of the polyp to submucosal tissues overlying the medial bony wall of the dorsolateral chamber is further supported by the common occurrence of a transient Horner's syndrome following avulsion/traction of both aural or nasopharyngeal polyps.[4,6]

Complicating Factors

Mucoid secretions are commonly noted in the middle ears of cats with middle ear polyps.[14] The epithelial lining of the middle ear contains mucus-containing goblet cells.[17,18] With chronic irritation, mucus-secreting glands are also noted to develop.[17,18] The presence of polyp material within the middle ear likely stimulates increased mucus production through irritation. It is also noted that occlusion of the auditory canal in normal cats results in the accumulation of a viscous, mucoid material which is of goblet cell and mucus gland origin.[17,18] These secretions normally exit the middle ear through the auditory canal. Polyp material partially obstructing the auditory canal likely results in mucoid-material retention in affected cats.

Secondary bacterial infections are also commonly noted in the middle ears of cats with aural polyps (17 of 22 reported cases).[5,6,19-21] Bacteria noted (in decreasing order of frequency) include *Pasturella multocida, Beta Hemolytic Streptococcus, Staphylococcus hominis, Bacteroides sp, Pseudomonas sp, and Sreptococcus zooepidemicus.*[6] The incidence of secondary infections warrants the routine practice of cytologic examination and culture and the use of postoperative antibiotics in the management of aural polyps.[6] This tendency toward the development of secondary infections is likely related to perforation of the tympanum and bacterial access from the ear canals.

It is uncommon to have secondary middle ear infections in cats with nasopharyngeal polyps (3 of 23 cases in one study[4]). In these cases, the bacteria isolated included *Bordetella sp, Pasturella sp,* and *Achromobacter sp.* Obstruction of the auditory canal is noted to predispose to secondary bacterial infection of the middle ear in the cat.[17] The middle ear of the cat has a normal, transient bacterial flora. Retained secretions associated with obstruction likely produce a microenvironment that is conducive to infection. Partial obstruction owing to nasopharyngeal growth may predispose to infection through a similar mechanism.

History and Clinical Signs

Initial clinical signs may be noted from days to years prior to presentation.[3,4,7] Polyps are most commonly unilateral at presentation. In one study of cats with only nasopharyngeal polyps, 21 were unilateral, 4 were bilateral.[4] In a group with only auricular polyps, 10 were unilateral, 2 were bilateral.[6]

Growth of the polyp from the middle ear is usually into the auditory canal or through the tympanum into the horizontal canal, or both. In one study of 28 cats, 50% were otic alone, 21% nasopharyngeal alone, and 29% a combination of both.[7] In another study of 37 cats, 51% had growth into the nasopharynx, 38% into the ear, and 11% of cats had both.[3]

At the time of presentation, polyps have almost always extended into the horizontal ear canal or the nasopharynx. It is difficult to say what clinical signs, if any, are associated with early polyp growth confined to the middle ear. It is likely that clinical signs at this point are minimal as supported by the lack of clinical signs of otitis media (head shaking, pain on opening mouth, neurologic signs) seen in a group of individuals with only nasopharyngeal polyps and radiographic and exploratory evidence of bulla involvement.[4]

The clinical signs associated with auricular polyps include debris accumulation within the ear canals, head shaking, scratching, and intermittent or consistent head tilting.[6] Intermittent head tilting is usually because of discomfort rather than neurologic dysfunction. These signs are likely products of perforation of the tympanum, irritation within the horizontal canal, and secondary bacterial and/or *Malassezia* colonization/infection within the canals. Debris accumulation in the canals is common and may be waxy to purulent.[5] These accumulations are a product of disruption of the normal "flushing" mechanism of the ear (lateral epithelial growth from the region of the tympanum), polyp irritation, and bacterial and/or *Malassezia* colonization/infection. Any source of irritation or inflammation within the ear canal results in increased ceruminous secretions. The actual incidence of bacterial and/or *Malassezia* colonization/infection has not been reported in affected cats; however, in the author's experience, they are common.

Neurologic signs of otitis media (Horner's syndrome, facial paresis, and paralysis) and otitis interna (head tilt, nystagmus, ataxia) are only uncommonly noted in patients with aural polyps.[5,8,19] These signs are most likely complications of secondary infections of the middle ear that could gain access to the inner ear through the membrane-covered oval or round window.[19] When infection is not present, it has been suggested that inner ear signs may be a product of increased pressure within the inner ear, mediated by pressure on the round and/or oval windows.[21]

The clinical signs associated with nasopharyngeal polyps are related to progressive growth down the auditory canal, occlusion of the auditory canal, or gradual growth and expansion into the posterior pharyngeal region. Most masses are visible within the posterior pharynx at the time of clinical presentation, both clinically and radiologically (30/31 cases in one study[4]). Visualization is facilitated by forward traction on the soft palate. Clinical signs of the expanding mass in the posterior pharynx include inspiratory stridor and snoring,[5] nasal discharge, gagging, and sneezing.[4,5] Nasal breathing may be compromised,[22] and sleep may be interrupted because of a need to mouth breath. Severe obstruction may result in dyspnea, cyanosis, and syncopal collapse.[15] Breathing difficulties and/or decreased ability to smell may result in significant inappetance. Large masses may impinge on the larynx and cause voice changes and may produce dysphagia. Affected cats may want to eat, but may have difficulty in swallowing. Halitosis may be significant.[3] These various problems may produce significant weight loss and loss of general bodily condition. Affected patients are prone to the development of secondary bacterial rhinitis or sinusitis. These signs may contribute to the symptoms and may be difficult to differentiate from the signs associated with polyps. Lower respiratory tract disease (pneumonia) can develop in chronic or severe cases, likely owing to compromise of large-airway clearance mechanisms. Neurologic signs associated with nasopharyngeal polyps are uncommon (noted in 3 of 31 cases in one study 4). These are most likely related to the development of secondary infection within the middle ear as suggested for aural polyps.

Factors Affecting Prognosis

Once polyps are clinically visible, the nature of the inflammatory process seems to make the masses relatively resistant to the effects of both anti-inflammatory and immunosuppressive dosages of oral glucocorticoids and topical glucocorticoids (for aural polyps).[8]

In those cases in which significant tissue is left within the bulla, regrowth is common.[4,6,7] In one study, mean time to regrowth was 3.5 months; range of 1 to 9 months.[3] This is most commonly noted with aural polyps treated with traction/avulsion[3,7] and is most likely related to the fact that, with this technique, significant polyp material remains within bulla. For this reason, many authors recommend VBO as the management of choice for both aural and nasopharyngeal polyps.[4,7] More recently, it has been noted that the use of a decreasing dosage regimen of oral glucocorticoids results in the lack of regrowth following partial removal via traction/avulsion of both aural and nasopharyngeal polyps.[3] Significant polyp remained within the bulla of affected patients and regrowth would have been expected in several. No regrowth was noted in 8 of 83 and 6/6 cases.[23] These observations would suggest that, even with significant polyp material left in the bulla, the creation of an acute inflammatory microenvironment through traction/avulsion allows the anti-inflammatory effects of glucocorticoids to be effective in causing residual polyp tissue to regress.

References

1. Allen HS, Broussard J, Noone K: Nasopharyngeal diseases in cats: a retrospective study of 53 cases (1991-1998). J Am Anim Hosp Assoc 35:457, 1999.

2. Rogers KS: Tumors of the ear canal. Vet Clin North Am 18:59, 1988.

3. Anderson DM, Robinson RK, White RA: Management of inflammatory polyps in 37 cats. Vet Rec 147:684, 2000.

4. Kapatkin A, Mattheisen DT, Noone KE, et al: Results of surgery and long-term follow-up in 31 cats with nasopharyngeal polyps. J Am Anim Hosp Assoc 26:387, 1990.

5. Trevor PB, Martin RA: Tympanic bulla osteotomy for treatment of middle ear disease in cats: 19 cases (1984-1991). J Am Vet Med Assoc 202:123, 1993.

6. Faulkner JE, Budsberg SC: Results of ventral bulla osteotomy for the treatment of middle ear polyps in cats. J Am Anim Hosp Assoc 26:496, 1990.

7. Veir JK, Lappin MR, Foley JE, Getzy DM: Feline inflammatory polyps: historical, clinical and PCR findings for feline calici virus and feline herpes virus-1 in 28 cases. J Fel Med Surg 4:195, 2002.

8. Harvey CE, Goldschmidt MH: Inflammatory polypoid growths in the ear canals of cats. J Small Anim Pract19:669, 1978.

9. Lane JG, Orr CM, Lucke VM, Gruffydd-Jones TJ: Nasopharyngeal polyps arising in the middle ear of the cat. J Small Anim Pract 22:511, 1981.

10. Bradley RL, Noone KE, Sauders GK, Patnaik AK: Nasopharyngeal and middle ear polypoid masses in five cats. Vet Surg 14:141, 1985.

11. Parker NR, Binnington AG: Nasopharyngeal polyps in cats: three case reports and a review of the literature. J Am Anim Hosp Assoc 21:473, 1985.

12. Muilenburg RK, Fry TR: Feline nasopharyngeal polyps. Vet Clin North Am Small Anim Pract 32:839, 2002.

13. Baker GJ: Nasopharyngeal polyps in cats. Vet Rec 111:43, 1982.

14. Little CJ: Nasopharyngeal polyps. *In* August JR (ed). Consultations in Feline Internal Medicine, 3rd ed. Philadelphia:WB Saunders, 1997, p. 310.

15. LeCouteur RA, Vernau KM: Feline vestibular disorders. Part 1: Anatomy and clinical signs. J Fel Med Surg 1:71, 1999.

16. Stanton ME, Wheaton LG, Render JA, Blevins WE: Pharyngeal polyps in two feline siblings. J Am Vet Med Assoc 186:1311, 1985.

17. Majima Y, Jin CS, Takeuch K, et al: Rheological properties of middle ear mucus in relation to goblet cell populations in the cat. Acta Otolaryngol (Stockh) 483:11, 1991.

18. Tos M, Wiederhold M, Larsen P: Experimental long-term tubal occlusion in the cat. A quantitative histopathological study. Acta Otolaryngal (Stockh) 97:580, 1984.

19. Cook LB, Bergman RL, Bahr A, Boothe HW: Inflammatory polyps in the middle ear with secondary suppurative meningoencephalitis in a cat. Vet Rad Ultras 44:648. 2003.

20. Remedios AM, Fowler JD, Pharr JW: A comparison of radiographic versus surgical diagnosis of otitis media. J Am Anim Hosp Assoc 27:183, 1991.

21. Seitz SE, Losonsky JM, Marretta SM: Computed tomographic appearance of inflammatory polyps in three cats. Vet Rad Ultras 37:99, 1996.

22. Bacmeister C: Dyspnea in a cat with otitis. Feline Pract 19:5, 1991.

23. Rosychuk RAW, Personal Communication, 2006.

Part VIII

Skin/Integument

Chapter 61

Skin Wound Healing

Tannaz Amalsadvala
Steven F. Swaim

A wound is defined as any interruption in the continuity of the body's tissue.[1,2] After injury, a wound immediately begins a complex process of healing, which involves sophisticated synchronization of molecular and biochemical events at the cellular level, to bring about tissue repair and regeneration. Wound healing is this fine-tuned process that restores anatomic and physiologic integrity to the tissue and culminates in the formation of a scar.[3]

Wound healing may be compartmentalized into four stages, i.e., inflammation, debridement, repair/proliferation, and maturation/remodeling.[3-6] These stages exhibit a significant degree of overlap and occur as a continuum from start to finish. Thus, more than one stage of healing can occur at one time and, regardless of wound size, all normally healing wounds undergo all stages of healing.

Etiologic factors for wounds are numerous and varied, ranging from mechanical trauma to physical agents such as extreme temperatures, chemicals, neoplastic processes, microbial infection, and surgery.[3]

Inflammation and Debridement Stages

The inflammatory stage of healing is the body's vascular and cellular defensive response.[7,8] It is separated into early and late phases.[4,5] The early phase consists of immediate responses including vascular tone dynamics and hemostasis, whereas the late phase is characterized by vascular responses as well as recruitment and activation of inflammatory cell populations.[7,8]

Tissue Reactions

The first response to any injury is hemorrhage, with the magnitude varying in accordance with the insult. Vasoconstriction occurs in an attempt to control hemorrhage. This is accompanied by an immediate enlargement of the defect, owing to inherent cutaneous elasticity and external muscle tension that retracts wound edges, causing wound gaping.[4] As a result, a wound may appear large; however, manipulation of the tissues may reveal that much of the enlargement is a result of tissue retraction.

Hemostasis, Lymphatic Reaction, and Scab

Torn blood vessels have exposed basement membranes containing subendothelial collagen, which when in contact with platelets bring about platelet activation and aggregation and initiate the intrinsic path of the coagulation cascade,[3,4,7,9] culminating in thrombus formation and hemorrhage control, i.e., a fibrin clot in the wound. The clot not only attenuates hemorrhage, but also occludes ruptured lymphatics, thereby preventing drainage, promoting edema, and localizing inflammation.[4] Later in the healing process, fibrinolysis dissolves fibrin plugs in the lymphatics, and lymphatic drainage resumes. When exposed to the external environment, the clot desiccates to form a scab.[3,4] A tightly adhered scab acts as a biologic bandage, beneath which wound contraction and epithelialization can progress undisturbed.[4,5]

Vascular and Humoral Events and Cellular Movement

The initial vasoconstriction is closely followed by reflex vasodilation and increased vascular permeability, resulting in plasma exudation[4,5] and the escape of inflammatory mediators and cellular components from blood vessels. Initiation of the arachidonic acid cascade results in production of prostaglandins, thromboxanes, and leukotrienes.[3,4,7,8] These humoral factors, along with histamine, serotonin, bradykinin, and complement activation, help perpetuate inflammation.[8] Mast cell-derived serotonin and histamine cause rounding of vascular endothelium, thereby causing loss of tight cellular junctions and promoting extravasation of plasma and other inflammatory mediators into the surrounding tissues.[8]

Surface receptors for leukocytes on endothelial cells become activated, with resultant leukocyte margination and eventual migration into interstitial tissues.[5,8]

Endothelial cells within blood vessels adjacent to the wounded tissue exhibit cellular adhesion molecules (CAMs), which bind inflammatory cells and assist in their passage between endothelial cells to the wound.[7] Further cellular migration is brought about with the help of proteinases (serine, metallo-, cysteine, and aspartic) which, by catabolizing ground substance and extracellular matrix, create a path for the cells.[7] Fibrin polymers are cross-linked to form a scaffold over which neutrophils and macrophages migrate toward the wound after diapedesis from the blood vessels.[3]

Polymorphonuclear leukocytes are the first responders to various chemotactic signals and appear at the site within hours of trauma.[4,8,9] They are followed closely by macrophages, and finally, T-lymphocytes.[8] Neutrophils are generally short-lived whereas macrophages persist for a significantly longer period.[5]

Cellular Functions

Besides playing a major role in coagulation, platelets also produce several cytokines and growth factors important to the progression of healing. Platelet activation results in release of platelet-derived growth factor (PDGF), transforming growth factor-α and -β (TGF-α and -β), and tumor necrosis factor-α (TNF-α)[2-4,7] from platelet alpha granules.[2,8] These signaling molecules are chemotactic for neutrophils, macrophages, and T-lymphocytes, which migrate toward the wound.[3,7] Platelet alpha granules contain four adhesive glycoproteins: fibrinogen, fibronectin, von Willebrand factor, and thrombospondin.[8] These glycoproteins participate in coagulation as well as temporary matrix synthesis.

Neutrophils and macrophages debride the wound of necrotic, devitalized tissue. Later, macrophages coordinate tissue proliferation.

Neutrophils are not essential to wound healing, despite being the first to arrive in the wound.[3,9] Neutrophils phagocytose bacteria and kill them by generating toxic reactive oxygen species or free radicals.[2,7] Their granules contain various proteinases, among which cathepsin G, urokinase-type plasminogen activator, collagenase, and elastase are predominant.[2,7] These proteinases can digest extracellular matrix components including elastin, fibrin, fibronectin, vitronectin, laminin, collagen, and proteoglycans. Proteinase inhibitors protect normal healthy tissues from the action of proteinases. Once spent, neutrophils are removed from the wound by macrophages or via wound exudate.[4]

Monocytes are transformed into macrophages once they are out of circulation and sequestered within tissue. Macrophage numbers reach their peak within 24 hours.[8,9] Macrophages are capable of phagocytosis as well as of discharging proteinases, specifically matrix metalloproteinases (MMPs), both of which are crucial during wound debridement and subsequent healing. Debridement and tissue proliferation are decelerated in wounds devoid of macrophages.[7] Tissue inhibitors of metalloproteinases (TIMPs) protect healthy tissue from the indiscriminate action of MMPs. Macrophages are activated to synthesize signaling molecules, including colony-stimulating factor, TNF-α, PDGF, interleukin-1, TGF-α and -β, fibroblast growth factor (FGF), and insulin-like growth factor-1, which induce cell proliferation, especially of keratinocytes, fibroblasts, and endothelial cells.[2,7] Therefore, macrophages are the bridge between the inflammatory and repair phases of wound healing.[7]

T-lymphocytes play a regulatory role in wound healing. They are not vital; however, their absence retards the healing process. Lymphocytes produce growth and regulatory factors that govern functions of other cells. The role of lymphocytes in healing is generally associated with a foreign antigen or secondary infection. They arrive in the wound at the same time as macrophages and interact with them in producing an immune response. Macrophages process foreign antigens, and these modified antigens are presented to the lymphocytes. The lymphocytes produce cytokines such as interferon-gamma (IFN-γ) and interleukins 2 to[2,4] Lymphocytes also produce TGF-β.[4]

The role of eosinophils in wound healing has not yet been elucidated. They are present in healing wounds and peak around 1 week post injury.[8] A rabbit cutaneous wound healing model demonstrated that eosinophils appeared to be responsible for secreting TGF-α after day 7,[8] however, eosinophils may delay wound re-epithelialization.[7]

Repair/Proliferation Stage

The repair/proliferation phase is composed of fibroblast proliferation and migration with production of wound extracellular matrix, neovascularization, and epithelial proliferation and migration.[2-6,8] Fibroblast activity and neovascularization result in granulation tissue formation.

Macrophages play a significant role in this stage of healing. They become activated in response to growth and chemotactic factors released from platelets during the latter part of the inflammatory and debridement phases. Digestion of fibronectin and collagen further potentiates macrophage activation and release of additional mediators of fibroplasia and angiogenesis, such as nitric oxide, which is essential for granulation tissue synthesis.[3,4] Macrophages recruit lymphocytes, which release lymphokines (interleukins and interferons) responsible for further reactivating macrophages, to ensure adequate levels of molecular mediators and vasoactive peptides throughout the proliferative phase.

Granulation Tissue – Production and Functions

Granulation tissue is composed primarily of fibroblasts, capillaries, macrophages, and collagen.[3,4,10] and appears in the wound between three and six days after commencement of healing.[5] Granulation tissue provides a mechanical barrier against microbial infection of the wound and a biologic barrier owing to the presence of granulocytes and macrophages on its surface.[3] It is also a source of collagen, which is required for wound repair and remodeling. Granulation tissue brings about wound contraction and serves as a foundation across which epithelial migration takes place.[4]

Fibroblasts are a predominant component of this stage of healing and a major constituent of granulation tissue. Sources of wound fibroblasts include pericytes and undifferentiated perivascular mesenchymal cells found in connective tissue.[4,6,8,9,11] Under the influence of factors such as PDGF, epidermal growth factor (EGF), FGF, IGF-1, and TGF-β, this quiescent cell population becomes activated, proliferates, and develops cytoplasmic extensions called ruffled membranes.[9] Fibroblasts secrete IGF-1, β-FGF, TGF-β, PDGF and keratinocyte growth factor (KGF).[4] Contact guidance, haptotaxis,[8,10] chemotaxis, and the use of ruffled membranes assist fibroblast movement along the fibrin meshwork within the wound.[4,8] As fibroblasts repopulate the wound bed, they continue synthesizing intercellular matrix constituents, including fibronectin, proteoglycans, collagen, and elastin.[4,8]

Neovascularization

The second component of the repair stage is neovascularization. Endothelial cell proliferation and subsequent migration occur in the presence of interstitial matrix or the absence of an intact basement membrane, resulting in capillary buds sprouting from pre-existing venules.[3,4,6,10] and capillary loop formation.[8,10] Once canalized, blood flow begins and circulation is established. New blood vessels grow at an approximate rate of 0.4 to 1.0 mm per day. In vitro studies have demonstrated that endothelial cells cultured on collagen types IV and V, the components of basement membranes,[8,12] form tubular structures instead of confluent monolayers, which are observed when cells are cultured on collagen types I and II.[8] Capillary buds that do not form lumens regress.[3,4,6] Lymphatics, although much slower to re-establish, follow a pattern similar to that of the capillaries and, therefore, lymphatic drainage during the early phases of wound healing is inadequate, contributing to edema formation.[3,4,8]

Wound pH and oxygen are important factors for fibroblast function and neovascularization. Optimal collagen synthesis is achieved when the microenvironment of the wound maintains a mildly acidic pH.[8] Oxygen tension at the wound periphery is almost 90 mm Hg, whereas in the center of the wound bed it falls to almost zero.[2,11] Under these hypoxic conditions, glycolysis–derived energy is sufficient to initiate fibroplasia. However, to sustain collagen production, molecular oxygen is vital for post-translational hydroxylation of proline and lysine moieties and cross-linkage of collagen fibrils.[11] Twenty mm Hg appears to be the critical oxygen tension for fibroplasia and collagen synthesis;[8,9] however, another report suggests that oxygen tension below 40 mm Hg impairs fibroplasia.[11]

Despite its deleterious effects on wound healing, a hypoxic environment and the oxygen tension gradient act as a stimulus for fibroblast mitosis, angiogenesis, and sustained secretion of growth factors from macrophages.[3,4,11] An oxygen tension gradient is a prerequisite for neovascularization.[8]

Angiogenic growth factors include PDGF, vascular endothelial growth factor (VEGF), tumor necrosis factor (TNF), and endothelin-1.[2,11] Upregulation of these angiogenic factors in endothelial cells increases cellular mitotic activity and thereby promotes neovascularization. Endothelial cells demonstrate a phenomenon called dynamic reciprocity, whereby they respond to environmental influences, such as cellular and chemical signals, and are capable of transforming their environment to induce changes beneficial to wound healing.[11]

As healing progresses, early components of the process regress as repair components increase. Fibrinolysis by plasmin disrupts the clot in the wound bed.[4] Gradually, neutrophils and lymphocytes are cleared from the wound by apoptosis or phagocytosis by macrophages. Fibrin, proteoglycans, tropocollagen, and protocollagen are substituted by collagen fibrils synthesized by the wound fibroblasts.

Collagen is a major component of granulation tissue.[10] Fibroblasts, under the influence of TGF-α and -β, EGF, PDGF, β-FGF, IL-1, and TNF, synthesize collagen fibrils and the viscoelastic extracellular matrix.[9,12] Collagen biosynthesis is a complicated process that involves gene transcription and translation, intracellular, intercellular, and extracellular transformation, and fibril assembly and cross-linkage.[12] Collagen includes two specific amino acids, hydroxylysine and 4-hydroxyproline.[12,13] These amino acids, along with glycine, form alpha peptide chains. These alpha peptide chains are intertwined to form a triple helix.[2,6,12,13] which is further convoluted to form a supercoiled helix.[13] Galactose is added to the superhelix before being extruded from the fibroblast as procollagen, which is further cleaved to produce tropocollagen.

Increase in wound strength is due to collagen deposition and collagen maturation. Tropocollagen is aggregated and cross-linked to produce collagen filaments. Collagen filaments are cross-linked to form collagen fibrils, which, when cross-linked together, form collagen fibers. On maturation, collagen type III becomes collagen type I[3,4,6,10] which as it matures and reorients within the wound increases the tensile strength of the wound.[4] In the first 2 weeks of wound healing, fibroblasts, fibrin, and collagen are vertically arranged between the wound edges, and the increase in tensile strength of the wound is due to an increase in collagen deposition.[9] In the late repair stage, the fibers are aligned horizontally.[3,4,8] Early strength of the wound is attributed to its collagen content, whereas late wound strength is associated with collagen type, maturation, and three-dimensional remodeling. As the collagen content of a wound increases, collagen synthesis balances collagen lysis. Extracellular proteoglycan matrix decreases proportionately as collagen increasingly occupies space.[4] This signals the beginning of the maturation phase.

Wound Contraction

Granulation tissue also contributes to wound contraction. Wound contraction is the centripetal force by which a wound achieves a reduction in size,[3,4,6,10] which may or may not culminate in complete wound closure. This phenomenon is especially important in open wound healing. Wound contraction does not involve synthesis of new skin, but rather centripetal movement of skin around the wound.[4,10]

One theory on wound contraction states that a sub-population of fibroblasts from the granulation tissue develop a higher percentage of actin-rich fibers, thereby transforming them into myofibroblasts.[2] These fibers are called stress fibers and contain myosin and tropomyosin.[8] TGF-β is thought to play a role in differentiation.[3,4,10] This response is an attempt to counteract by the inherent elastic nature of skin the retractive forces exerted by the wound edges.[4,10] Fibronexus is the interconnection between myofibroblasts and extracellular matrix. It plays a role in mediating wound contraction by reorienting the ground substance.[8] Additionally, fibronexus links myofibroblast stress fibers with collagen via fibronectin.[8]

A second theory on wound contraction suggests that regular fibroblasts use cell membrane tractional forces to reorganize and rearrange collagen fibrils.[4,6,10] As the fibroblast traverses the collagen, the cell membrane pulls collagen fibrils toward the center of the wound. This is best explained by the "toy tank moving over loose carpet" comparison.[4,10] This process is enhanced by PDGF, which stimulates extracellular matrix contraction, whereas FGF and IFN-γ inhibit the process.

Wound contraction is terminated by contact inhibition, that is, when one edge of the wound meets the other or when tensions exerted by skin elasticity at the wound edges and fibroblasts and myofibroblasts within the wound are equal.[4,10] The number of myofibroblasts present in any wound is proportional to the size of the wound and the tension on the wound edges; large, open wounds demonstrate higher numbers, whereas wounds that have undergone primary closure have significantly fewer myofibroblasts.[9]

Epithelialization

Epithelialization protects against external infection and fluid loss.[3] For epithelialization to occur, the wound must be free of infection and must maintain a moist, oxygen-rich microenvironment.[8] Epithelialization occurs independently of wound contraction and, in open wounds, occurs after granulation tissue has been laid down, i.e., after a lag phase of four to five days;[4] whereas in closed-wound healing, it begins almost immediately and is complete within two days.

Epithelial cells are influenced by β-FGF, EGF, IL-1, PDGF, and TGF-α and β. When up-regulated, these factors induce accelerated mitotic activity of epithelial cells. Mitotic activity and migration are not interdependent factors.[8] Epithelial cells develop microvilli within cell membranes. They then extend pseudopodia that facilitate migration.[3] Two theories elucidate epithelial migration. One theory proposes that desmosomal and hemidesmosomal attachments of basal epithelium to the basement membrane and adjacent epithelial cells at the wound edge are lost, thereby promoting migration of cells across the wound bed in monolayers.[2,3] This is known as the sliding theory.[4,8] The second hypothesis is called the leapfrog theory. This states that basal epithelial cells at the wound edge migrate on to the granulation tissue and implant. The epidermal cells just behind them migrate over the newly implanted epithelial cells and attach once they contact granulation tissue.[4,8] Epithelial migration is terminated by contact inhibition and desmosomal attachments are re-formed.[3,4,8] Epithelial cells also possess phagocytic activity, which is potentiated by fibronectin. This facilitates epithelialization over the wound bed under the scab or through wound exudate.[8]

Maturation/Remodeling Stage

Early wound strength increases as quickly as within the first 24 hours of wounding. The fibrin clot is the first contributor toward wound strength; however, strength does not reach a significant degree until 6 days.[4] Between days 5 and 15, continued deposition of collagen fibrils is reflected in a gain in wound tensile strength.[9] As healing progresses, extracellular matrix, collagen fibrils, capillary growth, and adhesive forces of epithelial cells add to building early wound strength.

Late wound strength starts only after wound healing has continued undisturbed for at least 21 days.[4] Once the rate of collagen synthesis is on par with that of collagen lysis, collagenases and matrix metalloproteinases digest extraneous material and preserve appropriately oriented collagen fibers. Collagen type III is replaced by collagen type I, which increases the tensile strength of the wound. As maturation progresses, the newly formed collagen bundles and the preexisting dermal collagen coalesce such that differentiation between the two is extremely difficult. No matter how complete the wound healing or how minimal the scar formation, it is always about 20% weaker than the adjacent uninjured tissue.[3,4,11]

As practitioners and their clients observe wound healing progress, certain visible processes will appear that have significance as to what is occurring. These can be helpful to the practitioner in explaining wound healing to the client and in management of the wound (Table 61-1).

Table 61-1. Clinical Relevances of the Visible Wound Healing Process

Process	Relevance
Wound hemorrhage	May help cleanse the wound of foreign material and toxins.
Wound edge retraction	A wound may appear larger than it actually is. Manipulate the edges to ascertain if tissue is absent, and to get an idea of what will be required for reconstruction.
Blood clot/scab	Provides a scaffold base for granulation tissue formation. Scab is a surface beneath which healing occurs.
Exudate, hyperemia, heat, edema, pain	Necessary parts of the inflammatory- debridement stage. Often wounds will appear (look and smell) worse before they start to improve (repair). Often at its peak at 3-5 days after wounding.
Granulation tissue	The first visible sign that the wound is progressing into the repair stage.
Wound contraction	A "friendly" process on the trunk of a dog and cat. Some large wounds may heal completely by this process. Weekly tracing on clear acetate can monitor its progress.
Epithelialization	Provides a temporary wound cover while contraction occurs. Indicates a granulation tissue bed is healthy enough to graft (if grafting is indicated). Provides poor durability if it is the final cover for a wound (reconstructive surgery is indicated).

Conclusion

The physiology of wound healing is an intricately woven, delicately balanced process involving fine-tuned communication between cellular players and various cytokines, vasoactive peptides, and chemical signals. The process of wound healing can be compared to the performance of a symphony orchestra. When each instrument plays its part in conjunction with other instruments at the appropriate time, beautiful music is the result. The same is true of wound healing. When each component performs its function in conjunction with other components at the proper time, uncomplicated wound healing takes place. The slightest upset of this fine-tuned equilibrium is capable of impairing it. Although we have come to learn so much about wound healing, more discoveries await around the corner.

References

1. Wysocki AB: Skin anatomy, physiology and pathophysiology. Nurs Clin North Am 34 (4):777, 1999.
2. Hosgood G: Wound repair and specific tissue response to injury. *In* Textbook of Small Animal Surgery. Vol 1. Slatter DH (ed). Philadelphia: WB Saunders, 2003.
3. Gregory CR: Wound healing and influencing factors. *In* BSAVA Manual of Canine and Feline Wound Management and Reconstruction. Fowler D, Williams JM (eds). Cheltenham, U.K: BSAVA, 1999.
4. Swaim SF, Henderson RA Jr: Wound healing. *In* Small Animal Wound Management. Philadelphia: Williams & Wilkins, 1997.
5. Swaim SF: The Effects of dressings and bandages on wound healing. Semin Vet Med Surg (Small Anim) 4(4):274, 1989.
6. Pavletic MM: Atlas of Small Animal Reconstructive Surgery. Philadelphia: WB Saunders, 1999.
7. Hart J: Inflammation 1: Its role in the healing of acute wounds. J Wound Care: 11(6):205, 2002
8. Fowler D: Principles of wound healing. *In* Surgical Complications and Wound Healing in the Small Animal Practice. Harari J (ed). Philadelphia: WB Saunders, 1993.
9. Nwomeh BC, Yager DR, Cohen KI: Physiology of chronic wounds. Clin Plast Surg 25(3):341, 1998.
10. Wilhelmi BJ, Blackwell SJ, Mancoll JS, Phillips LG: Creep vs. stretch: A review of the viscoelastic properties of skin. Ann Plast Surg 41(2):215, 1998.
11. Muller GH, Kirk RW: Structure and function of the skin. *In* Small Animal Dermatology. Muller GH (ed). Philadelphia: WB Saunders, 2001.
12. Swaim SF, Hinkle SH, Bradley DM: Wound contraction: basic and clinical factor . Comp Cont Edu Pract Vet 23(1):20 2001.
13. Fowler D: Wound healing: an overview. Semin Vet Med Surg (Small Animals) 4(4):256, 1989.

Chapter 62

Burns

Mark W. Bohling
Steven F. Swaim

Small animal burn injuries can be some of the most challenging cases that the veterinarian will be called upon to manage, and a thorough understanding of the pathophysiology of burn injury is crucial to maximizing the chance of successful treatment. Fortunately, our knowledge of burn pathophysiology has greatly increased in the past decade, and much of this knowledge has already been put into practice in the clinical management of burn cases. As with many other areas of veterinary medicine, much of the clinical and basic science literature comes from human medicine, and this chapter draws heavily from those resources. For purposes of clinical application, it is fortunate that many advances in the treatment of human burns are based largely on data derived from animal experimentation, in which the dog is a common model. This fact gives relevance for veterinary application of the human literature; however, care must still be exercised in the interpretation and application of the human literature to animals owing to the important anatomic and physiologic differences between humans and animals. This chapter reviews historical and recent advances in the understanding of burn pathophysiology and identifies areas for application of this information to the clinical management of burns in small animal practice.

Classification of Burn Injuries

Burns are classified into one of four types based on etiology:[1,2] *Thermal burns* are caused by exposure to temperature extremes (either high or low) sufficient to cause cellular damage. *Chemical burns* are caused by exposure to chemicals that cause tissue necrosis via chemical reactivity or thermal effects. *Electrical burns* are suffered when electrical current of sufficient amperage and voltage to cause cell death passes through the patient. *Radiation burns* are caused by exposure to ionizing radiation at levels that cause acute cell death; this injury is most commonly seen either from exposure to solar radiation, or as a side effect of radiation therapy for neoplastic disease, and will not be specifically discussed in this chapter. Knowledge of the source of the burn and the mechanism by which it inflicts injury is vital to the proper initial care of the burn patient; e.g., copious lavage for many chemical burns, rapid cooling of tissues exposed to high heat, gentle rapid rewarming of frozen tissues, etc.

With few exceptions, the primary organ system involved is the integument. Some types of burn injuries, notably chemical, electrical, and radiation, may have gastrointestinal or other primary sites of injury, and thermal burns that primarily involve the integument often have systemic effects, but the skin is normally the first and most important site of injury because it is usually the location where the initial damage occurs that leads to systemic sequelae and, therefore, is the focus of most of the investigation in burn pathophysiology and therapeutics.

Thermal Burns

Technically, thermal burns include injuries caused by exposure to either excessive heat (hyperthermic burns) or excessive cold (hypothermic burns). In this chapter, the use of the term "thermal burns" will deal with the former, whereas the term "frostbite" will be used for the latter. Thermal burns are subclassified according to the heat source, i.e., a flame or fire, scalds from hot liquids or gases, and burns from direct contact with a hot object.[3] Thermal burns occur when heat is transferred to the tissues in one of three ways: via conduction, convection, or radiation. Conduction is the most common source of thermal injury and occurs when the body is in direct contact with a hot object such as a heating pad or boiling water. Convection is the transfer of heat via airborne currents, such as the superheated air that comes from a fire. In radiation burns, energy in the form of electromagnetic radiation travels through the air until it strikes the body and is converted into heat; heat lamps can produce burns via this process.[1] Burn severity has historically been classified according to the depth of tissue destruction; this classification system has proven useful for treatment planning and prognostication. *Partial-thickness* burn injuries can be divided into two categories. *First-degree* burns are superficial injuries involving only the epidermis, with erythema as the only observable change. Because the dermis is not involved, skin integrity is maintained, with no blistering or open wounds, and rapid, scar-free healing occurs without medical intervention. First-degree burns are painful, because nociceptors in the epidermis are stimulated at the time of the injury. *Second-degree* burns are partial-thickness injuries of the skin that involve the dermis. In addition to pain and erythema, these injuries are characterized by blister formation and exudation of fluid (note: blisters are common in humans, but rare in dogs and cats owing to differences in dermal histologic structure). Partial-thickness burns can vary from superficial to deep, but at least some of the dermis and adnexa survive the injury so that scarring is usually absent. Complete healing usually requires 2 to 3 weeks in uncomplicated cases. Full-thickness burns can be further divided into three categories. *Third-degree* burns extend through the skin to the level of the subcutaneous tissues; some classification schemes recognize two further categories; *fourth-degree* burns, extending to the underlying muscle, and *fifth-degree* burns involving bone.[2] Depth of tissue destruction is directly proportional to factors that concentrate heat in the area of the injury; i.e., temperature to which the tissue is heated, and duration of exposure or contact.[4] Failure of cellular function and tissue necrosis follow a predictable progression as the temperature of the skin increases. Between 40 and 44°C cellular enzymatic activity is affected, resulting in sodium pump failure. Epidermal sloughing (partial-thickness burn) results if skin is heated to 60°C for more than 1 second, and skin temperatures above 70°C produce full-thickness burns.[5]

Local Response to Thermal Burn Injury

The local burn injury has been divided into three functional and anatomic areas; moving outward from the center of the burned area, the innermost area is the *zone of coagulation* (also known as the zone of necrosis or destruction). Complete loss of tissue viability occurs within this zone; the therapeutic goal in this area is debridement. The next area is the *zone of stasis*; in this area, heat-induced changes in erythrocytes reduce their deformability and reduce their ability to flow through microscopic vessels. This is compounded by reduction in microvessel luminal area owing to increased extraluminal pressure from tissue edema brought about by inflammation and subsequent increase in capillary permeability. The increase in local capillary permeability in response to burn injury is not an all-or-none phenomenon, but rather is a graded response based on the severity of the injury. In a scalded canine hindlimb model, the capillary permeability, as measured by local lymph flow and protein content, increased with increasing scald temperature.[6] Taken together, these changes cause sluggish blood flow and tissue hypoxia; in this intermediate zone, tissue either proceeds to necrosis or healing depending on further insults sustained and/or the effectiveness of treatment, making this area the principle focus of burn therapy. Finally, the outer *zone of hyperemia* is the area of the local inflammatory response to the burn. Tissue in the zone of hyperemia remains viable and will proceed to healing if no further insult is sustained.[7]

The local response to burn injury is similar to that of other inflammatory lesions, and is characterized by local vasodilation, an increase in vascular permeability, edema, and migration of inflammatory cells into the injured area.[8] The burned tissue and resident inflammatory cells at the time of injury are the primary source of chemokines that initiate the inflammatory response, including endotoxin,[9] prostaglandin E_2,[10] histamine, and activated complement.

Immediately after thermal injury, an upregulation of blood flow to the burned area occurs. Administration of the autonomic blocker hexamethonium ablates this response, indicating that this regional arteriolar vasodilation appears to be at least partly under postganglionic autonomic control.[12] Local upregulation of nitric oxide (NO) production also plays an important role in the regional vasodilatory response to burn. Several studies have demonstrated an increase in NO production in thermally injured tissue,[13] and in the surrounding nonburned skin as well.[14] NO is well known as a potent vasodilator that increases blood flow in local tissue beds in response to a variety of inflammatory stimuli including burns. NO has been demonstrated to act directly and also indirectly, by potentiating the release of other vasodilatory molecules such as substance P.[15]

Vascular permeability also increases in the periwound tissues after burn injury. The increase in permeability is mediated by the activation of the inflammatory cascade and is a graded phenomenon, i.e., transvascular flux of fluid and protein is directly proportional to the severity of the burn.[6] Increased vascular permeability, coupled with increased blood flow, leads to burn wound edema. Extravascular migration of neutrophils is partly a consequence of increased vascular permeability and partly mediated via direct effects on neutrophil diapedesis. Expression of the adhesion molecules CD11b/CD18 and adhesion to vascular endothelium are enhanced in neutrophils that are incubated in the presence of burn serum; this effect is blocked by the administration of monoclonal antibodies to the adhesion molecules.[16]

Interestingly, burn wounds seem to lack the ability of normal surgical wounds to stimulate their own healing. When angiogenic activity of wound fluid from surgical wounds, skin graft (donor) wounds, and burn wounds was compared, burn wound fluid was found to be completely lacking in ability to stimulate endothelial cell migration or proliferation, and contained less than 5% of the levels of fibroblast growth factor-2 (FGF-2) of surgical wound fluid.[17]

Most of the interest in the local burn response concerns the acute post-burn period, because so many life-threatening side effects begin with the acute burn wound. For those patients that survive, the burn wound enters a chronic stage that may result in wound healing problems as the skin attempts repair. In first- and second-degree burns the epidermis may be damaged but the basement membrane remains intact, and skin healing is generally rapid and uncomplicated. Third- and higher-degree burns present a problem, because necrosis of the dermis means that the overlying basement membrane is gone. The basement membrane is a necessary surface to direct the migration of stem cells onto the wound from the stratum basale of the surrounding unburned skin. As with any injury involving loss of the basement membrane, healing is by scar formation as fibroblasts enter the wound and lay down a collagenous matrix. Two chronic pathophysiologic processes that may affect burn wounds in small animals are scar contracture and post-burn blistering.

Wound contraction is the process by which motility of fibroblasts and myofibroblasts within the matrix exerts force that reduces the open wound area. This is a generally beneficial process, especially in dogs and cats that have more abundant skin on the body. It reduces the amount of tissue exposed to dehydration and contamination, and it stops when the burn is completely covered with new epithelium.[18] In contrast, *scar contracture*, although involving the same underlying mechanisms, is considered a pathologic process because it continues after the wound has been epithelialized.[18] Scar contracture results in pain and loss of mobility, and can be particularly debilitating when it is extensive or occurs over a joint or in an area with minimal skin mobility.[19] The degree of contracture appears to be proportional to the amount of scar tissue; therefore, prevention of contracture is directed toward prevention of excessive scar formation. Treatment of contracture is accomplished by surgical excision of the existing scar and application of a graft or flap to the resultant defect.[20]

Post-burn blistering is a relatively common complication in human burn patients.[21] Although uncommon in animals, we have also observed this phenomenon in a dog. After a large burn wound has healed by second intention, blisters may spontaneously appear, rupture, and heal in a continuous cycle. Immunohistochemical and ultrastructural analysis of the blisters reveals that the basement membrane displays areas of discontinuity and detachment from the dermis.[22] One hypothesis is that defective reorganization of the basement membrane may be associated with observed ultrastructural aberrations of dermal fibroblasts.[23]

Systemic Response to Thermal Burn Injury

Pulmonary System

The most important and far-reaching effect of thermal burn injury on the pulmonary system is from smoke inhalation.

Smoke inhalation occurs commonly as an intercurrent injury with thermal burn. Besides the often serious and even fatal local (pulmonary) effects, smoke inhalation also profoundly exacerbates the systemic sequelae of burn injury. The pathophysiologic response of the lung to smoke inhalation can be divided into several components: pulmonary edema, atelectasis, increased alveolar pressure, and deactivation of pulmonary surfactant.[24] These highly interdependent events combine to lead to the development of the acute respiratory distress syndrome (ARDS) that is one of the major complications of burn injury.[25]

The etiologic agents of smoke inhalation injury are numerous and interrelated, and include cytokines, eicosanoids, activated neutrophils, nitric oxide (NO), free radicals, and neurotransmitters such as substance P.[26,27] Three major sources of cytokines appear to be involved in the cytokine-mediated pulmonary injury and dysfunction following a burn. The first source is cytokines released from the burned tissue; the second source is the lung, which has been damaged by smoke inhalation; the third is the intestinal tract, which conveys cytokines to the lungs via the mesenteric lymphatics. These cytokines appear to act synergistically with bacteria and endotoxin to maximize increases in pulmonary vascular permeability and apoptosis of alveolar cells.[28]

Pulmonary edema begins to develop soon after smoke inhalation, as fluid, mucus, and neutrophils accumulate within alveoli and airways.[29,30] The eicosanoid thromboxane A2, synthesized and released from pulmonary tissue in response to smoke inhalation, plays a major role in the pathophysiology of smoke inhalation. Increased pulmonary lymph concentration of thromboxane A2 post-smoke exposure is associated with a parallel increase in pulmonary transvascular flux and vascular resistance, both systemic and pulmonary. The increased pulmonary vascular resistance appears to be primarily caused by an intense but transient venoconstriction.[24] Inhibition of thromboxane A2 with a thromboxane A2 synthase inhibitor significantly attenuates these changes.[29]

Nitric oxide (NO) is another systemic mediator of inflammation that is involved in pulmonary edema after burn injury.[31,32,26] Significant increases in NO in plasma and pulmonary lymph are seen within 24 hours post-burn owing to upregulation of inducible NO synthase and are associated with increases in pulmonary microvascular permeability, cardiac depression, and hemoconcentration.[32] NO appears to affect vascular permeability differently between species: in an ovine model, leakage of fluid increased while protein flux remained at normal levels,[33] while in the rat, transvascular albumin flux increased by 100%. Pulmonary compliance also decreases after a burn; this effect is caused partially by pulmonary edema and partly by reduction in production of pulmonary surfactant.[34]

Part of the complexity of smoke inhalation injury stems from the complex chemical composition of the inhaled smoke. Most burned small animals with smoke inhalation are exposed in an indoor environment such as a house fire. The smoke from house fires contains over 200 toxic substances.[35] Principal among these are carbon monoxide (from incomplete combustion of wood), hydrogen cyanide (from combustion of nitrogen-containing products, i.e., nylon, formica, melamine, wool), and inorganic acids HCl, HF, and HBr (from polyvinyl chloride, teflon, neoprene, and various plastics). Carbon monoxide toxicity occurs via three mechanisms: 1) binding to hemoglobin and reducing its oxygen carrying capacity; 2) carboxyhemoglobin formation, which results in a leftward shift of the oxyhemoglobin dissociation curve, reducing oxygen delivery to the tissues; and 3) binding with myoglobin to reduce oxygen availability to muscle, especially cardiac and skeletal. Hydrogen cyanide binds with mitochondrial cytochrome oxidase, thereby preventing oxygen utilization by cells. Hydrogen chloride and the other diatomic halide acids are all intensely irritating to respiratory mucous membranes, producing laryngospasm and bronchospasm at concentrations found in smoke.[36] Smoke inhalation also causes a dose-dependent injury to tracheobronchial epithelium and lung parenchyma via free hydroxyl and carbon radicals contained in the smoke and also via the accompanying neutrophilic infiltration.[35]

Cardiovascular System

Hypovolemia and Vascular Dysfunction

Loss of fluid volume from the vascular space is one of the early pathophysiologic changes seen with severe burns. Within 10 minutes after a burn, systemic vascular permeability to fluid and albumin increases, via myosin-mediated contraction of vascular endothelial cells, which increases the intercellular gap size in the endothelium.[37] Direct damage to endothelial cells, mediated by complement activation, histamine, and oxygen free radicals from the burn site,[11] exacerbates the process and causes further interstitial edema and loss of vascular fluid volume.[38]

The burn wound is another source of fluid loss via evaporative losses that are 4 to 20 times greater than for normal intact skin.[39] These losses can constitute a significant source of the fluid loss that leads to hypovolemia in large burns. The cumulative effect of hyperpermeability and fluid loss is to create profound hypovolemia within the first few hours after a large burn. Hypovolemia and reduced RBC deformability combine to cause hyperviscosity of the blood. This problem is compounded by systemic vasoconstriction, which is mediated by the sympathetic response to baroreceptor and nociceptor afferents[40,41] and is proportional to the severity of the burn.[42,43] The combined effects of hypovolemia, hyperviscosity, and vasoconstriction in turn lead to hypoperfusion and metabolic acidosis.[44,45]

Myocardial Effects

Direct myocardial effects also constitute a portion of the pathophysiology of burn shock. Left ventricular contractility was significantly decreased during the 6-hour post-burn observation period in dogs after a 50% total body surface area burn.[46] This impaired contractility is paralleled by a significant increase in intracellular Ca++ of cardiac myocytes.[47] At least a portion of this post-burn myocardial Ca++ influx and contractile dysfunction is mediated via the increased translocation of gut bacteria, endotoxin, and cytokines, and the ensuing systemic inflammatory response syndrome.[48] In one experiment, depopulation of the gut with oral antibiotics reduced post-burn myocardial levels of TNF-α and other cytokines and improved myocardial contractility.[49] Increased sympathetic input is another stimulus that causes cardiomyocytes to synthesize and release increased levels of TNF-α and other cytokines, resulting in defects in cardiac contraction and relaxation.[50]

Smoke inhalation also causes decreased cardiac output[51,29] and myocardial damage via the toxic effects of carbon monoxide, which decreases myocardial oxygen delivery and utilization. In a canine model, smoke inhalation caused an increase in carboxyhemoglobin, decreased ATP production by cardiomyocytes, and zymographic and histopathologic evidence of myocardial necrosis.[52]

Gastrointestinal System

The GI system can be profoundly affected by large burns, and in turn, is a major effector organ for the syndrome of shock, sepsis, and multiple organ failure that follows severe burns. Studies have demonstrated that, after a severe burn, loss of GI barrier function occurs, with translocation of gut bacteria, endotoxin, and cytokines, leading to septic shock.[53-56] Burn injury has been demonstrated to increase the rate of apoptosis of gut mucosal cells, with no effect on mucosal proliferation; this may be an important aspect of the loss of GI mucosal integrity seen after burns.[57] Post-burn GI motility is also impaired via a nitric oxide-dependent mechanism; inducible NOS expression by neurons of the myenteric plexus appears to play a significant role.[58]

The liver is also affected by burn injury. Burns cause increased oxidative stress in hepatocytes, marked by a decrease in liver glutathione level and increases in malondialdehyde (MDA) and myeloperoxidase (MPO) activity at 24 hours post-burn.[59] Hepatocyte turnover is also increased post-burn, as demonstrated by increases in both apoptosis and proliferation.[60] Liver synthetic function is also affected. Upregulation of certain products such as acute-phase proteins and downregulation of others has been noted by 3 days post-burn.[61]

Renal System

The incidence of acute renal failure in seriously burned human patients ranges from 1.3% to 38% and is associated with a high mortality rate, between 73% and 100%.[62] Burn severity (as percentage of total body surface area) is an independent predictor of the likelihood of acute renal failure and associated mortality.[63] A number of contributory factors including hypotension,[63] hypoalbuminemia,[63] hemoglobinemia, myoglobinemia,[63] sepsis,[63,64] reduced cardiac output, and systemic vasoconstriction have been identified, with elevated levels of stress hormones (catecholamines, vasopressin, angiotensin, and aldosterone) implicated in the mechanism.[65] Atrial natriuretic peptide (ANP), which is also elevated in post-burn patients, may play a protective role by increasing renal blood flow and urine output. Dogs receiving a constant norepinephrine infusion responded to exogenous ANP administration with improvement in renal and hemodynamic parameters.[65]

Acute renal failure may also develop as a late consequence of burn injury. The etiology is thought to be multifactorial, including late effects of renal ischemia, sepsis, nephrotoxic effects of antibiotics or other drugs, and renal glomerular deposition of proteins such as hemoglobin and myoglobin and other cellular debris from necrotic cells.[1,64]

Hematologic Responses

Burn injury produces an immediate and long-lasting reduction in circulating erythrocyte numbers. This so-called "burn anemia" results from increase in red cell loss coupled with decreased erythropoiesis. Up to 10% of the circulating red cell mass may be trapped and destroyed in a large burn,[66] but this only accounts for a portion of the total red cell losses – human burn patients average 12% loss of red cell mass within 6 hours of a large (15 to 40% TBSA) burn and may lose up to 18% of their red cell mass within 24 hours.[67] Within 1 hour of a burn injury, plasma free hemoglobin levels increase. Increased hemolysis occurs owing to a combination of factors. First, increased osmotic fragility appears to be caused by damage to the RBC membrane from activated complement, neutrophils, and oxygen free radicals.[68] Second, a decrease in erythrocyte deformability is caused by oxidative stress and subsequent lipid peroxidation of the red cell membrane.[69,70] In spite of the loss of RBC mass, which stimulates an appropriate elevation in erythropoietin release from the kidneys, erythropoiesis is nonetheless depressed.[71,72] Reduced erythropoiesis appears to be caused by an erythroid inhibitory protein[73] and as a secondary effect of decreased iron availability.[72] Administration of supplemental exogenous erythropoietin helps restore red cell mass after a burn.[74]

Burn injury also produces significant negative effects on leukocyte production and function. For example, lymphoid apoptosis is upregulated after burn injury, and may be linked to a parallel upregulation of TNF-α.[75] Burn injury also caused a downregulation of chemotactic cytokine production by mouse T cells, resulting in increased susceptibility to sepsis. This effect appears to be mediated via the sympathetic nervous system. Chemically sympathectomized mice had normalized cytokine production and improved resistance to sepsis. In vitro, T cells from burned mice or from normal mice treated with norepinephrine also demonstrated reduced cytokine production.[76]

Neurologic System

Effect of Pain on Burn Wound Response

Burns cause intense pain; even full-thickness burns, in which cutaneous nociceptors are destroyed, can still be painful because the full-thickness burn is surrounded by tissue that is damaged but not completely destroyed.[77] In this area of damaged tissue, peripheral nociceptors are activated by the burn injury, sending afferent input along A delta and C fibers.[78] Cellular damage and the ensuing inflammatory response also cause the release of chemical mediators of pain (kinins, prostaglandins), which further sensitize local nociceptors, causing a hyperalgesic state.[77] The intense pain stimulates a massive sympathetic discharge, which in turn drives many of the cardiovascular changes of burn shock. Even after the initial burn shock has been treated, chronic pain in burn patients continues to stimulate a chronic, albeit lower level of catecholamine release that mediates a number of the metabolic and organic derangements seen in burn patients.[78]

Other Neuromodulators of the Burn Wound Response

Besides the modulation of burn pain and its secondary effects, the peripheral nociceptor system is also involved in the initiation of the local inflammatory response to burn injury through its effect on vasomotor tone and chemotaxis of inflammatory cells. Scald injury of the rat hindpaw induced release of substance P and calcitonin gene-related peptide (CGRP) from peripheral sensory neurons. Both of these substances induced vasodilation in the injured tissue. In addition, neuropeptides have been demonstrated to induce chemotaxis and activation of neutrophils, eosinophils, mast cells, and monocytes following tissue injury,[79] and have been demonstrated to play a role in the development of ARDS following smoke inhalation.[27]

Metabolic and Endocrine Changes

Burn injury induces profound changes in energy and protein metabolism. These changes are initiated by two primary events: local effects, i.e., release of pro-inflammatory cytokines (TNF-α, IL-6, IL-8) and oxidant stress from cell lysis, and systemic effects from increased release of catabolic hormones (primarily cortisol and catecholamines).

Post-burn metabolism follows a biphasic course. There is a period of hypometabolism immediately after injury (the "ebb phase," which occurs during the shock), followed by a hypermetabolic state (the "flow phase"), during which basal energy expenditure increases by over 100% compared with pre-burn.[80,81] This change is caused by several conditions at the local and systemic levels. Loss of the barrier function of skin means that large amounts of body water are lost to evaporation; along with the water loss, significant heat is lost as the heat of evaporation. The hypothalamic "set point" is also elevated post-burn by 1 to 2°C in response to the release of cytokines and eicosanoids as part of the inflammatory process. The energy "cost" of this increased thermogenesis is paid via increases in non-productive metabolic work that consumes energy and produces heat. For instance, there is a 450% increase in triglyceride-fatty acid cycling and a 250% increase in glycolytic-gluconeogenic cycling in post-burn patients.[82]

Protein and carbohydrate metabolism are also altered in the post-burn state. Amino acid utilization for energy production is increased, producing a decline in lean body mass as body protein is catabolized. This negative energy and nitrogen balance differs significantly from that of simple starvation. In simple starvation, body adipose stores supply 90% of the basal energy requirement, and lean body mass accounts for only 5% to 8% of the body's energy needs. In the postburn state, relative insulin resistance caused by increased catabolic hormones (glucagon, cortisol, and catecholamines) results in a completely different energy consumption profile, in which only 50% of the body's energy needs are supplied by adipose tissue and lean body mass accounts for 30%.[83] Upregulation of hepatic gluconeogenesis and relative insulin resistance results in a persistent hyperglycemic/catabolic state marked by glucose intolerance and hyperinsulinemia, with reduced rate of glucose extraction by peripheral tissues (muscle, fat, etc.). Increased glucose uptake is limited to the burn wound, which has a high energy requirement for anaerobic glycolysis by inflammatory and endothelial cells and fibroblasts.[82] This so-called "burn diabetes" is a serious complication of burns in both the acute and chronic stages, as prognosis deteriorates with increasing loss of lean body mass.[83]

Application of Burn Pathophysiology to Treatment

The treatment of human patients with burns over a large percentage of the body surface area has gone through an interesting progression. Initially, the entire focus was on the burn site, and various bandaging, enzymatic, and other local treatments were developed for non-surgical debridement. The problem with the local therapy focus was that a high percentage of patients died of systemic complications of their burns, so attention was turned to developing treatments for burn shock and the other systemic complications of burn injuries.

More recently, the focus of treatment for patients with large full-thickness burns has once again turned to the local site, as the connection between the burned area and systemic pathophysiology has become clear. Today, large full-thickness burns are treated by complete surgical excision of the burn eschar as soon as the patient can be made stable enough for surgery. The benefit of this strategy is obvious: the burn eschar is the stimulus that drives the inflammatory reaction, leading to the entire cascade of local and systemic events described above. Early complete escharectomy removes this stimulus and effectively converts the burn - a major physiologic threat - into a comparatively benign, large, clean, open wound. Systemic post-burn levels of endotoxin and E-selectin (but not TNF-α or interleukin-10) were significantly reduced at 1 and 3 days after escharotomy in human burn patients.[9]

In one clinical study of severely burned children, administration of the anabolic agent oxandrolone improved net nitrogen balance, lean body mass, and expression of genes for muscle protein synthesis when compared with controls.[84]

Early enteral feeding has been demonstrated to ameliorate some of the GI effects of burns. By reversing the increased rate of apoptosis seen in mucosal epithelium after burn injury, early enteral feeding helps to maintain mucosal integrity.[57] This may be particularly important owing to the connection between loss of mucosal integrity and post-burn septic shock.

Frostbite

Frostbite may be seen when animals suffer lengthy exposure to cold, especially those that are injured or debilitated. Under these conditions, the extremities are most often affected, particularly the pinnae[85] and digits. The flank folds are also predisposed to frostbite owing to the extreme thinness of the skin in this region. Frostbite may also be encountered as an iatrogenic condition when cryotherapy is delivered improperly.[86] Three pathophysiologic mechanisms cause the tissue damage seen in frostbite: tissue freezing, hypoxia, and release of inflammatory mediators. These events occur simultaneously and work synergistically, as the pathologic changes caused by one exacerbates the others.[87,88]

Tissue freezing causes cell damage in two ways. Freezing causes formation of ice crystals, both intracellularly and extracellularly. Initially, extracellular ice crystals damage the cell membrane, leading to disruption of the osmotic gradient and intracellular dehydration. As tissue temperature continues to fall, intracellular ice crystals form and expand, causing direct physical disruption of the cell membrane and cell death. Freezing also causes direct cell damage via denaturation of cell membrane lipid-protein complexes.[87,88]

Local hypoxia is induced by cold-induced vasoconstriction. Initially, as tissues cool, local vascular beds respond with alternating cycles of vasoconstriction and vasodilation, the "hunting reaction."[87] Vasoconstriction causes decreased blood flow via decreasing vessel diameter; also blood viscosity increases. The vasodilatory phase brings partial thawing of frozen tissue and the reestablishment of blood flow. This is the freeze-thaw cycle that causes the greatest amount of tissue damage. After repeated cycles, vessel thrombosis occurs, leading to a continuous hypoxic state. The combined effects of direct cellular damage and tissue hypoxia stimulate the release of inflammatory cytokines (prostaglandins, thromboxanes, bradykinin, histamine) and activation of the inflammatory cascade, much the same as that seen in thermal burn injury. Activation of the inflammatory cascade leads in turn to clotting activation and intravascular thrombosis, completing the "vicious cycle."[87,88]

Current concepts in frostbite treatment focus on taking advantage of knowledge of the mechanisms of injury. Treatment includes 1) rapid rewarming of the frozen tissues, but not under "field conditions" where re-freezing may occur and exacerbate injury; 2) fluid therapy to improve local circulation; and 3) NSAIDs to combat activation of the inflammatory and clotting cascades.[87]

Chemical Burns

Chemical burns occur either through chemical reaction with cellular components, or via thermal effects when the chemical(s) in question produces an intense exothermic or endothermic reaction. The degree of tissue damage is proportional to the toxicity of the chemical, its quantity and concentration, and the duration of exposure.[1] Chemical burns tend to continue until the chemical in question is neutralized by reaction with tissue components (or by another externally applied chemical), or is washed off or sufficiently diluted during first aid treatment. Different classes of chemicals have different modes of tissue toxicity. Acids act as powerful oxidizing agents that disrupt protein structure and function by insertion of oxygen atoms into peptide bonds. Alkalis are reducing agents that denature protein through reduction of amide bonds that crosslink polypeptide chains; these reactions can be intensely exothermic, causing simultaneous thermal burns. Hydrocarbons act as lipid solvents that disrupt the cytoplasmic membrane.[1] Vesicants are chemical agents that cause blistering; therefore, the definition for this group of compounds is a functional rather than chemical one.[89] One agent in this group, the chemotherapeutic agent doxorubicin, is of special interest and concern because of its common use in veterinary medicine and high level of tissue toxicity when extravasated during administration. The exact mechanism of doxorubicin tissue toxicity is not known. One theory is that it may be a result of intercalation of doxorubicin with cellular DNA. Another theory is that enzymatic reduction of doxorubicin results in the formation of free radicals, which are the actual toxic constituents.[89] Doxorubicin is particularly toxic to tissues because, unlike many other chemical agents, it is not neutralized during the course of reaction with cellular constituents. Therefore, after doxorubicin causes cellular necrosis, it is released with the lysis of the cell and is able to continue its local tissue toxicity.[89] Current recommendations for doxorubicin extravasation include surgical excision, local injection with hyaluronidase to promote vascular uptake of the drug, thereby diluting it, and infiltration of the site with DMSO or other free radical scavengers such as dexrazoxane. The latter, a metal ion chelator, was developed as a cardioprotectant to reduce doxorubicin-induced cardiomyopathy. It has also shown promise as a treatment for doxorubicin extravasation in humans and has also been used in veterinary patients.[90] The proposed mechanism of action is that dexrazoxane protects tissues against free radical damage by iron-doxorubicin complexes by binding iron and thus making it unavailable.

Electrical Burns

Electrical burns in small animal patients are not common; most occur as oral burns, owing to chewing of electrical cords, or as a result of improper grounding of the patient when electrocautery is used. Heat, generated from the resistance of the tissues to current flow, is the major component of electrical injury. Joule's law ($J = I^2RT$) describes these relationships and indicates that heat production is directly proportional to tissue resistance and time of exposure, and proportional to the square of the amperage.[1,91] Tissue resistance is particularly important in determining the distribution and severity of the wound, with more resistant tissues suffering greater damage than less resistant ones. In particular, bone has a much higher electrical resistance than the surrounding muscle and fascia and also dissipates heat more slowly owing to its higher density. The net effect is that the superficial skin injury in electrical burns can appear to be relatively minor, while muscle, fascia, and neurovascular structures adjacent to bone have sustained severe damage.[91] This is an important consideration in prognostication and treatment of injuries where bone lies close beneath the area of visible burn, such as with electrical burns of the oral cavity.

Conclusions

Burns, particularly large ones, are among the most physically devastating and clinically challenging wounds that the veterinarian will treat. Virtually all body systems are impacted to one degree or another, with many complex interactions between systems. Although many of the critical pathophysiologic events begin at the local level, systemic sequelae often are the ultimate determinants of patient morbidity and mortality, and the application of the knowledge of these processes can have a major impact on burn mortality rates. Reported mortality rates from human burn centers have declined dramatically in the past 30 years. For example, a recent review of 1818 patient records at the Boston Shriners Burns Hospital compared mortality from two time periods, 1974 to 1980 and 1991 to 1997. The study showed an overall 88% reduction in mortality and a 57% reduction in mortality for the most severely burned (60 to 100% TBSA) patients.[92] These gains have been attributed to the adoption of aggressive fluid resuscitation, early escharectomy, improvements in sepsis prevention and pain control, and nutritional support.[92-94] Similar application of burn pathophysiologic principles may well yield comparable results for veterinary medicine.

References

1. Rutan RL: Physiologic response to cutaneous burn injury. *In* Burn Care and Therapy, Carrougher GJ (ed). St. Louis: Mosby, 1998, pp. 5-9.
2. Supple KG: Physiologic response to burn injury. Crit Care Nurs Clin North Am 16:119, 2004.
3. Hettiaratchy S, Dziewulski P: ABC of burns: pathophysiology and types of burns. Br Med J 328:1427, 2004.
4. Mortiz AR, Henriques FC: Studies of thermal injury. II. The relative importance of time and surface temperature in the causation of cutaneous burns. Am J Pathol 23:695, 1947.
5. Lawrence JC, Bull JP: Thermal conditions which cause skin burns. Engineer Med 5:61, 1976.
6. Ferrara JJ, Dyess DL, Collins JN, et al: Effects of graded thermal injury on microvascular permeability at the site of injury. J Surg Res 57:420, 1994.
7. Jackson DM: The diagnosis of the depth of burning. Br J Surg 40:558, 1953.
8. Gibran NS, Heimbach DM: Current status of burn wound pathophysiology. Clin Plast Surg 27:11, 2000.
9. Han TH, Lee SY, Kwon JE, et al: The limited immunomodulatory effects of escharectomy on the kinetics of endotoxin, cytokines, and adhesion molecules in major burns. Mediators Inflamm 13:241, 2004.
10. Hahn EL, Gamelli RL: Prostaglandin E2 synthesis and metabolism in burn injury and trauma. J Trauma 49:1147, 2000.
11. Friedl HP, Till GO, Trentz O, Ward PA: Roles of histamine, complement and xanthine oxidase in thermal injury of skin. Am J Pathol 135(1):203, 1989.
12. Taheri P, Choe E, Lippton H, et al: Autonomic control of the regional hemodynamic response to scald. Life Sci 56:701, 1995.
13. Rawlingson A: Nitric oxide, inflammation and acute burn injury. Burns 29:631, 2003.
14. Oliveira GV, Shimoda K, Enkhbaatar P, et al: Skin nitric oxide and its metabolites are increased in nonburned skin after thermal injuries. Shock 22:278, 2004.
15. Yonehara N, Yoshimura M: Interaction between nitric oxide and substance P on heat-induced inflammation in rat paw. Neurosci Res 36(1):35, 2000.

16. Fang Y, Chen Y, Ge S: The role of PMN CD11b/CD18 on the increasing PMN adhesion to endothelial cells induced by severe burn injury. Zhonghua Wai Ke Za Zhi 35:504, 1997.

17. Nissen NN, Gamelli RL, Polverini PJ, DiPietro LA: Differential angiogenic and proliferative activity of surgical and burn wound fluids. J Trauma 54:1205, 2003.

18. Rudolph R, Vande Berg J, Ehrlich HP: Wound contraction and scar contracture. *In* Wound Healing – Biochemical and Clinical Aspects. Cohen IK, Diegelman RF, Lindblad WJ (eds). Philadelphia: Saunders, 1992, p. 96-97.

19. Swaim SF, Henderson RA: Small Animal Wound Management, 2nd ed. Baltimore: Williams & Wilkins, 1997, p. 28.

20. Pavletic MM: Atlas of Small Animal Reconstructive Surgery, 2nd ed. Philadelphia: Saunders, 1999, p. 49.

21. Compton CC: The delayed postburn blister. A commonplace but commonly overlooked phenomenon. Arch Dermatol 128:249, 1992.

22. Bergman R, David R, Ramon Y, et al: Delayed postburn blisters: an immunohistochemical and ultrastructural study. J Cutan Pathol 24:429, 1997.

23. Chetty BV, Boissy RE, Warden GD, Nordlund JJ: Basement membrane and fibroblast aberration in blisters at the donor, graft, and spontaneously healed sites in patients with burns. Arch Dermatol 128:181, 1992.

24. Nieman GF, Clark WR Jr, Paskanik A, Feldbaum D: Segmental pulmonary vascular resistance following wood smoke inhalation. Crit Care Med 23:1264, 1995.

25. Enkhbaatar P, Traber DL: Pathophysiology of acute lung injury in combined burn and smoke inhalation injury. Clin Sci (Lond.) 107:137, 2004.

26. Murakami K, Traber DL: Pathophysiological basis of smoke inhalation injury. News Physiol Sci 18:125, 2003.

27. Wong SS, Sun NN, Lantz RC, Witten ML: Substance P and neutral endopeptidase in development of acute respiratory distress syndrome following fire smoke inhalation. Am J Physiol Lung Cell Mol Physiol 287:L859, 2004.

28. Magnotti LJ, Xu DZ, Lu Q, Deitch EA: Gut-derived mesenteric lymph: a link between burn and lung injury. Arch Surg 134:1333, 1999.

29. Westphal M, Noshima S, Isago T, et al: Selective thromboxane A2 synthase inhibition by OKY-046 prevents cardiopulmonary dysfunction after ovine smoke inhalation injury. Anesthesiology 102:954, 2005.

30. Cox RA, Burke AS, Soejima K, et al: Airway obstruction in sheep with burn and smoke inhalation injuries. Am J Respir Cell Mol Biol 29(3 Pt 1):295, 2003.

31. Enkhbaatar P, Murakami K, Shimoda K, et al: The inducible nitric oxide synthase inhibitor BBS-2 prevents acute lung injury in sheep after burn and smoke inhalation injury. Am J Respir Crit Care Med 167:1021, 2003.

32. Soejima K, Schmalstieg FC, Sakurai H, et al: Pathophysiological analysis of combined burn and smoke inhalation injuries in sheep. Am J Physiol Lung Cell Mol Physiol 280:L1233, 2001.

33. Soejima K, Traber LD, Schmalstieg FC, et al: Role of nitric oxide in vascular permeability after combined burns and smoke inhalation injury. Am J Respir Crit Care Med 163:745, 2001.

34. Martini WZ, Irtun O, Chinkes DL, et al: Surfactant phosphatidylcholine in thermally injured pigs. Crit Care Med 29:1417, 2001.

35. Park MS, Cancio LC, Jordan BS, et al: Assessment of oxidative stress in lungs from sheep after inhalation of wood smoke. Toxicology 195:97, 2004.

36. Alarie Y: Toxicity of fire smoke. Crit Rev Toxicol 32:259, 2002.

37. Huang Q, Xu W, Ustinova E, et al: Myosin light chain kinase-dependent microvascular hyperpermeability in thermal injury. Shock 20:363, 2003.

38. Enkhbaatar P, Murakami K, Shimoda K, et al: Inducible nitric oxide synthase dimerization inhibitor prevents cardiovascular and renal morbidity in sheep with combined burn and smoke inhalation injury. Am J Physiol Heart Circ Physiol 285:H2430-H2436, 2003.

39. Gordon MD, Winfree JH: Fluid resuscitation after a major burn. In Burn Care and Therapy Carrougher GJ (ed).. St. Louis: Mosby, 1998, pp. 5-23.

40. Cassuto J, Tarnow P, Yregard L, et al: Regulation of postburn ischemia by alpha- and beta- adrenoreceptor subtypes. Burns 31(2):131, 2005.

41. Sedowofia K, Barclay C, Quaba A, et al: The systemic response to thermal injury in children. Clin Endocrinol (Oxf) 49:335, 1998,

42. Sharar SR, Heimbach DM, Green M, et al: Effects of body surface thermal injury on apparent renal and cutaneous blood flow in goats. J Burn Care Rehabil 9(1):26, 1988.

43. Smith A, Barclay C, Quaba A, et al: The bigger the burn, the greater the stress. Burns 23(4):291, 1997.

44. Lowe GD: Blood rheology in general medicine and surgery. Baillieres Clin Haematol 1(3):827, 1987.

45. Kawakami M, Endoh Y, Orringer EP, Meyer AA: Improvements in rheologic properties of blood by fluid resuscitation after burn injury in rats. J Burn Care Rehabil 13(3):316, 1992.

46. Suzuki K, Nishina M, Ogino R, Kohama A: Left ventricular contractility and diastolic properties in anesthetized dogs after severe burns. Am J Physiol 260(5 Pt 2):H1433, 1991.

47. Xia ZF, Zhao P, Horton JW: Changes in cardiac contractile function and myocardial. Am J Physiol Heart Circ Physiol 280:H1916, 2001.

48. Yatani A, Xu DZ, Kim SJ, et al: Mesenteric lymph from rats with thermal injury prolongs the action potential and increases Ca2+ transient in rat ventricular myocytes. Shock 20:458, 2003.

49. Horton JW, Tan J, White DJ, et al: Selective decontamination of the digestive tract attenuated the myocardial inflammation and dysfunction that occur with burn injury. Am J Physiol Heart Circ Physiol 287:H2241, 2004.

50. Ballard-Croft C, Maass DL, Sikes P, et al: Activation of stress-responsive pathways by the sympathetic nervous system in burn trauma. Shock 18(1):38, 2002.

51. Quinn DA, Moufarrej R., Volokhov A, et al: Combined smoke inhalation and scald burn in the rat. J Burn Care Rehabil 24:208, 2003.

52. Qi S, Sun W: The effects of inhaled nitric oxide on cardiac pathology and energy metabolism in a canine model of smoke inhalation injury. Burns 30:65, 2004.

53. Deitch EA: The role of intestinal barrier failure and bacterial translocation in the development of systemic infection and multiple organ failure. Arch Surg 125:403, 1990.

54. Jones WG Jr, Minei JP, Barber AE, et al: Bacterial translocation and intestinal atrophy following thermal injury and burn wound sepsis. Ann Surg 211:399, 1990.

55. Ziegler TR, Smith RJ, O'Dwyer ST, et al: Increased intestinal permeability associated with infection in burn patients. Arch Surg 123:1313, 1988.

56. Gosain A, Gamelli RL: Role of the gastrointestinal tract in burn sepsis. J Burn Care Rehabil 26(1):85, 2005.

57. Jeschke MG, Debroy MA, Wolf SE, et al: Burn and starvation increase programmed cell death in small bowel epithelial cells. Dig Dis Sci 45:415, 2000.

58. Gan HT, Chen JD: Roles of nitric oxide and prostaglandins in pathogenesis of delayed colonic transit after burn injury in rats. Am J Physiol 288:R1316, 2005.

59. Ocal K, Avlan D, Cinel I, et al: The effect of N-acetylcysteine on oxidative stress in intestine and bacterial translocation after thermal injury. Burns 30:778, 2004.

60. Jeschke MG, Low JF, Spies M, et al: Cell proliferation, apoptosis, NF-kappaB expression, enzyme, protein, and weight changes in livers of burned rats. Am J Physiol Gastrointest Liver Physiol 280:G1314, 2001.

61. Jeong J, Adamson LK, Hatam R, et al: Alterations in the expression and modification of histones in the liver after injury. Exp Mol Pathol 75:256, 2003.

62. Schiavon M, Di Landro D, Baldo M, et al: A study of renal damage in seriously burned patients. Burns Incl Therm Inj 14(2):107, 1988.

63. Kim G, Oh KH, Yoon JW, et al: Impact of burn size and initial serum albumin level on acute renal failure occurring in major burn. Am J Nephrol 23:55, 2003.

64. Holm C, Hörbrand F, von Donnersmarck GH, Mühlbauer W: Acute renal failure in severely burned patients. Burns 25:171, 1999.

65. Aikawa N, Wakabayashi G, Ueda M, Shinozawa Y: Regulation of renal function in thermal injury. J Trauma 30:S174, 1990.

66. Loebl EC, Baxter CR, Curreri PW: The mechanism of erythrocyte destruction in the early post-burn period. Ann Surg 178(6):681, 1973.

67. Topley E, Jackson DM, Cason JS, Davies JW: Assessment of red cell loss in the first two days after severe burns. Ann Surg 155:581, 1962.

68. Hatherill JR, Till GO, Bruner LH, Ward PA: Thermal injury, intravascular hemolysis, and toxic oxygen products. J Clin Invest 78:629, 1986.

69. Bekyarova G, Yankova T: Alpha-tocopherol and reduced glutathione deficiency and decreased deformability of erythrocytes after thermal skin injury. Acta Physiol Pharmacol Bulg 23:55, 1998.

70. Bekyarova G, Yankova T, Kozarev I, Yankov D: Reduced erythrocyte deformability related to activated lipid peroxidation during the early postburn period. Burns 22(4):291, 1996.

71. Vasko SD, Burdge JJ, Ruberg RL, Verghese AS: Evaluation of erythropoietin levels in the anemia of thermal injury. J Burn Care Rehabil 12:437, 1991.

72. Andes WA, Rogers PW, Beason JW, Pruitt BA Jr: The erythropoietin response to the anemia of thermal injury. J Lab Clin Med 88(4):584, 1976.

73. Wallner S, Vautrin R, Katz J, Murphy J: The anemia of thermal injury: partial characterization of an erythroid inhibitory substance. J Trauma 27:639, 1987.

74. Sheldon GF, Sanders R, Fuchs R, et al: Metabolism, oxygen transport, and erythropoietin synthesis in the anemia of thermal injury. Am J Surg 135(3):406, 1978.

75. Cho K, Adamson LK, Greenhalgh DG: Parallel self-induction of TNF-alpha and apoptosis in the thymus of mice after burn injury. J Surg Res 98:9, 2001.

76. Takahashi H, Kobayashi M, Tsuda Y, et al: Contribution of the sympathetic nervous system on the burn-associated impairment of CCL3 production. Cytokine 29:208, 2005.

77. Gallagher G, Rae CP, Kinsella J: Treatment of pain in severe burns. Am J Clin Dermatol 1:329, 2000.

78. Stoddard FJ, Sheridan RL, Saxe GN, et al: Treatment of pain in acutely burned children. J Burn Care Rehabil 23(2):135, 2002.

79. Khalil Z, Helme R: Sensory peptides as neuromodulators of wound healing in aged rats. J Gerontol A Biol Sci Med Sci 51:B354, 1996.

80. Cartwright MM: The metabolic response to stress: a case of complex nutrition support management. Crit Care Nurs Clin North Am 16(4):467, 2004.

81. Cuthbertson DP, Zagreb H: The metabolic response to injury and its nutritional implications: retrospect and prospect. J Parenter Enteral Nutr 3(3):108, 1979.

82. Herndon DN, Tompkins RG: Support of the metabolic response to burn injury. Lancet 363:1895, 2004.

83. Demling RH, Seigne P: Metabolic management of patients with severe burns. World J Surg 24:673, 2000.

84. Wolf SE, Thomas SJ, Dasu MR, et al: Improved net protein balance, lean mass, and gene expression changes with oxandrolone treatment in the severely burned. Ann Surg 237:801, 2003.

85. Henderson RA, Horne R: The Pinna. *In* Textbook of Small Animal Surgery, 3rd ed. Slatter DH (ed). Philadelphia: Saunders, 2002, p. 1745.

86. Withrow SJ: Cryosurgery. *In* Small Animal Clinical Oncology, 3rd ed. Withrow SJ, MacEwen EG (eds). Philadelphia: Saunders, 2001, p. 79.

87. Reamy BV: Frostbite: review and current concepts. J Am Board Fam Pract 11(1):34, 1998.

88. Murphy JV, Banwell PE, Roberts AH, McGrouther DA: Frostbite: pathogenesis and treatment. J Trauma 48(1):171, 2000.

89. Vargel I, Erdem A, Ertoy D, et al: Effects of growth factors on doxorubicin-induced skin necrosis: documentation of histomorphological alterations and early treatment by GM-CSF and G-CSF. Ann Plast Surg 49(6):646, 2002.

90. Garrett LD: Beyond the lymphoma: paraneoplastic syndromes and more. Proceedings 23rd Annual Forum American College of Veterinary Internal Medicine. Baltimore, 2005.

91. Luce EA: Electrical burns. Clin Plast Surg 27:133, 2000.

92. Sheridan RL, Remensnyder JP, Schnitzer JJ, et al: Current expectations for survival in pediatric burns. Arch Pediatr Adolesc Med 154:245, 2000.

93. Sheridan RL: Burn care. Results of technical and organizational progress. JAMA 290:719, 2003.

94. Herruzo-Cabrera R, Fernandez-Arjona M, Garcia-Torres V, et al: Mortality evolution study of burn patients in a critical care burn unit between 1971 and 1991. Burns 21:106, 1995.

Chapter 63

Congenital Skin Diseases

Mark W. Bohling
Steven F. Swaim

Congenital cutaneous disease accounts for only a small percentage of veterinary surgical cases; nonetheless, a few congenital skin disorders are noteworthy in that they may benefit from surgical intervention or may drastically affect an animal's response to surgical treatment. The congenital dermatopathies of greatest importance to the veterinary surgeon are cutaneous asthenia, dermoid sinus, nasal dermoid sinus cyst, and aplasia cutis. Other congenital skin diseases of minor surgical importance that are briefly discussed in this chapter include Chediak-Higashi syndrome, cutaneous mucinosis, acral mutilation syndrome, and inherited disorders of keratinization. Congenital dermatoses are skin conditions present at birth. Although the exact cause of all congenital dermatoses is not known, most are thought to be the result of genetic defects. True congenital dermatoses are uncommon; more common are hereditary defects that manifest later in life.

Cutaneous Asthenia

Definitions and Mechanisms

Cutaneous asthenia has also been called Ehlers-Danlos syndrome, "rubber puppy" disease, dermal fragility syndrome, dominant collagen dysplasia, and dermatosparaxis.[1,2] Cutaneous asthenia is a group of inherited congenital connective tissue diseases that affect man and a number of animal species including dogs, cats, horses, cattle, sheep, rabbits, and mink.[1-5] The disease complex resembles Ehlers-Danlos syndrome in humans, which has at least eleven different variations that may be distinguished clinically, genetically, and biochemically.[1,3] In general, the condition is inherited as a simple autosomal dominant trait in dogs and cats,[1,2,4-7] although it has been reported to be a recessive trait in Himalayan cats.[1,2,8-10]

The condition is characterized by skin fragility, hyperextensibility (Figure 63-1), and laxity, with fragility being the primary feature of the condition.[1-5,11-13] The lack of tensile strength and decreased stiffness of the skin may be related to the organization or cross-linking of collagen molecules in the dermis.[3,13] The tensile strength of affected skin has been reported to be anywhere from one third to one fortieth that of normal skin.[1,11,12,14] In cats, a nine-fold reduction in tensile strength has been reported.[1,12] The collagen abnormality in Himalayan cats is due to a deficiency of procollagen peptidase.[8,10]

Histopathologically, the dermis of affected dogs has been reported to be normal in thickness,[15] or thinner than that of normal dogs (1.21 vs. 1.71 mm, respectively).[12] No significant difference in dermal thickness was noted between affected and normal cats in one study (1.41 and 1.44 mm, respectively);[12] another study reported significantly thinner dermis between affected and normal cats (0.25 vs. 1.71mm, respectively).[15] Epidermal thicknesses of both affected and unaffected dogs and cats ranged between 0.02 and 0.03 mm.[1,3,12]

Histopathologic abnormalities in the dermis are related to collagen, which gives tensile strength to the skin. In general, in affected animals, dermal collagen bundles are irregular in size and fibrillar in nature, and they lack the normal characteristic interweaving pattern of collagen bundles.[3,12] In addition, collagen bundles appear to be fine, often fragmented, with a lack of orientation and have a whorled appearance.[3,5,12,14] Mature collagen bundles are also lacking, and in some areas collagen fibers are surrounded by mucinous degeneration.[3,14]

The dermis of affected cats has fine, fibrillar collagen with collagen bundles of varying sizes, some of which appear to be unraveled. Large, short, whorled collagen bundles appear in the deep dermis.[12] The wrapping of collagen fibers around blood vessels and a coiled arrangement of fibers around sweat glands has also been reported in cats.[16] Electron microscopy reveals disorganization of collagen fibrils, with variation in fibril size and shape and irregular orientation resulting in a "moth-eaten" appearance.[1,5]

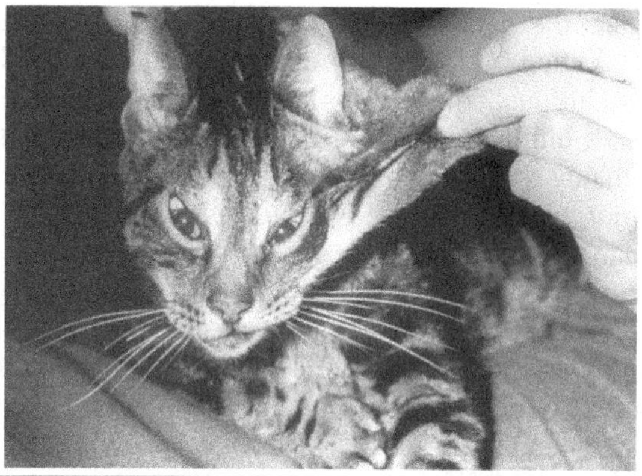

Figure 63-1. This cat with cutaneous asthenia has typical hyperextensibility of the skin.

Surgical Significance

The fragility of skin presents clinically significant factors for the veterinary surgeon. The incidence of lacerations is increased in affected animals, owing to the ease with which skin tears. Lacerations should be sutured promptly.[1] When manipulating skin for wound closure, excessive forceps tension on the wound edges should be avoided to prevent tearing the tissue, and careful undermining of the skin may be necessary to allow closure without tension.[8,12,17]

Mattress sutures, specifically a horizontal mattress pattern with or without stents of rubber tubing, has been recommended to help prevent the sutures from tearing through the skin.[1,8] However, cruciate sutures placed 5 mm from the wound edge have been found to be less likely to tear through the skin than simple interrupted, vertical, or horizontal mattress sutures.[12,13] Small tapered-point needles with swaged-on suture material have been advocated to help prevent skin tearing.[12,17] Because of the thin dermis, the skin tends to evert when it is sutured.[17]

Wound Healing

Delayed wound healing has been reported as a complication in Ehlers-Danlos syndrome in humans,[13,17] but using clinical and histologic criteria, wound healing in dogs and cats with cutaneous asthenia appears to be similar to that in unaffected animals.[17] In dogs with cutaneous asthenia, healed scar tissue has greater tensile strength than adjacent skin; in affected cats, however, the tensile strength of scar tissue is no different from adjacent skin.[13] The increased tensile strength reported in dogs was speculated to be caused by (1) a greater degree of intra- and intermolecular cross-linking of collagen fibrils in the scar, (2) amplified production of type I collagen in the scar, or (3) reduced collagenolysis, or a greater degree of collagen ground substance interaction in the scar.[13]

Dermoid Sinus and Nasal Dermoid Sinus Cyst

Definition and Mechanism

A dermoid sinus (pilonidal sinus) is a neural tube defect that results from incomplete separation of the skin and neural tube during embryonic development.[1,2,18-24] The sinus is a tubular skin indentation that extends as a blind sac from the dorsal midline to varying depths in the underlying tissues.[1] Dermoid sinuses have been classified by their depth of penetration (Figure 63-2).[20,21] Classes I through IV have an opening to the skin surface; in addition, a fifth type (Class V) has been reported and is a true cyst with no skin opening.[21,23,24] The sinuses occur in the cervical, craniothoracic, and sacrococcygeal regions (i.e., craniad and caudad to the area of the ridge of hair on Rhodesian ridgebacks). The sinuses occur most frequently in the cervical area and less often in the sacrococcygeal area.[20] One or more sinuses may be present on the same animal.[18-20,23] In the cervical area, the sinus is generally attached in the area of the dorsal spinous process of the second cervical vertebra and seldom extends any deeper. Class IV sinuses, which communicate with the dura mater, are seen mainly in the sacrococcygeal region, extending cranioventrad to the last sacral vertebra.[20] Dermoid sinuses occur by far most commonly in the Rhodesian ridgeback (Figure 63-3).[18-21,24] Cases have also been reported in the golden retriever,[25] shih tzu, boxer,[26] Yorkshire terrier,[22] springer spaniel,[27] chow-chow,[23] and Siberian husky.[28] In Rhodesian ridgebacks the condition may be caused by a gene complex.[1,21] Most historical data on inheritance of dermoid sinus suggests that the condition may be inherited as a simple recessive trait;[18-20] a more recent study suggested a more complex dihybrid mode of inheritance with differential penetrance.[21]

Nasal dermoid sinus cyst is unique from dermoid sinus and has been reported in the Golden retriever,[29] English bull terrier,[30] and Brittany, springer, and cocker spaniels.[29,31] In this condition, a sinus tract of invaginated keratinized epithelium with adnexal structures (hair follicles and glands) extends from a dorsal midline opening just caudal to the nasal planum (the so-called "nasal pit"), caudally into the nasal septum.[29] The condition is congenital and in man is caused by a neuroectodermal remnant in the prenasal space located between the nasal and frontal bones and the cartilaginous nasal capsule in the embryo.[29]

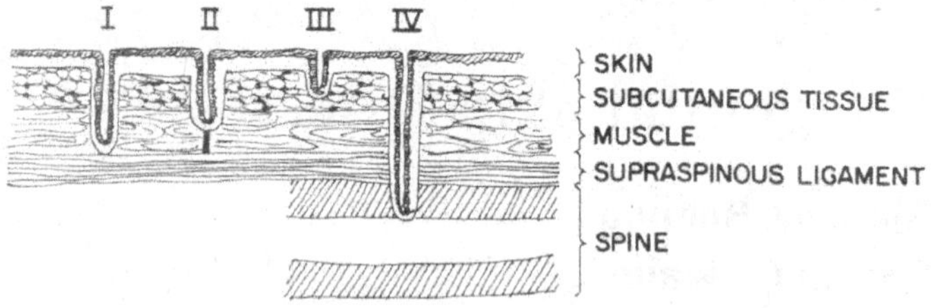

Figure 63-2. Classes of dermoid sinus. Class I, sinus extends to the supraspinous ligament where it is attached. Class II, sinus extends into muscular or subcutaneous tissue and is connected to the supraspinous ligament by a fibrous band. Class III, sinus extends into muscular or subcutaneous tissue but is not connected to the supraspinous ligament. Class IV, sinus extends to the spinal canal and is attached to the dura mater. Class V, (not illustrated) is a true cyst with no connection to the skin. (Adapted from Mann GE, Stratton J: Dermoid sinus in the Rhodesian ridgeback. J Small Anim Pract 7:631, 1966.)

Surgical Significance

Surgical excision is the treatment of choice for dermoid sinus and nasal dermoid sinus cyst;[1,18,20,29] however, observation without treatment has been described if the lesion is quiescent. When drainage or neurologic signs are present, surgery should be performed.[1] Careful dissection of all sinus structures is important; introduction of a small (3.5 Fr) urinary catheter into the sinus may help with identification of the sinus as dissection progresses. In dermoid sinus, deep fibrous attachments, possibly to the dura mater, may make complete excision impossible.[1,18] Incomplete sinus removal may result in recurrence of clinical signs.[18] Meningitis often complicates cases in which the dermoid sinus is attached to the dura mater;[1] therefore, extreme care and aseptic technique are indicated.[1,19] When dermoid sinuses communicate with the dura mater, hemilaminectomy or craniotomy with removal of part of the dura mater and associated abnormal tissue may be necessary to ensure complete removal of all sinus tissue.[20,26]

Aplasia Cutis

Definition and Mechanism

Aplasia cutis is a rare congenital disorder characterized by focal discontinuity of the epidermis. The condition has also been referred to as epitheliogenesis imperfecta. Most of the reports of this disease in the veterinary literature have been in cattle, horses, sheep, and pigs. In these species aplasia cutis is thought to be an autosomal recessive disorder.[32] There have been only isolated case reports in puppies and kittens.[33-35] The cause of the disease in these species is unknown.

Surgical Significance

Small lesions may be corrected by surgical repair or may heal by contraction and epithelialization. It has been suggested that in cattle the disease is not only an inherited defect in epidermal development but a more complex disorder of fibroblast metabolism.[36] Cultured fibroblasts from affected cattle have several metabolic disturbances, including a decrease in biosynthesis of

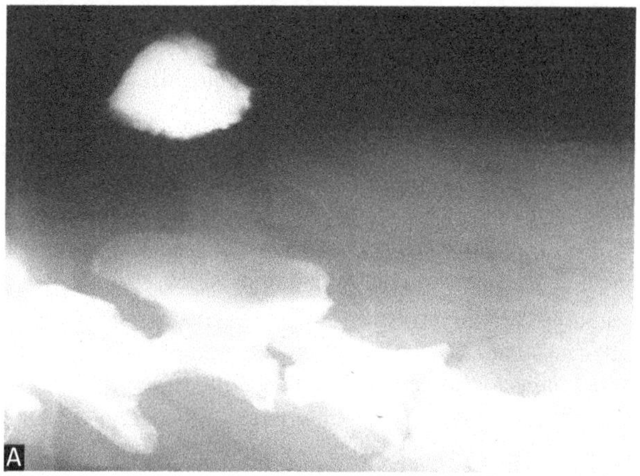

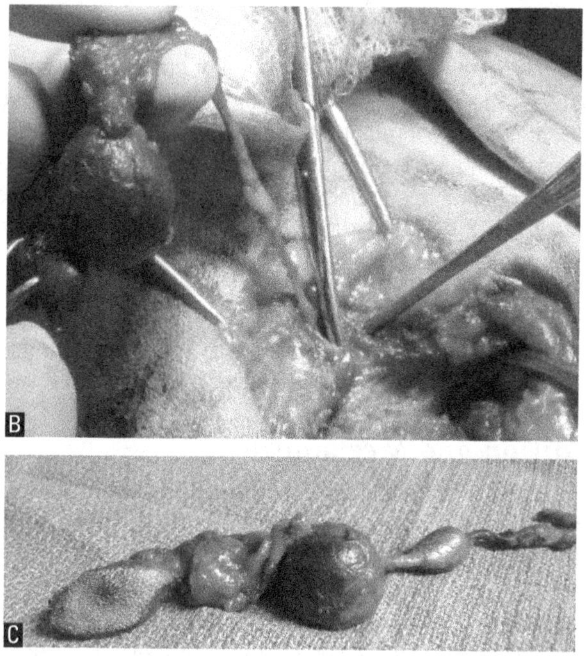

Figure 63-3. A. fistulogram of a cervical dermoid sinus in a Rhodesian ridgeback. Note the superficial cyst-like structure and extension of the contrast (delineating the sinus) to the spinous process of the third cervical vertebra. B. Surgical resection of the sinus. C. The excised sinus tract. Note the slightly darker area in the center of the ellipse of excised skin; this was the location of the sinus communication with the skin surface.

both collagen and lipids. If the same is true in other species, the probability of normal wound healing following surgical repair is decreased.

Chediak-Higashi Syndrome

Definition and Mechanism

The Chediak-Higashi syndrome is a rare autosomal recessive genetic defect that has been seen in several species, including humans and Persian cats.[37,38] Affected individuals have a structural defect that results in abnormally large granules in neutrophils, monocytes, and eosinophils. Melanin granules are likewise enlarged. The cellular abnormalities of affected animals include increased fragility of leukocyte granules, defective granular fusion, and enzyme deficiencies. These abnormalities may result in cellular rupture and tissue damage, defective chemotactic responsiveness, and reduced intracellular killing.[38,39] Affected animals may succumb to recurrent infections or lymphoid neoplasia.[38]

Surgical Significance

The distinct coat and eye color of affected Persian cats should alert the veterinary surgeon to the possibility of Chediak-Higashi syndrome. Knowledge of this syndrome may prevent unnecessary surgery, which could be complicated by excessive postoperative bleeding and infections. Recombinant canine granulocyte colony-stimulating factor has been shown to enhance neutrophil function in affected cats and may be a useful adjunct to reduce risk of infection when surgery is required.[39]

Cutaneous Mucinosis

Definition and Mechanism

In dogs both discoid lupus erythematosus[40] and hypothyroidism[41,42] have been shown to increase dermal mucin deposition. The Chinese Shar pei appears to be unique in its propensity to have cutaneous mucinosis, and this dermal abnormality appears to be inherited, and "normal" to some degree, in all Shar peis. In extreme cases, a Shar pei may develop severe myxedema and mucoid vesicles.[43,44] Cutaneous mucinosis is manifested histologically by wide separation of dermal collagen bundles by mucin. Even the "normal" Shar pei has more mucin deposition between collagen bundles than other breeds.

The cause of this increase in dermal mucin is unclear, but the source is thought to be the dermal fibroblast.[40] Myxedema may be the result of an increase in the synthesis or a decrease in the degranulation of mucopolysaccharides.[45] The mucopolysaccharides that accumulate in the dermis are chondroitin sulfate and hyaluronic acid.

Surgical Significance

Incision into the skin of the Shar pei will reveal a gelati¬nous material that tends to form beads or threads. It has been suggested that in severely affected Shar peis maturation of dermal fibroblasts may be delayed,[43] which could result in poor wound healing.

Acral Mutilation Syndrome

Definition and Mechanism

The acral mutilation syndrome is not a congenital anomaly but rather an inherited disease. This disease of self-mutilation has been reported in English pointers and French spaniels in North America, German short-haired pointers in Europe, and English springer spaniels in Australia.[46-48] Pedigree examination in each affected breed indicates that the condition is probably inherited as an autosomal recessive sensory neuropathy. Biochemical studies of affected pointers have demonstrated a reduction in substance P-like immunoreactivity,[49] while histologic examination has shown a reduction in the size of spinal ganglia as well as a deficiency of ganglionic neurons.[47]

Surgical Significance

Affected animals are difficult to maintain because of their persistent determination to chew their paws. Chronic wound management with topical medications and bandages, and constant use of muzzles or other forms of restraint are required. Even after healing, many dogs relapse as soon as restraints are removed; faced with this discouraging situation, many owners elect euthanasia.[46-48]

Inherited Defects of Keratinization

Definition and Mechanism

This category of rare diseases is grouped together because all share the feature of abnormal keratinization. Footpad hyperkeratosis has been described as a familial condition in the Irish terrier[50] and Dogue de Bordeaux;[51] related individuals of several other breeds (Labrador and golden retrievers, Kerry blue terriers, and mixed breed dogs) have also been reported.[1] A heritable defect of keratin filament formation causing increased epidermolysis was reported in 7 related Norfolk terriers; autosomal recessive inheritance is suspected.[52] Epidermolytic hyperkeratosis, a congenital condition in man characterized by collapse of the keratin filament cytoskeleton, has been reported in a single canine patient, a 6 month-old Labrador-retriever mix.[53]

Surgical Significance

The aforementioned keratinization defects appear to be rare in dogs, and although specific information regarding surgical complications is lacking, several reasonable inferences can be made. In each of these conditions, the cytologic and biochemical abnormalities appear to be limited to the superficial layers of the epidermis (superficial to the stratum basale);[50,52,53] therefore, primary healing should not be impacted to any great extent. However, the greatly thickened and cracked skin predisposes to bacterial and mycotic infections,[52] so superficial wound infection may be expected to be a problem. Appropriate therapy should be instituted prior to elective procedures to improve the condition of the epidermis and, thereby, minimize infection risk. In addition, while not confirmed, second intention healing might be impacted owing to possible effects of abnormal keratinization on wound epithelialization. A moist wound environment and judicious use of mild desquamating agents may prove beneficial.

Conclusion

Although the exact mechanism for the development of all of the congenital skin diseases is unknown, most have been found to have a genetic basis. In many instances, the condition is inherited as an autosomal recessive trait. With this in mind, it must be recommended that not only should affected animals be withdrawn from the breeding pool, but in most instances, the parents, and perhaps siblings, should not be used for breeding purposes. In some cases, test mating to affected animals may provide evidence that a particular animal does not carry the abnormal gene.[1,2,54]

References

1. Scott DW, Miller WH, Griffin CE: Small Animal Dermatology, 6th ed. Philadelphia: WB Saunders, 2001.

2. Foil CS: The skin. *In* Veterinary Pediatrics: Dogs and Cats From Birth to Six Months. Hoskins JD (ed). Philadelphia: WB Saunders, 1990.

3. Hegreberg GA, Padgett GA, Henson JB: Connective tissue disease of dogs and mink resembling Ehlers-Danlos syndrome in man. III. Histopathologic changes of the skin. Arch Pathol 90:159, 1970.

4. Hegreberg GA, Padgett GA, Gorham JR, Henson JB: A connective tissue disease of dogs and mink resembling the Ehlers-Danlos syndrome in man: II. Mode of inheritance. J Hered 60:249, 1969.

5. Paciello O, Lamagna F, Lamagna B, Papparella S: Ehlers-Danlos-like syndrome in 2 dogs: clinical, histologic, and ultrastructural findings. Vet Clin Pathol 32:13, 2003.

6. Patterson DF, Minor RR: Hereditary fragility and hyperextensibility of skin of cats: a defect in collagen fibrillogenesis. Lab Invest 37:170, 1977.

7. Minor RR, et al: Defects in fibrillogenesis causing hyperextensible, fragile skin in dogs. J Am Vet Med Assoc 752:142, 1983.

8. Collier LA, Leathers CW, Counts DF: A clinical description of dermatosparaxis in a Himalayan cat. Feline Pract 70:25, 1980.

9. Counts DF, Byers PH, Holbrook KA, Hegreberg GA: Dermatosparaxis in a Himalayan cat: I. biochemical studies of dermal collagen. J Invest Dermatol. 74:96, 1980.

10. Holbrook KA, Byers PH, Counts DF, Hegreberg GA: Dermatosparaxis in a Himalayan cat. II. Ultrastructural studies of dermal collagen. J Invest Dermatol 74:100, 1980.

11. Hegreberg GA, Padgett GA, Ott RL, Henson JB: A heritable connective tissue disease of dogs and mink resembling Ehlers-Danlos syndrome of man. I. Skin tensile strength properties. J Invest Dermatol 54:311, 1970.

12. Freeman LJ, Hegreberg GA, Robinette ID: Ehlers-Danlos syndrome in dogs and cats. Semin Vet Med Surg 2:221, 1987.

13. Freeman LJ, Hegreberg GA, Robinette JD, Kimbrell, JT: Biochemical properties of skin and wounds in Ehlers-Danlos syndrome. Vet Surg 18(2):97, 1989.

14. Hegreberg GA, Padgett GA, Henson JB, Ott RL: Cutaneous asthenia in Dogs. *In* Proceedings of the 16th Annual Meeting, Gaines Veterinary Symposium. Philadelphia, 1966.

15. Ducatelle R, Charlier G, Cornelissen F, et al: A morphometric classification of dermatosparaxis in the dog and cat. Vlamaams Diergen. Tudschrift 56(2) :107, 1987.

16. Rest JR: Pathology of two possible genodermatoses. J Small Anim Pract 30:230, 1989.

17. Freeman LJ, Hegreberg GA, Robinette JD: Cutaneous wound healing in Ehlers-Danlos syndrome. Vet Surg 18(2):88, 1989.

18. Gammie JS: Dermoid sinus removal in a Rhodesian ridgeback dog. Can Vet J 27:250, 1986.

19. Hathcock JT, Clampett EG, Broadstone RV: Dermoid sinus in a Rhodesian ridgeback. Vet Med Small Anim Clin 74:53, 1979.

20. Leyh R, Carithers RW: Dermoid sinus in a Rhodesian ridgeback. Iowa State Univ Vet 7:36, 1979.

21. Hillbertz NHCS: Inheritance of dermoid sinus in the Rhodesian ridgeback. J Small Anim Pract 46: 71, 2005.

22. Fatone G, Brunetti A, Lamagna F, Potena A: Dermoid sinus and spinal malformations in a Yorkshire terrier: diagnosis and follow-up. J Small Animal Pract 36:178, 1995.

23. Booth MJ: Atypical dermoid sinus in a chow chow dog. J South. Afr Vet Assoc 69: 102, 1998.

24. Tshamala M, Moens Y: True dermoid cyst in a Rhodesian ridgeback. J Small Anim Pract 41:352, 2000.

25. Cornegliani L, Jommi E, Vercelli A: Dermoid sinus in a golden retriever. J Small Anim Pract 42:514, 2001.

26. Selcer EA, Helman RG, Selcer RR: Dermoid sinus in a Shih Tzu and a boxer. J Am Anim Hosp Assoc 20:634, 1983.

27. Pratt JN, Knottenbelt CM, Welsh EM: Dermoid sinus at the lumbosacral junction in an English springer spaniel. J Small Anim Pract 41:24, 2000.

28. Cornegliani L, Ghibaudo G: A dermoid sinus in a Siberian husky. Vet Dermatol 10:47, 1999.

29. Anderson DM, White RAS: Nasal dermoid sinus cysts in the dog. Vet Surg 31:303, 2002.

30. Burrow RD: A nasal dermoid sinus in an English bull terrier. J Small Anim Pract 45:572, 2004.

31. Bailey TR, Holmberg DL, Yager JA: Nasal dermoid sinus in an American cocker spaniel. Can Vet J 42:213. 2001.

32. Scott DW: Large Animal Dermatology. Philadelphia: WB Saunders, 1988.

33. Gupta BN: Epitheliogenesis imperfecta in a dog. Am J Vet Res 34:443, 1973.

34. Hewitt MP, Mills JHL, Hunter B: Epitheliogenesis imperfecta in a black Labrador puppy. Can Vet J 76:371, 1975.

35. Munday BL: Epitheliogenesis imperfecta in lambs and kit¬tens. Br Vet J 726:47, 1970.

36. Frey J, Chamson A, Gourreau, JM, Gillet JP: Col¬lagen and lipid biosynthesis in a case of epitheliogenesis imperfecta in cattle. J Invest Dermatol 93:83, 1989.

37. Kramer JW, Davis WC, Prieur DJ: The Chediak-Higashi syndrome of cats. Lab Invest 36:554, 1977.

38. Tizard I: Veterinary Immunology: An Introduction, 7th ed. Philadelphia: WB Saunders, 2004.

39. Colgan SP, Gasper PW, Thrall MA, et al: Neutrophil function in normal and Chediak-Higashi syndrome cats following administration of recombinant canine granulocyte colony stimulating factor. Exp Hematol 20:1229, 1992.

40. Rosenkrantz WS, Griffin CE, Barr RJ, Walder EJ: Histological evaluation of acid mucopolysaccharide (mucin) in canine discoid lupus erythematosus. J Am Anim Hosp Assoc 22:577, 1986.

41. Scott DW: Histopathologic findings in endocrine skin disease of the dog. J Am Anim Hosp Assoc 75:173, 1982.

42. Miller WH, Buerger RG: Cutaneous mucinous vesiculation in a dog with hypothyroidism. J Am Vet Med Assoc 796:757, 1990.

43. Rosenkrantz WS, Griffin CE, Walder EJ, Froehlich PS: Idiopathic cutaneous mucinosis in a dog. Companion Anim Pract., 7:39, 1987.

44. Johnson GR: Cutaneous mucinosis in the Shar Pei. Proceedings of the American Academy of Veterinary Dermatology and American College of Veterinary Dermatology. New Orleans, 1986.

45. Freinkel RK, Freinkel N: Cutaneous manifestations of endocrine disorders. *In* Dermatology in General Medicine, 3rd ed. Fitzpatrick TB, et al (eds). New York: McGraw-Hill, 1987.

46. Cummings JF, de Lahunta A, Braund KG, Mitchell WJ: Nociceptive loss and acral mutilation in pointer dogs: canine hereditary sensory neuropathy. Am J Pathol 772:136, 1983.

47. Cummings JF, de Lahunta A, Winn SS: Acral mutilation and nociceptive loss in English pointer dogs: a canine sensory neuropathy. Acta Neuropathol (Berlin), 53:119, 1981.

48. Paradis M, de Jaham C, Page N, et al: Acral mutilation and analgesia in 13 French spaniels. Vet Dermatol 16:87, 2005.

49. Cummings JF, de Lahunta A, Simpson ST, MacDonald JM: Reduced substance P-like immunoreactivity in hereditary sensory neuropathy of pointer dogs. Acta Neuropathol. (Berlin) 63:33, 1984.

50. Schleifer SG, Versteeg SA, van Oost B, Willemse T: Familial footpad hyperkeratosis and inheritance of keratin 2, keratin 9, and desmoglein 1 in two pedigrees of Irish terriers. A.JVR 64: 715, 2003.

51. Paradis M: Footpad hyperkeratosis in a family of Dogue de Bordeaux. Vet Dermatol 3:75, 1992.

52. Barnhart KF, Credille KM, Ambrus A, Dunstan RW: A heritable keratinization defect of the superficial epidermis in Norfolk terriers. J Comp Pathol 130: 246, 2004.

53. Mecklenburg L, Hetzel U, Ueberschär S: Epidermolytic ichthyosis in a dog: clinical, histopathological, immunohistochemical and ultrastructural findings. J Comp Pathol 122: 307, 2000.

54. Pidduck H: Is this disease inherited? A discussion paper with some guidelines for canine conditions. J Small Anim Pract 26:279, 1985.

Part IX

Urinary System

Chapter 64

Renal Failure: Surgical Considerations

Don R. Waldron

The kidneys receive approximately 20 to25% of cardiac output and regulate the composition of extracellular fluid by filtration, reabsorption, secretion, and hormone production.[1] Many important systemic parameters are influenced by the kidneys, including acid-base status, electrolyte balance, the concentration of waste products of bodily metabolism, and red blood cell mass.[1-3] The diagnosis of renal failure implies sufficient loss of renal function to cause elevated levels of metabolic waste products, possible abnormalities in fluid and electrolyte balance, and loss of renal biosynthetic function.

The loss of function is reflected in laboratory tests as an increase in nonprotein nitrogenous waste products (blood urea nitrogen (BUN) and creatinine), a condition called azotemia. The inability to excrete nonprotein nitrogenous waste products may be caused by prerenal, primary (intrinsic renal), or postrenal mechanisms. Prerenal azotemia is caused by renal hypoperfusion states such as dehydration or hypotension. Postrenal azotemia is associated with obstruction of urine flow or disruption of urinary tract structure, resulting in leakage of urine into tissues or body cavities. Azotemia caused by prerenal or postrenal mechanisms may progress to cause renal damage and thus primary renal failure. Azotemia that is caused by primary renal disease has been classified based on duration as acute or chronic; in either case, the biochemical abnormalities associated with renal failure may cause profound changes in the animal's ability to maintain a normal homeostatic state.

In surgical patients, it is important to recognize prerenal or postrenal azotemia early in the course of disease, as early correction may prevent progression to primary renal failure. Patient factors such as age, cardiac status, and the concurrent administration of nephrotoxic drugs may compound other prerenal factors and influence the progression to primary renal disease. Postrenal azotemia is readily diagnosed by a good history plus physical examination with particular attention to palpation of the bladder and urethra. Some cases however, may require urethral catheterization, abdominocentesis, or imaging techniques such as radiographic contrast studies or ultrasound to confirm azotemia as postrenal and to identify the specific anatomic defect.

Acute renal failure (ARF) is an abrupt deterioration of renal function that occurs over hours to days, resulting in azotemia and decreased ability of the kidneys to regulate water and solute balance.[4] Differentiating ARF from chronic renal failure (CRF) can be difficult; however, correct diagnosis is important as ARF is potentially reversible whereas CRF is not.[5] ARF affecting surgical patients is most likely to occur in a hospital setting. The incidence of hospital-acquired ARF in animals appears to be relatively low. However, a previous study has documented a survival rate of only 40% in such cases; thus prevention of ARF is critical.[6] ARF in small animal species usually is caused by nephrotoxins; in humans, the cause is usually hypoperfusion.[6,7] Either nephrotoxins or hypoperfusion states may cause tubulointerstitial nephritis, glomerular or vascular disease, or renal tubular necrosis. Because prerenal azotemia may progress to ARF, early recognition is imperative, so that it can be corrected and primary renal damage prevented. Primary or intrinsic renal failure has been subdivided into phases and may or may not be reversible. During the induction phase of ARF, if causative factors are removed when tubule cell dysfunction may predominate over cell necrosis, recovery of cell function is possible and more likely than when the maintenance phase of ARF is reached. Evidence of early renal damage includes low specific gravity (less than 1.030 in dogs, less than 1.035 in cats), renal tubular cells and granular casts in urine sediment, failure of BUN and creatinine to return to normal after correction of hypoperfusion, and glucosuria in the normoglycemic patient.

The maintenance phase of ARF is characterized by irreversible renal tubular cell injury, with cellular necrosis. Correction of hypoperfusion during this phase has little effect if any on BUN and creatinine concentrations, and oliguria is often present after correction of hypovolemia or hypoperfusion. Oliguria in the dog is defined as urine production of less than 0.27 ml/kg/hour.[8] Patients with ARF that are nonoliguric may have a quicker recovery. This is not always the case, however, because ARF associated with aminoglycoside toxicity may or may not be reversible but is often nonoliguric. In a recent study, 39% of animals with ARF were nonoliguric.[9] If loss of nephrons with interstitial inflammation and fibrosis occurs, recovery of adequate renal function may be impossible. Adequate healing of renal tissue, however, may occur, initiating the recovery phase of ARF. This may not occur for two to three weeks after the onset of the maintenance phase. The recovery phase is characterized by an increase in urine production, and often polyuria. If oliguria was not present, the recovery phase is characterized by resolution of azotemia.[7]

Clinical consequences of ARF include disorders of fluid balance, inadequate urine production, and electrolyte and acid-base imbalance.[4] Other body tissues such as gastrointestinal, pulmonary, and cardiac systems may also be affected by renal failure.

Multiple factors often contribute to the decreased glomerular filtration rate (GFR) seen in cases of ARF. Hemodynamic factors are probably most important during the induction phase, involving a reduction in renal perfusion pressure or vasoconstriction of afferent arterioles. Possible mechanisms include response to adrenergic stimulation, failure of intrarenal autoregulation from lack of prostaglandin production, endothelial cell swelling, activation of the renin-angiotensin system, and a decrease in glomerular permeability. Tubular factors that cause decreased GFR may be more important during the maintenance phase of ARF. Obstruction of tubules with cells, cellular debris, and precipitated protein, leads to increased back pressure, thereby reducing GFR. Damage to tubular cells may also allow leakage of glomerular filtrate into interstitial tissues, reducing urine flow and allowing reabsorption of fluid and solute.[4,10]

Chronic renal failure or dysfunction is a more common clinical entity than ARF. The prevalence of CRF has been estimated to range between 0.5% and 7% in dogs and 1.6% and 20% in cats.[11,12] Causes of CRF are multifactorial and include familial, congenital, or acquired diseases. Renal lesions are most often tubulointerstitial or glomerular. In most cases, a specific initiating cause is not identified.[13] Recognition of CRF in a patient prior to anesthesia and surgery is necessary to avoid the potential for postoperative complications, prolonged hospitalization, or onset of acute renal failure. Ultimately, recognition of potential causes or risk factors for ARF in the perioperative period is important so that it may be prevented or treated early, when renal damage is least severe and potentially reversible, and metabolic complications can be avoided or minimized. Similarly, identification of patients with chronic renal disease already present is important for prognostic reasons and to prevent decompensation to a clinical diseased state or ARF after an anesthetic and/or surgical procedure. In this chapter, potential causes and risk factors for ARF in surgical patients are discussed with the goal of prevention or early treatment. The effects of uremia on the surgical patient are also discussed so that potential surgical complications may be prevented or minimized.

Etiology and Risk Factors for ARF in the Perioperative Patient

Hospital-acquired renal insufficiency is not uncommon in humans. In one study, iatrogenic factors were implicated in the majority of such episodes.[14] The most common inciting causes in 29 dogs with hospital-acquired acute renal failure were exposure to nephrotoxins and advanced age.[6] Chronic heart disease, preexisting renal disease, and anesthesia were identified as apparent contributors to ARF in these dogs. Those patients that do recover from ARF require lengthy and expensive treatment.[2] A number of risk factors and diseases have been described for the development of ARF in both the human and veterinary literature but it is unclear how many of the factors have been documented in animals (Table 64-1). Many factors have been identified in gentamicin-induced ARF in dogs, and it has been stated that those same predisposing factors likely affect the development of ARF in other cases as well.[2] Some of these factors are potentially correctable prior to an anesthetic and/or surgical treatment; thus, attention should be focused on identification and treatment of those factors. In a retrospective review of acute renal failure in dogs, pancreatitis, shock, sepsis and disseminated intravascular coagulation (DIC) were classified as ischemic disease states associated with ARF.[9]

Hypoperfusion States

Renal hypoperfusion may be caused by dehydration, hemorrhage, or shock. Dehydration has been sited as the most common and most important risk factor for ARF.[2] In humans, renal hypoperfusion associated with hemorrhage, surgery, or dehydration is a common cause of ARF.[15] In normal dogs, however, renal hypoperfusion by itself may not lead to persistent renal damage and ARF.[16] The canine kidney appears to be more resistant to ARF occurring secondary to shock or other hypotensive states. In contrast to animals with normal renal function, it has been shown experimentally that, after a hypotension episode, dogs with reduced renal mass had decreased GFR and mild histologic lesions compatible with ARF.[17] Similarly, it is thought that hypotension as a result of third-space disease (ascites or pleural effusion), decreased oncotic pressure (hypoalbuminemia), decreased cardiac output (cardiac failure), or an anesthetic episode may predispose the small animal surgical patient to ARF, particularly if clinical or subclinical renal disease already exists. Pancreatitis has been reported as a cause of ARF in animals, however, the pathophysiology is unclear. Possible causes include hypovolemic or septic shock, DIC, or the direct effects of trypsin or vasopressors released by the pancreas on glomerular capillaries.[18,19]

Table 64-1. Disease or Risk Factors for Acute Renal Failure in Dogs and Cats

Preexisting renal disease	Sepsis
Advanced age	Decreased cardiac output
Hypotension/Shock	Dehydration
Hypertension	Sodium, Potassium, Calcium deficiency or excess
DIC	Acidosis
Pancreatitis	Hyperviscosity syndromes
Nephrotoxic Drugs	

Modified from Grauer G: Prevention of acute renal failure. Vet Clin North Am 1996, and Grauer GF: Prevention of acute renal failure. *In* Textbook of Small Animal Surgery, 3rd ed. Slatter DH (ed). Philadelphia: Saunders, 2003.

Hypoperfusion may also potentiate the effects of nephrotoxic agents such as nonsteroidal anti-inflammatory drugs (NSAID), aminoglycoside antibiotics, anesthetic agents, and myoglobin (Table 64-2).[20] It appears that risk factors are additive in nature, and although a specific agent may not cause clinical problems in the normal animal, dehydration will potentially initiate nephrotoxicity of an otherwise safe drug such as Cox-2 selective NSAID. In surgical patients, hypoperfusion associated with an anesthetic episode may cause renal decompensation, especially if the animal has borderline or sublcinical renal disease.

Sepsis

Sepsis is a clinically important complication in perioperative patients that may lead to acute renal failure. Sepsis leads to ARF through a variety of mechanisms, including renal hypoperfusion owing to redistribution of renal blood flow, deposition of microthrombi in renal vasculature, or from direct toxic damage to tubular cells by bacteria or endotoxin.[21] Appropriate volume expansion and antibiotic therapy in septic patients may prevent ARF.

Canine pyometra has been associated with a variety of renal lesions. Renal defects include antigen-antibody-mediated-membranoproliferative glomerulonephritis, tubulointerstitial nephritis, and nephrogenic diabetes insipidus.[22,23] Many patients, however, have decreased GFR not associated with renal lesions or hypovolemia. Decreased GFR may occur in animals with or without azotemia, suggesting that some factor associated with pyometra causes a decrease in renal perfusion. Acute renal failure in dogs with pyrometra has been associated with *Escherichia coli* endotoxin although not all dogs with pyometra and renal failure have *Escherichia coli* infection.[2] Many animals with pyometra also have urinary tract infections including pyelonephritis.[24] Because of polyuria and lack of water consumption owing to malaise, prerenal azotemia may also be present. Renal hypoperfusion, glomerulonephritis, tubular damage, and pyelonephritis may all contribute to the development of ARF in patients with pyometra as may disseminated intravascular coagulation (DIC), sepsis, or septic shock. In geriatric patients with pyometra, azotemia may be present from prerenal and/or a combination of acute and chronic renal failure. The chronicity of renal disease may be difficult to determine until the pyometra is corrected.[24] Renal biopsy may assist in diagnosing the extent of renal dysfunction in such cases.

Table 64-2. Therapeutic/Diagnostic Agents with Nephrotoxic Potential

Antibacterial Agents
Aminoglycosides
Nafcillin
Cephalosporins
Sulfonamides
Fluoroquinolones
Tetracyclines
NSAIDS
Cancer Chemotherapeutics
Cisplatin, Carboplatin
Methotrexate
Doxorubricin
Adriamycin
Azathioprine
Ace Inhibitors
Antifungal Drugs
Amphotericin
Immunosuppressive Drugs
Cyclosporin
Interleukin (IL)-2
Radiocontrast Agents
Miscellaneous
Methoxyflurane
Acetaminophen
Penicillamine
Dextran 40
Methylene Blue
Allopurinol

Modified from Cowgill LD: Acute uremia. *In* Textbook of Veterinary Internal Medicine. Ettinger SJ, Feldman EC (eds). St. Louis: Elsevier Saunders, 2005

Toxins

Myoglobin is an uncommon but potential nephrotoxic cause of ARF, especially in the face of dehydration. Myoglobinuria can occur in the perioperative patient from malignant hyperthermia, exertional rhabdomyolyis, or prolonged grand mal seizures.[25-28] Early recognition and treatment will minimize potential renal damage from these diseases. Malignant hyperthermia is an acquired metabolic myopathy and has been related to exercise or general anesthesia (particularly halothane anesthesia). Greyhounds seem predisposed to the disease.[26,29]

Hemoglobin is not nephrotoxic in well hydrated patients, however hemolysis of whole blood is known to be toxic in humans. Conditions that could lead to hemolysis and possibly acute renal failure in small animal patients include burns, rapid intravenous infusion of large volumes of hypotonic solutions, transfusion reactions or hemolysis of whole blood during improper administration, immune-mediated hemolytic disease, infection by red blood cell parasites such as Babesia or Hemobartonella, or administration of acetaminophen, particularly in cats. In addition, methylene blue, which has been used in animals during surgery to aid in identification of neoplasia of the pancreas, may cause hemolysis in dogs and cats. Acute renal failure following burns is likely multifactor and caused by both hemolytic and red blood cell membrane fragmentation as well as hemo-concentration and catecholamine response leading to redistribution of blood flow.[30] Avoidance of these conditions or early recognition of hemolysis followed by appropriate fluid therapy to maintain renal blood flow and urine output may prevent renal damage from hemoglobinuria.

Electrolyte imbalances can increase the risk of acute renal failure. Hypercalcemia in the adult dog is often associated with neoplasms, most commonly lymphosarcoma but also anal sac apocrine gland adenocarcinoma, adenocarcinoma of the mammary gland or nasal cavity, thyroid carcinoma, and parathyroid gland tumors.[31] In a review of 29 dogs with primary hyperparathyroidism, 13 dogs had high blood urea nitrogen levels at initial presentation. Postoperatively, 7 dogs suffered from renal failure, 4 of which had elevated BUN preoperatively. Dogs that developed renal failure had significantly higher preoperative total calcium levels compared with animals that had normal renal function.[32] Hypercalcemia can contribute to prerenal azotemia because of decreased water consumption and polyuria from the direct effects of calcium on tubular concentrating ability. Chronic hypercalcemia causes tubular and interstitial damage that can lead to renal failure.[33] Acute hypercalcemia can cause defects in urine concentrating ability but does not lead to a decrease in GFR until the calcium concentration exceeds 16 mg/dl.[34] Damage caused by acute hypercalcemia may include direct tubular cell toxicity as well as ischemic injury from vasoconstriction. Early recognition of hypercalcemia in surgical patients (so that appropriate saline volume diuresis can reduce the serum calcium value) may help prevent renal damage, particularly in the face of possible renal hypoperfusion associated with anesthesia and surgery. For patients refractory to saline diuresis alone, corticosteroid and diuretic therapy may be needed to reduce serum calcium concentration to an acceptable level.

Other electrolyte abnormalities may contribute to acute renal failure concurrent with other risk factors. Hyponatremia is reported to potentiate contrast-media-induced acute renal failure in dogs.[35] Hypocalcemia, hypomagnesemia, and hypokalemia may potentiate the nephrotoxic effects of aminoglycoside antibiotics.[2]

Drug-Induced ARF

Many therapeutic agents have the potential to be nephrotoxic and thus may be predisposing factors to ARF in the surgical patient (Table 64-2).

Nonsteroidal anti-inflammatory drug (NSAID) use in dogs has grown markedly in the past 10 years. This class of drugs is now commonly used in dogs for treatment of pain related to osteoarthritis and in the perioperative period to decrease pain associated with both orthopedic and soft tissue surgical procedures. Renal toxicity is the second most important NSAID toxicity, after gastrointestinal effects.[36] The primary action of NSAID is to block expression of cyclooxygenase (COX) in cell membranes. Cyclooxygenase exists as both COX 1 and COX 2 isoforms; these have roles in normal homeostasis and are induced by proinflammatory stimuli. During periods of hypotension and reduced renal perfusion, prostaglandins are important for autoregulation to maintain renal blood flow and glomerular filtration, and thus are protective in nature. NSAIDs have the potential to cause prerenal renal impairment by depleting the kidney of vasodilatory prostaglandins.[37] The introduction of selective COX-2 inhibiting NSAIDs has decreased the prevalence of gastrointestinal toxicity, but because the kidney has both COX-1 and COX-2 isoforms, there may be little difference in the incidence of renal toxicity associated with the various NSAIDs. Any NSAID may cause renal toxicity especially if in the presence of preexisting renal disease. The exact mechanisms of renal impairment are unknown, but primary effects on the renal parenchyma may include acute interstitial nephritis, which may progress to papillary necrosis.[37] It appears that the overall occurrence of ARF owing to use of the newer NSAID (carprofen, deracoxib, and meloxicam) in dogs is low. Most dogs that develop ARF as a result of these NSAIDs either ingest excessive quantities of the drug or have a concurrent disease predisposing them to ARF.[38]

Specific antibiotics, particularly gentamicin, have known nephrotoxic potential. Gentamicin may cause an idiosyncratic acute renal tubular cell necrosis in humans and animals.[39,40] Several factors are known to predispose to gentamicin toxicity including dehydration, concurrent administration of furosamide, and hypokalemia.[41] It is known that measurements of BUN and creatinine levels are not good early indicators of renal damage from aminoglycoside toxicity. Glycosuria, proteinuria, hematuria, cylindruria, or decreased specific gravity are better indicators of renal damage.[42] Measurement of gamma glutamyl transpeptidase (GGT) activity in the urine or use of the urine GGT-to-creatinine ratio are more sensitive indicators of early nephrotoxicity from gentamicin therapy.[40,43] Nafcillin used as prophylactic antibiotic therapy in surgical patients was suspected of causing ARF in seven dogs at one institution. None of the dogs had preexisting renal disease and none had suffered a hypotensive episode. Six dogs recovered following intensive therapy for ARF.[44]

Radiographic contrast agents are often used parenterally for diagnostic purposes in surgical patients. Contrast agents used for excretory urography are hyperosmolar and cause an osmotic diuresis after administration. Possible pathogenic mechanisms for ARF caused by contrast agents include direct tubule injury, tubule precipitation of urinary proteins with contrast media causing obstruction, vasoconstriction of renal vessels leading to ischemic injury, or idiosyncratic reaction.[45] The prevalence of contrast-agent-induced renal failure in small animals appears to be very low but has been described in two case reports.[46,47] In one of the reported cases, preexisting renal disease was present prior to contrast administration. Correction of sodium or potassium imbalances is recommended prior to administration of intravenous contrast agents and the presence of preexisting renal disease should dictate caution in their administration.[35] Correction of dehydration and administration of fluids during and after the contrast study should be considered.

Vascular Disorders

Disseminated intravascular coagulation (DIC) is a clinicopathologic condition that can cause both a hemorrhagic diathesis and thrombosis of vasculature. DIC is always a secondary disease and has been associated with or caused by infectious, inflammatory, neoplastic, and toxic conditions. DIC may be seen in up to 50% of dogs with hemangiosarcoma.[48] Laboratory evidence of DIC includes thrombocytopenia, prolonged coagulation times, and decreased concentration of antithrombin III in plasma. A more recent test for the detection of elevated D-dimer protein in serum is a sensitive marker of clot lysis and strongly suggests DIC when elevated; a negative test all but excludes DIC as a diagnosis.[48] Acute renal failure from renal ischemia associated with renal vasculature thrombosis occurs in some cases of DIC. Because sluggish vascular flow, metabolic or respiratory acidosis, and shock can enhance DIC,[49] it is important to recognize and correct these predisposing conditions early in perioperative patients.

Anesthesia/Surgery

Anesthesia, surgery, and renal function may interact by several mechanisms. Renal disease may cause changes in fluid homeostasis, electrolyte levels, or acid-base status. These changes along with renal disease may affect the pharmacokinetics of drugs used in anesthesia. Ketamine is eliminated almost unchanged by the kidneys in the cat; thus renal disease in cats may result in prolonged duration of effect of ketamine in that species. Azotemia causes an increased sensitivity to thiobarbiturates; a decreased dose is advised for animals with renal disease.[50]

Anesthetic agents may affect renal function either by direct toxic effects or by changes produced in physiologic function. Anesthetic agents depress renal arterial pressure and the resultant hypotension causes release of renin by the juxtaglomerular apparatus. Renin, in turn, activates the angiotensin cascade, which stimulates the adrenal gland to increase aldosterone production. Aldosterone causes increased reabsorption of sodium, thereby promoting water retention, which helps maintain blood volume. Anesthetic agents such as halothane and isoflurane stimulate the renin-angiotensin system.[51] The stress of anesthesia and surgery also stimulates the renin-angiotensin system via sympathetic pathways. Hypovolemia as a result of intraoperative hemorrhage is also a potent stimulus for renin release. Glomerular afferent arteriolar vasoconstriction caused by the effects of angiotensin II and ADH in response to increased renin release is a proposed mechanism of decreased GFR in acute renal failure. Anesthesia, therefore, may contribute to the development of ARF through this mechanism.

Anesthesia and surgery may adversely affect normal renal function by causing increased release of ADH from the posterior pituitary. ADH causes vasoconstriction in the splanchnic and renal circulation while increasing the tubular reabsorption of water. Restricting the oral intake of water prior to anesthesia and/or administration of halothane or thiopental causes a mild elevation in ADH concentration. ADH secretion is a protective mechanism in most instances, but it may compound ischemia caused by hypovolemic shock.

The only anesthetic agent with direct nephrotoxicity that is commonly used in veterinary practice is the inhalant methoxyflurane.[50] This agent is now essentially obsolete because of lack of availability and because agents exist with safer and more desirable characteristics. The liver metabolizes methoxyflurane to free fluoride and oxalate. The fluoride ion is a potent nephrotoxic agent but by itself uncommonly caused renal disease in dogs.[52,53] A combination of methoxyflurane anesthesia, preexisting renal disease, and/or concurrent use of another nephrotoxic drug such as an NSAID makes methoxyflurane potentially dangerous.[54] Sevoflurane metabolism also produces fluoride ion; however, it has been determined that the potential for nephrotoxicity in dogs is low.[55] Sevoflurane also decomposes to the nephrotoxic agent Compound A in the carbon dioxide absorbent of a circle system. Low oxygen flow rates may raise the concentration of Compound A; thus it is recommended to avoid oxygen flow rates of less than 20 ml/kg/minute with this agent, especially in animals with renal disease.[50]

Chronic Renal Failure

Chronic renal disease/dysfunction (CKD) is the most common kidney disease in dogs and cats.[13] CKD is characterized by renal damage that has existed for 3 months or more or by a decrease in GFR of more than 50% from normal persisting for 3 months.[13] Many disease processes including neoplastic, infectious, and immune-related have been identified as causes of chronic renal failure in dogs and cats. When considering dogs with primary renal azotemia, tubulointerstitial nephritis, glomerulonephropathy, and amyloidosis are the most common lesions. The clinical magnitude of renal disease in animals with CKD varies considerably as the disease may or may not affect renal function. In early chronic renal disease, the animal is not azotemic and may have few clinical or laboratory abnormalities associated with disease. As the condition progresses, animals with chronic renal failure may have anemia, systemic hypertension and electrolyte and mineral imbalances. Hyperphosphatemia, hypercalcemia, or hypocalcemia are also seen in animals, depending on the stage of renal failure. Azotemia causes metabolic acidosis and may progress to uremia and anorexia and vomiting.

Identification of patients with chronic renal disease is important during the preoperative workup. The animal may be presented for a surgical problem unrelated to the urinary tract; however, the outcome of treatment for the primary surgical problem may depend on accurate assessment and awareness of problems related to renal disease.

Effects of Renal Failure on Surgical Patients

Wound Healing

Uremia has a detrimental effect on wound healing. Experimentally, azotemic and uremic rats show delayed gain of tensile strength in healing wounds.[56] The decreased wound strength may be a result of synthesis of poor quality collagen or increased collagen degradation.[57,58] Depressed formation of granulation tissue and division of epithelial cells have also been reported in uremic mice.[59]

The effects of uremia on wound healing may be theoretically clinical as wounds in azotemic and uremic patients proceed to heal normally, although more slowly. Selection of appropriate suture materials in view of potential slower wound healing is advised.

Hemostasis

Platelet function may be abnormal in animals with renal failure.[3,13] It is thought that uremia and one or more uremic toxins cause impairment of platelet adhesiveness and aggregation.[13,61] Diminished thromboxane–A2 production, abnormal intracellular calcium mobilization, and increased intracellular cAMP have been described in uremic platelets.[61] Coagulation factors are normal, so the most practical test of hemostasis in the uremic patient is a buccal mucosal bleeding time.

Administration of desmopressin acetate (DDAVP) has been reported to shorten bleeding times in uremic humans. Hemorrhagic diathesis of chronic renal failure is likely clinically insignificant in animals unless other coagulation disorders are present.[3]

Anemia

Patients with chronic renal failure frequently have mild to severe nonregenerative anemia. The anemia is characterized by normochromic, normocytic red blood cells. Although the anemia of chronic renal failure is often multifactorial, the most important cause of the anemia is a relative erythropoietin deficiency.[63] The lack of sufficient erythropoietin results in hypoplasia of erythroid precursors in the bone marrow; leukocyte and platelet production are not affected.

Other factors suggested to contribute to anemia in animals with renal failure are shortened red blood cell survival, platelet dysfunction, nutritional abnormalities, and gastrointestinal hemorrhage from mucosal ulceration.[13,62] Serum iron concentrations are also frequently below normal.

Cardiopulmonary Function

Pulmonary function can be impaired in animals with renal failure, thus potentially compromising their ability to tolerate anesthesia and surgery. Interstitial pneumonitis has been reported in a group of 10 dogs with chronic renal failure.[63] Of these dogs, 4 had respiratory signs and 3 had alveolar infiltrates within the lungs. Pulmonary arterial thromboembolism leading to dyspnea has occurred in canine patients with the nephrotic syndrome associated with glomerular disease.[66] This appears to be caused by a hypercoagulable state associated with excessive urinary loss of antithrombin III or with abnormal platelet function associated with hypoalbuminemia.[64,65] The clinical significance of pulmonary disease secondary to uremia for the anesthetized veterinary patient is unknown and seems questionable.

Cardiovascular abnormalities may occur as co-morbidities in animals with renal failure. Clinically, the most important potential abnormality is systemic hypertension. Systemic hypertension may be a cause or a consequence of chronic kidney disease.[13] The incidence of hypertension in dogs with chronic disease is reported to be from 30% to 90%.[66,67] Apparently, the condition is much more common in the cat, occurring in up to 66% of animals affected with renal disease.[68] The presence of a high initial systolic blood pressure (164 to 217 mm Hg) in dogs with renal disease increases the risk of having a uremic crisis and also seems to be a predictor of a faster decline in renal function in affected animals.[66] Hypertension also impairs the ability of the kidney to autoregulate renal perfusion, thus potentially complicating an anesthetic episode.[69] Pericardial effusion has been described in two clinically affected dogs secondary to renal disease.[70,71] In a further review of necropsy records from another 150 dogs with renal disease, 11 dogs had varying amounts of clear or hemorrhagic pericardial fluid.[70] The clinical significance of pericardial effusion as a result of renal failure in dogs is unknown but its occurrence seems uncommon.

Nutrition or Malnutrition

Anorexia and weight loss are nonspecific but common clinical signs associated with advanced kidney disease. Nausea and vomiting leading to malnutrition are also common, especially as uremia becomes advanced. Uremic gastropathy and gastrointestinal mucosal ulceration associated with gastric hyperacidity and histamine release from mast cells within mucosa contribute to nausea and vomiting. Oral lesions such as ulcers or stomatitis may be associated with anorexia especially in cats.

The importance of proper nutrition for prevention or treatment of disease in animals is well recognized. Protein-energy malnutrition can further intensify the catabolic state associated with general anesthesia and surgery. Deleterious effects of protein-energy malnutrition that are of particular importance to the surgical patient include impaired immune function, increased susceptibility to infection, and delayed wound healing.[72] Inadequate energy intake leads to use of body protein for energy, which worsens azotemia (and perhaps uremia) in animals with renal failure and reduces the protein available for renal repair in ARF.[73] Animals that have remained anorectic for more than 3 days or that have lost more than 10% of their body weight should receive nutritional supportive therapy.[73]

References

1. Brown SA: Physiology of the urinary tract. *In* Textbook of Small Animal Surgery, 3rd ed. Slatter DH (ed). Philadelphia: Saunders, 2003.
2. Grauer GF: Prevention of acute renal failure. *In* Textbook of Small Animal Surgery, 3rd ed. Slatter DH (ed). Philadelphia: Saunders, 2003.
3. Brown SA: Pathophysiology and therapeutics of urinary tract diseases. *In* Textbook of Small Animal Surgery, 3rd ed. Slatter DH (ed). Philadelphia: Saunders, 2003.
4. Cowgill LD, Francey T: Acute uremia. *In* Textbook of Veterinary Internal Medicine. 6th ed. Ettinger SJ, Feldman EC (eds). St Louis: Elsevier Saunders, 2005.
5. Dibartola SP: Renal disease: Clinical approach and laboratory evaluation. *In* Textbook of Veterinary Internal Medicine. 6th ed. Ettinger SJ, Feldman EC (eds). St Louis: Elsevier Saunders, 2005.
6. Behrend EN, et al: Hospital-acquired acute renal failure in dogs: 29 cases (1983-1992). J Am Vet Med Assoc 208:537, 1996.
7. Chew DJ, DiBartola SP: Diagnosis and pathophysiology of renal disease. *In* Textbook of Veterinary Internal Medicine. 3rd edition. Ettinger SJ (ed). Philadelphia: WB Saunders, 1989.
8. Grauer GF, Lane I: Acute renal failure: Ischemic and clinical nephrosis. *In* Canine and Feline Nephrology and Urology. Osborne CA, Finco DR (eds). Baltimore, Williams & Wilkins, 1995.
9. Vaden SL, et al: Retrospective case-control of acute renal failure in 99 dogs. J Vet Intern Med 11:58, 1997
10. Burnier M, Schirer RW: Pathogenesis of acute renal failure. *In* Acute Renal Failure Clinical and Experimental., Amerio A, et al (eds). New York, Plenum Press, 1987.
11. Lund E, et al: Health status and population characteristics of dogs and cats examined at private veterinary practices in the United States. J Am Vet Med Assoc 214: 1336-1341, 1999.
12. Watson A: Indicators of renal insufficiency in dogs and cats presented at a veterinary teaching hospital. Aust Vet Practi 31:54-58, 2001.
13. Polzin DJ, Osborne CA, Ross S: Chronic kidney disease. *In* Textbook of Veterinary Internal Medicine, 6th ed. Ettinger SJ, Feldman EC (eds). St Louis: Elsevier Saunders, 2005.
14. Hou SH, et al: Hospital acquired renal insufficiency: a prospective study. Am J Med 74: 243, 1983.
15. Brezis M, et al: Acute renal failure. *In* The Kidney, 3rd ed. Edited by Brennerard BM, Rector FC Jr (eds). Philadelphia: WB Saunders, 1986.
16. Phillips RA, et al: Effects of acute hemorrhagic and traumatic shock on renal function of dogs. Am J Physiol 145: 314, 1946.
17. Stone EA, et al: Renal function after prolonged hypotensive anesthesia and surgery in dogs with reduced renal mass. Am J Vet Res 42: 1675, 1981.
18. Hall JA, Macy DW: Acute canine pancreatitis. Comp Cont Educ Pract Vet 10:4 403-417, 1988.
19. Pitchumoni CS, Agarwal N, Jain NK: Systemic complications of acute pancreatitis. Am J Gastroenterol 83 (6):597-606, 1988.
20. Mandel AK, et al: Myoglobinuria exacerbates ischemic renal damage in the dog. Nephron 53:261, 1989.
21. Hardi EM, Rawlings CA: Septic shcok. Part I. Pathophysiology. Comp Cont Educ Pract Vet 5:369, 1983.

22. Hardy RM, Osborne CA: Canine pyometra: pathophysiology, diagnosis, and treatment of uterine and extrauterinelesions. J Am Anim Hosp Assoc 10:245, 1974.

23. Stone EA, et al: Renal dysfunction in dogs with pyometra. J Am Vet Med Assoc 193:457, 1988.

24. Stone EA: Ovary and uterus. *In* Textbook of Small Animal Surgery, 3rd ed. Slatter DH (ed). Philadelphia: WB Saunders, 2003.

25. Leary SL, et al: Recurrent malignant hyperthermia in a greyhound. J Am Vet Med Assoc 182: 521, 1983

26. Gannon JR: Exertional rhabdomyolysis (myoglobinuria) in the racing greyhound. *In* Current Veterinary Therapy VII. Small Animal Practice. Kirk RW (ed). Philadelphia: WB Saunders, 1980.

27. Howard EW, McCrindle MW. Acute renal failure in a dog following exertional rhabdomyolysis. J South Afr Vet Assoc 52:115, 1982.

28. Spangler WL, Maglie FM: Seizure induced rhabdomyolysis accompanied by acute renal failure in a dog. J Am Vet Med Assoc 172:1190, 1978

29. Shell LG: Diseases of periperal nerve, neuromuscular junction, and muscles. *In* Practical Small Animal Internal Medicine. Leib MS, Monroe WE (eds). Philadelphia: WB Saunders, 1997.

30. Norman TE, Chaffin MK, Johnson MC, et al: Intravascular hemolysis associated with severe cutaneous burn injuries in five horses. J Am Vet Med Assoc 226:2039, 2005.

31. Bergman PJ: Paraneoplastic syndromes. *In* Small Animal Clinical Oncology, 3rd ed. Withrow SJ, MacEwen EG (eds). Philadelphia: WB Saunders, 2001.

32. Gear RNA, et al: Primary hyperparathyroidism in 29 dogs: diagnosis, treatment, outcome and associated renal failure. J Sm Anim Pract 46 (1):10-16, 2005

33. Chew DJ, Capen CC: Hypercalcemic nephropathy and associated disorders. *In* Current VeterinaryTherapy VII, Small Animal Practice. Kirk RW (ed). Philadelphia: WB Saunders, 1980.

34. Lin LE: Renal function in hypercalcemic dogs during hydropenia and during saline infusion. Acta Physiol Scan 106:177, 1979.

35. Margulies KB, et al: Induction and prevention of radiocontrast-induced nephropathy in dogs with heart failure. Kidney Int 38:1101, 1990.

36. Lascelles DB, et al: Guidelines for safe and effective use of non-steroidal anti-inflammatory drugs in dogs. Pfizer Animal Health Technical Bulletin, November, 2004.

37. Huerta C, et al: Nonsteroidal anti-inflammatory drugs and risk of ARF in the general population. Am J of Kid Dis 45(3):531-539, 2005.

38. Stokes JE, et al: New and unusual causes of acute renal failure in dogs and cats. Vet Clin North Am 34(4): 909-922, 2004.

39. Englehart JA, et al: Drug-related nephropathies. Part II. Commonly used drugs. Comp Cont Educ Pract Vet 9:281-289, 1987.

40. Rivers BJ, et al: Evaluation of urine gamma-glutamyl transpeptidase-to-creatinine ratio as a diagnostic tool in an experimental model of aminoglycoside-induced acute renal failure in the dog. J Am Anim Hosp Assoc 32:323-336, 1996.

41. Adelaman RD: Furosemide enhancement of experimental gentamicin toxicity: comparison of functional and morphological changes with activities of urinary enzymes. J Infect Dis 140:342, 1979

42. Brown SA, et al: Gentamicin associated renal failure in the dog. J Am Vet Med Assoc 186: 686, 1985.

43. Greco DS, et al: Urinary gamma-glutamyl transpeptidase activity in dogs with gentamicin-induced nephrotoxicity. Am J Vet Res 46:2332-2335, 1985.

44. Pasco PJ, Ilkiw JE, Cowgill LD: Concerned about renal failure after anesthesia/surgery (letters). J Am Vet Med Assoc 204:1734, 1994.

45. Campese VM, Iseki K: Contrast induced acute renal failure. *In* Acute Renal Failure Clinical and Experimental. Amerio A, et al(eds). New York: Plenum, 1987.

46. Ihle SK, Kostolich M: Acute renal failure associated with contrast medium administration in a dog. J Am Vet Med Assoc 199:899, 1991.

47. Daley C, Finn-Bodner ST, Lenz SD: Contrast-induced renal failure documented by color-Doppler imaging in a dog. J Am Anim Hosp Assoc 30:33, 1994.

48. DuFort RM, Matros L: Acquired coagulopathies. *In* Texbook of Veterinary Internal Medicine, 6th ed. Ettinger SJ, Feldman EC (eds). St. Louis: Elsevier Saunders, 2005.

49. Slappendel RJ: Disseminated intravascular coagulation. *In* Current Veterinary Therapy X, Small Animal Practice. Kirk RW. Philadelphia: WB Saunders, 1989.

50. Mason DE: Urinary system. *In* Textbook of Small Animal Surgery, 3rd ed,. Slatter DH (ed). Philadelphia: Saunders, 2003.

51. Trim CM: Anesthesia and the urinary system. *In* Textbook of Small Animal Surgery. Slatter DH (ed). Philadelphia: WB Saunders, 1985.

52. Sawyer D: The anesthetic period. *In* The Practice of Small Animal Anesthesia. Piermattei D (ed). Philadelphia: WB Saunders, 1982.

53. Muir WW, Hubbell JA: Handbook of Veterinary Anesthesia. St. Louis: CV Mosby, 1989.

54. Matthews K, et al: Nephrotoxicity in dogs associated with methoxyflurane anesthesia and flunixin meglumine analgesia. Can Vet J 31:766, 1990.

55. Branson KR, Quandt JE, Martinez EA, et al: A multisite case report on the clinical use of sevoflurane in dogs. J Am Anim Hosp Assoc 37:420-432, 2001.

56. Peacock EE: Wound Repair, 3rd ed. Philadelphia: WB Saunders, 1984.

57. Hosgood G: Wound healing. *In* Textbook of Small Animal Surgery, 3rd ed. Slatter DH (ed). Philadelphia, Saunders, 2003.

58. Colin JF, Ellis H: The effect of uremia upon wound healing: an experimental study. Br J Surg 66:793, 1979.

59. Colin JF, Ellis H: The effect of uremia upon wound healing; histology and autoradiography in the mouse. Ann Surg 168:142, 1968.

60. Anagnostu A, Kurtzman NA: Hematological consequences of renal failure. *In* The Kidney, 3rd ed. Brenner BM, Rector FC (eds). Philadelphia: WB Saunders, 1986.

61. Himmelfarb J: Hematolological manifestations of acute renal failure. *In* Primer on Kidney Diseases. San Diego: Academic Press, 1998.

62. Cowgill L: Pathophysiology and management of anemia in chronic progressive renal failure. Semin Vet Med Surg (Small Anim) 7(3):175-182, 1992.

63. Moon ML, Grenlee PG, and Burk RL: Uremic pneumonitis-like syndrome in ten dogs. J Am Anim Hosp Assoc 22:687, 1986.

64. Green RA, Kabel AL: Hypercoagulable state in three dogs with nephrotic syndrome: role of acquired antithrombin III deficiency. J Am Vet Med Assoc 181: 914, 1982.

65. Green RA, et al.: Hypolabuminemia-related platelet hypersensitivity in two dogs with nephritic syndrome. J Am Vet Med Assoc 186: 485, 1985.

66. Jacob F, Polzin DJ, OsborneCA, et al: Association between initial systolic blood pressure and risk of developing a uremic crisis or dying in dogs with chronic renal failure. J Am Vet Med Assoc 222:322-329, 2003.

67. Michell A, et al: Absence of hypertension in dogs with renal insufficiency. Ren Fail 19: 61-68, 1997.

68. Syme H, et al: Prevalence of systolic hypertension in cats with chronic renal failure. J Am Vet Med Assoc 220:1799-1804, 2002.

69. Finco DR: Association of systemic hypertension with renal injury in dogs with induced renal failure. J Vet Intern Med 18:289-294, 2004.

70. Madewell BR, Nordin RW: Renal failure associated with pericardial effusion in a dog. J Am Vet Med Assoc 167:1091, 1975.

71. Berg RJ, Winfield W: Pericardial effusion in the dog: a review of 42 cases. J Am Anim Hosp Assoc 20:721, 1984.

72. Crowe DT: Enteral nutrition for critically ill or injured patients. Part I. Comp Cont Educ Pract Vet 8: 603, 1986.

73. Lewis LD, Morris ML, Hand MS: Small Animal Clinical Nutrition, 3rd ed. Topeka: Mark Morris Assoicates, 1987.

Chapter 65

Bacterial Urinary Tract Infections

Carl A. Osborne
Jody P. Lulich

In context of surgery, conceptual understanding of alterations in interactions between host defenses and pathogenic microbes that result in bacterial urinary tract infections (UTI) are important for at least two reasons. First, many surgical procedures designed to correct noninfectious disorders of the urinary tract may partially or totally interfere with local host defenses that normally prevent or impair development of UTI. Second, surgical correction of abnormalities that affect host defense mechanisms may be a prerequisite to preventing recurrent or persistent bacterial UTI.

Why is it Important to Recognize that Bacterial Urinary Tract Infection is not a Primary Diagnostic Entity?

Although the urinary tract communicates with an external environment loaded with bacteria and other potentially pathogenic agents, most of it is normally sterile and all of it is normally resistant to infection. As with all systems of the body, resistance to urinary tract infection is dependent on the interaction of several host defense mechanisms.[1] The pathogenesis of UTIs is related to the relationship between the virulence of uropathogenic infectious agents (analogous to seeds) and the functional status of host defense mechanisms (analogous to soil; Table 65-1). Growth of bacteria (seeds) usually will not occur unless abnormalities of host defenses (suitable soil) are present. Therefore, in context of diagnosis, prognosis, and therapy, a bacterial urinary tract infection (UTI) may be viewed as a secondary (or complicating) rather than a primary (or definitive) diagnostic entity.

CAVEAT--In addition to focusing on antimicrobial treatment of bacterial pathogens (which are usually secondary causes of urinary tract disease), it is also important to consider detection and treatment of abnormalities in host defenses that allow bacteria to colonize and invade tissues of the urinary tract (Tables 65-1 and 65-2). If UTIs are managed inappropriately, one or more sequelae may occur (Table 65-3). Early detection followed by proper treatment and follow-up evaluation will minimize the occurrence and severity of these sequelae.

What Diagnostic Classification will Facilitate Treatment of Bacterial Utis?

Bacterial UTI encompass a wide variety of clinical entities whose common denominator is microbial invasion of any of its components. Urinary tract infections may be classified on the basis of 1) anatomic location (i.e., kidney, ureter, bladder, and/or urethra), 2) etiology (*Escherichia coli, Staphylococcus intermedius,* etc.), 3) complexity (uncomplicated or complicated), and/or 4) response to therapy (persistent, relapse, reinfection, or superinfection).[1-3]

Anatomic localization of infections within the urinary tract should be considered because it may influence the prognosis; type, dosage, and dose interval of antimicrobial agent selected; and duration of therapy. Classification of UTIs based on complexity is also of prognostic and therapeutic significance because it allows differentiation of uncomplicated (or simple) urinary tract infections from complicated urinary tract infections (Tables 65-1 and 65-2).

Table 65-1. Natural and Acquired Urinary Tract Defenses against Bacterial Infection

I. Normal Micturition
- A. Adequate urine volume
- B. Frequent voiding
- C. Complete voiding

II. Anatomic Structures
- A. Urethral high pressure zones
- B. Surface characteristics of urethral urothelium
- C. Urethral peristalsis
- D. Prostatic secretions (antibacterial fraction and immunoglobulins)
- E. Normal length of urethra
- F. Ureterovesical flap valves
- G. Ureteral peristalsis
- H. Glomerular mesangial cells?
- I. Extensive renal blood supply and flow

III. Mucosal Defense Barriers
- A. Local antibody production
- B. Surface layer (hydrophilic glycosaminoglycans)
- C. Intrinsic mucosal cell antimicrobial properties
- D. Exfoliation of cells
- E. Commensal microbes (normal flora) of distal urethra and distal genital tract that interfere with infection by uropathogens

IV. Antimicrobial Properties of Urine
- A. Extremes (high or low) of urine pH
- B. Hyperosmolality (highly concentrated urine)
- C. High concentration of urea
- D. Organic acids
- E. Small molecular weight carbohydrates
- F. Tamm-Horsfall mucoprotein
- G. Leukocyte esterase-like substances (cats)?

V. Systemic Immunocompetence
- A. Cell-mediated immunity
- B. Humoral-mediated immunity

Table 65-2. Some Predisposing Causes of Complicated UTI

I. Interference with Normal Micturition
- A. Mechanical obstruction to outflow
  - 1. Uroliths, neoplasms and strictures (especially of urethra)
  - 2. Herniated urinary bladder
  - 3. Prostatic cysts, abscesses, or neoplasms
- B. Incomplete emptying of excretory pathway
  - 1. Damaged innervation
    - a. Vertebral fractures, luxations, subluxations, anomalies
    - b. Neoplasia
    - c. Reflex dyssynergia
  - 2. Anatomic defects
    - a. Diverticula of urethra, bladder, ureters, and renal pelves.
    - b. Vesicoureteral reflux

II. Anatomic Defects
- A. Congenital or inherited
  - 1. Urethral anomalies
  - 2. Ectopic ureters
  - 3. Persistent urachal diverticula
  - 4. Vulvar abnormalities predisposing to perivulvar dermatitis
- B. Acquired
  - 1. Diseases of the urinary tract, especially lower portions
  - 2. Urethrostomy and other surgical diversion procedures

III. Alteration of Urothelium
- A. Trauma
  - 1. Catheterization and other instrumentation
  - 2. Urolithiasis
- B. Metaplasia
  - 1. Administration of estrogens
  - 2. Estrogen-producing sertoli cell neoplasms
- C. Neoplasia
- D. Urinary excretion of cytotoxic drugs such as cyclophosphamide
- E. Alteration of normal flora of distal urethra, prepuce, and vagina

IV. Alterations in the Volume, Frequency, or Composition of Urine
- A. Decreased urine volume
  - 1. Negative water balance
  - 2. Primary oliguric renal failure
- B. Voluntary or involuntary retention
- C. Glucosuria
- D. Formation of dilute urine

V. Impaired Immunocompetence
- A. Diseases
  - 1. Congenital immunodeficiency?
  - 2. Acquired
    - a. Hyperadrenocorticism?
    - b. Uremia
- B. Corticosteroids; immunosuppressant drugs

Uncomplicated UTI

An uncomplicated UTI is defined as an infection in which an underlying structural, neurologic, immunologic, or functional abnormality cannot be identified. Although useful, this classification may be misleading in that it implies that bacterial infection is the primary rather than a secondary abnormality. However, most bacteria survive and multiply only when host defenses are compromised. Many simple UTIs encompass transient and potentially reversible defects in the patient's innate defense mechanisms, even though the underlying cause may escape detection. Others occur when normal host defenses are overwhelmed by virulent uropathogens. For example, nosocomial UTI could occur as a result of improper transurethral catheterization in a hospital intensive care unit harboring resistant uropathogens. Uncomplicated UTIs might also be caused by replacement of the normal microbial flora (so-called good bacteria) of the distal urethra and genital tract with uropathogenic microbes that have emerged as a consequence of prior treatment of the patient with antibiotics. Uncomplicated UTIs are usually associated with a better prognosis for recovery.

Complicated UTI

Complicated UTIs occur as a result of bacterial invasion of the urinary system secondary to an identifiable disease that interferes with one or more defense mechanisms (Table 65-2).[1,2,4] A relationship exists between the severity of host defense abnormality and the frequency and severity of UTI. In general, the abnormality in host defenses must be corrected or removed if secondary bacterial infection is to be completely eradicated and prevented from recurring. Failure or inability to do so is a common cause of persistent or recurrent UTI (relapse or reinfection).

CAVEAT--Differentiation of uncomplicated from complicated UTIs and anatomic localization of UTI require appropriate diagnostic evaluation, which may include transrectal palpation of the genitourinary tract, ultrasonography, survey and contrast radiography, cystoscopy, and aspiration, punch, or surgical biopsy.

Why is it Important to Differentiate UTIs According to whether they are Persistent, Relapses, Reinfections, or Superinfections?

Relapses

Recurrent bacterial UTIs that occur following withdrawal of therapy may be classified as relapses or reinfections (Table 65-4). Relapses (i.e., relapse of a persistent pathogen) are defined as recurrences of clinical signs caused by the same species (and serologic strain) of microbe. In this situation, remission of clinical signs and eradication of bacteria from the urine are not associated with eradication of pathogenic bacteria from tissues of the urinary tract. Although viable bacteria remain sequestered in sites inaccessible to bacteriocidal concentrations of antimicrobics, results of the culture of urine samples obtained by cystocentesis during antimicrobic therapy are likely to be negative if the drug is eliminated in high concentration in urine. Relapses of clinical signs usually occur within several days to a few weeks after interruption of antimicrobic therapy. The bacteria may become more resistant to antimicrobial agents than prior to therapy. The pathogenesis of relapsing UTI likely involves failure to completely eliminate pathogenic bacteria before antimicrobic therapy is withdrawn. Relapses represent antimicrobial treatment failures associated with one or more causes, and affect both male and female dogs throughout their lifespan (Table 65-5). Relapses have the potential to cause significant morbidity if mismanaged (Table 65-3).

Table 65-3. Potential Sequela to Untreated or Improperly Treated Bacterial Urinary Tract Infections

1. Lower urinary tract dysfunction (acute or chronic)
   a. Dysuria, pollakiuria
   b. "Urge" incontinence
   c. Damage to the detrusor muscle
   d. Damage to the urethra
2. Prostatitis (acute or chronic)
3. Struvite urolithiasis and its sequelae
4. Infertility
5. Renal dysfunction (acute or chronic)
   a. Pyelonephritis
   b. Renal failure
   c. Septicemia (especially in patients with concomitant obstruction to urine outflow)
6. Anemia of chronic inflammation
7. Lumbosacral discospondylitis

Reinfections

Reinfections are defined as recurrent UTI caused by one or more different pathogens (Table 65-4). In this situation, bacteria have been eradicated from urine and surrounding tissue, but persistent dysfunction of one or more host defense mechanisms predisposes to reinfection with different uropathogens (Tables 65-2 and 65-6). If superficial damage to tissues of the urinary tract induced by bacteria by the initial infection have time to heal, recurrence of clinical manifestations of reinfections often occur at a longer interval following cessation of therapy than relapses. Reinfections appear to be more common in female dogs and young to middle-aged cats with lower urinary tract disease.

Superinfections

Superinfections are defined as infections with one or more additional pathogens during the course of antimicrobial therapy.[1] They are most likely to occur in association with in-dwelling transurethral catheters; as a sequela to urinary diversion techniques (i.e., antepubic urethrostomy, tube cystostomy, percutaneous nephropyelostomy); and because of anatomic abnormalities that promote ascending migration of bacteria into the urinary tract.

CAVEAT--The therapeutic plan for relapses often differs from the therapeutic plan for reinfections. Therefore, it is important to compare results of bacterial culture of urine obtained prior to initiation of therapy to bacterial cultures of urine obtained during and/or after withdrawal of therapy.

Why is Diagnostic Urine Culture the Gold Standard of Diagnosis of Bacterial UTI?

Because UTI encompasses a spectrum of underlying abnormalities in host defense mechanisms in addition to bacterial pathogens, diagnostic and therapeutic requirements vary from case to case. No pathognomonic history, physical examination, radiographic, or ultrasonographic findings are associated with bacterial UTI.

In addition to bacterial infection, many diverse noninfectious disease processes, including neoplasia and urolithiasis, result in inflammatory lesions of the urinary tract characterized by exudation of RBC, WBC, and protein into urine. The resultant hematuria, pyuria, and proteinuria suggest inflammatory urinary tract disease, but do not indicate its cause or location within the urinary tract. Diagnosis of bacterial UTI solely on the basis of urinalysis and detection of inflammatory cells in urine sediment will result in over-diagnosis. Therefore, it is essential to distinguish between inflammation and infection related to urinary tract disease. Although detection of bacteria in fresh urine sediment should prompt consideration of UTI, it should be verified by urine culture. Non-bacterial "look-alikes" in urine sediment are often confused with bacteria.[4]

Quantitative urine culture is considered to be the gold standard for diagnosis of bacterial UTI.[18] In addition to facilitating differ-

Table 65-4. Examples of Patterns of Bacteriuria Detected by Sequential Urine Cultures Performed to Monitor Response to Antimicrobial Treatment of UTI

Time and Status of Culture of Urine for Bacteria					
Prior to Treatment	**3 to 5 Days After Initiating Treatment**	**3 to 5 Days Before Finishing Treatment**	**7 to 14 Days After Treatment Discontinued**	**More Than 2 Weeks After Treatment Discontinued**	**Interpretations**
Positive	Positive	Does not apply	Does not apply	Does not apply	Persistent UTI; Treatment failure
Positive	Negative	Negative	Positive for same microbe	Does not apply	Relapse (Table 65-5)
Positive	Negative	Negative	Negative	Negative	Cure
Positive	Negative	Negative	Negative	Positive for different microbe	Reinfection (Table 65-6)

Table 65-5. Checklist of Potential Causes of Recurrent UTIs Owing to Relapses

Use of Ineffective Drugs

1. Mixed infections with more than one type of pathogen in which all pathogens were not eradicated by antimicrobial therapy
2. Bacteria are resistant to drug selected
3. Antimicrobic does not attain therapeutic concentration in urine
4. Antimicrobic does not achieve therapeutic concentrations at infection sites (especially kidneys, prostate gland, and infection-induced uroliths)
5. Patient does not absorb a portion or all of an orally administered drug because of ingesta, gastrointestinal dysfunction, or interaction with other drugs
6. Initiation of therapy at an advanced state in the course of the disease
7. Acquired drug-resistant bacteria, including L-forms
8. Host factors detrimental to drug efficacy

Ineffective Use of Drugs

1. Use of improper antimicrobial susceptibility tests and/or misinterpretation of results
2. Prescription of antimicrobics for an insufficient period to eradicate uropathogens
3. Failure to prescribe a proper dosage and/or maintenance interval for an antimicrobic that would otherwise be effective
4. Lack of compliance characterized by failure or inability of owners to give the prescribed dosage of antimicrobic at the proper maintenance intervals and for sufficient a duration
5. Inappropriate use of combination of drugs that interfere with their ability to eradicate uropathogens
6. Premature assessment of therapeutic response

entiation of bacterial contaminants from bacterial pathogens, accurate identification of specific bacterial species aids in selection of antimicrobial drugs. Also recall that recurrent UTIs owing to relapses cannot be distinguished from recurrent UTIs owing to reinfections without comparison of pretreatment bacterial culture results to follow-up culture results.

CAVEAT--Failure to perform bacterial urine cultures or failure to correctly interpret the results of urine cultures may lead not only to diagnostic errors but therapeutic failures as well. Although detection of bacteria in properly collected urine samples is highly indicative of bacterial UTI, further information is required to confirm and localize the site(s) of infection.

Table 65-6. Checklist of Potential causes of Recurrent UTIs owing to Reinfections

1. Invalid culture results caused by:
   a. Contamination of specimen during collection, transport, storage, or handling
   b. Improper technique of bacterial culture of urine
2. Continued dysfunction of host defense mechanisms (Tables 65-1 and 65-2)
3. Failure or inability to recognize and eliminate predisposing causes
4. Iatrogenic infection, especially associated with transurethral catheterization
5. Sequelae to surgical techniques that have impaired host defense function, especially urethrostomies and urine diversion procedures
6. Spontaneous reinfection

How should Urine Samples be Collected for Diagnostic Culture?

We prefer to collect urine samples for bacterial culture by cystocentesis to eliminate problems of differentiating contaminants from pathogens.[3] Detection of bacteria, even in low numbers, in urine aseptically collected by cystocentesis is indicative of UTI. However, false positive results may occur if the needle penetrates a loop of intestine during cystocentesis, or if the sample is contaminated during transfer to culture media. For this reason, quantitative urine culture is routinely recommended, even for samples collected by cystocentesis. Urine culture results should be interpreted in context of other clinical findings (Table 65-7).[5]

CAVEAT--Catheter-induced UTIs (nosocomial infections) are common in patients with urinary tract diseases, and could even result in iatrogenic pyelonephritis, renal failure, and septicemia. Therefore, transurethral catheterization of patients at increased risk for UTI should be evaluated in context of risks and benefits.

Table 65-7. Checklist of Factors Influencing Interpretation of Qualitative Bacterial Cultures of Urine

- Method of urine collection?
- Time lapse between urine collection and bacterial culture?
- Method of preservation if urine is not cultured within 30 minutes?
- Pure or mixed culture of bacteria?

1 isolate	in about 75% of UTI
2 isolates	in only 20% of UTI
3 isolates	in only 5% of UTI

- Magnitude of inflammatory response (if any) detected by urinalysis?
- Light microscopic detection of bacteria in uncontaminated fresh unspun urine?

How should Urine Samples be Preserved Prior to Culture?

If diagnostic bacterial cultures are to be performed, urine should be collected for culture before antibacterial therapy is initiated. If the patient is currently being treated with an antimicrobic, it should be discontinued for approximately 3 to 5 days prior to diagnostic urine culture in order to minimize inhibition of in vivo and in vitro bacterial growth.

Because urine may be a good culture medium at room temperature (bacterial counts may double every 20 to 45 minutes), it should be cultured within 15 to 30 minutes from the time of collection.[6] Another indication for culture of fresh urine samples is that destruction of some fastidious bacteria may be detectable within an hour of collection. If for any reason culture of freshly collected urine samples is not possible, the samples should be kept in a sealed sterile container and immediately refrigerated following collection. Refrigerated samples may be stored for 6 to 12 hours without significant additional growth of bacteria.[6] However, it is emphasized that fastidious organisms may be killed in the urine environment if refrigeration storage time is prolonged.

Alternatively, commercially manufactured collection tubes combined with refrigeration may be used to preserve samples for up to 72 hours. Commercially manufactured urine culture and susceptibility test kits are also available (IndicatoRx, Idexx Laboratories, Westbrook , Maine).

CAVEAT--Transport of urine specimens to a commercial microbiology laboratory results in increased time between urine collection and aerobic culture and, therefore, adds a potential source of error, especially if the samples are not properly preserved. Freezing urine samples may also destroy bacteria.

Why are Quantitative Bacterial Urine Cultures a Standard of Practice in the Management of Utis?

The gold standard for diagnosis of UTI is isolation of bacteria in a properly collected urine sample. However, the presence of bacteria in urine per se is not synonymous with UTI because urine may be contaminated with bacteria as it flows through the urethra, and after it is removed from the patient, but before it is cultured. Quantitative urine culture includes determination of the number of bacteria (colony-forming units) per milliliter of urine in addition to isolation and identification of bacteria. Because it facilitates differentiation of bacteria that have contaminated the urine sample from bacteria that are likely to be causing UTI, quantitative culture is the preferred method of diagnostic culture for urine samples obtained by any collection method.

The concept of significant bacteriuria was introduced to aid differentiation between harmless bacterial contaminants of urine and pathogenic bacteria causing infectious disease of the urinary system.[1,2,7] A high bacterial count in a properly collected and cultured urine sample indicates the high probability of UTI (Table 65-8). Small numbers of bacteria obtained from untreated patients usually indicate contamination.

The lower limit of numbers of bacteria isolated from feline urine that indicate infection (so-called cutoff values) has not been precisely determined. However, it is usually less than that in dogs because feline urine appears to be less conducive to bacterial growth than urine of dogs (Table 65-8).[8]

CAVEAT--When interpreting bacterial cultures, several variables should be considered (Table 65-7). In up to 20% of canine patients, bacterial UTI may be present with less than 10,000 colony-forming units per milliliter of urine.[2,3] In this circumstance, samples collected by catheterization or during voiding might erroneously be interpreted as contaminants (Table 65-8). This observation emphasizes the importance of cystocentesis as the preferred method of collection for diagnostic urine culture.

How can Routine Quantitative Aerobic Cultures of Urine be Adapted to a Primary Care Veterinary Practice?

Many veterinarians do not routinely perform urine cultures because of the time and expertise required to specifically identify bacteria. However, all individuals can recognize lack of growth of bacteria on culture plates. Therefore, we recommend that veterinarians quantitatively culture urine on microbiology plates (such as blood agar and MacConkey agar) utilizing calibrated microbiologic loops.[9] If no growth occurs after incubation of the culture plates at 37° for approximately 24 hours, or if only small numbers of bacteria grow (contaminants), further efforts to identify bacterial species is unnecessary, and treatment with an antimicrobial drug is usually not warranted (Table 65-8). If significant numbers of bacteria (colony-forming units) are isolated, the microbiologic plates, or swab cultures from the plates, can then be sent to commercial laboratories for species identification and antimicrobial susceptibility tests. Therapy with an appropriate antimicrobial drug (refer to next section on empirical choices of antimicrobics) may be initiated pending results from the commercial laboratory.

We routinely use calibrated bacteriologic inoculating loops (available from Veterinary Lab Supply, 120 S. 1st Ave., Winterset Iowa 50237) or microliter mechanical pipettes that deliver exactly 0.01 or 0.001 milliliters of urine to culture plates. To facilitate culture, urine is streaked over the surface of agar plates with the inoculating loops by conventional methods. The plates are placed in an incubator upside down at 37°C for 18 to 24 hours, and then examined for bacterial growth. Blood agar will support growth of most aerobic organisms encountered in patients with UTI. MacConkey agar provides information that aids in tentative identification of bacteria and prevents "swarming" of microbes.

This strategy of in-hospital bacterial culture of urine not only fosters appropriate diagnosis and therapy, it is also financially sound. The fee normally paid to the diagnostic laboratory for a sterile urine culture can be rightfully earned by the veterinary

Table 65-8. Interpretation-Quantitative Urine Cultures in Dogs and Cats*

Collection Method	Significant		Suspicious		Contaminant	
	Dog	Cat	Dog	Cat	Dog	Cat
Cystocentesis	≥ 1000†	≥ 1000	100 to 1000	100 to 1000	≤ 100	≤ 100
Catheterization	≥ 10,000	≥ 1000	1000 to 10,000	100 to 1,000	≤ 1000	≤ 100
Voided midstream	≥ 100,000‡	≥ 10,000	10,000 to 90,000	1000 to 10,000	≤ 10,000	≤ 1000

***The data represent generalities. On occasion, bacterial UTI may be detected in dogs and cats with the fewer numbers of organisms (i.e., false negative results).**

† Numbers represent colony-forming units of bacteria per milliliter of urine.

‡Caution: Contamination of midstream samples may result in colony counts of 10,000/ml or higher in some cats, and especially female dogs (i.e., false positive results). Therefore, they should not be used for routine diagnostic culture of urine.

hospital. This strategy also enhances use of urine cultures to monitor the effectiveness of therapy (so-called "test of effectiveness").

CAVEAT--Before culture, urine should not be kept at room temperature or frozen. Also, urine should not be placed in enrichment broth immediately following collection to enhance bacterial growth, as this will invalidate the results of quantitative culture.

References

1. Osborne CA: Bacterial Infections of the Canine and Feline Urinary Tract: Cause, Cure, and Control. *In* Disease Mechanisms In Small Animal Surgery. Bojrab MJ (ed). Philadelphia: Lea & Febiger, 1993, p. 426.

2. Barsanti JA: Genitourinary infections. *In* Infectious Diseases of the Dog and Cat, 3rd ed. Greene CE (ed). St. Louis: Saunders Elsevier, 2006, p. 934.

3. Osborne CA, Lees GE: Bacterial infections of the canine and feline urinary tract. *In* Canine and Feline Nephrology and Urology. Osborne CA, Finco DR (eds). Malvern: Williams & Wilkins, 1995, p. 759.

4. Osborne CA, Stevens JB: Urinalysis: A clinical Guide To Compassionate Care. Shawnee Mission, Kansas: Bayer Corporation, 1999.

5. Ling, GV, Norris CR, Franti CE, et al: Interrelations of organism prevalence, specimen collection method, and host age, sex, and breed among 8,354 canine urinary tract infections (1969-1995). J Vet Internal Med 15: 341, 2001.

6. Padilla, J, Osborne CA, Ward GE: Effects of storage time and temperature on quantitative culture of canine urine. JAVMA 178:1077-1081, 1981.

7. Osborne CA, Lees GE: Diagnostic urine culture. *In* Canine and Feline Nephrology and Urology. Osborne CA, Finco DR (eds). Malvern: Williams & Wilkins, 1995, p. 206.

8. Lees GE, Osborne CA: Antibacterial properties of urine. A comparative review. J Am Anim Hosp Assoc 15:125, 1979.

9. Osborne CA: Three steps to effective management of bacterial urinary tract infections: diagnosis, diagnosis, diagnosis. Comp Cont Educ Vet Med 17:1233, 1995.

Chapter 66

Canine and Feline Urolithiasis: Pathophysiology, Epidemiology and Management

Jodi L. Westropp
Annette L. Ruby
Scott J. Campbell
Gerald V. Ling

Overview of Urolithiasis

Uroliths are organized concretions found in the urinary tract that contain primarily organic or inorganic crystalloid (ionic component of crystals) and a much smaller amount of organic matrix. When urine becomes supersaturated with minerals, and other parameters are conducive to crystallization, minerals can precipitate and individual crystals can be observed in the urine. Crystalluria does ***not*** mean that the patient is at risk for urolithiasis. Crystalluria is not a disease and no particular treatment is necessary unless a urolith is currently present or a urolith or urethral plug has formed in the past.

Supersaturation of urine with crystalloids depends on the interaction of dozens of crystalloid species formed by common mineral elements in the urine derived from the amount of each solute ingested and excreted in the volume of urine produced.[1] Organic molecule contributions, such as protein inhibitors or promoters of crystallization, may also influence crystal and stone formation.[2] Urine samples should be analyzed within 1 hour of collection to minimize temperature- and time-dependent in vitro crystallization.[3]

Urine pH also affects crystal formation: Struvite, calcium carbonate, and calcium phosphate are less soluble in alkaline urine; cystine, uric acid, and silica are less soluble in acid urine. Depending on which salt of uric acid is present, the solubility of the urate stone may be pH dependent. For example, ammonium urate is more soluble in an alkaline pH, but other salts of uric acid may not be influenced by urine pH to the same extent. Further research is required to properly identify the exact salts present in these calculi. Urine pH does not appear to have a major effect on the solubility of calcium oxalate (CaOx), and CaOx calculi can be observed over a wide spectrum of urine pH. In addition to urinary pH, factors that predispose to urinary stasis play an important role in urolithiasis, because crystals that remain in the urinary tract for a sufficient time to allow aggregation may allow urolith formation.

Relative Supersaturation

The most frequently reported method for evaluating the crystallization potential in canine and/or feline urine is the calculation of relative supersaturation (RSS),[4-6] although many other methods of assessment have been reported in humans.[7-9] Concentrations of lithogenic substances and urine pH are used to calculate the urinary RSS values for particular crystal types. A validated computer program is used to calculate the concentrations of numerous soluble ion complexes and the activity products of the stone-forming ion complexes.[6] The RSS for a particular crystal type is then calculated from the ratios of the activity products to the thermodynamic solubility products for each complex. A RSS less than 1 indicates that the urine is undersaturated with the ion complex evaluated, whereas a RSS greater than 1 indicates that the urine is supersaturated with the ion complex evaluated.

Imaging the Animal with Urolithiasis

Radiographs should be taken prior to stone removal and should include the entire urinary tract. CaOx, apatite, struvite, and silica stones are generally radioopaque. Most urate and cystine stones cannot be identified on plain radiography. Immediately after stone removal, additional radiographs should be assessed to be certain that no stones were inadvertently missed. CaOx stones oftentimes occur as multiple, small calculi and can be difficult to flush from the urethra. Contrast studies or ultrasound should be used to determine the presence or absence of residual urate or cystine stones after surgery. Periodic imaging (every 3 to 4 months) is essential to monitor for recurrent urolithiasis. This will enable the clinician to institute non-invasive therapy while stones are small and surgical interventions may be prevented.

Removal of Calculi

Removal of cystic calculi can be performed by various methods. Oftentimes, a cystotomy is performed. If clinically warranted, at the time of stone removal, a bladder biopsy can be obtained for histologic evaluation and culture. Alternatively, for larger cystic calculi in dogs and cats, laser lithotripsy is available at some referral institutions. Holmium:YAG laser lithotripsy can fragment stones by means of a photothermal process and the laser energy is absorbed in less than 0.5 mm of fluid, making it safe for urologic procedures.[10] The Ho:YAG laser has been reported to fragment all types of canine uroliths in vitro,[11] but more studies are needed to evaluate the time required to fragment canine and feline stones in vivo. Once the stones are fragmented, a basket can be inserted through the cystoscope and the largest fragment can be grasped to ensure that it will pass easily through the urethra. The larger pieces should be included for stone analysis to properly identify all the layers of the stone. This is important to subsequently initiate proper management strategies. All other fragments can be removed by voiding urohydropropulsion. Urohydropropulsion is also useful when the animal presents with small cystic calculi. If "sand and debris" or even small stones (3 to 5 mm) are seen in the urinary bladder, surgery is often not necessary and voiding urohydropropulsion may be a less invasive procedure for stone removal. For a complete review of this technique, the reader is referred to the literature.[12]

When to perform surgery in cats with ureteroliths is often a topic of debate among surgeons and internists. Results from a larger retrospective study of ureteral calculi in cats suggests that medical and surgical management are associated with high morbidity and mortality rates.[13] Medical management with aggressive fluid diuresis, parenteral diuretic therapy, analgesia, and even hemodialysis is recommended prior to any surgical intervention. When the ureteral calculus remains lodged in the ureter, despite medical therapy, and is causing renal compromise or significant discomfort to the cat, surgery should be performed to remove the obstruction. Ureterotomy or ureteroneocystostomy can be done to remove the ureterolith, with the latter procedure performed most often when the ureterolith is in the distal third of the ureter. Recurrent ureterolithiasis is reported to be as high as 40% in cats that were evaluated with serial abdominal imaging. Most of the ureteroliths we analyze at our laboratory are CaOx,[14] but we have noted an increased incidence of dried solidified blood calculi in the ureters of cats.[15]

Struvite Urolithiasis in Dogs

Struvite-containing calculi comprise about 45% of all canine uroliths analyzed at the UC-Davis Urinary Stone Analysis Laboratory. Almost three quarters of all struvite calculi occurred in female dogs. A strong statistical association between the female sex and increased risk of struvite-containing calculi in dogs has been documented.[16] An increased risk for struvite-containing calculi has been reported in Cocker spaniels, springer spaniels, and Labrador retrievers. A lower risk for struvite-containing calculi in dogs that were subject to stone formation was noted in both sexes of Dalmatians, Pomeranians, and Maltese.[17] We have reported a trend change in the proportion of canine urinary calculi composed of struvite from 1981 to 2001.[18] For both sexes, a 20-year statistically significant decrease was observed in the proportion of calculus specimens that contained struvite. This decrease in proportion was greater in males than in females. The change in trend may depend on breed, age, gender, and on the interaction among these three factors.

Struvite uroliths are most commonly found in the lower urinary tract, but occasionally are found in the renal pelves and ureters. Struvite uroliths come in a variety of shapes and sizes and other minerals such as calcium and phosphate can be incorporated into the stone because of secondary urine pH changes.

In dogs, virtually all struvite calculi are infection-induced, and the causative organism is usually *Staphylococcus intermedius* or, less commonly, *Proteus mirabilis.* These bacteria have the ability to hydrolyze urea into ammonia, bicarbonate, and carbonate. The resulting increase in the urine pH results in urinary supersaturation of the ions. The elevated pH is also thought to be a contributory factor in causing damage to the underlying uroepithelial glycosaminoglycan layer. It has been reported in humans, that non-urease-producing bacteria, may also influence the formation of urinary stones,[19] but this has not been evaluated in dogs. Occasionally, in the absence of infection, the urine can become supersaturated with the minerals that compose struvite uroliths, and stone formation can occur in the absence of infection. The solubility of struvite increases when the urine pH is less than 6.8.

Struvite Urolithiasis in Cats

Based on previously published epidemiology studies, struvite was the most common stone reported in cats until approximately 1993, when the incidence of CaOx began to increase.[20] Between 1998 and 2003, struvite was the second most common stone type at another laboratory.[21] We have also noted that struvite is the second most common mineral type found in calculi submitted to the UC-Davis Urinary Stone Analysis Laboratory, and the number of struvite stones has significantly decreased when evaluating the past 15 years.[22] However, the proportion of struvite stones analyzed in the past few years appears to be increasing, whereas the proportion of CaOx-containing uroliths is declining (Figure 66-1). We have noted a change in feline urolithiasis trends beginning in 1993, when 53% of the stones *contained* CaOx, while only 47% contained struvite. The proportion of CaOx-containing uroliths continued to increase over the next 8 years, while the proportion of struvite-containing uroliths decreased during that same period. Stones not containing CaOx or struvite appeared to be static during that same period. One hypothesis for this apparent change in trend could be that less highly acidifying diets are being prescribed by veterinarians, but diet histories were not available from these records to confirm or deny this hypothesis.

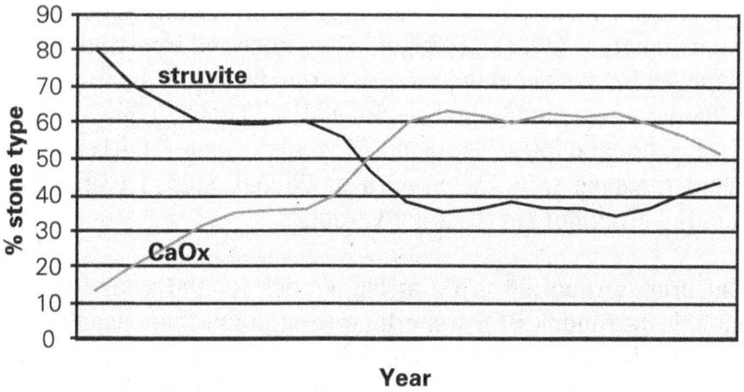

Figure 66-1. Average of struvite and calcium oxalate stones in cats over 3 years.

In 2000, the University of Minnesota Urolith Center reported that the foreign shorthair, ragdoll, Chartreux, Oriental shorthair, domestic shorthair, and Himalayan were breeds at risk for the formation of struvite calculi.[20] The Rex, Burmese, Abyssinian, Russian blue, Birman, Siamese, and mixed breed cats had a significantly lower risk of developing struvite uroliths. Table 66-1 provides a table of relative breed risks for struvite and CaOx formation that we have seen at The UC-Davis Urinary Stone Analysis Laboratory.[22] The bladder is the most common site for struvite urolith retrieval, and approximately 90% of the struvite uroliths submitted to our laboratory are removed from this site. Struvite stones were also submitted after being removed from the urethra (7%) and the upper urinary tract (0.34%) or after the stones were voided (2.5%). Ureteral stone submittals have significantly increased over the past 15 years.[22]

In cats, struvite stone formation usually occurs in sterile urine. This is in contrast to dogs in which struvite stones are usually associated with a urease-producing bacterial infection. Epidemiologic studies on diet and struvite formation in cats have been published,[23] but the pathophysiology of struvite urolith formation in cats is not yet completely understood. Struvite urolith formation likely results from a combination of breed, sex, and dietary factors. Struvite is more soluble in slightly acidic urine ($pH < 6.8$). Therefore, factors that may be associated with the formation of alkaline urine (e.g., family history of struvite stones, a diet low in animal protein, or distal renal tubular acidosis) should also be considered in cats with struvite urolithiasis.

Table 66-1. Relative Breed Risks for Struvite and CaOx

Breed	Calcium oxalate (n)	Risk ratio	95% confidence interval	Struvite (n)	Risk ratio	95% confidence interval
DSH	1731	1.06	1.03-1.09	1406	1.01	0.97-1.04
DLH	313	0.73	0.65-0.81	349	0.95	0.86-1.05
Himalayan	213	4.39	3.77-5.12	579	2.30	1.86-2.84
Persian	204	2.82	2.43-3.27	132	2.14	1.79-2.56
Siamese	132	1.13	0.95-1.34	176	1.76	1.52-2.05
DMH	115	0.72	0.60-0.87	131	0.97	0.81-1.15
Maine Coon	16	0.54	0.33-0.89	21	0.83	0.53-1.28
Tonkinese	5	0.95	0.38-2.35	2	0.44	0.11-1.82
British Shorthair	3	17.91	2.99-107.17	0	0	NE
Abyssinian	2	0.09	0.02-0.34	0	0	NE
Balinese	0	0	NE	0	0	NE
Bengal	0	0	NE	0	0	NE
Burmese	0	0	NE	0	0	NE
Birman	0	0	NE	0	0	NE
Scottish Fold	0	0	NE	0	0	NE

Calcium Oxalate Urolithiasis in Dogs and Cats

The exact mechanism of CaOx stone formation is unknown and likely involves interrelationships among gender, genetics, breed, diet, and environmental factors. In either species with proven or suspected CaOx urolithiasis, serum should be evaluated to assess the calcium concentrations. Elevated calcium from various causes (neoplastic, primary, or secondary hyperparathyroidism, or idiopathic hypercalcemia in cats) can predispose the animal to CaOx stone formation. In humans, approximately 75% of kidney stones are composed predominantly of CaOx, and oxalate metabolism is thought to play a crucial role in stone development. Hyperoxaluria can occur from increased dietary intake as well as a loss or diminished activity of oxalate-degrading bacteria in the colon (*Oxalobacter formigenes*).[24] Primary hyperoxaluria type I is an inborn error of glyoxylate metabolism and can lead to marked increases in hepatic oxalate production in humans.[25] Human beings are also much more prone to developing nephrolithiasis, particularly in industrialized nations, whereas bladder stones are found most frequently in developing countries[26] (as well as in dogs and cats). Although urinary supersaturation with crystals is implicated in stone formation in humans, several studies have investigated the possibility that the urine is not the initial site of stone development. A vascular etiology for nephrolithiasis in humans has been proposed,[26] suggesting that vascular abnormalities (e.g., hypertensive vascular injury, atherosclerosis) can lead to Randall's plaques (papillary lesions that are usually associated with calcium and phosphate or CaOx).[27] Stoller et al, hypothesized that the primary event in CaOx nephrolithiasis in humans may begin in the vascular bed at the tip of the renal papilla. Still other studies have investigated a role for elevated lipids in CaOx urolith formation in rats and humans.[28] Therefore, the primary site of urolithiasis may be unrelated to urinary stasis, infection, or other secondary causes for urinary stones, and novel treatment regimens may need to be investigated. No studies investigating these disorders or hypotheses have been published for cats and dogs and what, if any, relationships can be made between these species remains to be seen.

CaOx is one of the most common mineral types present in specimens of calculi that are obtained from dogs. The incidence of CaOx stones appears to be increasing over the past 20 years (with a reciprocal decrease in the proportion of struvite uroliths).[18] CaOx calculi appear to be more common in older, castrated male dogs.[16,29] Other risk factors for CaOx uroliths in dogs include obesity[29] and breed. Several small-breed dogs, including the miniature schnauzer, a breed that is recognized to also be at risk for hypertriglyceridemia, have a higher risk of CaOx urolith formation. Elevated cholesterol[26] and triglycerides have been evaluated in other species with CaOx uroliths, and research in rats suggests that elevated lipids may play a role in CaOx urolith formation.[26,28] However, the pathogenesis of stone formation in dogs and cats may differ from that in rats and humans.

CaOx stones are the most common urolith type found in people, and during the past 15 years the incidence of CaOx urolith formation has been increasing in cats.[20] CaOx stones are composed of calcium oxalate monohydrate (whewellite) or calcium oxalate dihydrate (weddellite). The exact cause of CaOx stone formation in the cat is unknown. The concern regarding struvite stone disease in cats seems to have led pet food manufacturers to restrict the magnesium content of feline diets and has also has resulted in the formulation of diets with greater urinary acidifying potential. Unfortunately, an increase in the frequency of CaOx urolithiasis appears to have occurred since these dietary modifications began. Between 1984 and 1995 the percentage of stones submitted to the University of Minnesota Urolith Center that were found to be composed of CaOx increased from 2% to 40%.30 We reported a similar trend from our laboratory.[14] Although dietary acidification can enhance the solubility of struvite crystals in the urine of cats, it also promotes the release of calcium carbonate from bone as a metabolic buffer, and hypercalciuria results.[31] Results have shown that differences in age, sex, breed, and reproductive status did not contribute to the apparent reciprocal relationship between occurrences of CaOx and struvite uroliths in cats.[20] However, as mentioned earlier in the struvite section, we, and others[21] have also noted a decrease in the proportion of CaOx stones submitted over the past few years. CaOx uroliths can occur anywhere in the urinary tract, and when ureteroliths are present in cats, the mineral composition is likely to be CaOx. Approximately 73% of CaOx stones we analyzed from cats were removed from the bladder, 7.3% were removed from the ureter(s), 4.3% were removed from the kidney(s), 13% were removed from the urethra and 2% were voided. Most of the time, if CaOx stones were removed from the urethra or voided, stones were also located elsewhere in the urinary tract.

Cat breeds reported to be at higher risk for CaOx urolithiasis include the ragdoll, British shorthair, foreign shorthair, Himalayan, Havana brown, Scottish fold, Persian, and exotic shorthair. The Birman, Abyssinian, Siamese, and mixed breed cats were at significantly lower risk for developing CaOx uroliths.[20] As mentioned, cats with CaOx urolithiasis are generally older than cats with struvite urolithiasis. Cats between 7 and 10 years of age are reported to be 67 times more likely to develop CaOx uroliths than are cats between one and two years of age.[20] Male cats were reported to be 1.5 times more likely to develop CaOx uroliths than were female cats, while neutered cats were seven times more likely to develop CaOx uroliths as compared with sexually intact cats.

Urate Urolithiasis in Dalmatian Dogs

Unlike most other breeds of dogs, Dalmatian dogs have well described alterations in purine metabolism that lead to the excretion of urate (salts of uric acid) or, much less commonly, uric acid in the urine rather than the more soluble metabolite, allantoin.[32] In Dalmatians, the liver does not completely oxidize available uric acid, even though it contains a sufficient concentration of uricase, the enzyme necessary to convert uric acid to allantoin. It is hypothesized that the hepatic cellular membranes are partially impermeable to uric acid.[33] In addition, Dalmatians are reported to excrete excessive amounts of uric acid from the kidneys, which is the result of a combination of reduced tubular reabsorptive capacity and increased tubular secretion.[34] Increased uric acid excretion appears to be a risk factor for urate stones, but not the only cause. All Dalmatians excrete relatively high amounts of uric acid (400 to 600 mg of uric acid per day as compared with 10 to 60 mg per day in non-Dalmatian dogs); however, not all Dalmatians form urate stones. It is likely that a combination of breed and other factors, such as a lack of urinary inhibitors,[35] may play a role in the pathogenesis of urate stone formation. It has been reported that most Dalmatians that form calculi are males.[17] Reasons for this sex difference could be that there is a contributing X-linked genetic trait, or that stones become lodged in the smaller diameter urethra of male dogs. Genetic studies have reported that the mode of inheritance is not X-linked and the prevalence of the clinical disease in male Dalmatians ranges form 26% to 34%.[32]

Depending on which salt of uric acid is present, the solubility of the urate stone may be pH dependent. For example, ammonium urate is more soluble in an alkaline pH, but other salts of uric acid may not be influenced by urine pH to the same extent. Further research is required to properly identify the exact salts present in these calculi.

Urate Urolithiasis in Non-Dalmatian Dogs

A high incidence of ammonium urate stones have been reported in dogs with portal vascular anomalies. Portal vascular shunts provide communication between systemic vasculature and the systemic circulation, bypassing the liver and resulting in decreased hepatic function. As a result, uric acid accumulates and may predispose the animals to urate stone formation. It is hypothesized that surgically correcting the underlying problem and eliminating the hyperuricosuria can prevent urate stone prevention for dogs with portovascular anomalies. Allopurinol is generally not recommended in dogs with portovascular anomalies, because of alterations in metabolism of this drug.

Other canine breeds (without hepatic dysfunction) have been reported to have an increased incidence for urate urolithiasis, particularly the English bulldog. The pathogenesis of the urate stone formation in this breed has not been determined and evaluation of eight male English bulldogs with stones revealed mild elevation in serum uric acid concentrations. Hepatic function was normal when assessed.[33] The miniature schnauzer, Shih tzu, and Yorkshire terriers,[33] and perhaps the Russian black terrier,[36] are also over represented.

Feline Urate Urolithiasis

We have evaluated the mineral composition of 4933 feline uroliths submitted to the UC-Davis Urinary Stone Analysis Laboratory from 1986 to 2003. Of these, 10.4% contained urate. Approximately half of these stones were composed of 100% urate. Others were mixed with struvite or CaOx, and of these, 49% were from female cats and 51% were from males. When evaluating data from our laboratory, the incidence of urate calculi in cats does not appear to have changed over the past 20 years; therefore, the occurrence of these calculi does not appear to be influenced by the dietary changes that occurred to minimize struvite stone formation. CaOx may be a secondary component of some urate stones, and urate stones found in cats with portosystemic shunts often also contain struvite.[30] Often, the pathophysiology of urate urolith formation in cats is unknown.

Cystine and Silica Urolithiasis in Dogs and Cats

Cystine uroliths account for a small percentage of uroliths we analyze at the UC-Davis Urinary Stone Analysis Laboratory. Other laboratories in the United States also report this stone type infrequently.[37] Cystinuria can occur in some dogs and cats and appears to be a heterogeneous disease. Cystinuria is an inherited renal transport disorder characterized by excessive urinary excretion of cystine as well as the other dibasic amino acids ornithine, arginine, and lysine. Dibasic aminoaciduria has also been reported with cystinuria. Concurrent excess carnitine has also been reported in the urine of five dogs with cystinuria that were studied.[38] The molecular basis of cystinuria has been investigated in Newfoundland dogs, and the cloning and sequencing of the canine SLC3A1 gene (the amino acid transport gene) and the identification of a nonsense mutation in exon 2 of this gene have been reported.[39] Cystine is insoluble in urine and the solubility of this amino acid decreases further in acidic urine. Generally cystine uroliths are not visible on plain radiography, unless they are exceptionally large. Cystine uroliths are rare in cats; they accounted for only 0.2% of uroliths from cats at the Minnesota Urolith Center[40] and 0.15% of the feline uroliths analyzed at our laboratory.

A diet that is high in moisture and reduced in dietary protein has the potential for minimizing the recurrence of stone formation in dogs with cystine uroliths. If protein is restricted in a dog excreting excessive sulfur amino acids, taurine supplementation is recommended. The effects of sodium on cystine excretion have not been evaluated in dogs, however, sodium has been reported to enhance cystinuria in humans.[41] The thiol–containing drugs (e.g., n-(2-mercaptopropionyl)-glycine (2-MPG)) can decrease the concentration of cystine in the urine by participating in a thiol-disulfide exchange reaction. In one retrospective study of 88 dogs,[42] the most common breeds with cystine urolithiasis were dachshunds, Tibetan spaniels, and basset hounds. Cystine excretion appeared to decrease as the animal aged. According to this study in dogs with recurrent cystine urolithiasis, dissolution was induced by increasing the tiopronin dosage to 40 mg/kg body weight per day. Adverse effects were found using the thiol-containing drugs and included aggressiveness and myopathy. All signs disappeared when treatment was stopped. In addition to the use of the thiol-containing drugs, increasing water intake should also be initiated.

Silica urolithiasis is uncommon in dogs and rare in cats. These uroliths account for approximately 0.1 to 2.0% of the uroliths seen each year from the Minnesota Urolith Center[43] as well as from the UC-Davis Urinary Stone Analysis Laboratory. Most dogs with silica uroliths are older, and male dogs appear to be predisposed. The most common breeds associated with silica urolithiasis at our laboratory include the German shepherd, Labrador retriever, and Australian shepherd. The hypothesized pathophysiology of silica stones is reviewed nicely elsewhere and the reader is referred to the literature for information pertaining to management.[43]

References

1. Robertson WG, Jones JS, Heaton MA, et al: Predicting the crystallization potential of urine from cats and dogs with respect to calcium oxalate and magnesium ammonium phosphate (struvite). J Nutr 132:1637S-1641S, 2002.

2. Walton RC, Kavanagh JP, Heywood BR: The density and protein content of calcium oxalate crystals precipitated from human urine: a tool to investigate ultrastructure and the fractional volume occupied by organic matrix. J Struct Biol 143:14-23, 2003.

3. Albasan H, Lulich JP, Osborne CA, et al: Effects of storage time and temperature on pH, specific gravity, and crystal formation in urine samples from dogs and cats. J Am Vet Med Assoc 222:176-179, 2003.

4. Lulich JP, Osborne CA, Sanderson SL: Effects of dietary supplementation with sodium chloride on urinary relative supersaturation with calcium oxalate in healthy dogs. Am J Vet Res 66:319-324, 2005.

5. Stevenson AE, Hynds WK, Markwell PJ: Effect of dietary moisture and sodium content on urine composition and calcium oxalate relative supersaturation in healthy miniature schnauzers and labrador retrievers. Res Vet Sci 74:145-151, 2003.

6. Stevenson AE, Blackburn JM, Markwell PJ, et al: Nutrient intake and urine composition in calcium oxalate stone-forming dogs: comparison with healthy dogs and impact of dietary modification. Vet Therap 5:218-231, 2004.

7. Laube N, Hergarten S: Can the Bonn Risk Index be replaced by a simple measurement of the urinary concentration of free calcium ions? J Urol 173:2175-2177, 2005.

8. Hussain F, Billimoria FR, Singh PP: Predictive value of some biochemical indices in stone formers. Int Urol Nephrol 22:25-31, 1990.

9. Pak CY, Hayashi Y, Finlayson B, et al: Estimation of the state of saturation of brushite and calcium oxalate in urine: a comparison of three methods. J Lab Clin Med 89:891-901,.1977;

10. Vassar GJ, Chan KF, Teichman JM, et al: Holmium:YAG lithotripsy: photothermal mechanism. J Endourol 13:181-190, 1999.

11. Wynn VM, Davidson EB, Higbee RG, et al: In vitro effects of pulsed holmium laser energy on canine uroliths and porcine cadaveric urethra. Lasers Surg Med 33:243-246, 2003.

12. Lulich JP, Osborne CA, Carlson M, et al: Nonsurgical removal of urocystoliths in dogs and cats by voiding urohydropropulsion. J Am Vet Med Assoc 203:660-663, 1993.

13. Kyles AE, Hardie EM, Wooden BG, et al: Management and outcome of cats with ureteral calculi: 153 cases (1984-2002). J Am Vet Med Assoc 226:937-944, 2005.

14. Westropp JL: Epidemiology of feline urolithiasis. *In* Feline Urinary Calculi: The New Stone Age. Montipillier, France 2005.

15. Westropp JL, Ruby AL, Bailiff N, et al: Dried solidified blood calculi in cats. JVIM 2005; *In press.*

16. Ling GV, Franti CE, Ruby AL, et al: Urolithiasis in dogs. I: Mineral prevalence and interrelations of mineral composition, age, and sex. Am J Vet Res 59:624-629, 1998.

17. Ling GV, Franti CE, Ruby AL, et al: Urolithiasis in dogs. II: Breed prevalence, and interrelations of breed, sex, age, and mineral composition. Am J Vet Res 59:630-642,.1998;

18. Ling GV, Thurmond MC, Choi YK, et al: Changes in proportion of canine urinary calculi composed of calcium oxalate or struvite in specimens analyzed from 1981 through 2001. J Vet Intern Med 17:817-823, 2003.

19. Kaya S, Poyraz O, Gokce G, et al: Role of genital mycoplasmata and other bacteria in urolithiasis. Scand J Infect Dis 35:315-317, 2003.

20. Lekcharoensuk C, Lulich JP, Osborne CA, et al: Association between patient-related factors and risk of calcium oxalate and magnesium ammonium phosphate urolithiasis in cats. J Am Vet Med Assoc 217:520-525, 2000.

21. Houston DM, Moore AE, Favrin MG, et al: Feline urethral plugs and bladder uroliths: a review of 5484 submissions 1998-2003. Can Vet J 44:974-977, 2003.

22. Cannon AB, Westropp JL, Kass PH, et al: Trends in feline urolithiasis: 1985-2004. *In* Proceedings of ACVIM, Louiville, KY 2005.

23. Lekcharoensuk C, Osborne CA, Lulich JP, et al: Association between dietary factors and calcium oxalate and magnesium ammonium phosphate urolithiasis in cats. J Am Vet Med Assoc 219:1228-1237, 2001.

24. Mittal RD, Kumar R: Gut-inhabiting bacterium Oxalobacter formigenes: role in calcium oxalate urolithiasis. J Endourol 18:418-424, 2004.

25. Monico CG, Rossetti S, Olson JB, et al: Pyridoxine effect in type I primary hyperoxaluria is associated with the most common mutant allele. Kidney Int 67:1704-1709, 2005.

26. Stoller ML, Meng MV, Abrahams HM, et al: The primary stone event: a new hypothesis involving a vascular etiology. J Urol 171:1920-1924, 2004.

27. Ohman S, Larsson L: Evidence for Randall's plaques to be the origin of primary renal stones. Med Hypotheses 39:360-363, 1992.

28. Lenin M, Thiagarajan A, Nagaraj M, et al: Attenuation of oxalate-induced nephrotoxicity by eicosapentaenoate-lipoate (EPA-LA) derivative in experimental rat model. Prostaglandins Leukot Essent Fatty Acids 65:265-270, 2001.

29. Lekcharoensuk C, Lulich J, Osborne C, et al: Patient and environmental factors associated with calcium oxalate urolithiasis in dogs. JAVMA 217:515-519, 2000.

30. Osborne CA, Lulich JP, Thumchai R, et al: Feline urolithiasis. Etiology and pathophysiology. Vet Clin North Am Small Anim Pract 26:217-232, 1996.

31. Dibartola SP: Metabolic acid-base disorders. *In* Fluid Therapy in Small Animal Practice. Dibartola SP (ed). Philadelphia: WB Saunders, 2000, pp. 211-240.

32. Bannasch DL, Ling GV, Bea J, et al: Inheritance of urinary calculi in the Dalmatian. J Vet Intern Med 18:483-487, 2004.

33. Bartges JW, Osborne CA, Lulich JP, et al: Canine urate urolithiasis. Etiopathogenesis, diagnosis, and management. Vet Clin North Am Small Anim Pract 29:161-191, xii-xiii, 1999.

34. Collins RL, Birchard SJ, Chew DJ, et al: Surgical treatment of urate calculi in Dalmatians: 38 cases (1980-1995). J Am Vet Med Assoc 213:833-838, 1998.

35. Carvalho M, Lulich JP, Osborne CA, et al: Role of urinary inhibitors of crystallization in uric acid nephrolithiasis: Dalmatian dog model. Urology 62:566-570, 2003.

36. Bende B, Nemeth T: High prevalence of urate urolithiasis in the Russian black terrier. Vet Rec 155:239-240, 2001.

37. Osborne CA, Sanderson SL, Lulich JP, et al: Canine cystine urolithiasis. Cause, detection, treatment, and prevention. Vet Clin North Am Small Anim Pract 29:193-211, xiii, 1999.

38. Sanderson SL, Osborne CA, Lulich JP, et al: Evaluation of urinary carnitine and taurine excretion in 5 cystinuric dogs with carnitine and taurine deficiency. J Vet Intern Med 15:94-100, 2001.

39. Henthorn PS, Liu J, Gidalevich T, et al: Canine cystinuria: polymorphism in the canine SLC3A1 gene and identification of a nonsense mutation in cystinuric Newfoundland dogs. Hum Genet 107:295-303, 2000.

40. Osborne CA, Kruger JM, Lulich J, et al: Feline lower urinary tract diseases. *In* Textbook of Veterinary Internal Medicine. Ettinger SJ, Feldman E (eds). Philadelphia: WB Saunders, 2000, pp. 1710-1747.

41. Jaeger P, Portmann L, Saunders A, et al: Anticystinuric effects of glutamine and of dietary sodium restriction. N Engl J Med315:1120-1123, 1986.

42. Hoppe A, Denneberg T: Cystinuria in the dog: clinical studies during 14 years of medical treatment. J Vet Intern Med 15:361-367, 2001.

43. Osborne CA, Jacob F, Lulich JP, et al: Canine silica urolithiasis. Risk factors, detection, treatment, and prevention. Vet Clin North Am Small Anim Pract 29:213-230, xiii, 1999.

Chapter 67

Feline Lower Urinary Tract Diseases

Carl A. Osborne
Jon M. Kruger
Jody P. Lulich

Terminology

Feline Urologic Syndrome (FUS)

In 1970, the term "feline urologic syndrome" and the acronym "FUS" were first used and soon became widely adopted as a diagnostic umbrella to refer to naturally occurring and experimentally induced feline lower urinary tract disease (FLUTD) with different sites of involvement, different combinations of clinical signs, and fundamentally different underlying causes.[1] The common denominator of all of these disorders was varying combinations of recurrent dysuria, pollakiuria, stranguria, hematuria, periuria (urinating in inappropriate locations), and/or urinary outflow obstruction. The similarity of clinical signs of FLUTD caused by diverse causes is understandable since the urinary tract can respond to various diseases in only a limited and predictable fashion. Unfortunately, use of the acronym FUS to lump all FLUTDs together, rather than separating them on the basis of specific underlying causes, fostered fundamental errors in the design of experimental, epidemiologic, and clinical studies designed to investigate the biologic behavior and diagnosis of this problem.[2] In addition a diagnosis of FUS based solely on history and physical examination findings resulted in a stereotyped approach to medical and surgical treatment and prevention of obstructive and nonobstructive LUTD, regardless of underlying cause.

Feline Lower Urinary Tract Disease (FLUTD)

In the early 1980's we advanced the concept that FUS was a poor synonym for a heterogeneous group of FLUTD that resulted from fundamentally different causes.[3,2] The causes may be single, multiple, and interacting or unrelated. This change in perspective with which we consider the naturally occurring forms of feline lower urinary tract disorders is of fundamental clinical significance because it helps to eliminate the stereotyped approach to treatment and prevention fostered by use of FUS as a diagnostic endpoint. We continue to urge our colleagues to substitute a clinical diagnosis of FUS with refined diagnostic terms pertaining to sites (e.g., urethra, bladder), causes (e.g., anomalies, urolithiasis, bacteria, fungi, parasites, neoplasms, metabolic disturbances, idiopathic forms), morphologic changes (e.g., inflammation, neoplasia), and pathophysiologic mechanisms (e.g., obstructive uropathy, reflex dyssynergia) whenever possible. If the cause of FLUTD cannot be identified after appropriate evaluation, we suggest that it be called idiopathic FLUTD with the understanding that not all cases of idiopathic FLUTD have the same underlying cause. Idiopathic FLUTD is an exclusion diagnosis.

Feline Idiopathic Cystitis and Feline Interstitial Cystitis

In the early and mid 1990's, investigators hypothesized that cats with idiopathic forms of LUTD had interstitial cystitis because they observed that some cats had abnormalities similar to those reported in humans with interstitial cystitis.[4,5] Human interstitial cystitis is a nonmalignant neuro-inflammatory disorder of humans of unknown etiology.[6] The disease is characterized by dysuria, pain above the pubic region which is relieved by voiding; dysuria; pyuria, hematuria, and/or proteinuria detected by urinalysis; distinctive petechial hemorrhages in the submucosa (called glomerulations) detected by cystoscopy; and decreased urine concentrations of glycosaminoglycans. In subsequent pilot studies of cats, decreased urine concentrations of glycosaminoglycans and increased urinary bladder permeability were also reported.[7] Therefore, they recommended that idiopathic LUTD be renamed feline interstitial cystitis (FIC). Since that time they have stated that use of the term feline interstitial cystitis as an umbrella term for all cats with idiopathic FLUTD is inappropriate. They reserve use of the term feline interstitial cystitis for cats that have persistent or frequent recurrence of clinical signs of lower urinary tract disease. Idiopathic FLUTD can be acute or chronic, but interstitial cystitis by definition is an idiopathic chronic inflammatory process. Currently the terms idiopathic FLUTD and feline idiopathic cystitis are often used as synonyms.

Incidence and Proportional Morbidity of LUTD

Incidence

The incidence of disease is defined as the annual rate of appearance of new cases of disease among the entire population of individuals at risk for the disease. The overall incidence of feline FLUTD in the United States and Great Britain has been estimated to be 1.5% per year.[8,9] Although idiopathic disease currently accounts for the majority of these cases,[5,10] the actual incidence of idiopathic disease, its rate of recurrence, and frequency of sequelae are unknown. There have been no contemporary controlled epidemiologic studies designed to evaluate subsets of cats with LUTDs defined on the basis of specific diagnostic criteria.

Proportional Morbidity Rates

The incidence of naturally occurring hematuria, dysuria, and/or urethral obstruction in domestic cats should not be confused with the frequency that such cats are seen in veterinary hospitals (so-called proportional morbidity rates). As apparent in the following discussion, proportional morbidity rates for FLUTD are not a reliable index of FLUTD incidence, since they may be affected by factors such as local population economics, geography, season, type of veterinary practice, and the interest and training of veterinarians.

Results of a recent retrospective study indicate that the proportional morbidity of FLUTD at Veterinary Teaching Hospitals from 1980 to 1997 was 8%, with significant variation between hospitals

(3%-13%)[11]. The wide variance reported by veterinary teaching hospitals emphasizes the need for caution in formulating generalities about proportional morbidity rates of LUTD on the basis of reports from one center. Lower urinary tract disease is more commonly encountered and/or recognized in Veterinary Teaching Hospitals with special interests in FLUTD. Although proportional morbidity rates reported by these centers are unlikely to be representative of veterinary hospitals without a special interest in urology , the frequency with which specific causes of LUTD are recognized by contemporary diagnostic evaluation suggests that specific causes of LUTD are "under-diagnosed".

Results of prospective studies performed at two Veterinary Teaching Hospitals indicate that the most commonly encountered forms of FLUTD are idiopathic LUTD (~65 %) and urolithiasis (~25%).[5,10] Diseases encountered less frequently include bacterial urinary tract infections, congenital defects, neurogenic disorders, neoplasia, and trauma.[9,11]

Priority of Diagnostic and Therapeutic Plans for Lower Urinary Tract Diseases

Logically, in order to localize and define different causes of diseases of FLUTD, the need for contemporary diagnostic evaluation of each patient becomes indisputable. In addition to an appropriate history and physical examination, complete urinalysis performed on samples that have not been altered by reverse flushing solutions, and evaluation of the urinary tract by survey abdominal radiography or ultrasonography should be performed. Screening quantitative urine cultures are indicated if pyuria is identified by urinalysis. Contrast radiography and/or endouroscopy may be required to aid in localization of problems in addition to identifying the underlying cause(s) of persistent or recurrent clinical signs. Localizing the site(s) and cause(s) of urethral obstruction is especially important if urethral surgery is being considered. A neurologic examination may also be helpful. Patients with renal dysfunction caused by urethral obstruction should be evaluated with the aid of complete blood cell counts, and serum chemistry profiles (especially potassium and bicarbonate concentrations), and perhaps electrocardiograms (for evaluation of the toxic effect of elevated serum potassium concentration on the heart). Quantitative mineral analysis of uroliths and urethral plugs should be routine. Tissue removed surgically should be evaluated routinely by light microscopy.

If the cause of feline lower urinary tract disease cannot be identified after appropriate evaluation, the terminology idiopathic FLUTD or feline idiopathic cystitis (FIC) is recommended.

Developmental Abnormalities

As with other species, congenital abnormalities of the lower urinary tract may be associated with hematuria, dysuria, urinary incontinence, and/or urethral obstruction[9]. However, these causes of FLUTD are uncommonly recognized. Vesicourachal diverticula are an exception to this generality as they have been diagnosed in as many as 1 of 4 cats with lower urinary tract disease. They are worthy of further discussion.

Vesicourachal Diverticula

Function and Dysfunction of the Urachus

The urachus is a fetal conduit that allows urine to pass from the developing urinary bladder to the placenta. It becomes nonfunctional at birth. Microscopic remnants of the fetal urachus characterized by microscopic lumens lined by transitional epithelium have been detected at the bladder vertex in adult healthy cats. In a study of 80 feline urinary bladders, more than 40% had microscopic urachal diverticula.

Microscopic remnants persisting in the urinary bladder vertex after birth usually are clinically silent, but represent a risk factor for development of development of macroscopic diverticula of the urinary bladder in adult cats.[12] Abnormal and/or sustained increase of bladder intraluminal pressure associated with feline lower urinary tract disorders may cause enlargement and/or tearing of microscopic diverticula leading to development of self-limiting macroscopic diverticula of varying size.

Congenital and Acquired Vesicourachal Diverticula

In our experience, radiographically detectable diverticula affecting the vertex of the urinary bladder wall occur in almost 1 of 4 adult cats with hematuria, dysuria, and/or urethral obstruction.[12,13] They occur twice as often in male (27%) as female (14%) cats. We have not observed a breed predisposition. The mean age of affected cats at the time of diagnosis in our series was 3.7 years (range = 1 to 11 years); clinical signs of LUTD were not observed when the cats were younger than one year of age. The higher frequency of occurrence of vesicourachal diverticula in males compared to females is likely related to the higher prevalence of urethral outflow obstruction in males.

There are two etiologically distinct forms of macroscopic vesicourachal diverticula. In cats with the most common form, microscopic remnants of the urachus located at the bladder vertex remain clinically silent until lower urinary tract disease develops. Radiographically detectable diverticula may develop at the bladder vertex as a result of enlargement of these microscopic vesicourachal remnants following onset of increased intraluminal pressure caused by acquired urethral obstruction and/or detrusor hyperactivity induced by inflammation. This hypothesis is supported by the observation that many macroscopic diverticula in cats resolve within 2 to 3 weeks after amelioration of clinical signs of lower tract disease.[13]

The second uncommon form consists of congenital macroscopic vesicourachal diverticula.[12] Although the exact sequence of events resulting in their formation has not been defined, they appear to be caused by disorders that cause abnormally high or sustained pressure in the bladder lumen. Congenital macroscopic vesicourachal diverticula typically are associated with signs of LUTD in immature cats. In our experience, they do not spontaneously resolve. Persistent congenital macroscopic diverticula predispose to bacterial urinary tract infections. If infections are caused by urease producing calculogenic microbes (especially staphylococci), infection induced struvite uroliths often develop.

Urachal diverticula are an uncommon primary factor in development of feline lower urinary tract disease. Most macroscopic diverticula of the bladder vertex are a sequela of lower urinary tract dysfunction. Furthermore, most macroscopic diverticula may be self limiting if the urinary bladder and urethra return to a normal state of function.[12,13] Acquired diverticula usually heal within 2 to 3 weeks following elimination of the underlying cause of increased intraluminal pressure.[13]

Uroliths and Urethral Plugs

The urinary system is designed to dispose of waste products in soluble form. However, some waste products are sparingly soluble and occasionally precipitate out of solution to form crystals. Growth or aggregation of microscopic crystals may lead to formation of macroscopic uroliths. Urolithiasis may be conceptually defined as the formation of uroliths from less soluble crystalloids of urine as a result of multiple genetic and/or acquired physiologic and pathologic processes. If such crystalloids become trapped ion the urinary system, they may grow to sufficient size to cause clinical signs.

Urolithiasis should not be thought of as a specific disease, but as a sequelae to one or more underlying abnormalities. Epidemiologic studies indicate numerous pathophysiologic, demographic, and environmental risk factors may be associated with the clinical expression of urolithiasis. Therefore, detection of uroliths is only the beginning of the diagnostic process. Determination of their mineral composition narrows etiologic possibilities. Knowledge of the patient's age, gender, diet, environment, and urine concentrations of calculogenic minerals, crystallization promoters, crystallization inhibitors, and their interactions provide additional insight into the diagnosis and management of uroliths.

Terminology

There are physical and probable etiopathogenic differences between feline uroliths and urethral plugs. Therefore, these terms should not be used as synonyms.

Uroliths are polycrystalline concretions composed primarily ($\geq$ ~95%) of minerals (organic and inorganic crystalloids) and smaller quantities ($\leq$ ~5%) of matrix. Unlike urethral plugs, uroliths are not disorganized precipitates of crystalline material, but are comprised of crystal aggregates with a complex internal structure.

Feline urethral plugs commonly are composed of large quantities ($\geq$ ~50%) of matrix mixed with minerals.[15] However, some urethral plugs are composed primarily of matrix, some consist of sloughed tissue, blood, and/or inflammatory reactants, and a few are composed primarily of aggregates of crystalline minerals. They may form a cast of the urethral lumen, implying a rapid rate of formation.

The mineral composition of uroliths and urethral plugs should be used to describe them since most therapeutic regimes have been based on their mineral composition. A variety of different minerals have been identified in uroliths and urethral plugs of cats.

Epidemiology of Uroliths and Urethral Plugs

Uroliths

In 2004, 8711 feline uroliths were submitted by veterinarians to the Minnesota Urolith Center for mineral analysis. Struvite was the primary component in 45 percent of the uroliths, calcium oxalate was the primary component in 44%, and salts of uric acid were the primary component in 5%. Less than 1% of the uroliths were composed of calcium phosphate and cystine.

Urethral Plugs

In 2004, 524 feline urethral plugs were submitted by veterinarians to the Minnesota Urolith Center for mineral analysis. Struvite was the primary component in 87 percent of the uroliths, while 10% of the plugs contained noncrystalline matrix. Less than 1% of the uroliths were composed of calcium oxalate and calcium phosphate.

Uroliths

Biologic Behavior of Uroliths

Overview: Detection of a urolith is not always justification for surgical management. In cats, small uroliths may remain asymptomatic within the urinary tract (especially the renal pelvis and urinary bladder) for months or years. However, the underlying cause(s) of uroliths and the sequela of uroliths (partial or total obstruction, urinary tract infection) remain potential hazards. In those situations in which uroliths are fortuitously detected in asymptomatic patients without significant bacteriuria, minimizing risk factors by medical management and monitoring urolith activity by appropriate procedures is an accepted alternative to surgery. If the urolith(s) remain inactive, therapy designed to dissolve or remove them is not mandatory. If the urolith(s) become active, appropriate medical and/or surgical therapy are recommended.

Rate of Formation: The rate of formation of uroliths varies from days to months, being influenced by mineral composition, and a variety of risk factors. Once crystals of one mineral type form in urine, they may reduce the amount of lithogenic substances required for other mineral types of crystals to form. The principle involved is called heterogeneous nucleation (or "seeding") and operates in the same way as when foreign substances like suture material or catheters predispose to formation of uroliths. Viewed in this context, a crystal of one mineral type serves as a risk factor for formation of crystals of other types, and provides one explanation of why macroscopic uroliths may contain more than mineral.

Movement of Uroliths: Small uroliths that form in the urinary bladder may pass into the urethra of male or female cats. Because of the tendency of uroliths to change in size and position, radiographic evaluation of the urinary system should be repeated if there has been a significant time lapse between diagnosis and surgery scheduled to remove them.

Recurrence: Cats that have formed uroliths are at increased risk for recurrent stone formation. In our experience, sterile struvite uroliths have recurred within weeks to several months after elimination. Cystine uroliths also may recur within a few weeks to several months following removal. Calcium oxalate, calcium phosphate and ammonium urate uroliths also have an unpredictable tendency to recur, typically within months or years (rather than weeks) following removal.

Pseudorecurrence: Because many feline uroliths are small, complete surgical removal of all uroliths may be difficult. In a retrospective clinical study performed at the University of Minnesota, uroliths were detected by radiographs taken within 14 days following cystotomies in 20 percent of the patients.[16] We call this phenomenon pseudorecurrence. Results of this study emphasize the importance of postsurgical radiography, ultrasonography, or uroendoscopy to assess urolith status prior to evaluating recurrence and/or therapeutic efficacy.

Ammonium Urate Uroliths

In the series of feline uroliths from the Minnesota Urolith Center, ammonium urate and uric acid collectively called purines comprised approximately 6 percent of the total. The urinary bladder and urethra were the most common sites of purine uroliths (99%), while kidneys and ureters (< 1%) were less common sites. In our series, males were affected as often as females. The mean age of affected cats was 6.1 ± 3.1 years (range = 5 months to 15 years).

Although portovascular anomalies associated with hyperammonemia and hyperuricemia have been confirmed as the underlying cause in a few cases of urate uroliths in cats, the cause(s) of formation of most urate uroliths has not been established. However, formation of ammonium urate uroliths is likely to be associated with several risk factors (Table 67-1).

Calcium Oxalate Uroliths

The underlying cause(s) of calcium oxalate urolith formation has not been defined. Risk factors incriminated include age, gender, breed, hypercalciuria, hyperoxaluria, decreased urine concentration of crystallization inhibitors, hypocitrituria, hypomagnesuria, acidosis, increased urine concentration, decreased urine volume, and urine retention (Table 67-2). Several nutritional risk factors have also been incriminated.

The frequency of detection of calcium oxalate urolithiasis in cats has increased in recent years. In 2004, calcium oxalate uroliths comprised approximately 44% percent of the feline uroliths submitted to the Minnesota Urolith Center. Although calcium oxalate uroliths were located primarily in the urinary bladder

Table 67-1. Potential Risk Factors Associated with Ammonium Urate Urolithiasis

Risk Factor	Etiopathologic Disorder	Pathophysiologic Mechanism
Hyperuricosuria	Hepatic portal vascular anomaly and other forms of hepatic failure	Reduces availability and/or function of hepatic urate oxidase and thereby minimizes conversion of uric acid to allantoin, which is more water soluble
Hyperuricosuria	Excess dietary purine	Promotes hyperuricemia and hyperuricosuria
Hyperuricosuria	Increased nucleic acid breakdown (e.g., lymphoma, leukemia, diffuse tissue destruction)	Results in accelerated metabolism of purines, which are further metabolized to uric acid
Hyperammonuria	Excess dietary protein	Provides additional urea for metabolism to NH_3, and glutamine for conversion to NH_4
Hyperammonuria	Metabolic acidosis	Promotes metabolism of glutamine to NH_4
Hyperammonuria	Aciduria	Ionizes NH_3 that has diffused into renal tubule lumens; trapped NH_4^{+1} is subsequently excreted
Hyperammonuria	Hypokalemia	Produces intracellular acidosis and subsequent NH_4 excretion
Hyperammonuria	Urinary tract infection by microorganisms that produce urease	Promotes conversion of urea in urine to NH_3 and NH_4
Aciduria	Aciduria	Decreases solubility of urine uric acid
Decreased urine volume	Intravascular volume depletion	Conservation of water promotes increased urine concentration and urine supersaturation of uric acid. Urine retention provides additional time for crystal nucleation and growth.

(72%), they were also found in various combinations in the kidneys, ureters, and urethra.

Calcium oxalate uroliths may occur at any age. However, they are recognized more frequently in older cats. In one study, cats older than 7 years, but less than 10 years were 67 times more likely to develop calcium oxalate uroliths than cats 1-2 years of age.[17] In our series, male cats (57%) were affected more than females (43%). Neutered cats were 7 times more likely to form uroliths than sexually intact cats. Case control epidemiologic studies indicate increased risk of calcium oxalate uroliths in Burmese, Himalayan, and Persian, British and exotic shorthair, Havana brown, ragdoll, and Scottish fold breeds suggesting that genetic factors may enhance risk in some cats.[9,17,18,19]

In most cats with calcium oxalate uroliths, serum concentrations of minerals, including calcium, have been normal. The sequence or sequences of events that promote initiation and growth of calcium oxalate uroliths in normocalcemic cats have not been defined. However, epidemiologic studies have identified several probable risk factors (Table 67-2).[20,21] Mild hypercalcemia (11.1 to 13.5 mg/dl) has been observed with sufficient frequency (35%) to warrant routine evaluation of serum total calcium concentration in affected patients.[21] The mechanism(s) of hypercalcemia has not been identified in most cats. Hypercalcemia promotes urinary calcium excretion, and may result in precipitation of calcium oxalate crystals. If hypercalcemia is confirmed in serially obtained serum samples, serum ionized calcium, parathormone, and vitamin D concentrations should be evaluated.

Cats with calcium oxalate urolithiasis typically have acid (urine pH of 6.3 to 6.7) urine. Pretreatment blood pH and total carbon dioxide concentration are often reduced (pH = 7.3). However, the solubility of calcium oxalate crystals is apparently not directly influenced by urine pH within the physiologic range. The indirect association between aciduria, acidemia, and calcium

Table 67-2. Potential Risk Factors Associated with Calcium Oxalate Urolith Formation

Risk Factor	Possible Cause(s)	Proposed Pathophysiologic Mechanisms
Hypercalciuria	Excess dietary calcium	May result in hypercalciuria
Hypercalciuria	Hypercalcemia	Results in increased renal clearance of calcium and hypercalciuria
Hypercalciuria	Excess vitamin D	Augments intestinal calcium absorption. By suppressing parathyroid hormone, promotes hypercalciuria.
Hypercalciuria	Acidosis; consumption of urine acidifying diets	Promotes skeletal mobilization of calcium, and reduces renal tubular reabsorption of calcium
Hypercalciuria	Hypophosphatemia (e.g., reduced dietary consumption or hyperparathroidism)	Stimulates calcitriol production, which augments intestinal calcium absorption
Hyperoxaluria	Reduced dietary calcium	May enhance intestinal absorption and renal excretion of oxalic acid
Hyperoxaluria	Excess dietary oxalate	Results in hyperoxaluria
Hyperoxaluria	Excess vitamin C	May be a precurser of oxalic acid
Hyperoxaluria	Pyridoxine deficiency	Promotes increased endogenous production of oxalic acid
Hyperoxaluria	Primary hyperoxaluria	Results in increased endogenous production of oxalic acid
Hypocitraturia	Idiopathic	Increases urine concentration of calcium ions available to bind with oxalate
Hypocitraturia	Acidemia (e.g., renal tubular acidosis)	Promotes renal tubular utilization of citrate and reduced excretion of citrate
Decreased macromolecular inhibitors?	Inherited disorder?	Minimizes production of glycoproteins capable of inhibiting calcium oxalate crystal growth and aggregation
Decreased volume of concentrated urine	Decreased water consumption; consumption of dry foods	Conservation of water promotes increased urine concentration and urine supersaturation of calcium oxalate. Urine retention provides additional time for crystal nucleation and growth.

oxalate urolithiasis may be that acidemia promotes mobilization of carbonate and phosphorus from bones to buffer hydrogen ions. Concomitant mobilization of bone calcium may result in hypercalciuria. Hypercalciuria in turn is a risk factor for calcium oxalate crystals. In addition, low urine pH decreases urinary citrate concentration by promoting renal tubular reabsorption of citrate. Results of epidemiologic studies support this association inasmuch that cats with calcium oxalate uroliths were 3 times more likely as hospitalized cats to have been fed diets that promote urine pH values less than 6.3.[18,22]

Several diet related risk factors may be associated with calcium oxalate uroliths. Urine acidifying potential and the effect of water consumption on urine volume and concentration are especially important.

Although reduction of urine calcium and oxalic acid concentrations by reduction of **dietary calcium** and oxalic acid appears to be logical goals, they are not necessarily a harmless maneuvers. Reducing consumption of only one of these constituents (such as calcium) may increase the availability of the other (such as oxalic acid) for intestinal absorption and subsequent urinary excretion.[9,20,22] Based on recent epidemiologic information suggesting that marked dietary calcium restriction is associated with increased risk for calcium oxalate urolith formation, the general consensus of opinion is that restricting dietary calcium is inadvisable. Moderate levels of dietary calcium are recommended in normocalcemic cats.

In one study, consumption of higher levels of **sodium** augmented renal excretion of calcium in healthy cats, but reduced supersaturation of urine with calcium oxalate.[20] The explanation of this paradox may be that the effects of oral sodium on water intake and its diluting effect on urine calcium concentration were greater than the effect of sodium on promoting urine calcium excretion. However, studies of cats with naturally occurring calcium oxalate uroliths revealed that consumption of a low sodium diet designed to minimize recurrence of calcium oxalate uroliths was associated with reduced urine calcium concentration and reduced supersaturation of urine with calcium oxalate.[23] Based on this evidence, moderate dietary restriction of sodium would be a logical recommendation for active calcium oxalate urolith formers.

Dietary phosphorus should not be restricted in patients with calcium oxalate urolithiasis because reduction in dietary phosphorus may be associated with activation of vitamin D, which in turn promotes intestinal calcium absorption and subsequent urinary calcium excretion. In addition, pyrophosphate is an inhibitor of calcium oxalate urolith formation.[22]

Increased urine **magnesium** concentration reduces formation of calcium oxalate crystals in vitro.[9] For this reason, supplemental magnesium has been used to minimize recurrence of calcium oxalate uroliths in man. However, supplemental dietary magnesium may contribute to formation of magnesium ammonium phosphate uroliths and hypercalciuria in cats. On the other hand, epidemiologic studies suggest that cats fed foods with reduced magnesium and urine acidifying capabilities are at risk for developing calcium oxalate uroliths. Pending further studies, we do not recommend dietary magnesium restriction or supplementation for cats with calcium oxalate uroliths.[20,24]

Ingestion of foods that contain high quantities of animal **protein** may contribute to calcium oxalate urolithiasis by increasing urinary calcium and oxalic acid excretion, and by decreasing urinary citric acid excretion. Some of these consequences result from obligatory acid excretion associated with protein metabolism. However, because cats are obligatory carnivores, dietary protein restriction is not recommended.

Epidemiologic studies performed at the University of Minnesota revealed that cats consuming canned diets had one third the risk for calcium oxalate urolith formation compared to other dietary formulations.[22] Increased urine volume could minimize formation of uroliths by reducing the concentration of calculogenic substances in urine, and also by promoting voiding before crystals have an opportunity to grow of sufficient size to cause clinical disease. Total **water** consumption is often less in cats fed dry diets resulting in formation of a lower volume of highly concentrated urine.

In summary, based on contemporary knowledge, diets that minimize calcium oxalate urolithiasis should be formulated to minimize acidosis, and should not contain excessive oxalic acid precursors. Likewise, excessive levels of vitamin D (which promote intestinal absorption of calcium), ascorbic acid (a precursor of oxalate), and sodium should be avoided. They should contain adequate, but not excessive, quantities of calcium, phosphorus, magnesium, potassium, and citrate. The diet should be adequately fortified with vitamin B_6 since vitamin B_6 deficiency promotes endogenous production and subsequent urinary excretion of oxalic acid. Canned diets are preferred over dry formulations to enhance formation of less concentrated urine and to promote increased micturition.

Struvite Uroliths

Results of our clinical and experimental studies indicate that two distinct etiologic mechanisms may be responsible for development of uroliths containing large quantities of struvite.[9] Formation of sterile struvite uroliths (perhaps in association with dietary risk factors) is the most common type. Formation of "infected" or "urease" struvite uroliths as a sequela to urinary tract infection with urease producing bacteria is a second type.

In 2004, approximately 45 percent of the naturally occurring feline uroliths submitted to the Minnesota Urolith Center were primarily struvite. Although the exact percentage of sterile versus infection-induced struvite uroliths in this series could not be precisely determined, we estimate that at least 90 percent to 95 percent were composed of sterile struvite. The remainder of this discussion pertains to sterile struvite uroliths. Information about infection induced struvite is described elsewhere.[2]

Compared to cats that develop calcium oxalate uroliths, cats with struvite uroliths tend to be younger. Cats $\geq$ 4 years of age but $\leq$ 7 years of age had the highest risk for developing struvite uroliths.[17] Struvite uroliths occur more commonly in females (55%) than males (45%). A case control comparison performed at the University of Minnesota revealed increased risk in domestic shorthair, foreign shorthair, oriental shorthair, ragdoll, Chartreux, and Himalayan breeds.[17] Neutered cats were 3.5 times more likely to develop struvite uroliths as sexually intact cats. The urinary bladder was the most common site of detection of struvite uroliths, while the kidneys, ureters, and urethra were less common sites.

Data derived from cats with induced sterile struvite uroliths indicate that several dietary factors play a role in the etiopathogenesis of naturally occurring sterile struvite uroliths. Of these, factors affecting urine magnesium concentration, urine pH, and urine concentration are of major therapeutic importance.[9,20] A decrease is urine volume and increase in urine specific gravity secondary to decreased water consumption would be a logical risk factor for urolith formation (Table 67-3). Likewise, excessive consumption of food (perhaps associated with ad libitum feeding) would be expected to result in obesity and excretion of excess minerals (some of which could be calculogenic) in urine. Cats maintain magnesium homeostasis by excreting excessive dietary magnesium in their urine.

Urethral Plugs

Urethral plugs contain varying quantities of minerals in proportion to large quantities of matrix. Although a variety of different minerals have been identified in urethral plugs of cats, struvite is the most common. Of 524 feline urethral plugs submitted to the Minnesota Urolith Center in 2004, the primary mineral composition of approximately 87% was struvite. Less than 1% were composed of calcium oxalate or calcium phosphate.

Risk factors associated with the formation of calcium oxalate, calcium phosphate, and magnesium ammonium phosphate crystals found in urethral plugs are probably similar to those associated with mineral formation in classic uroliths. The mineral composition of urethral plugs should be used to describe them, at least in part, since therapeutic regimes are often influenced by knowledge of their mineral composition.

Compared to uroliths, urethral plugs contain large quantities of matrix. Some urethral plugs do not contain crystalline components; 10% of the plugs evaluated in 2004 contained only noncrystalline matrix. The question about specific composition of urethral plug matrix has not yet been answered. However, it appears as though the amorphous matrix traps crystals and non- crystalline structures (including red blood cells, white cells, epithelial cells, spermatozoa, virus-like particles, and bacteria) in a manner analogous to the formation of fruit jello.[25]

Bacterial Urinary Tract infections

Initial episodes of LUTD in young adult cats usually occur in absence of significant numbers of detectable aerobic bacteria.[26,27] In prospective diagnostic studies of male and female obstructed and nonobstructed cats, aerobic bacterial urinary tract infections were identified in less than 3% of patients.[5,10] The infrequency with which aerobic bacteria have been isolated from urine of young adult and middle age cats during the initial phases of LUTD is related to highly effective local host defense mechanisms in this species.[26]

Table 67-3. Potential Risk Factors Associated with Sterile Struvite Urolith Formation

Risk Factor	Possible Cause(s)	Pathophysiologic Mechanism
Hypermagnesuria	Excess dietary magnesium	Results in increased renal clearance of magnesium and hypermagnesuria
Hyperammonuria	Excess dietary protein	Provides additional urea for metabolism to NH_3 and glutamine for conversion to NH_4
Hyperammonuria	Metabolic acidosis	Promotes metabolism of glutamine to NH_4
Hyperammonuria	Aciduria	Ionizes NH_3 that has diffused into renal tubule lumens; trapped NH_4 is subsequently excreted
Hyperammonuria	Hypokalemia	Produces intracellular acidosis and subsequent NH_4 excretion
Hyperphosphaturia	Excess dietary phosphorus	Results in increased renal clearance of phosphorus and hyperphosphaturia
Alkaline urine	Diet related factors	Increases urine concentration and saturation of PO_3^{-3} by removing hydrogen ions from $H_2PO_4^{-1}$ and HPO_4^{-2}
Decreased volume of concentrated urine	Decreased water consumption; consumption of dry foods	Conservation of water promotes increased urine concentration and urine supersaturation of calcium oxalate. Urine retention provides additional time for crystal nucleation and growth.

Although bacterial UTI is encountered in only 1 to 3% of young adult cats, the prevalence of UTI increases to 10% or greater in cats 10 years of age or older.[11,28] The frequency with which bacterial UTI has been recognized in geriatric cats with LUTD should prompt appropriate diagnostic evaluation in this population of clinical patients.

When bacterial UTI has been detected in cats, it usually is a secondary or complicating factor rather than as a primary etiologic factor. Local urinary tract defenses against bacterial infection are frequently compromised in cats with various forms of naturally occurring nonbacterial LUTD, especially if the episode is associated with urethral obstruction.

Use of indwelling transurethral catheters is associated with a high prevalence of secondary or complicating bacterial urinary tract infection. In studies of normal cats, and cats with induced LUTD, catheter-induced bacteriuria was detected in 33% of cats after 1 day of catheterization, and in 50% to 83% of cats after 5 days of indwelling catheterization.[29] Bacterial UTI is also a common sequelae in cats following perineal urethrostomies. Consult the chapter entitled, "Bacterial urinary tract infections: Diagnostic and therapeutic caveats for further information.

Idiopathic Feline lower Urinary Tract Disease

Etiopathogenesis

In approximately 65% of naturally occurring cases of LUTDs, the exact cause(s) of hematuria, pollakiuria, stranguria, periuria, and/or urethral obstruction are still unknown. After appropriate diagnostic evaluation, these cats are classified as having idiopathic FLUTD, feline idiopathic cystitis (FIC), or feline interstitial cystitis. Because there is no pathognomonic test or diagnostic procedure diagnosis of idiopathic LUTD is dependent on exclusion of other known causes.

Clinical observations suggest that stress may play a role in precipitating or exacerbating signs associated with idiopathic cystitis.[30,31,32] Neuroendocrine abnormalities identified in cats with chronic idiopathic cystitis are indicative of increased activity of the sympathetic nervous system and diminished adrenocortical responsiveness.[33,34] Based on these observations, strategies designed to normalize reactivity of the stress response system have been advocated to minimize recurrence of feline idiopathic cystitis.

Clinical Manifestations

Nonobstructive idiopathic FLUTD occurs in males and females of all ages, but more commonly in young to middle aged cats (mean 3.5 years, range 0.5-17.5 years).[5,10]

It is uncommon in cats less than one year and less common in cats older than 10 years. There are no apparent breed predilections.

Periuria, pollakiuria, stranguria, and gross hematuria are the most common clinical signs observed in cats with nonobstructive idiopathic FLUTDs and often precede the obstructive form of the disorder.

Unless complicated by concurrent illness, results of CBCs and biochemistry profiles of cats with nonobstructive idiopathic FLUTDs are usually normal. Urine obtained from cats with idiopathic FLUTDs is usually concentrated and acid. Hematuria and proteinuria in the absence of pyuria or bacteriuria are typical urinalysis findings.[9,35] Although microscopic hematuria may be a consequence of cystocentesis-induced trauma, the observation of gross hematuria in 81% and microscopic hematuria in 95% of nonobstructed cats with idiopathic FLUTDs suggests that hematuria is a prevalent feature of idiopathic FLUTDs.

The prevalence, magnitude, and type of crystalluria are variable in cats with idiopathic FLUTDs and do not appear to differ from unaffected control cats.[10] Struvite crystals have been the most common crystal type identified in urine of cats with idiopathic FLUTDs. Undoubtedly, some instances of struvite crystalluria in these patients represent in vitro rather than in vivo formation.

Results of urine culture from cats with idiopathic FLUTDs have been negative for aerobic bacteria, mycoplasma, ureaplasma, and viruses. Most cats with idiopathic FLUTDs are seronegative for FIV antibodies and FeLV antigen.[10,35]

Survey abdominal radiographs of cats with nonobstructive idiopathic FLUTD are usually normal. Contrast cystourethrography may be normal or may reveal thickening of the bladder wall, mucosal irregularities, urachal diverticula, and/or urethral narrowing. Ultrasonographic findings of idiopathic FLUTDs have not been characterized; however, blood clots and mural irregularities or thickening may be detected.

Cystoscopic examination of cats with nonobstructive idiopathic LUTDs may reveal increased mucosal vascularity, superficial urothelial desquamation, and petechial hemorrhages in the submucosa (so called "glomerulations").[7] Glomerulations are nonspecific and may be associated with other urinary bladder disorders.[6] In addition, cystoscopy induced urothelial trauma may be confused with primary pathologic lesions. Pending results of additional studies, detection of glomerulations by cystoscopy should be interpreted in the context of the results of other diagnostic evaluations.

Exploratory cystotomy has been commonly used for diagnostic evaluation of idiopathic FLUTDs. With the advent of less invasive means of evaluating the lower urinary tract, the need for cystotomy and surgical biopsy of the urinary bladder for the sole purpose of establishing a diagnosis has largely been eliminated. Even when performed most biopsy samples reveal mucosal erosions and ulcerations, and varying degrees of submucosal hemorrhage, edema, and fibrosis. These light microscopic findings are nonspecific, and rarely lead to improved therapy. Therefore, we cannot recommend cystotomy over less invasive diagnostic procedures for establishing a diagnosis of idiopathic FLUTDs.

Biologic behavior of Idiopathic LUTD

Clinical signs of hematuria, dysuria, and pollakiuria in many untreated nonobstructed males and females with acute idiopathic FLUTDs frequently subside within 5-7 days. These signs may recur after variable periods of time and again subside without therapy. Our impression is that recurrent episodes of acute idiopathic LUTDs tend to decrease in frequency as the cats become older.[37,38]

Though recurrent clinical signs in patients with idiopathic FLUTDs are often assumed to be recurrence of the original disease, recurrent signs may also be the result of a delayed manifestation of the original disease (for example, spontaneous or iatrogenic urethral stricture). In addition, onset of a different disease associated with clinical manifestations similar to those of the original disorder (such as urolithiasis) may occur.

Occasionally we have encountered cats with hematuria and dysuria that have persisted for weeks to months and for which a specific cause was not identified. Whether chronic idiopathic FLUTDs represent one extreme in the spectrum of clinical manifestations associated with similar etiologic factors, or whether it represents an entirely different mechanism of disease than that associated with acute self-limiting idiopathic disease is unknown.

Since clinical signs associated with this form of the disease are frequently self-limiting and of short duration, any form of therapy might appear to be beneficial, as long as it is not harmful. The self-limiting nature of clinical signs in many cats with idiopathic FLUTDs underscores the need for controlled prospective double-blind clinical studies in order to prove the efficacy of various forms of therapy.

References

1. Osbaldiston GW, Taussig RA: Clinical report on 46 cases of feline urological syndrome. *Vet Med Sm Anim Clin* 65: 461, 1970.

2. Osborne CA, Kruger JM, Lulich JP et al: Feline urologic syndrome, feline lower urinary tract disease, feline interstitial I cystitis: What's in a name? *JAVMA* 214: 1470, 1999.

3. Osborne CA, Johnston GR, Polzin DJ et al: Redefinition of the feline urologic syndrome. Feline lower urinary tract disease with heterogeneous causes. *Vet Clin N Amer* 14: 409, 1984.

4. Buffington CA, Chew DJ, Dibartola SP: Lower urinary tract disease in cats: Is diet still a cause? *JAVMA* 205: 1524, 1994.

5. Buffington CAT, Chew DJ, Kendall MS et al: Clinical evaluation of cats with nonobstructive urinary tract diseases. *JAVMA* 210: 46, 1997.

6. Hanno PM. Interstitial cystitis and related syndromes. In Walsh PC et al (eds), Campbell's Urology. 8th ed. Philadelphia, Saunders, 2002, p 631.

7. Buffington CAT, Chew DJ, DiBartola SP: Interstitial cystitis in cats *Vet Clin N Amer* 26: 317, 1996.

8.Lawler DF, Jolin DW, Collins JE: Incidence rates of feline lower urinary tract disease in the United States. *Feline Practice* 15: 13, 1985.

9. Osborne CA, Kruger JM, Lulich JP et al: Feline lower urinary tract diseases. In Ettinger SJ, Feldman EC (eds).: Textbook of Veterinary Internal Medicine. Vol. 2. 5th ed. Philadelphia, W.B. Saunders, 2000, p. 1710.

10. Kruger JM, Osborne CA, Goyal SM et al: Clinical evaluation of cats with lower urinary tract disease. *JAVMA* 199: 221, 1991.

11. Lekcharoensuk C, Osborne CA, Lulich JP. Epidemiologic study of risk factors for lower urinary tract diseases in cats. *JAVMA* 218; 1429, 2001.

12. Osborne CA, Johnston GR, Kruger JM et al: Etiopathogenesis and biological behavior of feline vesicourachal diverticula. Don't just do something--Stand there. *Vet Clin N Amer* 17: 697, 1987.

13. Osborne CA, Kroll RA, Lulich JP et al: Medical management of vesicourachal diverticula in 15 cats with lower urinary tract disease. *J Small Anim Pract* 30: 608, 1989.

14. Osborne CA, Kruger JM, Lulich JP et al: Feline lower urinary tract disease: Relationships between crystalluria, urinary tract infections, and host factors. In, August JR, ed.: Consultations In Feline Internal Medicine. Philadelphia, WB Saunders, 1994, p 351.

15. Osborne CA, Kruger JM, Lulich JP et al: Feline matrix-crystalline urethral plugs: A unifying hypothesis if causes. *J Small Anim Practice* 33: 172, 1992.

16. Lulich JP, Osborne CA, Polzin DJ et al: Incomplete removal of canine and feline urocystoliths by cystotomy. In, Proceedings 11th ACVIM Forum, Washington DC, 1993, p 397.

17. Lekcharoensuk C, Lulich JP, Osborne CA et al. Association between patient-related factors and risk of calcium oxalate and magnesium ammonium phosphate urolithiasis in cats. *JAVMA,* 217: 520, 2000.

18. Kirk CA, Ling GV, Franti CE, et al: Evaluation of factors associated with development of calcium oxalate urolithiasis in cats. *JAVMA* 207: 1429, 1995.

19. Thumchai R, Lulich JP, Osborne CA et al: Epizootiology evaluation of 3498 feline uroliths: 1982-1992. *JAVMA* 208: 547, 1996.

20. Kirk CA, Ling G, Osborne CA et al. Clinical guidelines for managing calcium oxalatee uroliths in cats: medical therapy, hydration, and dietary therapy. In, managing urolithiasis in cats: recent updates and practice guidelines. Lenexa KS, Thompson veterinary healthcare communications. 2003, p 10.

21. Osborne CA, Lulich JP Thumchai R et al: Diagnosis, medical treatment, and prognosis of feline urolithiasis. *Vet Clin N Amer* 26: 589, 1996.

22. Lekcharoensuk C, Lulich JP, Osborne CA et al. Association between dietary factors and feline calcium oxalate and magnesium ammonium phosphate urolithiasis. *JAVMA* 219; 1228, 2001.

23. Lulich JP, Osborne CA, Lekcharoensuk C: Effects of diet on urine composition of cats with calcium oxalate urolithiasis. *J Amer Anim Hosp Assoc* 40: 185, 2004.

24. Markwell PJ, Buffington CAT, Chew DJ, et al. Clinical evaluation of commercially available urinary acidification diets in the management of idiopathic cystitis in cats, *JAVMA* 214:361, 1999.

25. Osborne CA, Lulich JP, Kruger JM et al: Feline urethral plugs: Etiology and pathophysiology. *Vet Clin N Amer* 26: 233, 1996.

26. Lees GE: Bacterial urinary tract infections. *Vet Clin N Amer* 26: 297, 1996.

27. Kruger JM and Osborne CA: The role of uropathogens in feline lower urinary tract disease. *Vet Clin N Amer* 23: 101, 1993.

28. Bartges JW. Lower urinary tract disease in geriatric cats. In, Proceedings of the 15th American College of Veterinary Internal Medicine Forum, Orlando 1997, p322.

29. Barsanti JA, Shotts EB, Crowell WA, et al: Effect of therapy on susceptibility to urinary tract infection in male cats with indwelling urethral catheters. *J Vet Int Med* 6: 64, 1992.

30. Caston HT. Stress and the feline urological syndrome. *Feline Practice* 4:14, 1973.

31. Cameron ME, Casey RA, Bradshaw JWS, et al. A study of environmental and behavioural factors that may be associated with feline idiopathic cystitis. *J Small Anim Pract* 45:144, 2004.

32. Kalkstein TS, Kruger JM, Osborne CA. Feline idiopathic lower urinary tract disease. Part II. Potential causes. *Compend Cont Ed Pract Vet* 21:148, 1999.

33. Buffington CAT. External and internal influences on disease risk in cats. *JAVMA* 220, 994, 2002.

34. Westropp JL, Welk KA, Buffington CAT. Small adrenal glands in cats with feline interstitial cystitis. *J Urol* 170:2494, 2003.

35. Kruger JM, Osborne CA Lulich JP: Management of nonobstructive idiopathic feline lower urinary tract disease. *Vet Clin N Amer* 26: 571, 1996.

36. Barsanti JA, Brown J, Marks A, et al. Relationship of lower urinary tract signs to seropositivity for feline immunodeficiency virus in cats. *J Vet Int Med* 10:34, 1996.

37. Osborne CA, Kruger JM, Lulich JP: Feline lower urinary tract disease: The Minnesota Experience. In, Proc 15th Annual ACVIM Forum, San Antonio Texas 1997, p 338.

38. Kruger JM and Osborne CA: Recurrent nonobstructive idiopathic feline lower urinary tract disease: An illustrative case report. *J Amer Anim Hosp Assoc* 31: 312, 1995.

Chapter 68

Ureteral Ectopia

Mary A. McLoughlin

Anatomy of the Ureter

Ureters are fibromuscular tubes that transport urine through the retroperitoneal space from the renal pelvis to the urinary bladder.[1,2] Vascular supply to the ureter is derived from the cranial and caudal ureteral arteries that travel longitudinally and anastomose alongside the ureter. In males, the ureter passes dorsal to the ductus deferens, whereas in females, the ureter travels through the base of the broad ligament. Ureters exit the retroperitoneal space between the two-layer folds of peritoneum forming the lateral ligaments of the urinary bladder. Urine moves progressively through the ureters owing to organized peristaltic motion. Size of the ureter varies with species and patient size Ureters are considered to be larger than normal in dogs if the diameter is greater than 0.09 times the length of the second lumbar vertebrae. Enlarged ureters are usually greater than 3.0 mm.[3] Ureters attach to the dorsolateral surface of the bladder in the region of the bladder neck and pass through the bladder wall at an oblique angle creating a functional valve-like effect. The vesicoureteral junction can take on a "j"-shaped appearance.[3]

Embryologic Development

Understanding the complex embryologic development of the urogenital system forms a foundation for the understanding of some of the congenital abnormalities encountered in clinical medicine. Developmental abnormalities of the ureteral bud do not typically occur as an isolated event, but instead impact the development of the kidneys, bladder wall, trigone, vesicourethral junction, proximal urethra, internal sphincter mechanism, and some of the reproductive structures.

Development of the "normal" kidney and drainage system is classically described as proceeding through three successive yet integrated renal systems, pronephros, mesonephros, and metanephros, that share developmental components with the reproductive systems.[2,4-8] The most primitive form of the excretory system recognized in vertebrate animals is the pronephros. It is nonfunctional and quickly replaced by the mesonephros. However, a major portion of the pronephric duct is retained and later referred to as the mesonephric or Wolfian duct. The mesonephric duct system represents the second stage of excretory system development.[2,4,5] This will become the mature excretory system in amphibians, but only parts of this system are retained in the development of the excretory system of vertebrate animals. The mesonephric ducts are paired structures that fuse with the ventrolateral aspect of the cloaca.[5] As the cloaca divides to form the rectum and the urogenital sinus, the site of attachment of the mesonephric ducts differentiates, forming the posterior or dorsal wall of the urinary bladder. In males, parts of the mesonephric duct give rise to the ductus deferens. Close to their openings into the urethra, the seminal vesicles form.[2,4,5,8] In females, the reproductive structures actually arise and differentiate from the paramesonephric or Müllerian ducts. The Müllerian ducts arise separately in the mesoderm in close apposition to the mesonephric ducts (during the period of migration of the ureteric bud to the metanephros). It has been demonstrated that the Müllerian ducts arise inside the basal membrane of the mesonephric duct and may be derived from the same cells.[5] As, the Müllerian ducts migrate toward the urogenital sinus, they fuse together forming the uterus and vagina. The site of fusion between the Müllerian ducts and urogenital sinus forms the vestibulovaginal junction. A small layer of paramesonephric tissue referred to as the hymen is positioned between the membranes of the urogenital sinus and parametanephric duct.[8] This hymenal membrane usually ruptures at birth. Ultimately, the developing mesonephric ducts are resorbed leaving only scattered Gartner's glands as the only remnant in mature females.[2,4,5,8]

On the dorsal surface of the mesonephric duct, close to its attachment to the cloaca, the metanephric diverticulum or ureteral bud first arises.[2,4-8] Development of the metanephric system represents the third phase in the developmental progression. The ureteric bud extends dorsally to contact the developing metanephric blastemal ridge in the intermediate mesoderm and ultimately becomes the ureter. This contact or interaction between the ureteric bud and metanephric blastema is essential for the normal development of both the kidney and ureter, referred to as induction.[2,4,5-10] Within the metanephric blastema differentiation of the glomeruli, proximal and distal convoluted tubules, and the loops of Henle are initiated and maintained, forming the renal cortical structures. The proximal portion of the developing ureteral bud undergoes sequential division to form three major calyces, which, in turn, divide to form the minor calyces, papillary ducts, and collecting tubules, composing the medullary portion of the mature kidney. Synchronous migration of the kidney and ureter is occurring during this process of differentiation (Figure 68-1). Cranial migration of the kidney occurs to assume its final sublumbar position. Concurrently, the distal end of the ureteral bud is drawn toward the urogenital sinus.[4,5-9] The region of the mesonephric duct located between the urogenital sinus and the proximal region of the ureteral bud is referred to as the common excretory duct.[8] Migration or absorption of the common excretory duct into the wall of the urogenital sinus results in caudal migration of the ureteral bud. The future bladder neck and internal urethral meatus forms at the site of contact between the ureteral bud and urogenital sinus. The ureteral bud is positioned medial to the common excretory duct at the site of contact with the urogenital sinus. Cranial lateral migration of the ureter and caudal medial migration of the opening of the mesonephric duct occurs. Following migration, the ureteral orifice and the mesonephric duct opening (future deferent duct opening in males) are located equidistant from the neck of the bladder.[5,6,8] The common excretory duct extending between these openings develops into the trigonal base plate and ultimately the deep and superficial muscle layers of the trigone and proximal urethra in females and pelvic urethra in males, forming the internal urethra sphincter mechanism.[5-9]

Dysembryogenesis of the ureteral bud is the underlying cause of many congenital malformations of both the upper and lower urinary system.[6,7,10] Failure of the ureteral bud to arise from the mesonephric duct or failure of the bud to contact the metanephric blastema results in renal agenesis and may also result in failure of reproductive structures to develop. Abnormal positioning or lateral displacement of the ureteral bud on the mesonephric duct results in an altered migration pathway as the common excretory duct migrates or is absorbed into the wall of the urogenital sinus.[6-8] This subsequently results in distal displacement of the ureteral orifice, resulting in ectopic ureters and malformation of the structural integrity of the trigone (Figure 68-2). Bifurcation of the ureteral bud or formation of multiple ureteral buds will result in the formation of the duplex collecting system as the bud contacts and induces the metanephric blastemia.[6,7,9]

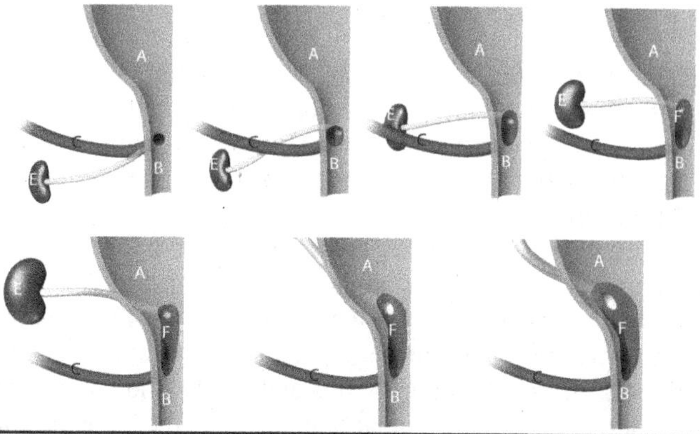

Figure 68-1. Migration of the ureteral bud and mesonephric opening through extrophy of the common excretory duct. A and B. Urogenital sinus (A to become the urinary bladder, B to become the urethra). C. Mesonephric duct. D. Ureteric bud. E. Metanephric mass to become the kidney. F. Region of common excretory duct (to form the trigone). (Adapted from: Cannizzo, K.L.: Uroendoscopic evaluation of ureteral ectopia in female dogs. Master's of Science Thesis, The Ohio State University 2001).

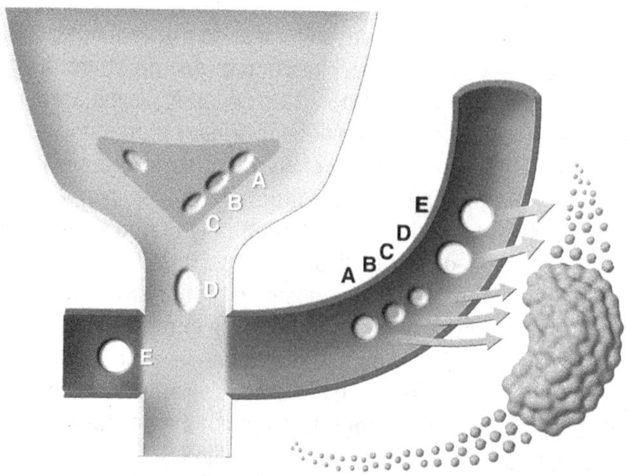

Figure 68-2. Association of ureteral bud position on the mesonephric duct and the resultant final position of the ureteral orifice. A. Normal position. B and C. Intravesicular ureteral ectopia. D. Urethral ureteral ectopia. E. Vestibular ureteral ectopia. (Adapted from: Cannizzo, K.L.: Uroendoscopic evaluation of ureteral ectopia in female dogs. Master's of Science Thesis, The Ohio State University 2001)

Ureteral Ectopia

Ureteral ectopia is a well-recognized congenital anomaly that may encompass a variety of malformations of both the urinary and reproductive systems. Ureteral ectopia is hallmarked by distal displacement of one or both ureteral orifice(s) to sites distal to the expected anatomic position at the tip of the trigone, frequently resulting in urinary incontinence.[11-16] Ureteral ectopia has been reported in dogs, cats, rats, horses, cattle, camilids, poultry, and humans.[2,4,8-23] The majority of the scientific literature pertaining to this developmental anomaly is focused on dogs and children. Distinct differences in the anatomy, morphology, and clinical presentation of ureteral ectopia exit between dogs and people. In humans, approximately 80% of all ectopic ureters are associated with a duplex collecting system, defined as a single kidney with complete duplication of the pyeloureteral system.[24,25] The ectopically displaced ureter is virtually always associated with the drainage of the upper moiety of the duplex system. Reports of duplex kidneys in veterinary patients are rare.[22,26]

The exact incidence of ureteral ectopia is unclear. Documentation of this anomaly is usually based on clinical signs of urinary incontinence in juvenile patients evident since birth or in adult female patients after ovariohysterectomy. Two previous studies have attempted to characterize the incidence of ureteral ectopia in a clinical population of dogs. One study reviewed a total of 67,721 small animal patients over a 7-year period, identifying 11 dogs with a confirmed diagnosis of ureteral ectopia. A second study reviewed 106,790 small animal patients, identifying a total of 18 affected dogs. An identical percentage incidence of occurrence was calculated at 0.016% for both studies.[4,27]

The specific locations of the displaced ureteral orifices have been well documented in both female and male dogs. Common sites of ectopically displaced ureteral orifices in females include sites within the trigone or bladder neck, vesicourethral junction, along the entire length of the urethra, or within the vagina or vestibule. However, in males the majority of displaced ureteral orifices are identified at the vesicourethral junction or pre-prostatic urethra in dogs.[4,12,13,15-18] Ureteral ectopia is frequently associated with intermittent, continuous or positional urinary incontinence and is considered to be the most common cause of urinary incontinence in young female dogs.[18] Affected females are identified approximately 4 to 20 times more frequently than affected male dogs.[4,13,15,16,18] This disparity likely reflects both a true sexual predisposition and under-diagnosis in continent male dogs. Urinary incontinence in male dogs with ectopic ureters may occur less frequently owing to the relative length of the urethra and increased pressure in the prostatic urethra and external sphincter mechanism that together oppose the passage of urine distally, resulting in retrograde bladder filling.[13,23]

Ureteral ectopia is reported in both purebred and mixed-breed dogs. It has been documented with greater frequency in specific breeds including Labrador retriever, Golden retriever, Siberian husky, Newfoundland, Skye terrier, West Highland white terrier, wire-haired fox terrier, and soft-coated Wheaten terrier, as well as standard and miniature poodles.[3,4,8,11-18] The specific etiology of this developmental anomaly remains unclear. A heritable basis for ureteral ectopia has been repeatedly suggested based on an increased incidence in predisposed breeds and potentially within family lines, identification of multiple affected littermates, and a single report of parent to offspring transmission.[5-8,16, 28-31] However, a genetic basis determined by a controlled breeding study, pedigree analysis, DNA analysis, or evaluation for gene mutations has not been performed. Hypervitaminosis A, deficiency in vitamin A and folic acid, and irradiation have been shown to result in urinary tract anomalies, including ureteral ectopia in rats but not in dogs.[32] Supplementation with vitamin A during gestation was also shown to eliminate these developmental defects.[4,5,7,8,32] At this point, no evidence suggests that diet or other specific environmental factors play a role in the development of ureteral ectopia.

Ectopic ureters are characterized as extramural or intramural based on their anatomic pathway. Extramural ectopic ureters bypass the urinary bladder and open directly into the vesicourethral junction, urethra, uterus, vagina, or vestibule.[4,8,11-13,15-18] Once considered to be a common finding, with improved diagnostic modalities it is now recognize that the incidence of extramural ectopic ureters in dogs is rare.[33,34] Intramural ectopic ureters attach to the serosal surface of the bladder in the expected dorsolateral position in the region of the bladder neck, but fail to open into the bladder lumen at the tip of the trigone. Intramural ureters tunnel distally below the submucosal layer to open at sites within the trigone, vesicourethral junction, urethra, vagina, or vestibule.[3,4,12,15,18,33-35] A number of anatomic variations of the terminal ureteral segment have been reported, including variations in the size and shape of the orifice, ureteral troughs, two ureteral openings on one or both ureters, multiple fenestrated openings along the submucosal tunnel, two submucosal tunnels opening through a single orifice, and presence of an ectopic ureterocele.[4,13,15,18,28,33-35] Ureteral ectopia is commonly associated with additional anomalies of the urinary system, including absent, small, or irregularly shaped kidneys, renal dysplasia, hydronephrosis, dilated ureter, tortuous ureter, pelvic bladder, shortened urethra, indistinct vesicoureteral junction, urachal remnants, and abnormal shape of the ureterovesical junction.[3,5,7,10]

Hydroureter is the most frequently reported abnormality associated with ureteral ectopia. It results from intermittent or partial urinary outflow obstruction. Ureteral dilation is most commonly associated with intramural ureters that are displaced to the distal aspect of the urethra or vestibule.[3,4,13,28,33,34] Intraluminal pressure within the urethra is increased between periods of micturition to maintain urinary continence. As urethral pressure increases and the lumen collapses, the ureteral remnant tunneling below the urethral mucosa also collapses, obstructing urine outflow. It is important to note that not all intramural ureters are dilated. Ureters that are minimally displaced, located within the trigone or vesicourethral junction, submucosal tunnels with multiple fenestrated openings, and ureters associated with a "trough-like" orifice are dilated less frequently.[4,12,13,33]

Clinical Presentation

Ureteral ectopia is the most common cause of urinary incontinence in young female dogs.[18] Ureteral ectopia should also be considered as a primary rule-out for patients with history of urinary incontinence developing after ovariohysterectomy, especially in breeds with a known predisposition for this anomaly. Normal voiding patterns and behavior can also be observed in affected patients. The cause of urinary incontinence associated with ureteral ectopia is considered multifactorial. Incontinence results from ureteral discharge of urine distal to the bladder neck and urethral sphincter mechanism or from functional and structural abnormalities of the vesicourethral junction and urethra, which result in primary sphincter mechanism incompetence.[4,12,13] The degree of urinary incontinence and patterns of urination cannot be used to confirm the diagnosis of ureteral ectopia nor determine if unilateral or bilateral disease exists.[4,12,13,16] Physical examination findings are often normal with the exception of moist or urine stained hair in the perivulvar or prepucial region. Secondary dermatitis or urine scalding may be observed. Abdominal palpation may detect marked abnormalities in kidney size or structure that can result from hydronephrosis or dysplasia. Hematologic and serum biochemical evaluations are normal unless associated abnormalities that diminish renal function exist. Urinary tract infections resulting from ascending bacterial pathogens are frequently identified.[2,36]

Methods of Diagnosis

The specific diagnosis of ureteral ectopia is based on identification of the ureteral orifice(s) distal to the expected position at the tip of the trigone. Historically, the diagnosis of ureteral ectopia has focused on the use of contrast radiographic procedures.

Plain and contrast radiography are frequently used to evaluate the upper and lower urinary tract of patients with suspected congenital anomalies and/or urinary incontinence. Excretory urography (IVU) and retrograde urethrography have long been considered the primary methods of diagnosis for ureteral ectopia in small animal patients.[4,11-13,16,33] These methods have been shown to provide a positive and anatomically accurate diagnosis in 62% to 77% of the confirmed cases of ureteral ectopia.[33] However, a variety of factors has been shown to compromise the diagnostic utility of these contrast procedures, including patient positioning and preparation, caudal displacement of the bladder (pelvic bladder syndrome), obscured visualization of the trigone and proximal urethra by overlying pelvic structures, degree of ureteral dilation or retrograde contrast accumulation.[33]

Intravenous urography provides valuable information regarding the upper urinary tract including renal structure and function, location, size and morphology of the ureters, and has the potential to determine location of the ureteral orifices. Lateral, ventrodorsal, and oblique radiographic views are necessary to assist in delineating the distal ureteral segment in the pelvic region. However, the diagnosis of ureteral ectopia often remains elusive following appropriate radiographic evaluation.[12,13,33]

Retrograde urethrography or vaginourethrography may provide additional information regarding length of the urethra, structure of the vesicourethral junction, identification of the ureteral orifices, and distal ureteral morphology.[33,37,38] One study demonstrated that retrograde ureteral filling with iodinated contrast was not observed in patients diagnosed with ectopic ureters unless the ureters were abnormally dilated. Dilation of the displaced ureters is reported in only 59% of the affected patients.[33]

Contrast-enhanced computed tomography (CT) is now considered the method of choice for evaluating ureteral ectopia in humans.[33] Improved spatial and temporal resolution characteristics of helical or axially acquired transverse imaging allows a more detailed evaluation of the anatomy because it is not obscured by overlying structures. A study to determine the diagnostic utility of helical CT for the diagnosis of ureteral ectopia was performed in 24 incontinent dogs with suspected ureteral ectopia. CT imaging reliably and accurately diagnosed ureteral ectopia and the specific location of the displaced ureteral orifices compared with traditional methods in 17 affected dogs.[33] Although CT imaging may be more costly, the superior diagnostic information obtained with CT as compared with other established techniques warrants its use. CT image interpretation does require experience and can be made more difficult by the need for systematic review of multiple image frames.[33]

Direct visualization of the lumenal surface of the lower urinary and reproductive tracts using a rigid or flexible endoscope can be performed in patients larger than 3 kg. Uroendoscopy has dramatically improved our ability to accurately diagnose ureteral ectopia and associated malformations of the ureteral orifices, vesicourethral junction, trigone, urethra, vestibule and vagina. This procedure also provides additional information regarding the anatomic pathway and morphology of the terminal ureteral segment.[12,13,16,28] Endoscopic evaluation of the distal segment of a dilated ureter can also be performed by gently passing an appropriately sized endoscope through the ureteral orifice into a dilated ureter. Radiographic evaluation of the upper urinary system should also be performed when the diagnosis of ureteral ectopia has been made by means of uroendoscopy. Contrast radiography, ultrasonography, or CT can be performed to assess the kidneys and ureters. Ultrasonographic examination is noninvasive and has been shown to be a reliable method of diagnosing ureteral ectopia when performed by a skilled operator. The confirmation of ureteral ectopia is made by identifying the location of the ureteral jet in addition to evaluating the size and structure of the ureter.[39,40]

Urodynamic evaluation, including cystometrogram and urethral pressure profile (UPP), has been shown to be a useful tool in the evaluation of the function of the bladder and urethra in patients with urinary incontinence and other voiding disorders. Results of urodynamic measurements have been reported in nine incontinent female dogs diagnosed with ureteral ectopia prior to surgical correction. Reduced bladder capacity and abnormalities in the urethral pressure profile consistent with urethral incompetence were noted in 89% of the dogs. Urodynamic assessment of dogs with ureteral ectopia may be valuable in identifying concurrent functional abnormalities of the lower urinary tract, but it may have limited use in predicting postoperative continence.[41]

Treatment

The goal of medical or surgical treatment of ureteral ectopia is resolution of urinary incontinence, re-establishment of anatomic integrity of the lower urinary system, and preservation of renal function. The treatment of ureteral ectopia is based on location and morphology of the ectopic ureter(s), and associated abnormalities of the urogenital systems.[4,12,13,16,35] Evaluation of renal function is necessary prior to instituting any type of therapy. Ultrasonographic evaluation of the kidneys and ureters combined with either IVU or renal nuclear scintigraphy is used to characterize renal function. Nephroureterectomy is performed when a kidney is determined to be nonfunctional and contralateral renal function is normal. A renal biopsy and culture are obtained if structural abnormalities of a functional kidney are noted or pyleonephritis is suspected.

Medical Treatment

Urinary incontinence associated with ureteral ectopia often is unresponsive or minimally responsive to accepted medical therapies, including the alpha-adrenergic agonists ephedrine sulfate or phenylpropanolamine, anticholinergic therapy such as oxybutinin, or hormonal therapy such as diethylstilbesterol (DES) in females or testosterone cypionate in males.[42,43]

Minimally Invasive Treatments

The treatment of primary sphincter mechanism incompetence using submucosal urethral bulking with bovine gluteraldehyde cross-linked collagen has been shown to be successful in female dogs with clinical signs of urinary incontinence.[44] The use of collagen injected both periurethrally and submucosally to treat urinary incontinence in women has been reported.[44] Urologic collagen is composed of highly purified bovine dermal collagen that is cross-linked with gluteraldehye in phosphate buffered saline. This product is composed of approximately 95% Type I collagen with 5% or less Type III collagen. A 14 or 19 French rigid endoscope with a 30-degree angle and a 4 French biopsy channel is used for uroendoscopy and placement of submucosal urethral bulking agents.

Complete evaluation of the lower urinary tract is performed prior to the injection of collagen. The tip of the endoscope is positioned to visualize the bladder neck and proximal urethra. The injection instrument is passed through the biopsy channel of the endoscope. The sites for injection are located approximately 1.5 cm. distal to the vesicourethral junction. Positioning of the endoscope facilitates inserting the beveled tip of the injection device below the urethral mucosa. Collagen is injected slowly while visualizing the distention of the urethral mucosa into the urethral lumen. Three to four sites are usually injected in a circular manner.[44] The procedure is considered complete when the injection sites appose one another. Complete urethral obstruction has not been reported in dogs.

Submucosal collagen implants have also been used to successfully treat selected dogs with proximally displaced ureteral ectopia without surgical intervention. The submucosal injection sites are positioned 1 to 1.5 cm distal to the displaced ureteral orifices, resulting in reflux of urine into the bladder lumen as well as creating obstruction to urine outflow. Ectopic ureter patients with moderate or severe ureteral dilatation or diminished renal function would not be consider a candidate for this noninvasive procedure.

Surgery

Evaluation of the upper and lower urinary tract is performed following a ventral midline celiotomy extending to the pubis. A stay suture placed in the apex of the bladder provides manipulation and retraction during the surgical exploratory and corrective procedures. The intrapelvic aspect of the female urethra can be exposed into the abdominal cavity by gentle traction on the apex of the bladder. A ventral midline cystotomy and urethrotomy are performed for direct visualization of the lumenal surface of the trigone, bladder neck, and urethra permitting identification of intramural ureters, submucosal tunnels, ureteral troughs, and most of the ectopically displaced ureteral orifices. Ureteral orifices located at the extreme terminal aspect of the urethra or vestibule may not be visualized from this approach without performing an osteotomy of the pubis to extend the urethral incision.

Ureteral Reimplantation/ Transposition

Transposition of a displaced ureter and ureteral orifice is indicated if the site of ureteral attachment is distal to the bladder neck. Surgical conformation of extramural ureters is infrequently reported.[12,13,28,33] Persistent urinary incontinence may result because the ureteral orifice is positioned distal to the bladder neck and urethral sphincter mechanism. Repositioning the distal segment of the ureter and ureteral orifice directly into the bladder may restore urinary continence if additional structural and/or functional abnormalities of the primary sphincter mechanism do not exist.

A ventral midline celiotomy is performed, and the extramural ureter is isolated distally where it attaches to the dorsal or dorsolateral surface of the bladder neck, vesicourethral junction, urethra, vagina, or uterus. The ureter is ligated at its most distal point of attachment with an absorbable suture and transected cranial to the ligature. The distal ureteral segment is isolated from the retroperitoneal space, respecting the ureteral blood supply that is positioned longitudinally within the fascial attachment. A ventral midline cystotomy is performed and the site of ureteral transposition is identified. This site can be located at any point between the apex of the bladder and the trigone. A mosquito hemostat is passed through a mucosal defect at an oblique angle and gently passed through the bladder wall. A small stay suture placed through the incised edge of the ureter is grasped to manipulate the ureter through the bladder wall. Once positioned within the bladder lumen, the terminal aspect (3-4 mm) of the ureter is excised and discarded. Intravesicular ureteral anastomosis is performed by suturing the ureteral mucosa to the bladder mucosa with a 5-0 absorbable monofilament suture material in an interrupted pattern. Surgical magnification may be necessary to accurately position these sutures. The bladder is closed in a routine manner.[2,4,12,13,35,45,46]

Neoureterostomy and Urethral/Trigonal Reconstruction

Intramural ectopic ureters pass through the bladder wall but fail to terminate and open into the bladder lumen at the tip of the trigone. This type of ectopic ureter continues to tunnel submucosally through the trigone to open at a site within or distal to the bladder neck. Urinary incontinence results owing to the ectopic location of the ureteral orifice and/or disruption of the smooth muscle layer of the urethral sphincter mechanism by the submucosal pathway of the ureteral remnant. Historically, surgical repair of intramural ectopic ureters has focused on the creation of a new ureteral opening within the bladder lumen and ligation of the distal submucosal ureteral segment, redirecting urine flow into the bladder lumen.[2,4,12,13,35,45-47] Persistent or recurrent urinary incontinence has been frequently reported after surgery.[2,12,13,35] To restore the functional anatomy of the internal urethral sphincter mechanism to improve continence after surgery, the terminal segment of the intramural ureter is resected from the surrounding tissues of the bladder neck and urethra. Surgical apposition of the mucosa and smooth muscle layers of the remaining defect are performed to realign the smooth muscle layer of the internal urethral sphincter mechanism.[12,13]

A ventral midline cystotomy and urethrotomy are performed, identifying the displaced ureteral orifices within the bladder neck and urethra. However, if a displaced ureteral orifice is located distally beyond the extent of this approach, in the terminal aspect of the urethra, a small incision is made through the distal urethral mucosa directly into the lumen of the submucosal ureter creating an orifice and avoiding the surgical morbidity of pelvic osteotomy. An appropriately sized urethral catheter (5, 8, or 10 French) is passed retrograde through each displaced ureteral orifice or distal ureterotomy incision. The catheter is passed retrograde to the site where the ureter passes through the bladder wall. It is essential to determine that this site is appropriately positioned near the tip of the trigone; if not, ureteral transposition should be performed. With the catheter in place, the submucosal ureter is sharply dissected from the surrounding urethral tissues including the mucosa, submucosa, and muscularis. Primary closure of the remaining defect in the bladder neck and urethra is performed using a 5-0 synthetic absorbable, monofilament suture material in a continuous or interrupted pattern. Closure of the urethral mucosa including a deep bite of the underlying smooth muscle layer is performed. Local hemorrhage is controlled by placement of the suture pattern to close the urethral defect. It may be necessary to dissect a portion of the submucosal ureter, immediately followed by closure of the defect to control hemorrhage before continuing with the complete dissection. The ureteral remnant is completely dissected from its submucosal position distally to the site where the ureter passes through the bladder wall. The ureter is transected approximately 0.5 cm from this site and sutured to create a new permanent ureteral opening within the bladder. Ureteral mucosa is sutured to the bladder mucosa using a 5-0 absorbable monofilament suture in an interrupted pattern. A balloon-tipped urethral catheter is passed into the bladder lumen, and a closed urine collection system is maintained for 24 to 36 hours after surgery. The cystotomy and urethrotomy are closed using 4-0 absorbable monofilament suture in a single or double layer continuous or interrupted pattern. Following removal of the urinary catheter, stranguria is frequently noted for several weeks after surgery.[12,13]

Nephroureterectomy

Removal of a nonfunctional kidney and associated ureter is indicated as a salvage procedure provided renal function in the contralateral kidney is normal. Aerobic bacteriologic cultures from the renal pelvis are obtained if a urinary tract infection has been documented or pyelonephritis is suspected. The ureter is sharply dissected from the ureteral fascia and retroperitoneal space to its termination. The ureter is ligated at its most distal point of attachment and transected cranial to the ligature. Removal of a nonfunctional kidney without the removal of an associated intramural ureter remnant will likely result in persistent urinary incontinence after surgery. The submucosal portion of the ectopic ureter is excised as previously described.

Post-Surgical Considerations

Persistent urinary incontinence is the most common complication after surgical repair of unilateral or bilateral ectopic ureters. Urinary incontinence has been reported to occur in 44% to 67% of patients after surgery.[2-4,15,18,27,35,36,41] Incontinence has been reported after ureteral reimplantation of extramural ectopic ureters as well as with neoureterostomy of intramural ectopic ureters and nephroureterectomy of a nonfunctional kidney associated with an ectopic ureter.[36] Associated primary sphincter mechanism incompetence is hypothesized to be an underlying cause of persistent urinary incontinence. Identification and treatment of urinary tract infection are the first steps in the management of any patient with persistent or recurrent urinary incontinence. Standard medical treatments with alpha-adrenergic agonist or anticholinergic drugs may have improved success in some patients with mild incontinence after surgery. Endoscopic injection of glutaraldehyde cross-linked collagen submucosally within the urethra has also been used successfully to treat persistent urinary incontinence.[1,2,44]

References

1. Christensen GC: The urogenital apparatus. *In* Miller's Anatomy of the Dog, 2nd ed. Evans HE , Christensen GC (eds). Philadelphia: WB Saunders, 1979, p. 551.

2. Alexander LG: Ectopic ureter and ureterocele. *In* Bojrab MJ (ed). Disease Mechanisms In Small Animal Surgery, 2nd ed. Malvern: Lea & Febiger, 1993, p. 515.

3. Mason LK, Stone EA, Biery DN, et al: Surgery of ectopic ureters: Pre- and postoperative radiographic morphology. J Am Anim Hosp Assoc 26:73, 1990.

4. Dean PW, Bojrab MJ, Constantinescu GM: Canine ectopic ureter. Comp Cont Educ Pract Vet 10(2):146, 1988.

5. Owen RR: Canine ureteral ectopia – a review. 1. Embryology and etiology. J Small Anim Pract, 14:407, 1973.

6. Tanagho E: Embryologic basis for lower ureteral abnormalities: a hypothesis. Urology 7:451, 1976.

7. Mackie GG: Abnormalities of the ureteral bud. Urol Clin North Am, 5:162, 1978.

8. Cannizzo KL: Uroendoscopic evaluation of ureteral ectopia in female dogs. Master's of Science Thesis, The Ohio State University, 2001.

9. Williams JL, Sago AL: Ureteral ectopia into seminal vesicle: embryology and clinical presentation. Urology 22(6):594,1983.

10. Li J, Hu T, Wang M, et al: Single ureteral ectopia with congenital renal dysplasia. J Urol 170:558, 2003.

11. Owen RR: Canine ureteral ectopia – a review. 2. Incidence, diagnosis and treatment. J Small Anim Pract 14:419, 1973.

12. McLoughlin MA, Chew DJ: Diagnosis and surgical management of ectopic ureters. Clin Tech Small Anim Pract 15:17, 2000.

13. McLoughlin MA, Bjorling DE: Surgery of the ureter. *In* Textbook of Small Animal Surgery, 3rd ed. Slatter D (ed). Philadelphia: WB Saunders, 2003, p. 1619.

14. Holt PE: Ectopic ureter in the bitch. Vet Rec 98:299, 1976.

15. Holt PE., Gibbs C, Pearson H: Canine ectopic ureter- A review of twenty-nine cases. J Small Anim Pract 23:195, 1982.

16. Sutherland-Smith J, Jerram RM, Walker AM, et al: Ectopic ureters and ureteroceles in dogs: presentation, cause and diagnosis. Comp Cont Educ Pract Vet, 4:303, 2004.

17. Hayes HM: Breed associations of canine ectopic ureter: a study of 217 female cases. J Small Anim Pract 25:501, 1984.

18. Holt PE, Moore AH: Canine ureteral ectopia: an analysis of 175 cases and comparison of surgical techniques. Vet Rec 136:345, 1995.

19. Blikslager AT, Green EM: Ectopic ureters in horses. Comp Cont Educ Pract Vet 14:802, 1992.

20. Cardwell JM, Thorne MH: Hydronephrosis and ureteral duplication in a young alpaca. Vet Rec 145(4):104, 1999.

21. Carrig CB, Grandage J, Ruth GR, et al: Ectopic ureter, ureteral stricture, and hemivertebrae in a heifer. J Am Vet Med Assoc 155(2):143, 1969.

22. Benko L: Cases of bilateral and unilateral duplication of ureters in the pig. Vet Rec 84(6):139, 1969.

23. Rutgers C, Chew DJ, Burt JK: Bilateral ectopic ureters in a female cat without urinary incontinence. J Am Vet Med Assoc 184:1394, 1984.

24. Gotoh T, Morita H, Tokunaka S, et al: Single ectopic ureter. J Urol 129:271,1983.

25. Wünsch L, Hübner U, Halsband H: Long-term results of treatment of single-system ectopic ureters. Pediatr Surg Int 16:493, 2000.

26. O'Handley P, Carrig CB, Walshaw R: Renal and ureteral duplication in a dog. J Am Vet Med Assoc 174:484, 1979.

27. Smith CW, Stowater JL, Kneller SK: Ectopic ureter in the dog-a review of cases. J Am Anim Hosp Assoc 17:245,1981.

28. Cannizzo KA, McLoughlin MA, Mattoon JS, et al: Transurethral cystoscopy and intravenous pyelography for the diagnosis of ectopic ureters in 25 female dogs. (1992-2000). J Am Vet Med Assoc 223:475, 2003.

29. Hayes HM Ectopic ureters in dogs: epidemiologic features. Teratology 10(2):129, 1974.

30. Musselman BC, Barry JJ: Varying degrees of ureteral ectopia and duplication in 5 siblings. J Urol 110:476, 1973.

31. Deweerd JH, Feeney DP: Bilateral ureteral ectopia with urinary incontinence in a mother and daughter. J Urol 98:335, 1967.

32. Kalter P, Warkany J: Experimental production of congenital malformations in strains of inbred mice by maternal treatment with hypervitaminosis A. Am J Pathol 38:1, 1961.

33. Samii VF, McLoughlin MA, Mattoon JS, et al: Digital fluoroscopic excretory urography, helical computed tomography and cystoscopy in 24 dogs with suspected ureteral ectopia. J Vet Intern Med 18:271, 2004.

34. Hosgood G, Salisbury SK, Blevins WE, et al: Unusual anatomic variation of bilateral ectopic ureters in a dog. J Am Vet Med Assoc 195:1591, 1989.

35. Stone EA, Mason LK: Surgery of ectopic ureters: types, method of correction, and postoperative results. J Am Anim Hosp Assoc 26:81, 1990.

36. McLaughlin R, Miller CW: Urinary incontinence after surgical repair of ureteral ectopia in dogs. Vet Surg 20:100, 1991.

37. Holt PE, Gibbs C, Latham J: Evaluation of positive contrast vaginourethrogram as a diagnostic aid in the bitch. J Small Anim Pract 25:531, 1984.

38. Leveille R, Atilola MA: Retrograde vaginocystography: a contrast study for evaluation of bitches with urinary incontinence. Comp Cont Educ Pract Vet 13:934, 1991.

39. Nyland TG, Samii VF: Radiographic and ultrasonographic imaging of the urinary tract and prostate. *In* Lower Urinary Tract Diseases in Dogs and Cats. Ling GV (ed). St. Louis: Mosby-YearBook, 1995, p. 70.

40. Lamb CR, Gregory SP: Ultrasonographic findings in 14 dogs with ectopic ureter. Vet Radiol Ultrasound 39(3):218, 1998.

41. Lane IF, Lappin MR, Seim HB: Evaluation of results of preoperative urodynamic measurements in nine dogs with ectopic ureters. J Am Vet Med Assoc 206:1348, 1995.

42. Rosen AE, Ross L:Diagnosis and pharmacological management of disorders of urinary incontinence in the dog. Comp Cont Educ Pract Vet 3:601, 1981.

43. Gregory SP: Developments in the understanding of the pathophysiology of urethral sphincter mechanism incompetence in the bitch. Br Vet J 150:135, 1984.

44. Arnold S, Hubler M, Lott-Stolz G, et al: Treatment of urinary incontinence in bitches by endoscopic injection of glutaraldehyde cross-linked collagen. J Small Anim Pract 37:163, 1996.

45. Sutherland-Smith J, Jerram RM, Walker AM, et al: Ectopic ureters and ureteroceles in dogs: treatment. Comp Cont Educ Pract Vet 4:311, 2004.

46. Rawlings CA: Repair of ectopic ureter. *In* Current Techniques in Small Animal Surgery, 2nd ed. Bojrab MJ (ed). Philadelphia: Lea & Febiger, 1983, pp. 308-312.

47. Dingwall JS, Eger CE, Owen RR: Clinical experiences with the combined technique of ureterovesicular anastomosis for treatment of ectopic ureters. J Am Anim Hosp Assoc 12:406, 1976.

Chapter 69

Canine Urethral Sphincter Mechanism Incompetence

Peter E Holt

During urine storage, urethral resistance is maintained by a complex mechanism of factors. These include tone in the urethral smooth muscle (the "internal" sphincter), tone in the urethral striated muscle (the "external" sphincter), the natural elasticity of the urethral wall tissues (not only musculature), the physical properties of the urethra (length and diameter), and the degree of engorgement of suburothelial venous plexuses. Because no true bladder neck sphincter exists in the bitch and continence is maintained by a complex mechanism of interacting factors, the term "urethral sphincter mechanism incompetence" was suggested to describe a weakness of the urinary sphincter.[1] This term has been widely adopted.

The neuromuscular function of the lower urinary tract in the dog is complex and not completely understood. A summary is provided in Figure 69-1.

Urethral sphincter mechanism incompetence occurs in dogs and cats, although it is rare in the latter. In dogs referred for the investigation of urinary incontinence, urethral sphincter mechanism incompetence is the most common diagnosis made in adults and is second only to ureteral ectopia in juveniles, particularly in females.[2-4]

It can present as a congenital or acquired condition. The acquired form is rare in the cat; in that species, most cases of urethral sphincter mechanism incompetence are congenital.[5] Although urethral pressure profilometry can be used to demonstrate incompetence of the urethral sphincter mechanism,[6] this technique is not readily available in general practice and is predisposed to a number of artefacts that can make interpretation difficult.[7,8] In general practice, therefore, the diagnosis is usually made on the basis of the breed and the history, and by the elimination of other possible diagnoses using imaging and laboratory techniques.

Congenital Urethral Sphincter Mechanism Incompetence in Bitches

This tends to be a problem of large breeds of dog, predominantly bitches. Leakage of urine is more copious compared with animals with ureteral ectopia and occurs predominantly when the dogs are recumbent. The urethra may be abnormally short or even absent, especially in cats, and urethral diverticula and dilations may be present in juvenile male dogs.[9] In many bitches,

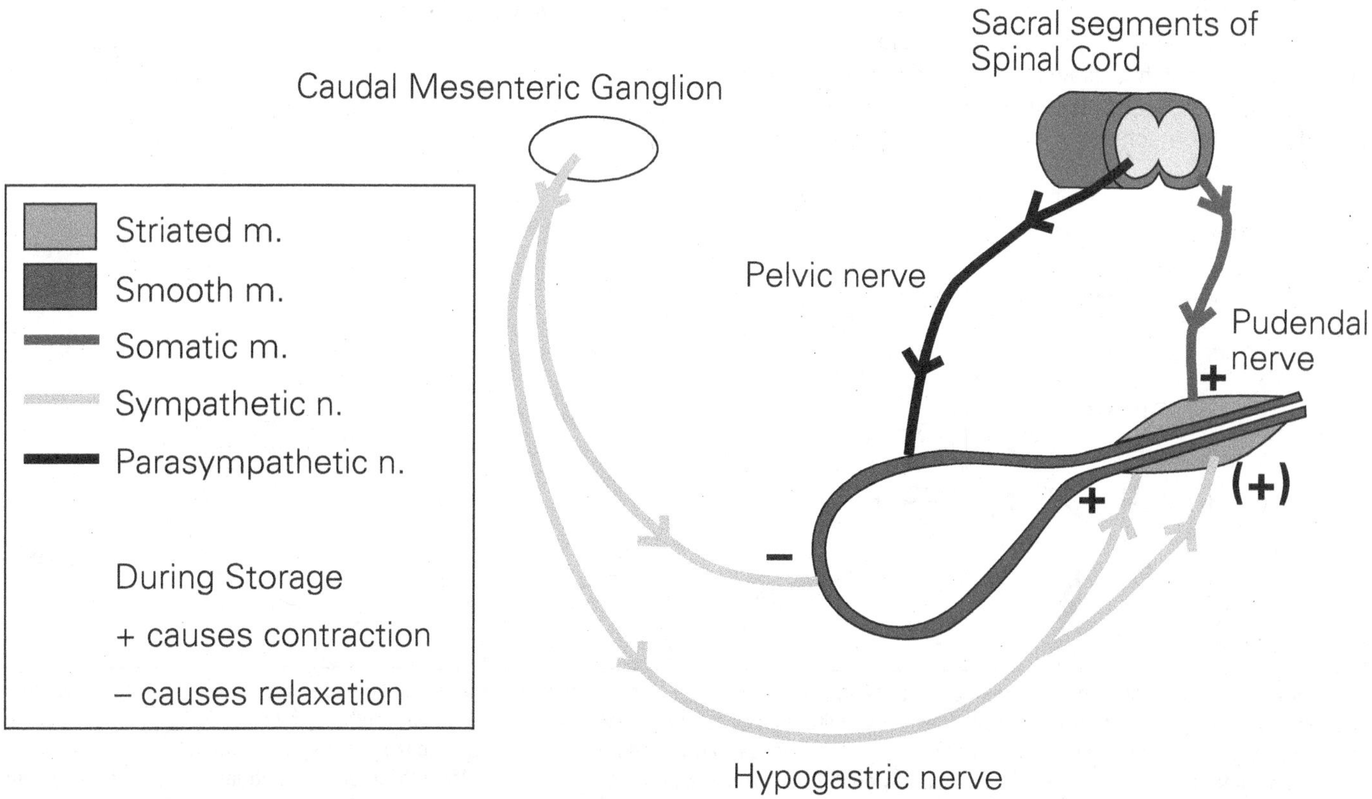

Figure 69-1. The neuromuscular control of urinary continence. During storage, the sympathetic innervation exerts a β (relaxation) effect on the bladder and an α-adrenergic (contractile) effect on urethral smooth muscle. In some species such as humans and cats, the sympathetic innervation also acts on the urethral striated muscle, but this has not yet been shown to occur in the dog. Urethral striated muscle provides additional tone during times of stress and is under voluntary control via the pudendal nerve.

no gross abnormalities are detected on contrast radiographic investigations, apart from a caudally positioned bladder. The diagnosis frequently relies on the history and elimination of other possible causes of incontinence. Approximately half of affected bitches become continent following their first estrus. Those that do not may be candidates for medical or surgical management. Estrogens are contraindicated in juvenile bitches with this condition because of possible adverse "feed-back" effects on the pituitary, but alpha-adrenergics such as phenylpropanolamine could be used, pending estrus.

Acquired Urethral Sphincter Mechanism Incompetence in Bitches

Acquired urethral sphincter mechanism incompetence usually (but not always) follows spaying in the bitch.[10,11] and castration in male dogs.[12] Before treatment can be contemplated, an understanding of the pathophysiology of urethral sphincter mechanism incompetence is required. The exact abnormality leading to urethral sphincter mechanism incompetence and the region of the urethra in which it occurs are unknown. It is a multifactorial problem and various factors are known or suspected to contribute to its clinical manifestation of urinary incontinence. These factors include urethral tone, urethral length, bladder neck position, body size and breed, ovariohysterectomy/ovariectomy, hormones, and obesity.

Urethral Tone

The introduction of urethral pressure profilometry as an investigative aid in the bitch has allowed confirmation of the belief that poor urethral tone is implicated in urinary incontinence owing to urethral sphincter mechanism incompetence.[6] Urethral tone is maintained by a complex interaction of neuromuscular, vascular, and passive elastic components, and it is unclear which of these is deficient in sphincter mechanism incompetence.

Urethral Length

Considerable variation exists in urethral length among bitches of different sizes. However, taking body size into consideration, bitches with urethral sphincter mechanism incompetence tend to have shorter urethras than do continent animals.[13]

Bladder Neck Position

Several authors recorded the radiographic finding of a "pelvic bladder" during the investigation of incontinent animals. The significance of this finding was disputed in the past but good evidence exists that an intrapelvic bladder neck contributes significantly to urinary incontinence owing to urethral sphincter mechanism incompetence.[13] The caudal bladder position in affected dogs is associated with the shorter urethral length and also the fact that the bladder moves caudally when a bitch moves from a standing to a relaxed recumbent position. This movement is more pronounced in bitches with urethral sphincter mechanism incompetence than in normal animals, suggesting a deficiency in supporting mechanisms in the lower urinary tract of affected animals.[14] The role of bladder neck position in bitches with urethral sphincter mechanism incompetence is thought to be due to changes in transference of abdominal pressures to the urethra (Figure 69-2).[13,15,16]

Body Size and Breed

Body size appears to be a factor because large and giant breeds are particularly at risk. Urethral sphincter mechanism incompetence is most common in the United Kingdom in Dobermans and

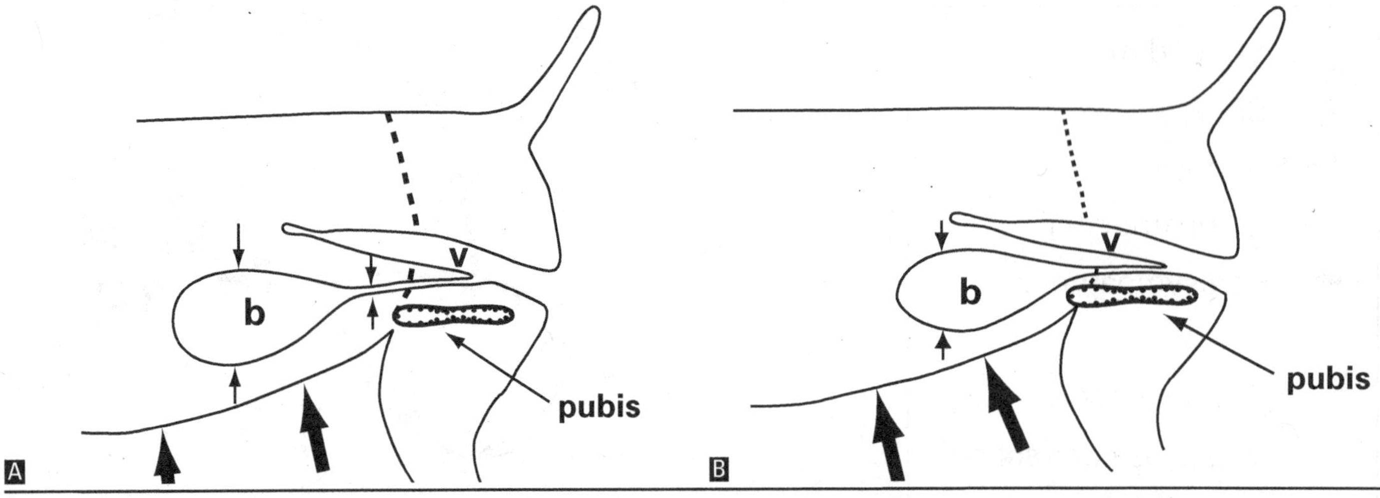

Figure 69-2. The effect of bladder neck position on continence control. In an animal with an intraabdominal bladder neck (A), increases in abdominal pressure are transmitted not only to the bladder but simultaneously to the bladder neck and proximal urethra. Thus any increase in intravesical pressure may be counteracted by an increase in urethral resistance. If the bladder neck is intrapelvic (B), however, abdominal pressure increases act predominantly on the bladder and less efficiently on the bladder neck and proximal urethra. If urethral tone is adequate, bladder neck position is of little relevance but, if urethral sphincter mechanism incompetence exists, the bitch with the anatomy illustrated in Figure 69-2B is more likely to leak urine at times of intraabdominal pressure increases (e.g., recumbency). Unfortunately for affected bitches and male dogs, the intrapelvic bladder neck is a common finding in animals with urethral sphincter mechanism incompetence. Retroperitoneal accumulations of fat in obese animals are likely to worsen this situation by displacing the caudal extent of the abdominal cavity cranially.
v – vagina; b – bladder; the dotted line represents the caudal extent of the abdominal (peritoneal) cavity.

Old English sheepdogs, and evidence exists that these breeds as well as Rottweilers, Weimaraners, springer spaniels, and Irish setters are particularly at risk.[10]

Ovariohysterectomy / Ovariectomy and Hormones

Aan association exists between spaying and urinary incontinence.[11] This is probably caused by a lack of circulating estrogens,[17] although one study suggests that an excess of gonadotrophins may also be a factor.[18] In general terms, spayed animals are nearly 8 times as likely to develop this form of urinary incontinence as are intact bitches.[11] However this should be considered in terms of dog years. In simple terms, if 100 bitches were not spayed, 10 years later, two of them would be incontinent. If 100 bitches were spayed, about 16 of them would be incontinent after 10 years. Spaying before the first season may increase the risk, although this could not be proved conclusively in a prospective study,[11] probably because of the low number of animals examined. One study suggested that, if early gonadectomy of female dogs is practiced, it should be delayed until the animal is at least three months of age.[19] The function and morphometry of the lower urinary tract are affected by the changes in hormone balance that occur during the estrus cycle.[20]

Obesity

Although not a cause of the condition, obesity may worsen the degree of incontinence, and weight loss may improve the situation.

Vestibulovaginal Stenosis in Relation to Urethral Sphincter Mechanism Incompetence in Bitches

Vestibulovaginal stenosis (owing to a true stricture or persistent perforate hymen) has been linked to urinary incontinence by some authors.[21-23] Holt and Sayle suggested that the incontinence might be associated with urine accumulating cranial to the stenosis during micturition and subsequently dribbling out.[21] However, Holt later demonstrated no difference in the prevalence of vestibulovaginal stenosis between normal and incontinent bitches.[13] The author now believes that vestibulovaginal stenosis per se is not a cause of incontinence, although if a bitch is already incontinent and leaking urine into the vagina, some may accumulate cranial to the stenosis, exacerbating the signs and predisposing to vaginitis. Experience suggests that the incontinence is a result of other causes such as urethral sphincter mechanism incompetence and that, if the incontinence owing to these other causes can be cured, the vestibulovaginal stenosis is irrelevant.

Urethral Sphincter Mechanism Incompetence in Male Dogs

Urethral sphincter mechanism incompetence in male dogs is uncommon.[9] As in the bitch, the condition can occur as either a congenital or acquired condition. The congenital condition is often associated with gross prostatic/pelvic urethral deformities (urethral dilatations and prostatic urethral diverticulae) and is unlikely to be successfully treated. As in the bitch, the acquired form is associated with neutering,[12] and larger breeds appear to be at risk. Incontinence is likely to occur when intraabdominal pressure increases (e.g., during recumbency). Affected animals tend to have intrapelvic bladder necks, although a short urethra does not appear to be a factor in males.[12] Conservative management is frequently disappointing. In comparison with the bitch, the condition is less likely to respond to medical therapy. The pathophysiology of male urethral sphincter mechanism incompetence is poorly understood, making rational treatment difficult. Drugs used in its management include androgens, estrogens, and alpha-adrenergics. Of these, alpha-adrenergics gave the best results but, even then, more than half of the dogs failed to respond to therapy.[9] Attempts have been made to relocate the intrapelvic bladder neck to an intraabdominal position. These have mainly involved pexy of the deferent ducts to the abdominal wall.[24,25] although the author has used prostatopexy (in castrated males) to the prepubic tendon.[26] As with medical treatment, the impression in a limited number of cases is that surgical treatment alone of urethral sphincter mechanism incompetence is less successful in males than in bitches.

Practical Applications

The treatment of sphincter mechanism incompetence may be difficult and most therapies correct only one of the factors discussed. It is unlikely, therefore, that any one form of treatment alone will cure 100% of cases in the long term.

In theory, sympathomimetic or parasympatholytic agents should improve continence control by increasing urethral tone or reducing intravesical pressure, respectively (Figure 69-1), but the results of clinical trials are variable and possible long-term adverse systemic effects have not been evaluated. Currently, the most popular medical treatment is the alpha-adrenergic, phenylpropanolamine.[27-30] Affected spayed bitches may also respond to therapy with estrogens such as estriol.[31] In some animals that respond initially to alpha-adrenergics or estrogens, the response ceases eventually. In the case of estrogens, this is possibly a result of desensitization of estrogen receptors. Estrogens sensitize the urethral smooth muscle to alpha-adrenergic stimulation and so a combination of estrogen and alpha-adrenergic therapy may be useful and reduce the dose of each individual drug, lessening the chances of side effects. Androgens have been employed in castrated male dogs but, in the author's experience, the results are disappointing.

The main options for surgical treatment are to attempt to:

- **increase urethral resistance** - e.g., peri-urethral surgical slings[32,33] or artificial sphincters;[34] intra-urethral injection of bulking agents;[35-37]
- **increase urethral length**, using bladder neck reconstruction techniques;[38]
- **re-locate the bladder neck to an intraabdominal position** by means of colposuspension,[39-43] vas deferentopexy,[24,25] urethropexy,[44,45] or prostatopexy.[26]

The potential problem with techniques intended to increase urethral resistance is that they may increase the morbidity by making an incontinent animal dysuric. Urethral bulking agents have been used most commonly to increase urethral resistance. Similarly, increasing urethral length carries potentially serious surgical risks and, in the author's view, should be reserved for animals with severe congenital urethral hypoplasia. In the author's opinion, the technique least likely to lead to serious complications is relocation of the bladder neck to an intraabdominal position by means of colposuspension. The greater experiences of medical urologists treating incontinent women suggests that colposuspension provides firmer anchorage of the lower urogenital tract than urethropexy and avoids urethral trauma. It may also prevent the caudal movement of the bladder that occurs during recumbency and is more pronounced in bitches with urethral sphincter mechanism incompetence.[14] However, a review of urethropexy as a treatment for urethral sphincter mechanism incompetence in 100 bitches revealed similar results to colposuspension,[45] although the prevalence and severity of urethral complications was higher. The reviewer believes that cystopexy is contraindicated in these cases because it may result in detrusor instability, a further cause of urinary incontinence.

Colposuspension is intended to move the intrapelvic bladder neck of bitches with urethral sphincter mechanism incompetence to an intraabdominal position so that increases in intraabdominal pressure can act simultaneously on the bladder and urethra. Thus, any increase in intravesical pressure is counteracted by an increase in urethral resistance (Figure 69-2).

Although great progress has been made over the past three decades in our understanding of the pathophysiology and, thus, the treatment of canine urethral sphincter mechanism incompetence, a recent editorial by one of the world's most respected urologists suggests we still have a great deal to learn.[46] Despite over 200 procedures being described for the treatment of human stress incontinence, the author was left asking, when it comes to his own patients, what should he do?

References

1. Holt PE: Urinary incontinence in the dog. In Pract 5:162, 1983.

2. Holt PE: Urinary incontinence in the bitch due to sphincter mechanism incompetence: prevalence in referred dogs and retrospective analysis of sixty cases.

J Small Anim Pract 26:181, 1985.

3. Holt PE: Urinary incontinence in dogs and cats. Vet Rec 127:347, 1990.

4. Holt PE: FECAVA LECTURE. Investigation and therapy of incontinent animals.

Eur J Comp Anim Pract 10:111, 2000.

5. Holt PE, Gibbs C: Congenital urinary incontinence in cats: a review of 19 cases. Vet Rec 130:437, 1992.

6. Holt PE: "Simultaneous" urethral pressure profilometry: comparisons between continent and incontinent bitches J Small Anim Pract 29:761, 1988.

7. Holt PE, Gibbs C, Wathes CM: Simultaneous urethral pressure profilometry using a microtip transducer catheter in the bitch: effects of bitch position and transducer orientation Neurourol Urodyn 9:281, 1990.

8. Holt PE, Gregory SP: Resting urethral pressure profilometry in bitches: artefact or reality? Comp Cont Educ Pract Vet 15:1207, 1993.

9. Aaron A, Eggleton E, Power C, Holt PE: Urethral sphincter mechanism incompetence in male dogs: a retrospective analysis of 54 cases. Vet Rec 139:542, 1996.

10. Holt PE, Thrusfield MV: Association in bitches between breed, size, neutering and docking, and acquired urinary incontinence due to incompetence of the urethral sphincter mechanism. Vet Rec 133:177, 1993.

11. Thrusfield MV, Muirhead RH, Holt PE: Acquired urinary incontinence in bitches: its incidence and relationship to neutering practices. J Small Anim Pract 39:559, 1998.

12. Power SC, Eggleton KE, Aaron AJ, et al: Urethral sphincter mechanism incompetence in the male dog: importance of bladder neck position, proximal urethral length and castration. J Small Anim Pract 39:69, 1998.

13. Holt PE: Importance of urethral length, bladder neck position and vestibulovaginal stenosis in sphincter mechanism incompetence in the incontinent bitch. Res Vet Sci 39:364, 1985.

14. Atalan G, Holt PE, Barr FJ: Ultrasonographic assessment of bladder neck mobility in continent bitches and bitches with urinary incontinence attributable to urethral sphincter mechanism incompetence. Am J Vet Res 59:673, 1998.

15. Gregory SP, Holt PE: Comparison of stressed simultaneous urethral pressure profiles between anesthetized continent and incontinent bitches with urethral sphincter mechanism incompetence. Am J Vet Res 54:216, 1993.

16. Holt PE, Jones A: In vitro study of the significance of bladder neck position in incontinent bitches. Vet Rec 146:437, 2000.

17. Nickel RF: Oestriol: pharmacology and effects on lower urinary tract function.

ESVIM Newsletter 9:13, 1999.

18. Reichler IM, Hubler M, Jöchle W, et al: The effect of GnRH analogs on urinary incontinence after ablation of the ovaries in dogs. Theriogenol 60:1207, 2003.

19. Spain CV, Scarlett JM, Houpt KA: Long-term risks and benefits of early-age gonadectomy in dogs. J Am Vet Med Assoc 224:380, 2004.

20. Hamaide AJ, Verstefen JP, Snaps FR, et al: Influence of the estrous cycle on urodynamic and morphometric measurements of the lower portion of the urogenital tract in dogs. Am J Vet Res 66:1075, 2005.

21. Holt PE, Sayle B: Congenital vestibulo-vaginal stenosis in the bitch. J Small Anim Pract 22:67, 1981.

22. Kyles AE, Vaden S, Hardie EM, Stone EA: Vestibulovaginal stenosis in dogs: 18 cases (1987-1995). J Am Vet Med Assoc 209:1889, 1996.

23. Crawford JT, Adams WM: Influence of vestibulovaginal stenosis, pelvic bladder, and recessed vulva on response to treatment for clinical signs of lower urinary tract disease in dogs: 38 cases (1990-1999). J Am Vet Med Assoc 221 995, 2002.

24. Weber UT, Arnold S, Hubler M, Kupper JR: Surgical treatment of male dogs with urinary incontinence due to urethral sphincter mechanism incompetence. Vet Surg 26:51, 1997.

25. Salomon JF, Cotard JP, Viguier E: Management of urethral sphincter mechanism incompetence in a male dog with laparoscopic-guided deferentopexy. J Small Anim Pract 43:501, 2002.

26. Holt PE, Coe RJ, Hotston Moore A: Prostatopexy as a treatment for urethral sphincter mechanism incompetence in male dogs. J Small Anim Pract (accepted for publication), 2005.

27. Richter KP, Ling GV: Clinical response and urethral pressure profile changes after phenylpropanolamine in dogs with primary sphincter incompetence. J Am Vet Med Assoc 187:605, 1985.

28. White RAS, Pomeroy CJ: Phenylpropanolamine: an α-adrenergic agent for the management of urinary incontinence in the bitch associated with urethral sphincter mechanism incompetence. Vet Rec 125:478, 1989.

29. Scott L, Leddy M, Bernay F, Davot JL: Evaluation of phenylpropanolamine in the treatment of urethral sphincter mechanism incompetence in the bitch. J Small Anim Pract 43:493, 2002.

30. Bacon N.J, Oni O, White RAS: Treatment of urethral sphincter mechanism incompetence in 11 bitches with a sustained-release formulation of phenylpropanolamine hydrochloride. Vet Rec 151:373, 2002.

31. Mandigers PJJ, Nell T: Treatment of bitches with acquired urinary incontinence with oestriol. Vet Rec 149:764, 2001.

32. Muir P, Goldsmid SE, Bellenger CR: Management of urinary incontinence in five bitches with incompetence of the urethral sphincter mechanism by colposuspension and a modified sling urethroplasty. Vet Rec 134:38, 1994.

33. Nickel RF, Wiegand U, Van Den Brom WE: Evaluation of a transpelvic sling procedure with and without colposuspension for treatment of femlae dogs with refractory urethral sphincter mechanism incompetence. Vet Surg 27:94, 1998.

34. Dean PW, Novotny MJ, O'Brien DP: Prosthetic sphincter for urinary incontinence: results in three cases. J Am Anim Hosp Assoc 25:447, 1989.

35. Arnold S, Jager P, DiBartola SP, et al: Treatment of urinary incontinence in dogs by endoscopic injection of Teflon. J Am Vet Med Assoc 195:1369, 1989.

36. Arnold S, Hubler M, Lott-Stolz G, Rusch P: Treatment of urinary incontinence in bitches by endoscopic injection of glutaraldehyde cross-linked collagen. J Small Anim Pract 37:163, 1996.

37. Barth A, Reichler IM, Hubler M, et al: Evaluation of long-term effects of endoscopic injection of collagen into the urethral submucosa for treatment of urethral sphincter mechanism incompetence in female dogs: 40 cases (1993-2000). J Am Vet Med Assoc 226:73, 2005.

38. Holt PE: Surgical management of congenital urethral sphincter mechanism incompetence in eight female cats and a bitch. Vet Surg 22:98, 1993.

39. Holt PE: Urinary incontinence in the bitch due to sphincter mechanism incompetence: surgical treatment. J Small Anim Pract 26:237, 1985.

40. Holt PE: Long-term evaluation of colposuspension in the treatment of urinary incontinence due to incompetence of the urethral sphincter mechanism in the bitch. Vet Rec 127:537, 1990.

41. Gregory SP, Holt PE: The immediate effect of colposuspension on resting and stressed urethral pressure profiles in anaesthetized incontinent bitches Vet Surg 23:330, 1994.

42. Rawlings CA, Mahaffey MB, Chernosky AC, Huzella L: Immediate urodynamic and anatomic response to colposuspension in female Beagles. Am J Vet Res 61:1353, 2000.

43. Rawlings CA, Barsanti JA, Mahaffey MB, Bement S: Evaluation of colposuspension for treatment of incontinence in spayed female dogs. J Am Vet Med Assoc 219:770, 2001.

44. Massat BJ, Gregory CR, Ling GV, et al: Cystourethropexy to correct refractory urinary incontinence due to urethral sphincter mechanism incompetence. Preliminary results in ten bitches. Vet Surg 22:260, 1993.

45. White RN: Urethropexy for the management of urethral sphincter mechanism incompetence in the bitch. J Small Anim Pract 42:481, 2001.

46. Blavais JG: What to do? Neurourol Urodyn 24:201, 2005.

Chapter 70

Urethral Disease and Obstructive Uropathy

Cheryl S. Hedlund
Giselle Hosgood

Urethral disease usually induces urinary incontinence or obstruction and produces characteristic clinical signs, including dysuria, stranguria, hematuria, pollakiuria, and urethral discharge. Urethral disease may be congenital or acquired and cause a functional or mechanical lesion (Table 70-1).

Table 70-1. Urethral Abnormalities Identified According to Predominant Clinical Characteristic

Urethral Abnormalities	
Urethral Incompetence	**Urethral Obstruction**
Neurogenic	Functional
Non-neurogenic	Mechanical
Congential	Calculi, plug
Hypospadia	Neoplasm
Epispadia	Polyp
Fistula	Granuloma
Stricture	Stricture
Ectopic ureter	Malpositioning
Ureterocele	Penile fractures
Acquired	Clots
Paradoxical incontinence	
Urethritis	
Sphincter mechanism incompetence	
Other Abnormalities	
Prolapse	
Disruption	

Normal Urethra

Anatomy

The urethra is the tube that conveys urine from the urinary bladder to the exterior of the body.[1] The male urethra is divided into prostatic, membranous, and spongiose or penile portions.[1,2] The prostatic portion extends from the urinary bladder to the caudal edge of the prostate, where the membranous portion begins. The membranous portion ends at the point of the bulb of the penis, where the spongiose portion continues to the external urethral orifice.[1,2] The vascular erectile tissue of the spongiose portion is continuous with the corpus spongiosum of the penis.[1] The female urethra corresponds to that portion of the male urethra cranial to the prostate.[1] The urethral mucosa is thrown into folds (rugae) that disappear with urethral distention. A prominent dorsomedian fold remains, known as the dorsal urethral crest.[1,2] In the male, the colliculus seminalis, an oval enlargement located in the middle of the urethral crest that projects into the urethral lumen, contains the minute openings of the uterus masculinus and is closely associated with the deferent ducts, which open on either side.[1,2]

The wall consists of four layers, mucosa, submucosa, muscularis, and adventia. The mucosa of both male and female urethras is predominantly transitional epithelium; it gradually changes to stratified squamous epithelium near the external urethral orifice. Stratified cuboidal, stratified columnar, or simple columnar epithelium is interspersed between these two sites.[2,3]

The propria submucosa consists of loose connective tissue with many elastic fibers and smooth muscle cells. The urethra in bitches is 68% to 78% connective tissue by volume.[4] Diffuse lymphatic tissue and nodules are also present in dogs.[2,3] Male cats also have simple tubular urethral glands.[2] Cavernous spaces in the submucosa and lamina propria along the entire length of the male and female urethra give the appearance of erectile tissue.[1-3] The quantity and size of cavernous spaces increase in the penile urethra where it becomes the corpus spongiosum.[2]

The urethral muscle is composed of three inner layers of smooth muscle and an outer layer of striated muscle and is continuous proximally with the detrusor muscle of the urinary bladder wall.[1] The amount of smooth versus striated muscle varies at sites along the urethra. In females, the proximal urethra is predominantly smooth muscle with a thick inner circular layer interspersed with thin, oblique fibers[5] and covered by a thin outer longitudinal layer.[3] Proximal smooth muscle has sphincter-like properties but is not a true anatomic sphincter and not under conscious control. Distally, the smooth muscle fibers become intermixed with striated muscle fibers and are replaced principally by circular striated bundles and a few longitudinal fibers. Terminally, a thin layer of circular smooth muscle lies on the inner side of predominant striated muscle bundles.[3] In males, smooth muscle predominates in the proximal urethra and striated muscle becomes dominant in the post-prostatic urethra.[6] In bitches, skeletal muscles is located in the distal half of the urethra.[7] Unlike dogs, cats have well organized circular and longitudinal smooth muscle fibers in the proximal urethra which shorten and widen the urethra during voiding.[7] Female cats have skeletal muscle in the distal third of the urethra.[7] The distal striated urethral muscle is functionally more efficient in males than in females and is under voluntary control.[8] Smooth muscles in the lower urinary tract are electrically coupled, exhibit spontaneous action potentials, contract when stretched, and are under autonomic control. Urethral muscle is surrounded by an adventitia of loose or dense irregular connective tissue.[2]

The blood supply to the urethra is by branches of the internal pudendal artery and vein.[1] Nerves leaving the pelvic and sacral plexuses (pelvic, pudendal, and hypogastric nerves) control functions involving the urethra.[1] Lymphatic drainage occurs through the medial iliac (formerly external iliac), hypogastric (formerly internal iliac), and sacral lymph nodes.[1]

Physiology

The primary functions of the urethra are (1) to maintain continence by providing resistance to urine flow in the nonvoiding state,[9] (2) to allow unhindered passage of urine during urinations,[9] and (3) to contribute to the normal host defenses against urinary tract infection.[10,11]

Micturition and Continence

Urinary continence is maintained by smooth and striated muscle tone, urethral wall elastic tension, and intraabdominal pressure and is influenced by urethral length. During voiding, simultaneous contraction of the urinary bladder and relaxation of the urethra allow urination.[12] It is triggered either by reflex or voluntarily. In reflex micturition, bladder afferent fibers excite neurons that project to the brainstem and activate the micturition center in the rostral pons and inhibit sympathetic preganglionic fibers that prevent voiding. Commands from the micturition center reach the sacral spinal cord through a reticulospinal pathway.[13] In voluntary micturition, the external sphincter is voluntarily relaxed by cortical inhibition of the pudendal nerve, which allows urine to flow through the meatus. With either mechanism, contraction of the destrusor muscle causes a vigorous discharge of the mechanoreceptors in the urinary bladder wall, which further activate the supraspinal loop and cause complete emptying of the urinary bladder.[14] During these phases, the urethra and the urinary bladder function interdependently and rely on the cerebral cortex for voluntary control.[9,12,14]

Micturition involves coordination of autonomic and somatic afferent and efferent activities. Postganglionic sympathetic innervation is via the hypogastric nerve, with preganglionic branches from the first and second lumbar spinal cord segments (L1, L2) in dogs or the second and third segments (L2, L3) in cats.[12,14] Parasympathetic innervation via the pelvic nerve originates from the first, second, and third sacral spinal cord segments (S1, S2, S3).[12,14] Somatic innervation of the striated urethral muscle is via the pudendal nerve originating from sacral cord segments S1 to S3.[12,14] Autonomic sympathetic impulses are mediated by acetylcholine at preganglionic synapses and norepinephrine at postganglionic synapses. Norepinephrine excites both alpha receptors (for contraction of smooth muscle; excites trigone and internal urethral sphincter) and beta receptors (for relaxation of smooth muscle; inhibits detrusor muscle).[12,14] Autonomic parasympathetic impulses activate cholinergic receptors of the urinary bladder and induce contraction of the detrusor smooth muscle.[12,14] The somatic innervation of the striated urethral muscle involves a single synapse between the motor nerve and the muscle, mediated by acetylcholine.[12,14]

Sympathetic autonomic activity dominates the storage phase: β-adrenergic stimulation facilitates relaxation of the detrusor muscle and α-adrenergic stimulation produces contraction of the trigone and proximal urethral smooth muscle to maintain continence. There is also α-adrenergic-mediated inhibition of parasympathetic transmission, decreasing cholinergic stimulation of the detrusor muscle and allowing relaxation.[8,12]

The primary adrenergic receptor within the prostatic urethra is the α_{1A} subtype (which is responsive to phenylephrine in a dose-dependent manner).[13] The striated urethral muscle plays a minimal role in maintaining continence, but somatic stimulation can cause temporary rapid contraction should increased resistance to urine flow be required.[8,12] The fibroelastic tissue of the urethra is also responsible for a significant component of resting urethral tone.[8,12]

The voiding phase is dominated by parasympathetic autonomic activity. Distention of the urinary bladder stimulates preganglionic parasympathetic sensory receptors through the pelvic nerve and initiates the micturition reflex.[12] Transmission through the parasympathetic ganglia in the pelvic plexus to postganglionic fibers stimulates the detrusor muscle and produces a wave of depolarization and subsequent strong, complete contraction of the urinary bladder. Simultaneously, sympathetic inhibition of the trigone and proximal urethra via the hypogastric nerve allows the smooth muscle to relax.[12] Pelvic nerve sensory neurons also send collaterals to inhibit interneurons in the sacral spinal cord. These in turn inhibit cell bodies of the pudendal nerve innervating the striated external urethral muscle.[12] When the urinary bladder is empty, discharges from the pelvic nerve cease, allowing for loss of inhibition of the hypogastric nerve (sympathetic) and the pudendal nerves (somatic) and closure of the urethra.[12]

Central control of micturition resides in the brain stem, at the level of the pons, and receives sensory stimulus from stretch and pain receptors in the urinary bladder. Voluntary control of the brain stem micturition center includes the cerbral cortex, basal gangia, thalamus, and cerebellum, and these components exert mostly an inhibitory influence over micturition.[12]

The Role of the Urethra in Host Defense

Some of the natural defense mechanisms of the urinary tract to prevent infection include the length of the urethra, the high pressure zones within the urethra, urethral and ureteral peristalsis, the vesicoureteral flaps that prevent urine reflux from the urinary bladder into the ureters, and the extensive renal blood supply and flow.[10,15] Other host defenses include the antimicrobial properties of urine, renal defenses, and systemic defenses. Most of the urinary tract is sterile; however, bacteria normally reside in the lower genitourinary tract. In dogs, these bacteria include species of *Staphylococcus, Streptococcus, Corynebacterium, Pasteurella, Proteus, Klebsiella, Mycoplasma, Escherichia coli* and others.[10] This resident population of bacteria may decrease establishment of a uropathogen or may emerge as a uropathogen if normal host defenses are altered. The uropathogenicity of each organism varies. The majority of urinary tract infections (UTI) result from ascending migration of pathogens.[10] The most common canine uropathogens are *Escherichia coli* (44.1%), *Staphylococcus spp* (11.6%), *Proteus* (9.3%), *Klebsiella spp* (9.1%), *Enterococcus spp* (8.0%) and *Streptococcus spp* (5.4%).[16] The identification of bacteria in the urine is not indicative of a urinary tract infection. An infection exists if a high number of bacteria exist in a properly collected and cultured sample.[10] The urethra contributes to the local host defenses involving normal micturition, anatomic barriers, and mucosal defense barriers.

Normal Micturition

Mechanical washout induced by unimpeded frequent and complete voiding of an adequate urine volume inhibits bacterial colonization of the urinary tract by rapidly eliminating organisms that reach the proximal urethra and urinary bladder.[10] Urination also reduces the microbial population of urethral mucosa by flushing the urethra with sterile urine. Washout is aided by distention of the urethra, which obliterates mucosal folds that could harbor bacteria.[10] The effectiveness of voiding depends on the rate of urine production, the frequency and completeness of voiding, and the rate of bacterial proliferation.[10] Urine composition also helps to prevent infections. Urine contains substances that inhibit bacterial colonization, including a high urea concentration, organic acids, low molecular weight carbohydrates and Tamm-Horsfall mucoprotein.[10,15] Cell-mediated and humoral immunity within the urine or urinary tract also give protection.[10,15] Antimicrobial properties of urine include extreme high or low urine pH, hyperosmolality, high urea concentration, organic acids, low molecular weight carbohydrates, Tamm-Horsfall mucoproteins, and perhaps others.[10,15]

Anatomic Barriers

A functional high-pressure zone in the mid-urethra of female dogs, corresponding to an area of smooth and striated muscle, has been hypothesized to inhibit the migration of bacteria along the urethra.[10] Surface characteristics of the urethral epithelium differ in the proximal and distal urethra and correlate, respectively, with absence or presence of bacteria. The normally sterile proximal urethra contains longitudinal folds called microplicae, which flatten when the lumen expands. The distal urethra contains microplicae, but it also has randomly arranged fingerlike projections called microvilli.[10] Urethral peristalsis, beginning in the proximal urethra and moving distally, may be important in maintaining unidirectional urine flow and inhibiting ascension of bacteria.[10] The incidence of cystitis is lower in males than in females, perhaps because of the gram-positive and gram-negative bactericidal fraction of prostatic fluid.[10] Nevertheless, in some dogs the prostate may act as a reservoir for bacteria.[17] In addition, the longer male urethra may provide greater resistance to bacterial access to the proximal urethra and urinary bladder.[10]

Mucosal Defense Barriers

Urinary tract mucosal defense barriers prevent bacterial migration and colonization. These barriers include a glycosaminoglycan layer, antibodies, intrinsic mucosal antimicrobial properties, cell exfoliation, and bacterial interference by commensal microbes of the distal urethra and distal genital tract.[15] Bacterial adherence to urethral epithelial surface is essential to subsequent tissue invasion and colonization.[11] The normal negative electric charge of both the bacterial cell wall and the urethral epithelium tends to repel the bacteria and prevent contact. Bacterial adherence is achieved by molecular bonding between molecular structures known as adhesins and specific receptor sites on the urethral epithelial surface.[11] Adhesins are present on bacterial cell wall fimbriae of gram-negative bacteria or on fibrillae of gram-positive bacteria. Although the mucosa has few direct antibacterial properties, a surface mucopolysaccharide glycosaminoglycan layer provides a barrier to bacterial adherence.[10] The urethral mucosa may also produce secretory immunoglobulin A (IgA).[10] Most of the IgA in the urine orginates from this source and inhibits bacterial ascent from the urethra to the urinary bladder.[10] Disruption of the surface glycosaminoglycan layer by acid or povidone-iodine, allows bacterial adherence to the urethral epithelium.[11] Exfoliation of urethral epithelial cells is a natural phenomenon that may be accelerated by abnormal conditions. This may expedite the removal of bacteria from the urethra during voiding.[10]

Urethral Dysfunction

Loss of normal urethral function usually results in urinary incontinence or obstruction. Urinary incontinence occurs when the intravesicular pressure exceeds the intraurethral pressure, resulting in uncontrolled loss of urine from the body. Incontinence may also occur owing to anatomic abnormalities that bypass the normal continence mechanisms (ectopic ureters). Such urinary incontinence is primarily caused by incompetence, and may be non-neurogenic or neurogenic. Urethral dysfunction causing urinary tract obstruction may be functional (neurogenic) or mechanical (intraluminal or extraluminal obstruction or loss of integrity). Urethral disease may also affect the ability of the urethra to contribute to host defenses against UTI. UTI is often a concurrent finding with urethral dysfunction, causing either incontinence or obstruction.

Urethral Incompetence

Non-Neurogenic Urethral Dysfunction as a Cause of Incontinence

Congenital or acquired urethral abnormalities may result in incontinence, including urethral malformations and conditions that cause urethral incompetence. In addition, urethral obstruction that leads to urinary bladder over-distention may cause detrusor damage and atony leading to overflow incontinence.

Congenital urethral disorders are infrequent. Urethral agenesis, urethral duplication, hypospadias, epispadias, diverticula, stricture, fistula, urethral ectopia, hermaphroditism, and pseudohermaphroditism have been reported. These conditions sometimes result in incontinence or abnormal flow of urine from the urethra.

Ectopic ureters may be associated with anatomic and functional abnormalities of the bladder and urethra.[18,19] Anatomic abnormalities of the urethra and vaginal vestibule are common in dogs with ectopic ureters and may result in continued incontinence after surgical repair if they are not treated concurrently. Urethral troughs, fenestrations, tenting, striping, and the intramural ureter in the dorsal urethral wall may affect the ability of the urethra to generate adequate closure pressure.[18,19] Congenital urethral incompetence that does not resolve after surgical treatment for ectopic ureters may also be a result of persistent ureteral malpositioning, vestibulovaginal malformation, or a congenital neuromuscular deficit on the proximal urethra.

For a discussion of acquired urethral incompetence see Chapter 69: Canine Urethral Sphincter Mechanism Incompetence

Paradoxical Urinary Incontinence

Paradoxical urinary incontinence mimics urethral obstruction without a physical obstruction.[20] Affected animals have a large urinary bladder and attempt to urinate without success. They may develop postrenal azotemia and uremia. Obstruction is believed to be caused by spastic contraction and inflammation secondary to chronic urethritis.[20] It is difficult to catheterize awake animals but anesthetized animals are catheterized without impedence. As the urinary bladder fills, intravesicular pressure eventually exceeds the resistance caused by the urethral lesion, resulting in urinary incontinence.

Urethritis

Chronic inflammation of the lower urinary tract may produce a syndrome of incontinence characterized by frequent, uncontrolled, involuntary detrusor contractions. It is a disorder of the storage phase of urination and is often referred to as urge incontinence. Inflammation of the urethra may be infectious or noninfectious. Urethritis is not a common clinical entity and is often associated with other urogenital inflammatory diseases, including prostatitis, cystitis, and vaginitis.[20] Noninfectious causes of urethritis, including trauma, chemicals, neoplasms, and urolithiasis, may predispose to bacterial urethritis. The normal urethra is not sterile, and resident bacteria normally populate the distal urethra.[10] Infectious urethritis may also occur secondary to infection elsewhere in the urogential tract (e.g., cystitis, prostatitis, or vaginitis).[20] Catheterization may induce urethritis through trauma, bacterial contamination, and reaction to the material of an indwelling catheter.[21]

Acute urethritis may induce stranguria or pollakiuria.[20] Gross hematuria may be present at the beginning of micturition. Urethral discharge must be differentiated from preputial or vaginal discharge.[20] Chronic urethritis may lead to urethral incompetence owing to fibrotic changes in the tissue. Similarly, infiltrative diseases such as neoplasms or granulomatous urethritis may also cause urethral incompetence.[22,23] As the intravesicular pressure increases, the damaged or diseased urethra is unable to prevent the flow of urine, and urinary incontinence results. Chronic urethritis with stricture or infiltrative disease can progress to cause urethral obstruction (see discussion of mechanical urethral obstruction later in this chapter).[22,23]

Neurogenic Urethral Dysfunction as a Cause of Incontinence

Lesions of the sacral spinal cord, sacral roots, or pudendal nerve decrease urethral pressure. Urethral muscle hypotonicity is commonly associated with lower motor neuron lesions at or caudal to the level of the L5 vertebrae (L6 in the cat). These lesions damage the sacral spinal cord segments or nerve roots (pudendal nerve and pelvic nerve).[24] Detrusor areflexia, with or without complete loss of urethral tone, usually results. With complete lesions, the striated urethral muscle is denervated but the hypogastric nerve innervating the proximal urethral smooth muscle remains intact, because it originates from lumbar spinal cord segments.[25] The sacral lesion abolishes normal sensory input from the stretch receptors in the detrusor muscle. As a result, the proximal urethral smooth muscle does not relax in response to the increased pressure of urinary bladder filling and remains fixed.[25] Manual expression of the urinary bladder may be easy or may meet resistance. Once the urinary bladder fills, the intravesicular pressure overcomes the proximal urethral smooth muscle resistance and overflow incontinence results. Some pain receptors in the hypogastric nerve may remain intact, and the animal may show discomfort and make unsuccessful attempts to urinate.[25]

Consequences of Urethral Incompetence

Urinary incontinence owing to urethral dysfunction results in urine soiling of the environment and pet, particularly causing skin irritation and scalding of the hind limbs, perineum, and ventral abdomen.[10,15] Overdistention of the urinary bladder may damage the muscle cells and also cause separation of the tight junctions between the detrusor muscle fibers, preventing excitation-contraction coupling (see discussion of consequences of chronic urethral obstruction later in this chapter). Increased capacity and incomplete emptying of the urinary bladder can result in large amounts of residual urine and predispose to recurrent urinary tract infection. Bacterial elimination from the urinary bladder is impaired after overdistention of the urinary bladder. Possible consequences of UTI include septicemia, discospondylitis, urolithiasis, incontinence, prostatitis, pyelonephritis, renal failure, and urinary bladder neoplasms. Long-standing urinary bladder distention and chronic UTI cause hypertrophy, hyperplasia, and connective tissue infiltration of the urinary bladder wall or urethra. This results in poor contractile function of these structures, and it reduces the capacity of the urinary bladder, thereby exacerbating the problem of urinary incontinence.

Urethral Obstruction

Urethral obstruction may be mechanical or functional. Diseases of the urethra frequently result in partial or complete obstruction of urine outflow. Calculi, neoplasia, granuloma, stricture, or urethral malpositioning can cause urethral obstruction. Occasionally, neurologic disease, prostatic disease, or blood clots may cause obstruction. The condition may be life-threatening and animals should be evaluated for hyperkalemia and metabolic acidosis. Total obstruction is an emergency as it quickly leads to uremia (two to three days) and death (three to six days) if untreated. Additionally, urethral obstruction can result in prolonged bladder distention, which causes temporary or permanent detrusor contractile dysfunction.

Functional Urethral Obstruction

Functional obstruction results from failure of coordination of urethral relaxation with detrusor contraction. Upper motor lesions of the urinary bladder with spinal lesions above L5 affect the suprasacral spinal cord segments.[12] The micturition reflex is lost, and detrusor areflexia with hypertonus of the urethra is the result of lack of inhibition of the hypogastric and pudendal nerves.[12] The urethral hypertonus causes increased resistance to urine flow, and manual urinary bladder expression is difficult. The animal does not perceive vesicle fullness, owing to loss of conscious sensation and cerebral motor control.[12] Micturition can be initiated by spinal reflexes, and a reflex bladder may develop over several days to weeks after the injury.[12] Once a threshold bladder capacity is reached, a "myotactic-like" reflex is initiated via stretch receptors in the bladder wall. These receptors send afferent impulses via the pelvic nerve to the sacral spinal cord. Depolarization of the pelvic nerve efferents contracts the detrusor muscle, but voiding is interrupted, involuntary, and incomplete, owing to failure of urethral relaxation.[12]

Partial suprasacral lesions may result in inappropriate contraction or relaxation failure of the urethral muscle, coincident with detrusor contraction. This condition is termed detrusor-urethral or reflex dyssynergia. The animal makes voluntary attempts to urinate but micturition is incomplete, giving the appearance of mechanical urethral obstruction.[12] The major resistance to urine flow is where the distal striated urethral muscle overlaps the proximal smooth muscle--approximately in the mid-urethra of females and the postprostatic membranous urethra of males. The primary cause of obstruction is thought to be over-discharge of the sympathetic nerve impulses to both the smooth and striated urethral muscle, causing increased intraurethral pressure during attempts at voiding.[12] Abnormalities of the somatic innervation to the urethral striated muscle may also contribute to the dyssynergia. Accompanying problems might include urinary tract infection, bladder atony, prostatic enlargement, urolithiasis, and priapism.[26,27]

Mechanical Urethral Obstruction

Intraluminal urethral obstruction may result from congenital or acquired urethral strictures, urethroliths, neoplasms, polyps, proliferative urethritis,[22] foreign bodies, blood clots, malpositioning, or penile fractures.[20,28-31] Urethral strictures may form secondary to previous urethral injury such as surgery, urethroliths, external trauma, or urethral catheterization. Urethral uroliths originate in the urinary bladder and cause urethral obstruction more frequently in male dogs, although this is reported in females. The most frequent site of urethral obstruction is the caudal end of the os penis, but uroliths can lodge elsewhere in the urethra. Clinical signs include stranguria and complete inability to urinate.

Primary urethral tumors are reported more frequently in older female dogs. Transitional cell carcinoma and squamous cell carcinoma are most common.[32-34] Other reported tumors include leiomyoma, leiomyosarcoma, prostatic adenocarcinoma, hemangiosarcoma, rhabdomyosarcoma, myxosarcoma, and lymphoma.[32-35] Metastases localize in regional lymph nodes and lungs.[32,33,35] Clinical signs vary and include stranguria associated with partial to complete obstruction. Hematuria and urinary incontinence are also reported.[34]

Proliferative urethritis (granulomatous infiltrative urethritis) is poorly defined in dogs. It is clinically indistinguishable from urethral neoplasms; typical clinical signs are stranguria, hematuria, and urinary obstruction.[22,23] Proliferations are often bands of tissue that are attached to the mucosa on both ends rather than being pedunculated or papillary. The mucosal proliferations can cause a one-way valve effect that causes outflow obstruction but often permits retrograde passage of urethral catheters. The urethra can be palpated as thickened and firm. Older female dogs appear predisposed to proliferative urethritis. The cause is unknown but the tissue reaction may represent a specific, cell-mediated reaction to antigens, organisms, or foreign bodies. Histologic findings include lymphoplasmacytic and neurotophic inflammation of the urethra.[22,23] The urethral epithelium becomes mildly to moderately hyperplastic. Multifocal, nodular, and coalescing aggregates of lymphocytes, plasma cells, macrophages, and neutrophils are observed in the mucosal and submucosal layers.[22,23]

Urethral obstruction in cats with idiopathic lower urinary tract disease may occur. Reasons for obstruction may include urethral inflammatory swelling, muscular spasms, reflex dyssynergia, luminal accumulation of sloughed tissue, inflammatory cells or erythrocytes, and formation of matrix-crystalline plugs.[36]

Extraluminal urethral obstruction can occur secondary to adjacent compressive masses or swelling. Fractures and tumors of the os penis have been reported to cause urethral obstruction.[37,38] Traumatic loss of urethral integrity from poor catheterization technique, pelvic fracture, and gunshot or bite wounds can lead to failure of urine outflow and signs consistent with outflow obstruction.

Consequences of Urethral Obstruction[8,39]

The consequences of urethral obstruction depend on whether the obstruction is acute or chronic and partial or complete. Partial or early outflow obstruction may not impair renal function sufficiently to cause uremia; however, complete obstruction causes signs of uremia within 24 hours. As functional renal mass decreases or as intravesical, ureteral, and renal pressure increases, urine concentrating ability is lost. Additionally, urethral obstruction may lead to detrusor atony, mucosal damage, urinary tract infection, and urethral or urinary bladder rupture. Acute complete or severe partial obstruction produces postrenal azotemia and uremia that, if not corrected, is fatal in 3 to 6 days. In contrast, chronic partial obstruction causes excessive pressure in the excretory pathway as the urinary bladder's capacity is exceeded. This increase in pressure causes progressive dilatation of the urinary tract, and damage to renal parenchyma may be sufficient to cause chronic renal failure.

Acute Complete Urethral Obstruction

Acute complete urethral obstruction manifests as anuria and results in overdistention of the urinary bladder. Local pressure at the obstruction site damages the muscosa, causing swelling, hemorrhage, and epithelial denudation. Overdistention of the urinary bladder causes similar changes. Outflow obstruction results in increased pressure in the urinary bladder and urethra proximal to the site of obstruction. As intravesicular pressure increases, damage occurs to the urothelium and detrusor muscle. Nerves in the urinary bladder wall are damaged and inflammatory cells infiltrate. The kidneys and ureters are affected if back pressure persists. As the urinary bladder's capacity is exceeded, intraureteral and renal intratubular pressures increase.[40] Normal pressure in the renal pelvis and ureters of the dog ranges from zero to 10 mm Hg.[41] With complete ureteral obstruction during saline diuresis, ureteral pressure in dogs reach 50 to 150 mm Hg within 5 to 15 minutes.[42,43] After 4 hours of obstruction, intratubular pressure declines but can still be as much as 3 times normal.[44-46] The decline in intratubular pressure is thought to result from a reduction in fluid volume in the tubular system because of decreased glomerular filtration rate (GFR), increased tubular reabsorption, or increased capacity of a compliant renal pelvis.[40]

Reduced Glomerular Filtration Rate

The GFR is determined by (1) the net ultrafiltration pressure across the glomerular capillaries (the difference between the hydrostatic pressure in the glomerular capillaries and the sum of the plasma oncotic pressure in the glomerular capillaries plus the hydrostatic pressure in Bowman's space); (2) the permeability of the glomerular capillary wall to water and small solutes; and (3) the surface area of the capillaries.[40] Urinary tract obstruction can affect one or more of these factors, significantly decreasing GFR.

As intratubular pressure increases, a decrease occurs in the effective filtration pressure (the difference between intraglomerular capillary pressure and the pressure in Bowman's space or intratubular pressure). This decrease is mainly due to a reduction in hydrostatic pressure in the glomerular capillaries and is accompanied by a marked decrease in renal blood flow after 24 hours' obstruction.[47-49] Progressive preglomerular constriction occurs with obstruction for longer than 5 hours, with a decrease in GFR of approximately 80% after 24 hours' obstruction.[50-52] Obstruction results in heterogeneous nephron function. Some nephrons cease to function and others show decreased GFR; they are, respectively, known as nonfiltering and filtering nephrons.[40] The GFR of outer, cortical nephrons is less affected than that of the inner, juxamedullary nephrons: after 24 hours' obstruction, decreases are 60% to 70% and 50% of normal, respectively.[52] After 24 hours, GFR decreases further owing to the major vasoconstricting agents thromboxane A_2, angiotensin II, and maybe the endothelial-derived relaxing factor.[39] The obstructed kidney may prevent further decrements in GFR by the production of vasodilatory prostaglandins such as prostaglandin E_2 and prostacyclin which antagonize the vasoconstrictive effects of thromboxane A_2 and angiotensin II.[39] Recovery of GFR following relief of obstruction decreases as the duration of obstruction increases.

Renal Hemodynamics

During obstructive uropathy, changes in renal blood flow can be divided into 3 phases.[40] During the first phase, 1 to 2 hours after obstruction, renal cortical blood flow actually increases above normal, in association with a decrease in intrarenal resistance and gradually increasing intraureteral pressure.[53-57] However, inner medullary blood flow decreases from the onset of obstruction, reaching less than 30% of normal within 6 hours.[85]

The initial increase in blood flow may be the result of augmented production of vasodilatory prostaglandins (prostaglandin E_2 [PG E_2] and prostacylin) by the obstructed kidney.[59-60] Increased renal prostaglandin production by the interstitial medullary cells is thought to be the result of a decline in the inner medullary blood flow secondary to the increase in ureteral pressure. The prostaglandin synthesis causes abrupt changes in vascular resistance with an overshoot in renal blood flow, seen in the fist phase.[40] During the second phase, 2 to 5 hours after obstruction, the renal blood flow decreases to normal and intraureteral pressure continues to increase. The second phase may be the result of an increase in renal resistance, a direct effect of increasing ureteral pressure on the interstitium. Finally, in the third phase, ureteral pressure begins to decrease but renal blood flow continues to decline progressively with time. The final, chronic phase is the result of an increase in resistance at the preglomerular level.[40] The progressive decrease in blood flow may be a result of increased production of thromboxane A_2, a metabolite of arachidonic acid and a powerful vasoconstrictor.[40] Persistent renin secretion and angiotensin production may also play a role in vasoconstriction, although the evidence is conflicting.[61-62] Renin initiates the production of angiotensin, a potent vasoconstrictor. Cells of the outer cortical nephrons have a higher concentration of renin than those of the juxtamedullary nephrons.[41] Increased renal nerve activity or high levels of catecholamines at critical sites in the kidney might also contribute to vasoconstriction and decreased renal blood flow.[63-65]

Soon after the onset of acute ureteral obstruction, an influx into the kidney occurs of leukocytes, primarily macrophages and T lymphocytes.[39] This influx is associated with a relative depletion of macrophages from the glomeruli. After relief of obstruction, the macrophage and T-lymphocyte infiltrate decreases over days.

Tubular Effects

The degree and duration of obstruction determine the degree and nature of tubular effects and their recovery.[39] Tubular abnormalities include a concentrating defect, altered reabsorption of solutes and water, and impaired excretion of hydrogen and potassium. Sodium, potassium, phosphate, magnesium, and proton retention may occur during obstruction. Tubular dysfunction may continue after relief of the obstruction owing to tubular damage.

Electrolytes

Complete urinary obstruction can lead to death from uremia in 3 to 6 days. Death is a result of combined abnormalities in fluid, electrolyte, and acid-base balances that result in accumulation of metabolic waste products.[39] Characteristically, hyperkalemic metabolic acidosis occurs, and serum phosphorous and calcium values may be elevated. Fractional excretion of potassium increases after relief of obstruction and hypokalemia may occur postobstruction.[39] This may be caused by increased delivery of sodium to the distal tubule where sodium-potassium exchange occurs.

Acidifying Defect

Metabolic acidemia associated with urethral obstruction results from retention of metabolic acids, consumption of bicarbonate to stabilize plasma and compartmental pH, generation of lactate associated with hypovolemia and hypoxia, and decreased conservation of bicarbonate in the obstructive and postobstructive periods.[39]

Direct effects of acidemia include decreased myocardial contractility, stroke volume, and cardiac output; excitable membrane alterations leading to dysrhythmias; central nervous system depression; and dysfunction of metabolic pathways.[39] Indirect effects of acidemia include alterations in transcellular potassium distribution, plasma protein binding, ionization of pharmacologic agents, oxygen transport, tissue catabolism, and increased parasympathetic activity. Whereas animals with urinary tract obstruction have hyperkalemic metabolic acidosis, a urine acidifying defect is apparent and may persist after relief of the obstruction.[40] Two defects have been isolated, a selective aldosterone deficiency and distal renal tubular acidosis, or the two may be combined. Two mechanisms are proposed. First, bicarbonate excretion increases markedly, owing to altered proximal tubule reabsorption.[40] Second, the kidney's ability to acidify urine at distal sites is impaired. The ability of outer cortical nephrons to secrete hydrogen ions appears intact, and the defect is most likely in the collecting duct or juxtamedullary nephrons.[66]

Sequela after Release of Obstruction

The decrease of GFR associated with 24 to 36 hours of obstruction is completely reversible.[67] Most early alterations in the kidney are functional and do not result in permanent loss of nephrons.[68] Complete obstruction for more than 6 days does result in permanent loss of nephrons.[68] Dogs with unilateral ureteral obstruction showed 39% recovery of renal function after 2 weeks of obstruction, 10% after 4 weeks, and 2% after 6 weeks.[40] Urinary tract obstruction, even after release, alters the kidney's ability to modulate water and electrolyte excretion. One of the first abnormalities in kidney function following obstruction is a decrease in the urinary concentrating ability. Following release of urinary tract obstruction a dramatic loss of water and solute occurs, a phenomenon referred to a postobstructive diuresis.[40,41] The factors presumed to be involved in the concentrating defect of obstructive uropathy include decreased removal of solute from the thick ascending limb of the loop of Henle, decreased total number of juxtamedullary nephrons, washout of solutes from the medulla owing to increased medullary blood flow, and decreased hydro-osmotic response of the cortical collecting duct to antidiuretic hormone.[69]

Factors contributing to this phenomenon include the volume status of the animal before release of the obstruction. Animals often receive intravenous fluids and undergo volume expansion. In part, the increased urine flow and sodium excretion after release of obstruction is a physiologic response to volume expansion.[70] Accumulation of urea and other relatively nonabsorbable solutes during obstruction can promote solute diuresis and result in loss of much sodium and water after release.[40]

The inappropriate increase in urine output after urinary obstruction release may also result from an intrinsic defect in renal tubular function. Studies have demonstrated a defect along the proximal and distal tubules of outer cortical nephrons and to the level of the loop of Henle in the juxtamedullary nephrons.[51,67] Other studies suggest the medullary collecting duct may be the site of altered water and sodium reabsorption.[41]

The medullary interstitial cells, responsible for prostaglandin synthesis, show proliferative changes by 5 days after obstruction.[39] Increased medullary prostaglandin synthesis decreases the reabsorption of sodium chloride by the medullary ascending limb of the loop of Henle and the medullary solute content.[40] Increased prostaglandin secretion may also increase blood flow in the vasa recta and cause persistent increase in blood flow in the vasa recta and cause persitent washout of the medulla. A decrease in medullary solute content has the end result of decreasing the diffusion of water out of the collecting duct.[40]

An increase in medullary prostaglandin production may antagonize the effect of vasopressin, reducing the permeability of the collecting tubules to water and contributing to the decrease of urine osmolality.[40] After obstruction, vasopressin-dependent cAMP production may also be impaired.[71,72]

Chronic Urethral Obstruction

Chronic partial obstruction is not immediately life threatening but results in pathologic changes in the urinary bladder, ureters, and kidneys. Chronic overdistention of the urinary bladder owing to resistance to urinary outflow may cause varying degrees of hydroureter and hydronephrosis.

During the early phases of obstruction, functional and morphologic changes in the ureter and renal pelvis include muscular hypertrophy and hyperplasia. Later, collagen and elastic connective tissue are produced by the smooth muscle cells, which impairs myogenic impulse transmission and distrupts normal peristalsis.[39]

Structural renal changes during hydronephrosis can result in chronic renal failure. Experimental urethral obstruction in the rat, rabbit, and dog cause initial changes in the proximal tubules, which show a transient dilatation over several days, and then undergo atrophy.[8] By 14 days postobstruction, there is progressive dilatation of the distal and collecting tubules with atrophy of the proximal tubular cells.[8] By 28 days, medullary thickness is reduced by 50%, anddilatation and atrophy of the distal and collecting tubules continues.[8] The cortex becomes thinner and the proximal tubules are markedly atrophic. Glomerular changes are noted after 28 days. By 8 weeks, only a thin parenchymal strip of connective tissue and small glomeruli remains.[8]

During chronic hydronephrosis with high intratubular pressures, 80% to 90% of the urine is reabsorbed into the tubules and exits via the renal veins.[8] A small portion of urine is reabsorbed into the hilar lymphatic vessels, and some fluid is extravasated into the perirenal spaces.[8]

Chronic Urinary Bladder Distention

Urinary bladder outlet obstruction with distention produces significant alterations in detrusor structure and function.[73] Chronic urinary bladder outlet obstruction causes increased thickness of the urinary bladder wall owing to muscle hypertrophy, hyperplasia, and collagen deposition by the smooth muscle cells.[74] Hypertrophy is the predominant response to moderate obstruction, whereas hyperplasia with more collagen deposition is the predominate response to severe obstruction.[74]

Although the urinary bladder enlarges, its compliance and capacity decrease.[73] This is demonstrated by a sharp incline in the filling limb of the cystometrogram.[73] Chronic obstruction results in reduced detrusor contractility and evidence of partial denervation is reported.[75-77] Postjunctional supersensitivity secondary to partial denervationcontributes to detrusor instability,[75,76] characterized by frequent, inappropriate detrusor contractions. Obstruction can cause rapid changes, and muscarinic receptor density is reduced by 50% after 24 hours' distention.[73] The defect in contractile mechanism is not solely due to low muscarinic receptor density.[78] Other factors in reduced contractility include a decrease in the myofilaments of hypertrophic smooth muscle cells; weak contractions of hyperplastic, immature muscle cells; weak contractions of hyperplastic, immature muscle cells;[74] increased noncontractile elements in the urinary bladder wall;[73] and decreased propagation of action potentials through the detrusor muscle secondary to intercellular disruption.[79] Electron microscopy studies of rabbit detrusor muscle after urinary bladder distention have shown acute disruption of intercellular junctions with secondary intercellular fibrosis.[80] Two months after urinary bladder distention, intracellular separation of the cytoplasm from the plasma membrane of the detrusor muscle fibers was demonstrated.[79] Results of another study question whether these changes are significant and really represent "disruption" of junctions. Gosling and coworkers reported similar findings in distended bladders and those of normal control subjects.[81] They proposed that these junctions represent normal "intermediate" junctions, as opposed to "close" or tight junctions. In their study, neither junction type was affected by distention.[81]

Urinary bladder outlet obstruction also alters the metabolic function of the urinary bladder, which may contribute to altered contractility.[82] After 2 weeks of obstruction, urinary bladder tissue showed a decrease in aerobic metabolism and an increase in anaerobic metabolism.[82] The ability of the urinary bladder to maintain a contraction and empty may be directly related to aerobic metabolism. Subsequently, the decrease in aerobic metabolism, even in the presence of increased anaerobic metabolism, may contribute to the decreased ability of the obstructed urinary bladder to empty.[82] Another study found that urinary bladder tissue shows a marked decrease in ATP concentration after obstruction, which may be attributed to the ischemic conditions created by distention.[81] Distention of the dog's urinary bladder for 2 hours reduced blood flow in the mucosa, muscularis, and total bladder tissue by 25% to 30% in each component.[81] In addition, the increase in connective tissue in the urinary bladder wall lowers the overall intracellular concentration of ATP in the smooth muscle.[81]

Sequelae after Release of Chronic Obstruction

Outflow obstruction predisposes to bacterial infections. Contributing factors include catheterization, urine stasis, vesicoureteral reflux and pre-existing infections. Detrusor atony and urethral swelling or spasm may contribute to urine stasis.[39]

After release of chronic urinary obstruction, postobstruction diuresis and concentrating defects are observed. The amount of function recovered depends on the duration of obstruction.[8] Release of obstruction within 6 days may allow full return of function. Release after 14 days may restore 50% to 65% function. Release after 30 days of obstruction may restore up to 30% of function. Obstruction for more than 4 weeks may result in permanent damage.[41]

Postobstruction renal failure may occur as a result of renal parenchymal loss owing to sustained increased intrarenal pressure, cytokine production by infiltrating leukocytes, electrolyte imbalances, fibrosis of damaged renal parenchyma, and renal ischemia owing to dehydration.[69] Death may be associated with fluid and electrolyte imbalances as a result of cardiopulmonary failure.

Other Abnormalities

Urethral prolapse

Urethral prolapse is an eversion or prolapse of mucosa from the tip of the penis. Dogs present for signs of preputial or penile bleeding. It is seen most often in young male brachycephalic dogs and can be associated with sexual excitement or stranguria associated with urethral infection or urolithiasis.[83,84] The exact cause is unknown but theories speculate a genetic predisposition or an increased abdominal pressure secondary to chronic upper airway obstruction.[84] In people, poor attachment between the muscle layers of the urethra associated with episodic increases in abdominal pressure is proposed as a cause.[84]

Urethral Trauma

Urethral injury may be associated with catheterization, obstruction or external trauma, especially abdominal, pelvic, or perineal trauma. Types of trauma include urethral contusions, tears, avulsion, or os penis fracture. Contusions may be asymptomatic or may cause hematuria, dysuria, and pollakiuria. Those with tears or avulsion may be unable to urinate or may have hematuria. Trauma resulting in disruption of urethral integrity results in urine leaking into the surrounding tissues or abdomen, causing a chemical-type irritation. Leakage into the subcutaneous tissues results in severe swelling, discoloration, and sometimes tissue necrosis. Urine contact with tissues for more than 12 to 24 hours results in inflammation, edema, and cellulitis, which delays healing and promotes fibrosis.[85] Uroabdomen results in profound dehydration, life-threatening hyperkalemia, severe postrenal azotemia, chemical peritonitis, and metabolic acidosis.[85] Manifestations of uroabdomen include lethargy, anorexia, vomiting, dehydration, abdominal distention, and pain. Additional complications of urtheral injury include stricture formation and urinary incontinence.

Urine is hyperosmolar and an accumulation in the abdominal cavity creates a concentration gradient across the peritoneum from the extracellualr fluid compartment to the abdominal cavity. Large molecules such as creatinine pull water into the abdomen whereas smaller solutes such as urea and electrolytes (potassium) diffuse into the extracellular fluid compartment. Sodium and chloride diffuse into the abdomen. Dehydration results from a combination of fluid shifts, fluid losses from vomiting, and a decrease in fluid intake. Dehydration leads to a decrease in glomerular filtration and a subsequent decrease in excretion of urea and creatinine. Retention of urine in the abdomen with accumulation of excretory products also results in increased serum urea and creatinine. The body's normal buffer system is depleted as hydrogen retained in abdominal urine is reabsorbed through peritoneal capillaries, leading to metablolic acidosis. The production of lactic acid secondary to poor tissue perfusion resulting from dehydration and hypovolemic shock also contribute to metabolic acidosis.

Urine accumulation in the abdomen causes a chemical peritonitis that results in functional ileus and pain. Septic peritionitis may occur if a urinary tract infection existed or a penetrating injury had occurred. Peritionitis contributes to a shift of fluid from the extracellular space into the abdomen with a concurrent loss of albumin into the abdominal effusion.[85]

References

1. Evans HE, Christensen GC: The urogenital sytem. *In* Miller's Anatomy of the Dog, 3rd ed. Evans HE (ed). Philadelphia: WB Saunders, 1993, p. 494.

2. Wrobel KH: Male reproductive system. *In* Textbook of Histology, 5th ed. Dellman HD, Eurell JA (eds). Philadelphia: Williams & Wilkins, 1998, p. 226.

3. Hendricks C: Urinary system. *In* Textbook of Histology, 5th ed. Dellman HD, Eurell JA (eds). Philadelphia: Williams & Wilkins, 1998, p. 203.

4. Augsburger HR, Cruze-Orive LM: Stereological analysis of the urethra in sexual intact and spayed female dogs. Acta Anat 154:135, 1995.

5. Cullen WC, Fletcher TF, Bradley WE: Histology of the canine urethra. I. Morphology of the female urethra. Anat Rec 199:177, 1981.

6. Cullen WC, Fletcher TF, Bradley WE: Histology of the canine urethra. II. Morphology of the male urethra. Anat Rec 199:187, 1981.

7. Goodkin JL, Stone EA, Sharp NJ: Urinary incontinence in dogs and cats. Part I. Urethral pressure profilometry. Comp Cont Educ 18(4):407, 1996.

8. Hosgood G, Hedlund CS: Urethral disease and obstructive uropathy. *In* Disease Mechanisms in Small Animal Surgery, 2nd ed. Bojrab MJ (ed). Philadelphia: Lea & Febiger, 1993, p. 528.

9. Filippich LJ, Read RA, Riesz G: Functional urethral obstruction in a cat. Aust Vet Pract 19:202, 1990.

10. Osborne CA, Lees GE: Bacterial infections of the canine and feline urinary tract. *In* Canine and Feline Nephrology and Urology. Osborne CA, Finco DR (eds). Baltimore: Williams & Wilkins, 1995, p. 759.

11. Senior DR: Bacterial urinary tract infections: Invasion, host defenses, and new approaches to prevention. Comp Cont Educ 7:334, 1985.

12. Lane IF: Disorders of micturition. *In* Canine and Feline Nephrology and Urology. Osborne CA, Finco DR (eds). Baltimore: Williams & Wilkins, 1995, p. 693.

13. Brune ME, Katwala SP, Milicic I, et al: Effects of selective and nonselective alpha-1-adrenoceptor antagonists ion intraurethral and arteriole pressures in intact and conscious dogs. Pharmacology 53:356, 1996.

14. Labato MA: Micurition disorders. *In* Textbook of Veterinary Internal Medicine: Diseases of Dogs and Cats, 6th ed. Ettinger SJ, Feldman EC (eds). St Louis: Elsevier Saunders, 2005, p. 105.

15. Bartges JW: Urinary tract infections. *In* Textbook of Veterinary Internal Medicine: Diseases of Dogs and Cats, 6th ed. Ettinger SJ, Feldman EC (eds). St Louis: Elsevier Saunders, 2005, p.1800.

16. Ling GV, Norris CR, Franti CE, et al: Interrelations of organism prevalence, specimen collection method and host age, sex and breed among 8,354 canine urinary tract infections (1969-1995). J Vet Intern Med 15:341, 2001.

17. Rogers KS, Lees GE, Simpson RB: Effects of single-dose and three-day trimethoprim-sulfadiazine and amikacin treatment of induced E. coli urinary tract infections in dogs. Am J Vet Res 49:345, 1988.

18. Cannizzo KL, McLoughlin MA, Mattoon JS, et al.: Evaluation of transurethral cystoscopy and excretory urography for diagnosis of ectopic ureters in female dogs: 25 cases (1992-2000). J Am Vet Med Assoc 223:475, 2003.

19. Lane IF, Lappin MR, Seim HB: Evaluation of results of preoperative urodynamic measurements in nine dogs with ectopic ureters. J Am Vet Med Assoc 206:1348, 1995.

20. Krawiec DR: Urethral diseases of dogs and cats. *In* Canine and Feline Nephrology and Urology. Osborne CA, Finco DR (eds). Baltimore: Williams & Wilkins, 1995, p. 718.

21. Lees GE, Osborne CA, Stevens JB, et al.: Adverse effects caused by polypropylene and polyvinyl feline urinary catheters. Am J Vet Res 41:1836, 1980.

22. Moroff SD, Brown BA, Matthiesen DT, et al: Infiltrative urethral disease in female dogs: 41 cases (1980-1987). J Am Vet Med Assoc 199:247, 1991.

23. Hostutler RA, Chew DJ, Eaton KA, et al: Cystoscopic appearance of proliferative urethritis in 2 dogs before and after treatment. J Vet Intern Med 18:113, 2004.

24. Gookin JL, Stone EA, Sharp NJ: Urinary incontinence in dogs and cats; Part II Diagnosis and management. Comp Cont Educ 18:525, 1996.

25. McGuire EJ: The innervation and function of the lower urinary tract. J Neurosurg 65:278, 1986.

26. Lane IF: Diagnosis and management of urinary retention. Vet Clin North Am 30(1):25, 2000.

27. Lane IF, Fischer JR, Miller E, et al: Function urethral obstruction in three dogs: Clinical and urethral pressure profile findings. J Vet Intern Med 14:43, 2000.

28. Breitschwerdt EB, Olivier NB, King GK, et al: Bilateral hydronephrosis and hydroureter in a dog associated with congenital urethral stricture. J Am Anim Hosp Assoc 18:799, 1982.

29. Rawlings CA: Extraperitoneal urinary bladder rupture and urinary fistula in a dog. J Am Anim Hosp Assoc 115:123, 1969.

30. Adams LG, Syme HM: Canine Lower urinary tract diseases. *In* Textbook of Veterinary Internal Medicine: Diseases of Dogs and Cats, 6th ed. Ettinger SJ, Feldman EC (eds). St Louis: Elsevier Saunders, 2005, p. 1850.

31. Elwick KE, Melendez LD, Higbee RG, et al: Neodymium:Yttrium-aluminum-garnet (Nd:YAG) laser ablation of an obstructive urethral polyp in a dog. J Am Anim Hosp Assoc 39:506, 2002.

32. Tarvin G, Patnaik A, Greene R: Primary urethral tumors in dogs. J Am Vet Med Assoc 172:931, 1978.

33. Wilson GP, Hayes HM, Casey HW: Canine urethral cancer. J Am Anim Hosp Assoc 15:741, 1979.

34. Stone EA: Urogenital tumors. Vet Clin North Am 15:597, 1985.

35. Davies RV, Read HM: Urethral tumors in dogs. J Small Anim Pract 31:131, 1990.

36. Kalkstein TS, Kruger JM, Osborne CA: Feline idiopathic lower urinary tract disease. Part 1. Clinical manifestations. Comp Cont Educ 21(1):15, 1999.

37. Mirkovic TK, Shmon CL, Allen AL: Urinary obstruction secondary to an ossifying fibroma of the os penis in a dog. J Am Anim Hosp Assoc 40:152, 2004.

38. Bradley RL: Complete urethral obstruction secondary to fracture of the os penis. Comp Cont Educ 7:759, 1985.

39. Bartges JW, Finco DR, Polzin DJ, et al.: Pathophysiology of urethral obstruction. Vet Clin North Am 26(2):255, 1996.

40. Klahr S: Pathophysiology of obstructive nephropathy. Kidney Int 23:414, 1983.

41. Brace JJ: Urinary tract obstruction. *In* Pathophysiology of Small Animal Surgery, Bojrab MJ (ed). Philadelphia, Lea & Febiger, 1981, p. 288.

42. Taylor MG, Ulmann E: Glomerular filtration after obstruction of the ureter. J Physiol 157:38, 1961.

43. Papdopoulou ZL: Glomerular filtration during stop flow. Proc Soc Exp Biol Med 130:1206, 1969.

44. Jaenike JR: The renal response to ureteral obstruction: A model for the study of factors which influence glomerular filtration pressure. J Lab Clin Med 76:373, 1970.

45. Yarger WE, Aynedjian HS, Bank N: A micropuncture study of postobstructive diuresis in the rat. J Clin Invest 51:625, 1972.

46. DalCanton A, Corradi A, Stanziale R, et al.: Glomerular hemodynamics before and after release of 24-hour bilateral ureteral obstruction. Kidney Int 17:491, 1980.

47. DalCanton A, Corradi A, Stanziale R, et al.: Effects of 24 hour unilateral ureteral obstruction on glomerular hemodynamics in rat kidney. Kidney Int 15:457, 1979.

48. Vaughan ED, Sorenson EJ, Gillenwater JY: The renal hemodynamic response to chronic unilateral complete ureteral occlusion. Invest Urol 8:78, 1970.

49. Hsu CH, Kurtz TW, Rosenzweig J, et al: Intrarenal hemodynamics and ureteral pressure during ureteral obstruction. Invest Urol 14:442, 1977.

50. Harris RH, Yarger WE: Renal function after release of unilateral obstruction in rats. Am J Physiol 227:806, 1974.

51. Buerkert J, Head M, Klahr S: Effects of acute bilateral ureteral obstruction on deep nephron and terminal collecting duct function in the young rat. J Clin Invest 59:1055, 1977.

52. Buerkert J, Martin D, Head M, et al.: Deep nephron function after release of acute unilateral obstruction in the young rat. J Clin Invest 62:1228, 1978.

53. Moody TE, Vaughan ED, Gillenwater JY: Comparison of the renal hemodynamic response to unilateral and bilateral ureteral occlusion. Invest Urol 14:455, 1977.

54. DalCanton A, Stanziale R, Corradi A, et al: Effects of acute ureteral obstruction on glomerular hemodynamics in rat kidney. Kidney Int 12:403, 1977.

55. Selkurt EE: Effects of ureteral blockade on renal blood flow and urinary concentrating ability. Am J Physiol 205:286, 1963.

56. Gilmore JP: Influence of tissue pressure on renal blood flow autoregulation. Am J Physiol 206:707, 1964.

57. Schramm LP: Influence of tissue pressure on renal vasoconstriction by elevated ureteral pressure. Am J Physiol 228:1126, 1975.

58. Solez K, Ponchak S, Buono RA, et al.: Inner medullary plasma flow in the kidney with ureteral obstruction. Am J Physiol 231:1315, 1976.

59. Allen JT, Vaughan ED, Gillenwater JY: The effect of indomethacin on renal blood flow and ureteral pressure in unilateral ureteral obstruction in awake dogs. Invest Urol 15:324, 1978.

60. Blackshear, JL, Wathen RL: Effects of indomethacin on renal blood flow and renin secretory responses to ureteral occlusion in the dog. Miner Electrolyte Metabol 1:271, 1978.

61. Yarger WE, Schocken DD, Harris RH: Obstructive nephropathy in the rat. Possible roles for renin-angiotensin system, protaglandins and thromboxanes in postobstructive renal function. J Clin Invest 65:400, 1980.

62. Moody TE, Vaughan ED Jr, Wyker AT, et al: The role of intrarenal angiotensin II in the hemodynamic response to unilateral obstructive uropathy. Invest Urol 14:390, 1977.

63. Wilson DR, Honrath U, Sole M: Effect of acute and chronic renal denervation on renal function after release of unilateral ureteral obstruction in the rat. Can J Physiol Pharmacol 57:731, 1979.

64. DiBona GF, Rios LL: Renal nerves in compensatory renal response to contralateral adaptation to ureteral occlusion. Am J Physiol 238:F26, 1980.

65. Francisco LL, Hoversten LG, DiBona GF: Renal nerves in the compensatory adaptation to ureteral occlusion. Am J Physiol 238:F229, 1980.

66. Thirakomen K, Kozlov N, Arruda JAL, et al.: Renal hydrogen ion secretion after release of unilateral ureteral obstruction. Am J Physiol 231:1233, 1976.

67. McDougal WS, Wright FS: Defect in proximal and distal sodium transport in postobstructive diuresis. Kidney Int 2:304, 1972.

68. Kerr WS: Effects of complete ureteral obstruction in dogs on kidney function. Am J Physiol 184:521, 1956.

69. Saphasan S, Sorrasuchart S: Factors inducing post-obstructive diuresis in rats. Nephron 38:125, 1984.

70. Muldowney FP, Duffy GJ, Kelly DG, et al: Sodium diuresis after relief of obstructive uropathy. N Engl J Med 274:1294, 1966.

71. Beck N, Webster SK: Impaired urinary concentrating ability and vasopressin-dependent cyclic AMP in post-obstructive kidneys (abstr.). Kidney Int 8:455, 1975.

72. Weber H, Schlondoroff D, Trizna W: The adenylate cyclase system in obstructive uropathy: a model for the mechanism of altered end-organ responsiveness (abstr.). Kidney Int 8:464, 1975.

73. Malkowicz SB, Wein AJ, Elbadawi A, et al: Acute biochemical and functional alterations in the partially obstructed rabbit urinary bladder. J Urol 136:1324, 1986.

74. Ghoniem GM, Regnier CH, Biancani P, et al: Effect of vesical outlet obstruction on detrusor contractility and passive properties in rabbits. J Urol 135:1284, 1986.

75. Sibley GNA: The physiological response of the detrusor muscle to experimental bladder outflow obstruction in the pig. Br J Urol 60:332, 1987.

76. Speakman MJ, Brading AF, Gilpin CJ, et al: Bladder outflow obstruction: a cause of denervation supersensitivity. J Urol 138:1461-1466, 1987.

77. Seki N, Karim OM, Mostwin JL: The effect of experimental urethral obstruction and its reversal on changes in passive electrical properties of detrusor muscle. J Urol 148:1957, 1992.

78. Levin RM, High J, Wein AJ: The effect of short-term obstruction on urinary bladder function in the rabbit. J Urol 132:789, 1984.

79. Lloyd-Davies RW, Hinman F: Structural and functional changes leading to impaired bacterial elimination after overdistension of the rabbit bladder. Invest Urol 9:136, 1971.

80. Lloyd-Davies RW, Clark AE, Prout WG, et al.: The effects of stretching the rabbit bladder. Invest Urol 8:145, 1970.

81. Gosling JA, Dixon JS, Dunn M: The structure of the rabbit urinary bladder after experimental distension. Invest Urol 14:386, 1977.

82. Kato K, Lin ATL, Haugaard N, et al: Effects of outlet obstruction on glucose metabolism of the rabbit urinary bladder. J Urol 143:844, 1990.

83. McDonald RK: Urethral prolapse in a Yorkshire terrier. Comp Cont Educ 11(6):682, 1989.

84. Kirsch JA, Hauptman JG, Walshaw R: A urethropexy technique for surgical treatment of urethral prolapse in the male dog. J Am Anim Hosp Assoc 38:381, 2002.

85. Gannon KM, Moses L: Uroabdomen in dogs and cats. Comp Cont Educ 24: 604, 2002.

Chapter 71

Organ Transplantation – Clinical Renal Transplantation in the Dog and Cat

Clare R. Gregory
Andrew E. Kyles
Margo Mehl

Clinical Renal Transplantation in Cats

Criteria for the Renal Recipient

Renal transplantation is one method of treatment for renal insufficiency.[1-5] It cannot be regarded as an emergency treatment or "last-ditch" effort to save the life of a critically ill, malnourished patient. Surgical intervention has to take place before all medical means of therapy have been exhausted. The authors consider body weight to be an important indication of the status of the renal transplant candidate. If a cat has been in compensated renal failure and starts to lose body weight, or presents in renal failure with a history of chronic weight loss, transplantation should be considered as an option before further weight loss occurs. In the critically ill human surgical patient, maximum physical performance deteriorates after a 10% loss in normal body weight. Greater than a 40% weight loss is usually lethal. Previous attempts by the authors to alter the course of physical deterioration resulting from decompensated renal failure via enteral or parenteral alimentation prior to transplantation have failed. Hemodialysis, however, is highly effective in managing severely uremic patients several days prior to surgery. The authors use hemodialysis to correct electrolyte and acid/base imbalances and lower the blood urea nitrogen concentration to 100 mg/dl or less. Blood urea nitrogen concentrations greater than 100 mg/dl predispose cats to postoperative cerebral edema and seizures owing to rapid clearance of the blood urea nitrogen by a normally functioning renal graft. Age, plasma creatinine, blood urea nitrogen, and other clinical pathologic assessments of renal function cannot in themselves indicate a suitable patient for transplantation. All physical and biochemical parameters must be assessed to determine the overall suitability of a candidate.

Feline candidates for renal transplantation should be free of feline leukemia virus infection and active acquired immunodeficiency syndrome and free of other complicating diseases. It appears that renal insufficiency can produce systemic hypertension in the feline patient, leading to congestive heart failure. Cats in renal failure often have systolic murmurs secondary to anemia that may not represent significant cardiac disease. Cardiac enlargement determined by ultrasonographic examination, gallop rhythms, and/or electrocardiographic abnormalities are possible indications to decline a candidate for transplantation. An abdominal ultrasonographic examination and intestinal biopsies should be performed if neoplasia or inflammatory bowel disease is suspected. Immunosuppression often enhances tumor growth, and inflammatory bowel disease appears to promote acute allograft rejection.

The feline renal donor/recipient pair do not have to be related or tissue matched, but they must be blood cross-matched. The antigens present on red blood cells are also present on the endothelium of the graft blood vessels. Preformed antibodies to these antigens will cause clotting of the graft vessels and infarcts of the organ at the time of surgery. The feline renal recipient must also be blood cross-matched to 2 to 3 blood donor cats. The primary reason for this is the anemia that accompanies chronic renal failure. Following rehydration of a patient prior to surgery, packed red blood cell volumes may fall as low as 12% to 15%. To attain a packed red blood cell volume of 30% in the renal recipient prior to surgery may require 180 to 250 milliliters of whole blood. Also, in our experience, some cats in chronic renal failure are unable to accept blood transfusions, i.e., all cross-match assays show agglutination of donor red cells. In two instances, the renal disease was secondary to Lupus erythematosus. In one other, however, no cause for the coagulopathy could be found. All cats were of the same blood type (A). This is an important consideration if the transplant patient is traveling a great distance to the transplant clinic. Cross matching should be done locally to ensure transfusions can be given prior to surgery. Erythropoietin can be helpful in controlling the anemia associated with renal failure. Administration of erythropoietin starting one to two months prior to surgery can greatly reduce the need for blood products.

Renal diseases successfully treated by renal transplantation in the cat include membranous glomerulonephropathy, chronic tubulointerstitial nephritis, polycystic renal disease, and ethylene glycol toxicosis. Cats with a suspected history of bacterial urinary tract infection should have a renal biopsy performed and be subject to a 2-week cyclosporine challenge prior to surgery. Cyclosporine is administered orally at 4 mg/kg twice daily, and urine cultures are performed 7 and 14 days following the initiation of cyclosporine treatment. Latent infections will often become active once cyclosporine is administered. We currently recommend renal transplantation for cats whose renal failure was secondary to obstruction by calcium oxalate uroliths; however, clients must be warned that some of these cats may form additional uroliths following transplantation that may obstruct and injure or destroy the transplanted kidney. Cats with renal failure whose kidneys are of normal or increased size should have a biopsy performed to rule out lymphosarcoma.

In the past, cats that had positive serum titers for toxoplasmosis, either IgG or IgM, were not considered candidates for immunosuppression and transplantation. Both cats and dogs have developed fatal toxoplasmosis infections following renal transplantation and immunosuppression.[6] Currently, animals with positive serum titers that undergo transplantation are administered clindamycin or trimethoprim/sulfadiazine prior to surgery and for the life of the patient. (LR Aronson, University of Pennsylvania, personal communication). Trimethoprim/sulfadiazine must be used with care because this drug can enhance cyclosporine nephrotoxicity.

Criteria for the Renal Donor

The renal donor should be in excellent health and have no evidence of renal insufficiency based on clinical pathologic testing: complete blood count, serum chemistry panel, urinalysis, and urine bacterial culture. An intravenous pyelograph is performed to assure that the donor has two normally shaped and well vascularized kidneys. The feline donor should be free of feline leukemia virus infection and be blood cross-match compatible and of similar weight and body size of the recipient. The renal donor should have a normal life expectancy following unilateral nephrectomy.[7] Elevation in serum creatinine levels and proteinuria have been reported in human kidney donors, and long-term monitoring of renal function has been recommended.

Preoperative Preparation of the Recipient

Prior to surgery, the renal recipient is given balanced electrolyte solutions subcutaneously or intravenously at 1.5 to 2 times daily maintenance requirements. Whole blood or packed red blood cell transfusions are administered until a packed red cell volume of 25% to 30% is achieved. Hemodialysis is employed for cats that maintain a blood urea nitrogen concentration equal to or greater than 120 mg/dl despite aggressive fluid diuresis. Cyclosporine oral solution (Neoral) is administered 48 hours prior to surgery at a dose of 3 to 5 mg/kg every 12 hours. The cyclosporine oral solution should be placed in gelatin capsules prior to administration. Capsule sizes #0 or #1 work well for most cats. Cyclosporine oral solution has an unpleasant taste that causes some cats to salivate profusely, resulting in partial loss of the dose. Clindamycin is administered to animals with positive serum titers for toxoplasmosis.

The morning of surgery, a blood sample is taken from the recipient 12 hours following the last oral dose of cyclosporine. This will give a 12-hour trough blood concentration. The authors follow whole-blood concentrations of cyclosporine assayed by high pressure liquid chromatography. In cats, a concentration of 500 ng/ml is maintained for the first 30 postoperative days, reducing to 250 ng/ml by 3 months after transplantation. Prednisolone, 1 mg/kg/12 hours, orally, is also started the evening following surgery and is reduced to 0.5 to 1 mg/kg/24 hours by 1 month postoperatively if renal function is normal. If renal function starts to deteriorate in the first weeks to months following transplantation, i.e., serum creatinine concentrations begin to rise above 2 mg/dl, azathioprine (0.3 mg/kg/72hours) is added to the immunosuppressive protocol. Cats receiving azathioprine should have blood cell counts and serum chemistry profiles performed weekly until a safe and effective dose is found. White blood cells counts should be maintained at higher than 3000/µl and serum chemistry profiles should be evaluated for evidence of hepatitis or pancreatitis.

Surgery

Two teams perform renal transplantation: One team harvests the donor kidney and closes the abdominal wound, and one team prepares the recipient vessels and receives the kidney.[2,3,5,8] The two-team approach minimizes the warm ischemia time of the donor kidney, which should be kept to less than 60 minutes, unless preservation protocols are employed.[9] The authors have not used perfusion solutions to maintain the kidney prior to vascularization, but iced heparinized saline solution is used to flush blood from the kidney following harvest. It is important to thoroughly cool the kidney immediately following excision from the donor. Cold sponges should be placed on the kidney during the implantation procedure to keep it from prematurely warming.

Anesthesia protocols vary with each patient. In general, the recipient receives atropine (0.03 mg/kg) and oxymorphone (0.05 mg/kg) subcutaneously prior to induction. The cat is mask- or boxed–induced, and anesthesia is maintained using isoflurane or sevoflurane inhalant anesthesia and oxygen. During the procedure, balanced electrolyte solutions and/or whole blood or packed red blood cells are administered intravenously. Systemic arterial pressure is monitored by direct arterial catheterization or by indirect measurement using Doppler ultrasonography. Hypotension can be managed using dopamine (5 µg/kg/minute intravenously) and fluid boluses as necessary. Both cats receive broad-spectrum antibiotics administered intravenously just prior to surgery. As the abdominal incision is made, the donor cat should receive mannitol (0.5 g/kg as a bolus followed by a constant infusion of 1 mg/kg/minute) to protect the kidney to be transplanted during harvest. Mannitol significantly reduces the incidence and duration of acute tubular necrosis associated with warm ischemia.

The donor nephrectomy is performed via a ventral midline celiotomy. Magnifying loupes providing 3.3x to 4.5x magnification are recommended for the vascular dissection. The vascular pedicle of the donor kidney can contain only one artery. Renal arteries may bifurcate close to the aorta. A length of 0.5 cm or more is required for arterial anastomosis. If two or more veins are present, the largest is saved for venous anastomosis. The vascular pedicle should contain the longest vein possible, so the left kidney is explored first.

Once the kidney to be harvested is selected, the recipient team should be informed so they can prepare the recipient vessels. It is extremely important to clean the donor renal artery and vein of as much fat and adventitia as possible. The large fat pad in the renal pelvis should be removed, being careful not to damage the ureter. Removal of the fat and adventitia from the vessels prior to nephrectomy reduces warm ischemia time. The diameter of the renal vein is measured and a sterile paper template is made to guide the size of the venotomy in the recipient's caudal vena cava. The ureter is isolated to the the level of the bladder. Donor nephrectomy is performed when the recipient team is prepared to receive the kidney. Anastomosis of the renal vessels and the ureter in the small dog and cat requires 3x to 10x magnification. The higher magnification is necessary to suture the ureter to the bladder. The authors use an operating microscope.

The recipient's post renal aorta and vena cava are isolated via a ventral midline celiotomy. The kidney is implanted between the left renal artery and the caudal mesenteric artery. First, the aorta is occluded using vascular occlusion clamps. Using an arterotomy clamp, a 1.5 to 2 mm defect is created in the aortic wall. The lumen of the aorta is flushed with heparinized saline solution. The caudal vena cava is then occluded adjacent to the arterotomy site in the aorta. Using the template created by measuring the donor renal vein, an oval defect is created in the caudal vena cava. The vena cava is flushed with heparinized saline solution.

Once the recipient vessels have been prepared for implantation of the graft, the donor kidney is harvested. The kidney is flushed with iced heparinized saline. The renal artery is gently dilated and adventitia is excised from the distal end. The artery is anastomosed to the aorta, end-to-side, using 8-0 nylon in a simple continuous pattern. The renal vein is then anastomosed to the vena cava using 7-0 silk or 8-0 nylon, depending on the size of the vein, in a simple continuous pattern. Owing to a lack of visibility of the wall adjacent to the aorta, the first side of the vein closest to the aorta is sutured inside the lumen of the vessels (back-wall technique). Once the first side is sutured, the side away from the artery is sutured in a conventional manner.

As soon as both the renal artery and vein are sutured, the venous occlusion clamp is removed, followed by the arterial occlusion clamp. Hemorrhage is controlled by pressure, or by the addition of simple interrupted sutures if needed.

The ureter is sutured to the bladder in the following manner.[1,10,11] A 1-centimeter incision is made in the seromuscular layer of the bladder on the ventral surface. The mucosa will bulge through the incision. A 3- to 4-mm incision is made in the mucosa at the caudal aspect of the seromuscular incision. The periureteral fat is excised from the distal 5 mm of the ureter, and the end of the ureter is spatulated. Using 8-0 vicryl in a simple interrupted pattern, the mucosa of the ureter is sutured to the mucosa of the bladder. The proximal and distal sutures are placed first. A 5-0 polypropylene stent is used to check patency of the stoma. Once the mucosal layers are opposed, the seromuscular layer is closed over the ureter using 4-0 absorbable suture in a simple interrupted pattern.

The kidney capsule is fixed to the abdominal wall by creating a peritoneal/transversus abdominus muscle flap based on a ventral pedicle. The flap is sutured to the renal capsule using simple interrupted sutures of 5-0 polypropylene. Fixing the kidney to the abdominal wall prevents torsion of the kidney on its pedicle with resulting ischemia and loss of the graft. To provide nutritional support during the postoperative period, a gastrostomy or esophagostomy tube is placed prior to recovery from anesthesia.

In dogs, the transplanted kidney can be placed in the iliac fossa of the recipient. The renal vein is anastomosed end-to-side to the external iliac vein, using 4-0 or 5-0 silk in a continuous pattern. The renal artery is anastomosed end-to-end with the external iliac artery, using 4-0 or 5-0 polypropylene suture in a simple interrupted pattern. As in the cat, a peritoneal/muscle flap is used to secure the kidney to the abdominal wall. The iliac vessels are no longer used as recipient vessels for feline transplant patients. While not a problem in dogs, loss of the iliac blood supply in cats can result in ipsilateral hind limb weakness, paralysis, and ischemia.[8]

Unless evidence exists of bacterial nephritis or severely enlarged polycystic kidneys, the authors do not remove the recipient's native kidneys at the time of transplantation. These kidneys are available to provide some support if the transplanted organ should fail, and can be removed at a later date if indicated.

Postoperative Care of the Renal Recipient

During and following surgery, it is imperative to keep the transplant patient warm and the hematocrit and systolic blood pressure within normal limits. Avoid unnecessary stress and handling. Postoperative pain is controlled by the administration of oxymorphone (0.05 mg/kg subcutaneously) as needed. The recipient receives balanced electrolyte solutions supplemented to correct electrolyte or acid/base abnormalities.[1,11] Urine specific gravity is followed twice daily via free catch of the urine. Urine specific gravity is usually greater than 1.020 by the third postoperative day. Packed blood cell volume, total plasma protein level, serum electrolyte levels, and the plasma creatinine concentration are assessed 3 to 4 times daily until renal function is stable. During the early postoperative period needless venapuncture, blood sampling, and patient handling should be avoided. If the surgery is a technical success, the urine specific gravity will be increased, and the plasma creatinine will be decreased by the third postoperative day. The recipient will look clinically improved. Normal appetite usually returns by postoperative day 3 to 5. If the graft has failed or has delayed function, the recipient will be depressed and anorectic. The urine will remain isosthenuric. Approximately three days following surgery, an ultrasonographic examination of the transplanted kidney and ureter can be performed if renal function is not returning to normal. If perfusion of the graft is good without evidence of hydronephrosis or hydroureter secondary to obstruction, the graft may have suffered acute tubular necrosis consistent with delayed graft function. As long as the kidney remains perfused, function can start as late as 3 weeks following surgery.

Hypertension is a common complication that can occur within the first 72 hours after surgery.[13,14] Cats can develop hypertension (systolic blood pressure $\geq$ 170 mm/Hg) and are at higher risk for neurologic disorders such as ataxia, blindness, seizures, and stupor. Occasionally, uncontrollable seizures and death can result. Controlling hypertension has significantly reduced the frequency of these complications. Indirect, systolic blood pressure is measured by ultrasonic Doppler every hour for at least 24 hours after surgery, and then at decreasing intervals over the next 48 hours. When the systolic blood pressure is equal to or higher than 170 mm/Hg, hydralazine (2.5 mg total dose/subcutaneously) is given. If the systolic blood pressure has not decreased to normal within 15 to 20 minutes, a second dose is given. In the rare case that the hypertension is refractory to hydralazine therapy, acetylpromazine (0.01 mg/kg, intravenously, subcutaneously) is administered. Rarely, transplant patients can develop a lethal sensitivity to cyclosporine; this is termed hemolytic uremic syndrome.[15] Cats become uremic with a coexisting hemolytic anemia and thrombocytopenia. The transplanted kidney is lost to ischemia produced by diffuse vascular thrombosis. No treatment currently exists for this syndrome in cats.

If the transplant recipient is not eating well by 24 hours following surgery, feedings are begun using the gastrostomy or esophagostomy tube. Normal caloric intake is attained over 24 to 48 hours. Cyclosporine is administered at levels necessary to achieve trough whole blood concentrations of 500 ng/ml. Prednisolone is administered at 1 mg/kg/12 hours, orally, and is tapered to 0.5 to 1 mg/kg/24 hours by 4 weeks postoperatively. Erythropoietin can be administered if the hematocrit remains below 25%.

Transplant recipients are discharged from the hospital when they have achieved an adequate nutritional intake and the cyclosporine blood level has stabilized. The feeding tube is left in place until the cat has completely acclimated at home.

Long-Term Management of the Renal Recipient

Management of the transplant patient must be coordinated with the client, the local veterinarian(s), and the transplant center. Examinations are initially performed weekly by the local veterinarian. Measurements of packed blood cell volume, total serum protein concentration, plasma creatinine concentration, and whole blood cyclosporine concentration, and a urinalysis are performed. Periods between examinations are gradually extended to 3 or 4 weeks. The authors recommend that a complete blood count should be performed monthly, and a serum chemistry panel, urinalysis with urine culture, and cardiac consult be performed 3 times a year.

During the first year after transplantation, the most common complications that occur are acute rejection, infections, and the development of cancers.[6,16-20] Acute rejection can often be attributed to poor owner compliance in giving medications and having cyclosporine blood concentration assays performed on a regular basis. Acute rejection is an emergency situation that must be treated quickly and aggressively with injectable cyclosporine (Sandimmune [Norvartis AG, Basel, Switzerland], 6.6 mg/kg once daily over 4 to 6 hours), corticosteroids, and the intravenous administration of balance electrolyte solutions. Cats do not show illness associated with acute rejection, so rising creatinine concentrations are considered grounds for treatment unless obstructive uropathy can be proven by ultrasonographic evaluation of the kidney and ureter.[21,22] In cats, slow, chronic elevations of serum creatinine, in the presence of adequate blood levels of cyclosporine, are treated with the addition of azathioprine (0.3 mg/kg/72 hours) to the immunosuppressive protocol. The white blood cell count and hepatic enzyme concentrations must be monitored and the dose adjusted as necessary to prevent severe leukopenia (< 3000 cells/μl) or hepatitis.

Transplant patients are susceptible to infections. Viral, bacterial, parasitic, coccidian, protozoal, and fungal infections can all develop. When treating bacterial infections, aminoglycoside and trimethoprim/sulfa antibiotics must be avoided as they are nephrotoxic when combined with cyclosporine. When adding any medication to the immunosuppressive protocol, check the drug insert that is provided with cyclosporine for possible interactions. Many agents can raise or lower cyclosporine whole blood concentrations by interfering or promoting cytochrome P-450 enzyme activity.

Immunosuppressed patients are also at an increased risk for the development of cancer. The most common types are lymphoma and squamous cell carcinoma. Transplant recipients also develop diabetes mellitus with an increased frequency. Diabetes can be a temporary or a chronic problem. Insulin therapy can provide long-term control.

Clinical Renal Transplantation in the Dog

There are only few differences in the technical aspects of renal transplantation between the dog and the cat. Most dogs, owing to their size, do not require magnification for anastomosis of the vessels, although 2x to 3x magnifying loops are helpful. In addition to implanting the graft on the terminal aorta and vena cava, the external iliac artery and vein can be used as recipient vessels for the transplanted kidney. The iliac vessels should not be used for the recipient vessels in cats because loss of the iliac blood supply in cats can result in rear limb weakness, paralysis, or ischemia.[8]

For ease of anastomosis, a left donor kidney is placed in the right iliac fossa of the recipient, and a right donor kidney should be placed in the left iliac fossa. If necessary, a donor kidney can be placed in the ipsilateral iliac fossa of the recipient; however, the arterial anastomosis will be more difficult to perform. The chosen iliac fossa is prepared for end-to-end anastomosis of the renal artery to the iliac artery and end-to-side anastomosis of the renal vein to the iliac vein. The iliac artery is isolated, and a bulldog or other vascular clamp is used to occlude it near the aortic bifurcation. The iliac artery is then ligated distally, near the femoral ring, and is severed. The free length of the artery is flushed clean of blood using heparinized saline solution. The end of the artery is gently dilated and the adventitia is excised from the proximal 3 to 5 mm. The iliac vein lies deep to the artery in fat and adventitia. It is isolated over the same area as the artery, gaining as much free length as possible. The iliac vein has multiple tributary veins in this region that must be ligated. Careful inspection dorsal and caudal to the vein will reveal these branches. Once the tributary veins have been ligated, two vascular clamps are placed on the iliac vein as far apart as possible. The first is placed distally, and the second is placed proximately. A section of the wall is excised from the iliac vein that is slightly larger than the diameter of the donor renal vein. It is important to create a defect in the vein wall and not just a slit. The vein is flushed clean of blood using heparinized saline solution.

Two 4-0 to 6-0 sutures of silk are placed at each end of the defect in the vein wall. Each suture is subsequently placed at the cranial or caudal aspect of the renal vein and tied. The renal vein is then anastomosed to the iliac vein using a simple continuous pattern on both the medial and lateral sides of the vessels.

Following completion of the venous anastomosis, the renal artery and iliac artery are isolated near the midline of the recipient. The arteries are anastomosed using 5-0 to 8-0 nylon or polypropylene in a simple interrupted pattern. Once arterial anastomosis is complete, the vascular clamps are removed from the vein and then the artery. Some hemorrhage is expected, can be controlled with light pressure, and should stop within a few minutes. Large defects in the arterial anastomosis have to be controlled by placement of additional sutures. Ureteroneocystostomy is performed using the same method as described for the cat. The kidney capsule is attached to the adjacent abdominal wall using simple interrupted sutures of 3-0 polypropylene or a peritoneal/ transversus abdominis muscle flap.

Following renal transplantation, dogs are highly likely to develop intestinal intussusceptions. Two treatments have resulted in the prevention of this condition that develops postoperatively. First, morphine, 0.5 mg/ml, is administered subcutaneously as a premedication and postsurgically at 0.5 mg/kg subcutaneously every 3 to 4 hours to control pain.[23] Second, enteroplication is performed after the renal transplant procedure is completed. The seromuscular layers of the bowel are joined using simple interrupted sutures of 3-0 polydioxanone.[24]

Owing to the difficulty of immunosuppressing the dog's rejection response, few renal transplants have been performed clinically for canine patients with renal failure. The primary difference in transplantation between the dog and cat is selection of the donor. Using cyclosporine and prednisolone to achieve immunosuppression, the authors will only use mixed-lymphocyte-response matched, related donors. The new formulation of cyclosporine, with conventional or newly developed agents, has proven to successfully control the canine rejection response.[25,26] With the use of MHC-nonmatched donors, the authors employ one of two immunosuppressive protocols: 1) cyclosporine and leflunomide (4-6 mg/kg/24 hours) or 2) cyclosporine (Neoral), azathioprine (1-5 mg/kg every 48 hours), and prednisolone (1 mg/kg/24 hours). Cyclosporine is administered at a dose that will achieve a trough whole-blood level of 500 ng/nl. Leflunomide is administered at a dose necessary to maintain a trough plasma blood concentration of 20 μg/ ml. Azathioprine dosage is adjusted to avoid leukopenia and hepatitis. The dose of prednisolone is reduced over 1 to 3 months, depending on the serum creatinine concentration and degree of side effects suggestive of Cushing's syndrome. In a long on-going study, Mathews et al[27] employed antithymocyte serum, cyclosporine, azathioprine, and prednisolone for immunosuppression of unrelated dog donor-recipient pairs. A median survival time of eight months was achieved with two dogs surviving more than two years.[27] In a completed clinical study, the authors found that the combination of cyclosporine, azathioprine, and prednisolone prevented renal allograft rejection in 15 dogs. Of these, three dogs are alive 24 to 50 months following surgery, five of the dogs died in the perioperative period owing to the development of systemic thromboembolism, and four of the dogs died owing to the development of lethal bacterial infections. Renal allograft rejection can be controlled in the dog; however, a balance must be maintained between the control of rejection and the development of lethal infections. Owing to the hypercoagulable state present in the canine renal failure patient, perioperative anticoagulation therapy must be employed (Gregory CR, et al. Unpublished paper in review).

Canine renal transplantation is still in the development phase. The work of Mathews et al[27] and our own studies have been invaluable in highlighting the techniques and the difficulties, both clinically and financially. Over the next several years, case selection, immunosuppressive management, and anticoagulation strategies will be further refined, and outcomes will improve.

Client Education

Before performing renal transplantation for the dog or cat, clients must be fully informed of the risks, responsibilities, and costs associated with the procedure. Clients must be able to administer medications orally 2 times a day for the life of their pet. Fractious cats and dogs are not good candidates because of the extensive nursing required in the perioperative period and the need for regular examinations by the local veterinarian. Clients must have access to a 24-hour emergency facility. Finally, clients must understand that no matter how carefully selected and managed, their cat or dog may die owing to the stress of the procedure or failure of the graft to function.

Feline and canine renal transplantation is becoming more widely available in the United States and is also performed in Australia, Japan, and Europe. Survival rates have improved with careful patient selection, better perioperative care and monitoring, and the introduction of the microemulsified form of cyclosporine (Neoral). Renal transplantation can offer long-term survival with a normal quality of life for cats and dogs with renal failure.

References

1. Bernsteen L, et al: Renal transplantation in cats. Clin Tech Small Anim Pract 15:40, 2000.
2. Gregory CR: Renal transplantation in the cat. Comp Cont Educ Pract Vet15:1325, 1993.
3. Gregory CR, Gourley IM: Organ transplantation in clinical veterinary medicine. *In* Textbook of Small Animal Surgery, 2nd ed. Slatter D (ed). Philadelphia: WB Saunders, 1993, pp. 95-101.
4. Kochin E.J. and Gregory CR: Renal transplantation:patient selection and postoperative care. *In* Consultations in Feline Internal Medicine, 2nd ed, WB Saunders Company, Philadelphia, 1993 pp. 339-342.
5. Gregory CR, Bernsteen L: Organ Transplantation in Clinical Veterinary Practice. *In* Textbook of Small Animal Surgery, 3rd ed. Slatter D (ed). Philadelphia: WB Saunders, 2003, p. 122.
6. Bernsteen L, et al: Acute toxoplasmosis following renal transplantation in three cats and a dog. JAVMA 215:1123, 1999.
7. Lirtzman RA, Gregory CR: Long-term renal and hematologic effects of uninephectomy in healthy feline kidney donors. JAVMA 207:1044,1995.
8. Bernsteen L, et al: Comparison of two surgical techniques for renal transplantation in cats. Vet Surg 28:417, 1999.
9. McAnulty JF: Hypothermic storage of feline kidneys for transplantation: successful ex vivo storage up to 7 hours. Vet Surg 27:312, 1998.
10. Kochin E.J. and Gregory CR. Evaluation of a method of ureteroneocystostomy in the cat. JAVMA 202: 257,1993.
11. Gregory CR et al: A mucosal apposition technique for ureteroneocystostomy after renal transplantation in cats. Vet Surg 25:13, 1995.

12. Wooldridge JD, Gregory CR: Ionized and total serum magnesium concentrations in feline renal transplant recipients. Vet Surg 28:31, 1999.

13. Gregory CR, et al: Central nervous system disorders after renal transplantation in cats. Vet Surg 26:386, 1997.

14. Kyles A E, et al: Management of hypertension controls postoperative neurologic disorders after renal transplantation in cats. Vet Surg 28:436, 1999.

15. Aronson LR, Gregory CR: Possible hemolytic uremic syndrome in three cats after renal transplantation and cyclosporine therapy. Vet Surg 28:135, 1999.

16. Gregory CR et al: Preliminary results of clinical renal allograft transplantation in the dog and cat. J Vet Int Med 1:53, 1987.

17. Gregory CR et al: Feline leukemia virus-associated lymphosarcoma following renal transplantation in a cat. Transplantation 52(6):1097, 1991.

18. Gregory CR et al: Renal transplantation for treatment of end-stage renal failure in cats. JAVMA 201:285, 1992

19. Gregory CR, et al: Oxalate nephrosis and renal sclerosis after renal transplantation in a cat. Vet Surg 22:221, 1993.

20. Mathews KG, Gregory CR: Renal transplants in cats: 66 cases (1987-1996). JAVMA 211:1432, 1997.

21. Nyland TG, et al: Ultrasonographic evaluation of renal size in dogs with acute allograft rejection. Vet Radiol Ultrasound 38:55, 1997.

22. Pollard R, et al: Ultrasonographic evaluation of renal autografts in normal cats. Vet Radiol Ultrasound 40:380-385, 1999.

23. McAnulty JF, Southard JH, Belzer FO: Prevention of postoperative intestinal intussusception by prophylactic morphine administration in dogs used for organ transplantation research. Surgery 105:494, 1989.

24. Kyles AE, Gregory CR, Griffey SM, et al: Modified noble plication for the prevention of intestinal intussusception after renal transplantation in dogs. J Invest Surg 16:161, 2003.

25. Bernsteen L, Gregory CR, Kyles AE, et al: Microemulsified cyclosporine-based immunosuppression for the prevention of acute renal allograft rejection in unrelated dogs: preliminary experimental study. Vet Surg 32:213, 2003.

26. Kyles AE, Gregory CR, Griffey SM, et al: Immunosuppression with a combination of the leflunomide analog, FK778, and microemulsified cyclosporine for renal transplantation in mongrel dogs. Transplantation 27:1128, 2003.

27. Mathews KA, et al: Kidney transplantation in dogs with naturally occurring end-stage renal disease. JAAHA 36:294, 2000.

Part X

Genital System

Chapter 72

Prostate

Richard Wheeler

Prostate diseases, with few exceptions other than neoplasia, are diseases of intact male dogs. Most of these diseases evolve from endocrine-induced changes to the structure and integrity of the prostate. Resolution can often be achieved by medical management, hormone manipulation, or surgical intervention–including castration.

Anatomy

The canine prostate is a bilobed encapsulated organ composed of stromal cells, smooth muscle cells, and epithelial cells. It is closely associated with the neck of the urinary bladder, and encircles a portion of the urethra (prostatic urethra). Vasculature is supplied by the prostatic artery–a branch of the internal pudendal artery–and the prostatic vein.[1] Parasympathetic innervation, which stimulates glandular secretions, is supplied by the pelvic nerve.[1] Sympathetic innervation, which stimulates smooth muscle contraction during ejaculation, derives from the hypogastric nerve.[1] The blood vessels and nerves approach the prostate from the craniodorsal aspect.

The prostate is located at the cranioventral edge of the pelvic inlet. Post-pubertal maturation and advanced disease result in enlargement of the prostate and advancement cranioventrally into the abdomen where it is accessible to surgery. The prostate is a pharmacologically privileged organ protected by a blood-prostate barrier imposed by gap junctions between epithelial cells.

Physiology

The prostate is the only accessory sex gland in the dog. It produces ejaculatory fluid to increase seminal volume. The prostatic fluid may have some antibiotic effects and may play a role in activating spermatozoa for fertilization. Ironically, prolonged exposure to prostatic fluid is detrimental to sperm viability.

The canine ejaculate can be collected in three distinct fractions. The first fraction is of prostatic origin and is often an insignificant volume. The second fraction is concentrated sperm, derived from the epididymus. The third fraction is again prostatic and constitutes the most voluminous portion of the ejaculate. The total volume of the third fraction varies depending on the individual, breed, and duration of coitus (or collection); it can range from 1 milliliter to more than 20 milliliters. Normal prostatic fluid is clear, serous, and has a neutral to slightly acidic pH.

Clinical Presentation

The presentation of prostatic disease is primarily attributable to prostatic enlargement. The magnitude of space-occupying effects determines the type and severity of clinical signs. Dramatic enlargement of the prostate by hypertrophy or mass lesions may cause dorsal displacement of the colon, resulting in tenesmus or "ribbon-like" feces. Cranioventral displacement of the bladder may cause dysuria, increased urgency, and compromise of urinary tract defense mechanisms, predisposing to ascending cystitis and its associated clinical signs.

Other clinical signs are attributable to hyperplasia of the parenchyma and stroma. Increased vascularity and decreased stromal integrity predispose to microvascular hemorrhage, evidenced as hematospermia, hematuria, or hemorrhagic urethral discharge.[1] Occlusion of efferent ducts obstructs glandular secretions, forming cystic glands. These dilated acini may rupture, contributing to urethral discharge,[1] or they may coalesce into large cavitations that contribute to the mass effect. Hyperplasia compromises natural defense mechanisms and immunity, predisposing to bacterial infection.[1]

Finally, duration of onset of disease plays a major role in clinical presentation. Acute prostatic inflammation is often associated with severe rectal or abdominal pain as the prostatic capsule is unable to accommodate rapid swelling. Chronic disease is often asymptomatic as the body accommodates to the insidious course of disease; however, once a critical mass is attained (i.e., obstructive enlargement), space-occupying effects become evident.

Diagnosis

Thorough history and physical examination of the dog will provide important information for the interpretation of further diagnostic procedures. The presence of pain or pyrexia implicates an acute or septic disease process. Castrated dogs are at decreased risk of infectious disease and this may direct differential diagnosis toward neoplasia.

Rectal palpation is a highly subjective and nonspecific determinant of prostatic enlargement as only the caudal pole can be palpated. As the prostate enlarges and moves cranially and ventrally into the abdomen, abdominal palpation in conjunction with rectal palpation may be necessary in order to feel the prostate.[1] Symmetry of the bilobed prostate should be evaluated.

Cytologic evaluation of prostatic fluid can identify erythrocytes, neutrophils, bacteria, and normal or neoplastic epithelial cells (Figure 72-1). Prostatic fluid is most easily obtained by manual ejaculation, isolating the third fraction. If the dog is not amenable to collection, prostatic massage and urethral flushing or the urethral brush method can be performed.[1] Blood or smegma from the prepuce or penis may contaminate the sample, complicating interpretation.

Culture of prostatic fluid must be interpreted carefully. Prostatic fluid is collected as described above for cytologic evaluation. It must be noted that these techniques do not provide an aseptic means of fluid collection;[1] normal bacterial flora of the urethra or prepuce may contaminate the sample.

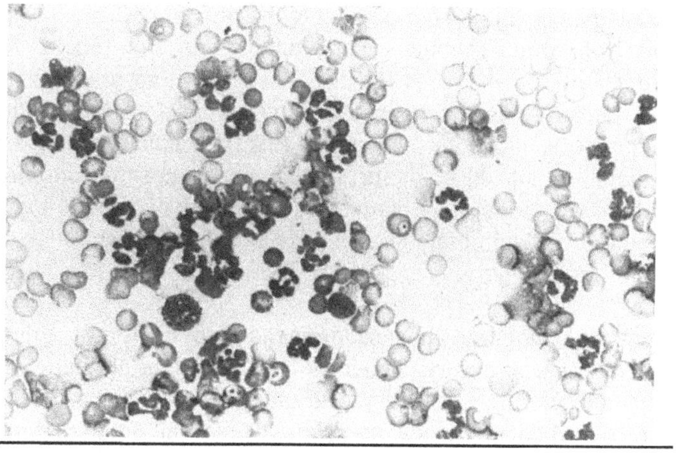

Figure 72-1. Prostatic fluid

Survey radiographs are often nondiagnostic for mild to moderate prostatic disease.[1] With advanced prostatic disease and significant enlargement, radiographs may demonstrate a soft-tissue density in the caudal abdomen, space-occupying lesion of the urinary bladder, or dorsal displacement of the colon.[1] However, they do not localize the lesion to the prostate or differentiate prostatic pathologies.

Retrograde cystourethrograms may more readily demarcate the borders of the prostate and its association to the bladder. Infiltration of contrast media into the prostate via the prostatic urethra may implicate specific prostatic diseases.[1]

Ultrasonography is the most effective, noninvasive technique to differentiate prostatic diseases. Evaluation of prostatic size, symmetry, and echogenicity implicates specific disease processes; however, definitive diagnosis cannot be made by ultrasonography alone.

Ultrasound-guided fine-needle aspiration (US-FNA) of prostatic lesions may provide the most definitive diagnosis of prostatic disease. One study demonstrated 80% agreement in diagnosis comparing US-FNA to histopathologic findings at necropsy.[2] Potential complications include seeding bacteria along the needle tract and leakage of suppurative material into the abdomen.[2]

Prostatic biopsy can be performed via laparotomy, transabdominally by ultrasound guidance, or by perirectal biopsy.[1] Again concerns arise for seeding bacteria along the needle tract and abdominal contamination.

Serology and hematology have limited application in diagnosing prostatic disease other than to rule out systemic infection. Mild elevations in alkaline phosphatase (ALP) are commonly seen, but are nonspecific for prostate disease.[3]

Prostate-specific markers have been used extensively in human medicine for early diagnosis of prostate cancer. To date, no such substance has been shown to reliably diagnose or differentiate prostatic diseases in the dog. The most promising marker, canine prostate-specific arginine esterase (CPSE), is produced by epithelial cells in response to androgens and is secreted in prostatic fluid.[3] CPSE serum levels are increased in dogs with benign prostatic hypertrophy compared with those in normal dogs; however this does not differentiate prostatic neoplasia.[3]

Pathophysiology

Benign Prostatic Hypertrophy (Hyperplasia)

Benign prostatic hyperplasia/hypertrophy (BPH) is a normal, senile, usually asymptomatic condition of aging, intact dogs. Fifty percent of intact dogs over the age of 5 years, and 95% of intact dogs older than 9 years have gross or histologic signs of BPH.[1]

Enlargement of the prostate is hormonally driven, as evidenced by prostatic atrophy after castration. The hypothalamic-pituitary-testicular axis is predominantly responsible for the production of male sex hormones. The hypothalamus produces gonadotropin releasing hormone (GnRH), which induces pituitary secretion of the gonadotropins–luteinizing hormone (LH) and follicle stimulating hormone (FSH). LH stimulates testicular Leydig cell production of testosterone. Dihydrotestosterone (DHT) is the primary mediator of prostate growth.[1,4] It is synthesized in the prostate by the metabolism of testosterone under the influence of the enzyme 5a-reductase.[1,4] Both testosterone and DHT induce growth factors in stromal and epithelial (glandular) cells, which increase cell size (hypertrophy) and cell numbers (hyperplasia), and decrease normal rates of apoptosis (programmed cell death).[1,4,5] However, DHT binds to the cells with 10 times greater affinity and dissociates much slower, exerting exponentially greater effects on prostatic growth than does testosterone.[1,4] Estrogen (E2) plays a significant, yet uncertain role in the development of BPH.[1,4] It may increase receptors or receptor affinity to DHT.[4]

BPH is generally eccentric (away from the center), so the prostatic urethra is not occluded, and stranguria is rarely seen as a presenting complaint in dogs.[1] BPH induces symmetrical enlargement that, if extreme enough, will produce symptoms of space occupying effects. Hematospermia is often an incidental finding during routine semen evaluation.

On ultrasound evaluation, BPH is diagnosed when the prostate exceeds normal parameters. In some cases of BPH, prostate size can be within normal parameters; however, changes in the appearance of the stroma and parenchyma indicate pathologic changes consistent with BPH.[1] These changes include diffuse echogenicity ("moth eaten appearance") or the presence of parenchymal cysts.[1]

Castration is the definitive treatment for BPH.[1] Elimination of testosterone induces complete regression of prostatic growth to near pre-pubertal size.[1,4] In valuable breeding animals, or when castration is not an option, life-long hormonal regulation aimed at decreasing concentrations of testosterone or DHT can dramatically reduce BPH. Finasteride ("Proscar", Merck; 5 mg PO daily) blocks the enzyme 5a-reductase, preventing conversion of testosterone to DHT.[1,5] It has demonstrated good efficacy in reducing prostatic size.[1,5] It has a high margin of safety, maintains fertility, and has no reported side effects.[1,5]

Megestrol acetate (MGA, "Ovaban," Schering 0.5 mg/kg PO daily), a synthetic progestin, inhibits gonadotropin release (LH) by negative feedback inhibition to the pituitary, resulting in decreased levels of testosterone and E2 production.[1] Lower levels of testosterone correlate to lower levels of DHT and reduction of BPH. No detrimental effects on fertility or side effects have been reported. A gonadotropin releasing hormone (GnRH) vaccine ("Canine Gonadotropin Releasing Factor (GnRF) Immunotherapeutic," Pfizer Animal Health; 1 ml SQ, repeat in 4 to 6 weeks, booster every 6 months) has recently received conditional licensing for the treatment of BPH in dogs. Preliminary studies show an increase in anti-GnRH antibodies, a decrease in serum testosterone concentration, and a decrease in prostate and testicular size.[6] Effects on fertility have not been evaluated, but the decrease in testicular size is suggestive of decreased sperm production.

Prostatitis

BPH is the inciting cause of prostatitis.[1,4] BPH disrupts the integrity of the prostate and affects natural immunity and resistance to infection, lymphatic drainage, and the normal vascularity of the gland.[1,4] Two distinct forms of prostatitis are recognized: aseptic prostatitis and septic prostatitis.[4] Aseptic prostatitis is a noninfectious inflammatory reaction characterized by prostatic infiltration with neutrophils. Septic prostatitis develops as bacteria from the normal flora of the urogenital tract opportunistically invade the prostate.[1,4] *Escherichia coli* is the most common isolate; *Pseudomonas, Staphylococcus, Streptococcus,* and *Proteus* are other common pathogens.[1,4] Septic prostatitis can further be categorized as acute or chronic. The fundamental difference is duration of onset and presenting clinical signs. Chronic prostatitis is often subclinical or symptomatic of low-grade infection.[1] Acute prostatitis presents as a sudden onset of severe abdominal pain and pyrexia.[1]

Diagnosis of prostatitis is made by demonstration of inflammatory cells in prostatic fluid. In the case of septic prostatitis, presence of intracellular bacteria or a positive bacterial culture should be confirmed. Culture and histology of a prostatic biopsy or fine-needle aspirate may provide definitive diagnosis.

Successful treatment of prostatitis requires resolution of any infectious component and removal of the inciting cause, BPH. First, treatment of the bacterial infection requires use of antibiotics that are able to penetrate the prostatic barrier. Appropriate antibiotics must be lipophilic to penetrate the lipid bilayer, slightly basic as the normal and infected pH of the prostate is usually neutral to slightly acidic, and should have low protein-binding affinity to dissociate from the circulation.[1] Current antibiotic options (enrofloxacin, trimethoprim-sulfa, erythromycin, and chloramphenicol)[1] should be selected based on safety and antibiotic sensitivity. Secondly, effective treatment of chronic prostatitis requires treatment of BPH (see above).

Prostatic Abscess

Septic prostatitis may progress to purulent vacuolization of the prostate or infection of parenchymal cysts.[1,4,7] The vacuoles or cysts may coalesce and form large intracapsular abscesses, causing asymmetric enlargement of the prostate.[1] Clinical signs vary from chronic, nondescript symptoms to acute onset with abdominal pain and pyrexia. If an abscess ruptures, presentation may be an acute abdomen and septic shock.[1] A presumptive diagnosis is made by sonogram. History, clinical signs, and hematology help differentiate prostatic abscesses from intraprostatic cysts. Conclusive diagnosis is made by demonstration of suppurative fluid obtained by biopsy, fine-needle aspiration, or exploratory surgery.[1]

Treatment requires abscess drainage and long-term antimicrobial therapy and resolution of BPH. Surgical drainage and omentalization is the preferred surgical technique.[1] Other surgical options include complete or partial prostatectomy, marsupialization, or placement of Penrose drains. Successful, nonsurgical drainage by ultrasound-guided aspiration has been reported.[8] Regardless of the treatment method, concurrent castration is highly recommended.

Cystic Lesions of the Prostate

Prostatic abcesses must be differentiated from prostatic cysts. Parenchymal (retention) cysts are diffuse hypoechoic structures within the parenchyma of the prostate that develop subsequent to BPH and are the most common cystic condition seen in the canine prostate.[1,7] "Squamous metaplasia," epithelial hyperplasia in response to estrogen exposure, is responsible for formation of some parenchymal cysts.[1,7] Epithelial hyperplasia and stromal fibrosis block the efferent ductules of the glands, resulting in the accumulation of serosanguinous fluid and subsequent dilatation and destruction of the acini.[1,4,7,8] Cysts are lined by a single layer of epithelial cells.[1,4,7] Chronic prostatitis may lead to fibrosis and dissolution of the cystic lining, forming giant cavities (cavitary prostatitis) (Figure 72-2).[7]

Extremely large parenchymal cavities may extend beyond the margins of the prostate. Cavities or cysts may be asymptomatic or they may contribute to symptoms of hematuria or hematospermia if they rupture. They may cause space-occupying symptoms or predispose to prostatic abcessation from ascending or hematogenous spread of bacteria.

Treatment of parenchymal cysts requires treatment of BPH pharmacologically or by castration. In squamous metaplasia, elimination of the estrogen source (e.g., exogenous estrogen therapy or endogenous estrogen production by Sertoli cell or adrenal tumors) is necessary.[1,7] Small cysts may regress, but large cysts and cavities may require surgical drainage if they are clinically significant. Drainage by US-FNA has been described.[8] Surgical excision and omentalization is the procedure of choice when surgery is warranted.[1]

Paraprostatic cysts (müllerian duct cysts) lie outside the prostatic capsule, distinguishing them from parenchymal cysts. They are not hormonally controlled, are not associated with BPH, and do not regress post-castration. They develop late in life from the remnants of the müllerian (paramesonephric) duct.[1,7] During embryogenesis, male sexual differentiation induces regression of the müllerian duct by secretion of müllerian inhibiting

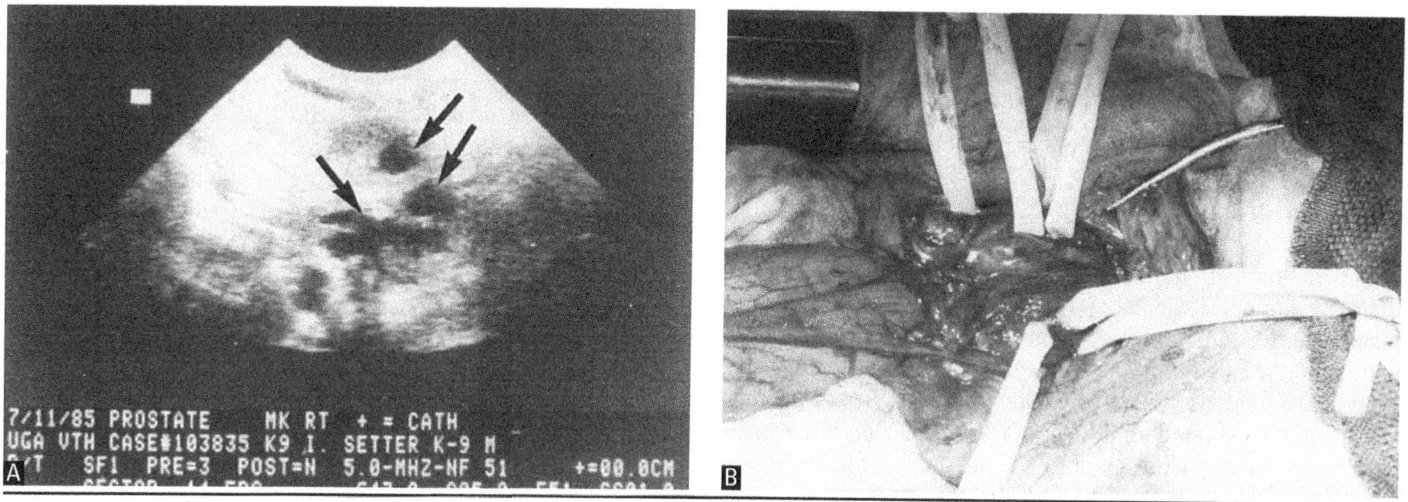

Figure 72-2A & B. Prostatic cyst in ultrasound (A) and in surgery (B).

substance (MIS).[1] In females, the müllerian duct gives rise to the oviducts, uterus, and cranial vagina.[1] Incomplete regression of the müllerian duct can result in fluid-filled cysts located adjacent to the prostate, with variable degrees of prostatic involvement. The cysts generally do not communicate with the prostate or the urethra. Paraprostatic cysts require drainage or surgical resection only if they are symptomatic.

Prostatic Neoplasia

The highest incidence of prostatic neoplasia occurs in castrated dogs.[9,10] There does not appear to be any association with age at time of castration.[10] Adenocarcinoma is the most commonly diagnosed neoplasia.[9,10] Transitional cell carcinoma is also common, presumably from the close association of the prostate to the bladder.[9]

Presenting complaints may include stranguria, which is more common with prostatic neoplasia than with other prostatic conditions because of the invasive nature of the tumor into the lumen of the urethra.[1] Rectal palpation or ultrasonography commonly demonstrates asymmetry of the prostate. Ultrasonography may also identify echogenic mass lesions within the parenchyma. Definitive diagnosis is made by biopsy or fine-needle aspiration.

Prostatic cancers are highly malignant and metastasis has usually occurred by the time of diagnosis.[1,9,10] Prognosis is grave to guarded at diagnosis and treatment is generally palliative, focusing on maintaining a patent urethra.[11] Therapeutic options that have been described include complete prostatectomy, chemotherapeutic and radiation therapy,[12] and transurethral resection (TUR).[11] All treatment modalities have been associated with significant side effects including incontinence and death; and none have prolonged or maintained the patients' quality of life.

References

1. Johnston SD, Root Kustritz MV, Olson PNS: Disorders of the Canine Prostate. *In* Canine and Feline Theriogenology. Philadelphia: WB Saunders, 2001, p. 337.

2. Powe JR, Canfield PJ, Martin PA: Evaluation of the cytologic diagnosis of canine prostatic disorders. Vet Clin Pathol 33:150, 2004.

3. Gobello C, Castex G, Corrada Y: Serum and seminal markers in the diagnosis of disorders of the genital tract of the dog: a mini-review. Theriogenology 57:1285, 2002.

4. Epstein JI: The lower urinary tract and male genital system *In* Robbins and Cotran Pathologic Basis of Disease, 7th ed. Kumar V, et al (eds). Philadelphia: Elsevier Saunders, 1999, p. 1023.

5. Sirinarumitr K, Sirinarumitr T, Jhonson SD, et al. Finasteride-induced prostatic involution by apoptosis in dogs with benign prostatic hypertrophy. AJVR 63:495, 2002.

6. Trettien A: New Treatment Option for Canine Benign Prostatic Hyperplasia. Pfizer Animal Health Technical Bulletin, Sept 2006.

7. Nghiem HT, Kellman GM, Sandberg SA, Craig BM: Cystic lesions of the prostate. RadioGraphics 10:635, 1990.

8. Boland LE, Hardie RJ, Gregory SP, Lamb CR: Ultrasound-guided percutaneous drainage as the primary treatment for prostatic abscesses and cysts in dogs. JAAHA 39:151, 2003.

9. McEntee M: Reproductive oncology. Clin Tech Small Aim Pract 17:133, 2002.

10. Teske E: Canine prostate carcinoma: epidemiological evidence of an increased risk in castrated dogs. Molec Cell Endocrinol 197:251, 2002.

11. Liptak JM, Brutscher SP, Monnet E, et al: transurethral resection in the management of urethral and prostatic neoplasia in 6 dogs. Vet Surg 33:505, 2004.

12. Lucroy MD, Bowles MH, Higbee RG, et al: Photodynamic therapy for prostatic carcinoma in a dog. J Vet Intern Med 17:235, 2003.

Chapter 73

Disorders of the Testes

Cheri A. Johnson

In the absence of genetic and hormonal influences to the contrary, normal mammalian sexual differentiation will be female. In the embryo, cells from the genital ridge become bipotential, or indifferent, gonads. The single most important factor that determines the development of a testis from the indifferent gonad is located on the short arm of the Y chromosome. This has been termed the sex-determining region Y, the Sry gene. Other genes on the autosomes and the sex chromosomes are also involved in determination of testis or ovary.[1] The hormones produced by the fetal testis in turn are responsible for the differentiation into the male phenotype. Fetal Sertoli cells produce müllerian-inhibiting substance (MIS), which, with its receptor, causes regression of the müllerian ducts that would otherwise have developed into the oviduct, uterus, and cranial vagina. Fetal Leydig cells produce testosterone, which, with androgen receptor, causes the Wolffian ducts to stabilize and develop into the ductuli deferentes and epididymes.[2,3] Dihydrotestosterone causes the urogenital sinus, the genital tubercle, and the genital swelling to differentiate into the urethra and prostate, penis, and scrotum, respectively.[3] Testicular differentiation is observed in the canine fetus at day 36 of gestation. Müllerian duct regression is complete by day 46.[4]

Factors produced by the fetal testis also cause testicular descent from its fetal position near the caudal pole of the kidney, through the inguinal canal, into the scrotum. The transabdominal testicular descent is mediated by insulin-like 3 ligand (Insl3) and its receptor. Insl3 is produced by pre- and postnatal Leydig cells and induces growth and differentiation of the gubernaculum from the caudal suspensory ligament. The transabdominal migration is androgen-independent, whereas, the inguinoscrotal descent is mediated by testosterone. Testosterone causes regression of the cranial suspensory ligament.[2,5] During the inguinoscrotal phase of migration, shortening of the gubernaculum and eversion of the cremaster muscle occurs. Normal testicular descent is a prenatal event in cats, and is normally complete by 10 to 42 days of age in dogs.[6]

Cryptochidism

Failure of normal testicular descent is referred to as cryptorchidism, which means hidden or covered testes. The condition can be bilateral or unilateral. The undescended, or "retained" testes may be in an intraabdominal location anywhere along the line from the caudal pole of the kidney to the inguinal canal. Undescended testes can also be located in the inguinal canal or the subcutaneous tissue between the external inguinal ring and the scrotum. On rare occasions, a unilateral cryptorchid testis is found in the perineal subcutis just caudal or lateral to the scrotum.

The neonatal testes in puppies and kittens are mobile and easily move out of the scrotum back toward the inguinal area. For this reason, it is sometimes difficult to confidently diagnose cryptorchidism in young animals. By 6 to 8 weeks of age, a typical age for puppies and kittens to be acquired and presented for their first vaccinations, both testes should be palpable in the scrotum. Anecdotal reports exist in dogs of testicular descent occurring as late as 6 months of age, but this is not normal. Some authors have recommended that a diagnosis of cryptorchidism not be made until a dog is 6 months old.[6] Whether these reports represent exceptionally mobile scrotal testes rather than truly delayed descent is not known.

Cryptorchid testicles continue to produce testosterone. Therefore, secondary sexual characteristics, and typical male libido and behavior are seen. Spermatogenesis is impaired by the higher temperature to which non-scrotal testes are exposed, and also by other factors such as hormone receptor defects in the cryptorchid testis. Bilaterally cryptorchid animals are expected to be sterile. Monorchidism, the condition of unilateral testicular aplasia, is rare in dogs and cats.

The prevalence of cryptorchidism in the general population is not known. Of 1345 cats presented to a veterinary teaching hospital for castration, 23 (1.7%) were cryptorchid.[7] Of these, 18 were unilateral cryptorchids, with no difference in left- verses right-sided involvement. All five cases with bilaterally cryptorchid testes were intraabdominal. Of 3038 male feral cats trapped for neutering, 35 (1.2%) were cryptorchid, and 46 (1.5%) were thought to have previously been neutered based on physical examination.[8] The prevalence of cryptorchidism in canine hospital populations is reported from 1.2 to 5 %.[6] Although the mode of inheritance is not known in either species, it is well accepted that cryptorchidism is associated with familial lineage. Therefore, the prevalence is likely to vary according to breed. For example, the incidence of cryptorchidism in a study of 2929 boxer dogs was 10.7%.[9] The heritability estimates in that study indicated that the mode of inheritance was complex, but that genetic selection would be successful in changing the prevalence of cryptorchidism in the boxer breed.

Careful palpation of the scrotum is usually sufficient to establish the diagnosis of cryptorchidism in dogs and cats older than 6 to 8 weeks, keeping in mind the mobility of the testes. If doubt exists in such young animals, they should be re-examined at a later date. Occasionally, adult animals with no scrotal testes are adopted without knowledge of previous surgeries. In such cases, a question may exist as to whether the animal is cryptorchid or has been castrated. Behavior typical of intact males, or the typical odor of tom cat urine, might raise the index of suspicion of cryptorchidism. The physical examination findings of penile spines in a cat, or a well developed prostate gland in a dog provide indirect evidence of the presence of a testis because both structures are androgen-dependent. Both involute or regress promptly after castration.

Other diagnostic tests for cryptorchidism include determination of serum concentrations of luteinizing hormone (LH) or testosterone, and ultrasonography. Following castration, serum concentrations of LH increase because negative feedback from testosterone no longer occurs. Therefore, the finding of high serum LH in a male with no scrotal testes is indicative of previous castration, whereas low serum LH indicates the presence of androgen. The nidar of the episodic secretion of testosterone in intact male dogs and cats may be below the detection threshold of some testosterone assays. Therefore, serum concentrations of testosterone should be measured before and after the administration of gonadotropin-releasing hormone (GnRH) or human chorionic gonadotropin (hCG). Castrated animals have low resting testosterone and no response to GnRH or hCG. A single, random determination of testosterone in an intact male dog or cat may also be low or undetectable, depending on the assay. High resting testosterone or an increase in serum concentrations in response to GnRH or hCG confirms the presence of a testis. Ultrasound may identify the presence and location of a cryptorchid testicle. This might be helpful in planning the surgical approach. Negative ultrasound findings do not necessarily exclude the possibility of cryptorchidism because the undescended testis can be small.

Castration is the recommended treatment because in dogs the risk of testicular neoplasia in the cryptorchid testis is significantly greater than in scrotal testes. Although testicular neoplasia is uncommon in cats, it has been reported in cryptorchid testes.[10] If, at the time of surgery, the ductus deferens, testicular vessels, and/or the epididymis are found, it is highly likely that a testis also exists on the ipsilateral side. Monorchidism (testicular aplasia) is rare. When testicular aplasia is suspected, it is important to confirm the true absence of testicular tissue with appropriate hormonal testing as described above. Medical management to cause descent of intraabdominal testes has been unsuccessful. To date, results of treatment for testes in the inguinal subcutis have been largely anecdotal in veterinary medicine and highly variable in human and veterinary medicine. Some have argued that the reported successful cases could have descended spontaneously or that they represented highly mobile, otherwise normal testes.[11]

Testicular Neoplasia

Testicular tumors are common in dogs but rare in cats. They may be incidental findings during physical examination, castration, or necropsy, or they may cause clinical signs. The most common testicular tumors are Sertoli cell tumors, Leydig (interstitial) cell tumors, and seminomas. They occur with about equal frequency except in intraabdominal testes in which the tumor is most often of Sertoli cell origin. Sertoli and Leydig cell tumors can produce hormones and cause paraneoplastic syndromes.[12]

The most common clinical sign of testicular neoplasia is enlargement of the testis. Paraneoplastic syndromes commonly occur with testicular tumors that produce hormones. These syndromes include atrophy of the contralateral testis, alopecia, and hyperpigmentation, gynecomastia, pendulous prepuce, squamous metaplasia of the prostate, and bone marrow suppression. The bone marrow toxicity caused by estrogen can result in anemia, thrombocytopenia, and/or leukopenia. Therefore, the clinical signs may be referable to anemia or bleeding. Intraabdominal testicular tumors may cause mechanical interference with other abdominal organs. Infertility is also a possible result of testicular neoplasia, but most affected dogs are past their breeding years.

Several risk factors for testicular neoplasia have been identified in dogs. Age is probably the most important. Testicular tumors are unlikely in dogs younger than 6 years of age but are fairly common in dogs 10 or more years old. In dogs older than 6, the incidence of testicular cancer has been calculated to be 68.1/1000 dog-years at risk.[13] Cryptorchidism is also a significant risk factor. In a study of 1266 dogs, testicular cancer was diagnosed 10.9 times more commonly in cryptorchid testes than in scrotal testes.[14] Environmental carcinogens[15] and certain gene expressions[16] are also risk factors.

Neoplasia should be suspected for any testicular mass in an old dog. Gynecomastia and pendulous prepuce have been referred to as feminization. Feminization is caused by estrogen alone, or by an imbalance of estrogen and androgens.[17] These findings in an intact male, especially if alopecia is also present, should make one highly suspicious of an estrogen-producing testicular tumor. In a dog with an enlarged prostate, squamous metaplasia is suspected on the basis of finding excessive numbers of squamous cells in the ejaculate or in fine-needle aspirate samples from the gland. Estrogen is the cause of prostatic squamous metaplasia. The presence of excess estrogen can be confirmed by exfoliative cytology of the prepucial mucosa, which cornifies under the influence of estrogen just as does the vaginal epithelium. A testicular tumor is the most likely source of excess estrogen in a male dog.

The diagnosis of testicular neoplasia is often made on the basis of palpation of a testicular mass. Tumors are usually more firm than the surrounding testicular tissue. If a testicular tumor is not palpable in a dog with feminization or prostatic squamous metaplasia, or other situations where testicular neoplasia is a likely diagnostic consideration, testicular ultrasound should be performed. Ultrasound is useful in identifying small tumors, especially when they are deeper in the parenchyma and difficult to feel. Although fine-needle aspiration or biopsy could be used to confirm the diagnosis of neoplasia and to differentiate testicular tumors from one another, this is rarely indicated because the treatment for all is surgical removal of the affected testis. Because of possible bone marrow toxicity from estrogen production by the tumor, preoperative evaluation should include a complete blood count. Because most affected dogs are geriatric, a preoperative biochemical panel and urinalysis are also appropriate.

If the dog still has value as a stud, unilateral castration should be performed. If not, both testes could be removed. The affected testis is then submitted for histopathologic evaluation. In contrast to the situation in men, most canine testicular tumors are benign. Therefore, complete staging of the disease could reasonably be delayed until histopathologic confirmation of malignancy. Intraabdominal metastasis is more likely than pulmonary. Treatment options for malignant and metastatic tumors should be considered in consultation with a veterinary oncologist.

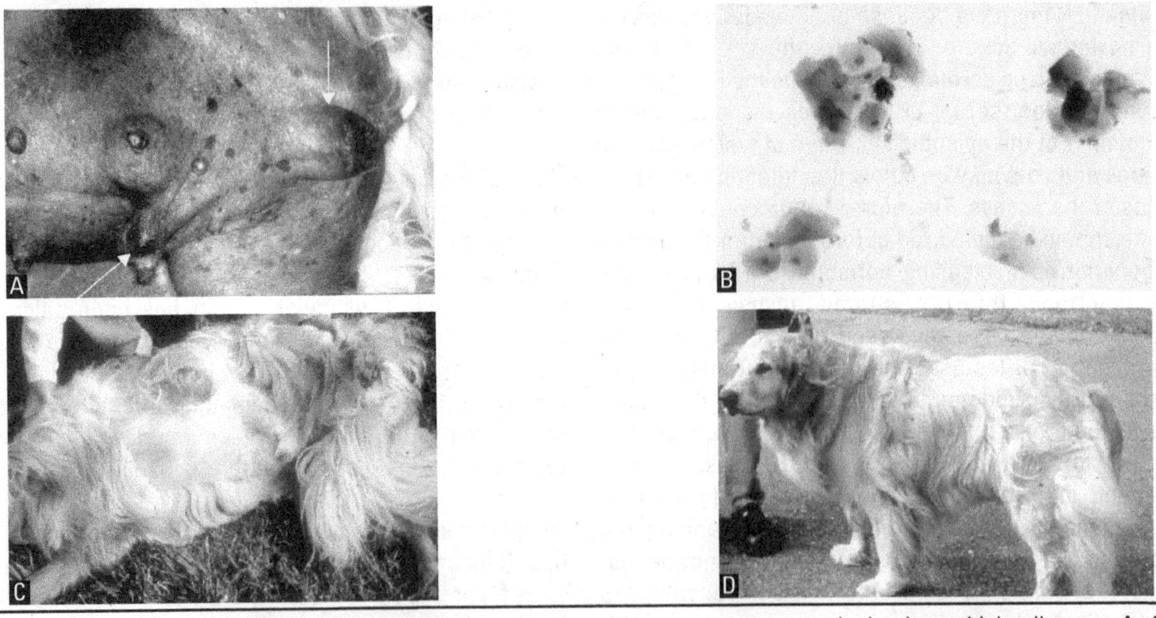

Figure 73-1A-D 10-year-old golden retriever with paraneoplastic syndrome from an estrogen-producing interstitial cell tumor. A. Alopecia and hyperpigmentation, mammary and nipple development, pendulous prepuce (white arrow), asymmetric testes (black arrow). B. Cornification of prepucial mucosal epithelium. C. and D. Resolution of alopecia, hyperpigmentation and feminization following castration.
(Courtesy of Dr. William Schall, Michigan State University.)

Relative to cryptorchidism and neoplasia, other testicular disorders are much less commonly seen in general small animal practice. Testicular masses other than neoplasia include spermatocele, granuloma, and cysts. Although abscesses can form in the testis, with testicular infection it is more common to have diffuse involvement than a focal mass. Owners may assume that an enlarged scrotum must be due to testicular enlargement. Other causes of scrotal enlargement include epididymal or spermatic cord enlargement (including scirrhous cord), scrotal herniation of omentum or small bowel, hydrocele, or edema of the scrotal skin. Hydrocele is the accumulation of fluid between the visceral and parietal vaginal tunics in the scrotum. The fluid may be a transudate in the case of lymphatic obstruction of the spermatic cord, or it may be blood or exudate in the case of trauma or infection. In addition to careful palpation, ultrasound of the scrotal contents is extremely helpful in differentiating among the causes of scrotal enlargement.

Spermatocele/Sperm Granuloma

Spermatocele is a cystic dilation of the ductal system that is caused by stasis and accumulation of sperm.[18] It is much more likely to occur in the ductus deferens or epididymis than in the testis. Spermatoceles may cause a local inflammatory reaction with infiltration of monocytes and macrophages and the development of a sperm granuloma. Conversely, preexisting testicular inflammation, orchitis, may cause the obstruction and formation of a spermatocele. Spermatoceles also occur as a result of trauma, including that induced by fine-needle aspiration or biopsy. Some spermatoceles are congenital in origin. Spermatocele may be an incidental finding causing no clinical signs, or it may cause swelling and/or a palpable mass. If it is associated with an inflammatory condition, the animal may also experience discomfort.

Cysts occasionally arise from the seminiferous tubules or rete testis. These may be incidental findings during testicular ultrasonography, or the cysts may be large enough to alter the size or shape of the testis. Cysts involving the rete testis may completely obstruct the movement of sperm into the epididymis.

Whenever a lesion is found in one testis, both should be thoroughly evaluated to determine if the disorder is unilateral or bilateral. Differentiation of focal testicular lesions such as tumors, granulomas, or cysts can be accomplished by ultrasound and fine-needle aspiration. Samples should be submitted for cytologic evaluation and culture, if appropriate. When cysts or spermatoceles are incidental findings causing no clinical signs, further evaluation is not necessary. Biopsies could also be obtained but fine-needle aspiration is usually sufficient for focal lesions. Surgical removal of the affected testis is often a more cost-effective approach than biopsy because it is potentially therapeutic as well as obtaining samples for histopathologic and microbiologic evaluation.

Orchitis

Infectious or inflammatory conditions of the testes are relatively uncommon in dogs, and rare in cats. When they occur, the epididymis is often also affected. Infections may be of hematogenous origin or from penetrating wounds. Of the infectious agents, *Brucella canis* is of particular concern in dogs because of its insidious nature and devastating effect on reproduction.[19] *Brucella canis* infection usually does not cause signs of systemic illness in dogs. The transient fever and testicular swelling following infection often go unnoticed. Although *B. canis* can cause epididymal and testicular enlargement, it is often not of a magnitude to be found by casual observation. Scrotal dermatitis associated with the epididymitis has been reported, but this is certainly not a consistent finding. Only after dogs have become infertile do owners become aware of a problem. Occasionally *B. canis* infects nonreproductive organs including the eyes and intervertebral discs. When it does, there are associated clinical signs. With chronic infection the testes atrophy. Other bacteria and mycotic agents such as *Blastocymes* can also cause orchitis. Lymphocytic orchitis has been reported and is suspected to have an immune-mediated basis.[20] Testicular trauma can cause hemorrhage, edema, and inflammation.

Orchitis is suspected when swelling, heat, and pain are found during examination of the testis. If other signs of illness are present, these should be pursued as well. *Brucella canis* serology should be performed in every dog with orchitis or epididymitis. The rapid slide agglutination test (RSAT) is an excellent screening test. It is highly sensitive; therefore, a negative result is good evidence <u>against</u> the diagnosis, assuming that the infection has been present for at least 8 to 12 weeks and the animal has not been receiving antibiotic therapy. The RSAT is not specific. False-positive results are common. If the RAST for *B. canis* result is positive, antibiotic therapy must be withheld until confirmatory tests are complete. If the RSAT for *B. canis* is negative, additional diagnostic tests for orchitis can be pursued. These could include ultrasound, seminal fluid cytology and culture, and/or fine-needle aspiration to obtain samples for cytologic evaluation and culture. Empiric treatment with antibiotics may be initiated pending the results. If trauma is the suspected cause, cold compresses may be considered to reduce swelling because pressure will have a negative effect on spermatogenesis. In the case of unilateral orchitis in a valuable stud, the fate of the contralateral testis must be considered. Spermatogenesis can be adversely affected by the heat, pressure, and/or direct extension of infection. To save the unaffected side, hemicastration might be consider if response to treatment is not prompt.

Torsion of the Spermatic Cord

Other causes of testicular enlargement include spermatic cord torsion and spermatic cord occlusion. Torsion of the spermatic cord has often been referred to as testicular torsion, but torsion of the spermatic cord is more accurate. Torsion of the spermatic cord occurs more often in intraabdominal testes than in scrotal testes.[21] Often the intraabdominal testis also has a tumor. The most prominent clinical sign of spermatic cord torsion is the acute onset of severe pain. The clinical signs may be typical of an acute abdomen when an intraabdominal testis is involved. The pain with intrascrotal spermatic cord torsion may be manifest by reluctance to walk.[22] Torsion of the spermatic cord causes swelling and firmness of the cord, the epididymis, and the testis. The spiral nature and dilation of the testicular vessels within the torsed spermatic cord may be recognized by ultrasound.

Treatment is castration of the affected intraabdominal testis. Castration is also usually recommended for intrascrotal spermatic cord torsion because irreparable damage to spermatogenesis may occur within hours. A scrotal hernia can also cause occlusion of the spermatic cord,[23] in which case, the clinical signs are identical to torsion of the cord. More commonly, however, scrotal hernias do not occlude the spermatic cord or affect the testes. The usual signs of scrotal hernia are unilateral scrotal enlargement with minimal pain.

Testicular Hypoplasia

A variety of congenital disorders results in testicular hypoplasia or hypogonadism. Often abnormal genitalia are an associated finding. Hypoplasia and hypogonadism are recognized in young animals as they reach puberty. As discussed earlier, genetic and hormonal factors are necessary for normal determination of the indifferent gonad into a testis and subsequent sexual differentiation into a phenotypic male. Therefore, abnormalities in expression of genes that determine the differentiation of the testis, in the testicular production of hormones, and/or in hormone receptors may be involved.[24-26] Determining the specific cause of testicular hypoplasia in an individual animal usually requires extensive evaluation, particularly if the external genitalia are a normal male phenotype. An exception is the calico or tortoiseshell tom cat.

Because both the orange and the black coat color require an X chromosome to be expressed, male cats, having only one X, should not be able to show both colors. The calico or tortoiseshell coat color is therefore a marker for XXY or a chimeric state. At least 7 different chromosomal compliments have been described for male calico/tortoiseshell cats.[6] Some of these cats are fertile, phenotypically normal males with normal spermatogenesis found on testicular histopathology. Presumably these are chimeras with the normal feline 38, XY karyotype in the gonadal tissue. Some calico/tortoiseshell toms have testicular hypoplasia. Testicular histopathology may be normal in some areas; some or all seminiferous tubules without spermatogonia; or, some or all tubules with Sertoli cells only.

In other animals with testicular hypoplasia, abnormalities anywhere along the hypothalamic-pituitary-gonadal axis, as well as disorders of sexual differentiation, must also be considered. The finding of concomitant abnormalities in the external or internal genitalia, such as ambiguous or female external genitalia, hypospadia, or persistent müllerian ducts, helps define the factors that might be involved.[27,28] Sometimes, straightforward karyotyping provides the answer.

Because animals with testicular hypoplasia are unlikely to have normal semen quality and usually are otherwise not desirable for breeding, extensive workup may not be warranted for the benefit of the individual. However, if more than one animal in the lineage is similarly affected, workup may be worthwhile for the breed. Physical examination will confirm the abnormally small testes. If need be, the functional ability of hypoplastic testes could be evaluated by measuring testosterone before and after the administration of GnRH or hCG, and by evaluating semen. The results are unlikely to be normal, but if they were, some owners might elect not to have the animal castrated.

Testicular Atrophy

In contrast to hypoplasia, testicular degeneration and atrophy are acquired conditions. Testicular atrophy is common in geriatric dogs, especially those over 10 years of age. The American Kennel Club will not register puppies sired by dogs older than 12 years without documentation of normal semen. The testis is easily damaged and atrophy often results. The spermatogonia are usually more sensitive to damage than are Sertoli and interstitial cells. Therefore, testosterone production may continue even when spermatogenesis is lost. Heat, pressure, infection, certain toxins and drugs (including glucocorticoids), radiation, nutritional deficiencies, and trauma (including biopsy) are a few of the many causes. By the time a male is presented with atrophic or degenerate testes, it may be difficult to determine the initiating cause. If a dog still has value as a stud, testicular function should be evaluated over longer than a 2-month period because the canine spermatogenic cycle is 62 days.[6] The prognosis for atrophic or degenerate testes to recover fertility is guarded, even if the cause can be found and corrected. If the condition is unilateral, submitting the affected side for culture and histopathologic evaluation would be reasonable.

Azoospermia

Male animals may be presented for evaluation of functional, rather than physical, abnormalities of the testes. A thorough history and physical examination should be performed. *Brucella canis* serology should be done in any dog presented for infertility. The first step in evaluating the endocrine function of the gonad is to determine serum concentrations of testosterone before and after GnRH or hCG. The first step in evaluating spermatogenesis is to perform a semen evaluation. Readers are referred to the textbook Canine and Feline Theriogenology[6] for a complete discussion of the diagnostic approach to infertility in the stud. Our discussion will be limited to the absence of sperm, azoospermia, in the ejaculate because this is a situation that often warrants testicular biopsy. In animals that still have sperm in the ejaculate, biopsy is often recommended as the last diagnostic test because damage to the testicular parenchyma will be done in the process. Although in the absence of complications, testicular biopsy of normal testes apparently does not have an adverse effect on semen quality in dogs,[29] the same may not be true for testes wherein spermatogenesis is already marginal.

The absence of sperm in the ejaculate may reflect retrograde ejaculation, incomplete ejaculation, obstruction to sperm outflow, or lack of spermatogenesis. Retrograde ejaculation of a few spermatozoa into the urinary bladder is normal in dogs and cats. The magnitude is greater when electroejaculation is the technique used for semen collection.[30] Although it has been considered by some to be a potential cause of azoospermia, the author has not observed retrograde ejaculation of such magnitude to explain a complete lack of sperm in the seminal fluid. To evaluate the possibility, the number of spermatozoa in the seminal fluid collected is compared with the number obtained from the urinary bladder after ejaculation.

The canine epididymis produces alkaline phosphatase. Therefore, the concentration of alkaline phosphatase in seminal fluid can be used as a marker for the presence of epididymal fluid in the ejaculate. Fluid originating from the epididymis should also contain motile spermatozoa. When it does not, but alkaline phosphatase concentrations are high, either bilateral obstruction to outflow of sperm from the testes to the epididymes exists, or the testes are not producing sperm. If an azoospermic sample has low concentrations of alkaline phosphatase, two possibilities exist. One is that only the first fraction (pre-sperm) of the ejaculate, which originates from the prostate, was collected. The other possibility is bilateral obstruction to outflow of sperm from the epididymes.

In dogs and cats, samples obtained by fine-needle aspiration of the testis may be used to assess the presence or absence of spermatozoa. However, biopsy specimens will be necessary to fully assess the spermatogenic cycle.[31] Meticulous surgical technique and the postoperative application of cold compresses to the scrotum will help minimize post-biopsy swelling.[32]

References

1. Silversides DW, Pilon N, Behdjani R, et al: Genetic manipulation of sex differentiation and phenotype in domestic animals. Theriogenology 55:51, 2001.

2. Hughes IA: Female development – all by default? N Engl J Med 351:8, 2004.

3. Melniczek JR, Dambach D, Prociuk U, et al: Sry-negative XX sex reversal in a family of Norwegian Elkhounds. J Vet Intern Med 13:564, 1999.

4. Meyers-Wallen VN, Manganaro TF, Kuroda T, et al: The critical period for Müllerian duct regression in the dog embryo. Biol Reproduc 45:626, 1991.

5. Gorlov IP, Kamat A, Bogatcheva NV, et al: Mutations of the GREAT gene case cryptorchidism. Hum Molec Gen 11:2309, 2002.

6. Johnston SD, Root Kustritz MV, Olson PN: Sexual differentiation and normal anatomy of the dog. Sexual differentiation and normal anatomy of the tom cat. *In* Canine and Feline Theriogenology, Philadelphia: WB Saunders, 2001, pp. 275; 497.

7. Millis DL, Hauphman JG, Johnson CA: Cryptorchidism and monorchidism in cats. 25 cases (1980-1989) J Am Vet Med Assoc 200:1128, 1992.

8. Williams LS, Levy JK, Robertson SA, et al: Use of the anesthetic combination of tiletamine, zolazepam, ketamine and xylazine for neutering feral cats. J Am Vet Med Assoc 220:1491, 2002.

9. Nielen AL, Janss LL, Knol BW: Heritability estimations of diseases, coat color, body weight, and height in a birth cohort of Boxers. Am J Vet Res 62:1198, 2001.

10. Yasuda MN, Kamimura Y, et al: Teratoma in a feline unilateral cryptorchid testis. Vet Pathol 38:729, 2001.

11. Rafer J, Handelsman DJ, Swerdloff RS, et al: Hormonal therapy of cryptorchidism. N Engl J Med 314:466, 1986.

12. Peters MA, de Jong FH, Teerds KJ, et al: Ageing, testicular tumors and the pituitary-testis axis in dogs. J Endocrinol 166:153, 2000.

13. Reif JS, Maguire TG, Kenney RM: A cohort study of canine testicular neoplasia, J Am Vet Med Assoc 175:719, 1979.

14. Pendergrass TW, Hayes HM: Cryptorchidism and related defects in dogs: epidemiologic comparisons to man. Teratology 12:51, 1975.

15. Hayes HM, Tarone RE, Casey HW: A cohort study of the effects of Vietnam service on testicular pathology of US military working dogs. Military Med 160:248, 1995.

16. Peters MA, Mol JA, van Wolferen ME, et al: Expression of insulin-like growth factor (IGF) system and steroidogenic enzymes in canine testis tumors. Reprod Biol Endocrinol 1:22, 2003.

17. Mischke R, Meurer D, Hoppen HO, et al: Blood plasma concentration of oestradiol-17β, testosterone and testosterone/oestradiol ratio

in dogs with neoplastic and degenerative testicular diseases. Res Vet Sci 73:267, 2002.

18. Mayenco Aguirre AM, Garcia Fernandez P, Sanchez Muela M: Sperm granuloma in the dog: Complications of vasectomy. J Small Anim Pract 37:392, 1996.

19. Johnson CA, Walker RD: Clinical signs and diagnosis of Brucella canis infecture. Comp Cont Edu 14:763, 1992.

20. Fritz TE, Lombard LS, Tyler SA, et al: Pathology and familial incidence of orchitis and its relationship to thyroiditis in a closed beagle colony. Exper Molec Pathol 24:142, 1976.

21. Naylor RW, Thompson SM: Intra-abdominal testicular torsion – a report of two cases. J Am Animal Hosp Assoc 15:763, 1979.

22. Young ACB: Two cases of intrascrotal torsion of a normal testicle. J Small Anim Pract 20:229, 1979.

23. Dorn AS: Spermatic cord occlusion in a dog. J Am Vet Med Assoc 173:82, 1978.

24. Flier JS, Underhill LH: Androgen resistance – the clinical and molecular spectrum. N Engl J Med 326:611, 1992.

25. Peter AT, Markwelder D, Asem EK: Phenotypic feminization in a genetic male dog caused by nonfunctional androgen receptors. Theriogenol 40:1093, 1993.

26. Knighton EL: Congenital adrenal hyperplasia secondary to 11β-hydroxylase deficiency in a domestic cat. J Am Vet Med Assoc 225:238, 2004.

27. Meyers-Wallen VN, Donahue PK, Ueno S, et al: Müllerian inhibiting substance is present in testes of dogs with persistent Müllerian duct syndrome. Biol Reproduct 41:881, 1989.

28. King GJ, Johnson EH: Hypospadias in a Himalayan cat. J Small Anim Pract 41:508, 2000.

29. Attia KA, Zaki AA, Eilts BE, et al: Anti-sperm antibodies and seminal characteristics after testicular biopsy or epididymal aspiration in dogs. Theriogenol 53:1355, 2000.

30. Dooley MP, Pineda MH: Effect of method of collection on seminal characteristics of the domestic cat. Am J Vet Res 47:286, 1986.

31. Dajlbom M, Mäkinen A, Suominen J: Testicular fine needle aspiration cytology as a diagnostic tool in dog infertility. J Small Anim Pract 38:506, 1997.

32. Johnson CA, Olivier NB, Nachreiner RF, et al: Effect of 131I-induced hypothyroidism on indices of reproductive function in adult male dogs. J Vet Intern Med 13:103, 1999.

Chapter 74

Pathophysiology of the Penis

Michelle Anne Kutzler

Development

Normal reproductive development in male dogs and cats is dependent on exposure of the embryologic urogenital sinus and mesonephric (Wolffian) ducts to androgens during the middle third of gestation (between 20 and 40 days before birth). At this stage of development, the urogenital sinus consists of a pelvic portion that extends from the bladder to the ischial arch and from which the urethra is derived and also a phallic portion that is associated with the genital tubercle. The epithelial lining of the phallic portion expands along the genital tubercle as a solid cord called the urethral plate and hollows to form a canal. Mesenchymal proliferation on both sides of the urethral plate enlarges the urogenital folds, leading to the establishment of a median urethral groove on the ventral surface of the genital tubercle. The elongating genital tubercle develops into the penis and the urogenital folds fuse ventrally along the entire length of the genital tubercle, establishing the penile urethra. The erectile tissue of the corpus spongiosum is formed by differentiation of mesodermal tissues within the urethral folds, and it advances along the urethra as fusion of the urethral folds progresses. The scrotal swelling that arises lateral to the urogenital folds gradually moves caudomedially and the caudal parts enlarge and fuse in the midline to form the scrotum and the scrotal raphe. The prepuce develops from a separation of two layers of ectodermal cells that originate on the distal tip of the penis. In prepubertal dogs, the separation of ectodermal layers forms an incomplete ring with a ventral connection between the under surface of the glans of the penis and prepuce, known as the frenulum. In contrast to dogs, the prepuce of prepubertal cats is circumferentially adhered to the glans. In both species, this penile-preputial attachment prevents extension of the glans from the prepuce during erection. The normal preputial mucosa is composed of stratified squamous epithelium. When substitutes for preputial mucosa are needed during a surgical repair, buccal or intestinal mucosa has been successfully used as a substitute.[1]

During embryonic development, the urethra is reported to arise from the fusion of paired free edges of the urethral folds, resulting in a closure of the urethral fossa after rupture of the urethral membrane.[2] However, subsequent research was unable to detect either fusion of the urethral folds or rupture of the urogenital membrane so the precise embryologic development of the urethra remains unclear.[3] What is not in dispute is that, in the absence of androgens (testosterone or dihydrotestosterone) or androgen receptors, the mesonephric ducts, penis, and penile urethra do not develop.[4] In addition, prenatal androgen exposure in female fetal dogs and cats masculinizes the urogenital sinus and allows persistence of the mesonephric ducts.[5]

Anatomy and Physiology

The prepuce is a fold of skin that covers the glans penis when the penis is not erect. The prepuce consists of an external lamina and an internal lamina, which are continuous at the preputial opening. The internal lamina terminates at the fornix, where it becomes continuous with the skin of the glans, while the external lamina is the haired skin of the outer surface. The prepuce is suspended from the ventral abdomen by preputial ligaments and muscles. These modified cutaneous muscles keep the prepuce over the glans of the penis in the retracted state. The penis is attached to the ischial arch by the crura and ischiocavernosus muscles. The penis consists of the root, body, and glans. The root is not externally visible. The body of the penis is made up of cavernous tissue. The distal corpus cavernosum is ossified (os penis) and extends distally from just behind the bulb to the tip of the glans.[6] A ventral groove within the os penis accommodates the urethra, the proximal end of which is a common site of urethral obstruction with urinary calculi.[4] The glans penis of the dog is divided into two principal parts: the pars longa glandis and the bulbus glandis. Applying pressure behind the bulbus glandis results in contraction of the ischiourethralis muscle, which inserts onto a fibrous ring that encircles the common trunk of the left and right dorsal veins of the penis. Contraction of the ischiourethralis muscle occludes the dorsal vein, resulting in engorgement of the cavernous tissues within the penis. Additionally, the caudal twisting of the penis during tail-to-tail position taken during the genital lock in dogs occludes the emissary veins.[7] Transection of the ischiourethralis muscle prevents canine erection, including partial penile erection of the bulbus glandis.[8] Detumescence requires relaxation of these muscle fibers, which allows drainage through the pudendal veins.

On the glans of the adult intact cat penis is a band about 4 mm wide, consisting of 120 to 150 backward-pointing keratinized spines encircling the glans and forming 6 to 8 circular rows.[9] These spines are androgen-sensitive and an indirect indicator of the presence of male hormones in cats.[9] The spines completely regress 13 to 24 weeks after castration.[9] The spines are an adaptation to provide additional stimulation during breeding to induce ovulation.[9] However, the smooth penis of the castrated male will still cause ovulation.[9] The urethral epithelium is also androgen-sensitive in male cats and is significantly higher with a lower fibrocyte density than in castrates.[4] The presence of penile spines can be used to identify incompletely castrated males.[10] Additional endocrine stimulation testing can be used to confirm a diagnosis of incomplete castration beginning with a venous blood sample collected for baseline testosterone concentration. Post-stimulation blood samples are collected 30 and 120 minutes after intravenous (500 IU/cat) administration of human chorionic gonadotropin (HCG).[10] Testosterone concentrations increase by 5- and 10-fold in 30 and 120 minutes, respectively.[10] HCG administration by intravenous injection produces a more consistent stimulation than intramuscular or subcutaneous administration.

The vascular supply of the prepuce is through the dorsal artery and vein of the penis and a branch of the external pudendal vessels. The lymphatic drainage is to the preputial and superficial inguinal lymph nodes. The blood supply to the corpus cavernosum penis is by the deep and dorsal penile arteries. Erection occurs when an increase in cavernosal arterial blood flow is coupled with a decrease in venous outflow from the corpora via the dorsal penile vein, resulting in sinusoidal relaxation and filling of the corpora cavernosum.

The corpus cavernosum is a conglomeration of venous sinusoids that functions as erectile tissue. The caudal epigastric artery can serve as a donor vessel to increase blood flow to the corpus cavernosa when flow has been reduced to the dorsal penile artery.[11] In the dog, the rapid engorgement of the bulb also depends on dilation of helicine arteries in the erectile tissue along with venous blood from the pars longa glandis. An elaborate venous drainage system connects the corpora to the iliac veins, and leakage in this system is an important cause of impotence in man. The circumflex vein drains into the deep dorsal vein and provides additional drainage to the distal two thirds of the cavernous bodies. Minor cavernous vein leakage in the presence of normal arterial flow has minimal effect on the development of erection.[12] However, penile rigidity can be prevented by excessive cavernous vein outflow resulting from pathologic changes in the cavernous smooth muscles, abnormal local venous drainage, insufficient neurotransmitter release, and alteration of the cavernous endothelium.[13] The corporal bodies are easily accessible to percutaneous needle punctures and can be used as an emergency vascular access in dogs with severe hypovolemia.[14]

The spinal nuclei for control of erection are located in the intermediolateral gray matter at the S1-S3 and T12-L3 in dogs.[15] The sacral nuclei axons fuse to form the pelvic nerve (nervus erigens), whose visceral parasympathetic efferent fibers (cavernous nerves) are located on the lateral aspect of the urethra.[15] The cavernous nerves penetrate the tunica albuginea of the corpora cavernosa alone and enter with the deep penile artery and cavernous vein.[15] These nerves can be damaged easily during urogenital surgery. Desensitization of the glans penis results in genital disorientation during mating and also intromission failure in cats16 but not in dogs.[17] In the dog, thoracolumbar sympathectomy results in reduced mating frequency, but when copulation does occur, the genital lock, which is highly dependent on vasomotor changes in the penis, remains unaltered.[18] Erection can be induced via electrostimulation of the cavernous nerves along the posterolateral aspect of the prostate.[11] Erection can also be induced in castrated males, but a higher threshold level of energy is needed. The minimum voltage required to induce erection in intact dogs (0.2 – 4.0 V) was half of that of castrates (0.6 – 12 V).[19]

The hypogastric nerve is a peripheral sympathetic nerve that plays a crucial role in the transport of sperm through the vas deferens, secretion of accessory gland fluid, and bladder neck closure. Pressure receptors for ejaculation are located in the body of the penis beneath the surface of the epithelium. Ejaculation failure occurs when sympathetic pathways from the lumbar splanchnic nerve are injured bilaterally in the retroperitoneum or within the pelvis, resulting in impaired bladder neck closure but unimpaired seminal emission.[20] Bilateral transection of the hypogastric nerves in dogs results in retrograde ejaculation, as the hypogastric nerves are the sole pathway of efferent signals for active bladder neck contraction at ejaculation.[20] The function of the hypogastric nerve can be returned after hypogastric nerve-hypogastric nerve reattachment.[20]

The male dog has two ejaculatory reflexes that are mainly controlled by somatic signals via the pudendal nerve from which the dorsal nerve of the penis arises. The first ejaculatory reflex occurs following intromission, lasts for 15 to 30 seconds, and is characterized by intense pelvic movement, alternate stepping of the back legs, rapid engorgement of the glans penis, contraction of the bulbospongiosus muscle, and expulsion of the sperm-rich fraction of the ejaculate. The second ejaculatory reflex occurs during the genital lock, lasts for 10 to 30 minutes, and is characterized by rhythmic contraction of the urethral muscles, bulbospongiosus muscle, and ischiocavernosus muscle, and expulsion of prostatic fluid.

Congenital Penile and Preputial Abnormalities

Hypospadias

Hypospadias is an uncommon congenital abnormality of male external genitalia in dogs and cats.[21] The exact frequency is unknown because severe cases result in neonatal death and mild cases may go undiagnosed.[21] Few reports have been published of this condition in cats and a review of 2.2 million canine medical records from 17 veterinary teaching hospitals yielded only 66 cases.[21] Hypospadias occurs when development of the urethra is incomplete. Hypospadias is defined by the location of the urethral orifice: glandular, penile, penoscrotal, scrotal, and perineal.[1] Hypospadias may result from fetal androgen deficiency, 5-α-reductase deficiency, or tissue resistance to androgens.[22] Hypospadia also occurs frequently with intersex conditions. Affected individuals are genetically male (XY) with abnormally formed external genitalia and bilateral cryptorchidism. In addition, a familial genetic component to hypospadias in dogs may exist as the Boston terrier breed is overrepresented with this condition.[21] Developmental preputial defects, such as those occurring with hypospadias, can be surgically corrected by manipulation of the preputial muscles to provide cranial advancement of the prepuce over the penis. A caudal superficial epigastric arterial pedicle flap has been suggested as a source of skin for preputial reconstruction.[23] Blood supply to the flap site, skin availability, type and size of defect, and restoration of function following reconstruction all must be considered before surgery.

Persistent Frenulum

Persistence of the penile frenulum occurs infrequently in dogs and cats. Common clinical signs of a persistent frenulum include pain during erection, intromission failure, balanoposthitis, and dysuria.[24] In non-breeding animals, no clinical signs may be associated with the condition. Surgical ligation and sectioning of the frenulum are curative and the prognosis is excellent.[24]

Phimosis

Phimosis, a rare disorder in dogs and cats, is the inability to extend the glans penis beyond the preputial orifice and is characterized by a narrow preputial opening.[25] Few published reports exist on abnormally small preputial openings in dogs. Clinical signs of phimosis vary from an asymptomatic narrowing of the preputial orifice, to preputial urine retention with posthitis, to complete occlusion of the preputial orifice with signs of urinary obstruction. Surgical repair of phimosis includes resection of a small wedge of the dorsal preputial margin followed by apposition of the ipsilateral preputial skin and mucosal edges.[26] Care must be taken that the new preputial opening is not made too large so as to allow continual protrusion of the penis.

Acquired Penile and Preputial Abnormalities

Paraphimosis

Paraphimosis is an inability to completely withdraw the penis into the prepuce.[27] It is most commonly seen in young intact males and may occur secondary to trauma, masturbation, sexual hyperactivity or the presence of a female in estrus, constriction of preputial hair around the penis, inability of the preputial muscles to pull the prepuce back over glans penis after erection, pseudohermaphroditism, neurologic deficits in dogs with posterior paresis, or as an idiopathic event. Prolonged exposure of the glans penis causes vascular engorgement, epithelial drying, edema, and inflammation, thus exacerbating the paraphimosis.[27] The condition becomes worse with time and may progress to corporal thrombosis.

The conservative treatment is to replace the penis in the prepuce as soon as possible with the aid of regional anesthesia. Penile edema can be relieved by massage. A preputiotomy may be necessary to accommodate replacement of the penis. If a preputiotomy is performed, the tissues should be carefully closed to the original state. In cases where nonsurgical management has failed, preputial lengthening (preputioplasty), preputial muscle myorrhaphy (shortening of the preputial muscles), and penile amputation with concurrent urethrostomy have been reported to correct the paraphimosis.[28] To amputate the penis, the prepuce is reflected caudally following excision of the suspensory structures and ligation of the preputial blood supply. The dorsal and deep arteries of the penis, both branches of the perineal artery, are ligated when the penis is amputated from the ischial attachments.[29] A segment of the urethra should be retained for urethrostomy.

Phallopexy is another method for treatment of paraphimosis that results from the creation of a permanent adhesion between the dorsal surface of the penis and the preputial mucosa.[27] Phallopexy should be performed on the dorsal surface of the penile shaft to avoid the urethra and the looser preputial tissues present on the ventral side.[27] During this procedure, care must be taken to avoid incising into the underlying cavernous tissue.[27] Urine pooling and balanoposthitis may result if this procedure is performed too far caudally in the prepuce.[27] The penile tip should be retained inside the preputial orifice 5 to 10 mm when the penis is in the nonerect state.[25]

Priapism

Priapism, an uncommon disorder in cats and dogs, is a persistent penile erection in the absence of sexual excitation that results in pain and dysuria. Priapism is most likely to develop secondary to trauma during mating or during castration, genitourinary infection or inflammation, or constipation resulting in persistent pelvic nerve stimulation, neurologic dysfunction (e.g., distemper-associated inflammatory lesions within the spinal cord), or from decreased venous outflow resulting from an occlusive thromboembolism or mass.[30] This form of priapism (low-flow priapism) is associated with a poorer prognosis as the damage from the ischemia is more severe.[31] In low-flow priapism, the danger is not in the priapism itself, but in the reduction of oxygen and an elevation of carbon dioxide partial pressure resulting from the hemostasis within the cavernous tissues.[32] High-flow priapism results from a persistent increase in blood flow from a neuroarterial disturbance or the development of arteriovenous fistulae.[31]

Arteriovenous fistulae are reported infrequently dogs and cats. Occasionally, arteriovenous fistulae develop on the prepuce.[33] Clinically, a preputial arteriovenous fistula manifests as a network of large tortuous pulsating blood vessels that enlarge gradually over several months.[33] Diagnosis can be made using angiography. Angiography is the optimal technique for planning treatment of arteriovenous communications. Characteristic angiographic findings of arteriovenous fistulae include premature venous filling, absence of the normal capillary phase, and reduced distal arterial flow.[34] Conservative surgical treatment for arteriovenous fistulae involves ligating the proximal supplying vessels to reduce blood flow through the fistula.[33] The prognosis for dogs with arteriovenous fistulae depends on the size and site of the fistula and the degree of cardiovascular failure at the time of diagnosis.[34]

A penile cavernogram can be used to identify thromboemboli or masses resulting in decreased venous outflow as well as the extent of venous outflow impairment.[35] Dynamic cavernosography consists of infusing heparinized saline at increasing rates (3-25 ml/minute) until the intracavernous pressure plateaus at 80 mm Hg (full erection pressure) followed by infusion of 60% Hypaque meglumine contrast medium to opacify abnormally draining veins.[13] Butterfly needles (21-gauge) can be inserted into the corpora cavernosa and connected to a pressure transducer. Dynamic cavernosometry should be performed following erection induction with administration of intracavernous papaverine (2-10 mg).[11,36] Papaverine decreases arterial resistance and increases venous resistance. Intracavernosal injection of epinephrine, norepinephrine, or phenylephrine prevents penile erection.[37]

Regardless of the primary cause, stagnation of blood containing a decreased concentration of oxygen and an increased concentration of carbon dioxide in the cavernous tissues results in edema formation with further venous occlusion and eventual irreversible fibrosis in the main venous outflow tracts of the penis. Histologically, severe cavernosal congestion with large hemoglobin crystals and organizing fibrin thrombi develop.[30] Conservative treatment consists of various combinations of cold water compresses, penile lubrication, corticosteroids, antibiotics and diuretics. Because the penis cannot be manually reduced into the prepuce, it becomes congested, dry, and eventually necrotic. Medical treatment with intravenous benzotropine mesylate (0.015 mg/kg), an anticholinergic and antihistaminergic drug, has been used successfully in horses but must be administered within 6 hours after the onset of priapism.[38] Increasing venous outflow via drainage and flushing of the cavernous tissues with heparinized saline (0.9% NaCl) solution in combination with infusion of phenylephrine[39] or epinephrine[40] has also been reported for the treatment of low-flow priapism. However, the penis may be irreparably damaged at the time of initial presentation, necessitating amputation and urethrostomy.

Trauma

Traumatic lesions of the penis and prepuce may result from bite wounds or automobile accidents, in association with a pelvic injury or during sexual activity while the penis is erect. Treatment of traumatic lesions of the penis varies depending on the damage. Emergency therapy should be directed at controlling hemorrhage and maintaining patency of the urethra. If the tip of the penis is lacerated, it can be debrided and sutured. A tourniquet around the proximal penis will decrease the amount of blood in the field and improve the precision with which sutures are placed. If damage is extensive, it may be necessary to amputate larger parts of the traumatized penis. A wedge-shaped incision should be made through the corpora tissues, and the os penis distal to the lesion is removed with a rongeur.[29] The cavernous body of the penis is sutured and the urethral orifice is re-established on the ventral body of the penis. Following preputial reconstruction, daily penile extrusion should be carried out to prevent adhesions between the penis and the prepuce.

The os penis can be fractured as a result of trauma; however, this injury is rare.[41] Fracture of the os penis may result in occlusion or disruption of the penile urethra. Presenting clinical signs include dysuria, stranguria, pollakiuria, and hematuria. In acute cases, pain can be elicited over the fracture site. Urethral catheterization may also indicate an obstruction at the level of the os penis. If a urinary catheter can be passed and the os penis fragments are well aligned, the fracture may heal satisfactorily with placement of an indwelling catheter for 5 to 21 days after the injury.[42] Distraction of the fracture fragments or swelling-associated trauma can result in urethral occlusion, which necessitates a urethrostomy to re-establish urine flow. A prescrotal urethrotomy will allow catheterization of the bladder if a urethral catheter will not pass through the penile urethra and will preserve the male's reproductive function.[29] The retractor penis muscle should be reflected to one side because splitting the retractor penis muscle will result in muscle contraction and premature closure of the urethrostomy site.[29]

Radiography is necessary for definitive diagnosis of an os penis fracture.[43] Surgical repair of the fracture is indicated if urethral obstruction is occurring. A rubber tourniquet is placed caudal to the os penis to minimize bleeding during surgery and a longitudinal incision is made through the epithelium on the lateral aspect of the penis.[43] A small periosteal elevator should be passed along the urethral groove in order to separate the corporal bodies from the os penis. Ventral ridges of the os penis can be debrided using bone-cutting forceps to allow expansion of the urethra within the urethral groove during healing of the fracture to prevent urethral narrowing. A finger plate[41] and Kirschner wires[44] have been used in the surgical repair of os penis fractures. Dorsal positioning of the screws through the os penis will prevent occlusion of the urethra.[43] In chronic cases of os penis fractures, palpation of the penis may reveal slight thickening over the fracture site.[41] Chronic dysuria or complete urethral obstruction following bone callus formation along the fracture site impinging the urethra may occur within 2 years of the trauma.[41,43,45] A retrograde urethrogram using a contrast agent will confirm location of urethral narrowing.[43] Surgical repair is accomplished by removing excess bone and fibrous tissue.[43] The effect of a fracture of the os penis on breeding ability has not been reported.

Neoplasia

Neoplasms of the glans penis and penis are not common.[28] Neoplasia common to skin will occur on the penis and prepuce; this includes papilloma, hemangioma, melanoma, and histiocytoma.[28] The transmissible venereal tumor can be found on the glans penis and prepuce. It is a contagious, neoplastic disease, transmitted by transplantation of viable tumor cells during mating.[46] Malignant neoplasms include mast cell sarcoma, reticulum cell sarcoma, melanoma, hemangiosarcoma, squamous cell carcinoma, and venereal sarcoma. Squamous carcinoma may be seen on the epithelium of the glans; a hemangiosarcoma of the cavernous tissues may occur.[28] Clinical signs include persistent or intermittent preputial discharge with the presence of solitary or multiple cauliflower-like, papillary, multilobulated or pedunculated masses. Any of these lesions should be widely excised and identified, and chemotherapy and/or radiation therapy should be instituted if indicated based on tumor identification.

References

1. Smith MM, Gourley IM: Preputial reconstruction in a dog. J Am Vet Med Assoc 196:1493-1496, 1990.
2. Glenister TW: A correlation of the normal and abnormal development of the penile urethra and of the infraabdominal wall. Br J Urol 30:117-126, 1958.
3. Kluth D, Lambreact W, Reich P: Pathogenesis of hypospadias – more questions than answers. J Pediatr Surg 23:1095-1101, 1988.
4. Herron MA: The effect of prepubertal castration on the penile urethra of the cat. J Am Vet Med Assoc 160:208-211, 1972.
5. Beach FA, Kuehn RE, Sprague RH, et al: Coital behavior in dogs. XI. Effects of androgenic stimulation during development on masculine mating responses in females. Horm Behav 3:143-168, 1972.
6. Beach FA: Hormonal modulation of genital reflexes in male and masculinized female dogs. Behav Neurosci 98(2):325-332, 1984.
7. Grandage J: The erect dog penis: a paradox of flexible rigidity. Vet Rec 91:141-147, 1972.
8. Hart BL: The action of extrinsic muscles during copulation in the male dog. Anat Rec 173:1-6, 1972.
9. Aronson LR, Cooper ML: Penile spines of the domestic cat: their endocrine-behavior relations. Anat Rec 157:71-78, 1967.
10. Memon MA, Ganjam VK, Pavletic MM, et al: Use of human chorionic gonadotropin stimulation test to detect a retained testis in a cat. J Am Vet Med Assoc 201:1602, 1992.
11. Floth A, Paick JS, Suh JK, et al: Hemodynamics of revascularization of the corpora cavernosa in an animal model. Urol Res 19:281-284, 1991.
12. Aboseif SR, Wetterauer U, Breza J, et al: The effect of venous incompetence and arterial insufficiency on erectile function: an animal model. J Urol 144:790-793, 1990.
13. Stief CG, Diederichs W, Benard F, et al: The diagnosis of venogenic impotence: dynamic or pharmacologic cavernosometry? J Urol 140:1561-1563, 1988.
14. Stein M, Gray R: Corpus cavernosum as an emergency vascular access in dogs. Acad Radiol 2:1073-1077, 1995.
15. Lue TF, Zeineh SJ, Schmidt RA, et al: Neuroanatomy of penile erection: its relevance to iatrogenic impotence. J Urol 131:273-280, 1984.
16. Aronson LR, Cooper ML: Mating behaviour in sexually inexperienced cats after desensitization of the glans penis. Anim Behav 17:208-212, 1969.
17. Hart BL: Reproductive system. *In* The Beagle As An Experimental Dog. Andersen AC (ed). Ames: Iowa State University Press, 1970, pp. 296-312.
18. Beach FA: Coital behavior in dogs: VII. Effects of sympathectomy in males. Brain Res 15:243-245, 1969.
19. Takahashi Y, Hirata Y, Yokoyama S, et al: Loss of penile erectile response to intracavernous injection of acetylcholine in castrated dog. Tohoku J Exp Med 163:85-91, 1991.
20. Kihara K, Sato K, Ando M, et al: A mechanism of retrograde ejaculation after bilateral hypogastric nerve transections in the dog. J Urol 148:1301-1309, 1992.
21. Hayes HM., Wilson GP: Hospital incidence of hypospadias in dogs in North America. Vet Rec 118:605-606, 1986.
22. Svensson J: Male hypospadias, 625 cases, associated malformations and possible etiological factors. Acta Paediatric Scand 68:587-592, 1979.
23. Paveltic MM: Caudal superficial epigastric arterial pedicle grafts in the dog. Vet Surg 9:103-107, 1980.
24. Barrand KR: Persistent penile frenulum. J Small Anim Pract 40:105, 142, 1999.
25. Proescholdt TA, DeYoung DW, Evans LE: Preputial reconstruction for phimosis and infantile penis. J Am Anim Hosp Assoc 13:725-727, 1977.
26. Bright SR, Mellanby RJ: Case report: Congenital phimosis in a cat. J Fel Med Surg 6:367-370, 2004.
27. Somerville ME, Anderson SM: Phallopexy for treatment of paraphimosis in the dog. J Am Anim Hosp Assoc 37:397-400, 2001.
28. Ndiritu CG: Lesions of the canine penis and prepuce. Mod Vet Pract 60:712-715, 1979.
29. Wilson GP: Surgery of the male reproductive tract. Vet Clin North Am 5:537-550, 1975.
30. Swalec KM, Smeak DD: Priapism after castration in a cat. J Am Vet Med Assoc 195:963-964, 1989.
31. Pohl J, Pott B, Kleinhans G: Priapism: a three phase concept of management according to aetiology and prognosis. Br J Urol 58:113-118, 1986.
32. Hashmat AL, Macchia RJ, Waterhouse K: Treatment of priapism by corporoglans shunt. A report on 20 cases. J Urol 125:A234, 1981.

33. Trower ND, White RN, Lamb CR: Arteriovenous fistula involving the prepuce of a dog. J Small Anim Pract 38:455-458, 1997.

34. Hosgood G: Arteriovenous fistulas: pathophysiology, diagnosis and treatment. Comp Cont Educ Pract Vet 11:625-636, 1989.

35. Root Kustritz MV, Olson PN: Priapism or paraphimosis. J Am Vet Med Assoc 214:1483-1484, 1999.

36. Lue TF, Hricak H, Schmidt RA, et al: Functional evaluation of penile veins by cavernosography in papaverine-induced erection. J Urol 135:479-482, 1986.

37. Lue TF: Intracavernous drug administration: its role in diagnosis and treatment of impotence. Semin Urol 8:100-106, 1990.

38. Wilson DV, Nickels FA, Williams MA: Pharmacologic treatment of priapism in two horses. J Am Vet Med Assoc 199:1183-1184, 1991.

39. Sidi AA: Vasoactive intracavernous pharmacotherapy. Urol Clin North Am 15:95-101, 1988.

40. Moon DG, Lee DS, Kim JJ: Altered contractile response of penis under hypoxia with metabolic acidosis. Int J Impot Res 11:265-271, 1999.

41. Stead AC: Fracture of the os penis in the dog–two case reports. J Small Anim Pract 13:19-22, 1972.

42. Robertson JJ: Management of miscellaneous orthopedic conditions. In Current Techniques *In* Small Animal Surgery, 3rd ed. Bojrab MJ (ed). Philadelphia: Lea & Febiger, 1990, pp. 894-895.

43. Kelly SE, Clark WT: Surgical repair of fracture of the os penis in a dog. J Small Anim Pract 36:507-509, 1995.

44. Jeffrey KL: Fracture of the os penis. J Am Anim Hosp Assoc 10:41-44, 1974.

45. Bradley RL: Complete urethral obstruction secondary to fracture of the os penis. Comp Cont Educ Pract Vet 7:759-763, 1985.

46. Páramo RM: Transmissible venereal tumors. *In* Veterinary Clinical Advisor. Coté E (ed). St. Louis: Elsevier, 2007, pp. 1191-1192.

Chapter 75

Dystocia in the Bitch

Catharina Linde Forsberg

Some of the more challenging but also most rewarding cases in the busy general practice are the bitches presenting with suspected, or confirmed dystocia, or where the owners ask for an elective Cesarean section. Often both the welfare of the mother and the chances for survival of the pups are dependent on the accurate assessments and informed decisions made by the veterinarians and the staff at the clinic. To diagnose dystocia, a thorough appreciation of the various stages of the normal parturition – eutocia - in the bitch is vital.

Physiologic Changes During Pregnancy Start

Metabolic demands are increased during pregnancy. Blood volume increases by 40%, primarily composed of plasma, resulting in a hemodilution and a hematocrit of around 30% at term. This is thought to facilitate placental perfusion. Cardiac output is increased owing to enhanced heart rate and stroke volume. Oxygen consumption during pregnancy increases by 20%, while the functional residual capacity of the lungs is decreased owing to anterior displacement of the diaphragm by the enlarged uterus. Pregnant animals also may have delayed gastric emptying owing to decreased gastric motility and displacement of the stomach.

Gestation Length

Gestation length in the bitch averages 63 days, but can vary from 56 to 72 days if calculated from the first mating.[1] This large variation is mainly owing to the long and variable period of behavioral estrus of the bitch. Gestation length is highly predictable when calculated either from the pre-ovulatory surge of luteinizing hormone (LH), when it is 65 ± 1 days; from the day of ovulation, when it is 63 ± 1 days;[2] or from the time of fertilization of the oocytes, when it is 60 ± 1 days.[1,3]

The ability to determine gestational age and to predict the day of parturition in the bitch is of considerable clinical importance especially in case of suspected prolonged gestation, as well as in a bitch that is scheduled for elective Caesarean section. Some of the methods discussed here are applicable only in the bitch that has been examined in advance in anticipation of dystocia, whereas others are useful also in acute cases of dystocia.

B-mode Ultrasonography

B-mode ultrasound can be used throughout pregnancy to assess the diameter of pregnancy structures and to estimate fetal size.[4-6] Inner chorionic cavity diameter on days 18 to 37 from ovulation and fetal head diameter on day 38 to parturition show the best correlation to gestational age and to predicting parturition day.

Other fetal structures used to time pregnancies are fetal limb buds, first detectable at days 33 to 35; eyes, kidney, and liver at days 39 to 47; and intestines at days 57 to 63.

Radiography

Using radiography, the fetal skeleton is visible rarely before day 42; the skull on days 45 to 49; pelvic bones on days 53 to 57; and teeth on days 58 to 63.

Serum Progesterone

Serum progesterone concentration can be a useful predictor of the day of parturition. It is becoming increasingly more common that breeders determine the optimal day of mating of the bitch by checking the serum progesterone during proestrus and estrus. Progesterone rises sharply from near basal levels to ≥ 4.5 nmol/l (≥ 1.5 ng/ml) at the time of the LH peak, and parturition can be expected to occur 65 ± 1 days later. The accuracy of prediction of parturition day within a ± 1, ± 2, and ± 3 day interval using pre-breeding serum progesterone concentrations was 67%, 90%, and 100%,[7] and was not seen to be influenced by either body weight or litter size. The serum progesterone level is also useful in predicting the parturition day in the bitch at term, as it decreases sharply from 12 to 15 nmol/l (4-5 ng/ml) to below 6 nmol/l (2 ng/ml) starting 24 hours before the onset of whelping.

Other Clinical Signs

Relaxation of the pelvic and abdominal musculature is a consistent but subtle indicator of impending parturition. It is, therefore, usually best observed by the owner of the bitch.

The drop in rectal temperature in most bitches is a good predictor of the day of parturition. During the final week of pregnancy the rectal temperature of the bitch fluctuates, as a consequence of the fluctuations in the (thermoregulatory) progesterone level, but it then drops sharply 8 to 24 hours before parturition, which is 10 to 14 hours after the concentration of progesterone in peripheral plasma has declined to less than 6 nmol/l (2 ng/ml). To properly assess the prepartum drop in body temperature, however, measurements should be made every 1 to 2 hours as long as the temperature decreases, but can be done less frequently when the temperature is seen to increase again. The degree of the drop in rectal temperature varies between 1° C (33.8° F) and 3.5° C (38.3° F), probably as an effect of surface area/body volume ratio. Thus, in short-haired miniature breed bitches it can fall to 35° C (95° F), in medium-sized bitches to around 36°C (96.8° F), whereas it seldom falls below 37°C (98.6° F) in bitches of the giant breeds or bitches with a thick hair coat. In bitches with uterine inertia, a distinct drop in body temperature may not be seen to occur.

Behavioral changes may be manifested. Several days before parturition the bitch may become restless, seek seclusion, or be excessively attentive, and may refuse food. She may exhibit nesting behavior 12 to 24 hours before parturition concomitant with increasing frequency and force of uterine contractions. Shivering is a response to the drop in body temperature.

In primiparous bitches, **lactation** may be established less than 24 hours before parturition, whereas, after several pregnancies, colostrum can be detected as early as 1 week pre-partum.

Normal Parturition

Stress produced by the reduction of the nutritional supply by the placenta to the fetus stimulates the fetal hypothalamic-pituitary-adrenal axis, resulting in release of adrenocorticosteroid hormone, and is thought to be the trigger for parturition. An increase in fetal and maternal cortisol is believed to stimulate the release of prostaglandin F_{2a}, which is luteolytic, from the fetoplacental tissue, resulting in a decline in plasma progesterone concentration. Withdrawal of the progesterone blockade of pregnancy is a prerequisite for the normal course of canine parturition; bitches given long-acting progesterone during pregnancy fail to deliver.[2] Concurrent with the gradual decrease in plasma progesterone concentration during the last 7 days before whelping is a progressive qualitative change in uterine electrical activity. A significant increase in uterine activity occurs during the last 24 hours before parturition, with the final fall in plasma progesterone concentration to below 6 nmol/l (2 ng/ml).[2,8,9] In the dog, estrogens have not been unambiguously shown to increase before parturition as they do in many other species. Sensory receptors within the cervix and vagina are stimulated by the distention created by the fetus and the fluid-filled fetal membranes. This afferent stimulation is conveyed to the hypothalamus and results in release of oxytocin during second stage labor. Afferents also participate in a spinal reflex arch with efferent stimulation of the abdominal musculature to produce abdominal straining. Relaxin causes the pelvic soft tissues and genital tract to relax, which facilitates fetal passage. In the pregnant bitch, this hormone is produced by the ovary and possibly also by the placenta and uterus and rises gradually over the last two thirds of pregnancy.[10]

First Stage

The duration of the first stage usually is between 6 and 12 hours. It may last 36 hours, especially in a nervous primiparous animal, but for this to be considered normal the rectal temperature must remain low. Vaginal relaxation and dilation of the cervix occur during this stage. Intermittent uterine contractions, with no signs of abdominal straining, are present. The bitch may appear uncomfortable, and the restless behavior may become more intense. Panting, tearing up and rearranging of bedding, shivering, and occasional vomiting may be seen. Some bitches show no behavioral evidence of first-stage labor. The inapparent uterine contractions increase both in frequency, duration, and intensity toward the end of the first stage. Inexperienced breeders may not fully understand the function of this preparatory stage of parturition during which the recurrence of uterine tones, the softening of the birth canal, and the opening of the cervix take place.

During pregnancy, the orientation of the fetuses within the uterus is 50% heading caudally and 50% cranially, but this changes during first-stage labor as the fetus may rotate on its long axis and extend its head, neck, and limbs. This results in 60% to 70% of pups being born in anterior and 30% to 40% in posterior presentation.[11,12] The fluid-filled fetal membranes are pushed ahead of the fetus by the uterine propulsive efforts and dilate the cervix.

Second Stage

It is crucial that the veterinarian is able to determine whether the bitch is in the second stage or still in the first stage of labor. If one or more of the following signs have been observed the bitch is in second-stage labor:

- The rectal temperature has been down and is returning to normal level
- Visible abdominal straining is observed
- Fetal fluids are passed

The duration of the second stage is usually between 3 and 12 hours; in rare cases, it has lasted 24 hours. At the onset of second-stage labor the rectal temperature rises to normal or slightly above normal. The first fetus engages in the pelvic inlet, and the subsequent intense, expulsive uterine contractions are accompanied by abdominal straining. On entering the birth canal the allantochorionic membrane may rupture and a discharge of some clear fluid may be noted. Covered by the amniotic membrane, the first fetus is usually delivered within 4 hours after onset of second-stage labor.[13] Normally, the bitch will break the membrane, lick the neonate intensively, and sever the umbilical cord. At times, the bitch will need some assistance to open the fetal membranes to allow the newborn to breathe, and sometimes the airways will have to be emptied of fetal fluids. The umbilicus can be clamped with a pair of hemostats and cut with a blunt scissors to minimize hemorrhage from the fetal vessels, leaving about 1 cm of the umbilicus. In case of continuing hemorrhage, the umbilicus should be ligated.

In normal labor the bitch may show infrequent and/or weak straining for up to 2, and at the most, 4 hours before giving birth to the first fetus. If the bitch is having strong, frequent but nonproductive straining, this indicates the presence of some obstruction. Veterinary advice should be sought after no more than 20 to 30 minutes.

Expulsion of the first fetus usually takes the longest. The interval between births in normal uncomplicated parturition is from 5 to 120 minutes.[11,12] As long as pups remain in both uterine horns the fetuses are mostly delivered alternately from each side. When giving birth to a large litter a bitch may accumulate lactic acid in the myometrium and stop straining. Such a rest between the deliveries of two consecutive fetuses may last for more than 2 hours. The second-stage straining will then resume, until all the fetuses are born. A normal parturition stimulates fetal circulation, empties airways of fetal fluids, and thereby, facilitates breathing.

Parturition is usually completed within 6 hours after the onset of secondstage labor, but it may last up to 12 hours. It should not be allowed to last for more than 24 hours considering the risks involved both for the bitch and the fetuses.

Third Stage

Expulsion of the placenta and shortening of the uterine horns usually follows within 15 minutes of the delivery of each fetus. Two or three fetuses may, however, be born before the passage of their placentas occurs. Should the bitch ingest more than one or two of the placentas, she may develop diarrhea. The greenish postpartum discharge of fetal fluids and placental remains (lochia) will be seen for up to 3 weeks or more. They are most profuse during the first week. Uterine involution is normally completed after 12 to 15 weeks.

Dystocia

Dystocia, defined as difficult birth or the inability to expel all fetuses through the birth canal without assistance, is a frequent problem in the dog. The over all incidence is probably below 5%, but in some breeds may amount to almost 100%, especially those of the achondroplastic type and those selected for large heads.[11,14,15] Dystocia in the bitch in around 75% of cases is of maternal origin, and in 25% of fetal origin (Table 75-1).[14]

Table 75-1. Causes of Dystocia in Bitches (182 cases) (Darvelid and Linde-Forsberg, 1994)

	Frequency (percent)
Maternal causes	75.3
Primary complete inertia	48.9
Primary partial inertia	23.1
Narrow birth canal	1.1
Uterine torsion	1.1
Uterine prolapse	–
Uterine strangulation	–
Hydrallantois	0.5
Vaginal septum formation	0.5
Fetal causes	24.7
Malpresentations	15.4
Malformations	1.6
Fetal oversize	6.6
Fetal death	1.1

Clinical Assessment

When a bitch with dystocia is presented, taking an accurate history and performing a thorough physical examination are important prerequisites for proper management. In the absence of an obvious cause for the dystocia, such as an obstructed fetus visible in the vagina, the three criteria for being in second-stage labor, namely body temperature returned to normal, visible abdominal straining, and passage of fetal fluids, should be assessed. An evaluation of the bitch's general health status should be made and signs of any adverse effects of parturition noted. Observation should be made of the bitch's behavior and the character and frequency of straining. The vulva and perineum should be examined, noting color and amount of vaginal discharge. Mammary gland development including congestion, distention, size, and presence of milk should be evaluated. Palpation of the abdomen and estimating the degree of distention and the uterine tone should be carried out. Digital examination of the vagina using aseptic technique should be undertaken to detect obstructions and determine the presence and presentation of any fetus in the pelvic canal. In most bitches, it is not possible to reach the cervix during first stage, but an assessment of the degree of dilation and tone of the vagina may give some indication of the status of the cervix and the tone of the uterus. Pronounced tone of the anterior vagina may indicate satisfactory muscular activity in the uterus, whereas flaccidity may indicate uterine inertia.[16] The character of the vaginal fluids also indicate whether the cervix is closed, with the production of a fluid that is scant and sticky, creating a certain resistance to the introduction of a finger, or open, when fetal fluids lubricate the vagina, making exploration easy. When the cervix is closed, the vaginal walls also fit tightly around the exploring finger, whereas with an open cervix the cranial vagina appears more open.

Radiographic examination is valuable to assess gross abnormalities of the maternal pelvis and the number and location of fetuses, to estimate fetal size, and to detect signs of fetal death. Intrafetal gas will appear 6 hours after fetal death and can be detected radiographically, whereas overlapping of cranial bones and collapse of the spinal column will be seen after 48 hours. Ultrasound examination will determine fetal viability or distress, with normal heart rate being 180 to 240 beats per minute, decelerating in the compromised fetus.

Diagnosis

The range of normal variations observed in dogs at parturition makes recognition of dystocia difficult. Although strict time limits are not applicable in all cases, and the intensity, duration, and frequency of the uterine contractions are also crucial factors, the following criteria may serve as rules of thumb, both in the discussions with the dog owners and to assist in the diagnosis:

- The rectal temperature has been down by 1 to 3° C and has returned to normal with no signs of labor.
- Fetal fluids were observed 2 to 3 hours ago but there are no signs of labor.
- Labor is absent for more than 2 hours or has been weak and infrequent for more than 2 to 4 hours.
- Labor has been normal but is becoming increasingly more infrequent and weak.
- Strong and persistent non-productive labor has been occurring for more than 20 to 30 minutes.
- A green vulvar discharge is present but no fetuses have been delivered. (This discharge emanates from the marginal hematoma of the placentas and indicates that at least one placenta is becoming separated from the maternal blood supply. It is normal once birth is underway).
- An obvious cause of dystocia is evident such as pelvic fracture or a fetus stuck in the birth canal and partially visible.
- The bitch has been in second-stage labor for more han 12 hours.

Signs of toxemia (disturbed general condition, edema, shock) are noted when parturition should be occurring.

Causes of Maternal Dystocia

Uterine Inertia

Uterine inertia is by far the most common cause of dystocia in dogs. In primary inertia, a normal uterus may fail to respond to the fetal signals because there are only one or two pups and, thus, insufficient stimulation to initiate labor (the single pup syndrome) or because of overstretching of the myometrium by a large litter, excessive fetal fluids, or oversized fetuses. Other causes of primary inertia may be an inherited predisposition, dehydration, or a nutritional imbalance, fatty infiltration of the myometrium, age-related changes, deficiency in neuroendocrine regulation, or systemic disease in the bitch. Primary complete uterine inertia is the failure of the uterus to begin labor at full term. Primary partial uterine inertia is said to occur when uterine activity is enough to initiate parturition but is insufficient to complete a normal birth of all fetuses in the absence of an obstruction. Secondary uterine inertia implies exhaustion of the normal uterine myometrium caused by obstruction of the birth canal. The pathogenesis of secondary inertia is thus different and medical treatment is seldom effective. Therefore, secondary intertia should be clearly distinguished from primary inertia.

Management of Uterine Inertia

It is not unusual that pups are born in the car on the way to the veterinarian. Most of these pups would probably have been delivered in the calm and quiet of home had the owners tried to induce straining in the bitch themselves, thereby giving the pup a better start in life and possibly also resulting in the whole litter being born without further intervention. In cases of primary uterine inertia with a bright and alert bitch, therefore, the owners should initially be instructed to try to induce straining by actively exercising the bitch for 10 to 15 minutes, for instance by running around the house or up and down the stairs. Another means to induce straining in the bitch with insufficient labor is by inserting two fingers into the vagina and pushing or "walking" with them against the dorsal vaginal wall, thus inducing an episode of straining (the Ferguson reflex). This method can also be effective in initiating labor after successful correction of the position or posture of an obstructed fetus. Gentle massaging of the mammary glands will induce oxytocin release and may enhance labor progress. Owners should also be advised to provide the bitch with sufficient fluids and energy, e.g., glucose, to avoid dehydration and hypoglycemia during labor.

Psychological stress may lead to nervous voluntary inhibition of labor, mainly in a nervous primiparous animal. Reassurance by the owner or administration of a low dose tranquilizer may remove the inhibition.[17] Once the first fetus is born, parturition will usually proceed normally.

The bitch with complete primary uterine inertia is usually bright and alert, has a normal rectal temperature, and has no evidence of labor. The cervix is often dilated, and vaginal exploration is easy to perform owing to the presence of fetal fluids, but the fetus may be out of reach because of the flaccid uterus. Before initiation of medical treatment of uterine inertia, obstruction of the birth canal must be excluded. Per oral or intravenous fluids and glucose should be administered.

Calcium solutions and oxytocin are the drugs of choice in cases of primary uterine inertia. Oxytocin has a direct action on the rate of calcium influx into the myometrial cell, which is essential for myometrial contraction. Some 10 minutes before the administration of oxytocin, 10% calcium borogluconate, 0.5 to 1.5 ml/kg bodyweight, should be given by slow intravenous infusion (1 ml/min) with careful monitoring of the heart rate. The calcium can also be administered subcutaneously, which eliminates the risk for arrhythmia but presents a small risk for granuloma formation at the injection site. Hypoglycemia may occur, particularly after prolonged straining. In such cases, a dilute (10 to 20%) glucose solution can be added to the infusion or given intravenously in doses of 5 to 20 ml. The recommended dose of oxytocin for the bitch is 1 to 5 IU given IV or 2.5 to 10 IU IM, and it can be repeated at 30-minute intervals. The response to treatment will, however, be reduced with each repeated administration. Higher doses than recommended or too frequent administration may result in prolonged contracture of the myometrium, preventing fetal expulsion and impeding uteroplacental blood flow, causing hypoxia in the fetuses. The disadvantages of oxytocin administration also include a tendency to cause premature induction of placental separation and cervical closure. If there is no response to treatment after a second administration of oxytocin, the pups should be delivered without further delay, either with the aid of obstetrical forceps, if only one or two pups remain and are within easy reach in the uterine corpus, or by cesarean section. The long-acting ergotamines should never be used in connection with parturition.

The treatment regimen includes:

- A 10% solution of calcium gluconate is given slowly intravenously while carefully checking the bitch's heart rate.
- The bitch is given 30 minutes to respond to treatment. If straining begins, the treatment can be repeated if necessary or continued with oxytocin.
- If the calcium infusion has no effect within 30 minutes, oxytocin is given intravenously or intramuscularly.
- The bitch is again given 30 minutes to respond to treatment. If straining begins, the treatment can be repeated if necessary, although each additional administration will elicit a weaker response.
- If no response occurs within 30 minutes, further treatment is not likely to be successful. The fetuses should be delivered, either by forceps, if only one or two fetuses remain and are within easy reach, or by cesarean section.

Obstruction of the Birth Canal

Some maternal causes for obstruction are listed below:

Uterine Torsion and Uterine Rupture

These are acute, life-threatening conditions occurring either during late pregnancy or at the time of parturition. The condition of the bitch may quickly deteriorate. Surgery is always required and a quick diagnosis is essential for survival of the bitch.

Uterine Inguinal Herniation

Uterine inguinal herniation is often detected during the fourth week of pregnancy when the fetal uterine enlargements are 2 to 2.5 cm in size. The early stages may be mistaken for mastitis of the rear mammary glands. The condition is corrected by surgery, repositioning the uterine horns, and suturing the herniation. In case of circulatory disturbance and substantial tissue damage, the uterus may have to be removed.

Soft Tissue Abnormalities

Soft tissue abnormalities such as vaginal septa and neoplasms or fibrosis of the birth canal may cause obstructive dystocia. Vaginal septa usually are remnants of the fetal müllerian duct system, but may also occur secondary to vaginal trauma or infection. If extensive, both septa and neoplasms may prevent the passage of the fetuses. Often, however, prepartum the vagina is relaxed enough to allow the fetuses to pass. Cervical or vaginal fibrosis is seen in rare cases and is usually secondary to trauma or inflammatory processes and may in severe cases cause dystocia. Tumors and septa formations may be surgically removed, preferably during anestrus and before mating; but in cases of fibrosis, surgery is seldom successful because of new scar tissue formation during the healing process.

Narrow Pelvic Canal

Narrow pelvic canal causing obstructive dystocia may result from immaturity, congenital malformation of the pelvis, or pelvic fractures. The normal canine pelvis usually has a vertical diameter greater than the horizontal. Congenitally narrow birth canals exist in some terrier and brachycephalic breeds, e.g., Boston terriers and Scottish terriers. In addition, fetuses of those breeds have comparatively large heads and wide shoulders. In the achondroplastic Scottish terrier, dorsoventral flattening of the pelvis modifies the normal pelvic inlet, and creates an obstruction to the engagement of the fetuses. Significant differences were found in Scottish terrier bitches whelping normally compared with those with dystocia owing to a too-narrow birth canal caused by a dorsoflattening and a shortening of the pelvis.[15] In Boston terrier bitches a significantly greater inner pelvic height was found in normally whelping bitches. In this breed also, the size of the pups, and especially of their heads, was important because the weight of the pup was related to the size of its head. The English bulldog has a large, deep chest and pronounced waist. The fetuses, therefore, are presented at a relatively acute angle to the pelvic inlet. Bulldogs also may have slack abdominal musculature, leading to insufficient uterine contractions and abdominal straining to lift the fetus up into the pelvic cavity. In cases of pelvic obstructions, usually a cesarean section is necessary. Genetic counseling to breeders is also important in these cases.[15]

Causes of Fetal Dystocia

Fetal causes of dystocia include malpresentations/malorientations and oversized fetuses or monstrosities, e.g., those with hydrocephalus, edema, or duplications. Fetal death may result in dystocia owing to malpositioning or inadequate stimulation for parturition to begin. A healthy fetus is active during expulsion, extending its head and limbs, twisting, and rotating to get through. In most breeds, the greatest bulk of the fetus lies in its abdominal cavity, whereas the bony parts, the head and the hips, are comparatively small. The limbs are short and flexible and rarely cause serious obstruction to delivery in the normally sized fetus.

Posterior Presentation

Posterior presentation is considered normal in dogs, occurring in 30% to 40% of fetal deliveries.[11,12] Posterior presentations have, however, been related both to higher pup mortality[11] and to a predisposition for dystocia, particularly where this involves the first fetus to be delivered, because mechanical dilation of the cervix may be inadequate. In addition, expulsion is rendered more difficult because the fetal chest instead of being compressed becomes distended by the pressure from the abdominal organs through the diaphragm and because the fetus is being delivered against the direction of its hair coat. Occasionally, the fetus may have the elbows hooked around the pelvic brim, preventing further expulsion. When a fetus becomes lodged in the pelvic canal, pressure on the umbilical vessels trapped between the fetal chest and the maternal pelvic floor may cause hypoxia and reflex inhalation of fetal fluids.

Breech Presentation

Breech presentation (i.e., posterior presentation with hindlegs flexed forward) can be a serious complication, especially in medium- and small-sized breeds. Vaginal exploration will reveal a tail tip and maybe the anus and the bony structure of the pelvis of the fetus.

Lateral or Downward Deviation of the Head

These are two of the most common malpositionings in the dog. Downward deviation is seen in brachycephalic breeds and long-headed breeds such as Sealyham and Scottish terriers whereas lateral deviation is most common with long-necked breeds such as rough collies. In downward deviation of the head, either both front legs and sometimes the nape of the neck of the fetus can be palpated, or both front legs may be flexed backwards and only the skull of the fetus be reached. In lateral deviation, vaginal exploration will demonstrate just one front leg, the one contralateral to the direction of the deviation of the head (i.e., when the head is deviated to the left, the right front paw will be found and vice versa).

Backward Flexion of Front Legs

This condition is especially common when the fetus is weak or dead and is sometimes seen in combination with deviation of the head, especially downward. For bitches of the larger or even medium-sized breeds, it may be possible to deliver a puppy with one or both front legs flexed.

Bicornual or Transverse Presentation

A fetus, instead of progressing from the uterine horn through the cervix to the vagina, may sometimes proceed into the contralateral uterine horn. This may be owing to some obstruction, or the fetus may have been implanted close to the body of the uterus. These cases always require surgery, because no room exists for manual correction.

Two Fetuses Presented Simultaneously

Sometimes one fetus from each horn is presented at the same time, jamming the birth canal. If one is coming backwards this one should when possible be removed first, because it occupies more space.

Oversized Fetuses

A pup weight of 4% to 5% of the weight of the bitch is considered the upper limit for an uncomplicated birth. Oversized fetuses are often associated with small litter size. In brachycephalic breeds such as the Boston terrier and the Scottish terrier, dystocia occurs from the combination of a flattened pelvic inlet and puppies having a large or a long head. Obstructive dystocia was found to occur at pup weights of 2.5% to 3.1% of the adult weight in these breeds.[15]

Management of Fetal Malpresentations

If a fetus is present in the birth canal, manipulation by hand or by obstetrical forceps may be attempted before a decision is made to proceed with a cesarean section. This is relevant in cases where it is assumed that, by removing the obstructed pup, the birth of the remaining pups may proceed without problems.

Fetal position must be assessed. If the fetus has advanced partly through the pelvic canal, it will create a characteristic bulge of the perineal region. Easing the vulvar lips upward may reveal the amniotic sac and the position of the fetus. Vaginal exploration and radiographic examination will aid in making a diagnosis in the cases when the fetus has not advanced as far. Having an assistant holding the bitch so that it is standing upright on the hind legs or with the bitch sitting on his lap facing forward takes advantage of the force of gravity to get the fetus within reach for palpation. In bitches of the giant breeds it may even be possible to insert one hand through the vagina into the uterus to extract the pup.

During natural birth the pup will almost make a full somersault, emerging from the loop of the uterine horn, progressing upward to pass through the pelvic canal, and then down through the long vagina and vestibulum of the bitch, to reach the vulva placed some 5 to 15 cm below the level of the pelvic floor. Thus, after the fetus is seized, a traction should be gently applied in posteroventral direction.

If external manipulation is to be attempted, generous application of obstetrical lubricant (liquid paraffin, petroleum jelly, or a sterile water-soluble lubricant) is helpful, especially if the bitch has been in second-stage labor for some time. The narrowest part of the birth canal is within the rigid pelvic girdle. The fetus that cannot be easily pulled out may have to be pushed cranially in front of the pelvic girdle, where corrections of its position or posture are easier to perform. This should be done between periods of straining of the bitch, never working against the uterine contractions. The widest part of the pelvic girdle usually is on the diagonal; thus, rotating the fetus 45 degrees may create sufficient room for passage.

Depending on the position and posture of the fetus, its head and neck should be grasped, from above or below whichever is most convenient, or its pelvis, or legs. Care should be taken because the neck and limbs of the fetus are easily torn when pulled. Correction of posture may be more easily accomplished by manipulation of the fetus through the abdominal wall with one hand and concurrent transvaginal manipulation with the other. A finger may be introduced into the mouth of the fetus to help in correcting a downward deviation of the head. Should it be necessary to change the postures of the limbs, a finger should be inserted past the elbow or knee and the limb moved medially under the fetus and corrected.

A gently applied alternating right-to-left traction of the puppy, gently rocking it back and forth or from side to side and possibly twisting it to a diagonal position within the pelvis, will help free the shoulders or the hips one at a time. By applying a slight pressure over the perineal bulge the fetus may be prevented from sliding back in again between strainings.

Obstetrical forceps should only be used for assisted traction of a relatively oversized fetus when the rest of the pups in the litter are likely smaller or when just one or two fetuses remain. The forceps is guided with a finger and never introduced further than to the uterine body because of the risk of getting part of the uterine wall within the grip, and thus causing serious damage. If the head of the fetus can be reached, the grip should be applied around the neck (Pålssons forceps) or across the cheeks. In posterior presentation the grip should be around the fetal pelvis. If the legs can be reached, the grip should be around those, not around the feet.

Outcome of Obstetrical Treatment

Digital manipulation including forceps delivery and/or medical treatment for dystocia is successful in only 27.6% of the cases.[14] Around 65% of bitches with dystocia, thus, end up having a cesarean section. Early diagnosis and prompt treatment are crucial to reduce pup death rate in cases of dystocia.

Criteria for Cesarean Section

The indications for Cesarean section include the following:

- Abnormalities of the maternal pelvis or soft tissues of the birth canal
- Primary, complete or partial, uterine inertia that does not respond to medical treatment
- Secondary uterine inertia with inadequate resumption of labor after removal of the obstruction
- Fetal absolute or relative oversize, or fetal monstrosity
- Excess or deficiency of fetal fluids
- Fetal malposition unamendable to manipulation
- Fetal death with putrefaction
- Pregnancy toxemia
- Neglected dystocia
- Prophylactic/elective (history of previous dystocia).

Once a decision has been made to deliver the litter by cesarean section, surgery should be carried out without delay. The bitch has often endured hours of more or less intensive labor and may be suffering from physical exhaustion, dehydration, acid-base disorders, hypotension, hypocalcaemia, and often, hypoglycemia. The prognosis for both bitch and offspring is good if surgery is performed within 12 hours after the onset of second-stage labor; it continues to be fairly good for the bitch after 12 hours but guarded for the fetuses. If more than 24 hours have passed after the onset of second-stage labor the entire litter is usually dead and further delay compromises the life of the bitch.

The decision to perform an elective Cesarean section should be made by the veterinarian based on a well founded presumption that if surgical intervention was not provided the bitch would experience dystocia. The veterinarian may, however, also have to take into consideration that it may be better for practical purposes and for the safety of the bitch to do an elective cesarean section on a Friday afternoon rather than during the week-end when the clinic may not be fully staffed. Performing elective cesarean sections in a line of dogs that cannot reproduce successfully without intervention, or for the convenience of the breeder, may be questioned on ethical grounds.

The bitch submitted for an elective cesarean section should be at term, and preferably have entered first stage of parturition, so that the fetuses are mature and have enough surfactant for normal lung function. Pre-surgery treatment with methylprednisolone 0.5, 1 or 2 mg/kg bw or dexamethasone preferably 24 to 48 hours and at least 1 hour pre-surgery to advance fetal lung maturation (especially of the brachycephalic breeds) and for maternal preparation is advocated by some, although not scientifically documented in the dog.

If peripheral plasma progesterone was determined at the time of mating, this is a good help in making the decision when to perform the elective cesarean section. C-section on a bitch before day 62 past the LH surge (defined as the initial raise in serum progesterone concentrations two times that of basal, i.e., in the range of 4.5 to 7.5 nmol/l [1.5 – 2.5 ng/ml]) is likely to result in a high percentage of neonatal losses owing to fetal immaturity. Elective cesarean sections, therefore, should be made at the earliest 62 to 64 days after the LH-surge (i.e., 58-60 days post fertilization). Progesterone at this time is usually less than or about 6 nmol/l (2 ng/ml).

Postpartum

The postpartum bitch should be examined if:

- Severe genital hemorrhage is continuous.
- All placentas have not been expelled within 4 to 6 hours after the birth of the last pup.
- The lochia are putrid and/or foul smelling.
- The rectal temperature is higher than 39.5°C (103 °F).
- The general condition of the bitch is affected.
- The general condition of the pups is affected.

Postpartum Hemorrhage

True hemorrhage should be distinguished from normal vaginal post-parturient discharge and from cases of subinvolution of the placental sites (SIPS). SIPS occurs predominantly in the young, primiparous bitch and is observed as a scant vaginal hemorrhage over many weeks or even months. This is no cause for alarm, as long as the bitch does not become anemic or develop a uterine infection. No effective treatment exists and the condition in the vast majority of cases heals spontaneously, and it usually does not recur at subsequent parturtitions.

Excessive hemorrhage after parturition may, in contrast, indicate uterine or vaginal tearing or vessel rupture or may be evidence of a coagulation defect. The hematocrit should be checked, remembering that 30% is normal for the bitch at term. Inspection of the vulva and vagina should be performed in an attempt to locate the source of the bleeding. Oxytocin can be administered to promote uterine involution and contraction of the uterine wall. In more severe cases of uterine hemorrhage, an exploratory laparotomy may be necessary. The bitch should be monitored closely for signs of impending shock, and blood transfusion may be required while attempting to determine the cause of hemorrhage.

Retained Placentas/Fetuses

Retained placentas in the bitch may cause severe problems, especially when accompanied by retained fetuses or infection. Clinical signs of retained placenta include a thick dark vaginal discharge. Retained fetuses can be identified by palpation or ultrasonographic or radiographic examination. The examination should also encompass the corpus uteri and the vagina for the presence of partly expelled fetuses or fetal membranes. A retained placenta is often palpable in the uterus, depending on the size of the bitch and the degree of uterine involution. Extraction of retained tissue, by careful "milking" of the uterine horn or by using forceps, is sometimes possible. Treatment with 1 to 5 IU oxytocin per dog SC or IM 2 to 4 times daily for up to 3 days can help expulsion of retained placentas. The long-acting ergot alkaloids should not be used because they may cause closure of the cervix. Antibiotic treatment is advisable if the bitch is showing signs of illness.

References

1. Holst PA, Phemister RD: Onset of diestrus in the beagle bitch: Definition and significance. Am J Vet Res 35:401-406, 1974.

2. Concannon PW, et al: Biology and endocrinology of ovulation, pregnancy and parturition in the dog. J Reprod Fertil 39(Suppl.):3-25, 1989.

3. Linde-Forsberg C, Ström Holst B, Govette G: Comparison of fertility data from vaginal vs intrauterine insemination of frozen-thawed dog semen: a retrospective study. Theriogenol 52:11-23, 1999.

4. Luvoni GC, Beccaglia M: The prediction of parturition date in canine pregnancy. Reprod Dom Anim, 41:27-32, 2006.

5. Kutzler MA, Yeager AE, Mohammed HO, Meyers-Wallen VN: Accuracy of canine parturition date prediction using fetal measurements obtained by ultrasonography. Theriogenol 60(7):1309-1317, 2003.

6. Son C, Jeong K, Kim J, Park I, et al: Establishment of the prediction table of parturition day with ultrasonography in small pet dogs. J Vet Med Sci 63(7):715-721, 2001.

7. Kutzler MA, Mohammed HO, Lamb SV, Meyers-Wallen VN: Accuracy of canine parturition date prediction from the initial rise in preovulatory progesterone concentration. Theriogenol 60:1187-1196, 2003.

8. Concannon PW: Canine pregnancy: Predicting parturition and timing events of gestation. *In* Recent Advances in Small Animal Reproduction. Concannon PW, England G, Verstegen J, Linde-Forsberg C (eds). International Veterinary Information Service (www.ivis.org).

9. van der Weyden GC, et al: Physiological aspects of pregnancy and parturition in the bitch. J Reprod Fertil Suppl 39:211-224, 1989.

10. Steinetz BG, et al: Diurnal variation of serum progesterone, but not relaxin, prolactin or oestradiol-17beta in the pregnant bitch. Endocrinol 127:1057-1063, 1990.

11. Johnston SD, et al: Canine pregnancy length from serum progesterone concentrations of 3-32 nmol/l (1 to 10 ng/ml) (abstract). *In* Proceedings, Symposium on Canine and Feline Reproduction, Sydney, 1996.

12. van der Weyden GC, et al: The intrauterine position of canine fetuses and their sequence of expulsion at birth. J Small Anim Pract 22:503-510, 1981.

13. Wallace MS: Management of parturition and problems of the periparturient period of dogs and cats. Semin Vet Med Surg (Small Anim) 9:28-37, 1994.

14. Darvelid AW, Linde-Forsberg C: Dystocia in the bitch: A retrospective study of 182 cases. J Small Anim Pract 35:402-407, 1994.

15.. Eneroth A, et al: Radiographic pelvimetry for assessment of dystocia in bitches: a clinical study in two terrier breeds. J Small Anim Pract 40:257-264, 1999.

16. Jackson PGG: In Handbook of Veterinary Obstetrics. 2nd ed. PGG Jackson (ed). London:WB Saunders, 2004.

17. Freak MJ: The whelping bitch. Vet Rec 60:295-301, 1948.

Chapter 76

Diseases of the Uterus

Bronwyn Crane
Michelle Kutzler

Uterine Prolapse

Prolapse of the uterus is rare in the bitch but can occur just prior to or following parturition when the cervix is open. The prolapsed tissue may include one or both uterine horns. If both horns have prolapsed, the diagnosis is relatively simple. If only one horn has prolapsed, vaginoscopy may be required to differentiate the prolapsed tissue. In cases where only one horn has prolapsed, the bitch may present with abdominal discomfort and straining. The broad ligament may tear, resulting in hemorrhage from the uterine vessels. If hemorrhage occurs, the patient may present with hemoperitoneum or die quickly from exsanguination. In some cases of vaginal prolapse, the uterus can be included, along with other structures, in the prolapsed tissue.[1] Once the diagnosis of uterine prolapse is made, treatment aims are to replace it and to prevent infection. If the tissue has been severely traumatized and devitalized, the best treatment is ovariohysterectomy. Laparotomy is often required to replace the prolapsed uterus. Another option is amputation without laparotomy, taking care to avoid the bladder and urethra.

Subinvolution of Placental Sites

Subinvolution of placental sites (SIPS) is characterized by prolonged hemorrhagic vaginal discharge that persists beyond the expected emission of lochia following parturition. Serosangineous vaginal discharge is normal for the first 4 to 6 weeks postpartum during the period of endometrial reconstruction. In cases of SIPS, trophoblast cells invade deep areas of the endometrium and myometrium following placental separation during third-stage labor, resulting in frank intrauterine hemorrhage. The condition is considered to be self-limiting and there is no proven treatment. Administration of broad-spectrum systemic antibiotics does not shorten the disease course, but it is often used prophylactically to reduce the risk of concurrent endometritis. Bitches are clinically normal, afebrile, and have normal postpartum hematologic parameters. In rare cases, bitches can experience severe hemorrhage, necessitating a blood transfusion and/or ovariohysterectomy.

Uterine Infection

Endometritis is an infection and inflammatory reaction within the endometrium, whereas metritis is an infection with inflammatory changes in both the endometrium and myometrium. These conditions occur as a result of the introduction of bacteria following parturition and less commonly, following breeding. During the postpartum period, bacteria are able to ascend from the vagina to the uterus through an open cervix. Subsequently, the bitch may develop septicemia or endotoxemia. Metritis can occur in a bitch of any age and is not influenced by hormones as in the case of cystic endometrial hyperplasia (CEH)-pyometra. A bitch is more likely to develop metritis postpartum following a retained fetus, retained placenta, obstetrical manipulations, or infectious abortion, but metritis may also occur following a normal parturition. The clinical signs of metritis are those of general systemic illness, such as vomiting, anorexia, lethargy, agalactia, and hyperthermia. A malodorous vaginal discharge is usually present that is distinct from and persists longer than normal lochia. Ultrasonographic evaluation of the uterus would reveal an increase in uterine wall thickness and in luminal diameter. Fluid may or may not be present in the uterus. In the case of a retained fetus, organized areas of hyperechogenicity would be present.[2] A complete blood count would show a leukocytosis with a left shift. Radiography can also be used to detect retained fetuses and double-contrast hysterography can be used to identify a retained placenta. Histologic evaluation of the uterus following hysterectomy would show inflammatory cell infiltration into the endometrium and myometrium and an overall increase in thickness. If the bitch is not intended for breeding, or the condition is severe and a retained fetus is present, the best treatment is ovariohysterectomy. Otherwise, medical management includes the use of broad-spectrum systemic antibiotics and ecbolics to stimulate uterine evacuation. Administration of PGF2α 0.01 to 0.1 mg/kg SQ every 2 to 4 hours is continued until uterine clearance is achieved.

Cystic Endometrial Hyperplasia-Pyometra

Cystic endometrial hyperplasia (CEH)-pyometra is the most common uterine disease in older and middle-aged intact bitches and queens, with an average age of 9.36 years.[3] CEH is infrequently diagnosed in dogs younger than 4 years old and occurs slightly more often in maiden bitches. In colony-raised beagle bitches, the incidence of CEH was 15.2%.[3] However, this incidence may be an over-estimation of the occurrence in the general population as colony raised queens had a significantly higher incidence of CEH compared with feral queens.[4]

CEH is a subclinical disease characterized by the proliferation and hypersecretion of endometrial glands resulting in the formation of fluid-filled cysts. Alone, CEH is not associated with any clinical signs other than infertility. CEH is generally considered to be the initiating stage that progresses into pyometra after uterine bacterial colonization occurs. Pyometra is a life-threatening illness involving the accumulation of intraluminal purulent exudate within the uterus and inflammatory cell infiltration into the layers of the endometrium and myometrium. Although CEH generally precedes pyometra, pyometra can occur without CEH.

CEH-pyometra is an endocrine disease. The condition occurs during diestrus when corpora lutea are present and progesterone concentrations are high. The average interval from the onset of proestrus to diagnosis of CEH-pyometra is 35 days (range 20-70 days).

Progesterone stimulates endometrial growth and glandular secretory activity. Progesterone also reduces myometrial contractility and maintains cervical closure. In addition, progesterone diminishes immune function by decreasing neutrophil chemotaxis and phagocytosis and increases endometrial bacterial adherence. Despite this, peripheral serum progesterone concentrations in bitches with pyometra are not higher than in normal diestrus bitches. Estrogens also have a role in the pathogenesis of CEH through the up-regulation of endometrial progesterone and estrogen receptors. However, in studies in which CEH has been experimentally induced, estrogens alone were ineffective at inducing disease. Administration of estrogens followed by progesterone or progesterone alone will induce CEH. In cases of spontaneously occurring CEH, estrogen receptor (ER) and progesterone receptor (PR) expression are increased within the surface epithelium, endometrial glands, stromal fibroblasts, and myometrium.[5] Clinically, CEH-pyometra are reported sequelae following the use of exogenous estrogens for pregnancy termination, exogenous progestins for contraception, anovulatory (cystic) follicles, and ovarian neoplasia. The use of medroxyprogesterone acetate for population control increases the prevalence of pyometra in treated bitches to 45% over a prevalence of only 5% in untreated bitches.[6]

Bacteria gain access to the uterus via ascension during cervical dilation that occurs with estrus. Bacteria found in healthy uteri and the uteri of bitches with pyometra are representative of the normal microflora of the vagina and cervix. The most common bacteria isolated in cases of pyometra is *Escherichia coli.* Infusion of *E. coli* isolates obtained from bitches with pyometra into the uteri of healthy bitches resulted in the development of pyometra.[7] Certain serotypes of *E. coli* are more commonly associated with pyometra, indicating that these strains may possess increased virulence or arise from a concurrent urinary tract infection. The presence of the K antigen is common feature of *E. coli* isolates from cases of pyometra.[8] In addition, approximately 50% of *E. coli* isolates from cases of pyometra contain cytotoxic necrotizing factor (CNF), which reduces the integrity of the endometrial epithelium. Other less common bacteria isolated from cases of pyometra include *Streptococcus sp., Enterobacter sp., Proteus sp., Klebsiella sp.,* and *Pseudomonas sp.* The mechanical irritation of bacteria within the endometrium provides a stimulus for CEH. In fact, any stimuli, from an embryo to a piece of silk thread, will stimulate local proliferation of endometrial glands and hyperplastic changes within the endometrium. In cases of mechanically induced CEH and pyometra, ER and PR expression are reduced in the surface epithelium and endometrial glands, whereas PR expression is slightly increased in the stromal fibroblasts and myometrium.[5] This may be partly due to a loss of cellular integrity caused by damage to the endometrium or due to an increased response to progesterone, which naturally causes down-regulation of the two receptor types.

Histologic criteria and gross pathologic lesions for CEH have been categorized into five groups in an effort to classify the disease based on severity.[9] Bitches in group 1 have a slightly enlarged and rounded uterus and a histologic diagnosis of endometrial hyperplasia without endometritis. Bitches in group 2 have enlargement of the uterus less than or equal to 3 cm in diameter and a histologic diagnosis of hyperplastic endometrium with irregular cysts. Bitches in group 3 have enlargement of the uterus and uterine horns greater than or equal to 7 cm and histologic lesions consisting of a roughened endometrial surface, cysts, and endometrial ulceration. Group 4 animals are subdivided depending on the patency of the cervix. Bitches in group 4 with an open cervix (group 4A) have enlargement of the uterus and uterine horns less than or equal to 3 cm with histologic evidence of endometrial fibrous, hypertrophic myometrium and cysts. Bitches in group 4 with a closed cervix (group 4B) have enlargement of the uterus with thinning of the uterine wall and a histologic diagnosis of atrophic cysts within the endometrium and myometrium.

De Bosschere and colleagues developed a histomorphometric classification for CEH-pyometra.[10] CEH can be categorized as mild or severe based on the number of cysts and the percentage of the uterus affected. CEH is recognized by an increased endometrium-to-myometrium ratio. Pyometra is distinguished from CEH by the presence of inflammatory exudate. Pyometra can be categorized as hyperplastic or atrophic. In hyperplastic pyometra, a severe inflammatory reaction exists, and more than 25% of the endometrium is occupied by luminal endometrial glands. Many large cysts are present, with an increase in endometrium-to-myometrium ratio and moderate fibroblast proliferation. With atrophic pyometra, a severe inflammatory reaction also exists, but no cysts are present, the endometrium-to-myometrium ratio is decreased, and no fibroblast proliferation occurs.

The clinical signs of pyometra include vaginal discharge (80%), fever (47%), polydipsia, polyuria, and vomiting.[11] Other symptoms include lethargy and anorexia. Uterine exudate in the form of vaginal discharge may be purulent, mucoid, or hemorrhagic. Many clinical signs of pyometra result from the effects of bacterial toxins. Neutrophilia is a common hematologic finding, ranging from 15,000 to 60,000 cells/ml. Hyperproteinemia and hyperglobulinemia may occur secondary to dehydration and antigenic stimulation. Impaired renal function (hyposthenuria and proteinuria) results from *E. coli* lipopolysaccharide endotoxin on distal convoluted tubules and collecting ducts causing insensitivity to antidiuretic hormone. Cytotoxic necrotizing factor positive *E. coli* will also cause hepatocellular damage and/or hypoxia owing to dehydration and decreased circulation resulting in increased aspartate transaminase (AST) and alanine transaminase (ALT).

Diagnosis of CEH-pyometra is made by clinical signs, abdominal palpation of an enlarged uterus, hematologic and biochemical results, and radiographs or ultrasonography revealing uteromegaly. Ultrasonography is particularly useful as it can be used to evaluate endometrial integrity, uterine wall thickness, uterine distention (Figure 76-1) and the presence of cystic endometrial glands. In CEH without pyometra, endometrial glands are increased in size and number, appearing as 1- to 2-mm anechoic areas within the endometrium.[11] Subclinical CEH has also been identified in queens using fluoroscopy and scintigraphy, with hysterograms showing a corkscrew appearance to the uterus with irregular filling defects in the lumen.[12] It is important to note that the corkscrew appearance is normal for diestrus in both queens and bitches (Figure 76-2). When fluid in the uterus is detected, pyometra may be differentiated from CEH with mucometra by measuring circulating prostaglandin-F metabolites (PGFM). Concentrations of PGFM ≥ 3054 pmol/l, ≥ 2388 pmol/l, or ≥ 1666 pmol/l indicate a 95%, 90%, or 80% probability of pyometra, respectively.[13] Combining PGFM results with percentage of band neutrophils present on hematologic evaluation increases the sensitivity of differentiating pyometra from mucometra to 100%. However, PGFM determination is not clinically available.

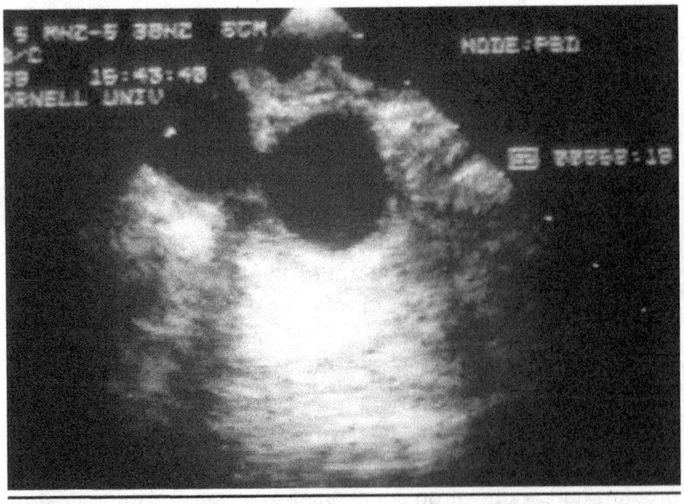

Figure 76-1. Anechoic intraluminal fluid distension of several loops of uterine horn in a bitch with a pyometra.

The recommended treatment for pyometra in most bitches and queens is ovariohysterectomy. Prior to surgery, the patient should be stabilized, especially if endotoxemia is present. For less severe cases of pyometra in animals intended for breeding, patients can be treated medically with $PGF_{2\alpha}$ and systemic antibiotics. Prostaglandin $F_{2\alpha}$ causes myometrial contractility, which expels the luminal contents. It also causes luteolysis, which decreases progesterone concentrations. Side effects of $PGF_{2\alpha}$ are associated with the dose administered and include panting, salivation, anxiety, vomiting, diarrhea, urination, abdominal contractions, and ataxia within 15 minutes of administration. Side effects may last for up to 120 minutes. Therapeutic regimens using high dosages of $PGF_{2\alpha}$ with infrequent treatment schedules are associated with the most severe side effects and least effective treatments. It is important to remember that the therapeutic index for $PGF_{2\alpha}$ in dogs is narrow, with a lethal dose of 5.13 mg/kg for dinoprost (natural $PGF_{2\alpha}$). Low doses (0.01-0.10 mg/kg) of $PGF_{2\alpha}$ administered subcutaneously every 2 to 4 hours until complete uterine evacuation and luteolysis have occurred is a highly effective treatment. Tolerance, in the form of fewer side effects, develops after repeated treatments. In addition, most side effects of $PGF_{2\alpha}$ can be avoided if it is administered intravaginally. $PGF_{2\alpha}$ administered at a dose of 0.15 mg/kg in an intravaginal infusion every 12 hours for up to 12 days effectively alleviated the disease in 9 of 11 bitches treated.[14] Meyers-Wallen and coworkers reported that 40% of bitches treated for pyometra produced a litter within 1 year after treatment.[15] However, case selection for medical treatment is critical as bitches categorized in Dow's group 3 or 4 had a 40% recurrence rate of pyometra during the first post-treatment diestrus. Of treated bitches, 77% will redevelop pyometra within 27 months post-treatment.

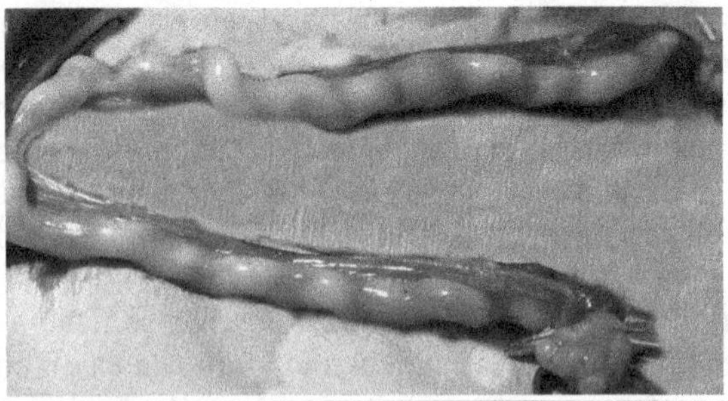

Figure 76-2. Corkscrew appearance of the diestrus uterine horns in a queen during a routine ovariohysterectomy surgery.

Mucometra

Mucometra can occur as a sequela of CEH and as a precursor to pyometra. Glandular hyperplasia causes accumulation of mucoid or serous fluid in the uterine lumen. Mucometras typically are incidental findings at ovariohysterectomy in clinically normal bitches. Diagnosis is made using ultrasonography and hematologic evaluation. Treatment for bitches not intended for breeding is ovariohysterectomy. Medical treatment for bitches intended for breeding and with mild forms of CEH is similar to that for pyometra.

Uterine Stump Pyometra

Uterine stump pyometra has a similar pathogenesis as pyometra with the exception that the patient was previously believed to have had the uterus and ovaries completely removed. In patients with a uterine stump pyometra, remnants of ovarian tissue with a variable amount of uterine tissue have been left behind following ovariohysterectomy (OHE).[16] The clinical signs are similar to CEH-pyometra and include vulvar discharge, depression, and anorexia. Diagnosis is made by retrograde vaginography and ultrasonography that reveal single or multiple fluid-filled areas adjacent to the bladder. Treatment involves surgical resection of all remaining uterine and ovarian tissue. Simultaneous vaginopexy should be performed as a higher incidence of post-surgical urinary incontinence resulting from pelvic adhesions has been reported following this condition.

Uterine Neoplasia

Uterine neoplasia is uncommon in the bitch. Reported incidences for reproductive tract tumors range from 1% to 19%.[16] Uterine neoplasia occurs most commonly in bitches older than 10 years with no established breed predisposition. The most common benign uterine neoplasia is a leiomyoma. Uterine leiomyoma often exists without clinical signs and is an incidental finding during routine OHE. Other benign uterine tumors reported include fibroma, fibroleiomyoma, fibromyoma, fibroadenoma, adenoma, lipoma, angiolipoleiomyoma, and endometrial polyps. Malignant uterine tumors reported in the dog include adenocarcinoma, endometrial carcinoma, lymphosarcoma, hemangiosarcoma, metastatic transmissible venereal tumor, and metastatic dysgerminoma. The clinical signs of malignant uterine adenocarcinoma include a bloody or purulent vaginal discharge, dysuria, hematuria, lethargy, anorexia, and abdominal distention. Presumptive diagnosis is based on clinical signs and radiographic and ultrasonographic findings. A definitive diagnosis requires excisional biopsy with histopathologic evaluation. The treatment for all uterine neoplasms is ovariohysterectomy. The prognosis depends on the degree of local invasion and the presence of metastasis.

Uterine neoplasia is also rare in the queen. One survey of 4402 neoplasms in cats found that only 13, or 0.29%, involved the uterus.[17] In this study, the age at diagnosis ranged from 3 to 16 years (median age nine years). Among cats with uterine neoplasia, more than half are purebred. However, the over-representation of purebred cats is likely owing to an increased proportion of intact purebred queens. The most common uterine neoplasias reported in queens are leiomyomas, leiomyosarcomas, and adenocarcinomas. Concurrent mammary adenocarcinomas have been reported with cases of uterine leiomyoma and adenocarcinoma. The presenting clinical signs of queens with uterine neoplasia are variable and ranged from asymptomatic with incidental discovery at ovariohysterectomy, to infertility, weight loss, palpable abdominal mass, stranguria, hematuria, constipation, pyometra, lethargy, anorexia, and malodorous vaginal discharge. By the time of diagnosis, half of the queens with uterine adenocarcinoma had metastases and few lived longer than five months following ovariohysterectomy.

References

1. McNamara P, Harvey H, Dykes N: Chronic vaginocervical prolapse with visceral incarceration in a dog. J Am Anim Hosp Assoc 33:533-536, 1997.

2. Grundy SA, Davidson AP: Acute metritis secondary to retained fetal membranes and a retained nonviable fetus. J Am Vet Med Assoc 224:844, 2004.

3. Fukuda S: Incidence of pyometra in colony-raised beagle dogs. Exp Anim 50:325, 2001.

4. Perez J, Conley A, Dieter J, et al: Studies on the origin of ovarian interstitial tissue and the incidence of endometrial hyperplasia in domestic and feral cats. Gen Comp Endocrinol 116:10, 1999.

5. De Bosschere H, Ducatelle R, Tshama M: Is mechanically induced cystic endometrial hyperplasia (CEH) a suitable model for study of spontaneously ocurrung CEH in the uterus of the bitch? Reprod Dom Anim 37:152, 2002.

6. Von Berky A, Townsend WL: The relationship between the prevalence of uterine lesions and the use of medroxyprogesterone acetate for canine population control. Aust Vet J 70:249, 1994.

7. Hagman R, Kuhn I: Escherichia coli strains isolated from the uterus and urinary bladder of bitches suffering from pyometra: comparison by restriction enzyme digestion and pulsed-field gel electrophoresis. Vet Microbiol 84:143, 2002.

8. Noakes DE, Dhaliwal GK, England GCW: Cystic endometrial hyperplasia/pyometra in dogs: a review of the causes and pathogenesis. J Reprod Fertil Suppl 57:395, 2001.

9. Dow C: The cystic hyperplasia-pyometra complex in the bitch. Vet Rec 70:1102, 1958.

10. De Bosschere H, Ducatelle R, Vermeirsch H, et al.: Cystic endometrial hyperplasia- pyometra complex in the bitch: should the two entities be disconnected? Theriogenol 55:1509, 2001.

11. Bigliardi E, Parmigiani E, Cavirani S, et al: Ultrasonography and cystic hyperplasia-pyometra complex in the bitch. Reprod Dom Anim 39:136, 2004.

12. Chatdarong K, Kampa N, Axner E, et al: Investigation of cervical patency and uterine appearance in domestic cats by fluoroscopy and scintigraphy. Reprod Dom Anim 37:275, 2002.

13. Hagman R, Kindahl H, Fransson B, et al: Differentiation between pyometra and cystic endometrial hyperplasia/mucometra in bitches by prostaglandin $F_{2\alpha}$ metabolite analysis. Theriogenol 66:198, 2006.

14. Gabor G, Siver L, Szenci O: Intravaginal prostaglandin $F_{2\alpha}$ for the treatment of metritis and pyometra in the bitch. Acta Vet Hung 47:103, 1999.

15. Meyers-Wallen V, Goldschmidt M, Flickinger G: Prostaglandin $F_{2\alpha}$ treatment of canine pyometra. J Am Vet Med Assoc 189:1557, 1986.

16. Johnston SD, Root Kustritz MV, Olson PNS: Disorders of the canine uterus and uterine tubes (oviducts). *In* Canine and Feline Theriogenology. Johnston SD, Root Kustritz MV, Olson PNS (eds). Philadelphia: WB Saunders, 2001, p 206.

17. Miller A, Ramos-Vara J, Dickerson M, et al: Uterine neoplasia in 12 cats. J Vet Diagn Invest 15:575-522, 2003.

Chapter 77

Surgical Disease of the Vulva and Vagina

Beverly J. Purswell
Kara A. Kolster

Anatomy

The vulva is the external portion of the reproductive tract. The vertical opening of the vulva is formed by the labia or lips, which meet at the dorsal and ventral commissures. The clitoris, a homolog of the male penis, lies within the clitoral fossa just inside the ventral commisure of the vulva.

The vestibule lies dorsal and cranial to the clitoral fossa, and opens to the exterior at the vulva. The vestibule is oriented dorsally and turns 90° to horizontal as it clears the ishial arch. The urethral tubercle containing the external urethral orifice lies on the ventral floor of the vestibule, near the vaginovestibular junction. The portion of the tubular tract caudal to this point is shared by the reproductive and urinary systems. Lymph nodules are present in the subepithelial tissue of the vestibule, particularly in the area opposite the urethral tubercle.

The vagina extends from the vestibule to the external cervical os. It is highly distensible except for the portion immediately surrounding the cervix. There is extensive longitudinal folding of the vaginal mucosa. A dorsal longitudinal fold is present leading toward the cervix. The external cervical os projects ventrally into the vaginal lumen and is undercut by a ventral fornix.

Vaginal Examination

Inspection of the vaginal tract is made through the vulva. It should begin with visual inspection of vulvar conformation, perivulvar skin, and labia. The size and turgidity of the vulva should be related to the stage of estrous cycle. The presence and character of any discharge should be noted. The clitoris and vaginal mucosa are examined by parting the labia. The normal clitoris is relatively small and has a mucosal surface. The mucosa should appear smooth and pink along the entire length of the tract.

The cranial vestibule and caudal vagina can be examined visually and digitally. Visual inspection is aided by use of an otoscope or vaginal speculum. Digital examination with a lubricated, gloved finger is necessary to evaluate the texture of the mucosa and identify physical abnormalities such as vaginal bands or strictures. Irritation of the vestibular mucosa leads to hyperplasia of the subepithelial lymph nodules, which is identified as a "sandpaper" texture to the mucosa.

Vaginoscopy is necessary for visual evaluation of the cranial vagina. The vaginal mucosa is edematous during proestrus. Edema decreases and the folds become angulated as estrogen levels fall and progesterone levels increase during estrus. Mucosal pallor increases during estrus. The cervix protrudes into the vagina and is directed ventrally. It is differentiated from the surrounding vaginal folds by its characteristic cobblestone appearance. The external os is located in the midst of the cobblestones. If vaginoscopy is performed during estrus, serosanguinous discharge can be seen discharging from the external os. At the onset of diestrus and throughout diestrus and anestrus, the vaginal folds are flattened. A longitudinal striped appearance is apparent in early diestrus.

Exfoliative vaginal cytology is a useful technique to examine the vagina and determine the nature of vaginal conditions and discharges. Vaginal cytology can determine the presence or absence of estrogen influence and inflammation. Estrogen influence is evidenced by a large percentage of cornified squamous epithelial cells, usually more than 50%. Inflammation is indicated by the presence of large numbers of degenerate and nondegenerate neutrophils. The only exception to this is early diestrus when large numbers of nondegenerate neutrophils are considered normal. This technique is useful in identifying the stage of the estrous cycle and as a diagnostic tool for vaginal discharges.

Episiotomy

Episiotomy is indicated to provide better exposure of the vestibule and distal vagina in conjunction with other surgical procedures. A vertical incision is made from the dorsal commissure directly on the midline to extend the vulvar opening and provide increased exposure to pelvic tissues that are not accessible via laparotomy.

Episioplasty

Episioplasty is a reconstructive procedure that is indicated when the vulva is concealed by redundant perivulvar skin.[1-3] Turbulent urine flow and moisture retention lead to recurrent perivulvar pyoderma, vaginitis, vestibulitis, and urinary tract infections. The condition is commonly seen in bitches spayed prepubertally that have a juvenile vulva that is recessed within skin folds. In episioplasty, excess skin is removed dorsally and laterally to expose the vulva (Figure 77-1). If vaginal discharge is present and not completely resolved by surgery, estrogen therapy may be considered. Treatment with estrogen thickens the vaginal epithelium, thus helping to resolve the chronic inflammation. Fatal bone marrow suppression is a risk of chronic estrogen use; therefore, low-dose therapy is used and tapered off over time, thus identifying the lowest effective dose. Weight loss is recommended prior to surgery in obese patients. Weight gain following surgery may cause the redundant skin fold to recur.

Vaginal Fold Prolapse (Vaginal Hyperplasia)

Vaginal fold prolapse results from an individual's exaggerated response to estrogen stimulation during estrus.[2,4,5,6] Historically, this condition has been referred to as vaginal hyperplasia, which is a misnomer. Occurring only during proestrus and

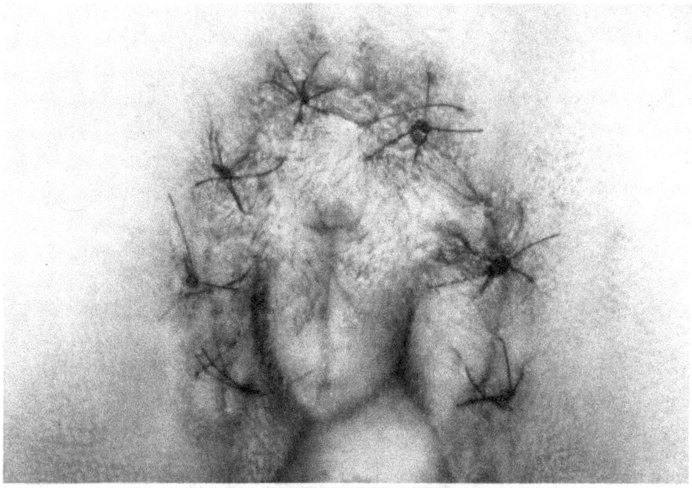

Figure 77-1. Postsurgical appearance of the vulva after episioplasty as treatment for chronic urinary tract infections and perivulvar inflammation. (From Textbook of Veterinary Internal Medicine, 6th ed. Ettinger SJ, Feldman EC (eds). Philadelphia: Elsevier, 2005, p.1689, with permission from the publisher.)

estrus, the vaginal epithelium thickens normally owing to the effect of estrogen, a protective mechanism for the vagina during copulation. In cases of vaginal fold prolapse, the protruding mass has pronounced edema in the underlying tissues overlaid by multiple layers of cornified squamous epithelial mucosa, thus leading to the description of hyperplasia. With vaginal fold prolapse, a mass can be observed when the vulvar lips are parted or it can be seen protruding from the lips of the vulva. The tissue involved usually originates from the vaginal floor cranial to the urethral papilla. The vaginal lumen is dorsal to the mass, which differentiates vaginal fold prolapse from vaginal prolapse, which usually presents as a circular doughnut-shaped mass. Biopsy shows hyperplastic, cornified epithelium characteristic of estrus. The mass usually regresses spontaneously following estrus but recurrence rates during subsequent estrous cycles is high. In some cases the mass is present throughout diestrus or pregnancy. Permanent resolution is achieved by ovariohysterectomy. Surgical removal of the protruding mass is indicated if it is large or if extensive mucosal damage is present.[4,6] The external urethral orifice should be identified on the ventral aspect of the mass and catheterized to prevent damage during surgery. Approximately 25% of surgical cases recur in animals that have not had ovariohysterectomy. Potential complications include dysuria if the weight of the mass impinges on the urethra or if urethral damage occurs during surgery. Vaginal fold prolapse is most commonly seen in young, brachycephalic, and large breed dogs. Breeding of affected dogs is not recommended as the condition may be hereditary.

Vaginal Prolapse

Vaginal prolapse is less common than vaginal fold prolapse. It is identified as a doughnut-shaped eversion of the entire vaginal circumference, with the vaginal lumen in the center. Prolapse typically occurs during estrus or parturition, when excessive straining occurs in the presence of relaxed perivulvar tissue. It may occur as a result of forced separation of a copulatory tie, protracted labor, or constipation. It is heritable and is most common in brachycephalic breeds. Surgical correction consists of reducing the prolapse. Resection may be necessary if significant tissue damage is present. Episiotomy, manual compression to reduce edema, and traction on the uterus through a ventral midline incision may aid reduction. Reduction is maintained in the immediate postoperative period by placing nonabsorbable sutures across the labia. Cervipexy may decrease the incidence of recurrence. This is accomplished by tacking the cervix to the prepubic tendon. Care must be taken not to involve the urethra.

Vaginal Tumors

Vaginal tumors in the bitch are typically benign.[7] The common signalment is an older, intact female with a history of straining to urinate and defecate, vulvar discharge, or a mass protruding from the vulva. The most common tumor types are leiomyomas, fibromas, lipomas, and transmissible venereal tumors (TVT). TVT can metastasize via lymphatics or be spread to the mouth by licking. Malignant leiomyosarcomas are seen rarely. Intraluminal tumors are usually pedunculated and may protrude from the vulva. These can typically be excised. Extraluminal tumors may cause bulging of the perineum. Extensive dissection may be required to remove extraluminal masses. TVT is most common in free-roaming dogs. Some TVTs can regress spontaneously after several months. Multiple masses are common and complete excision is difficult. Recurrence is common unless the tumors are also treated with radiation and chemotherapy. Chemotherapy with vincristine (0.025 mg/kg, IV, weekly, for 2-8 treatments) is considered the treatment of choice. Debulking of the tumor(s) may assist in therapy.

Clitoral Enlargement

Clitoral enlargement occurs owing to abnormalities of sexual differentiation (male pseudohermaphrodism), exposure to exogenous androgens, or excess sex hormone production secondary to hyperadrenocorticism (Figure 77-2). The bitch may present for excessive licking of the vulvar area, reluctance to sit, vulvar discharge, or appearance of a mass protruding from the vulva. An os clitoris may be present in cases of abnormal sexual differentiation. Friction between the enlarged clitoris and vulva may cause inflammation and vaginitis. The tissue may also be traumatized from exposure if it protrudes from the vulva. Surgery is indicated if the enlarged clitoris is causing clinical signs or if an os clitoris is present. The clitoris will not regress with removal of androgen influence if an os clitoris is present. Accurate location of the urethra is critical prior to surgery.

Trauma

Trauma to the vulva and vagina may occur as a result of dogfights, breeding injuries, attempts to disrupt a coital tie, dystocia, malicious acts, or be iatrogenic. Lacerations are usually longitudinal. Contusions or puncture wounds may also occur. Treatment is usually not necessary for minor injuries. Surgical correction is indicated for large lacerations or puncture wounds. Estrual bitches should be confined to prevent mating and reinjury.

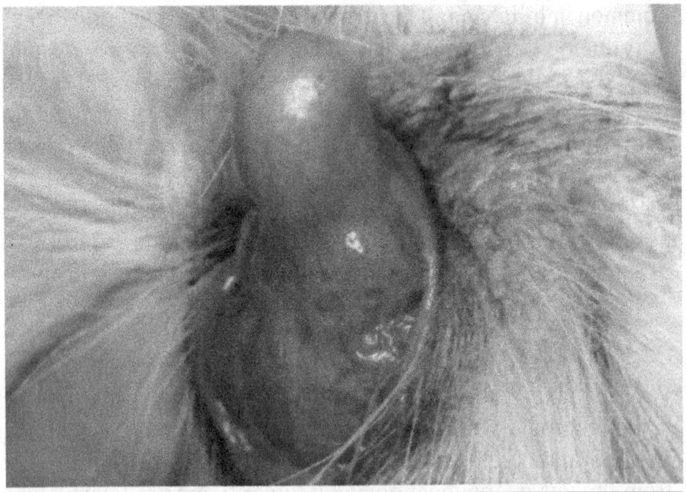

Figure 77-2. Clitoris of a male pseudohermaphrodite, showing penis-like anatomy. (From Textbook of Veterinary Internal Medicine, 6th ed. Ettinger SJ, Feldman EC (eds). Philadelphia: Elsevier, 2005, p.1689, with permission from the publisher.)

Developmental Abnormalities

A variety of congenital developmental abnormalities may occur that partially obstruct the vagina or vestibule and require surgical correction, especially in breeding animals. The paired müllerian (paramesonephric) ducts fuse embryologically to form the tubular reproductive tract in the female. The urogenital sinus fuses with the ducts and develops into the vestibule. The hymen forms at the vaginovestibular junction. Congenital abnormalities arise from incomplete fusion of these embryologic structures or from incomplete perforation of the hymen. Abnormalities manifest as vertical bands or circumferential strictures and most commonly occur in the area of the vaginovestibular junction. The true incidence of congenital vaginal abnormalities is unknown because many cases are asymptomatic until breeding is attempted. Vaginal bands and strictures cause partial obstructions that can prevent natural mating and/or whelping. Other possible signs include chronic vaginitis and vulvar discharge. Digital examination, vaginoscopy, and contrast vaginography are useful diagnostic tools. Vertical bands can be small enough to break down digitally or may be thicker and require surgical resection (Figure 77-3). Strictures can be dilated or surgically resected but scarring and recurrence are common. Partial vaginectomy has been reported as the most successful procedure for resolving clinical signs.

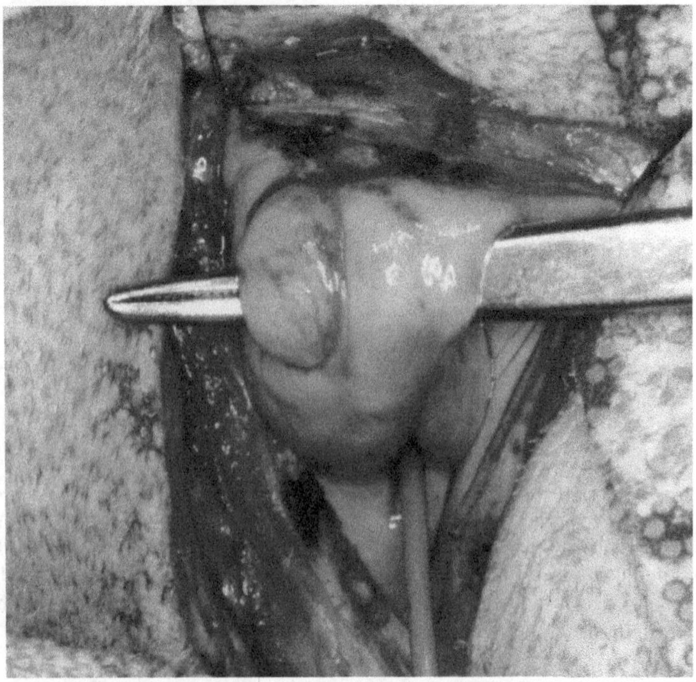

Figure 77-3. An instrument is used to demonstrate a large dorsoventral vaginal septum. The urethra is catheterized and an episiotomy increases surgical exposure.

Bibliography

1. Hammel SP, Bjorling DE: Results of vulvoplasty for treatment of recessed vulva in dogs. J Am Anim Hosp Assoc 38:79, 2002.

2. Johnston SD, Kustritz MVR, Olson PNS: Canine and Feline Theriogenology. Philadelphia: Saunders, 2001, p. 4.

3. Lightner BA, McLoughlin MA, Chew DJ, et al: Episioplasty for the treatment of perivulvar dermatitis or recurrent urinary tract infections in dogs with excessive perivulvar skin folds: 31 cases (1983-2000). J Am Vet Med Assoc 219:1577, 2001.

4. Pettit GD: Vagina and vulva. *In* Current Techniques in Small Animal Surgery. Bojrab MJ (ed). Philadelphia: Lippincott Williams & Wilkins, 1998, p. 503.

5. Purswell BJ: Vaginal disorders. *In* Textbook of Veterinary Internal Medicine. Ettinger SJ, Feldman EC (eds). St. Louis: Elsevier, 2005, p. 1686.

6. Wykes PM, Olson PN: Vagina, vestibule, and vulva *In* Textbook of Small Animal Surgery, 3rd ed. Slatter D (ed). Philadelphia: Saunders, 2003, p. 1502.

7. Mello Martins MI, Ferreira de Souze F, Gobello C: Canine transmissible veneral tumor: etiology, pathology, diagnosis and treatment. *In* Recent Advances in Small Animal Reproduction. Concannon PW, England G, Verstegen J III, and Linde-Forsberg C (eds). International Veterinary Information Service, Ithaca NY (www.ivis.org), 2005.

Chapter 78

Mammary Gland Disorders of the Dog and Cat

Mitch Robbins

Mammary Gland Anatomy

The mammary glands are highly modified and enlarged sweat glands. The gland itself consists of epithelial glandular tissue, and the supporting connective tissue.

Although the number and location of mammary glands is variable, most dogs will have 5 bilaterally symmetric pairs. The glands are named based on their location as: cranial thoracic, caudal thoracic, cranial abdominal, caudal abdominal, and inguinal. Most cats will have 4 bilaterally symmetric pairs of glands (cranial and caudal thoracic, abdominal, and inguinal).[1,2]

Blood supply to the individual mammary glands is based on location. The thoracic glands receive their primary arterial supply from the perforating sternal branches of the internal thoracic artery. Abdominal and inguinal glands are supplied by mammary branches of the epigastric arteries. The cranial superficial epigastric artery is located at the level of the costal arch. It supplies the cranial abdominal gland and joins the caudal superficial epigastric artery. The caudal superficial epigastric artery is a branch of the pudendal artery. It runs cranially under the inguinal mammary gland to supply the inguinal gland and the caudal abdominal gland. Cranial to this, it joins the terminal branches of the cranial superficial epigastric artery.[1]

Lymphatic drainage of the mammary glands is bilaterally symmetric and is variable. The cranial thoracic glands drain directly to the axillary node. The inguinal gland drains directly into the inguinal lymph node. Drainage of the caudal thoracic and abdominal mammary glands can be to either or both the inguinal or axillary lymph nodes. Communication between left and right sides has also been documented.[3]

Disorders of the Mammary Gland

Pseudopregnancy

Pseudopregnancy is a normal physiologic syndrome seen during diestrus in nonpregnant bitches; usually occurring 6 to 8 weeks after estrus. Clinical signs associated with pseudopregnancy include behavioral changes (nesting and maternal behavior) as well as physical changes (weight gain, mammary enlargement, lactation, and contractions). The cause of pseudopregnancy is thought to be the rapid decrease in serum progesterone that stimulates synthesis and secretion of prolactin. Some nonpregnant bitches may be more sensitive to prolactin, causing an exaggerated response and leading to marked mammary gland enlargement and lactation.[4]

Bitches that present with exaggerated pseudopregnancy may be treated conservatively if the signs are mild. Pseudopregnancy is self-limiting and signs will usually subside within 3 weeks. An Elizabethan collar can be used to decrease mammary gland stimulation.

If a more aggressive therapy is necessary, treatment with prolactin inhibitors has been reported.[5,6] Cabergoline was used at a dose of 5 μg/kg orally once daily for 5 to 7 days or as a subcutaneous injection at a dose of 1.5 to 5 μg/kg every 48 hours for 2 to 3 treatments. The outcome of treatment was successful, with 95% to 100% of cases having resolution of mammary swelling and lactation within 5 to 7 days of the start of administration.[5,6] The most common side effects were vomiting, lethargy, and anorexia. Other prolactin inhibitors that have been used to treat pseudopregnancy include bromcriptine 10 to 100 mg/kg/day for 10 to 14 days and metergoline 0.2 mg/kg/day for 8 to 10 days.[4]

While ovariohysterectomy is the treatment of choice for the long-term prevention of pseudopregnancy in bitches that are not intended for breeding, its use as a primary treatment for pseudopregnancy is not advocated.[4] Ovariohysterectomy will lead to a sudden and severe decrease in progesterone levels and can exacerbate the rapid increase in serum prolactin concentration. For this reason, many surgeons will delay ovariohysterectomy for several months after estrus.

Mastitis

Mastitis is uncommon in lactating bitches. Patients will present to the veterinarian with systemic clinical signs such as lethargy, anorexia, and mammary gland pain of variable intensity. Diagnosis is based on history and physical examination findings of a large, swollen, hot, and painful mammary gland. Culture and sensitivity tests are helpful in identification of specific pathogens. *Escherchia coli*, beta-hemalytic streptococci, and staphylococci are most common.[4] Although antibiotic therapy (ampicillin or oxacillin[4]) are usually effective treatments, occasionally, severely infected glands may become necrotic and require surgical debridement.

In some cases, swollen, enlarged, and painful mammary glands can arise from nonseptic inflammation and milk stasis. Often, this will follow acute weaning of puppies from an actively lactating bitch. Treatment may be either to reintroduce the puppies to nursing or to try to stop lactation.[4] Surgery is not necessary for these patients because there is no progression to abscessation and necrosis of the glands.

Mammary Gland Neoplasia

Canine Mammary Gland Tumors

Mammary gland tumors are among the most common tumors in female dogs. The average age for the development of mammary gland neoplasia is 8 to 10 years, with young dogs having a higher incidence of benign tumors.[7] Several factors have been shown to increase the risk of mammary gland tumor formation. These factors include obesity at 1 year of age, obesity 1 year prior to the diagnosis of the mammary gland tumors, intake of home-made versus commercial diets,8 and ovariohysterectomy.[9]

The influence of female hormones has been well established. Ovariohysterectomy at a young age reduces the risk of development of mammary gland tumors. Compared with an intact female dog, the risk of developing mammary gland tumors in a dog that has an ovariohysterectomy before the first heat cycle is 0.05%. That risk increases to 8% if the ovariohysterectomy is performed after the first heat cycle and 26% if the ovariohysterectomy is performed after the second heat cycle. There is no protective benefit if ovariohysterectomy is performed after the third heat cycle.[9]

The presence of estrogen and progesterone receptors in canine mammary tumors has been established. Almost 100% of normal canine mammary tissue contains receptors for progesterone and estrogen. These receptors are found on 70% of benign mammary tumors and 50% of malignant mammary tumors.[10]

Tumor Types and Behavior

Approximately 50% of mammary tumors in dogs are benign. Benign tumor types include fibroadenomas, benign mixed tumors, simple adenomas, and benign mesenchymal tumors.[11]

The most common malignancies (the other 50% of tumors) are carcinomas (solid carcinoma, tubular adenocarcinoma, papillary adenocarcinoma, and anaplastic carcinoma).

Sarcomas comprise approximately 10% of malignancies. Reported sarcomas include osteosarcoma, fibrosarcoma, and osteochondrosarcoma. Extraskeletal osteosarcoma commonly occurs in the mammary gland. These osteosarcoma are typically seen in older female dogs. The reported metastatic rate for mammary gland osteosarcoma is 63% with a median survival of 90 days.[12]

Mixed malignant mammary gland tumors have histologic characteristics of mesenchymal and epithelial cell origin. They comprise approximately 8% of malignancies and behave similarly to carcinomas.

Inflammatory mammary gland tumors are rare in dogs. Inflammatory mammary gland tumors are characterized by rapid growth, edema, erythema, and firmness and warmth of the tissue. Inflammatory mammary gland tumors must be differentiated from inflammatory and infectious diseases of the mammary gland. Fine-needle aspirate of inflammatory mammary gland tumors is usually suggestive of carcinoma. Prognosis for patients with inflammatory mammary gland tumors is poor. Distant metastasis is often present at the time of diagnosis and hemostatic abnormalities consistent with disseminated intravascular coagulation are present in 30% of patients.[13]

Diagnosis and Clinical Staging

Patients with mammary tumors may present to the veterinarian with clinical signs referable to the mass(es) in the mammary chain or signs related to lymphatic obstruction or metastasis.

Biopsy with histopathologic evaluation is the most accurate method of diagnosis of canine mammary tumors. Fine-needle aspiration is discouraged owing to the insensitivity of cytology to differentiate malignant from benign tumors.[14]

Staging of patients with mammary tumors should always include thoracic radiographs and a minimum data base of information including complete blood count, serum chemistry profile, and urinalysis. Nuclear bone scans may be helpful in the identification of dogs with osseous metastasis. Pulmonary metastasis may be present in up to 50% of patients with malignant mammary tumors. When present, pulmonary metastasis may appear as well define nodules (64%), as poorly differentiated interstitial nodules (18%), or as pleural effusion with no evidence of pulmonary lesions (18%).[15,16]

Treatment

Treatment can ensue once a histologic diagnosis has been obtained and staging has been performed. Surgery is the first line of treatment for mammary tumors. Effective surgical planning requires knowledge of anatomy, vascular and lymphatic supply, and the behavior of the tumor being treated.

In canine patients, surgical dose has not been associated with improved survival,[17] but has theoretical implications based on lymphatic drainage for invasive tumors. Options for surgical treatment include simple lumpectomy, mammectomy, regional mastectomy and radical mastectomy.

Performing ovariohysterectomy concurrent with the removal of mammary gland tumors in intact females is controversial. In two studies, concurrent ovariohysterectomy improved survival 45%;[11,18] however, other studies indicate no difference in survival.[17,19]

Prognosis

Several prognostic indicators have been identified in canine mammary gland malignancy (Table 77-1). Among these are tumor size, tumor fixation to underlying tissue, skin ulceration, tumor type, tumor grade, evidence of vascular or lymphatic invasion, lymphoid infiltration into the tumor, lymph node involvement, and the presence of estrogen or progesterone receptors.[20]

Feline Mammary Gland Tumors

Mammary gland tumors are the third most common cancer in cats.[21] Of mammary gland tumors in cats, 80% are malignant (adenocarcinoma), 25% of cats have ulcerated masses, and more than 50% have more than one gland involved. More than 80% of cats with mammary cancer will develop metastasis; 49% of cats have lymph node metastasis.[22]

Prognosis for cats with mammary gland carcinoma is dependent on tumor size. Overall median survival is approximately 12 months. Cats with tumors less than 2 centimeters in diameter have a median survival of 2 years. Cats with tumors between 2 and 3 centimeters have a median survival of 2 years. Cats with tumors larger than 3 centimeters have a median survival of 6 months. Cats with histologically well differentiated tumors with no evidence of lymphatic invasion have a better prognosis than those with higher grade tumors.[22]

Table 78-1. Prognostic Factors in Canine Mammary Gland Cancer

Tumor Size		
	> 3cm diameter	30% recurrence
	> 3cm diameter	85% recurrence
Fixation to underlying skin or skin ulceration		Poorer prognosis
Grade/differentiation		
	Low grade	20% recurrence
	High grade	80% recurrence
Lymphoid infiltration into tumor		Better prognosis
Histologic type		
		Sarcomas worse than carcinomas
		Mixed same as carcinomas
Lymph node status	No histologic metastasis	20% recurrence
	Histologic metastasis	80% recurrence
Histologic evidence of lymphatic or vascular invasion		Poorer prognosis
Progesterone/estrogen receptors		Better prognosis

Surgery is the most effective means of treatment of feline mammary tumors. Radical mastectomy is recommended to decrease the chances of local recurrence. Local recurrence with conservative surgery is 66%.[22]

Feline Mammary Fibroadenomatous Hyperplasia

Fibroadenomatous hyperplasia is an important differential diagnosis for mammary gland neoplasia in cats. Fibroadenomatous hyperplasia is a progestogen-dependent ductal hyperplasia. While the most common occurrence is in intact young female cats within 2 weeks of estrus, it has been reported in male and spayed female cats after treatment with megesterol acetate.[23] Clinically, cats present with large, red, and swollen mammary glands. Although most cases will respond to ovariohysterectomy or resolve spontaneously within 4 to 6 weeks, there have been reports of the use of the prosterone antagonist aglepristone for the treatment of cats with fibroadenomatous hyperplasia that does not respond to ovariohysterectomy. Aglepristone was used at a dose of 10 to 20 mk/kg in variable frequency (1 to 2 times weekly). With this treatment, tumor regression was rapid in all cats within 1 to 2 weeks. Pregnant cats had a high tendency to abort and develop endometritis.[24,25]

References

1. Christensen GC: The mammae. *In* Miller's Anatomy of the Dog. Evans HE, Christensen GC (eds). Philadelphia: WB Saunders, 1979, p. 101.

2. Dyce KM: Textbook of Veterinary Anatomy. Philadelphia: WB Saunders, 1987, p. 367.

3. Morrison WB: Canine and feline mammary tumors *In* Cancer in Dogs and Cats Medical and Surgical Management. Morrison WB (ed). Jackson: Teton NewMedia, 2002, p. 565.

4. Feldman EC and Nelson RW: Canine and Feline Endocrinology and Reproduction. St. Louis: Saunders, 2004, p. 808.

5. Harvey MJ, Cauvin A, Dale M, et al: Effect and mechanisms of the anti-prolactin drug cabergoline on pseudopregnancy in the bitch. J Small Anim Pract 38:336, 1997.

6. Arbeiter K, Brass W, Ballabio R, Jochle W: Treatment of pseudopregnancy in the bitch with cabergoline, an ergoline derivative. J Small Anim Pract 29:781, 1988.

7. MacEwen EG, Withrow SJ: Tumors of the mammary gland. *In* Small Animal Clinical Oncology. Withrow SJ, MacEwen EG (eds). Philadelphia: WB Saunders, 1996, p. 356.

8. Sonnenschein EG: Body conformation, diet and risk of breast cancer in pet dogs: a case controlled study. Am J Epidemiol 133:694, 1991.

9. Hahn KA, Richardson RC, Knapp DW: Canine malignant mammary neoplasia: biologic behavior, diagnosis, and treatment options. J Am Anim Hosp Assoc 28:251,1992.

10. MacEwen EG, Patnaik AK, Harvey HJ, et al: Estrogen receptors in canine mammary tumors. Cancer Res 42:2255-2259.

11. Johnston SD: Reproductive systems. *In* Textbook of Small Animal Surgery 2nd ed. Slatter D (ed). Philadelphia: WB Saunders, 1993, pp. 2177-2200.

12. Lagenbach A, Anderson MA, Dambach DM, et al: Extraskeletal osteosarcoma in dogs: a retrospective study of 169 cases (1986-1996). J Am Anim Hosp Assoc 34:113-120, 1998.

13. Perez-Alenza D, Tabanera E, Pena L: Inflammatory mammary carcinoma in dogs: 33 cases (1995-1999). J Am Vet Med Assoc 219:1110-1114, 2001.

14. Allen SW, Prasse KW, Mahaffey EA: Cytologic differentiation of benign from malignant mammary tumors. Vet Pathol 23:649-655, 1986.

15. Forest LJ, Graybush CA: Radiographic appearance of pulmonary metastasis in 25 cats. Vet Radiol 39:4-8, 1998.

16. Tiemessen I: Thoracic metastasis of canine mammary tumors- A radiographic study. Vet Radiol 30:249-252, 1989.

17. Allen SW, Mahaffey EA: Canine mammary neoplasia: Prognostic indicators and response to surgical therapy. J Am Anim Hosp Assoc 25:540-546, 1989.

18. Sorenmo KU, Shofer FS, Goldschmidt MH: Effect of spaying on survival of dogs with mammary carcinoma. J Vet Intern Med 14:266-270, 2000.

19. Yamagami T, Kobayashi T, Takashi K, et al: Influence of ovariectomy at the time of mastectomy on the prognosis for canine malignant mammary tumors. J Small Anim Pract 37:462-464, 1996.

20. Robbins M: Reproductive oncology. *In* Textbook of Small Animal Surgery 3rd ed. Slatter D (ed). Philadelphia: WB Saunders, 2003, pp. 2437-2444.

21. Hayes A: Feline mammary gland tumors. Vet Clin North Am 7:205-212, 1977.

22. MacEwen EG, Withrow SJ: Tumors of the mammary gland. *In* Small Animal Clinical Oncology. Withrow SJ, MacEwen EG (eds). Philadelphia: WB Saunders, 1996, pp. 356-372.

23. Chastain CB, Panciera D: Mammary fibroadenomatous hyperplasia associated with megesterol acetate. Small Anim Clin Endocrinol 14:39-40, 2004.

24. Chastain CB, Panciera D: Aglepristrone treatment of fibroadenomatous hyperplasia of the mammary glands. Small Anim Clin Endocrinol 13:38-39, 2003.

25. Gorlinger S, Kooistra HS, van den Broek A, Okkens AC: Treatment of fibroadenomatous hyperplasia in cats with aglepristone. J Vet Intern Med 16:710-713, 2002.

Part XI

Endocrine System

Chapter 79

Diseases of the Thyroid Gland

Janet R Kovak

Anatomy

The thyroid glands are paired lobular glands lying adjacent to the tracheal rings, connected by an isthmus in the dog but independent in the cat. The normal size of each thyroid gland in the dog is approximately 2 cm x 1 cm x 0.5 cm and approximately 2 cm x 0.5 cm x 0.3 cm in the cat.[1,2] The blood supply varies slightly between the two species. The blood supply in the dog is derived from the cranial and caudal thyroid artery; the cat thyroid lobes are supplied solely from the cranial thyroid artery. Venous drainage is via the cranial and caudal thyroid veins. Efferent lymphatic drainage in the dog is into the cervical lymphatic trunk or internal jugular vein.[2] Ectopic thyroid tissue can be present anywhere along the cervical region to the base of the heart.[1]

Thyroid Hormone Metabolism

The thyroid gland regulates basal metabolism. Two molecules, tyrosine and iodine, are important for thyroid hormone synthesis. Tyrosine is a part of a large molecule (MW 660,000) called thyroglobulin, which is formed within the follicle cell and secreted into the lumen of the follicle. Iodine is converted to iodide in the intestinal tract and transported to the thyroid where the follicle cells trap the iodide through an active transport process. The tyrosyl ring can accommodate two iodide molecules: if one iodide attaches, it is called monoiodotyrosine (MIT), if two iodide molecules attach to the tyrosyl ring, it is called diiodotyrosine (DIT). The coupling of two iodinated tyrosines results in the formation of the main thyroid hormones. Two DIT molecules form tetraiodothyronine (T_4), whereas one MIT coupled with one DIT molecule forms triiodothyronine (T_3). Thyrotropin, or thyroid stimulating hormone (TSH), is the most important regulator of thyroid activity. TSH secretion is regulated by thyroid hormones by way of negative feedback inhibition of the synthesis of thyrotropin releasing hormone (TRH) at the level of the hypothalamus and by inhibition of the activity of TSH at the level of the pituitary.

Thyroxine (T_4) is the major storage form of thyroid hormone, whereas T_3 is the active form of the hormone. The majority of T_3 formation occurs outside of the thyroid gland by the deiodination of T_4. Another type of T_3 is formed when an iodide molecule is removed from the inner phenolic ring of T_4. This compound is called reverse T_3 and has few of the biologic effects of thyroid hormones. Reverse T_3 increases in non-thyroidal illness and is responsible for the decrease in total serum T_4 (T T_4) seen in "euthyroid sick" syndrome. As for all lipid soluble hormones that are transported in plasma, T_3 and T_4 are bound to plasma proteins. The amount of thyroid hormone that is free in plasma is remarkably low, e.g., in dogs, the amount of free hormone is a little less than 1.0% for T_4 and slightly greater than 1.0% for T_3.[2-4]

Canine and Feline Hypothyroidism

Primary canine hypothyroidism is the most common cause of naturally occurring hypothyroidism, accounting for more than 95% of all cases.[3] The two histologic forms are lymphocytic thyroiditis or idiopathic thyroid atrophy. Congenital hypothyroidism may be caused by thyroid dysgenesis, dyshormonogenesis, T_4 transport defects, and goitrogens, or rarely, by iodine deficiency. Secondary hypothyroidism may be acquired, as in German shepherd dogs with cystic Rathke's pouch, or secondary to pituitary tumors, radiation therapy, or endogenous or exogenous glucocorticoids.[2,5] Congenital causes of secondary hypothyroidism include hereditary TSH deficiency as observed in the giant schnauzer breed. Tertiary hypothyroidism can be acquired, for example, with hypothalamic tumors, or can be congenital as a result of defective TRH or TRH receptor defects.[5]

Feline hypothyroidism is generally iatrogenic, occurring after surgical or radioactive iodine treatment. This condition is usually transient, resolving when ectopic thyroid tissue resumes production of normal thyroid hormone concentrations.[6]

The signalment of hypothyroid dogs carries a distinct breed predisposition, with high-risk breeds presenting as early as 2 to 3 years of age and low-risk breeds presenting at a slightly older age (4 to 6 years). Breeds predisposed to hypothyroidism include golden retrievers, Doberman pinschers, and dachshunds.[7]

Clinical Signs

Clinical signs of hypothyroidism are gradual and subtle in onset, with lethargy and obesity being most common. Owners are often not aware of the onset of signs and think that their dog is just becoming "older." Dermatologic evidence of hypothyroidism is the most common clinical finding after lethargy and obesity. Symmetric truncal or tail head alopecia is a classic finding in hypothyroid dogs. The skin is often thickened because of myxedematous accumulations in the dermis.[5,7]

Cardiovascular signs of hypothyroidism, including bradycardia, decreased cardiac contractility, and electrocardiographic abnormalities, are rare presenting complaints.[3] Neuromuscular signs such as myopathies and megaesophagus are also uncommon manifestations of canine hypothyroidism. Neuropathies including bilateral or unilateral facial nerve paralysis, vestibular disease, and lower motor neuron disorders are occasionally seen in hypothyroid dogs. Myxedema coma is an unusual finding in hypothyroid dogs and manifests as stupor and coma secondary to myxedematous fluid accumulations in the brain and severe hyponatremia.[4,5,7]

Diagnosis

The clinicopathologic finding of a normocytic normochromic anemia resulting from erythropoeitin deficiency, decreased bone marrow activity, and decreased serum iron and iron binding capacity may be seen in many hypothyroid dogs. Even more commonly seen is hypercholesterolemia, seen in approximately 75% of hypothyroid dogs, owing to altered lipid metabolism, decreased fecal excretion of cholesterol and decreased conversion of lipids to bile acids.[3] Other findings include hyperlipidemia, presence of target cells, and rare mild hypercalcemia in cases of congenital hypothyroidism.[3]

Diagnosis is based on measurement of serum basal total thyroxine (T_4) and triiodothyronine (T_3) concentrations, serum free T_4 and T_3 concentrations, endogenous canine serum TSH levels, and/or dynamic thyroid function tests including the TRH and TSH stimulation tests. Variables that affect T_4 are many and include age, breed, environmental and body temperature, diurnal rhythm, obesity, and malnutrition. Euthyroid-sick syndrome is characterized by a decrease in serum T T_4 and increase in reverse T_3 (see above). Concurrent illnesses such as diabetes mellitus, chronic renal failure (CRF), hepatic insufficiency, and infections can cause euthyroid-sick syndrome, resulting in decreases in serum T T_4 concentrations. Drugs such as anesthetics, phenobarbital, primidone, diazepam, trimethoprim-sulfas, quinidine, phenylbutazone, salicylates, and glucocorticoids can also decrease serum basal T T_4 concentrations.[3,5,7]

Free thyroid (FT) hormone concentrations, or unbound thyroxine and triiodothyronine, are used in human medicine to differentiate between euthyroid sick syndrome and true hypothyroidism. In humans, the diagnostic accuracy of a single FT_4 measurement is approximately 90%.[8] Measurement of FT_4 concentrations is achieved by equilibrium dialysis (gold standard) or analogue immunoassays. Theoretically, FT_4 is not subject to spontaneous or drug-induced changes that occur with T T_4. Early studies, classifying dogs as hypothyroid based on TSH-stimulation tests, indicated that FT_4 by equilibrium dialysis was 90% accurate whereas other FT_4 assays (analogue assays) were no better than T T_4.[8]

With the advent of the endogenous canine TSH assay, veterinarians now have a method of assessing the thyroid-pituitary axis in dogs without dynamic testing. With thyroid gland failure, decreases in serum FT_4 and T T_4 are sensed by the pituitary gland, resulting in an increase in serum endogenous TSH concentration. As FT_4 concentration falls, a logarithmic increase occurs in serum endogenous TSH concentration making it the most sensitive test for the detection of early hypothyroidism. However, nonthyroidal disease can affect endogenous TSH concentrations as well as FT_4 and T T_4 concentrations; therefore, the use of endogenous TSH alone is not recommended as a method of assessing thyroid function.[8,9]

Feline Hyperthyroidism

Hyperthyroidism is the most common endocrinopathy of cats. Middle-aged to older cats are typically affected, and no breed or sex predilection exists. Hyperthyroidism is characterized by hypermetabolism; therefore, polyphagia, weight loss, polydipsia, and polyuria are the most prominent features of the disease.[6] Activation of the sympathetic nervous system is also seen with hyperactivity, tachycardia, pupillary dilatation, and behavioral changes. Long-standing hyperthyroidism leads to hypertrophic cardiomyopathy, high-output heart failure, and cachexia, which may lead to death.[2,6]

Diagnosis

Clinicopathologic features of hyperthyroidism include erythrocytosis and an excitement leukogram (neutrophilia, lymphocytosis) caused by increased circulating catecholamine concentrations. Increased catabolism of muscle tissue in hyperthyroid cats may result in increased BUN, but not creatinine.[10] Increased metabolic rate results in liver hypermetabolism; therefore, serum activities of liver enzymes increase (ALT, AST) in 80% to 90% of hyperthyroid cats. Serum cholesterol decreases, not as a result of decreased synthesis, but rather as a result of increased hepatic clearance mediated by thyroid hormone excess.[6,10,11]

Diagnosis of feline hyperthyroidism is achieved by measurement of total serum concentrations of thyroxine (T T_4); total serum triiodothyronine (T T_3) is generally noncontributory to a diagnosis.[10,11] Because the disease has become more common and recognized in its early stages, serum free-thyroxine concentrations (FT_4) have recently been shown to be more diagnostic of early or "occult" hyperthyroidism.[8] Diagnosis may be challenging in cats with occult hyperthyroidism that demonstrate clinical signs suggestive of hyperthyroidism (polyphagia, polyuria, polydipsia, weight loss, goiter) but who have normal (usually high-normal) T T_4 concentrations. In cases of suspected occult hyperthyroidism, dynamic endocrine testing using the T3-suppression test or the TRH-stimulation test may be beneficial.[10,12,13,14]

Treatment Options

Options for treatment of feline hyperthyroidism include oral supplementation, radioactive iodine treatment, or surgical thyroidectomy. Radioactive iodine (^{131}I) is the optimal therapy for feline hyperthyroidism. It is safe and effective with minimal side effects or complications. Approximately 80% of cats become euthyroid within 3 months after a single treatment. Radiation safety procedures must be strictly followed.[15-17] Oral methimazole is given by supplementation daily and may be associated with side effects including anorexia, vomiting, pruritis, and uncommonly, more serious effects such as thrombocytopenia and agranulocytosis.[18] Surgical excision is a potentially definitive treatment. Patients may be high-risk candidates for anesthesia; when possible, euthyroid status is achieved prior to treatment with oral methimazole.

Surgical Techniques

Surgery is performed via a ventral midline cervical approach, and the thyroid glands are excised via an intracapsular, modified intracapsular, extracapsular, or modified extracapsular technique. A modified extracapsular approach has been associated with the lowest number of hypocalcemia-related complications. The patient should be monitored carefully after surgery for complications including hypocalcemia, hypothyroidism, and laryngeal paralysis.[2,19] Hyperthyroidism can reoccur if inadequate excision was performed or if hypertrophy of ectopic thyroid tissue exists. Recurrent disease may be treated with re-exploratory surgery, medication, or ideally, ^{131}I therapy.[15]

Thyroid Neoplasia

Whereas benign adenomatous changes of the thyroid gland are most common in cats, a larger percentage of dogs have malignant disease. Although carcinoma in cats is often associated with clinical signs of hyperthyroidism, dogs have typically nonfunctional tumors.[2,4] In feline patients, treatment of thyroid carcinoma involves a combination of surgical and radioiodine therapy. Although complete excision may be curative for nonmetastatic disease, the rate of metastasis may be as high as 71%.[20]

Canine thyroid carcinoma is typically more aggressive than feline thyroid carcinoma. Of canine tumors, 90% are malignant; they are only rarely functional and associated with clinical signs associated with hyperthyroidism.[4,21] Dogs may present asymptomatically or with a palpable mass in the cervical region. Definitive diagnosis is based on histologic evaluation. Owing to the highly vascular nature of the tumor, coagulation parameters should be assessed prior to biopsy and open, rather than needle, biopsy is recommended. Ultrasound, nuclear scintigraphy, and CT scan have all been evaluated to better delineate the extent of tumor invasion.[22-24] Surgical resection of the tumors has been associated with the best response if the mass is freely moveable, small in size, nonmetastatic, and completely resected.[25] Radiation or chemotherapy may be elected to treat masses that are incompletely resected or not amenable to resection.[26] Surgical complications include hemorrhage, damage to regional structures including the recurrent laryngeal nerve, as well as postoperative hypocalcemia or, rarely, hypothyroidism.[2,4,21,25] Long-term survival may be achieved in dogs depending on the histologic features of the tumor and whether early diagnosis is made before local invasion or metastatic spread of the disease.[21]

References

1. Hullinger RL: The endocrine system. *In* Miller's Anatomy of the Dog, 4th ed. Evans HE (ed). Philadelphia: WB Saunders, 1993, p. 559.

2. Ehrhart N: Thyroid. *In* Textbook of Small Animal Surgery, 3rd ed. Slatter D (ed). Philadelphia: WB Saunders, 2002, p. 1700.

3. Feldman EC, Nelson RW: Hypothyroidism. *In* Canine and Feline Endocrinology and Reproduction. Feldman EC, Nelson RW (eds). Philadelphia: WB Saunders, 2004, p. 86.

4. Feldman EC, Nelson RW: Canine thyroid tumors and hyperthyroidism. *In* Canine and Feline Endocrinology and Reproduction. Feldman EC, Nelson RW (eds). Philadelphia: WB Saunders, 2004, p.219.

5. Chastin CB, Panciera DL: Hypothyroid diseases. *In* Ettinger SJ, Feldman EC (eds). Textbook of Veterinary Internal Medicine. Philadelphia:WB Saunders, 1995, p. 1487.

6. Peterson ME: Feline hyperthyroidism: Pretreatment clinical and laboratory evaluation of 131 cases. J Am Vet Med Assoc 183:103-110, 1983.

7. Panciera DL: Conditions associated with canine hypothyroidism. Vet Clin North Am Small Anim Pract. 31(5):935, 2001.

8. Ferguson DC, et al: Free thyroid hormone measurements in the diagnosis of thyroid disease. J Vet Intern Med 3:121, 1989.

9. Dixon RM, Mooney CT: Evaluation of serum free thyroxine and thyrotropin concentrations in the diagnosis of canine hypothyroidism J Small Anim Pract. 40(2):72, 1999.

10. Peterson ME: Feline hyperthyroidism. Vet Clin North Am 14(4):809, 1984.

11. Meric SM: Diagnosis and management of feline hyperthyroidism. Comp Cont Educ Pract 11:1053, 1989.

12. Graves T: Complications of treatment and concurrent illness associated with hyperthyroidism in cats. *In* Current Veterinary Therapy XII. Kirk RW, Bonagura JA (eds). Philadelphia: WB Saunders, 1994, p. 369.

13. Peterson ME, Graves TK, Gamble DA: Triiodothyronine (T3) suppression test: an aid in the diagnosis of mild hyperthyroidism in cats. J Vet Intern Med 4:233, 1990.

14. Peterson ME, Broussard JD, Gamble DA: Use of the thyrotropin releasing hormone stimulation test to diagnose mild hyperthyroidism in cats. J Vet Intern Med 8(4):279, 1994.

15. Kintzer PP, Peterson ME: Nuclear medicine of the thyroid gland. Scintigraphy and radioiodine therapy. Vet Clin North Am Small Anim Pract 24(3):587, 1994.

16. Slater MR, Geller S, Rogers K: Long-term health and predictors of survival for hyperthyroid cats treated with iodine 131. J Vet Intern Med 15 (1):47, 2001.

17. Peterson ME: Radioactive iodine (radioiodine) treatment for hyperthyroidism in cats. *In* Current Veterinary Therapy XII. Kirk RW, Bonagura JA (eds). Philadelphia: WB Saunders, 1994, p.373.

18. Peterson ME, Kintzer PP, Hurvitz AI: Methimazole treatment of 262 cats with hyperthyroidism. J Vet Intern Med 2(3):150, 1988.

19. Flanders JA, Harvey HJ, Erb HN: Feline thyroidectomy. A comparison of postoperative hypocalcemia associated with three different surgical techniques. Vet Surg 16(5):362, 1987.

20. Turrel JM, et al: Thyroid carcinoma causing hyperthyroidism in cats: 14 cases. J Am Anim Hosp Assoc 193:359, 1988.

21. Flanders JA: Surgical therapy of the thyroid. Vet Clin North Am Small Anim Pract 24 (3): 607, 1994.

22. Weisner ER, Nyland TG: Ultrasonography of the thyroid and parathyroid glands. Vet Clin North Am Small Anim Pract 24:973, 1994.

23. Marks SL, Koblick PD, Hornof WJ, et al.: 99mTc-pertechnetate imaging of thyroid tumors in dogs: 29 cases (1980-1992). J Am Vet Med Assoc ,204(5):756, 1994.

24. Slensky KA, Volk SW, Schwarz T et al.: Acute severe hemorrhage secondary to arterial invasion in a dog with thyroid carcinoma. J Am Vet Med Assoc 223(5):649, 2003.

25. Klien MK, Powes BE, Withrow SJ, et al: Treatment of thyroid carcinoma in dogs by surgical resection alone: 20 cases (1981-1989). J Am Vet Med Assoc 206(7):1007, 1995.

26. Brearley MJ: Hypofractionated radiation therapy for invasive carcinoma in dogs: A retrospective analysis of survival. J Small Anim Pract 40:206, 1999.

Chapter 80

Diseases of the Parathyroid Glands

Janet R. Kovak

The control of calcium and phosphate metabolism is vital as these ions play an important role in many physiologic processes. Calcium is necessary for intracellular reactions, including muscle contraction, nerve cell activity, the release of hormones through the process of exocytosis, and activation of numerous enzymes.[1] Inorganic phosphate also functions as an important hydrogen ion buffering system in blood. Organic phosphate is an important part of the cell, including the plasma membrane and intracellular components including nucleic acids, ATP, and AMP. The regulation of calcium involves control of the movement of calcium between the extracellular fluid and three body organs: bone, gastrointestinal tract, and kidneys.[2]

Parathyroid Hormone

The main endocrine organ involved in the control of calcium and phosphate metabolism is the parathyroid gland. Four parathyroid glands are present in the cat and the dog. The external parathyroid lies at the cranial-lateral pole of the thyroid gland, and the internal parathyroid gland rests medially within the thyroid parenchyma. Vascular supply to the parathyroid glands is provided via branches of the thyroid artery and vein.[3] During embryologic development, fragments of parathyroid tissue may migrate and be present ectopically in peritracheal fascia to the thoracic inlet or cranial mediastinum.[4] Parathyroid hormone (PTH), primarily an 84-amino acid, single-chain polypeptide, is synthesized, stored, and secreted by the chief cells of the parathyroid glands.[1]

The effect of PTH is to increase calcium and decrease phosphate concentrations in extracellular fluids. PTH has direct effects on bone and kidney metabolism of calcium and indirect effects on gastrointestinal metabolism of calcium.[5] The initial effect of PTH on bone is to promote the transfer of calcium across the osteoblast osteocyte membrane. PTH acts on the distal convoluted tubules of the kidneys to increase absorption of calcium and decrease renal phosphate reabsorption through an effect on the proximal tubules. PTH is involved also in the activation of vitamin D at the kidney level. PTH mediates the absorption of calcium from the gut indirectly through its effect on vitamin D. PTH secretion is controlled by free (ionized) calcium concentrations in blood; decreases in calcium stimulate PTH secretion, and increases in calcium turn off secretion.[1]

Hyperparathyroidism

Hypercalcemia can be caused by a variety of etiologies including hypercalcemia of malignancy, hyperparathyroidism, granulomatous disease, osteoporosis, hypoadrenocorticism, chronic renal disease, and hypervitaminosis D.[5] The initial signs of hypercalcemia are polydipsia and polyuria resulting from impaired response of distal renal tubules to antidiuretic hormone (ADH). Listlessness, depression, and muscle weakness result from depressed excitability of neuromuscular tissue. Mild gastrointestinal signs of hypercalcemia include inappetence, vomiting, and constipation.[6] In cats, neoplasia, renal failure, and urolithiasis are the most common conditions associated with hypercalcemia.[7]

The diagnostic approach to hypercalcemia consists of ruling out the most common cause, which is hypercalcemia of malignancy. Lymphosarcoma and adenocarcinoma of the anal sac, tumors that are commonly associated with hypercalcemia, secrete a PTH-like hormone that increases bone resorption and inhibits renal tubular reabsorption of phosphorus.[1,8] A thorough history and physical examination including lymph node and rectal examination, CBC, serum chemistry profile, urinalysis, and chest/abdominal radiographs are necessary to search for underlying neoplastic processes. Once a diagnosis of neoplasia has been excluded, the next differential for hypercalcemia is chronic renal failure. This is the most difficult to exclude because other causes of hypercalcemia may result in renal damage owing to soft tissue mineralization of the kidneys. Therefore, an animal with hypercalcemia, azotemia, and hyperphosphatemia could suffer from primary hyperparathyroidism or primary renal failure with secondary renal hyperparathyroidism. Furthermore, patients with hypercalcemia secondary to renal disease may also exhibit elevations in intact PTH. Diagnosis of primary hyperparathyroidism is based on the findings of hypercalcemia (preferably ionized), hypophosphatemia, high-normal to elevated serum parathormone concentrations, and a mass in the cervical region. Intact PTH, using a sandwich assay validated for use in the dog and cat, should be measured.[9] It should be emphasized that a normal PTH concentration in the presence of elevated total and/or ionized calcium is "inappropriate" for the calcium level and would be considered diagnostic for primary hyperparathyroidism. For suspected cases of hypercalcemia of malignancy in which the diagnostic approach has failed to identify a neoplastic process, PTH-related protein (PTH-rp) concentrations may be measured.[6,9]

Primary Hyperparathyroidism

Dogs with primary hyperparathyroidism may present asymptomatically or with polydipsia, polyuria, and weakness as well as with urinary tract signs attributable to urolithiasis and infection.[10-12] The most common clinical signs observed in cats with hypercalcemia are anorexia and lethargy.[13] The majority of dogs have parathyroid adenomas or parathyroid hyperplasia with rare carcinomas reported.[14] If primary hyperparathyroidism is suspected, several imaging modalities, including ultrasonography, CT scan and scintigraphy may be utilized if a palpable neck mass is not present. Parathyroid scintigraphy has been shown to have poor sensitivity and specificity.[15] Ultrasonography may better delineate the side and size of parathyroid mass present.[16] Additionally, percutaneous ultrasound-guided techniques may be used to ablate masses. Radiofrequency as well as chemical ablation have been reported. Although these techniques have proven to be safe and effective, the potential risk factors include hypocalcemia and laryngeal paralysis. Additionally, repeat injections may be required for successful treatment.[17,18]

Prior to surgical intervention, diuresis with normal saline may be instituted to lower serum calcium levels. For severe hypercalcemia, furosemide (in a well hydrated animal), glucocorticoid, or calcitonin therapy may be indicated.[5] Administration of glucocorticoids should be delayed until a definitive diagnosis has been made as administration may interfere with the ability to confirm lymphosarcoma histologically.[1] Bisphosphonates have been used to slow hypercalcemia in humans; they function by inhibiting osteoclast function and viability.[19]

Surgery requires a full ventral neck exploration to evaluate both external and internal parathyroid glands bilaterally. Additionally, the whole cervical region to the thoracic inlet should be evaluated for ectopic parathyroid tissue. If all four glands are enlarged owing to parathyroid hyperplasia, excision of one to three of the glands may reduce the associated hypercalcemia.[3] Visualization of the abnormal parathyroid tissue may be aided with intravenous new methylene blue infusion, although Heinz body anemia is a risk factor of administration.[20] Patients should be monitored postoperatively for renal failure and signs of hypocalcemia, which include panting, twitching, or tremors. Development of postoperative renal failure in dogs has been found, in one study, to be more likely to develop in dogs with a higher initial calcium level.[12] Hypocalcemia occurs in up to 58% of dogs after surgery owing to negative feedback and suppression of the remaining glands from elevated PTH levels.[14] Dogs with higher initial calcium levels (> 14 mg/dl) are more likely to become clinically hypocalcemic after surgery.[1] Calcium, in the form of vitamin D (dihydrotachysterol) or calcitriol (1,25$(OH)_2D_3$), supplementation should be instituted pre- or postoperatively and continued until calcium levels normalize over 2 to 8 weeks. Long-term prognosis after parathyroidectomy, if renal damage has not occurred, is favorable.[11-14]

Hypoparathyroidism

The classic biochemical findings in animals with hypoparathyroidism are hypocalcemia (both total and ionized) and hyperphosphatemia with an inappropriately low PTH level. Other causes of hypocalcemia include iatrogenic (post-thyroidectomy) hypoparathyroidism, chronic and acute renal failure, acute pancreatitis, hypoalbuminemia, puerperal tetany (eclampsia), ethylene glycol intoxication, intestinal malabsorption, and nutritional secondary hyperparathyroidism.[21] The absence of PTH results in urinary calcium loss, decreased calcium mobilization from bone, and decreased intestinal absorption of calcium.[22] The majority of clinical signs are attributable to low circulating ionized calcium, leading to neuromuscular excitability.[21] Early signs of hypocalcemia are nonspecific and include anorexia, facial rubbing, nervousness, and a stiff gait. Later signs progress to cardiac arrhythmias, hyperventilation, and finally, generalized tetany and/or seizures.[21]

Diagnosis of primary hypoparathyroidism is achieved by obtaining a complete blood count, chemistry profile, urinalysis, ionized calcium and magnesium levels, as well PTH level. Serum or plasma PTH concentrations should be measured on a freshly drawn sample in a fasted animal. Handling of the sample is crucial to appropriate diagnosis, as PTH is prone to degradation if subjected to warm temperatures.[9]

Treatment of hypoparathyroidism is directed at the underlying cause. In animals that undergo bilateral thyroidectomy, it is possible to autotransplant parathyroid tissue by sectioning the glands and implanting them within adjacent neck musculature.[3] Glands maybe functional within 2 weeks of transplantation.[23] Medical therapy for hypoparathyroidism may require intravenous calcium administration for an acute crisis or permanent vitamin D supplementation in chronic cases.[24]

References

1. Feldman EC, Nelson RW: Hypercalcemia and primary hyperparathyroidism. *In* Canine and Feline Endocrinology and Reproduction, 3rd ed. Feldman EC, Nelson RW (eds). Philadelphia:WB Saunders, 2004, p. 661.

2. Meuten DJ: Hypercalcemia. Vet Clin North Am Small Anim Pract 14:411, 1982.

3. Flanders JA: Parathyroid gland. *In* Slatter D (ed). Textbook of Small Animal Surgery, 3rd ed. Philadelphia: WB Saunders, 2002, p. 1711.

4. Hullinger RL: The endocrine system. *In* Miller's Anatomy of the Dog, 4th ed. Evans HE (ed). Philadelphia: WB Saunders, 1993, p. 559.

5. Flanders JA: Parathyroid glands. *In* Bojrab MJ (ed). Disease Mechanisms in Small Animal Surgery, 2nd ed. Philadelphia: Lea & Febiger, 1993, p.583.

6. Refsal KR, Provencher-Bollinger AL, Graham PA, et al.: Update on the diagnosis and treatment of disorders of calcium regulation. Vet Clin North Am Small Anim Pract 31(5):1043, 2001.

7. Savary KC, Price GS, Vaden SL: Hypercalcemia in cats: A retrospective study of 71 cases (1991-1997). J Vet Intern Med 14:184, 2000.

8. Weir EC: Humoral hypercalcemia of malignancy in canine lymphosarcoma. Endocrinol 122:602, 1988.

9. Chew DJ, Nagode LA, Rosol TJ, et al: Utility of diagnostic assays in the evaluation of hypercalcemia and hypocalcemia: parathyroid hormone, vitamin D metabolites, parathyroid hormone-related peptide, and ionized calcium. *In* Current Veterinary Therapy XII. Kirk RW, Bonagura JA (eds). Philadelphia: WB Saunders, 1995, p. 378.

10. Feldman EC, Hoar B, Pollard R, et al: Pretreatment clinical and laboratory findings in dogs with primary hyperparathyroidism: 210 cases (1987-2004). J Am Vet Med Assoc 227:756, 2005.

11. Devries SE, Feldman EC, Nelson RW, et al: Primary parathyroid gland hyperplasia in dogs: six cases (1982-1991). J Am Vet Med Assoc 202(7): 1132, 1993.

12. Gear RN, Neiger R, Skelly BJ, et al: Primary hyperparathyroidism in 29 dogs: diagnosis, treatment, outcome and associated renal failure. J Small Anim Pract 46 (1):10, 2005.

13. Kallet AJ, Richter JP, Feldman EC, et al. Primary hyperparathyroidism in cats: seven cases (1984-1989). J Am Vet Med Assoc 199(12): 1767, 1991.

14. Berger B, Feldman EC: Primary hyperparathyroidism in dogs: 21 cases (1976-1986). J Am Vet Med Assoc 191:350, 1987.

15. Matwichuk CL, Taylor SM, Daniel GB, et al: Double-phase parathyroid scintigraphy in dogs using technetium-99M-sestamibi Vet Radiol Ultrasound 41(5):461, 2000.

16. Weisner ER, Penninck D, Biller DS, et al: High-resolution parathyroid sonography. Vet Radiol Ultrasound 38 (6):462, 1997.

17. Long CD, Goldstein RE, Hornof WJ, et al: Percutaneous ultrasound-guided chemical ablation for treatment of primary hyperparathyroidism in dogs. J Am Vet Med Assoc 215 (2):217, 1999.

18. Pollard RE, Long CD, Nelson RW, et al: Percutaneous ultrasonographically guided radiofrequency heat ablation for treatment of primary hyperparathyroidism in dogs. J Am Vet Med Assoc 218(7):1106, 2001.

19. Fleish H: Bisphosphonates: A new class of drug in diseases of bone and calcium metabolism. *In* Bisphosphonates and Tumor Osteolysis. Bruner KW, et al (eds). Berlin: Springer-Verlag, 1989 p.1.

20. Fingeroth JM, Smeak DD: Intravenous methylene blue infusion for intraoperative identification of parathyroid gland tumors in dogs. Part III: Clinical trials and results in three dogs. J Am Anim Hosp Assoc 24:673, 1988.

21. Feldman EC, Nelson RW. Hypocalcemia and primary hypoparathyroidism. *In* Canine and Feline Endocrinology and Reproduction, 3rd ed. Feldman EC, Nelson RW (eds). Philadelphia: WB Saunders, 2004, p. 716.

22. Henderson AK, Mahony O: Hypoparathyroidism: Pathophysiology and diagnosis. Comp Cont Educ Small Anim Pract 27(4):270, 2005.

23. Padgett SL, et al: Efficacy of parathyroid gland autotransplantation in maintaining serum calcium concentrations after bilateral thyroidectomy in cats. J Am Anim Hosp Assoc 34:219, 1998.

24. Henderson AK, Mahony O: Hypoparathyroidism: Treatment. Comp Cont Educ Small Anim Pract 27(4):280, 2005.

Chapter 81

Surgical Diseases of the Endocrine Pancreas

Emily Soiderer
S. Kathleen Salisbury

Anatomy

The pancreas is a lobulated structure adjacent to the duodenum that consists of a body and two lobes or limbs. The body lies adjacent to the pylorus, whereas the right limb is closely associated with the descending duodenum on its dorsomedial aspect, enclosed by the mesoduodenum. The left limb of the pancreas lies between the peritoneal layers of the deep leaf of the greater omentum. It is caudal to the stomach and found dorsally in the abdomen adjacent to the left kidney and transverse colon.

The blood supply to the majority of the pancreas originates from the celiac artery via the hepatic and splenic arteries. The gastroduodenal branch of the hepatic artery gives off the cranial pancreaticoduodenal artery, which supplies the body of the pancreas and the cranial half of the right limb. The splenic artery supplies branches that enter the distal end of the left limb. The caudal pancreaticoduodenal artery originates from the cranial mesenteric artery and supplies the remainder of the pancreas. Innervation of the pancreas is derived either from the vagus and splanchnic nerves or is intrinsic to the gland.[1]

Physiology of the Endocrine Pancreas

The endocrine function of the pancreas stems from specialized cells of the islets of Langerhans. These islets are ovoid collections of cells scattered throughout the parenchyma of the pancreas, making up a small portion of the pancreatic volume compared with the exocrine portion.[2,3] The origin of islet cells is believed by some to be neuroectodermal, however this theory is controversial.[4-6] Islet cells are functionally grouped as amine precursor uptake and decarboxylation (APUD) cells.[2] These cells concentrate the amino acid precursors of certain amines and decarboxylate them to form the amines, which function as regulators and neurotransmitters. Functional tumors arising from these cells are termed APUDomas.

The cells of the islets are further categorized based on their hormonal production. Four distinct cell types have been described, each secreting a single hormone: A cells (alpha), B cells (beta), D cells (delta), and F (or P) cells.[2,7] A cells surround the centralized B cells and produce glucagon.[2,8] B cells secrete insulin and account for 60% to 75% of the islet cell population.[2,9] They are located within the center of the islet.[2] D cells produce somatostatin and occupy an intermediate position within the islet between the A and B cells. F cells secrete pancreatic polypeptide and are found in low numbers.[9]

Disorders of the endocrine pancreas are usually a result of either an excess or deficiency in production of one of these hormones. Knowledge of the normal actions of each of these hormones, and the clinical signs and significance of their inappropriate production, is vital to understanding diseases of the endocrine pancreas. Diseases related to excessive or deficient production of insulin are the most common disorders of the endocrine pancreas.

Insulin

The main metabolic function of insulin is to regulate serum glucose concentration and promote the conversion of glucose, fatty acids, and amino acids to their storage forms (glycogen, triglycerides, and protein). The stimulus for insulin release from B cells is high serum glucose concentration. Insulin is made in the rough endoplasmic reticulum of the B cells and is then packaged in the Golgi apparatus into membrane-bound granules. The granules move to the plasma membrane via a process involving microtubules, and their contents are then expelled through exocytosis.[2] Other stimuli for insulin release include other sugars (fructose, mannose, ribose), amino acids, hormones (glucagon, secretin, gastric inhibitory peptide, cholecystokinin, growth hormone, adrenocorticotropin (ACTH), progesterone, and estrogen), drugs, fatty acids, potassium, acetylcholine, and ketones.[2] Glucose enters cells via facilitated diffusion or by secondary active transport with sodium (Na+) (intestine and kidneys).[2] Insulin facilitates glucose entry into cells by increasing the number of glucose transporters in the cell membrane, particularly in muscle, fat, and some other tissues.[2] Glucose penetrates only a few tissues readily, such as the brain, liver, and red and white blood cells.

Insulin facilitates glucose utilization via glycolysis and promotes glycogen production in the liver, adipose tissue, and skeletal muscle by increasing glycogen synthase activity. Insulin also decreases gluconeogenesis because of the promotion of protein synthesis in peripheral tissues, thereby decreasing the amount of amino acids available for gluconeogenesis.[2]

In adipose tissue, insulin functions to increase glucose entry, fatty acid synthesis, glycerol phosphate synthesis, triglyceride deposition, and potassium uptake.[2] It also activates lipoprotein lipase and inhibits hormone-sensitive lipase. In muscle, insulin increases glucose entry, glycogen synthesis, amino acid uptake, protein synthesis in ribosomes, ketone uptake, and potassium uptake. It decreases protein catabolism, and release of gluconeogenic amino acids. In the liver, insulin increases protein and lipid synthesis, decreases ketogenesis, and decreases glucose output owing to decreased gluconeogenesis, increased glycogen synthesis, and increased glycolysis.[2]

Glucagon

Glucagon is primarily a counter-regulatory mechanism hormone that restores plasma glucose levels in states of hypoglycemia by increasing gluconeogenesis, glycogenolysis, and protein-lipid flux in the liver.[10] It has an additional function in gastrointestinal smooth muscle relaxation.[10]

Somatostatin

Somatostatin inhibits the secretion of islet hormones, including insulin, glucagon, and pancreatic polypeptide. It also inhibits the secretion of gut peptides, including gastrin and secretin. Finally, it inhibits pancreatic exocrine secretion and gastric acid secretion, and reduces splanchnic blood flow, intestinal motility, and carbohydrate absorption, while increasing water and electrolyte absorption.[10]

Pancreatic Polypeptide

Pancreatic polypeptide reduces cholecystokinin-induced gastric acid secretion, increases intestinal transit times by reducing gastric emptying and upper intestinal motility, and inhibits postprandial exocrine pancreas secretion via a vagal-dependent pathway.[10]

Specific Disorders of the Endocrine Pancreas

Diabetes Mellitus

Diabetes mellitus (DM) is the most common disorder of the endocrine pancreas in the dog and cat. Therefore, it is important for the surgeon to understand the anesthetic and perioperative management of the diabetic patient.

DM may be caused by failure of insulin production, failure of insulin release, excessive degradation of circulating insulin, or resistance to insulin effects by target tissues.[11] In people, DM is classified as type 1, type 2, gestational diabetes, and other specific types of diabetes.[12] Presently, no classification system exists for veterinary patients; however, the most common cause of DM in dogs and cats is failure of insulin production and secretion by the B cells of the pancreas. Type 1 diabetes in humans is characterized by B cell destruction leading to an absolute insulin deficiency.[12] The cause of this destruction is usually a cellular-mediated autoimmune response.[13] Humans have multiple genetic predispositions to autoimmune destruction of B cells. B cell destruction in humans is also related to environmental factors that are still poorly defined.[13] The cause of B cell destruction in dogs and cats is unknown, however, evidence supports a role for immune-mediated processes. Inflammatory cell infiltration of pancreatic islets occurs in 46% of dogs with DM.[14] Anti-beta cell antibodies have been found in approximately 50% of dogs with insulin-dependent diabetes mellitus.[15] Islet cell destruction secondary to pancreatitis has also been proposed as a cause of diabetes mellitus. The pancreas has a large functional reserve, however, and progressive destruction of pancreatic tissue by recurrent or chronic pancreatitis is a rare cause of exocrine pancreatic insufficiency and diabetes in dogs.[16]

When surgery is considered in a diabetic patient, the status of the patient's diabetes must be determined and the goals of the surgery should be considered.[11] Ideally, surgery should be delayed until the diabetes is well regulated. This is not always possible, however,as occasions may arise in which an urgent condition necessitates surgical intervention before diabetes can be regulated, or a patient's previously well-regulated state may become disrupted owing to the onset of a new condition. The benefit of surgery must be weighed against the risk of pursuing it with the patient in an unregulated state. Surgery may be elective and independent of the diabetes itself, it may be part of long-term management of the diabetic state, or it may be emergent.[11]

Pathophysiology

In diabetes mellitus, the deficiency of or resistance to insulin results in an inability to maintain a euglycemic state. Glucose transport into cells fails and despite high levels of glucose in the bloodstream, an intracellular glucose deficiency results: "starvation in the midst of plenty."[2] This state of starvation leads to inappropriate signaling by cells to increase hepatic gluconeogenesis and glycogenolysis, and decrease glycogenesis. Glycogen stores are quickly depleted and the liver signals for alternate substrates for glycolysis. Energy requirements can only be satisfied by using protein and fat reserves. Lipolysis of fat stores begins and fatty acids are metabolized, leading to the production of ketone bodies. The fatty acids are catabolized to acetyl-coA. The supply of acetyl-coA exceeds the capacity of the tissues to catabolize the acetyl-coA and the excess is converted to ketone bodies.[2] Muscle proteins are catabolized to amino acids for gluconeogenesis. The net effect of accelerated protein catabolism is a negative nitrogen balance, protein depletion, and wasting.

Diabetic patients may be complicated surgical patients owing to the various effects of their persistently hypoinsulinemic state. These patients may suffer from hepatic lipidosis because of excessive fatty deposition in their livers from mobilization of fat stores as a substitute glucose source.[2,17] Fatty acids are transported to the liver and the triglyceride depot is expanded. At the same time, insulin deficiency decreases the release of triglycerides from the liver, leading to hepatic lipidosis and hepatomegaly. This is often a problem in poorly regulated patients, but even well regulated diabetic patients may still have compromised hepatic function. This will have bearing upon anesthetic protocols, and dosages for anesthetic agents metabolized by the liver may need to be reduced.[18]

Pancreatitis is another potential and serious consequence of diabetes.[19-21] Many diabetic animals are prone to pancreatitis and may have a history of it. Anesthesia and manipulation of the pancreas can cause hypotension and subsequently result in decreased perfusion of the pancreas, leading to an acute bout of pancreatitis upon the patient's recovery.[18,21] This will complicate the management of the patient postoperatively and the need to withhold food from that patient will complicate the clinician's ability to regulate the diabetes.

Although rare, diabetic nephropathy is an additional complication that may occur.[22] Histologic findings include membranous glomerulonephropathy, glomerular and tubular basement membrane thickening, glomerular fibrosis, and glomerularsclerosis. Severe proteinuria develops followed by azotemia, and eventually, uremia. Oliguric and anuric renal failure may ensue. The histopathologic findings are dependent on duration of the disease and control of hyperglycemia.[22] Other concurrent endocrinopathies may complicate management. Hyperadrenocorticism and acromegaly contribute to insulin resistance and may be causes for poor regulation of patients with diabetes mellitus.

Increased susceptibility to bacterial infections is a concern for the diabetic surgical patient.[23] Prolonged hyperglycemia predisposes to infection, and risk of infection may increase with increasing glucose concentrations.[23,24] Defective function of polymorphonuclear leukocytes has been demonstrated in diabetes mellitus.[23,25] Chemotaxis, phagocytosis, serum opsonic activity, and bactericidal function of neutrophils of diabetic patients are all diminished. Abnormalities in antibody formation, complement system, and cell-mediated immunity also have been found in poorly controlled diabetic patients.[25] Perioperative antibiotic therapy is advisable in diabetic patients.

Preoperative Evaluation of the Diabetic Patient

A thorough diagnostic evaluation should be completed prior to any surgical procedure in a diabetic patient. A thorough history and physical examination are essential. A minimum data base, including a complete blood count, serum chemistries, urinalysis and urine culture, is essential to identify concurrent problems. Urine culture should be performed owing to the susceptibility of diabetic patients to urinary tract infections. Evaluating the skin for evidence of dermatitis is important for identifying potential sources of infection that should be resolved prior to surgery. Radiographs, electrocardiogram, ultrasound examination, etc., should be completed prior to surgery if indicated based on history, physical examination findings and laboratory analysis. If the determination is made that the patient is poorly regulated, elective surgical procedures should be postponed until appropriate control of the diabetic state is attained.

Perioperative Management of the Diabetic Patient

Management during surgery requires special attention. If the animal's disease is well regulated, food is withheld after midnight the night before the surgical procedure, and blood glucose concentration is measured on the morning of surgery. If the blood glucose concentration is greater than 150 mg/dl, one half of the regular dose of intermediate- or long-acting insulin is administered.[26] If the blood glucose concentration is less than 150 mg/dl, insulin is not given and the blood glucose concentration is re-evaluated postoperatively. Transient hyperglycemia is much less dangerous than hypoglycemia. Intravenous fluids containing 2.5% or 5% dextrose are started at induction and administered throughout anesthesia at 10 ml/kg/hour, unless there are indications to adjust this rate. For procedures of less than 1 hour, blood glucose can be measured postoperatively. Patients that have longer procedures and patients that are less well controlled should have their blood glucose concentration measured every 30 minutes. The dextrose drip should be adjusted as needed to prevent hypoglycemia. If the blood glucose concentration drops below 100 mg/dl, the rate of the dextrose drip (or its concentration for patients at risk of fluid overload) should be increased. If the blood glucose concentration is greater than 300 mg/dl, then 0.25 units/kg of regular insulin is administered subcutaneously.

Postoperative management is aimed at returning the patient to a normal routine and eating habits. Blood glucose concentration is measured every 4 to 6 hours with the goal of maintaining it between 150 and 250 mg/dl. If it increases above 250 mg/dl, regular insulin may be administered subcutaneously. A small meal should be offered the evening of surgery. Fluid therapy is continued overnight and if the patient eats the following morning, fluids are discontinued and the normal intermediate-acting insulin regimen is re-instituted. Transient hyperglycemia and glucosuria may occur for a few days after discharge from the hospital. The owner should be notified of this and advised not to change the insulin dose.

Unregulated or ketoacidotic diabetic patients requiring emergency procedures should be assessed via immediate evaluation of blood glucose concentration with reagent strips, hematologic and biochemical analysis, and urinalysis. Blood gas analysis is ideal if available. Appropriate stabilization with fluid therapy and correction of ketoacidosis is vital to restore acid-base and electrolyte balance and to counteract dehydration. Regular insulin is administered following guidelines of an established protocol for diabetic ketoacidotic patients. The goal is to lower the blood glucose concentration to less than 300 mg/dl and resolve ketonuria. The animal may exhibit Kussmal breathing as it attempts to blow off carbon dioxide and compensate for its metabolic acidosis. This should be recognized, particularly when the animal is under anesthesia, and not be mistaken for too light a plane of anesthesia. Falsely interpreting this breathing pattern and increasing the depth of anesthesia can have adverse consequences. Timing of surgery is determined by the patient's response to therapy and the nature of the emergency. Gradual restoration of imbalances is best tolerated rather than attempting to normalize them all at once.

Ovariohysterectomy in the Diabetic Patient

Intact female dogs are especially prone to becoming unregulated as estrogen concentrations rise during proestrus and estrus and directly antagonize the effects of insulin. During the long luteal phase of diestrus, progesterone predominates and stimulates growth hormone secretion.[27] Growth hormone causes a decrease in the number of insulin receptors on target cell membranes and may also lower the affinity of the remaining receptors for insulin.[11] This leads to prolonged and possibly severe insulin resistance. The animal is at higher risk for developing ketoacidosis as well as a uterine infection. Intact diabetic females are at risk for pyometra owing to the elevated progesterone concentrations and increased susceptibility to infection. The diabetic patient should undergo ovariohysterectomy before beginning her next estrus. If the patient presents in a ketoacidotic state, ovariohysterectomy may prove to be urgent in order to successfully control the diabetes. Postoperatively, insulin resistance will improve and the patient's insulin requirements may markedly decrease. Careful serial monitoring of blood glucose concentration should be done.

Pregnancy also can disrupt the diabetic patient's regulated state. Again, high concentrations of progesterone and growth hormone lead to insulin resistance. The placenta and fetus increase the demands for energy and hyperglycemia persists, possibly leading to ketoacidosis. Increased fetal growth hormone may lead to large feti which can cause dystocia and necessitate emergency cesarean section in an unregulated diabetic patient. The feti may also develop fetal beta-cell hyperplasia owing to high circulating levels of glucose, plasma amino acids, and fats from the poorly regulated mother.[11] If they are carried to term, puppies and kittens may be prone to hypoglycemic seizures. It should also be recognized that the mother's insulin requirement will decrease by 50% when the placenta separates from the uterus if a cesarean section is performed. Owing to the difficulties with blood glucose regulation associated with the estrous cycle and pregnancy, the increased susceptibility to developing pyometra, and the possibility of passing on diabetes mellitus to offspring, all intact females with diabetes should be spayed.

Pancreatic Transplantation for Treatment of Diabetes Mellitus

Pancreatic transplantation as a means of treating diabetes mellitus has been investigated for 4 decades. Whole pancreas transplantation has been successfully performed in dogs exclusively for research purposes. The first pancreatic transplantation in a human was performed in 1966. The major goal of transplantation is prevention or reduction of long-term complications of diabetes (such as heart disease, renal failure, blindness, and stroke). Successful transplantation appears to stop the progression of diabetic nephropathy and diabetic neuropathy; however, it requires major surgery and potentially lifelong immunosuppression to prevent rejection of the transplant.[28] The value of pancreatic transplantation in diabetic pets is problematic because diabetic dogs and cats do not live long enough (even with normal life expectancy) to develop the long-term complications seen in people. Ethical considerations are also a factor because one donor dog would have to be euthanized to provide a healthy pancreas for one recipient. Owners may find the side effects of immunosuppression more difficult to deal with than daily insulin administration. However, as technology improves, pancreatic transplantation may become a more viable option for pets.

Transplantation of pancreatic islets is a promising alternative to whole pancreas transplantation. Donor tissue can be altered to reduce immunogenicity, cost is moderated, and a larger number of patients can be treated. However, many islets must be transplanted because the duration of graft survival can be correlated with the number of islets transplanted.[28,29] This often requires utilization of several donors, which may lead to a need for levels of immunosuppression that can be harmful to the recipient.[28] This has led to the development of immunoprotected islet transplantation through microencapsulation. This process completely encloses each islet within a semipermeable membrane made of a nontoxic polysaccharide that is permeable to small molecules such as insulin and glucose, but is completely impermeable to large molecules such as immunoglobulins. This makes them "invisible" to the recipient's immune system. Microencapsulated pancreatic islets have been transplanted free into the peritoneal cavity of 12 pet dogs with naturally occurring diabetes mellitus. Blood glucose concentration decreased to normal or below normal within 8 to 12 hours. Euglycemia was present for 1 to 6 months, with a mean of 3 months.[28]

Insulinoma

The most common tumor of the endocrine pancreas in the dog is insulinoma, a functional tumor of the pancreatic beta cell. Insulinoma is diagnosed in middle-aged to older dogs (average age 9 years, range 3-15 years).[30] It occurs primarily in large breed dogs including Irish setters, Labrador retrievers, German shepherds, and golden retrievers. No gender predilection is associated with insulinomas in dogs.[31] Insulinoma is considered rare in cats as few cases have been reported.[32-34] Of these reports, all cats were of older age (range 12-17 years) and 3 of 5 were Siamese.

Pathophysiology

Insulinomas secrete insulin independently of the normal suppressive effects of hypoglycemia. Although insulin is the most abundant hormone produced by these tumors, evidence exists of multihormonal production, including pancreatic polypeptide, glucagon, somatostatin, serotonin, and gastrin.[35,36] Clinical signs associated with insulinomas result from the hypoglycemic effects of hyperinsulinemia, leading to neuroglycopenia, and stimulation of the sympathetic nervous system, leading to an increase in circulating catecholamines.[30,37,38] Clinical signs caused by neuroglycopenia include lethargy, weakness, ataxia, collapse, seizures, posterior paresis, and depression.[13,34] Clinical signs resulting from stimulation of the sympathoadrenal system include muscle tremors, nervousness, restlessness, and hunger.[37,38] Clinical signs are usually episodic because of the counter-regulatory mechanisms that enable recovery from hypoglycemic episodes.[38] Clinical signs can be present for days to months, with most dogs being symptomatic for 1 to 6 months prior to presentation.[30,38] The onset of clinical signs is related to the degree of hypoglycemia and the rate at which it occurs.[30,38] Gradual blood glucose changes are less likely to cause clinical signs of hypoglycemia than an acute drop. Dogs that have a slowly decreasing glucose concentration over a prolonged period of time (i.e., weeks) may be able to adjust without showing clinical signs until the blood glucose concentration reaches a point at which the animal can no longer adapt to the hypoglycemia and signs of neuroglycopenia result.[38] These dogs can typically adjust to blood glucose concentrations as low as 20 to 30 mg/dl. However, if the hypoglycemia develops acutely, perhaps over a few hours, clinical signs will develop quickly. Because of the failure of insulin secretion to drop during periods of hypoglycemia, dogs with insulinoma are predisposed to developing clinical signs during fasting and exercise.[38] In addition, insulin-secreting tumors remain responsive to many of the stimuli that promote insulin secretion in healthy dogs, such as eating, but the secretory response may be exaggerated, so severe hypoglycemia can occur.[38]

Normally, B cells of the pancreatic islets maintain the primary control of blood glucose concentrations. When blood glucose concentration rises above 110 mg/dl, insulin is secreted and the glucose concentration decreases into the normal physiologic range. When the blood glucose concentration falls below 60 mg/dl, insulin synthesis and secretion are inhibited and blood glucose returns to normal as tissue utilization slows and blood glucose concentration increases.[38] With insulinoma, insulin secretion is not inhibited and hypoglycemia results. Hypoglycemia triggers the production of counter-regulatory hormones including glucagon, epinephrine, growth hormone, and cortisol. Glucagon, epinephrine, and norepinephrine concentrations increase at the onset of the counter-regulatory response; growth hormone and cortisol increase later.[38] Glucagon is the main counter-regulatory hormone in acute hypoglycemia. Glucagon secretion is stimulated by hypoglycemia and by beta-adrenergic nervous system stimulation and adrenomedullary catecholamines.[38] Glucagon is secreted into the portal circulation and activates glycogenolysis and gluconeogenesis in the liver. Hypoglycemia stimulates growth hormone secretion, which decreases glucose uptake into some tissues, increases hepatic production of glucose, and possibly decreases tissue binding of insulin.[2] Adrenocorticotropic hormone and cortisol are increased by direct stimulation of the pituitary gland and stimulation of the pituitary-adrenocortical axis by the sympathetic nervous system. Long-term elevation of cortisol aids lipolysis, promotes protein catabolism and the conversion of amino acids to glucose by the liver and kidney, and limits utilization of glucose by tissues. The effects of increased cortisol and growth hormone do not occur for hours and are more effective in countering chronic hypoglycemia than acute hypoglycemia.

The autonomic nervous system response to hypoglycemia has alpha- and beta-adrenergic effects. Hypoglycemia stimulates catecholamine secretion by the adrenal medulla. Alpha-adrenergic effects result in inhibition of endogenous insulin secretion and stimulation of peripheral vasoconstriction, causing an increase in cerebral blood flow in the healthy dog. Epinephrine stimulates hepatic glycogenolysis and gluconeogenesis, mobilizes muscle glycogen and gluconeogenic precursors, stimulates lipolysis, and inhibits glucose utilization by insulin-sensitive tissues. Beta-adrenergic effects include stimulation of hepatic and muscle glycogenolysis, increased plasma glucagon secretion, stimulation of lipolysis, inhibition of glucose uptake by muscle, and increased cerebral blood flow secondary to an increase in cardiac output. Cholinergic effects lead to stimulation of pancreatic polypeptide secretion, increased gastric motility, and hunger stimulation.[38]

The counter-regulatory response to hypoglycemia can be effective in controlling hypoglycemia; however the continued production and secretion of insulin from an insulinoma will eventually overwhelm the ability of these mechanisms to counteract the hypoglycemia. Without surgical or medical intervention, the patient will succumb to the effects of hypoglycemia.

Hypoglycemia can affect most cells, but the cells of the central nervous system (CNS) are the most vulnerable. The carbohydrate storage ability of these cells is minimal and glucose is their primary energy source. A continuous supply of glucose from the blood is essential. Glucose enters the cell via diffusion, independent of insulin. When the blood glucose concentrations are inadequate for intracellular oxidative processes, a decline in energy-rich phosphorylated compounds (adenosine triphosphate

[ATP]) occurs in neurons.[38] The lack of energy results in cellular dysfunction and cellular changes similar to hypoxia: increased vascular permeability, vasospasm, vascular dilation, and edema. This is followed by neuronal death.[11,38] Owing to varying metabolic rates in the CNS, the most active sites are affected first. In mammals this is the cerebral cortex. The least metabolically active area is the brain stem and, therefore, it is more resistant to hypoglycemia.[11,38] The majority of damage occurs in the brain, but peripheral nerve degeneration and demyelination can occur.[38] Other major organ systems are dependent on glucose for energy, but the CNS will show signs of an acute drop in blood glucose long before organ failure develops.[38]

Differential and Definitive Diagnosis

A thorough diagnostic workup must be performed to make a diagnosis of insulinoma. This begins simply with an accurate and thorough history from the owner as well as a thorough physical exam. A patient-side glucose test strip should be run at presentation, but results of serum chemistries will help most in identifying hypoglycemia as the primary or sole cause of the clinical signs. Hypoglycemia is defined as a blood glucose concentration below 60 mg/dl. The presence of hypoglycemia narrows the differential list, but does not establish insulinoma as the cause. Whipple's triad has classically been used as a criterion for diagnosis: (1) presence of neurologic signs associated with hypoglycemia, (2) fasting blood glucose concentration below 60 mg/dl, (3) resolution of clinical signs with feeding or administration of glucose.[38-40] Whipple's triad however only confirms hypoglycemia as the cause of the neurologic signs. It does not yield a diagnosis of insulinoma, because any cause of hypoglycemia could fulfill Whipple's triad.[38-39,41]

Hypoglycemia results from excessive glucose utilization, impaired hepatic gluconeogenesis and glycogenolysis, deficiency of counter-regulatory hormones, inadequate dietary intake of glucose and/or its substrates, and iatrogenic hypoglycemia.[38] Hepatic-induced hypoglycemia can be a result of congenital causes such as portosystemic shunts or acquired causes such as cirrhosis and acquired portosystemic shunting. Insufficient hepatic glycogen stores and inadequate hepatocellular function to support gluconeogenesis are responsible for the hypoglycemia associated with liver disease.[38] Any severe insult to the liver that results in decreased hepatocellular function, such as infection, toxic insult, or necrosis, can lead to hypoglycemia. Hypoglycemia can be caused by starvation or sepsis, or may be idiopathic in neonates, toy breed dogs, and hunting dogs.[42] Endocrinopathies such as adrenocortical insufficiency, hypopituitarism, ACTH deficiency, glucagon deficiency and non-beta cell-derived hyperinsulinism can cause hypoglycemia. Glycogen-storage disease, renal failure, cardiac disease, and polycythemia are also associated with hypoglycemia. Artifactual hypoglycemia can occur from prolonged blood storage prior to separation of the red cells from the serum or plasma. Continuing metabolism of glucose by the red blood cells will decrease the glucose concentration in a whole-blood sample. Iatrogenic hypoglycemia can occur owing to insulin or oral sulfonylurea drug overdosage. Finally, extrapancreatic neoplasia, such as leiomyosarcoma and hepatic adenocarcinoma, has been associated with hypoglycemia. Hepatic tumors may grow large enough that they utilize a large amount of glucose as well as interfere with gluconeogenesis. These tumors can also secrete insulin and insulin-like peptides that contribute to hypoglycemia. Often, patients with hypoglycemia not associated with hyperinsulinism will have other clinical pathologic abnormalities that will help to narrow the differential diagnosis list and guide further diagnostics.

The diagnosis of insulinoma is supported by finding an inappropriately elevated serum insulin concentration in the presence of hypoglycemia. The insulin concentration must be compared with the concurrent blood glucose concentration. The serum insulin concentration in a healthy fasted dog is usually between 5 and 20 μU/ml. Blood glucose concentration is normally between 70 and 110 mg/dl. A serum insulin concentration that exceeds 20 μU/ml in a dog with a blood glucose concentration less than 60 mg/dl, along with clinical signs, strongly supports the diagnosis of an insulin-secreting tumor.[38] However, an insulin-secreting tumor is also possible with a serum insulin concentration in the high normal range (10–20 μU/ml). Animals with other causes of hypoglycemia as well as those with insulin-secreting tumors may have a serum insulin concentration between 5 and10 μU/ml. In 85 dogs with blood glucose concentrations less than 60 mg/dl, 73% had a serum insulin concentration greater than 20 μU/ml, 21% had a serum insulin concentration between 10 and 20 μU/ml, and 6% had a concentration between 5 and10 μU/ml.[38] Several different insulin:glucose ratios have been used to further assess the likelihood of an insulin-secreting tumor. Although these ratios are controversial, the amended insulin:glucose ratio is considered to be the most reliable.[38] The amended insulin:glucose ratio consists of the following formula:

$$\frac{\text{plasma insulin } (\mu\text{U/ml}) \times 100}{\text{plasma glucose (mg/dl)} - 30}$$

Based on the human literature, an amended insulin:glucose ratio greater than 30 is diagnostic for an insulin-secreting tumor. However, in dogs this test is not specific for insulinoma. Other causes of hypoglycemia, such as hepatic tumors and sepsis, may result in abnormal amended insulin-glucose ratios.[38] Because of this, the absolute serum insulin concentration during hypoglycemia should be evaluated in concert with the history, physical examination findings, and clinical pathologic test results.[38,39]

Provocative tests, including the glucagon tolerance test, L-leucine test, tolbutamide and ethanol response test, oral glucose tolerance test, epinephrine stimulation test, calcium infusion test, C-peptide suppression test, and diazoxide infusion test, have been reported.[11,38,39] These tests are not considered more sensitive than the insulin-glucose pair, can be expensive and inefficient, and can potentiate significant hypoglycemia dangerous to the animal, so they are not recommended.

The disease process is further characterized with diagnostic imaging. Abdominal radiographs are usually unremarkable owing to the small size of insulinomas and their location within the pancreas; a visible mass or visceral displacement is extremely rare.[38] Although metastasis can occur to the liver, lymph nodes, and peripancreatic omentum, these lesions are not likely to be detectable on radiographs. Pulmonary metastasis is rare, and thoracic radiographs are usually unremarkable until late in the disease. Abdominal ultrasonography is likely to be more useful than radiography, but can still be unrewarding. Detection of a mass in the pancreas is helpful in supporting a diagnosis of insulinoma in animals that have the appropriate clinical picture. It is common to be unable to identify a lesion in the pancreas and, therefore, the lack of an identifiable mass via ultrasonography does not rule out its presence. Ultrasonography may also detect metastatic lesions in the liver and peripancreatic tissue.

The use of computed tomography (CT) for identifying insulinomas has recently been investigated. In one study of 14 confirmed insulinomas, ultrasonography, CT, and single-photon emission CT (SPECT) were evaluated for detecting and localizing canine insulinoma.[43] Five primary insulinomas were correctly identified with ultrasonography, 10 with CT, and 6 with SPECT.[43] CT identified 2 out of 5 lymph node metastases, but also showed 28 false-positive lesions.[43] The authors concluded that ultrasonography could be used for initial evaluation of dogs with hypoglycemia, and although CT identified most primary tumors, intraoperative inspection and palpation were still superior. SPECT appeared as effective as ultrasonography and CT.[43] Scintigraphy has also been used as an additional imaging modality. In one study, 5 dogs with insulinomas were imaged using[111] In-pentetrotide scintigraphy to identify somatostatin receptors. All insulinomas expressed high-affinity somatostatin receptors.[44] However, scintigraphy was able to accurately predict the anatomic location of the primary tumor in only 1 out of 4 dogs, and was unable to differentiate a right- from left-pancreatic lobe tumor.[44,111] In-pentetrotide scintigraphy was concluded to be a useful diagnostic adjunct but was unable to localize the tumor in some cases.[44]

Treatment

Surgical exploration of the abdomen offers the best results in terms of diagnosis, therapy, and prognosis. Most dogs with insulin-secreting tumors have visible nodules present upon inspection of the pancreas.[38] Definitive diagnosis is based on histopathologic evaluation of lesions resected or biopsied at the time of surgery. A solitary nodule within the pancreas is likely to be resectable and will afford long-term control of hypoglycemia, however, cure is unlikely. The goal of surgery is to remove as much neoplastic tissue as possible; debulking of gross metastatic disease may afford a significant therapeutic effect. The blood glucose concentration should be stabilized as well as possible prior to anesthesia and surgery. Manipulation of an insulinoma may result in release of insulin and a further drop in blood glucose concentration.

Localization of a pancreatic mass is based on careful inspection and gentle palpation of the entire pancreas. Primary lesions are distributed equally between the two limbs of the pancreas, and an identifiable mass was located approximately 92% of the time in one source.[38] Another source reported inability to identify a mass in 20% of cases.[45] If a mass is not identified, special methods, such as intravenous administration of methylene blue and intraoperative ultrasonography, can be used to assist in identification of the lesion.[46-48] Methylene blue is an azo dye that concentrates in the parathyroid glands and endocrine pancreas. Intravenous infusion of this dye has been recommended for identification of primary nodules and differentiation of metastatic versus nonmetastatic lesions.[46-48] Methylene blue stains normal pancreatic endocrine tissue a dusky slate blue, whereas hyperfunctioning tissue is stained a reddish-violet.[34] Side effects include Heinz body hemolytic anemia, acute renal failure, pseudocyanosis, green-tinged urine, and possibly pancreatitis.[46-49] Intraoperative ultrasonography in humans has a success rate of greater than 95% for finding insulinomas; this modality may prove useful in dogs.[50]

Thorough exploration of the abdomen is vital to identifying the extent of metastatic disease. Gross metastasis is identifiable at the time of surgery in approximately 36% of cases.[51] Metastasis most commonly occurs to the liver, regional lymph nodes, and peripancreatic tissue. Lesions should be biopsied or resected if possible. Ideally, all of the abnormal tissue should be removed and submitted for histopathologic evaluation.

Palpation may reveal a thickened pancreas, or the pancreas may feel completely normal.

Successful surgery depends on the location of the tumor. A tumor in the left or right limb at the distal aspect is the most amenable to resection. Tumors at the body or in the region of the common bile duct are the most difficult to remove and increase the risk of postoperative pancreatitis owing to the potential for disrupting pancreatic blood supply. The extensive manipulation necessary to remove tumors in this area and the likelihood of incomplete resection may warrant a decision to leave the mass. If nonresectable disease is present, biopsy of the mass is the minimum the surgeon should accomplish. Closing the abdomen and pursuing medical therapy is advisable.

Intravenous fluids should be administered for 12 to 24 hours prior to, during, and after surgery to ensure adequate perfusion of the pancreas. Manipulation and dissection of the pancreas during surgery results in inflammation and predisposes the animal to postoperative pancreatitis. Hypotension will result in poor perfusion of the pancreas and may potentiate pancreatitis. Aggressive fluid support may help avoid hypotension and minimize the severity of the pancreatitis. Dextrose therapy is often needed to counteract clinical signs of hypoglycemia. Administration of a 2.5% or 5% dextrose solution is usually adequate. Maintenance of normal blood glucose concentration intraoperatively is extremely important. It should be measured every 30 to 60 minutes during surgery with a goal of maintaining it above 40 mg/dl, but not to necessarily reach a normal blood glucose concentration. It is rare to need more than a 5% dextrose solution, and if needed, a constant rate infusion of glucagon can help raise the blood glucose concentration when dextrose alone is inadequate.

Postoperative care is aimed at controlling pancreatitis, hypoglycemia, and if it occurs, hyperglycemia. Serum electrolytes and blood glucose concentration should be measured twice daily. If pancreatitis is recognized, intravenous fluid therapy is continued (routinely 120 ml/kg/day) and food and water are withheld for 24 to 48 hours. Plasma administration is advisable and parenteral nutrition is started.

If persistent hypoglycemia occurs postoperatively, functional metastatic disease is present. Medical therapy to prevent clinical signs should be instituted as well as frequent feeding (every 4 to 6 hours) with a diet appropriate for pancreatitis. Feeding frequency is increased to at least 3 to 6 times per day. A variety of medical therapies can help to control hypoglycemia. Glucocorticoid therapy (prednisone or prednisolone 0.25 mg/kg PO every 12 hours) is often the first medication used when frequent feedings are not adequate. The glucocorticoid dose can be increased as needed to control clinical signs, keeping in mind the adverse side effects of this drug. Increasing doses of glucocorticoids will result in signs of hyperadrenocorticism and possibly gastric ulceration. When these side effects become unacceptable, the glucocorticoid dose should be decreased and another therapy added to control the clinical signs of hypoglycemia.

Diazoxide (5 mg/kg PO every 12 hours) is a benzothiadiazide that is used alone or in combination with glucocorticoids. Diazoxide inhibits insulin secretion, promotes hepatic gluconeogenesis and glycogenolysis, and inhibits tissue use of glucose. Diazoxide can be difficult to obtain and is expensive. It is reported to be 70% effective in controlling hypoglycemia but does not have any antineoplastic effects.[52] The dose can be increased to 30 to 40 mg/kg PO every 12 hours if necessary. Side effects include hyperglycemia, bone marrow suppression, cardiac arrhythmias, hypernatremia, cataracts, and gastrointestinal disturbances.[52,53]

Octreotide is a somatostatin analog that inhibits insulin secretion and has been used with varying success in humans.[54,55] Doses up to 40 μg every 8 to 12 hours are reported to be effective without causing adverse side effects.[56] In one study, the endocrine effects of a single subcutaneous dose of 50 μg of octreotide were studied in healthy dogs in the fasting state and in dogs with insulinoma. After octreotide administration to dogs with insulinomas, baseline plasma insulin concentrations decreased significantly and plasma glucose concentrations increased.[57] However, evaluation of octreotide in a study of 3 dogs with insulinoma showed that octreotide had no benefit over placebo and little effect on circulating glucose and insulin concentrations.[58]

Streptozocin is a nitrosurea alkylating agent that is directly cytotoxic to pancreatic beta cells. It had previously not been advisable to use in dogs owing to its association with acute renal failure from renal tubular necrosis.[59-61] Other side effects are vomiting, which can be severe, and increases in hepatic enzyme activities. These toxicities are dose-dependent, with vomiting and hepatic enzyme increases occurring at lower dosages. Acute renal tubular necrosis occurs at higher doses. A diuresis protocol has met with some success.[62] Normal saline was administered at 18.3 ml/kg/hour intravenously for 3 hours prior to streptozocin administration. The dose (500 mg/m^2) was diluted to the appropriate volume and administered over the next 2 hours at the same rate. Normal saline was then administered for another 2 hours after the streptozocin infusion was complete. Butorphanol (0.4 mg/kg IM) was given as an antiemetic immediately after streptozocin administration. Treatments were repeated every 3 weeks until there was no evidence of tumor progression (> 50% increase in tumor dimensions), recurrence of hypoglycemia, or development of a streptozocin-induced toxicosis. Mean duration of euglycemia was 163 days compared with 90 days for the control group, although this was not statistically significant. Two dogs had measurable reductions in size of metastases, and the clinical signs of 2 of 3 dogs with polyneuropathy resolved. Side effects of the drug were minimal with the diuresis protocol.[62]

Prognosis

Long-term prognosis for insulinoma in dogs is guarded to poor owing to the malignant behavior of these tumors. They are malignant in terms of their metastatic potential; microscopic or gross metastasis at the time of diagnosis is almost certain. Mean survival time from the onset of clinical signs has been reported to be 12 months for dogs treated medically.[63] However, Tobin reported a median survival time of 74 days for dogs treated medically and a median of 381 days for those that underwent surgery.[64] It should be noted that the medically treated dogs had advanced disease and may have had shorter survival times because of this and the owners' possible feelings of hopelessness leading to euthanasia. Prognosis also depends on age at the time of onset of clinical signs, with younger dogs having significantly shorter survival times than older dogs. Dogs that have a solitary pancreatic nodule (stage I) have significantly longer disease-free intervals (mean 14 months) after surgery than those with metastatic spread to the liver, regional lymph nodes (stage II), or distant sites (stage III).[65] High preoperative serum insulin concentrations are also associated with shorter survival times.[65] Approximately one third of dogs undergoing surgery die or are euthanized within 1 month as a result of severe metastatic disease, uncontrollable hypoglycemia, or postoperative pancreatitis. Another one third die or are euthanized within 6 months of surgery owing to severe metastatic disease and recurrence of clinical hypoglycemia. The final one third live beyond 6 months without recurrence of hypoglycemia and many of these survive well beyond 1 year.[63]

Gastrinoma (Zollinger-Ellison Syndrome)

Gastrinomas are pancreatic islet cell tumors that secrete excessive amounts of gastrin. They were first identified in humans in 1955 by Zollinger and Ellison.[66] The Zollinger-Ellison syndrome consists of hypergastrinemia, a neuroendocrine tumor, and gastrointestinal ulceration. These tumors are rare in veterinary patients with only a few reports in the literature.[67-70] They occur in middle-aged dogs (range: 3-12 years, mean 7.5 years) and older cats (mean 11 years).[38] No breed predilection has been identified. Female dogs and cats may be overrepresented.[71]

The most common clinical signs of gastrinoma are vomiting, anorexia, and weight loss owing to gastroduodenal ulceration.[9,23,67-69] Other signs that may occur include lethargy, depression, hematemesis, hematochezia, diarrhea, melena, and abdominal pain. These animals are at risk for gastrointestinal perforation and peritonitis from the ulcerative disease, and may experience collapse and shock secondarily. Physical examination may be unremarkable or may reveal an extremely sick animal if perforation has occurred.[9,30,67-69] Physical examination findings depend on the severity and duration of disease. Animals may be lethargic, thin to emaciated, febrile, dehydrated, and in shock.[38]

Pathophysiology

Gastrin is a polypeptide hormone produced by G cells in the lateral walls of the glands of the antral portion of the gastric mucosa.[2] It is also found in the pancreatic islets in fetal life. Gastrinomas are found in the pancreas, but it is uncertain if gastrin is found in the pancreas in normal adults.[2] The main actions of gastrin are stimulation of gastric acid secretion and pepsin secretion, as well as stimulation of the growth of gastric mucosa and small and large intestinal mucosa.[2]

The stimulus for gastrin secretion is related to the contents of the stomach, with secretion increased by the presence of the products of protein digestion (amino acids) that act directly on G cells. Luminal distention is also a stimulus for gastrin secretion. Gastrin inhibition occurs via the direct effect of acid in the antrum on G cells and by release of somatostatin, a gastrin-secretion inhibitor.[2] In patients with gastrinoma, hypergastrinemia induces excessive gastric secretion of hydrochloric acid, which is responsible for the development of esophageal, gastric, and duodenal ulcers, the disruption of intestinal digestive and absorptive functions, and the development of clinical signs.[38] With excessive gastrin secretion, hydrochloric acid secretion is increased and this hyperacidity leads to ulceration. Reflux esophagitis may occur, and as the excessive acid moves through the GI tract, it can cause direct ulceration of the duodenum and jejunum. Intestinal hyperacidity may also lead to intestinal inflammation, mucosal edema, villous atrophy, and inactivation of pancreatic lipase and bile salts.[38,72] Gastrinomas may also secrete other hormones including insulin, ACTH, and pancreatic polypeptide.

Diagnosis

Diagnostic workup includes a minimum database consisting of a complete blood count, serum chemistries, and urinalysis. CBC abnormalities seen with gastrinoma include neutrophilia, hypoproteinemia, and regenerative anemia, likely resulting from inflammation and blood loss. Serum chemistry abnormalities may include hypoalbuminemia, hypocalcemia, and increases in alanine aminotransferase and alkaline phosphatase. Hypochloremia, hypokalemia, and metabolic alkalosis may occur from frequent vomiting. Tumor secretion of other hormones such as ACTH and insulin may occur and possibly lead to hyper- or hypoglycemia. Sudan staining of fecal material may reveal steatorrhea; melena is usually present. Urinalysis is unremarkable.

Abdominal radiographs are usually unremarkable. However, if an ulcer has perforated, loss of abdominal contrast consistent with peritonitis may be present. Contrast radiography can identify gastric and duodenal ulcers and thickening of the gastric rugal folds, pyloric antrum, and/or intestine.[38] Increased gastrointestinal transit time as well as esophagitis and secondary megaesophagus may be present. Abdominal ultrasonography may find thickened gastric and intestinal walls, gastric ulcers, a pancreatic mass, and/or metastatic lesions.[38] Gastrinomas can be difficult to identify because of their potentially small size; failure to identify a mass by ultrasonography does not rule it out. Scintigraphy with radiolabeled somatostatin analogues may be useful owing to a high concentration of somatostatin receptors in gastrinomas in people.[70] A positive scan can also help identify patients that may benefit from medical therapy with somatostatin analogues like octreotide, which decrease gastrin release.[67-70]

Gastroduodenoscopy may reveal ulcerative lesions in the stomach and duodenum as well as esophagitis. Gastric rugal folds may be thickened. Histologic evaluation of the gastric mucosa may reveal mild to severe inflammation with lymphocytic, neutrophilic, eosinophilic, or plasma cell infiltrates as well as mucosal hypertrophy.

Definitive diagnosis of gastrinoma is based on histopathologic and immunocytochemical evaluation of the mass excised at surgery. Baseline serum gastrin concentrations are useful prior to surgical exploration, particularly if a pancreatic mass is not visualized by ultrasonography. Demonstration of persistent hypergastrinemia with appropriate clinical signs is supportive of a diagnosis of gastrinoma. Fasting serum gastrin concentration is measured with multiple blood samples drawn after an overnight fast. The reference range for gastrin concentration will vary among laboratories, but the upper limit is usually less than 100 pg/ml in dogs and cats.[70,73] The majority of reported cases of histologically confirmed gastrinoma in dogs and cats have gastrin concentrations greater than three times higher than the upper normal value. Normal gastrin concentrations have been documented in humans with gastrinoma, and so it is likely that dogs and cats with normal gastrin concentrations may still have a gastrinoma. It is also important to note that an elevated fasting serum gastrin concentration is not pathognomonic for gastrinoma. Other syndromes associated with hypergastrinemia include chronic renal failure, chronic gastritis, gastric outflow obstruction, liver disease, achlorhydria, and administration of H_2-receptor antagonists.[38] Once hypergastrinemia is documented and other causes are ruled out, a presumptive diagnosis of gastrinoma can be made.

Treatment

Treatment is aimed at surgical excision of the tumor and control of gastric acid hypersecretion. The decision as to when exploratory surgery is performed depends on the clinical status of the animal. Prior to undertaking anesthesia, the animal must be stabilized. Medical therapy with gastric acid blockers should be instituted first with the goal of reducing gastric hyperacidity and controlling its secondary effects. Surgical goals include identification of a pancreatic mass and definitive diagnosis, as well as successful resection of the tumor. Because approximately 80% of animals with gastrinomas have gastrointestinal ulcers, the stomach and bowel should be evaluated for evidence of deep or perforated ulcers, and resection of these areas should be performed when necessary.[7] Surgery also offers an opportunity to stage the disease by identifying and biopsying gross metastatic lesions. Approximately 70% of animals have metastasis at the time of initial diagnosis.[38]

Medical therapy for gastrinomas involves blocking gastric acid hypersecretion with H_2-receptor antagonists and the H^+-K^+ ATPase inhibitor, omeprazole. For maximal hydrochloric acid secretion from parietal cells to occur, three receptor sites must be activated. These receptor sites bind gastrin, histamine, and acetylcholine. H_2-receptor antagonists bind to the H_2-receptor and block gastrin's stimulatory effect on hydrochloric acid secretion because all three receptor sites are not occupied by their respective peptides.[38] H_2-receptor antagonists include famotidine (0.5 – 1.0 mg/kg PO every 12-24 hours), ranitidine (2.2 mg/kg PO every 12 hours) and cimetidine (10 mg/kg every 6-8 hours). Dosages may need to be increased as the disease progresses to control hyperacidity.

Omeprazole is the preferred drug for gastrinoma in humans.[38] It acts as a proton pump inhibitor (inhibits parietal cell H^+-K^+ ATPase), which is the last common step in gastric acid secretion. Omeprazole is considered to be more effective than H_2-receptor antagonists because it inhibits gastric acid secretion stimulated by any of the secretagogues, while the H_2-receptor antagonists inhibit only the actions of histamine. Omeprazole has a long duration of action and is effective at controlling the clinical signs of gastrinoma in dogs.[73] Dosage is 0.7 to 1.0 mg/kg PO every 24 hours.

Octreotide, a long-acting somatostatin analogue, is occasionally used in humans with gastrinoma refractory to H_2-receptor antagonists and omeprazole. It has been used in dogs.[70] Dosing ranges between 5 to 20 μg subcutaneously every 8 hours.

Prognosis

The long-term prognosis for gastrinoma is poor owing to its highly malignant nature with 76% of cases having gross metastasis at the time of diagnosis.[74] In previous studies, surgical and/or medical treatment resulted in survival times of 1 week to 18 months.[75] With the availability of drugs to reduce gastric hypersecretion and to promote healing of ulcers, the short-term prognosis is improving.

Glucagonoma

Glucagonoma is a tumor of the A cells of the pancreatic islets in which excessive amounts of glucagon are inappropriately secreted. Glucagon-secreting tumors are rare in both humans and animals, with only a few reported cases in dogs.[76-82] Dogs typically present with a characteristic dermatitis involving the foot pads that is consistent with superficial necrolytic dermatitis (SND). High levels of glucagon are thought to be involved in the development of these skin lesions, although the mechanism is poorly understood. Patients may also develop diabetes mellitus caused by stimulation of gluconeogenesis and glycogenolysis from excessive secretion of glucagon.[76] DM usually occurs when insulin production cannot match the increased glucagon secretion.[77] Other clinical signs include cheilosis, normocytic-normochromic anemia, venous thrombosis, weight loss, polyuria, polydipsia, glossitis, stomatitis, and diarrhea. Three dogs with glucagonoma ranged in age from 8 to 11 years and had a chief complaint of chronic dermatitis. Skin lesions occur particularly in areas of trauma and involve hyperkeratosis of the foot pads; erythematous, erosive, and crusting lesions on the muzzle, external genitalia, perineum, and periocular region. Other common historical complaints included weight loss, polydipsia, and polyuria. Weight loss is likely a result of the catabolic effects of glucagon on fat and protein metabolism.[83]

Diagnosis

A baseline complete blood count, serum biochemistries, and urinalysis should be obtained. Clinical pathologic abnormalities can include a mild nonregenerative anemia, hypoalbuminemia, hepatic enzyme elevations, low blood urea nitrogen, and possibly persistent hyperglycemia. Elevated serum glucagon concentration in the absence of hypoglycemia is suggestive of the presence of a glucagonoma.[38,80] Other syndromes associated with mildly elevated glucagon concentrations include diabetic ketoacidosis, renal failure, hepatic failure, sepsis, and starvation.[30] Hypoaminoacidemia may also be a feature of this disease, and supplementation of amino acids may improve dermatologic conditions.[30] Skin biopsies are necessary to diagnose superficial necrolytic dermatitis, which is characterized by diffuse parakeratotic hyperkeratosis, acanthosis, vacuolar changes of keratinocytes, and epidermal edema.[76-79] Submission of multiple biopsy samples from the edges of early skin lesions is most useful.[80] Diagnostic imaging of the thorax and abdomen may show evidence of local or metastatic disease. Abdominal ultrasonography may reveal hepatic lesions or a pancreatic mass, however, of 9 dogs with glucagonomas that had ultrasonography performed, a pancreatic mass was visualized in only one dog.[76-82] Abdominal computerized tomography has been used in one dog to identify a pancreatic mass and was also successful in identifying multiple liver masses.[77]

Treatment and Prognosis

Surgical resection is the treatment of choice. Histologic evaluation of pancreatic masses in dogs has demonstrated pancreatic carcinomas with glucagon immunoreactivity.[77-79] Metastasis is common, and if present, tumor debulking may be helpful in palliating clinical signs. Chemotherapy has been attempted in humans with some success.[84-85] Dietary supplementation with essential fatty acids, zinc, and amino acids may improve skin lesions, and has shown success as an infusion in one case report in a man.[86] Long-term prognosis is poor. Most canine patients are diagnosed late in the course of the disease, preventing the possibility of a cure. Short-term palliation of signs can be successful with early surgical and medical treatment.

Pancreatic Polypeptidoma

Pancreatic polypeptide (PP) is a common component of pancreatic islet cell tumors. It is well documented that the majority of endocrine tumors contain multiple hormones, and pancreatic polypeptide is the second most common hormone identified by immunocytochemistry in canine pancreatic endocrine tumors.[87] This rare pancreatic islet cell tumor has been documented to produce clinical signs in only one dog. This 7-year-old spayed female cocker spaniel presented with a history of chronic vomiting, anorexia, and weight loss.[87] Elevated serum PP concentration was documented. Serum gastrin concentrations were also elevated but provocative testing was normal. Necropsy revealed a pancreatic adenocarcinoma with metastasis to the liver, gastric hypertrophy, and multiple duodenal ulcers. Immunocytochemical staining of the tumor for gastrin was negative. Serum PP concentrations were extremely elevated and both the tumor and its metastases stained strongly positive for PP. The authors proposed that the high serum concentrations of PP contributed to the dog's gastrointestinal ulceration and vomiting.[87]

VIPoma and Somatostatinoma

VIPomas are pancreatic islet cell tumors that have been identified in humans, but have not been documented in dogs and cats.[38] Intestinal secretion of fluid and electrolytes secondary to high circulating concentrations of vasoactive intestinal polypeptide (VIP) causes clinical signs of profuse watery diarrhea, fecal loss of potassium and bicarbonate, and low or absent gastric acid secretion. This may lead to a severe metabolic acidosis secondary to bicarbonate loss in the diarrhea. VIPomas are diagnosed based on measurement of serum fasting VIP concentrations by radioimmunoassay and histologic confirmation of a non-beta-cell pancreatic tumor with a high content of VIP.[88] Surgical excision is the treatment of choice, with 50% achieving remission when metastasis is not present.[89] Medical therapy with streptozocin plus fluorouracil has been used in humans with nonresectable or metastatic carcinoma. Octreotide has been used to lower plasma concentrations of VIP in patients refractory to other treatment modalities.

Somatostatinomas have also been recognized in humans, but not in dogs and cats. Somatostatin has been found to be present in canine islet cell tumors.[32,35,36] In humans, excess secretion of somatostatin from D cells of the pancreas causes glucose intolerance, cholelithiasis, diarrhea, steathorrhea, hypochlorhydria, and weight loss.[90] Diagnosis is based on clinical features, documentation of increased serum concentrations of somatostatin, and histologic examination of the tumor. Metastasis occurs to the liver and adjacent lymph nodes and is usually present at the time of diagnosis of these slow-growing tumors. Surgical excision is the treatment of choice, but chemotherapy with streptozocin has been attempted.[38]

Conclusion

The endocrine pancreas is a complex organ that presents multiple challenges for the veterinary surgeon. Its production of various hormones and their effects on the body require an understanding of the normal physiology of the endocrine pancreas as well as the pathophysiology of its disorders. These disorders can be challenging to diagnose and a thorough understanding of endocrine function is necessary to correlate the clinical picture with its etiology. Diagnosis and appropriate management of affected cases relies on knowledge of the mechanism of disease, the potential for perioperative complications, and the long-term outcome with medical or surgical management.

References

1. Guilford WG: Strombeck's Small Animal Gastroenterology 3rd ed. Philadelphia: WB Saunders, 1996.
2. Ganong WF: Endocrine functions of the pancreas and regulation of carbohydrate metabolism. *In* Review of Medical Physiology. New York: McGraw Hill, 2003, p. 336.
3. Dyce KM, Sack WO, Wensing CJ: Textbook of Veterinary Anatomy. Philadelphia: WB Saunders, 1987.
4. Pearse AG, Takor TT: Neuroendocrine embryology and the APUD concept. Clin Endocrinol 5 Suppl:229S-244S, 1976.
5. Teitelman G: Insulin cells of pancreas extend neurites but do not arise from the neuroectoderm. Dev Biol 142:368, 1990.
6. Madsen OD, Jensen J, Blume N, et al: Pancreatic development and maturation of the islet B cell. Studies of pluripotent islet cultures. Eur J Biochem 242:435, 1996.
7. Nelson RW: Diabetes mellitus *In* Textbook of Veterinary Internal Medicine. Ettinger SJ (ed). Philadelphia: WB Saunders, 1995, p. 1510.
8. Hawkins KL, Summers BA, Kuhajda FP, et al: Immunocytochemistry of normal pancreatic islets and spontaneous islet cell tumors in dogs. Vet Pathol 24:170, 1987.
9. Lurye JC, Behrend EN: Endocrine tumors. Vet Clin North Am Small Anim Pract 31:1083-1110, 2001.
10. Boushey RP, Drucker DJ: Gastrointestinal hormones and gut endocrine tumors *In* Williams Textbook of Endocrinology. Williams RH (ed). Philadelphia: WB Saunders, 2003, p. 1777.
11. Fingeroth JM: Endocrine pancreatic disease *In* Disease Mechanisms in Small Animal Surgery, 2nd ed. Bojrab J (ed). Philadelphia: Lea & Febiger, 1993, p. 589.
12. Fleeman LM, Rand JS: Management of canine diabetes. Vet Clin North Am Small Anim Pract 31(5):855, 2001.
13. Clinical Practice Recommendations 2005. Diabetes Care. Jan 28 Suppl 1:S1-79, 2005.
14. Alejandro R, Feldman EC, Shenvold FL, et al: Advances in canine diabetes mellitus research: etiopathology and results of islet transplantation. J Am Vet Med Assoc. 193:1050, 1988.
15. Hoenig M, Dawe DL: A qualitative assay for beta cell antibodies. Preliminary results in dogs with diabetes mellitus. Vet Immunol Immunopathol 32:195, 1992.
16. Williams DA: Exocrine pancreatic disease *In* Textbook of Veterinary Internal Medicine. Ettinger SJ (ed). Philadelphia: WB Saunders, 1995, p. 1381.
17. Greco DS: Diagnosis of diabetes mellitus in cats and dogs. Vet Clin North Am Small Anim Pract 31(5):845, 2001.
18. Trim CM: Anesthesia and the endocrine system *In* Textbook of Small Animal Surgery, 2nd ed. Slatter D (ed). Philadelphia: WB Saunders, 1993, p. 2290.
19. Nelson RW: Diabetes mellitus *In* Textbook of Veterinary Internal Medicine. Ettinger SJ (ed). Philadelphia: WB Saunders, 1995, p. 1517.
20. Hess RS, Kass PH, Shofer FS, et al: Evaluation of risk factors for fatal acute pancreatitis in dogs. J Am Vet Med Assoc 214:46, 1999.
21. Cook AK, Breitschwerdt EB, Levine JF, et al: Risk factors associated with acute pancreatitis in dogs: 101 cases (1985-1990). J Am Vet Med Assoc 203:673, 1993.
22. Nelson RW: Diabetes mellitus *In* Textbook of Veterinary Internal Medicine. Ettinger SJ (ed). Philadelphia: WB Saunders, 1995, p. 1536.
23. Aragon D, Ring CA, Covelli M: The influence of diabetes mellitus on postoperative infections. Crit Care Nurs Clin North Am 15:125, 2003.
24. Golden SH, Peart-Vigilance C, Kao WH, et al: Perioperative glycemic control and the risk of infectious complications in a cohort of adults with diabetes. Diabetes Care 22:1408, 1999.

25. Schaer M: Surgery in the diabetic patient. Vet Clin North Am Small Anim Pract 25(3):651-660, 1995.

26. Paddleford RR: Manual of Small Animal Anesthesia, 2nd ed. Philadelphia: WB Saunders, 1999, p. 306.

27. Kooistra HS, den Hertog E, Okkens AC, et al: Pulsatile secretion pattern of growth hormone during the luteal phase and mid-anoestrus in beagle bitches. J Reprod Fertil 119:217, 2000.

28. Feldman EC, Nelson RW, Soon-Shiong P: Transplantation as a means of treating diabetes mellitus. *In* Kirk's Current Veterinary Therapy XII. Small Animal Practice. Bonagura JD (ed). Philadelphia: WB Saunders, 1995, p. 398.

29. Street CN, Lakey JR, Shapiro AM, et al.: Islet graft assessment in the Edmonton protocol: implications for predicting long-term clinical outcome. Diabetes 53: 3107, 2004.

30. Waters CB, Scott-Moncrieff JCR: Cancer of endocrine origin *In* Cancer in Dogs and Cats: Medical and Surgical Management. Morrison WB, (ed). Jackson, WY: Teton NewMedia, 2002, p. 573.

31. Nelson RW: Insulin-secreting islet cell neoplasia *In* Textbook of Veterinary Internal Medicine. Ettinger SJ (ed). Philadelphia: WB Saunders, 1995, p. 1501.

32. O'Brien TD, Norton F, Turner TM, et al.: Pancreatic endocrine tumor in a cat: clinical, pathological, and immunohistochemical evaluation. J Am Anim Hosp Assoc 26:453, 1990.

33. McMillan FD, Barr B, Feldman EC: Functional pancreatic islet cell tumor in a cat. J Am Anim Hosp Assoc 21:741, 1985.

34. Hawks D, Peterson ME, Hawkins KL, et al: Insulin-secreting pancreatic (islet cell) carcinoma in a cat. J Vet Intern Med 6:193, 1992.

35. Hawkins KL, Summers BA, Kuhajda FP, et al: Immunocytochemistry of normal pancreatic islets and spontaneous islet cell tumors in dogs. Vet Pathol 24:170, 1987.

36. Minkus G, Jutting U, Aubele M, et al: Canine neuroendocrine tumors of the pancreas: a study using image analysis techniques for the discrimination of metastatic versus nonmetastatic tumors. Vet Pathol 34:138, 1997.

37. Nelson RW: Insulin-secreting islet cell neoplasia *In* Textbook of Veterinary Internal Medicine. Philadelphia: Ettinger SJ (ed). WB Saunders, 1995, p. 1502.

38. Feldman EC, Nelson RW: Canine and Feline Endocrinology and Reproduction. St. Louis: WB Saunders, 2004, p. 616.

39. Nelson RW: Insulin-secreting islet cell neoplasia *In* Textbook of Veterinary Internal Medicine. Ettinger SJ (ed). Philadelphia: WB Saunders, 1995, p. 1505.

40. Whipple AO, Grantz VK: Adenoma of islet cells with hyperinsulinism. A review. Ann Surg 101:1299, 1935

41. Fossum TW: Small Animal Surgery. St. Louis: Mosby, 1997, p. 401.

42. Nelson RW: Insulin-secreting islet cell neoplasia *In* Textbook of Veterinary Internal Medicine. Ettinger SJ (ed). Philadelphia: WB Saunders, 1995, p. 1504.

43. Robben JH, Pollak YW, Kirpensteijn J, et al: Comparison of ultrasonography, computed tomography, and single-photon emission computed tomography for the detection and localization of canine insulinoma. J Vet Intern Med 19:15, 2005.

44. Garden OA, Reubi JC, Dykes NL, et al: Somatostatin receptor imaging in vivo by planar scintigraphy facilitates the diagnosis of canine insulinoma. J Vet Intern Med 19:168, 2005.

45. Steiner JM, Bruyette DS: Canine insulinoma. Comp Cont Educ Pract Vet 18:31, 1996.

46. Smeak DD, Fingeroth JM, Bilbrey SA: Intravenous methylene blue as a specific stain for primary and metastatic insulinoma in a dog. J Am Anim Hosp Assoc 24:478, 1988.

47. Fingeroth JM, Smeak DD, Jacobs RM: Intravenous methylene blue infusion for intraoperative identification of parathyroid gland and pancreatic islet-cell tumors in dogs. Part I: experimental determination of dose-related staining efficacy and toxicity. J Am Anim Hosp Assoc 24:165, 1988.

48. Fingeroth JM, Smeak DD: Intravenous methylene blue infusion for intraoperative identification of pancreatic islet-cell tumors in dogs. Part II: Clinical trials and results in four dogs. J Am Anim Hosp Assoc 24:175, 1988.

49. Osana DJ, Armstrong PJ, Duncan DE, et al: Acute renal failure after methylene blue infusion in a dog. J Am Anim Hosp Assoc 26:410, 1990.

50. Hiramoto JS, Feldstein VA, LaBerge JM, et al: Intraoperative ultrasound and preoperative localization detects all occult insulinomas; discussion 1025-1026. Arch Surg 136:1020, 2001.

51. Elie MS, Zerbe CA: Insulinoma in dogs, cats, and ferrets. Comp Cont Educ 17:51, 1995.

52. Leifer CE, Peterson ME, Matus RE: Insulin-secreting tumor: diagnosis and medical and surgical management in 55 dogs. J Am Vet Med Assoc 188:60, 1986.

53. Plumb DC: Veterinary Drug Handbook, 3rd ed. White Bear Lake, MN: Pharma Vet Publishing, 1999, p.187.

54. Vezzosi D, Bennet A, Rochaix P, et al: Octreotide in insulinoma patients: efficacy on hypoglycemia, relationships with Octreoscan scintigraphy and immunostaining with anti-sst2A and anti-sst5 antibodies. Eur J Endocrinol 152:757, 2005.

55. Arnold R, Simon B, Wied M: Treatment of neuroendocrine GEP tumors with somatostatin analogues: a review. Digestion 62 Suppl 1:84, 2000.

56. Nelson RW: Insulin-secreting islet cell neoplasia *In* Textbook of Veterinary Internal Medicine. Ettinger SJ (ed). Philadelphia: WB Saunders, 1995, p. 1508.

57. Robben JH, van den Brom WE, Mol JA, et al.: Effect of octreotide on plasma concentrations of glucose, insulin, glucagon, growth hormone, and cortisol in healthy dogs and dogs with insulinoma. Res Vet Sci In press, 2005.

58. Simpson KW, Stepien RL, Elwood CM, et al: Evaluation of the long-acting somatostatin analogue octreotide in the management of insulinoma in three dogs. J Small Anim Pract 36:161, 1995.

59. Meyer DJ: Pancreatic islet cell carcinoma in a dog treated with streptozotocin. Am J Vet Res 37:1221, 1976.

60. Meyer DJ: Temporary remission of hypoglycemia in a dog with an insulinoma after treatment with streptozotocin. Am J Vet Res 38:1201, 1977.

61. Kaneko JJ, Mattheeuws D, Rottiers RP, et al: Renal function, insulin secretion, and glucose tolerance in mild streptozotocin diabetes in the dog. Am J Vet Res 39:807, 1978.

62. Moore AS, Nelson RW, Henry CJ, et al: Streptozocin for treatment of pancreatic islet cell tumors in dogs: 17 cases (1989-1999). J Am Vet Med Assoc 221:811, 2002.

63. Nelson RW: Insulin-secreting islet cell neoplasia *In* Textbook of Veterinary Internal Medicine. Ettinger SJ (ed). Philadelphia: WB Saunders, 1995, p. 1509.

64. Tobin RL, Nelson RW, Lucroy MD, et al: Outcome of surgical versus medical treatment of dogs with beta cell neoplasia: 39 cases (1990-1997). J Am Vet Med Assoc 215:226, 1999.

65. Caywood DD, Klausner JS, O'Leary TP, et al.: Pancreatic insulin-secreting neoplasms: clinical, diagnostic, and prognostic features in 73 dogs. J Am Anim Hosp Assoc 24:577, 1988.

66. Zollinger RM, Ellison EH: Primary peptic ulcerations of the jejunum associated with islet cell tumors of the pancreas. Ann Surg 142:709, 1955.

67. Green RA, Gartrell CL: Gastrinoma: a retrospective study of four cases (1985-1995). J Am Anim Hosp Assoc 33:524, 1997.

68. Fukushima U, Sato M, Okano S, et al: A case of gastrinoma in a Shih-Tzu dog. J Vet Med Sci 66:311, 2004.

69. Fukushima R, Ichikawa K, Hirabayashi M, et al: A case of canine gastrinoma. J Vet Med Sci 66:993, 2004.

70. Altschul M, Simpson KW, Dykes NL, et al.: Evaluation of somatostatin analogues for the detection and treatment of gastrinoma in a dog. J Small Anim Pract 38:286, 1997.

71. Waters CB, Scott-Moncrieff JC: Cancer of endocrine origin. *In* Cancer in Dogs and Cats: Medical and Surgical Management. Morrison WB (ed). Baltimore, Williams & Wilkins, 1998, p. 599.

72. Zerbe CA, Washabau RJ: Gastrointestinal endocrine disease *In* Textbook of Veterinary Internal Medicine. Ettinger SJ (ed). Philadelphia: WB Saunders, 1995, p. 1597.

73. Brooks D, Watson GL: Omeprazole in a dog with gastrinoma. J Vet Int Med 11:379, 1997

74. Zerbe CA, Washabau RJ: Gastrointestinal endocrine disease *In* Textbook of Veterinary Internal Medicine. Ettinger SJ (ed). Philadelphia: WB Saunders, 1995, p. 1600.

75. Zerbe CA: Islet cell tumors secreting insulin, pancreatic polypeptide, gastrin, or glucagon. In: Current Veterinary Therapy XI. Kirk RW, Bonagura GD (eds). Philadelphia: WB Saunders, 1992, p. 368.

76. Gross TL, O'Brien TD, Davies AP, et al: Glucagon-producing pancreatic endocrine tumors in two dogs with superficial necrolytic dermatitis. J Am Vet Med Assoc 197:1619, 1990.

77. Langer NB, Jergens AE, Miles KG: Canine glucagonoma. Comp Cont Educ 25:56, 2003.

78. Torres SM, Caywood DD, O'Brien TD, et al: Resolution of superficial necrolytic dermatitis following excision of a glucagon-secreting pancreatic neoplasm in a dog. J Am Anim Hosp Assoc 33:313, 1997.

79. Miller WH, Anderson WI, McCann JP: Necrolytic migratory erythema in a dog with a glucagon-secreting endocrine tumor. Vet Derm 2:179, 1991.

80. Allenspach K, Arnold P, Glaus T, et al: Glucagon-producing neuroendocrine tumor associated with hypoaminoacidemia and skin lesions. J Small Anim Pract 41:402, 2000.

81. Torres SM, Johnson K, McKeever P, et al: Superficial necrolytic dermatitis and a pancreatic endocrine tumor in a dog. J Small Anim Pract 38:246, 1997.

82. Bond R, McNeil PE, Evans H, et al: Metabolic epidermal necrosis in two dogs with different underlying diseases. Vet Rec 136:466, 1995.

83. Chastain MA: The glucagonoma syndrome: A review of its features and discussion of new perspectives. Am J Med Sci 321(5):306, 2001.

84. Brentjens R, Saltz L: Islet cell tumors of the pancreas: the medical oncologist's perspective. Surg Clin North Am 81:527, 2001.

85. Fiasse R, Pauwels S, Rahier J, et al: Use of octreotide in the treatment of digestive neuroendocrine tumours. Seven year experience in 20 cases including 9 cases of metastatic midgut carcinoid and 5 cases of metastatic gastrinoma. Acta Gastro Belgica 56:279, 1993.

86. Alexander EK, Robinson M, Staniec M, et al: Peripheral amino acid and fatty acid infusion for the treatment of necrolytic migratory erythema in the glucagonoma syndrome. Clin Endocrinol 57:827, 2002.

87. Zerbe CA, Boosinger TR, Grabau JH, et al.: Pancreatic polypeptide and insulin-secreting tumor in a dog with duodenal ulcers and hypertrophic gastritis. J Vet Intern Med 3:178, 1989.

88. Krejs GJ: VIPoma syndrome. Am J Med 82 (Suppl 5B):37, 1987.

89. Smith SL, Branton SA, Avino AJ, et al: Vasoactive intestinal polypeptide secreting islet cell tumors: a 15-year experience and review of the literature. Surgery 124:1050, 1998.

90. Krejs GJ: Non-insulin-secreting tumors of the gastroenteropancreatic system. *In* Williams Textbook of Endocrinology, 9th ed. Wilson JD, Foster DW, Kronenberg HM, Larsen PR (eds). Philadelphia: WB Saunders, 1998, p. 1663.

Chapter 82

Adrenal Glands

Andrew E. Kyles

Anatomy

The adrenal glands are paired, retroperitoneal structures located cranial and medial to the cranial pole of each kidney. The right adrenal gland lies dorsolateral to, and is intimately associated with, the caudal vena cava. The left adrenal gland is more caudal in location. The phrenicoabdominal vein courses over the ventral surface of each adrenal gland, while the phrenicoabdominal artery lies on the dorsal surface of the gland. The adrenal arterial blood supply is derived from branches of the aorta and phrenic, renal, accessory renal, phrenicoabdominal, and lumbar arteries. Venous drainage is into the caudal vena cava and renal and phrenicoabdominal veins. Malignant adrenal tumors sometimes invade these venous structures.

The adrenal gland consists of two separate endocrine components with distinct embryonic origins. The cortex is derived from the celomic epithelium and is of mesodermal origin. Histologically, the cortex is divided into an outer zona glomerulosa, the chief site of aldosterone production, and the zona fasciculata and the inner zona reticularis, which together are responsible for the production of glucocorticoids and sex hormones. The medulla is derived from the sympathetic ganglia and is ectodermal in origin. The adrenal medulla produces catecholamines, epinephrine, and norepinephrine.

Glucocorticoids

Physiology

The production of glucocorticoids is regulated via the hypothalamic-pituitary-adrenal axis. Corticotrophin-releasing hormone (CRH) is a 41 amino acid peptide hormone. CRH is secreted by neurons in the anterior portion of the paraventricular nuclei of the hypothalamus. CRH is delivered to the pituitary gland via a portal circulation and acts to stimulate the secretion of adrenocorticotrophic hormone (ACTH) from the anterior pituitary gland (adenohypothesis). ACTH is a 39 amino acid peptide hormone derived from a large precursor molecule, proopiomelanocortin. The primary function of ACTH is to stimulate the secretion of glucocorticoids from the adrenal cortex. Cortisol is the major glucocorticoid produced. Circulating cortisol and synthetic glucocorticoids produce a negative feedback inhibition of the hypothalamus and pituitary, thus inhibiting ACTH secretion. During severe stress, such as pain, trauma, acute hypoglycemia, and surgery, the suppressive effects of glucocorticoids are overridden, resulting in increased secretion of CRH, ACTH, and glucocorticoids.

Hyperadrenocorticism

Hyperadrenocorticism (Cushing's syndrome) is caused by chronic exposure to excessive concentrations of glucocorticoids. Of dogs with naturally occurring hyperadrenocorticism, 80% to 85% have pituitary-dependent hyperadrenocorticism (PDH). PDH causes excessive production of ACTH resulting in bilateral adrenocortical hyperplasia and excessive secretion of glucocorticoids. The majority of dogs with PDH have a small pituitary adenoma (microadenoma); 10% to 20% of dogs with PDH have large pituitary adenomas (macroadenoma). These tumors can compress and invade the overlying hypothalamus, resulting in clinical signs such as dullness, listlessness, inappetance, and disorientation, which can progress to neurologic signs such as aimless wandering, ataxia, head pressing, circling, and seizures. Pituitary carcinomas are rare in dogs.

Functional primary adrenocortical tumors secrete excessive amounts of cortisol independent of pituitary control. The excess gluocorticoid production suppresses hypothalamic CRH and plasma ACTH concentrations, resulting in cortical atrophy of the contralateral adrenal gland. Functional adrenocortical tumors commonly retain ACTH receptors and respond to exogenous ACTH administration by secreting cortisol. Histologic differentiation of adrenocortical adenomas and carcinomas is challenging; it would appear that the two tumor types occur with approximately equal frequency in dogs. Cases of simultaneous occurrence of PTH and an adrenocortical tumor or pheochromocytoma have been reported, as have bilateral adrenocortical tumors and simultaneous occurrence of an adrenocortical tumor and a pheochromocytoma. Naturally occurring hyperadrenocorticism should be differentiated from the iatrogenic form caused by chronic glucocorticoid therapy.

Signalment

The median age of dogs with naturally occurring hyperadrenocorticism is 11.4 years;[1] the disease is uncommon in dogs younger than 6 years of age. Hyperadrenocorticism is seen in a variety of breeds, with poodles, daschunds, various terrier breeds and German shepherd dogs being commonly represented. Approximately 75% of dogs with PDH weigh less than 20 kg, whereas 45% 50% of dogs with a functional adrenocortical tumor weigh more than 20 kg.[1] Females account for 55% to 60% of dogs with PDH and 60% to 65% of dogs with a functional adrenocortical tumor.[1] Hyperadrenocorticism is rarely diagnosed in cats. There are reports of cats with clinical signs of hyperadrenocorticism caused by a progesterone-secreting adrenal tumor.

History and Physical Examination Findings

Hyperadrenocorticism is one of the most common endocrinopathies in dogs. The clinical signs are largely attributable to chronic glucocorticoid excess, resulting in gluconeogenic, immunesuppressive, anti-inflammatory, protein catabolic, and lipolytic effects. Clinical signs include polydipsia and polyuria, polyphagia, bilateral symmetric alopecia and other skin abnormalities (hyperpigmentation, comedone formation, thin skin, thin hair coat, and calcinosis cutis), pendulous abdomen (owing to hepatomegaly, muscle wasting, and intraabdominal fat accumulation), muscle weakness, muscle atrophy, panting, heat intolerance, and anestrous or testicular atrophy. The number and severity of clinical signs vary markedly. PDH and a functional adrenocortical tumor cannot be differentiated based on clinical signs.

Medical Complications Associated with Hyperadrenocorticism

1. Hypertension
2. Pyelonephritis
3. Diabetes mellitus
4. Pulmonary thromboembolism

Clinicopathologic Findings

CBC: Excess glucocorticoids produce a stress leukogram in most dogs, consisting of a mature neutrophilia, lymphopenia, eosinopenia, and monocytosis.

Biochemistry profile: The most common abnormality is increased serum alkaline phosphatase (ALP) activity (a result in part of the induction of a glucocorticoid isoenzyme unique to dogs). Alanine aminotransferase (ALT) activity may also be increased associated with a steroid hepatopathy. Mild to moderate increases in cholesterol and triglyceride concentrations are common, and serum bile acid concentrations may be elevated. Serum bilirubin and albumin concentrations are usually within the reference ranges. Glucose concentration varies, with approximately 10% of dogs developing overt diabetes mellitus (interestingly, up to 80% of cats with hyperadrenocorticism are diabetic). Blood urea nitrogen and serum creatinine concentrations may be low as a result of diuresis.

Urinalysis: Urine specific gravity is often low, although most dogs retain an ability to concentrate urine with water deprivation. Urinary tract infections occur in 40% to 50%.[2] Proteinuria is common, associated with urinary tract infection or glomerular leakage. Glucosuria may occur if the renal glucose threshold is exceeded.

Thyroid function tests: Decreased basal serum T_4 and/or T_3 concentrations are common.

Diagnostic Imaging

Thoracic radiography: Mineralization of the tracheobronchial tree and pulmonary parenchyma is a nonspecific finding that is more common in dogs with hyperadrenocorticism. Radiographs should be evaluated for signs of pulmonary metastases and pulmonary thromboembolism.

Abdominal radiography: Findings include hepatomegaly, obesity, and mineralization of soft tissue structures. Adrenal gland mineralization occurs in approximately 50% of adrenocortical tumors.

Abdominal ultrasonography: Dogs with PDH usually have relatively equal sized adrenal glands with normal or enlarged dimensions. In dogs with a functional adrenocortical tumor, the affected adrenal gland is usually enlarged and irregular with mixed echogenicity, and a normal or atrophied adrenal gland is usually observed on the contralateral side. Compression or invasion of the phrenicoabdominal vein and/or caudal vena cava may have occurred, and intraabdominal metastases may be present. The liver is generally enlarged with increased echogenicity, and urinary calculi and dilated renal pelvises (caused by pyelonephritis) may be present.

CT or MRI: Used to rule out a pituitary macroadenoma. Abdominal imaging may provide additional information on adrenal anatomy, intraabdominal metastases, and vascular invasion.

Adrenal Function Tests

Screening tests are used to confirm the diagnosis of hyperadrenocorticism.

Basal plasma cortisol concentration: As cortisol is released episodically, this test has virtually no diagnostic value.

Urine cortisol:creatinine ratio: This test adjusts for fluctuating plasma concentrations of cortisol. Has high sensitivity but low specificity; may thus be a good test for ruling out hyperadrenocorticism.

ACTH stimulation test: This measures the response of the adrenal glands to maximal ACTH stimulation. It has a sensitivity of 60 to 85% and a specificity of 85 to 90%.[3] It cannot differentiate PDH from a functional adrenocortical tumor. This is the only test that can identify dogs with iatrogenic hyperadrenocorticism and is the only test in veterinary medicine for monitoring response to therapy.

Low-dose dexamethasone suppression (LDDS) test: Dexamethasone is a synthetic glucocorticoid that does not cross react in the cortisol assay. In normal dogs, the cortisol concentration decreases 2 to 3 hours after dexamethasone administration, whereas dogs with hyperadrenocorticism do not experience suppressed cortisol concentrations. For the LDDS test, dexamethasone is administered (0.01 mg/kg IV) and blood samples collected 4 and 8 hours later. The sensitivity of the test at 8 hours after administration is 85 to 95% and the specificity is 70 to 75%.[3]

Differentiating tests are used to differentiate PDH from a functional adrenocortical tumor.

High-dose dexamethasone suppression (HDDS) test: After administration of a high dose of dexamethasone (0.1 mg/kg IV), approximately 75% of dogs with PDH have suppressed cortisol concentrations, whereas in dogs with a functional adrenocortical tumor, even large doses of dexamethasone should not suppress plasma cortisol concentrations.[3]

Endogenous plasma ACTH concentration: In dogs with a functional adrenocortical tumor, the hypothalamic-pituitary axis is suppressed and the ACTH concentration is low or undetectable, whereas dogs with PDH usually have an ACTH concentration above the reference range.

Surgery

Adrenalectomy: Surgical removal is the treatment of choice for adrenal tumors. During surgery, hemostasis is a definite challenge. Adrenal tumors can cause a tumor thrombus in the caudal vena cava. In most dogs with a caval thrombus, the tumor invades the phrenicoabdominal vein and extends into the caudal vena cava.[4] This results in a pedunculated caval thrombus based around the insertion of the phrenicoabdominal vein that can be removed by temporary caval occlusion and a venotomy centered around the insertion of the phrenicoabdominal vein. After unilateral adrenalectomy, cortisol secretion from the contralateral, atrophied adrenal gland is suppressed and glucocorticoid supplementation is needed during and following surgery. Aldosterone secretion from the contralateral adrenal gland is usually adequate, although electrolyte concentrations should be closely monitored and mineralocorticoid therapy instituted if hyperkalemia and/or hyponatremia are observed. Bilateral adrenalectomy necessitates lifelong glucocorticoid and mineralocorticoid supplementation.

Dogs with hyperadrenocorticism are hypercoagulable and at increased risk of experiencing pulmonary thromboembolism after surgery; therefore, these patients should be maintained on anticoagulant regimens following surgery. Other surgical considerations include impaired wound healing, a greater propensity for wound infection, impaired respiratory function, and hypertension. Postoperative mortality rates are relatively high (21-28%).[4,5] Other serious postoperative complications include pancreatitis, pneumonia, sepsis, and acute renal failure.

Hypophysectomy: Transsphenoidal hypophysectomy is the treatment of choice for humans with PDH and has been shown to be an effective treatment in dogs with PDH.[6,7] Potential intraoperative complications include hemorrhage from the arterial circle during exploration of the fossa. Following hypophysectomy, dogs require lifelong therapy with glucocorticoids and thyroxine. Diabetes insipidus is normally transient, requiring short-term treatment with vasopressin. Reduced tear production is frequently reversible. Estimated survival rates at 2 and 4 years were 76% and 68%, and 2- and 4-year estimated relapse-free fractions were 75% and 58%.[7]

Medical Therapy

Mitotane (o,p'-DDD, Lysodren): Mitotane is a potent adrenolytic drug that causes selective destruction of the zona fasciculata and zona reticularis (site of glucocorticoid production) while sparing the zona glomerulosa (site of mineralocorticoid production). The drug is most commonly used to induce and maintain a state of partial adrenocortical destruction, with the goal of restricting glucocorticoid production to amounts needed for daily life. The ACTH stimulation test is used to monitor therapy. It can also be used to induce complete adrenocortical destruction, a state that requires lifelong glucocorticoid and mineralocorticoid therapy. The results of using mitotane in cats with hyperadrenocorticism have been disappointing.

Trilostane: Trilostane is an orally administered competitive inhibitor of the enzyme 3β-hydroxysteroid dehydrogenase. This enzyme converts pregnenolone to progesterone and 17-hydroxypregnenolone to 17-hydroxyprogesterone in the adrenal cortex. Trilostane thus inhibits the production of cortisol, aldosterone, and androstenedione. Similar to the use of mitotane, the aim is to restrict cortisol production and the dose of drug is altered based on the results of ACTH stimulation testing. Trilostane has been used successfully to manage PDH and functional adrenocortical tumors in dogs. Trilostane is reported to ameliorate the signs of feline hyperadrenocorticism.

Ketoconazole: Ketoconazole is a fungistatic drug that blocks several P-450 enzyme systems. It produces reversible inhibition of the synthesis of glucocorticoids and androgens, while sparing mineralocorticoid production. Trilostane has largely replaced ketoconazole for the management of hyperadrenocorticism. The use of ketoconazole in cats with hyperadrenocorticism has produced mixed results.

Mineralocorticoids

Physiology

The production of mineralocorticoids is primarily regulated by the renin-angiotensin system. Renin is produced by the juxtaglomerular cells, which surround the afferent arterioles of the renal glomeruli. The juxtaglomerular cells monitor renal perfusion. Volume depletion and hypotension stimulate renin production. Renin acts on a plasma α2-globulin produced by the liver, releasing angiotensin I. Converting enzyme in the lung converts angiotensin I to angiotensin II, a potent vasoconstrictor and the primary stimulant for aldosterone production. The primary site of action of aldosterone is the renal tubule, where it promotes the resorption of sodium and water and the excretion of potassium. This results in expansion of the extracellular fluid volume, and removes the stimulus for renin production.

Hyperaldosteronism

Primary hyperaldosteronism (Conn's syndrome) is caused by autonomous secretion of aldosterone by a tumor of the zona glomerulosa layer of the adrenal cortex. Hyperaldosteronism results in sodium retention, expansion of the extracellular fluid volume, and hypertension. The production of renin is suppressed. Increased potassium excretion leads to progressive depletion of body potassium and the development of hypokalemia and hypokalemic metabolic alkalosis.

The condition is rare in cats and dogs. Clinical signs include weakness, which may be episodic, cervical ventroflexion (cats), lethargy, polyuria, and/or polydipsia. The most common clinicopathologic abnormality is moderate-to-severe hypokalemia. The sodium concentration may be normal or slightly elevated. Definitive diagnosis requires demonstrating an inappropriately elevated aldosterone concentration with a low renin concentration. Adrenalectomy is the treatment of choice in animals with no detectable metastases. Medical therapy consists of potassium supplementation and spironolactone (an aldosterone antagonist) administration.

Adrenocortical Insufficiency

Hypoadrenocorticism is a syndrome that results from deficient secretion of glucocorticoids and/or mineralocorticoids by the adrenal cortices. Primary hypoadrenocorticism (Addison's disease) is caused by the destruction of more than 90% of adrenocortical tissue. Primary hypoadrenocorticism is rare in the dog and cat. The most common cause is idiopathic adrenocortical insufficiency, which is most likely a result of immune-mediated destruction of the adrenal cortices. Iatrogenic hypoadrenocorticism is a possible complication of mitotane therapy in dogs with hyperadrenocorticism. Although mitotane usually spares the zona glomerulosa and thus mineralocorticoid production, some dogs experience a permanent, complete adrenocortical failure. Other causes of primary hypoadrenocorticism include bilateral adrenalectomy, hemorrhage or infarction of the adrenal glands, granulomatous or neoplastic destruction of the adrenal glands, amyloidosis, and trauma. Secondary hypoadrenocorticism is caused by deficient production of ACTH, resulting in impaired secretion of glucocorticoids by the adrenal cortices; the production of mineralocorticoids is spared.

Deficiency of glucocorticoids causes a decreased tolerance to stress, including a reduced ability to mount a stress response to surgery. Other signs include inappetance, vomiting, diarrhea, abdominal pain, and lethargy. Aldosterone deficiency impairs the patient's ability to conserve sodium and water and causes a failure to excrete potassium, resulting in hyponatremia and hyperkalemia. Hyponatremia induces lethargy, depression, and nausea, whereas hyperkalemia results in muscle weakness and impaired cardiac conduction. These patients experience hypovolemia, hypotension, reduced cardiac output, and impaired renal perfusion.

Signalment

Female dogs account for approximately 70% of cases.[8] Hypoadrenocorticism can be diagnosed in dogs of any age, but is most common in young and middle-aged dogs. No breed predilection has been identified.

History and Physical Examination Findings

Acute hypoadrenocorticism (Addisonian crisis) causes hypovolemic shock. Dogs present in a state of collapse or they collapse when stressed, with a weak pulse, profound bradycardia, vomiting, diarrhea, dehydration, and hypothermia. The chronic form of hypoadrenocorticism causes vague, non-specific, and often episodic clinical signs. Signs include lethargy, anorexia, weight loss, vomiting, diarrhea, obtundation, shaking or shivering, muscle fasiculations, muscle weakness, and polyuria/polydipsia.

Clinicopathologic Findings

CBC: Changes can include lymphocytosis, eosinophilia, and a mild nonregenerative anemia.

Biochemistry profile: The most common abnormalities noted include hyponatremia, hyperkalemia, pre-renal azotemia, and metabolic acidosis. The normal sodium:potassium ratio is 27:1 to 40:1; most patients with hypoadrencorticism have a ratio below 25:1. In approximately 10% of dogs with primary hypoadrenocorticism, the serum electrolyte concentrations are within the reference ranges at initial examination.

Electrocardiographic Findings

Hyperkalemia impairs electrical conduction in the heart. An ECG can be used to evaluate patients with hypoadrencorticism. As a rough guide:

Modest hyperkalemia (5.5-6.5 mEq/L)	Peaking of T waves Shortening of Q-T interval
Moderate hyperkalemia (6.5-7.5 mEq/L)	Increased QRS duration P-wave amplitude decreases P-R interval prolonged
Severe hyperkalemia (> 7.5 mEq/L)	P wave disappears Severe bradycardia

Adrenal Function Tests

ACTH stimulation test: The gold standard for diagnosing hypoadrenocorticism. The resting cortisol concentration is low or nondetectable with a subnormal or negligible cortisol response to ACTH.

Endogenous plasma ACTH concentration: Used to differentiate primary from secondary hypoadrenocorticism. Dogs with primary hypoadrenocorticism have a markedly elevated ACTH concentration (owing to a lack of negative feedback of cortisol), whereas those with secondary hypoadrenocorticism have low or undetectable concentrations of ACTH.

Medical Therapy

Acute primary hypoadrenocorticism: Initial therapy consists of aggressive intravenous fluid therapy using normal saline (0.9% sodium chloride) at an initial rate of 60 to 80 ml/kg/hour for 1 to 2 hours. Urine output and, if possible, central venous pressure should be monitored. This therapy will correct the hypovolemia and hyponatremia. The serum potassium concentration decreases owing to dilution and improved renal perfusion, and specific therapy for hypokalemia is usually not required. Other therapies for hyperkalemia include intravenous glucose administration (addition of 5% dextrose to intravenous fluids), which can be combined with insulin therapy and intravenous calcium administration.

Intravenous glucocorticoid therapy (hydrocortisone sodium succinate, prednisolone sodium succinate, or dexamethasone sodium phosphate) is initiated early during treatment of acute hypoadrenocorticism. Mineralocorticoid therapy is not essential for the management of an Addisonian crisis, but administration of a mineralocorticoid is usually initiated.

Chronic primary hypoadrenocorticism: During maintenance therapy, a mineralocorticoid is administered. Fludrocortisone acetate (15 mg/kg PO once daily, adjusting the dose to keep the serum sodium and potassium concentrations within the reference ranges) has mainly mineralocorticoid effects, although it retains some glucocorticoid activity. Desoxycorticosterone pivalate (DOCP; 2.2 mg/kg IM or SQ every 25 days) has no glucocorticoid activity and should be combined with a low dose of prednisone or prednisolone (0.1-0.2 mg/kg/day).

Prognosis

The long-term prognosis for the management of hypoadrenocorticism is excellent with appropriate maintenance therapy. Animals should receive supplemental doses of glucocorticoids during periods of stress, such as when undergoing anesthesia and surgery.

Adrenal Medulla

Physiology

The adrenal medulla is essentially a large sympathetic ganglion that lacks postganglionic fibers. Catecholamines are the primary secretory product of chromaffin cells. Catecholamines are synthesized from the amino acid tyrosine. The first step in catecholamine synthesis, the conversion of L-tyrosine to L-DOPA, involves the enzyme tyrosine hydroxylase, and is the rate-limiting step. Secretory products are stored in cytoplasmic vesicles in the chromaffin cells. Stimulation of the chromaffin cell results in exocytosis of the vesicles and expulsion of their contents. The end product of catecholamine synthesis is predominately epinephrine in humans and dogs, and norepinephrine in cats. The half-life of catecholamines in the circulation is short (minutes). Catecholamine catabolism is mediated by two enzymes, catecholamine-O-methyltransferase (COMT) and monoamine oxidase (MAO). The predominant metabolite is vanillylmandelic acid (VMA), which, along with the catecholamines, is excreted in the urine.

Pheochromocytoma

Pheochromocytoma is a catecholamine-producing tumor derived from the chromaffin cells of the adrenal medulla. Neoplastic transformation of the chromaffin cells results in loss of regulatory control of catecholamine release. In the fetus, chromaffin cells are widely distributed and form paraganglia. Most extra-adrenal chromaffin cells involute after birth, although remnants remain, and tumors of the extra-adrenal chromaffin cells, paraganglionomas, are reported. A substantial portion of dogs with a pheochromocytoma also have another malignancy. Pheochromocytomas can occur in human patients with multiple endocrine neoplasia type 2 (MEN2) syndrome, and a similar syndrome has been reported in dogs.

History and Physical Examination Findings

Clinical signs are often vague and episodic. Clinical signs may relate to either excessive circulating catecholamine concentrations or the presence of an abdominal mass. The most common signs in dogs are weakness and collapse. Signs related to catecholamine excess include tachycardia and arrhythmias, panting, anxiety, pacing, seizures, blindness (from retinal hemorrhage), polyuria and polydipsia, vomiting, diarrhea, and anorexia. Signs related to the adrenal mass include hemoabdomen (associated with tumor rupture) and Budd-Chiari syndrome (owing to obstruction of the caudal vena cava producing ascites and hind limb edema and weakness). In some dogs, the pheochromocytoma is diagnosed as an incidental finding, for instance during performance of abdominal ultrasonography for an unrelated reason.

Clinicopathologic Findings

CBC and biochemistry panel: Findings are nonspecific.

Urinalysis: Proteinuria owing to hypertensive glomerulopathy may be present, as well as hyposethenuria or isothenuria.

Catecholamine concentrations: The measurement of basal plasma catecholamine concentrations and the urine concentrations of catecholamines and catecholamine metabolites is not routinely performed in veterinary medicine.

Arterial Blood Pressure Determination

Catecholamine secretion and systemic hypertension tend to be episodic in patients with a pheochromocytoma.

Diagnostic Imaging

Abdominal ultrasonography: Pheochromocytomas appear as adrenal gland mass lesions with variable echogenicity. The patient should also be assessed for the presence of intraabdominal metastases and vascular invasion.

CT or MRI: Abdominal imaging may provide additional information on adrenal anatomy, intraabdominal metastases, and vascular invasion.

Treatment

Adrenalectomy is the treatment of choice. Patients with a pheochromocytoma are a challenge to anesthetize. Dogs in which a pheochromocytoma is suspected are placed on phenoxybenzamine at least 2 weeks prior to surgery. Phenoxybenzamine is an α-adrenergic blocking drug with a long duration of action. It is considered the drug of choice for preoperative management of hypertension as it binds noncompetitively with the receptor, and thus, surges of catecholamine release cannot override the inhibition. A relatively high dose of phenoxybenzamine is recommended (up to 2.5 mg/kg b.i.d. PO). Management of hypertension prior to surgery allows reexpansion of the intravascular plasma volume by removing the vasoconstrictive effects of high catecholamine concentrations. Intraoperative hypertension is managed by intravenous administration of phentolamine, a short-acting, competitive α-adrenergic blocking drug (loading dose 0.1 mg/kg; CRI 1-2 μg/kg/min). Intraoperative hypotension is managed by decreasing the dose of or discontinuing phentolamine; administration of phenylephrine; or rapid expansion of the vascular volume by administration of crystalloid fluid, plasma volume expanders, or blood products. Phenylephrine is a short-acting α_1-adrenergic agonist that can displace phentolamine from the receptor. Esmolol, a short-acting β_1-adrenergic blocking drug, is administered intravenously (loading dose 0.1 mg/kg; CRI 50-70 μg/kg/min) in those cases with persistent tachycardia despite adequate α-adrenergic blockade and vascular volume expansion. Medications that stimulate catecholamine release should be avoided, including ketamine, morphine, and halothane. Moderate surface-induced hypothermia (esophageal temperature of 32° C) is recommended in case temporary caval occlusion is required.

References

1. Reusch CE, Feldman EC: Canine hyperadrenocorticism due to adrenocortical neoplasia. J Vet Intern Med 5:3, 1991.

2. Forrester SD, Troy GC, Dalton MN, et al: Retrospective evaluation of urinary tract infection in 42 dogs with hyperadrenocorticism or diabetes mellitus or both. J Vet Intern Med 13:557, 1999.

3. Behrend EN, Kemppainen RJ: Diagnosis of canine hyperadrenocorticism. *In* The Veterinary Clinics of North America, Small Animal Practice-Endocrinology. Behrend EN, Kemppainen RJ (eds). Philadelphia, WB Saunders, 2001, p. 985.

4. Kyles AE, Feldman EC, DeCock HEV, et al: Surgical management of adrenal gland tumors with and without associated tumor thrombi in dogs: 40 cases (1994-2001). J Am Vet Med Assoc 223: 654-662, 2003

5. van Sluijs FJ, Sjollema BE, Voorhout G, et al: Results of adrenalectomy in 36 dogs with hyperadrenocorticism caused by adreno-cortical tumour. Vet Q 17:113, 1995.

6. Meij BP, Voorhout G, van der Ingh TS, et al: Results of transsphenoidal hypophysectomy in 52 dogs with pituitary-dependent hyperadrenocorticism. Vet Surg 27:246, 1998.

7. Hanson JM, van'tHoofd MM, Voorhout G, et al: Efficacy of transsphenoidal hypophysectomy in treatment of dogs with pituitary-dependent hyperadrenocorticism. J Vet Intern Med 19:687, 2005.

8. Peterson ME, Kintzer PP, Kass PH: Pretreatment clinical and laboratory findings in dogs with hypoadrenocorticism: 225 cases (1979-1993). J Am Vet Med Assoc 208:85, 1996.

Part XII

Hematopoietic System

Chapter 83

Spleen

Brigitte A. Brisson

Anatomy and Function

The spleen lies along the left body wall within the superficial leaf of the greater omentum and is attached to the greater curvature of the stomach by the omentum, more specifically, the gastrosplenic ligament.[1] Although its shape, size, and position vary with species and breed as well as other factors such as drugs or pathologic conditions, the spleen is typically oblong and red-blue. Blood enters the spleen from the splenic artery, a branch of the celiac artery, and leaves through the splenic vein, which empties into the gastrosplenic vein and eventually into the portal vein.[1] Splenosis or accessory splenic nodules are commonly found within the omentum of small animals and likely represent small revascularized fragments of spleen that occur secondary to trauma.[1-4] Single nodules of ectopic splenic tissue embedded along the surface of the pancreas are described in cats but are not attributed to trauma.[4] Siderotic or siderofibrotic plaques are slightly raised, yellow to grey, irregularly sized deposits of calcium and iron that are commonly found along the margin of the splenic capsule of older dogs.[5] These plaques are thought to develop secondary to splenic trauma.[6,7] The spleen of dogs and cats is often visible radiographically. On the ventrodorsal view, the head of the spleen sits laterally on the left side and is often visualized as a triangular soft-tissue density just caudal to the gastric fundus and cranial to the left kidney. On a lateral radiographic projection, the tail of the spleen can be identified along the ventral body wall just caudal to the liver.

The spleen is composed of a capsule rich in elastic and smooth muscle fibers, a network of fibromuscular trabeculae, and the parenchyma, which is located between the capsule and trabeculae and consists of red and white splenic pulp.[1] The white pulp contains diffuse and nodular lymphoreticular tissue and the red pulp is primarily made of venous sinuses and cords of reticular cells.[1] Whereas the canine spleen is considered sinusoidal, the feline spleen has a poorly developed sinusoid system and is often referred to as nonsinusoidal. As whole blood filters through the trabecular meshwork of the spleen, plasma is skimmed off into the white pulp while red blood cells move toward the red pulp.[8] In dogs, a small portion of the blood that enters the spleen is delivered directly into the venous sinuses of the red pulp, bypassing the splenic cords and travelling rapidly through the spleen; this is known as a closed circulation. A larger portion of the blood that enters the spleen empties into the red pulp and circulates slowly through the fine trabecular meshwork of the splenic cords; this is known as the open circulation. Within the cords, red blood cells distort themselves to squeeze through small pores between the reticuloendothelial cells lining the sinus walls to be released into the venous circulation. This process slows the flow of red blood cells through the spleen and results in increased blood viscosity, low blood pH, and decreased blood concentrations of glucose and oxygen. These conditions cause increased mechanical and metabolic stress to older or damaged red blood cells. During their slow passage through the red pulp of the spleen, abnormal red blood cells, therefore, are culled or pitted as required and bacteria or unwanted debris are phagocytosed by the macrophages that line the trabeculae and venous sinuses.

Physiology – Normal Splenic Functions

Red Blood Cell Storage

The slow passage of red blood cells from the splenic cords to the splenic sinuses essentially traps red blood cells within the trabeculae and makes the red pulp of the spleen a reservoir for red cells. It has been shown that 10 to 20% of a dog's red blood cells may be sequestered in the spleen at any one time.[9] Smooth muscle fibers of the spleen contract in response to endogenous or exogenous catecholamines in order to rapidly release the stored red blood cells into the general circulation.[9] In fact, blood loss equal to 40% of the circulatory volume is fatal in splenectomized dogs.[10] In addition, approximately 30% of circulating platelets can be found within the normal spleen at any given time.[9,11]

Hematopoiesis

Although the spleen actively participates in red blood cell production during fetal development, hematopoeisis within the spleen stops at birth when the bone marrow takes over this task almost exclusively. In times of high demand, when the bone marrow is unable to produce enough red blood cells, foci of extramedullary hematopoiesis can develop within the spleen.[11,12] These foci are thought to be derived from pluripotent hematopoeitic stem cells present within the spleen. Extramedullary hematopoeisis is a comon cytologic and histologic diagnosis in dogs and cats.[3,13]

Red Blood Cell Maturation

Reticulocytes released into circulation by the bone marrow become trapped within the spleen where they spend a few days in order to complete their maturation. While in the spleen, remaining intracellular material and excessive cell membrane are removed. By this process, immature cells entering the spleen leave as mature, biconcave cells.[8]

Removal of Abnormal or Senescent Red Blood Cells

Red blood cells live approximatly 4 months, after which time they are no longer pliable enough to squeeze through the pores of the splenic sinuses. Older red blood cells either rupture as they attempt to pass through sinus pores or they simply become trapped within the spleen and are removed by the reticuloendothelial system; this is also known as culling.[8] During phagocytosis, the iron present in the red cells is recycled and released into circulation as plasma transferrin to be used by the bone marrow to produce new erythrocytes, or it is retained in the spleen and stored by the phagocyte as ferritin and hemosiderin.[14] Whereas normal red blood cells deform to pass through the fenestrations in the splenic sinuses, the passage of more rigid cells containing inclusion bodies is delayed. The increased contact time with the perisinusoidal phagocytic cells allows removal of inclusion bodies such as Heinz bodies and Howell-Jolly bodies; this process is known as pitting.[8]

Immune Function

Because of its architecture and sluggish blood flow, the spleen provides an excellent environment for phagocytosis and immune function. For this reason, the spleen is more effective at removing poorly oopsonized bacteria than is the liver.[11] The pulp of the spleen contains large reticuloendothelial cells that phagocytose circulating debris, microorganisms (bacteria and parasites), and antibody-coated cells. Removal of antibodies that coat the red blood cell surface (pitting) results in the formation of a smaller cell, a spherocyte. Because spherocytes are less pliable, they tend to get trapped within the spleen and are destroyed by phagocytosis.[8] The spleen is also thought to play a role in the complement pathways and in the the production of B and T lymphocytes, plasma cells, and antibodies (especially IgM).[8]

Other Functions

Other reported functions include the production of the tetrapeptide tuftsin, a potent stimulator of neutrophil and macrophage phagocytic activity in man; storage and activation of Factor VIII; regulation of the formation and degradation of angiotensin-converting enzyme; and modulation of plasma norepinephrine levels and/or prostaglandin E_2 activity.[8]

Diseases of the Spleen

Dogs and cats with splenic diseases have clinical signs and hematobiochemical changes that vary considerably depending on the underlying pathology.[15,16] Ventricular tachyarrhythmias are prevalent in dogs with splenic masses, particularly if the mass has ruptured.[17,18] Arrhythmias have also been described in dogs with splenic torsion[19,20] and have been commonly reported during and after splenectomy.[16,20] The mechanism of arrhythmias secondary to splenic disease is not well understood but may result from transient ischemic coronary episodes, shock, reduced cardiac output, acidosis, or toxemia.[20]

A study evaluating hematologic parameters in dogs with malignant and benign splenic lesions revealed that dogs with sarcomas have significantly higher total white blood cell counts compared with dogs with benign disease, and significantly higher neutrophil counts than do dogs with round cell tumors or benign disease.[21] Dogs with round cell tumors have significantly lower platelet counts than do dogs with benign disease and lower monocyte counts than do dogs with sarcomas or benign disease.[21] Although the degree of anemia and presence of schistocytes was not shown to vary with the disease process in one study,[21] another reported that anemia, nucleated red blood cells and abnormal cell morphology were asociated with splenic neoplasia.[22]

Treatment for most splenic disorders (splenic abscess, torsion, neoplasia, and trauma) involves splenectomy. Splenectomy is also indicated when medical management of immune-mediated diseases (immune-mediated hemolytic anemia [IMHA] and immune-mediated thrombocytopenia) has failed and for the detection of occult carriers of Ehrlichia, Babesia, or Hemobartonella in blood donors.[23] The effects of splenectomy are not completely understood but it is generally accepted that the spleen is not essential to life in dogs and cats. Following splenectomy, the functions of the spleen are carried out by the liver, lymph nodes, and bone marrow. However, since the spleen takes over hematopoeisis when the bone marrow is unable to do so, splenectomy is contraindicated in cases of bone marrow hypoplasia.

A study evaluating hematologic and biochemical changes at 3 and 10 days post splenectomy in dogs with splenic disease revealed no consistent changes in RBC, WBC, and platelet counts, or bone marrow samples or biochemical profiles.[16] Although not signicant, thrombocytosis (platelet count greater than 500,000/μl) was reported in 50% of patients 10 days after surgery.[16] Serum iron, transferrin, and IgM concentrations also remained normal after splenectomy.[16] These findings differ slightly from those previously reported for normal dogs, which included significant increases in platelet counts, minimal elevation in WBC count, and reduction in hematocrit, red cell volume, plasma volume, and iron turnover.[24] The exact cause for postsplenectomy thrombocytosis is unknown but it has been reported to resolve after 40 days in normal dogs.[25] Although postsplenectomy sepsis is commonly reported in people,[8,26] and a few cases have been reported in small animals,[9,27] this does not appear to be a common complication. A study reports that approximately 20% of patients undergoing splenectomy developed pyrexia in the postoperative period, but no correlation was found between pyrexia and positive bacterial culture of the splenic tissue.[16]

Because the spleen is no longer present to filter the blood, red blood cell inclusions such as Howell-Jolly bodies are more commonly seen and small animal patients are at higher risk for developing parasitic blood infections.[28,29] Other reported consequences of splenectomy include decreased exercise tolerance and response to shock or hemorrhage.[30,31] Retrospective evaluations of patients undergoing splenectomy for various conditions have identified no complications related to the procedure itself or to asplenism.[15]

Prevalence of Splenic Diseases

Significant discrepancy exists with regard to the incidence of neoplastic versus nonneoplastic splenic lesions in dogs and cats. Some studies report that benign splenic masses such as hematoma and nodular hyperplasia are most commonly diagnosed in dogs undergoing splenectomy,[3,9,15,32] whereas others describe neoplastic lesions, especially hemangiosarcoma as being most common.[22,33,34] Neoplastic splenic pathology, especially mastocytosis, is reported most commonly in cats.[4]

Splenomegaly

Splenomegaly is the term used to describe a uniformly enlarged spleen regardless of the cause. Splenic mass is the terminology used when an asymmetric enlargement of the spleen is noted. Dogs appear to develop splenic masses more commonly than diffuse splenic enlargement, whereas cats most commonly develop diffuse splenomegaly.[3,4,22]

Drug-induced splenomegaly is reported with the administration of phenothiazine barbituates such as acepromazine and ultra-short-acting barbituates such as thiopental.[35] These drugs result in significant pooling of blood within the spleen secondary to smooth muscle relaxation of the splenic capsule.[9] In fact, as much as 5 to 40% of a dog's red blood cells may become sequested in the spleen during anesthesia.[36,37] One study revealed that induction protocols containing thiopental and a combination of ketamine-diazepam caused significant splenic enlargement compared with induction protocols that used propofol.[38] Drug-induced splenomegaly has been shown to last more than 2 hours.[35,38] Other causes of congestive splenomegaly include portal hypertension, right-sided heart failure, and splenic torsion.[30]

Splenic Torsion

Splenic torsion is a rare condition that affects large, deep chested dogs and may occur as a primary entity or secondary to gastric dilation volvulus (GDV).[19,20] Great Danes and German shepherd dogs have been identified as breeds that are predisposed to splenic torsion; males are affected more frequently than females.[19] Although the etiology of spontaneous splenic torsion is uncertain, it has been suggested that the spleen retains a rotated position after spontaneous resolution of a GDV or that repeated gastric dilation stretches the gastrosplenic ligament, making the spleen more prone to torsion.[39,40] Torsion of the splenic vascular pedicle and obstruction of the venous outflow causes blood to accumulate in the sinusoids, eventually leading to thrombosis of splenic vessels. Clinical signs vary, depending on whether the torsion is acute or chronic, and include shock and abdominal pain in acute cases and anorexia, lethargy, vomiting, discolored urine, and polyuria/polydypsia in chronic cases.[19,20] A diagnosis of splenic enlargement is usually made by palpation and radiography.[19,41] Specific radiographic (C-shaped spleen) and ultrasonographic (generalized splenomegaly, hypoechoic pattern consistent with congestion and abnormal flow through the hilar splenic vessels) abnormalities have also been reported.[19,40-42] Splenectomy is the treatment of choice. Most surgeons recommend removal of the spleen without derotating the pedicle to prevent the release of thrombi, endotoxins, and free radicals,[19,20,43] although one report describes an acute case in which the pedicle was derotated in order to salvage the spleen of a racing greyhound.[44] A previous case report described a 180-degree splenic torsion that was initially untwisted but required complete splenectomy four days later owing to complete torsion of the splenic pedicle.[20] Montgomery suggested that splenopexy should be performed if the surgeon elects to preserve the spleen but a technique was not described.[45] Gastropexy is recommended following splenectomy for splenic torsion, to decrease the risk of gastric torsion in the future.[19,46] Although the prognosis is not always good, one study reported 100% survival in 19 cases of splenic torsion.[19]

Splenic Hyperplasia

Splenic hyperplasia represents a more physiologic form of diffuse splenic enlargement that typically remains asymptomatic. Hyperplasia can occur owing to immune stimulation, secondary to infection or septicemia (splenitis), or with splenic hyperactivity related to the active removal of abnormal red blood cells in patients with IMHA or blood parasites. Passive congestion secondary to portal hypertension caused by hepatic disease or right-sided heart failure are other potential causes. Nodular hyperplasia is common in older dogs and is characterized by single or multiple subcapsular nodules of various size. Nodular hyperplasia is of no clinical significance but must be differentiated from other less benign splenic masses.

Splenic Hematoma

Splenic hematoma can develop secondary to an underlying splenic pathology such as neoplasia, secondary to trauma, or as a spontaneous lesion.[5,34,47] An association has been made between splenic hematomas and nodular hyperplasia in the dog. Nodular hyperplasia results in distortion of the marginal splenic blood flow, causing an accumulation of blood within and around the hyperplastic nodules leading to the formation of a hematoma.[3] Splenic hematomas can present as multiple smaller masses or as a single mass that might be as large as 20 cm in diameter.[33] Splenic hematomas cannot be grossly differentiated from hemangiosarcomas but are often larger, firmer, and more organized than hemangiosarcoma lesions.[3] Splenic hematoma is treated by splenectomy and appears to have a good prognosis, with one study reporting that all dogs died of unrelated disease at a median of 14 months postsplenectomy.[47] A more recent study reported 83% and 64% survival rates at 2 and 12 months, respectively.[32]

Splenic Neoplasia

Infiltrative neoplastic diseases such as lymphoma, histiocytosis, and mastocytosis are common causes of splenomegaly.[48,49] Malignant histiocytosis is most commonly reported in Bernese Mountain dogs.[49] Mast cell neoplasia is most frequent in cats and represents the number one splenic condition diagnosed in this species.[4] Hemangioma and its malignant counterpart hemangiosarcoma (HSA) are tumours of endothelial origin that occur commonly in dogs and less commonly in cats.[3,4] Hemangiosarcoma has been reported by some as the most common splenic mass diagnosed in dogs,[22,33,34] but others have reported higher rates for benign lesions such as hemangioma, hematoma, and nodular hyperplasia.[3,9,15,32] Other neoplastic disorders such as leiomyoma, leiomyosarcoma, fibrosarcoma, lipoma, and liposarcoma as well as other sarcomas are associated with asymmetric splenic enlargement, resulting in a mass effect but these occur less frequently.[33,34,50,51]

Hemangiosarcoma has been described as the most common splenic tumor in dogs.[3,15,33,34] The heart, skin, and liver are other common sites of primary HSA.[52,53] Male, large breed dogs, particularly German shepherd dogs, Labrador and golden retrievers are predisposed to HSA.[3,15,22,34,52] Splenic HSA can present as single or multiple masses of variable diameter; these masses can rupture and develop omental attachments.[33] Gross distinction between HSA and splenic hematoma is not possible, although splenic HSA tends to be multifocal with nodules that are individually smaller and more cavitated than those seen in cases of hematoma.[3] Metastasis to the liver is most common, followed by the omentum and mesentery;[33,52,53] more than 50% of patients have metastatic lesions at the time of diagnosis.[52] Other commonly reported sites of metastasis include the kidney, regional lymph nodes, heart, and lungs.[33,52,53] When metastasis is not present, splenectomy is the treatment of choice. Lesions of nodular hyperplasia within the liver can easily be confused with metastasis; as such, hepatic nodules should be biopsied to confirm the diagnosis.[54] Partial splenectomy is not recommended even in cases where a localized mass is present.

Histologic differentiation between hematoma, hemangioma, and HSA can be difficult; multiple tissue sections should be examined to reduce the risk of misdiagnosis.[3,55] The interval between diagnosis and death is generally short (3 to 4 months) and does not appear to be affected by the stage of disease (presence or not of visible metastasis).[22,33,52,54] A large retrospective study reported 31% and 7% survival rates at 2 and 12 months, respectively.[32] In this last study, the presence of a single mass was associated with an increased survival rate (16%) at 12 months.[32] Newer chemotherapeutic protocols may hold promise in improving survival.[56]

Splenic Trauma

Splenic trauma is most commonly related to blunt abdominal trauma. Trauma commonly results in rupture of the splenic capsule and parenchyma, leading to abdominal hemorrhage. Iatrogenic trauma to the spleen is also possible during abdominal procedures and laparoscopy. Owing to its highly vascular nature, trauma to the spleen can lead to significant abdominal hemorrhage and possibly death. Surgical intevention may be required in cases where conservative treatment (abdominal pressure bandage, intravenous fluids, and blood transfusions) is not successful at controlling hemorrhage. Surgical treatment should aim to control hemorrhage and, if possible, to save the spleen. Hemostasis may be achieved by suturing the ruptured splenic parenchyma and capsule with mattress sutures and applying an omental patch or a hemostatic sponge such as Surgicel or Gelfoam to control residual oozing.[57-59] As in humans, if splenectomy is required, partial splenectomy is preferred in order to retain some splenic function.[59-60] Autotransplantation of resected splenic tissue in an attempt to maintain some splenic function has been studied in dogs as a model for human trauma patients.[60-62] Techniques described include the implantation of avascular "splenic chips" or slices within a pouch of the greater omentum; conflicting results regarding the success of this technique have been reported.[60-62] Although autogenous splenic transplants have been shown to grow and hypertrophy in dogs, the amount of splenic tissue required for normal function is unknown.

Splenic Abscess

Splenic abscessation is rarely reported but can occur as a single abscess[15,33] or as diffuse microabscesses spread throughout the entire organ.[4,33,34] Abscesses have been described secondary to sepsis (bacteremia) and penetrating foreign bodies.[4,33,63] Single splenic abscesses can be removed by partial[15] or complete splenectomy.[33] Diffuse abscessation is best treated by complete splenectomy.[33,34]

Splenic Thrombosis and Infarction

Splenic infarction is a condition that is most commonly associated with a coagulopathy and splenomegaly as well as other systemic disorders such as cardiac, liver, or renal disease, neoplasia, hyperadrenocorticism, sepsis, and DIC.[3,4,33,42] Splenic infarcts can have a nodular appearance that make them difficult to differentiate from nodular hyperplasia, hematoma, or HSA.[42] Treatment is generally aimed at correcting the primary condition. Splenectomy is reserved for patients with serious splenic complications such as hemoabdomen.[42] Splenic infarction secondary to splenic torsion (with or without GDV) is discussed elsewhere.

References

1. Bezuidenhout AJ: The lymphatic system. *In* Miller's Anatomy of the Dog, 3rd ed. Evans HE (ed). Philadelphia: WB Saunders, 1993, p. 749.

2. Patnaik AK, Lieberman PH, MacEwen EG: Splenosis in a dog. J Small Anim Pract 26:23, 1985.

3. Spangler WL, Culbertson MR: Prevalence, type, and importance of splenic diseases in dogs: 1,480 cases (1985-1989). J Am Vet Med Assoc 209:829, 1992a.

4. Spangler WL, Culbertson MR: Prevalence and type of splenic diseases in cats: 455 cases (1985-1991). J Am Vet Med Assoc 201:773, 1992b.

5. Hottendorf GH, Hirth RS: Lesions of spontaneous subclinical disease in beagle dogs. Vet Pathol 11:240, 1974.

6. Chapman WL: Diseases of lymph nodes and spleen. *In* Textbook of Veterinary Internal Medicine. Ettinger SJ (ed). Philadelphia: WB Saunders, 1975, p. 1671.

7. Ishmael J, McC Howell J: Siderofibrotic nodules of the spleen of the dog. J Small Anim Pract 8:501, 1967.

8. Sills RH: Splenic function: physiology and splenic hypofunction. Crit Rev Oncol Hematol 7:1, 1987.

9. Couto CG, Hammer AS: Diseases of the lymph nodes and the spleen. *In* Textbook of Veterinary Internal Medicine, 4th ed. Ettinger SJ, Feldman EC (eds). Philadelphia: WB Saunders, 1995, p. 1930.

10. Dillon AR, Hankes GH, Nachreiner RF, Redding RW: Experimental hemorrhage in splenectomized and non-splenectomized dogs. Am J Vet Res 41:707, 1980.

11. Pope ER, Rochat MC: Spleen. *In* Bojrab MJ (ed): Disease Mechanisms in Small Animal Surgery. Philadelphia: Lea & Febiger, 1993, p. 616.

12. Robertson JL, Newman SJ: Disorders of the spleen. *In* Schalms' Veterinary Hematology, 5th ed. Feldman BF, Zinkl JG, Jain NC (eds). Philadelphia: Lippincott Williams & Wilkins, 2000, p. 272.

13. O'Keefe DA, Couto G: Fine-needle aspiration of the spleen as an aid in the diagnosis of splenomegaly. J Vet Intern Med 1:102, 1987.

14. Andrews GA, Smith JE: Iron metabolism. *In* Schalms's Veterinary Hematology, 5th ed. Feldman BF, Zinkl JG, Jain NC (eds). Philadelphia: Lippincott Williams & Wilkins, 2000, p. 129.

15. Hosgood G: Splenectomy in the dog: a retrospective study of 31 cases. J Am Anim Hosp Assoc 23:275,1987.

16. Richardson EF, Brown NO: Hematological and biochemical changes and results of aerobic bacteriological culturing in dogs undergoing splenectomy. J Am Anim Hosp Assoc 32:199, 1996.

17. Knapp D, Aronsohn MG, Harpster NK: Cardiac arrhythmias associated with mass lesions of the canine spleen. J Am Anim Hosp Assoc 29:122, 1993.

18. Marino DJ, Matthiesen DT, Fox PR, et al: Ventricular arrhythmias in dogs undergoing splenectomy: a prospective study. Vet Surg 23:101, 1994.

19. Neath PJ, Brockman DJ, Saunders HM: Retrospective analysis of 19 cases of isolated torsion of the splenic pedicle in dogs. J Small Anim Pract 38:387, 1997.

20. Stevenson S, Chew DJ, Kociba GJ: Torsion of the splenic pedicle in the dog: a review. J Am Anim Hosp Assoc 17:239, 1981.

21. Elders R: Haematological parameters in dogs presenting with malignant and benign splenic lesions. Proceedings of the 21st Annual Forum of the American College of Veterinary Internal Medicine, 2003.

22. Johnson KA, Powers BE, Withrow SJ, et al: Predictors of neoplasia and survival after splenectomy. J Vet Intern Med 3:160, 1989.

23. Feldman BF, Handagama P, Lubberink AAME: Splenectomy as adjuctive therapy for immune-mediated thrombocytopenia and hemolytic anemia in the dog. J Am Vet Med Assoc 187:617, 1985.

24. Waldmann TA, Weissman SM, Berlin N: The effect of splenectomy on erythropoiesis in the dog. Blood 15:873, 1959.

25. Mandell CP: Essential thrombocytopenia and reactive thrombocytosis. *In* Schalms' Veterinary Hematology, 5th ed. Feldman BF, Zinkl JG, Jain NC (eds). Philadelphia: Lippincott Williams & Wilkins, 2000, p. 505.

26. Van Wyck DB: Overwhelming postsplenectomy infection (OPSI): the clinical syndrome. Lymphology 16:107, 1983.

27. Withrow SJ: Dental extraction as a probable cause of septicemia in a dog. J Am Anim Hosp Assoc 15:345, 1979.

28. Gaunt SD: Hemolytic anemias caused by blood rickettsial agents and protozoa. *In* Schalms' Veterinary Hematology, 5th ed. Feldman BF, Zinkl JG, Jain NC (eds). Philadelphia: Lippincott Williams & Wilkins, 2000, p. 154

29. Rogers KS: Anemia. *In* Textbook of Veterinary Internal Medicine, 5th ed. Ettinger SJ, Feldman EC (eds). Philadelphia: WB Saunders, 2000, p. 198.

30. Bartels P: Indications for splenectomy and the post-operative survival rate. J Small Anim Pract 10:781, 1970.

31. Crane SW: Spleen. *In* Canine and Feline Surgery. Archibald J, Catcott EJ (eds). Santa Barbara: American Veterinary Publications, 1984, p. 499.

32. Spangler WL, Kass PH: Pathologic factors affecting postsplenectomy survival in dogs. J Vet Intern Med 11:166, 1997.

33. Day MJ, Lucke VM, Pearson H: A review of pathological diagnoses made from 87 canine splenic biopsies. J Small Anim Pract 36:426, 1995.

34. Frey AJ, Betts CW: A retrospective survey of splenectomy in the dog. J Am Anim Hosp Assoc 13:730, 1977.

35. Hausner E, Essex HE, Mann FC: Roentgenologic observations of the spleen of the dog under ether, sodium amytal, pentobarbital sodium and pentothal sodium anesthesia. Am J Physiol 121: 387, 1938.

36. Hahn PE, Bale WF, Bonner JF: Removal of red cells from the active circulation by sodium pentobarbital. Am J Physiol 415:1942, 1938.

37. Merin RG, Hoffman WL, Kraus AL: The role of the canine spleen in cardiovascular homeostasis during halothane anesthesia. Circ Shock 4:241, 1977.

38. Wilson DV, Evans AT, Carpenter RE, Mullineaux DR: The effect of four anesthetic protocols on splenic size in dogs. Vet Anaesth Analg 31:102, 2004.

39. Hurley RE, Stone MS: Isolated torsion of the splenic pedicle in a dog. J Am Anim Hosp Assoc 30:119, 1994.

40. Konde, LJ, Wrigley RH, Lebel JK, et al: Sonographic and radiographic changes associated with splenic torsion in the dog. Vet Radiol 30:41, 1989.

41. Stickle RL: Radiographic signs of isolated splenic torsion in dogs: eight cases (1980-1987). J Am Vet Med Assoc 194:103, 1989.

42. Hardie EM, Vaden SL, Spaulding K, Malarkey DE: Splenic infarction in 16 dogs: a retrospective study. J Vet Intern Med 9:141, 1995.

43. Wright RP, Callahan KE: Surgically treating a case of splenic torsion. Vet Med 82:532, 1987.

44. Goldsmid SE, Davis P, Pechman R: Successful derotation of a splenic torsion in a racing greyhound. J Small Anim Pract 35:112, 1994.

45. Montgomery RD, Henderson RA, Horne RD, et al: Primary splenic torsion in dogs: literature review and report of five cases. Canine Pract 15:17, 1990.

46. Millis DK, Nemzek J, Riggs C, et al: Gastric dilatation-volvulus after splenic torsion in two dogs. J Am Vet Med Assoc 207:314, 1995.

47. Wrigley RH, Konde LJ, Park RD, Lebel JL: Clinical features and diagnosis of splenic hematomas in dogs : 10 cases (1980 to 1987). J Am Anim Hosp Assoc 25:371, 1989.

48. Brooks MB, Matus RE, Leifer CE, Patnaik AK: Use of splenectomy in the management of lymphoma in dogs: 16 cases (1976-1985). J Am Vet Med Assoc 191:1008, 1987.

49. Ramsey IK, McKay JS, Rudorf H, Dobson JM: Malignant histiocytosis in three Bernese mountain dogs. Vet Rec 138:440, 1996.

50. Spangler WL, Culbertson MR, Kass PH: Primary mesenchymal (nonangiomatous/nonlymphomatous) neoplasms occurring in the canine spleen: anatomic classification, immunohistochemistry, and mitotic activity correlated with patient survival. Vet Pathol 31:37, 1994.

51. Weinstein MJ, Carpenter JL, Schunk JM: Nonangiogenic and nonlymphomatous sarcomas of the canine spleen:57 cases (1975-1987). J Am Vet Med Assoc 195:784, 1989.

52. Brown NO, Patnaik AM, MacEwen EG: Canine hemangiosarcoma: retrospective analysis of 104 cases. J Am Vet Med Assoc 186:56, 1985.

53. Waters DJ, Caywood DD, Hayden DW, Klausner JS: Metastatic pattern in dogs with splenic haemangiosarcoma: clinical implications. J Small Anim Pract 29:805,1988.

54. Wood CA, Moore AS, Gilatto JM, et al: Prognosis for dogs with stage I or II splenic hemangiosarcoma treated by splenectomy alone: 32 cases (1991-1993). J Am Anim Hosp Assoc 34:417, 1998.

55. Prymak C, McKee LJ, Goldschmidt MH, Glickman LT: Epidemiologic, clinical, pathologic, and prognostic characteristics of splenic hemangiosarcoma and splenci hematoma in dogs: 217 cases (1985). J Am Vet Med Assoc 193:706, 1988.

56. Clifford CA, Mackin AJ, Henry CJ: Treatment of canine hemangiosarcoma: 2000 and beyond. J Vet Intern Med 14:479, 2000.

57. Buntain WL, Lynn HB: Splenorrhaphy: changing concepts for the traumatized spleen. Surgery 86:784, 1979.

58. Coln D, Horton J, Ogden ME, Buja LM: Evaluation of hemostatic agents in experimental splenic lacerations. Am J Surg 145:256, 1983.

59. Crane SW: Evaluation and management of abdominal trauma in the dog and cat. Vet Clin North Am Small Anim Pract 10:655, 1980.

60. Krasna IH, Thompson DA: Failure of autotransplantation of spleen in dogs: an anatomic, radionuclide imaging, and pathologic study. J Pediatr Surg 20:30, 1985.

61. Szendroi T, Miko I, Hajdu Z, et al.: Splenic autotransplantation after abdominal trauma in childhood, clinical and experimental data. Acta Chir Hung 36:349, 1997.

62. Visagie WJ, van Tonder E, Nell CJ: Autotransplantation of splenic tissue into the omentum: a method of preserving splenic tissue. S Afr J Surg 19:119, 1980.

63. Brisson BA, Bersenas A, Etue SM: Ultrasonographic diagnosis of septic arthritis secondary to porcupine quill migration in a dog. J Am Vet Med Assoc 224:1467-70, 2004.

Chapter 84

Thymus

David Biller
Meredith Esterline

Anatomy

The thymus is a gray to pink bilobed organ found in the precardiac mediastinum.[1] It extends from just cranial to the first rib to the fifth rib in dogs or sixth rib in cats, although the size and shape are highly variable.[2] It is divided into right and left lobes. The left lobe extends more caudally than the right to between the left thoracic wall and left ventricle, but composes only 40% of the weight of the thymus.[1] The larger right lobe is more laterally expanded and extends to the pericardial sac. Dorsally, the thymus is associated with the phrenic nerves, the trachea, and the cranial vena cava. The thymus is derived from the endoderm and ectoderm of the third pharyngeal pouch and the third branchial cleft.[3]

Nine arterial vessels have been identified that comprise the blood supply to the thymus.[4] The left lobe is supplied by several branches. Two branches of the brachiocephalic trunk supply the cranial and caudal poles of the left thymus. The left internal thoracic artery sends a large branch to the caudal pole, has three thymic arterial branches with two going to the cranial pole and one going to the caudal pole, and feeds the pericardiophrenic artery, which sends a thin branch to the cranial pole. The right lobe is supplied by a branch of the right internal thoracic artery, the pericardiophrenic artery, which forms one branch to each pole of the right lobe. Veins of the thymus are associated with the arteries. Four to six lymphatic vessels empty into the cranial mediastinal and sternal lymph nodes.[1] Parasympathetic and sympathetic nerve fibers supply the thymus.[1,2]

The thymus has a capsule of fibrous intralobular septae separating the two lobes. These are difficult to separate cranially, but caudally allow separation into the two distinct lobes. These septae allow passage for vessels, nerves, and lymphatics.[3] The septae end near the corticomedullary junction in a compartment called the perivascular space, where nutrient and waste exchange occurs between the lobules and the blood and lymphatic circulation.[3] B-cells, plasma cells, myeloid cells, eosinophils, and mast cells also accumulate within the perivascular space. The cortex, located peripherally, is made up of a large population of small, immature thymocytes, specialized cortical epithelial cells, and scattered macrophages. The centrally located medulla contains nearly mature and mature T-cells that are closely associated with medullary epithelial cells, dendritic cells, macrophages, and Hassall's corpuscles. Hassall's corpuscles appear onion like, with concentrically organized, highly keratinized epithelial cells. The medulla has a lower cell density than does the cortex. The cortex to medulla ratio is 1:1.[2] The most peripheral part of the thymus is the thin subcapsular zone, which is lined with a thin perivascular epithelium extending along the internal capsule and along the intralobular septae.[3]

Physiology

The thymus is responsible for seeding T-cells against foreign antigens while recognizing the tissues of the body as normal. T-cells begin formation in the bone marrow as common lymphoid precursor (CLP) cells, which may develop into T-cells, B- cells, or natural killer (NK) cells.[5] Some of the CLP cells enter the thymus and become immature thymocytes. These cells go through stages to become immature T- cells, making them positive for T-cell markers like CD4 and CD8.[3] Nurse cells in the cortex are thought to form protective environments for thymocyte differentiation. Each nurse cell is responsible for up to 200 thymoctyes. Positive selection occurs in the cortex, exposing the thymocytes to foreign antigens, resulting in recognition.[5] In the medulla, negative selection occurs, with dendritic cells designed to stimulate apoptosis of the cells with excessive self reactivity.[6] A large number of macrophages are present to help remove the unwanted T-cells. Hassall's corpuscles also contribute to removal of unwanted T cells.[3] Only 5% to 10% of T-cells survive positive and negative selection.[3,5] T-cells remain in the thymus for 4 to 5 days during this process.[6]

The thymus enlarges until the animal is 4 to 5 months of age, and then begins a rapid but never complete involution process.[2] It has been thought that increased adrenal corticosteroids coupled with a decrease in growth hormone may influence the involution process.[7] The thymic tissue is replaced by fat.

Neonatal thymectomy results in a loss of the cell-mediated immune response.[6] The number of circulating lymphocytes decreases dramatically, as do the lymphocytes in T-dependent areas. The number of plasma cells in lymphoid tissues, the amount of serum immunoglobulin, and antibody formation also decrease. Adult thymectomy results in a gradual decrease in the numbers of lymphocytes, suggesting that a reservoir of thymus-derived cells exists and must be exhausted.[6]

Pathophysiology

Although rare, some thymic-related diseases have been reported. In a review of thymic disease processes, 54 of the 66 cases reported in dogs and cats were thymoma or thymic lymphoma.[8]

Thymomas

Thymomas are tumors that originate from the thymic epithelium.[9] In dogs, large breeds and females are overrepresented.[10] In cats, purebreds (especially Siamese) and domestic shorthairs are commonly affected.[11,12] They usually occupy the cranial mediastium but may extend from the neck to the posterior mediastinum.[13] Thymomas are often nodular and encapsulated, causing compression of nearby structures. Cystic thymomas, more common in cats than in dogs, occur with distention and fusion of the perivasulcar space.[14] Variable degrees of lymphocyte infiltration may be present; small or heterogenous lymphocytes are usually found, although large lymphocytes predominate in one third of thymomas.[13] The epithelial cells of a thymoma are usually elongated, but occasionally may be round to oval. Epithelial cells are arranged in solid, trabecular, cribriform, whorled, rosette, or angiocentric patterns.[13] Other cells found within thymomas include mast cells, eosinophils, macrophages, melanocytes, plasma cells, and neutrophils. The results of fine-needle aspiration of thymomas may contain any of these cells, along with large numbers of lymphocytes; the epithelial cells may be present in smaller numbers. Cystic thymomas often yield a nondiagnostic sample.[9] Staining for cytokeratin positively identifies the epithelial cells of a thymoma.[13] The majority of thymomas are benign, with few metastasizing; however, thymomas are better categorized as invasive or noninvasive. Noninvasive thymomas are typically easy to resect. Invasive thymomas are nonresectable, and palliative partial resection can result in high morbidity. Approximately 70% of thymomas are resectable, and no diagnostic test has been proven to be predictive of resection preoperatively.[9] Most presenting clinical signs of thymoma involve the respiratory tract, with the most common presentation in the dog and cat being coughing and dyspnea, respectively.[11,15,16] Other clinical signs are often associated with general ill health and paraneoplastic syndromes.

Paraneoplastic processes are common in conjunction with thymomas. Acquired myasthenia gravis is the most common thymoma-associated paraneoplastic condition, caused by the production of autoantibodies against acetylcholine receptors in muscular tissue, leading to generalized weakness and megaesophagus.[2] The presence of megaesophagus is an important prognostic indicator, because patients with megaesophagus prior to surgery are at a high risk for aspiration pneumonia postoperatively. Isolated reports of resolution of megaesophagus and decline in acetylcholine antibodies after thymectomy exist.[10,17] Polymyositis may be linked to myasthenia gravis as well, with 29% of dogs with myasthenia gravis having polymyositis.[10] The cardiac muscle may also be affected. Autoantibodies to acetylcholine have been proposed to cause myocarditis or to attack the conducting tissue directly, resulting in third-degree atrioventricular heart block.[15,18] Hypercalcemia has been reported, and in one case parathyroid-related protein (PTHrP) was increased. Resection of thymoma caused calcium and PTHrP to return to normal levels.

Cats may present with exfoliative dermatitis characterized by auricular and periauricular reddening progressing to marked exfoliation over the head, neck, trunk, and limbs, with skin ulceration in the axillae and inguinal regions.[19,20] Brown waxy exudate is found in the interdigital region and in the claw beds.[21] Skin histopathology shows an interface dermatitis with CD3+ lymphocytes, mast cells, and plasma cells, and folliculitis.[22] The presence of CD3+ lymphocytes may be related to abnormal immune regulation that could occur with thymic disease. One cat with a thymectomy made a full recovery; other cats included in the study were euthanized. Other non-thymic tumors commonly occur in approximately 10% of human patients, and this is seen in dogs and cats as well.[23]

Prognosis with thymoma is varied, and few retrospective large-scale studies exist. If megaesophagus is not present, an 83% 1 year survival has been reported.[15] In 11 dogs that were treated with chemotherapy and/or radiation therapy, a wide range of survival times has been found, ranging from 61 days to over 1657 days, with a median of 180 days.[12] In a study of 12 cats, half of them survived after surgical excision for a median of 21 months.[11]

Thymic Lymphoma

Thymic lymphoma is the most common thymic disease in the cat. Siamese and feline leukemia-positive cats are overrepresented.[8] It is frequently accompanied by other findings associated with lymphoma, such as enlarged lymph nodes or paraneoplastic hypercalcemia.[9] Chemotherapy for lymphoma is the definitive treatment, and a rapid and complete response is common.[9] If the response is partial or if no response to chemotherapy is seen, thymoma is suspected. Radiation therapy can be used along with induction chemotherapy to improve the likelihood of rapid remission; it can be used if there is a delay in beginning chemotherapy; or if the patient is resistant to chemotherapy.[24]

Thymic Hemorrhage

Fatal thymic hemorrhage usually occurs within 2 years of birth during the involution process.[2] The etiology is uncertain, but several theories have been proposed. The vessels of the thymus are not well supported during involution, and relatively minor trauma to the neck may cause the fragile vessels to rupture.[25] Ingestion of anticoagulant medication may be linked; in a case series of 10 dogs, half of them had consumed rodenticide.[26] Sudden increases in blood pressure owing to excitement have been hypothesized to result in hemorrhage.[27] Epileptiform seizure activity has been linked to thymic hemorrhage and death.[28] There is some debate over whether thymic hemorrhage is considered to be a true pathogenic entity or if it is always secondary to another cause.[25] German shepherds and cocker spaniels may be overrepresented, and two Shetland sheepdog littermates were affected.[27,29] The mediastinum does not contain sufficient tissue for a hematoma to form, so bleeding can go unchecked and spill into the thoracic cavity. The mortality rate with thymic hemorrhage is high, but aggressive medical treatment with fluid support, blood transfusion, and vitamin K therapy if rodenticide toxicity is suspected, or rapid thoracotomy for control of bleeding and thymectomy if medical treatment is unrewarding.[27,30]

Thymic remnants in aberrant locations have also been implicated in thymic hemorrhage. Fatal hemopericardium has been reported secondary to bleeding from a heart base thymic remnant.[28]

Other Thymic Disorders

Premature thymic atrophy can be seen with viral disease (canine distemper, parvovirus, feline leukemia, feline immunodeficieny virus, and panleukopenia), zinc deficiency, and growth hormone deficiency in Weimerainers.[7] The absence of a thymus may be associated with fading puppy syndrome.[31] Thymic hypoplasia is associated with lethal acrodermatitis in bull terriers with zinc deficiency, with a severe reduction of lymphocytes in T-lymphocyte rich areas of lymphoid tissue.[32] Thymic hyperplasia has been reported in cats with laryngeal lymphoma and skin disease.[8] Other neoplastic conditions of the thymus may include carcinoma in conjunction with thymoma, germ cell tumor, and thymolipoma.[2]

References

1. Bezuidenhout AJ: The lymphatic system. *In* Miller's Anatomy of the Dog, 3rd ed. Evan HE (ed). Philadelphia: WB Saunders 1993, pp. 753-755.

2. Bellah JR, Smith AN: The thymus. *In* Textbook of Small Animal Surgery, 3rd ed. Slatter D (ed). Philadelphia: WB Saunders 2003, pp. 1083-1090.

3. Chaplin DD: Lymphoid tissues and organs. *In* Fundamental Immunology, 5th ed. Paul WE (ed). Philadelphia: Lippincott Williams & Wilkins, 2003, pp. 422-428.

4. Yalcin H, Tipirdamaz S: A macroanatomic investigation on the arterial vessels of the canine thymus. Rev Med Vet 153(3):173-175, 2002.

5. Bogen SA: Organs and tissues of the immune system. Immunol Infect Immun Washington, DC: ASM Press 2004, pp. 69-70, 316.

6. Tizard IR: Veterinary Immunology: An Introduction, 7th ed. Philadelphia: WB Saunders, 2004, pp. 61, 80-81, 223.

7. Davenport DJ: The lymphoid system. *In* Veterinary Pediatrics. Hoskins JD (ed). Philadelphia: WB Saunders, 1990, p. 405.

8. Day MJ: Review of thymic pathology in 30 cats and 36 dogs. J Small Anim Pract 38:393-403, 1997.

9. Withrow SJ: Thymoma. *In* Small Animal Clinical Oncology. Withrow SJ, MacEwen EG (eds). Philadelphia: WB Saunders, 2001, pp. 646-651.

10. Klebanow ER: Thymoma and acquired myasthenia gravis in the dog: a case report and review of 13 additional cases. J Am Anim Hosp Assoc 28:63-69, 1992.

11. Gores BR, Berg J, Carpenter JL, Aronsohn MG: Surgical treatment of thymoma in cats: 12 cases (1987-1992). J Am Vet Med Assoc 204(11):1782-1785, 1994.

12. Smith AN, Wright JC, Brawner WR Jr, et al: Radiation therapy in the treatment of canine and feline thymomas: a retrospective study (1985-1999). J Am Anim Hosp Assoc 37:489-496, 2001.

13. Jacobs RM, Messick JB, Valli VE: Tumors of the hemolymphatic system. *In* Tumors in Domestic Animals, 4th ed. Menten DJ (ed). Ames: Iowa State Press, 2002, pp. 165-166.

14. Patnaik AK, Lieberman PH, Erlandson RA, Antonescu C: Feline cystic thymoma: a clinicopathologic, immunohistologic, and electron microscopic study of 14 cases. J Feline Med Surg 5:27-35, 2003.

15. Atwater SW, Powers BE, Park RD, et al: Thymoma in dogs: 23 cases (1980-1991). J Am Vet Med Assoc 205(7):1007-1013, 1994.

16. Carpenter JL, Valentine BA: Squamous cell carcinoma arising in two feline thymomas. Vet Pathol 29:541-543, 1992.

17. Lainesse MFC, Taylor SM, Myers SL, er al: Focal myasthenia gravis as a paraneoplastic syndrome of canine thymoma: improvement following thymectomy. J Am Anim Hosp Assoc 32:111-117, 1996.

18. Hackett TB, Van Pelt DR, Willard MD, et al: Third degree atrioventricular block and acquired myasthenia gravis in four dogs. J Am Vet Med Assoc 206(8):1173-1176, 1995.

19. Forster-van Hijfte MA, Curtis CF, White RN: Resolution of exfoliative dermatitis and Malassezia pachydermatis overgrowth in a cat after surgical thymoma resection. J Small Anim Pract 38(11):451-454, 1997.

20. Smits B, Reid MM: Feline paraneoplastic syndrome associated with thymoma. NZ Vet J 51(5):244-247, 2003.

21. Scott DW, Yager JA, Johnston KM: Exfoliative dermatitis in association with thymoma in three cats. Feline Pract 23(4):8-13, 1995.

22. Rottenberg S, Von Tscharner C, Roosje PJ: Thymoma-associated exfoliative dermatitis in cats. Vet Pathol 41:429-433, 2004.

23. Rosenberg JC: Thymic neoplasms. *In* Cancer, Principles and Practice of Oncology, 4th ed. DeVita VT et al (eds). Philadelphia: JB Lippincott, 1993, p. 763.

24. Meleo KA: The role of radiotherapy in the treatment of lymphoma and thymoma. Vet Clin North Am Small Anim Pract 27(1):115-128, 1997.

25. van der Linde-Sipman JS, van Dijk JE: Hematomas in the thymus in dogs. Vet Pathol 24:59-61, 1987.

26. Liggett AD, Thompson LJ, Frazier KS, et al: Thymic hematoma in juvenile dogs associated with anticoagulant rodenticide toxicity. J Vet Diagn Invest 14(5):416-419, 2002.

27. Coolman BR, Brewer WG, D'Andrea GH, Lenz SD. Severe idiopathic thymic hemorrhage in two littermate dogs. J Am Vet Med Assoc 205(8):1152-1153, 1994.

28. Bradley GA, Tye J, Lozano-Alarcon F, et al: Hemopericardium in a dog due to hemorrhage originating in a heart base thymic remnant. J Vet Diagn Invest 4:211-212, 1992.

29. Klopfer U, Yakobson B, Nobel TA: Spontaneous fatal hemorrhage in the involuting thymus in dogs. J Am Anim Hosp Assoc 21:261-264, 1985.

30. Glaus TM, Rawlings CA, Mahaffey EA, Mahaffey MB: Acute thymic hemorrhage and hemothorax in a dog. J Am Anim Hosp Assoc 29:489-491, 1993.

31. Roth JA: Possible association of thymus dysfunction with fading syndromes in puppies and kittens. Vet Clin North Am Small Anim Pract 17:603, 1987.

32. Jezyk PF, Haskins ME, MacKay-Smith WE, Patterson DF: Lethal acrodermatitis in bull terriers. J Am Vet Med Assoc 188(8):833-839, 1986.

Part XIII

Orthopedic

Chapter 85

Primary Bone Healing

D.J. Griffon

General Aspects

Bone has a breaking strength similar to that of medium steel. Yet it is elastic and relatively light, representing only 10% of body weight.[1] A fracture occurs when a bone is subjected to forces greater than its ultimate failure load, resulting in a loss of continuity. In these instances, the main goal of orthopedic surgeons is to palliate the biomechanical functions of bone until its structural integrity has been regained. Bone assumes other vital functions such as storage of phosphorus and of approximately 99% of the body's calcium.[1] Its medullary cavity is a site of hematopoiesis and, in adults, a storage area for fat. However, the consequences of fractures on these functions are typically negligible compared with their impact on the biomechanical functions of bones. Indeed, structural integrity of the skeleton is essential to maintain locomotion and protection of vital organs. Bone serves as a frame for the origin and insertion of surrounding muscles and allows transmission of loads across the weight-bearing axis. Osteosynthesis was developed to restore these roles and promote early return to function of the patient.

The lack of callus formation between two bone fragments apposed under a rigid plate was first noted by Lane in 1914.[2] Krompecher later reported that a neutral biomechanical environment was required to allow primary angiogenic bone formation in embryonic intact bone. The lack of callus formation as seen on postoperative radiographs of fractures repaired with compression plates was documented by Danis in 1949.[3] He termed this mode of repair "internal welding," referring to direct filling of the fracture site with bone, without formation of mechanically relevant periosteal or endosteal callus. Schenk and Willenegger later confirmed that healing under these conditions occurred by direct osteonal proliferation.[4] Stable interdigitation of bone fragments is clinically achieved by application of rigid, nongliding implants, such as compression bone plates or lag screws. Precise reduction and rigid fixation appear to eliminate the biological signals that are known to attract osteoprogenitor cells from surrounding soft tissues and contribute to callus formation in secondary healing.[5] Even under these conditions, the microenvironment differs within the fracture site and influences the process by which bone is laid. Indeed, full congruency between the fragment ends is never achieved, even after meticulous reposition. Instead, contact and compression are obtained in circumscribed zones (contact points), separated by areas where fragment ends are separated by small gaps.[6]

Primary Healing of a Diaphyseal Fracture or Osteotomy

In the presence of normal blood supply and cell functions, accurate apposition and compression between bone fragments are prerequisites for primary healing. This may be achieved in clinical cases after anatomic reduction of a simple fracture and fixation with a compression plate. However, the application of a bone plate tends to create different biomechanical microenvironments within the fracture site. A compression plate applied across a transverse osteotomy generates high pressure and, therefore, improves contact in the cortex located directly under the plate (Figure 85-1). On the other hand, the far cortex becomes a tension side and is predisposed to gap healing.[7,8] Both gap and contact healing differ from secondary healing by their lack of resorption of the fracture ends, even if a high magnitude of compression is applied across the fracture site.

Contact Healing

Contact healing occurs between apposed cortical surfaces, when the defect between bone ends measures less than 0.01 mm and interfragmentary strain is less than 2%.[9,10] These conditions allow the defect to be filled by primary osteonal reconstruction. Lamellar bone is directly deposited in the normal axial direction of the bone.[8,10] The process is initiated by the formation of cutting cones at the ends of osteons located closest to the fracture site.[11]

Osteoclasts line the spearhead of the cutting cone, while osteoblasts form the rear of the cutting cones, so that bony union and Haversian remodeling occur simultaneously.[7,11] Osteoclasts advance across the fracture site, forming longitudinally oriented resorption cavities.[7] Perivascular osteoblastic precursors accompanying the capillary loops within these cavities differentiate into osteoblasts and produce osteoid.[10] Crossing osteons appeared at osteotomy sites 3 weeks after canine radii had been experimentally transected and stabilized with a plate.[6,7] Based on tetracycline labeling, the daily progress of these cutting cones across the fracture site has been calculated to vary between 70 and100 μm, which is about 3 times the size of each individual osteoclast.[12] Crossing osteons mature by filling with osteonal lamellar bone and become the "spot welds" that unite the two fragments, without formation of periosteal callus. The lamellar bone formed is immediately aligned parallel to the long axis of the bone, with Haversian canals deviating from this axis by less than 10°.[13] However, the newly formed bone is less dense than the intact cortex during the first few months; therefore, the fracture area remains visible on radiographs until complete remodeling, which takes a few months up to a few years, depending on the species.[8]

Gap Healing

A different process of primary bone healing has been observed in experimental defects, and later confirmed to occur across small gaps of rigidly fixed fractures. If interfragmentary deformation remains less than 2%, bone directly forms in gaps measuring less than 800 μm to 1 mm. This "gap healing" differs from the healing in contact areas as bony union and Haversian remodeling become separate sequential steps.[7] The fracture site fills directly by intramembranous bone formation, but the newly formed lamellar bone is oriented perpendicular to the long axis and later undergoes secondary osteonal reconstruction. A vascular loop from the medullary vasculature grows into the gap, and loose connective tissue fills the site.[9] Osteoprogenitor cells accompany the vascular loop and differentiate into osteoblasts. After two weeks, the blood supply is well established and osteoblasts deposit layer upon layer of lamellar bone on each surface of the gap, until the two fragment ends are united.[11] Woven bone may form initially in larger gaps, to subdivide the area into smaller compartments, subsequently filled with lamellar bone.[7] Although the fragment ends are united by lamellar bone, this area remains mechanically weak, as the bone is oriented perpendicular to the long axis and poorly connected to adjacent intact cortex. Haversian remodeling starts between three and eight weeks, when osteoclasts form longitudinally oriented resorption cavities (Figure 85-1).[11] These cutting cones are formed by new osteons within the fracture gap and by osteons originating from the surrounding intact bone. They advance across the fracture plane to unite the new lamellar bone deposited in the gap to each fragment end. The resorption cavities mature into longitudinally oriented lamellar bone, so that with time, the anatomical and mechanical integrity of the cortex is reestablished.

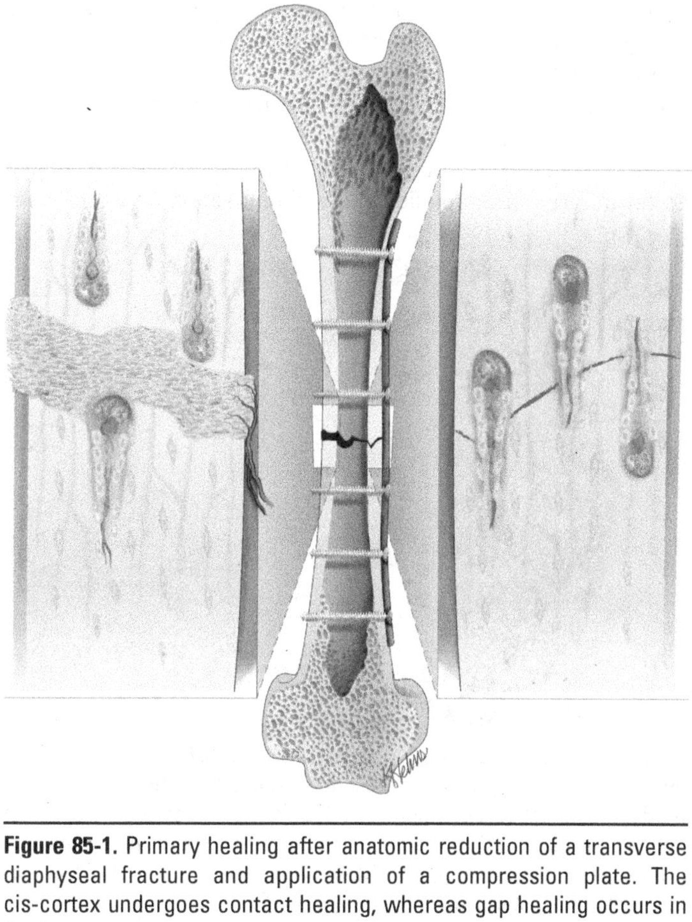

Figure 85-1. Primary healing after anatomic reduction of a transverse diaphyseal fracture and application of a compression plate. The cis-cortex undergoes contact healing, whereas gap healing occurs in the trans-cortex.

Primary Healing of Cancellous Bone

Cancellous bone has a lower volume-to-surface ratio, which makes it 25 to 100 times weaker than cortical bone.[14] In a long bone, this relative weakness is palliated by the greater cross-sectional area of metaphyseal or epiphyseal bone, compared with the diaphysis. This characteristic improves the stability of metaphyseal bone in bending and torsion and increases its tolerance to strain, compared with diaphyseal bone. Indeed, any deformation applied to the bone will be distributed over a larger area in the metaphysis than in the diaphysis. In addition, metaphyseal fractures often result in impaction of cancellous bone, thereby creating a mechanical environment minimizing interfragmentary motion.[15] Cancellous bone may consequently undergo primary healing, with new bone being deposited along the surfaces of the trabeculae.

Healing of cancellous bone has also been described in the context of bone grafting techniques. In dogs, the largest amounts of autogenous bone can be collected from the iliac crest, followed by the proximal humerus and medial proximal tibia.[16] Ribs and proximal femur have been used less commonly as donor sites.[17,18] Metaphyseal cancellous bone is typically harvested via a round hole created through the cortex with a pin or a trephine. The healing of these circular defects has been studied in the proximal tibia of dogs.[19] By two weeks, a hematoma and fibrovascular tissue fill the bone defect. An endosteal callus forms by four weeks, with foci of cartilage and woven bone later replaced with lamellar bone. The normal structural arrangement of lamellar bone and hematopoietic marrow was reestablished in the marrow cavity at 12 weeks. Healing of donor sites was later found to vary somewhat with location, but a second collection can be obtained from the same metaphyseal site 12 weeks after the first harvest.[16,17] Defects in the proximal tibia heal slower than do those located in the humerus and fill with more fibrous tissue.[17]

Primary Healing of Circular Bone Defects

The healing of circular bone defects occurs in a stable environment because the surrounding cortex remains continuous. However, the healing process varies with the diameter of the defect.

The healing of unicortical transverse burr holes has been described as similar to fracture gap healing by Schenk.[6] In this experiment, unicortical 200 μm diameter holes created in the tibia of rabbits initially contained well vascularized granulation tissue. Osteogenic cells in the periosteum and endosteum rapidly proliferated and differentiated, initiating a healing process along the walls of the defect. Osteoblasts subsequently formed a continuous layer and deposited lamellar bone in a concentric manner. This bone was gradually replaced by longitudinally oriented osteons over the next months. Larger holes, up to 1 mm in diameter, are initially filled with a primary scaffold of woven bone. This scaffold consists of randomly oriented trabeculae, creating 200 μm diameter compartments filled with granulation tissue. Osteoblasts form a film over these trabeculae and begin to fill intertrabecular spaces with lamellar bone. Within a month, these compartments have narrowed down to the size of cortical bone vascular channels. Remodeling then proceeds to restore the original microscopic appearance of the cortex within a couple of months. Schenk drew four important conclusions from these observations; 1) small bone defects heal by primary intention, under stable conditions; 2) bone is always deposited on a solid surface, consisting of the wall of the defect or the surfaces of trabeculae within the defect; 3) osteoclasts do not appear within the defect until 3 to 4 weeks, once remodeling is initiated; 4) the absence of osteoclasts within the first week after creation of small circular defects would imply that all signaling factors involved at this stage must influence osteprogenitor cells.

Filling of larger holes, such as screw holes, takes longer and may not be complete. Fibrous tissue is first formed along the surface of the walls (Figure 85-2).[20] Lamellar bone is then deposited into the fibrous network, proceeding from the periphery toward the center of the defect. Although remodeling gradually restores the orientation of the bone, the thickness of the cortex may not be regained. The prolonged radiographic visibility of these defects reflects both their decreased cortical thickness and the presence of less mineralized new bone. Increasing the diameter of the defect eventually reaches a critical point, beyond which the regenerative capacities of the bone are exceeded and the defect persists permanently. The dimension of these critical-size defects vary with the location, species, and other environmental conditions. These defects are especially relevant in the skull and mandible, where they provide nonunion models for evaluation of new agents stimulating bone healing. In the diaphysis of long bones, the size of a bicortical circular defect, such as a screw hole, is essentially limited by its stress-rising effect and potential for iatrogenic fractures. For example, defects measuring 20% of the diameter of the femur decreased the torsional strength of the bone by 34% in sheep.[21]

Evaluation of Bone Healing

Clinical assessment of fracture healing has traditionally been based on physical examination and radiographs. Current research focuses on improving existing imaging techniques and developing new tools for early detection of complications (such as infection and delayed healing) and objective guidance of postoperative fracture management (return to function and implant removal).[22-24] For example, the ultrasonographic appearance of healing has recently been described after biologic fracture fixation of long bones (e.g., external coaptation, external fixators, or interlocking nails) in dogs and cats. Ultrasonographic signs of bony union included a hyperechoic continuous line in three views and disappearance of intramedullary implants. In this clinical study, secondary fracture healing was diagnosed 20 days earlier via ultrasonography than it was radiographically.[25] Correlating these findings with a biomechanical evaluation of the callus would strengthen recommendations for implant destabilization or removal based on early ultrasonographic signs of healing. Indeed, fracture healing should intuitively be evaluated by the return of prefracture stiffness and ultimate strength, because the main goal of fracture management is to restore the structural functions of bone. Ultimate strength and stiffness of the bone defect are commonly measured to quantify healing in experimental fracture models used to study bone repair or evaluate fracture treatment modalities. For example, no refracture nor angulation were diagnosed in an experiment

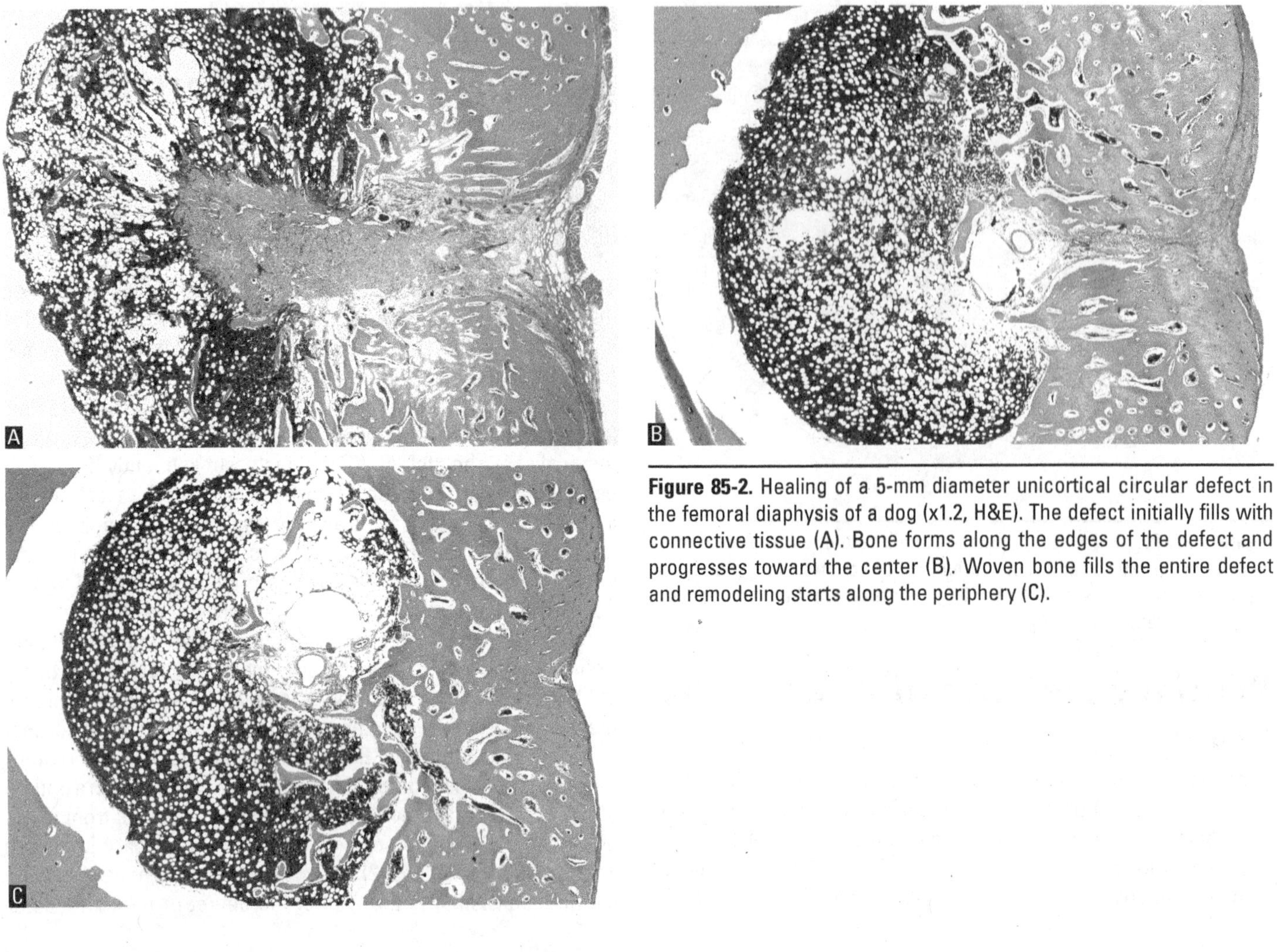

Figure 85-2. Healing of a 5-mm diameter unicortical circular defect in the femoral diaphysis of a dog (x1.2, H&E). The defect initially fills with connective tissue (A). Bone forms along the edges of the defect and progresses toward the center (B). Woven bone fills the entire defect and remodeling starts along the periphery (C).

where an external fixator was removed once the fracture gap had regained a stiffness equal to 10 Nm/degree.[26] Although measurement of fracture stiffness recently allowed early detection of human patients at risk for tibial nonunions, biomechanical testing of clinical cases remains impractical.[27] Instead, clinical assessments of fracture healing are based primarily on radiographic criteria. Experimental evaluation of fracture healing strives for added precision and objectivity, and often includes densitometry and/or histologic techniques.

Radiographic Evaluation

Danis was the first to characterize primary fracture healing based on its radiographic appearance.[3] The gradual disappearance of a fracture line without formation of an external callus defines direct healing on serial radiographs (Figure 85-3). Although no resorption of the fragment ends occurs with contact healing, the progression of cutting cones across the gap decreases the radioopacity of the zone around the fracture.[8,28]

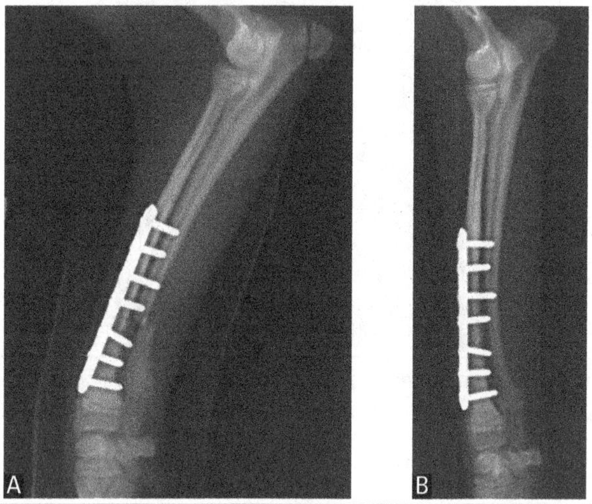

Figure 85-3. Radiographic appearance of primary healing. A. Postoperative lateral radiograph of transverse fractures of the distal diaphysis of the radius and ulna in a 6-month-old dog. The radial fracture has been managed with direct reduction and plate fixation. B. Similar projection obtained 8 weeks later. Cortical apposition and rigid fixation lead to bony union without formation of callus.

Complete remodeling of the fracture varies with the location and species from a few months up to a few years, during which the fracture site remains radiolucent compared with intact cortex.[8] Primary healing displays few radiographic signs compared with secondary bone formation, and the monitoring of fracture healing under these circumstances is indirectly based on the absence of adverse clinical and radiologic signs.[29] Radiographic evidence of callus formation and bone resorption after "rigid" fixation of a fracture is consistent with secondary bone healing. These signs are interpreted as evidence that the stability and/or reduction achieved did not match those intended.

Dual Energy X-Ray Absorptiometry

Dual energy X-ray absorptiometry (DEXA) quantifies the bone mineral content and density of the entire skeleton (whole body analysis) or of a specific region of interest within a bone. The first mode of analysis is most commonly used to diagnose and monitor human osteoporosis. The second mode of analysis has been used experimentally in animals to objectively evaluate healing of bone defects.[30-33] Based on the area of interest selected, the computer software allows analysis of another region of similar dimensions, to act as a control. This control may consist of an area of intact bone or the same region evaluated serially. Because the software measures areas rather than volumes, the thickness of samples should be standardized for meaningful comparison. DEXA can be repeated several times in small animals with no morbidity other than that of routine sedation. This lack of invasiveness makes DEXA especially relevant in longitudinal studies of unicortical bone defects and experimental osteotomies. DEXA measurements have been found to correlate with the torsional properties of healing canine tibial osteotomies.[30] These findings would support the use of DEXA as an objective guide for timing fracture fixation removal, recommendations related to exercise regimen, and prediction of abnormal fracture healing patterns. However, metal implants create artifacts preventing the evaluation of regions in contact with plates. Therefore, osteotomies and fractures suitable for DEXA include those that do not require fixation (single ulnar osteotomy for example) or can be managed by external fixation. In the future, DEXA may also be indicated in veterinary patients for early detection of bone pathology, such as sclerosis (as a marker for elbow dysplasia), neoplasia, and infection. Clinical trials may also support its use, to monitor local bone metabolism and response to therapy in patients with osteomyelitis or neoplasia. In the meantime, clinical applications of DEXA in veterinary medicine remain limited by the lack of indications and equipment cost.

Histology

Histologic evaluation of fracture sites has improved our understanding of the cellular mechanisms involved in primary healing. For example, gap and contact healing are essentially differentiated based on their microscopic appearance. Histology remains especially relevant when testing new therapies, where precise evaluation of the fracture site is required. Studies may focus on potential adjuncts to current fracture treatments, in which case, the agent must be found to accelerate the normal healing process of an uncomplicated fracture or osteotomy model. Experiments focusing on the treatment of fracture complications, such as nonunions, test whether novel agents promote healing of critical defects that would otherwise not fill with new bone. In both instances, histologic evaluation provides valuable information regarding the type and extent of healing occurring within the defect. Biocompatibility of new grafting materials may be determined by the degree of inflammation shortly after implantation in bone defects. However, serial histologic studies are required to evaluate the osteoconductive properties of an agent, its degree of incorporation, its rate of degradation, and cellular mechanisms involved in these processes.[34] Histologic evaluation of bone defect healing may be subjectively scored on 5-μm thick decalcified sections, stained with hematoxylin and eosin.[20,3] However the microscopic appearance of primary bone healing is best evaluated on thin sections of undecalcified bone.[14] These 50- to 80-μm thick sections may be obtained on fresh bone or bone defatted in xylene and embedded in methylmethacrylate.[20,35] Histomorphometric analysis of these sections generates quantitative data that can serve as a basis for objective evaluation of bone healing. Digital images of sections are captured with a digital camera and analyzed with image analysis software to quantify each type of tissue present within the defect. Nomenclature and calculations for bone histomorphometry have previously been standardized by the American Society of Bone and Mineral Research.[13] Four types of histomorphometric data may be directly measured on these images: area, length (such as a perimeter), distance (between points or lines), and number (of cells, for example). These measurements are indices of the amount of tissue examined and can only be compared between subjects when related to a common referent, such as a clearly defined area or perimeter within a section. For example, we have used the total area of standardized cortical defects as a referent to measure the percentage of this area filled with implant, fibrous tissue, and new bone.[20,36] These measurements were then used to compare the degradation rate and osteoproductive properties of bone graft substitutes. Two-dimensional histologic sections actually display profiles of three-dimensional bone defects. Histomorphometric criteria, therefore, may also be reported as three-dimensional terms, as long as consistency is maintained throughout the study. Three-dimensional data commonly derived from measurements of areas on histologic sections include bone volume, osteoid volume, and fibrosis volume. Bone and osteoid surfaces are calculated based on two-dimensional bone and osteoid perimeters, respectively. The fourth type of histomorphometric data, number measurements, can only be reported in two-dimensional analyses, thereby requiring a referent.

The origin of dynamic bone histomorphometry dates back to 1958, when Milch discovered the localization of tetracycline in bone.[37] A few years later, Frost developed the methodology to study the tetracycline-based histology of bone remodeling.[38] Since then, other fluorescent labels such as xylenol orange, calcein blue, and calcein green have been used instead of, or in addition to, tetracycline (Figure 85-4). Combining labels of different fluorescence within the same study facilitates the identification of individual lines and corresponding time of administration. The mineral apposition rate (MAR) is then calculated as the distance between the midpoints, or between corresponding edges of two consecutive labels, divided by the time between the midpoints of the labeling periods.[13] The MARs for resting lamellar bone in mammals range from 0.83 to 2.7 μm/day.[6,39] Histologic techniques based on fluorescent bone labeling have played a key role in improving our understanding of bone biology. These techniques provide crucial insights into the dynamic processes of activation, resorption, and formation (ARF) of the basic multicellular unit (BMU) responsible for the remodeling of cancellous and cortical bone.[40] Dynamic bone histomorphometry has contributed to numerous studies exploring the relationship between bone and various biomechanical or biologic factors. The findings of these studies supported mechanistic theories about the regulation of bone formation and maintenance, eventually leading to the Utah paradigm of bone physiology.[41] Dynamic histomorphometry is now commonly used to evaluate new therapies stimulating bone formation.[36,39] For example, the MAR of woven and lamellar bone nearly doubled during distraction osteogenesis of an experimental osteotomy in goats.[39] We have previously measured MARs in an ovine metaphyseal defect model designed to evaluate the biologic properties of impacted bone graft substitutes.[20] In this study, the MARs measured within circular defects were 50% greater than remodeling rates 4 weeks after surgery, and returned to resting levels by 12 weeks. The values obtained at the center of the defects at 4 weeks were also greater than those obtained at the periphery of the defects at the same time period. Measurements obtained along the edges of these defects appear to reflect a more mature phase of healing, with bone formation proceeding from the periphery toward the center of the defects. While these findings reflect the progression of healing in unicortical bone defects, they also stress the importance of standardizing techniques for histomorphometry. Measurements should be obtained on a representative number of sections and at standardized locations within bone defects to allow meaningful comparison of bone healing between treatment groups.

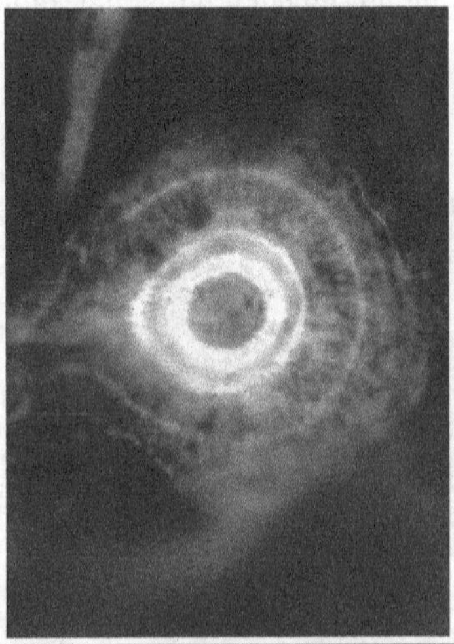

Figure 85-4. Fluorescence labeling for evaluation of bone healing in sheep. Bone labeling consisted of oxytetracycline (30 mg/kg) on days 23 and 35, and alizarin complexone (30 mg/kg) 84 days after creation of a metaphyseal bone defect.[36]

Advantages and Disadvantages of Rigid Internal Fixation

Primary fracture healing skips the intermediate steps of tissue differentiation and resorption of the fragment ends, leading directly, although not necessarily faster, to the final remodeling of Haversian canals. Direct healing is rarely a goal in itself but rather a product of maintained absolute stability.[29] Rigid fixation is one of the concepts laid out by the association for the study of internal fixation or AO (Arbeitsgemeinschaft fur Osteosynthesefragen), in order to promote early return to mobility and function of the fracture patient. In 1958, the AO recognized the advantages of anatomic fracture reduction, stable internal fixation, and preservation of the blood supply. At that time, the treatment of fractures involved mostly immobilization in plaster or by traction, often leading to prolonged healing and loss of function. In comparison, the pursuit of absolute stability, originally proposed for most fractures, immediately restored limb length and joint alignment. Rigid implants palliated the biomechanical function of bones and allowed early mobilization of joints adjacent to the fracture. Although AO principles still stand as fundamentals, their interpretation and clinical application have been adjusted in response to the knowledge emerging from experimental and clinical studies. Anatomic reduction, compression of articular fragments, and rigid immobilization remain golden standards in the management of joint fractures (Table 85-1). Eliminating gaps or steps in the articular surface and preventing callus formation facilitate cartilage healing and minimize postoperative joint disease. However, the emphasis in extraarticular fracture fixation has evolved in recent decades from mechanical to biologic priorities. This change has mainly been prompted by a better understanding of the effects of plating on the underlying bone and the influence of micromotion on closely apposed bone fragments.

Table 85-1. Advantages and Disadvantages of Rigid Internal Fixation

Advantages	Disadvantages
Early return to function	Increased surgical time
Lack of complications associated with callus formation, such as nerve entrapment or obstipation	Trauma to adjacent soft tissues
Simple postoperative care (compared with external fixators)	Contamination of the fracture site
Anatomic reduction of articular fractures minimizes post-operative degenerative joint disease	Slower gain in biomechanical strength compared with callus formation
	Disruption of the blood supply

Traditional plating techniques affect the blood supply of a fractured bone not only by the design and nature of fixation, but also by the soft tissue trauma associated with their placement. The surgical approach, elevation of soft tissues, and manipulation of bone fragments required to achieve anatomic reduction and plate fixation add to the traumatic event initially responsible for the fracture. Rigid immobilization of the plate and bone construct then relies on frictional hold. The extent of this interface and the rigidity of the plate correlate with the degree of osteoporosis of the underlying cortex.[42] This ischemic osteoporosis has been attributed to a blockade of the centrifugal flow of blood.[43] The vascular impairment is believed to be short-lived, with revascularization occurring four weeks after application of a plate and markedly increasing by eight weeks. Other studies failed to correlate bone necrosis of vascular origin with cortical porosis 8 and 24 weeks following plate application to intact canine femurs.[44] In fact, porosis was greater in the inner endosteal layer, away from the bone-plate interface, and in the absence of necrosis. If rigid fixation allows direct formation of bone, stress shielding develops when two components of different elastic moduli form one mechanical system. Adaptational osteopenia has therefore been suggested as another mechanism to explain the osteoporosis of the bone in contact with a plate. Although the structural changes of bone after plate fixation have been well characterized, the relative contribution of decreased cortical perfusion and stress redistribution to these changes remains controversial. The biphasic appearance of these changes is currently attributed to an initial osteonecrosis 8 to 12 weeks after plate fixation, resulting from cortical vascular disturbances, followed by osteopenia at 24 to 36 weeks, secondary to the mechanical environment.[45] These studies support the design of new implants minimizing contact with the fractured bone and/or providing a "less-than-rigid" fixation. The concept of "biologic fracture fixation" or "indirect fracture repair" has consequently gained acceptance among surgeons, affecting primarily the reduction techniques, method of fixation, and postoperative management of extraarticular comminuted fractures of long bones.[46]

References

1. Heppenstall RB: Fracture healing. *In* Fracture Treatment and Healing. Heppenstall RB (ed). Philadelphia: WB Saunders, 1980.

2. Lane WA: The operative treatment of fractures. London: The Medical Publishing Company, 1914.

3. Danis R: Theorie et pratique de l'osteosynthese. Paris: Masson, 1949.

4. Schenk R, Willenegger H: [on the Histological Picture of So-Called Primary Healing of Pressure Osteosynthesis in Experimental Osteotomies in the Dog.]. Experientia, 19:593-595, 1963.

5. O'Sullivan ME, Chao EYS, Kelly PJ: The effect of fixation on fracture healing. J Bone Joint Surg Am 71:306-310, 1989.

6. Schenk RK, Hunziker EB: Histologic and ultrastructural features of fracture healing. *In* Bone Formation and Repair. Brighton C, Friedlander G, Lane J (eds). Rosemont: American Academy of Orthopaedic Surgeons, 1994.

7. Kaderly RE: Primary bone healing. Semin Vet Med Surg (Small Anim) 6(1):21-25, 1991.

8. Rahn BA: Bone healing: histologic and physiologic concepts. *In* Bone in Clinical Orthopedics. Fackelman G (ed). New York: Thieme, 2002.

9. Shapiro F: Cortical bone repair. The relationship of the lacunar-canalicular system and intercellular gap junctions to the repair process. J Bone Joint Surg Am 70(7):1067-1081, 1988.

10. Mann FA, Payne JT: Bone healing. Semin Vet Med Surg (Small Anim), 4(4):312-321, 1989.

11. Hulse D, Hyman B: Fracture biology and biomechanics. *In* Textbook of Small Animal Surgery. Slatter D (ed). Philadelphia: WB Saunders, 1993.

12. Schenk RK: Histology of fracture repair and non-union. AO Bulletin: 19, 1978.

13. Parfitt AM, et al: Bone histomorphometry: standardization of nomenclature, symbols, and units. Report of the ASBMR Histomorphometry Nomenclature Committee. J Bone Miner Res, 2(6):595-610, 1987.

14. Perren SM: Primary bone healing. *In* Disease Mechanisms in Small Animal Surgery. Bojrab MJ (ed). Philadelphia: Lea & Febiger, 1993.

15. Rahn BA: Bone healing: histologic and physiologic concepts. *In* Bone in Clinical Orthopaedics - A study in comparative osteology. Sumner-Smith G (ed).Philadelphia: WB Saunders, 1982.

16. Penwick RC, Mosier DA, Clark D M: Healing of canine autogenous cancellous bone graft donor sites. Vet Surg 20(4):229-234, 1991.

17. Trevor PB, et al: Evaluation of the proximal portion of the femur as an autogenous cancellous bone donor site in dogs. Am J Vet Res 53(9):1599-1603, 1992.

18. Fox AM: Cancellous bone grafting in the dog: an overview (1984). J Am Anim Hosp Assoc 20:840-8, 1984.

19. Johnson KA: Histologic features of the healing of bone graft donor sites in dogs. Am J Vet Res 49(6):885-888, 1988.

20. Griffon DJ, et al: An ovine model to evaluate the biologic properties of impacted morselized bone graft substitutes. J Biomed Mater Res 56(3):444-451, 2001.

21. Edgerton BC, An KN, Morrey BF: Torsional strength reduction due to cortical defects in bone. J Orthop Res 8(6):851-855, 1990.

22. Southwood LL, et al: Evaluation of serum biochemical markers of bone metabolism for early diagnosis of nonunion and infected nonunion fractures in rabbits. Am J Vet Res, 64(6):727-735, 2003.

23. Southwood LL, et al: Use of scintigraphy for assessment of fracture healing and early diagnosis of osteomyelitis following fracture repair in rabbits. Am J Vet Res 64(6):736-45, 2003.

24. Hoesel LM, et al: Biochemical bone markers are useful to monitor fracture repair. Clin Orthop Relat Res 440:226-232, 2005.

25. Risselada M, et al: Ultrasonographic and radiographic assessment of uncomplicated secondary fracture healing of long bones in dogs and cats. Vet Surg 34(2):99-107, 2005.

26. Richardson JB, Kenwright J, Cunningham JL: Fracture stiffness measurement in the assessment and management of tibial fractures. Clin Biomech 7:75-79, 1992.

27. Claes L, et al: Monitoring and healing analysis of 100 tibial shaft fractures. Langenbecks Arch Surg 387(3-4):146-152, 2002.

28. Morgan JP, Leighton RL: Radiographic appearance of fracture healing. *In* Radiology of Small Animal Fracture Management. Morgan J, Leighton R. Philadelphia: WB Saunders, 1995.

29. Perren SM: Evolution of the internal fixation of long bone fractures. The scientific basis of biological internal fixation: choosing a new balance between stability and biology. J Bone Joint Surg Br 84(8):1093-1110, 2002.

30. Markel MD, Chao EY: Noninvasive monitoring techniques for quantitative description of callus mineral content and mechanical properties. Clin Orthop Relat Res (293): 37-45, 1993.

31. Griffon DJ, McLaughlin R, Hoskinson J: Effect of a bone inducing agent derived from a cultured human osteosarcoma cell line after orthotopic and heterotopic implantation in the dog. Vet Comp Orthop Trauma 9:22-28, 1996.

32. Grier SJ, Turner AS, Alvis MR: The use of dual-energy x-ray absorptiometry in animals. Invest Radiol 31(1):50-62, 1996.

33. Ehrart N, et al: Effect of cisplatin on bone transport osteogenesis in dogs. Am J Vet Res 63:703-711, 2002.

34. Griffon DJ: Evaluation of osteoproductive biomaterials. Helsinki: University of Helsinki, PhD Thesis, 2002.

35. Schenk R: [on the Histological Processing of Undecalcified Bone.]. Acta Anat (Basel), 60:3-19, 1965.

36. Pratt JN, et al: Impaction grafting with morsellised allograft and tricalcium phosphate-hydroxyapatite: incorporation within ovine metaphyseal bone defects. Biomaterials 23(16):3309-3317, 2002.

37. Milch RA, Rall DP, Tobie JE: Bone localization of the tetracyclines. J Natl Cancer Inst 19(1):87-93, 1957.

38. Frost HM: Measurement of human bone formation by means of tetracycline labeling. Can J Biochem Physiol 41:331-342, 1969.

39. Welch RD, et al: Histomorphometry of distraction osteogenesis in a caprine tibial lengthening model. J Bone Miner Res 13(1):1-9, 1998.

40. Jee WS: The past, present, and future of bone morphometry: its contribution to an improved understanding of bone biology. J Bone Miner Metab 23 Suppl:1-10, 2005.

41. Frost HM: The Utah paradigm of skeletal physiology: an overview of its insights for bone, cartilage and collagenous tissue organs. J Bone Miner Metab 18(6):305-316, 2000.

42. Field JR: The evolving concept of indirect fracture fixation. *In* Bone in Clinical Orthopedics. Sumner-Smith G, ackelman, GE (eds). New York: Thieme, 2002.

43. Rhinelander FW: The normal microcirculation of diaphyseal cortex and its response to fracture. J Bone Joint Surg Am 50(4):784-800, 1968.

44. Uhthoff HK, Boisvert D, Finnegan M: Cortical porosis under plates: reaction to unloading or to necrosis. J Bone Joint Surg Am 76(A): 1507-1512, 1994.

45. Field JR: Bone plate fixation: its relationship with implant induced osteoporosis. Vet Comp Orthop Trauma 10:88-94, 1997.

46. Aron DN, Palmer RH, Johnson AL: Biologic strategies and a balanced concept for repair of highly comminuted long bone fractures. Comp Cont Educ Pract Vet 17:35-49, 1995.

Chapter 86

Secondary (Indirect) Bone Healing

D.J. Griffon

Whereas primary bone healing proceeds with direct formation of bone across the fracture site, secondary bone healing is characterized by a succession of stages and formation of an intermediate callus prior to bone formation. This process shares similarities with the healing of soft tissues and has arbitrarily been divided into three overlapping phases: inflammation, repair, and remodeling (Figure 86-1).[1] Each of these healing phases has unique histologic features, and each can occur in isolation or in concert with the other to achieve bone union. This passage through intermediate tissues of increasing stiffness and strength gradually restores the mechanical stability required for bone formation. Ultimately, any tissue other than bone persisting within a fracture gap represents incomplete healing.[2]

Secondary healing is the most common type of healing encountered in clinical orthopedics, especially since the principles of biologic fracture fixation have gained popularity in man and small animals. The concept of "biologic osteosynthesis" emphasizes the role of soft tissue integrity in bone healing and "less than rigid" fixation of the fracture.[3] This concept contrasts with the "biomechanical approach" to fracture management, aiming for anatomic reduction and rigid fixation, potentially leading to primary bone healing. Instead, the goals of biologic fracture fixation are to restore the overall length and alignment of the bone while limiting surgical approach and manipulation of fragments. Applied to highly comminuted fractures of long bones, biologic fracture management accelerates healing and return of biomechanical strength, thereby lowering complication rates in man and small animals.[4,5] Once considered a sign of failure, callus formation has become a goal in the management of extraarticular fractures of long bones.

Staged Tissue Repair in Secondary Bone Healing

Inflammatory Phase

An inflammatory phase begins immediately after traumatic disruption of bone and surrounding soft tissues and persists until formation of cartilage or bone is initiated. This stage is essentially characterized by ischemic bone necrosis, hematoma formation, and formation of a fibrin mesh at the fracture line.

Fractures inevitably disrupt medullary vessels leading to hemorrhage. Although contraction and thrombosis of disrupted vessels minimize blood loss, interruption of blood flow leads to hypoxia and necrosis of bone, characterized histologically by the presence of empty lacunae. Radiographically, this resorption of fragment ends may be recognized as a local loss of radioopacity and widening of the fracture gap 5 to 7 days after injury.[6] Bone

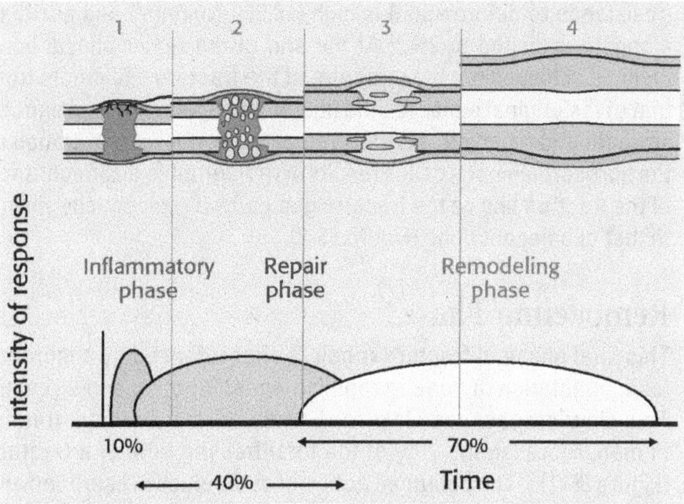

Figure 86-1. Phases of secondary bone healing. Inflammation (1) is the most intense and shortest phase of secondary bone healing. The fracture gap then fills with tissues of increasing stiffness and strength, eventually allowing bone formation. Granulation tissue (2) is replaced by a fibrocartilaginous callus (3) that mineralizes into a hard callus (4). Remodeling is the longest phase of secondary healing, resulting in gradual disappearance of the callus (Reproduced with permission from: Griffon DJ: Fracture healing. In Johnson AL, Houlton JEF, Vannini R (eds). AO Principles of Fracture Management in Small Animals. Davos: AO Publishing, 2005, pp. 72-98).

resorption is primarily mediated via prostaglandins E1 and E2, inflammatory mediators that may also stimulate angiogenesis and proliferation of osteoprogenitor cells.[7] Mononuclear phagocytes delivered by newly formed vessels assist in removal of necrotic bone and aid in construction of the callus. Macrophages are also believed to orchestrate the orderly sequence of wound healing and play a similar role in fracture repair. They contain several growth factors, including fibroblast growth factor (FGF), initiating fibroplasia in soft tissue as well as bone repair.[8-10] Resorption of fragment ends is particularly obvious in spontaneous fracture healing: the fracture gap widens, thereby lowering interfragmentary strain and minimizing the deformation of local tissues.[11]

The lack of mechanical support provided by the fracture hematoma is well established. Its biologic contribution to fracture healing, initially questioned, has gained general acceptance among surgeons. In fact, preservation of the fracture hematoma has become one of the goals of indirect reduction techniques and biologic fracture fixation. The main contribution of the hematoma is the release of growth factors, thereby setting the stage for the repair phase. Transplantation of fracture hematoma has been found to induce endochondral bone formation in ectopic sites, which is consistent with osteoinduction.[12] The hematoma also acts as an osteconductive spacer, providing a scaffold for cells, thereby guiding the size and shape of the callus.[11,13] Local acidity and vascular endothelial growth factor (VEGF) contained in the hematoma encourage vascular ingrowth.[14] The formation of new vessels is also stimulated by mast cells, which are abundant during this phase and release vasoactive substances.[8,15] Within hours, a transient extraosseous blood supply emerges from surrounding soft tissues, revascularizing the hypoxic fracture site.[16] The proliferative vascular response was enhanced by a muscle flap, thereby improving the healing of experimental tibial osteotomies in dogs.[17] This study illustrates the importance of preserving soft tissues around the fracture. Unless infection, excessive motion, or extensive necrosis of the surrounding soft tissues persists at the fracture site, the hematoma is resorbed by the end of the first week.[2] Clinically, the end of the inflammatory stage coincides with a decrease in pain and swelling.

Repair Phase

Granulation Tissue

Within a few days, capillary ingrowth, mononuclear cells, and fibroblasts contribute to the transformation of the hematoma into granulation tissue. This initial stage of the repair phase coincides with a slight gain in mechanical strength because granulation tissue can withstand a tension force up to 0.1 Nm/mm^2.[18] Yet, its tolerance to elongation (up to twice the original length) explains its formation at a stage where interfragmentary deformation remains high.

Connective Tissue

As granulation tissue matures into connective tissue, collagen fibers become more abundant; ultimate tension strength (to 1-60 Nm/mm^2) and resistance to elongation (17% maximum) increase. Types I, II, and III collagen are initially deposited, but as the maturation process continues, type I collagen predominates.[19] This interfragmentary fibrous tissue is organized in a diagonal pattern, optimizing its ablity to elongate.[11]

"Soft Callus"

Mesenchymal cells within the cambium layer of the periosteum, the endosteum, the bone marrow, and adjacent soft tissues start proliferating during the inflammatory phase and differentiate into chondrocytes during the repair phase (Figure 86-1). This proliferation and differentiation are triggered by several growth factors, among which bone morphogenetic proteins (BMPS) and transforming growth factor-β (TGF-β) play major roles. Periosteal stripping in immature animals results in production of a callus away from the bone as osteoprogenitor cells are pulled with the periosteum.[1] In mature patients, the periosteum has a tendency to tear rather than strip; osteoprogenitor cells remain attached to the bone and produce a callus in contact with the fracture site. Interfragmentary strain, local blood supply, and tissue oxygenation also affect the elaboration and size of the cartilaginous callus. Local hypoxia encourages mesenchymal cells to differentiate into chondrocytes rather than osteoblasts.[20-22] Whereas the external callus relies entirely on an extraosseous vascularization, the internal or medullary callus developing from the endosteal cell layer receives its blood supply from medullary arterioles.[22,23] The presence of a fibrocartilage layer within the medullary canal temporarily interrupts the medullary blood flow across the fracture gap. The external callus and the internal callus both constitute the "bridging callus."[24] The full extent of the bridging callus is underestimated on radiographs, because the cartilaginous portion is not visible (Figure 86-2).[6] This partly explains the discrepancy between palpation of a large callus and radiographic visualization of a relatively smaller ossified bridge.

This early "soft callus" formed during the first 3 weeks after injury resists compression but its ultimate tensile strength (4-19 Nm/mm^2) and elongation at rupture (10-12.8%) are similar to those of fibrous tissue.[25] Production of a prominent external callus is a common finding in well vascularized unstable fractures. The resulting enlargement of the cross-sectional diameter in the injured area greatly increases the resistance to bending: the strength efficiency increases by the third power of the distance to the neutral axis of the bone, and the rigidity increases by the fourth power.[26] Increasing proteoglycan concentrations within the fibrocartilage also contribute to the stiffening of the interfragmentary gap.[20]

"Hard Callus"

Callus formation does not become apparent on radiographs until mineralization proceeds. The periosteal component of the callus grows first and appears as a collar around the fracture site. The smaller internal callus forming within the medullary cavity is harder to visualize radiographically owing to superimposition with the external callus.[6] Mineralization of the soft callus proceeds from the fragment ends toward the center of the fracture site and forms a "hard callus," following a process similar to endochondral ossification of growth plates.[11] Mitochondria within chondrocytes first appear to accumulate calcium-containing granules.[27] Under hypoxia and anaerobic metabolism, these intramitochondrial deposits of calcium phosphate are released into the extracellular matrix and become the seeds for growth of apatite microcrystallites. Vascular invasion of fibrocartilage is then coupled with the degradation of nonmineralized matrix compartments by macrophages. Following this resorbing front, blood vessels and osteoprogenitor cells form new trabeculae. Although the mechanical properties of this calcified fibrocartilaginous tissue have not been reported, these structures contribute greatly to the restoration of strength and stiffness within the fracture gap, thus allowing formation of compact bone. The ultimate tensile strength of compact bone is around 130 Nm/mm^2, but its modulus of elasticity (resistance to deformation) is high (10,000 Nm/mm^2) and ability to elongate is limited to 2%.[11] At the end of the repair phase, bone union is achieved but the structure of the fracture site differs from that of the original bone. Yet, the injured bone has regained enough strength and rigidity to allow low-impact exercise.[28] Maturation of the fibrocartilaginous callus results in radiographic disappearance of the fracture line as the fracture gap gains a radioopacity similar to that of adjacent bone (Figure 86-2).

Remodeling Phase

This final phase of fracture repair is characterized by a morphologic adaptation of bone to regain optimal function and strength. This slow process may last for 6 to 9 years after initial trauma in man, representing 70% of the total healing time of a fracture (Figure 86-1).[29] The balanced action of osteoclastic resorption and osteoblastic deposition is governed by Wolff's law and modulated by piezoelectricity, a phenomenon by which electrical polarity is created by pressure exerted in a crystalline environment.[22,30,31] Axial loading of long bones creates an electropositive convex surface, onto which osteoclastic activity predominates. On the opposite, concave, surface electronegativity is associated with increased osteoblastic activity. The external callus becomes more fusiform and gradually disappears (Figure 86-2). Remodeling of the internal callus allows reestablishment of a continuous medullary cavity in the diaphysis of the bone. As medullary blood flow resumes, this extraosseous blood supply subsides.

Influence of the Biomechanical Environment on Bone Healing

If adequate vascularity is a prerequisite for bone healing, the biomechanical environment determines the pattern of repair.[1] Bone formation requires restoration of mechanical stability, which may be achieved by a natural process of healing or by osteosynthesis, with partial or complete stabilization of the fracture fragments. Whereas primary bone formation occurs under

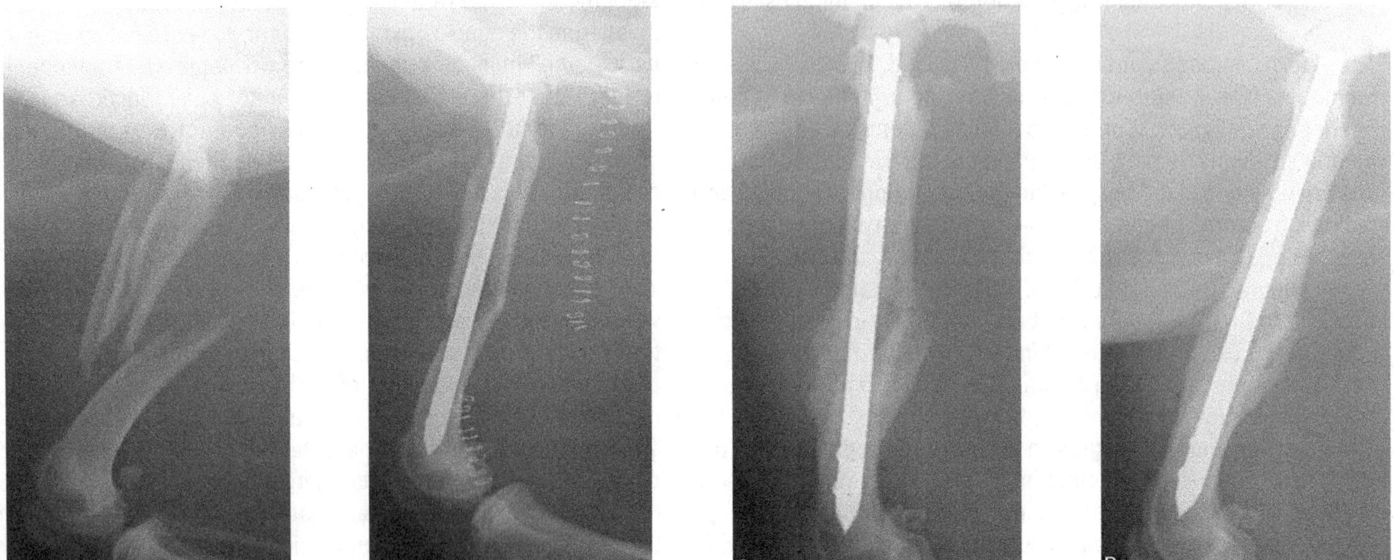

Figure 86-2. Radiographic appearance of secondary bone healing. Open lateral radiograph of the femur of a 10-month-old dog with a comminuted diaphyseal fracture (A). Radiograph obtained immediately after closed placement of an interlocking nail (B). A bridging callus is noted on radiographs obtained 6 weeks later (C). Remodeling of the callus can be appreciated 12 weeks after surgery, as the callus becomes more fusiform (D).

extreme conditions of reduction and immobilization, spontaneous healing represents the opposite end of the spectrum and best illustrates the mechanisms involved in secondary bone healing.

Spontaneous healing of complete fractures typically occurs in the presence of highly unstable fragment ends. Bone repair must develop in spite of high interfragmentary strain, defined as the deformation occurring at the fracture site relative to the size of the gap. However, bone formation can occur only in a stable biomechanical environment with an interfragmentary strain lower than 2%.[32,33] Nature's ways to deal with this unfavorable situation become especially obvious: initial contraction of muscles surrounding the fracture, resorption of fragment ends, orderly repair with tissues suitable for the mechanical environment, and formation of a prominent external callus. Progression from soft to hard callus depends on adequate blood supply and gradual increase in stability at the fracture site. If the fracture gap is well vascularized, uncontrolled interfragmentary motion will stimulate callus formation and the fracture will progress to a cartilaginous callus. However, if this callus is unable to stabilize the fragments, a hypertrophic nonunion and pseudoarthrosis will develop. A stable fracture with an adequate blood supply will allow formation of a mineralized callus; however, initial displacement of bone fragments owing to trauma and muscle contraction frequently results in malunions.

The pattern of healing after external coaptation or semi-rigid internal fixation of fractures is intermediate between the biologic stabilization by a callus formed in spontaneous healing and the callus-free repair obtained after absolute stabilization. Fracture healing after external coaptation resembles spontaneous bone repair except that misalignment of fragments is minimized by closed reduction. Gliding implants such as intramedullary pins and nails typically allow some motion, including axial micromotion during weight bearing and rotational shear between fracture fragments that do not interdigitate. The amount of callus produced after application of external fixators is highly variable, depending on the fracture configuration and the rigidity of the applied frame. Callus formation after plate fixation may occur when the implant is not placed on the tension side of the bone, fracture reduction is not perfect, or when the plate lacks rigidity.[34] These observations led to the concept of biologic fixation, which is especially relevant for comminuted fractures. In these cases, perfect apposition of fragments is unlikely and the surgeon privileges biologic factors over anatomic reduction and mechanical stability.[3,35] The general alignment of the joints is restored but manipulation of fragments and adjacent soft tissues is minimized. A buttress plate or a plate-rod combination is applied across the fracture gap, bridging the entire length of the bone. This "less-than-rigid" surgical fixation is less invasive than traditional plate fixation and results in increased callus production. In one study, the bone density and osteogenesis in comminuted fractures were increased 12 weeks after application of a bridging plate, an intramedullary nail, or an external fixator compared with application of lag screws and compression plate.[5] Similar results have been reported in clinical studies where biologic fixation of comminuted fractures increased callus production and accelerated radiographic union and gain of biomechanical strength, allowing earlier return to function in man and small animals.[36,37] More recently, the concept of "elastic plate osteosynthesis" has been applied to unilateral femoral shaft fractures in 24 immature dogs.[38] Each fracture was treated with a veterinary cuttable plate maintained to the bone with two screws placed as far as possible from the fracture site. Although care should be taken to restore the physiologic degree of femoral torsion, fractures were often bridged with callus by 4 weeks (Figure 86-3).

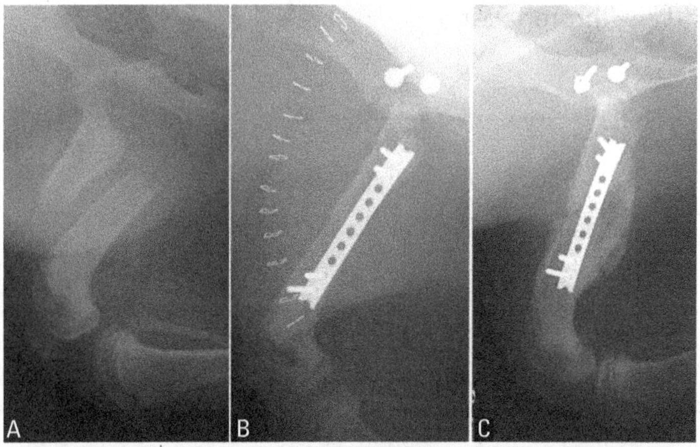

Figure 86-3. A femoral fracture in a 4-month-old dog. Elastic plating (A). A veterinary cuttable plate is maintained to the bone with two screws placed as far as possible from the fracture site (B). Note the amount of callus bridging the fracture 3 weeks after repair (C).

Role of Growth Factors and Inflammatory Mediators

Fracture healing is orchestrated by complex interactions between a cascade of growth factors, local cells, and their environment. Although our understanding of the sequence of growth factors involved in fracture healing has drastically improved over the last 50 years, the list of agents affecting bone formation is still growing. Research efforts currently focus on signals triggering the release of growth factors and defining the role of each factor within the sequential tissue differentiation characterizing secondary bone healing. Conflicting results regarding the roles of osteoinductive agents reflect the influence of numerous factors on their effects, including target cells, dose tested, species, and characteristics of the local environment. For example, the efficacy of osteoinductive preparations was initially questioned in primates, until further studies identified the dose-dependent effect of osteoinduction and the lower sensitivity of higher vertebrates compared with rodents.[39,40] In spite of these challenges, a general knowledge of growth factors is required to understand their impact on fracture management and their clinical applications as promoters of bone formation (Figure 86-4).[9,41]

The body of evidence supporting the role of growth factors in bone metabolism has led to the recognition of the inflammatory phase as an essential step in staging the subsequent phases of bone healing. The fracture hematoma, once considered a potential hindrance to fracture healing, is now preserved as an endogenous source of prostaglandins (PGs), kinins, and other noncollagenous proteins.[42] Platelets are the first source of mitogenic factors at the traumatized site.[43] In addition to coagulation factors, they release platelet-derived growth factor

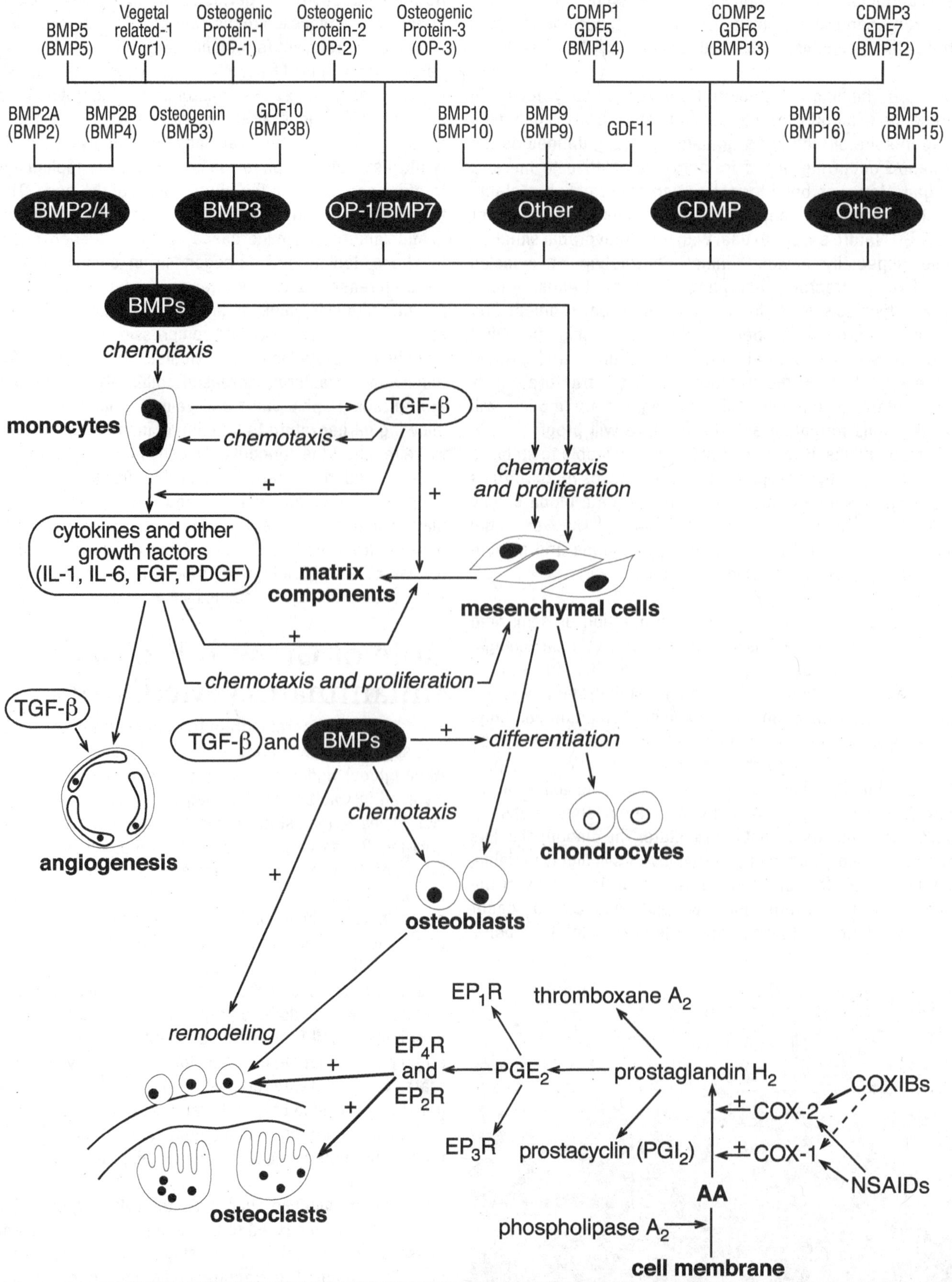

Figure 86-4. Biologic modulation of bone healing: bone morphogenetic proteins (BMPs) and prostaglandins (PGs). BMP: bone morphogenetic protein; TGF-β: transforming growth factor-β; GDF: growth differentiation factor; CDMP: cartilage-derived morphogenetic protein; FGF: fibroblast growth factor; PDGF: platelet-derived growth factor; IL: interleukin; AA: arachidonic acid; COX: cyclooxygenase; NSAIDs: nonsteroidal anti-inflammatory drugs; PGs: prostaglandins; $EP_{1\text{-}4}R$: prostaglandin receptors 1-4.[41,42,52]

(PDGF) and transforming growth factor-β1 (TGF-β1).[9] Although PDGF appears to stimulate osteoblastic proliferation in vitro, its exact role in fracture repair has not been clearly defined.[9] The fibrin seal forming between bone fragments provides a support for migration of inflammatory cells and their byproducts. Macrophages, neutrophils, and mast cells release growth factors (FGF, PDGF, TGFβ, and FGF), promoting angiogenesis and stimulating fibroblasts. The fibroblast growth factors (FGF) are part of a family of nine structurally related polypeptides, among which acidic FGF (FGF-1 or α-FGF) and basic FGF (FGF-2 or β-FGF) are the most abundant. Both factors encourage growth and differentiation of a variety of cells, including epithelial cells, osteoblasts, and chondrocytes. The mitogenic effects of FGF-1 have been associated with proliferation of chondrocytes, while osteoblasts express FGF-2 receptors.[44,45] Inflammatory cells also produce cytokines (interleukins such as IL-1, IL-6, and tumor necrosis factor or TNF), attracting mesenchymal cells to the fracture site (Figure 86-4). Pro-inflammatory stimuli and cytokines promote the formation of prostaglandins (PGs) by osteoblasts and osteoclasts. Among these, PG-E2 is the most abundant PG produced by osteoblasts and the most potent PG stimulating both bone formation and resorption.[42] These effects are mediated via interaction with four receptor subtypes (EP_1R, EP_2R, EP_3R, and EP_4R), especially EP_2R and EP_4R.[42] PGs increase the number and activity of osteoclasts.[46] These cells release proteases that dissolve bone mineral matrix and collagen and remove damaged bone, thereby contributing to bone resorption and release of growth factors contained in the matrix. Other studies have documented increased bone formation and turnover after subcutaneous injection of PGE2 in dogs.[47,48] This activity would result from mitogenic properties on osteoblasts and stimulation of undifferentiated cells to engage in osteogenic differentiation.[42,46] In humans, impact loading has been associated with an increased production of PG.[49] These findings support the theory according to which PGs mediate the physiologic response to mechanical loading.[42] Based on their range of activities, PGs are likely to contribute to all phases of fracture healing, including the remodeling phase of secondary bone healing.

In the repair phase, chemotaxis, proliferation, coordination, and differentiation of stem cells into chondrocytes or osteoblasts are orchestrated by numerous growth factors, among which TGF-β and bone morphogenetic proteins (BMPs) play a major role (Figure 86-4). Both are members of the TGF-β superfamily, a group of dimeric proteins, acting as growth and differentiation factors during embryogenesis and tissue repair in postnatal life. TGF-β1 is released by platelets immediately after a fracture, but the most intense staining occurs during cartilage cell proliferation and endochondral ossification.[50] Although the response to TGF-β varies with dose, species, and biologic environment, this agent stimulates the proliferation of undifferentiated mesenchymal stem cells and induces the expression of BMPs.[9,41] Since Urist discovered the phenomenon of osteoinduction and attributed it to a single protein in 1965, the structure of 16 BMPs has been identified.[51,52] All belong to the TGF-β superfamily, except BMP-1. Among these, BMP-2 through 7 and BMP-9 have been found osteoinductive, meaning that these proteins can provide the primordial signal for mesenchymal stem cells to engage into osteoblastic differentiation.[52] Each BMP exerts its effects by binding to a specific combination of membrane receptors (Type I and II serine threonine sulfate), and activating the intracellular Smad signaling pathway that eventually determines the outcome of the signal.[52] Numerous studies have described the typical sequence of endochondral ossification occurring after ectopic implantation (sites normally devoid of osteoprogenitor cells, such as the subcutaneous tissue) of these agents: recruitment and proliferation of monocytes and mesenchymal stem cells, differentiation into chondrocytes, hypertrophy of chondrocytes, and calcification of the matrix, followed by vascular invasion, osteoblastic differentiation, and bone formation. This sequence ends with remodeling of the new bone, leading to bone marrow formation.[53] This staged differentiation of tissues illustrates the roles of BMPs in natural fracture healing and eventually led to clinical trials of two recombinant proteins, rhBMP-2 and rhBMP-7, in open and nonunion fractures of the tibia in man.[54]

Effects of Nonsteroidal Anti-Inflammatory Drugs on Bone Healing

Much interest has been focused on the management of pain in small animals and its impact on bone healing. Nonsteroidal anti-inflammatory drugs (NSAIDs) are now routinely prescribed as part of the perioperative management of fracture patients for their antipyretic, analgesic, and antiphlogistic properties. Preoperative administration of NSAIDs can minimize peripheral and central sensitization to painful stimuli, thereby improving postoperative analgesia and preventing the development of chronic pain syndromes.[55] They do not cause sedation and appear to decrease the doses of opioids required in the multimodal analgesic approach most commonly used to manage trauma cases in the immediate perioperative phase. Combined, these benefits accelerate postoperative return to function, shorten hospitalization, and reduce associated costs for owners.[56] NSAIDs act essentially at the peripheral and regional levels, but are potent enough to justify their use as sole analgesics for patients discharged from the hospital. Their action relies on the inhibition of cyclooxygenase (COX), a catalyzer for the enzymatic conversion of arachidonic acid liberated from cell membranes into prostaglandins, prostacyclin, and thromboxane (Figure 86-4). This mechanism of action is responsible for the side effects of NSAIDs, including impaired platelet function, renal vasoconstriction, and gastrointestinal ulceration. These limitations have prompted the development of anti-inflammatory agents that inhibit preferentially the cyclooxygenase induced during inflammation (COX-2), while sparing the endogenous isoenzyme (COX-1). COX-2 preferential NSAIDS (coxibs) have a 2- to 100-fold difference in the concentration of drug necessary to inhibit COX-2 versus COX-1 in vitro.[57] These agents have essentially replaced nonselective cyclooxygenase inhibitors in small animal practice. Among these, carprofen has recently been evaluated in dogs undergoing fracture repair.[58] In this prospective study of 26 traumatized dogs, perioperative administration of carprofen did not cause clinically relevant adverse effects on hemostasis or renal function. Nonetheless, the perioperative use of NSAIDs in fracture patients has been tempered by concerns of potential deleterious effects on bone healing. Indeed, NSAIDs may theoretically inhibit bone formation because they interfere with the release of inflammatory mediators, including PGs. COX-2 has been found to be the rate-limiting enzyme in the synthetic pathway of PGs.[46] Any inhibition of COX-2 would be expected to affect the release of PGs and suppress their contribution to bone healing (outlined in the section on growth factors and bone healing). COX-2 expression naturally increases after fracture and suppression of this enzyme results in a relative reduction in osteoblastogenesis.[46] The effects of nonselective NSAIDs, such as indomethacin and aspirin, have been studied extensively, and the majority of experimental in vivo studies report a negative effect on bone healing.[59] Fewer studies have evaluated the effect of COX-1-sparing agents and several report conflicting results. Table 86-1 summarizes the results of selected experimental and all clinical studies published over the last 5 years regarding the effects of COX-2 selective NSAIDs on bone healing.[60-68] Among these, the effects of short-term (10 days) administration of celecoxib (3 and 6 mg/ kg) were compared with a negative control in rats with induced femoral fractures.[64] Celecoxib impaired fracture healing and increased the rate of nonunions (26%, 9/34) compared witih the negative control (0/41). The fracture callus at 8 weeks contained more cartilage in the treated group, decreasing its biomechanical properties. Using the same fracture model, other investigators tested the effects of another COX-2 preferential agent, valdecoxib (5 mg/kg/day) administered for 7 or 21 days after fracture.[63] They found no difference in physical, biomechanical, and histologic evaluations of healing after the shorter course of administration. In contrast, 21 days of treatment impaired healing at 21 days compared with the placebo group, but the difference disappeared by 35 days. The temporal effect of COX-2 selective NSAIDs on bone ingrowth was further evaluated using a bone chamber model in rabbits.[66] In this study, rofecoxib decreased bone production if administered continuously for 6 weeks, but had no adverse effect if administered for 2 weeks, whether early or late after implantation of the chamber in the tibia. The overall evidence derived from animal studies is that a short course of COX-1-sparing NSAIDS may alter the callus forming early in the repair phase but has no long-term effect on fracture healing. However, extrapolation to small animal practice warrants caution because these results were obtained on rodents with drug regimens differing from those applied clinically. Few clinical studies have attempted to address the effect of COX-1-sparing NSAIDs in fracture patients (Table 86-1), with a validity limited by their retrospective nature. Better evidence was recently provided in a prospective, randomized, double-blind study of human patients undergoing spinal arthrodesis.[68] In this study, patients receiving celecoxib 1 hour before induction and every 12 hours for 5 days after surgery had lower pain scores and a similar rate of nonunions at 1 year than did patients in the placebo group. Based on the current literature, no firm evidence-based recommendation can be made regarding the use of NSAIDs in fracture treatment. NSAIDs may theoretically delay bone healing, especially if long courses and/or high doses are prescribed in patients with compromised fracture healing. Even in these patients, the potential delay in bone repair must be weighed against the benefits of NSAIDs outlined earlier. In the future, large, randomized clinical trials of agents commercialized for small animals should be developed to assess their effects on objective signs of healing (bone mineral density, size of callus) as well as patient-oriented measures of outcome (removal of implant, return to unrestricted exercise).

References

1. Griffon DJ: Fracture healing. *In* AO Principles of Fracture Management in Small Animals. Johnson AL, Houlton JEF, Vannini R (eds). Davos: AO Publishing, 2005.

2. Schiller A: Bone and joints. *In* Pathology. Farber RE (ed). Philadelphia: Lippincott, 1988.

3. Aron DN, Palmer RH, Johnson A L: Biologic strategies and a balanced concept for repair of highly comminuted long bone fractures. Comp Cont Educ Pract Vet 17:35-49, 1995.

4. Dudley M, et al: Open reduction and bone plate stabilization, compared with closed reduction and external fixation, for treatment of comminuted tibial fractures: 47 cases (1980-1995) in dogs. J Am Vet Med Assoc 211(8):1008-1012, 1997.

5. Claes L, et al: Fixation technique influences osteogenesis of comminuted fractures. Clin Orthop Relat Res (365):221-229, 1999.

6. Morgan JP, Leighton,RL: Radiographic appearance of fracture healing. *In* Radiology of Small Animal Fracture Management. Morgan J, Leighton R (eds). Philadelphia: WB Saunders, 1995.

7. Millis DL: Bone- and non-bone-derived growth factors and effects on bone healing. Vet Clin North Am Small Anim Pract, 29(5):1221-1246, 1999.

8. Heppenstall RB: Fracture healing. *In* Fracture Treatment and Healing. Heppenstall R (eds). Philadelphia: WB Saunders, 1980.

9. Lieberman JR, Daluiski A, Einhorn TA: The role of growth factors in the repair of bone. Biology and clinical applications. J Bone Joint Surg Am 84-A(6):1032-1044, 2002.

10. Leibovich SJ, Ross R: The role of the macrophage in wound repair. A study with hydrocortisone and antimacrophage serum. Am J Pathol 78(1):71-100, 1975.

11. Rahn BA: Bone healing: histologic and physiologic concepts. *In* Bone in Clinical Orthopedics. Fackelman G (ed). New York: Thieme, 2002.

12. Mizuno K, et al: The osteogenetic potential of fracture haematoma. Subperiosteal and intramuscular transplantation of the haematoma. J Bone Joint Surg Br 72(5):822-829, 1990.

13. Hulse D, Hyman B: Fracture biology and biomechanics. *In* Textbook of Small Animal Surgery. Slatter D (ed). Philadelphia: WB Saunders, 1993.

14. Street J, et al: Is human fracture hematoma inherently angiogenic? Clin Orthop Relat Res (378):224-237, 2000.

15. Marks RM, et al: Mast cell granules cause proliferation of human microvascular endothelial cells. Lab Invest 55(3):289-294, 1986.

16. Wilson JW: Blood supply to developing, mature and healing bone. *In* Bone in Orthopedics. Fackelman GE (ed). New York: Thieme, 2002.

17. Richards RR, Schemitsch EH: Effect of muscle flap coverage on bone blood flow following devascularization of a segment of tibia: an experimental investigation in the dog. J Orthop Res 7(4):550-558, 1989.

18. Perren SM, Boitzy A: Cellular differentiation and bone biomechanics during the consolidation of a fracture. Anat Clin 1:13, 1978.

19. Lane WA: The operative treatment of fractures. London: The Medical Publishing Company, 1914.

20. Schenk RK, Hunziker EB: Histologic and ultrastructural features of fracture healing. *In* Bone Formation and Repair. Brighton C, Friedlander G, Lane J (eds). Rosemont: American Academy of Orthopaedic Surgeons, 1994.

21. Carter DR, et al: Mechanobiology of skeletal regeneration. Clin Orthop Relat Res (355 Suppl):S41-55, 1998.

22. Remedios A: Bone and bone healing. Vet Clin North Am Small Anim Pract 29(5):1029-1044, 1999.

23. Binnington AG: Bone remodeling and transplantation. *In* Canine Orthopedics. Wittick, WG (ed). Philadelphia: WB Saunders, 1990.

Table 86-1. Clinical Studies (2000-2005) and Selected Experimental Studies Evaluating the Effects of COX-2 Preferential NSAIDs on Bone Healing.[59]

Authors	Year	Experimental Animals	Fracture	Drugs	Outcome
Gerstenfeld et al[63]	2004	Rats	Femoral diaphyseal Fx	Valdecoxib, 5 mg/kg/d for 7 or 21 d post fracture, compared to placebo	No effect if Tx limited to 7 d. Tx for 10d affected healing at 21 days but not at 35 d.
Brown et al[62]	2004	Rats	Femoral diaphyseal Fx	Celecoxib 3mg/kg/d starting on d1 and administered for 4,8, or 12 weeks	Increased amount of fibrous tissue in the Fx gap notes at week 4, no effect on mechanical properties and radiographic evaluation at weeks 4,8,12.
Bergenstock et al[64]	2005	Rats	Femoral diaphyseal Fx	Celecoxib, 3 or 6 mg/kg/d for 10d post fracture, compared to placebo	Impaired healing at 18 wks, based on radiographs, mechanical testing and histology. NU in 26% fractures
Goodman et al[66]	2005	Rabbits	Bone chamber, longitudinal study	Control (6 weeks without tx) then Rofecoxib, 12.5 mg/d for first 2 of 6 weeks, wash out, Rofecoxib, 12.5 mg/d for last 2 of 6 weeks, wash out, Rofecoxib, 12.5 mg/d for 6 weeks	Bone ingrowth was affected only if NSAIDs were administered for 6 weeks.
Authors	**Year**	**Clinical Study Design**	**Procedure**	**Drugs**	**Outcome**
Giannoudis et al[61]	2000	Retrospective	ORIF femur	NSAIDs (patient recall)*	OR of NU with NSAID use: 10.74
Bhandari et al[60]	2003	Observational	ORIF tibia	NSAIDs (patient recall)*	No effect of NSAID on healing
Bhattacharyya et al[65]	2005	Retrospective	Humeral shaft	NSAIDs (prescription records)*	Relative risk of nonunion with NSAID use 61-90 days after fracture: 3.9.
Reuben and Ekman[68]	2005	Prospective randomized	Spinal arthrodesis	Celecoxib, 400 mg, 1 dose before surgery, then 200 mg every 12 h for 5 d	No difference between groups
Reuben et al[67]	2005	Retrospective	Spinal arthrodesis	Given for 5 consecutive postoperative days: Celecoxib, 50 mg/d, Ketorolac, 20-110 mg/d, or Ketorolac, 120-240 mg/d	OR of NU with high-dose ketorolac: 8.8 OR of NU with low-dose ketorolac: 3.0 No difference between placebo, celecoxib, rofecoxib

NU: nonunion; OR: odds ratio; Tx: treatment; Fx: fracture; NSAID: nonsteroidal anti-inflammatory drug.

*** Study did not distinguish types of NSAIDs administered, dose, timing, or duration**

24. Rhinelander FW, Wilson JW: Blood supply to developing, mature and healing bone. *In* Bone in Clinical Orthopaedics. Sumner-Smith, G (ed). Philadelphia, WB Saunders, 1982.

25. Mann FA, Payne JT: Bone healing. Semin Vet Med Surg (Small Anim) 4(4):312-321, 1989.

26. Perren SM: Physical and biological aspects of fracture healing with special reference to internal fixation. Clin Orthop Relat Res (138):175-196, 1979.

27. Ketenjian AY, Arsenis C: Morphological and biochemical studies during differentiation and calcification of fracture callus cartilage. Clin Orthop Relat Res (107):266-273, 1975.

28. Frost HM: The biology of fracture healing. An overview for clinicians. Part I. Clin Orthop Relat Res (248):283-293, 1989.

29. Wendeberg B: Mineral metabolism of fractures of the tibia in man studied with external counting of Sr85. Acta Orthop Scand Suppl 52:1-79, 1961.

30. Bassett CAL: Biophysical principles affecting bone structure. *In* Biochemistry and Physiology of Bone. Bourne, GH (ed). New York, Academic Press, 1971.

31. Cruess RL, Dumont J: Basic fracture healing. *In* Textbook of Small Animal Orthopaedics. Newton CD, Nunamaker DM (eds). Philadelphia: Lippincott, 1985.

32. Perren SM, Cordey J: The concept of interfragmentary strain. *In* Current Concepts of Intenal Fixation of Fractures. Uhthoff HK(ed). Berlin: Springer, 1980.

33. Rahn BA: Bone healing: histologic and physiologic concepts. *In* Bone in Clinical Orthopaedics - A Study in Comparative Osteology. Sumner-Smith G (ed). Philadelphia: WB Saunders, 1982.

34. Hutzschenreuter P, Perren SM, Steinemann S: Some effects of rigidity of internal fixation on the healing pattern of osteotomies. Injury 1:77-85, 1980.

35. Perren SM: Evolution of the internal fixation of long bone fractures. The scientific basis of biological internal fixation: choosing a new balance between stability and biology. J Bone Joint Surg Br 84(8):1093-1110, 2002.

36. Heitemeyer U, et al: Severely comminuted femoral shaft fractures: treatment by bridging-plate osteosynthesis. Arch Orthop Trauma Surg 106(5):327-330, 1987.

37. Johnson AL, Smith CW, Schaeffer DJ: Fragment reconstruction and bone plate fixation versus bridging plate fixation for treating highly comminuted femoral fractures in dogs: 35 cases (1987-1997). J Am Vet Med Assoc 213(8):1157-1161, 1998.

38. Cabassu J: Elastic plate osteosynthesis of femoral shaft fractures in young dogs. Vet Comp Orthop Trauma 14:40-45, 2001.

39. Aspenberg P, Lohmander LS, Thorngren KG: Monkey bone matrix induces bone formation in the athymic rat, but not in adult monkeys. J Orthop Res, 9(1):20-25, 1991.

40. Ripamonti U, et al: Initiation of bone regeneration in adult baboons by osteogenin, a bone morphogenetic protein. Matrix 12(5):369-380, 1992.

41. Zachos TA, Bertone AL: Growth factors and their potential therapeutic applications for healing of musculoskeletal and other connective tissues. Am J Vet Res, 66(4):727-738, 2005.

42. Radi ZA, Khan NK: Effects of cyclooxygenase inhibition on bone, tendon, and ligament healing. Inflamm Res 54(9):358-366, 2005.

43. Bolander MV: Regulation of fracture repair and synthesis of matrix macromolecules. *In* Bone Formation and Repair. Brighton CT, Friedlaender GE,. Lane JM (eds). Rosemont: American Academy of Orthopedic Surgeons, 1994.

44. Jingushi S, et al: Acidic fibroblast growth factor (aFGF) injection stimulates cartilage enlargement and inhibits cartilage gene expression in rat fracture healing. J Orthop Res 8(3):364-371, 1990.

45. Canalis E, Centrella M, McCarthy T: Effects of basic fibroblast growth factor on bone formation in vitro. J Clin Invest 81(5):1572-1577, 1988.

46. Raisz LG: Prostaglandins and bone: physiology and pathophysiology. Osteoarthritis Cartilage 7(4):419-21, 1999.

47. High WB: Effects of orally administered prostaglandin E-2 on cortical bone turnover in adult dogs: a histomorphometric study. Bone 8(6):363-373, 1987.

48. Li XJ, et al: Transient effects of subcutaneously administered prostaglandin E2 on cancellous and cortical bone in young adult dogs. Bone 11(5):353-364, 1990.

49. Thorsen K, et al: In situ microdialysis in bone tissue. Stimulation of prostaglandin E2 release by weight-bearing mechanical loading. J Clin Invest 98(11):2446-2449, 1996.

50. Rosier RN, O'Keefe RJ, Hicks DG: The potential role of transforming growth factor beta in fracture healing. Clin Orthop Relat Res (355 Suppl):S294-300, 1998.

51. Urist MR: Bone: formation by autoinduction. Science 150(698):893-899, 1965.

52. Termaat MF, et al: Bone morphogenetic proteins. Development and clinical efficacy in the treatment of fractures and bone defects. J Bone Joint Surg Am 87(6):1367-1378, 2005.

53. Reddi AH: Initiation of fracture repair by bone morphogenetic proteins. Clin Orthop Relat Res (355 Suppl):S66-72, 1998.

54. Friedlaender GE, et al: Osteogenic protein-1 (bone morphogenetic protein-7) in the treatment of tibial nonunions. J Bone Joint Surg Am 83-A Suppl 1(Pt 2):S151-158, 2001.

55. Perkins FM, Kehlet H: Chronic pain as an outcome of surgery. A review of predictive factors. Anesthesiology 93(4):1123-1133, 2000.

56. Crandell DE, Mathews KA, Dyson DH: Effect of meloxicam and carprofen on renal function when administered to healthy dogs prior to anesthesia and painful stimulation. Am J Vet Res 65(10):1384-1390, 2004.

57. Todhunter R, Johnston S: Osteoarthritis. *In* Textbook of Small Animal Surgery. Slatter D (ed). Philadelphia: WB Saunders, 2003.

58. Bergmann HM, Nolte IJ, Kramer S: Effects of preoperative administration of carprofen on renal function and hemostasis in dogs undergoing surgery for fracture repair. Am J Vet Res 66(8):1356-1363, 2005.

59. Koester MC, Spindler KP: Pharmacologic agents in fracture healing. Clin Sports Med 25(1):63-73, viii, 2006.

60. Bhandari M, et al: Predictors of reoperation following operative management of fractures of the tibial shaft. J Orthop Trauma 17(5):353-361, 2003.

61. Giannoudis PV, et al: Nonunion of the femoral diaphysis. The influence of reaming and non-steroidal anti-inflammatory drugs. J Bone Joint Surg Br 82(5):655-658, 2000.

62. Brown KM, et al: Effect of COX-2-specific inhibition on fracture-healing in the rat femur. J Bone Joint Surg Am 86-A(1):116-123, 2004.

63. Gerstenfeld LC, Einhorn TA: COX inhibitors and their effects on bone healing. Expert Opin Drug Saf 3(2):131-136, 2004.

64. Bergenstock M, et al: A comparison between the effects of acetaminophen and celecoxib on bone fracture healing in rats. J Orthop Trauma 19(10):717-723, 2005.

65. Bhattacharyya T, et al: Nonsteroidal antiinflammatory drugs and nonunion of humeral shaft fractures. Arthritis Rheum 53(3):364-367, 2005.

66. Goodman SB, et al: Temporal effects of a COX-2-selective NSAID on bone ingrowth. J Biomed Mater Res A 72(3):279-287, 2005.

67. Reuben SS, Ablett D, Kaye R: High dose nonsteroidal anti-inflammatory drugs compromise spinal fusion. Can J Anaesth 52(5):506-512, 2005.

68. Reuben SS, Ekman EF: The effect of cyclooxygenase-2 inhibition on analgesia and spinal fusion. J Bone Joint Surg Am 87(3):536-542, 2005.

Chapter 87

Enhancement of Fracture Healing

Erick Egger
Elizabeth Pluhar

Physical Stimulation of Bone Healing

It has long been known that the mechanical environment of a long-bone fracture can influence the biologic process of healing.[1] Classically this has been demonstrated by the development of a large periosteal callous through the pathway of endochondral ossification in fractures stabilized with relatively flexible fixation that allows some motion at the fracture site. This is opposed by healing with minimal periosteal callous formation by direct intramembranous ossification when fractures are rigidly fixed, allowing virtually no motion between fracture ends. Which of these two pathways is preferable has been debated extensively as reviewed in chapters 85 and 86 on "bone healing" in this text. More recently, researchers and clinicians have been manipulating these responses to mechanical environment to optimize or stimulate fracture healing. This section summarizes the current techniques being investigated and used clinically, and the proposed mechanisms of action of these techniques.

Induced Micromotion (IMM)

This concept has been extensively studied by Goodship and Kenwright in the sheep tibia model[2-3] and in at least one human clinical trial.[4] This scheme uses an external fixator with pneumatic driven activator that provides axial tension and compressive forces that can be controlled in displacement, speed, and duration. A positive effect was seen in an ovine 3-mm transverse osteotomy gap model in callous formation and increasing stiffness of healing if stimulated by 1 mm of induced displacement when compared with nonstimulated controls.[2] More recent work suggests that the positive effects of IMM are greatest at relatively moderate or higher rates of induced motion (40 and 400 mm/sec versus 2 mm/sec).[3] This positive effect was greatest when IMM was initiated 1 week postoperatively when compared with delayed initiation (after 6 weeks) and when studied at 12 weeks. Consequently, these authors feel IMM has the optimal positive effect on the early phases of the repair process, which in their model appears to be endochondral ossification. A subsequent clinical trial on 39 human tibial fractures treated with IMM did show a significant decrease in healing time compared with nonstimulated controls.[4] Another study[5] on externally induced motion was performed on 2-mm femoral osteotomies in rats. A specialized external fixator was used to provide cranial-caudal bending of the osteotomy from day 7 to day 18, 3 times a week. Finite element analysis found the cranial aspect of the healing osteotomy experienced approximately 7% tensile strain, while the caudal aspect of the osteotomy experienced 3.5% compressive strain. Overall, the tensile strains tended to promote endochondral ossification. They hypothesized by increasing the pool of mesenchymal progenitor cells and demonstrated increased bony bridging, whereas the compressive strains suppressed chondrogenesis and encouraged intramembranous ossification.

Dynamization

Dynamization is a concept that was initially described by De Bastiani and incorporated in the design of a human external fixator system (Orthofix™).[6] De Bastiani proposed providing initially rigid fixation to allow revascularization and initial fracture healing followed by releasing the axial stabilization while continuing bending and torsional stabilization. Whereas many human clinical cases have been treated using this technique, most experimental studies have failed to show an overall significant positive effect on osteotomy healing in dogs.[7] In one study that did report a positive overall affect with dynamization performed 7 days postoperatively, the effect may have reflected increased rigidity resulting from total osteotomy gap collapse.[8] Another study using a veterinary external fixator design suggested dynamization after two weeks tended to cause larger callous size and callous density, but may impede remodeling at the fracture gap.[9] Statistically significant differences were not found with densitometry, absorptiometry, or CT throughout the period of the study, and a lack of torsional stiffness or maximal strength difference was found at the end, 13 weeks postoperatively.

Destabilization

The basis of this concept is to provide stabilized fixation initially and decrease that fixation rigidity as the fracture heals and develops strength. It developed as an attempt to combine the early advantages of stable fixation, such as rapid reduction in postoperative pain and increasing speed to limb use while avoiding the potential long-term disadvantages of rigid fixation such as stress protection of the fracture. Destabilization, also known as "staged disassembly," developed as more rigid fixation was obtainable with external fixators through the use of more complex frames,[10] new components,[11] and threaded fixation pins.[12] Clinical observation of periodic atrophic delayed and nonunions occurring with these rigid devices stimulated attempts to optimize fracture healing by manipulating the fracture fixation mechanical environment. Early experiments with both transverse[13] and oblique[14] canine tibial osteotomies suggested that destabilization from rigid configurations of external fixator to much less rigid type I configurations (twofold in torsion, threefold in bending, and sevenfold in axial compression)[15] resulted in more callous production but a decreased healing strength when performed at 0, 2, and 4 weeks after osteotomy. Minimal callous production and more appearance of remodeling with greater fracture strength were seen when destabilized six weeks after osteotomy. No effect was seen when the osteotomies were destabilized 12 weeks after osteotomy and compared with contralateral rigidly stabilized controls. These results suggested that too great or early reduction in fixation rigidity can cause the fracture healing pathway to convert from primary intramembranous ossification to secondary endochondral ossification. Destabilization could result in greater fracture strength when performed at six weeks, probably by stimulating the hypertrophy and remodeling phase of primary bone healing. Late destabilization of that model provided no beneficial effect, either because the responsiveness of the healing tissue was inadequate at that time or the study did not go long enough (12 to 15 weeks). It was also noted that problems with fixation, pin loosening, and secondary lameness with infection developed as the fixation pin numbers decreased after destabilization. However, a similar, more recent and well controlled study performed by Dupuis' laboratory found no significant differences in healing of a 2-mm wide oblique osteotomy when destabilizing from a type II to a type I frame.[16] These authors concluded that the previous positive study results may have reflected excessively rigidly control osteotomies, essentially causing stress protection, and that destabilization from a type III may, in fact, be a return to normal bone healing rather than enhanced bone healing.[17-19] However, they also recognize that different clinical situations may require different approaches, and slow-healing fractures may still benefit from a gradual increase in loading by progressive removal of fixation.[16]

Increasing Stabilization

A final scenario of fracture fixation manipulation that has been discussed is that of allowing early motion at the fracture site to induce a large periosteal callous through the chondral precursor pathway, and then increasing rigidity to encourage the later stages of ossification. We performed a pilot study of this approach starting with a type I configuration for 4 weeks, followed by conversion to a rigid type III configuration after significant callous production. Overwhelming problems with fixation failure and pin loosening resulting in loss of reduction and poor limb use owing to pain caused the abandonment of this approach; however, with today's improvement in device design and threaded pin use, the concept deserves further study.

Direct Current Stimulation (DC)

DC uses a constant 20 μA to stimulate the fracture. The cathode is placed at the stimulation site and the anode/battery pack is buried in subcutaneous tissues. Brighton[15,20] showed that at the cathode, PO_2 is lower, which appears to favor bone formation; proteoglycan and collagen synthesis are increased. Currently, DC is approved for use in human established nonunions and spinal fusions,[21] with up to 83% success reported for tibial nonunions.[22] The implantable battery eliminates the problem of patient compliance, but usually requires removal after six months.

Pulsed Electromagnetic Fields (PEMF)

The PEMF signal was developed to induce electrical fields in bones similar in magnitude and time to the endogenous electrical fields produced in response to strain.[21] They may reflect the ability of bone to respond to change in mechanical environment known as Wolff's Law. The signal consists of bursts of EM pulses repeated at 15 Hz. Various in vivo studies have shown upregulation of TGF-B and a several fold increase in BMP mRNAs, which increased chondroneogenesis by enhancing differentiation of osteochondral precursor cells,[22] suggesting that PEMF will have optimal effect on endochondral bone production. That is consistent with the clinical observation that PEMF is more effective in treating hypertrophic nonunions than atrophic nonunions.[22] Currently PEMF is used in humans as an adjunct to standard fracture and delayed union therapy.

Capicitative Coupling (CC)

This approach uses 2 surface electrodes placed on alternate sides of the fracture; the induced field is driven by an oscillating electrical current.[21] Field strength is calculated to be 0.1 to 20 mV/cm continuously applied. Stimulation of bone cell proliferation has been observed but the physiology of how electrical signals stimulate has been difficult to demonstrate in the laboratory.[23] CC is typically used with casting in treatment of nonunions with a 60% to 77% success rate and improvement from 65% to 85% success rates in obtaining spinal fusion.[23]

Combined Magnetic Fields (CMF)

CMF appears to affect calcium ion transport across cell membranes and activate secretion of growth factors (insulin-like-growth factor-II), increasing cell proliferation.[23,24] However, more study is needed to fully explain its stimulation effect. Currently CMF is applied for 30 minutes a day in cases of nonunion and to stimulate spinal fusion.[21] Treatment of osteoarthritis and neuroarthropathy has been suggested but awaits more understanding of its mechanism of action.[21]

Low-Intensity Ultrasound (LIUS)

Low-intensity ultrasound with high-frequency short bursts has been shown to accelerate fracture healing, but no specific stage of healing appears to be more sensitive.[25] A minimal heating effect (less than 1 degree C) may increase some enzymatic activity. Ultrasound does affect the exchange rate of potassium ions and increases the release of intracellular calcium and appears to stimulate proteoglycan synthesis in rat chondrocytes.[26] Also a greater degree of blood flow has been shown in canine ulnar fracture models with a generalized stimulatory effect.[27] In humans it is applied for 20 minutes daily. Current clinical indications are aimed at reducing the healing time of fresh fractures to avoid delayed unions and subsequent loss of fracture reduction.[28] It has also been used in treatment of nonunions and increasing strength of the new bone produced by distraction osteogenesis.[21]

Shock-Wave Therapy

Shock wave uses a high-energy variable-frequency mechanical impulse applied with a transducer that can focus the impulses to concentrate on deeper structures. A rapid positive pressure wave is followed by a variable negative pressure that may cause cavitation of soft tissues or disruption of large structures. It was originally used as lithotripsy for the noninvasive fragmentation of kidney stones.[29] Several studies have shown positive and variable effects on the healing of nonunions,[28] and one clinical study found a positive effect on late healing of acute tibial osteotomies in dogs.[30] Although the mechanism of action has not been clarified, it is proposed that shock-wave application produces microtrauma with hematoma creation. Subsequently, the induced neovascularization stimulates connective tissue proliferation and activity.[31] Generally, 6000 to 12,000 shock impulses are applied at a treatment that may be repeated periodically. Currently, shock-wave therapy is recommended only as an adjunctive to traditional treatments for chronic nonunions, particularly those with compromised local circulation. A temporary weakening of the osseous structures may result from the trabecular microfractures produced. There also appears to be a significant analgesic effect so caution in post-treatment activity must be used to avoid catastrophic fracture until the treated bone has an opportunity to respond and strengthen.

Biologic Stimulation of Bone Healing

Most fractures in companion animals heal in an acceptable time period with adequate stabilization of the fracture fragments. Factors that contribute to delay or prohibition of fracture healing exist. Major categories of these factors are deficiencies of vascular supply, deficiencies in the vigor of the osteochondral response, and deficiencies in stability or physical continuity. Use of cells, bioactive factors, and/or supportive matrices can enhance fracture healing by providing or stimulating the deficient factor. Bioactive materials can be grouped based on their properties that enhance healing: osteogenesis, new bone formation; osteoinduction, recruitment and differentiation of bone-forming cells; and osteoconduction, mechanical support or scaffold for bone-forming cells. These therapeutic options can be used alone or in synergistic combinations. Some of the bioactive factors discussed here are available for clinical use; however others are not, and have only been used in experimental fracture or defect models.

Materials that are Primarily Osteogenic and Osteoconductive

Autogenous cancellous or corticocancellous grafts are frequently used by veterinary surgeons. These grafts are the gold standard for enhancing fracture healing against which bone substitutes are compared. Autograft is readily available from the metaphysis of several long bones or the ilium. The volume of graft is limited and donor site morbidity occurs. When handled properly, autograft provides mesenchymal stem cells and differentiated osteoblasts and osteocytes that can form new bone. The mineralized bone in the autograft provides osteoconductive surfaces on which bone-forming cells can lay down new matrix. Bone grafts are addressed more extensively in Chapter 88.

Mesenchymal stem cells (MSC) or multipotent adult progenitor cells (MAPC) are pluripotent cells that have a high replicative capacity and the potential to differentiate into many tissues including the osteogenic lineage.[30] Approximately 1 in 25,000 nucleated cells from an adult canine bone marrow aspirate is a MSC.[32] These cells can be directed to develop into an osteogenic lineage during culture expansion by exposing the cells to a number of substances, such as transforming growth factor-β (TGF-β), insulin-like growth factor (IGF), vascular endothelial growth factor (VEGF), dexamethasone, β-glycerophosphate, or ascorbic acid phosphate.[33,34] The MSCs in the marrow of an autogenous graft are exposed to these factors during the inflammatory response from the fracture and surgical intervention. Bone morphogenetic proteins or osteogenic proteins, BMP-2 or BMP-7/OP-1, are potent factors that induce MSC to differentiate into osteoblastic cells.[35-37] Local concentrations of bone morphogenetic protein (BMP) at a fracture site may increase as osteoclasts resorb bone matrix.[38] The multipotent cells that appear early in the fracture hematoma also appear to synthesize BMPs, which creates a cascade of events that results in greater numbers of multipotent cells and increased levels of BMPs.[39]

Two services currently purify and expand MSC from either bone marrow (VetCell Bioscience) or lipoaspirates (Vet-Stem). These concentrates have been used to enhance healing of equine tendons and ligaments. MSCs expanded in culture and exposed to an osteoinductive factor have been loaded onto an osteoconductive carrier. Although these osteogenic and osteoconductive combinations have been shown to enhance fracture and bone defect healing in many experimental animal models, they are not currently used in human or veterinary clinical fractures. The problems associated with clinical use of this treatment modality are that 1) 2 to 3 weeks are required to purify and expand the cells following the initial collection, causing a delay before sufficient amounts of patient-derived MSCs are available for re-introduction; 2) patient-derived MSCs may not be suitable for regeneration of damaged tissues if the patient is aged or if has bone marrow neoplasia; and 3) the cost of isolation, expansion, and safety and quality control must be covered for each patient and is cost-prohibitive.

Many surgeons are mixing unconcentrated bone marrow aspirates with osteoconductive material, such as bone allograft or hydroxyapatite to enhance bone healing. The osteogenic potential of concentrated MSCs has been shown to be significantly greater than fresh bone-marrow aspirate. Systems that concentrate MSCs from fresh bone-marrow aspirates instantly in the operating room are commercially available. CELLECT® (Johnson & Johnson) filters fresh marrow through a central chamber that holds osteoconductive material (i.e., cancellous bone or demineralized bone matrix) and concentrates the MSC three- to fourfold.

Periosteum is tissue that covers the external surface of most bones. It is composed of two microscopically distinct layers. An outer, fibrous layer is composed of fibroblasts, collagen, and elastin fibers with a neural and microvascular network.[40-42] The inner, cambium layer in contact with the cortical surface is highly cellular. It contains MAPC, osteogenic progenitor cells and osteoblasts, fibroblasts, tiny blood vessels, and sympathetic nerves.[41-43] Trauma activates the progenitor cells of the periosteum, although most studies have explored the use of periosteum to generate cartilage. Experimental models have shown that the osteogenic potential of this tissue can be stimulated by basic fibroblastic growth factor (bFGF), transforming growth factor-beta (TGF-β) and BMPs.[44-46] One study showed the powerful ability of periosteum to heal 5-cm tibial cortical defects in sheep with new bone production.[47]

Activated platelets in the fracture hematoma release several growth factors including platelet-derived growth factor (PDGF) and bFGF. These factors stimulate the proliferation of periosteum-derived cells and contribute to the mitogenic response of the periosteum during callus formation.[48-50] After proliferation these cells differentiate into osteoblasts or chondroblasts to form bone or cartilage to allow bridging of the fracture gap.

Materials that are Primarily Osteoconductive

Processed allogenic bone graft has no osteogenetic capacity and little osteoinductive activity. Its primary purpose is to provide structural integrity and act as a scaffold for new bone formation.[51] In order to minimize its immunogenicity, the graft must be processed in some way, which in turn compromises its mechanical properties. The advantages of allograft are that it is readily available in virtually unlimited amounts and engenders no donor site morbidity. Large cortical allografts are pieces of dead bone, and subsequently, are not completely replaced by new host bone and are more prone to infection. Veterinary Transplant Services Incorporated is a bone bank for canine and feline allograft bone in a variety of structures.

Synthetic bone graft substitutes consist of calcium sulfate or plaster of Paris; hydroxyapatite, tricalcium phosphate, and combinations of these minerals, known as ceramics; and synthetic glasses composed of SiO2, Na2O, CaO, and P2O5. The materials vary in fabrication technique, crystallinity, pore dimensions, mechanical properties, and resorption rate. All synthetic porous substitutes share numerous advantages over autograft and allograft including their unlimited supply, easy sterilization, and storage. However, the degree to which the substitute provides an osteoconductive structural framework for new bone ingrowth differs depending on material composition. Calcium sulfate as cement and pellets is commercially available and its affordability, resorbability, and biocompatibility make it an option for veterinary surgeons. Cerasorb Vet (New Generation Devices) is a veterinary product of pure tricalcium phosphate that is available in granular and block forms.

Hydroxyapatite (HA) porous implants are produced when coral carbonate in the exoskeleton of a marine invertebrate of the genus Porite is converted by a hydrothermal exchange. The new material is mechanically superior while maintaining the internal structure of the coral. It has parallel channels 230 μm in diameter with interconnecting fenestrations of 190 μm diameter that are similar to the structure of cortical bone. Fibrovascular tissue that initially invades HA implants is later replaced by mature lamellar bone.[52] Although some surface resorption of the bulk implant does occur by osteoclast-like cells, major remodeling is minimal owing to the inert, insoluble structure of the HA.

Many ceramic preparations are commercially available and are widely used in human orthopedic surgery. Disadvantages of ceramic implants include brittle handling properties, variable rates of resorption, poor performance in diaphyseal defects, and potentially adverse affects on normal bone remodeling. These shortcomings have restricted their primary use to bone graft extenders and carriers for pharmaceuticals. A particulate bioglass preparation marketed for veterinary use (Consil, Nutramax Laboratories Inc.) is indicated for use in infrabony pockets associated with dental and periodontal disease and defects. Bioactive glass may induce more osteoproduction than other ceramics, but it is slowly resorbed.

Materials that are Osteoconductive and Osteoinductive

Demineralized bone matrix (DBM) is allograft bone that has undergone acid extraction of the mineralized portion of the matrix that increases the availability of inductive proteins. Several osteoinductive proteins, including bone morphogenetic protein, may be present in physiologic and biologic concentrations and proportions. One of the advantages of DBM is that, with time and continued remodeling, it will be completely resorbed and replaced by new host bone. Veterinary Transplant Services Inc. markets canine and feline DBM powder alone or combined with cancellous allograft chips to provide an osteoconductive matrix.

As mentioned earlier, fresh bone marrow, that may be centrifuged or filtered to concentrate MSCs, can be mixed with DBM/cancellous chips to provide a graft material that has osteogenic as well as osteoinductive and osteoconductive properties. Another strategy that provides a synergistic effect among bioactive materials is to mix DBM or DBM and bone marrow aspirate with platelet concentrate. A platelet concentrating system, Symphony PCS (DePuy), uses an automated device to rapidly concentrate platelets from a relatively small volume of a patient's blood. The concentrate has three to six times the levels of PDGF, IGF, TGF-β, and VEGF. These factors are chemotactic for stem cells, osteoblasts, and chondrocytes and are mitogenic for MSCs and osteoblasts. There is also a graft delivery system, Symphony GDS (DePuy) or GPS (Biomet) that has a specially designed graft chamber and manifold for the delivery of graft materials to an orthopedic surgical site. The system facilitates premixing of graft materials with platelet concentrate, bone marrow, or blood that can then be placed into a fracture site or bone defect.

Materials that are Primarily Osteoinductive

Osteoinductive molecules promote bone formation mediated by cell signaling that prompts multipotent cells to differentiate into osteoblasts. The most widely studied of these cytokines are the BMPs. This family of proteins has several members, but BMPs 2, 4, 6, and 7 (also known as osteogenic protein-1, OP-1) have the most potent osteoinductive efficacy.[53] Experimental preclinical studies in a variety of species including dogs have demonstrated healing of bone defects, fractures, and spinal fusions with the application of different BMP-carrier systems. Early studies used DBM or highly purified BMP, and more recent studies use recombinant BMP, usually human recombinant BMP (rhBMP). These water-soluble proteins must be combined with a carrier to maintain sustained delivery of adequate protein concentrations in the desired site.

Much of the current research effort is to find the optimal carrier and optimal dose for different species and specific sites in every species. Bone morphogenetic protein 2 (Medtronic Sofamor

Danek) on an absorbable collagen sponge, and the OP-1 implant (Stryker Biotech), OP-1 in a purified bovine type 1 collagen particulate matrix, are the most heavily studied osteoinductive biomaterials. These two products are available for limited applications in human orthopedic surgery, including periodontal lesions, spinal fusions, and tibial nonunion fractures. Although these implants are not approved for veterinary use and their cost would most likely be prohibitive, they have had extra label use in a limited number of clinical cases of delayed or nonunion fractures in dogs. The latest method of delivery of BMPs and other bioactive cytokines to desired sites is by gene therapy. Delivery of the relevant DNA to host cells can be accomplished using nonviral, e.g, plasmid, or viral, e.g., adenovirus, vectors. The vectors can be delivered directly into the host tissues by in vivo transfer, or indirectly by in vitro transfer into harvested host cells that are then returned to the desired site. Bone morphogenetic proteins are addressed more extensively in Chapter 86.

The exact roles in bone formation of other growth factors that have been identified are less clear. Conflicting results in experimental studies using these cytokines for fracture healing and clinical applications of these bioactive factors have been reported. Unlike the BMPs, these growth factors are incapable of de novo bone formation in an ectopic site. Transforming growth factor-beta is a protein found in platelets, bone, and cartilage that may act synergistically with other cytokines to promote differentiation, proliferation, and matrix synthesis by osteoblasts. Osteoclasts degrade bone during fracture repair by acid hydrolysis of the matrix, creating an acidic environment that can activate latent TGF-β.[54] The TGF-β released from the bone matrix can activate osteoblasts to produce new bone matrix.

Basic fibroblast growth factor (bFGF) acts primarily as a mitogen, stimulating increased DNA synthesis and cell division. When injected into a fracture site on a fibrin or hyaluronan carrier, it increased callus size, mineral content, and mechanical strength of the healing bone.[55,56] Insulin-like growth factors I and II stimulate bone formation by promoting proliferation of osteoblastic precursors and matrix production by osteoblasts. Platelet-derived growth factor is released by platelets during fracture healing and is chemotactic for fibroblasts, monocytes, and osteoblasts and stimulates proliferation of mesenchymal cells. Growth and differentiation factor-5 (GDF-5) is a divergent member of the TGF-β superfamily required for normal skeletal development. When loaded on a collagen matrix, GDF-5 induced ectopic cartilage and bone formation, new bone formation in long-bone defects in non-human primates, and fusion of vertebral transverse processes in rabbits.[57,58]

References

1. Wu JJ, Shyr HS, Chao EYS, et al: Comparison of osteotomy healing under external fixation devices with different stiffness characteristics. J Bone Joint Surg 66A:1258, 1984.

2. Goodship AE, Cunningham JL, Kenwright J: Strain rate and timing of stimulation in mechanical modulation of fracture healing. Clin Orthop Rel Res 355S:S105, 1998.

3. Goodship AE, Kenwright J: The influence of induced micromovement upon the healing of experimental tibial fractures. J Bone Joint Surg 67B:650, 1985.

4. Kenwright J, Goodship AE, Kelly DJ, et al: Effect of controlled axial micromovement on healing of tibial fractures. Lancet 2:1185, 1986.

5. Smith-Adaline EA, Volkman SK, Ignelzi MA, et al: Mechanical environment alters tissue formation patterns during fracture repair. J Orthop Res 22:1079, 2004.

6. De Bastiani G, Aldegheri R, Renzi Brivio L: The treatment of fractures with a dynamic axial fixator. J Trauma 34:185, 1993.

7. Larsson S, Wookcheol K, Caja VL, et al: Effect of early axial dynamization on tibial bone healing: a study in dogs. Clin Orthop 388:240, 2001.

8. Egger EL, Gottsauner-Wolf F, Palmer J, et al: Effects of axial dynamization on bone healing. J Trauma 34:185, 1993.

9. Gorman SC, Kraus KH, Tidwell AS, et al: In vivo axial dynamization of canine tibial fractures using the Securos external skeletal fixation system. Vet Comp Orthop Traumatol 4:199, 2005.

10. Egger, EL: Static strength evaluation of six external skeletal fixation configurations. Vet Surg 12:130, 1983.

11. Kraus KH, Wotton HM, Rand WM: Mechanical comparison of two external fixator clamps designs. Vet Surg 27:224, 1998.

12. Clary EM, Roe SC: Enhancing external skeletal fixation pin performance: Consideration of the pin-bone interface. Vet Comp Orthop Traumatol 8:1, 1995.

13. Egger EL, Lewallen DG, Norrdin RW, et al.: Effects of destabilizing rigid external fixation on healing of unstable canine osteotomies. *In* Proceedings 34th Annual Meeting Orthopaedic Research Society, Atlanta, CA. 1988 (abstr); 302.

14. Egger EL, Histand MB, Norrdin RW, et al: Canine osteotomy healing when stabilized with decreasingly rigid fixation compared to constantly rigid fixation. Vet Comp Orthop Traumatol 6:182, 1993.

15. Brighton CT, McCluskey WP: Cellular response and mechanisms of action of electrically induced osteogenesis. *In* Peck WA (ed): Bone and Mineral Research, 4th ed. Amsterdam: Elsevier, 1986, p. 213.

16. Auger J, Dupuis J, Boudrealult F, et al: Comparison of multistage versus one-stage destabilization of a type II external fixator used to stabilize an oblique tibial osteotomy in dogs. Vet Surg 31:10, 2002.

17. Hente R, Cordey J, Rahn BA, et al: Fracture healing of the sheep tibia treated using unilateral external fixator. Comparison of static and dynamic fixation. Injury 30:SA44, 1999.

18. Kenwright J, Gardner T: Mechanical influences on tibial fracture healing. Clin Orthop 355S:S179, 1998.

19. O'Dougherty DM, Butler SP, Goodship AE: Stress protection due to external fixation. J Biomechanics 28:575, 1995.

20. Brighton CT, Friedenberg ZB, Mitchell EI, Booth RE: Treatment of nonunion with constant direct current. Clin Orthop 124:106, 1977.

21. Nelson FR, Brighton CT, Ryaby J, et al: Use of physical forces in bone healing. J Am Acad Orthop Surg 11:344, 2003.

22. Brighton CT, Black J, Friedenberg ZB, et al: A multicenter study of the treatment of non-union with constant direct current. J Bone Joint Surg Am 62:2, 1981.

23. Lorich DG, Brighton CT, Gupta R, et al: Biochemical pathway mediating the response of bone cells to capacitive coupling. Clin Orthop 350:246, 1998.

24. Fitzsimmons RJ, Baylink JT, Ryaby JT, Magee FP: EMF-stimulated bone-cell proliferation. *In* Bland M (ed): Electricity and Magnetism in Biology and Medicine. San Francisco: San Francisco Press, 1993, p. 889.

25. Azuma Y, Ito M, Harada Y, et al: Low-intensity pulsed ultrasound accelerates rat femoral fracture healing by acting on the various cellular reactions in the fracture callus. J Bone Miner Res 16:671, 2001.

26. Wu CC, Lewallen DG, Bolander ME, et al: Exposure to low intensity ultrasound stimulates aggrecan gene expression by cultured chondrocytes. Trans Orthop Soc 21:622, 1996.

27. Rawool D, Goldberg B, Forsberg F, et al: Power Doppler assessment of vascular changes during fracture treatment with low-intensity ultrasound. Trans Radiol Soc North Am 83:1185, 1998.

28. Kristiansen TK, Ryaby JP, McCabe J, et al: Accelerated healing of distal radial fractures with the use of specific, low-intensity ultrasound: A multicenter, prospective, randomized, double-blind, placebo-controlled study. J Bone Joint Surg Am 79:961, 1997.

29. Thiel M: Application of shock waves in medicine. Clin Orthop 387:18, 2001.

30. Haynesworth SE, Goshima J, Goldberg VM, Caplan AI: Characterization of cells with osteogenic potential from human marrow. Bone 13:81, 1992.

31. Odgen JH, Alvarex RG, Levitt R, Marlow M: Shock wave therapy (Orthotripsy®) in musculoskeletal disorders. Clin Orthop 387:22, 2001.

32. Bruder SP, Kraus KH, Goldberg VM, Kadiyala S: The effect of implants loaded with autologous mesenchymal stem cells on healing of canine segmental bone defects. J Bone Joint Surg 80A:985, 1998.

33. Jaiswal N, Haynesworth SE, Caplan AI, Bruder SP: Osteogenic differentiation of purified, culture-expanded human mesenchymal stem cells in vitro. J Cell Biochem 64:295, 1997.

34. Lennon DP, Haynesworth SE, Bruder SP, et al: Human and animal mesenchymal progenitor cells from bone marrow: identification of serum for optimal selection and proliferation. *In* Vitro Cell Devel Biol 32:602, 1996.

35. Rickard D, Sullivan T, Shenkar B, et al: Induction of rapid osteoblast differentiation in rat bone marrow stromal cell cultures by dexamethasone and BMP-2. Dev Biol 16(1):218, 1994.

36. Chen T, Shen W, Kraemer F: Human BMP-7/OP-1 induces the growth and differentiation of adipocytes and osteoblasts in bone marrow stromal cell cultures. J Cell Biochem 82:187, 2001.

37. Volk SW, Diefendorfer DL, Christopher SA, et al: Effects of osteogenic inducers on cultures of canine mesenchymal stem cells. Am J Vet Res 66(10):1729, 2005.

38. Yang LJ, Jin Y: Immunohistochemical observations on bone morphogenetic protein in normal and abnormal conditions. Clin Orthop 257:249, 1990.

39. Bostrom MPG: Expression of bone morphogenetic proteins in fracture healing. Clin Orthop 355S:116, 1998.

40. Taylor JF: The Periosteum and bone growth. *In* Bone Growth VI. Hall BK (ed). Boca Raton: CRC Press, 1992.

41. Ellender G, Feik SA, Caraach BJ: Periosteal structure and development in a rat caudal vertebra. J Anat 158:173, 1988.

42. Hohmann EL, Elde RP, Rysavy JA, et al: Innervation of periosteum and bone by sympathetic vasoactive intestinal peptide-containing nerve fibers. Science 232:868, 1986.

43. Aubin J, Triffitt J: Mesenchymal stem cells and osteoblast differentiation. *In* Principles of Bone Biology. Bilezkian J, Raisz J, Rodan GA (eds). San Diego: Academic Press, 2002.

44. Iwasaki M, Nakahara H, Nakata K, et al: Regulation of proliferation and osteochondrogenic differentiation of periosteum-derived cells by transforming growth factor-beta and basic fibroblast growth factor. J Bone Joint Surg 77A:543, 1995.

45. Joyce ME, Roberts AB, Sporn MB, Bolander ME: Transforming growth factor-beta and the initiation of chondrogenesis and osteogenesis in the rat femur. J Cell Biol 110: 2195, 1990.

46. Gruber R, Mayer C, Bobacz K, et al: Effects of cartilage-derived morphogenetic proteins and osteogenic protein-1 on osteochondrogenic differentiation of periosteum-derived cells. Endocrinology 142:2087, 2001.

47. Pluhar GE, Wheeler DL, Toth CA: Importance of periosteal removal on ovine critical sized defect healing. *In* Proceedings 52nd Annual Meeting, Orthopaedic Research Society, 2006.

48. Gruber R, Varga F, Fischer MB, Watzek G: Platelets stimulate proliferation of bone cells: involvement of platelet-derived growth factor, microparticles and membranes. Clin Oral Implants Res 13(5):529, 2002.

49. Gruber R, Karreth F, Frommlet F, et al: Platelets are mitogenic for periosteum-derived cells. J Orthop Res 21(5):941, 2003.

50. Slater M, Patava J, Kingham K, Mason RS: Involvement of platelets in stimulating osteogenic activity. J Orthop Res 13(5):655, 1995.

51. Burwell RG: The fate of bone grafts. *In* Recent Advances in Orthopaedics. Apley AG (ed). London: Churchill Livingstone, 1969.

52. Chapman MW, Bucholz R, Cornell CN: Treatment of acute fractures with a collagen-calcium phosphate graft material: A randomized clinical trial. J Bone Joint Surg 79A:495, 1997.

53. Wozney JM, Rosen V: Bone morphogenetic protein and bone morphogenetic protein gene family in bone formation and repair. Clin Orthop 346:26, 1998

54. Oreffo RO, Bonewald L, Kukita A, et al: Inhibitory effects of the bone-derived growth factors, osteoinductive factor and transforming growth factor-beta on isolated osteoclasts. Endocrinology 126:3069, 1990.

55. Kawaguchi H, Kurokawa T, Hanada K, et al: Stimulation of fracture repair by recombinant human basic fibroblast growth factor in normal and streptozotocin-diabetic rats. Endocrinology 135:774, 1994.

56. Nakamura K, Kawaguchi H, Aoyama I, et al: Stimulation of bone formation by intraosseous application of recombinant human basic fibroblast growth factor in normal and ovariectomized rabbits. J Orthop Res 15:307, 1997.

57. Spiro RC, Liu L, Heidaran MA, et al: Inductive activity of recombinant human growth and differentiation factor-5. Biochem Soc Trans 28(4):362, 2000.

58. Spiro RC, Thompson AY, Poser JW: Spinal fusion with recombinant human growth and differentiation factor-5 combined with a mineralized collagen matrix. Anat Rec 263(4):388, 2001.

Chapter 88

Bone Grafting

André Autefage
Loïc M. Dejardin

Bone grafting is used extensively in human and veterinary medicine. It is commonly utilized for treatment of delayed unions or nonunions, filling of bone defects, or joint arthrodesis. It is estimated that 500,000 to 600,000 bone grafting procedures are performed in humans annually in the United States alone.[1] No accurate estimates exist for the number of bone grafts performed in veterinary medicine.

Types of Bone Grafts – Terminology

Bone grafts are described based on the relationship between donor and recipient, on the type of bone harvested, and on the site of the application. **Autografts** are tissues that are transplanted from one site to another in the same individual. Because the genetic composition of the donor and recipient sites are identical, no immune response occurs. Cancellous bone autografts are the most commonly used bone grafts in veterinary medicine. **Allografts** are transplanted from one individual to another of the same species. Genetic differences between the donor and recipient may induce an immune reaction based on the recognition of foreign antigens from the graft by the host immune system. Most bone allografts require some form of processing or preservation prior to use. **Xenografts** are tissues transplanted from one individual to another of a different species. Xenografts often induce a more severe immune response.

Bone grafts are also defined according to the type of bone transplanted. **Cancellous bone** grafts are composed of the porous, highly cellular trabecular bone found in the long bone epiphyses and metaphyses as well as in the iliac wings and the sternebrae. The trabeculae are covered with a highly reactive endosteal membrane that includes osteoclasts, osteoblasts, and bone lining cells. The cavities between the trabeculae are filled with highly cellular bone marrow. **Cortical bone** grafts are composed of the dense, compact bone from the diaphyses of long bones. They are mechanically strong, but have a relatively low cellularity. **Corticocancellous bone** grafts are combinations of the two types of bone, which allow surgeons to take advantage of the benefits of both types of grafts. Ribs and the craniodorsal part of the iliac wings are the main sources of corticocancellous bone grafts in dogs. An allograft used with fresh cancellous bone or bone marrow is termed a **composite graft. Vascularized bone autografts or allografts** are harvested with their blood supply and microvascular anastomoses are necessary at the time of implantation. **Osteochondral** grafts include bone and articular cartilage.

A bone graft placed in its normal position (i.e., within bone tissue) is said to have been **orthotopically** transplanted. If the graft is transplanted to an abnormal anatomic site, it is said to have been **heterotopically** transplanted.

Function Of Bone Grafts

An ideal bone graft would perform four functions: osteogenesis, osteoinduction, osteoconduction, and mechanical support.[2,3] However, depending on the type, the most common bone grafts are able to provide only one or more of these functions (Table 88-1).

Osteogenesis

Osteogenesis is defined as the creation of new bone by bone-forming cells regardless of their origin. This function may be performed by donor cells (osteoblast precursors, osteoblasts, or chondroblasts) that survived the transplantation (fresh autogenous grafts only[2]) or by host cells stimulated by the graft or the grafting process. Cancellous bone has a much greater osteogenic potential than does cortical bone, in part because its copious porosity allows for fast and intense revascularization that contributes to cell survival.[4] Furthermore, cancellous bone is filled with bone marrow, which contains mesenchymal stem cells able to differentiate into osteoprogenitor cell lines. Finally, the trabeculae provide a large surface covered by lining cells and active osteoblasts. The survival of osteogenic cells in a graft depends on the nourishment they receive directly after transfer.[5] Although the percentage of cells surviving transfer of a fresh cancellous autograft is unknown, it has been shown that, in vitro, approximately 65% of the cells may survive up to 3 hours when the graft is maintained at room temperature in a saline solution.[6] However, it has been estimated that the survival rate of osteogenic cells in vivo does not exceed 5% following transplantation.[7] With cancellous bone autografts, early osteogenesis is characterized by active new bone formation in direct contact with the transplanted graft within 1 week following transplantation.[4] Similarly, with vascularized cortical grafts, more than 90% of the osteocytes may survive transplantation,[8] with new bone formation beginning as early as 24 hours after surgery.[9] In contrast, with nonvascularized cortical grafts, osteogenesis begins with vascular ingrowth, which does not occur until the sixth day after transplantation.[10]

Table 88-1. Functions of Types of Autologous Bone Grafts (Adapted from Finkemeier [12])

Function	Cancellous	Nonvascularized cortical	Vascularized cortical
Osteogenesis	+++	–	++
Osteoinduction	++	+/–	+/–
Osteoconduction	++++	+	+
Immediate mechanical support	–	+++	+++
Mechanical support at 1 year	+++	+++	+++

Osteoinduction

Osteoinduction refers to the recruitment of mesenchymal and pluripotent osteoprogenitor cells which later differentiate into bone- or cartilage-forming cells at the implantation site. Differentiation of mesenchymal cells is regulated via growth factors such as bone morphogenetic proteins, transforming growth factor-beta, insulin-like growth factors, fibroblast growth factors, platelet-derived growth factors, tumor necrosis factor, prostaglandin E2, and other cytokines.[11] Although these factors are produced by live cells and are present in the bone matrix, living graft cells are considered more osteoinductive than bone matrix. Because of the trabecular structure, cancellous bone matrix proteins are more readily accessible than are those of cortical bone. Osteoinductive factors may also be released during graft resorption, which in turn contributes to graft incorporation.[12] Despite the lack of evidence that inductive proteins and cytokines are active in autologous cancellous bone grafts, cancellous bone is widely believed to be osteoinductive.[12]

Osteoconduction

Osteoconduction refers to the three-dimensional process of tissue ingrowth within the graft, which acts as a scaffold. This process involves the invasion of the graft framework by capillaries as well as the migration of host osteoblasts, osteoclasts, and mesenchymal cells.[2,13] In porous cancellous bone grafts, initial fibrovascular invasion occurs quickly and is followed by bone ingrowth, characterized by direct apposition of new bone on the graft trabeculae. During subsequent graft remodeling, necrotic trabeculae are progressively resorbed and replaced by new bone. Although growth factors, collagens, and noncollagenous proteins participate in the regulation of this process, the three-dimensional trabecular structure of cancellous bone is the primary determinant of the speed and completeness of graft incorporation.[13] Histologic differences observed during cancellous versus cortical graft incorporation illustrate this phenomenon. Indeed, dense cortical grafts must undergo a resorptive phase, with removal of necrotic Haversian systems, before fibrovascular ingrowth into resorptive pores or channels can occur.[14] The process of initial bone resorption followed by fibrovascular invasion and appositional new bone formation as seen with cortical bone graft incorporation has been termed "creeping substitution." The differences between the incorporation of cancellous and cortical bone grafts suggest that the porosity and surface area of the pores directly influence the speed and rate of incorporation.

Mechanical Support

Mechanical or structural support describes the ability of a bone graft to act as a load-sharing space filler in the treatment of large bone defects, and its effectiveness depends on the nature of the graft. Although cancellous bone is an efficient space filler, it does not provide substantial structural support. In contrast, a cortical graft provides excellent early mechanical support. Importantly, the strength of a graft changes over time in response to the biomechanical environment. Local bone resorption and revascularization substantially increase porosity, causing nonvascularized cortical autografts to become weaker at the host-graft interface six weeks after grafting.[14-16] Conversely, vascularized cortical autografts do not undergo resorption and revascularization and, therefore, show superior strength six weeks postoperatively.[15] However, six months following transplantation, the strength of nonvascularized and vascularized cortical grafts is similar.[15] Regardless of the type, cortical grafts are unable to withstand substantial loads, and must be supported by adequate internal fixation during the incorporation process to prevent catastrophic failure.

Biology of Bone Graft Incorporation

The term *incorporation* is used to describe the biologic interactions between a bone graft and host tissue at the recipient site that result in bone formation with subsequent improvement in mechanical properties.[17] This process includes the host inflammatory reaction to the surgical trauma, the host inflammatory and/or immune reaction to the graft material, and the processes of cell proliferation, migration, differentiation, and revascularization, resulting in new bone formation and union between graft and host bone. The sequence of events leading to graft incorporation is relatively consistent, although some differences exist between incorporation of cancellous and cortical bone as well as vascularized and nonvascularized bone grafts.[15,18-20] The biologic events occurring at the graft site include: (i) hematoma formation; (ii) inflammation, migration, and proliferation of mesenchymal cells, and development of fibrovascular tissue in and around the graft; (iii) vascular invasion of the graft; (iv) resorption of graft surfaces; and (v) bone formation on the graft surface. The incorporation of nonvascularized bone grafts (cancellous or cortical) begins with the formation of a local hematoma. This hematoma is rich in growth factors and other cytokines and allows for the survival of transplanted cells near the trabecular or cortical surfaces up to one week after transplantation.[21] The associated inflammatory response leads to the formation of granulation tissue, which invades the grafted site and contributes to the revascularization of the graft. Revascularization and cell differentiation vary with the type of graft, surgical technique, mechanical environment, and quality of the recipient bed. Cancellous grafts are revascularized faster than are cortical bone grafts. Histocompatibility and immunogenicity of the graft also play an important role in the rate of vascularization. Incompatible bone grafts induce an immune reaction that delays or inhibits vascularization of the graft;[4] a major mismatch may induce resorption of a cancellous bone allograft and replacement by fibrocartilage.[22] Aseptic and atraumatic surgical techniques improve the success rate of graft incorporation. Fluid exudation, infection, or devascularization of the recipient bed will delay or prevent revascularization of the graft. The mechanical environment of the graft site also has a profound effect on revascularization and cell differentiation. Although instability at the host-graft interface induces local shear strains that may impede vascular invasion of the graft, the effect of the mechanical environment on graft incorporation varies between cancellous and cortical grafts. Cancellous grafts are less susceptible to shear strains owing to their porosity and use as loosely packed fragments. In contrast, the host-graft interface of dense, monolithic cortical bone grafts is highly vulnerable to instability because the proximity of the host and graft fragments induces large local shear strains that prevent vascular penetration of the narrow Haversian canals.[17] Accordingly, cancellous grafts do not require absolute stability, but cortical grafts must be rigidly stabilized. The quality of the tissues at the host site is also a primary factor in the incorporation process. Of particular importance is the vascularity in the graft bed and the abundance and competence of endothelial cell progenitors and connective tissue.[17] Excessive surgical trauma, the presence of necrotic tissue, systemic steroids, infection, and radiation therapy may compromise vascularization of the recipient bed and the pool of local progenitor cells.[17,23]

Incorporation of Autografts

Cancellous Autografts

Although the rate of cell survival remains unknown, the majority of transplanted cells probably die as a result of local ischemia or induction of apoptosis. However, bone marrow mesenchymal cells and endothelial cell progenitors are relatively resistant to ischemia and may survive transplantation and may even proliferate in response to changes in oxygen tension, pH, and cytokines.[17] Survival of these cells along with recruitment of host mesenchymal stem cells is the key to successful incorporation of cancellous bone autografts. Following cancellous bone autograft transplantation, vascular invasion of intertrabecular spaces and formation of abundant granulation tissue proceed from the host-graft interface. This process is usually complete within two weeks.[4] With vascular ingrowth, differentiation of osteoprogenitor cells into osteogenic cells (osteoblasts) occurs. Osteoblasts start laying down poorly mineralized new bone (osteoid) on the surface of the necrotic trabeculae,[24] while hematopoietic marrow elements accumulate within the graft.[10] By 12 weeks, cancellous bone chip grafts have the radiographic and histologic appearance of mature cancellous bone.[4] Eventually, the necrotic trabecular framework will be resorbed and remodeled via osteoclastic and osteoblastic activity. New bone may be remodeled in response to local stresses. Indeed, when cancellous bone grafts are used for filling of diaphyseal gaps, the remodeling process transforms cancellous bone into cortical bone. Osteogenic activity peaks around 6 to 8 weeks following transplantation, while "corticalization" of the graft in response to mechanical stresses requires up to 24 weeks.[24]

Nonvascularized Cortical Autografts

Two major differences exist between cancellous and cortical graft incorporation: (i) the rate of revascularization and (ii) the process of new bone formation. Whereas fresh cancellous autografts are revascularized as early as 1 week after surgery, vascular invasion of cortical autograft is postponed until 7 to 8 weeks.[25] This delay is due to the structure of cortical bone, with vascular penetration of the graft requiring peripheral osteoclastic resorption and vascular infiltration of Volkmann and Haversian canals.[14] In experimental studies, the resorptive activity was confined almost exclusively to the osteons, whereas resorption of interstitial lamellae was uncommon. As the Haversian canals reached a critical size, the resorptive process ceased in favor of new bone apposition.[10] By 8 weeks, only a third of the graft had been replaced with new bone, whereas the incorporation front showed increased porosity and the remaining core of the graft appeared as a necrotic mineralized matrix.[14,25] At 1 year, 40% of the original necrotic bone remained in cortical autografts.[14,19] It is not known whether the failure to repair nonosteonic lamellar bone persists indefinitely. It seems likely that the mixture of necrotic and viable bone in the cortical graft remains unaltered once the anabolic and catabolic stages of repair have been completed. Thus, cancellous grafts tend to be completely replaced by new bone, whereas cortical grafts remain as mixtures of necrotic and viable bone.[10] While consolidation of the host-graft interfaces with woven bone stabilizes the graft and allows vascular penetration into the cortex,[26] the delay between initial bone resorption and later bone deposition increases bone porosity at the incorporation front, locally reducing the strength of the graft by half between 6 and 24 weeks.[14,25] As a result, protection of the graft segment via rigid fixation is necessary for at least 6 to 12 months. Furthermore, in order to prevent graft site fractures, implant removal is not recommended.

Cortical bone autograft stabilization using rigid fixation favors its incorporation and influences the biologic events leading to its remodeling.[27] Lack of absolute stability at the host-graft interfaces delays graft incorporation. In a study using a canine ulnar diaphyseal segment model without stable internal fixation, only 22% percent were united at 12 weeks, 54% at 6 months and 66% at 1 year.[28] These results clearly contrast with another experimental study in which a cortical autograft was stabilized using internal fixation. By 3 months, both host-graft interfaces had healed.[26] Similarly another canine study showed that healing of a 4-centimeter femoral cortical autograft stabilized using rigid internal fixation was similar to bone healing under stable conditions.[27] New bone was deposited directly onto the surface of nonviable bone, and revascularization occurred from the recipient site medullary artery or a neonutrient artery traversing the cortical bone and reestablishing a medullary circulation. The graft was incorporated directly into the recipient site without local bone resorption and was used as a scaffold for new bone.[27] Incorporation, not resorption, was the prominent feature of the graft healing. Thus, resorption and replacement are not the fate of all devascularized cortical autografts.

Vascularized Cortical Autografts

A vascularized cortical graft involves bone that has been harvested with its nutrient artery and vein; the transplantation is obtained by transfer to another site with microvascular anastomosis of the two vessels. Incorporation of vascularized cortical autografts is achieved more predictably. Because the blood supply of the grafts is maintained, their incorporation may differ markedly from that of nonvascularized grafts. In particular, when the anastomosis is successful and the graft does not suffer intraoperative ischemia, up to 94% of osteocytes survive the transplantation procedure.[8] Such vascularized cortical grafts heal rapidly at the host-graft interface and their remodeling is similar to that of normal bone. Three months after surgery, vascularized grafts may be indistinguishable from normal bone.[25] Vascularized cortical grafts are stronger than nonvascularized grafts during the initial 6 weeks after transplantation because of the lack of resorption.[15] However, at 6 months, little difference exists in strength between vascularized and nonvascularized cortical autografts in the dog.[15] Although the vascularized cortical graft is not significantly weakened during the initial incorporation phase, appropriate internal fixation must be used until the graft can undergo hypertrophy in response to changes in local mechanical loading, according to Wolff's law. Although vascularized grafts are not commonly used in veterinary medicine owing to the financial challenges associated with the acquisition and maintenance of operating microscopes and microvascular instrumentation, vascularized grafts are better than nonvascularized grafts for large segmental bone defects.[12]

Incorporation of Cortical Allografts

Bone allografts have been used in human and veterinary surgery for decades and the histologic events in allograft incorporation have been well described.[9,10,16,18,20,26,29-35] The main differences between cortical autografts and cortical allografts are the slowness of incorporation, the process of revascularization, and the biologic events resulting from the immunogenicity of the graft.

Incorporation of cortical allografts occurs via healing at the host-graft interface, which involves the gradual formation of a callus extending from the host bone to the surface of the allograft without local resorption.[20,36] Union of the host-graft interface is generally obtained within 3 months,[26,31,37] although healing times may vary from 10 weeks to 37 weeks.[36] The principal determinants of host-graft union are stability of the construct and contact between host bone and the graft.[38] The process of revascularization and repair of the cortical allografts is controversial. In some studies, incorporation of cortical allografts followed a pattern similar to that seen with cortical autografts, albeit with slower and less extensive vascular penetration and slower new bone formation.[5,29,32] Revascularization and subsequent resorption were almost complete one year postoperatively, although a large amount of necrotic bone remained within the graft.[32] Other studies,[20,26,27,33] however, suggest that the pattern of revascularization and repair differs from that observed for cortical autografts involving the deposition of a thin layer of new bone (1 to 2 mm thick) over the necrotic cortex of the graft that remained intact. Whereas the outer bone was supplied by extraosseous vessels, the medullary cavity was avascular.[33] The repair process was slow, with less than 10% of the graft being incorporated at one year and only 20% at 5 1/2 years.[20] Although anecdotal reports have shown that a femoral cortical allograft can remain structurally intact for eight years and that it can assume the mechanical support of limb function for five years after plate removal,[33] from a mechanical standpoint, persistence of a large amount of necrotic bone in the allograft is likely to decrease strength in vivo over time. A 50% loss in allograft strength was noted after 10 years and was correlated with an increase in microfractures, probably related to mechanical stresses induced by weight bearing.[39] Because necrotic bone cannot repair itself, these microfractures may ultimately induce catastrophic allograft failure. In human medicine, the risk of these fractures (up to 19%) is significant in the third year after implantation.[40-42]

Immunogenicity of bone allografts has been demonstrated in experimental studies. The immunologic response of the host is predominantly a cell-mediated response to cell surface antigens carried by cells in the allograft, i.e., major histocompatability complex (MHC) class I and class II antigens. MHC class I antigens are found on all nucleated cells of the body and MHC class II antigens are expressed on the surface of macrophage-myeloid lineage cells, as well as osteoblasts.[43,44] Accordingly, because bone marrow cells represent a significant source of MHC I and MHC II antigens, removal of bone marrow in allografts is likely to decrease their immunogenicity.[45] Although both collagen and matrix can induce immune responses, they are considered relatively weak when compared with cell-mediated immunogenicity.[44] Evidence also exists that all types of allografts induce the production of graft-specific antibodies that can be detected as early as three weeks after transplantation.[46,47] Whereas the immune response depends on the MHC class I and class II disparities,[47] its duration and intensity also depend on graft treatment and size, with frozen mismatched allografts inducing a weaker response than fresh allografts.[46]

When the allografts are relatively small, the antidonor antibodies are detectable for a shorter period of time than when massive allografts are used.[47] Several studies on experimental animals have shown that the process of incorporation of bone allografts is negatively influenced by the degree of mismatch between major histocompatibility complex antigens.[29,30,35] However, even if antibodies are formed against bone allografts, no clear evidence exists that they are directly involved in the rejection process.[10] Despite the experimental evidence that allografts can induce a host immune reaction, the clinical significance of this reaction is unclear. In biopsy specimens obtained 9 to 78 months after transplantation of large frozen cortical allografts in humans, no clear relationship was demonstrated between the extent of graft incorporation and the degree of histocompatibility between graft and host.[48]

Although most cortical allografts heal via intramembranous bone formation, clinical and experimental studies have shown that incorporation and remodeling may vary extensively. Incorporation may involve complete revascularization, resorption, and repair,[29,32] or leave a large amount of necrotic bone, with biologic attachment of soft tissues to the allograft surface and good functional results for several years.[20,33] Similarly, remodeling may occur in response to mechanical stresses, according to Wolff's law.[9,49]

Incorporation of Processed Cortical Allografts

Allografts are often treated to decrease their immunogenicity and for long-term preservation. Such processing methods influence the degree of biologic reaction and/or mechanical properties. Freezing reduces the effects of histocompatibility mismatch and the biologic activity of the graft, most likely because of cellular destruction.[35] Likewise, freeze-drying reduces the graft immunogenicity,[16] but also substantially alters its material properties, making it more brittle[50] and susceptible to fractures.[37] Ethylene oxide (EO) sterilization allows storage of allografts for long periods of time and reduces the risk of infection from graft contamination. However, EO-sterilized bone develops structural alterations during storage at room temperature that decrease its compressive strength and screw pullout load.[51] Conversely, storage at -20°C for one year does not significantly modify a graft's resistance to compressive, bending, and torsional loads.[52] Although EO is an effective sterilization agent, it may have a deleterious effect on graft incorporation.[53-55]

Gamma irradiation is the most widely used method in human medicine. However, because irradiation alters collagen crosslinks[56] and destroys the bone matrix fibrillar network,[5] this process affects the material properties of the graft in a dose-dependent fashion.[50] Specifically, irradiation reduces graft strength and energy-absorbing capacity prior to failure.[57,58] However, experimental studies in rats have shown that low-dose irradiation followed by soaking in 70% ethanol and deep freezing does not compromise the natural course of graft incorporation.[59] Autoclaving induces protein denaturation, which significantly decreases the graft osteoinductive and osteoconductive properties.[11] Although experimental studies in dogs showed that autoclaved cortical autografts can be incorporated,[60] the process markedly delays incorporation.[5] In addition, a 43% complication rate has been associated with the use of autoclaved allografts in human medicine.[61] In an attempt to increase cortical graft revascularization, microperforations of the graft have been performed. Although a perforation pattern involving an array of 300 μm laser-made holes placed 3 mm apart did not significantly affect compression strength and flexural deformity,[62] perforation of cortical bone has been shown to substantially improve the amount of newly formed bone and enhance allograft incorporation.[63]

Incorporation of Osteochondral Grafts

Osteochondral grafts include shell grafts and massive grafts. Shell grafts include articular cartilage and 2 to eight mm of subchondral bone, and are generally used for joint resurfacing. Shell autografts are incorporated quickly and completely when fixation is adequate.[11] Bone healing is obtained within 3 months.[64-66] In fresh osteochondral autografts, articular cartilage remains viable. In an experimental study of mosaicplasty (multiple autologous osteochondral plugs implanted in articular cartilage defects) in dogs, host-graft cartilage interfaces healed with fibrocartilage; a continuity between graft and host cartilage was obtained as early as 16 weeks and maintained until 1 year.[67] Massive allogeneic osteochondral grafts are used to reconstruct joints in limb-sparing procedures after tumor resection. These grafts are composed of cortical bone, epiphyseal and metaphyseal cancellous bone, and articular cartilage. The pattern of bone incorporation is similar to that of bone allografts.[29] Although the cartilage of frozen osteochondral allografts undergoes significant cellular and structural alteration including chondrocyte death, thinning, and fibrillation,[68] it may provide adequate function for up to six years[55] before osteoarthritis becomes a problem.[42] Soft tissue including ligaments, tendons, and fascia may be firmly reattached to the surface of the allograft by a seam of appositional bone laid onto the graft.[55]

Use of Bone Grafts

The three principal indications for bone grafts are enhancement of bone healing, replacement of bone lost through trauma or surgical resection, and in joint surgery.

Cancellous Grafts

Cancellous bone autografts are the most commonly used bone grafts in veterinary orthopedics, particularly to enhance healing in the treatment of comminuted fractures of long bones. Biologic fracture stabilization can be achieved using: (i) an "open-but-do-not-touch" approach that permits viewing of the fracture fragments, realignment of the bone, and cancellous bone grafting.[69,70] or (ii) a closed reduction that involves alignment without surgically exposing the fracture site. Although any nonreconstructible fracture that requires open reduction and internal fixation may benefit from a cancellous autograft, use of minimally invasive techniques of fracture treatment, i.e., closed reduction without cancellous bone grafting, is more successful than open approaches.[71] In our experience, comminuted fresh fractures of long bones of dogs and cats treated with a minimally invasive approach and the use of a plate-rod construct without any cancellous graft heal successfully. Therefore, systematic use of cancellous bone autografts to enhance bone healing in comminuted fractures of long bones is questionable.

Treatment of delayed union or nonunion fractures includes the use of rigid fixation often associated with cancellous bone grafting. Although most nonunions are biologically viable and are adequately treated by rigid internal fixation with compression of bone fragments, fresh autologous cancellous bone packed into the nonunion site and around bone ends should be considered as part of the procedure. In biologically inactive nonunions, cancellous bone grafting is essential.[72] Another major indication for cancellous bone autografts is filling of bone defects after surgical excision of benign bone tumors or bone cysts, after debridement of open fractures, and following sequestrectomy in osteomyelitis. Regardless of the condition, the bone ends and the surrounding soft tissues must provide revascularization of the cancellous graft, and adequate stabilization must be achieved. If the soft tissue bed is poorly vascularized, delayed grafting is preferable to immediate grafting after debridement and wound lavage.[11]

Treatment of osteomyelitis requires excision of infected soft tissue and bone, which may result in significant bone loss, requiring filling of the defect with a bone graft or bone graft substitute. Because cortical grafts are likely to become infected and bone substitutes may act as foreign bodies, only fresh autologous cancellous bone should be used to fill such defects. However, because autologous cancellous bone undergoes significant resorption at the center of the graft,[73] cancellous bone autografts are usually not recommended for the treatment of large segmental bone defects.[73,74]

Masquelet et al [73] described a new procedure for the treatment of segmental defects using cancellous autografts. The first stage consisted of inserting a cement spacer into the defect.

This spacer has a mechanical role, preventing invasion of the recipient site with fibrous tissue, which may preclude further bone healing. It also has a biologic role, inducing formation of a richly vascularized pseudosynovial membrane around the cement plug. In the second stage, 1 month later, the membrane is incised and the cement spacer replaced with cancellous bone autograft, after which the membrane is sutured over the graft. This technique has been successfully used experimentally to treat large (3 cm) femoral diaphyseal and periosteal defects in sheep. In the group in which a cancellous graft was placed inside the induced membrane, the defects healed with restoration of the normal bone diameter. In contrast, graft resorption occurred in all animals when the autologous cancellous bone was placed after removal of the membrane.[73] This membrane, therefore, actively contributes to the revascularization of the bone graft, acting as an in situ delivery system for growth factors (VEGF, TGF-β) and osteoinductive factors (BMP-2).[73,75] In people, this technique allowed reconstruction of bone defects up to 25 cm in length.[75]

Joint arthrodesis requires stable fixation and use of cancellous bone graft (Figure 88-1). Several clinical reports and experimental studies have demonstrated the usefulness of autogenous cancellous graft in arthrodesis. Indeed, the use of autogenous cancellous graft has been shown to enhance the rate of new bone formation and joint fusion when compared with nongrafted joints, which allowed earlier removal of external coaptation devices.[76]

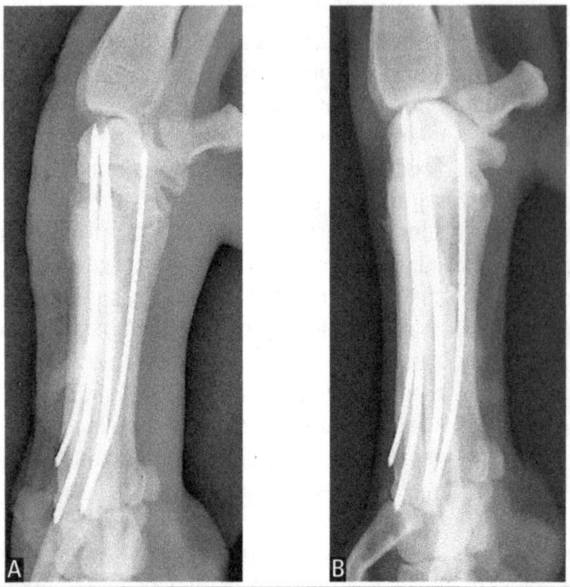

Figure 88-1. Partial carpal arthrodesis with a cancellous bone autograft. A: Day 0; B: follow up at 2 months showing graft incorporation and remodeling with complete bone fusion.

To optimize the incorporation and survival rate of graft osteogenic cells, fresh cancellous bone graft should be placed in the recipient site as soon as possible after being harvested. For example, storage of cancellous bone for three hours, using methods similar to those used for organ preservation, resulted in a 20% decrease in the number of viable cells.[6] Cancellous bone may be applied to the surgical site with or without compression. Compression of cancellous bone autograft does not enhance osteogenic capability[77] and may reduce the osteoconductive potential of the graft.[78] Although a larger quantity of autologous cancellous bone is often considered beneficial, overfilling does not enhance early osteogenesis and must be avoided if it necessitates the use of multiple harvest sites.[79] Small graft fragments (approximately 3 mm by 1 mm) have been shown to have the best rate of revascularization and the greatest rate of survival of osteogenic cells.[80]

Corticocancellous Grafts

Corticocancellous grafts obtained from the iliac crest or a rib may be used as either blocks or small chips. A block of corticocancellous graft may be used as a cortical graft in relatively small segmental defects (Figure 88-2). Whereas cortical bone provides mechanical support and volume expansion, cancellous bone enhances graft incorporation. Accordingly, corticocancellous grafts are often useful in neurosurgery to induce spinal fusion (e.g., in Wobbler syndrome) or when relatively large amounts of bone graft are required.[81] Incorporation of corticocancellous grafts is similar to that for cancellous bone grafts.

Cortical Grafts

Although cortical allografts have been widely used in the treatment of long-bone comminuted fractures in dogs and cats,[2,11,24,26,27,31-33,36,37,51,82,83] the recent increased reliance on biologic fracture-repair techniques have made the use of cortical grafts nearly obsolete. Cortical autografts may be used in opening wedge osteotomies to limit limb segment shortening in the treatment of angular deformities. A small piece of cortical bone is packed within the bone defect to provide mechanical support. With rigid fixation, incorporation of such a cortical autograft is obtained within 2 to 3 months. Cortical allografts, associated with autogenous fresh cancellous bone packed around the host-graft interfaces, are mainly used in limb-sparing surgeries for the treatment of bone tumors. Here, too, the use of distraction osteogenesis via bone transport or use of metal prostheses may contribute to the reduction of clinical use of cortical allografts.

Osteochondral Grafts

Neither massive osteochondral allografts nor mosaicplasty are routinely used in small animal surgery. Although massive osteochondral allografts could potentially be used in limb-salvage procedures, logistical difficulties in obtaining anatomically appropriate grafts to achieve good joint function makes the use of cortical allografts with arthrodesis a more effective option. Recession sulcoplasty (block or wedge) in the treatment of patellar luxation is the osteochondral autograft most commonly used in small animal surgery. With such an osteochondral autograft, healing between the grafted sulcus and the femoral condyle is generally complete by 10 weeks. The subchondral trabecular bone is slightly thickened and the articular cartilage of the graft is viable and appears histologically normal.[64]

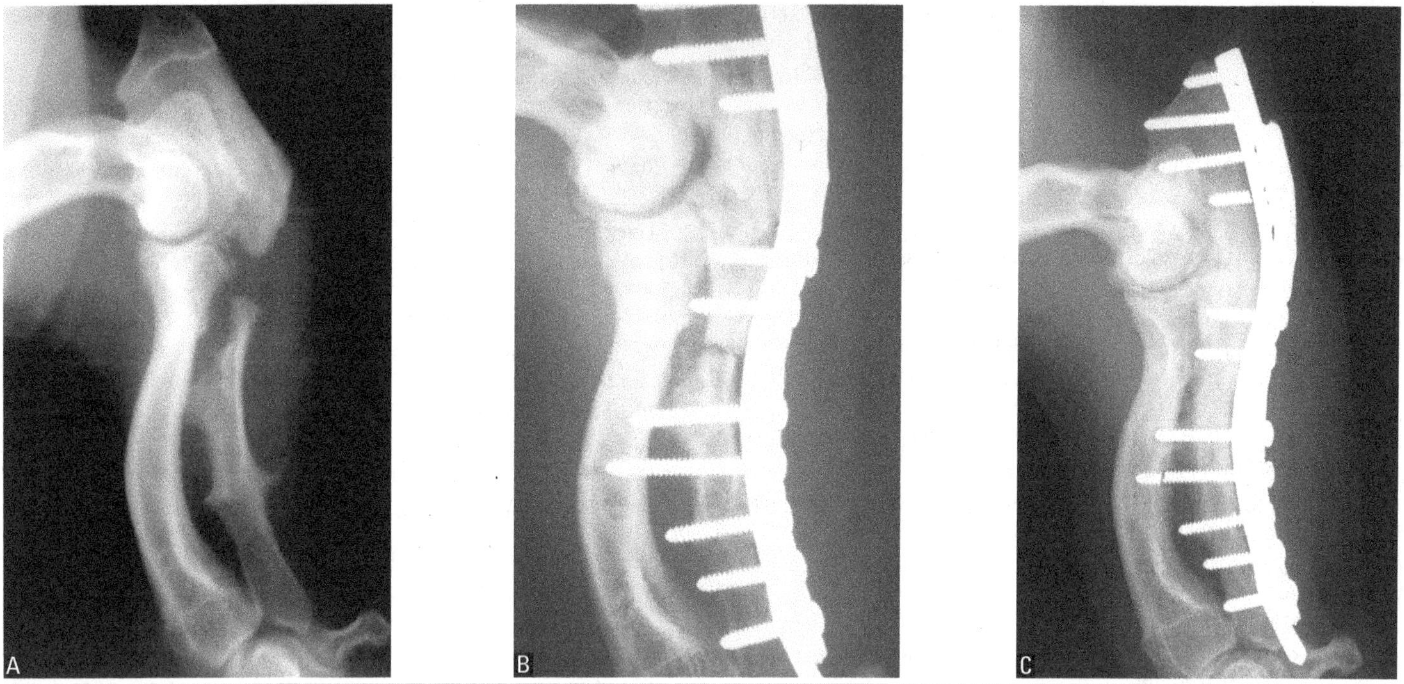

Figure 88-2. Use of a corticocancellous bone graft (iliac wing) for the treatment of a nonunion of the ulna. A: preoperative radiograph; B: postoperative radiograph; C: follow-up at 6 months.

References

1. Anker CJ, Holdridge SP, Baird B, et al: Ultraporous b-tricalcium phosphate is well incorporated in small cavitary defects. Clin Orthop Relat Res 434:251, 2005.

2. Millis DL, Martinez SA: Bone grafts. *In* Textbook of Small Animal Surgery. Slatter D (ed). Philadelphia: WB Saunders, 2003, p. 1875.

3. Sinibaldi KR: Bone grafting principles and techniques. *In* Current Techniques in Small Animal Surgery. Bojrab MJ, Ellison GW, Slocum B (eds). Baltimore: Williams & Wilkins, 1998, p. 901.

4. Wilson JW, Rhinelander FW, Stewart CL: Vascularization of cancellous chip bone grafts. Am J Vet Res 46(8):1691, 1985.

5. Brown KLB, Cruess RL: Bone and cartilage transpl antation in orthopaedic surgery. A review. J Bone Joint Surg 64-A(2):270, 1982.

6. McAnulty JF: Effect of various short-term storage methods on viability of cancellous bone fragments. Am J Vet Res 60(1):63, 1999.

7. Alexander JW: Bone grafting. Vet Clin North Am Small Anim Pract 17(4):811, 1987.

8. Doi K, Tominaga S, Shibata T: Bone grafts with microvascular anastomosis of vascular pedicles: an experimental study in dogs. J Bone Joint Surg 59-A(6):809, 1977.

9. Weiland AJ, Phillips TW, Randolph MA: Bone grafts: a radiologic, histologic, and biomechanical model comparing autografts, allografts, and free vascularized bone grafts. Plast Reconst Surg 74(3):368, 1984.

10. Burchardt H: The biology of bone graft repair. Clin Orthop Relat Res 174:28, 1983.

11. Stevenson S: Bone grafting. *In* Textbook of Small Animal Surgery. Slatter D (ed). Philadelphia: WB Saunders, 1993, p. 1694.

12. Finkemeier CG: Current concepts review - Bone-grafting and bone-graft substitutes. J Bone Joint Surg 84-A(3):454, 2002.

13. Cornell CN, Lane JM: Current understanding of osteoconduction in bone regeneration. Clin Orthop Relat Res 355S:S267, 1998.

14. Enneking WF, Burchardt H, Puhl JJ, et al: Physical and biological aspects of repair in dog cortical-bone transplants. J Bone Joint Surg 57-A(2):237, 1975.

15. Dell PC, Burchardt H, Glowczewskie FPJ: A roentgenographic, biomechanical, and histologic evaluation of vascularized and non-vascularized segmental fibular canine autografts. J Bone Joint Surg 67-A(1):105, 1985.

16. Friedlaender GE: Current concepts review - bone grafts. J Bone Joint Surg 69-A(5):786, 1987.

17. Bauer TW, Muschler GF: Bone graft materials - an overview of the basic science. Clin Orthop Relat Res 371:10, 2000.

18. Heiple KG, Chase SW, Herndon CH: A comparative study of the healing process following different types of bone transplantation. J Bone Joint Surg 45-A(8):1593, 1963.

19. Goldberg VM, Stevenson S: Natural history of autografts and allografts. Clin Orthop Relat Res 225:7, 1987.

20. Enneking WF, Mindell ER, Observations on massive retrieved human allografts. J Bone Joint Surg 73-A(8):1123, 1991.

21. Gould SE, Rhee JM, Tay BK-B, et al: Cellular contribution of bone graft to fusion. J Orthop Res 18(6):920, 2000.

22. Stevenson S, Hohn RB, Templeton JW: Effects of tissue antigen matching on the healing of fresh cancellous bone allografts in dogs. Am J Vet Res 44(2):201, 1983.

23. Weigel JP: Bone grafting. *In* Disease Mechanisms in Small Animal Surgery. Bojrab MJ (ed). Philadelphia: Lea & Febiger, 1993, p. 678.

24. Johnson AL: Principles of bone grafting. Semin Vet Med Surg (Small Anim), 6(1):90, 1991.

25. Goldberg VM, Stevenson S, Shaffer JW, et al: Biological and physical properties of autogenous vascularized fibular grafts in dogs. J Bone Joint Surg 72-A(6):801, 1990.

26. Johnson AL, Stein LE: Morphologic comparison of healing patterns in ethylene oxyde-sterilized cortical allografts and untreated cortical autografts in the dog. Am J Vet Res 49(1):101, 1988.

27. Wilson JW: Blood supply to developing, mature, and healing bone. *In* Bone in Clinical Orthopedics. Sumner-Smith G (ed). Stuttgart: Thieme, 2002, p.23.

28. Shaffer JW, Field GA, Goldberg VM, et al: Fate of vascularized and non-vascularized autografts. Clin Orthop Relat Res 197:32, 1985.

29. Stevenson S, Li XQ, Martin B: The fate of cancellous and cortical bone after transplantation of fresh and frozen tissue-antigen-matched and mismatched osteochondral allografts in dogs. J Bone Joint Surg 73-A(8):1143, 1991.

30. Bos GD, Goldberg VM, Powell AE, et al: The effect of histocompatibility matching on canine frozen bone allografts. J Bone Joint Surg 65-A(1):89, 1983.

31. Johnson AL, Shokry MM, Stein LE: Preliminary study of ethylene oxide sterilization of full-thickness cortical allografts used in segmental femoral fracture repair. Am J Vet Res 46(5): 1985.

32. Schena CJ, Graham DL, Hoefle WD: Segmental freeze-dried and fresh cortical allografts in the canine femur. II. A sequential histological comparison over a one-year time interval. J Am Anim Hosp Assoc 21:193, 1985.

33. Wilson JW, Hoefle WD: Diaphyseal allograft: eight-year evaluation in a dog. Vet Comp Orthop Trauma (3):78, 1990.

34. Stevenson S, Horowitz M: Current concepts review - the response to bone allografts. J Bone Joint Surg 74-A(6):939, 1992.

35. Stevenson S, Li XQ, Davy DT, et al: Critical biological determinants of incorporation of non-vascularized cortical bone grafts. J Bone Joint Surg 79-A(1):1, 1997.

36. Sinibaldi KR: Evaluation of full cortical allografts in 25 dogs. J Am Vet Med Assoc 194(11):1570, 1989.

37. Schena CJ, Mitten RW, Hoefle WD: Segmental freeze-dried and fresh cortical allografts in the canine femur. I. A sequential radiographic comparison over a one-year time interval. J Am Anim Hosp Assoc 20:911, 1984.

38. Stevenson S, Emery SE, Goldberg VM: Factors affecting bone graft incorporation. Clin Orthop Relat Res 324:66, 1996.

39. Wheeler DL, Enneking WF: Allograft bone decreases in strength in vivo over time. Clin Orthop Relat Res 435:36, 2005.

40. Berrey BH, Lord CF, Gebhardt MC, et al: Fractures of allografts. J Bone Joint Surg 72-A(6):825, 1990.

41. Thompson RC, Pickvance EA, Garry D: Fractures in large-segment allografts. J Bone Joint Surg 75-A(11):1663, 1993.

42. Mankin HJ, Gebhardt MC, Jennings C, et al: Long-term results of allograft replacement in the management of bone tumors. Clin Orthop Relat Res 324:86, 1996.

43. Chalmers J: Transplantation immunity in bone homografting. J Bone Joint Surg 41-B(1):160, 1959.

44. Friedlaender GE: Bone allografts: the biological consequences of immunological events. J Bone Joint Surg 73-A(8):1119, 1991.

45. Horowitz MC, Friedlaender GE: Induction of specific T-cell responsiveness to allogeneic bone. J Bone Joint Surg 73-A(8):1157, 1991.

46. Stevenson S: The immune response to osteochondral allografts in dogs. J Bone Joint Surg 69-A(4):573, 1987.

47. Stevenson S, Shaffer JW, Goldberg VM: The humoral response to vascular and nonvascular allografts of bone. Clin Orthop Relat Res 323:86, 1996.

48. Musculo DL, Caletti E, Schajowicz F, et al: Tissue-typing in human massive allografts of frozen bone. J Bone Joint Surg 69-A(4):583, 1987.

49. Kushner A: Evaluation of Wolff's law of bone formation. J Bone Joint Surg, 22(3):589, 1940.

50. Pelker RP, Friedlaender GE, Markham TC: Biomechanical properties of bone allografts. Clin Orthop Relat Res 174:54, 1983.

51. Roe SC, Pijanowski GJ, Johnson AL: Biomechanical properties of canine cortical bone allografts: effects of preparation and storage. Am J Vet Res 49(6):874, 1988.

52. Tshamala M, van Bree H, Mattheeuws D: Biomechanical properties of ethylene oxyde sterilized and cryopreserved cortical bone allografts. Vet Comp Orthop Trauma 7:25, 1994.

53. Johnson AL, Eurell JA, Schaeffer DJ: Evaluation of canine cortical bone graft remodeling. Vet Surg 21(4):293, 1992.

54. Thorén K, Aspenberg P: Ethylene oxyde sterilization impairs allograft incorporation in a conduction chamber. Clin Orthop Relat Res 318:259, 1995.

55. Stevenson S: Biology of bone grafts. Orthop Clin North Am 30(4):543, 1999.

56. Lietman SA, Tomford WW, Gebhardt MC, et al: Complications of irradiated allografts in orthopaedic tumor surgery. Clin Orthop Relat Res 375:214, 2000.

57. Hamer AJ, Strachan JR, Black MM, et al: Biomechanical properties of cortical allograft bone using a new method of bone strength measurement: a comparison of fresh, fresh-frozen and irradiated bone. J Bone Joint Surg 78-B(3):363, 1996.

58. Currey JD, Foreman J, Laketic I, et al: Effects of ionizing radiation on the mechanical properties of human bone. J Orthop Res 15(1):111, 1997.

59. Jinno T, Miric A, Feighan J, et al: The effects of processing and low dose irradiation on cortical bone grafts. Clin Orthop Relat Res 375:275, 2000.

60. Coupland BR: Experimental bone grafting in the canine: the use of autoclaved autogenous normal tibial bone. Can Vet J 10(6):170, 1969.

61. Asada N, Tsuchiya H, Kitaoka K, et al: Massive autoclaved allografts and autografts for limb salvage surgery. Acta Orthop Scand 68(4):392, 1997.

62. Lewandrowski K-U, Bonassar L, Uhthoff HK: Mechanical properties of perforated and partially demineralized bone grafts. Clin Orthop Relat Res 353:238, 1998.

63. Delloye C, Simon P, Nyssen-Behets C, et a:, Perforations of cortical bone allografts improve their incorporation. Clin Orthop Relat Res 396:240, 2002.

64. Boone EG, Hohn RB, and Weisbrode SE: Trochlear recession wedge technique for patellar luxation: an experimental study. J Am Anim Hosp Assoc 19:735, 1983.

65. Desjardins MR, Hurtig MB, Palmer NC: Incorporation of fresh and cryopreserved bone in osteochondral autografts in the horse. Vet Surg 20(6):446, 1991.

66. Van Vetchen BJ, Vasseur PB, Rodrigo JJ, et al: A comparison of four different methods of fixation of osteochondral fragments. Vet Comp Orthop Trauma 6:80, 1993.

67. Hangody L, Kish G, Kárpáti Z, et al: Autogenous osteochondral graft technique for replacing knee cartilage defects in dogs. Orthopedics, 5(3):175, 1997.

68. Stevenson S, Dannucci GA, Sharkey NA, et al: The fate of articular cartilage after transplantation of fresh and cryopreserved tissue-antigen-matched and mismatched osteochondral allografts in dogs. J Bone Joint Surg 71-A(9):1297, 1989.

69. Johnson AL, Hulse DA: Fundamentals of orthopedic surgery and fracture management. In Small Animal Surgery. Fossum TW (ed). St Louis: Mosby, 2002, p. 821.

70. Houlthon JEF, Dunning D: Perioperative patient management. *In* AO Principles of Fracture Management in the Dog and Cat. Johnson AL, Houlthon JEF, Vannini R (eds).. Stuttgart: Thieme, 2005, p. 1.

71. Leunig M, Hertel R, Siebenrock KA, et al: The evolution of indirect reduction techniques for the treatment of fractures. Clin Orthop Relat Res 375:7, 2000.

72. Rovesti GL: Nonunions. *In* AO Principles of Fracture Management in the Dog and Cat. Johnson AL, Houlthon JEF, Vannini R (eds). Stuttgart: Thieme, 2005, p. 402.

73. Masquelet AC, Fitoussi F, Muller GP: Reconstruction des os longs par membrane induite et autogreffe spongieuse. Ann Chir Plast Esthét: 45:346, 2000.

74. Pelissier P, Martin D, Baudet J, et al: Behavior of cancellous bone graft placed in induced membranes. Br J Plast Surg 55:596, 2002.

75. Pelissier P, Masquelet AC, Bareille R, et al: Induced membranes secrete growth factors including vascular and osteoinductive factors and could stimulate bone regeneration. J Orthop Res 22(1):73-79, 2004.

76. Johnson KA, Bellenger CR: The effects of autologous bone grafting on bone healing after carpal arthrodesis in the dog. Vet Rec 107:126, 1980.

77. Martinez SA, Probst CW, Hauptman JG, et al: Effects of fixed compression load on the osteogenic effect of autogenous cancellous bone grafts in dogs. Am J Vet Res 53(12):2381, 1992.

78. Tägil M, Aspenberg P: Impaction of bone grafts impairs osteoconduction in titanium chambers. Clin Orthop Relat Res. 352:231, 1998.

79. DeVries WJ, Runyon CL, Martinez SA: Effect of volume variations on osteogenic capabilities of autogenous cancellous bone graft in dogs. Am J Vet Res 57(10):1501, 1996.

80. Renegar WR: Autogenous cancellous bone grafts. *In* Current Techniques of Veterinary Surgery. Bojrab MJ (ed). Philadelphia: Lea & Febiger, 1983, p. 742.

81. Culvenor JA, Parker RJ: Collection of cortico-cancellous bone graft from the ilium using an acetabular reamer. J Small Anim Pract 37:513, 1996.

82. Bloomberg MS, Goring RL: Frozen diaphyseal bone allografts combined with external and internal pin splintage in small animal orthopedic surgery. J Am Anim Hosp Assoc 20:393, 1984.

83. Dueland RT, Trotter EJ, Aron DN, et al: Cryopreserved intercalary bone allografts: early experience (1975-1980) in eight canine cases. J Am Anim Hosp Assoc 25:305, 1989.

Chapter 89

Bone Substitutes

André Autefage
Loïc M. Dejardin

Rationale for Bone Substitutes

The ability of the skeletal system to heal is remarkable. When bone healing is impaired, however, the use of various types of bone grafts including cancellous autografts, vascularized cortical autografts, and cortical allografts, or bone transport techniques has been recommended. Owing to limitations inherent in each technique, the search for bone substitutes remains a medical necessity and has been the subject of extensive research.

Cancellous bone autografts, while considered the gold standard for bone repair, are fraught with limitations, including donor site morbidity (infection, pain, hematoma), limited availability, and high cost owing to increased surgical time. The impact of such limitations is exacerbated if several harvesting sites are required to obtain a sufficient graft volume. Furthermore, cancellous bone autografts are poorly suited for the treatment of segmental defects because of their tendency to undergo central resorption in cortical defects larger than 4 to 5 cm in people and ~3 cm in dogs.[1,2] Vascularized bone transplant, routinely used in specialized human surgical units, requires a major microsurgical operative procedure and a sophisticated infrastructure. Therefore, this technique is rarely used in veterinary medicine. Conversely, cortical allografts are widely used with many successes reported in both the human and veterinary orthopedic literature.[3-11] However, limited supply, high cost of bone banking, risk of rejection, and compromised mechanical properties make the continued reliance on cortical allografts a serious concern.[12,13] The early attraction of distraction osteogenesis techniques has been somewhat mitigated by their shortcomings including local morbidity, limited response of soft tissues to distraction, and cumbersome follow-ups.

Therefore, a critical need exists to develop artificial bone substitutes to act as replacements for biologic bone grafts. The ideal bone substitute should be biocompatible, osteoconductive, osteoinductive, osteogenic, structurally similar to the bone to be replaced, easy to use, and affordable.[14] Further, it is advantageous if the bone substitute is also bioresorbable; however, this is not a limiting factor.

Properties of a Bone Substitute

An **osteoconductive** material promotes bone apposition on its surface and functions as a three-dimensional scaffold supporting vascular and cellular ingrowth, leading to new bone formation. An **osteoinductive** scaffold material provides a biologic stimulus that induces the recruitment and differentiation of host and transplanted cells into osteoprogenitor cells and then into osteoblasts. An **osteogenic** material contains living cells directly capable of new bone formation. Bioactivity is defined as the ability of a material to develop a strong, direct bond with the neighboring bone tissue, without the formation of the fibrous interface typically induced by an implanted foreign body.[13]

Approaches to Bone Substitutes

The use of bone substitutes, or more generally, bone tissue engineering, is based on three strategies: (i) matrix-based approaches, (ii) cell-based approaches, and (iii) factor-based approaches.

Matrix-Based Approaches

Matrix-based approaches utilize structural scaffolds to replace the missing bone. Consequently, repair of osseous tissue depends on the recruitment of endogenous osteoprogenitor cells. Optimally, these tissue-engineered scaffolds have a porous structure that facilitates bony ingrowth; however, their lack of biologic activity can limit their use.

Biomaterials

Calcium Phosphate Ceramics

Calcium phosphate (CaP) ceramics are inorganic synthetic materials with no inherent osteoinductive or osteogenic properties. Because of their osteoconductive behavior in vivo, they have been shown to induce a biologic response similar to that of bone and are therefore deemed bioactive materials. For example, when implanted into healthy bone, osteoid and, subsequently, new bone are produced directly onto the surface of the CaP ceramic without any soft tissue interface. Calcium phosphate ceramics are extremely strong in compression but are also brittle and possess poor tensile strengths. Calcium phosphate scaffolds should be tightly packed in rigidly stabilized bone in order to protect them from shear and tensile stresses as well as to optimize bone incorporation.[15]

Hydroxyapatite ($Ca_{10}(PO_4)_6(OH)_2$, HA) is structurally similar to the apatite found in normal human bone and, along with beta tricalcium phosphate ($Ca_3(PO_4)_2$, β-TCP), is the most highly biocompatible and widely used calcium phosphate bioceramic. However, the behavior of HA and β-TCP after implantation is slightly different. The rate of biodegradation of β-TCP is much greater than that of HA. As β-TCP is resorbed, new bone formation fills the area once occupied by the β-TCP scaffold.[16] In contrast, biodegradation of HA is slow and although it may be osteointegrated, fragments may still be present in the bone several years after implantation. When β-TCP was implanted in a canine metaphysis, no inflammatory response occurred and direct bone apposition was noted at 4 to 6 weeks.[17] Because of its biocompatibility and bioresorbability, β-TCP is used as a filling material in defects where autografts are indicated or as a bone expander supplementing autologous cancellous bone grafts. The biocompatibility of HA has also been demonstrated in vivo, where incorporation occurs without inducing an inflammatory or foreign body response.[18] By three weeks, the HA surface is lined with fibroblasts and osteoblasts with an interposition layer of mineralized osteoid laid down directly by osteoblasts.[16] The precise chemical composition of macroporous CaP ceramics influences their osteointegration capability. Significant differences in the amount of new bone were observed depending on the ratio of HA to β-TCP in biphasic CaP (BCP) mixtures, where BCPs containing a higher volume of β-TCP induced better osteointegration when compared with pure HA ceramics.[19]

Calcium phosphate materials are osteoconductive but usually not osteoinductive. Under some conditions, however, CaP scaffolds may acquire osteoinductive properties owing to the binding of an optimum amount of endogenous bone morphogenetic protein (BMP) to the material.[13,20] This indirect osteoinductive property depends on both the type of CaP ceramic with different phasic composition and porous structure and the species of animal in which it is implanted.[20] When a BCP scaffold was implanted intramuscularly and subcutaneously, obvious bone formation was detected in dogs and pigs, but no bone formation was observed in rabbits, goats, and rats.[20]

CaP Cement

Calcium phosphate materials may also be used as bone cement. In an injectable bone cement, including particles of a BCP (60/40 HA/β-TCP) incorporated in a methyl cellulose carrier gel, bone ingrowth proceeded at a greater rate than in BCP blocks alone.[21] However, the major drawback of this system is the lack of significant initial mechanical properties, which imposes the requirement of an additional method of bone stabilization and leads to difficulty in maintaining the composite within the defect during surgery. To address these concerns, ceramic pastes may be used. This type of injectable CaP solidifies in situ after several minutes via a nonexothermic reaction to form a high compressive strength material. In the metaphysis of long bone in dogs, a cement composed of a monocalcium phosphate monohydrate, β-TCP and $CaCO_3$, was both osteoconductive and biocompatible. At 2 weeks, extensive apposition of woven bone and unmineralized osteoid had occurred on the cement, without interposition of fibrous tissue between bone and cement.[22] However, only a small proportion of the volume of this cement was resorbed and replaced by bone during the first 16 weeks. At 78 weeks, cement was not totally resorbed.[22]

The strength of macroporous CaP ceramics having interconnected porosity may be improved by filling the pores with a CaP cement. Using a highly soluble, self-setting calcium phosphate cement made of β-TCP and dicalcium phosphate dihydrate, it has been demonstrated that all the cement is replaced by bone after 4 months. Filling the macroporous ceramic pores with the CaP cement significantly improved the mechanical strength of these ceramics without modifying their integration in the healing bone or its biocompatibility.[23]

Coralline Hydroxyapatite

Coralline hydroxyapatite is a natural material derived from sea coral. Certain sea coral species produce a CaP porous structure that is close to normal human bone structure. Coralline substitutes may be natural, e.g., directly harvested from the sea or manufactured by conversion from natural coral. It is processed by a hydrothermal chemical exchange method that converts the coral calcium carbonate to a crystalline material. Goniopora and Porites species of sea coral may be used as biomaterials. Coralline HA-Goniopora has larger macropores, measuring 600 μm in diameter as well as 260-μm intercommunicating pores, a structure close to typical cancellous bone. In contrast, with smaller 230-μm macropores and 190-μm intercommunicating pores, the structure of coralline HA-Porites is similar to that of cortical bone.[24]

Coralline HA has a completely continuous three-dimensional pore structure with a high degree of uniformity in both macro- and micropore size. Coralline HA exhibits many of the criteria for a functional bone graft substitute: it is readily available, is easily contoured, has an adequate compressive strength, and allows ingrowth of new bone. However, no evidence exists of rapid degradation.[16]

Bioactive Glasses

Bioactive glasses are materials consisting of calcium, phosphorus, and silicone dioxide. They possess osteointegrative and osteoconductive properties. Their mechanical strengths are significantly greater than porous CaP ceramics. However, when drilling or shaping, they are susceptible to fracture and consequently are difficult to fix to the bone. Therefore, they are primarily used for filling bone cavities instead of as segmental bone replacements. Bioglasses have also found use as bone-graft expanders.[25]

Demineralized Bone Matrix

Demineralized bone matrix (DBM) is produced by acid extraction of the bone mineral phase. The preservation of the organic phase of the bone matrix confers DBM with some osteoconductive and osteoinductive properties. The osteoinductive capacity of DBM has been demonstrated by Urist.[26] Demineralized bone matrix has poor biomechanical strength and can have variable osteoinductive capability depending on the processing steps, the sterilization method, and the final formulation.[27] To date, the true osteoinductive potential of DBM, in humans, has been challenged because ectopically implanted DBM is not capable of reliably inducing bone formation.

Bone formation that takes place directly on DBM may start during the inflammatory phase of healing, indicating early differentiation and osteoblast activity. During this early phase of healing, osteoprogenitor cells are recruited from the bone marrow, the endosteum, the periosteum, and/or the vasculature.[28] This osteoinductive ability of DBM may be attributed to the presence of BMP 2 and BMP 7.[29] Growth factors such as insulin-like growth factors-1 (IGF-1) and transforming growth factor-beta 1 (TGF-β 1) have also been found in DBM.[30] Early new bone formation is also related to the osteoconductive capacity of DBM that allows osteoblast precursors to adhere to a collagen matrix similar to endogenous cortical bone matrix. Indeed, the surface of DBM looks like the surface of the injured bone, which is the site of bone deposition during healing.[28] A final advantage of DBM is its rapid resorption rate.

Polymer Composites

Polymer composites with CaP ceramics (HA and β-TCP), particularly polylactic (PLA) and/or polyglycolic acid (PGA), have been investigated. Generally, these composites are used as delivery vehicles or carriers for growth factors.

Porosity

Scaffolds for osteogenesis should mimic bone morphology, structure, and function in order to optimize integration into surrounding tissue. Pores are necessary for bone tissue formation because they allow migration and proliferation of osteoblasts and other mesenchymal cells, as well as vascularization via micropore channels. Some controversy exists in the literature over the optimum pore size for bone tissue engineering scaffolds. For coralline HA, scaffolds containing larger pores (~500 μm) have been associated with greater bone ingrowth than implants with smaller pore size (200 μm).[24] Similarly, when using macroporous biphasic CaP ceramics, it was shown that implants having larger, 565-μm sized pores, provided more abundant newly formed bone than those with smaller, 300-μm sized, pores.[30] Although pore sizes of approximately 100 μm are sufficient to allow cell migration into the implant, capillary invasion of the scaffold, which is essential to enhance new bone formation, requires pore sizes of 300 μm or greater. Indeed, while smaller pores (90-120 μm) may induce hypoxic conditions leading to osteochondral formation before osteogenesis, larger pores (~350 μm) will promote a more effective neoangiogenesis, leading to direct osteogenesis.[31,32] Interestingly, in some studies, the morphology of bone-formation porous HA blocks with 300 to 400 μm pores resembled that of the Haversian system in bone remodeling. This pore size coincides with the average diameter in the Haversian system (approximately 300 μm), indicating that the optimal pore size for bioceramic scaffolds should closely mimic the pore size of normal bone.[31]

Implant-Host Interactions

Biointegration of a bioceramic scaffold implant depends on its mechanical stabilization. Micromotion favors the formation of fibrous tissue and precludes biointegration even if the implant is bioactive, like CaP ceramics.[33] For CaP bioceramics, a strong chemical similarity exists between HA and the bone mineral crystals. These materials have the capability to initiate nucleation and crystal growth of CaP at their surface from biologic fluids by a dissolution/precipitation process. Thus, a layer of nanocrystalline carbonated apatite associated with specific bone proteins is deposited onto the CaP ceramic and enables osteoblast adhesion and activity.[33] This process is similar to bone remodeling. The neoformed layer would present a composition analogous to the cement line at the edge of an osteon.[33] Thus, the bond between implant and bone is strong and mechanical tests demonstrate that 4 weeks after implantation, fractures occurred within HA ceramic and not at the implant-bone interface.[34]

When a bioactive material is implanted, inside the connective tissue that has replaced the initial hematoma osteoblasts differentiate in close proximity to the biomaterial. Such osteoblasts are immobilized at the material surface as they would be at the surface of bone trabeculae. Owing to the polar activity of these cells, the extracellular matrix is synthesized by the cell pole in contact with the material, leading to the deposition of an osteoid matrix at the material surface. Both the immature bone formed in contact with the material and the scaffold itself are subject to remodeling and are subsequently degraded by osteoclasts and giant cells. New bone gradually replaces the de novo bone material, leading to osteointegration.

Incorporation

At 24 weeks following implantation of small cylinders of several types of ceramics into rabbit cortical bone, there was no degradation of coralline HA-Goniopora, 27% degradation of coralline HA-Porites, and 46% degradation of β-TCP. New bone occupied 56% of the coralline HA-Goniopora implant, 53% of coralline HA-Porites, and 45% of the β-TCP implant.[24] In large segmental diaphyseal defects, HA and β-TCP alone are not suitable as bone substitutes. In a 2.5-cm long segmental canine radial defect, use of these ceramics resulted in nonunions in many of the limbs 24 weeks postoperatively. In contrast, all the defects filled with autologous cancellous bone grafts achieved union.[35] This study clearly showed the limits of the inherent osteoconductive or osteoinductive capability of CaP ceramics. Osteointegration leading to healing of the bone defect requires active participation of host cells and a favorable recipient site environment that provides osteoprogenitor cells and neovascularization of the implant. In epiphyseal or metaphyseal cavities of relative small volume, CaP ceramics alone may be integrated because (i) packing of the ceramic may induce mechanical stabilization of the material, and (ii) the neighboring cancellous bone is well vascularized and contains mesenchymal stem cells capable of osteoblastic differentiation. In large segmental diaphyseal defects, the behavior may be different because (i) mechanical stabilization is difficult to obtain, and (ii) the recipient site is not capable of providing osteoprogenitor cells in a sufficient quantity to completely colonize the implant. With porous scaffold materials, osteogenic cells do not differentiate homogeneously within the biomaterial. The thickness of the scaffold may be critical as it may impair revascularization at the center of the biomaterial and, therefore, limit cell survival. Moreover, the number of cells supplied by the granulation tissue may be inadequate in the central area of extensive defects because of the remoteness of source tissues.[36]

Cell-Based Approaches

Cell-based therapies entail transferring cells that have osteogenic potential directly to the repair site to facilitate synthesis of new bone, thereby reducing the reliance on local osteoprogenitors. These cell-based strategies rely on the implantation of (i) fresh autologous bone marrow, (ii) purified, culture-expanded mesenchymal stem cells (MSCs), or (iii) differentiated osteoblasts. Mesenchymal stem cells and progenitor cells are present in almost all normal tissues. Stem cells are resting cells that can be activated by biochemical signals to divide and differentiate. This cell division provides two daughter cells that are not identical: one daughter cell returns to the original resting state of the mother cell while the second daughter cell proliferates, producing an abundance of progenitor cells. These progenitors are subsequently triggered to differentiate to form a mature tissue.[37] A heterogeneous population of cells, including actual stem cells and progenitors derived from these cells, is present in bone marrow, periosteum, bone trabeculae (within Haversian canals of cortical bone), adipose tissue, and muscle.

Of all potential sources of progenitor cells, the most readily available is the bone marrow, which can be harvested via percutaneous aspiration or as a small core of cancellous bone. Pluripotent progenitor cells may evolve according to several pathways such as cells from liver tissue, central nervous system tissue, or osteoblasts. The differentiation of these cells down one pathway depends on their biologic environment and is influenced by factors such as oxygen tension, nutrient concentration, neighboring cells, mechanical stimuli, and the chemical composition of the surrounding extracellular matrix.[37] In addition, the osteoblastic differentiation pathway is modulated by a broad range of inducible factors, such as IGF and members of the TGF-β superfamily, including BMP-2 and BMP-7.[37]

When a cell-matrix composite graft is used, it is essential to ensure that the environment created by the matrix, i.e., surface texture, pore size and geometry, three-dimensional architecture, and degradation properties, is compatible with the survival of the cells.[37] It is also important to consider the biologic environment of the implanted bone substitute. The survival of implanted cells depends on the capacity for oxygen and other nutrients to diffuse into and out of the site through the implant. Bone marrow harvested by aspiration contains on average from 350 to 1000 progenitors cells per milliliter.[38,39] Mesenchymal stem cells appear to be present at a frequency of approximately 1 in 10^5 to 10^6 nucleated marrow cells.[39,40] An increase in the volume of bone marrow aspirate from 1 to 4 ml decreases the concentration of progenitor cells by 50%. Thus, it has been suggested that, in humans, the maximum number of progenitor cells may be obtained in four 1-ml aliquots rather than in one 4-ml aliquot.[38] Aspirates of bone marrow may be mixed with carriers, such as CaP ceramics or DBM, and this composite graft packed into bone defects. Use of the composite bone marrow-DBM in canine nonunions has been shown to induce healing at a rate at least equal, if not superior, to that obtained using standard autologous bone grafting techniques.[41] The addition of bone marrow aspirate to HA or β-TCP dramatically improved the outcome of these scaffold implants in the treatment of experimentally induced segmental radial defect in dogs.[35] The biomechanical and radiographic parameters of β-TCP with bone marrow were roughly comparable to those of cancellous bone autografts at 12 and 24 weeks. At 12 weeks, 94% of defects filled with CaP augmented with bone marrow achieved union, whereas nonunion was observed in 90% of defects filled with CaP alone.[35] It has been estimated that the number of osteoprogenitors provided by bone marrow aspirates is only 20% of what would be needed to permit colonization of the entire implant by new bone;[37] however, it is possible to improve the efficacy of aspirated bone marrow by concentrating the marrow-derived cells.

Centrifugal density separation yields an approximately 4-fold concentration of marrow-derived cells, which has been shown to significantly increase bone formation.[42] Mesenchymal cells can be isolated from bone marrow and expanded ex vivo without any apparent modification in phenotype or loss of function.[43] Using culture systems, ex vivo expansion produces a significant increase in the number of MSCs that can be delivered back to the surgical site.[43] With a ceramic carrier, cultured MSCs promote faster and more extensive new bone formation than fresh bone marrow because of the 300-fold increase in the number of MSCs yielded by the culture expansion process.[44] In a critical-sized canine ulnar defect stabilized by internal fixation, porous HA beads loaded with cultured cells from cancellous bone cores were implanted. Invasion by bone tissue was found in the stromal cell-bearing implants but not in control implants containing only HA granules.[36,45] Similarly, when BCP cylinders augmented with cultured mesenchymal stem cells from bone marrow aspirates were implanted in a critical-sized (21 mm) canine femoral defect stabilized by internal fixation, bone healing was achieved in 12 to 16 weeks. In contrast, no substantial bone regeneration occurred over the 16 week period when ceramic cylinders alone were implanted.[44] Under appropriate culture conditions, these MSCs may differentiate into osteoprogenitor cells and grow as a monolayer culture. Next, the matrix may be loaded with these cells and implanted, constituting a hybrid bone substitute. Marrow cells grown in primary culture for 10 days and transferred to porous coralline HA for a 2-week culture have shown an enhanced rate and extent of bone formation when compared with samples implanted with undifferentiated marrow cells.[46]

Factor-Based Approaches

Factor-based therapies represent an attempt to overcome the limitation of ceramic scaffold implants used alone by directly providing osteoinductive stimuli. Growth and differentiation factors are carried by the implant that is inserted into the bone defect.

Growth factors and Bone Morphogenetic Proteins (BMPs)

Fibroblast growth factors (FGFs) play a role in angiogenesis and mesenchymal cell mitogenesis. Activity of both FGF-1 and FGF-2 has been identified during the early stages of fracture healing. Using basic FGF in tibia osteotomies in dogs accelerated all the stages of bone repair and stimulation of callus remodeling.[47] It is unclear what the therapeutic role of other growth factors such as insulin-like growth factor and platelet-derived growth factor play in fracture healing.[48] Among the growth factors that have been investigated, BMPs, which are members of the TGF-β superfamily, appear to have the most osteoinductive potential. Bone morphogenetic proteins initiate the bone healing cascade through the recruitment of mesenchymal cells from local bone and soft tissues and also guide the differentiation of mesenchymal cells into osteoblasts. To date, more than 15 BMPs have been described, but only a few seem active in the bone healing process[49] (Figure 89-1). Two BMPs are produced by recombinant gene technology and are commercially available: BMP-2 and BMP-7 (also known as OP-1). In veterinary medicine, experimental studies in dogs and clinical trials in dogs and cats have been performed to assess the efficacy of BMPs in the treatment of bone defects,[50,51] fracture nonunions, and arthrodesis.[52]

The efficacy of BMPs was evaluated in the healing of a critical-sized radial defect (2.5 cm) in dogs. In one study, the defect was filled with a cylinder of natural coral (calcium carbonate) alone or enhanced with bovine-derived bone protein and compared to autologous cancellous bone graft.[50] Coral alone did not allow bone union whereas coral implants enhanced with bone protein achieved rates of union, bone formation, and biomechanical

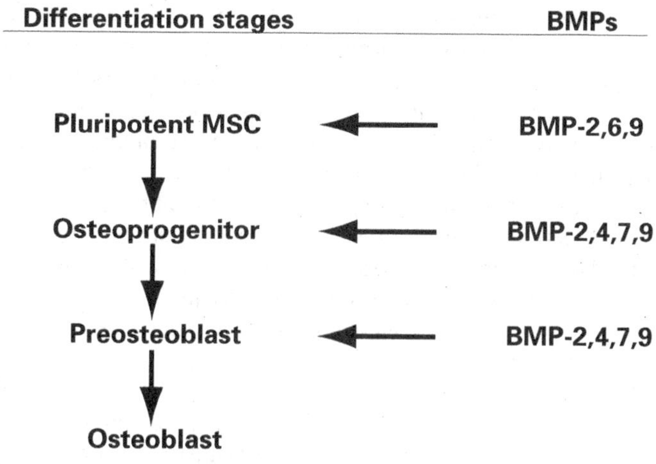

Figure 89-1. Main BMPs involved in the process of differentiation of Mesenchymal Stem Cells (MSC).

strength that were superior during the first 12 weeks, and comparable at 24 weeks with those of autogenous cancellous bone graft. In subsequent study, the effectiveness of recombinant human BMP-2 (rhBMP-2), delivered in a collagen sponge, was evaluated in the same segmental defect model in dogs.[51] None of the defects that were treated with a collagen carrier alone healed. From the day of surgery to 12 weeks postoperatively, the rhBMP-2 implants produced bone at a rate equivalent to cancellous bone autograft and were biomechanically comparable. However, defects treated with rhBMP-2 showed evidence of cyst-like bone voids, whose incidence appeared to be dose-related. The specific mechanism by which these voids developed was not determined, but it clearly appears that further research for the optimal dose of rhBMP-2 protein is needed prior to clinical applications. A nonglycosylated rhBM2/fibrin composite was applied in 41 sites in 38 dogs and cats requiring an arthrodesis or revision surgery for fracture nonunions.[52] Bone healing was obtained in 90% of the treated cases with rhBMP-2. Although cancellous bone autografts are the gold standard for the treatment of these clinical conditions, the number of animals showing radiographic bridging in pancarpal arthrodesis was higher in the group treated with rhBMP-2 than in the group treated with autografts at 17 weeks (100% vs. 59%).[53,54] Similar results have been obtained in the experimental treatment of segmental defects in animal models.

Gene Therapy

Gene therapy involves the transfer of genetic information to cells. When a gene is properly transferred to a target cell, the cell synthesizes the protein encoded by the gene. In general, the duration of protein synthesis depends on the technique used to transfer the gene to the cell. Gene therapy can be applied either systemically or regionally. For bone healing, in normal patients, gene therapy can be used regionally. The gene can be introduced directly to an anatomic site with use of an in vivo technique, or it can be introduced via an ex vivo approach. In ex vivo gene delivery, cells are harvested from the patient, the cDNA is transferred to the cells in tissue culture and the genetically modified cells are then administered back to the patient.

Appropriate vectors must be used to enhance the entry and expression of DNA into target cells. These vectors may be of viral or nonviral origin. Viruses are efficient vectors because DNA delivery is a critical aspect of their life cycle. However, several major concerns are related to the use of viral vectors. First, the possibility exists of recombination with other viruses in the host cell as well as replication and multiplication in the patient. Second, the duration of transgene product (protein) expression by the transduced cells may be limited owing to immune response to viral proteins.[48] Finally, the risk of malignant transformation following viral integration into the host genome is a serious concern.[55]

Gene therapy is considered as a tool in the treatment of bone defects because of the possibility of upregulating more biologic expression of individual proteins in specific tissues and cells. Although proteins used in bone tissue engineering can be manufactured, their life span is relatively short after being injected or surgically placed at the target site. Gene therapy provides the gene for the desired protein and then the transfected cells produce a biologically active protein in situ. This technique results in a higher and more constant level of protein production when compared with manufactured proteins. This is particularly important for proteins such as the BMPs.[56] One review reports the results of experimental and clinical studies evaluating use of growth factors using gene therapy for enhancing fracture healing.[57] Although the production of the protein has a relatively short duration (e.g., up to 6 weeks) because of associated immunologic response to the vector used for transduction, this duration is satisfactory and useful to boost healing in the treatment of fractures or bone defects. In small animal models, growth factors delivered by gene therapy resulted in better healing than those delivered as recombinant proteins.[57] Experimental studies in large animals have yet to demonstrate the benefits, without any deleterious side effects, of gene therapy for fracture healing and filling of bone defects.

Carriers for Delivering Growth Factors

Growth factors tend to rapidly diffuse away from the target site when administered alone. To limit this phenomenon and, therefore, to optimize their local osteoinductive potential, various carriers have been evaluated. The choice of the carrier or delivery system is essential to the success of growth-factor therapy. The ideal carrier should have several characteristics, including (i) the ability to deliver the growth factor at the appropriate time and at the proper dose, (ii) the ability to enhance cell recruitment and attachment, (iii) the presence of structural voids to allow for cell migration and angiogenesis, and (iv) be biodegradable without inducing an immune or inflammatory response and without producing toxic byproducts.[48] Matrix requirements for BMP carriers vary from simple delivery systems, such as minipellets, beads, or microspheres, to complex three-dimensional structures with a macro- and microporosity that attempt to mimic the matrix of the repair tissue. Optimally, carriers should be resorbable. The four major categories of BMP carriers are natural polymers, inorganic materials, synthetic polymers, and composite materials.[58] Table 89-1 illustrates their main properties.

The typical pharmacokinetic profile of BMP-2 release differs according to the delivery system. The initial burst delivery of BMP has a half-life of less than 10 minutes and appears to be carrier-independent. The secondary release of BMP is characterized by a half-life of 3 to 5 days with collagen carriers, whereas mineral-based delivery systems have a longer half-life, with BMP detected for up to 5 weeks.[58,59] In vitro and in vivo studies have shown the temporal sequence of BMP expression during membranous bone formation. Bone morphogenetic protein-6 appears first, followed by BMP-4 and later by BMP-2. Considerable overlap exists in the time of expression, suggesting codependency of these factors. This sequential expression shows that the BMPs are not necessarily interchangeable and that it is possible that different BMPs can influence the expression of other BMPs as part of a cascade.[60] Moreover, co-administration of BMP-2/BMP-7 or BMP-2/BMP-6 have been shown to be 5 to 10 times more potent in inducing bone formation than BMP-2 alone.[27]

To date, the best strategy for bone repair using growth factors has not been determined. The optimal dose of proteins required to achieve bone repair in clinical studies is not clearly established. The large variability in doses and experimental protocols among studies makes the determination of an optimal dose difficult. Moreover, the ideal delivery matrix for the appropriate factor has yet to be identified. There are three major obstacles to routinely using growth factors for bone repair: (i) the high costs of these growth factors, particularly BMPs, (ii) the selection of the optimal doses, and (iii) the optimization of the carrier matrix or delivery vehicle in order to allow vascular ingrowth, osteoprogenitor cell population, and invasion within the scaffold.

References

1. Masquelet AC, Fitoussi F, Muller GP: Reconstruction des os longs par membrane induite et autogreffe spongieuse. Ann Chir Plast Esthét 45:346, 2000.

2. Pelissier P, Martin D, Baudet J, et al: Behavior of cancellous bone graft placed in induced membranes. Br J Plast Surg 55:596, 2002.

3. Bloomberg MS, Goring RL: Frozen diaphyseal bone allografts combined with external and internal pin splintage in small animal orthopedic surgery. J Am Anim Hosp Assoc 20:393, 1984.

4. Schena CJ, Mitten RW, Hoefle WD: Segmental freeze-dried and fresh cortical allografts in the canine femur. I. A sequential radiographic comparison over a one-year time interval. J Am Anim Hosp Assoc 20:911, 1984.

5. Johnson AL, Stein LE: Morphologic comparison of healing patterns in ethylene oxyde-sterilized cortical allografts and untreated cortical autografts in the dog. Am J Vet Res 49(1):101, 1988.

6. Roe SC, Pijanowski GJ, Johnson AL: Biomechanical properties of canine cortical bone allografts: effects of preparation and storage. Am J Vet Res 49(6):874, 1988.

7. Sinibaldi KR: Evaluation of full cortical allografts in 25 dogs. J Am Vet Med Assoc 194(11):1570, 1989.

8. Wilson JW, Hoefle WD: Diaphyseal allograft: eight-year evaluation in a dog. Vet Comp Orthop Trauma (3):78, 1990.

9. Stevenson S: Bone grafting. *In* Textbook of Small Animal Surgery. Slatter D (ed). Philadelphia: WB Saunders, 1993, p. 1694.

10. Wilson JW: Blood supply to developing, mature, and healing bone. *In* Bone in Clinical Orthopedics. Sumner-Smith G (ed). Stuttgart: Thieme, 2002, p. 23.

Table 89-1. Main Carrier Materials used for BMP Delivery

Categories	Carrier materials	Formulations	Advantages/*Disadvantages*
Natural polymers	Collagen	Gelatin	Biocompatible
		Demineralized bone matrix	Bioresorbable
		Fibrillar collagen	Sourcing
	Hyaluronan	Gels, sponges, pads	*Processing*
	Fibrin	Adhesive glue	*Disease transmission*
	Chitosan	Hydrogels, sponges, pads	*Immunogenicity*
Inorganic materials	CaP cement	Injectable, implantable, solid	Biocompatible
			Bioresorbable
			Osteoconductive
			Phase separation during injection
			Lack of macroporosity
			Lack of mechanical strength
	Sintered CaP ceramics	Granules, blocks	Biocompatible
			Osteoconductive
			Prolonged residence time
			Lack of mechanical strength
			Slowness of bioresorption
Synthetic polymers	Polylactide	Highly porous tridimensional scaffold	Design flexibility
	Polyglycolide	Linear oriented scaffold	Elimination of disease transmission
	Polylactide-co-glycolide	Fibers	
		Sheets	*Potential decrease of pH*
		Microspheres	*Bulk degradation*
			Excessive inflammation
Composites	CaP ceramics/natural polymers		Improvement of mechanical strength
	Natural/synthetic polymers		Improvement of release property
	Ceramic/natural polymers/synthetic polymers		Improvement of handling, porosity and providing injectability

11. Millis DL, Martinez SA. Bone grafts. *In* Textbook of Small Animal Surgery. Slatter D (ed). Philadelphia: WB Saunders, 2003, p. 1875.

12. Bauer TW, Smith ST: Bioactive materials in orthopaedic surgery: overview and regulatory considerations. Clin Orthop Relat Res (395):11, 2002.

13. LeGeros RZ: Properties of osteoconductive biomaterials: calcium phosphates. Clin Orthop Relat Res (395):81, 2002.

14. Greenwald AS, Boden SD, Goldberg VM, et al: Bone-graft substitutes: facts, fictions, and applications. J Bone Joint Surg Am 83-A Suppl 2 Pt 2:98, 2001.

15. Finkemeier CG: Bone-grafting and bone-graft substitutes. J Bone Joint Surg Am 84-A(3):454, 2002.

16. Damien CJ, Parsons JR: Bone graft and bone graft substitutes: a review of current technology and applications. J Appl Biomater 2(3):187, 1991.

17. Cameron HU, Macnab I, Pilliar RM: Evaluation of biodegradable ceramic. J Biomed Mater Res 11(2):179, 1977.

18. Jarcho M: Calcium phosphate ceramics as hard tissue prosthetics. Clin Orthop Relat Res (157):259, 1981.

19. Frayssinet P, Trouillet JL, Rouquet N, et al: Osseointegration of macroporous calcium phosphate ceramics having a different chemical composition. Biomaterials 14(6):423, 1993.

20. Yang Z, Yuan H, Tong W, et al: Osteogenesis in extraskeletally implanted porous calcium phosphate ceramics: variability among different kinds of animals. Biomaterials 17(22):2131, 1996.

21. Gauthier O, Bouler JM, Weiss P, et al: Kinetic study of bone ingrowth and ceramic resorption associated with the implantation of different injectable calcium-phosphate bone substitutes. J Biomed Mater Res 47(1):28, 1999.

22. Frankenburg EP, Goldstein SA, Bauer TW, et al: Biomechanical and histological evaluation of a calcium phosphate cement. J Bone Joint Surg Am 80-A(8):1112, 1998.

23. Frayssinet P, Mathon D, Lerch A, et al: Osseointegration of composite calcium phosphate bioceramics. J Biomed Mater Res 50(2):125, 2000.

24. Shimazaki K, Mooney V: Comparative study of porous hydroxyapatite and tricalcium phosphate as bone substitute. J Orthop Res 3(3):301, 1985.

25. Giannoudis PV, Dinopoulos H, Tsiridis E: Bone substitutes: an update. Injury 36 Suppl 3:S20, 2005.

26. Urist MR: Bone: formation by autoinduction. Science 150(698):893, 1965.

27. Yoon ST, Boden SD: Osteoinductive molecules in orthopaedics: basic science and preclinical studies. Clin Orthop Relat Res (395):33, 2002.

28. Colnot C, Romero DM, Huang S, et al: Mechanisms of action of demineralized bone matrix in the repair of cortical bone defects. Clin Orthop Relat Res (435):69, 2005.

29. Han B, Tang B, Nimni ME: Quantitative and sensitive in vitro assay for osteoinductive activity of demineralized bone matrix. J Orthop Res 21(4):648, 2003.

30. Gauthier O, Bouler JM, Aguado E, et al: Macroporous biphasic calcium phosphate ceramics: influence of macropore diameter and macroporosity percentage on bone ingrowth. Biomaterials 19(1-3):133, 1998.

31. Kuboki Y, Jin Q, Takita H: Geometry of carriers controlling phenotypic expression in BMP-induced osteogenesis and chondrogenesis. J Bone Joint Surg Am 83-A Suppl 1(Pt 2):S105, 2001.

32. Karageorgiou V, Kaplan D: Porosity of 3D biomaterial scaffolds and osteogenesis. Biomaterials 26(27):5474, 2005.

33. Cazalbou S, Combes C, Rey C: Calcium phosphate ceramics. J Aust Ceram Soc 40(1):58, 2004.

34. Hong L, Hengchang X, de Groot K: Tensile strength of the interface between hydroxyapatite and bone. J Biomed Mater Res 26:7, 1992.

35. Johnson KD, Frierson KE, Keller TS, et al: Porous ceramics as bone graft substitutes in long bone defects: a biomechanical, histological, and radiographic analysis. J Orthop Res 14(3):351, 1996.

36. Frayssinet P, Autefage A: Hybrid materials for use as bone substitutes. Preliminary results and prospects for the future. Rev Rhum Engl Ed 60(5):302, 1993.

37. Muschler GF, Midura RJ: Connective tissue progenitors: practical concepts for clinical applications. Clin Orthop Relat Res (395):66, 2002.

38. Muschler GF, Boehm C, Easley K: Aspiration to obtain osteoblast progenitor cells from human bone marrow: the influence of aspiration volume. J Bone Joint Surg Am 79-A(11):1699, 1997.

39. McLain RF, Fleming JE, Boehm CA, et al: Aspiration of osteoprogenitor cells for augmenting spinal fusion: comparison of progenitor cell concentrations from the vertebral body and iliac crest. J Bone Joint Surg 87-A(12):2655, 2005.

40. Kadiyala S, Jaiswal N, Bruder SP: Culture-expanded bone marrow-derived mesenchymal stem cells can regenerate a critical-sized segmental bone defect. Tissue Eng 3(2):173, 1997.

41. Tiedeman JJ, Connolly JF, Strates BS, et al: Treatment of nonunion by percutaneous injection of bone marrow and demineralized bone matrix. An experimental study in dogs. Clin Orthop Relat Res (268):294, 1991.

42. Connolly J, Guse R, Lippiello L, et al: Development of an osteogenic bone-marrow preparation. J Bone Joint Surg Am 71(5):684, 1989.

43. Bruder SP, Fox BS: Tissue engineering of bone. Cell based strategies. Clin Orthop Relat Res (367 Suppl):S68, 1999.

44. Bruder SP, Kraus KH, Goldberg VM, et al: The effect of implants loaded with autologous mesenchymal stem cells on the healing of canine segmental bone defects. J Bone Joint Surg Am 80-A(7):985, 1998.

45. Frayssinet P, Primout I, Rouquet N, et al: Bone cell grafts in bioreactor: a study of feasibility of bone cell autograft in large defects. J Mater Sci Mater Med 2:217, 1991.

46. Yoshikawa T, Ohgushi H, Tamai S: Immediate bone forming capability of prefabricated osteogenic hydroxyapatite. J Biomed Mater Res 32(3):481, 1996.

47. Nakamura T, Hara Y, Tagawa M, et al: Recombinant human basic fibroblast growth factor accelerates fracture healing by enhancing callus remodeling in experimental dog tibial fracture. J Bone Miner Res 13(6):942, 1998.

48. Lieberman JR, Daluiski A, Einhorn TA: The role of growth factors in the repair of bone. Biology and clinical applications. J Bone Joint Surg Am 84-A(6):1032, 2002.

49. Cheng H, Jiang W, Phillips FM, et al: Osteogenic activity of the fourteen types of human bone morphogenetic proteins (BMPs). J Bone Joint Surg Am 85-A(8):1544, 2003.

50. Sciadini MF, Dawson JM, Johnson KD: Evaluation of bovine-derived bone protein with a natural coral carrier as a bone-graft substitute in a canine segmental defect model. J Orthop Res 15(6):844, 1997.

51. Sciadini MF, Johnson KD: Evaluation of recombinant human bone morphogenetic protein-2 as a bone-graft substitute in a canine segmental defect model. J Orthop Res 18(2):289, 2000.

52. Schmoekel HG, Weber FE, Hurter K, et al: Enhancement of bone healing using non-glycosylated rhBMP-2 released drom a fibrin matrix in dogs and cats. J Small Anim Pract 46:17, 2005.

53. Michal U, Fluckiger M, Schmokel H: Healing of dorsal pancarpal arthrodesis in the dog. J Small Anim Pract 44(3):109, 2003.

54. Schmoekel H, Schense JC, Weber FE, et al: Bone healing in the rat and dog with nonglycosylated BMP-2 demonstrating low solubility in fibrin matrices. J Orthop Res 22(2):376, 2004.

55. Bushman F, Lewinski M, Ciuffi A, et al: Genome-wide analysis of retroviral DNA integration. Nat Rev Microbiol 3(11):848, 2005.

56. Hannallah D, Peterson B, Lieberman JR, et al: Gene therapy in orthopaedic surgery. J Bone Joint Surg Am 84-A(6):1046, 2002.

57. Southwood LL, Frisbie DD, Kawcak CE, et al: Delivery of growth factors using gene therapy to enhance bone healing. Vet Surg 33(6):565, 2004.

58. Seeherman H, Wozney JM: Delivery of bone morphogenetic proteins for orthopedic tissue regeneration. Cytokine Growth Factor Rev 16(3):329, 2005.

59. Winn SR, Uludag H, Hollinger JO: Carrier systems for bone morphogenetic proteins. Clin Orthop Relat Res (367 Suppl):S95, 1999.

60. Boden SD: Bioactive factors for bone tissue engineering. Clin Orthop Relat Res (367 Suppl):S84, 1999.

Chapter 90

Salter Fractures

Dirsko von Pfeil
Charles E. DeCamp

In 1963 Salter and Harris described a system of categorizing fractures involving the growth plate in relationship to the epiphyseal plate, the epiphysis, and the metaphysis (Figure 90-1).[1] Today, these specific fractures involving the growth plate are commonly called "Salter Fractures." Fractures of the growth plate may cause partial or complete arrest of growth, which may result in the loss of bone length and/or subsequent development of angular limb deformities and gait abnormalities. It is imperative to understand the physiology of the growth plate and the possible consequences of trauma in order to properly assess the severity of damage, give an appropriate prognosis, and provide the correct treatment.

This chapter describes the basic anatomy of the growth plate, the relative contributions of the different growth plates to overall growth, the etiology and biomechanics of Salter fractures, and some diagnostic and prognostic guidelines.

Microscopic Anatomy

The growth plate consists of fibrous, cartilaginous, and bony components (Figure 90-1). The fibrous component surrounds the growth plate and is divided into an ossification groove, called the groove of Ranvier, and a perichondrial ring known as the ring of LaCroix. The groove of Ranvier contributes chondrocytes for growth in both the diameter and length of the growth plate.[2] The ring of LaCroix is located between the ossification groove and the periosteum of the metaphysis and provides mechanical support for the growth plate. A biomechanical study in rabbits suggested that this structure protects growth cartilage from shear forces.[3]

The cartilaginous component of the growth plate is divided into reserve (or germinal), proliferative, and hypertrophic zones. The hypertrophic zone is further divided into the zones of maturation, degeneration, and provisional calcification (Figure 90-1). It is important to remember that damage to the reserve zone is associated with destruction of the germinal cells and, therefore, carries a high risk of resulting growth abnormalities. The hypertrophic zone is the weakest part of the growth plate and is most commonly involved in Salter fractures.[1]

Immediately adjacent to the cartilaginous component is the bony component of the growth plate. This is the portion of the metaphysis in which cartilage cells are transformed into bone. The major cell type of the growth plate is the chondrocyte. Cell matrix, consisting of 70% water and 30% collagen fibrils, proteoglycans, and other noncollagenous proteins, is found as well.[4] Collagen fibers provide tension and shear resistance to the cartilage. Proteoglycans and water give resistance to pressure.[5]

Vascular Supply

An intact vascular supply is necessary for cell proliferation and cartilage resorption and calcification, which are all necessary for growth, and for healing of fractures. Injury that results in disruption of or changes in the vascular networks may cause abnormal growth or cessation of growth.[5] The arterial blood supply to the growth plate consists of branches of the vascular supply to the epiphysis and metaphysis (Figure 90-2). The multiple branches of the epiphyseal arteries arborize into the growth plate, providing vascularization to the first 4 to 10 cell columns of the proliferative zone. No vessels penetrate beyond the proliferative zone and, therefore, the hypertrophic zone is relatively avascular. Chondrocytes in the hypertrophic zone must use anaerobic glycolysis to furnish energy. Perichondrial arteries supply the fibrous structures of the growth plate. The nutrient artery provides four fifths of the metaphyseal blood supply. Branches of the metaphyseal arteries supply the remainder. Terminal branches of these vessels end in small vascular loops or capillary tufts below the last intact row of chondrocytes of the growth plate.[6] Venous drainage of the metaphysis occurs via the large central vein of the diaphysis.[7]

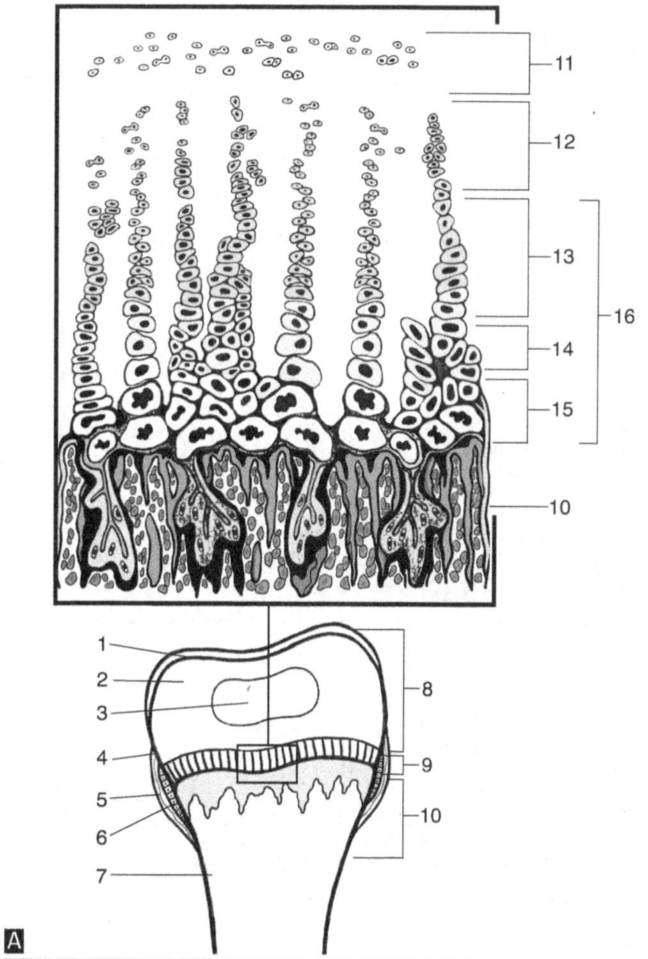

Figure 90-1A. Normal anatomy. 1) Articular cartilage; 2) Epiphyseal cartilage; 3) Secondary ossification center; 4) Groove of Ranvier; 5) Ring of LaCroix; 6) Periosteum; 7) Cortical bone; 8) Epiphysis; 9) Growth plate; 10) Metaphysis; 11) Reserve zone or germinal layer; 12) Zone of proliferation; 13) Zone of maturation; 14) Zone of degeneration; 15) Zone of provisional calcification; 16) Zone of hypertrophy.

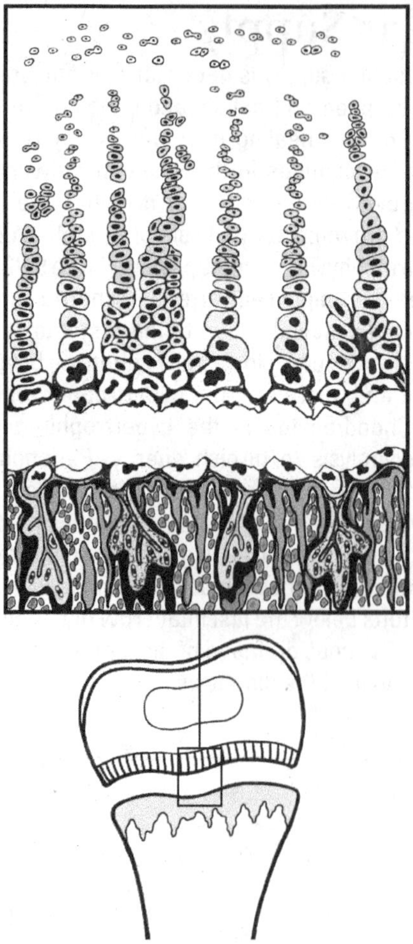

B

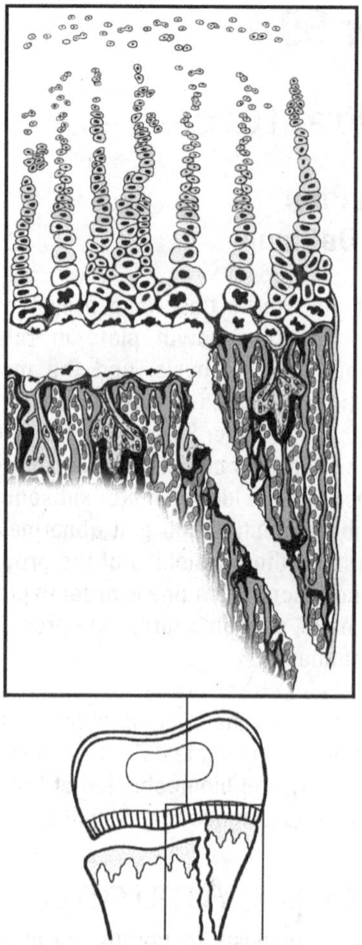

C

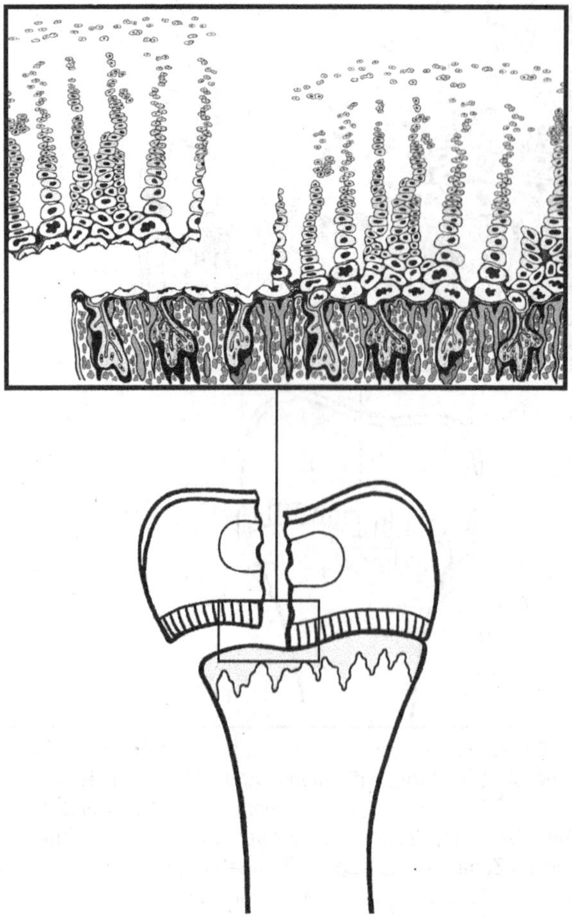

D

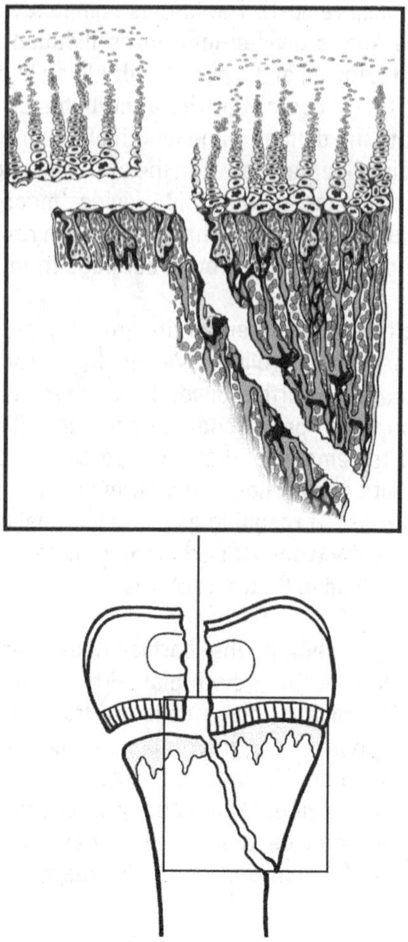

E

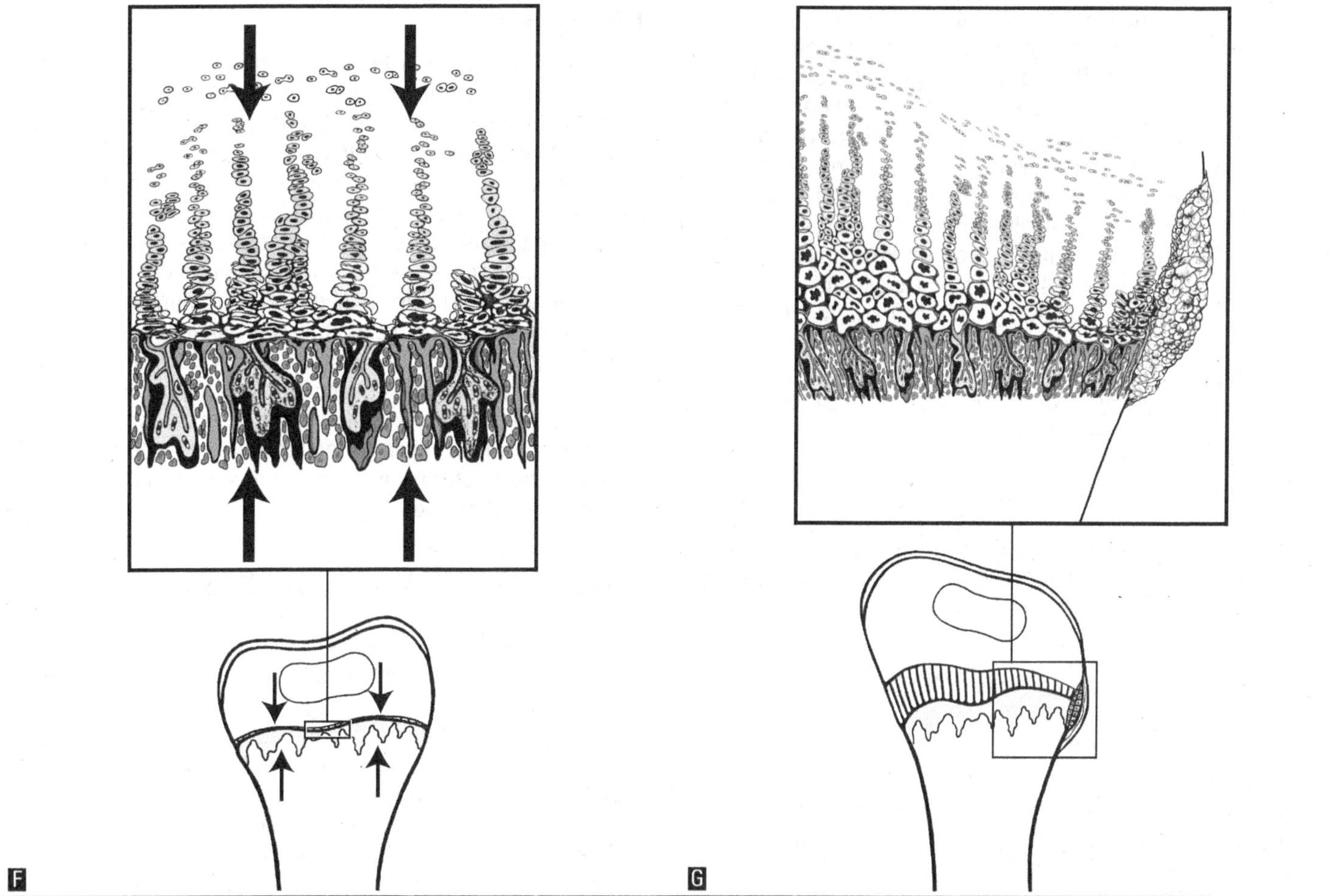

Figures 90-1B-G. Salter Fractures. 1b) Salter type 1 fracture through the hypertrophic zone of the epiphyseal plate; Figure 1c) Salter type 2 fracture through the epiphyseal plate and the metaphysis; Figure 1d) Salter type 3 fracture through the epiphyseal plate and the epiphysis; Figure 1e) Salter type 4 Fracture through the epiphysis and the metaphysis; Figure 1f) Salter type 5 fracture: Compression fracture of the epiphyseal plate; Figure 1g) Type 6 fracture: Lateral bone bridge formation.

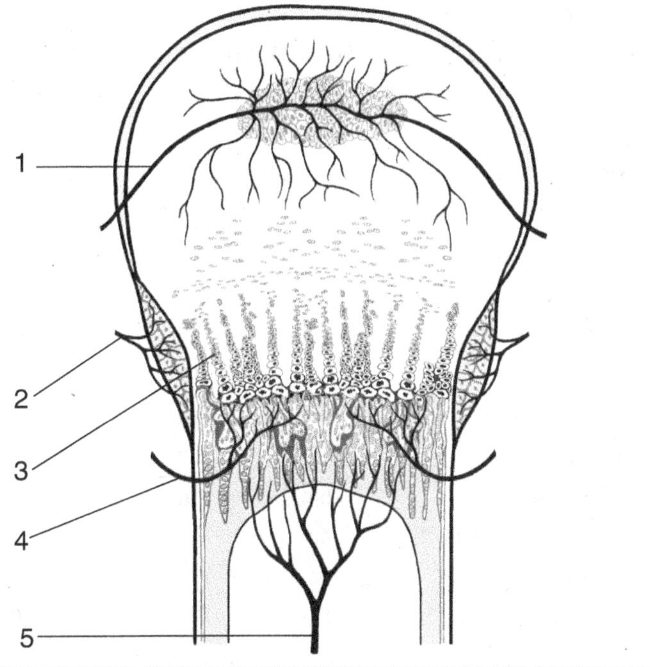

Figure 90-2. Blood supply of the growth plate. 1) Epiphyseal artery; 2) Perichondrial artery; 3) Growth plate; 4) Metaphyseal artery; 5) Nutrient artery.

In general, the blood supply to the growth plate does not enter through associated ligaments to the joint. However, it has been shown that in 28% of people, the femoral capital growth plate is supplied via branches of the artery of the ligament of the femoral head (epiphysis).[8] In contrast, no such blood supply is evident in the dog.[9]

Growth Plate Closure and Contribution of Different Growth Plates to Overall Growth

It is important to be aware of the closure times and the relative contribution of the different growth plates to overall growth in order to better assess the risk for possible secondary problems after a Salter fracture. It is generally agreed that the rapid growth period of the dog is between 3 to 6 or 7 months of age.[10,11] Most dogs achieve 90 to 95% of their adult size by the end of 7 to 9 months.[11] Growth plates of giant breed dogs may not close until 15 to 18 months of age. Studies on bone growth have shown significant individual and breed variations in the time of growth plate closure. These studies also report that longitudinal growth may stop prior to radiographic evidence of growth plate closure.[10-12] Radiographic evidence of growth plate closure occurs between 4 months and 12 months of age, depending on the specific anatomic site and breed of dog.[10-12] Table 90-1 shows a summary of the reported time frames of growth plate closure in the front and hind limbs of the average dog.[12,13] Growth plates that contribute a large percentage of the total axial growth of the long bones, such as the radius, ulna, and tibia, remain open longer compared with those of smaller bones, such as the carpal or tarsal bones. Cats have similar patterns of growth plate closure. Physeal closure begins at 4 months and is usually completed at 7 to 9 months of age. However, final closure of the distal radial physis in cats can occur as late as 20 months of age.[14] Studies in dogs have been performed to evaluate the relative contribution of each epiphyseal plate to total growth.[15,16] Table 90-1 summarizes the results of these studies.

Whenever the function of the growth plate is severely impaired, anatomic deformity is likely to develop. Trauma, dietary, hormonal, and genetic etiologies are clinically important to growth deformity in the dog. The following paragraphs will focus on the effect of trauma to the growth plate.

Fractures of the Growth Plate

Prevalence

Growth plate fractures are the result of trauma. Of dogs with fractures of long bones, 50 to 55% have been reported to be younger than 1 year of age.[17,18] Among the reported cases of long-bone fractures, 30% had trauma to the growth plate, and 7% subsequently developed growth deformities. In a study of 92 dogs with growth deformity as result of trauma, 75% showed a disturbance of the ulna or radius. The tibia had 4% and the femur 8% of the deformities reported.[19]

Biomechanics

Any material, including bone or a specific area of the bone such as the growth plate, can be exposed to disruptive forces such as tension, compression, torsion, shear, and bending (see chapter 126). Depending on the amount of applied stress, bone may deform and return to normal configuration when the stress is reduced. This is known as elastic deformation. If the stress exceeds the elastic limit, the deformation persists. This is known as plastic deformation. When the point of failure is surpassed, the material breaks. The growth plate of immature animals is more prone to failure than either the ligamentous structures supporting the joint or the relatively elastic bone in these young animals.[20] Therefore, it is common to see growth plate injury without distortion of the joint or fracture of the bone. Although Salter and Harris applied shear stress in their original experiments, Salter fractures can also be caused by bending, torsion, tension, or compression.[1,5,18,21]

Classification Systems

Salter-Harris Classification

Salter and Harris described a classification for fractures involving the growth plate, mostly intended for use in human patients, which categorizes fractures in relation to the epiphyseal plate, the epiphysis, and the metaphysis (Figure 90-1).[1] This same report explains results of an experimental study in rodents, demonstrating that fractures commonly developed through the zone of hypertrophy, which is mechanically the weakest zone of the growth plate. Salter and Harris also investigated healing of the different fracture types and suggested that the higher the fracture grade, the worse the prognosis for normal growth. They also postulated that interference with blood supply to the epiphysis is associated with a poor prognosis. The Salter-Harris classification is also commonly used in veterinary medicine.

Table 90-1. Closure Times and Contribution of Growth of the Different Growth Plates in the Canine Appendicular Skeleton

Forelimb				Hindlimb			
Growth Plate	Closure		Growth (%)	Growth Plate	Closure		Growth (%)
	Earliest	Latest			Earliest	Latest	
Scapular tuberosity	12w	5m		Greater trochanter	6m	11m	
Proximal humerus	10m	12m	80	Proximal femur	6m	12m	30-40
Distal humerus	5m	8m	20	Lesser trochanter	9m	12m	
Proximal ulna	5m	8m	0-15	Distal femur	6m	11m	60-70
Anconeal process	4m	5m		Proximal tibia	6m	12m	55
Distal ulna	6m	11m	85-100	Tibial tuberosity	11m	12m	
Proximal radius	5m	9m	25	Distal tibia	5m	11m	45
Distal radius	6m	11m	65	Medial malleolus	4m	5m	
Accessory carpal bone	10w	5m		Proximal fibula	6m	11m	60
Metacarpal bones	5m	7m		Distal fibula	5m	11m	40
Phalanges	4m	7m		Tuber calcaneous	11w	8m	
				Metatarsal bones	5m	8m	
				Phalanges	4m	8m	

w = weeks; m = months; % = percent.

Salter and Harris describe five types of fractures (Figure 90-1).[1,5,18,21,22] Type I represents complete epiphyseal separation through the zone of hypertrophy. The reserve zone (germinal layer of the growth plate) is usually intact.

In a type II injury, the fracture occurs partially through the growth plate and partially through the metaphysis. Type I and type II Salter fractures represent 65.5% of growth plate fractures in small animals and, therefore, are the most common types seen.[22]

Type III is an intraarticular epiphyseal fracture. The fracture line is not limited to the hypertrophic zone but also includes a small area of the reserve zone. Salter Type IV fractures are also intraarticular, but the fracture line extends into the metaphysis, thus completely crossing the growth plate. Type III and IV fractures often represent condylar fractures and occur most commonly in the distal humerus.[22] Salter types III and IV represent 25.5% of all growth plate fractures in the dog.[22]

Type V Salter fractures are characterized by partial or complete compression of the growth plate. This crushing injury is uncommon. It is difficult to diagnose on the basis of radiographs. It may help to compare the width of the growth plate with the contralateral side, and to repeat the radiographic study at 2-week intervals to better assess damage.

Some investigators have suggested adding a type VI fracture to the traditional Salter-Harris classification system.[21,23,24] A type VI fracture involves the peripheral region of the growth plate, the zone of Ranvier. More commonly, it results from a localized contusion or avulsion of that specific portion of the growth mechanism. Peripheral osseous bridge formation commonly occurs, leading to peripherally localized epiphysiodesis and subsequent angular deformity.[21,24,24]

Ogden Classification

The classification proposed by the human surgeon John Ogden is one concerned with injury to the growth mechanism rather than only physeal or epiphyseal injury. It is a more detailed scheme that permits further understanding of the injury to the growth mechanism as a whole. Ogden subdivided the Salter and Harris classification in order to better predict a prognosis for growth disturbances.[24] Salter type I lesions are divided into three subtypes (1A-C), type II lesions into four subtypes (2A-D), and type III lesions into three subtypes (3A-C), type IV lesions into four subtypes (4A-D). The subdivisions are made according to the injured zones and specific fracture pattern of the growth plate (Figure 90-3). For example, in contrast with type 1A where the fracture is primarily through the zone of hypertrophic cartilage, type 1B fractures occur through the zone of degenerating cartilage and primary spongiosa, whereas type 1C fractures are associated with injury to the germinal portion of the physis. Subdivisions for type two to four injuries are according to the size and amount of fragments, and specific location of the fracture. Ogden also introduced new lesions (types VI – IX), describing injury of the ossified or nonossified epiphyseal nucleus, the fibrous structures of the growth plate, and multiple fractures of the epiphysis. In people, this classification system has been shown to provide a better prognosis for injuries of the growth plates, compared with the Salter-Harris system.[25-27] While further description of this system is beyond the scope of this chapter, this grading scheme may help to predict more accurately a prognosis for small animals with growth plate injuries.[24]

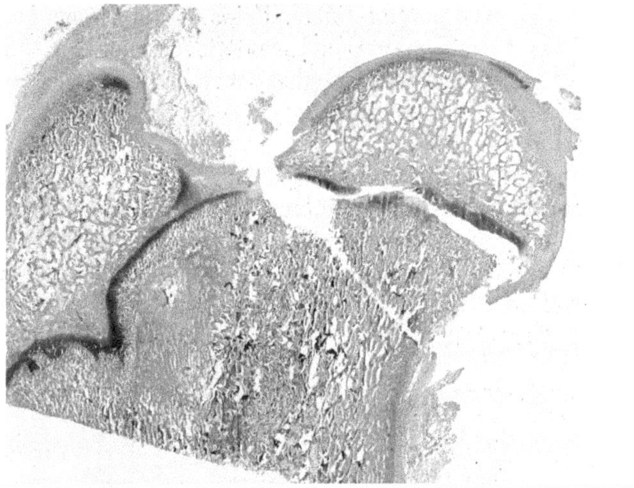

Figure 90-3. (Courtesy: Dr. Ann L. Johnson, University of Illinois). Fracture of the proximal femoral physis, showing the fracture line going through the zones of reserve, proliferation, and hypertrophy. Destruction of cells in the reserve zone and the zone of proliferation increases the risk for a poor prognosis.

Classification Based on Blood Supply

Although the Salter-Harris classification is useful for a radiographic description of the growth plate fracture, this system does not consistently correlate with the clinical and histologic findings, nor does it predict the normality or abnormality of future growth.[28] An additional classification for fractures of the epiphyseal plate has been suggested in human medicine.[15] This system is based on the integrity of epiphyseal and metaphyseal blood circulation. Radiography is used to assess displacement of the fracture fragments, and scintigraphy is used to assess the degree of vascular damage. Type A fractures are described as having the circulation intact, with no displacement of the fragments. Type A fractures are not expected to have a negative effect on subsequent growth. In type B1 fractures, there is mild displacement of the fragments but some areas are still in direct bony contact. Type B2 fractures show more severe fragment displacement. In type B1 and type B2 fractures, epiphyseal and metaphyseal vessels intermingle through vertical fissures across the epiphyseal plate. In these fractures, bony bridges may form and lead to cessation of longitudinal growth. Type C fractures are described as having complete disruption of the epiphyseal circulation. These fractures carry a poor prognosis for normal growth.[15,29]

Histologic Findings in Traumatic Growth Plate Injuries in Dogs

A study of the histologic appearance of traumatic canine physeal injuries that had been radiographically classified as Salter-Harris type I or type II fractures showed that in 10 of 13 cases, the fracture disrupted cells in the proliferative zone, rather than in the hypertrophic zone (Figure 90-4).[30] Destruction of cells in the proliferative zone may worsen the prognosis for continued growth, in contrast to the expected favorable outcome established by the Salter-Harris classification. Other experimental studies showed that the fracture sites do not always occur at the level of the hypertrophic zone, as described by Salter and Harris, but can also involve other zones of the growth plate.[31,32] These differences may be explained by the fact that force impact occurred from only one side in the Salter and Harris experiments, whereas in vivo, combined forces may be acting, resulting in a variety of fracture patterns through the growth plate. As a result of these histologic findings, it can be suggested that the Salter-Harris classification of fractures, as described for humans and rodents, may not be fully comparable to clinical and experimental evidence in dogs.

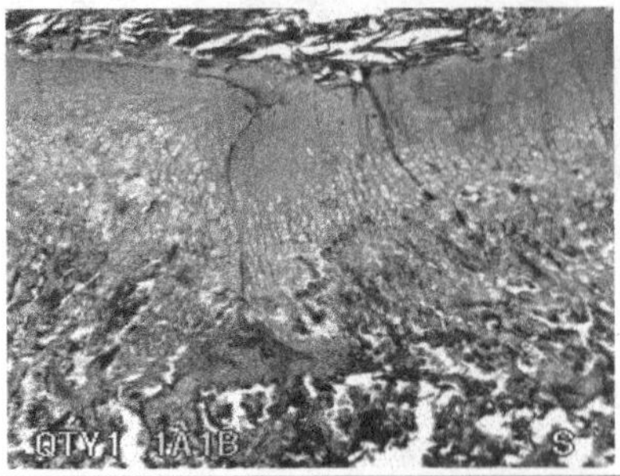

Figure 90-4. (Courtesy: J.M. Wattenbarger, M.D., OrthoCarolina, and Helen Gruber, PhD., Department of Orthopaedic Surgery, Carolinas Medical Center, Charlotte.). Vertical septa connecting the metaphysis and epiphysis at 6 days after trauma to the epiphyseal plate of a rat. These septa develop into bone bridges between the metaphysis and epiphysis, which can eventually lead to cessation of growth and the development of angular limb deformity.

Epiphyseal Bone Bridge Formation

Physeal bone bridges connect epiphyseal and metaphyseal marrow compartments, and are thought to be responsible for cessation of localized growth and development of angular limb deformities attributed to asymmetrical restriction of longitudinal growth across the physeal plate.[32-36] Although fracture healing generally occurs without complication when the fracture is contained within the cartilage of the physis, cellular debris and the formation of vertical septa followed by physeal bone bridge formation are seen when the fracture extends to the physeal–epiphyseal border. Experimental studies found that fractures may involve all regions of the growth plate.[32,37] In one study of 20 rats, the periosteum was elevated from the proximal tibiae.[37] A fracture through the growth plate was then created. The authors reported histologic evidence of vertical septa within the growth plate extending from the epiphysis to the metaphysis as early as 6 days after injury, (Figure 90-4), which were followed by the formation of bony bridges across the physis by days 10 and 21 in 65% and 75% of the rats, respectively. The presence of bone bridges after trauma to the epiphyseal plate has previously been described; however, it was not known that physeal bone bridge formation starts to occur so soon after injury.[32-36]

Diagnosis

Most types of Salter fractures can easily be diagnosed using radiography;[38] although sometimes it is difficult to determine the amount of damage, especially with Salter-Harris type V fractures. Whenever trauma to the growth plate is suspected, serial radiographs are recommended at 1- or 2-week intervals to detect abnormalities in growth. Magnetic resonance imaging (MRI) has been shown to be superior to plain radiographs and computed tomography as a means of diagnosing injuries to the growth plate.[39-41] MRI provides accurate mapping of physeal bone bridges and associated growth abnormalities that may have already developed.[39] It has been shown that an excellent correlation exists between MRI and histologic findings.[42] Knowledge obtained from MRI studies provides an accurate diagnosis that may change the initial treatment plan. Scintigraphy provides early and accurate evidence of disturbance of epiphyseal blood flow, which, in turn, may cause growth plate injury.[29] As described above, scintigraphy may be a useful alternative means for the classification of growth plate injuries.

Prognosis

About 5 to 17% of all growth plate injuries in dogs are reported to have clinically significant sequelae.[18,19,36,43] The sequelae in altered growth following growth plate fracture depend on many factors, including which physis is injured; the type and severity of injury, including displacement; the stage of physeal maturation (i.e., the age of the animal) at the time of injury; the promptness of proper diagnosis; and the method of treatment. In general, the younger the animal, especially those younger than 6 months of age, the more serious the consequences to longitudinal bone growth.[43] The degree of retardation in bone growth following physeal injury is roughly proportional to the degree of destruction to the region or zone of the epiphyseal plate.[36]

Clinical lameness as a sequala to growth plate injury occurs only if the length discrepancy between legs is more than 2 centimeters in animals under 20 kilograms or more than 3 centimeters in animals over 20 kilograms.[44]

Although the Salter-Harris classification system provides a good description of epiphyseal fractures, the prognosis should always be guarded. Although the majority of patients with types I and II fractures have an excellent prognosis for normal growth, radiographically undetectable physeal damage may exist that can only be diagnosed retrospectively. Damage to the epiphyseal vessels and to the fibrous component of the physis may occur in both Salter fracture types I and II, but when early reduction and fixation are possible, uncomplicated healing is expected within 3 to 4 weeks. The prognosis for type III fractures may be good if early reduction and good reconstruction of the joint surface are achieved, and if the epiphyseal blood supply is not severely disrupted. In contrast, more severe trauma carries a guarded prognosis because malalignment and arthritis may develop. Damage to the germinal layer, the joint cartilage, and to the vascular supply in type IV fractures is common, therefore, the prognosis is guarded. Type V fractures are always associated with a poor prognosis if they happen during a period of rapid growth, because of destruction of the cells in the germinal layer.[45] Partial or complete premature closure of the growth plate and the development of bone deformities are frequently observed.

In a study of distal femoral Salter I or II injuries in 17 dogs, 82.4% showed some degree of femoral growth disturbance, and the mean extent of decreased growth was 6.7%.[43] However, clinical lameness was observed in only 3 dogs evaluated.[43] The authors suggested that compression, injury to the blood supply of the germinal layer, and fissuring through the growth plate with secondary formation of bone bridges may have possibly contributed to the high incidence of decreased femoral growth. The results of this study showed that prognosis for normal growth cannot be based solely on the Salter-Harris classification system.

It has been shown that the initial displacement, number of reduction attempts, and treatment method did not significantly affect the incidence of premature closure of the growth plate in people.[46] However, it has also been shown that improved anatomic reduction decreases the incidence of premature physeal closure.[46] For example, evidence of a residual gap following reduction is associated with a 66% incidence of premature closure, whereas with no gap the incidence decreases to 17%.[46] Residual gaps may be due to entrapment of periosteum; therefore, open reduction to remove entrapped periosteum and thus prevent development of length discrepancies or angular limb deformation has been suggested.[46,47]

As a general guideline, patients with injuries to the growth plates should be reevaluated at 2-week intervals for least for 6 to 8 weeks following treatment or until complete closure of the growth plates occurs. This will ensure early detection and correction of abnormalities.[5]

Summary

Salter fractures involve the growth plate and may result in cessation of bone growth or development of angular limb deformities. This may lead to impaired joint function and abnormal gait. Salter and Harris developed a classification system based on radiographic appearance in order to better describe growth-plate fractures and better predict a prognosis. This radiographic description of growth-plate fractures is well accepted in veterinary medicine. However, it has been shown that the prognosis does not always correlate well with the Salter fracture type. Although it was believed in the past that the germinal layer and the zone of proliferation are not affected in types I or II Salter fractures, histologic studies have shown that injury to these zones can be found even in these "low grade" fracture types. Therefore, the initial prognosis for any Salter fracture should be guarded, and frequent reevaluation until healing and/or complete growth plate closure is recommended. Advanced imaging techniques such as MRI and scintigraphy may become useful diagnostic and prognostic tools for managing animals with Salter fractures.

References

1. Salter RB, Harris WR: Injuries involving the epiphyseal plate. J Bone Joint Surg Am 277:7-71, 1963.

2. Tonna EA: The cellular complement of the skeletal system studied autoradiographically with tritiated thymidine (H3TDR) during growth and aging.J Biophys Biochem Cytol 9:813-824, 1961.

3. Deppermann F, Dallek M, Meenen N et al: The biomechanical significance of the periosteum for the epiphyseal groove. Unfallchirurgie 15(4):165-173, 1989.

4. Heinegard D, Oldberg A: Structure and biology of cartilage and bone matrix noncollagenous macromolecules. FASEB J 3(9):2042-2051, 1989.

5. Prieur WD: Management of growth plate injuries in puppies and kittens. J Small Anim Pract 30:631-638, 1989.

6. Brookes M, Landon DN: The juxta-epiphyseal vessels in the long bones of foetal rats. J Bone Joint Surg Br 46:336-345, 1964.

7. DeMarneffe R: Recherches morphologiques et experimentales sur la vascularisation osseuese. Acta Chir Belg 50:681, 1951.

8. Chung SM: The arterial supply of the developing proximal end of the human femur. J Bone Joint Surg Am 58(7):961-970, 1976.

9. Kaderly RE, Anderson BG, Anderson WD: Intracapsular and intraosseous vascular supply to the mature dog's coxofemoral joint. Am J Vet Res 44(10):1805-1812, 1983.

10. Riser WH: Growth development of the normal canine pelvis, hip joint and femur from birth to maturity: A radiographic study. Am J Vet Rad Soc 14(2):24-34, 1973.

11. Smith RN: The developing skeleton. J Am Vet Rad Soc 9:30-36, 1963.

12. Sumner-Smith G: Observations on epiphyseal fusion of the canine appendicular skeleton. J Small Anim Pract 7(4):303-311, 1966.

13. Schebitz H, Wilkens H: Atlas der Röntgenanatomie bei Hund und Katze. Berlin: Parey, 1989.

14. Smith RN: Fusion of ossification centers in the cat. J Small Anim Pract 10:523-530, 1969.

15. Shapiro F: Epiphyseal disorders. NEnglJMed 31:1702-1710, 1987.

16. Conzemius MG, Smith GK, Brighton CT, et.al: Analysis of physeal growth in dogs, using biplanar radiography. Am J Vet Res 55(1):22-27, 1994.

17. Phillips IR: A survey of bone fractures in the dog and cat. J Small Anim Pract 20(11):661-674, 1979.

18. Maretta SM, Schrader SC: Physeal injuries in the dog: A review of 135 cases. J Am Vet Anim Assoc 182(7):708-710, 1983.

19. Ramadan RO, Vaughan LC: Disturbance in the growth of the tibia and femur in dogs. Vet Rec 104(19):433-435, 1979.

20. Harsha WN: Effects of trauma on epiphysis. Clin Ortho 10:140-147, 1957.

21. Newton CD, Nunamaker DM: Pediatric fractures. *In:* Textbook of Small Animal Orthopaedics. JB Lippincott: Philadelphia, 1985.

22. Carmichael S: Fractures in skeletally immature animals. *In* BSAVA Manual of Small Animal Fracture Repair and Management. British Small Animal Veterinary Association: Shurdington, 1998.

23. Llewellyn HR: Growth plate injuries: Diagnosis, prognosis and treatment. J Am Anim Hosp Assoc 12:77, 1976.

24. Ogden JA: Injury to the growth mechanisms of the immature skeleton.

Skeletal Radiol 6(4):237-53, 1981.

25. Cannata G, De Maio F, Mancini F, et.al: Physeal fractures of the distal radius and ulna: long-term prognosis. J Orthop Trauma. 17(3):172-179; discussion 179-180, 2003.

26. Wessel LM, Gunter SM, Jablonski M, et.al: Predicting growth patterns after supracondylar fracture of the humerus in childhood. Orthopade 32(9):824-832, 2003.

27. Mandalia V, Shivshanker V: Accessory ossicle or intraepihyseal fracture of lateral malleolus: are we familiar with these? Emerg Med J 22:149-152, 2005.

28. Lee BS, Esterhai JL Jr, Das M: Fracture of the distal radial epiphysis. Characteristics and surgical treatment of premature, post-traumatic epiphyseal closure. Clin Orthop Relat Res 5(185):90-6, 1984.

29. Neugebauer W, Kuper K, Flach A, et.al: Value of scintigraphic examination methods with 99mTechnetium in injuries of the epiphyseal cartilage. Aktuelle Traumatol 11(6):217-24, 1981.

30. Johnson JM, Johnson AL, Eurell JA: Histological appearance of naturally occurring canine physeal fractures. Vet Surg 23(2):81-86, 1994.

31. Dale GG, Harris WR: Prognosis of epiphyseal separation. An experimental study. J Bone Joint Surg [Br] 41:1221-1240, 1959.

32. Gomes LS, Volpon JB, Goncalves RP: Traumatic separation of epiphyses. An experimental study in rats. Clin Orthop Relat Res 236:286-295, 1988.

33. Aitken AP: The end results of the fractured distal tibial epiphysis. J Bone Joint Surg 18:685-691, 1936.

34. Aitken AP, Magill HK: Fractures involving the distal femoral epiphyseal cartilage. J Bone Joint Surg Am 34-A(1):96-108, 1952.

35. Brashear HR: Epiphyseal fractures. A microscopic study of the healing process in rats. J Bone Joint Surg Am 41:1055-1064, 1959.

36. Campbell CJ, Grisolia A, Zanconato G: The effects produced in the cartilaginous epiphyseal plate of immature dogs by experimental surgical traumata. J Bone Joint Surg Am 41-A:1221-1242, 1959.

37. Wattenbarger JM, Gruber HE, Phieffer LS: Physeal fractures, part I: histologic features of bone, cartilage, and bar formation in a small animal model. J Pediatr Orthop 22(6):703-709, 2002.

38. Kleine LJ: Radiographic diagnosis of epiphyseal plate trauma. JAAHA, 7:290-295, 1971.

39. Jaramillo D, Hoffer FA, Shapiro F et al: MR imaging of fractures of the growth plate. Am J Roentgenol 155(6):1261-1265, 1990.

40. Rogers LF, Poznanski AK: Imaging of epiphyseal injuries. Radiology 191(2):297-308, 1994.

41. Iwinska-Zelder J, Schmidt S, Ishaque N, et al: Epiphyseal injuries of the distal tibia. Does MRI provide useful additional information? Radiologe 39(1):25-29, 1999.

42. Jaramillo D, Kammen BF, Shapiro F: Cartilaginous path of physeal fracture-separations: evaluation with MR imaging-an experimental study with histologic correlation in rabbits. Radiology 215(2):504-511, 2000.

43. Berg RJ, Egger EL, Konde LJ, et al: Evaluation of prognostic factors for growth following distal femoral physeal injuries in 17 dogs. Vet Surg (13):172-180,1984.

44. Berzon JL: The classification and management of epiphyseal plate fractures. J Am Anim Hosp Assoc 16:651-658, 1980.

45. Strobino LJ, Colonna PC, Brodey RS et. al.: The effect of compression on the growth of epiphyseal bone. Surg Gynecol Obstet 103(1):85-93, 1956.

46. Barmada A, Gaynor T, Mubarak SJ: Premature physeal closure following distal tibia physeal fractures: a new radiographic predictor. J Pediatr Orthop 23(6):733-792, 2003.

47. Phieffer LS, Meyer RA Jr, Gruber HE, et al.: Effect of interposed periosteum in an animal physeal fracture model. Clin Orthop Relat Res 376:15-25, 2000.

Chapter 91

Nonunion, Delayed Union, and Malunion

Ross H. Palmer

Bone is unique in its tremendous ability for repair via regeneration rather than scarring. Indeed, fracture healing typically proceeds in an orderly fashion provided the necessary systemic factors and local environment are present.[1] In fact, bone healing often occurs without veterinary intervention, although the convalescent and long-term morbidity may not be ideal. It is, thus, the veterinarian's role to determine when and how to intervene so that patient morbidity is minimal and functional outcome is maximized. Simplistically, the veterinarian must provide the fracture zone with biologic and mechanical environments that are conducive to the natural reparative process. Failure to provide either of these prerequisites predictably results in failure to achieve bone union and restore limb function.

Union

Bony union refers to a healed fracture. Although it sounds simple enough, considerable "gray area" exists as to when union is achieved depending on the measurement tool being used. "Radiographic union" refers to a subjective assessment of radiographs where the evaluator is satisfied that adequate amounts of new reparative bone have been deposited to achieve bridging of the fracture. "Histologic union" and "mechanical union," where the healed bone is indistinguishable from the bone prior to injury, may take many months to years. A clinician often refers to "clinical union" where he or she is convinced by the radiographs, an appropriate healing time period, and the patient's use of the limb that functional healing has occurred.

Delayed Union

A delayed union is defined as slower than anticipated healing compared with similar fractures treated with similar methods in similar patients. This term is vague because numerous variables exist, including patient age, systemic health, degree of soft tissue injury, presence of concurrent injuries or disease, patient size, fracture configuration and location, treatment method, and surgeon expertise, that may all affect the healing rate.[2] When delayed union is diagnosed, the veterinarian must determine whether treatment intervention is indicated. This determination is based on serial evaluations of radiographic appearance, patient comfort, and limb function. Delayed union is a diagnosis of a dynamic process that may either progress to complete union or culminate in nonunion. Because delayed union can be a transitional state between injury and nonunion, the distinction between delayed union and nonunion may be subtle in some instances.

Nonunion

Delayed union may culminate in nonunion. A nonunion fracture is one in which progression of healing has ceased and union is unlikely without further intervention.[2,3] Nonunions are classified as viable or nonviable based on the biologic activity detected at the fracture site. This distinction directs subsequent treatment strategies.[2,3]

Terminology

Viable Nonunions

Viable nonunion (also called **reactive** or **vascular** or **biologically active** nonunions) are biologically active at the fracture site and have evidence of bone reaction and callus formation.[2-4] Because radiography is the traditional instrument used for assessment of fracture healing, viable nonunions are further subclassified based on the degree of radiographic callus present (Figure 91-1). **Hypertrophic nonunions,** often called "elephant's foot nonunion" have an abundant amount of radiographic callus and are often caused by inadequate fracture stabilization in a highly vascularized region of a young animal. **Moderately hypertrophic nonunions** are characterized by lesser degrees of radiographic callus formation, often referred to as "horse hoof callus," and are often associated with fracture instability in a bone with less soft tissue attachment and/or in a more skeletally mature animal. **Oligotrophic nonunion**, although considered biologically active, produces little callus and can be difficult to distinguish from nonviable nonunion. Nuclear scintigraphy may demonstrate biologic activity of the fracture zone where it is not evident on radiographs.[5,6] When scintigraphy is not readily available, it is clinically advisable to err toward classification as nonviable nonunion as these fractures are treated more comprehensively.

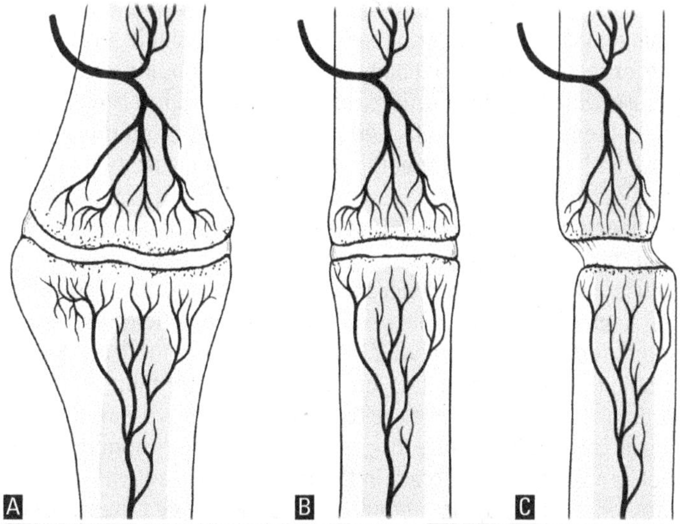

Figure 91-1. Types of viable nonunions. (A) Hypertrophic ("elephant's foot") have an abundant amount of radiographic callus; (B) Moderately hypertrophic ("horse-hoof") have a moderate amount of radiographic callus; and (C) Oligotrophic have minimal to no detectable radiographic callus (making them easy to confuse with nonviable nonunions).

Nonviable Nonunions

Nonviable nonunions (also called **biologically inactive** nonunions) have a severe interruption of blood supply and lack callus production and osteogenic potential. Nonviable nonunions are subdivided into four categories (Figure 91-2).[2,3] **Dystrophic nonunion** is nonunion in which the blood supply to an intermediate fragment is compromised. The fragment heals to one of the main fracture segments, but not to the other. The area of nonunion is biologically inactive as evidenced by a lack of callus, a persistent fracture gap, and rounded, sclerotic fracture ends.

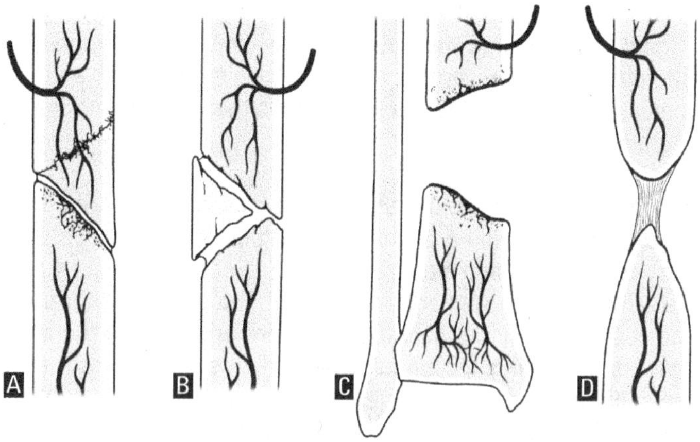

Figure 91-2. Types of nonviable nonunions. (A) Dystrophic nonunion has healing of an intermediate fragment to one of the main segments, but not the other; (B) Necrotic nonunions have one or more isolated, nonhealing, avascular bone fragments ("sequestra") that appear as radiodense fragments with sharp margins; (C) Defect nonunions have a large, nonhealing fracture gap; (D) Atrophic nonunions have defect filled with scar tissue and partial resorption of adjacent fractured bone ends.

Necrotic nonunions have one or more avascular bone fragments within the fracture zone. These avascular bone fragments, called *sequestra*, have no union with any surrounding bone and have sharp margins and sclerosis on radiographs. Necrotic nonunions in dogs and cats are nearly always the result of excessive elevation of soft tissues from a bone fragment combined with bacterial contamination and inadequate stabilization. Conversely, necrotic nonunion seldom occurs when closed or "open but do not touch" treatment strategies are employed to highly comminuted fractures. **Defect nonunions** occur when there is a large gap at the fracture site as a result of the original trauma or from bone fragment loss owing to sequestration, resorption, or surgical removal. Regardless of the specific cause of the defect nonunion, a critically sized defect exists and callus cannot bridge the gap. **Atrophic nonunion** is the end result of the preceding types of nonviable nonunion. The bony defect is filled with scar tissue and the fractured bones are partially resorbed. Poor limb use leads to osteoporosis and muscle atrophy.

A **pseudoarthrosis** may occur with time as a result of motion at the site of the nonunion.[2,3] The clinical conditions are sclerosis of the bone ends, formation of fibrocartilage between the bone ends, and a fibrous capsule filled with serum. Periarticular fibrosis may cause stiffness of the adjacent joint such that much of the motion is concentrated in the pseudoarthrosis, especially if it is near a joint.

Etiology

A complex array of local and systemic factors is necessary to achieve predictable bone healing.[1,7,8] Systemic factors include the patient's nutritional state, hormonal balance, age, general health, and medications. Local factors include the conditions within the fracture zone such as health of the soft tissues, size of the fracture gap, stability, contamination/infection, and foreign materials.

The local environment of the fracture zone must be suitably stable (mechanical environment) and viable (biologic environment) in order for bone healing to occur. Although many local and systemic factors may contribute to the development of nonunion, more often than not, an imbalance in the mechanical and/or biologic conditions of the fracture zone is the major contributor to nonunion.

Poor blood supply to the fracture zone is a common contributing cause of delayed union or nonunion. Blood supply to healthy, intact diaphyseal long bone is primarily from centrifugal flow outward from the intramedullary space.[9] The outer one third of bone is supplied by periosteal vasculature arising from the soft tissues surrounding the bone. When a bone is fractured, the normal blood supply is disrupted and the initial vascular supply for bone healing comes almost entirely from the surrounding extraosseous tissues. Being a viscoelastic material, bone is stiffer and capable of absorbing larger amounts of energy prior to failure when it is more rapidly loaded.[10] Once the failure point is reached, however, the bone fractures and releases this absorbed energy to the surrounding soft tissue envelope, disrupting the blood supply to the fracture zone. Such high energy absorbed to failure often produces a highly comminuted fracture pattern. A surgeon who attempts to anatomically reconstruct the highly comminuted fracture pattern often compounds the vascular compromise to the injured bone.[11] During the extensive manipulation of each fracture fragment, the soft-tissue envelope is further disrupted. If cerclage wire is used in these efforts, it must be used properly because improperly used wire typically loosens and cleaves off any developing extraosseous blood supply.[12] Because even the most delicately performed open approach to the fracture zone induces some injury to the fracture zone's blood supply, the surgeon should contemplate the biologic impact of the treatment plan before starting surgery. Poor blood supply may also be inherent to the region of the fracture. Whereas the femur has a strong muscular attachment along its caudal margin at the linea aspera, the distal tibia has minimal surrounding muscular envelope. Indeed, fractures of the tibia accounted for approximately 60% of all appendicular nonunions in cats in one study.[13] Toy and miniature breeds of dogs have decreased vascular density at the distal diaphyseal-metaphyseal junction of the radius as compared with large breeds of dogs.[14]

Fracture zone instability is another common contributing cause of delayed or nonunion in small animal patients. Strain is a measure of fracture zone motion. Osteoblastic cells have low strain tolerance, consequently direct bone union cannot progress in the presence of excessive fracture zone motion.[15] Callus and fibrocartilage are more strain tolerant and, logically, formation of these tissues is an intermediate step of callus bone healing. However, if formation of these tissues does not effectively reduce fracture gap strain down to tolerable levels, osteoblastic activity cannot occur and a nonunion develops. Indeed, persistence of fibrocartilage in the fracture zone produces a typical histologic appearance of a nonunion.[16] It is important for the surgeon to understand the forces acting on a fracture and the ability of the selected fixation to constrain those forces. A relatively common nonunion scenario arises when a single large Steinmann pin is used to stabilize a transverse, slightly interdigitating, femoral diaphyseal fracture.[17] What appears to be adequate rotational stability intraoperatively is soon discovered to be inadequate as the patient's recovery continues. The torsional moments induced during weight-bearing and muscular contraction exceed the torsional stability provided by the interdigitation of the fracture ends and the negligible frictional interaction of the smooth IM pin surface against the endosteal bone surface. The highly vascularized femoral diaphysis attempts to heal by developing exuberant periosteal callus, but is incapable of reducing strain levels down to a level conducive to osteoblastic activity. Predictably, a hypertrophic viable nonunion develops.

Conversely, fracture zone hyperstability may also contribute to nonunion.[2,3] Although the exact mechanical environment required for optimal bone healing is not known, axial micromotion appears to be beneficial in stimulating bone healing.[18,19] The desired mechanical environment is apparently dynamic, with rigid stability desired early in healing followed by controlled axial micromotion in later stages. It may well be that hyper-rigid fixations may delay or halt healing in these later stages. Indeed, one study suggested that the use of oversized, rigid type II external skeletal fixation contributed to the development of nonunion in cats.[13]

Large fracture gaps, which may result from inadequate fracture reduction or bone loss owing to the original trauma, excision at surgery, or removal of a sequestrum, may contribute to the development of nonunion. Recent emphasis in the treatment of highly comminuted fractures has been on the use of biologic strategies in order to maintain the viability of all bone fragments within the fracture zone.[11,20] These approaches certainly do not advocate surgical removal of vascularized bone fragments, and the development of sequestra appears rare when such strategies are employed in dogs and cats. However, one must be sure that, in the shift of emphasis away from anatomic reduction of these comminuted fractures, large fracture gaps do not remain. Surrounding soft tissues may become interposed within the fracture zone and impede callus formation. There is a species-specific critical-size bone defect greater than which bone healing is not likely. Key's hypothesis states that a long-bone defect greater than 1.5 times the diaphyseal diameter exceeds the regenerative capacity of bone in skeletally mature dogs, thereby causing nonunion.[21,22] Indeed, a 21-mm long defect in the femur stabilized with a bone plate induced atrophic nonunion in dogs.[23] Key's hypothesis appears to overestimate the regenerative capacity of bone in the adult cat.[22] When large fracture gaps are unavoidable, appropriate autogenous or allogeneic bone grafting is indicated to prevent soft-tissue interposition and provide some biologic stimulus for healing within the gap.[8,11,24-29] Alternatively, an osteotomy can be performed adjacent to the fracture gap, and bone transport combined with callus distraction used to fill the large fracture gap.[30-33]

Infection within the regional soft tissues or the bone itself is a relatively uncommon cause of delayed bone healing in dogs.[34] Nonetheless, appropriate aseptic surgical technique must be employed to minimize the incidence of surgical infection. Particular care should be given to the treatment of open fractures as they have a greater incidence of delayed and nonunion.[35] When adequately stabilized, bone can heal in the presence of infection, but healing may be delayed by bone lysis and/or implant loosening.[2,36] Neovascularization of the fracture zone, critical for bone healing, may be impeded by the presence of infection.

In addition to the basic clinical prerequisites for predictable bone healing (fracture zone stability and viability), a complex cascade of events must take place. Local and systemic mediators stimulate the differentiation of precursor mesenchymal cells into new fibroblasts, chondroblasts, osteoclasts, and osteoblasts needed for neovascularization, soft callus, and bone formation.[1,4] One study found fewer committed mesenchymal stem cells in the early stages of experimental nonunions and suggested that the differentiation of mesenchymal stem cells is inhibited in states of chronic nonunion.[37]

Although alterations in the local environment of the fracture zone are more frequently recognized contributors, systemic factors may also delay fracture healing. Hyperparathyroidism, whether primary or secondary to renal or nutritional causes, delays bone healing as a result of calcium and phosphorus imbalance. Hyperadrenocorticism, whether primary or iatrogenic, may alter calcium absorption and deposition enough to delay callus formation. Bone healing may be delayed by administration of corticosteroids, some antineoplastic agents, and possibly some fluoroquinolones and NSAIDs.[38-44] Elderly patients exhibit delayed bone healing as compared with younger, especially skeletally immature, patients.

Diagnosis

Patient signalment and fracture location influence the likelihood of a delayed or nonunion. A study of 2825 fractures in dogs showed a 3.4% incidence of nonunion. The incidence of nonunion was highest in the radius/ulna (40.6%) and femur (38.5%), whereas the humerus (12.5%) and tibia (4.2%) developed nonunion less commonly.[34] A study of 422 fractures in cats showed a 4.3% incidence of nonunions.[13] This fact highlights that, contrary to popular opinion, cats are every bit as prone to major complications of fracture healing as are dogs. Nonunion in cats was most common in fractures of the tibia/fibula (61.1%), radius/ulna (16.7%), and proximal ulna with intact radius (16.7%). Older cats, heavier cats, cats with open fractures, cats with comminuted fractures and cats with fractures stabilized with type II external skeletal fixation were more likely to develop nonunion.[13]

Although radiography is the principal assessment tool for bone healing, one should not lose sight of the importance of physical examination and history taking when making patient assessments and therapeutic decisions. Instances often arise where the radiographic progression of healing is slow, but patient function and comfort are optimal. In such instances, surgical intervention may not be warranted, particularly if fracture healing is progressive, albeit slower than anticipated. Conversely, some patients exhibit lameness, muscle atrophy, pain on fracture-site palpation, stiffness, and even gross fracture instability. These findings are usually associated with some loss of the original fixation through implant migration, implant breakage and/or ensuing fracture instability. Surgical site infection is usually associated with draining tracts originating from the fracture zone, swelling and pain on deep palpation of the fracture zone, or limb manipulation.

Radiographs made at 4- to 8-week intervals are commonly used to assess fracture healing, implant stability, and maintenance of bony apposition and alignment. Making a definitive diagnosis of delayed union is difficult. In delayed union, radiographs indicate progressive healing, but at a slower rate than initially expected. Radiographs may show early bone resorption of the fracture ends, periosteal bone reaction, endosteal and periosteal callus formation, and finally, bridging callus. The radiographic diagnosis of nonunion is based on the lack of progressive fracture healing during a period of 3 or more months and the persistence of a fracture gap. The characteristic radiographic appearance of a nonunion is varied as previously described for each classification. Viable nonunions have variable amounts of callus, but no callus bridging of the fracture zone. Nonviable nonunions lack callus formation. The distinction between viable and nonviable nonunion is critical as this directs the therapy. The distinction between an oligotrophic, viable nonunion and a nonviable nonunion can be particularly challenging. Alternative imaging modalities such as ultrasonography, nuclear scintigraphy, dual x-ray absorptiometry, computed tomography, and magnetic resonance imaging have each been used to assess fracture healing and may have roles in distinguishing viable from nonviable nonunions.[5,45-51] However, as with traditional radiography, each imaging modality has its limitations. Recent investigations have evaluated the predictive value of serum biomarkers in making an early diagnosis of nonunion.[52] In the absence of definitive distinction between viable and nonviable nonunions, clinicians should assume nonviability as this will direct a more aggressive and comprehensive course of action.

Treatment

Identification and treatment of all factors contributing to nonunion are the keys to effective management. Treatment of nonunion typically consists of removal of all loose implants, anaerobic and aerobic bacterial culture (of the fracture zone and/or removed implants/sequestra), and application of a fixation capable of providing long-term stability to the fracture zone. Sequestra, if present, should be removed. Nonviable nonunions require additional specific interventions to stimulate the biologic activity of the fracture zone. These traditionally include reestablishing the intramedullary canal of the main bone fragments, decortication/shingling of the regional main bone segments, and autogenous cancellous bone grafting.[2-4] One study described successful treatment of nonviable nonunions by limited en bloc ostectomy of the nonunion site and compression plate fixation.[53] In this report, autogenous cancellous bone grafting was only used if significant bony defect remained after ostectomy. Other modifications of the traditional treatment strategies for nonviable nonunions include use of demineralized bone matrix allografts, autogeneic and allogeneic mesenchymal stem cells, human recombinant bone morphogenetic protein – 2 (rhBMP-2), other growth factors, autologous bone marrow injections, pulsed electromagnetic fields, low-intensity pulsed ultrasound, extracorporeal shock-wave therapy, and hyperbaric oxygen administration.[24,25,54-71]

Malunion

A malunion fracture is a fracture that has healed in a nonanatomic position. Some degree of malunion is present in most instances of closed-fracture stabilization. Malunion may also be present when biologic strategies for spatial alignment are employed for treatment of highly comminuted fractures. Malunion can occur following anatomic reduction if implants fail prior to complete bone union. Mild degrees of malunion often are tolerated with no apparent short-term or long-term patient morbidity.

Terminology

Malunions are described by their displacement (Figure 91-3). **Overriding malunions** occur when the major bone segments have slid past one another, but normal axial and rotational alignment has been maintained. Minor overriding is usually well tolerated, especially in the pelvic limb, and surgical correction may not be warranted. One study showed that dogs can adapt to 23.5% loss of femoral length without inducing significant patient disability.[72] **Angular malunions** occur when deviation from normal axial alignment is significant. Angular malunion may be in the mediolateral plane (varus or valgus deviation) or the craniocaudal plane (recurvatum or antecurvatum deviation) or any plane in between. Minor recurvatum or antecurvatum is relatively well tolerated, but minor varus or valgus deviation can cause significant locomotor disability. Femoral varus malunion may cause medial patellar luxation and valgus malunion may cause lateral patellar luxation. **Rotational malunions** occur when torsional malalignment is present. Minor torsional malunion is often well tolerated, but excessive torsion can alter a patient's gait and place abnormal stresses on adjacent joints. Excessive femoral torsional malunion may cause patellar luxation or contribute to coxofemoral osteoarthritis.

Etiology

Gravitational, ground reaction forces and muscular pull on the bone segments determine the deviation that occurs with malunion formation. Collapse of the pelvic canal is relatively common when ilial body fractures are treated non-surgically or with insufficient internal fixation.[73-75] External torsional deformity of the proximal femur is common when the pull of the external hip rotator muscles (iliopsoas, gemelli, internal obturator, and quadratus femoris muscles) is not neutralized by intramedullary pin fixation or the rotational displacement is not recognized at the time of fracture reduction and rigid stabilization.[17] After fracture healing, patients tend to hold the hip in a normal position such that the distal limb is internally rotated. Valgus and external torsional deviation of the distal limb is common when applying closed fixation to fractures of the antebrachium and crus.[76,77] Hanging limb positioning has been advocated for surgical fixation of diaphyseal fractures of the radius/ulna and tibia/fibula. Using a large pointed reduction forcep anchored to the malleoli or talus seems to reduce the tendency for cranial angulation of the distal segment in tibial diaphyseal fractures.

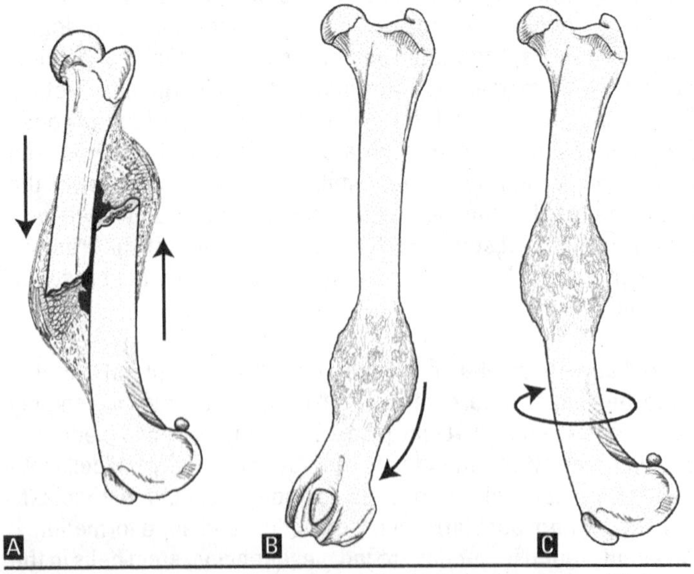

Figure 91-3. Malunions are described by their displacement. (A) Overriding malunion; (B) Angular malunion; (C) Rotational malunion.

Diagnosis and Treatment Plannning

Careful gait observation, physical examination, and radiographic assessment are needed prior to surgical corrective osteotomy procedures. Mild alterations in limb position during radiography can induce artifactual limb alignment measurements on radiographs because radiographs reduce a three-dimensional structure to a two-dimensional image.[78,79] Placement of the affected bone parallel to and as close to the radiographic cassette as possible should reduce radiographic artifact.[78] Care should also be taken to place the limb in neutral rotation and include the joints proximal and distal to the affected bone. It is advisable to perform repeated radiographs with the limb held in the proper position to be certain that malalignment measurements are repeatable. It is essential that the surgeon think three-dimensionally when studying the radiographs. Alternatively, computed tomography including three-dimensional reconstructions can be used.[79-82] In fact, three-dimensional models can be made commercially from these CT studies.[83]

Treatment

Surgery is indicated when the patient does not have acceptable function. The goals of surgical correction of malunion are to improve limb function by restoring more normal alignment and length, thereby correcting abnormal stresses in adjacent joints. If only minor improvements in alignment, limb length, and most importantly, limb function are anticipated, then the morbidity, risks, and costs of the procedure may preclude surgical treatment. When surgical treatment for malunion is indicated, a corrective osteotomy is usually performed at the point of maximal deformity. Ideally, the osteotomy would allow maximal bony contact at the osteotomy and preserve or restore normal limb length and limb alignment. Different forms of osteotomies can be performed, each with their own advantages, disadvantages, and indications. Commonly performed osteotomies include transverse, closing wedge, opening wedge, oblique, step, and dome osteotomies (Figure 91-4).

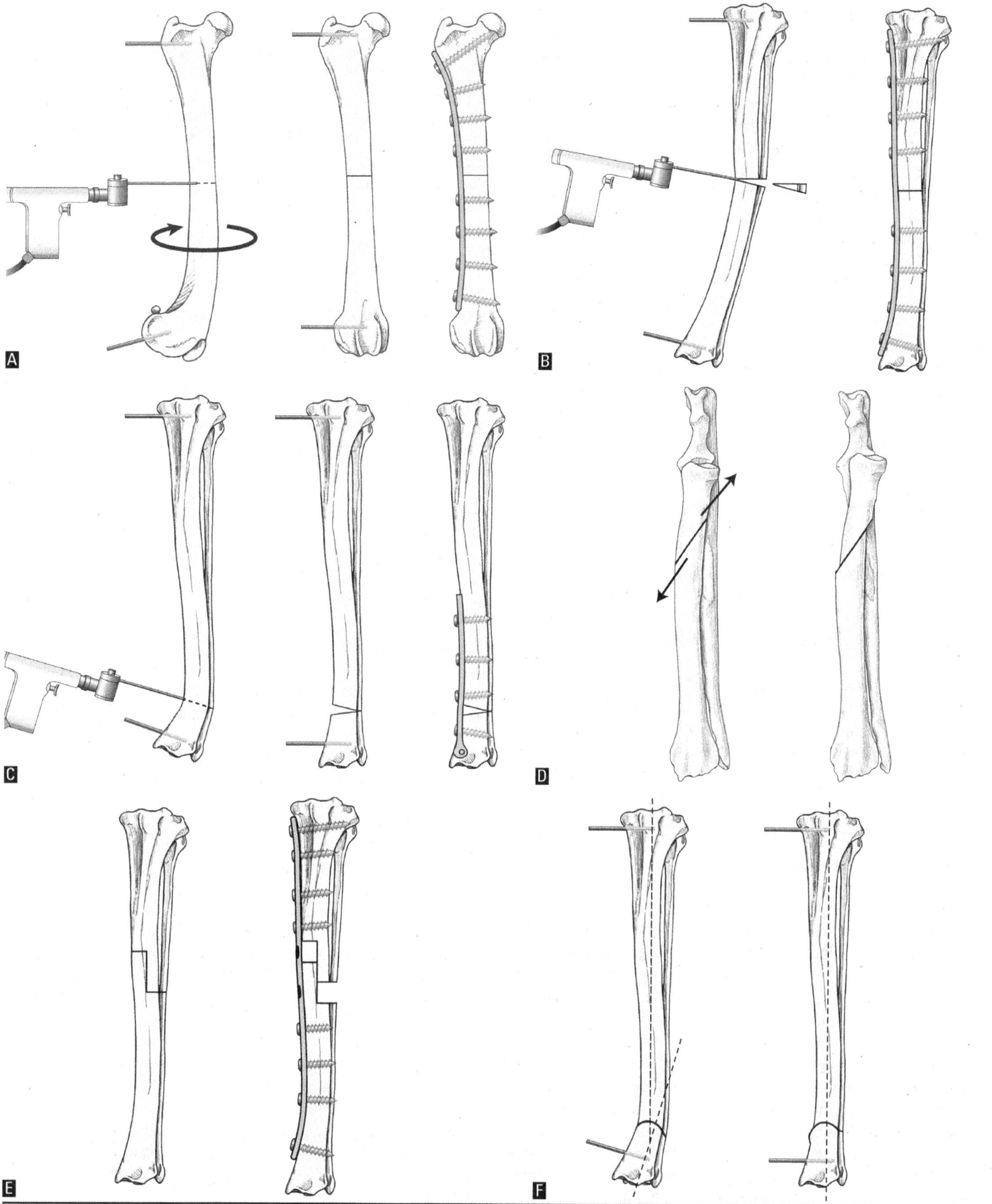

Figure 91-4. Corrective osteotomies. (A) Transverse; (B) Closing wedge; (C) Opening wedge; (D) Oblique; (E) Step; (F) Dome.

Transverse osteotomies are indicated for correction of simple torsional malunions. Closing and opening wedge osteotomies are used for correction of angular malunions. **Closing wedge osteotomies** maximize bony contact, but may result in some loss of limb length. **Opening wedge osteotomies** sacrifice bony contact at the osteotomy in favor of increasing limb length. Sliding of **oblique osteotomies** can be used to correct translational deformity and to achieve some lengthening (or shortening) of the limb. **Step osteotomies** are relatively complex and are, on rare occasions, used to obtain acute limb lengthening. **Dome osteotomies** are used to correct angular deformity while maximizing bony contact and preserving limb length. Dome osteotomies have been described for correction of malunions of the femur, radius and ulna.[84,85] Conceptually, a three-dimensional dome osteotomy would function similar to a ball-in-socket joint and would easily allow for three-dimensional corrections in limb alignment prior to application of the fixation. In reality, most dome osteotomies are made in two dimensions such that three-dimensional corrections sacrifice some bony contact at the osteotomy.

Osteotomies can be used for acute limb alignment correction with static fixation or for slow progressive limb alignment correction using dynamic fixation methods. Static fixation is most often obtained with external fixators, bone plates, or interlocking nails. External fixators offer several advantages for corrective osteotomies: (1) placement of the fixation pins parallel to the adjacent joints prior to osteotomy helps the surgeon visualize when the joints are properly aligned; (2) complex contouring of a bone plate is not required; (3) fixation pins can be placed into a relatively small bone segment.[76,86,87] Locking screw/plate designs may simplify the use of bone plate stabilization of corrective osteotomies because the interlock between the screw head and the plate obviates the need for precise plate contouring.[88] Bone plates and interlocking nails can be of limited use when the osteotomy leaves a relatively small bone segment. On occasion, cross-pin fixation can be used in young dogs in osteotomies performed in the metaphyseal region. Rarely, coaptation has been used with dome osteotomies.[84]

If significant limb lengthening and angular correction are required, progressive callus distraction (callotasis) is indicated.[89-91] Often correction of angular malalignment can be performed acutely, but restoration of large discrepancies in limb length must be performed gradually. Callus distraction involves stabilizing an osteotomy with a specially designed external fixator that utilizes linear motors to induce distraction. Ring fixators with linear motors are commonly employed for such osteotomy distractions and provide the surgeon with several key advantages: (1) the rings placed around the limb allow the surgeon to correct complex three-dimensional malalignment with relative ease; (2) corrections to alignment can be made after the fixation is applied; and (3) the use of small-diameter, tensioned fixation wires allows the system to be applied to small bone segments. After allowing a lag period for initial callus formation, the osteotomy is gradually distracted at a rate of approximately 1 mm per day. Once the desired limb length is achieved, daily distractions cease and the static fixation (1 month per cm distraction) allows regenerate bone in the osteotomy gap to consolidate.

References

1. Frost H: The biology of fracture healing: an overview for clinicians. Part I. Clin Orthop 248:283-293, 1989.

2. Piermattei DL FG: Delayed union and nonunion. *In* Handbook of Small Animal Orthopedics and Fracture Repair, 3rd ed. Piermattei DL FG (ed). Philadelphia: WB Saunders, 1997, pp. 154-162.

3. Sumner-Smith G: Delayed unions and nonunions. Vet Clin North Am (Small Anim Pract) 21:745-760, 1991.

4. Robello GT, Aron DN: Delayed and nonunion fractures. Semin Vet Med Surg (Small Anim) 7:98-104, 1992.

5. Southwood LL, Kawcak CE, McIlwraith CW, et al: Use of scintigraphy for assessment of fracture healing and early diagnosis of osteomyelitis following fracture repair in rabbits. Am J Vet Res 64:736-745, 2003.

6. Wahner H: Radionuclides in the diagnosis of fracture healing. J Nucl Med 19:1356-1358, 1978.

7. Palmer R: Decision-making in fracture treatment: the fracture-patient scoring system. American College of Veterinary Surgeons Symposium 1994;388-390.

8. Piermattei DL FG: Fractures: classification, diagnosis and treatment. *In* Handbook of Small Animal Orthopedics and Fracture Repair, 3rd ed. Piermattei DL FG (ed). Philadelphia: WB Saunders, 1997, pp. 24-146.

9. Rhinelander F: Normal bone anatomy. *In* Textbook of Small Animal Orthopaedics.Newton C, Nunamaker DM (eds). Philadelphia: JB Lippincott, 1985, p.12.

10. Nordin M, Frankel VH: Biomechanics of bone. *In* Basic Biomechanics of the Musculoskeletal System, 2nd ed. Nordin M, Frankel VH (eds). Lea & Febiger, Philadelphia, 1989.

11. Palmer RH: Biological osteosynthesis. Vet Clin North Am Small Anim Pract 29:1171-1185, vii, 1999.

12. Newton CD, Hohn RB: Fracture nonunion resulting from Cerclage appliances. J Am Vet Med Assoc 164:503-508, 1974.

13. Nolte DM, Fusco JV, Peterson ME: Incidence of and predisposing factors for nonunion of fractures involving the appendicular skeleton in cats: 18 cases (1998-2002). J Am Vet Med Assoc 226:77-82, 2005.

14. Welch JA, Boudrieau RJ, DeJardin LM, et al: The intraosseous blood supply of the canine radius: implications for healing of distal fractures in small dogs. Vet Surg 26:57-61, 1997.

15. Perren SM: Physical and biological aspects of fracture healing with special reference to internal fixation. Clin Orthop Relat Res 175-196, 1979.

16. Sumner-Smith G: A histological study of fracture nonunion in small dogs. J Small Anim Pract 15:571-578, 1974.

17. Braden TD, Brinker WO: Radiologic and gross anatomic evaluation of bone healing in the dog. J Am Vet Med Assoc 169:1318-1323, 1976.

18. Goodship AE, Kenwright J: The influence of induced micromovement upon the healing of experimental tibial fractures. J Bone Joint Surg Br 67:650-655, 1985.

19. Goodship AE, Watkins PE, Rigby HS, et al: The role of fixator frame stiffness in the control of fracture healing. An experimental study. J Biomech 26:1027-1035, 1993.

20. Perren SM: Evolution of the internal fixation of long bone fractures. The scientific basis of biological internal fixation: choosing a new balance between stability and biology. J Bone Joint Surg Br 84:1093-1110, 2002.

21. Key J: The effect of a local calcium depot on osteogenesis and healing of fractures. J Bone Joint Surg 16(A):176-184, 1934.

22. Toombs JP, Wallace LJ, Bjorling DE, et al: Evaluation of Key's hypothesis in the feline tibia: an experimental model for augmented bone healing studies. Am J Vet Res 46:513-518, 1985.

23. Kraus K, et al: Critically sized osteo-periosteal femoral defects: a dog model. J Invest Surg 12:115,1999.

24. Kawcak CE, Trotter GW, Powers BE, et al: Comparison of bone healing by demineralized bone matrix and autogenous cancellous bone in horses. Vet Surg 29:218-226, 2000.

25. Kraus KH, Kadiyala S, Wotton H, et al: Critically sized osteo-periosteal femoral defects: a dog model. J Invest Surg 12:115-124, 1999.

26. Lenehan T, Smith GK: Management of infected tibial nonunions with sequestration in the dog. Vet Surg 13:115-121, 1984.

27. Toombs JP, Wallace LJ: Evaluation of autogeneic and allogeneic cortical chip grafting in a feline tibial nonunion model. Am J Vet Res 46:519-528, 1985.

28. Vaughan L: The use of bone autografts in canine orthopedic surgery. J Small Anim Pract 1972;13.

29. Wilson JW, Rhinelander FW, Stewart CL: Vascularization of cancellous chip bone grafts. Am J Vet Res 46:1691-1699, 1985.

30. Claes L, Laule J, Wenger K, et al: The influence of stiffness of the fixator on maturation of callus after segmental transport. J Bone Joint Surg Br 82:142-148, 2000.

31. Kesemenli C, Subasi M, Kirkgoz T, et al: Treatment of traumatic bone defects by bone transport. Acta Orthop Belg 67:380-386, 2001.

32. Klotch DW, Ganey TM, Slater-Haase A, et al: Assessment of bone formation during osteoneogenesis: a canine model. Otolaryngol Head Neck Surg 112:291-302, 1995.

33. Raschke MJ, Mann JW, Oedekoven G, Claudi BF: Segmental transport after unreamed intramedullary nailing. Preliminary report of a "Monorail" system. Clin Orthop Relat Res 282:233-240, 1992.

34. Atilola M, Sumner-Smith, SG: Nonunion fractures in dogs. J Vet Orthop 3:21-24, 1984.

35. Stampley A, Delmain, KS: The results of internal fixation for the treatment of open fractures in 32 dogs. Canine Pract 16:22, 1991.

36. Stead A: Osteomyelitis in the dog and cat. J Small Anim Pract 25:1, 1984.

37. Boyan BD, Caplan AI, Heckman JD, et al: Osteochondral progenitor cells in acute and chronic canine nonunions. J Orthop Res 17:246-255, 1999.

38. Goodman S, Ma T, Trindade M, et al: COX-2 selective NSAID decreases bone ingrowth in vivo. J Orthop Res 20:1164-1169, 2002.

39. Hogevold HE, Grogaard B, Reikeras O: Effects of short-term treatment with corticosteroids and indomethacin on bone healing. A mechanical study of osteotomies in rats. Acta Orthop Scand 63:607-611, 1992.

40. Huddleston PM, Steckelberg JM, Hanssen AD, et al: Ciprofloxacin inhibition of experimental fracture healing. J Bone Joint Surg Am 82:161-173, 2000.

41. Sawin PD, Dickman CA, Crawford NR, et al: The effects of dexamethasone on bone fusion in an experimental model of posterolateral lumbar spinal arthrodesis. J Neurosurg 94:76-81, 2001.

42. Simon AM, Manigrasso MB, O'Connor JP: Cyclo-oxygenase 2 function is essential for bone fracture healing. J Bone Miner Res 17:963-976, 2002.

43. Waters RV, Gamradt SC, Asnis P, et al: Systemic corticosteroids inhibit bone healing in a rabbit ulnar osteotomy model. Acta Orthop Scand 71:316-321, 2000.

44. Zhang X, Schwarz EM, Young DA, et al: Cyclooxygenase-2 regulates mesenchymal cell differentiation into the osteoblast lineage and is critically involved in bone repair. J Clin Invest 109:1405-1415, 2002.

45. den Boer FC, Patka P, Bakker FC, et al: New segmental long bone defect model in sheep: quantitative analysis of healing with dual energy x-ray absorptiometry. J Orthop Res 17:654-660: 1999.

46. Markel MD, Bogdanske JJ, Xiang Z, et al: Atrophic nonunion can be predicted with dual energy x-ray absorptiometry in a canine ostectomy model. J Orthop Res 13:869-875, 1995.

47. Hendler A, Hershkop M: When to use bone scintigraphy. It can reveal things other studies cannot. Postgrad Med 104:54-56, 59-61, 65-56 passim, 1998.

48. Kim N: Evaluation of fracture healing in canine radius by bone scan with 99m Tc-MDP. Korean J Vet Clin Med 16:293-299, 1999.

49. Lynch JA, Grigoryan M, Fierlinger A, et al: Measurement of changes in trabecular bone at fracture sites using X-ray CT and automated image registration and processing. J Orthop Res 22:362-367, 2004.

50. Risselada M, Kramer M, de Rooster H, et al: Ultrasonographic and radiographic assessment of uncomplicated secondary fracture healing of long bones in dogs and cats. Vet Surg 34:99-107, 2005.

51. Schelstraete K, Daneels F, Obrie E: Technetium-99m-diphosphonate, gallium-67 and labeled leukocyte scanning techniques in tibial nonunion. Acta Orthop Belg;58 Suppl 1:168-172, 1992.

52. Southwood LL, Frisbie DD, Kawcak CE, et al: Evaluation of serum biochemical markers of bone metabolism for early diagnosis of nonunion and infected nonunion fractures in rabbits. Am J Vet Res 64:727-735, 2003.

53. Blaeser LL, Gallagher JG, Boudrieau RJ: Treatment of biologically inactive nonunions by a limited en bloc ostectomy and compression plate fixation: a review of 17 cases. Vet Surg 32:91-100, 2003.

54. Connolly JF, Guse R, Tiedeman J, et al: Autologous marrow injection as a substitute for operative grafting of tibial nonunions. Clin Orthop Relat Res 259-270, 1991.

55. Tiedeman JJ, Connolly JF, Strates BS, et al: Treatment of nonunion by percutaneous injection of bone marrow and demineralized bone matrix. An experimental study in dogs. Clin Orthop Relat Res 294-302, 1991.

56. Baylink DJ, Finkelman RD, Mohan S: Growth factors to stimulate bone formation. J Bone Miner Res 8 Suppl 2:S565-572, 1993.

57. Bodamyali T, Bhatt B, Hughes FJ, et al: Pulsed electromagnetic fields simultaneously induce osteogenesis and upregulate transcription of bone morphogenetic proteins 2 and 4 in rat osteoblasts in vitro. Biochem Biophys Res Commun 250:458-461, 1998.

58. Clark DM: The use of electrical current in the treatment of nonunions. Vet Clin North Am Small Anim Pract 17:793-798, 1987.

59. Dimitriou R, Tsiridis E, Giannoudis PV: Current concepts of molecular aspects of bone healing. Injury 36(12): 1392-1404, 2005.

60. Itoh T, Mochizuki M, Fuda K, et al: Femoral nonunion fracture treated with recombinant human bone morphogenetic protein-2 in a dog. J Vet Med Sci 60:535-538, 1998.

61. Kerwin SC, Lewis DD, Elkins AD, et al: Effect of hyperbaric oxygen treatment on incorporation of an autogenous cancellous bone graft in a nonunion diaphyseal ulnar defect in cats. Am J Vet Res 61:691-698, 2000.

62. Mayr E, Frankel V, Ruter A: Ultrasound - an alternative healing method for nonunions. Arch Orthop Trauma Surg 120:1-8, 2000.

63. Meskens M, Stuyck JA, Feys H, Mulier J: Treatment of nonunion using pulsed electromagnetic fields: a retrospective followup study. Acta Orthop Belg 56:483-488, 1990.

64. Millis DL: Bone- and non-bone-derived growth factors and effects on bone healing. Vet Clin North Am Small Anim Pract 29:1221-1246, 1999.

65. Millis DL, Wilkens BE, Daniel GB, et al: Radiographic, densitometric, and biomechanical effects of recombinant canine somatotropin in an unstable ostectomy gap model of bone healing in dogs. Vet Surg 27:85-93, 1998.

66. Paatsama S, Lindholm S, Oksanen J, et al: [The use of bone morphogenetic proteins in delayed fracture healing, pseudoarthrosis and in ulna osteotomy carried out because of elbow joint diseases]. Tierarztl Prax 24:164-168, 1996.

67. Rompe JD, Rosendahl T, Schollner C, et al: High-energy extracorporeal shock wave treatment of nonunions. Clin Orthop Relat Res 387:102-111, 2001:

68. Schaden W, Fischer A, Sailler A: Extracorporeal shock wave therapy of nonunion or delayed osseous union. Clin Orthop Relat Res 387:90-94, 2001.

69. Schmokel HG, Weber FE, Seiler G, et al: Treatment of nonunions with nonglycosylated recombinant human bone morphogenetic protein-2 delivered from a fibrin matrix. Vet Surg 33:112-118, 2004.

70. Suresh Kumar R, Ramakrishna O, Sreerman PK: Histologic changes during femoral fracture defect healing using demineralized bone matrix combinations in canines. Indian Vet J 76:38-41, 1999.

71. Warden S, Bennell KL, McMeeken JM, Ward JD: Acceleration of fresh fracture repair using the sonic accelerated fracture healing system (SAFHS): a review. Calcif Tissue Int 66:157-163, 2000.

72. Wagner SD, Desch JP 2nd, Ferguson HR, et al: Effect of distal femoral growth plate fusion on femoral-tibial length. Vet Surg 16:435-439, 1987.

73. Bertoy RW: Megacolon in the cat. Vet Clin North Am Small Anim Pract 32:901-915, 2002.

74. Ferguson JF: Triple pelvic osteotomy for the treatment of pelvic canal stenosis in a cat. J Small Anim Pract 37:495-498, 1996.

75. White RN: Surgical management of constipation. J Feline Med Surg 4:129-138, 2002.

76. Johnson AL, Kneller SK, Weigel RM: Radial and tibial fracture repair with external skeletal fixation. Effects of fracture type, reduction, and complications on healing. Vet Surg 18:367-372, 1989.

77. Fjeld T: [Surgical correction of angular deformities of the radius and ulna following malunion fractures]. Nord Vet Med 37:273-285, 1985.

78. Palmer R: Patellar luxation in large breed dogs. American College of Veterinary Surgeons Symposium 2004.

79. Kawakami H, Sugano N, Yonenobu K, et al: Effects of rotation on measurement of lower limb alignment for knee osteotomy. J Orthop Res 22:1248-1253, 2004.

80. Zannoni C, Cappello A, Viceconti M: Optimal CT scanning plan for long-bone 3-D reconstruction. IEEE Trans Med Imaging 17:663-666, 1998.

81. Apelt D, Kowaleski MP, Dyce J: Comparison of computed tomographic and standard radiographic determination of tibial torsion in the dog. Vet Surg 34:457-462, 2005.

82. Aper R, Kowaleski MP, Apelt D, et al: Computed tomographic determination of tibial torsion in the dog. Vet Radiol Ultrasound 46:187-191, 2005.

83. www.protomed.net. 2005.

84. MacDonald JM, Matthiesen D: Treatment of forelimb growth plate deformity in 11 dogs by radial dome osteotomy and external coaptation. Vet Surg 20:402-408, 1991.

85. Sikes R, Olds RB, Renegar W, Wayne S: Dome osteotomy for the correction of long bone malunions: case reports and discussion of surgical technique. J Am Anim Hosp Assoc 22:221-226, 1986.

86. Fox SM, Bray JC, Guerin SR, et al: Antebrachial deformities in the dog: treatment with external fixation. J Small Anim Pract 36:315-320, 1995.

87. Quinn MK, Ehrhart N, Johnson AL, et al: Realignment of the radius in canine antebrachial growth deformities treated with corrective osteotomy and bilateral (type II) external fixation. Vet Surg 29:558-563, 2000.

88. Wagner M: General principles for the clinical use of the LCP. Injury 34 Suppl 2:B31-42, 2003.

89. Rahal SC, Volpi RS, Vulcano LC: Treatment of segmental tibial defects using acute bone shortening followed by gradual lengthening with circular external fixator. J Vet Med A Physiol Pathol Clin Med 52:180-185, 2005.

90. Marcellin-Little DJ, Ferretti A, Roe SC, et al: Hinged Ilizarov external fixation for correction of antebrachial deformities. Vet Surg 27:231-245, 1998.

91. Yanoff SR, Hulse DA, Palmer RH, et al: Distraction osteogenesis using modified external fixation devices in five dogs. Vet Surg 21:480-487, 1992.

Chapter 92

Septic Arthritis

Loretta J. Bubenik

Septic arthritis refers to an active joint infection, usually bacterial in origin. It is not common in companion animals, but when it occurs, it can be devastating for the joint. Treatment and outcome depend on the source, organism involved, and duration of infection.

Etiology

Septic arthritis occurs from exogenous inoculation or hematogenous spread of bacteria to the joint. Penetrating injuries, surgical procedures, and intraarticular injections are common exogenous sources. Hematogenous infection occurs when bacteria from distant sites, such as the respiratory tract, oral cavity, umbilicus, genitourinary tract, or heart, localize in the joint.[1] Preexisting disease or conditions causing immunosuppression predispose to joint infection.[2,3] Young animals are often affected, although no breed or age predilection exists.[4]

Escherichia coli, Staphylococcus, Streptococcus, and *Pasteurella* species are commonly isolated from septic joints, with staphylococcal infections being most prevalent.[5,6] *Borrelia burgdorferi,* bacterial L-forms, *Mycoplasma spumans, Mycobacterium tuberculosis,* fungi, protozoa, and rickettsial organisms have also been implicated.[2]

Pathophysiology

Once exposed to bacteria, a cascade of events initiates the potentially destructive process within the joint environment. Bacterial infiltration results in synovial tissue edema, activation of the immune system, and initiation of the inflammatory cascade. Inflammation of the synovium, capillary rupture, and necrosis promote extravasation of fibrin, clotting factors, polymorphonuclear leukocytes, and proteinaceous fluid into the joint.[7] Intraarticular pressure increases, potentially leading to ischemia, subluxation, or avascular necrosis of intraarticular structures. Lysosomal enzymes and enzyme by-products released during activation of the inflammatory cascade degrade cartilage, disrupt synovial fluid dynamics, and impair cartilage nutrition.[7] Granulation tissue formed as a result of inflammation can penetrate and undermine the cartilage, causing further joint destruction.[8] As the process progresses and cartilage is destroyed, subchondral bone can also become involved.[8] Destruction of articular cartilage and degenerative joint changes combined with thickening and scarring of periarticular tissues leads to restricted joint mobility, and in severe cases, loss of joint function. Early therapeutic intervention is imperative to minimize destructive joint changes.[8,9]

Diagnosis

Isolation of bacteria from the joint in question is necessary for definitive diagnosis of septic arthritis, but this is not always possible and degree of suspicion plays a role. Attempt at bacterial isolation is made by aseptic arthrocentesis followed by cytologic evaluation and culture of the synovial fluid. Abnormal cytologic findings consistent with septic arthritis include increased numbers of white blood cells (40,000/μL or greater, mostly neutrophils that may or may not be degenerate), loss of fluid viscosity, presence of intracellular bacteria, and increased fluid turbidity (Table 92-1).[5,6,10] Direct plating of synovial fluid for culture is not ideal because this leads to frequent negative results.[11,12] Culture of the synovium has been clinically shown to be more beneficial than culture of synovial fluid alone,[5,13] but reports are conflicting in that experimental tests have not shown the same.[11] Submission of synovial fluid on a culture swab has the potential to inhibit some organisms, resulting in decreased yield,[14] although reasonable success can be achieved using the technique.[11] To facilitate bacterial growth, synovial fluid should immediately be placed in blood culture media at a 1:9 ratio. The synovial fluid-culture media combination is incubated for 24 hours at 37 C (98.6 F) before being plated for identification of organisms.[11]

Other diagnostics depend on the suspected type of infection. In all cases a complete blood count, chemistry panel, and urinalysis should be performed to evaluate the animal as a whole and to look for systemic disease, although yield might be low. In cases of aspergillosis, fungal hyphae might be seen and can be cultured from synovial fluid.[15] Special stains such as India ink, periodic acid-Schiff, and silver nitrate stains, or treatment of preparations with 10% potassium hydroxide can improve visualization of fungal organisms.[16,17] Synovial fluid from cats with calicivirus infection can be normal or can have elevated cell counts with a predominance of mononuclear cells; virus isolation is possible from synovial fluid and tissues of affected joints.[18] Polymerase chain reaction with DNA isolation can be useful in some cases

Table 92-1. Characteristics of Synovial Fluid from Normal and Septic Joints for Comparison.[5,6,10]

	Normal Joint	Septic Joint
Color	Clear to light straw	Pink-tinged to yellow/white
Turbidity	None	Turbid
Viscosity	Viscous, 2-5 cm string test	Low viscosity, < 2 cm string test
N. cell count	≤ 500 to 3,000 cells/μL	≥ 40,000 cells/μL
Cell type	10% Neutrophils 60-90% Mononuclear cells	> 80% Neutrophils, may or may not be degenerate
Volume	Minimal (< 0.25 to 1ml)	Large (often > 1ml)

N.= Nucleated

of septic arthritis in which definitive diagnosis is difficult, such as mycobacterial infections.[19] The source of infection should be isolated in cases of hematogenous seeding of the joint with bacteria.

Early radiographic changes associated with septic arthritis include joint effusion and soft-tissue swelling. With progression of disease, bone lysis, joint surface irregularity, bone sclerosis, ankylosis, and subluxation can be seen.[20] Nuclear scintigraphy provides earlier diagnostic information than does conventional radiography. Positive joints do not specifically indicate infection;[21-23] however, newer scintigraphic agents have the potential to differentiate infection from other forms of inflammation.[24] Advanced imaging through computed tomography or magnetic resonance imaging might also be beneficial in the diagnosis of joint infection.[20,25]

Clinical Findings

In animals suffering from septic arthritis, the affected joint is usually swollen and painful. Only one joint is typically involved. The joint might be warm to the touch and the animal is often severely lame or unable to bear weight. Systemic signs such as malaise, inappetence, and fever are variable in cases of exogenous disease, but with hematogenous infection, they are more likely to be present.[13] In addition to fever, anorexia, depression, and oral ulcerations, cats affected with calicivirus can exhibit acute swelling and pain of the distal joints and may be reluctant to move.[18,26]

Treatment

Therapy is directed at minimizing cartilage destruction and eradicating the infection. Antimicrobials are administered after synovial fluid for cytologic evaluation, culture, and susceptibility testing has been obtained. Intravenous administration of a broad spectrum, bactericidal antimicrobial is indicated initially, but a favorable initial response permits a change to oral antimicrobial administration within the first 3 to 5 days of therapy. Long-term antimicrobial administration is based on culture and bacterial susceptibility testing. If culture results are negative, antimicrobial therapy is continued based on positive clinical response to treatment. Antimicrobials should be continued for a minimum of 4 weeks or at least 2 weeks beyond the resolution of clinical signs.

Final antibiotic choice is based on culture and antimicrobial susceptibility testing. If empiric antibiotic administration is necessary, care should be taken in antibiotic selection because antimicrobial resistance of commonly isolated organisms is constantly changing. Staphylococci, in one report, showed 18% resistance to first-generation cephalosporins.[27] Clinical response to treatment should always be monitored. Common first-line defense antimicrobials would include first-generation cephalosporins and penicillins supplemented with β-lactamase inhibitors because Staphylococci are most commonly isolated from joint infections.[27] Tetracycline is recommended for those animals with infectious arthritis secondary to *Borrelia*, rickettsial infections, *Mycoplasma*, and bacterial L-forms.[2,13]

Antibiotic penetration into joint cavities and efficacy against the causative organism is necessary for resolution of infection. Synovial fluid and serum antibiotic kinetics are similar, with synovial fluid concentrations gradually increasing as serum concentrations rise.[28,29] Final synovial fluid concentration depends on the molecular size of the antibiotic and inflammation-dependent changes in synovial membrane permeability.[28,29] Synovial fluid antibiotic concentrations decrease as joint inflammation resolves, but therapeutic antibiotic concentrations within the joint likely remain.[12,30] Following equilibration, antibiotic concentration within the joint is the same or higher after systemic administration when compared with intraarticular injection, so systemic therapy alone is typically sufficient.[31] Furthermore, intraarticular injection of antibiotics can cause chemical synovitis with worsening of the pathologic process and should be avoided.[32,33]

Medical management consisting of appropriate antimicrobial therapy, passive range of motion exercises, and pain management can result in resolution of infection and return to function if the animal is treated aggressively and early in the course of disease.[34] However, joint lavage is essential to remove cellular and enzymatic constituents in some cases. In young animals, decompression can be especially important to reduce pressure within the joint and preserve epiphyseal vascularity.[7] Needle aspiration and lavage alone do not adequately remove deleterious materials from the joint, but can provide some benefit if surgical lavage is not an option.[34] Arthrotomy or arthroscopy with surgical debridement and copious lavage of the affected joint is indicated for postoperative joint infections, septic joints untreated for 72 hours or more, joints that have not responded to 72 hours of appropriate medical management, or joint infection secondary to penetrating wounds.[9,34] At the time of surgery, the joint is explored, cultured, debrided of necrotic debris, and lavaged with large volumes of an isotonic solution. Joints with healthy appearing tissues after debridement and lavage are closed primarily at the time of surgery. If the tissue appears unhealthy, open-joint management or ingress-egress systems may need to be utilized.

An ingress-egress flushing system allows for continued joint lavage during the postoperative period and is considered for animals with severe infections and extensive tissue damage. However, intraarticular drainage systems can be difficult to maintain. Open-joint management is an effective alternative. Open joints and lavage systems should be managed aseptically and the drains removed or the joint closed when drainage is minimal and less purulent to decrease the chance of nosocomial infection. Open joints should be kept moist until they are closed. Cytologic evaluation of exudate can be helpful in deciding when to remove the drain or close the joint.

Fluid therapy and nutritional supplementation should be instituted as needed. The inciting cause in cases of hematogenous seeding of the joint with bacteria must be found and treated appropriately. Pain medication is imperative to facilitate joint mobility and patient comfort. It is also important to maintain joint mobility through passive range of motion activity, yet limit heavy weight-bearing to prevent undue stress on the already weakened articular cartilage. Swimming or underwater treadmill activity would be beneficial because joint stress is reduced through these activities. In severe cases that have not responded to antibiotic therapy or surgery and in cases with irreversible, severe joint damage or stiffness, amputation is a feasible alternative. For some joints, arthrodesis is indicated if the infection, but not the severe destructive changes within the joint, can be eliminated.

Prognosis

Prognosis is variable and depends on the degree of cartilage destruction and duration of disease. Arthritis is expected following joint infection, but the severity and resulting disability are difficult to predict. Up to 50% of people suffer permanent joint dysfunction and 75% have residual disabilities after treatment of septic arthritis.[35,36] Many animals recover with minimal deficits, but others suffer permanent joint dysfunction.[6,34] Furthermore, some animals will have a residual lameness secondary to a continued immune response to lingering microbial antigens within the joint, even though the infection has been eradicated.[37] These animals might respond to corticosteroid therapy, but treatment should only be initiated after repeated negative joint cultures.[2] Calicivirus infection in kittens is usually self-limiting, but can be associated with a 25% mortality rate in adults cats.[18,26]

In summary, septic arthritis can lead to severe joint destruction and debilitation if not treated aggressively and early in the course of the disease. Parenteral antibiotic therapy followed by long-term oral antibiotic administration is imperative. Surgical intervention is necessary in some instances to decompress the joint, debride devitalized tissue, and lavage. Arthritis is expected after joint infection, but early treatment can minimize joint destruction.

References

1. Koch D: Management of infectious arthritis in the horse. Comp Cont Educ Pract Vet 1:545, 1979.

2. Bennett D, May C: Joint diseases of dogs and cats. *In* Textbook of Veterinary Internal Medicine. Ettinger SJ, Feldman EC (ed). Philadelphia: WB Saunders, 1995, p. 2032.

3. Gardner GC, Weisman MH: Pyarthrosis in patients with rheumatoid arthritis: A report of 13 cases and a review of the literature from the past 40 years. Am J Med 88(5):503, 1990.

4. Soontornvipart K, Kohout P, Proks P: Septic arthritis in dogs: A retrospective study of 20 cases (2000-2002). Acta Vet BRNO 72:405, 2003.

5. Bennett D, Taylor D: Bacterial infective arthritis in the dog. J Small Anim Pract 29:207, 1988.

6. Marchevsky AM, Read RA: Bacterial septic arthritis in 19 dogs. Aust Vet J 77(4):233, 1999.

7. Goldenberg DL: Septic arthritis. Lancet 351(9097):197, 1998.

8. Alderson M, Nade S: Natural history of acute septic arthritis in an avian model. J Orthop Res 5(2):261, 1987.

9. Brown S, Newton C: Infectious arthritis and wounds of joints. *In* Textbook of Small Animal Orthopaedics. Newton C, Nunamaker D (ed). Philadelphia: JB Lippincott, 1985, p.1047.

10. Duncan RJ, Prasse KW, Mahaffey EA: Veterinary Laboratory Medicine, Clinical Pathology. Ames: Iowa State University Press, 1994, p. 300.

11. Montgomery RD, Long IR, Milton JL, et al: Comparison of aerobic culturette, synovial membrane biopsy, and blood culture medium in detection of canine bacterial arthritis. Vet Surg 18(4):300, 1989.

12. Bertone AL, McIlwraith CW, Jones RL, et al: Comparison of various treatments for experimentally induced equine infectious arthritis. Am J Vet Res 48(3):519, 1987.

13. Budsberg S: Musculoskeletal infections. *In* Infectious Diseases of the Dog and Cat. Greene C (ed). Philadelphia: WB Saunders, 1998, p. 555.

14. Carr AP: Infectious arthritis in dogs and cats. Vet Med 92:786, 1997.

15. Day MJ, Penhale WJ, Eger CE, et al: Disseminated aspergillosis in dogs. Aust Vet J 63(2):55, 1986.

16. Jang SS, Biberstein EL: Fungal diseases. *In* Infectious Diseases of the Dog and Cat. Green C (ed). Philadelphia: WB Saunders, 1998, p. 349.

17. Marcellin-Little DJ, Sellon RK, Kyles AE, et al: Chronic localized osteomyelitis caused by atypical infection with Blastomyces dermatitidis in a dog. J Am Vet Med Assoc 209(11):1877, 1996.

18. Levy JK, Marsh A: Isolation of Calicivirus from the joint of a kitten with arthritis. J Am Vet Med Assoc 201(5):753, 1992.

19. Canvin JM, Goutcher SC, Hagig M, et al: Persistence of Staphylococcus aureus as detected by polymerase chain reaction in the synovial fluid of a patient with septic arthritis. Br J Rheumatol 36(2):203, 1997.

20. Owens JM, Ackerman N: Roentgenology of arthritis. Vet Clin North Am 8(3):453, 1978.

21. Gupta NC, Prezio JA: Radionuclide imaging in osteomyelitis. Semin Nucl Med 18(4):287, 1988.

22. Hoffer P, Newmann R: Diagnostic nuclear medicine. Baltimore: Williams & Wilkins, 1988.

23. Demopulos GA, Bleck EE, McDougall IR: Role of radionuclide imaging in the diagnosis of acute osteomyelitis. J Pediatr Orthop 8(5):558, 1988.

24. Appelboom T, Emery P, Tant L, et al: Evaluation of technetium-99m-ciprofloxacin (Infecton) for detecting sites of inflammation in arthritis. Rheumatology (Oxford) 42(10):1179, 2003.

25. Schlesinger AE, Hernandez RJ: Diseases of the musculoskeletal system in children: Imaging with CT, sonography, and MR. AJR 158(4):729, 1992.

26. Barr M, Olsen C, Scott F: Feline viral diseases. *In* Textbook of Veterinary Internal Medicine. Ettinger SJ, Feldman EC (eds). Philadelphia: WB Saunders, 1995, p. 409.

27. Prescott JF, Hanna WJ, Reid-Smith R, et al: Antimicrobial drug use and resistance in dogs. Can Vet J 43(2):107, 2002.

28. Wolfson JS, Hooper DC: Fluoroquinolone antimicrobial agents. Clin Microbiol Rev 2(4):378, 1989.

29. Hughes S, Fitzgerld RJ: Musculoskeletal Infections. Chicago: Year Book Medical Publishers, 1987, p. 697.

30. Bertone AL, Jones RL, McIlwraith CW: Serum and synovial fluid steady-state concentrations of trimethoprim and sulfadiazine in horses with experimentally induced infectious arthritis. Am J Vet Res 49(10):1681, 1988.

31. Errecalde JO, Carmely D, Marino EL, et al: Pharmacokinetics of amoxicillin in normal horses and horses with experimental arthritis. J Vet Pharmacol Ther 24(1):1, 2001.

32. Goldenberg DL, Brandt KD, Cohen AS, et al: Treatment of septic arthritis: Comparison of needle aspiration and surgery as initial modes of joint drainage. Arthritis Rheum 18(1):83, 1975.

33. Orsini JA: Strategies for treatment of bone and joint infections in large animals. J Am Vet Med Assoc 185(10):1190, 1984.

34. Fitch RB, Hogan TC, Kudnig ST: Hematogenous septic arthritis in the dog: Results of five patients treated nonsurgically with antibiotics. J Am Anim Hosp Assoc 39(6):563, 2003.

35. Cooper C, Cawley MI: Bacterial arthritis in an English health district: A 10 year review. Ann Rheum Dis 45(6):458, 1986.

36. Meijers KA, Dijkmans BA, Hermans J, et al: Non-gonococcal infectious arthritis: A retrospective study. J Infect 14(1):13, 1987.

37. Dow SW, Lappin, MR: Immunopathologic consequences of infectious disease. *In* Kirk's Current Veterinary Therapy xii-Small Animal Practice. Breitschwerdt E (ed). Philadelphia: WB Saunders, 1995, p. 554.

Chapter 93

Osteomyelitis

Loretta J. Bubenik

Osteomyelitis usually results from open fractures or open fracture repair. The term simply means inflammation of the bone and marrow contents, but bacterial infection is often implied when the word is used. Endogenous and exogenous modes of infection occur, with exogenous being more frequent. Treatment varies depending on the source of infection, the organism involved, and duration of infection.

Etiology

A variety of organisms has been implicated in bone infections. A single organism is usually involved.[1] Beta-lactamase-producing staphylococcal species, streptococcal species, and gram-negative aerobic bacteria are most commonly isolated,[2-4] with staphylococcal species, usually *Staphylococcus intermedius*, isolated 46 to 74% of the time.[2,4,5] Multiple organisms are isolated 33 to 66% of the time.[4,6]

Isolation of anaerobic bacteria can be difficult, but isolation rates as high as 70% have been reported.[1] Isolation of anaerobes is site–dependent, with the radius/ulna, mandible, and tympanic bulla commonly involved.[1] Anaerobic bacteria should be suspected in cases of apparent infection but lack of growth on culture, infection secondary to disruption of tissue normally inhabited by anaerobic bacteria, or when infection from an external source has occurred.[1,7-9] Common anaerobic isolates include *Bacteroides, Fusobacterium, Actinomyces, Clostridium, Peptococcus,* and *Peptostreptococcus* species.[1,8,10]

Mycotic bone infection also occurs, but usually results from hematogenous spread.[9] Isolated fungal organisms include *Cryptococcus neoformans, Coccidioides immitis, Aspergillus species, Penicillium species, Blastomyces dermatitidis, Histoplasma capsulatum,* and *Phialemaenium.*[11-16]

Pathophysiology

Osteomyelitis comes from endogenous or exogenous sources. Acute hematogenous osteomyelitis is the endogenous form; bone infection develops from an infectious focus at a distant site within the body such as the skin, respiratory system, heart, oral cavity, or genitourinary tract. Alternatively, exogenous bone infection (infection from nonhematogenous routes) may occur from direct inoculation (e.g., bites, punctures, or surgery), open fractures, foreign body migration, or gun shot wounds. Osteomyelitis from exogenous sources is divided into acute and chronic forms.

Acute hematogenous osteomyelitis typically affects the metaphyseal region of long bones, but diaphyseal infections can occur.[2,17] Bacteria lodge in the metaphysis where the capillary endothelium is discontinuous and blood flow slows in the veins.[18,19] After localizing in the metaphysis, bacteria and activated platelets cause inflammation and thrombus formation, producing an ischemic environment that is conducive to bacterial proliferation.[19] Infection either progresses or is walled off by the immune response.[20] Cellular debris, inflammatory by-products, and bacteria cause thrombosis, abscessation, and compromise of blood supply to the bone. Sequestration, formation of a walled off, devitalized portion of bone, can occur when exudate reaches the outer cortex and elevates the periosteum, compromising cortical blood supply to that area of bone.[19] The isolated bone fragment is usually surrounded by purulent debris (lacuna) and can form an opening for escape of purulent material outside the walled off area (cloaca). Chronic osteomyelitis can result when the infection is walled off, but not eliminated by the body.

Fungal organisms typically gain entrance to the body via inhalation or spread from the gastrointestinal tract. Hematogenous dissemination occurs after localization of the organisms in areas away from the bone.[11,14-16,21-23] Hence, fungal osteomyelitis is usually considered hematogenous in origin, although primary fungal osteomyelitis and direct bone inoculation occur on occasion.[15]

Nonhematogenous acute and chronic osteomyelitis occur when an organism invades osseous tissue by overwhelming the immune system or by seeding compromised tissue. Normal bone is resistant to infection, but soft-tissue injury, bone devitalization, surgical implants, instability of bone fragments, prolonged wound exposure, and immunosuppression increase the risk of infection.[24,25]

Acute nonhematogenous osteomyelitis is usually a complication of surgical fracture repair and clinical signs are typically apparent 5 to 7 days after surgery. Long bones are more often affected than axial bones, probably owing to increased occurrence of fracture in long bones.[2,4,6] The degree of soft-tissue devitalization, fracture stability, type of fracture repair, organism virulence, and immune system competence influence development of fracture site infection.[6,9,24] Trauma from fracture generation and/or surgery and implants applied during fracture repair disrupt blood supply and provide foreign material for bacterial adherence and proliferation.[24] Implants decrease the quantity of bacteria needed to establish an infection and provide a site for bacterial adherence that can escape immunosurveillance and antibiotics.[24,26] Moreover, devitalized bone fragments increase the risk of infection for both virulent and nonvirulent strains of bacteria.[27] Bullet penetration and bites cause soft-tissue injury and are a means of bacterial inoculation. Shrapnel, migrating foreign bodies, and occasionally bites leave material behind that allow bacteria to evade host immune responses and proliferate.[9]

Nonhematogenous, chronic osteomyelitis develops from inadequate treatment of acute osteomyelitis, hidden infections associated with implants or other foreign material, and/or isolation of bacteria from the immune system.[24,28,29] In fractures with prolonged infection, granulation and fibrous tissue isolate devitalized bone (sequestration) and cause delayed healing and/or persistent infection.[19,27] The sequestration of fracture fragments occurs because the fragment of bone is devitalized at the time of fracture owing to trauma and is walled off instead of being resorbed or incorporated into the fracture callous. However, devitalization and sequestration of bone after fracture can also occur through the same mechanism as with acute hematogenous osteomyelitis. Persistent, chronic infection is enhanced by the presence of metallic implants/foreign material and through bacterial biofilm production, which protects bacteria from immunosurveillance.[24,26,30]

Clinical Findings

Acute hematogenous osteomyelitis is not common but most often affects young animals.[2,4] Findings can include soft-tissue swelling over the affected site, moderate to severe lameness, inappetence, malaise, fever, and debilitation. The source of bone infection may or may not be found during initial examination, but the animal should be examined for such. The oral cavity, integument system, urogenital tract, lungs, and heart should be carefully examined. Draining tracts occur uncommonly.[19]

Acute osteomyelitis of nonhematogenous sources has no breed or sex predilection and typically occurs after fracture repair. In such cases, the surgical wound may be edematous, erythematous, and warm, and the limb is painful during manipulation. Animals are often febrile and have a substantial lameness. Draining tracts are not common during the acute phase, but incisional drainage might be obvious. Signs of systemic illness such as inappetence and lethargy might also be apparent.[9]

Animals suffering from chronic nonhematogenous osteomyelitis usually present with an insidious lameness and varying degrees of pain at the fracture site. If the fracture is not healed, the degree of fracture instability can influence the degree of pain and lameness. Moderate to severe muscle atrophy is usually present in the affected limb and a draining tract might be apparent. It is common for drainage to dissipate with antimicrobial administration only to return once antimicrobials are discontinued. Muscle fibrosis and contracture owing to the effects of long-standing infection on the soft tissues might contribute to the lameness.[9] Signs of systemic involvement, such as fever and inappetence, are less likely to be present than with acute infections.

The clinical presentation of animals suffering from fungal osteomyelitis is similar to those suffering from bacterial osteomyelitis. Signs include lameness, swelling, and pain associated with the affected area, and the presence of draining tracts. However, animals with fungal osteomyelitis often have disseminated disease and systemic signs such as general malaise, inappetence, respiratory compromise, lymphadenopathy, weight loss, and fever.[11,31] Any age, breed, and sex can be affected, but German shepherd dogs may be overrepresented, possibly owing to genetic factors involving altered immune function.[11]

Diagnosis

History and signalment play a role in diagnosis of bone infection. Concurrent or prior infection elsewhere in the body in conjunction with sudden lameness, pain, heat, and swelling over the affected bone is suggestive of acute hematogenous osteomyelitis. For acute nonhematogenous osteomyelitis, a history of recent fracture repair, animal bite, evidence of foreign body migration, or puncture wound is more suggestive. Chronic osteomyelitis is usually associated with a history of previous fracture repair or implantation of foreign material and may also be linked to a previous diagnosis of osteomyelitis.

Radiography is commonly employed in the evaluation of suspected osteomyelitis. Radiographs alone have a sensitivity of only 62.5% and a specificity of 57.1% for diagnosis of osteomyelitis, but are commonly used in conjunction with clinical signs to make a diagnosis.[32] For an acute infection, soft-tissue swelling without alteration in bone architecture predominates,[9,33] but with chronic infection, periosteal new bone proliferation, cortical bone resorption, cortical thinning, implant loosening, and bone sequestration might be apparent (Figure 93-1).[2,4,33,34] Osteolytic and proliferative changes generally lag behind the actual time of infection by 10 to 14 days, so obtaining a second radiograph several days later may aid in diagnosis of questionable cases.[35] Radiographic evidence of sequestration may be delayed by several weeks, but in chronic situations, the presence of a sequestrum can be common (Figure 93-2).[36] Contrast radiography (fistulography) of draining tracts might help identify sequestra or foreign bodies.[9] Scintigraphy with Technetium-99 methylene diphosphonate can provide early information regarding active bone and joint remodeling; however it is not specific for infection.[33,37] New scintigraphic techniques offer distinction between infection and other inflammatory processes and might hold some benefit in the future.[38] Magnetic resonance imaging and computed tomography can also aid in early diagnosis of osteomyelitis.[34,39,40]

To obtain a definitive diagnosis, tissue samples, direct swabs, and/or needle aspirates should be aseptically collected from the affected area for cytology, aerobic and anaerobic culture, and antimicrobial susceptibility testing. Gram staining of samples can provide early information for empiric treatment while awaiting

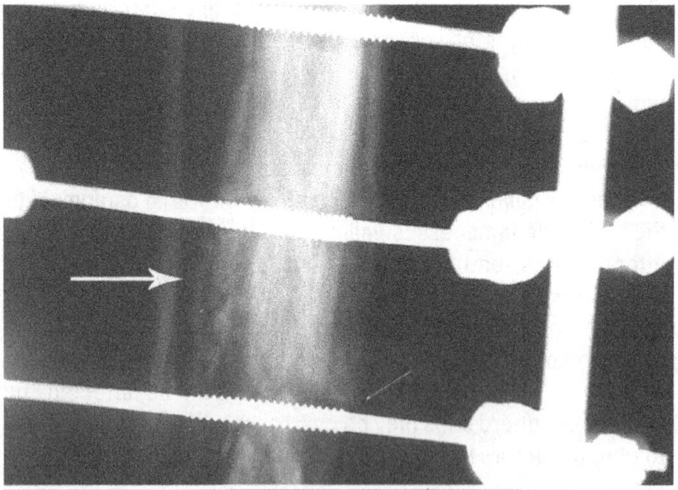

Figure 93-1. Chronic Osteomyelitis. This is a radiograph from a 2-year-old dog that developed osteomyelitis from an open fracture sustained 1 month earlier. Note the periosteal proliferation (solid white arrow) and the radiolucent line along the fixators pin (small line arrow) indicating implant loosening.

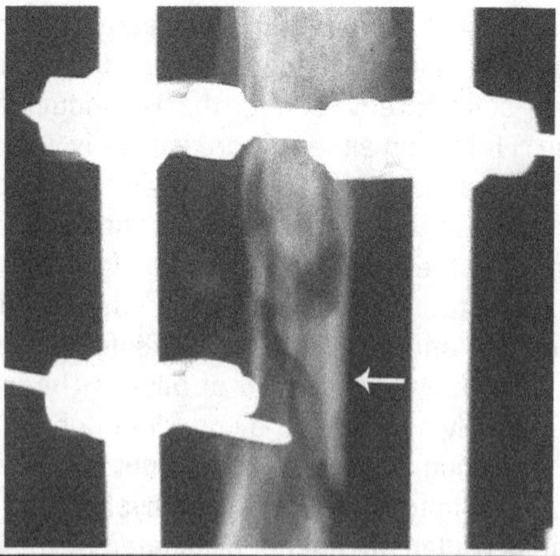

Figure 93-2. Sequestrum. This is a radiograph from a 2-year-old dog that developed osteomyelitis from an open fracture sustained 1 month earlier. Note the lack of periosteal reaction and remodeling of the devitalized portion of bone (solid white arrow).

culture results. Percutaneous aspiration of tissues around and in the affected site can have isolation rates as high as 86%,[41] although some reports do not concur with that high a rate.[2,4] If an abscess is present, the chances of obtaining organisms is likely higher. Tissue culture or direct swabbing through a surgical approach might be more likely to result in a positive culture. In chronic cases, needle aspiration might be less rewarding because bacteria can adhere tightly to surrounding structures with minimal exfoliatation.[24,29,42] Ideally, antibiotics should be withheld for at least 24 hours before sample collection to improve yield in chronic cases and should be initiated after sample collection in acute cases unless the animal's condition dictates otherwise.[43] Culturing draining tracts should be avoided because contaminants rather than the causative organism are often isolated.[44] If systemic involvement or hematogenous osteomyelitis is suspected, blood cultures should be performed.[45] In people with hematogenous osteomyelitis, approximately 50% of blood cultures grow the causative organism.[46]

Supportive diagnostics including a complete blood count, biochemistry panel, and urinalysis might show other organ-system involvement, be suggestive of infection, or not reveal anything of significance. For acute infections, especially hematogenous osteomyelitis, thoracic and abdominal radiographs, abdominal ultrasound, and/or echocardiogram can elucidate the source of infection and determine the animal's systemic condition.

A diagnosis of fungal osteomyelitis is often made from cytologic or histologic evaluation of affected tissues. Cytology of affected areas mostly consists of pleocellular infiltration, including macrophages, lymphocytes, plasma cells, neutrophils, and multinucleated giant cells; lesions are pyogranulomatous in nature.[31] Fungal hyphae or intracellular organisms are often apparent on preparations.[11,14-16,21-23] Special stains such as India ink, periodic acid-Schiff, and silver nitrate stains, or treatment of preparations with 10% potassium hydroxide can improve visualization of organisms.[21,31] Serologic testing is helpful to identify exposure.[31] Fungal culture is necessary for definitive diagnosis. In cases of aspergillosis, fungal hyphae can be seen in the urine sediment and can be cultured from urine of some infected animals.[11] Bone biopsy should be performed to rule out neoplasia and to obtain samples for culture and histopathology. Radiographic changes include soft-tissue swelling, periosteal and endosteal bone proliferation, and bone lysis. Lesions are typically below the elbow and stifle, but may be anywhere and must be differentiated from bone tumors.[11,14-16,21-23] Complete blood count and biochemistry profiles are not specific for fungal disease, but findings include nonregenerative anemia, leukocytosis, hyperglobulinemia, and eosinophilia.[11,14-16,21-23]

Treatment

Antibiotic penetration into bone and efficacy against the causative organism are necessary for resolution of infection. Ultimately, antibiotic choice is based on culture and antimicrobial susceptibility testing. Empiric therapy is initiated while culture and antimicrobial susceptibility are pending or when cultures fail to offer an appropriate therapeutic strategy. If the causative organism cannot be identified, continued antimicrobial administration is based on appropriate response to the initial therapeutic regimen. Intravenous therapy is always initiated for acute infections, and a favorable initial response permits a change to oral antimicrobial administration within the first 3 to 5 days of therapy. Oral therapy is appropriate in chronic cases, but is typically combined with surgical intervention. In cases of severe soft-tissue destruction, microvascular muscle flaps can provide increased blood supply and improved delivery of antibiotics and healing factors to the wound bed.[47]

Care should be taken in antibiotic selection because antimicrobial resistance of commonly isolated organisms is constantly changing and antibiotic effectiveness is dependant on many factors. Penicillins and penicillin-combination drugs, cephalosporins, and aminoglycosides readily penetrate normal and infected bone.[48-52] Staphylococci isolated from canine infections are often resistant to pure penicillins because of β-lactamase production, so β-lactamase-resistant drugs are preferred.[53] Staphylococci showed 18% resistance to first generation cephalosporins in one report,[54] although cephalosporins are a commonly used antibiotic in the first line of defense against bone infections.[54] Aminoglycosides lose some effectiveness in hypoxic or acidotic conditions and in the presence of white blood cells, so efficacy should be monitored during treatment.[55] Fluoroquinolones have good bone penetration and are beneficial for many gram-negative infections.[56] However, fluoroquinolones are not effective under anaerobic conditions and should be avoided in immature animals owing to potential deleterious effects on cartilage.[57,58] Clindamycin penetrates normal bone and is useful for gram-positive and anaerobic osteomyelitis.[59-61]

Duration of antimicrobial therapy depends on the severity of the infection, but antibiotics should be continued for at least 2 weeks beyond radiographic and clinical resolution of infection, which typically requires weeks to months of therapy.[55,62-66] Recurrence is lower in people with acute osteomyelitis if antibiotics are continued for a minimum of 30 days.[63] Owners should be warned that treatment will likely require long-term commitment and can be expensive.

Surgery is a necessary component of treatment in some cases of osteomyelitis. Palpable abscesses must be drained, cultured, debrided, and lavaged. In animals with nonhematogenous osteomyelitis, loose implants and foreign material must be removed.[64] For chronic osteomyelitis, surgery is often necessary to promote resolution of infection and involves aggressive debridement of devitalized bone fragments and necrotic soft tissue, removal of sclerotic bone occluding the medullary canal, and removal of loose implants or foreign material.[65] If debridement is adequate and the wound bed is healthy, closure over an active drain can be considered, otherwise the wound should be left open and closed at a later time once the tissues appear healthy. Multiple operations might be necessary to resolve infection in refractory cases of osteomyelitis.[6]

Stabilization of an unstable fracture is essential in nonhematogenous osteomyelitis. For amendable fractures, external fixators can be applied with minimal disruption of blood supply and have an added advantage of being easily removed.[66] If the soft tissues are healthy and the surgical procedure has consisted primarily of sequestrectomy and debridement of a fistulous tract, internal fixation can be considered.[67,68] However, all implants should be removed once the fracture is healed because they can harbor organisms and lead to recurrent osteomyelitis.[26] In fracture cases, bone grafting should be considered, but delayed grafting might be necessary in excessively exudative wounds because graft resorption can occur.[5,20]

Fluid therapy, nutritional supplementation, and analgesics should be instituted as needed and when systemic involvement is present. The inciting cause in cases of hematogenous osteomyelitis must be found and treated appropriately. Rehabilitation of the affected limb is also important, especially in chronic osteomyelitis, because inflammation of the soft tissues secondary to infection can lead to considerable muscle atrophy, fibrosis, and contracture, and prevent return to function. In severe cases that have not responded to antibiotic therapy or surgery and in cases with irreversible muscle damage and excessive joint stiffness, amputation might be necessary.

Although systemic antibiotic therapy is essential in the treatment of orthopedic infections, local antibiotic therapy provides another means of treatment that has some advantages when combined with systemic therapy.[41,69-71] Local antibiotic administration maintains a higher local drug concentration at the site of infection for a prolonged period of time with reduced systemic toxicity.[72-75] Local delivery of antibiotics usually involves temporary implantation of antibiotic-impregnated polymethylmethacrylate (AIPMMA) at the site of infection, but biodegradable delivery systems have also been investigated.[76-79] Local antibiotic delivery systems work by gradual release of antibiotics to the site of infection via antibiotic elution out of the implanted material. Tissue antibiotic concentration and elution rate depend on multiple factors including the antibiotic used, cement configuration, type of antibiotic carrier, and tissue environment.[69,73-75,80-83] AIPMMA is most often used in the form of preformed beads that are bought or handmade. The beads are placed at the site of infection and are left there for a duration based on the expected elution rate of the impregnated antibiotic.

Beads can be replaced serially to maintain an adequate local antibiotic concentration, but implanted cement should ultimately be removed from the infected site because it can harbor bacteria and result in recurrent osteomyelitis.[84]

Treatment of fungal osteomyelitis is difficult and expensive. Animals require long-term antifungal therapy (months) and are treated at least a month beyond resolution of clinical signs.[85] Some animals require life-long therapy[85] or amputation.[21] Antifungals include fluconazole, ketoconazole, amphotericin B, and itraconazole, but itraconazole is associated with fewer side effects.[85] Amputation is a reasonable alternative to therapy for fungal osteomyelitis if the systemic fungal disease is under control but the local bone infection cannot be cured.

Prognosis

Osteomyelitis typically carries a favorable prognosis unless fungal organisms are involved. Most animals respond favorably to treatment if antibiotic therapy is appropriate and the inciting cause is treated. Most infected fractures will heal in the face of infection so long as appropriate antibiotic therapy is used and the fracture is stable. For acute osteomyelitis, aggressive early intervention is necessary for resolution and prevention of chronic osteomyelitis. The inciting cause must be eliminated in cases of hematogenous spread or foreign body migration for complete resolution of disease.[6,62] In chronic cases, a favorable response to treatment occurs in up to 90% of affected dogs, but recurrence is possible.[6,62]

For fungal disease, prognosis is guarded to poor, although some animals respond to therapy. Systemic disease worsens the prognosis. Recurrence is possible[16,85] and varies from 20 to 25% in cases of blastomycosis.[85] On the other hand, histoplasmosis infection in cats often responds favorably to itraconazole.[85]

Although uncommon, complications can also affect the ultimate prognosis in cases of osteomyelitis. For acute cases, recurrence and progression to chronic disease can occur. Infections near the epiphysis can rarely lead to concurrent joint infection, and septicemia can result from inappropriate local bacterial control. Finally, chronic osteomyelitis, and some cases of acute osteomyelitis, can lead to refractory or recurrent osteomyelitis, nonunion, restricted joint motion, and loss of limb function.

In summary, many factors contribute to the formation, progression, and prognosis of osteomyelitis. The cause must be identified and treated appropriately. Diagnosis is based on culture and suspicion of disease, whereas treatment depends on the severity and type of infection present. For bacterial infections, the prognosis is favorable as long as treatment is appropriate for the type of disease, but fungal osteomyelitis carries a guarded to poor prognosis.

References

1. Muir P, Johnson KA: Anaerobic bacteria isolated from osteomyelitis in dogs and cats. Vet Surg 21(6):463, 1992.

2. Caywood DD, Wallace LJ, Braden TD: Osteomyelitis in the dog: A review of 67 cases. J Am Vet Med Assoc 172(8):943, 1978.

3. Griffiths GL, Bellenger CR: A retrospective study of osteomyelitis in

4. Smith CW, Schiller AG, Smith AR, et al: Osteomyelitis in the dog: A retrospective study. J Am Anim Hosp Assoc 14:589, 1978.

5. Bardet JF, Hohn RB, Basinger R: Open drainage and delayed autogenous cancellous bone grafting for treatment of chronic osteomyelitis in dogs and cats. J Am Vet Med Assoc 183(3):312, 1983.

6. Braden TD: Posttraumatic osteomyelitis. Vet Clin North Am Small Anim Pract 21(4):781, 1991.

7. Dow SW, Jones RL, Adney WS: Anaerobic bacterial infections and response to treatment in dogs and cats: 36 cases (1983-1985). J Am Vet Med Assoc 189(8):930, 1986.

8. Johnson KA, Lomas GR, Wood AK: Osteomyelitis in dogs and cats caused by anaerobic bacteria. Aust Vet J 61(2):57, 1984.

9. Johnson KA: Osteomyelitis in dogs and cats. J Am Vet Med Assoc 204(12):1882, 1994.

10. Walker RD, Richardson DC, Bryant MJ, et al: Anaerobic bacteria associated with osteomyelitis in domestic animals. J Am Vet Med Assoc 182(8):814, 1983.

11. Day MJ, Penhale WJ, Eger CE, et al: Disseminated aspergillosis in dogs. Aust Vet J 63(2):55, 1986.

12. Legendre AM, Walker M, Buyukmihci N, et al: Canine blastomycosis: A review of 47 clinical cases. J Am Vet Med Assoc 178(11):1163, 1981.

13. Lomax LG, Cole JR, Padhye AA, et al: Osteolytic phaeohyphomycosis in a German Shepherd dog caused by Phialemonium obovatum. J Clin Microbiol 23(5):987, 1986.

14. Shelton GD, Stockham SL, Carrig CB, et al: Disseminated histoplasmosis with bone lesions in a dog. J Am Anim Hosp Assoc 18:143, 1982.

15. Wigney DI, Allan GS, Hay LE, et al: Osteomyelitis associated with Penicillium veruculosum in a German shepherd dog. J Small Anim Pract 31:449, 1990.

16. Brearley MJ, Jeffery N: Cryptococcal osteomyelitis in a dog. J Small Anim Pract 33:601, 1992.

17. Emmerson TD, Pead MJ: Pathological fracture of the femur secondary to haematogenous osteomyelitis in a Weimaraner. J Small Anim Pract 40(5):233, 1999.

18. Whalen JL, Fitzgerald RH Jr, Morrissy RT: A histological study of acute hematogenous osteomyelitis following physeal injuries in rabbits. J Bone Joint Surg [Am] 70(9):1383, 1988.

19. Kahn DS, Pritzker KP: The pathophysiology of bone infection. Clin Orthop 96:12, 1973.

20. Resnick C, Resnick D: Pyogenic osteomyelitis and septic arthritis. *In* Radiology, Diagnosis, Imaging, Intervention. Traveras J, Ferucci J (ed). Philadelphia: JB Lippincott, 1986, p. 229.

21. Marcellin-Little DJ, Sellon RK, Kyles AE, et al: Chronic localized osteomyelitis caused by atypical infection with Blastomyces dermatitidis in a dog. J Am Vet Med Assoc 209(11):1877, 1996.

22. Moore AH, Hanna FY: Mycotic osteomyelitis in a dog following nasal Aspergillosis. Vet Rec 137(14):349, 1995.

23. Wolf AM: Histoplasma capsulatum osteomyelitis in the cat. J Vet Int Med 1(4):158, 1987.

24. Gristina AG, Costerton JW: Bacterial adherence and the glycocalyx and their role in musculoskeletal infection. Orthop Clin North Am 15(3):517, 1984.

25. Scheman L, Janota M, Lewin P: The production of experimental osteomyelitis. J Am Med Assoc 117:1525, 1941.

26. Smith MM, Vasseur PB, Saunders HM: Bacterial growth associated with metallic implants in dogs. J Am Vet Med Assoc 195(6):765, 1989.

27. Evans RP, Nelson CL, Harrison BH: The effect of wound environment on the incidence of acute osteomyelitis. Clin Orthop (286):289, 1993.

28. Marrie TJ, Costerton JW: Mode of growth of bacterial pathogens in chronic polymicrobial human osteomyelitis. J Clin Microbiol 22(6):924, 1985.

29. Mayberry-Carson KJ, Tober-Meyer B, Smith JK, et al: Bacterial adherence and glycocalyx formation in osteomyelitis experimentally induced with Staphylococcus aureus. Infect Immunol 43(3):825, 1984.

30. Petty W, Spanier S, Shuster JJ, et al: The influence of skeletal implants on incidence of infection. Experiments in a canine model. J Bone Joint Surg [Am] 67(8):1236, 1985.

31. Jang SS, Biberstein EL: Fungal diseases. *In* Infectious Diseases of the Dog and Cat. Green C (ed). Philadelphia: WB Saunders, 1998, p. 349.

32. Braden T, Tvedten H, Motosky U: The sensitivity and specificity of radiology and histopathology in the diagnosis of post-traumatic osteomyelitis. Vet Comp Orthop Traumatol 3:98, 1989.

33. Mandell GA: Imaging in the diagnosis of musculoskeletal infections in children. Curr Probl Pediatr 26(7):218, 1996.

34. Gold RH, Hawkins RA, Katz RD: Bacterial osteomyelitis: Findings on plain radiography, CT, MR, and scintigraphy. Am J Roentgenol 157(2):365, 1991.

35. Gupta NC, Prezio JA: Radionuclide imaging in osteomyelitis. Semin Nucl Med 18(4):287, 1988.

36. Tumeh SS, Aliabadi P, Seltzer SE, et al: Chronic osteomyelitis: The relative roles of scintigrams, plain radiographs, and transmission computed tomography. Clin Nucl Med 13(10):710, 1988.

37. Willis RB, Rozencwaig R: Pediatric osteomyelitis masquerading as skeletal neoplasia. Orthop Clin North Am 27(3):625, 1996.

38. Appelboom T, Emery P, Tant L, et al: Evaluation of technetium-99m-ciprofloxacin (Infecton) for detecting sites of inflammation in arthritis. Rheumatol (Oxford) 42(10):1179, 2003.

39. Schlesinger AE, Hernandez RJ: Diseases of the musculoskeletal system in children: Imaging with CT sonography and MR. Am J Roentgenol 158(4):729, 1992.

40. Erdman WA, Tamburro F, Jayson HT, et al: Osteomyelitis: Characteristics and pitfalls of diagnosis with MR imaging. Radiology 180(2):533, 1991.

41. Dernell W, Withrow S, Straw R, et al: Clinical response to antibiotic impregnated poly methyl methacrylate bead implantation of dogs with severe infections after limb sparing and allograft replacement-18 cases (1994-1996). Vet Comp Orthop Traumatol 11:94, 1998.

42. Geissler WB, Purvis JM: Hematogenous osteomyelitis and septic arthritis in children: A ten year review. J Miss State Med Assoc 30(3):71, 1989.

43. Hall BB, Rosenblatt JE, Fitzgerald RH: Anaerobic septic arthritis and osteomyelitis. Orthop Clin North Am 15(3):505, 1984.

44. Mackowiak PA, Jones SR, Smith JW: Diagnostic value of sinus-tract cultures in chronic osteomyelitis. J Am Med Assoc 239(26):2772, 1978.

45. Dunn JK, Dennis R, Houlton JEF: Successful treatment of two cases of metaphyseal osteomyelitis in the dog. J Small Anim Pract 33:85, 1992.

46. Waldvogel FA, Medoff G, Swartz MN: Osteomyelitis: A review of clinical features, therapeutic considerations and unusual aspects. N Engl J Med 282(4):198, 1970.

47. Basher A, Presnell, KR: Muscle transposition as an aid in covering traumatic tissue over the canine tibia. J Am Anim Hosp Assoc 23:617, 1987.

48. Cunha BA, Gossling HR, Pasternak HS, et al: The penetration characteristics of cefazolin, cephalothin, and cephradine into bone in patients undergoing total hip replacement. J Bone Joint Surg [Am] 59(7):856, 1977.

49. Fitzgerald RH Jr: Antibiotic distribution in normal and osteomyelitic bone. Orthop Clin North Am 15(3):537, 1984.

50. Darouiche RO, Green G, Mansouri MD: Antimicrobial activity of antiseptic-coated orthopaedic devices. Int J Antimicrob Agents 10(1):83, 1998.

51. Hall BB, Fitzgerald RH Jr: The pharmacokinetics of penicillin in osteomyelitic canine bone. J Bone Joint Surg [Am] 65(4):526, 1983.

52. Rosin H, Rosin AM, Kramer J: Determination of antibiotic levels in human bone. I. Gentamicin levels in bone. Infection 2(1):3, 1974.

53. Love D: Antimicrobial susceptibility of Staphylococci isolated from dogs. Aust Vet Practit 19(4):196, 1989.

54. Prescott JF, Hanna WJ, Reid-Smith R, et al: Antimicrobial drug use and resistance in dogs. Can Vet J 43(2):107, 2002.

55. Hughes S, Fitzgerld RJ: Musculoskeletal infections. Chicago: Year Book Medical Publishers, 1987, p. 697.

56. Fong IW, Ledbetter WH, Vandenbroucke AC, et al: Ciprofloxacin concentrations in bone and muscle after oral dosing. Antimicrob Agents Chemother 29(3):405, 1986.

57. Paton JH, Reeves DS: Fluoroquinolone antibiotics. Microbiology, pharmacokinetics and clinical use. Drugs 36(2):193, 1988.

58. Wolfson JS, Hooper DC: Fluoroquinolone antimicrobial agents. Clin Microbiol Rev 2(4):378, 1989.

59. Braden TD, Johnson CA, Gabel CL, et al: Physiologic evaluation of clindamycin, using a canine model of posttraumatic osteomyelitis. Am J Vet Res 48(7):1101, 1987.

60. Norden CW, Shinners E, Niederriter K: Clindamycin treatment of experimental chronic osteomyelitis due to Staphylococcus aureus. J Infect Dis 153(5):956, 1986.

61. Smilack JD, Flittie WH, Williams TW Jr: Bone concentrations of antimicrobial agents after parenteral administration. Antimicrob Agents Chemother 9(1):169, 1976.

62. Budsberg SD, Kemp DT: Antimicrobial distribution and therapeutics in bone. Comp Cont Educ Pract Vet 12(12):1758, 1990.

63. Fitzgerald RH Jr, Peterson LF, Washington JA, et al: Bacterial colonization of wounds and sepsis in total hip arthroplasty. J Bone Joint Surg [Am] 55(6):1242, 1973.

64. Nunamaker D: Osteomyelitis. *In* Textbook of Small Animal Orthopaedics. Newton C and Nunamaker D (ed). Philadelphia: JB Lippincott, 1985.

65. Nunamaker DM: Management of infected fractures. Osteomyelitis. Vet Clin North Am 5(2):259, 1975.

66. Marcellin-Little DJ: External skeletal fixation. *In* Textbook of Small Animal Surgery. Slatter D (ed). Philadephia: WB Saunders, 2003, p. 1818.

67. Kaltenecker G, Wruhs O, Quaicoe S: Lower infection rate after interlocking nailing in open fractures of femur and tibia. J Trauma 30(4):474, 1990.

68. Muir P, Johnson KA: Interlocking intramedullary nail stabilization of a femoral fracture in a dog with osteomyelitis. J Am Vet Med Assoc 209(7):1262, 1996.

69. Calhoun JH, Mader JT: Antibiotic beads in the management of surgical infections. Am J Surg 157(4):443, 1989.

70. Fitzgerald RH Jr: Experimental osteomyelitis: Description of a canine model and the role of depot administration of antibiotics in the prevention and treatment of sepsis. J Bone Joint Surg [Am] 65(3):371, 1983.

71. Ostermann PA, Seligson D, Henry SL: Local antibiotic therapy for severe open fractures. A review of 1085 consecutive cases. J Bone Joint Surg [Br] 77(1):93, 1995.

72. Eckman JB, Henry SL, Mangino PD, et al: Wound and serum levels of tobramycin with the prophylactic use of tobramycin-impregnated polymethylmethacrylate beads in compound fractures. Clin Orthop (237):213, 1988.

73. Klemm KW: Antibiotic bead chains. Clin Orthop (295):63, 1993.

74. Adams K, Couch L, Cierny G, et al: In vitro and in vivo evaluation of antibiotic diffusion from antibiotic-impregnated polymethylmethacrylate beads. Clin Orthop (278):244, 1992.

75. Wininger DA, Fass RJ: Antibiotic-impregnated cement and beads for orthopedic infections. Antimicrob Agents Chemother 40(12):2675, 1996.

76. Gerhart TN, Roux RD, Hanff PA, et al: Antibiotic-loaded biodegradable bone cement for prophylaxis and treatment of experimental osteomyelitis in rats. J Orthop Res 11(2):250, 1993.

77. Jacob E, Setterstrom JA, Bach DE, et al: Evaluation of biodegradable ampicillin anhydrate microcapsules for local treatment of experimental staphylococcal osteomyelitis. Clin Orthop (267):237, 1991.

78. Mackey D, Varlet A, Debeaumont D: Antibiotic loaded plaster of paris pellets: An in vitro study of a possible method of local antibiotic therapy in bone infection. Clin Orthop (167):263, 1982.

79. Mehta S, Humphrey JS, Schenkman DI, et al: Gentamicin distribution from a collagen carrier. J Orthop Res 14(5):749, 1996.

80. Nijhof M, Dhert W, Tilman P, et al: Release of tobramycin from tobramycin-containing bone cement in bone and serum of rabbits. J Mater Sci 8:799, 1997.

81. Buchholz HW, Elson RA, Heinert K: Antibiotic-loaded acrylic cement: Current concepts. Clin Orthop (190):96, 1984.

82. Fish DN, Hoffman HM, Danziger LH: Antibiotic-impregnated cement use in U.S. Hospitals. Am J Hosp Pharm 49(10):2469, 1992.

83. Popham GJ, Mangino P, Seligson D, et al: Antibiotic-impregnated beads. Part ii: Factors in antibiotic selection. Orthop Rev 20(4):331, 1991.

84. Tobias KM, Schneider RK, Besser TE: Use of antimicrobial-impregnated polymethyl methacrylate. J Am Vet Med Assoc 208(6):841, 1996.

85. Legendre AM: Antimicrobial therapy. *In* Current Veterinary Therapy. Kirk R (ed). Philadelphia: WB Saunders, 1995, p. 327.

Chapter 94

Hypertrophic Osteodystrophy in Dogs

Ron Montgomery

Hypertrophic osteodystrophy (HOD) is a readily diagnosed, inflammatory, and osteoclastic disease process on the metaphyseal side of active physes, predominantly of large and giant breeds.[1-21] The distal radius and ulna are the most often and most severely affected sites with clinical signs. HOD was first reported in dogs in 1935 and was initially called Barlow's disease.[2,7] HOD has had the synonyms of metaphyseal osteopathy, idiopathic osteodystrophy, osteodystrophy II, canine skeletal scurvy, Barlow's disease, and Moeller-Barlow disease.[1,2,7] The first two synonyms are accurate descriptors, whereas canine skeletal scurvy is not accurate based on comparison of clinical signs, pathophysiology, and etiologies.[2]

Etiology

HOD has a cryptogenic etiology despite extensive investigation. Etiologies considered include excessive dietary vitamins and minerals,[1-14] vitamin C deficiency,[2,10] infectious agents (viral and bacterial)[10,14] immune-mediated inflammatory disease,[10,11] a form of osteochondrosi,[10] vascular anomalies,[8,10] and genetic or familial predisposition.[3,10,12] Whether the etiology is from exogenous (e.g., infectious agents), endogenous (e.g., abnormal metabolism), or a combination of influences is unclear.[1,2,10] However, many proposed etiologies have been ruled out or determined to be unlikely as sole causes.

Dietary causes of HOD that are unlikely include excessive vitamin D, excessive mineral supplementation, excessive calories, and deficient vitamin C (only primates and guinea pigs require dietary vitamin C).[1,2] Abnormal metabolism of vitamin C remains a possibility.[1,2] Many dogs with HOD have not had vitamin and mineral supplementation, and many dogs on high levels of vitamin and mineral supplementation do not develop HOD. High calorie diets are also much more common among young dogs than is HOD. It appears that, at most, diets that promote rapid growth and/or affect bone formation may contribute to, but not cause, HOD.

Respiratory and/or gastrointestinal disease a few weeks prior to some cases of HOD has prompted consideration of infectious agents as etiologies.[2,12] Distemper and distemper vaccination (modified-live) have been prominent etiologic considerations.[2,12,18,19] Experimentally, evidence of canine distemper virus in bone cells of the metaphyseal region of dogs has been reported.[18,19] However, Koch's postulates have never been satisfied with regard to HOD. A comparison of multiple risk factors for HOD and canine distemper virus infection based on a Veterinary Medical Database (VMDB) survey concluded that the risk factors were not similar.[3] Although dogs less than 6 months old were identified to be at greatest risk for both diseases, distemper cases occurred over 12 times more often than HOD.[3]

Nevertheless, specific vaccination protocols using killed virus, or modified-live measles instead of modified-live distemper virus, or vaccinating separately for distemper, parvovirus, and adenovirus have been proposed for Weimaraners.[12,13] Bacterial infection has also been reported in conjunction with HOD.[14] Which came first was undeterminable, although the debilitating effects of HOD were speculated to allow an opportunistic E. coli bacteremia.[14] An autoimmune or hyper-inflammatory etiology has also been proposed, perhaps initiated by infection.[11] The relative infrequency of HOD compared with suspected infectious agents plus the predominant clinical signs being at the distal radius and ulna make an infectious agent difficult to explain, at least as a sole etiology.

When considering osteochondrosis as an etiology for HOD, details of endochondral bone formation should also be considered. Osteochondrosis affects all physes and includes microscopically visible loss of distinct chondrocyte columns and excessive thickness of the zone of chondrocyte hypertrophy. HOD affects a later step of in endochondral osteogenesis the process than osteochondrosis affects and has a different pathophysiology. HOD pathology occurs in the metaphysis immediately adjacent to the physis where primary spongiosum is located and transformation to the secondary spongiosum begins. The area affected by HOD normally has rapid growth, high lysosomal enzymatic activity, and high osteoblast and osteoclast activity.[5] Although vessels do not cross the physis, the metaphyseal side of the physis has an extremely rich blood supply from the nutrient artery and peripherally from metaphyseal arteries (Figure 94-1A).[2,8] The normal vascularity of this region is so extreme during rapid bone growth that the distinction between normal and inflammatory is subtle, and based mainly on the lack of pathology. A multitude of small arterioles approach perpendicular to the physis, then make a "hairpin" turn away from the physis (Figure 94-1B),[8] which affects laminar blood flow. The hairpin turns have been postulated to be "clinically important in growth deformities."[8] Capillary structure here also includes "buds" or dead end capillaries with endothelium that lacks a basement membrane and in places may be open, which allows extravasation of blood into the inter-trabecular sinuses immediately adjacent to the physis (Figure 94-1C).[5,6] Ironically, the area immediately adjacent to the last transverse septum of the physis is reported to have low oxygen tension and localized vascular stasis,[5] despite the nearby hypervascularity.

Rapid endochondral bone formation ostensibly plays a role in HOD, based on the disease's location and the signalment of affected individuals. HOD occurs only in dogs with open physes.

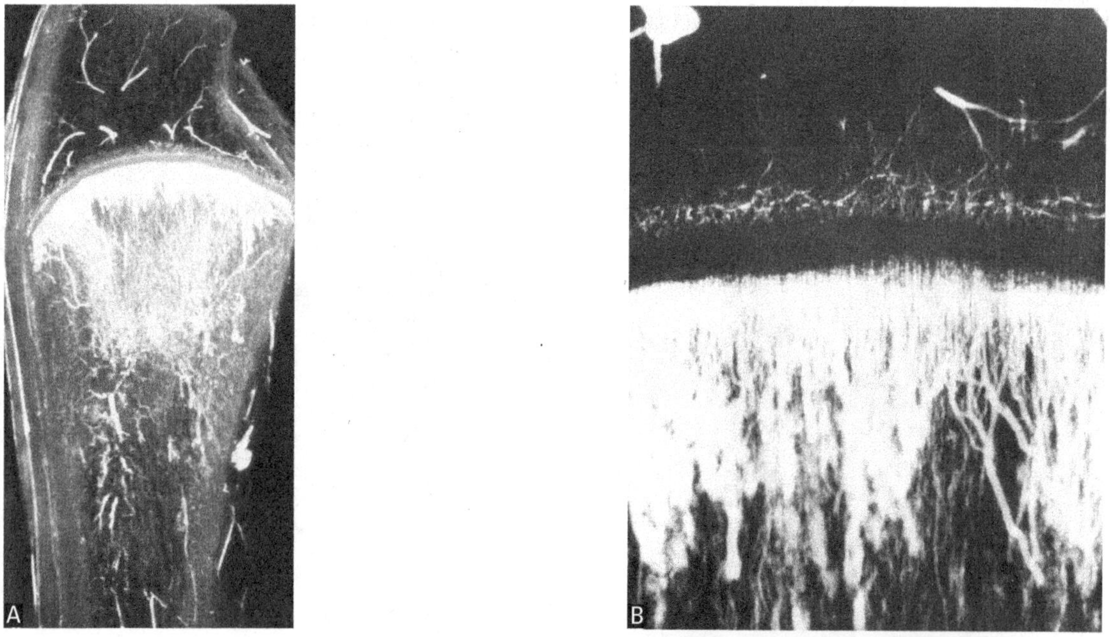

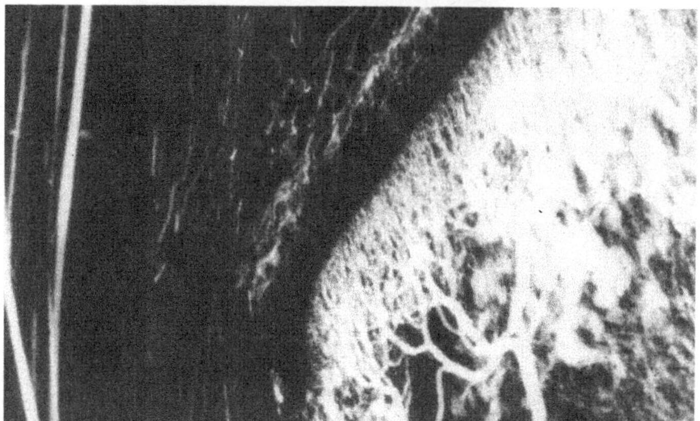

Figure 94-1. Microangiograms of normal immature canine radius. A. Note the extreme hypervascularity in the normal growing dog at the area where HOD occurs. B. Higher magnification shows vascular vessels make a 1800 turn at the physis, which slows laminar blood flow. C. Higher magnification demonstrates some vessels appear to be "open-ended" to sinusoidal space of relatively stagnant blood.

Furthermore, HOD tends to coincide with peak metabolic activity of the physis, i.e., at 3 to 5 months of age, in large and giant breeds, and more often in males.

Predispositions for breed and gender were determined for this chapter by a retrieval from the Veterinary Medical Data Base including all participating institutions and from 1994-2004 inclusively (Table 94-1). Seven breeds (Great Danes, Weimaraners, Labrador retrievers, golden retrievers, German shepherd dogs, mixed breed dogs, and boxers) accounted for about two thirds (64%) of all reported cases. The 20 breeds listed in Table 94-1 accounted for almost 90% of all cases of HOD, the majority of which were large or giant breeds. Nineteen other breeds had 1 case of HOD each. The number of HOD cases per breed is influenced by the breed's popularity.

Great Danes and Weimaraners appear to be greatly overrepresented, whereas mixed breed dogs appear to be under represented, based on HOD cases/100,000 of the breed, which does adjust for breed popularity (calculated for breeds with > 1000 in the survey). For example, the VMDB survey had 2460 Great Danes, 2510 standard poodles, and 2336 border collies, yet Great Danes had 1016/100,000 whereas the latter two breeds had 80/100,000 and 171/100,000 respectively. Weimaraners had 1279/100,000, while 4 breeds with a comparable number of individuals did not exceed 186/100,000. Mixed breed dogs were ostensibly under represented with only 17/100,000. Labrador retrievers (63/100,000) accounted for 30,248 individuals in the VMDB survey (~10% of all dogs), second only to mixed breeds with 63,974 individuals (Table 94-1). Two publications based on the VMDB, but using different methods and different years surveyed, also reported a strong predisposition for Great Danes to have HOD, both in number of cases presented and at high risk when adjusted for breed popularity.[3,4] These articles also reported the 7 breeds listed above as having predilection for HOD between 1980-1989, and 1986-1995.[3,4]

Males are slightly more likely to develop HOD, which is irrelevant to diagnosis. However, predisposition toward males may relate to etiology, e.g., males tend to be slightly larger, hence endochondral osteogenesis is more rapid. The male:female ratio was 48:52 for the total population, and was 53:47 for cases with HOD in the VMDB 1994-2004 survey for this chapter. Most other reports indicate no gender predilection, or a slight predilection for males. A study of the VMDB study from 1980-1989 reported males were 2.3 times more likely to develop HOD than were females.[3]

Pathology

Inflammation is the overwhelming characteristic seen in HOD. HOD affects a transverse zone of the metaphysis immediately adjacent to the physis, which corresponds to the radiolucent line referred to as a pseudophyseal line (Figure 94-2). This diseased area consists of massive infiltration of neutrophils and mononuclear cells, hemorrhage, osteoclastic resorption of trabeculae, fibrosis, and necrotic trabeculae (Figure 94-2C).[2] Osteoid, which should be developing on the calcified cartilage spicules, is absent.[2] In a few cases, the physis may be of irregular width or abnormally wide, owing to increased length of the zone of hypertrophy.[2] In more severe cases, subperiosteal hemorrhage beginning near the affected metaphysis can occur.

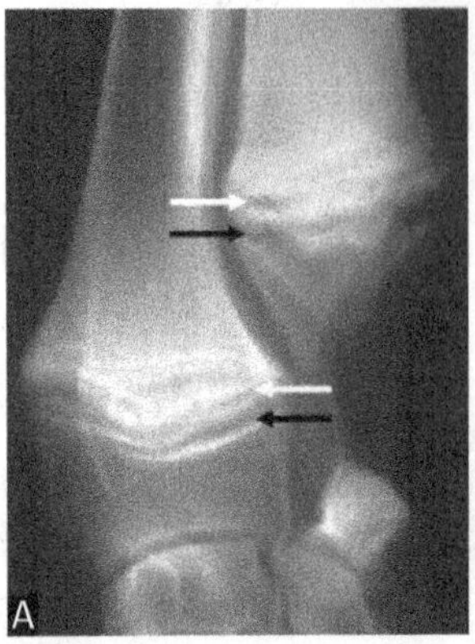

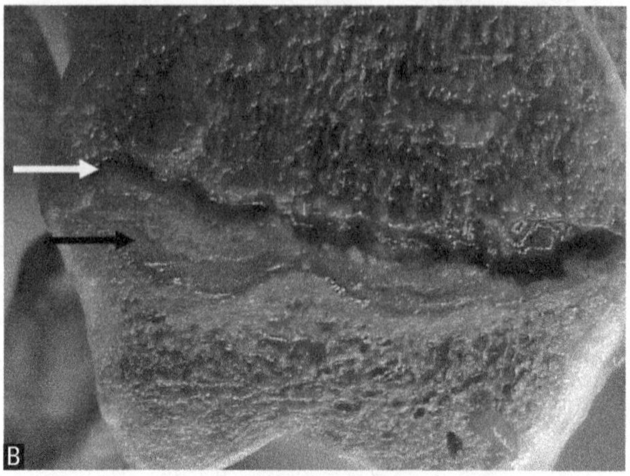

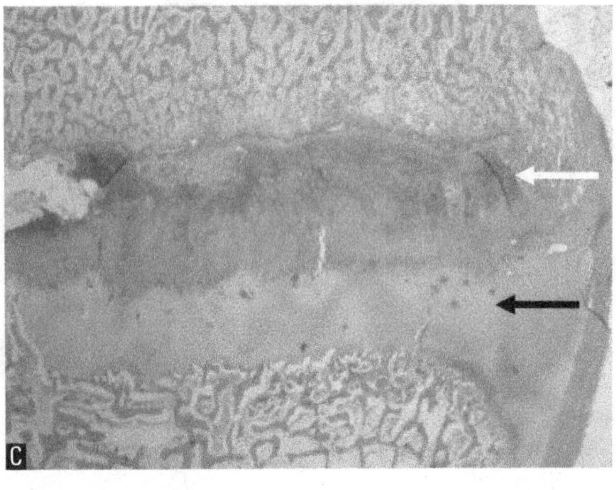

Figure 94-2. A. Pseudophyseal line (solid arrow) just proximal to the physis (hollow arrow) is pathognomonic for HOD. B. Gross sagittal section showing area of bone lysis (solid arrow) on the metaphyseal side of the physis (hollow arrow) which corresponds to the radiolucency of the pseudophyseal line. C. Microscopic section (low magnification/H & E stain) of same area showing necrosis of mineralized primary spicules and massive inflammation (solid arrow) adjacent to the normal physis (hollow arrow).

Table 94-1. Breeds with Multiple Cases of Hypertrophic Osteodystrophy from the Veterinary Medical Data Base, 1994-2004.

Breeds	Total Individuals	Total H.O.D. Cases	% of All H.O.D. Cases	H.O.D. cases/100,000 dogs
All Breeds	307,168	166	100.0%	54
Great Dane	2,460	25	15.1%	1,016
Labrador Retriever	30,248	19	11.4%	63
Weimaraner	1,485	19	11.4%	1,279
Golden Retriever	18,167	14	8.4%	77
German Shepherd	12,617	11	6.6%	87
Mixed Breed	63,974	11	6.6%	17
Boxer	5,002	7	4.2%	140
Irish Setter	820	6	3.6%	< 1,000 of breed
Rottweiler	9,287	6	3.6%	65
Border Collie	2,336	4	2.4%	171
Kuvasz	167	4	2.4%	< 1,000 of breed
Blue Heeler	1,641	3	1.8%	183
German Shorthaired Pointer	1,875	3	1.8%	160
Irish Wolfhound	514	3	1.8%	< 1,000 of breed
Anatolian Shepherd	82	2	1.2%	< 1,000 of breed
Bullmastiff	698	2	1.2%	< 1,000 of breed
Chesapeake Bay Retriever	1,075	2	1.2%	186
English Springer Spaniel	3,736	2	1.2%	54
Mastiff	1,122	2	1.2%	178
Poodle (Standard)	2,510	2	1.2%	80

New bone formation can occur subsequent to subperiosteal hemorrhage, which elevates the periosteum (Figure 94-3). The new bone may persist as permanent deformity (abnormally enlarged metaphyseal region, valgus deformity) (Figure 94-4). The extent of subperiosteal hemorrhage and periosteal new bone formation can be extensive, but this is rare. All bones that develop primarily via endochondral ossification (i.e., long bones, metacarpi) can potentially be affected by HOD.[2] Bone remodeling after HOD results in normal bones in the vast majority of cases. Necropsies performed on fatal cases have reported HOD lesions at the ends of other long bones, ribs, and vertebrae plus diffuse mineralization of pleura, pericardium, aorta, and lungs.[10] Hypertrophic bone lesions concurrent with classic HOD have also been reported in the axial skeleton (calvarium, maxilla, mandible, scapula, vertebrae, costochondral junction of ribs, and ilial wing).[2,10,15,20,21]

Clinical Diagnosis

Signalment

HOD typically occurs in 3- to 5-month-old (range 2 to 8 months old), large-breed dogs of either gender.[1] The age at clinical presentation for HOD is typically younger than for other juvenile bone and joint diseases of large-breed dogs, although there is overlap.[1,2] Great Danes have a greater incidence of HOD than any other breed, and along with Weimaraners are at greatest risk when adjusted for breed popularity (1016 HODs/100,000 Great Danes and 1279 HODs/ 100,000 Weimaraners). Great Danes, Weimaraners, Labrador retrievers, golden retrievers, German shepherd dogs, mixed breed dogs, and boxers account for the majority of HOD cases. Mixed breed dogs ostensibly have a lower risk, with only 17 HOD cases/100,000 mixed breed dogs (Table 94-1).

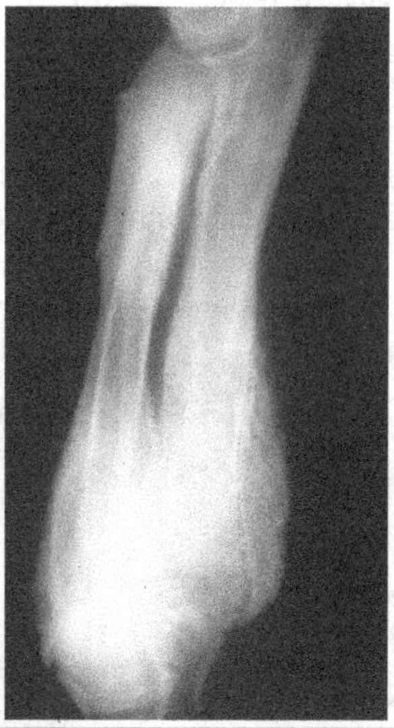

Figure 94-3. Severe case of HOD which, in addition to pseudophyseal line, has subperiosteal hemorrhage and subsequent osseous metaplasia.

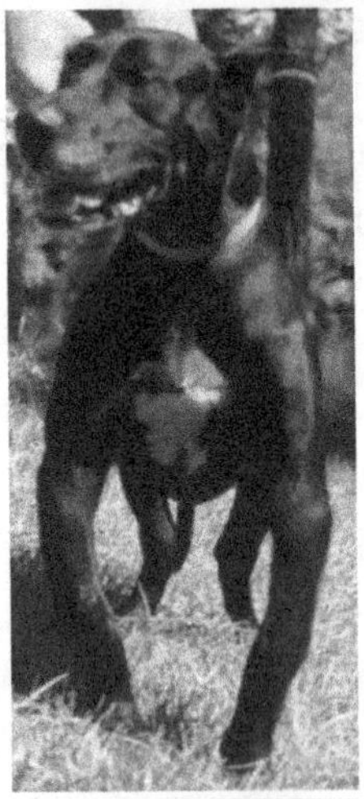

Figure 94-4. Mature Great Dane with deformity owing to severe HOD as a juvenile, which included extensive periosteal hemorrhage and subsequent new bone formation.

Patient History

Dogs with HOD typically present with either acute or peracute onset of signs, often of a day or less duration. Mild HOD cases occur, with less severe clinical signs and longer duration prior to presentation; however, mild HOD cases are uncommon in the author's experience. History typically includes malaise, pain (vocalization), reluctance or inability to stand, and anorexia. HOD is most often a single event in a dog's life, but can be episodic until skeletal maturity. Because clinical signs of HOD are obvious to owners, a diagnosis of HOD as a juvenile would be expected in the history of the rare adult dog with musculoskeletal deformity due to HOD (Figure 94-4).

Examination Findings

Bilaterally symmetrical swelling of the distal radius/ulna area is obvious via palpation and often readily visible (Figure 94-5A). Swelling of the distal tibia/fibula area may also be present but is typically less severe (Figure 94-5B). Other locations (see **Pathology**) are uncommon or unnoticed owing to less clinically detectable signs. Gentle palpation of the swollen areas results in a painful to extremely painful response, and excessive warmth of the area is often appreciated. Core body temperature in excess of 104° F is a consistent finding. Dehydration is often present as a consequence of malaise and reluctance or inability to stand. Arthrocentesis of the carpii will yield inflammatory synovial fluid indicative of and owing to the extreme inflammation of the adjacent area; the adjacent joints (carpii and perhaps tarsii) are otherwise not involved in the pathophysiology. Arthrocentesis is not indicated but, if HOD is not recognized, may be performed owing to suspicion of infectious arthritis (infectious arthritis typically occurs in older dogs, affects one joint, and has less pronounced swelling, which is centered over the joint).

Radiographic Findings

A pseudophyseal line is pathognomonic for HOD (Figure 94-2) and is located adjacent to and on the diaphyseal side of the physis of the distal radius and ulna (and distal tibia if affected). The radiolucency is due to the attending osteoclasia and osteonecrosis plus the increased fluid density of inflammation characteristic of HOD's pathophysiology. Subperiosteal hemorrhage and/or calcification may be observed in the metaphyseal area adjacent to the pseudophyseal line (Figure 94-3). Pseudophyseal lines can potentially be identified on the metaphyseal side of any physis. Osteopathy at other locations (see **Pathology**) when classic HOD lesions are present may be identified radiographically.

Treatment

Treatments ranging from nothing to corticosteroids have been reported, depending on the severity of clinical signs.[2,21] Treatments limited to correcting diet, symptomatic supportive care, and/or nonsteroidal anti-inflammatory drugs tend to be unacceptably slow or completely ineffective. The author prefers intravenous prednisolone sodium succinate (Solu-Delta-Cortef; Pharmacia & Upjohn Company, Kalamazoo, Michigan 49001 USA) because of its speed and reliability in reversing clinical signs. Other injectable corticosteroids are acceptable, including long-acting corticosteroids. However, it is often unnecessary to repeat even the short-acting prednisolone sodium succinate. Such short-term use of corticosteroids makes side effects unlikely. Nonsteroidal anti-inflammatory drugs may be adequate for mild cases, but are not preferred over corticosteroids.

Supportive care is indicated for severe or refractory cases until clinical signs abate, including adminstering intravenous fluids, providing a well padded area to lie on, and alternating sides of

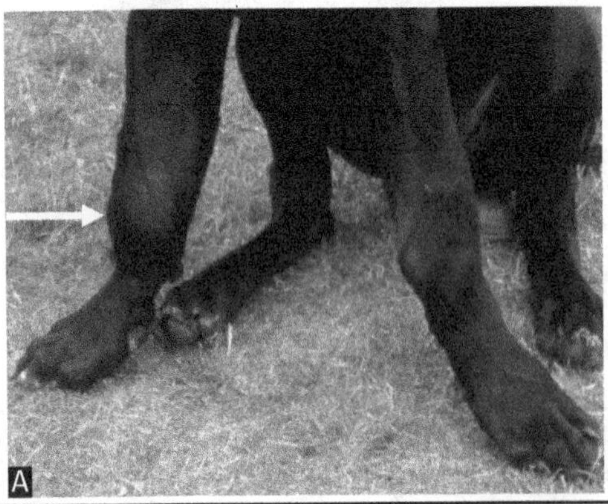

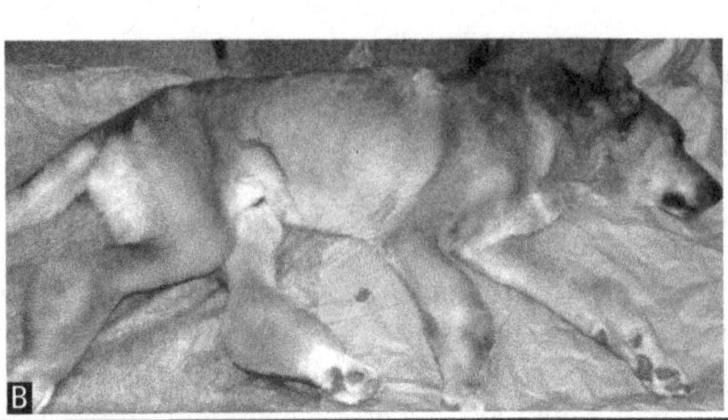

Figure 94-5. A. A 4-month-old Labrador retriever with HOD. Note the bilateral enlargement just proximal to the carpii. B. A 6-month-old golden retriever with atypical clinical presentation of HOD affecting the distal tibia more prominently than the radius/ulna.

recumbency at 2-3-hour intervals. Refractory cases may dictate forced feeding. Stress and anorexia may potentiate opportunistic bacterial infections, so blood cultures and/or antibiotics may be warreanted.[14] Stopping excessive dietary supplements is probably appropriate. Dietary supplementation with vitamin C and vitamin D may be contraindicated for HOD because of the possibility of promoting dystrophic calcification.[2,9,10]

Prognosis

HOD is a single-episode, completely reversible disease in the vast majority of cases. Relapses are infrequent and are treated in the same manner as described above. HOD only occurs while physes are present, primarily in rapidly growing dogs (a function of age and the breed's size). Cases that develop after 8 months of age are unknown in the author's experience. Death in treated cases is exceedingly rare. Euthanasia, although uncommon and usually unjustified, is the most common cause of death.

Deformity owing to HOD is rare (Figure 94-4), but when present is accompanied by lameness. Lameness is caused by mechanical dysfunction, valgus deformity, and perhaps degenerative arthritis caused by the malformations (ostensibly not directly owing to HOD affecting the joint). The acute pain and other signs associated with HOD are not present in adult dogs with deformity caused by HOD.

References

1. Montgomery RD: Miscellaneous orthopaedic diseases. *In* Textbook of Small Animal Surgery. Slatter DH (ed). Philadelphia: Saunders, 2003, p. 2251.

2. Lenehan TM, Fetter AW: Hypertrophic osteodystrophy. *In* Textbook of Small Animal Orthopaedics. Newton CD, Nunamaker DM (eds). Philadelphia: Lippincott, 1985, p. 597.

3. Munjar TA, Austin CC, Breur GJ: Comparison of risk factors for hypertrophic osteodystrophy, craniomandibular osteopathy and canine distemper virus infection. Vet Comp Ortho Traumatol 11:37, 1998.

4. LaFond E, Greur GJ, Austin CC: Breed susceptibility for developmental orthopedic diseases in dogs. J Am Anim Hosp Assoc 38:467, 2002.

5. Brighton CT: Epiphyseal bone formation. *In* Textbook of Small Animal Orthopaedics. Newton CD, Nunamaker DM (eds). Philadelphia: Lippincott, 1985, p. 21.

6. Anderson CE, Parker J: Invasion and resorption in endochondral ossification: An electron microscopic study. J Bone Joint Surg 48:899, 1966.

7. Morell G: La maladie de Barlow spontanee chez le chin. Vet Bull 6:68, 1935.

8. Rhinelander FW, Wilson JW: Blood supply to developing, mature and healing bone. *In* Bone in Clinical Orthopaedics. Sumner-Smith G (ed). Philadelphia: Saunders, 1982, p. 81.

9. Hedhammer A, Fu-ming Wu, Krook L, et al: Overnutrition and skeletal disease: An experimental study in growing Great Dane dogs. Cornell Vet 64 (Suppl 5):9, 1974.

10. Trostel CT, Pool RR, McLaughlin RM: Canine lameness caused by developmental orthopedic diseases: panosteitis, Legg-Calve'-Perthes disease, and hypertrophic osteopathy. Compendium 25:282, 2003.

11. Bohning R, Suter P, Hohn RB, et al: Clinical and radiographic survey of canine panosteitis. JAVMA 156:870, 1970.

12. Abeles V, Harrus S, Angles JM, et al: Hypertrophic osteodystrophy in six Weimaraner puppies associated with systemic signs. Vet Rec 145:130, 1999.

13. Harrus S, Waner T, Aizenberg I, et al: Development of hypertrophic osteodystrophy and antibody response in a litter of vaccinated Weimaraner puppies. J Small Anim Pract 43:27, 2002.

14. Schulz KS, Payne JT, Aronson *E: Escherichia coli* bacteremia associated with hypertrophic osteodystrophy in a dog. JAVMA 199:1170, 1991.

15. Muir P, Dubielzig RR, Johnson KA: Hypertrophic osteodystrophy and calvarial hyperostosis. Compendium 18:143, 1996.

16. Bohning RH, Suter PF, Hohn RB, Marshall J: Clinical and radiologic survey of canine panosteitis. JAVMA 156:870, 1970.

17. Cook JL: Foreleg lameness in the young patient. Vet Clin North Am 31:55, 2001.

18. Mee AP, Webber DM, May C, et al: Detection of canine distemper virus in bone cells in the metaphysis of distemper infected dogs. J Bone Miner Res 7:829, 1992.

19. Mee AP, Gordon MT, May C, et al: Canine distemper virus transcripts detected in the bone cells of dogs with metaphyseal osteopathy. Bone 14:59, 1993.

20. Appeldoorn AM, Schrauwen EMJ: Hypertrophic osteodystrophy in a toy breed. VCOT 8:210, 1995.

21. Bellah JR: Hypertrophic osteodystrophy. *In* Bojrab MJ (ed). Disease Mechanisms in Small Animals, 2nd ed. Philadelphia, Williams & Wilkins, 1993, p. 859.

Chapter 95

Panosteitis

Ron Montgomery

Panosteitis is one of the most common causes of lameness in young, large breed dogs, and is common worldwide.[1-20] Panosteitis is a self-limiting disease of the bone marrow of long bones in which the adipose and hematopoietic tissue is temporarily replaced by fibrous tissue.[1-20] Osseous changes also occur affecting the trabeculae, endosteum, and in more severe cases, the cortex and periosteum.[4,15] Pain and lameness of the affected limb(s) are the consistent clinical signs that last 2 weeks or less.[4,15] Panosteitis typically recurs episodically, and is the classic cause of "shifting leg lameness."[4,15] It is unusual for panosteitis to affect the same bone twice (1%), but it can affect the same leg multiple times.[4] Clinical signs of panosteitis are uncommon after 18 months of age, although in one study 18% of the patients were older than 18 months.[4] Panosteitis spontaneously regresses, so treatment is usually limited to short-term administration of NSAIDs or corticosteroids as needed for adequate pain control.

Synonyms for panosteitis include: enostosis, eosinophilic panosteitis, juvenile osteomyelitis, and canine panosteitis.[9,15] Enostosis is defined as "morbid bony growth of endosteum or within the medullary cavity."[14] This, along with fibrosis and destruction of normal medullary cellularity, describes the most common pathologic features of panosteitis.[4,15] Early reports of panosteitis were associated with eosinophilia, but subsequent reports indicate only 1% to 5% have eosinophilia.[4,9,15] Juvenile osteomyelitis is a misleading nomen (see etiology). Canine panosteitis is redundant because, to the authors knowledge, it has only been reported in dogs.[15] Panosteitis is the commonly used name. One sage author has proposed that any name change should await definitive identification of the etiology.[4]

Panosteitis was first described in 1951 in young German shepherd dogs in Europe.[15] Panosteitis was reported in the United States in 1960, and was reported to spread rapidly.[15] However, the "spread" of panosteitis is thought to be a result more of increased awareness than epidemiologic spread.[15]

Etiology

The etiology of panosteitis is unknown.[2,15] Along with HOD and cranial mandibular osteopathy, panosteitis is a disease of unknown etiology in juvenile dogs that is characterized by osseous proliferation and excessive bone remodeling.[9] However, panosteitis is a unique disease with characteristics unlike any other known disease.[4]

Proposed etiologies for panosteitis include bacterial infection, viral infection (e.g., distemper), genetics, stress, metabolic disease, vascular anomalies, allergy, hyperestrinism, parasite migration, autoimmune reaction after viral infection, and hemophilia.[3,13,15] Some reports of potential etiologies had convincing circumstantial evidence, but subsequent cases did not support the connection. Medical advances (e.g., improved microbiology diagnostics, parasite control, vaccines, etc.) have made several proposed etiologies unlikely. Other proposed etiologies remain possible, but proof is lacking. Attempts to isolate causative infectious agents from dogs with panosteitis have been unsuccessful.[20]

Bacterial infection was the originally proposed etiology.[15] Panosteitis was thought to be a result of purulent hematogenous osteomyelitis caused by streptococcus.[15] However, necropsy of 18 dogs failed to identify any bacteria at the lesions.[9,18] Other studies also reported negative cultures associated with panosteitis lesions.[4] The few blood and bone marrow cultures have been negative for aerobic and anaerobic bacteria.[15] Histopathology consistently fails to implicate a bacterial etiology, and WBC counts are typically normal.[4,15] Antibiotic therapy is ineffective.[15] Furthermore, the long clinical history with panosteitis does not support a readily contagious agent as the sole cause.[1-20]

Viral etiology has been strongly supported by some authors,[9] and it remains a potential cause. Initial reports of panosteitis in 1951 roughly corresponded to the common use of live distemper vaccination, and a connection was suspected.[9] Most dogs are vaccinated against canine distemper and never develop panosteitis. Nevertheless, some authors recommend vaccination with killed distemper or adenovirus vaccine rather than modified live which may still "allow transcription into messenger RNA."[9,19] Viral etiology of panosteitis was suggested by a report of successfully inducing panosteitis via medullary aspirates (filtered or unfiltered to remove bacteria) from dogs with panosteitis and injected intramedullary into unaffected dogs.[18] Panosteitis-like lesions were reported in the inoculated bones 2 to 3 weeks later and also developed in one bone of a marrow recipient that was not inoculated.[18] Transmission was reported to be more readily accomplished in male dogs;[18] however, the validity of this report has been questioned.[15] Host response to inoculated foreign material likely caused the observed lesions. In addition, bone marrow and buffy coat samples from dogs with panosteitis were placed in kidney cell lines without cytotoxic effects, which would refute a viral etiology.[15,20] Reports of panosteitis with concurrent clinical findings of pyrexia, tonsillitis and leukocytosis also suggest viral infection;[9] however, the numerous cases of panosteitis without pyrexia, tonsillitis, and/or leukocytosis makes it likely that these signs were coincidental.

Genetic influence or cause of panosteitis is a consideration because of predilection for certain breeds (Table 95-1). Panosteitis is most common in German shepherd dogs, but can occur in almost any large breed.[11] A purely genetic cause is doubtful because so many breeds are affected (n=59 in our VMDB[1] survey. The VMDB does not give number of cases at every month, or year, of age. Cases within an age range are reported as "0-2 wks; 2wks-; 2mn; 2-6mn; 6-12mn; 1-2yr; 2-4yr; 4-7yr; 7-10yr; 10-; 15yr; and 15yr+." The number of cases for VMDB data in Figure 95-1 was placed at the center of the age ranges, with cases > 4 years old placed at 60 months on the chart).[9] One report stated that English pointer pups and German shepherd pups were raised in the same pen, yet only German shepherds routinely developed panosteitis.[15] This limited report supports lack of an infectious agent even more than it suggests genetic influence.

Hemophilia A was reported in three male German shepherd dogs with panosteitis. Histopathologic and gross pathologic studies showed typical panosteitis plus hematomas. The signalment is the same for both diseases. However, the author stated it was "unwarranted to conclude that all dogs suffering from enostosis have bleeding disorders," but suggested that "bleeding disorders should be considered when discussing the etiology of enostosis."[13]

A frequent correlation exists between the first estrus and the first episode of panosteitis, which has led to speculation of hyperestrinism as a cause of panosteitis. Stress is thought to often precipitate panosteitis episodes.[15] Stress is a common factor in estrus, metabolic disease, allergy, parasite migration, and autoimmune reaction after viral infection, all of which have been speculated as causes of panosteitis. The inability to identify a single cause of panosteitis over 5 decades suggests that panosteitis may be caused by the confluence of multiple factors.

Pathology

Panosteitis is a self-limiting disease of the metaphysis and diaphysis of long bones of juvenile dogs, predominantly large breeds.[4,15] Panosteitis has never been reported to affect the epiphysis.[15] Panosteitis begins with loss of medullary adipose tissue, followed by fibrous proliferation, intramembranous ossification, osteoclastic removal of trabeculae, and in more severe cases, periosteal proliferation and cortical changes.[9,11,15] The process then regresses to normal or near normal architecture in the vast majority of cases.[15] This cycle is typically 60 to 90 days, but may be up to 190 days.[3,15,16]

Panosteitis has been characterized as a disease of adipose bone marrow with secondary osseous effects.[15] As supportive evidence, the reaction to fractures and to irradiation to remove bone marrow are examples given of adipose bone marrow damage, with histologic and radiographic responses similar to panosteitis.[15] In addition, these events also follow a 90-day pattern.[15] Pathology begins with vascular leakage of protein-rich edema from congested medullary blood vessels and degeneration of adipose tissue.[3,9,11,15,16] Increased leucocytes and plasma cells are typically not observed.[2,4,9,17]

As the edema quickly organizes, fibroblastic reticular cells of bone marrow stroma produce a marked and highly cellular fibrosis in the medullary canal.[2,4] Hematopoietic tissue is replaced by massive amounts of fibrous tissue, which is rich in fibroblast, osteocytes, osteoblast, and osteoclast, but which is usually not inflammatory.[4,9] Osteoclasts remove much of the preexisting trabeculae, which are replaced by formation of a haphazard trabecular system of woven bone.[4,9,15] These new trabeculae tend to be short and thick, and may obliterate the medullary canal.[9] In addition, areas of acellular calcified material and intramembranous woven bone are scattered throughout the medullary cavity.[2,4,15] High osteoblast and fibroblast activity also occurs along the endosteum, and in some cases, the cortex and periosteum.[3,4,16] Cortical bone may be replaced with woven bone, especially around the nutrient foramen, and appear as a zone of decreased density.[9] Hyperemia of periosteum and adjacent soft tissues commonly provokes a mild periosteal reaction that may not be detected in most dogs, but can result in periosteal new bone a few millimeters thick.[2]

During late stages, woven bone trabeculae are replaced by fewer lamellar bone trabeculae, which tend to be fewer and thicker than normal.[15] Remnants of the pathologic changes may persist for months.[2,4] Components of the histologic appearance of panosteitis are not unique or pathognomonic (e.g., also seen at borders of bone tumors and focal bone infections);[2] however, no evidence of inflammatory cell exudate, necrosis, or neoplasia exists.[2,17] The amount of remodeling varies between dogs and even between episodes.[9] Repeated attacks make marrow aplastic, with little to no hematopoietic bone marrow.[15]

Clinical Diagnosis

Signalment

The quintessential case of panosteitis is a 10-month-old male German shepherd dog. Although the signalment has strong predispositions, the range of breeds and ages represented is broad. Ranges of and predispositions for age, breed, and gender were determined for this chapter by literature review and a retrieval from the Veterinary Medical Data Base, including all participating institutions, and from 1994-2004 inclusively. Cases per 100,000 were calculated for breeds with more than 1000 in the total population.

Age

The majority of panosteitis patients are 5 months to 12 months old; however, the age range is 2 months to 5 years old and older. The VMDB survey for this chapter had 662 cases of panosteitis, of which 380 dogs (57%) were 6 to 12 months old.* This VMDB survey further indicated that 64% were ≤ 12 months old, and 89% were ≤ 2 years old (n=590). The VMDB survey had a case at 2 months old, but also reported 14 cases between 7 years old to more than 15 years old (2%) (Figure 95-1).

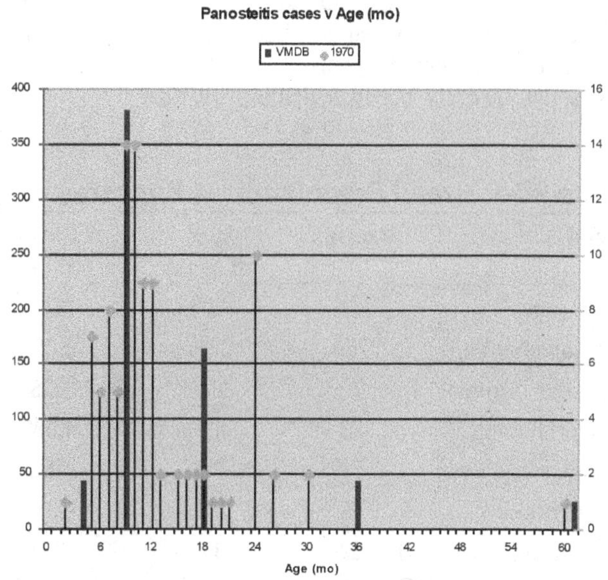

Figure 95-1. Age distribution of dogs with panosteitis from VMDB (662 dogs) and Bohning et al report (100 dogs) indicates panosteitis is predominantly a juvenile disease.

The literature cites age ranges typical for panosteitis from 5 months to 12, 18, 20, or 24 months old.[3,4,11,15] An excellent 1970 study of 100 consecutive cases of panosteitis reported the peak occurrence was at 9 months and 10 months (n=14 each month) (Figure 95-1). This study also reported that 71% were 5 to 12 months old, 82% were ≤ 18 months old, and 95% were ≤ 2 years.[4] The reported mean age at initial diagnosis was 12 months 2 weeks old, but the mean calculated from their data by this author was 10 months old.[4] Female German shepherds accounted for the single cases at 2 months and 5 years old.[4] The second youngest was 5 months old (n=7), and the second oldest was 30 months old (n=2).[4] Hence, the age range or mean that constitutes "typical" depends on what percentage of cases is included. Results of the VMDB survey for this chapter and the 1970 study of 100 dogs with panosteitis are comparable (Figure 95-1).

Breed

German shepherds are most commonly afflicted with panosteitis, whether based on number of cases, % of all cases, or cases per 100,000 of the breed (Table 95-1). Our VMDB survey indicated German shepherds had the most cases (n = 259), the highest percentage of cases (39%), and the highest risk (2053 cases of panosteitis/100,000 German shepherds). A 1970 study of 100 consecutive cases of panosteitis had 79% German shepherds.[4] An earlier VMDB survey is the only report with German shepherds having the second highest number of cases (n=648); mixed breed dogs had the most cases (n=945).[1]

Basset hounds had the second highest risk (1999 cases / 100,000 bassets), were tied for 3rd most cases with 53 (Table 95-1), and accounted for 8% of all cases in our VMDB survey. Labrador retrievers had the second highest number of cases with 72 and accounted for 11% of all cases, but had lower risk with 238 cases / 100,000 Labrador retrievers (Table 95-1).

Eight breeds (Table 95-1) account for 81% of all cases of panosteitis in our VMDB survey. These or similar lists of prevalent breeds being previously reported.[1-4,8,9,15] Panosteitis occurred in 59 breeds in our VMDB survey, but 25 breeds had only 1 case. Twelve breeds, including mixed breeds, had fewer than 100 cases/100,000 of the breed, indicating low risk.

Table 95-1. Breed Prevalence of Panosteitis

Breed	# cases	% of all cases	# Cases / 100,000 of breed
All Breeds	666	100%	217
German shepherd	259	39%	2,053
Labrador retriever	72	11%	238
Bassett hound	53	8%	1,999
Golden retriever	53	8%	292
Mixed breed	53	8%	83
Rottweiler	22	3%	237
Great Dane	16	2%	650
Doberman pinscher	14	2%	297

81% of all cases are in one of these 8 breeds.

Small breeds with panosteitis had a total of 12 cases, or 1.8% of all dogs with panosteitis, in our VMDB survey. Cardigan Welsh corgis had the most cases with 3, blue heelers accounted for 2 cases, whereas the American cocker spaniel, Maltese, Norwich terrier, miniature schnauzer, Shetland sheepdog, Pembroke Welsh corgi, and wirehaired pointing griffon had 1 case of panosteitis each. A previous study likewise reported 99% of dogs with panosteitis were large breed (miniature schnauzer was the exception).[4]

Gender

The predilection for males to have panosteitis is consistent and noteworthy. Our VMDB study showed males accounted for 70% of all cases of panosteitis, yet the overall population was only 48% males. Males account for 67% to 84% of all cases of panosteitis based on the literature.[3,4,6,11,12,15] One study of 100 dogs with panosteitis had 79% males, with German shepherds and 1 Saint Bernard accounting for all the females.[4] Panosteitis recurrences have been reported to be more predictable in males.[15] Females usually have the first episode of panosteitis associated with the first estrus.[15]

Patient History

An acute onset of mild to moderate lameness is the typical history, although severe lameness is also commonly reported.[4,9,11,15] Duration of lameness is up to 14 days (rarely, 3 weeks in severe cases), although lameness from panosteitis is often as short as 2 days.[2,4,9,15] Decreased appetite and activity may be reported coinciding with the lameness.[2,3,4,11,12] Lameness is not affected by rest or exercise, but lameness usually increases during the first few days of an episode.[15] Pain is most likely from stimulation of pain receptors in the periosteum and/or owing to medullary hyperemia and congestion.[2] The initial episode of panosteitis most often affects a front leg, followed by rear leg, then returns to a front leg.[15] "Shifting leg lameness" is a classic historical description for panosteitis (see Prognosis for more detail).[2,3,9,11,12] Lameness can also affect one or more legs simultaneously or sequentially (Figure 95-2).[2,4,15] The initial onset of lameness owing to panosteitis is uncommon (~10%) over 2 years of age (see Signalment for more detail).[4,15]

Examination Findings

Lameness ranges from mild to non-weight bearing.[15] Diagnosis is primarily via palpation.[15] Pain of affected bone is exacerbated and localized by deep palpation of the bone, with painful responses ranging from mild to severe.[2-4,9,11,12,15] Panosteitis tends to start at the nutrient foramen (approximately at the junction of the proximal third with the distal two thirds of long bones), but panosteitis can also occur elsewhere in the diaphysis or metaphysis.[4,9,12,15] Care should be taken not to compress soft tissues, other than skin, to avoid a false positive response. Panosteitis is easily overlooked, and probably often, unless direct palpation of long bones is a routine part of the orthopedic examination for dogs at risk.[4] Muscle atrophy is rarely present owing to panosteitis because of its acute onset and short duration of clinical signs.[4] Confirmation via radiographs is recommended, although initial radiographs may only rule out other etiologies.[3,4] One report indicated

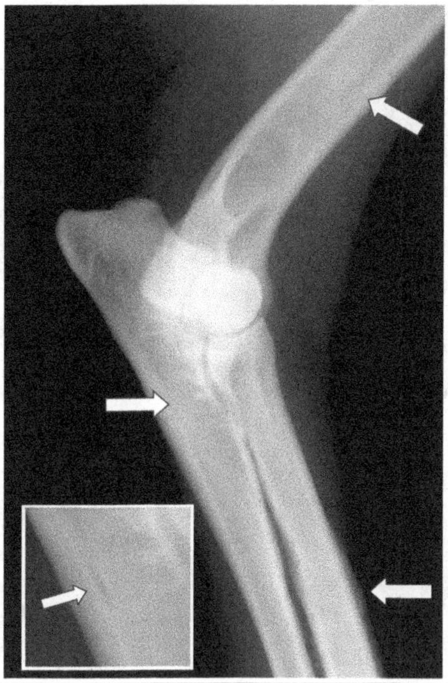

Figure 95-2. Radiographic signs of panosteitis evident in ihe humerus, radius and ulna of the same leg (arrows). The ulna has the earliest radiographic signs (see insert) of radiolucency at the endosteal surface. The later radiographic sign, which is most often the first appreciated, is radiodensity of the medullary canal which is patchy (humerus) or generalized (radius).

minimal radiographic signs in 5 of 100 dogs with panosteitis.[4] In addition, radiographic signs of panosteitis may not be observed for 10 to14 days after onset of clinical signs, yet there may be more sensitivity during the first few days (i.e., the patient may be more likely to be presented for examination).[2,12,15] A poor correlation exists between severity of clinical signs and radiographic changes with panosteitis.[2,4,9,11,15]

The most commonly affected bone differs among reports. One report lists in descending order the ulna (42%), radius (25%), humerus (14%), femur (11%), and tibia (8%).[15] A different report lists the most commonly affected bones as the humerus (68%), femur (68%), ulna (54%), radius (27%), and tibia (24%).[4] The latter reported panosteitis of the contralateral bone in 31% (humerus) to 60% (tibia) of the cases, with only 1 of 100 dogs having panosteitis in the same bone more than once.[4] Different phases of the disease may be occurring concurrently in the same dog at the same time (Figure 95-2).[15]

Concurrent orthopedic diseases are common (26% in one report)[4] in dogs with panosteitis.[2-4,9,11,15] Hence, a complete orthopedic examination, and radiography as indicated, should always be performed. Other findings are rare, but may include pyrexia, anorexia, tonsillitis, eosinophilia, muscle atrophy, and elevated white blood cell counts, none of which are unique to panosteitis.[3,4,9,15] Fever, anorexia, tonsillitis, and eosinophilia have each been reported to occur in only about 1% of panosteitis cases.[4,9] Most cases of panosteitis are in otherwise healthy dogs.[3]

Radiographic Findings

Four radiographic stages are associated with panosteitis, three of which are commonly observed. These stages are in reality a continuum of pathology, and various authors differ on the arbitrary points of delineating stages. The radiographic stages of panosteitis are 1) radiolucency of the medullary canal, 2) radiopacity of the medullary canal, 3) endosteal, cortical, and periosteal reaction, and 4) recovery.

The earliest radiographic sign of panosteitis is increased radiolucency of the medullary canal (Figure. 95-2).[4,8,12,15] The radiolucency corresponds to the early pathologic changes to medullary adipose tissue, occurs early, and is rarely observed.[2,12,15] Radiolucency can be recognized 10 to 14 days after onset of clinical signs.[12] High quality radiographs are necessary to see changes that are present when clinical lameness begins.[9] If uncertain, additional radiographs should be taken 2 to 3 weeks later to show more obvious changes.[9]

The second stage of radiographic change, and typically the first observed, is increased density of the medullary canal in a patchy or mottled pattern, most frequently starting near the nutrient foramen (Figure 95-3).[4,11,12,15] The radiopacity corresponds to the pathologic changes of proliferating stromal and adventitial cells in the medullary canal, and their subsequent calcification and intramembranous bone formation.[2,9,12,15] This radiographic stage typically begins 10 to 14 days after initial clinical signs.[15] Initially, these changes can be subtle (Figure 95-2).[9] Radiographic changes of this stage usually last 4 to 6 weeks.[4] Consistent early changes in this stage are loss of normal trabecular pattern, loss of medullary-cortical contrast (owing to increased medullary radiodensity), plus a variable number of intramedullary granular densities.[3,4,9] Early changes that may also be observed are accentuation of the trabecular pattern prior to or adjacent to increased medullary radiodensity, and the cortical changes around the nutrient foramen which accentuates the foramen (Figures 95-2 and 95-3).[4,9] Midway in this radiographic stage the appearance is patchy or mottled, with sclerotic densities of various size and extent.[3] Granular density can be seen in the medullary canal early to late in this stage.[4] Homogenous radiodensity fills the medullary canal in some cases.[4] As this stage progresses toward the next, the endosteal surface becomes roughened, with coarse trabeculae extending into the medullary canal.[4] In about a third of cases, usually those with extensive medullary involvement, periosteal roughening is followed by periosteal new bone (Figure 95-4).[4]

The third radiographic stage, typically the second observed, includes endosteal, cortical and periosteal reaction (Figures 95-2 and 95-4). The radiographic signs of endosteal, cortical, and periosteal bone changes correspond to the pathologic changes described for the previous stage and formation of woven bone that progress to affecting cortical bone.[9] There is continuation of the obvious patchy or mottled radiodensity, and often an increased radiodensity approaching that of the cortex.[4,9] Endosteal roughening and then periosteal roughening may precede new bone formation, and a coarse trabecular pattern may be present.[9,15] Periosteal new bone is seen in 15 to 25% of affected cases, ostensibly the more severe cases.[2] Periosteal and endosteal new bone yields the appearance that the cortex

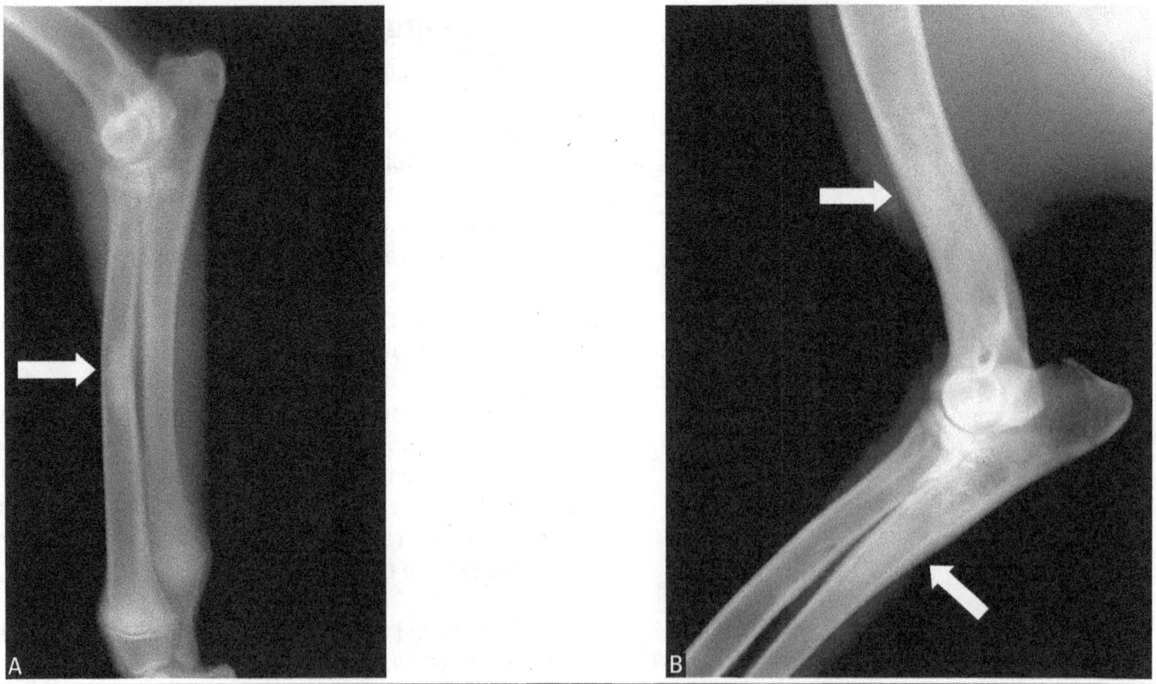

Figure 95-3A. Discrete patchy area of medullary radiodensity characteristic of panosteitis which is later than seen in the ulna of Figure 95-2.
Figure 95-3B. Radiodensity of the medullary canal of the radius is patchy and limited in area, compared to the more advanced humerus which is patchy but nearing gerneralized radiodensity of the entire diameter and over a larger area.

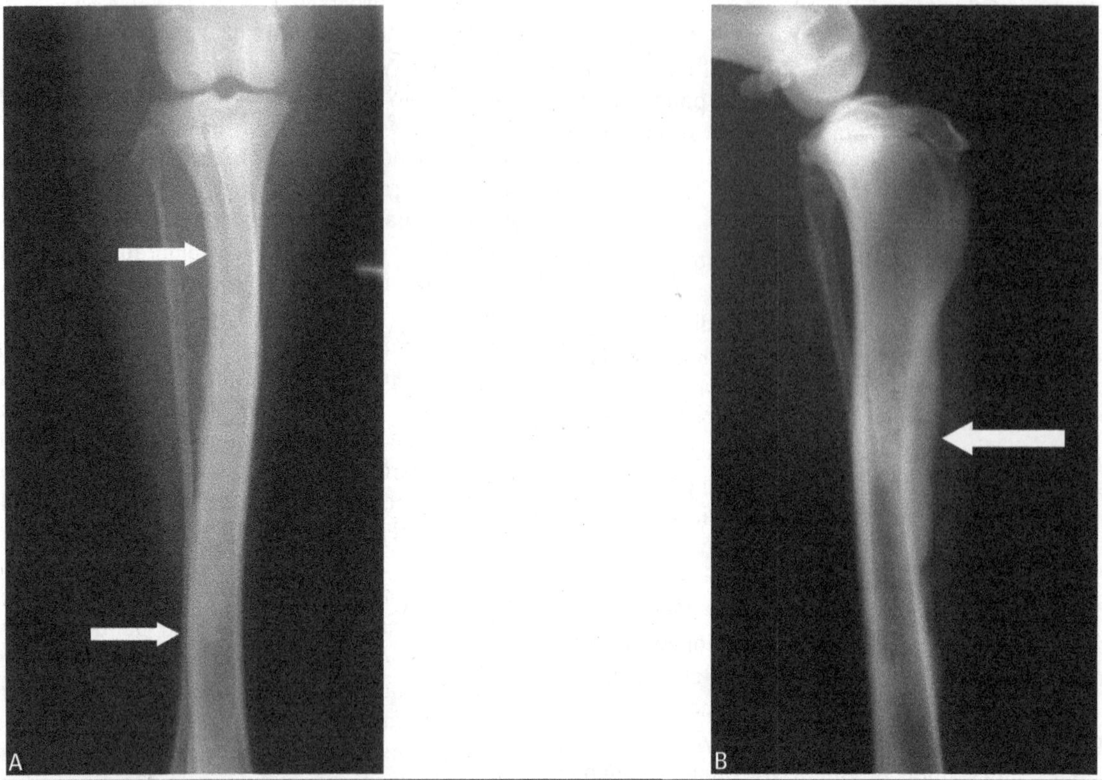

Figure 95-4A. Radiodensity of the medullary canal typical of panosteitis has progressed from patchy and limited areas, as seen in figure 95-3, to involve almost the entire length of this tibia.
Figure 95-4B. This tibia has medullary radiodensity plus the perioosteal proliferation, indicating even further progression compared to figures 92-94A. Not all dogs with panosteitis progress to this severity of radiographic changes.

is thicker in that region and margins are indistinct.[9] Cortical bone may be replaced with woven bone in some areas.[9] Cortical osteoporosis, if seen, is due to enlargement of the osteonal canals.[15] Thickening of areas of the cortex occurs in about a third of cases.[4] Radiographic diagnosis of panosteitis is easiest in this stage.[4]

The fourth radiographic stage, typically the third observed, is recovery. The radiographic signs correspond to the reversal of the pathologic changes, plus evidence of residual changes. These changes include a decreased number of granular densities, return to normal medullary appearance, and cortical and trabecular remodeling, with regression toward the nutrient foramen (reverse order of formation).[2,3] The medullary canal progresses to a more normal appearance over a 2- to 3-month period.[9] Regression of bony changes is via osteoclastic removal of trabeculae that do not serve a biomechanical function, and requires months.[2] Persistent changes can include slightly increased density of the medullary canal, granular densities, fewer and coarser trabecular bone, roughened endosteum, and increased cortical thickness (Figure 95-5).[2,4]

The severity and extent of radiographic changes with panosteitis varies greatly.[2,4,15] The overall cycle of radiographic changes for a given bone with panosteitis is typically 60 to 90 days, but may last up to 190 days.[3,15,16] Different stages of panosteitis often occur concurrently in the same dog at the same time (Figure 95-2).[2,4,15] One study reported radiographic changes consistent with panosteitis in 2 or more bones at the same time in 24 of 25 dogs that had radiographs of all limbs.[4] As many as 7 bones have been affected at one time by panosteitis.[15] Radiographic changes owing to panosteitis often center around the nutrient foramen.[4,9,12,15] One report stated that changes affect the diaphysis only in 75% of dogs, with extension to include the metaphysis in 25% of dogs.[4] There has not been a report of panosteitis affecting the epiphysis.[15] Panosteitis affecting the same bone twice is rare (1%).[4] Repeat episodes of panosteitis can result in bones becoming cuboidal and "lose their graceful appearance" owing to repeated remodeling.[15] Although panosteitis almost always affects the long tubular bones, 1 dog was reported to have radiographic lesions typical of panosteitis in the ilium.[4]

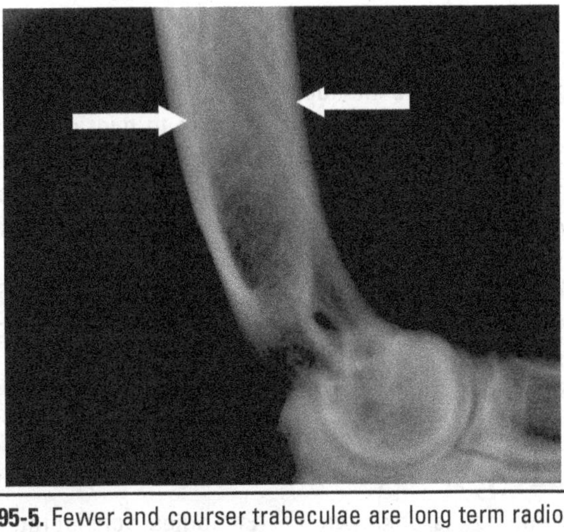

Figure 95-5. Fewer and courser trabeculae are long term radiographic indicators of prior panosteitis in this humerus. NOT all episodes of panosteitis have as severe, or any, chronic radiographic changes. These changes are seen after the clinical signs of panosteitis.

Treatment

Because panosteitis is self-limiting, with clinical signs limited to lameness because of pain, appropriate therapy is typically limited to NSAIDs. Treatment can be on an as-needed basis for the duration of clinical signs, which may be a short as 2 days to as long as 3 weeks.[2,4,9,15] Aspirin has been frequently recommended, but other NSAIDs would also be appropriate.[4,9,15] Corticosteroids may be used in refractory or severe cases.[2,15] Other analgesics may be used but are rarely necessary.[15] Exercise or rest does not affect the severity of lameness,[15] although two reports suggest restricted activity as part of the treatment.[2,9] Concurrent orthopedic problems or other signs (e.g., anorexia) are treated separately.[2,3]

Other treatments that have been tried with minimal success include antibiotics, vitamin and mineral supplements, dietary changes, and irradiation of diseased bone and adrenal glands.[15]

Prognosis

The prognosis for a given episode of panosteitis is excellent. Lameness and pain last from 2 days up to 3 weeks, with or without treatment.[2,4,9,11,15] However, pain may be severe, and even less than severe cases warrant pain relief. Medication such as NSAIDs or corticosteroids almost always provide excellent relief from clinical signs. The severity of attacks tends to decrease as age increases.[15]

The long-term prognosis for panosteitis is also excellent.[2,4,9,11] However, recurrences are common in dogs up to about 18 months old.[2-4,15] Approximately 5 to11% of panosteitis cases occur in dogs over 2 years old (Figure 95-1).[4] Although it is rare for panosteitis to afflict the same bone a second time (1%), panosteitis will often afflict one or more other long bones in the same or different legs.[4]

The initial episode of panosteitis most often affects a front leg, followed by rear leg, then returns to a front leg.[15] "Shifting leg lameness" is a classic historical description for panosteitis.[2,3,9,11,12] In many cases lameness shifts every 2 to 4 weeks, with lapses of up to 1 month or more.[4,9,15] The frequency of recurrence has been reported to be more predictable in males.[15] It is not uncommon for a dog to have 1 or just a few episodes, rather than repeated and frequent episodes up to age 18 to 24 months; at least not enough episodes affecting the dog for veterinary attention to be sought. In a report of 100 consecutive dogs with panosteitis, multiple leg involvement occurred in 49%, and multiple bone involvement in 53%.[4] Multiple leg involvement was equally distributed between front and rear legs.[4] Lameness can also affect one or more legs simultaneously.[4] The frequency and severity of clinical lameness tend to decrease with age.[15]

References

1. LaFond E, Breur GJ, Austin CC: Breed susceptibility for developmental orthopedic diseases in dogs. J Am Anim Hosp Assoc 38:467, 2002.

2. Trostel CT, Pool RR, McLaughlin RM: Canine lameness caused by developmental orthopedic diseases: panosteitis, Legg-Calve'-Perthes disease, and hypertrophic osteopathy. Compendium 25:282, 2003.

3. Cook JL: Foreleg lameness in the young patient. Vet Clin North Am 31:55, 2001.

4. Bohning RH, Suter PF, Hohn RB, Marshall J: Clinical and radiologic survey of canine panosteitis. JAVMA 156:870, 1970.

5. Munjar TA, Austin CC, Breur GJ: Comparison of risk factors for hypertrophic osteodystrophy, craniomandibular osteopathy and canine distemper virus infection. Vet Comp Ortho Traumatol 11:37, 1998.

6. Schwarz T, Johnson VS, Voute L, Sullivan M: Bone scintigraphy in the investigation of occult lameness in the dog. J Small Anim Pract 45:232, 2004.

7. Wallace JM: Meloxicam. Compendium 25:64, 2003.

8. Barrett RB, SchallWD, Lewis RE: Clinical and radiographic features of canine eosinophilic panosteitis. JAAHA 4:94, 1968.

9. Muir P, Dubielzig RR, Johnson KA: Panosteitis. Compendium. 18:29, 1996.

10. Weinstein MJ, Rhodes WH, Mongil CM, Smith GK: Orthopedic conditions of the Rottweiler. Compendium 17:925, 1995.

11. McLaughlin RM: Hind limb lameness in the young patient. Vet Clin North Am 31:101, 2001.

12. Lewis DD, McCarthy RJ, Pechman RD: Diagnosis of common developmental orthopedic conditions in the canine patients. Compendium 14:287, 1992.

13. Grodalen J, Sjaastad O, Teige J: Enostosis (Panosteitis) in three dogs suffering from hemophilia A. Canine Pract 16:10, 1991.

14. Dorland's Illustrated Medical Dictionary (28th Edition). Philadelphia: Saunders,1994, p. 557.

15. Lenehan TM, Fetter AW: Canine panosteitis. *In* Newton CD, Nunamaker DM (eds). Textbook of Small Animal Orthopaedics. Philadelphia: Lippincott, 1985, p. 591.

16. Van Sickle DC, Hohn RB: Selected orthopedic problems in the growing dog. Am Anim Hosp Assoc 1975.

17. Milton JL: Panosteitis. A review of the literature and 32 cases. Auburn Vet 35:11, 1979.

18. Zeskov B: A contribution to "eosinophilic panosteitis" in dogs. Zentralbl Veterinarmed 7:671, 1960.

19. Mee AP, Gordon MT, May C, et al: Canine distemper virus transcripts detected in the bone cells of dogs with metaphyseal osteopathy. Bone 14:59, 1993.

20. Turnier JC: A case study of canine panosteitis: comparison of radiographic and radioisotopic studies. Am J Vet Res 39:35, 1978.

Chapter 96

Craniomandibular Osteopathy

Ron Montgomery
Brenda Austin Simmons

Craniomandibular osteopathy (CMO) is an uncommon inflammatory disease of juvenile dogs characterized by bone proliferation and remodeling of the mandibles.[1-31] The temporomandibular joint is often affected, and involvement (thickening) of other bones of the cranium is common. Pain associated with CMO is typically moderate to severe. Difficulty eating, deformity, and/or pain when opening the mouth are common presenting complaints. West Highland terriers and Scottish terriers are the predominant breeds affected. Long bones may also infrequently be affected, with or without clinical signs of lameness and/or pain with palpation. CMO typically regresses as normal bone formation ends at about 1 year of age.[1]

CMO was first reported in 1958 in five West Highland terriers, and in 1959 in West Highland white and Scottish terriers.[1,2] Clinical and radiographic diagnosis was initially neoplasia. However, histopathology indicated non-neoplastic mandibular periostitis with osseous and chondromyxomatous proliferation.[1] Synonyms for CMO include mandibular periostitis, calvarial hyperostosis, idiopathic hyperostosis of the calvaria, and lion jaw.[1,3,4]

A Veterinary Medical Data Base (VMDB) survey was perform for this chapter from 1994-2004 and reported a total of 29 CMO cases. Review of the literature reported 65 CMO cases,[4-24] some of which predated the years of the VMDB survey whereas others may have also been included in the VMDB study. In addition, cases have been reported in the literature that may be atypical CMO cases. Pastor et al reported a disease he termed calvarial hyperostotic syndrome (CHS).[4] Five unrelated bull mastiff males between 5 and 9 months old had asymmetrical bony proliferation of the frontal, temporal, and occipital bones, with one dog having bony proliferation of the tympanic bullae.[4] All dogs with CHS recovered. Trowald-Wigh reported 12 Irish setters with confirmed canine leucocyte adhesion deficiency (CLAD).[23] The pathogenesis of CLAD includes absence of granulocyte adhesion proteins and the inability of neutrophils to migrate from blood vessels into the tissues.[23] Similar diseases have been reported in humans and bovines.[23] CMO-like lesions were reported; however, CLAD lesions also include various osteopathies of long bones, purulent infections, and multi-organ involvement. These 12 Irish setters with CLAD were between 8 weeks and 15 weeks old at the onset of clinical signs, and all were euthanized owing to the severity and recurrence of clinical signs.[23] Two litters each had 4 CLAD dogs, the remaining 2 were unrelated.[23]

Etiology

CMO's etiology is unknown.[1,27-31] Etiologies considered include congenital,[1,25] and infectious,[21,26] and inherited.[1,25] Neither case histories nor the literature indicate that CMO is present at birth, which by definition means it is not a congenital disease.[27] Rather, CMO ostensibly develops at 3 to 9 months of age (Figure 96-1). Infection does not appear to be the cause of CMO. Microscopic evaluation of affected tissues does not show infectious organisms. Bacterial cultures (n=26) from 4 West Highland white terriers were negative.[22] Antibiotics used in CMO cases have not be reported as an effective treatment.[1-31] Schulz reported E. coli was cultured from a boxer's mandible affected with CMO,[13] which was probably incidental. The predominance of CMO cases occurring in terriers, especially West Highland and Scottish, strongly suggest a genetic etiology. Conversely, CMO occurring in multiple other breeds, including some large breed dogs, causes some doubt regarding a genetic etiology, assuming these other breeds were pure bred and that CMO was not confused with a similar disease.

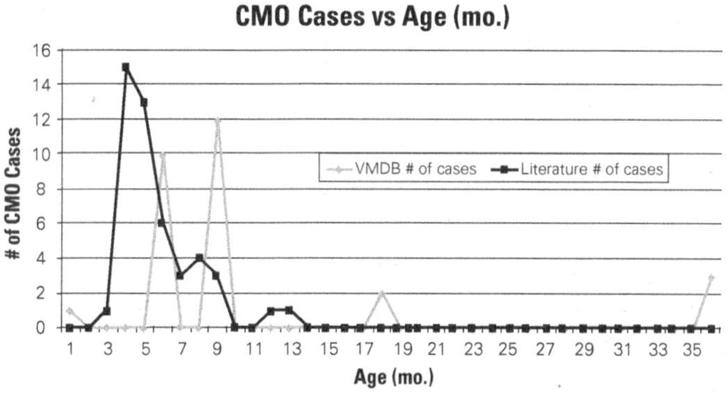

Figure 96-1. The VMDB does not give number of cases at every month, or year, of age. Cases within an age range are reported as "0-2 wks; 2 wks-; 2 mn; 2-6 mn; 6-12 mn; 1-2 yr; 2-4 yr; 4-7 yr; 7-10 yr; 10-; 15 yr; and 15 yr+". The number of cases for VMDB data in Figure 96-1 was placed at the center of the age ranges, with cases $\geq$ 4 years old placed at 60 months on the chart. 8 West Highland terriers with CMO reported by Riserx did not report age, but were included in breed assessments.

Pathology

Normal lamellar bone is removed by osteoclasts and may be accompanied by massive numbers of inflammatory cells (predominantly lymphocytes, plasma cells, and neutrophils). Muscle and connective tissue along the normal bone surface are also destroyed by this pathologic process. New bone formation is coarse and/or woven, and extends well beyond the normal periosteum. The marrow spaces are filled with highly vascular fibrous tissue, and occasionally, islets of cartilage. The new bone can have a "mosaic pattern...indicating the sporadic and rapid deposit and resorption of the abnormal bone."[1] Similar pathologic changes can be observed with some osteosarcomas, hyperparathyroidism, and callous formation.[1] The pathologic changes vary with the bone involved. Mandibular changes are characterized by large, irregular exostosis, whereas changes of the calvarium and tympanic bullae most often result in thickening while maintaining a relatively smooth inner and outer surface.[1]

Gross changes are readily apparent, especially of the mandibles (Figure 96-2). Visible and palpable enlargement of the mandibles is hallmark for CMO. Bilateral symmetry is the rule, but there are many exceptions. The tympanic bullae are usually involved, with

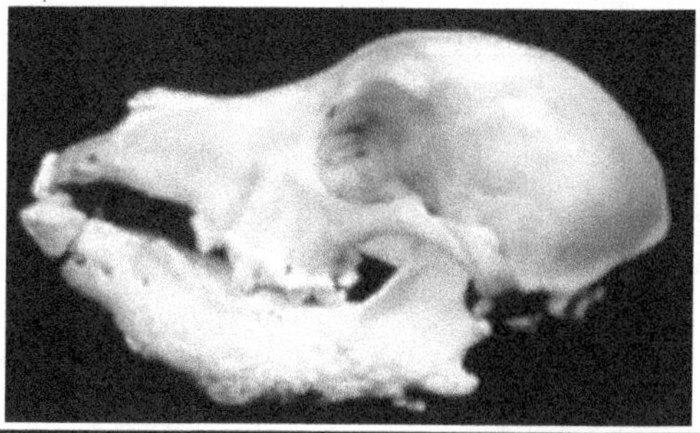

Figure 96-2. Gross bony changes owing to CMO. Note the large amount of irregular bony proliferation of the mandibles. In some cases, the tympanic bullae, temporomandibular joint, and flat bones of the calvarium may also be affected.

enlargements by 2 to 3 times normal size caused by massive amounts of new bone.[1] In addition, variable amounts of fusion between the enlarged tympanic bullae and the angle of the mandible are common.[1]

Clinical Diagnosis

Signalment

The quintessential case of CMO is an intact male Scottish terrier or West Highland white terrier up to 12 months old.

Age

Dogs aged up to 12 months accounted for 82% of the cases in our VMDB survey (Figure 96-2). The age range was from 0 to 2 weeks to 15 years old (one dog in each) (Figure 96-1). CMO is generally considered a juvenile disease, with cessation of clinical signs with osseous maturity. Because similar pathologic changes can be observed with some osteosarcomas, hyperparathyroidism, and callous formation,[1] misdiagnosis is a possibility for the 5 mature dogs indicated to have CMO out of a total population over 300,000 dogs.

The age of the 65 dogs with CMO reported in the literature ranged from 3 months to 13 months old at presentation, plus 1 dog at 24 months old with bone proliferation of the frontal sinus and polyarthritis.[4-24]

Breed

West Highland white terriers and Scottish terriers were by far the most common breeds to have CMO, and had the greatest risk per 100,000 of the breeds (Table 96-1). Although West Highland white terriers had the most cases of CMO, Scottish terriers had the highest risk based on number of CMO cases per 100,000 of the breed. Mixed breed dogs had the lowest number of cases (n=2) and the lowest risk (2 CMO cases / 100,000 mixed breed dogs). However, the risk for CMO overall was low, as indicated by only 9 CMO cases per 100,000 of all breeds. In addition, the low number of CMO cases per 100,000 for the breeds at highest risk was also low compared witih risk factors for other diseases (i.e., hypertrophic osteodystrophy and panosteitis). Terriers accounted for 16 of the 29 CMO cases (55%) reported in the literature.[4-24] However, large breed dogs such as the bulldog, bassett hound, Weimaraner, bull mastiff and Great Dane were also reported to have had CMO (Table 96-1).[4-24]

Table 96-1. CMO Cases from VMDB Survey 1994-2004 and Reported in the Literature

Breeds	total of Breed	CMO Cases	per 100,000	Literature
All Breeds	307,168	29	9	
West Highland White Terrier	2,039	8	392	35
Scottish Terrier	1,374	6	437	16
Labrador Retriever	30,248	4	13	1
Bulldog	2,808	3	107	0
Cairn Terrier	957	1	*104*	2
Boston Terrier	2,465	1	41	1
Basset Hound	2,651	1	38	0
Welsh Corgi, Cardigan	569	1	*176*	0
Mixed Breeds	63,974	1	2	0
Weimaraner	1,485	1	67	0
Bullmastiff	698	1	*143*	1
Great Dane	2,460	1	41	1
English Mastiff				1
Doberman Pinscher				2
Catahoula				1
Redbone Hound				1
Boxer				1
Shetland Sheepdog				1
Pyrenean M				2

The numbers italicized under "per 100,000" indicates < 1,000 of breed in the VMDB survey.

Gender

Males are more likely to have CMO based on the VMDB survey for this chapter (Table 96-2). The male:female ratio was 48:52 for all dogs, while those with CMO had a male:female ratio of 64:36. A strong predilection appears to exist for intact dogs to have CMO (85%) (Table 96-2). However, the vast majority of dogs with CMO were 12 months old or younger, and for all dogs up to 12 months old the percentage of intact dogs (76% of males and 69% of females) was closer to the percentage of dogs with CMO that were intact.

Patient History

CMO has an insidious onset. The dog's presenting complaint(s) are most often pain when a person opens the dog's mouth and decreasing ability to open the mouth (decreased range of motion of the temporomandibular joint). More advanced cases also have visible enlargement of the mandible, decreased eating, and perhaps weight loss. Other dogs of that litter may also be affected.

Examination Findings

The presenting complaints are confirmed. Palpation of the mandibles can reveal an irregular surface and enlargement. The animal has pain on attempting to open the mouth and an inability to open the mouth to a normal widtheven with sedation/anesthesia. A complete examination should be performed to rule out retrobulbar abscess, fracture, and oral lesions (e.g., tooth disease, foreign body, etc.).

Radiographic Findings

Enlargement of the mandibles is the earliest and most obvious radiographic abnormality (Figure 96-3) and may be extreme in advanced cases. Enlargement of the tympanic bullae is predomi-

Table 96-2. Number of Dogs with CMO Based on VMDB Survey

	All dogs	CMO cases	Ratio All	Ratio M:F
Male	150,665	18	48	64
Female	161,119	10	52	36
	All dogs	**CMO cases**	**% of All Dogs**	**% of CMO**
Intact	121,331	23	39	85
Neutered	190,267	4	61	15

Whether or not a female was spayed was unknown for 186 dogs of the total population, and for 0 cases of CMO. A dog's gender was unknown for 1700 dogs of total population and for 1 case of CMO. For dogs ≤ 12 months old, 76% of males were intact and 69% of females were intact.

nantly via thickening of the bony wall and may be several times normal size. Radiodensity and/or bone proliferation between the tympanic bullae and the angle of the mandible may be observed. Flat bones of the calvarium (especially the frontal and parietal bones) may be markedly thicker, but tend to maintain smooth cortical surfaces.

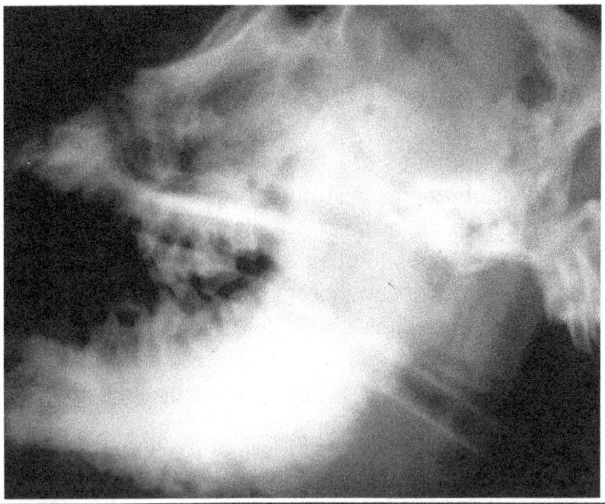

Figure 96-3. Radiographs of CMO. Note the large amount of bony proliferation of the mandibles. The tympanic bullae, temporomandibular joint, and flat bones of the cranium may also be involved in some cases.

Treatment

Corticosteroids titrated against the clinical signs are the primary treatment for CMO. Various analgesics have also reportedly been used for pain control; however, aspirin has been specifically and repeatedly reported to be ineffective. Antibiotic use has been reported infrequently and shown to be without notable effect. Soft, high-caloric diets are indicated to decrease the pain associated with eating and to maintain body weight. Supportive care, especially fluids and caloric supplementation, may be necessary. Physical therapy aimed at maintaining temporomandibular range of motion has not been reported, but could potentially be beneficial.

Prognosis

Outcome of the disease in 42 dogs has been reported in the literature. Thirty (30) dogs survived, ostensibly with resolution of the CMO lesions. Age at resolution was given in only one dog, at 11 months old.[5] Five dogs with CMO were euthanized.[6-9] Two dogs died, one during the first night of hospitalization and the other after 9 weeks of treatment.[10,14] Fourteen other dogs had follow up examinations between 10 weeks and 9 years after initial treatment, and had lesions that were ostensibly either resolved or resolving.[6,8-13] Insufficient information exists to determine whether prognosis is related to age at onset, age at which treatment begins, severity of clinical signs at the time of initiating treatment, speed of progression of clinical signs, or other factors.

References

1. Riser WH, Newton CD: Craniomandibular osteopathy. *In* Textbook of Small Animal Orthopaedics. Newton CD, Nunamaker DM (eds). Philadelphia: JB Lippincott, 1985, p. 621.

2. Littlewort MCG: Tumor-like exostosis on the bones of head in puppies. Vet Rec 70:977, 1958.

3. Muir P, Dubielzig RR, Johnson KA: Hypertrophic osteodystrophy and calvarial hyperostosis. Compendium 18:143, 1996.

4. Pastor KF, Boulay JP, Schelling SH, Carpenter JL: Idiopathic hyperostosis of the calvaria in five young bullmastiffs. J Am Anim Hosp Assoc 36:439, 2000.

5. Riser WH: What is your diagnosis? JAVMA 148:1543, 1966.

6. Watson ADJ, Adams WM, Thomas CB: Craniomandibular osteopathy in dogs. Compendium 17:911, 1995.

7. Watkins JD, Bradley R: Craniomandibular osteopathy in a Labrador puppy. Vet Rec 79:262, 1966.

8. Franch J, Cesari JR, Font J: Craniomandibular osteopathy in two Pyrenean mountain dogs. Vet Rec 142:455, 1998.

9. Taylor SM, Remedios A, Myers S: Craniomandibular osteopathy in a Shetland sheepdog. Can Vet J 36:437, 1995.

10. Watson ADJ, Huxtable CRR, Farrow BRH: Craniomandibular osteopathy in Doberman Pinschers. J Small Anim Pract 16:11, 1975.

11. Huchkowsky SL: Craniomandibular osteopathy in a bullmastiff. Can Vet J 43:883, 2002.

12. Hudson JA, Montgomery RD, Hathcock JT, Jarobe JM: Computed tomography of craniomandibular osteopathy in a dog. Vet Rad Ultrasound 35:94, 1994.

13. Dennis R, Barnett KC, Sansom J: Unilateral exophthalmos and strabismus due to craniomandibular osteopathy. J Small Animal Practice 34:457, 1993.

14. Broome CJ: Concurrent craniomandibular osteopathy and polyarthritis in a dog. Aust Vet Pract 33:146, 2003.

15. Pagett GA, Mostosky UV: Animal model: The mode of inheritance of craniomandibular osteopathy in West Highland White terrier dogs. Am J Med Genet 25:9, 1986.

16. Battershell D: What is your diagnosis? JAVMA 155:1735, 1969.

17. Geissler M: What is your diagnosis? JAVMA 171:369, 1977.

18. Hathcock JT: Craniomandibular osteopathy in an English bulldog. JAVMA 181:389, 1982.

19. Schulz S: A case of craniomandibular osteopathy in a Boxer. J Small Anim Pract 19:749, 1978.

20. Burk RL, Broadhurst JJ: Craniomandibular osteopathy in a Great Dane. JAVMA 169:635, 1976.

21. Carithers RW, Mitten RW, Taylor J: Craniomandibular osteopathy. JAVMA 171:369, 1977.

22. Riser WH, Parkes LJ, Shirer JF: Canine craniomandibular osteopathy. J Am Vet Radiol Soc 8:23, 1967.

23. Trowald-Wigh G, Ekman S, Bansson K, et al: Clinical, radiological and pathological features of 12 Irish Setters with canine leucocyte adhesion deficiency. J Small Anim Pract 41:211, 2000.

24. Alexander JW: Selected skeletal dysplasias: craniomandibular osteopathy, multiple cartilaginous exostosis, and hypertrophic osteodystrophy. Vet Clin North Am (SA) 13:55, 1983.

25. Putnam RW, Archibald J: Skeletal diseases in the dog. Mod Vet Pract 49:59, 1968.

26. Munjar TA, Austin CC, Breur GJ: Comparison of risk factors for hypertrophic osteodystrophy, craniomandibular osteopathy and canine distemper virus infection. Vet Comp Ortho Traumat 11:37, 1998.

27. Montgomery R: Miscellaneous orthopaedic diseases. *In* Textbook of Small Animal Surgery, 3rd ed. Slatter DH (ed). Philadelphia: WB Saunders, 2003, p. 2251.

28. LaFond E, Breur GJ, Austin CC: Breed susceptibility for developmental orthopedic diseases in dogs. J Am Hosp Assoc 38:467, 2002.

29. Riser WH: Canine craniomandibular osteopathy. *In* Disease Mechanisms in Small Animal Surgery, 2nd ed. Bojrab MJ, Smeak DD, Bloomberg MS (eds). Philadelphia: Lea & Febiger , 1983, p. 892.

30. Alexander JW, Kallfeiz FA: A case of craniomandibular osteopathy in a Labrador retriever. Vet Med 70:560, 1975.

31. Baker JR: Bone disease in a dog similar to infantile cortical hyperostosis (Caffey's disease). Vet Rec 75: 1975.

Chapter 97

Canine Angular Limb Deformities

Denis Marcellin-Little

Epidemiology

Angular limb deformities are common in dogs. They are seen primarily in dogs of chondrodystrophic breeds. Chondrodystrophic dogs have a genetic make-up that leads to variable impairment of the growth of their appendicular skeleton and skull.[1] Their axial skeleton is spared. Most chondrodystrophic dogs have symmetrically deformed forelimbs and pelvic limbs. The forelimbs of chondrodystrophic dogs initially and primarily have a premature closure of the distal ulnar physes that may lead to a valgus (i.e., abaxial or lateral) deformity, caudal angulation, and slight external rotation of the distal portion of the antebrachia originating at the distal radial physes. Most likely as a consequence of that primary closure, chondrodystrophic dogs often have a varus (i.e., axial or medial) deformity originating at the proximal radial physes (Figure 97-1). The pelvic limbs of chondrodystrophic dogs also have angular and rotational deformities, specifically varus and caudal angulation and external rotation originating from the proximal portion of the tibiae, coxa vara, and medial patellar luxation. Breeders and owners of chondrodystrophic dogs anticipate a certain degree of curvature in the limbs of their dogs and they may not seek medical care to treat the consequence of these deformities unless the dogs are limping consistently.

Angular deformities occur as a result of injuries, most often injuries to growing long-bone physes but also as a result of fracture malunions. Most angular limb deformities or traumatic origins affect the antebrachium. These deformities represent approximately 1% of the orthopedic problems of dogs,[2] and

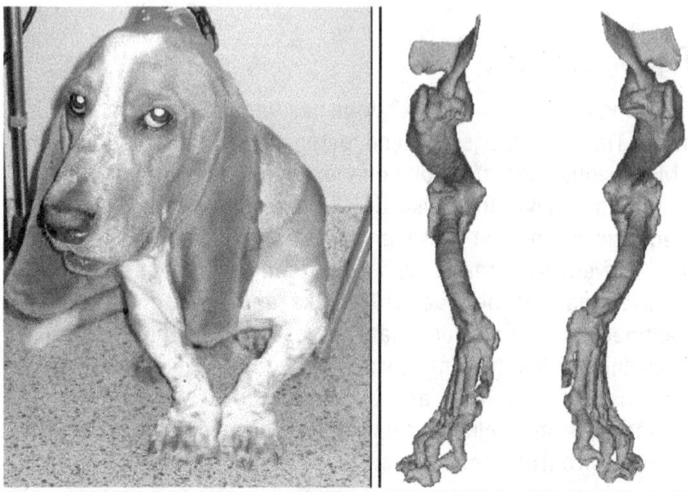

Figure 97-1. This 1-year-old basset hound (left) has a deformity of both forelimbs that includes valgus angulation of the distal portion of his antebrachia and varus angulation of the proximal portion of his antebrachia. These angulations are visible on a 3D rendering of his forelimbs that is based on a computed tomography scan (right).

may include valgus or varus angulation of variable severity. The purpose of this chapter is to review the assessment, therapeutic decision-making, and surgical management of canine angular limb deformities, particularly antebrachial deformities.

Preoperative Assessment

The preoperative assessment of patients with limb deformities is complex and includes a variety of factors: limb use and cosmesis, range of motion, static rotation, pronation, supination, mediolateral (ML) and craniocaudal (CC) angulation, length deficit, joint effusion, pain, and osteoarthritis (OA) in the joints adjacent to the deformity. It is important to proceed with a complete assessment of deformity in patients as rapidly as possible because growth and time will negatively impact the deformed limb. In a study, the average delay before the time of a deformity was noticed and the time corrective osteotomies were performed was 18 weeks.[3] Some clinicians have the misguided impression that monitoring (i.e., reevaluating every few weeks) a deformity is a valid form of management. This form of conservative management is rarely medically advisable.

The owners' motivation when bringing in patients with limb deformities is primarily enhancing limb use and function, but also enhancing overall mobility, alleviating limb pain, and improving limb cosmesis. Limb use, cosmesis, and overall mobility may be graded (Table 97-1).[3] It is critically important to make sure that these grades are agreed upon by owner and clinician to avoid discrepancies in perceived severity of the problem. Some owners underestimate the severity of the problem, others overestimate it. Angular limb deformities, for example, tend to be noticed later in life and underestimated in dogs with long or curly hair compared with dogs with short hair. Owners may underestimate the severity of a developmental humeroradial (caudolateral) luxation in a young puppy because they may perceive limb use as acceptable. Some owners are primarily motivated by limb cosmesis of their pets (i.e., show dogs). The optimal management of limb deformities will improve both function and cosmesis of treated patients.[3] Poor limb use per se is not a clear indication for surgery or does not mean that one specific surgery should be performed. For example, a dog with an antebrachial deformity and a developmental humero-ulnar luxation leading to absence of ulnar trochlear notch may have poor limb function but may not be a candidate for a corrective osteotomy. A dog with severe OA combined with an angular limb deformity may not function better if the deformity is corrected because of the presence of OA-induced pain.

All measurements from the affected limb should be compared with measurements from the opposite limb, with measurements of dogs of similar age and conformation, or with values reported in the scientific literature.[4] The range of motion of affected limbs should be carefully assessed before surgery, and the cause of any anomaly of motion should be understood before therapy is initiated (Figure 97-2).[4] Range of motion is an important aspect of the assessment of the affected limb because loss of joint motion may have a profoundly negative impact on limb use. For example, a dog with loss of carpal extension may not be able to bear weight on his forelimb. Loss of motion is common with developmental antebrachial deformities, particularly loss of carpal flexion as a result of a developmental subluxation and loss of elbow flexion as a result of humero-ulnar or humeroradial subluxation or OA.[3]

Angulation

Limb (radial) angulation is assessed in patients with limb deformities.[5] Valgus and varus ML deformities have a more significant impact on limb use than do CC deformities. The forelimb has few adaptive options in adjusting for the presence of ML deformities compared with CC deformities, where an increase of decrease in elbow and shoulder joint flexion may offset a deformity. When standing and walking, dogs most likely load their forelimbs so the center of their shoulder joint and the metacarpal pad form a vertical line, as seen from the front of the dog. That line is named the ML mechanical axis of the limb (Figures 97-2 and 97-3). Having a vertical mechanical axis leads to the lowest energy expenditure and optimizes the effectiveness of locomotion. Valgus deformities are often visually more striking than varus deformities and may have a higher negative impact on limb use because the normal limb most often has 5° to 10° of valgus. For example, a medial deformity of 20° in a dog with an initial valgus of 10° will lead to a manus orientation of approximately 10°, a reasonably discrete deformity; but a lateral deformity of 20° will lead to approximately 30° valgus, a significant deformity. It is not possible to accurately assess CC angulation of the antebrachium during stance or palpation. It is assessed on radiographs. ML angulation should be assessed while the patient is not sedated and is bearing weight on his affected limb. ML angulation during stance overestimates the actual angulation of the antebrachium, particularly in patients with valgus deformities, because joint subluxation may occur in addition to bone angulation when the joint is loaded asymmetrically. Angulation may also occur when patients place their limbs in pain-relieving positions, to decrease the load placed on a joint or on part of a joint. ML angulation is also assessed when the patient is relaxed (often under sedation).

Table 97-1. Assessment of Limb use, Cosmesis, and Overall Mobility in Patients with Limb Deformities

	Limb use (lameness)	Cosmesis (difference with opposite limb)	Mobility (activity level, performance)
Excellent	None	None	Normal
Good	Mild, intermittent	Minor	Mild restriction
Fair	Constant	Significant	Severe restriction
Poor	Toe-touching to NWB	Major	Very limited mobility

Abbreviation: NWB = non weight-bearing.

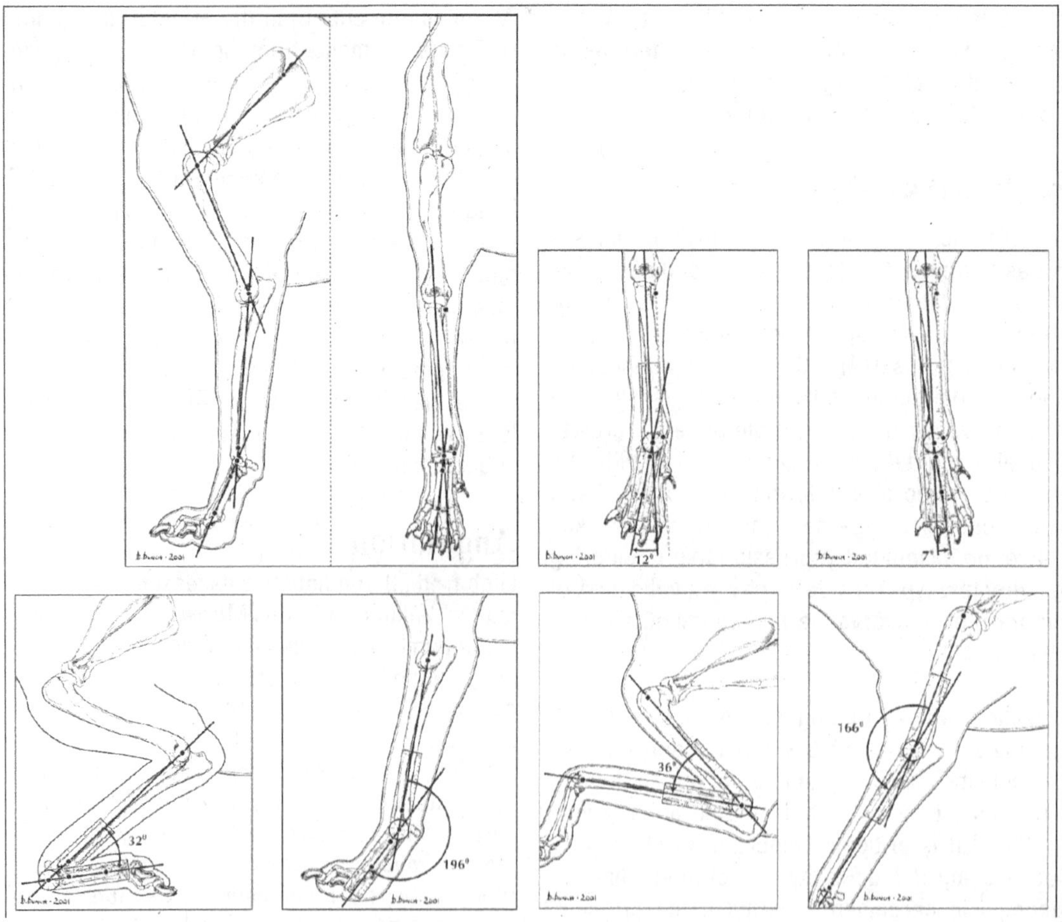

Figure 97-2. Normal range of motion of the carpus and elbow joint in Labrador retrievers as measured using a plastic goniometer aligned with the metacarpal, craniocaudal midpoint of the distal portion of the antebrachium, lateral epicondyle, cranio-caudal midpoint of the proximal portion of the humerus, and spine of the scapula (upper left). Nineteen degrees of motion are available in a mediolateral direction (upper right), 164° in a craniocaudal direction for carpal motion (lower left), and 130° of elbow motion. (From Jaegger G, Marcellin-Little DJ, Levine D: Am J Vet Res 63:979-986, reproduced with permission < requested from AVMA, pending >).[4]

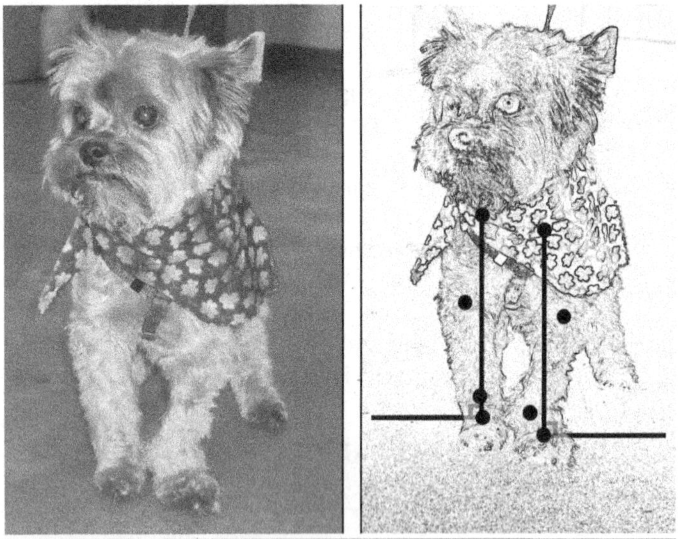

Figure 97-3. This Yorkshire terrier has valgus deformity of the distal portion of the radius. On the right, dots have been placed on the approximate centers of the shoulder, elbow, carpus, and metacarpal pad. The centers of the shoulder joints and metacarpal pads appear to form a line perpendicular to the ground.

ML angulation measured on a relaxed limb tends to be the most accurate assessment of limb angulation. Whereas many patients have a single (unifocal) angular limb deformity, some patients have two (bifocal, Figures 97-1 and 97-4) or more complex angular deformities (Table 97-2). Others have a uniformly angled bone, resembling a bow, described as multifocal deformities.[5]

Rotation

Pronation (internal rotation) and supination (external rotation) are assessed preoperatively. This is primarily done to evaluate the antebrachium for the presence of restrictions in motion and synostoses. Synostoses are confirmed on radiographs. Synostoses, when present in patients with growth potential, may have devastating consequences on elbow joint congruity and, to a lesser extent, on carpal joint congruity. Synostoses are unusual in dogs with developmental antebrachial deformities resulting from premature closure of the distal ulnar and radial physis or resulting from chondrodystrophy. Synostoses are much more common in patients who previously underwent segmental ulnar ostectomies or in patients with prior radio-ulnar shaft fractures. Pronation and supination may also be used as a predictor of rotational deformities. Dogs have approximately 45° of rotational motion in their antebrachium, with a pronation of 0° and a supination of 45°. Cats have twice as much supination as dogs.

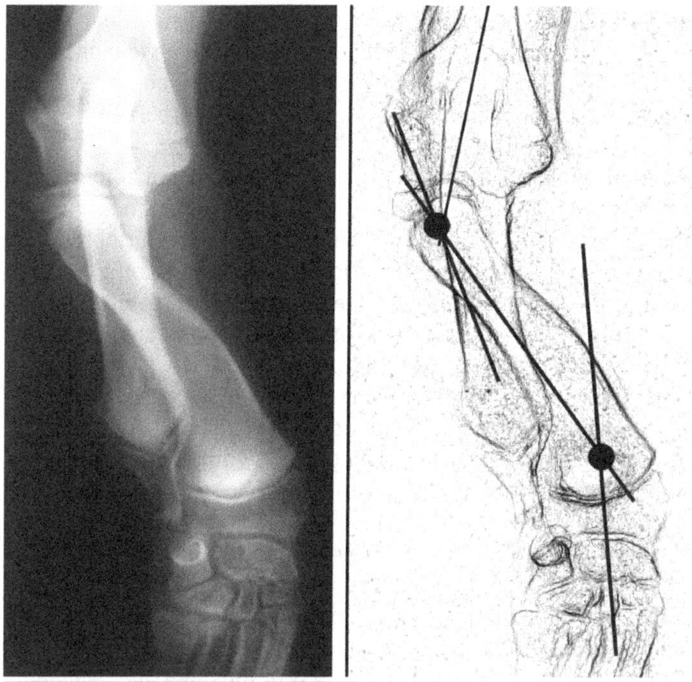

Figure 97-4. This dog has a bifocal angular radial deformity with a valgus deformity of the distal portion of the radius and a varus deformity of the proximal portion of the radius. The radial and ulnar physes do not appear closed.

Rotational deformities are assessed preoperatively. Rotation is a common component of antebrachial deformities: valgus deformities are often associated with external rotation and varus deformities with internal rotation. Rotation is difficult to assess because the presence of angulation influences the perceived angulation of an extremity and because dogs may use their available pronation or supination to enhance their limb function and decrease their perceived pain. Dogs with severe valgus, for example, tend to purposefully rotate their limbs externally to improve the contact of their digits on the ground during stance. Looking at the direction of the footfall as a sole measure of rotational deformity is inappropriate because it greatly overestimates the rotation present in the antebrachium. Instead, rotation should be assessed on a relaxed (or sedated) patient by comparing the direction of the plane formed during flexion and extension of the carpus with the direction of the plane formed during flexion and extension of the elbow joint.[5] Rotational deformities cannot be assessed reliably on radiographs.

Length Deficits

Radial-length deficit is assessed on the patient by comparing the distance between the radial head, palpable proximally and laterally, with the medial styloid process of the radius, palpable distally and medially. Ulnar-length deficit is assessed on the patient by comparing the distance between the olecranon, proximally and caudally, with the lateral styloid process, medially and distally. Length deficits are assessed more accurately on radiographs. Compensatory humeral overgrowth may be assessed on the patient by comparing the distance between the greater tubercle, proximally and cranially, with the lateral humeral epicondyle, laterally and distally. If a humeral-length discrepancy between the affected and control limb is suspected, it may be assessed more accurately on radiographs.

Translation

Translation is a displacement of a limb segment in relation to another limb segment in a direction parallel to the long axis of that limb. Translation may be present as a consequence of a fracture malunion. It is rare in dogs. Dogs with severe caudad deformity of the radius originating in the distal portion of the bone compensate for these deformities by hyperextending their carpus. This results in a perceived caudal translation of the carpus in relation to the radius.

Joint Subluxation

Careful assessment of the joints adjacent to the deformity should be performed. Joint effusion may be present as a consequence of a severe subluxation or cartilage damage. Crepitus may be present as a consequence of cartilage wear or osteophytes at the

Table 97-2. Common Components of Classic Canine Antebrachial Deformities

Type of deformity	Length deficit	Angulation	Rotation	Other components*
Chondrodystrophy (mild)	None	U valgus, distal radius	External	Distal HU subluxation
Chondrodystrophy (severe)	None	U valgus, distal radius U varus, proximal radius	External	Distal HU subluxation
Chondrodysplasia	None	U valgus, distal radius U varus, proximal radius	External	Distal HU subluxation
Traumatic PPC, distal ulna	Mild	U valgus, distal radius	External	Distal HU subluxation
Traumatic PPC, distal radius, medial	Moderate	U varus, distal radius	Internal	Distal HR subluxation
Traumatic PPC, distal radius, lateral	Moderate	U valgus, distal radius	None	Distal HR subluxation
Traumatic PPC, distal radius, complete	Severe	None	None	Distal HR subluxation
Radial fracture malunion	Moderate	U valgus, radial midshaft	External	Synostosis
Osteochondrodystrophy†	Severe	M valgus, radial midshaft	External	None

Abbreviations: U = Unifocal; PPC = premature physeal closure; HU = humero-ulnar; HR = humeroradial.
*** Other components assessed include elbow and carpal subluxation and synostoses.**
† Deformity associated with retained dwarfism, retained cartilaginous core, and hypertrophic osteodystrophy in skeletally immature dogs of giant breeds.

articular margins. A pain response may be suspected based on activity level, weight shift toward the opposite forelimb or away from the forelimbs, or during manipulation (flexion, extension, pronation, supination, valgus, or varus stress). Assessing pain is critically important because the presence of pain suggests articular damage (cartilage erosion, synovitis, subluxation, OA) and that damage should be assessed as objectively as possible and factored in the preoperative planning and surgical recommendations made to the owner. Subluxation and OA are confirmed on radiographs.

Radiographs are an important step in the assessment of antebrachial deformities. CC and ML views of the antebrachium are made and compared.[3] A magnification marker or object with known length should be placed along the antebrachium and be parallel to the plate when these radiographs are made using digital radiography in order to accurately calibrate these radiographs and assess length deficits. Radial- and ulna-length deficits are measured in millimeters and as a percentage of radial and ulnar length.[3] Dogs in which a premature closure of the radius or the ulna precedes a premature closure of the other antebrachial bone have a larger deficit present in the bone responsible for the initial closure. For example, a dog with primary closure of the distal ulnar physis and secondary closure of the distal radial physis may have a 10% length deficit in the ulna and a 4% length deficit in the radius. Understanding the primary closure site impacts the therapeutic decision. Radiographs are used to assess the shape of the radius and the ulna and the type (i.e., uni-, bi-, or multifocal) and origin (i.e., proximal physis, shaft, or distal physis) of the angular deformity in the ML plane. The radial angular deformities as in the ML and CC planes often have different origins. The classic angular deformity that results from chondrodystrophy, for example, includes a unifocal valgus deviation originating at the distal radial physis and a multifocal caudal deformity involving the radial midshaft. Priority will be given to the ML angulation when planning the correction of antebrachial deformities because dogs can compensate for CC angulation much more than for ML angulation. The radiographic appearance of the radial and ulnar physes should be assessed on radiographs. Partial or complete closure may be seen. Interestingly, the correlation between growth potential and radiographic appearance of the physes is low. Some physes appear open but do not appear to lead to bone growth. Other physes appear closed but have appeared to contribute to bone growth (unpublished data). Radiographs are assessed for the presence of carpal and elbow joint subluxation or luxation (Table 97-3). Elbow (sub)luxation appears to have a larger impact on limb use than does carpal subluxation and is easier to assess on radiographs. In experimental models of antebrachial deformities caused by premature physeal closure of the distal ulnar physis induced by submitting the distal portion of the ulna to high doses of radiation, cartilage damage in the elbow joint occurs within 2 weeks of ulnar premature physeal closure (Figure 97-5).

Because conservative and surgical management of antebrachial deformities has a limited power in improving joint geometry (with the exception of circular external fixation, see further on for additional information), it is critically important to address joint subluxation as rapidly as possible in skeletally immature patients with antebrachial deformities. The presence and severity of OA are also assessed on radiographs. Severe OA is irreversible and may limit the positive impact of corrective osteotomies. Its presence should be taken into account when choosing therapy. The presence, location, and length of a radio-ulnar synostosis should be assessed on the ML radiograph.

Computed tomography (CT) may be used to further assess the shape of a deformed antebrachium. The digital information contained in cross-sectional CT may be imported into computer-aided design (CAD) software to make 3D renderings (Figure 97-1). CAD is used to enhance the contrast of these images, eliminate data collection artifacts (i.e., beam hardening in CT scans), and select specific information for the creation of specific 3D renderings (Figure 97-1). The 3D rendering is oriented in space, and a support structure may be created. These 3D renderings may be kept at their original size or may be resized. Making half-sized models requires only one eighth of the material required to make a full-sized model because length, width, and depth are halved in a smaller model. Decreasing the size of the model may be necessary to make a model of a structure too large for specific manufacturing methods or to decrease the model cost. The creation of physical models based on 3D renderings is named free-form fabrication (FFF). Approximately 25 different types of FFF methods are used, making models ranging from wax to titanium. Stereolithography apparatus (SLA) was the first commercially available FFF method (Figure 97-6). SLA relies on an ultraviolet laser to cure a photopolymer. SLA is slow but precise. Its speed depends on the power of its laser beam. The maximal size of prototypes in SLA machines ranges from 250 x 250 x 250 mm to 500 x 500 x 500 mm (VIPERsi SLA, 3D Systems, Valencia, CA).

Treatment Decisions

Several options are available to help manage antebrachial deformities, ranging from conservative management to corrective osteotomies. The decision tree for management of limb deformities is complex.

Table 97-3. Common Joint Anomalies resulting from Abnormal Antebrachial Growth

Joint Anomaly	Cause	Potential Consequences
Distal humero-ulnar subluxation	PPC distal ulna	Nonunited anconeal process, severe elbow OA
Distal humeroradial subluxation	PPC proximal radius	Fragmentation of the medial coronoid process
	PPC distal radius	Severe elbow OA
Caudolateral radial luxation	Unknown	Severe elbow incongruity, loss of elbow flexion
Proximal radio-ulnar subluxation	PPC distal ulna	Loss of carpal flexion, mild carpal OA

Abbreviations: PPC = premature physeal closure; OA = osteoarthritis.

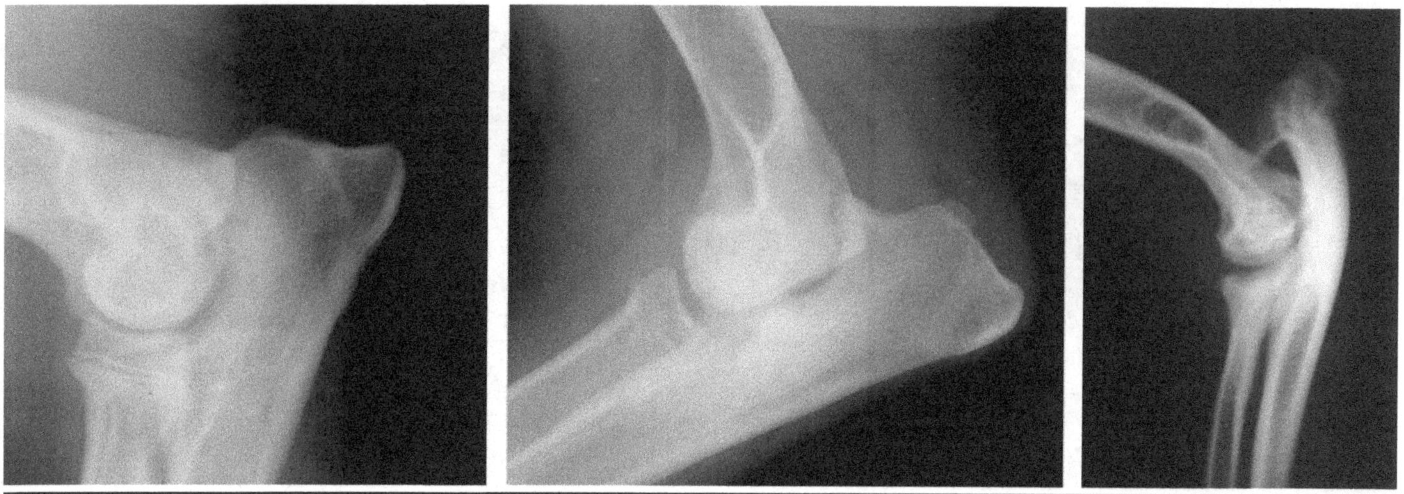

Figure 97-5. A distal humero-ulnar subluxation is present in the dog on the left with a premature closure of the distal ulnar physis. The dog in the center has a distal humeroradial subluxation with a premature closure of the proximal radial physis. The dog (on the right) with a premature closure of the proximal radial physis has a severely abnormal trochlear notch.

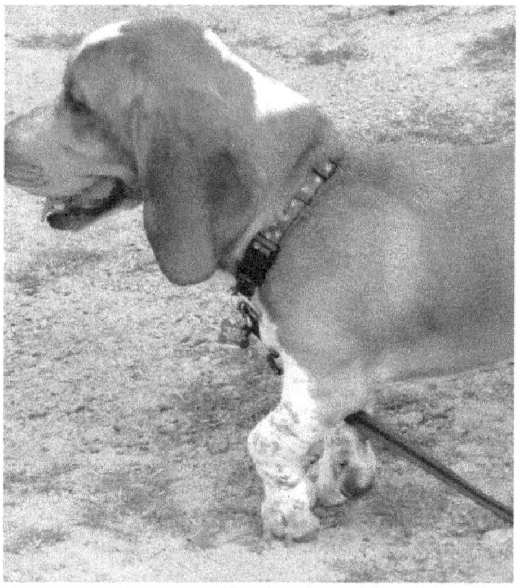

Figure 97-6. Side view of the basset hound seen on Figure 97-1. Although his antebrachial deformities are similar in angulation and rotation between left and right forelimbs, his left forelimb is often held in a position incompatible with comfortable weight bearing (right). While the right side may be managed conservatively, the left side will benefit from a corrective osteotomy.

Conservative Management

Conservative management may be a valid option for the management of an antebrachial deformity if the patient has little or no residual growth potential, if joint subluxation is minimal, and if current limb use is deemed acceptable. As a general rule, conservative management is ineffective at improving limb deformities. Splinting is sometimes used with the intent to positively affect an angular limb deformity by protecting limbs from impact or limiting their future angulation or rotation. Splinting, however, has not been proven effective and does not appear to offer clinical benefits to patients with angular limb deformities. Splinting also has side effects: it limits limb use, promotes muscle atrophy, and may lead to skin abrasions or necrosis. We do not recommend splinting patients with limb deformities. Specific thresholds that could be used to recommend conservative management over surgical management are sometimes reported (i.e., 20% of limb length deficit) but do not have practical benefits in clinical patients because specific impairment to limb use results from the complex combination of angulation, length deficit, rotation, and joint subluxation associated with the patient's size, body conformation, and fitness level. It would be beneficial to determine the specific influences of these factors on limb use to predict whether surgical management would be indicated in dogs with developing deformities. For example, most basset hounds have severe antebrachial deformities resulting from their chondrodystrophic appendicular skeleton. Some basset hounds, however, have a combination of angular and rotational deformities that lead to hyperextension of their digits combined with a flexion of their carpus that lead to a significant impairment of these affected limbs (Figure 97-7). Whereas their specific deformities most often resemble a classic form of chondrodystrophy, a small increase in angulation or rotation may lead to a dramatic decrease in limb use. Although most basset hounds are managed successfully without surgery, some will benefit dramatically from a corrective osteotomy. Conservative management should be avoided in dogs with joint subluxation, even in the presence of seemingly acceptable limb use, because the negative impact of joint subluxation on the articular cartilage is profound and occurs within 2 weeks after the occurrence of that subluxation.

Surgical Management

Conservative management should also be avoided in dogs with deformities and with a large remaining growth potential because growth will most likely to lead to joint subluxation and to the increase in the severity of the deformity. The presence of an angular limb deformity, even in without limb disuse, predisposes the adjacent joints to the development of OA even in the absence of joint subluxation. This is likely because with an angular deformity abnormal stresses are placed on the articular cartilage of the adjacent joint. The development of OA as a result of bone angulation has been reported in people with proximal tibial (varus) deformities and within seven months after the experimental creation of angular deformities in young dogs. Therefore, it seems indicated to discuss the consequence of angulation on the potential development of OA with owners, especially in large and giant breeds when large abnormal forces placed on articular cartilage may lead to OA.

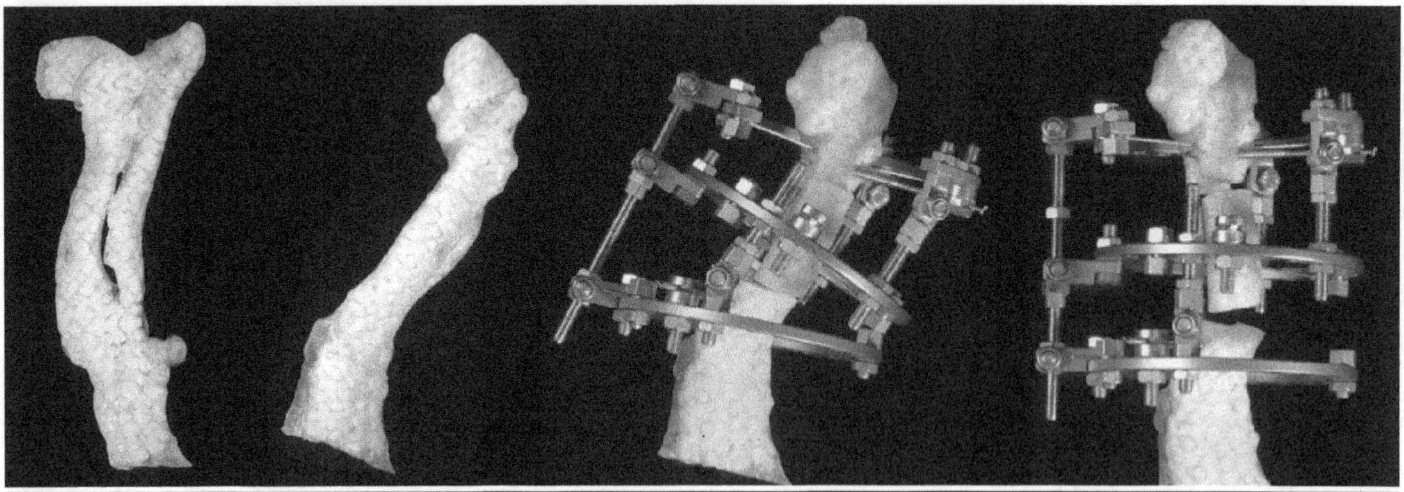

Figure 97-7. The 3D rendering in Figure 97-1 was used to make a full-sized stereolithography model of the left forelimb of the basset hound using rapid protyping methods. The model is used to assess the components of the deformity and to rehearse a corrective osteotomy. A circular external skeletal fixation frame with two sets of hinges allowing a simultaneous correction of both deformities with a single angular motor adjustment is placed on the model and adjusted to correct the antebrachial deformity.

Some surgeries are performed with the intent to promote corrective or compensatory growth. They generally rely on release osteotomies. Corrective growth is growth that leads to a decrease in abnormal limb angulation. It occurs when limb angulation occurs early in life. For example, if a 3-month-old puppy has a green-stick fracture leading to a 30° angulation of his radius, corrective growth will occur to decrease that angulation over time. To be effective, corrective growth requires a large growth potential. It appears ineffective in puppies more than five months old. Compensatory growth is growth that leads to a decrease in joint subluxation or limb-length deficit. For example, in a puppy with premature closure of the distal radial physis occurring late in growth when growth potential is less than 5% of final bone length. Compensatory growth in the proximal radial physis may prevent the occurrence of a distal humeroradial subluxation. Compensatory overgrowth also occurs in bones adjacent to the bones with length deficits. For example, a dog with a short radius and ulna could have overgrowth of his humerus. In humans, overgrowth is a routine complication after fracture of long bones in children. Overgrowth after fracture has not been reported in dogs, to our knowledge. Ulnar osteotomies are a convenient, minimally invasive surgical option allowing corrective growth in young dogs with deformities and with a large remaining growth potential. The ostectomy should not be made near the elbow joint, where it could lead to a caudal displacement of the distal aspect of the proximal ulnar segment that would lead to elbow subluxation. The osteotomy should not be made too distally where it could lead to a weakness in the site of origin of the lateral collateral ligament. When an ulnar ostectomy is performed in a very young patient, the surgery should be minimally traumatic because a future surgery may take place in that site and minimal tissue changes will facilitate the future surgery, and because a radio-ulnar synostosis should be avoided. Bone healing will occur after most ulnar ostectomies. This healing may be delayed or stopped through removal of the periosteum during the procedure and through placement of a fat graft collected from the axilla. If the osteotomy heals prematurely, a prompt decision should be made as to whether the premature healing predisposes the patient to long-term problems and interferes with future bone growth. A second osteotomy may be performed based on these factors. Short segmental ulnar ostectomies are most effective at addressing distal humeroulnar subluxations compared with distal humeroradial subluxations. In my experience, distal humeroulnar subluxations of up to three mm may be addressed though ulnar ostectomies. The corrective growth that occurs after an ulnar ostectomy is the result of the growth potential remaining in the radius at the time of the procedure. This means that ulnar ostectomies should be performed as early as possible when a premature closure of the distal portion of the ulna is diagnosed. Some surgeons perform radial osteotomies or ostectomies with the intent to decrease distal humeroradial subluxations. I do not recommend them because they may lead to limb disuse or additional angular deformities owing to malunion, or they may fail to improve elbow joint congruity.

Periosteal stripping is more popular in horses than in dogs. The information regarding the specific benefits of periosteal stripping in dogs with deformities is scant. Periosteal stripping is based on the fact that the thick periosteum present in puppies (the younger, the thicker) restricts longitudinal bone growth. Dogs may be candidates for periosteal stripping if they have a significant angular deformity in the absence of severe rotation or joint subluxation. I have personally used periosteal stripping in two patients with acceptable results (unpublished data).

Surgical stapling has been used to restrict the longitudinal growth of one aspect of a distal physis, while the opposite aspect of that physis still grows. Staples are curved metal implants that bridge the physis. Staples are removed after a few weeks to avoid permanent growth cessation of the stapled side. Stapling has been effective in specific patients to induce corrective growth. These patients must be very young at the time of initial diagnosis; they must have a partial premature closure; and they must not have subluxation of the joints adjacent to the deformity. They should be followed carefully after the procedure to avoid under- or over-correction and to monitor complications.

Linear fixators may be used to correct deformities, when the deformity does not include a significant length deficit, when angulation and rotation may be acutely corrected during the procedure, and when subluxation is not present in the joint adjacent to the deformity. When acute corrections are performed, lengthening is often limited to the length gained through the angular correction. Anatomically, that length roughly equals half of the maximal gap present at the transcortex. Functionally, though, a limb may be longer once an angular correction is performed because the anatomic and functional axes of the limb are realigned after the correction of an angular deformity. Linear fixators do not appear to be effective at correcting the cranio-caudal component of an angular limb deformity when treating antebrachial deformities. Attempting to distract a linear fixator may place a large amount of stress on the fixator and on the patient's soft tissue. The creation of a gap will also require the fixator to function as a buttress; therefore, increasing the bending and axial loads present at the osteotomy site. The practical consequences of that are that frames used for acute angular corrections should have flawless mechanical properties.

Bone plates may be used to treat antebrachial deformities when significant lengthening is not necessary and when the subluxation of adjacent joint does not require specific treatment. Bone plates are deceivingly simple in theory: the radius and ulna are osteotomized, the angular, rotational, and minor length deficits are corrected, and the bone is fixed in place with a plate. In large dogs, a plate may also be placed on the ulna. Like linear ESF frames, plates often have to be used in buttress fashion when correcting antebrachial deformities because the contact between bone ends is likely minimal after deformity correction. Unfortunately, the irregular nature of the bone surface requires complex contouring of the plate. This is a process easier to achieve in relatively small and thin plates, but the buttress use of that plate requires a relatively large and thick (i.e., stiff) plate. Bone plate fixation has significant limitations in patients with bifocal (varus, proximally, and valgus, distally) deformities because the optimal correction of these deformities requires a proximal and distal osteotomy, whereas the optimal plate placement requires a single midshaft osteotomy.

Circular external skeletal fixation frames are the most versatile method used to treat antebrachial deformities in dogs. This is because circular ESF may be used to simultaneously correct angulation in one or two locations in a deformed bone, eliminate a length deficit, eliminate a rotational deformity, and decrease the subluxation present in adjacent joints.

In some patients with limb deformities, however, simpler management methods may be used. With circular ESF, the frame consists of rings connected together by threaded rods. The method for placement of circular ESF frames is termed the Ilizarov method, from the name of the Russian surgeon who popularized it. The frame is fixed to the bone with tensioned small-diameter wires and, potentially, with half-pins. Circular ESF offer unlimited geometric adaptability. The ring size and number, threaded rod size, length, and number, and wire size, number, and orientation can be tailored to the purpose of fixation and the anatomy of the patient. The circular ESF systems with widest use are the small bone fixator and the circular external skeletal fixation systems.[5,6] Linear and circular ESF frames may be combined to form hybrid ESF frames. Unifocal deformities are the simplest deformities to treat. Multifocal deformities tend to be treated like unifocal deformities by focusing or realigning the proximal and distal joints.[5] Bifocal deformities are most challenging to address because they are generally the combination of a proximal and distal physeal deformity, usually in short bones. Their treatment potentially requires making two independent juxta-articular osteotomies and angular corrections (Figure 97-6).

Circular external fixators are made of individual parts that can be assembled into an unlimited number of configurations. Ilizarov frames can be used to treat bone deformities and fractures, to perform arthrodeses, to transport bone segments, and to treat joint contractures, with varying frame configurations. Ilizarov frames have been used in multiple species ranging in size from the rat, used as an animal model for research, to the horse. Most frame components remain constant, regardless of the use of the frame and the size of the patient. These components include fine wires, fixation elements, supporting elements, connecting elements, assembly elements, and sliding elements. Tensioning devices and wrenches complete the Ilizarov instrumentation.[7,8] The fines wires used with the Ilizarov method have a diameter ranging from 1.0 to 1.6 mm in animals and 1.5 to 2.0 mm in humans. One-millimeter-diameter wires are used in dogs weighing less than 10 kg, 1.2-mm-diameter wires in dogs weighing 10 to 20 kg, and 1.5-mm-diameter wires in dogs weighing more than 20 kg. Different wire points are available: half point, bayonet point, or trocar point. Wires with optimal bone penetration should be used in order to minimize thermal trauma to the limb. In our clinical experience, the half-point wires have the best bone penetration. Half-point wires, olive wires, also called stopper wires, have a larger diameter ball in their midpoint. They can be used to prevent translation of the bone fragment on the wire. When two olive wires are placed on opposite sides of the bone across a fracture site, the bending strength of the bone-frame construct is increased. Twisted wires or bent wires can potentially be used as an alternative to olive wires. However, they have several disadvantages: they are weaker and may be difficult to remove once bone healing is complete and bone growth surrounds the twisted portion of the wire.

Fixation elements allow wire fixation onto the Ilizarov frame. They include cannulated bolts, with a central hole or slotted bolts with an eccentric slot. The wires should always be kept straight to avoid frame migration, wire rupture, bone stress, or potential fracture during wire tensioning. When placing a wire, a cannulated bolt is used on the near side, the wire is then placed through the limb, and a cannulated or slotted bolt is used on the far side. Washers can be used to offset the wire from the ring by one mm or more or to potentially connect a wire to a connecting rod. The supporting elements include rings, plates, and posts, where the bolts attach. The rings are currently available with inside diameters ranging from 40 mm to 120 mm. For the small bone fixator system (SBF, Hofmann srl., Monza, Italy), nine ring sizes are available in 10-mm increments. For the circular fixator system (IMEX, Inc., Longview, TX), four ring sizes are available. They are made of stainless steel, aluminum, or carbon composite material. A space of no less than one cm should be present between the inside edge of the rings and the skin. Partial rings should be used on the flexion side of joints to allow unrestricted range of motion after frame placement. Plates and posts are used to offset wires from rings to fix short bone fragments. The connecting elements connect the supporting elements. They include threaded and telescopic rods. The diameter of the rods determines the size of all other Ilizarov elements. Rods of 4-, 5-, or 6-mm-diameter are commercialized. Their pitches are 0.66, 0.8, and 1 mm, respectively. Their length ranges from 30 to 200 millimeters. Systems of five mm can be used in cats and dogs of all sizes. Systems of six mm can be used in man and in medium to giant dog breeds. At least three connecting rods are used to connect the rings. With hinged fixation, two connecting elements have hinges and a third element, used for distraction, is named the angular motor. Hinged connecting rods are made with two male posts rotating around a bolt. The angular motor is connected to the ring with two twisted plates.

With conventional, straight Ilizarov fixation, all connecting rods can be used as linear motors for distraction. The assembly elements include bolts and nuts used to assemble supporting elements and connecting elements. Some nuts have dots or marks on their faces to facilitate adjustments. With hemispherical washers, the direction of the connecting rods in relation to the rings can vary. This feature is helpful when ring fixators are used for fracture repair. Nylon-insert nuts may be used to secure hinges and other points of rotation. The sliding elements include buckles. Originally, the buckle was Ilizarov's first fixation element. Buckles now are used mainly as points of rotation between two rings. Tensioners are used to tension the wires. They come in multiple forms: mechanical and pneumatic. They are a critical part of the Ilizarov instrumentation. No tension is placed in animals weighing less than one kg. Twenty to 30 kg of tension are placed in animals weighing 5 to 10 kg, 30 to 60 kg in animals weighing 10 to 20 kg, and 60 to 90 kg in animals weighing more than 20 kg.[9] Graduated and nongraduated tensioners are available, but only graduated tensioners provide information on the amount of tension placed on the wires.

Box wrenches and flat wrenches are used to perform frame adjustments. Wrenches of 7, 8, and 10 mm are used with 4-, 5-, and 6-mm systems, respectively. Although they were not part of the original Ilizarov instrumentation, fixation cubes have been developed to connect half-pins to the rings, creating hybrid frames. Half-pins can be added to the frames to enhance fixation of short bone fragments or to fix partial rings to the proximal part of the humerus and femur, where full rings cannot be used. To our knowledge, five manufacturers make circular external fixation systems of various complexity for canine use. Four systems are made in Europe (two in Italy, one in France, and one in England) and one in the United States.

Ilizarov frames should be built so dogs can bear normal weight after frame placement. The frames should have four rings, whenever possible. The outer rings should span the bone and the inner rings should be close to the fracture or osteotomy site, creating a "far-near-near-far" pattern. The specific frame design has been described in detail in several reports.[3,5,8] This includes choosing the number of rings, their size, their type, the type of hinge or hemispheric washers, their location, the number and location of osteotomy, the type and location of wire and pin fixation, and the presence of sliding or traction components for correction of elbow joint subluxation. Partial rings, placed on the flexion side of joints, decrease the interference of the frame with normal joint range of motion. The rings should have the smallest diameter that maintains a centimeter-wide gap between their inside edge and the skin.

Circular external fixators are particularly complex. Having a comprehensive preoperative plan enhances case management by: 1) requiring a full understanding of the current pathophysiology and its anticipated evolution; 2) requiring evaluation of all anatomic constraints 3) requiring evaluation of the biomechanical characteristics of the situation; 4) ensuring availability of frame components; and 5) decreasing surgical time. The preparation of hinged frames ideally includes a drawing showing a cross-section of the limb at the level of the planned osteotomy, the ring, the hinges, the angular motor, and the wires.[3] With advances in 3D data collection and rapid manufacturing methods, digital images of affected bones may be collected and used to make models. These models may be used for operative rehearsal. We currently make models for complex multifocal bone deformities using helical CT scanning and stereolithography, ink-jet, or electron-beam melting rapid prototyping methods (Figure 97-6).[10] These models appear to improve the accuracy of diagnosis and the precision of the surgical placement and postoperative corrections. They also appear to decrease the duration of surgery. Silicon molds of first-generation models may be made to reproduce bones of interest for educational or experimental use.

Ilizarov frames have the advantage of relying on tensioned fine wires with a diameter ranging between 1.0 to 1.6 mm in small animals and between 1.5 to 2.0 mm in humans. Even though these fine wires are less disruptive than conventional external fixation pins with a larger diameter, they have to be placed carefully to optimize the biomechanics of fixation while minimizing soft-tissue interference or potential injury. As a general rule, patients should be able to function normally while the fixator is in place. This is only possible when the fixator is stable and when neurovascular bundles and major muscle groups are unaffected by the transosseous wires. The frames should not interfere with the skin of the limbs, axilla, or groin, during locomotion. It is imperative to leave at least a one cm space between the skin and the inside edge of the rings to avoid skin irritation and necrosis. In small animals, the placement of full rings around the limbs is limited to the radius and tibia, and, in some instances, the distal portion of the humerus and femur. As a consequence, the use of conventional Ilizarov frames, with two rings above and below the osteotomy or fracture site, is limited to the radius and tibia. Partial rings are often used on the flexion side of joints, with a cranial opening for the proximal aspect of the radius and caudal opening on the proximal aspect of the tibia. The principles of Ilizarov fixation can be applied to the femur and humerus but the frames have to be modified to include arches, plates, and cubes for half-pin fixation. These hybrid frames are challenging to conceive, to place, and to maintain.

Few reports provide information about wire placement in small animals. Marti and Miller reported on safe, hazardous, and unsafe corridors for placement of linear external fixators.[11,12] Putod described the cross-sectional anatomy of dog limbs. Software packages with cross-sectional and 3D anatomic representations are becoming available for human anatomy and, to a lesser extent, for dogs. The medial aspect of the radius is safe, distal to the insertion of the pronator teres muscle (distal two thirds of the bone). Laterally, the radial head can be palpated subcutaneously. The lateral aspect of the radial shaft is a hazardous corridor, because of the presence of the extensor muscles. The radial nerve is on the caudomedial aspect of the limb. Practically, wire placement in the radius is craniomedial to caudolateral and caudomedial to craniolateral, with wire angles of 90° in the distal third and 45° to 60° in the proximal two thirds. When hybrid fixation is made necessary by the presence of a short bone fragment, half-pins can be placed in the distal part of the radius, caudomedially, medially, or craniomedially, or in the proximal part of the radius, laterally. Wire placement through the proximal part of the radius in a craniocaudal direction, in a slightly laterally offset position, has been described (by Dr. Yves Latte), but is not used by the author. This wire placement has several drawbacks: transfixation of the extensor muscles and transfixation of the ulna, eliminating the ability to pronate and supinate. In our experience, the clinical function is better if transfixation of the ulna is avoided, because the elimination of pronation and supination appears to negatively impact limb use and also appears to lead to premature loosening of the pins and wires. The ulna has two safe zones: the olecranon, proximally and caudally, and the lateral styloid process, distally and laterally. Wire placement in the ulna is generally limited to wires used for displacement of the ulna in relation to the radius. One or two wires can be placed on posts, from a medial to lateral direction, across the caudal aspect of the proximal portion of the ulna. The posts can be adjusted progressively to treat proximal or distal humero-ulnar subluxations.

Ferretti designed the SBF fixator and was the first clinician who used the Ilizarov method in veterinary medicine. He established guidelines for wire size and tension. Wire tension should not exceed 30 kg when the wires are placed on partial rings or posts, away from the rings. Several biologic factors strongly influence the stability of Ilizarov frames. For correction of deformity, the preservation of the periosteum helps stability at the osteotomy site. The regeneration of callus or new bone helps to create an internal support for the bone (bio-buttress). The bone healing rate at the osteotomy site is enhanced by the presence of an increased blood supply at the osteotomy site (in young dogs, with large bone, and metaphyseal osteotomy). It is also enhanced by a minimally traumatic osteotomy, a long resting period after osteotomy and before distraction, a small amount of daily distraction, and a high frequency of distraction.

For fracture treatment, bone healing seems enhanced when fractures are treated closed. Enhanced bone healing also creates a beneficial bio-buttress. Sharp wires are used to decrease thermal trauma to the limb. The wires are placed with a low-speed power drill. A 2- to 3-mm-long skin incision may be made at the entry and exit sites of the wires to decrease skin trauma. The author has abandoned the use of such incisions. Drilling is generally started on the side of the bone that provides maximal control for wire positioning and safest wire placement - the medial aspect of the radius and tibia. Once the transcortex has been pierced, the wire can be tapped with a mallet to avoid rotation of the wire through the tissues on the opposite side of the limb. The use of a drill with an oscillating function also helps to protect soft tissues. The soft tissues can be gently reflected by digital pressure. Tension should not be present on the skin after wire placement. If tension is present, the wires may be moved below the skin surface and a new hole in the skin may be made with a more relaxed skin placement. A releasing incision may also be made in the skin to eliminate a minor amount of tension.

Postoperative Management

The postoperative management of dogs after surgical correction of antebrachial deformities focuses on wound care, maintaining limb use, avoiding excessive stress placed on the bone and external fixation frame, and maintaining range of motion in the carpus and elbow joints.

It is important to maintain limb use during the early postoperative period by giving pain medications, rapidly eliminating swelling, using protected weight-shifting and weight-bearing exercises, and avoiding trauma. Swelling may be present in the extremity and around the surgical site in the early postoperative period, particularly in patients undergoing intraoperative derotation of the extremity. Swelling is controlled by enhancing lymphatic and venous drainage through elevation of the extremity, passive range of motion of the carpus, gentle finger massage (effleurage), and cold therapy. Swelling is most often eliminated in 2 to 3 days. In patients with circular external fixators undergoing distraction osteogenesis, distraction starts on the third day after surgery.[3] Distraction tends to increase tissue tension and leads to loss of range of motion, particularly carpal joint motion, in the late treatment stages. The distraction rate is often decreased when tissue tension increases, and activities promoting joint motion and stretching are routinely performed. Bandages and braces may be used to regain joint motion in specific instances.

The soft-tissue complications of Ilizarov fixation are comparable to the soft-tissue complications of conventional external fixation. In most cases, the complications are a consequence of improper surgical technique. Neuropraxia results from nerve trauma. Hemorrhage can result from a vascular injury. In most cases, hemorrhage is intraoperative, but it may occur several weeks after surgery, when wires abrade blood vessels. Skin irritation or necrosis can result from ring placement in contact with the skin or from the contact of the frame with the groin or axilla. Focal drainage occurs at the skin wire interface, especially when wires are loose. Muscle contracture may result from decreased limb use or from the tension generated during limb lengthening. In our experience, the soft-tissue complications associated with Ilizarov fixation are common, but they are generally minor and rarely affect the outcome of surgery.

Rotation is most often corrected acutely, intra-operatively. Angulation is most often corrected first, progressively after surgery. Mild lengthening is combined with angular correction in dogs likely to heal rapidly (i.e., young dogs). Lengthening is accelerated after angular correction is complete, generally 15 to 30 days after surgery. The distraction rate is often 1 to 2 mm per day at the point of maximal distraction, divided in 2 to 4 increments.[3] Radiographic follow-up is done at the end of angular correction, and every 3 to 4 weeks afterward until bone healing is complete. Circular external fixation frames are removed under sedation. The long-term outcome of the correction of antebrachial deformities has been good to excellent, from cosmetic and functional standpoints.[3,8] Circular ESF has been used to treat antebrachial deformities that include a severe elbow joint subluxation, a limb-length deficit, and an angular limb deformity of the distal portion of the radius and ulna. Placing a circular external fixator with a single set of hinges and making two osteotomies (one used to correct angulation and limb length and one to eliminate elbow joint subluxation) had lead to excellent clinical results. Distal humeroradial subluxations of up to 13 mm have been reduced using this method in 5 dogs. Circular ESF has been used to treat bifocal antebrachial deformities that include a severe varus defornity of the proximal portion of the radius and a valgus (generally combined with a multifocal caudal deformity) of the distal portion of the radius (Figure 97-6).

References

1. Sande RD, Bingel SA: Animal models of dwarfism. Vet Clin North Am Small Anim Pract 13:71-89, 1983.
2. Johnson JA, Austin C, Breur GJ: Incidence of canine appendicular musculoskeletal disorders in 16 veterinary teaching hospitals from 1980 to 1989. Vet Comp Orthop Traumatol 7:56-69, 1994.
3. Marcellin-Little DJ, Ferretti A, Roe SC, et al: Hinged Ilizarov external fixation for correction of antebrachial deformities. Vet Surg 27:231-245, 1998.
4. Jaegger G, Marcellin-Little DJ, Levine D: Reliability of goniometry in Labrador Retrievers. Am J Vet Res 63:979-986, 2002.
5. Marcellin-Little DJ: Treating bone deformities with circular external skeletal fixation. Comp Cont Educ Pract Vet 21:481-491, 1999.
6. Marcellin-Little DJ: Fracture treatment with circular external fixation. Vet Clin North Am Small Anim Pract 29:1153-1170, 1999.
7. Marcellin-Little DJ, Ferretti A: Improving bone healing with the circular external fixation method. Vet Forum 14:40-47, 1997.
8. Marcellin-Little DJ: External skeletal fixation. *In* Slatter DH (ed). Textbook of Small Animal Surgery, 3rd ed. Philadelphia: WB Saunders, 2003, pp.1818-1834.
9. Lewis DD, Bronson DG, Samchukov ML, et al: Biomechanics of circular external skeletal fixation. Vet Surg 27:454-464, 1998.
10. Harrysson OLA, Cormier DR, Marcellin-Little DJ, et al: Rapid prototyping for treatment of canine limb deformities. Rapid Prototyping J 9:37-42, 2003.
11. Marti JM, Miller A: Delimitation of safe corridors for the insertion of external fixator pins in the dog. 2: Forelimb. J Small Anim Pract 35:78-85, 1994.
12. Marti JM, Miller A: Delimitation of safe corridors for the insertion of external fixator pins in the dog. 1: Hindlimb. J Small Anim Pract 35:16-23, 1994.

Chapter 98

Miscellaneous Orthopaedic Diseases

Ron Montgomery

Asynchronous Growth of the Radius And Ulna

Normal synchronous growth of the radius and ulna yields a straight antebrachium with normal articular surfaces at the elbow and carpus. Growth in length of the radius and ulna comes from the physes, or growth plates. The distal radial physis accounts for 60% to 70% of the radius length, while the distal ulnar physis accounts for 100% of the ulna length distal to the elbow (80% - 85% of the overall ulna length).[1,2] Therefore, the diaphyses of the radius and ulna must slide past each other to maintain a straight antebrachium (Figure 98-1).[1]

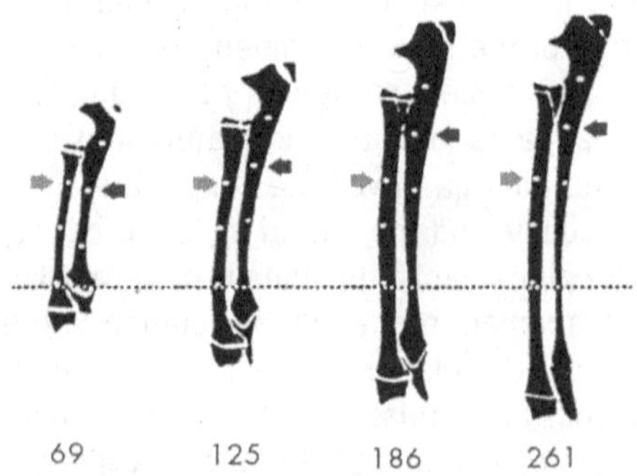

Figure 98-1. Adapted from Carrig CB, Vet Clin N Am 13,91, 1983 (Ref 2). Growth of the radius and ulna is depicted at ~2 months, ~4 months, ~ 6 months, and ~9 months of age. Following the radiographic markers (arrows) as age increases shows that the radial and ulnar cortices must slide past each other during growth. Also noteworthy: the fastest growth occurs between 4 months and 6 months of age; the vast majority of growth is complete by 6 months of age; from the level of the elbow distally (note proximal ulnar marker) virtually 100% of the ulnar length comes from the distal ulnar physis.

Asynchronous growth of the radius and ulna (AGRU) results in an antebrachium that is shortened and has angular, rotational and/or bowing deformity (Figure 98-2).[1-5] Less obvious, but more significant, are the articular malformations of the elbow and/or carpus.[1-6] The articular surfaces are sculpted for each individual during growth via Wolff's law.* Forces that are normal in direction and proportion yield a congruent, healthy, and mechanically effective joint. Abnormal forces, as occur with AGRU, yield an incongruent, unhealthy, and mechanically ineffective joint that cannot be corrected and often not even significantly improved with contemporary techniques.[6] AGRU has numerous etiologies, each with specific clinical abnormalities reflecting which part(s) of the synchronous growth is abnormally effected.[1-6] Regardless

*Wolff's law: *"a bone, normal or abnormal, develops the structure most suited to resist the forces acting upon it."* Dorland's Medical Dictionary, 28th ed. Philadelphia: Saunders.

of the specific etiology, however, all forms of AGRU have the pathologies described above to some extent.

The most recognized form of AGRU is premature closure of the distal ulnar physis, also referred to as radius curvus (Figure 98-2).

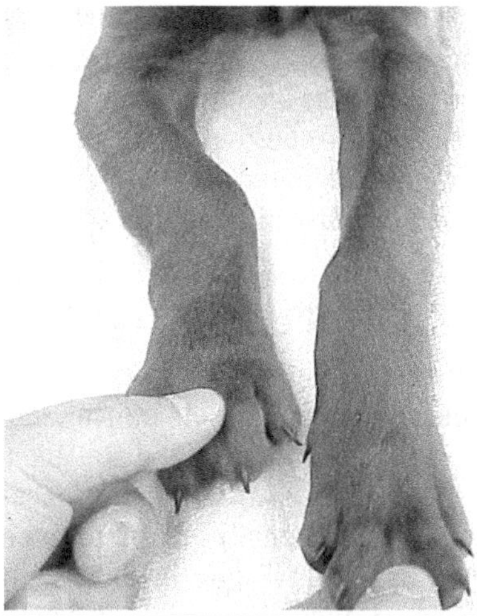

Figure 98-2. Puppy with AGRU of the right foreleg which is shortened, bowed, and externally rotated.

The distal ulnar physis is cone shaped, which concentrates compressive forces. Excessive compressive forces, i.e., when a dog jumps down from a relatively high place and lands first and most forcefully on its front leg(s), can result in Salter-Harris V (compression) fractures. (Other Salter-Harris fracture types can also occur.) This inciting trauma is often not witnessed by the owner, or is soon forgotten because the duration of lameness is short. If radiographs are taken soon after the trauma, the nondisplaced Salter-Harris V fracture is not detectible. Radiographs when AGRU is present, but before normal physeal closure, show premature closure of the distal ulnar physis. The distal ulnar physis stops growing and becomes an anchoring point for the distal radius, tethered via fibrous connective tissue. The pathology is mechanically analogous to a moving boat tethered to an anchor caught on the bottom. Premature closure of the distal ulnar physis results in the radius deviating laterally with supination (remember the distal ulna is caudolateral to the distal radius). Additionally, there is cranial bowing of the distal radius (the radius is growing in length while the ulna is not), malarticulation of the radiocarpal joint with valgus deformity, humeroulnar subluxation with varus deformity, and shortening of the antebrachium (Figure 98-3). Similar deformity occurs if the lateral part of the distal radial physis stops growing prematurely (partial closure), which is the second most commonly observed form of AGRU.[6]

Complete closure of the distal radial physis results in relatively minor angular deformity, decreased length of the antebrachium, and malarticulation of the carpus and elbow. Premature closure of the proximal radial physis results in a substantial widening of the radiohumeral joint, radioulnar malarticulation, and shortening of the antebrachium (Figure 98-4). An additional but uncommon cause of AGRU is a radius and ulna fracture that heals in a single mass (synostosis), which prevents the sliding of the diaphyses (Figure 98-5).

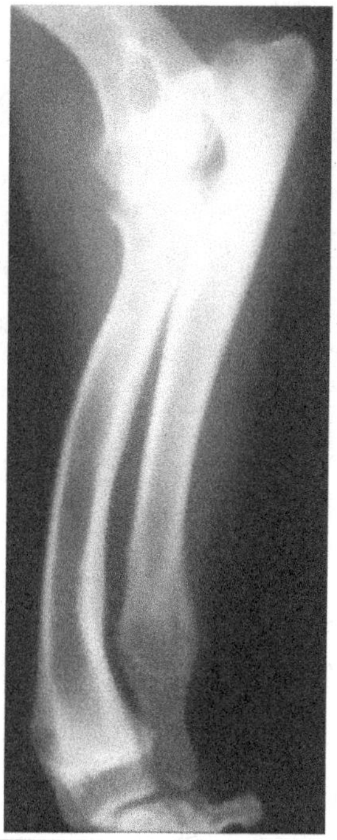

Figure 98-3. Radiograph showing premature closure of the distal ulnar physis causing antebrachial shortening, substantial curvature and humeroulnar subluxation.

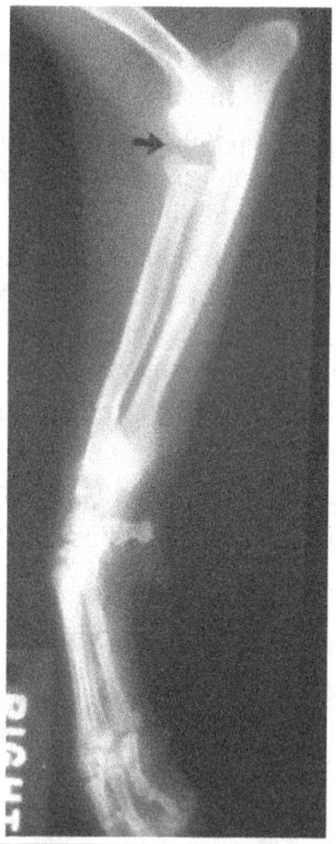

Figure 98-4. Radiograph showing premature closure of the proximal radial physis resulting in substantial widening of the radiohumeral joint (arrow), radioulnar malarticulation and shortening of the antebrachium.

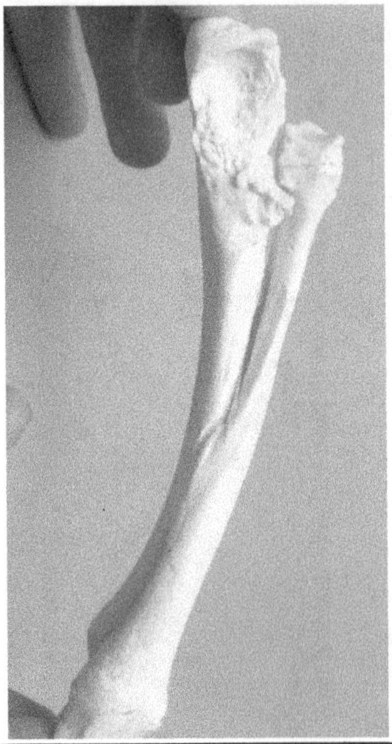

Figure 98-5. Photo of synostosis due to prior fracture and subsequent union of the radius and ulna to each other. Note the large step deformity of the radial head and coronoid processes with accompanying degenerative joint disease.

The severity of deformity depends on the potential growth remaining at the time of physeal damage (premature closure). Potential growth is a combination of the dog's age and adult size. Approximately 90% of bone length is obtained by 6 months of age in all but giant breed dogs, with the most active growth occurring between 3 and 4 months of age. A 3-month-old dog has more potential bone growth than a 5-month-old dog of the same adult size. Similarly, a 4-month-old Labrador retriever has more potential growth than a 4-month-old Chihuahua. The more potential bone growth, the worse the deformity will be if left untreated. The most effective treatment is removal of a section of the ulna (anchor rope) on the same side of the interosseous ligament as the pathology as soon as AGRU begins. Ulnar osteotomy is most effective if performed early and enough potential bone growth remains to correct the pathologies.

Atraumatic etiologies of AGRU also exist.[4,5] The most common cause of AGRU is selective breeding, which creates and perpetuates achondroplastic/chondrodysplastic breeds such as basset hounds, English bulldogs, and dachshunds. Although the condition is generally accepted in these breeds, the pathologies exist nevertheless. AGRU is also present in dogs with dwarfism, an inherited condition reported in the Labrador retriever, malamute, Norwegian elkhound, and Samoyed breeds.[4] A mild form of AGRU also occurs with retained cartilaginous core.[4,5]

Retained Cartilaginous Core

Retained cartilaginous core (RCC) is an abnormality of endochondral ossification in which conversion from physeal cartilage to bone is delayed at the distal ulnar physes. The etiology is most likely a clinical manifestation of osteochondrosis. Clinical abnormalities are usually limited to lateral deviation of the carpii, usually up to 10° (Figure 98-6). Radiographically, the distal ulnar physis extends an excessive distance proximally. RCC predominantly affects juvenile Great Danes, although the condition may persist into adulthood and/or affect other large breeds. Treatment is typically not indicated.[4,5]

Puppy Carpal Laxity Syndrome

Puppy carpal laxity syndrome is carpal hyperextension or hyperflexion in the absence of an identifiable cause (e.g., tendon rupture or fractures) (Figure 98-7).[7] Puppies with this condition are not in pain and have a full range of motion of the carpus. The condition can be unilateral or bilateral, and typically occurs at 2 to 5 months of age. Multiple puppies in a litter may be affected, suggesting an etiology of nutrition, environment, husbandry, or inheritance. A breed predilection is not recognized, however, and mixed breeds are affected at least as often as pure breeds. The etiology is unknown. The pathophysiology appears to be an imbalance in muscle tone between the extensor and flexor

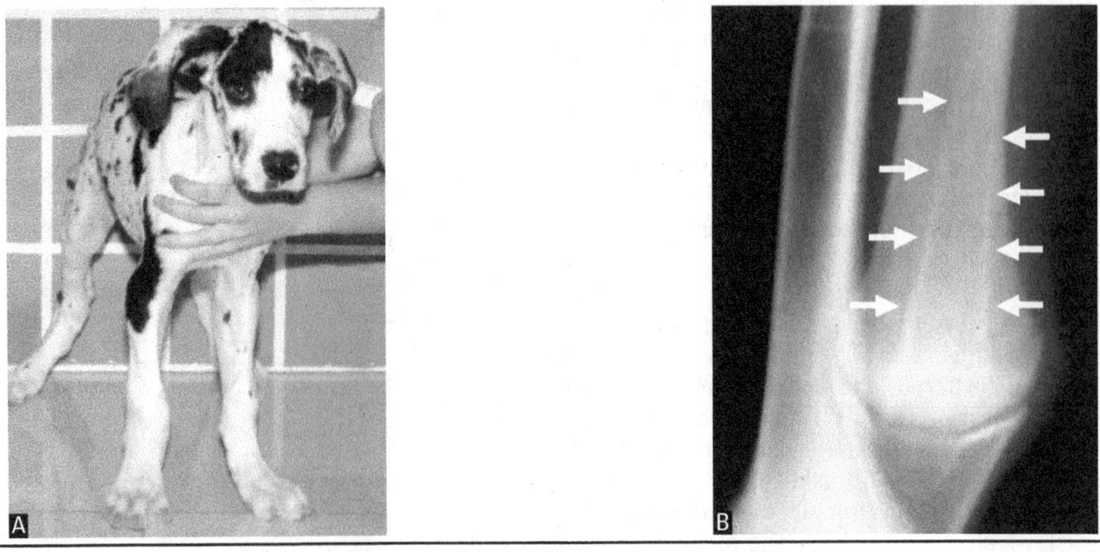

Figure 98-6. (A) Retained cartilaginous core (RCC) of distal ulna causing slight carpus valgus. (B) Radiograph of distal antebrachium showing RCC, seen as excessive proximal extension of the distal ulnar physis (arrows) in shape of a flame.

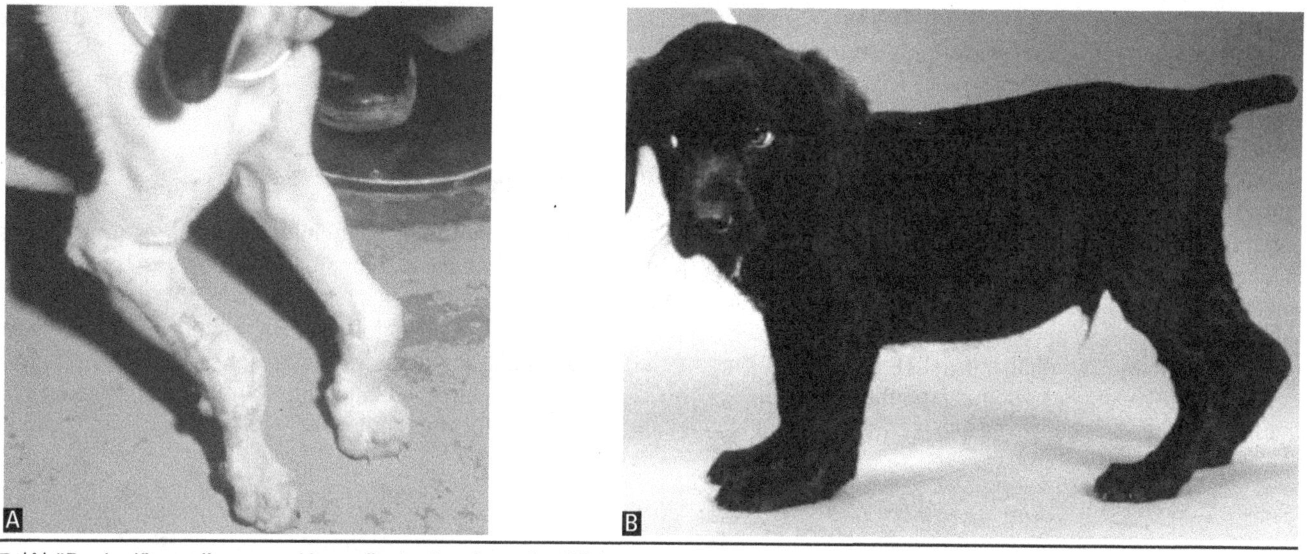

Figure 98-7. (A) "Bucked" carpii or carpal hyperflexion in a juvenile. (B) "Dropped" carpii or carpal hyperextension in a juvenile.

muscles of the carpus. Correction of the condition occurs spontaneously in the vast majority of dogs in less than or up to 2 weeks, although the condition will persist into adulthood in rare cases. Encouraging exercise has been recommended. Treatment with splints prolongs correction to about 6 weeks.[4-6]

Ectrodactyly

Ectrodactyly is a true congenital deformity (present at birth) wherein the paw's shape is that of two large toes rather than four normal sized toes (Figure 98-8), giving rise to the synonyms of "lobster claw" and "split-hand deformity."[4,5,8] Typically only one front paw is affected. Subluxation of the ipsilateral elbow occurs in slightly less than half the cases of ectrodactyly. Radiographs of the foot reveal various bizarre combinations of fused and absent metatarsal and phalanges bones. Ectrodactyly has been proven to be of an inherited etiology in humans and cats, and is probably inherited in dogs as well. Medium and large breed dogs (especially mixed breed dogs) have been reported with ectrodactyly thus far in the literature. Treatment is usually not necessary, as most dogs with ectrodactyly have few if any clinical signs other than the anatomic deformity.

Dwarfism

The most common form of "dwarfism" in dogs is intentional selection of the autosomal dominant trait to create and perpetuate "toy" and "miniature" breeds, as well as breeds such as the basset hound. The term "dwarf" is not conventionally used to describe intentional dwarfism, and the condition is not generally considered pathologic. However, clinical problems do occur that are attributable to the selective breeding owing to conformation (especially joint malarticulation). Dwarfism will refer to unintentional.

Dwarfism has been reported in the beagle, cocker spaniel, English pointer, French bulldog, Great Pyrenees, Labrador retriever, malamute, Norwegian elkhound, miniature poodle, Samoyed, Scottish deerhound, and Scottish terrier.[4,5] The author

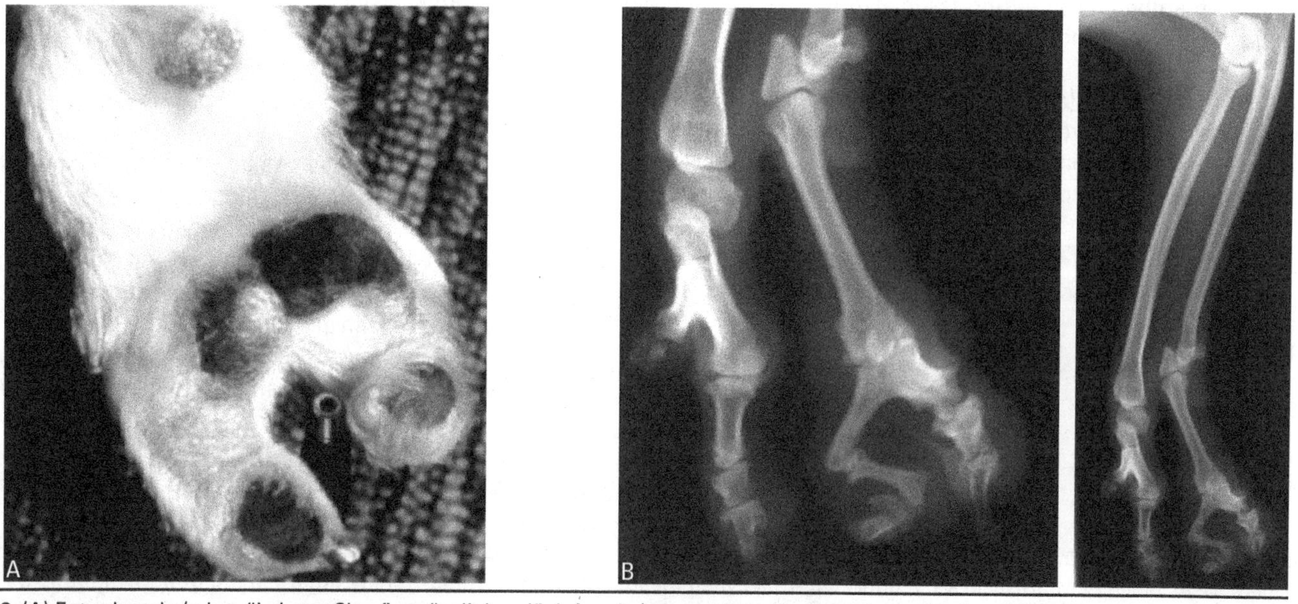

Figure 98-8. (A) Ectrodactyly (a.k.a. "Lobster Claw", or "split hand" deformity) shown from the ventral perspective. (B) Radiograph of ectrodactyly showing bizarre combination of fusion and absence of bones.

has observed dwarfism most often in the Labrador retriever, almost certainly influenced by the breed's current popularity (i.e., number of Labrador retrievers and ill advised breeding practices). Dwarfism can occur owing to a variety of anomalies and modes of inheritance, each yielding a characteristic phenotype and associated pathologies. Achondroplastic dwarfism is the term used for humans. It results in a phenotype of short limbs and a normal trunk, which is the most common form of dwarfism in dogs (Figure 98-9). Autosomal recessive inheritance is the etiology in breeds in which the mode has been studied.[4] Dogs with dwarfism appear normal at birth, but the condition becomes obvious in a few months. Individual bones can be affected equally or unequally, resulting in straight or curved legs, and/or the front legs versus rear legs being equal or unequal in length. characteristic is the failure of an adult hair coat (primary hairs) to develop, and easy epilation of the puppy (secondary) hair, resulting in alopecia in areas of high friction such as the caudal thighs, caudal forearms, and around the collar.[5]

Hemimelia/Amelia

In dogs and cats, congenital agenesis of the diaphysis of the radius is the most common form of this rare condition.[4,5] Conventional nomenclature indicates the affected bone first (i.e., radius, ulna, tibia, fibula), followed by amelia (complete agenesis) or hemimelia (complete agenesis of the diaphysis). In addition to dogs and cats, humans, goats, rats, and chickens have been reported to have hemimelia.

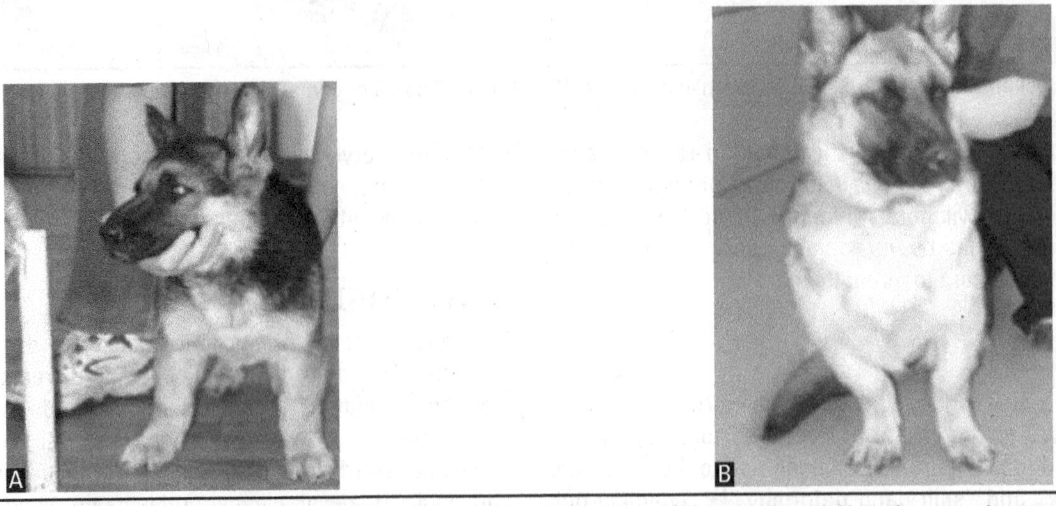

Figure 98-9. Achondroplastic dwarfism in German Shepherd dog at (A) 3 months old and (B) 9 months old. Note the normal appearance of the trunk and abnormally short legs. Photographs courtesy of Mr. Fred Lanting, AKC Judge, Willow Wood Consulting.

Associated pathologies include retinal dysplasia (Labrador retriever), retinal detachment and cataracts (Labrador retriever and Samoyed), and hemophilia (malamute). Owners are often unaware the conformation is abnormal (if the dog is pure breed) and should be informed. In addition, owners should be advised to have the dog evaluated for associated pathologies and the reasons that neutering the dog is important.

Pituitary dwarfism (also called hypophyseal infantilism) is caused by under secretion of growth hormone and gonadotropin deficiency, resulting in a proportional dwarfism with retention of infantile characteristics (Figure 98-10). The most obvious infantile

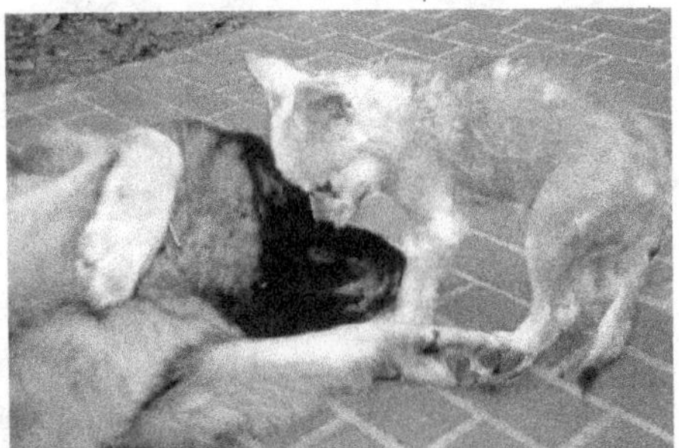

Figure 98-10. Pituitary dwarfism in a 1 year old dog-wolf hybrid (right), with a normal dog (left). Photograph courtesy of Mr. Fred Lanting, AKC Judge, Willow Wood Consulting.

The pathogenesis of hemimelia is failure of the radius to develop in utero. The etiology is unconfirmed, although inheritance is generally postulated. One breeding pair of cats reproduced kittens with amelia over multiple litters (three of eight kittens affected). Other proposed etiologies include accidents in utero, irradiation, drug toxicities, vaccines, and dietary deficiencies (especially minerals, e.g., zinc, copper, manganese). Unilateral occurrence being more common than bilateral obscures the proposed etiologies.

Cats are reported to have radial hemimelia more often than dogs. No size or breed predilection exists. History indicates that the owners noticed the deformity (Figure 98-11) (shortened antebrachium with varus deformity and/or carpus valgus) at or soon after birth. In older dogs, the appearance of the deformity could be confused with one form of AGRU (distal radius closure), although palpation reveals the lack of a radius diaphysis. Radiographs confirm the diagnosis. Limb function is commensurate with the deformity, ranging from not weight-bearing to good (albeit abnormal). Effective treatment has not been devised, nor is heroic surgery indicated as the condition is ostensibly not painful. Amputation can be performed for cosmesis or treatment of chronic decubital ulcers. Neutering affected animals is recommended, and arguably others in the genetic lineage as well.

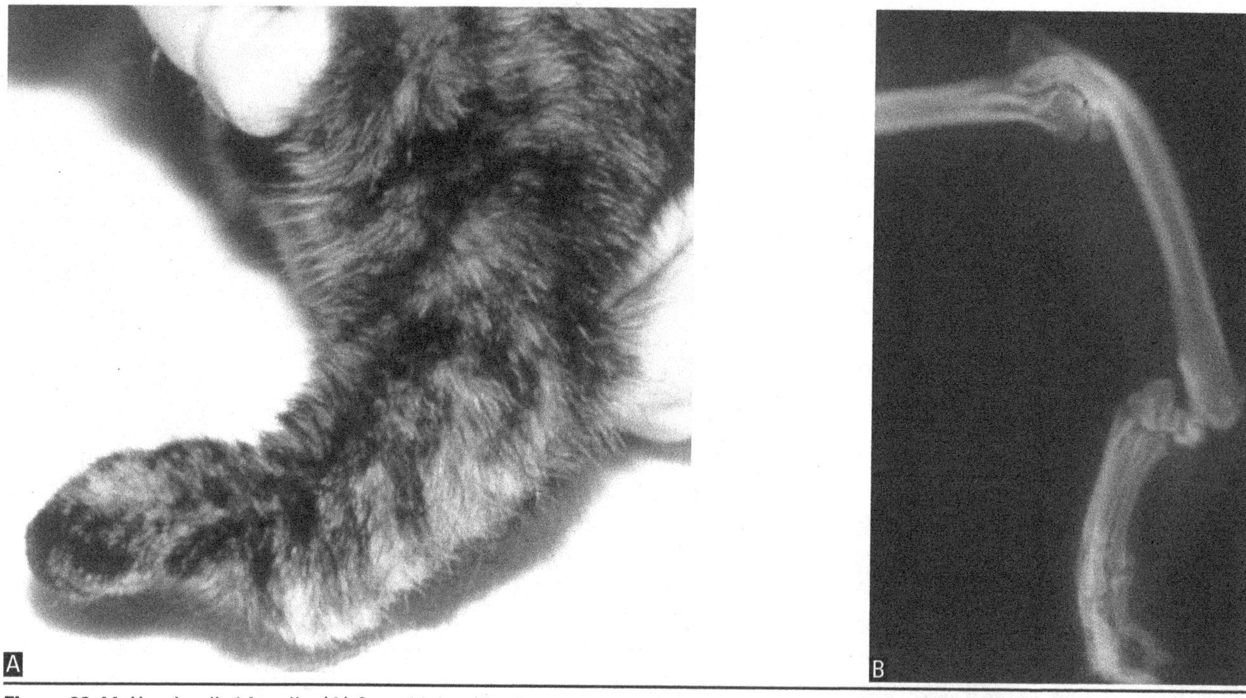

Figure 98-11. Hemimelia/ Amelia. (A) Cat with hemimelia showing carpal subluxation and gross deformity of foreleg (thumb is on shoulder and other hand is behind the elbow). (B) Radiograph showing absence of the radius with malarticulation of the carpus and elbow.

Rickets and Osteomalacia

Osseous deformity and hypomineralization owing to abnormal metabolism of vitamin D, calcium, and phosphorus from various etiologies is referred to as "rickets." Osteomalacia is the adult onset form, although conventional use often substitutes the term rickets. "Renal rickets" is probably the form seen most often clinically in dogs. Inappropriate all-meat diets in "big cats" (tigers, lions, etc.), especially juveniles, causes severe hypomineralization. A group of related juvenile vizslas (Figure 98-12) was studied at Auburn University's College of Veterinary Medicine over a period of several months. Affected dogs had pronounced curvature and shortening of the long bones, which also affected range of motion of adjacent joints. Nutritional and concurrent renal failure were effectively eliminated as causes, and rickets was tentatively diagnosed.

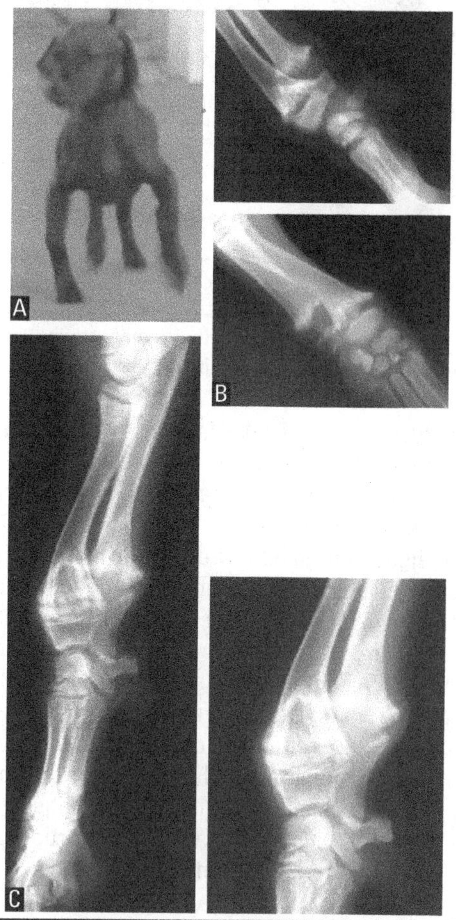

Figure 98-12. Vizsla with rickets. (A) Note the curvature of the front legs and shortened stature. (B) In these radiographs of the distal radius and ulna at approximately 8 weeks of age, there is the characteristic marked widening of the physis in the distal radius and ulna. (C) Several months later there continues to be abnormal appearing metaphysis though the physis have a more normal appearing physeal width.

Bone Cyst

Bone cysts in dogs are rare and include subchondral, simple (cystic), and aneurysmal forms.[4,5] Subchondral bone cysts are relatively small and identified radiographically. Simple and aneurysmal bone cysts are relatively large and often readily palpable. Differential diagnosis between neoplasia and simple bone cyst or aneurysmal bone cyst can be difficult. Therefore, confirming a diagnosis and case management should be performed with due diligence.

Subchondral bone cysts are an osteochondrosis lesion most commonly identified in horses. Subchondral bone cysts are lined with synovial membrane and contain serosanguineous fluid, myxoid, or fibrous tissue. Forage obliterates the cyst and establishes a new blood supply to initiate healing. It is performed if the cyst is large enough or causing a clinical problem and prior to development of significant degenerative joint disease.

Simple bone cysts contain serosanguineous fluid and are lined with fibrous tissue. They can occur in the metaphysis of any long bone or multiple long bones (polyostotic). The most common presentation is a single simple bone cyst (monostotic) located in the distal radius or distal ulna of a juvenile or young adult, large breed dog. Doberman pinchers and German shepherd dogs appear to be over-represented. The etiology of simple bone cysts is uncertain, although the typical signalment of juvenile or young adult dogs suggest an aberration of, or insult during, bone growth. A hereditary predisposition has been suggested for Doberman pinschers. Clinical signs include lameness and painful swelling of the affected metaphysis (with or without pathologic fracture of the bone cyst). Radiographs image a large, expansile mass, absence of osteolysis and/or osteogenesis, variable amounts of cortical thinning, and a fluid density center (Figure 98-13).

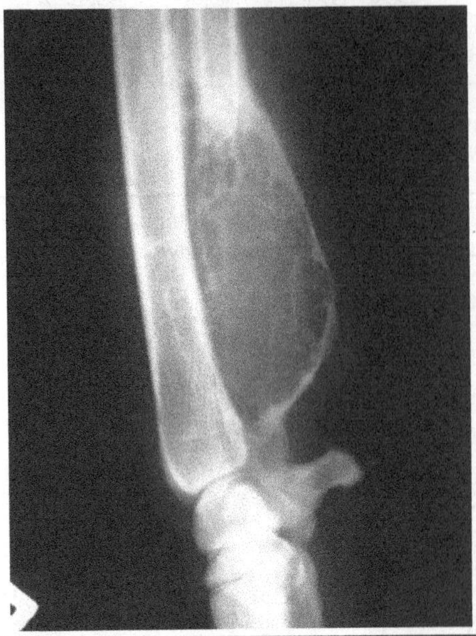

Figure 98-13. Bone cyst in the distal ulna demonstrating an expansile, multi-trabeculated appearance with thin cortices.

Simple bone cysts do not usually cross the physis or involve the epiphysis. A bone cyst may also be asymptomatic and identified as an incidental finding. Asymptomatic cases of simple bone cyst may not require surgery, especially if the ulna is involved as it is not a major weight bearing bone. Surgery is indicated if biopsy is desired to confirm the diagnosis, the simple bone cyst is causing clinical problems (e.g., lameness), and/or if preemptive intervention to avoid a pathologic fracture is desirable (especially a bone bearing significant weight such as the radius). Surgical correction can be via forage of the cyst and into the adjacent medullary cavity, or curettage and bone grafting. With either technique, fracture stabilization devices such as bone plates or external fixators minimize the risk of pathologic fracture. In humans, injection of simple bone cyst with corticosteroid has been reported as a successful treatment.

Aneurysmal bone cysts contain large vascular sinusoids, are expansile, osteolytic and locally invasive of adjacent bone and soft tissue. Aneurysmal bone cysts have been classified as probably intraosseous arteriovenous shunts, but have also been classified as neoplastic. Aneurysmal bone cysts have been diagnosed in young adults to geriatric dogs. Clinical signs are localized pain and swelling, usually of several months' duration. A predilection exists for the axial skeleton, although any bone can be affected. Treatments are intended to decrease vascularity while maintaining structural strength, and include debridement with bone grafting, radiation therapy, and cryotherapy. Aneurysmal bone cysts have been reported in dogs, cats, horses, and people.

Congenital Shoulder Luxation

Congenital shoulder luxation is a disease of small and toy breed dogs that, in the author's opinion, is in many ways analogous to congenital medial patella luxation, albeit much less common. Clinical signs are first observed when the puppy begins to walk, or in young adults, depending on severity. Clinical signs range from non-weight-bearing and constant luxation, to the more common intermittent luxation and associated intermittent lameness (Figure 98-14). Palpation may reveal a medial luxation. Applying medial pressure on the proximal humerus and abducting the elbow with one hand while palpating the relative position of the acromion process with the other hand should diagnose medial shoulder luxation or subluxation. Radiographs are indicated to access the changes to the glenoid cavity and humeral head, with craniocaudal stress radiographs if used for the purpose of diagnosis or documentation.

The condition is presumed not to be of traumatic etiology, and by convention is called congenital, but may be developmental. Medial luxation or subluxation of the shoulder dictates coexisting insufficiency of the medial collateral ligament and joint capsule, with possible involvement of the subscapularis muscle/tendon. Because congenital shoulder luxation involves abnormal forces in a juvenile, Wolff's law dictates that the glenoid cavity and humeral head develop an abnormal shape. The glenoid cavity may be more shallow, flat, or even convex, with or without identifiable erosion of the medial brim; the humeral head is flattened to varying extents.

Treatment should be proportional to the severity. Various surgical techniques have been described to stabilize the luxation, with relatively low success rates. A flat or convex glenoid cavity would logically predict poorer results of medial stabilization, as would complete luxation and the presence of osteoarthritis. Shoulder arthrodesis is a reasonable option in dogs owing to the high mobility of the scapula. However, the presence of the infraspinatus nerve and the sparse amount of scapular bone (i.e., decreased ability of implants to hold) makes arthrodesis problematic in these small and toy breed dogs. Dogs with infrequent intermittent lameness that appears to the owner to be non-painful may be harmed more by surgery than helped.[4,5]

Congenital Elbow Luxation

Congenital elbow luxation occurs predominantly in English bulldogs, basset hounds, Yorkshire terriers, Pekingese, and other small and toy dogs.[4,5] A hereditary etiology has been suggested, but not confirmed. The pathogenesis has been speculated to be an in utero insufficiency of the elbow's medial collateral ligament and perhaps annular ligament. The luxation is lateral in all but

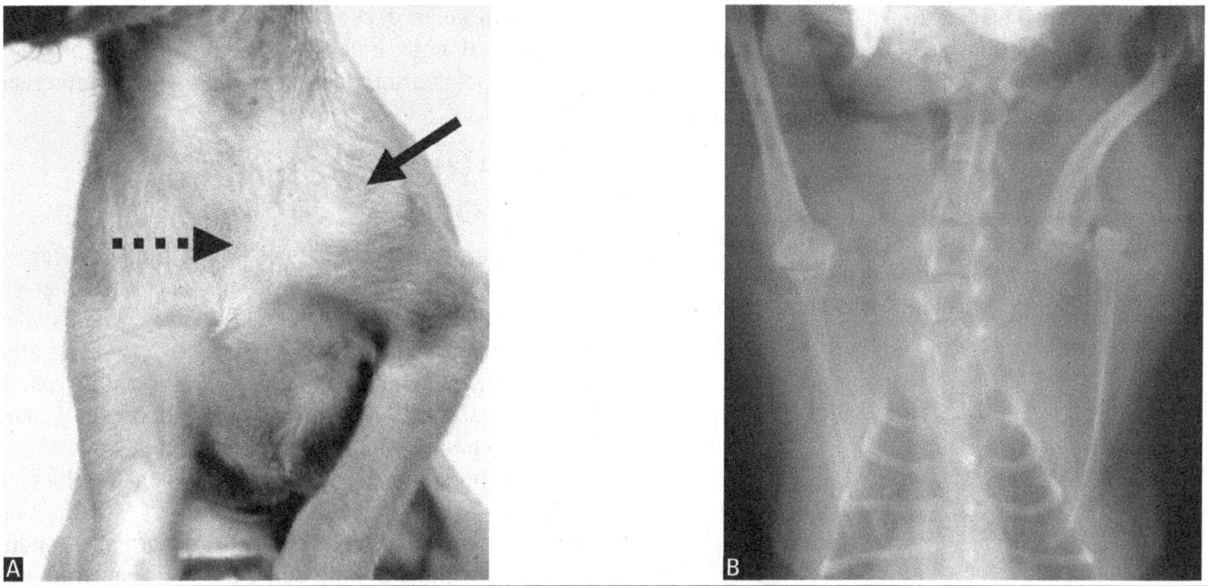

Figure 98-14. Congenital shoulder luxation (left) in a puppy. (A) Note the Abduction of the arm, with lateral position of elbow, prominent acromial process (solid arrow) and medial placement of humeral head (dashed arrow). (B) Radiograph showing congenital medial shoulder luxation. Note the flat to convex shape of the affected glenoid cavity.

one documented case,[9] and can be unilateral or bilateral. The critical pathologies with congenital elbow luxation are the lateral location of the triceps muscle insertion (hence, contraction does not extend the elbow), and malarticulation in a young dog, causing gross osseous deformities of the joint (see Wolff's law). Congenital elbow luxation causes an obvious deformity (Figure 98-15) consisting of lateral luxation, flexion of the elbow, and pronation of the antebrachium. Appearance of affected dogs has been compared to the praying mantis insect. Gait is likewise overtly abnormal, since inability to extend the elbow(s) causes the dog to crawl (Figure 98-16). A craniocaudal radiograph of the affected leg yields a Cr-Cd image of the humerus and a lateromedial image of the radius and ulna (Figure 98-17), as opposed to adult dogs with traumatic elbow luxation in which the radius and ulna are not typically rotated.

Satisfactory treatment of congenital elbow luxation depends on age at the time of surgery and adult weight of the dog. If treated when only a few weeks old, a modified external fixator (Figure 98-18) typically results in a functional joint (although radiographically abnormal). A small K-wire (e.g., 0.062") is placed mediolaterally through the olecranon near the triceps insertion;

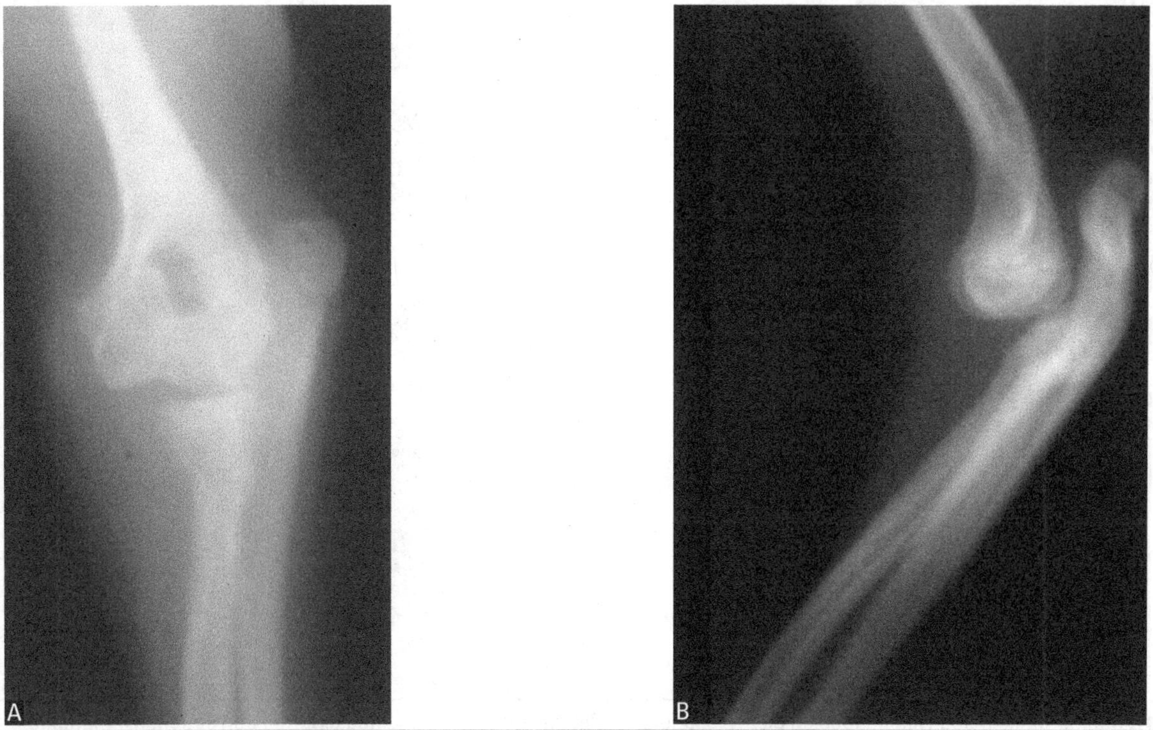

Figure 98-15. Congenital elbow luxation. Note that in the craniocaudal radiograph of the elbow there is a lateromedial view of the radius and ulna. (B) In mediolateral radiograph of the elbow there is a craniocaudal view of the radius and ulna.

a second K-wire is likewise placed transcutaneously across the distal humeral epicondyles, and a rubber band of appropriate tension is placed externally from the lateral tip of the olecranon pin to the medial tip of the transepicondylar pin, which rotates the olecranon to the correct functional position caudally. The dog is encouraged to walk on the leg normally (i.e., not splinted) until reduction is maintained without the rubber band present (typically a couple of weeks).[9,10] Success of this technique is fairly reliably predicted based on the ease of manually reducing the luxation. For older dogs, in which the luxation is not readily reduced, transposition of the olecranon can yield reasonable function in some cases. Heavier dogs (e.g., English bulldogs), especially if not treated early, have a poor prognosis for a functional joint; arthrodesis is an option for unilateral cases.

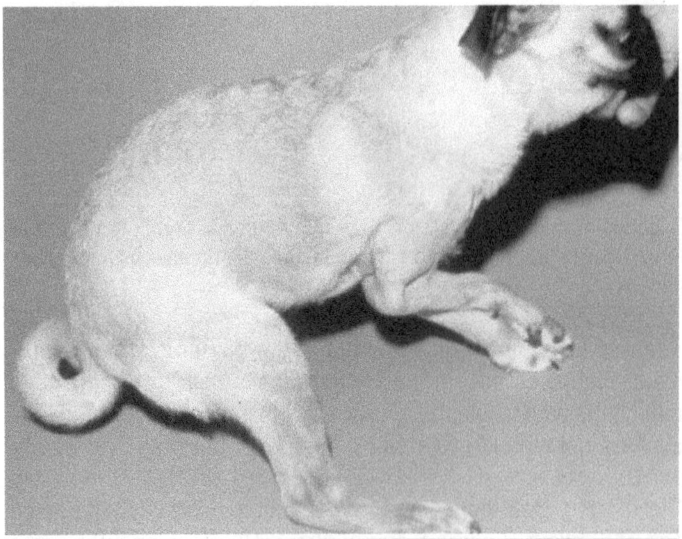

Figure 98-16. Congenital elbow luxation is a juvenile. Note the "Praying Mantis" appearance of the front legs due to inability to extend the elbows. There is also internal rotation of the antebrachii and abnormal topographic anatomy of the elbows.

Multiple Cartilaginous Exostosis

Multiple cartilaginous exostosis (MCE) is a rare disease with the interesting pathogenesis of extra physes or articular-epiphyseal complexes* that are aberrantly located on, and usually perpendicular to, cortical bone (Figure 98-19).[5,11,12] The pathogenesis most widely accepted is that the MCE originated from the physis before separating. Any bone of the axial or appendicular skeleton formed by endochondral osteogenesis may have MCE, with the involvement of multiple bones being typical. As the juvenile dog grows, so do the cartilaginous exostoses. MCEs are mushroom shaped, with the stalk consisting of bone formed by endochondral osteogenesis, and the top being cartilage covered and comparable histologically to an A-E complex. Growth continues until osseous maturity, when the MCEs, the normal physes, and A-E complexes cease growth and ossify. Onset of clinical signs is predictably while the dog (and exostoses) are undergoing rapid growth (2 to 5 months of age). Clinical signs associated with MCE depend on their location and what damage (primarily via pressure) the exostoses cause to adjacent tissue. Clinical signs range from a palpable mass, to lameness (pressure on muscle, nerve and/or vessels) to paralysis (compression of the spinal cord). Diagnosis is confirmed via radiographs of multiple bones with characteristic bone lesions. The bone lesions show bone of variable shape and size extending perpendicular to the metaphysis with radiolucent areas (hyaline cartilage) capping the end. Biopsy results indicate a typical physis consistent with

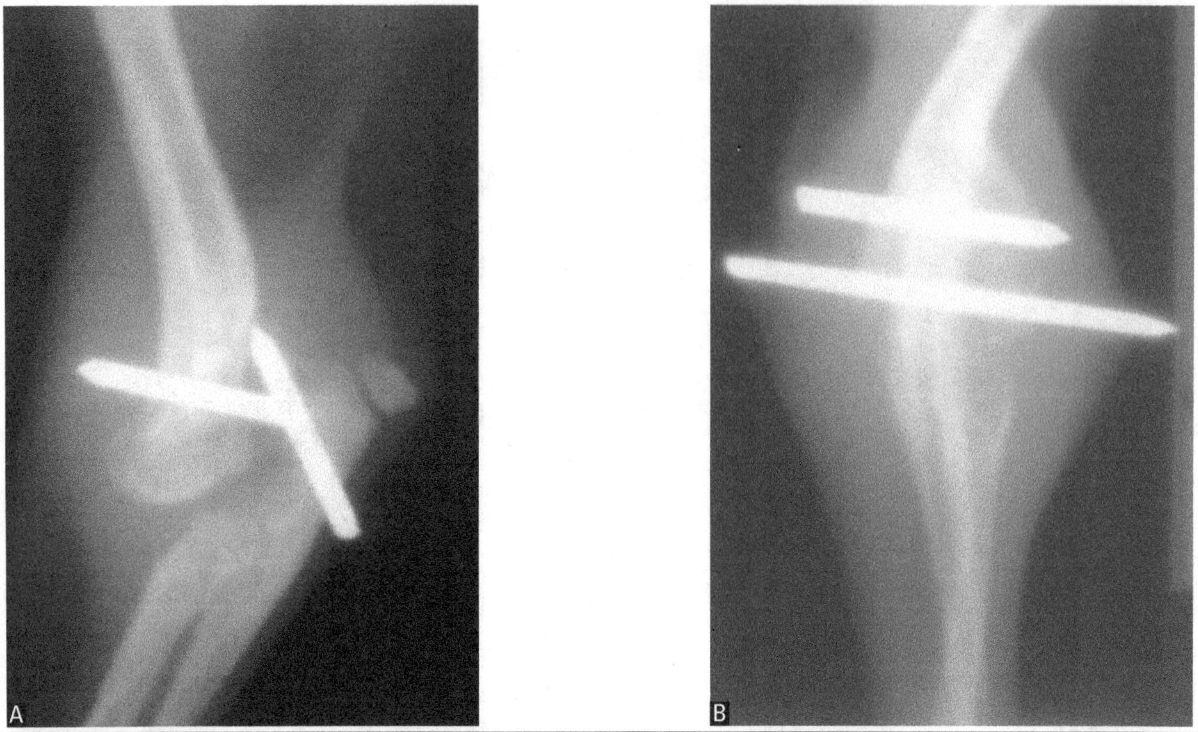

Figure 98-17. Radiographs of dog with congenital elbow luxation. (A) Pin placement for modified external correction. (B) Placement of rubber band on the pin tips (external to the skin) of appropriate tension reduces the luxation while allowing flexion and extension of the elbow joint necessary for juvenile joint health.

* Articular-epiphyseal complexes are histologically and functionally analogous to physes, with the difference being that the cartilage of A-E complexes remains in the mature dog as the articular cartilage.

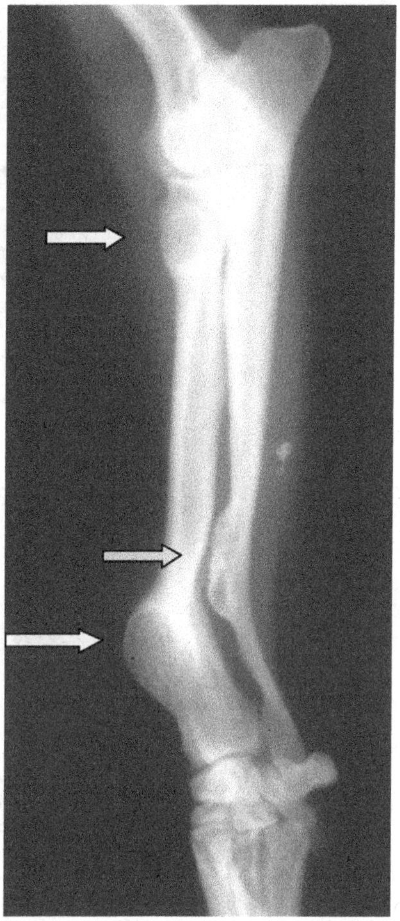

Figure 98-18. Multiple cartilaginous exostosis occurred in multiple other locations in this dog. Cartilage covering the exostosis (arrow) was visible on histopathology.

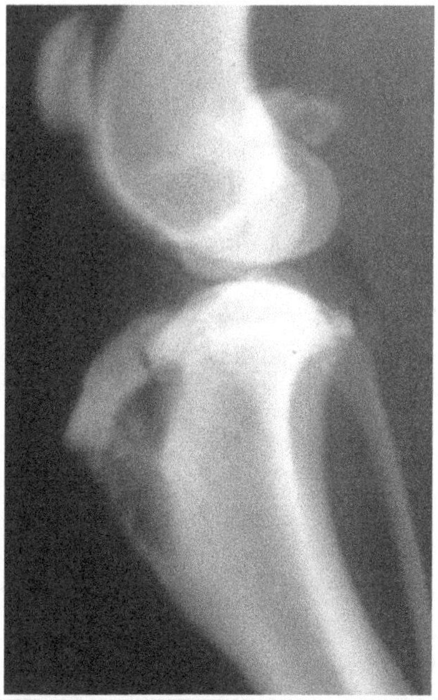

Figure 98-19. Osgood-Schlatter disease in a hunting dog. There is an increased width of the physis of the tibial crest.

the age of the animal. The marrow portion of the MCE (stalk) contains adipose or hematopoietic marrow. Most cases of MCE have good outcomes unless the MCE has caused irreparable damage (e.g., to the spinal cord), because the MCE ceases growth when the normal physes cease growth. Multiple cases of MCE metamorphosis into chondrosarcomas or osteosarcomas have been reported in the literature; hence, monitoring or removal would be judicious.

Osgood-Schlatter's

Osgood-Schlatter's disease is a physitis of the tibial crest.[5,13] It has been observed in juvenile dogs, specifically active hunting breeds (e.g., pointers). Osgood-Schlatter's disease is a condition in juvenile boys (~8-15 years old) also called "football knee". It most commonly occurs in larger, athletically active boys. The physes of the tibial crests become inflamed, painful, and radiographically abnormal (i.e., widened and irregular) (Figure 98-20).[17] Adjacent soft tissues are also inflamed in the acute phase. Osteochondrosis has been a proposed etiology. The more likely and more widely accepted etiology is repetitive trauma. Tension from the patellar tendon, especially strong and repetitive forces, can overload the adjacent physis, resulting in physitis. Rest is the preferred treatment for most cases, followed by avoiding the causative activity until skeletal maturity. Fixation is required only for a displaced tibial crest (determined by flexing the stifle and palpating a lax patellar tendon and unstable tibial crest).

Hypertrophic Osteopathy

Hypertrophic osteopathy (HO) is the only disease reviewed in this chapter that occurs typically in mature dogs. The most common cause of HO is a mass within the thorax. The likely pathogenesis is stimulation of the vagus nerve, which subsequently alters vascularity to the periosteum of the distal limbs, which promotes periosteal proliferation.[14] This proposed pathogenesis is supported by research in which transection of the vagus nerve resulted in reversal of the periosteal lesions of the distal limbs. HO was originally called hypertrophic pulmonary osteoarthropathy (HPOA). Rhabdomyosarcomas of the urinary bladder have also been reported to cause HO, and the joint is not directly effected.[15-17]

Dogs with HO are typically presented for a firm, non-painful swelling of the metacarpus, metatarsus, and phalanges. The swelling may progress more proximally in some cases. Radiographs show a characteristic, if not pathognomonic, periosteal proliferation characterized as "palisades" (columns, similar to numerous tall buildings) (Figure 98-20B). HO is not treated per se. Rather, treatment is directed toward the underlying cause. Although neoplasia (metastatic or primary) in the thorax is the most common inciting cause of HO, other diseases have been reported to result in HO (e.g., spirocerca lupi parasitism, emphysema, etc).[4]

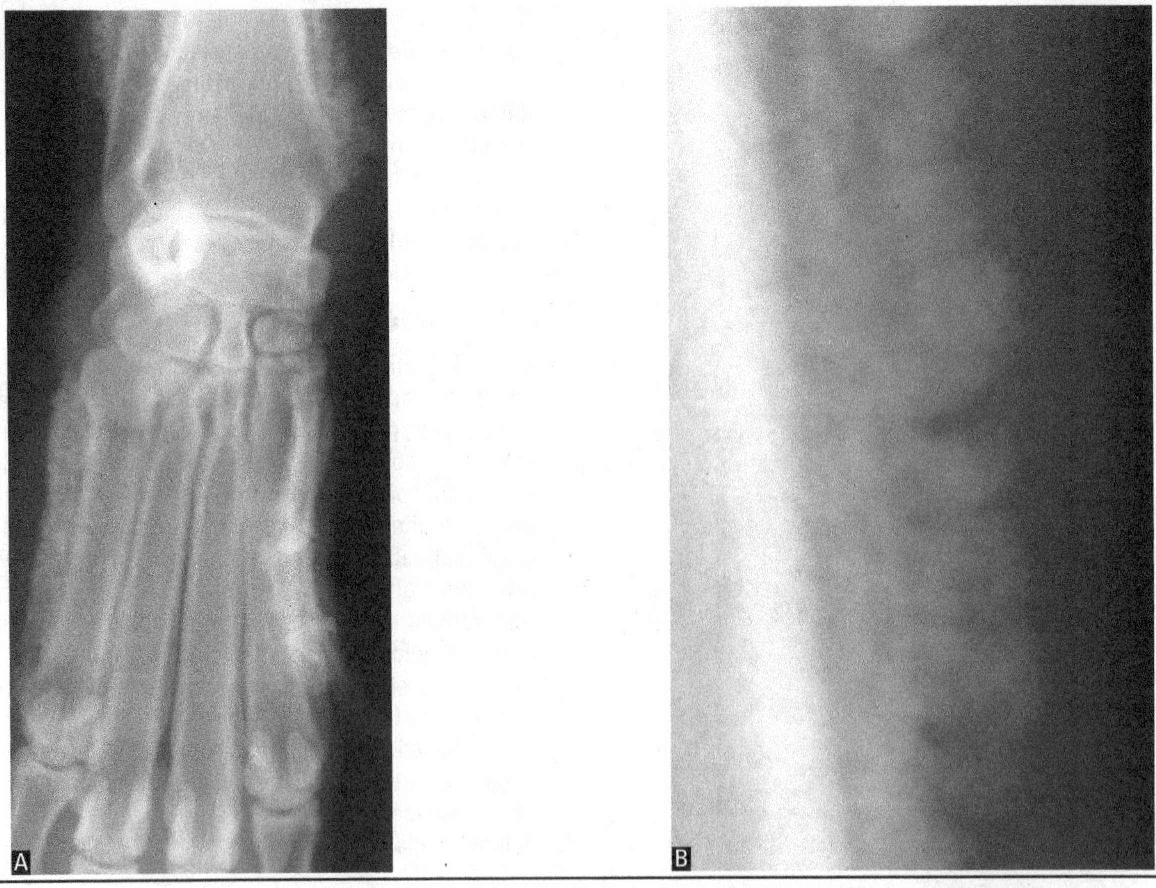

Figure 98-20. Hypertrophic Osteopathy in an adult dog with lung tumors. (A) Periosteal reaction is present along the metacarpi and distal radius and ulna. Note that the joints are unaffected. (B) Close up of the unique "Palisades" periosteal reaction associated with HO.

References

1. Newton CD: Radial and ulnar osteotomy. *In* Textbook of Small Animal Orthopaedics. Newton CD, Nunamaker DM (eds). Philadelphia: JB Lippincott, 1985, p. 533.

2. Carrig CB: Growth abnormalities of the canine radius and ulna. Vet Clin North Am 13:91, 1983.

3. Fox SM: Premature closure of the distal radial and ulnar physes in the dog. Parts I & II. Comp Cont Educ 6:128, 212, 1984.

4. Milton JL, Montgomery RD: Diagnosis of foreleg lameness. *In* Clinical Signs and Diagnosis in Small Animals. Ford RB (ed). New York: Churchill Livingstone,1988, p. 351.

5. Montgomery RD: Miscellaneous orthopaedic diseases. *In* Textbook of Small Animal Surgery, 3rd ed. Slatter D (ed). Philadelphia: Saunders, 2002, p. 2251.

6. Theyse LFH, Voorhout G, Hazewinkel HAW: Prognostic factors in treating antebrachial growth deformities with a lengthening procedure using circular external skeletal fixation system in dogs. Vet Surg 34:424, 2005.

7. Shires PK, Hulse DA, Kearney MT: Carpal hyperextension in two month old pups. JAVMA 186:49, 1985.

8. Carrig CB, et al: Ectrodactyly in the dog. Vet Radiol 22:123, 1981.

9. Montgomery RD, Milton JL, Hudson JA, Finn-Bodner ST: Medial congenital elbow luxation in a dog. Vet Comp Ortho Traumatol 6:1, 1993.

10. Milton JL, Montgomery RD: Congenital elbow dislocations. Vet Clin North Am (SA) 17:873, 1987.

11. Gambardella PC, Osborne CA, Stevens JB: Multiple cartilagenous exostosis in the dog. JAVMA 166:761, 1975.

12. Alexander JW: Solitary and multiple cartilagenous exostosis in the dog. Canine Pract 5:43, 1978.

13. Ehrenborg G, Engfeldt B, Olsson SE: On the aetiology of the Osgood-Schlatter lesion, and experimental study in dogs. Acta Chir Scand 122:445, 1961.

14. Halliwell WH: Tumor like lesions of bone. *In* Pathophysiology in Small Animal Surgery, 2nd ed. Bojrab MJ (ed). Philadelphia: WB Saunders, 1993, p. 933

15. Rendano VT, Slauson DO: Hypertrophic osteopathy in a dog with prostatic adenocarcinoma and without thoracic metastasis. JAAHA 18:905, 1982.

16. Caywood DD, Osborne CA: Urinary System. *In* Textbook of Small Animal Surgery, 1st ed. Slatter D (ed). Philadelphia: WB Saunders, 1985, p. 2561.

17. Jaffe JL: Metabolic, Degenerative and Inflammatory Diseases of Bones and Joints. Philadelphia: Lea & Febiger, 1972.

Chapter 99

Metabolic, Nutritional, and Endocrine Bone Disorders

Herman A.W. Hazewinkel

Metabolic diseases of the skeleton can be due to inborn errors of metabolism or be acquired. The former includes abnormalities in collagen synthesis and, as a consequence, abnormal growth or mineralization of the skeleton, whereas the latter includes a variety of hormonal diseases with or without a nutritional cause. Here we will limit ourselves to three examples of collagen disease, which are important to recognize as the differential diagnoses of diseases of endogenous and of nutritional origin.

Multiple Epiphyseal Dysplasia

Although different types exist, the major features of multiple epiphyseal dysplasia are irregular epiphyseal growth, with little vertebral involvement and a mild dwarfism, and an irregularly shaped acetabulum.[1] In humans, this genetic trait is autosomal dominant as well as recessive, whereas in dogs it seems to be autosomal recessive.

The clinical signs become obvious at the age of 2 to 3 months and are seen in a variety of breeds including Labrador retrievers, viszlas, and Rottweilers. The owner will notice that the dog does not grow as fast as the litter mates. The elbow joints may be abducted and the gait abnormal in cases with joint deformities, however, this is not always the case. The dog will have short legs and a normal skull and vertebral column. Radiology will reveal shortening of the long bones when compared with litter mates and, in some cases, abnormal joint alignment (Figure 99-1A). Concomitantly, osteochondrosis and other developmental diseases can be present, but so far we have not seen it in conjunction with ocular diseases like retina dysplasia.

In cases of abnormal joint alignment, the prognosis is extremely poor. In other cases, the disturbed growth will not have a major impact on the dog's well being.[2]

Osteogenesis Imperfecta

The disorder is first noticed at about 3 to 4 weeks of age, when dogs with osteogenesis imperfecta (OI) reveal a reluctance to move. They are well proportioned, with blue sclera, translucent and fragile teeth, and legs with hyperlaxity at different joints and possibly with multiple fractures. Blood biochemistry and calciotropic hormone plasma levels are normal. The etiology is a genetic defect, probably autosomal recessive, which encodes for procollagen molecules of collagen type I, resulting in an abnormal collagen structure affecting the formation and stability of bone mineral associated with this collagen.[3] Because collagen type I represents 90% of the organic substance of bones, teeth, and tendons, this genetic defect has consequences for osteoid and dentin mineralization, and for connective-tissue strength at multiple sites including the chordae tendiniae. The rupture of the latter may cause sudden death of the patient. The disease has been reported in golden retrievers, collies, poodles, beagles, Bedlington terriers, dachshunds, and domestic cats.[4]

The diagnosis can be made by a clinical and radiologic investigation. Radiographs show poorly mineralized bones (long bones and ribs) with only some contrast in the area bordering the growth plates, which are of normal width, and fractures of long bones and ribs (Figure 99-1B). The diagnosis can be confirmed by pathologic investigation, which reveals regular growth plates, with some disturbed mineralization of the primary mineralization zone, but with absence of secondary spongiosa, as well as with irregularly arranged woven bone without Haversian systems in lamellar bone.[4] Sometimes dentinogenesis imperfecta, owing to poor mineralization of collagen type I of the dentine, is concomitantly present. Differential diagnoses include (1) alimentary

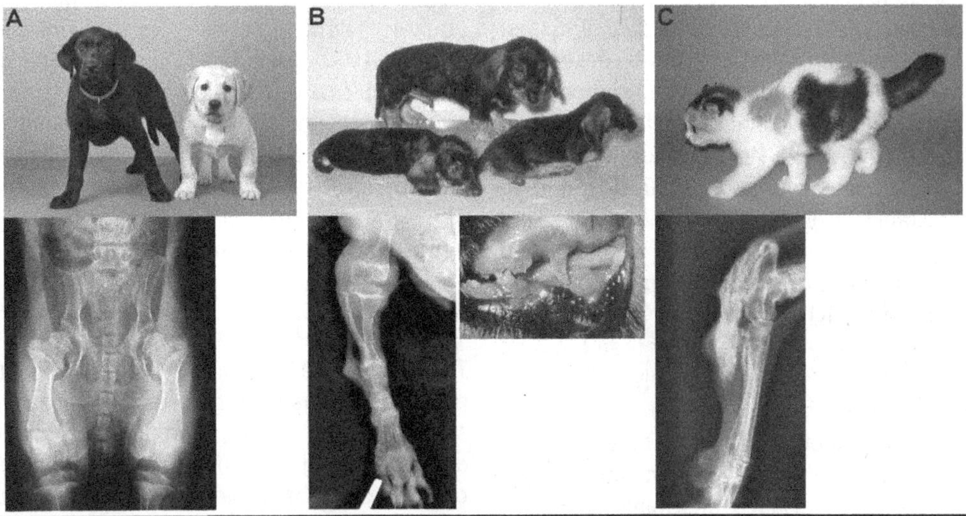

Figure 99-1. Metabolic bone disorders. (A) Disproportional Labrador pup with multiple epiphyseal dysplasia revealing short long-bones, abnormal physeal growth, and irregularly shaped acetabulum with normally shaped vertebrae. (B) Dachshund pup with osteogenesis imperfecta with poor mineralization of long bones and slight widening of growth plates. (C) Offspring of Scottish fold cat with osteochondrodysplasia revealing short misshapen distal limbs with exostosis plantar to and distal of the calcaneus.

secondary hyperparathyroidism (discussed later), although this does not go together with flexible joints, blue sclera, or transparent teeth, and the diet of the patient does not differ from that of its normal litter mates; (2) hypovitaminosis D, although that is characterized by the increased width of growth plates; (3) hypothyroidism, although these patients are mobile, do not have fractures, and reveal delayed skeletal maturation with otherwise normal mineralization.

Treatment of osteogenesis imperfecta for human patients includes biphosphonate supplementation to strengthen the bone, and allogeneic mesenchymal stem cell or bone-marrow transplantation with acceptable success;[5] but for companion animals, the prognosis is poor.

Osteochondrodysplasia in Cats

Osteochondrodysplasia is a generalized skeletal disease characterized by short, misshapen distal limbs; exostosis plantar to the calcaneus; and round joints of distal limbs with diffuse osteopenia of adjacent bone; and short, thick inflexible tails (Figure 99-1C). It occurs in offspring of both genders originating from the mating of a Scottish fold with a normal cat. The Fold-ear is a dominant trait but does not always coincide with these skeletal abnormalities. The patient reveals lameness, a stiff gait, and a reluctance to jump, starting at a young age. Histologically, cartilage maturation seems to be disturbed.[6] Differential diagnosis is hypervitaminosis A, although this reveals exostosis around the proximal joints.

Treatment of single cases varies from expectative, radiation of exostosis,[7] and pantarsal arthrodesis,[8] to injections with pentosan with oral dosage of glucosaminoglycans,[6] all of which have been described as producing some success. However, breeding with Fold-eared cats can be prevented, because prognosis of this disease is poor.

Vitamin A

Vitamin A is essential in bone metabolism, especially in reducing chondrocyte proliferation in growth plates, decreasing periosteal osteoblast activity, and stimulating osteoclast activity, in addition to a variety of functions in reproduction, epithelization, and retina integrity. Vitamin A is present in animal fat, for example in ground beef (1400 IU/kg dm), raw egg (40,000 IU/kg dm), bovine liver (1,500 000 IU/kg dm), and cod liver oil (850,000 IU/kg dm). In dogs, but not in cats, vitamin A ($C_{20}H_{29}OH$) can be synthesized out of β-carotene ($C_{40}H_{56}$) by cleavage with the aid of carotenase present in the intestinal mucosa and liver cells. Approximately 1 μg of carotene is equivalent to 0.5 IU of vitamin A. Therefore, the dietary requirement of vitamin A for cats is higher than for dogs (10,000 IU and 5000 IU per kg dm food, respectively). The upper limit of vitamin A for cats is reported to be 100,000 IU/ kg dry matter (i.e., 10 times the requirement). Another difference between dogs and cats regarding vitamin A metabolism is in inactivation; dogs but not cats can form retinyl esters to inactivate vitamin A and are able to excrete 15 to 60% of the daily intake as retinyl palmitate in the urine. Therefore, hypervitaminosis A is seen more frequently in cats than in dogs, especially at an older age (3 to 13 years).[9]

Hypervitaminosis A

Hypervitaminosis A can be caused in kittens and puppies after several weeks of over-supplementation. They reveal reduced growth in length and osteoporosis of long bones together with flaring of metaphyseal regions. Hypervitaminosis A in dogs results in anorexia, decreased weight gain, narrowing growth plate cartilage, decreased new bone formation, and thin cortices. Concentrations of vitamin A in plasma serum exceed the normal ranges for dogs (i.e., 1800-18,000 IU/L).

Hypervitaminosis A in cats may produce a stiff neck and/or enlarged joints in the front and hind legs (mainly elbow and stifle joint) owing to ankylosis, dull hair coat, change in character (probably owing to hypersensitivity and/or bone pain), anorexia, and weight loss (see Figure 114-3 in Chapter 114, Nutrition in Orthopedics). To confirm the diagnosis bone biopsies can be taken, but a liver biopsy, which is easier, will show fatty infiltration.[9] In addition, retinol levels of the liver are increased, in contrast to plasma retinol levels, which were normal in 20% of the cases in a study in cats with hypervitaminosis A.[10]

In dogs, a history of supplementation with cod liver oil will help to make the diagnosis. In cats, the history can indicate a prolonged preference for raw fish, raw liver, or supplements, but this is not always the case, suggesting an individual predisposition.[9] On the other hand, a diet with 10^6 IU vitamin A per kg given to adult cats failed to produce the classic skeletal signs of hypervitaminosis A in 2 years' time.11 Both 0.5* 10^6 and 10^6 IU vitamin A per kg diets (92% dm) given to pregnant queens coincided with a 1.7- and 9-fold incidence increase of kittens with malformations, including neural tube defects, cleft palate, and pelvic hypoplasia, when compared with controls receiving 19,800 IU vitamin A per kg food.[11]

The therapy should be instituted as soon as the diagnosis is made and includes analgesia and food adaptation. Because all commercially available balanced foods include at least the required amount of vitamin A, it is better to prescribe a balanced home-made diet without vitamin A added to it. Such a diet should have a low animal-fat content (lean meat such as veal, lamb, or poultry, or cottage cheese). Per 100 g of cooked meat (including its boiling water with taurine in it) and 60 g of cooked rice should be added 2 tsp of corn oil, 0.5 tsp iodized salt, and 1 tsp bone meal to prevent deficiencies.[12] Because cats will often have hepatic lipidosis, the dosage of analgesia should be on the lower side. General improvement can be seen 4 weeks after the start of the therapy; ankylosis will not disappear so the cats will stay lame, although not from pain.[9]

Vitamin D

The importance of vitamin D (vitD) for skeletal development was reported in dogs even before it was described in humans.[13] The skeletal abnormalities, including thin cortices, curved bones, and enlarged growth plates, that developed in dogs raised on oatmeal could be prevented and cured by the administration of cod liver oil. Sunlight was found to prevent rickets in children and to cure rickets in a goat based on the ability to synthesize cholecalciferol in the skin under the influence of ultraviolet-B light. This ability has been developed in amphibians, reptiles, birds, herbivores, and omnivores, but not in dogs and cats.[14] The cutaneous level of the vitamin D_3 precursor 7-dehydrocholesterol (7-DHC) is low,[14] because of a high level of 7-DHC reductase, an enzyme with high activity converting 7-DHC into cholesterol.[15] Thus, dogs and cats are solely dependent on dietary resources to meet their vitamin D requirement. Balanced dog and cat food does not need any vitamin D supplementation, irrespective of the season or the latitude.

Vitamin D_3 is absorbed in the intestine by passive diffusion, transported in plasma bound to chilomicrons, lipoproteins, and vitD-binding proteins (DBP), and routed to the liver where 40% to 60% will be absorbed.[16] Here vitD_3 is hydroxylated into 25-hydroxy-cholecalciferol (25OHvitD_3). Eventually, this metabolite is further hydroxylated at different places, thus forming a variety of metabolites with different or no activity. Two metabolites are considered to be the most active: 1,25dihydroxy-cholecalciferol (1,25 $(OH)_2$vitD_3) and 24,25dihydroxy-cholecalciferol (24,25$(OH)_2$vitD_3). Other metabolites are considered metabolites of the oxidation pathway and can be increased in case of vitamin D intoxication.[17] A 1000-fold difference in plasma concentration exists between 25OHvitD_3 (nmol/L) and 24,25$(OH)_2$vitD_3 (nmol/L), versus 1,25$(OH)_2$vitD_3 (pmol/L), but the latter is the most active metabolite. Under normal circumstances, only 0.4% of the latter is not bound to transport proteins and thus it is biologically active. In vitD intoxication, 1,25$(OH)_2$vitD_3 is freed from the binding protein, resulting in high vitD activity without a severe increase of the total plasma concentration of 1,25$(OH)_2$vitD_3.[18] The hydroxylation into 24,25 or 1,25$(OH)_2$vitD_3 in the kidneys is reflected in the plasma concentration, whereas other hydroxylation sites (such as intestine, growth plates, and placenta) are not. A variety of factors, related to breed, age, and dietary contents, influence the plasma concentrations of these main metabolites (Table 99-1).[19-27] The main role of 1,25$(OH)_2$vitD_3, the biologically most active metabolite, is the mineralization of newly formed cartilage and osteoid. Its increase of active intestinal

Table 99-1. Factors Influencing the Subsequent Steps of VitD Hydroxylation

VitD_3 → 25OHvit D_3

- The amount of vitD_3 in the plasma and thus the vitD_3 intake. Dogs raised on a diet deficient of vitD_3, revealed significant lower plasma levels of 25OHvitD_3.[19] In cats, a linear correlation could be demonstrated between vitD_3 intake and plasma levels of 25OHVitD_3.[15] In young Great Danes, however, an 8-fold increase of vitD_3 was not reflected in the plasma concentration 25OHvitD_3, whereas a 100-fold intake was.[20]
- Growth hormone (GH) plasma level: in miniature poodles (MPs) the 25OHvitD_3 plasma levels were significantly lower than in MPs injected daily with GH or in Great Danes with known juvenile acromegaly, all on the same diet.[21]
- Influenced by the further hydroxylation process and thus by the calcium requirement, i.e., an excessive calcium intake in dogs with hypoparathyroidism causes an increased plasma 25OHvitD level, without changes in plasma levels of the dihydroxylated metabolites.[19] Calcium supplementation in alimentary secondary hyperparathyroidism increases 25OHvitD_3 synthesis.[22]
- A disturbance in the enterohepatic cycle and/or intestinal fat absorption coincides with a decreased level of 25OhvitD.[23]

25OHVIT D_3 → 24,25$(OH)_2$VIT D_3

- Amount of vitD in the food: in vitD deficiency, the plasma level of 24,25$(OH)_2$vitD_3 is extremely low (3% of normal value),[19] whereas if the intake of vitD is 100 times the recommended dosage for 3 months, the plasma level of 24,25$(OH)_2$vit increases to 16-fold.[24]
- Breed differences, mainly owing to GH plasma levels. In Great Danes the ratio is between 25OHvitD: 24,25$(OH)_2$vitD_3 = 1-3: 1, whereas this ratio in MPs is 1:1-3 owing to a down-regulating effect of GH and/or IGF-I on 24-hydroxylase activity.[19,21]
- Calcium status of the animal. In case of nutritionally induced hyperparathyroidism, plasma 1,25$(OH)_2$vitD_3 levels are increased and 24,25$(OH)_2$vitD_3 levels are decreased, both in large and small breed dogs.[19] This is due to decreased activity of renal (but not intestinal) 24-hydroxylase.[25]
- Dietary restriction of phosphorous decreases renal 24-hydroxylase activity.[26]

25OHVITD → 1,25$(OH)_2$VITD

- Insufficient amount of vitD in the diet will moderately decrease total plasma 1,25$(OH)_2$vitD_3 concentration.[19] Based on the 1000 concentration difference, only a small amount of 25OHvitD_3 is necessary to produce an adequate amount of 1,25$(OH)_2$vitD_3, especially because the 24-hydroxylation is almost stopped.[19] However, an increased protein-binding percentage of 1,25$(OH)_2$vitD_3 can be anticipated, and thus less biologically active 1,25$(OH)_2$vitD_3 is available.
- An increased vitD_3 intake will stimulate 1,25$(OH)_2$vitD_3 synthesis and as a consequence, 24-hydroxylase activity will increase, leading to an augmented hydroxylation of 1,25$(OH)_2$vitD_3 into 1,24,25$(OH)_3$vitD_3, as has been shown by Tryfonidou et al. (2003) in a study in 2 groups of Great Danes with 100-fold difference in vitD_3 dietary intake.[20]
- The breed and age of the animal; young, fast-growing dogs with their increased levels of GH and insulin-like growth factor I, reveal a higher 1,25$(OH)_2$vitD_3 plasma concentration than small breed dogs, even when raised on the same diet.[19,21]
- Calcium can directly or via parathyroid hormone (PTH) influence the 1α-hydroxylation of 25OHvitD_3. PTH stimulates 1,25$(OH)_2$vitD_3 production. Hypophosphatemia can stimulate 1α-hydroxylase directly and thus form a positive feedback loop with increased 1,25$(OH)_2$vitD_3 production, and as a consequence, an increase in phosphate absorption in the intestine, reabsorption in the kidneys, and resorption from the bone.[27]

and renal calcium and phosphorous absorption and its stimulation of the parathyroid hormone-induced osteoclastic bone resorption should be seen in the light of making calcium and phosphorous available for the mineralization process. The main role of 25OHvitD_3, the most abundant metabolite in plasma, is to become hydroxylated, although it has biologic activity, which mainly increases active calcium absorption. The main roles of 24,25$(OH)_2$vitD_3 are decreasing the actions of 1,25$(OH)_2$vitD_3 on the intestine, but working in concert in cartilage maturation and possibly suppression of osteoclast activity.[19]

Hypovitaminosis D

Hypovitaminosis D in young growing animals is called rickets. It is characterized by thin cortices, wide growth plates, broad osteoid seams, and a low plasma concentration of most of the vitamin D metabolites. Rickets is seen only under extreme circumstances, including in dogs fed unsupplemented vegetarian food, in dogs with an inability to absorb fat and thus also vitamins soluble in fat,[23] and in dogs with inborn errors of vitamin D_3 metabolism.

The diagnosis can be made with radiographs, revealing thin cortices and wide ("mushroom shaped") growth plates (see Figure 114-1C of Chapter 114, Nutrition in Orthopedics). Because active calcium and phosphorous absorption will be decreased in hypovitaminosis D, plasma concentrations of these minerals will be lowered. As a consequence, more PTH will be synthesised and secreted, thus increasing activity of 1α-hydroxylase. However, owing to the lack of sufficient substrate, the total 1,25$(OH)_2$vitD_3 plasma concentration will be lowered (with even less unbound, biologically active metabolite). Under the influence of hyperparathyroidism, the osteoclasts will increase bone resorption to compensate for the decreased active calcium absorption, and thus osteoblasts will increase osteoid production as well. Osteoid will seal off the mineralized bone, preventing osteoclasts from resorbing more bone; the decreased bone and increased amount of collagen explain the bowing of the legs rather than the pathologic fracturing seen in hyperparathyroidism.

Treatment depends on the underlying cause. Because the vegetarian diet is often unbalanced at multiple points, a balanced diet is the treatment of choice. Restoration of the skeleton can be noticed in 3 weeks' time because cartilage and osteoid are present and ready to become mineralized.[14] Atresia of the bile bladder can be corrected surgically.[23] Inborn error of vitamin D metabolism is resistant to even prolonged vitamin D therapy.

Hypovitaminosis D in mature dogs is called osteomalacia. It can be expected in mature dogs raised on a vegetarian diet (without sufficient vitD supply) or in case of severe kidney failure with decreased 1α-hydroxylation of the 25-OHvitD metabolite. The latter can occur despite the renal secondary hyperparathyroidism. Because of hypovitaminosis D, newly formed osteoid will not mineralize, but in older animals this activity is reduced, leaving alone the osteoclast activity. Generalized osteoporosis will occur. This will seldom cause clinical problems, because the animal will already be suffering from its renal failure, but microscopically widened osteocyte lacunae can be noticed. Especially in the jaw, bone resorption can cause noticeable weakening (the "rubber jaw syndrome") with loosening of elements.

Hypervitaminosis D

Hypervitaminosis D in dogs is not easy to induce. Dogs developed an efficient 24-hydroxylase-induced mechanism to increase hydroxylation of 1,25$(OH)_2$vitD_3 in case of its overproduction owing to increased vitD intake.[20] Only after 3 months of very high levels of dietary vitD content (100 times the required amount of 500 IU/ kg food) was the 24-hydroxylation mechanism not efficient, eventually leading to increased calcium absorption. In the dogs with the excessive vitD intake, bone trabecules were thicker, bone remodelling was decreased, and endochondral ossification was severely disturbed, the latter even before calcium absorption increased (Figure 99-2A).[20] This led to the conclusion that excessive vitD intake is a direct cause of disturbance of endochondral ossification, and that the mechanism is not via hypercalcemia as was hypothesised earlier.[20] Disturbance of endochondral ossification in distal growth plates of the ulna caused radius curvus syndrome in most of these dogs.

Parathyroid Hormone

Parathyroid hormone (PTH) is synthesized in and secreted from the four parathyroid glands, lying in or near the thyroid glands. Its synthesis is increased by decreasing plasma concentrations of calcium; chronic calcium deficiency causes enhanced synthesis per chief cell as well as hyperplasia of chief cells. Phosphorus does not have a direct effect on chief cell activity, whereas 1,25$(OH)_2$vitD_3 executes a negative feedback on chief cell activity. In case of decreasing plasma 1,25$(OH)_2$vitD_3 concentration, PTH acts directly on bone and kidneys to mobilize and reabsorb calcium, respectively. The second phase is increased osteoclast activity; PTH has no direct effect on osteoclasts but acts indirectly via the shrinkage of osteoblasts, thus exposing bone to the osteoclasts. Osteocytes under the influence of PTH enlarge their lacunae, indicating osteocytic osteolysis.[27] Owing to coupling of osteoclast and osteoblast activity, mediated by local factors, osteoblast activity eventually increases. An important effect of PTH on renal tubuli is the decrease of the tubular maximum for phosphorus.

Alimentary Secondary Hyperparathyroidism (or All-Meat Syndrome)

In fast growing animals the calcium requirement is much higher than in mature animals. Insufficient chronic calcium intake, owing to imbalanced food (especially meat based) will induce hyperparathyroidism with increased osteoclastic and osteocytic bone resorption and increased osteoblast activity: bone turnover is severely increased. This explains the radiologic and pathologic findings in the skeleton: normal growth in width of the bone, but an excessively increased osteoclastic bone removal especially in the endosteum and in the areas of cancellous bone (i.e., metaphyses, diaphyses, vertebrae). The cortex can become so thin that it cannot withstand normal muscle contraction or the bodyweight of the animal, leading to pathologic fractures (i.e., greenstick and compression fractures) (see Figure 114-1B in chapter 114, Nutrition in Orthopedics). Compression fractures of vertebrae can cause paralysis and can determine the prognosis of the animal, although complete restoration can occur when

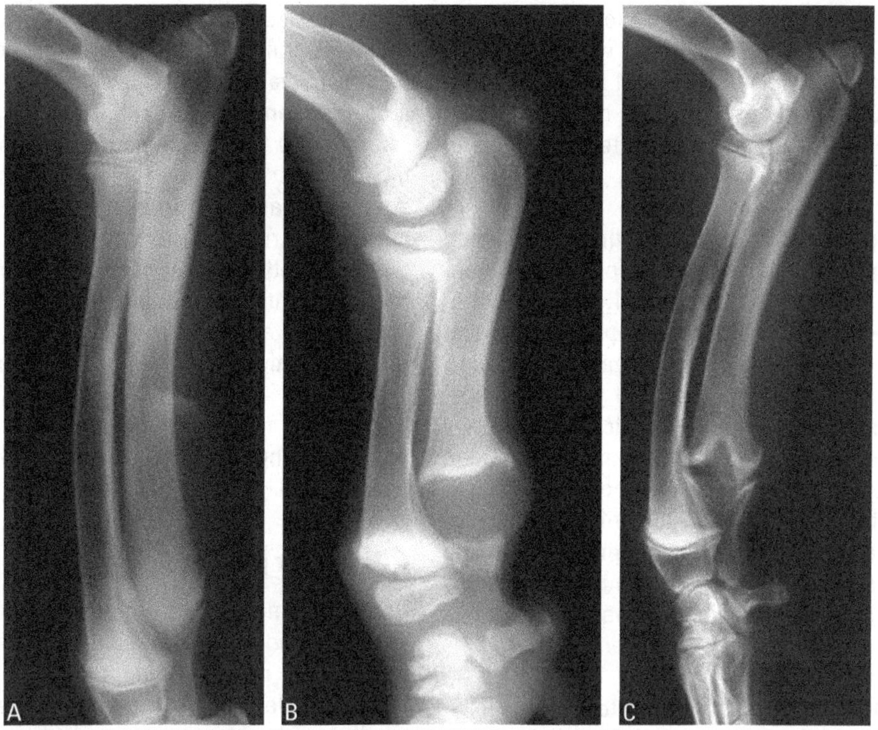

Figure 99-2. Nutritional bone disorders. (A) Young dogs with access at weaning to food with high calcium content developed panosteitis at the age of 4 months, characterized radiologically by increased mineral density in the medulla at different sites.[32] (B) Excessive calcium intake causing hypophosphatemia and hypoparathyroidism with decreased activation of $25OHvitD_3$ caused rickets-like disease with poorly mineralized cortical and cancellous bone and increased width of growth plates.[33] (See also Figure 114-1C of Chapter 114, Nutrition in Orthopedics). (C) Excessive vitamin D intake causes disturbances of endochondral ossification including retained cartilage cones in (especially fast growing) growth plates, even before it causes increased calcium absorption with hypercalcemia.[20] (See also Figure. 114-1D of Chapter 114, Nutrition in Orthopedics).

additional trauma is prevented and adequate therapy is instituted.[9] The increased $1,25(OH)_2vitD_3$ plasma level in alimentary secondary hyperparathyroidism (ASH) explains the normal mineralization of the growth plate cartilage, visible as a white area bordering the growth plates of normal width.[16] This is the most important clinical finding to differentiate between rickets (wide growth plates) and ASH (narrow growth plates), both with thin cortices and possibly greenstick fractures.

The therapy includes strict rest to prevent more damage and normalization of the diet. Normalization of the diet can be accomplished with a complete, balanced food; extra calcium carbonate (50 mg calcium per kg body weight per day) can be added. Because the endogenous $1,25(OH)_2vitD_3$ is increased in hyperparathyroidism, calcium absorption is highly efficient and extra vitamin D is contraindicated in order to avoid further increasing osteoclast activity.[9]

Fractures should be treated only conservatively, i.e., even splints cannot be applied, because the bone will break at the proximal margin of the splint. After mineralization of the skeleton, which is completed within a month, corrective surgery can be considered.

Differential diagnoses are rickets, osteogenesis imperfecta, and renal hyperparathyroidism.

Calcitonin

In the dog calcitonin (CT) is synthesized mainly in the parafollicular or C-cells in the thyroid glands. The synthesis of calcitonin is increased in case of calcium intake and gastrin. Chronic excessive calcium intake, especially at a young age, caused hyperplasia of C-cells.[28] Phosphorus has no known effect on the C-cells, whereas $1,25(OH)_2vitD$ suppresses CT gene expression.[29]

The main function of CT is the storage of calcium in the skeleton. thus preventing (post-)prandial hypercalcemia. It does so via an instant release of secretory granulae filled with CT after stimulation by calcium or gastrin followed by instant retraction of the ruffle border of osteoclasts. Chronic hypercalcemia causes hypercalcitoninism, characterized by an increased CT plasma concentration and/or increased response on calcium intake, not directly related to the total amount of absorbed calcium.[30] As a consequence, osteoclast activity is decreased. In addition, chronic hypercalcemia will suppress parathyroid synthesis and activity, including suppressed osteoclasia.

Nutritional Hypercalcitoninism

Induction of hypercalcitoninism depends on the growth rate of the dog, the age of the animal when the excessive calcium intake starts, and the duration of the period the excessive calcium intake lasts.

Miniature poodles (MPs) raised on a diet with excessive calcium content (3.3% calcium on dry matter base [dmb], which is 3 times the calcium requirement according to NRC 1974 and 6 times the requirement of NRC 1985 (based on an average growing beagle puppy) developed no clinical or radiologically detectable skeletal abnormalities.[31]

Great Dane (GDs) puppies with access to the bitch's diet, which had increased calcium (3.3% on dmb) in order to prevent eclampsia puerperalis (milk fever), during only the period of partial weaning (i.e., 3-6 weeks of age) developed hyperplasia of C cells with excessive response of CT release following a calcium bolus injection. Despite the fact that at 6 weeks of age all pups got standard food (with 1.1% calcium), the dogs with access to the calcium supplanted food at partial weaning revealed this excessive response until 4 months of age. All these dogs developed enostosis (panosteitis eosinofylica) characterized by shifting lameness and white confluent areas in the medullary cavities (Figure 99-2B), whereas the pups with access to the control food from partial weaning onward had normal skeletal development.[32]

GDs with access to the above described bitch's diet (3.3% calcium on dmb) during partial weaning and continued thereafter, developed severe hypercalcemia, hypophosphataemia, and hypoparathyroidism. Calcification of newly formed osteoid and cartilage was much disturbed both as a result of the hampered phosphate absorption causing hypophosphataemia and the disturbed vitamin D metabolism owing to hypoparathyroidism (Figure 99-2C). The skeleton revealed rickets-like abnormalities with thin cortices and wide growth plates. After normalization of the diet, the chief cells became active again and the skeleton mineralized completely.[33]

GDs raised on food with an increased calcium or calcium plus phosphorous content (i.e., 3.3% calcium and 0.9% phosphorous or 3.3% calcium and 3.0% phosphorous, respectively) starting at weaning (i.e., 6 weeks of age) revealed decreased bone remodeling owing to decreased osteoclast activity and disturbances in endochondral ossification, i.e., osteochondrosis. Decreased remodeling was not expressed as a proportional widening of foramina in the cervical area, leading to the so-called wobbler syndrome, as was also described by Hedhammar et al. (1974) who raised GDs with excessive food intake and compared them with restrictedly fed dogs.[34] The disturbances of endochondral ossification were noticed as osteochondrosis in joint cartilage (in the centrocaudal area of the humeral head) and as retained cartilage in the growth plates of ribs, distal ulnae, distal radius, and crus. Disturbances in growth in length developed in these dogs with radius curvus syndrome, elbow incongruities, and deviation of the hind paws[33,35] (see Figure 114-1D and Figure 114-4 of Chapter 114, Nutrition in Orthopedics).

The diagnosis of hypercalcitoninism can only be confirmed by a provocation test with determination of the plasma calcitonin concentration, which warrants a homologous radioimmunoassay for CT.[36] A thorough history with special emphasis on diet composition will not even be informative in many cases, because the calcium intake at pre-weaning is not known to many owners. After weaning calcium intake is often not known either because labels of commercial dog food usually state the "minimal content" rather than the actual content of calcium, unlike special diets with a maximum-claim for calcium (per kg food or per energy content). The diagnosis of hypercalcitoninism refers to the known cause of a series of entities characterized by decreased skeletal remodelling (panosteitis, canine wobbler syndrome) and disturbed endochondral ossification (osteochondrosis, retained cartilage cones) in growth plates and joint cartilage. Although genetics may play a role in the occurrence of these entities (although this is not yet proven), high calcium intake plays an important role in their expression and so far no other causative factor has been indicated.

Therapeutic measures should include normalization of the diet. With osteochondrosis and radius curvus syndrome surgery may be indicated.

Growth Hormone

Growth hormone (GH) originates from the somatotrophic cells in the anterior lobe of the pituitary. Its release is characterized by rhythmic pulses, reflecting the pulsatile delivery of growth hormone-releasing hormone, and intervening troughs. The GH level is under primary control of somatotropin-release inhibiting factor, both of which originate from the hypothalamus. The effects of GH can be divided into rapid or metabolic and slow or hypertrophic actions. The rapid effect includes insulin resistance, inducing enhanced lipolysis and restricted glucose transport across cell membranes. The slow effects are mediated through insulin-like growth factor I (IGF-I), which is synthesized in the liver and in other GH-target cells including chondrocytes. At growth plate level, GH stimulates cell differentiation after clonal expansion through the locally produced IGF-I. IGF-I reached higher levels in growing dogs fed free choice compared with restricted feed controls, whereas dietary protein or carbohydrate content fed iso-energetically to growing dogs did not influence IGF-I levels.[37,38]

GH Excess

Basal plasma concentrations of GH are significantly higher in young dogs of large breeds than in dogs of the same age but of small or miniature breed.[39] The levels of GH in large breed dogs decrease during maturation and are not significantly different from that of small breed dogs at 6 months of age 38 and reach the level range for adult dogs.[38] Prior to that time the pups of giant breed dogs go through a period of plasma GH concentrations comparable with those known to cause acromegaly in adult dogs. The plasma IGF-I levels are higher in large breed young dogs and, although decreasing during life, stay higher in large than in small breed dogs.[38] The heavy overgrowth features known in young puppies of giant breeds are the result of transient juvenile gigantism.[39]

Research dogs, receiving supraphysiologic doses of porcine GH (which has a structure identical to canine GH) in a dosage of 0.5 IU per kg body per day, revealed a steep 2.5- to 3.5-fold increase in plasma IGF-I levels immediately after starting administration of GH at the age of 13 weeks. In addition, a significant increase in weight gain (112 ± 15 vs. 76 ± 10 g in controls [$p < 0.05$]), in alkaline phosphatase, and in mineralization but not in bone resorption could be noticed at 21 weeks of age.[21] This uncoupling of mineralization and resorption may be the cause that, in 2 out of 5 GH-treated dogs and none of the controls, panosteitis-like lesions were noticed on the radiographs. The length of the radius and ulna were 10% greater in the GH-treated dogs than in the controls at 21 weeks of age, with microscopically noticeable thickening of the growth plates without any signs of osteochondrosis. This finding makes it likely that it is not the physiologic transient juvenile gigantism in puppies of large breeds that makes them susceptible to osteochondrosis.[21] Long-term administration of IGF-I did not result in increased body size in miniature poodles.[40]

GH-excess is known as acromegaly and occurs in middle-aged female dogs and middle-aged and elderly, predominantly male, cats. Acromegaly in companion animals is characterized by soft-tissue overgrowth rather than by bony overgrowth, as is characteristic for acromegaly in humans. In dogs, endogenous progesterone or exogenous progestogens induce GH secretion from hyperplastic ductular epithelium in the mammary gland. In dogs, soft-tissue hypertrophy of the mouth, tongue, and pharynx may cause snoring, thickening of the skin, and prognatism, and owing to that, wide interdental spaces.[37,38] In cats, GH excess originates from primary pituitary adenomas and reveals less pronounced physical changes than in dogs with GH excess. In cats, acromegaly may be complicated by diabetes mellitus, neurologic signs owing to tumor growth, and degenerative arthritis with periarticular periosteal reaction.[38] The diagnosis is made by measuring plasma GH concentrations or, even better, by measuring the less fluctuating plasma IGF-I concentration, although hyperglycemia (in cats) and high alkaline phosphate levels in mature dogs can be indicative. The medical history in dogs and imaging techniques in cats can support the diagnosis. Discontinuation of exogenous progestins and/or ovario(hyster)ectomy in dogs, and hypophysectomy in cats are indicated.[33, 41]

GH Deficiency

Congenital growth hormone deficiency causes a retardation of growth. This genetic disease, with autosomal recessive inheritance, is seen in different dog breeds but mainly German shepherd and Carelian bear dogs, as well as in cats.[38] A deficiency exists in both GH and thyroid-stimulating hormone, resulting in short but proportional statue (Figure 99-3A) with growth-plate closure before 1 year of age. Owing to concomitant deficiency of luteinizing hormone and follicle-stimulating hormone, female dwarfs come frequently into heat without ovulating, thus preventing breeding, whereas males produce motile sperm. Owing to developing hypothyroidism, the hair coat is lost and the dogs become dull and inactive at a later age.[37,38]

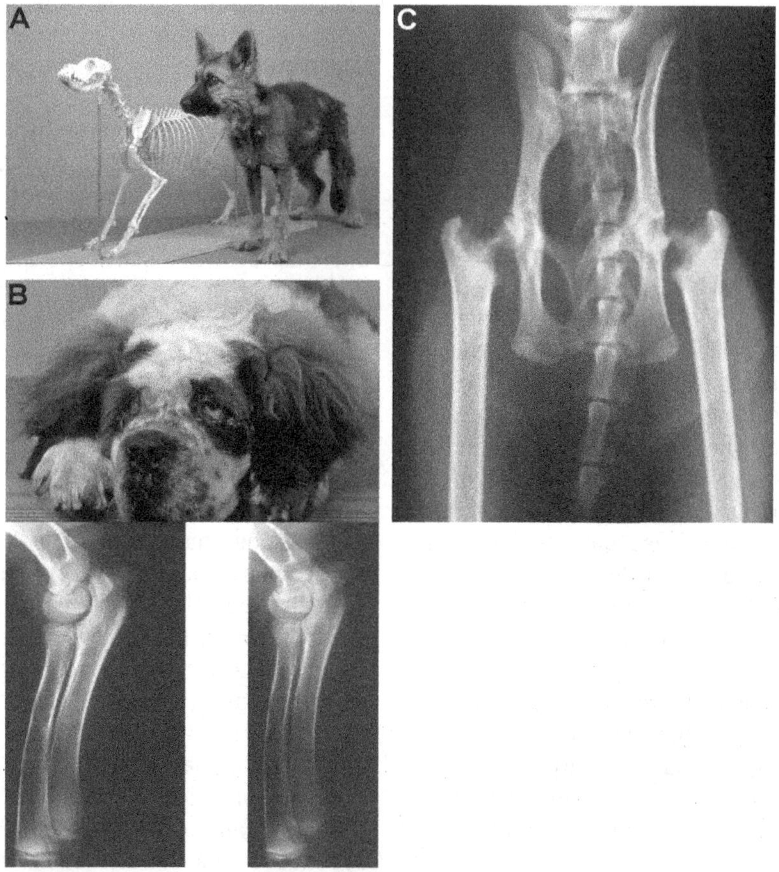

Figure 99-3. Endocrine bone disorders. (A) Congenital growth-hormone deficiency results in proportional dwarfism as revealed from the skeleton and phenotype, respectively, of two adult German shepherd dogs with this genetic disease. (B) Hypothyroidism in a 6-month-old St.Bernard with mental retardation, puffy facial features, and a skeleton with delayed maturation. Skeletal development normal for its age could be reached in 1 month of thyroxine therapy (see anconeal process which should be fused at 6 months of age). (C) Bilateral femoral neck metaphyseal osteopathy in a 14-month-old, early castrated, male cat with gradual progression of lameness and radiologically demonstrated lucency in the femoral necks, which may result in pathologic fractures.

The diagnosis is made based on the typical habitus, and the low GH- and IGF-I-plasma levels. Differential diagnosis is cretinism owing to hypothyroidism (but those dwarfs are disproportional (legs too short), dull, and have a retarded skeletal maturation) and a variety of cardiac, hepatic, gastrointestinal, and renal diseases causing growth failure.[42] Treatment with porcine GH is advocated, but limited experience is available. Progestins, known to induce GH secretion in the mammary gland in both genders with release into systemic circulation, can be used with growth-stimulating effects on the skeleton and hair coat.[37] Without therapy, the prognosis is poor because most dwarfs die at an average age of 4 years from a variety of dysfunctions.

Thyroid Hormones

The thyroid glands secrete tetraiodothyronine (L-thyroxine or T_4) and triiodothyronine (T_3) in a ratio of 5:1, with T3 being 3 to 4 times more biologically potent than T_4. Iodine is actively transported from the extracellular fluid into the thyroid follicular cells. In iodine excess, organic binding in the thyroids is blocked, whereas in iodine deficiency thyroid function is increased. Thyroid hormone in circulation is coupled to binding proteins. The iodine content of meat is less than 10 μg per 100 gram on dmb and decreases even more after cooking, whereas dry dog food has an iodine content of 50 to 100 μg per 100 gram on dmb; for cats the requirement is at least 100 μg per 100 gram on dmb.[7,38]

Hypothyroidism in Young Animals

Hypothyroidism at a young age is characterized by disproportional dwarfism and mental retardation (cretinism). It can be caused by iodine deficiency (owing to a strict carnivore diet without supplementation), lymphocytic thyroiditis, or congenital hypothyroidism (owing to thyroid dysgenesis or defective thyroid hormone synthesis) as described in dogs and cats.[38] In complete athyrosis, symptoms manifest at 2 to 2 months of age with hypoactivity, hypothermia, puffy and retarded facial features, retarded growth in length, and delayed loss of puppy hair (Figure 99-3B). The skull is broadened, the tongue may be too big for the mouth, and mental dullness and retardation are reported by the owners. Since thyroid hormone influences both the activity of chondrocyte progenitors and the maturation of chondrocytes during endochondral ossification, hypothyroidism leads to skeletal abnormalities. Radiographic investigation of long bones and vertebral bodies reveal retarded skeletal maturation with delayed appearance of secondary ossification centers, delayed growth in length, but normal cortices and growth plates.[43]

Differential diagnoses can include dwarfism (although proportional and lively), owing to GH deficiency, rickets (with thin cortices, wide growth plates), secondary hyperparathyroidism (thin cortices, normal growth plate) and chondrodysplasia (normal cortices, normal growth plate, abnormal alignment and/or joint congruities).

The diagnosis can be made by measuring plasma concentrations of thyroid hormone, thyroid scintigraphy, measuring an increased endogenous thyroid-stimulating hormone plasma level, and by comparing radiographs of the patient with breed- and age-matched controls.[38]

The therapy includes normalization of the diet (in case of iodine deficiency) or thyroxine therapy at a dose rate of 10 μg/kg body weight twice daily for dogs and half that dosage for cats.[38] After 1 month the skeleton is expected to reach the stage of the biologic age of the animal (Figure 99-3B), although radiologic control may reveal pathologic abnormalities, and mental retardation can stay manifest.

Hypothyroidism in Adults

Often as a result of autoimmune disease, thyroid tissue disappears, leading to a slowly occurring hypothyroidism, characterized by slowing of mental and physical activities, disinterest, thin hair coat, thick skin with puffy appearance owing to myxedema. The patient can reveal lameness because of myositis in the skeletal muscles and increased plasma creatinine kinase activity.[38] It has been demonstrated that skeletal muscle in a hypothyroid cat is more fatigable, with changes in the isometric twitch speed properties.[44] In addition, lameness characteristic for osteoarthrosis can be seen owing to mucopolysaccharide accumulation in the joint capsules; often this occurs in multiple joints, leading to a stiff gait rather than to lameness. In some cases severe front leg lameness, eventually non-weight bearing, is seen owing to myxedema formation in the carpal tunnel, with median nerve entrapment as can occur around the facial nerve. It is the author's experience that the front legs are never equally affected. The diagnosis is made by excluding tumor (e.g., osteosarcoma, neurofibroma) in the affected leg and by diagnosing hypothyroidism.[43]

With medical treatment of hypothyroidism (see earlier) the prognosis for animals with myositis and nerve impingement is good, whereas it is guarded for those with osteoarthrosis. In fact, the dog will improve mentally earlier than its joint capsules heal, and thus over-use can make the complaint of osteoarthrosis even worse. In the healing period, the dog should be leash restricted.[43] Other neurologic disorders that may coincide with hypothyroidism (including myasthenia gravis, vestibular disease, laryngeal paralysis) may not result in resolution of the signs.[45]

Sex Hormones

Skeletal growth and puberty are connected as the sex hormones testosterone and estrogen play a role in cartilage growth and endochondral ossification. Although both hormones are not essential, they play a role in growth, skeletal development, and maintenance of the adult skeleton. Androgens stimulates both chondrocyte hyperplasia and maturation. The anabolic effects of testosterone are associated with augmentation of pulsatile GH secretion. This drives longitudinal bone growth and epiphyseal growth-plate maturation, which culminates in cessation of skeletal elongation. The effect of estrogens (following aromatization of androgens and stimulation of estrogen receptors) depends on its concentration: low concentration stimulates cartilage growth, whereas high concentration stops cartilage growth. It has been demonstrated that many of the growth-promoting effects of the sex steroids are mediated through estrogens rather than androgens. In addition, skeletal maturation with growth-plate closure is also estrogen-dependent in both sexes.[46] Androgens stimulate osteoblast proliferation and antagonize osteoclast-activating effects of PTH, leading to increased cortical bone formation. Estrogens repress osteoclastogenesis and stimulate endosteal and trabecular bone formation, both increasing bone strength.[46]

Sex Hormone Deficiency

Estrogen or testosterone deficiency owing to castration occurs soon after surgery. Especially in female dogs, investigations have been performed to study bone strength and composition following ovariohysterectomy, as a model for osteoporosis in postmenopausal women. However, dogs differ considerably in this regard, perhaps owing to the mean estric cycle of 6 months in dogs. In a study in beagle dogs it revealed that 10 months postovariohysterectomy, cancellous bone remodeling was not significantly different from presurgical levels.[47] No reports show that early castration will cause osteoporosis or its related pathologic fractures in companion animals.

In a study comparing early (at 7 weeks), late (at 7 months), and no castration in dogs, it revealed that growth-plate closure was postponed in case of castration, even more so in early castration. Because growth velocity did not differ among groups, but the growth period was elongated, the final bone length was increased in both sexes especially in the early castrated dogs.[48] Similarly, in cats, gonadectomy in both genders either at 7 weeks or 7 months of age revealed a delayed closure of the distal radial physis compared with the intact cats.[49] In cats, the growth plates of the proximal femur normally close at 7 to10 months of age, but this occurs much later in early gonadectomized males. This can increase the vulnerability of early castrated cats for physeal fractures in the proximal or distal femur even at adult age.

Femoral neck metaphyseal osteopathy is seen incidentally, mainly in early castrated male cats. The cat has a vague onset of hind-limb lameness with progression to severe lameness with pain on extension of the hip. Radiologic investigation reveals lucency in the proximal metaphyseal area of the femur with pathologic fracture in a limited number of cases (Figure 99-3C). Histopathologic evalutaion may reveal thickening and splitting of the articular cartilage with necrotic bone and vascular congestion at the epiphysis, with an increased number of osteoclasts. Damage to the blood supply of the femoral head and neck is hypothesized with secondary osteoporosis and pathologic fracture,[50] although the pathophysiology of this entity needs to be further elucidated.

References

1. Jezyk PF: Constitutional disorders of the skeleton in dogs and cats. *In* Textbook of Small Animal Orthopedics. Newton CD, Nunamaker DM (eds). Philadelphia: JB Lippincott, 1985, p. 637.

2. Brocks BAW, Hazewinkel HAW: Abnormal skeletal growth in the Labrador retriever: a case report of 5 dogs. Vet Comp Orthop Traum 18:25, 2005.

3. Casella JP, Barber P, Catterall AC, et al: A morphometric analysis of osteoid collagen fibril diameter in osteogenesis imperfecta. Bone 15:329, 1994.

4. Seliger F, Leeb T, Peters M, et al: Osteogenesis imperfecta in two litters of Dachshunds. Vet Pathol 40:530, 2003.

5. Millington-Ward S, McMahon HP, Farrar GJ: Emerging therapeutic approaches for osteogenesis imperfecta. Trends Mol Medicine 11:299, 2005.

6. Malik R, Allan GS, Howlett CR, et al: Osteodysplasia in Scottish Fold cats. Aust Vet J 77:85, 1999.

7. Hubler M, Volkert M, Kaser-Hotz B, et al: Palliative irradiation of Scottish Fold osteochondrodysplasia. Vet Radiol Ultrasound 45:582, 2004.

8. Mathews KG, Koblik PD, Knoeckel MJ, et al: Resolution of lameness associated with Scottish fold osteodystrophy following bilateral ostectomies and pantarsal arthodesis; a case report. J Am Anim Hosp Assoc 31:280, 1995.

9. Hazewinkel HAW, Mott J: Osteoarticular affections in puppies and adult dogs; nutritional approach. *In* Royal Canine Health Nutrition Encyclopaedia. Paris: Diffomedia, 2005.

10. Pobisch R, Onderscheka K: Die Vitamin A-hypervitaminose bei der Katz. Wiener Tierärztliche Monatschrift 63:334, 1976.

11. MacDonald ML, Rogers QR, Morris JG: Teratogenic effects of chronic ingestion of high levels of vitamin A in cats. J Anim Physiol Anim Nutr (Berl) 87:42, 2003.

12. Donoghue S, Szanto J, Kronfeld DS: Hypervitaminosis A in a dog; an example of hospital dietics. *In* Nutrition, Malnutrition and Dietetics in the Dog and Cat. Edney ATB (ed). Waltham Center Press, 1987, p. 94.

13. Mellanby T: The part played by an "accessory factor" in the production of experimental rickets. J Physiol 52:1, 1918.

14. How KL, Hazewinkel HAW, Mol JA: Dietary vitamin D dependen¬ce of cat and dog due to inadequate cutaneous synthesis of vitamin D. J Gen Comp Endocr 96:12, 1994.

15. Morris JG, Earle KE, Anderson PA: Plasma 25-hydroxyvitaminD in growing kittens is related to dietary intake of cholecalciferol. J Nutr 129:909, 1999.

16. Gascon-Barré M, Huet PM: Role of the liver in the homeostasis of calciferol metabolism in the dog. Endocrinology 110:563, 1982.

17. Shepard RM, DeLuca HF: Plasma concentrations of vitamin D_3 and its metabolites in the rat as influenced by vitamin D3 or 25-hydroxyvitamin D3 intakes. Arch Biochem Biophys 202:43, 1980.

18. Pettifor JM, Bikle DD, Cavaleros M, et al: Serum levels of free 1,25 dihydroxyvitaminD in vitamin D toxicity. Ann Intern Med 122:511, 1995.

19. Hazewinkel HAW, Tryfonidou MA: Vitamin D3 metabolism in dogs, Mol Cell Endocrinol 197:23, 2002.

20. Tryfonidou MA, Holl MS, Stevenhagen JJ, et al: 135-fold vitamin D_3 supplementation severely disturbs the endochondral ossification in growing dogs. Domest Anim Endocrinol 24:265, 2003.

21. Tryfonidou MA, Hazewinkel HAW: Different effects of physiologically and pharmacologically increased growth hormone levels on cholecalciferol metabolism at prepubertal age. J Steroid Biochem Mol Biol. 89-90:49, 2004.

22. Haddad P, Gascon-Barré M, Brault G, et al: Influence of calcium or 1,25 dihydroxyvitamin D_3 supplementation on the hepatic microsomal and in vivo metabolism of vitamin D_3 in vitamin D depleted rat. J Clin Invest 78:1529, 1986.

23. Schulze C, Rothuizen J, van Sluijs FJ, et al: Extrahepatic biliary atresia in a border collie. J Small Anim Pract 41:27, 2000.

24. Tryfonidou MA, Oosterlaken-Dijksterhuis MA, Mol JA, et al: 24-hydroxylase: potential key regulator in hypervitaminosis D_3 in growing dogs. Am J Physiol Endocrinol Metab 284:E505, 2003.

25. Shinki T, Jin CH, Nishmura A, et al : Parathyroid hormone inhibits 25-hydroxyvitamin D_3 mRNA expression stimulated by 1α,25-dihydroxyvitamin D_3 in rat kidney but not in intestine. J Biol Chem 267:13757, 1992.

26. Goff JP, Reinhardt TA, Engstrom GW, et al: Effect of dietary calcium or phosphorus restriction and 1,25-dihydroxyvitamin D administration on rat intestine 24-hydroxylase Endocrinol 131:101, 1992.

27. Weisbrode SE, Capen CC: The ultrastructural effects of parathyroid-hormone, calcitonin, and vitamin D on bone. *In* Bone and Cartilage in Health and Disease. Bonucci E, Motta PM (eds). Dordrecht: Kluwer Academic Publishers, 1990, p. 253.

28. Goedegebuure SA, Hazewinkel HAW: Morphological findings in young dogs chronically fed a diet containing excess calcium. Vet Pathol 23:594, 1986.

29. Gagel RF, Peleg S: Thyroid C cells and medullary carcinoma as target tissues for vitamin D action. *In* Vitamin D. Feldman D, Glorieux FH, Wesly J (eds). San Diego: Academic Press, 1997, p. 369.

30. Cooper CH, Bolman RM, Lineman WM: Interrelationship between calcium, calcemic hormones and gastrointestinal hormones. Recent Prog Hormone Res 34:259, 1978.

31. Hazewinkel HAW, Schoenmakers I: Influence of protein, minerals and vitamin D on skeletal developments of dogs. Vet Clin Nutr 2:93, 1995.

32. Hazewinkel HAW, Nap RC, Schoenmakers I, et al: Dietary influence on development of enostosis in young dogs. Vet Surg 29:279, 2000.

33. Schoenmakers I, Hazewinkel HAW, Voorhout G, et al: Effect of diets with different calcium and phosphorus contents on the skeletal development and blood chemistry of growing great danes. Vet Rec 147:652, 2000.

34. Hedhammar A, Wu FM, Krook L, et al: Over nutrition and skeletal disease. An experimental study in growing Great Dane dogs. Cornell Vet 64 (Suppl 5):5, 1974.

35. Hazewinkel HAW, Goedegebuure SA, Poulos PW, et al: Influ¬ences of chronic calcium excess on the skeleton of growing Great Danes. J Am Anim Hosp Assoc 21:377, 1985.

36. Hazewinkel HAW, Schoenmakers I, Pelling D, et al: Biological potency and radioimmunoassay of canine calcitonin. Domest Anim Endocrinol 17:333, 1999.

37. Kooistra HS: Acromegaly and pituitary dwarfism. *In* Textbook of Veterinary Internal Medicine. 6th ed. Ettinger SJ, Feldman EC (eds). St Louis: Elsevier, 2005, p. 1497.

38. Rijnberk A: Clinical endocrinology of dogs and cats. Dordrecht: Kluwer Academic Publishers, 1996.

39. Nap RC, Hazewinkel HAW, Mol JA: Prepubertal differences in plasma growth hormone and IGF-I concentrations related to adult body size in the dog. J Endocrinol Invest 15:91, 1992.

40. Guler HP, Binz K, Eigenmann JE, et al: Small stature and insulin-like growth factors: prolonged treatment of mini-poodles with recombinant human insulin-like growth factor. Acta Endocrinol 121:456, 1989.

41. Meij BP: Hypophysectomy as a treatment for canine and feline Cushing's disease. Vet Clin North Am / SAC 31:1015, 2001.

42. Gelens HC, Ihle SL: Failure to grow Vet Clin North Am / SAC 29:989, 1999.

43. Hazewinkel HAW, Nap RC: Hormonelle Erkrankungen des Skelettsystems. *In* Kleintierkrankheiten Band 3, Orthopädische Chirurgie und Traumatologie. Bonath KH, Prieur WP (eds). Stuttgart: Ulmer Verlag, 1998, p. 487.

44. Roy RR, Zhong H, Hodgson JA, et al: Effect of altered thyroid state on the in situ mechanical properties of adult cat soleus. Cells Tissues Organs 173:162, 2003.

45. Jaggy A, Oliver JE, Ferguson DC, et al: Neurological manifestations of hypothyroidism; a retrospective study of 29 dogs. J Vet Intern Med 8:328, 1994.

46. Vanderschueren D, Vandenput L, Boonen S: Reversing sex steroid deficiency and optimizing skeletal development in the adolescent with gonadal failure. Endocr Dev 8:150, 2005.

47. Boyce RW, Franks AF, Jankowsky ML, et al: Sequential histomorphometric changes in cancellous bone from ovariohysterectomized dogs. J Bone Miner Res 5:947, 1990.

48. Salmeri KR, Bloomberg MS, Scruggs SL, et al: Gonadectomy in immature dogs: effects on skeletal, physical, and behavioural development. J Am Vet Med Assoc 198:1193, 1991.

49. Root MV, Johnston SD, Olson PN: The effect of prepubertal and postpubertal gonadectomy on radial physeal closure in male and female domestic cats. Vet Radiol Ultrasound 37:363, 1996.

50. Queen J, Bennett D, Carmichael S, et al: Femoral neck metaphyseal osteopathy in the cat. Vet Rec 142:159, 1998.

Chapter 100

Canine Osteochondrosis

Jennifer L. Lansdowne
Curtis W. Probst

Osteochondrosis (OC) is a disorder affecting the process of endochondral ossification in growing people and animals including dogs, horses, pigs, and chickens.[1] Although the clinical manifestations associated with OC are well described, the etiology and pathogenesis are not yet completely understood. Osteochondrosis affects the articular-epiphyseal and physeal cartilage cells and can be expressed clinically as osteochondritis dissecans lesions, fragmentation of the medial coronoid process of the ulna (FCP), ununited anconeal process (UAP), retained cartilage cores, Osgood-Schlatter syndrome (OC of the tibial tuberosity), slipped epiphysis, or incomplete ossification of the humeral condyle. All these conditions are considered to have a similar pathogenesis. Osteochondrosis is a common cause of secondary osteoarthritis in people and domestic animals.[2] Osteochondritis dissecans (OCD) is the most common clinical manifestation of osteochondrosis. Although osteochondritis is a misnomer because it implies inflammation of bone and cartilage, it has become entrenched in veterinary medical terminology. Synonyms for OCD found in the literature include osteochondrosis dissecans and dyschondroplasia. Regardless of the terminology, to the veterinarian OCD indicates a dissecting cartilaginous lesion between the bone epiphysis and articular surface. Lesions of canine OCD have been described on the cervical vertebrae, glenoid surface of the scapula, proximal humerus, distal humerus, distal radius, femoral head, distal femur, tibial tarsal bone, and most recently, the lumbosacrum.

This chapter is an overview of the normal growth and ossification of the canine appendicular skeleton, followed by an in-depth review of the pathology and pathogenesis of osteochondrosis. Pathogenic factors specific to the shoulder, elbow, stifle, tarsus, lumbosacrum, and incomplete ossification of the humeral condyle are also described.

Normal Growth and Ossification of the Canine Skeleton

The growing canine skeleton is composed of cartilage and bone. Three distinct embryonic lineages are responsible for the formation of the skeleton.[3,4] The craniofacial skeleton arises from cranial neural crest cells, the vertebral skeleton is derived from paraxial mesoderm (somites), and the limb skeleton is formed from the lateral plate mesodermal cells.[3,4] Cells from each lineage migrate to locations in the embryo where bone will eventually form and there they develop into characteristic mesenchymal condensations of high cell density.[3,4] These condensations develop into osteoblasts or chondrocytes.[3,4] The cells in the region of the craniofacial skeleton develop into osteoblasts and directly form bone by intramembranous ossification. In the remaining skeleton, chondrocytes develop first and provide a framework of cartilage models. The cartilage models are replaced by bone and bone marrow through the endochondral ossification process.

The cartilage models of future appendicular bones grow by appositional and interstitial growth and quickly resemble the future bone in shape and relative size.[3,5] As capillaries enter and supply the surrounding perichondrium, osteoblasts are formed from circulating progenitor cells and begin to lay down a thin layer of bone around the cartilage. At the same time, the chondrocytes in the center become hypertrophic. As the collar of bone and area of hypertrophy continue to enlarge, the matrix surrounding the hypertrophic chondrocytes begins to calcify by incorporating hydroxyapatite. This results in a network of trabeculae with a cartilaginous core, called primary spongy bone. Primary spongy bone is rapidly resorbed and secondary spongy bone with new trabeculae is formed. The actual process of replacing calcified cartilage (endochondral ossification) occurs in the mid-diaphysis of long bones first. The initial area of ossification is called the primary ossification center and extends in each direction toward the end of the cartilage model. As the process continues, secondary ossification centers develop in each epiphysis. A plate of cartilage remains between the ossified secondary and primary centers and is responsible for the longitudinal growth of long bones.[3] This plate is called the physeal growth plate (Figure 100-1). The cartilage on the end of the secondary ossification center that is closest to the joint is termed the articular-epiphyseal cartilage complex (AECC). Epiphyseal cartilage of this complex is responsible for growth of the epiphysis and the development of its shape. At maturity in normal dogs, articular cartilage is all that remains on the surface of the bony epiphyses.

The process of ossification starts at weeks 3 to 4 in the canine fetus, but cannot be detected radiographically until 3 weeks prior to parturition. When a puppy is born, the epiphyses are still cartilaginous with no or only small secondary centers of ossification present. By 2 to 4 months of age, depending on breed, only the physeal growth plates and articular cartilages remain unossified.[6]

Normal Growth of the Articular-Epiphyseal Cartilage Complex

Articular cartilage is divided into three regions: superficial, middle and deep (Figure 100-2).[7] The superficial region is immediately under the surface of the joint and consists of the lamina splendens (composed of filamentous proteins that bind proteinaceous material and provide lubrication for joint surfaces) and the gliding zone (cells are parallel to the surface).[8] The middle region has cells arranged perpendicularly to the surface of the articular cartilage and is divided into the transitional zone (characterized by cell activity and interstitial growth, allowing the articular cartilage to cover the epiphysis during growth) and the radial zone (composed of cells lined up in irregular columns).

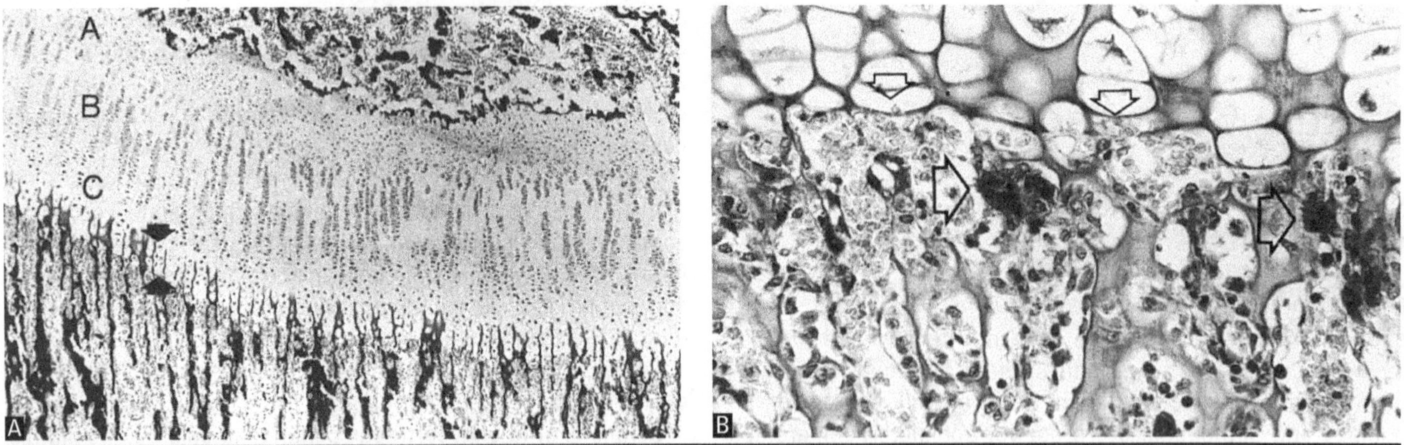

Figure 100-1. Histologic sections that demonstrate the mechanism of longitudinal growth as seen morphologically in the growth plate and the metaphysis. (A) Undecalcified section of the proximal tibial metaphyseal growth plate with part of the epiphysis (above) and the metaphysis (below) from a 9-day-old rabbit. In the growth plate, the zone of germinal (resting) cells (A), proliferating (columnar) cells (B), transitional (hypertrophying) cells (C), and vesiculated cells (between arrows) are seen. The matrix in the longitudinal bars separating the columns of vesiculated cells is calcined (von Kossa's stain; 50x). (B) Section of the junction between the proximal tibial metaphyseal growth plate (top) and the metaphysis (bottom) in a newbom puppy. It illustrates how the horizontal bars of the cartilage matrix are eroded by vascular sprouts (small arrows) and how chondroclasts (large arrows) resorb calcified matrix in the longitudinal bars (Hematoxylin and eosin (H&E) stain; 250x). (From Summer-Smith, G. (Ed.): Bone in Clinical Orthopedics. Philadelphia, W.B. Saunders, 1982.)

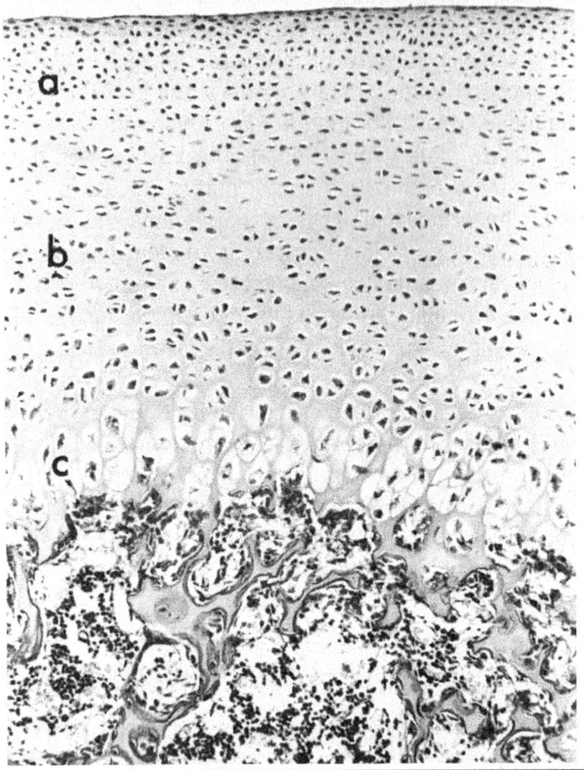

Figure 100-2. Histologic section of the articular cartilage of the proximal humerus from a 9-day-old rabbit. The immature joint cartilage is the growth cartilage of the epiphysis. The germinal (resting) cells (a) are located about four or five cell layers away from the joint surface. Deeper in the cartilage is the zone of proliferating cells (b), and then the zone of hypertrophying (vesiculated) cells (c), where the cartilage is invaded by vessels paving the way for ossification (H&E stain; 50x). (From Summer-Smith, G. (Ed.): Bone in Clinical Orthopedics. Philadelphia, W.B. Saunders, 1982).

The superficial and middle regions are responsible for the expansion of the articular surface during development. The deep region is composed of calcified cartilage and subchondral bone supporting the articular cartilage. Vascular invasion of calcified tissue occurs here, followed by endochondral ossification. The deep region is responsible for the development of epiphyseal bone. A thin wavy hematoxylin-stained line called the tidemark can be seen histologically separating the non-calcified tissue of the middle region from the calcified tissue of the deep region in adults.[5]

Normal Growth of the Physeal Growth Plate

The physeal growth plate and the epiphyseal component of the AECC differentiate into four morphologically and chemically distinct zones during development (Figure 100-3). From the epiphysis toward the metaphysis, they are the resting (reserve or germinal), proliferative, hypertrophic, and calcifying zones; orderly maturation of cells in these zones is required for proper endochondral ossification.[1,3] The cells of the resting zone are small and relatively inactive. The proliferative adjacent zone has both local and systemic growth factors that stimulate chondrocyte proliferation. In this zone clonal expansion of proliferated cells takes place toward the metaphysis (cartilage-bone junction) where the cells enlarge, arrange in columns and eventually hypertrophy.[3] The cells of the hypertrophic zone are highly metabolically active, but do not divide. The matrix surrounding the hypertrophic cells continues to calcify, and the lowermost cells undergo apoptosis (regulated cell death).[3] Osteoclasts and osteoblasts, which have developed from progenitor cells brought in by invading blood vessels, remove the calcified cartilage and deposit bone, respectively. When maturity is reached, the metaphyses and diaphysis are united and the cartilaginous portion is completely replaced by bone. With few exceptions, in mature animals the only remaining cartilage is the hyaline cartilage of the joint surfaces.

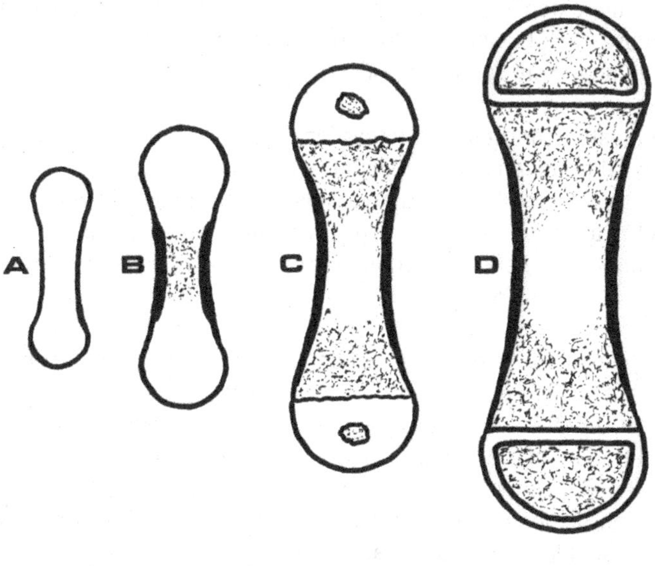

Figure 100-3. Schematic drawing of the development of a long bone. A, Early in fetal life, the long bone consists only of cartilage. B, When the fetus is about 30 days old, it has some cortical and trabecular bone at midshaft. The cortical bone is formed by periosteal apposition, whereas the trabecular bone is formed by endochondral ossification. C, In the newbom puppy, the entire diaphysis (which includes the two metaphyses) is made of cortical and trabecular bone including bone marrow, while the epiphyses have just begun to ossify. D, When the puppy is a few months old, the only cartilage left in the long bone is the one in the growth plates and in the immature joint.

Vascular Supply and Nutrition of Epiphyseal Cartilage

The epiphyseal cartilage of both the physeal growth plate and the AECC have a well developed blood supply through a network of cartilage canals.[1,9,10] The cartilage canals regress as the animal ages and the growth cartilage becomes thinner. The physiologic process of this regression is termed chondrification.[10] Chondrification causes the vessels, nerve fibers, and stromal cells within the canals to be substituted with cartilage without pathologic effects on the surrounding tissue.[10] Nutrition is supplied to the AECC by these blood vessels, in addition to synovial fluid.[1] The contribution of each source depends on age, species, and anatomic location.[1] In the adult, articular cartilage receives a minor contribution from vessels of the subchondral bone, obtaining most of its nutrients from the synovial fluid.

Pathophysiology

Pathology and Morphology

Osteochondrosis is characterized by failure of normal differentiation of cartilage to bone during endochondral ossification; neither matrix calcification nor vascular penetration occurs in focal areas of the growing epiphyseal/articular cartilage, resulting in retention of cartilage rather than conversion to bone.[1] Although abnormal focal regions of retained cartilage are avascular, they receive nutrients from diffusion of synovial fluid and continue to grow. This results in focal abnormally thickened cartilage, which is less resistant (more compliant) to mechanical stresses. The increased thickness eventually prevents adequate diffusion of nutrients and results in a disturbance of the metabolism of the basal layer. Degeneration and necrosis of the chondrocytes at the base of the OC lesion are the ultimate outcome, which can lead to the separation of the retained cartilage from the underlying calcified tissue. This phenomenon occurs along the tidemark and rarely involves subchondral bone.[11] The resulting fragments are characteristic of OCD lesions when they develop in the AECC.

In the AECC the earliest identifiable histologic lesion is termed *osteochondrosis latens* and is identified as focal necrosis of the cartilage canal vessels and the surrounding cartilage of the resting zone of the epiphyseal cartilage.[10] If the necrotic cartilage resists resorption and persists as a cone of dead tissue surrounded by bone it is termed *osteochondrosis manifesta* and appears grossly as an area of delayed endochondral ossification.[10] Because this necrotic cartilage is soft and friable, it does not provide a suitable foundation for the over-laying AECC; thus, even minimal trauma can lead to fissure and fracture formation. When these fissures and fractures extend from the necrotic tissue to the articular surface it is termed *osteochondritis dissecans*.[10] In pigs and horses, early lesions of OC of the AECC have been associated with abnormalities in cartilage canal blood vessels.[10,12-15] These abnormalities have been hypothesized to cause local ischemia and chondronecrosis.

Spontaneous repair attempts of the OCD lesions usually occur beneath the cleft with granulation tissue production, fibrogenesis, and osteoblastic and osteoclastic activity. Subchondral bone formation occurs at the base of the granulation tissue, but does not extend past the tidemark. The granulation tissue undergoes chondrification and may even develop some hyaline cartilage. Continuous passive motion during healing may encourage hyalinization of the fibrocartilage.[5] The success of the reparative process is related to the size and extent of the defect as well as time from development. Small defects can completely heal through matrix flow and intrinsic repair (chondrocytes, proliferation and increased extra-cellular matrix production). In large defects, however, fibrocartilage degenerates within one year, which leads to secondary osteoarthritis from release of breakdown products.[5,16]

Osteochondrosis of the AECC can lead to OCD lesions in the shoulder, elbow, stifle, hock, and vertebral articular facets, and FCP.[17] Two types of OCD lesions of the AECC exist. Type I OCD lesions are the classic form and occur when the lesion is in or near the center of a convex joint surface. In these cases, the cartilage flap does not have contact with any vascular tissue, such as the joint capsule. As a result, the flap eventually becomes detached and floats in the joint. This flap may be resorbed or may increase in size as a result of nourishment from synovial fluid. When the flap is free in the joint and becomes ossified it is termed a loose body or "joint mouse." These lesions typically occur in the humeral head, medial condyle of the humerus, and the lateral and medial femoral condyles.

Type II OCD lesions occur at the periphery of the joint surface providing contact between the cartilage flap and the joint capsule or ligament. Eventually the flap will undergo endochondral ossification and not produce a joint mouse. Osteochondritis dissecans lesions of the medial or lateral ridge of the talus and sacrum, as well as fragmented coronoid process and ununited anconeal process, are typically type II lesions.[6]

Clinically, OC lesions can be divided into four grades, with grade I the most mild and grade IV the most severe. Grade I classification is given in cases with grossly normal articular cartilage and a small defect in the subchondral bone, whereas grade IV is given when a cartilage flap is separated from the bone. Grades II and III are given subjectively to cases that fall between mild and severe. Because animals are not in pain until the fissure reaches the articular cartilage, grade IV (OCD lesion) is the most common form diagnosed by veterinarians.

In the physeal growth plate, early lesions of OC are much less obvious than in the AECC until after failure of endochondral ossification has occurred. In the growth pate, retained cartilage is composed of viable hypertrophic chondrocytes. Retention of cartilage in the growth plate usually does not lead to necrosis, probably owing to the presence of vessels in the cartilage. The majority of these lesions heal uneventfully. Clinical signs may manifest if a pathologic fracture occurs within the thickened cartilage or, more importantly, if it occurs at the distal end of the ulna. Incongruity of the radius and ulna can occur owing to slowed growth of the ulna relative to the radius. Occasionally, incongruity can be seen as a result of OC of the distal radial growth plate. Osteochondrosis of the physeal growth plate can result in UAP, retained cartilaginous cores of the distal ulna, and genu valgum (knock-knee).[17]

Pathogenesis

The underlying lesions of osteochondrosis occur in the growing animal, although they may not show clinical signs until adulthood.[1] The primary lesion of OCD is a dissecting cartilaginous separation between calcified and noncalcified tissues.[5] The necrotic base of the OC lesion is the starting point for fissures. If the necrotic cartilage is large enough and/or there is sufficient trauma has occurred, a cleft will form from the articular cartilage to the subchondral bone. This results in synovitis from release of inflammatory mediators, joint effusion, and clinical evidence of lameness. It has been suggested that premature disruption of the nutritional function of the vasculature of the cartilage canals results in cartilage necrosis (osteochondrosis latens).[18] Recently it has been shown that there is premature cessation of blood supply to the epiphyseal growth cartilage caused by focal interruption of the vessels leading from the bone marrow into the cartilage canals.[10] This study proposed that OC occurs secondary to ischemic necrosis caused by microtrauma to the vessels of the cartilage canals in the transition zone between bone and cartilage.[10] It has also been suggested, based on the finding of an increased amount of lipid in OCD cartilage flaps, that delayed calcification may be a result of a lipid metabolism defect.[19]

The effects on the subchondral bone adjacent to the OCD lesion are typically myelofibrosis and trabecular remodeling. It can be quite extensive, but necrosis of the bone is not a prominent feature of OCD. Subchondral bone cyst formation is a possible, but uncommon, sequela to OCD.

Suggested contributing factors for OC development are trauma, familial/hereditary predisposition, ischemia, rapid growth, and dietary factors.[1] The etiology is likely multifactorial, with no single factor accounting for all aspects of the disease. Our current understanding of the contributions of trauma and genetic factors is discussed below.

Trauma is the most widely considered factor in all species regarding the etiology of OC[1] and is important in the progression of OC to OCD. Trauma does not have to be severe to cause separation of cartilage and bone in the abnormal cartilage of OC. The gross and histologic appearances of the chronic lesions (lesions with a cartilaginous flap) support this theory. The usual locations are in areas with increased biomechanical stresses.[1] It has been hypothesized that epiphyseal cartilage is inherently weaker and thus more vulnerable to trauma than articular cartilage,[20] however, no research currently supports this concept. Research in swine has shown that, although both the medial and lateral condyle can be affected with OC, the most clinically relevant lesions occur on the medial condyle.[21] Indeed, the medial condyle receives most of the weight-bearing forces. Most cases of OC have an insidious onset and although purely traumatic osteochondral fractures can occur, particularly in people following severe automobile accidents, they are not considered to be OC. Olsson hypothesized that local traumatic factors within joints, which vary with location, was a principal cause of canine OC.[6] He theorized that repeated microtrauma in predilection sites was crucial to the development of OC.[22] Examples of local microtrauma include impingement of the dorsolateral area of the humeral head in the shoulder joint or forced contact between the medial aspect of the lateral femoral condyle and lateral part of the intercondylar eminence in the stifle joint of animals with genu valgum. Olsson also hypothesized that transient incongruence in growth rates between the radius and ulna was a factor in ununited coronoid and ununited anconeal process as well as distal humeral OC. Further support for local microtrauma comes from studies performed in calves, which found that when they were housed on hard surfaces the prevalence and severity of OC was increased.[23] Another study compared pigs that were loaded into crates by dropping them from varying heights under 1 meter to pigs that were not loaded.[24] This study found that OC lesions were more severe and prevalent in pigs that were loaded. Unfortunately these theories have only been evaluated in the chronic stages of the disease and not in the early stages, thus the true pathogenesis remains unknown. However, because most early lesions heal, it is possible that, if joints are protected from trauma during the vulnerable development stage, clinically relevant disease could be reduced.[1] Trauma may be influenced by heritable factors, such as anatomic conformation and/or quality of the surrounding bone and cartilage, and facilitated and/or aggravated by mechanical stress to the area in the limited time period that important blood vessels exist.[10]

Familial cases of OC have been reported in people, including cases in identical twins.[1] Domestic pigs, which have been genetically selected for certain traits, have a high prevalence of OC, regardless of breed, whereas wild and miniature pigs do not.[25] A polygenetic mode of inheritance of elbow joint OCD in Labrador retrievers has been shown.[26] Dog breeds that reach a mature weight of more than 20 kg tend to be more commonly affected with OC.[1] This prevalence appears to be increased in animals in which rapid growth is emphasized. There also tends to be a greater male incidence, possibly owing to a more rapid growth rate when compared with females. It has been proposed that low serum concentrations of the main metabolites of vitamin D3 found in growing large-breed dogs fed standard dog food may play a role in disturbances in endochondral ossification.[27,28] Thus, other contributing factors result in OC, not just overall growth rate and feeding regimen. It is unlikely that nutrition, hormonal influences, and trauma alone could account for the development of OC.

In general, the larger the defect the more likely a dog is to have a persistent lameness. In addition, the larger the lesion the more likely the opposite joint surface is to develop a "kissing lesion." The kissing lesion occurs as a result of lack of normal physiologic compression on the opposite articular surface, which is necessary for maintenance of healthy cartilage. If motion is present between the bone and cartilage flap, synovitis and pain will ensue. Healing will not take place owing to the motion and the presence of synovial fluid between the flap and bone. Healing will only occur if the flap is stabilized or removed.

Specific Osteochondritis Dissecans Lesions

In most cases, diagnosis is based on signalment, history, clinical signs, and physical and orthopedic examination, and confirmed with bilateral radiographs of the affected joint. Not uncommonly, advanced imaging such as computed tomography or exploratory arthroscopy or arthrotomy is required to make a definitive diagnosis. Contrast arthrography is rarely necessary.

Although most cases are presented as young dogs, any aged dog can be seen. Lameness ranges from sudden to insidious onset, from barely appreciable to non-weight bearing. Dogs can present with any degree of joint effusion, reduced range of motion, muscle atrophy, and pain associated with the OCD lesion. In most cases, regardless of treatment, development of secondary osteoarthritis is inevitable.

Shoulder Joint

Osteochondritis dissecans of the scapulohumeral joint is a common cause of lameness and is the most commonly seen form of OC in dogs in the United States.[17] Surgical removal of the cartilage flap is the preferred method of treatment in dogs with clinical signs. Long-term prognosis following surgery is good to excellent.

The most common site for OC lesion development in the shoulder is the caudal central or caudal-central-medial region of the humeral head (Figure 100-4). Lesions of the glenoid occur rarely.[29] Although the particular susceptibility of the caudal central aspect of the humeral head is not fully understood, it has been suggested that it is due to the increased thickness of cartilage normally present in that area in dogs.[30,31] It has been suggested that trauma from contact between the humeral head and the glenoid cavity of the scapula predisposes any abnormally developed cartilage to vertical fractures.[30,31] In 1965, it was proposed that the particular location of the OC lesion of the shoulder was caused by the repeated impingement of the caudal part of the humeral head by the scapula during full extension.[6,32] Olsson later suggested that this could be supported by the finding in dogs with shoulder osteoarthritis that osteophytes on the caudal region of the humeral head are often attached to the scapula by fibrous tissue, indicating a dynamic component to their development.[6,32]

Many cases of shoulder OCD heal spontaneously.[6] The pedicle of the cartilage flap may rupture, thereby dislodging the flap and allowing fibrocartilage to grow from the floor of the defect. The dislodged flap may develop into a joint mouse, become resorbed, or continue to grow. It is possible that the flap(s) can become a large calcified body/bodies in the caudal pouch of the joint. If the calcified body remains in the caudal pouch it may not give rise to clinical signs; however, if it becomes entrapped between the scapula and humerus it can cause sudden pain and locking of the shoulder joint. If the calcified piece migrates to the sheath of the biceps tendon it can cause persistent lameness.

Humeral head OCD most commonly affects large and giant breed dogs with 56 different breeds being identified in a study of 626 affected dogs.[33] While some large breeds such as the Swiss mountain dog, Great Dane, German shepherd, Newfoundland, Rottweiler, Labrador retriever, golden retriever, and Bernese mountain dog, are at a high risk of developing OCD of the humeral head,[34,35] some large breeds such as the doberman pinscher, collie and Siberian husky are considered to be at low risk.[33] Small and medium-sized breeds can also be affected.[33,36-39]

Although most dogs present for unilateral lameness, approximately 50% (range 20% to 85%) have radiographically detectable lesions bilaterally.[5,31,33] In one study, only 24% of dogs diagnosed with bilateral lesions on radiographs had clinically bilateral disease.

Elbow Joint

Several lesions of the elbow joint can be classified as manifestations of OC including fragmented coronoid process (FCP), OCD, and ununited anconeal process (UAP) (See Chapter on elbow dysplasia). Of all these, the most common cause of elbow arthrosis is some abnormality of the coronoid process (fragmented or fissured) and, less commonly, OCD of the humeral condyle.[17] The most common site for OCD in the elbow is along the medial aspect of the humeral condyle (Figure 100-5). Careful examination must be performed to definitively diagnosis OC or OCD. Long-term prognosis following surgical treatment for OC of the elbow is guarded. Early treatment may decrease lameness, but will not prevent progression of secondary osteoarthritis.

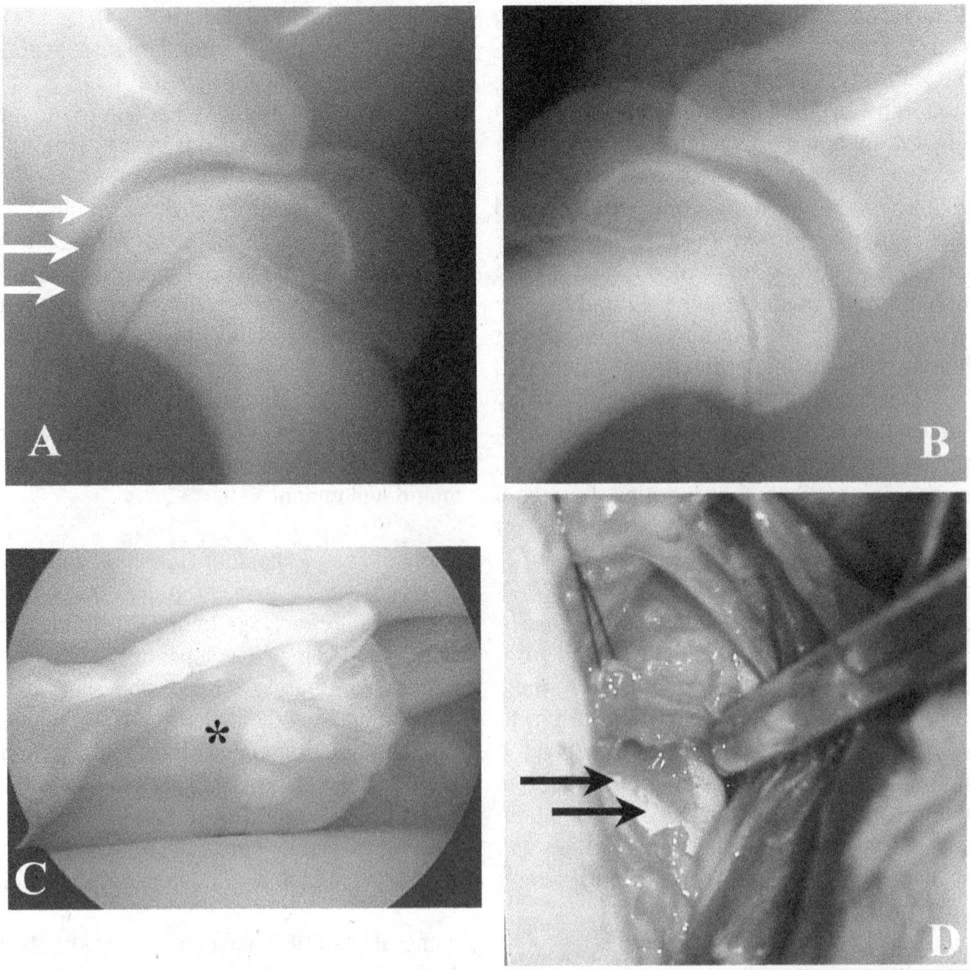

Figure 100-4. A series of images illustrating OCD of the caudal humeral head. (A) Lateral radiographic view of the affected side. Note the flattened area of subchondral bone (white arrows). (B) Lateral radiographic view of the normal side. Note the curved, smooth surface of the caudal humeral head. (C) An arthroscopic view of a cartilage flap (asterisk) involving the caudal humeral head. (D) An intra-operative view of the caudal humeral head showing the subcondral bone (black arrows) after flap removal.

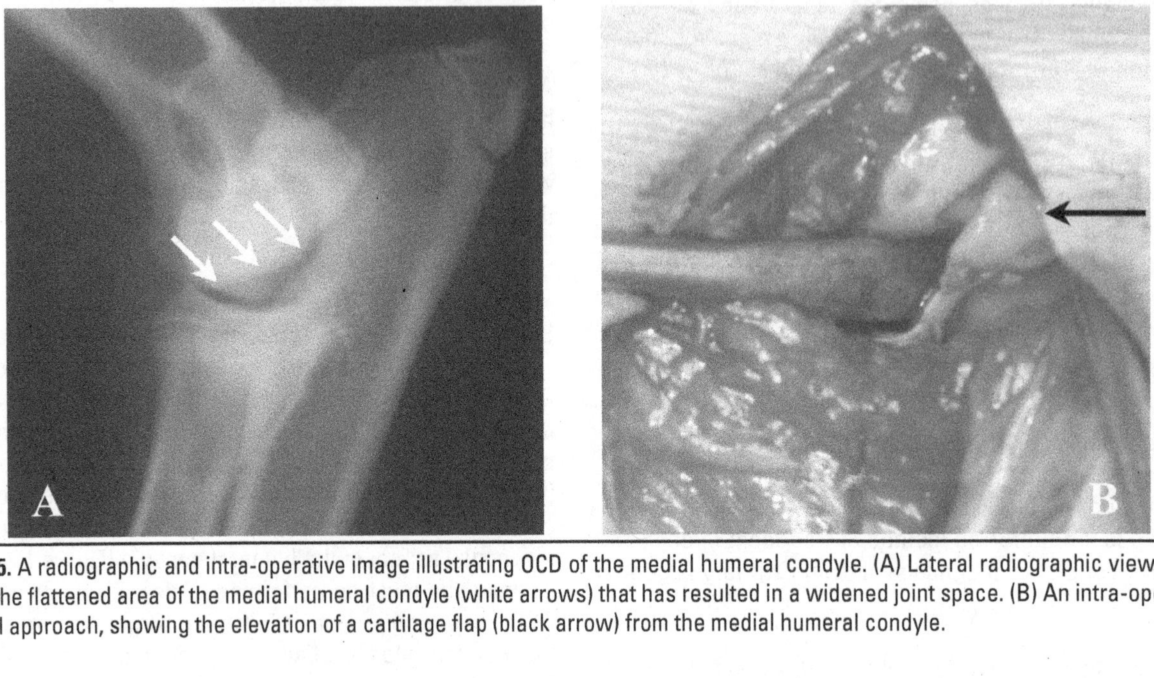

Figure 100-5. A radiographic and intra-operative image illustrating OCD of the medial humeral condyle. (A) Lateral radiographic view of an elbow joint. Note the flattened area of the medial humeral condyle (white arrows) that has resulted in a widened joint space. (B) An intra-operative view, via a medial approach, showing the elevation of a cartilage flap (black arrow) from the medial humeral condyle.

Osteochondrosis of the elbow occurs less commonly tha; shoulder OC, however, the signalment is similar. Large- and giant-breed dogs are most commonly affected, with the highest prevalence in Bernese mountain dogs, golden retrievers, Labrador retrievers and Rottweilers. In a study on 1247 Labrador retriever puppies in an Australian breeding colony producing guide dogs, 15% had OC of the elbow.[40] The Newfoundland, flat-coated retriever, chow chow, Great Dane, and German shepherd have also been found to be over-resented breeds with elbow OC.[6,34,35] Most dogs are presented when they are less than 1 year of age, however ages ranging from 4 months to 12 years have been reported.[41-43] Males are affected more often than females (2:1). Right and left elbows are affected equally, with bilateral disease in 20 to 50% of patients.[41,44]

Stifle Joint

Osteochondrosis of the femorotibial joint is uncommon in dogs.[42,45] It occurs most commonly along the lateral femoral condyle, but can also occur on the medial femoral condyle (Figure 100-6). Surgical treatment of stifle OCD is required, and although prognosis depends on the size of the lesion, it is generally only fair.

Young, large-breed dogs usually present between 4 and 9 months. Breeds at risk include: boxers, Great Danes, German shepherds, Labrador retrievers, Rottweilers, bullmastiffs, bulldogs, Irish wolfhounds, golden retrievers, and Newfoundlands.[34,35] Approximately 66% of cases occur in male dogs and approximately 72% of cases are bilateral.[45]

Tibiotarsal Joint

Osteochondritis dissecans of the tibiotarsal joint is well known, but uncommon. It occurs along the medial or lateral talar ridge in a cranial to caudal direction (Figure 100-7). The medial ridge is more commonly affected. Prognosis is guarded and lameness is likely to persist even without strenuous exercise. Prognosis is improved in cases with small lesions that are treated early. Moderate to severe osteoarthritic changes are expected.

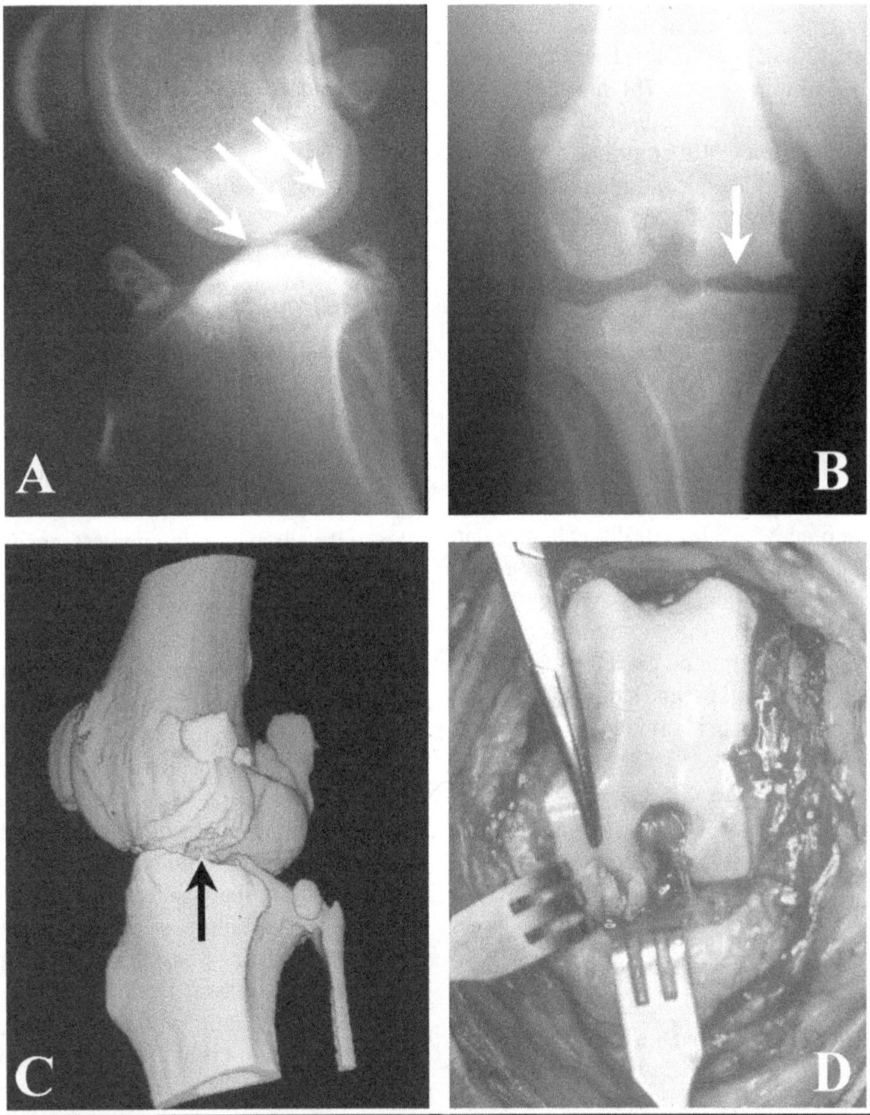

Figure 100-6. A series of images illustrating OCD of the femoral condyle. (A) A lateral radiographic view showing flattening of the lateral femoral condyle (white arrows) and a mineralized joint mouse in the cranial aspect of the fat pad. (B) A caudocranial radiographic view showing a flattened area of the medial femoral condyle (white arrow). (C) A CT scan three-dimensional reconstruction showing the extent of a medial femoral condyle OCD lesion (black arrow). (D) An intra-operative photo showing an OCD flap (hemostat is pointing to the flap) involving the medial femoral condyle.

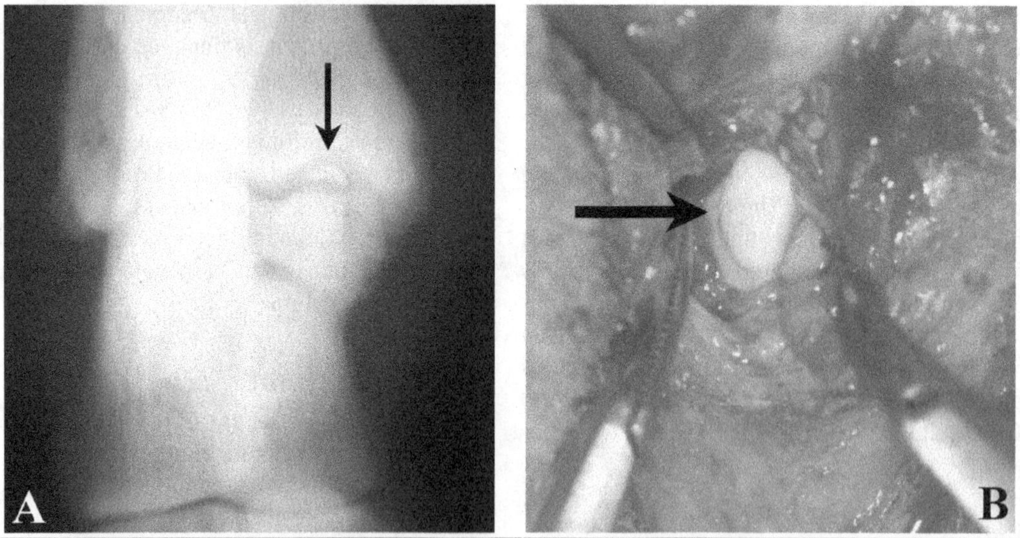

Figure 100-7. Radiographic and intra-operative images illustrating OCD of the troclear ridge of the talus. (A) A caudocranial radiographic view of the tarsus showing the OCD lesion (black arrow) of medial trochlear ridge and secondary osteoarthritis. (B) An intra-operative view showing a nondisplaced OCD lesion (black arrow) of the lateral trochlear ridge of the talus.

A histologic study of 38 OCD flaps removed surgically from the hock joint concluded that OCD of the talus follows the same sequence of events as OCD of other joints. The one difference is that the cartilage flaps do not only undergo calcification, but also ossify and attach to the synovial membrane and/or the collateral ligament (Type II). This is likely owing to the relatively rich vascular supply from the surrounding synovial membrane and collateral ligament. Olssen suggested that the reason for the increased incidence on the medial trochlear ridge is local pressure by the tendon of the flexor hallucis longus muscle and pull by the short branch of the medial collateral ligament.[6]

Most dogs present when they are less than 1 year of age, although a range of 4 months to 4 years has been reported.[46] The incidence in males and females is almost equivalent.[44] Large-breed dogs, particularly the Labrador retriever, Rottweiler, and bullmastiff are over represented.[34,35,44,46] Tarsal OCD is bilateral in approximately 60% of cases (range 54% to 69%).[45,46] Most tarsal OCD lesions (79%) occur on the medial trochlear ridge of the talus.[44,47] Of these lesions, 80% occur on the plantar aspect of the ridge. Conversely most lesions that occur on the lateral trochlear ridge are present on the dorsal aspect of the ridge.[44] It has been reported that lesions of the lateral trochlear ridge occur more often in Rottweilers than in other breeds.[48,49]

Lumbosacrum

Lumbosacral OCD is a form of cauda equina syndrome.[50] Lesions of vertebral OCD vary from cartilaginous overgrowth to flaps of cartilage that separate from the underlying bone and cavitation of the vertebral epiphysis.[51] Sacral OCD is a developmental disturbance of the sacral end plate, with subsequent separation of hyaline cartilage with a bone center from the dorsal corner.[52,53] Lesions are usually on the craniodorsal corner of the sacral body, or less commonly, on the caudal endplate of the seventh lumbar vertebra (91% and 9%, respectively).[51] Of dogs presenting with cauda equina neuropathy, 15 to 30% have been reported to have lumbosacral OCD.[51,54]

Lumbosacral OCD lesions most commonly affect German shepherds, with male dogs being over represented (4:1, male:female).[51] Dogs are usually diagnosed when they are older than 14 months (range 14 months to 13 years; mean 6.3 years).[51] It has been suggested that despite radiographic evidence, clinical signs do not appear until dogs are over 18 months of age.

Incomplete Ossification of the Humeral Condyle

Forelimb lameness caused by a radiographically visible radiolucent line in the center of the humeral condyle was first described by Meutstege in 1989.[55] It subsequently became known as incomplete ossification of the humeral condyle (IOHC) and is an uncommon cause of forelimb lameness in dogs.[56]

The pathogenesis of incomplete ossification of the distal intercondylar humerus epiphyseal plate (IOHC) is unknown. In normal dogs, two separate centers of ossification appear in the humeral condyle at 14 +/- 8 days after birth.[57] One ossification center includes the capitulum and the lateral aspect of the humeral condyle and one ossification center develops into the trochlea and the medial aspect of the condyle. The two centers of ossification normally unite at 70 +/- 14 days after birth.[56] The fissure line seen in IOHC of adult dogs coincides precisely with the cartilaginous remnant between the lateral and medial centers of ossification of the humeral condyle present in immature dogs (Figure 100-8).[56] For this reason it is thought that the source of the problem is failure of complete ossification of the humeral condyle.[56] Another possible cause is a form of stress fracture, in which the condylar fissure develops after ossification of the condyle is complete.[58] It has been proposed that incongruency in the elbow joint creates stress within the humeral condyle that either prevents ossification or promotes a stress fracture.[58] If an incongruency is the underlying factor, then IOHC may be a manifestation of elbow dysplasia. Fragmented coronoid process and OCD lesions have been found to co-exist in some cases of non-fractured condyles, suggesting that the pathogenesis

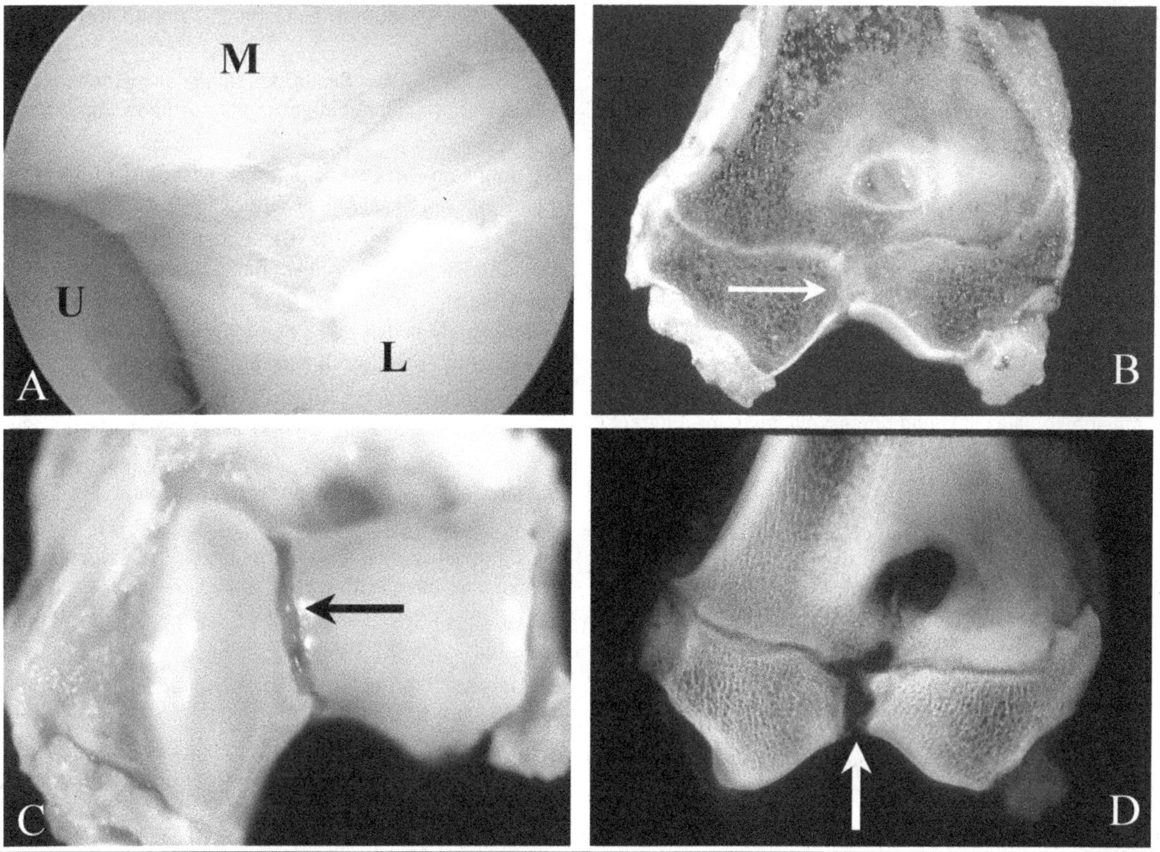

Figure 100-8. A series of images illustrating incomplete ossification of the humeral condyle. (A) An arthroscopic view showing the incomplete disruption in the articular surface between the medial humeral condyle (M) and the lateral humeral condyle (L). A portion of the ulnar notch (U) can be seen. (B) A postmortem specimen showing the retained cartilage (white arrow) between the medial and lateral humeral condyles. (C) A postmortem specimen showing complete disruption of the articular surface (black arrow) of the humeral trochlea. (D) A faxitron radiograph showing the retained cartilage (white arrow) between the medial and lateral humeral condyles.

is linked.[56,59] It is suspected that IOHC has a genetic basis with a recessive mode of inheritance in spaniels.[56] It has also been suggested that chondrodystrophic dogs are at greater risk;[58] however, normotrophic dogs can also be affected.[59,60] Biopsies taken from the intercondylar area during surgery usually reveal fibrous tissue, with high osteoclastic activity and plasma cell numbers suggesting chronic inflammation.[56,59] Regardless of the etiology, dogs with IOHC are predisposed to humeral condylar fractures, particularly following minor trauma. Most dogs present with a humeral condylar fracture following major or minor trauma, or following normal activity such as jumping from a height of 1 meter or less, climbing stairs, or running.[56] A radiolucent line between the condyles of the contralateral humerus is reported to be present in 44% to 86% percent of dogs,[56,59] indicating that bilateral disease is common.

Spaniel breeds are at highest risk of developing IOHC, however it has been described in several other breeds. It has been reported in cocker spaniels, Brittany spaniels, springer spaniels, Cavalier King Charles spaniels, clumb er spaniels, and a pug, a Yorkshire terrier, a Tibetan mastiff, a Rottweiler and several Labrador retrievers.[56,58,60-62] A recent study from Germany also reported the German wachtell, German shepherd, and mixed breed dog as being at high risk.[59] Interestingly, although spaniels were well represented at the practice in this study, none were presented for IOHC.[59] Regardless of breed, males have been found to be at higher risk than females.[56,59]

Age of animals that present for associated non-fracture lameness range from 4 months to 5 years, with 54% presented when they are younger than 1 year.[59] Duration between first clinical signs and presentation in dogs with non-fracture lameness was 4 weeks to 12 months, with an average of 4 months.[59]

References

1. Ekman S, Carlson CS: The pathophysiology of osteochondrosis. Vet Clin North Am Small Anim Pract 28:17-32, 1998.

2. Kuroki K CJ, Tomlinson JL, Kreeger JM: In vitro characterization of chondrocytes isolated from naturally occurring osteochondrosis lesions of the humeral head of dogs. Am J Vet Res 63:186-193, 2002.

3. Mundlos S, Olsen BR: Heritable diseases of the skeleton. Part I: Molecular insights into skeletal development-transcription factors and signaling pathways. Faseb J 11:125-132, 1997.

4. Olsen BR, Reginato AM, Wang W: Bone development. Annu Rev Cell Dev Biol 16:191-220, 2000.

5. Probst CW, Johnston SA: Osteochondrosis. *In* Textbook of Small Animal Surgery, 2nd ed. Slatter D (ed). Philadelphia: WB Saunders, 1993, p. 1944.

6. Olsson S: Pathophysiology, morphology, and clinical signs of osteochondrosis in the dog. *In* Disease Mechanisms in Small Animal Surgery, 2nd ed. Bojrab MJ (ed). Philadelphia: Lea & Febiger, 1993, p. 777.

7. Silberberg R, Silberberg M, Vogel A, et al: Ultrastructure of articular cartilage of mice of various ages. Am J Anat 109:251-275, 1961.

8. Kincaid SA, Van Sickle DC: Bone morphology and postnatal osteogenesis. Potential for disease. Vet Clin North Am Small Anim Pract 13:3-17, 1983.

9. Hayashi K: Three-dimensional organization of the cartilage canal--a scanning electron-microscopic study by vascular cast of the rabbit's femoral head. Nippon Seikeigeka Gakkai Zasshi 66:548-559, 1992.

10. Ytrehus B, Ekman S, Carlson CS, et al: Focal changes in blood supply during normal epiphyseal growth are central in the pathogenesis of osteochondrosis in pigs. Bone 35:1294-1306, 2004.

11. Cordy DR, Wind AP: Transverse fracture of the proximal humeral articular cartilage in dogs. (So-called osteochondritis dissecans). Pathol Vet 6:424-436, 1969.

12. Carlson CS, Cullins LD, Meuten DJ: Osteochondrosis of the articular-epiphyseal cartilage complex in young horses: evidence for a defect in cartilage canal blood supply. Vet Pathol 32:641-647, 1995.

13. Carlson CS, Hilley HD, Meuten DJ: Degeneration of cartilage canal vessels associated with lesions of osteochondrosis in swine. Vet Pathol 26:47-54, 1989.

14. Carlson CS, Meuten DJ, Richardson DC: Ischemic necrosis of cartilage in spontaneous and experimental lesions of osteochondrosis. J Orthop Res 9:317-329, 1991.

15. Ytrehus B, Andreas Haga H, Mellum CN, et al: Experimental ischemia of porcine growth cartilage produces lesions of osteochondrosis. J Orthop Res 22:1201-1209, 2004.

16. Hamerman D: The biology of osteoarthritis. N Engl J Med 320:1322-1330, 1989.

17. Piermattei DL, Flo GL: Brinker, Piermattei, and Flo's Handbook of Small Animal Orthopedics and Fracture Repair, 3rd ed. Philadelphia: WB Saunders, 1997.

18. Kincaid SA, Allhands RV, Pijanowski GJ: Chondrolysis associated with cartilage canals of the epiphyseal cartilage of the distal humerus of growing pigs. Am J Vet Res 46:726-732, 1985.

19. Kincaid SA, Rudd RG, Evander SA: Lipids of normal and osteochondritic cartilage of the immature canine humeral head. Am J Vet Res 46:1060-1065, 1985.

20. Nakano T, Aherne FX: The pathogenesis of osteochondrosis--a hypothesis. Med Hypotheses 43:1-5, 1994.

21. Della Salda L, Borghetti P, Maltarello MC, et al: Superficial and deep defects in dyschondroplastic and degenerated pig articular cartilage. J Submicrosc Cytol Pathol 29:51-58, 1997.

22. Olsson SE: General and local [corrected] aetiologic factors in canine osteochondrosis. Vet Q 9:268-278, 1987.

23. White SL, Rowland GN, Whitlock RH: Radiographic, macroscopic, and microscopic changes in growth plates of calves raised on hard flooring. Am J Vet Res 45:633-639, 1984.

24. Nakano T, Aherne FX: Involvement of trauma in the pathogenesis of osteochondritis dissecans in swine. Can J Vet Res 52:154-155, 1988.

25. Ytrehus B, Grindflek E, Teige J, et al: The effect of parentage on the prevalence, severity and location of lesions of osteochondrosis in swine. J Vet Med A Physiol Pathol Clin Med 51:188-195, 2004.

26. Padgett GA, Mostosky UV, Probst CW, et al: The inheritance of osteochondritis dissecans and fragmented coronoid process of the elbow joint in labrador retrievers. J Am Anim Hosp Assoc 31:327-330, 1995.

27. Hazewinkel HA, Tryfonidou MA: Vitamin D3 metabolism in dogs. Mol Cell Endocrinol 197:23-33, 2002.

28. Tryfonidou MA, Holl MS, Vastenburg M, et al: Hormonal regulation of calcium homeostasis in two breeds of dogs during growth at different rates. J Anim Sci 81:1568-1580, 2003.

29. Milton JL, Rumph PF, Reed AO: Osteochondritis dissecans of the shoulder in the racing greyhound: a report of two cases and a survey of 109 greyhound anatomy specimens. J Am Anim Hosp Assoc 17:617-622, 1981.

30. Kincaid SA, Van Sickle DC: Regional histochemical and thickness variations of adult canine articular cartilage. Am J Vet Res 42:428-432, 1981.

31. Johnston SA: Osteochondritis dissecans of the humeral head. Vet Clin North Am Small Anim Pract 28:33-49, 1998.

32. Craig PH, Riser WH: Osteochondritis dissecans in the proximal humerus of the dog. J Am Vet Radiol Soc 6:40, 1965.

33. Rudd RG, Whitehair JG, Margolis JH: Results of management of osteochondritis dissecans of the humeral head in dogs: 44 cases (1982-1087). J Am Anim Hosp Assoc 26:173-175, 1990.

34. LaFond E, Breur GJ, Austin CC: Breed susceptibility for developmental orthopedic diseases in dogs. J Am Anim Hosp Assoc 38:467-477, 2002.

35. Slater MR, Scarlett JM, Kaderly RE: Breed, gender, and age as risk factors for canine osteochondritis dissecans. Vet Comp Orthop Traum 4:100-106, 1991

36. Dingwall JS, Staples JW, Pennock PW: Osteochondritis dissecans in a miniature poodle. Mod Vet Pract 53:47-48, 1972.

37. Griffiths RC: Osteochondritis dissecans of the canine shoulder. J Am Vet Med Assoc 153:1733-1735, 1968.

38. Johnson KA, Dennis KA: Osteochondritis dissecans in a beagle. Aust Vet J 54:364, 1978.

39. Knecht CD, Van Sickle DC, Blevins WE, et al: Osteochondrosis of the shoulder and stifle in 3 of 5 Border Collie littermates. J Am Vet Med Assoc 170:58-60, 1977.

40. Studdert VP, Lavelle RB, Beilharz RG: Clinical features and heredity of osteochondrosis of the elbow in Labrador retrievers. J Small Anim Pract 32:557, 1991.

41. Boudrieau RJ: Osteochondritis dissecans of the elbow in the dog. J Am Anim Hosp Assoc 19:627, 1983.

42. Denny HR, Gibbs C: Osteochondritis dissecans of the canine stifle joint. J Small Anim Pract 21:317-322, 1980.

43. Olsson SE: The early diagnosis of fragmented coronoid process and osteochondritis dissecans of the canine elbow joint. J Am Anim Hosp Assoc 19:616, 1983.

44. Trostel CT, McLaughlin RM, Pool RR: Canine lameness caused by developmental orthopedic diseases: osteochondrosis. Comp Cont Educ Pract Vet 24:836-852, 2002.

45. Montgomery RD, Milton JL, Henderson RA, et al: Osteochondritis dissecans of the canine stifle. Comp Cont Educ Pract Vet 11:1199-1205, 1989.

46. Smith MM, Vasseur PB, Morgan JP: Clinical evaluation of dogs after surgical and nonsurgical management of osteochondritis dissecans of the talus. J Am Vet Med Assoc 187:31-35, 1985.

47. Beale BS, Goring RL, Herrington J: A prospective evaluation of four surgical approaches to the talus of the dog used in the treatment of osteochondritis dissecans. J Am Anim Hosp Assoc 27:221-229, 1991.

48. Fitch RB, Beale BS: Osteochondrosis of the canine tibiotarsal joint. Vet Clin North Am Small Anim Pract 28:95-113, 1998.

49. Weinstein MJ, Mongil CM, Rhodes WH, et al: Orthopedic conditions of the rottweiler. Comp Cont Educ Pract Vet 17:925-939, 1995.

50. Glyde M, Doyle R, McAllister H, et al: Magnetic resonance imaging in the diagnosis and surgical management of sacral osteochondrosis in a mastiff dog. Vet Rec 155:83-86, 2004.

51. Hanna FY: Lumbosacral osteochondrosis: radiological features and surgical management in 34 dogs. J Small Anim Pract 42:272-278, 2001.

52. Lang J, Hani H, Schwalder P: A sacral lesion resembling osteochondrosis in the German shepherd dog. Vet Radiol Ultrasound 33:69-78, 1992.

53. Snaps FR, Heimann M, Saunders J, et al: Osteochondrosis of the sacral bone in a mastiff dog. Vet Rec 143:476-477, 1998.

54. Lang J, Jaggy A: The radiographic examination on the canine cauda equina. Eur J Companion Anim Pract 3:40-47, 1993.

55. Meutstege FJ: Incomplete humeral condylar fracture inthe canine humerus as a cause of obvious elbow lameness. Veterinary Orthopedic Society Proceedings, 1989; 11.

56. Marcellin-Little DJ, DeYoung DJ, Ferris KK, et al: Incomplete ossification of the humeral condyle in spaniels. Vet Surg 23:475-487, 1994.

57. Hare WC: The ages at which the centers of ossification appear roentgenographically in the limb bones of the dog. Am J Vet Res 22:825-835, 1961.

58. Butterworth SJ, Innes JF: Incomplete humeral condylar fractures in the dog. J Small Anim Pract 42:394-398, 2001.

59. Meyer-Lindenberg A, Heinen V, Fehr M, et al: Incomplete ossification of the humeral condyle as a cause of lameness in dogs. Vet Comp Orthop Traum 15:187-194, 2002.

60. Robin D, Marcellin-Little DJ: Incomplete ossification of the humeral condyle in two Labrador retrievers. J Small Anim Pract 42:231-234, 2001.

61. Rovesti GL, Fluckiger M, Margini A, et al: Fragmented coronoid process and incomplete ossification of the humeral condyle in a rottweiler. Vet Surg 27:354-357, 1998.

62. Cook JL, Tomlinson JL, Reed AL: Fluoroscopically guided closed reduction and internal fixation of fractures of the lateral portion of the humeral condyle: prospective clinical study of the technique and results in ten dogs. Vet Surg 28:315-321, 1999.

Chapter 101

Conditions of the Adult Canine Shoulder

Derek B. Fox
James L. Cook

Several conditions can affect the canine shoulder joint. Often the signalment of the animal helps to distinguish those diseases that typically occur in the juvenile patient, such as osteochondritis dessicans, from those that are more common in adult animals. This chapter discusses four disease conditions that are sources of shoulder lameness more commonly affecting the adult, large-breed dog.

The Rotator Cuff

Many of the conditions of the adult canine shoulder involve components of the rotator cuff. The term "rotator cuff" was initially used in reference to four muscles of the human shoulder that are responsible for the motion of the brachium and for providing active shoulder stability. The four muscles include the supraspinatus, infraspinatus, teres minor, and subscapularis. The canine shoulder differs in form and function from the human shoulder owing to the quadripedal nature of the dog, however the presence and importance of these four muscles persist. Whereas in the human, the cuff muscles are largely responsible for abduction and rotation of the brachium, these muscles serve predominantly to flex and extend the canine shoulder, in addition to providing active stability to the joint.

Calcification of the Supraspinatus

Calcification or mineralization of the supraspinatus tendon of the canine shoulder is a well documented condition, yet it remains controversial with respect to its etiopathogenesis, relationship to clinical signs, and treatment. The supraspinatus muscle originates from the supraspinous fossa of the scapula and inserts on the greater tubercle of the humerus, extending to the medial aspect of the tubercle through a broad tendon. The muscle acts to extend the shoulder. Microangiographic studies have revealed an area of the central tendon of the insertion over the greater tubercle that is completely devoid of blood vessels.[1]

Etiopathogenesis

Much of what is known about the etiopathogenesis of rotator cuff calcific tendinopathy must be extracted from the human literature. The two causative agents that are discussed most frequently are tissue hypoxia and localized pressure.[2] Most researchers concur with a theory describing the process of calcification to be reactive in nature rather than primarily degenerative.[2] Furthermore, it has been suggested that the disease evolves in various stages: precalcific, calcific, and postcalcific. During the precalcific stage, fibrocartilaginous metaplasia occurs in avascular areas of the tendon and the new chondroid cells produce glycosaminoglycan-rich extracellular matrix.[2,3] The calcific stage is subdivided into three phases: formative, resting, and resorptive.[4] The hallmark of the formative phase is the formation of chalky deposits of coalescing matrix vesicles containing calcium crystals.[2] Histopathologic analysis will reveal positive staining of the calcific clumps with Von Kossa's stain. The resting phase of the calcific stage marks the cessation of calcium deposits that are surrounded by fibrocartilagenous tissue without evidence of inflammation. The resorptive phase may occur nonpredictably following the resting phase, and is so named for the presence of macrophages and multinucleated cells that begin to phagocytose the calcified deposit, resulting in a granulomatous appearance to the lesion.[3] The chalky clumps previously detected change into a toothpaste-like substance during the resorptive phase. The postcalcific stage is one of remodeling that occurs through the formation of granulation tissue, neovascularization, and deposition of type III collagen in an attempt to heal the void left after the resorption of calcium deposits.[2]

Clinical Relevance

Several reports now document the occurrence of calcification of the supraspinatus tendon in dogs.[5-8] Adult Labrador retrievers, Rottweilers and German shepherd dogs are the most frequently reported affected animals, however this may indicate breed popularity rather than true prevalence.[5-8] Other than the speculation of localized tissue hypoxia within the avascular portion of the supraspinatus tendon, no definitive risk factors have been determined in reported canine populations. The relationship between clinical signs and the presence of calcific deposits in the supraspinatus is not clear. Supraspinatus calcifying tendinopathy may be an incidental finding and result in no clinical signs.[6,8] Interestingly, Bardet reports that 11% of dogs affected with shoulder instability concurrently possess supraspinatus calcification.[9] In another study assessing 13 dogs positively diagnosed with calcification of the supraspinatus that also underwent radiographic examination of the elbows, 69% had evidence of fragmented coronoid processes, elbow osteoarthritis, or both.[6] What cannot be determined from these studies is if the diagnosis of supraspinatus calcification is related to other orthopedic conditions within the same joint or limb, or if its incidence reflects coincidence. From reports of humans who are symptomatic from calcific tendinopathy of the supraspinatus alone and the successful resolution of clinical signs following calcific deposit dissolution or removal in some dogs, one may conclude that the presence of the disorder is responsible for lameness in a certain percentage of dogs. However, concurrent sources of forelimb pain should always be pursued and addressed appropriately.

Diagnosis

Pain may or may not be elicited on palpation of the tendon of insertion of the supraspinatus over the greater tubercle and on shoulder flexion.[5,7] Because of the concurrence of supraspinatus calcification and other shoulder pathology, the biceps tendon should also be palpated for evidence of pain or inflammation, and the joint examined for signs of instability. Similarly, the elbow should be thoroughly palpated to examine for signs of pain, effusion, and decreased range of motion.

The most common diagnostic tool is radiography. However, mineralization of the supraspinatus may be indistinguishable from that of the biceps tendon if only mediolateral radiographs are taken. Therefore, a flexed cranioproximal-craniodistal tangential view of the intertubercular groove, or "skyline" view, should also be taken to distinguish the location of the calcific density (Figure 101-1).[8] Depending on the stage of the disease process, the affected area of the tendon may not be detectable with radiographs. Ultrasonography can be used successfully to detect disruption or inflammation within tendon fibers. Furthermore, if present, calcification is easily recognized as hyperechoic foci with distal acoustic shadowing.[10] If magnetic resonance imaging is used, T1-weighted images will show calcifications as areas of decreased signal intensity and T2-weighted images may demonstrate a perifocal band of increased signal intensity associated with edema.[2]

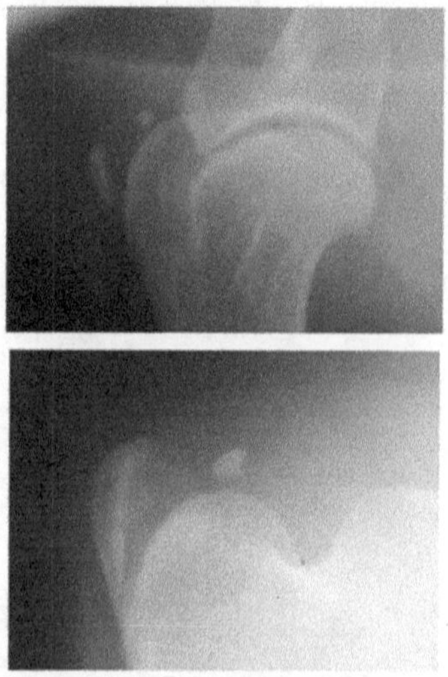

Figure 101-1. Lateral and craniproximal – craniodistal or "skyline" radiographic views showing two calcific deposits in the supraspinatus tendon. The skyline view allows localization of the pathology to the supraspinatus tendon versus the biceps tendon. (photos courtesy of Dr. Loic Dejardin)

Treatment

Various treatments have been described for lameness attributable to calcification of the supraspinatus in the dog, including conservative management, surgical removal of the calcific deposits and extracorporeal shock-wave therapy. Surgery consists of accessing the deposits through longitudinal incisions in the tendon for their subsequent removal. Interestingly, in a long-term follow-up study of four operated cases, Laitinen noted that that the calcific depositis had reoccurred in all the dogs after a mean follow-up time of 5.1 years after surgery.[6] However, despite the reformation of the calcium-based deposits, resolution of lameness has been reported following their surgical removal in the majority of cases.[6-8] In the human, conservative management is the favored initial treatment and surgery is indicated only if 1) clinical signs progress, 2) the pain appears to be consistent and interfering with quality of life, and 3) if conservative management fails.[11] Current opinions from veterinary orthopedic researchers have become similar, recommending a period of conservative management including rest, administration of nonsteroidal anti-inflammatory drugs (NSAIDs), and physical therapy for 3 months from the time of diagnosis before attempting surgery.[6] Lameness attributable to calcification of the suprapinatus has been shown to resolve in some dogs with conservative management.[6] Another advantage of this approach is to allow other sources of underlying lameness to manifest and be appropriately diagnosed because the incidental occurrence of supraspinatus calcification appears to be high and may serve as the proverbial red herring.

Another treatment strategy that has been reported in the dog is extracorporeal shock-wave therapy, which employs low-frequency, high-pressure pneumatic impulses that are generated outside of the body but delivered to the affected area through a hand-held applicator in a noninvasive, but site-specific fashion.[5] Success with this technique in alleviating clinical signs has been demonstrated in a small population.[5]

Other techniques described in the human literature include ultrasound-guided needle aspiration and lavage, and arthroscopic-assisted aspiration and debridement.[2] These authors have had success with using arthroscopy to assist in the debridement of focal calcium deposits in a small population of dogs. However, the use of needle aspiration has not been described in the dog to the knowledge of the authors.

Infraspinatus Contracture

The infraspinatus is a fusiform muscle of the shoulder rotator cuff that originates from the infraspinous fossa of the scapula and inserts on the lateral aspect of the greater tubercle over a small bursa. It can either flex or extend the shoulder depending on the joint's position when the muscle contracts.

Etiopathogenesis

Contracture of the infraspinatus represents a chronic process by which initial injury to the muscle and tendon eventually results in severe fibrosis and adherence to the underlying joint capsule. The condition was first described in 1970,[12] and is a well recognized disorder occurring in medium- to large-breed working dogs.[13] The initiation of the process can either be self-inflicted through vigorous activity or a result of a traumatic event. Most typically, affected dogs present with acute pain and swelling over the lateral aspect of the shoulder after a period of strenuous activity, although this phase of the disease frequently goes unnoticed. Palpation of the supraspinatus and infraspinatus muscle groups during this acute injury phase reveals swelling and elicits a painful response. During the ensuing weeks, the dog is typically reluctant to bear weight and flex or extend the affected limb at the level of the scapulohumeral joint. Over time, the tendon can undergo irreversible and severe contraction with marked concomitant muscle atrophy. The result is the adoption of a classic posture of the affected forelimb consisting of adduction of the elbow, abduction of the antebrachium, and external rotation of the limb with extension at the level of the shoulder (Figure 101-2). Research has demonstrated that the suprascapular nerve is not involved in this process and that fibrous tissue eventually replaces the vast majority of affected normal muscle fibers.[14,15] The supraspinatus muscle can be simultaneously or independently involved in a similar process.[16]

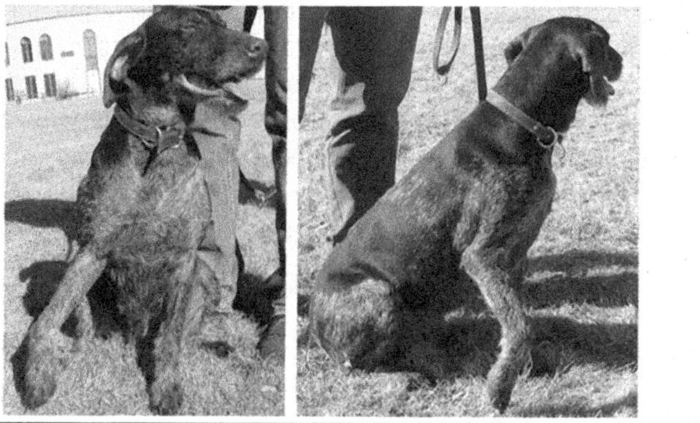

Figure 101-2. A dog affected by infraspinatus contracture with classic position of the limb. (photos courtesy of Dr. James Tomlinson)

Diagnosis

A presumptive diagnosis can be made based on patient history, the characteristic positioning of the affected limb, and orthopedic examination. Dogs affected by this condition will carry the limb in a similarly characteristic fashion during ambulation in which the lower limb swings out in a circumducted fashion while advancing the foot forward. Careful palpation will reveal atrophy of the infraspinatus and possibly the supraspinatus muscles with subsequent prominence of the scapular spine and acromial process. Attempts to internally rotate or adduct the proximal humerus will result in noticeable scapular excursion away from the thoracic wall. Radiographs of the shoulder may be normal or reveal a narrowing of the scapulohumeral joint space, particularly evident on the craniocaudal view. Ultrasonographic examination of the infraspinatus muscle and tendon can be completed to substantiate the diagnosis, as findings associated with both the early and late stages of the disease have been described.[17]

Treatment

If the disorder can be diagnosed in the early stages, in which the tendon has been strained prior to any secondary fibrotic response, conservative management consisting of rest and NSAIDs has been reported to be successful.[17] Ultrasound examination of these injuries will greatly assist with this early intervention.[17] However, if pursuing conservative management, owners should be advised about the risk for contracture to occur. Once the muscle and tendon have undergone fibrosis and contracture, only surgical release has been shown to be successful. The infraspinatus is released through tenotomy and partial excision of the tendon close to its insertion on the lateral aspect of the greater tubercle. Adhesions to the underlying joint capsule must be examined for and freed. A dramatic release and recession of the proximal myotendinous junction with immediate restoration of joint range of motion should be detected once the tendon is completely released. Prognosis with this treatment appears to be good to excellent.

Biceps Tendon Pathology

Pathologic conditions of the biceps tendon reported to occur in dogs include tenosynovitis, partial or complete rupture, avulsion, tendinitis, tendinosis, displacement, and bipartite tendon.[18-25] Most often, these conditions occur in middle-aged medium- and large-breed dogs that participate in athletic activities. No documented gender predisposition exists to the authors' knowledge. Apart from rupture or avulsion, dogs with biceps tendon pathology are presented for unilateral forelimb lameness of insidious onset. Dogs typically bear weight on the affected limb. Rupture or avulsion may result in more acute and more severe lameness.

Etiopathogenesis

Bicipital tenosynovitis (also called tendinitis or tendinosis), with or without partial tearing, appears to be the most common pathologic condition of the biceps tendon in dogs.[18-25] The etiology likely involves chronic overuse with superimposed "micro" or "macro" traumatic episodes involving the tendon. The problem is chronic inflammation of the portion of the biceps tendon that crosses the shoulder joint. Histologically, synovial villous hypertrophy, hypervascularity, and lymphocytic-plasmacytic infiltration are noted.[21,24] Long-term, this condition can result in tendon fibrosis, necrosis, fibril disruption, collagenolysis, metaplasia, and calcification; enthesiophytosis; and secondary osteoarthritis.[21,24]

Avulsion or rupture of the biceps tendon can occur at the tendon's origin at the supraglenoid tubercle or can include avulsion of the tubercle from the scapula.[18,19,26,27] Avulsion of the tubercle can occur as a Salter-Harris fracture at the supraglenoid ossification center in immature dogs.[26,27] Rupture of the tendon can also occur at mid-substance or the musculotendinous junction. Avulsion and ruptures of all types are most often associated with trauma from jumping, falling, or blunt impact (i.e., vehicular trauma).

The etiology and significance of displaced and bipartite biceps tendons are not known.[18,19] These conditions may involve genetically based anatomic variations and appear to have a variety of manifestations from incidental findings to overt pain and lameness.

Diagnosis

Physical examination of dogs with biceps tendon pathology is similar regardless of specific cause. The most consistent examination findings reported include lameness, mild to moderate atrophy of the affected spinatus muscles, pain on shoulder flexion (especially with the elbow extended), and pain on direct palpation of the biceps tendon, and/or manual tensioning of the biceps muscle.[18-25,28,29]

Definitive diagnosis and characterization of the type of pathology of the biceps tendon typically requires more advanced imaging modalities such as contrast arthrography, ultrasonographic evaluation, and/or arthroscopic visualization.[18-25,28,29] Plain radiographic views of the affected shoulder joint provide relevant information regarding secondary bone and soft tissue changes and should be included in the diagnostic database. "Skyline" radiographic views may aid in evaluating the biceps groove.[20,23] In cases of bicipital tenosynovitis, radiographs may show evidence of osteophytosis and enthesiophytosis associated with the biceps tendon and groove (Figure 101-3). Contrast arthrography provides additional information regarding the anatomy and integrity of the biceps tendon. Contrast arthrography is reported to be sensitive for identifying biceps tenosynovitis,[23] but generally does not delineate type or extent of the pathology or give information regarding changes within the tendon tissue.[18-25]

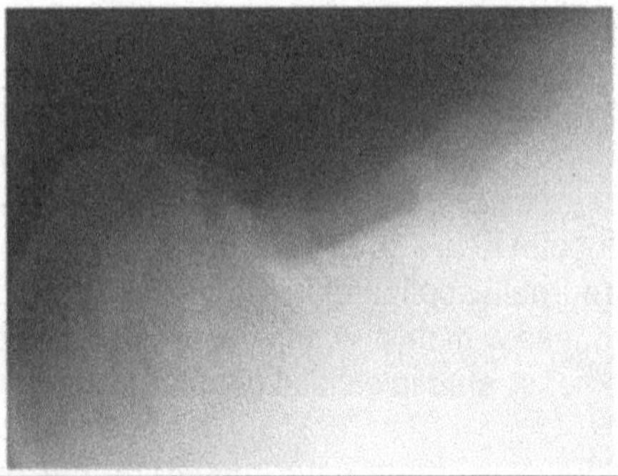

Figure 101-3. "Skyline" radiographic view showing reactive osseus proliferation within the intertubercular groove commonly seen with biceps tenosynovitis.

Ultrasonography of the biceps tendon, performed by an experienced individual, provides for assessment of intratendinous pathology, associated effusion, and pathologic changes of the biceps groove (Figure 101-4).[23,25,29] Ultrasonography is helpful for determining the type and severity of the pathology in the majority of cases.[25,29] Arthroscopic evaluation of the shoulder joint allows for visualization and assessment of all intra-articular structures, providing definitive evidence of visible biceps pathology as well as involvement of other tissues (Figure 101-5). More advanced imaging techniques such as computed tomography and magnetic resonance imaging are currently being investigated for their usefulness for diagnosis of shoulder joint pathology in dogs.

It is critical to perform a comprehensive diagnostic evaluation of dogs suspected, or even confirmed, to have biceps tendon pathology. Biceps tendon pathology can be a secondary or incidental finding. Many dogs with biceps tendon problems also have elbow pathology, neurologic dysfunction, or neoplasia. It is vital to look for other pathology in every dog diagnosed with biceps tendon disorders as these other problems are often more clinically important and will greatly affect treatment and

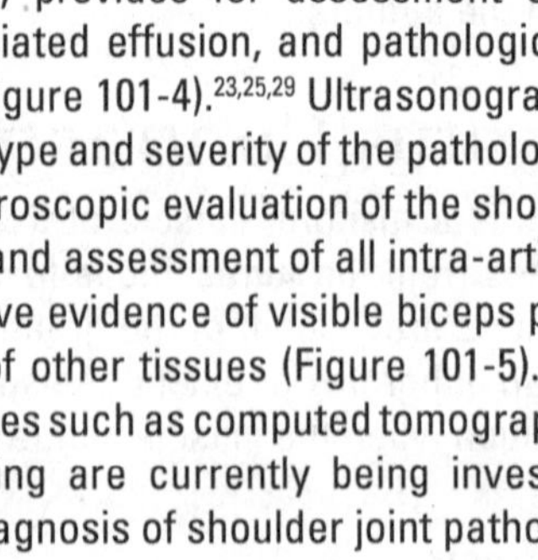

Figure 101-4. Ultrasonographic image showing a transverse view of a biceps tendon with disruption of normal tendon architecture and associated effusion indicating biceps tenosynovitis from a partial tear.

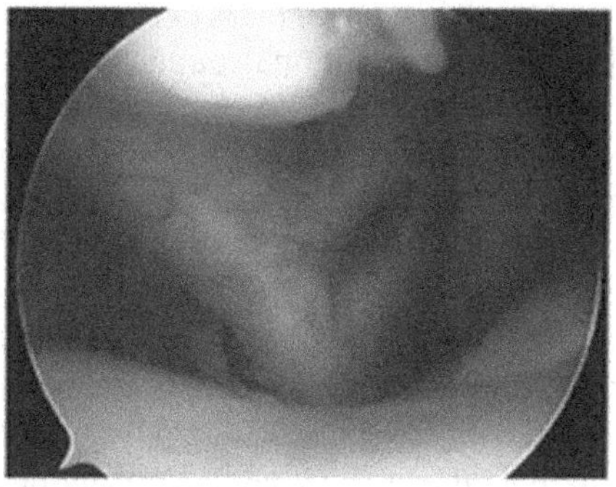

Figure 101-5. Arthroscopic views of a biceps tendon with tenosynovitis and partial avulsion.

prognosis. The authors recommend performing a complete neurologic examination and obtaining radiographs of the elbows in all cases.

Treatment

When biceps tendon pathology is determined to be a significant cause of pain, lameness, and/or dysfunction in dogs, treatment is indicated. Nonsurgical management of biceps tendon pathology consisting of activity modification, nonsteroidal anti-inflammatory drugs, analgesics, and/or intra-articular injections may be effective in many cases.[18-20,22,25] Exercise restriction appears to be a critical component of successful nonsurgical management. Success rates for nonsurgical treatment of biceps tenosynovitis range from 41% to 73%.[20,25] This variability in outcome is likely due in part to the inability to fully assess the cause and severity of tendon pathology preoperatively. Optimizing comprehensiveness and consistency in diagnosis and characterization of biceps tendon pathology in dogs may lead to more definitive algorithms for decision-making regarding indications for various treatments in these patients.

Surgical management is deemed necessary in a significant number of dogs with biceps tendon pathology.[18-20,22-26,28-30] The reported surgical treatment options for biceps tendon disease include tenodesis, tenotomy, primary repair, debridement, transposition, and lavage.[18-20,22-26,28-30] In the authors' experience, primary repair, debridement, and transposition are rarely indicated for primary lesions of the biceps tendon. However, these treatment options have been reported to result in successful outcomes, and may warrant consideration in selected cases. Avulsions that include an adequate portion of supraglenoid tubercle can be successfully treated using open or closed reduction techniques and stabilized with internal fixation, such as pin and tension band wiring, divergent pinning, and/or lag screw fixation (Figure 101-6).[26,27]

For surgical treatment of biceps tenosynovitis with or without partial tears, biceps tenodesis via an open approach and open or arthroscopic biceps tendon release (tenotomy) are the most common surgical procedures used to treat biceps tendon problems in dogs.[18-20,22,25,28-30] Each of these techniques has been reported to be a successful means of treatment for biceps disorders in dogs. Arthroscopic biceps tenotomy was reported to result in good to excellent results in 5 dogs in a series based on subjective measures over a 6-month follow-up period.[28] Open tenodesis has been be associated with good and excellent outcomes in more than 90% of dogs treated.[20,22] Six dogs treated by arthroscopic tenodesis were judged to have good or excellent outcomes in another reported series.[29]

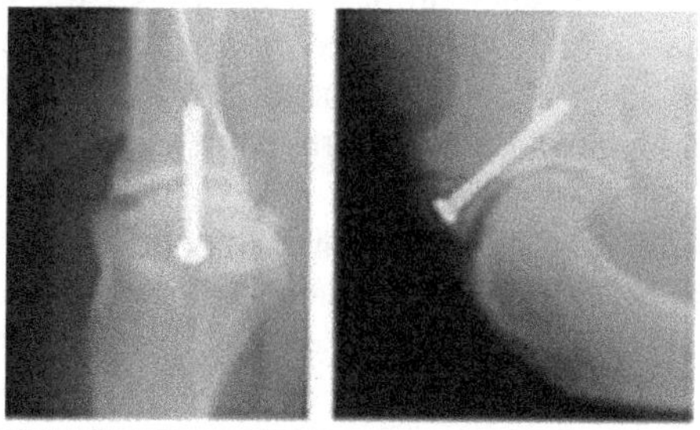

Figure 101-6. Postoperative radiographic views of a dog with avulsion of the biceps tendon origin at the supraglenoid tubercle treated by lag screw fixation after arthroscopically and fluoroscopically guided and performed reduction.

The published literature regarding surgical treatment of biceps tendon pathology suggests that postoperative protection of the repair or treatment, weight management, and physical rehabilitation are critical for a successful outcome when treating biceps tendon problems using any modality.[18-20,25,28-30] It is important to counsel owners that maximal function may not be reached until 6 months following surgery in the majority of cases, and that these are typically chronic problems requiring compliance in treatment, careful monitoring, and most of all, patience. However, when these factors are addressed, the prognosis for the vast majority of biceps tendon disorders is good to excellent for pain-free, "pet-level" function, and guarded to good for high-level athletic function.

Shoulder Instability

Shoulder instability owing to periarticular soft-tissue pathology is a commonly diagnosed problem in humans. Bardet has described a shoulder instability syndrome in dogs.[9] Although lateral and multidirectional shoulder instabilities have been described,[9,31] medial shoulder instability (MSI) appears to be the predominant type of shoulder instability seen in dogs.[9,32,33] Characterization of epidemiology, pathology, diagnosis, indications for treatment, treatment options, outcomes, and prognosis for MSI are currently a major focus in veterinary medicine. Dogs diagnosed with MSI are most commonly middle-aged, large-breed dogs with a history of chronic unilateral forelimb lameness.[32,33] Dogs with MSI typically have an intended purpose of work, performance, or active pet-level function.[32,33]

Etiopathogenesis

The etiology of MSI is not known, but available data suggest that this problem occurs as a result of chronic overuse injury with episodes of "micro" trauma to the shoulder occurring during the development of disease. The pathology associated with MSI includes lameness, shoulder joint laxity, pain on manipulation of the shoulder, and abnormalities of the medial joint capsule, subscapularis tendon, and medial glenohumeral ligament observed via arthroscopy.[9,32-34]

Diagnosis

Signalment, complete history, complete orthopedic and neurologic examination, blood work, radiographs, and ultrasonography are integral to the comprehensive diagnostic approach. Ultrasonographic evaluation is recommended for all potential MSI patients to rule out primary or concurrent musculotendinous pathology. Definitive diagnosis of MSI is based primarily on palpation and exploratory arthroscopy.

Palpation under sedation is a key component of preoperative diagnosis of MSI. Range of motion in flexion, extension, and rotation, the "shoulder drawer sign" as described by Bardet,[9] and the shoulder abduction test[32,33] should be assessed in each limb. Shoulder abduction angles measured under sedation have been reported to provide objective data for diagnosis of MSI in dogs.[32,33] Shoulders with clinical and arthroscopic evidence of MSI have significantly higher angles (53.7 ± 4.7°) compared with shoulders considered normal (32.6 ± 2.0°).[33]

Currently, arthroscopic exploration provides the most definitive diagnosis of MSI and allows assessment of cartilage damage and other key structures in the shoulder joint. Arthroscopic identification of tearing and laxity of the subscapularis tendon, medial glenohumeral ligament, and joint capsule are consistent findings in reported cases of MSI (Figure 101-7).[32,33]

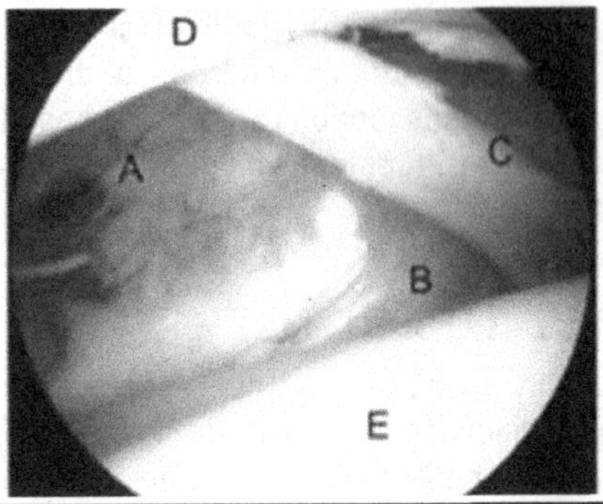

Figure 101-7. Arthroscopic view of the pathology of the medial joint capsule (A), subscapularis tendon (B), and medial glenohumeral ligament (C) typically seen in dogs diagnosed with medial shoulder instability. The distance between glenoid (D) and humeral head (E) also appears excessive.

It is vitally important to rule out separate or concurrent causes of shoulder lameness. Dogs with MSI may also have elbow pathology, neurologic dysfunction, or neoplasia. It is vital to look for other pathology in every dog presumptively diagnosed with MSI as these other problems are often more clinically important and will greatly affect treatment and prognosis. The authors recommend performing a complete neurologic examination and obtaining radiographs of the elbows in all cases.

Treatment

Few data are available regarding indications for treatment, treatment options, and prognosis for shoulder MSI in dogs. Treatment recommendations are based on extent and severity of instability, concurrent shoulder pathology, concurrent orthopedic problems, the overall health of the patient, the intended use of the patient, and the commitment of the owner.[9,31-35] The use of radiofrequency-induced thermal capsulorrhaphy (RITC) for treatment of MSI in dogs has been reported to be successful.[32,34] RITC treatment resulted in improved clinical function in 93% of cases, with 79% considered to have excellent outcomes and 7% considered to be failures.[32] Appropriate postoperative care appears to be a critical factor in realizing success in these cases. It is imperative that the dogs be kept in a non-weight-bearing sling for 3 to 4 weeks after RITC treatment in order to protect the treated tissue. It is vital that careful attention to sling and limb management is employed during this period. Severe complications, primarily skin wounds and carpus and elbow contracture, can occur if the sling is not properly cared for and range of motion exercises are not performed at the time of sling change (at least once weekly). For the subsequent 6 weeks, strict exercise restriction with physical rehabilitation is recommended, followed by a progressive return to full function. Dogs do not reach improved function until 12 to 16 weeks after treatment and do not reach full post-treatment function until 5 to 6 months after treatment.[32] Bilateral shoulder instability, complete tears of the MGL, a single major traumatic episode as the cause of the MSI, concurrent forelimb orthopedic pathology, neurologic dysfunction, and shoulder osteoarthritis are reported to be contraindications for RITC treatment of MSI.[32] For complete tears of the MGL, ST, or MJC, open or arthroscopic reconstruction of the medial compartment by direct tissue reapposition and tissue anchor and suture or imbrication suture reinforcement is recommended.[35] Excision arthroplasty and arthrodesis may also be viable options in a subset of patients with severe MSI. For those cases that do not fit the inclusion criteria for any surgical treatment, non-surgical treatment consisting of weight management, activity modification, and medical therapy is recommended. No study in which any of these treatments for MSI were compared has been reported to date.

Shoulder instability appears to be a documented problem in dogs that can result in pain and lameness. However, our understanding of etiopathogenesis, clinical versus subclinical pathology, optimal diagnostic tools, indications for treatment, surgical decision making, and prognostication for shoulder instability in dogs is lacking, and a significant amount of work needs to be done to further characterize and make definitive recommendations regarding this entity.

References

1. Kujat R: The microangiographic pattern of the rotator cuff of the dog. Arch Orthop Trauma Surg 109:68, 1990.

2. Uhthoff HK, Loehr JW: Calcific tendinopathy of the rotator cuff: Pathogenesis, diagnosis and management. J Am Acad Orthop Surg 5:183, 1997.

3. Archer RS, Bayley JIL, Archer CW, et al: Cell and matrix changes associated with pathological calcification of the human rotator cuff tendons. J Anat 182:1, 1993.

4. Uhthoff HK, Sarkar K, Maynard JA: Calcifying tendinitis: A new concept of its pathogenesis. Clin Orthop 118:164, 1976.

5. Danova NA, Muir P: Extracorporeal shock wave therapy for supraspinatus calcifying tendinopathy in two dogs. Vet Rec 152:208, 2003.

6. Laitinen OM, Flo GL: Mineralization of the supraspinatus tendon in

dogs: A long-term follow up. J Am Anim Hosp Assoc 36:262, 2000.

7. Muir P, Johnson KA, Cooley AJ, et al: Force-plate analysis of gait before and after surgical excision of calcified lesions of the supraspinatus tendon in two dogs. Vet Rec 139:137, 1996.

8. Flo GL, Middleton D: Mineralization of the supraspinatus tendon in dogs. J Am Vet Med Assoc 197:95, 1990.

9. Bardet JF: Diagnosis of shoulder instability in dogs and cats: A retrospective study. J Am Anim Hosp Assoc 34:42, 1998.

10. Long CD, Nyland TG: Ultrasonographic evaluation of the canine shoulder. Vet Radiol Ultrasound 40:372, 1999.

11. Gschwend N, Scherer M, Löhr J: Tendinits calcarea of shoulder joint (T.c.). Orthopade 10:196, 1981.

12. Meutstege FJ: Contracuctuur van de M. Infrapsinatus als oorzaak van boegkreupelheid bij een hond. Tijdschr Diergeneeskd 95:24, 1970.

13. Pettit GD: Infraspinatus muscle contracture in dogs. Mod Vet Pract 61:451, 1980.

14. Pettit GD, Chatburnn CC, Hegreberg GA, et al: Studies on the pathophysiology of infraspinatus muscle contracture in the dog. Vet Surg 7:8, 1978.

15. Bennet RA: Contracture of the infraspinatus muscle in dogs: A review of 12 cases. J Am Anim Hosp Assoc 22:481, 1986.

16. Bennet D, Campbell JR: Unusual soft tissue orthopaedic problems in the dog. J Small Anim Pract 20:27, 1979.

17. Siems JJ, Breuer GJ, Blevins WE, et al: Use of two-dimensional real-time ultrasonography for diagnosing contracture and strain of the infraspinatus muscle in a dog. J Am Vet Med Assoc 212:77, 1998.

18. Bardet JF: Shoulder diseases in dogs. Vet Med Dec:909, 2002.

19. Bardet JF: Lesions of the biceps tendon – diagnosis and classification. Vet Comp Orthop Traumatol 12:188, 1999.

20. Stobie D, Wallace LJ, Lipowitz AJ, et al: Chronic bicipital tenosynovitis in dogs: 29 cases (1985-1992). J Am Vet Med Assoc 207:201, 1995.

21. Gilley RS, Wallace LJ, Hayden DW: Clinical and pathologic analyses of bicipital tenosynovitis in dogs. Am J Vet Res 63:402, 2002.

22. Lincoln JD, Potter K: Tenosynovitis of the biceps brachii tendon in dogs. J Am Anim Hosp Assoc 20:385, 1984.

23. Rivers B, Wallace L, Johnston GR: Biceps tenosynovitis in the dog: Radiographic and sonographic findings. Vet Comp Orthop Traumatol 5:51, 1992.

24. Davidson EB, Griffey SM, Vasseur PB, et al: Histopathologic, radiographic, and arthrographic comparison of the biceps tendon in normal dogs and dogs with biceps tenosynovitis. J Am Anim Hosp Assoc 36:522, 2000.

25. Bruce WJ, Burbidge HM, Bray JP, et al: Bicipital tendonitis and tenosynovitis in the dog: a study of 15 cases. NZ Vet J 48:44, 2000.

26. Deneuche AJ, Viguier E: Reduction and stabilization of a supraglenoid tuberosity avulsion under arthroscopic guidance in a dog. J Small Anim Pract 43:308, 2002.

27. Cook JL, Cook CR, Tomlinson JL, et al: Scapular fractures in dogs: Epidemiology, classification, and concurrent injuries in 105 cases (1988-1994). J Am Anim Hosp Assoc 33:528, 1997.

28. Wall CR, Taylor R: Arthroscopic biceps brachii tenotomy as a treatment for canine bicipital tenosynovitis. J Am Anim Hosp Assoc 38:169, 2002.

29. Cook JL, Kenter K, Fox DB: Arthroscopic biceps tenodesis: Technique and results in six dogs. J Am Anim Hosp Assoc 41:121, 2005.

30. Adamiak Z, Szalecki P: Treatment of bicipital tenosynovitis with double tenodesis. J Small Anim Pract 44:539, 2003.

31. Mitchell RAS, Innes JF: Lateral glenohumeral ligament rupture in three dogs. J Small Anim Pract 41:511-514, 2000.

32. Cook JL, Tomlinson JL, Fox DB, et al:. Treatment of dogs diagnosed with medial shoulder instability using radiofrequency-induced thermal capsulorrhaphy. Vet Surg 34:469-475, 2005.

33. Cook JL, Renfro DC, Tomlinson JL, Sorensen JE: Measurement of angles of abduction for diagnosis of shoulder instability in dogs using goniometry and digital image analysis. Vet Surg 34:463-468, 2005.

34. O'Neill T, Innes JF: Treatment of shoulder instability caused by medial glenohumeral ligament rupture with thermal capsulorrhaphy. J Small Anim Pract 45:521-524, 2004.

35. Fitch RB, Breshears L, Staatz A, Kudnig S: Clinical evaluation of a prosthetic medial glenohumeral ligament repair in the dog (ten cases). Vet Comp Orthop Traumatol 14:222-228, 2001.

Chapter 102

Elbow Dysplasia

Stéphane Bureau
Jean-François Bardet

Originally, the term "elbow dysplasia" was introduced to describe a generalized osteoarthritis of the elbow joint in which an ununited anconeal process occurred in some but not in all of the affected joints.[1] Later, fragmentation of the medial coronoid process of the ulna and osteochondritis dissecans of the medial aspect of the humeral condyle were recognized to also be associated with this generalized osteoarthritis.[2] The modern concept of elbow dysplasia means a complex of polygenic hereditary developmental abnormalities of the elbow, including ununited anconeal process (UAP), fragmented medial coronoid process (FMCP), osteochondrosis of the medial humeral condyle (OCD), and elbow incongruity (EI).[3-5] The term elbow dysplasia has been accepted to describe all conditions resulting in arthrosis of the elbow joint regardless of the underlying cause (1990, International Elbow Working Group meeting, San Francisco).

The same form of dysplasia may be found in both elbows or a combination of forms may be observed, such as FMCP and OCD.[6-11] Breeds may be predisposed to a particular form of elbow dysplasia. The German shepherd dog suffers more from UAP.[12-14] FMCP and incongruity are the most common findings in the Bernese mountain dog.[15-16] Rottweilers most frequently have FMCP but are rarely affected by OCD.[6,8,11] The Labrador retriever is most likely to have OCD and FMCP.[11,17] The suggestion that different patterns of disease exist within breeds or within families is extremely important in gaining a complete understanding of this complicated syndrome.[18]

The pathogenesis of this disease remains poorly understood and controversial.[4,19] The finding of all forms of dysplasia within both elbows of a single dog, plus the finding of various forms of elbow dysplasia within the same elbow suggests a common etiology.[18] Incongruity exists in the different forms of elbow dysplasia.[20] Three major pathogenetic mechanisms proposed to explain the development of elbow dysplasia are asynchronous growth of the radius and ulna, osteochondrosis, and trochlear notch dysplasia.

Ununited Anconeal Process

The pathogenesis of UAP is controversial. The heritability in the German shepherd dog was reported early and conclusively.[1,21,22] The lesion in other breeds has not been so well studied; however, it is thought that it is probably inherited in these dogs as well.[18]

Ununited anconeal process has been described as a manifestation of osteochondrosis.[3] Osteochondrosis (OC) is disturbed endochondral ossification of articular or physeal cartilage.[23,24] The cartilage continues to grow and it becomes abnormally thick and obviously less resistant to mechanical stress.[23,24] In other cases, OC causes retarded growth or premature closure of a growth plate.[24] Retention of cartilage in the distal ulna may occasionally lead to retarded growth of the ulna; overgrowth of the radius with a relatively shorter ulna could be the cause of UAP (Figure 102-1).[24,25] The radius that is too long relative to the ulna forces the trochlea of the humerus in a proximal direction, which exerts more pressure than normal on the anconeal process, resulting in damage to the joint cartilage and to the ossification center of the anconeal process.[3,25] If OC is present, the entire structure is less resistant to trauma and a tear in the weakened cartilage prevents osseous bridging of the gap.[3] Measurements made of the olecranon in German shepherd dogs with UAP showed a significantly shorter olecranon in affected limbs.[12] The UAP may be completely separated or joined to the ulna by fibrous or fibrocartilaginous tissue.[19] In large-breed puppies, deformed anconeal processes with degenerated articular surfaces have lesions such as ischemia, degeneration, and multifocal dystrophic mineralization, which were apparently a result of pressure exerted by an upward thrust of the condylar surface of the humerus.[4] In a study on dogs with UAP this pressure on the anconeal process was eliminated by lengthening the ulna through osteotomy.[19]

Although asynchronous growth of the radius and ulna may play a role in the pathogenesis of UAP, breeds of dogs having secondary centers of ossification at that location are most likely predisposed to develop that lesion. In the German shepherd dog, the separate ossification center of the anconeal process appears at 11 to 14 weeks and the anconeal process is united with the olecranon at 20 to 22 weeks.[9] In the greyhound, UAP is unknown; this is assumed to be because the anconeal process of the ulna ossifies more rapidly than that in the German shepherd dog.[26] Bony union is completed in approximately 2 to 3 weeks in the greyhound against 6 to 8 weeks in the German shepherd dog.[26] Surgical specimens of UAP from breeds with secondary centers of ossification of the anconeal process had a well formed articular surface of the proximal trochlear notch in which the articular cartilage was supported by an oriented cancellous bony base.[4] The fracture line travelled along what appeared to be a fenestrated closing growth plate. By contrast, surgical specimens of UAP from large-breed dogs that did not have separate secondary centers of ossification of this process were deformed, had less ordered cancellous bone architecture, and did not have the remnants of a closing growth plate along the base. The fracture lines of these specimens had the disordered appearance of a fatigue or stress fracture.[4]

Fragmented Medial Coronoid Process – Osteochondritis Dissecans

Fragmented medial coronoid process is commonly seen with OCD or erosive lesions.[2,7,11] Nevertheless, the lesions can occur independently and one does not lead on to the other.[27] Olsson proposed that both FMCP and OCD are manifestations of OC and could result in overgrowth of the ulna.[3,9] No histologic evidence was found that the medial coronoid process of the ulna has a separate center of ossification.[28] The cartilaginous medial

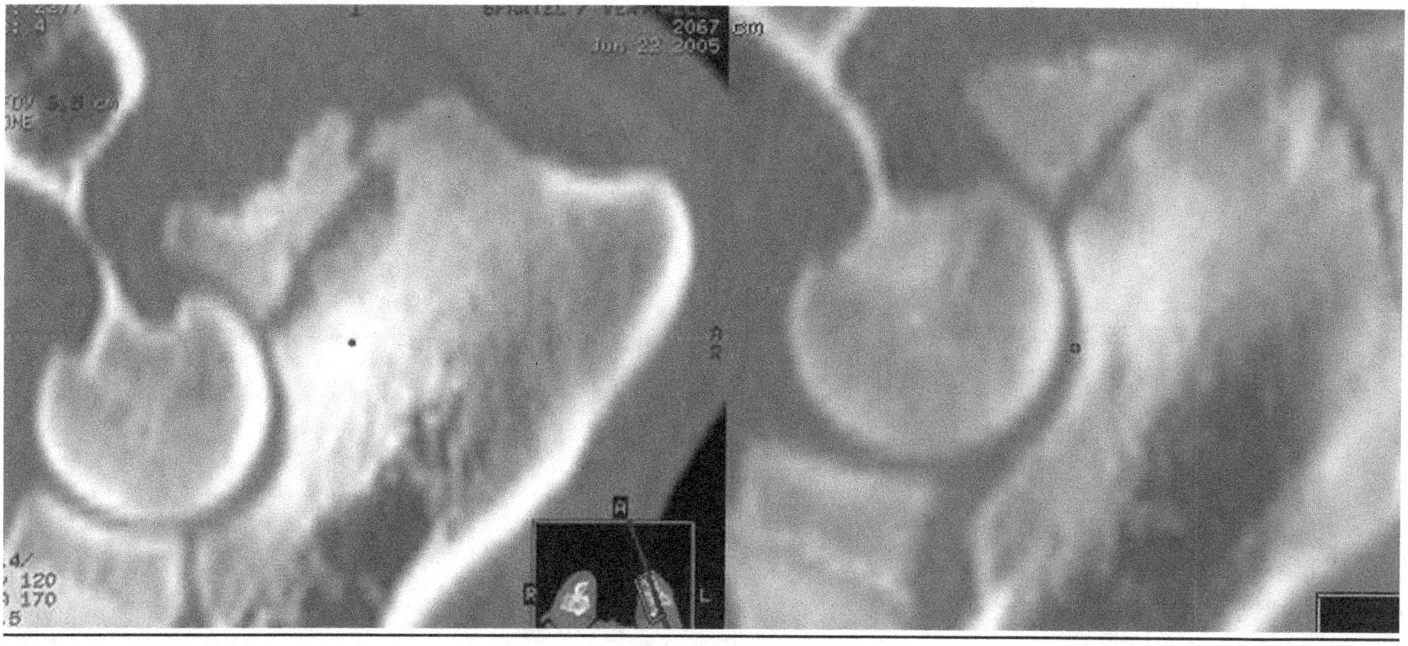

Figure 102-1. CT scan of two dogs affected by UAP. Overgrowth of the radius with a relatively shorter ulna could be the cause of UAP (right) but is not systematically observed (left).

coronoid process ossifies from its base to the tip and ossification is completed at 20 to 22 weeks.[9] This delay in ossification of the medial coronoid process may predispose it to fragmentation when mechanical stresses are applied.[25] There is no step between the coronoid process and the radius during the stance phase of the gait cycle.[29] A study of the distribution of forces between the articular surface of the humerus and radius, and between the humerus and ulna in normal canine joints shows that the ulna is an important structure in the transfer of load. The ratio of the mean forces between the proximal articular surfaces of the radius and ulna remained close to a 50:50 distribution regardless of the applied load.[30] In human elbow joints the coronoid process appears to be an essential osseous block to prevent posterior subluxation.[31]

In puppies up to 5 months of age, the bones would move past one another along the longitudinal axis over a distance of about 1 to 2 mm. In puppies older than 5 months, longitudinal movement of the radius and ulna was limited. No movement could be elicited in any of the specimens older than 6 to 7 months. This may be due in part to the natural slowing of longitudinal bone growth as skeletal maturity is approached, but it may also be due in part to the restraining effect on growth plates exerted by the maturing intraosseous membrane and the ligament that begins to mature and resist longitudinal movement at about this time.[4]

Overgrowth of the ulna places an abnormal load on the medial coronoid process and the medial condyle of the humerus; FMCP, OCD, or both in combination could appear.[3] The resulting malalignment of the proximal ulna and radius caused much of the weight that was transferred from the humeral condyle to the antebrachium to be transmitted through the small, elevated medial coronoid process, leading to fragmentation or abnormal ossification of the coronoid process.[3,29] Owing to mechanical stress, fissures can result within the thickened cartilage of medial condyle that eventually leads to the formation of a cartilage flap or OCD lesion.[25] If the overgrowth of the ulna develops late, the development of the skeleton has reached a stage of near maturity that does not provide the ground for the appearance of FMCP and OCD. In that case, the increased load on the humeroulnar compartment of the elbow joint leads only to erosion, or "kissing lesion" that may extend into the underlying bone.[3]

The split line reveals the prevailing alignment of collagen fibers in subchondral bone. An interrelation exists between development and differentiation of connective and supporting tissues and the load acting on them.[32] The orientation of the split line denotes the direction of maximal tensile strength. Three main types of split-line pattern could be differentiated and correspond well with the different fissure and fragmentation line pattern of the medial coronoid process.[32] These similarities may indicate an association between orientation of the split line and type of lesion.[32]

Up to seven types of lesions of the medial coronoid process are described, with articular cartilage of the medial coronoid process at the same level as that of the radial head or elevated (Figure 102-2).[33] A decrease of the height of the step between the articular surface of the coronoid and radial head is obtained after a proximal ulna sliding osteotomy.[33,34] The damage to the medial coronoid process varies widely. It may remain cartilaginous, have a delayed ossification, or may ossify at a more normal time. The lesion may appear as a fissure within the cartilage with complete separation of the cartilage fragment or it may appear as a fissure within the bone, with an incomplete fracture or complete separation of a bony fragment.[18] A FMCP might be separated from the fracture bed and remain viable because it is loosely attached to the joint capsule from which it continues to maintain its blood supply. Thus, if displaced, the fragments may remain unchanged or, because of a persistent blood supply, the fragments of cartilage may become larger and may ossify or fragments of bone may enlarge.[9] The OCD lesion lies opposite

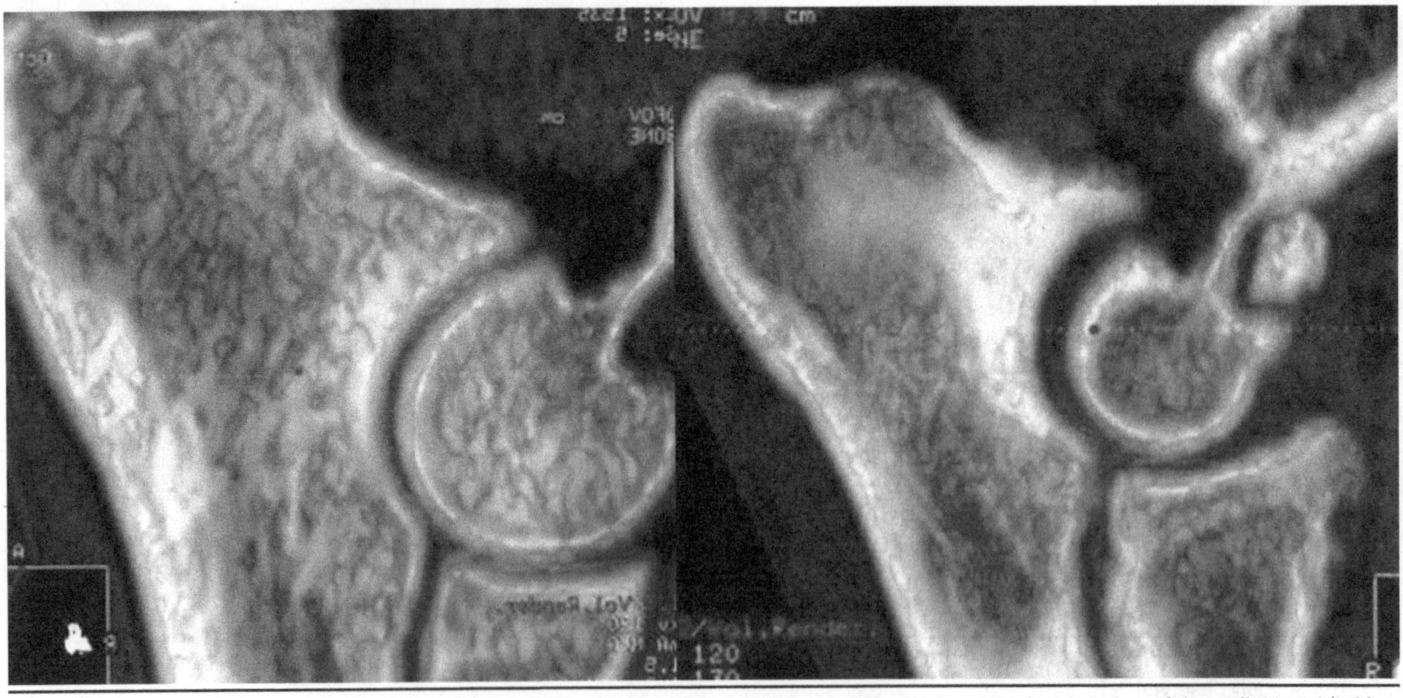

Figure 102-2. CT scan of two 2 dogs affected by FMCP. The medial coronoid process could be at the same level as that of the radial head (left) or could be elevated (right).

the medial coronoid process. The fragment may remain in situ. If it is not removed surgically, it gradually becomes free but rarely mineralizes; it may detach and form a joint mouse.[9]

Medial compartment osteoarthritis with eburnation of the medial humeral condyle is currently diagnosed by arthroscopy. The canine medial compartment osteoarthritis is similar to medial compartment osteoarthritis of the human knee.[35] Research shows an association of the medial compartment osteoarthritis with a varus deformity of the elbow similar to what is described in the knee in people. The humeroulnar angle in normal dogs measured on craniocaudal radiographs varies from 0.53° to 9.09°.[35] Dogs with medial compartment osteoarthritis have a varus deformity with this angle greater than 7°.[36]

The cartilaginous growth disturbance is likely to have genetic and environmental, and mainly nutritional and traumatic causes.[23,25] However, the theory that the lesions are caused by OC is not supported by consistent findings of histologically defective cartilage at early lesion sites. Histologic evidence of thickened degenerated cartilage is reported in less than 20% of 120 dogs with elbow dysplasia.[37] In a multiyear necropsy study, histologic lesions consistent with OC lesions are observed in elbows from 3- to 5-month-old puppies.[4] Both the medial humeral condyle and medial coronoid process have compressed the subchondral capillary bed, disrupted subchondral spongiosa, and focally thickened cartilage lesions. In puppies older than 5 months of age, focal lesions on the medial humeral condyle were roughened and fibrillated but had an intact articular surface. Although the lesions in these older puppies were located at the same site on the medial condyle as were the lesions in the younger puppies, they more closely resembled osteoarthritis than OC.[4] Differences in the histologic and ultrastructural appearance of the OCD and FMCP lesions tend to suggest that they are two separate disease entities. It is hypothesised that OCD results from incorrect cartilage maturation and endochondral ossification, and the etiology of FMCP is subchondral fracture with an ineffective fibrous repair in some cases.[27]

Joint Incongruity

The normal canine joint showed a continuous arc formed by the central ridge of the trochlear notch and the proximal radial articulation.[20] Specific areas of articular contact were identified on the radius, the craniolateral aspect of the anconeal process, and the medial coronoid process.[29] The medial coronoid and radial contact areas were continuous across the radioulnar articulation.[29] The incongruity observed between the radius and the ulna suggests either a lagging growth rate of the radius or an ulnar trochlear notch of smaller diameter.

The most obvious abnormality was the finding that the distal edge of the trochlear notch of the ulna with its medial coronoid process lay approximately 2 mm proximally to the articular surface of the radius.[20] Measurements of radial and ulnar length have indicated a statistically significant relative increase in length of the proximal ulna in middle-size and large-breed dogs during a vital period of limb development (before 16 to 20 weeks of age). The ulna was temporarily up to 3 mm longer than the paired radius.[38] Incongruity may not always be evident owing to compensatory adjustment during growth.[38] Examples of bilateral FMCP were found in which a 1- to 2-mm elevation of the medial coronoid process above the radial articular surface remained in one elbow joint.[4] This degree of incongruity, although compatible with a lagging radial growth, is in itself insufficient to explain the relative increase in the length of the proximal ulna.

Disparity in radial and ulnar lengths were noted in both normal and lame dogs and failed to correlate with obvious radiographic joint incongruity.[39] This indicates that variation in the length of these bones may be a normal variation of growth and a common finding in large-breed dogs. Only 5 of 15 lame dogs demonstrated obvious disparity in radial and ulnar length, although it is possible that joint incongruity might have temporarily occurred during growth yet was not apparent at presentation.[39]

Another explanation for the incongruity between the radius and ulna is an abnormal development of the ulnar trochlear notch, resulting in a slightly elliptic joint surface with an arc of curvature insufficient to encompass the humeral trochlea. This creates a joint with major contact points in the areas of the anconeal process and medial coronoid process but without a point of contact between the trochlear notch and the humeral trochlea (Figure 102-3).[20] Underdevelopment of the trochlear notch may be temporary or persistent and becomes evident between the ages of 4 to 6 months.[20] If the incongruity is present at the age of 4 to 6 months, the skeleton at that time is as yet incompletely ossified. Fracture, fragmentation, or fissure of the medial coronoid process could occur owing to the increased weight-bearing forces on the too-high lying parts of the ulna.[20] For the same reason, the

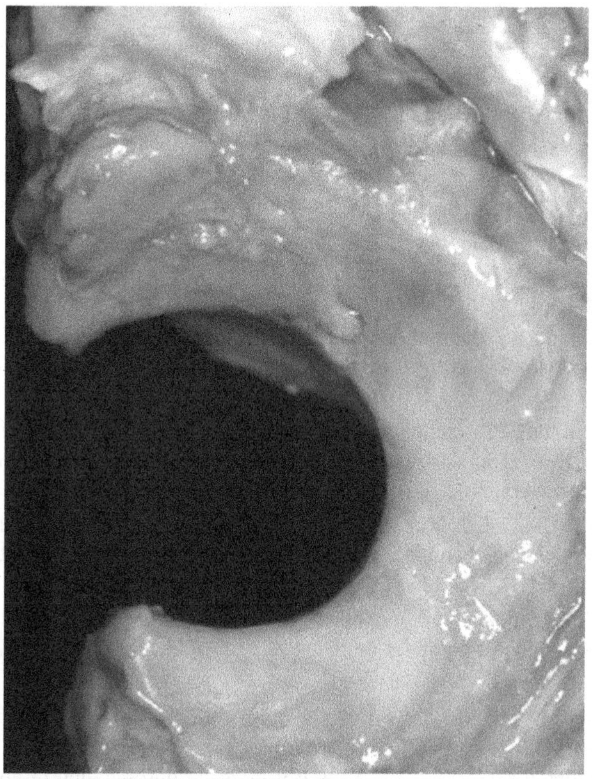

Figure 102-3. An abnormal development of the ulnar trochlear notch with an arc of curvature insufficient to encompass the humeral trochlea creates a joint with major contact points in the areas of the anconeal process and medial coronoid process.

lesion could be an OCD lesion.[20] The humeral condyle is pressed against the anconeal process and causes micromovement of the cartilage bridge and partial to complete separation of the articular process.[20,38] If the incongruity is present after 6 months, it may be present on its own and interferes with the formation of the articular surfaces and the manner in which they articulate; consequently, with time, osteoarthritis develops as a secondary joint disease.[20] Nevertheless, the grade of arthrosis is not always higher in the older dog than in the young dog. Dogs over 5 years of age were identified suffering from FMCP even in the absence of osteophyte formation.[40] It is possible that a different etiopathogenesis such as traumatic fracture or persistent physeal cartilage may have been involved.[40]

The increase in the relative size of the proximal ulna in heavier breeds could be necessary to accommodate a larger trochlear notch for articulation with a heavier humerus.[38] This need for rapid growth may also be a contributing factor for the failure of the trochlear notch to reach the required arc of curvature to encompass the humeral trochlea.[38]

In severe cases, it is obvious that the increased load on the medial coronoid process has led to remodelling of the ulnar part of the elbow joint, leading to a more open trochlear notch.[3] This observation however does not support the hypothesis that an elliptic trochlear notch makes it too small for the trochlea of the humerus. Moreover, the hypothesis of an abnormally developed, slightly elliptical trochlear notch seems unlikely to be a major contributing factor, as combined UAP and FMCP should then occur in much larger numbers of dogs and ulnar ostectomy would have no effects in cases with UAP.[3,19]

One study compared the radius of curvature of the ulnar trochlear notch of the Rottweiler, a breed predisposed to FMCP, to that of greyhound, a breed that has never reported be affected by this disease.[41] The greater radius of curvature within the distal part of the trochlear notch in the Rottweiler results in a more open elliptical shape. It may result in dynamic or positional instability of the cubital joint, increasing stress leading to FMCP. It may also be formed as a result of asynchronous growth of the radius and ulna.[41]

Heritability

Elbow dysplasia is inherited as multifactorial or polygenic traits.[5,42,43] Osteochondritis dissecans and FMCP were found to be inherited independently as polygenic traits.[17] Fragmented coronoid process and incongruity were found to be genetically separate diseases.[16] If elbow dysplasia is the phenotypic effect of independent genetic diseases, the phenotype may behave polygenetically even though the underlying components are monogenous.[16] The incidence of elbow dysplasia was found to be strongly breed-specific statistically and was higher in intermediate and heavy-set breeds when compared with sight hounds and setter-type breeds.[38] The exact nature of the environmental contribution to the disease remains unclear, although several putative factors have been put forward such as nutrition and exercise.[5,16]

Males generally are more frequently affected.[7,10,11,42,44] Heritability in Labrador retrievers was 0.77 for males and 0.45 for females.[45] In Rottweilers, estimation of heritability for elbow dysplasia was 0.34 +/- 0.04.46 Reported incidence for this breed in Norway was 40%.[8] In Bernese mountain dogs and Rottweilers, heritability based on regression of sons on sires was 0.34, and the estimated heritability based on regression of daughters on dams was 0.28 and 0.4 respectively.[43] An inherited basis for elbow osteochondrosis has also been reported in the Labrador retriever with a greater contribution of the dam suggesting a "maternal effect."[10] The differences in the prevalence can be explained by a direct effect of genes on the sex chromosomes or by an effect of secondary sex characteristics such as differences in growth rate, sex hormones, or behavioral patterns. For a polygenic trait such as arthrosis in the elbow joint, the effect of secondary sex characteristics is a more plausible explanation.[43]

Conclusion

Elbow dysplasia describes all conditions (UAP, FMCP, OCD, EI) resulting in arthrosis of the elbow regardless of the underlying cause. A genetic predisposition is widely recognized. All forms of elbow dysplasia were initially thought to be secondary to osteochondrosis but the research of the last 20 years using histology, traumatic tactile pressure sensor, computed tomography, and subchondral split-line patterns clearly indicates a biomechanical basis as the major pathophysiologic mechanism of UAP, FMCP, and EI. Differences in the pathology and ultrastructural appearance of the OCD and FMCP lesions tend to suggest that they are two separate diseases. The proximal joint surface of the ulna contributes substantially to load transfer through the canine elbow joint. Anomalies that increase this load appear to contribute to canine elbow dysplasia, mainly fragmentation of the medial coronoid process. Because of the great interest in this common invalidating pathology and the modern tools of investigation, we share a better understanding on how elbow dysplasia might appear, but more research is needed to refine the latest knowledge and to design prevention techniques for elbow osteoarthritis.

References

1. Carlson WD, Severin GA: Elbow dysplasia in the dog: a preliminary report. J Am Vet Med Assoc 138:295, 1961.

2. Olsson SE: En ny typ av armbagsledsdysplasi hos hund ? En preliminary rapport [A new type of elbow dysplasia in the dog? A preliminary report] Svensk Vet Tidn 26:152, 1974.

3. Olsson SE: Pathophysiology, morphology, and clinical signs of osteochondrosis in the dog. *In* Disease Mechanisms in Small Animal Surgery, 2nd ed. Bojrab MS, Smeak DD, Bloomberg MS (eds). Philadelphia: Williams & Wilkins, 1993, p. 777.

4. Trostel CT, McLaughlin RM, Pool RR: Canine elbow dysplasia: anatomy and pathogenesis. Comp Cont Educ Pract Vet 25(No. 10):754-762, 2003.

5. Bedford PGC: Control of hereditary elbow disease in pedigree dogs. J Small Anim Pract 35:119, 1994.

6. Grondalen J: Arthrosis with special reference to the elbow joint of young rapidly growing dogs. II. Nord Vet Med 31:69, 1979.

7. Bennet D, Duff SRI, Kene RO, Lee R: Osteochondrosis dissecans and fragmentation of the coronoid process in the elbow joint of the dog. Vet Rec 109:329, 1981.

8. Grondalen J: Arthrosis in the elbow joint of young rapidly growing dogs. VII. Occurrence in the rottweiler dogs. Nord Vet Med 34:76, 1982.

9. Olsson SE: The early diagnosis of fragmented coronoid process and osteochondritis dissecans of the canine elbow joint. J Am Anim Hosp Assoc 19:616, 1983.

10. Studdert VP, Lavelle RB, Beilharz RG,et al: Clinical features and heritability of osteochondrosis of the elbow in Labrador retrievers. J Small Anim Pract 32:557, 1991.

11. Guthrie S: Use of a radiographic scoring technique for the assessment of dogs with elbow osteochondrosis. J Small Anim Pract 30:639, 1989.

12. Guthrie S: Some radiographic and clinical aspects of ununited anconeal process. Vet Rec 124:661, 1989.

13. Corley EA, Carlson WD: Radiographic, genetic and pathologic aspects of elbow dysplasia. J Am Vet Med Assoc 147:1651, 1965.

14. Cawley AJ, Archibald J: Ununited anconeal processes of the dog. J Am Vet Med Assoc 10:454, 1959.

15. Wind AP: Incidence and radiographic appearance of fragmented coronoid process. Calif Vet 6:19, 1982.

16. Ubbink GJ, Hazewinkel HAW, Van de Broek J, Rothuizen J: Familial clustering and risk analysis for fragmented coronoid process and elbow joint incongruity in Bernese Mountain dogs in the Netherlands. Am J Vet Res 60:1082, 1999.

17. Padget GA, Mostosky UV, Probst CW, et al.: The inheritance of osteochondritis dissecans and fragmented coronoid process of the elbow joint in Labrador retrievers. J Am Anim Hosp Assoc 31:327, 1995.

18. Morgan JP, Wind A, Davidson AP: Hereditary Bone and Joint Diseases in the Dog. Osteochondroses. Hip Dysplasia. Elbow Dysplasia. Vet Schlutersche, 2000, p. 41.

19. Sjostrom L, Kasstrom H, Kallber M: Ununited anconeal process in the dog. Pathogenesis and treatment by osteotomy of the ulna. Vet Comp Orthop Traumatol 8:170, 1995.

20. Wind AP: Elbow incongruity and developmental elbow diseases in the dog: Part 1. J Am Anim Hosp Assoc 22:711, 1986.

21. Corley EA, Sutherland TM, Carlson WD: Genetic aspect of canine elbow dysplasia. J Am Vet Med Assoc 153:543, 1968.

22. Hayes HM, Selby LA, Wilson GP, Hohn RB: Epidemiologic observations of canine elbow disease. J Am Anim Hosp Assoc 14:449, 1979.

23. Nap RC: Pathophysiology and clinical aspects of canine elbow dysplasia. Proceedings of the 7th International Elbow Working Group Meeting, Constance, Germany, July 1, 1995.

24. Olsson SE: Osteochondritis dissecans in the dog. Proceedings of Annual Meeting of the American Animal Hospital Association 42:362, 1975.

25. Scharwz PD: Canine Elbow dysplasia. *In* Kirk's Current Veterinary Therapy XIII, Small Animal Practice. Bonagura JD (ed). Philadelphia: WB Saunders, 2000, p. 1004.

26. Van Sickle DC: A comparative study of the postnatal elbow development of the Greyhound and the German shepherd dog. J Am Vet Med Assoc 147(11):1650, 1965.

27. Guthrie S: Aetiopathogenesis of canine elbow osteochondrosis: a study of loose fragments removed at arthrotomy. Res Vet Sci 52:284, 1992.

28. Guthrie S, Vaughan LC: Post natal development of the canine elbow joint: a light and electron microscopical study. Res Vet Sci 52:67, 1992.

29. Preston CA, Schulz KS, Kass PH: In vitro determination of contact areas in the normal elbow joint of dogs. Am J Vet Res 61:1315, 2000.

30. Mason DR, Schulz KS, Fujita Y, et al.: In vitro force mapping of normal canine humeroradial and humeroulnar joints. Am J Vet Res 66:132, 2005.

31. Johnson JA, King GJW: Anatomy and biomechanics of the elbow. *In* Shoulder and Elbow Arthroplasty. Williams GR, Yamaguchi K, Ramsey ML, Galatz LM (eds). Philadelphia: Lippincott Williams & Wilkins, 2005, p. 279.

32. Kunzel W, Breit S, Probst A: The subchondral split line patterns of the medial coronoid process in canine ulnae. Anat Histol Embryol 33:339, 2004.

33. Bardet JF: Arthroscopy of the elbow in dogs. Part II: the cranial portals in the diagnosis and treatment of the lesions of the coronoid process. Vet Comp Orthop Traumatol 10:60, 1997.

34. Bardet JF, Bureau S: La fragmentation du processus coronoide chez le chien. Etude rétrospective de 83 coudes traités par ostéotomie ulnaire proximale de raccourcissement. Prat Med Chir Anim Comp 31:451, 1996.

35. Besancon MF, Schultz KS, Filipowicz DE, Johnson EG: Standing radiographs of the Canine Elbow. Proceedings Veterinary Orthopaedic Society, Keystone 2005; 22.

36. Olivieri M: Personal Communication, Sept. 2005.

37. Grondalen J: Arthrosis with special reference to the elbow joint of young rapidly growing dogs. A pathoanatomical investigation. Nord Vet Med 33:1, 1981.

38. Wind AP, Packard ME: Elbow incongruity and developmental diseases in the dog: Part II J Am Anim Hosp Assoc 22:725, 1986.

39. Thomson MJ, Robins GM: Osteochondrosis of the elbow: a review of the pathogenesis and a new approach to treatment. Aust Vet J 72(10):375, 1995.

40. Meyer-Lindenberg A, Langhann A, Fehr M, Nolte I: Prevalence of fragmented medial coronoid process of the ulna in lame adult dogs. Vet Rec 151:230, 2002.

41. Collins KE, Cross AR, Lewis DD, et al: A comparison of the radius of curvature of the ulnar trochlear notch of rottweiler and greyhound using three dimensional digitization. Vet Surg 28(5):389, 1999.

42. Grondalen J, Lingaas F: Arthrosis in the elbow joint of young rapidly growing dogs: a genetic investigation. J Small Anim Pract 32:460, 1991.

43. Swenson L, Audell L, Hedhammar A: Prevalence and inheritance of and selection for elbow arthrosis in Bernese mountain dogs and rottweiler in Sweden and benefit : cost analysis of a screening and control program. J Am Vet Med Assoc 210:215, 1997.

44. Grondalen J, Lingaas F: Arthrosis in the elbow joint among Rottweiler dogs. Results from investigations into hereditary disposition. Tijdschrift voor Diergeneeskunde 133: Supplement 1, 1988.

45. Guthrie S, Pidduck HG: Heritability of elbow osteochondritis within a closed population of dogs. J Small Anim Pract 31:93, 1990.

46. Maki K, Liinamo AE, Ojala M: Estimates of genetic parameters for hip and elbow dysplasia in Finnish Rottweilers. J Anim Sci 78:1141, 2000.

Chapter 103

Legg-Calve-Perthes Disease

Michael G. Conzemius
Peter Lotsikas

History

In 1910, Legg, Calve, and Perthes independently described a condition of the hip in children.[1-3] Calve thought that the condition was due to rickets.[2] Perthes thought that it was related to degenerative arthritis, probably of an infectious nature.[3] Legg, however, hypothesized that impairment of blood supply to the femoral epiphysis was the cause of the condition; a hypothesis that parallels our current understanding of the pathogenesis.[1] Of historical interest, Waldenstrom described a case of tuberculosis of the hip in 1909 that may have actually been a case of Legg-Calve-Perthes (LCP) disease.[4] In 1935, LCP disease was first described in the veterinary literature by Tutt.[5] Later, Spicer (1936), Schnelle (1937), and Moltzen-Nielsen (1938) described the condition, using some form of a synonym of LCP disease, in the veterinary literature.[6] Common synonyms for this condition are avascular necrosis of the femoral neck, aseptic necrosis, osteonecrosis, coxa plana, osteochondritis deformans juvenilis, and osteochondrosis.

Pathogenesis

The main histologic feature of LCP disease in both dogs and humans has been described as ischemic necrosis of the center of ossification of the femoral head.[7] Ponseti et al described histologicl, histochemical, and ultrastructural observations of biopsy specimens from the lateral aspect of the femoral head and neck of children with LCP disease.[7] They reported that beneath normal cartilage was thickened epiphyseal cartilage that contained areas of hypercellular and fibrillated cartilage with prominent blood vessels.[7] Ultrastructural examination of these areas revealed irregularly oriented collagen fibers and variable amounts of proteoglycan granules. Hypercellular areas suffered from a decrease in proteoglycans, glycoproteins, and collagen compared with that of normal epiphyseal cartilage. These findings suggest that the disease could be a localized expression of a generalized transient disorder of epiphyseal cartilage that is responsible for delayed skeletal maturation. The collapse of the femoral head likely results from a mechanical failure of this necrotic area that heals as a disorganized epiphyseal cartilage matrix with abnormal ossification. The severe deformity of the femoral head is a consequence of collapse of this mechanically inferior repairing cartilage. What remains unclear is whether the abnormalities of the epiphyseal cartilage are primary or secondary to ischemic events.[8]

In the dog, three histologically distinct stages of the disease have been described: ischemic, early repair, and advanced repair.[9]

The ischemic (necrosis) stage is characterized by empty osteocyte lacunae and the absence of viable marrow. The chondrocytes of the articular and physeal cartilages are histologically and ultrastructurally normal during this stage. The metaphyseal trabeculae may be thickened, but the process of endochondral ossification is generally uninterrupted.

In the early repair stage, the articular cartilage develops clefts and fissures as the subchondral bone begins to collapse beneath it, and the overall shape of the femoral head appears flattened (coxa plana). The repair process begins with revascularization at the periphery of the epiphysis. Fibrovascular tissue composed of capillaries, macrophages, fibroblasts, and histiocytes advances toward the center, resorbing the necrotic marrow debris and dead trabeculae. The articular cartilage appears thickened, especially in the zone of calcification, and the physeal cartilage becomes invaded with fibrovascular repair tissue.

In the advanced repair stage, the articular cartilage becomes markedly thickened with clefts and infolding, and the entire femoral head appears enlarged, with eventual loss of its normal spherical shape. Areas of osteoclastic absorption and extensive new bone formation can be seen histologically at this stage. The disease is considered irreversible at this point because the collapse and repair permanently change the contour of the femoral head. Ultimately, progressive osteoarthrosis develops. The etiology for the ischemia, subsequent fragmentation, and protracted reformation of the femoral head observed in this disorder remain unknown.[7]

Etiology

Many theories as to the etiology of LCP disease have been proposed and disproved since the disease was first described in the dog in 1935. Because the disease affects primarily small and toy breeds, heritability or anatomic variations in small breeds would seem to be factors contributing to the development of the clinical disease. Indeed, Vasseur et al[9] demonstrated that LCP disease was a heritable condition in the Manchester terrier. To understand the exact pattern of inheritance for LCP disease, additional investigation of affected pedigrees must be performed. Intuitively, this condition is likely heritable in similar dog breeds. Supporting information is found in a study comparing the vascular anatomy of the hip in a miniature dog with that in a normal-sized mongrel.[10] This study demonstrated a distinct difference between the two groups in the channel of the superior retinacular vessels. In the miniature dog, the vessels coursed through a shallow neck and appeared as a suspended bridge as compared with a deep fossa of the femoral neck in the mongrel dog.[10] The consequence of the difference in vascular supply may be that the femoral heads of miniature dogs are more susceptible to vascular compromise or insults from trauma, synovitis, or vascular abnormalities.

A more recent suggestion is that LCP disease arises after ischemic infarction, venous or arterial, of the capital femoral epiphysis. Vascular compromise leading to LCP disease has been experimentally demonstrated in animal models by several authors.[11-13] Coagulation disorders as a source of infarction were examined in both humans and dogs. Evidence of thrombocytosis and hypofibrinolysis secondary to a protein C and S deficiency was reported in 1997 by Glueck et al.[14] However, other investigators have failed to reproduce their findings.[13] The largest study that evaluated coagulation abnormalities involved a population of 139 children in Northern Ireland with LCP disease. Of the children afflicted with the condition, 38% had a prolonged activated partial thromboplastin time compared with 5.9% in a control group of 220 children.[13] However, no significant differences existed in antithrombotic factors protein C, protein S, or antithrombin (AT) III, or resistance to activated protein C. An association between the prolonged partial thromboplastin time and a clotting factor deficiency was not demonstrated.[13] Likewise, Brenig et al were unable to demonstrate any alterations in protein C, protein S, activated protein C, factor II, factor V, factor VIII:C, or AT III activities in plasma samples of 18 dogs with histopathologically confirmed LCP disease.[15] The cause for prolonged activated partial thromboplastin time in some of these patients remains unknown. Genomic DNA from 15 dogs affected with LCP disease has also been evaluated for mutations in the protein C gene, however no mutations were found.[16]

Diagnosis

Patients generally present in the first year of life with the owner complaining that the dog has a limp. High-risk breeds include terriers, toy poodles, chihuahuas, Lhasa Apsos, miniature pinschers, pugs, and other toy breed dogs.[17] Although LCP disease in people affects males more often than females, no sex predilection has been identified in the dog. Depending on the stage of the disease, the severity of lameness can range from subtle to non-weight bearing. Clinical signs can also vary if the disease is bilateral, which reportedly occurs in 12 to 16% of cases.[18,19] Physical examination findings generally include lameness, muscle atrophy, and pain on extension and abduction of the affected hip joint(s). Given the breeds affected with LCP disease, medial patellar luxation is also a common incidental finding.

Confirmation of examination findings can be performed using radiography. Radiographic findings depend on disease stage (Figure 103-1). Early findings can include evidence of an increase in radiopacity as new bone is laid down on empty lacunae. Progression of the disease includes resorption of necrotic bone. Loss of bone is faster than the production of new bone in this pathologic process and radiographic evidence of osteolysis will be present as the disease progresses. As the femoral head begins to collapse, it will lose its spherical shape and an increase in the joint space may be present. Following collapse, osteoarthritis will rapidly form and osteophytes will be present on radiographs. If both LCP disease and a medial patellar luxation are present and one needs to identify which is most likely causing the clinical signs, nuclear scintigraphy can be performed. Empirically, LCP disease is almost always a bigger contributor to clinical lameness than is a medial patellar luxation. If the etiology of the radiographic findings is in question, arthrocentesis with cytology and a culture should be performed. However, given the infrequency of idiopathic septic arthritis in the dog, this is rarely needed.

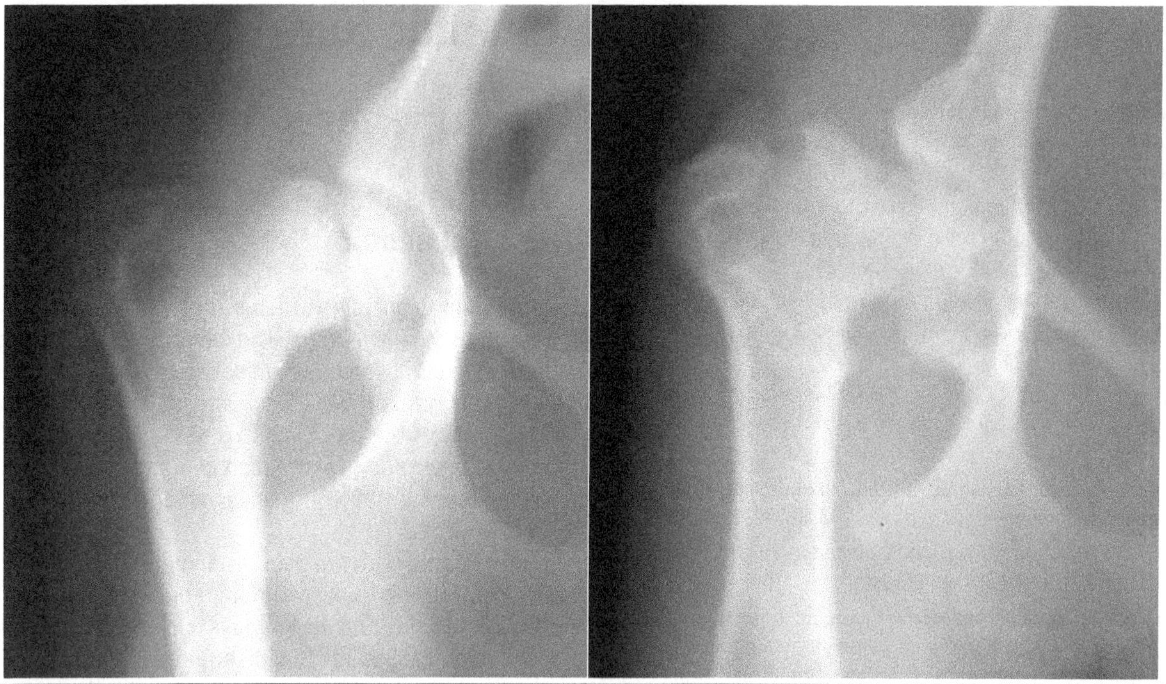

Figure 103-1. Hip-extended radiographs of a 10-month-old Cairn terrier (left) with evidence of sclerosis in the femoral neck and collapse of the femoral head. Radiographic progression of the disease is evident when the dog is 14 months old (right) with complete collapse of the femoral head and severe osteoarthritis.

Treatment

Nonsurgical management consists of strict exercise restriction. In an effort to enforce exercise restriction of unilateral LCP disease a non-weight-bearing sling can be applied. The authors would suggest the use of a Robinson sling, however, the use of an Ehmer sling has been reported to be successful in at least one case report.[20] The duration of exercise restriction varies, but it has been reported that if nonsurgical management is going to be successful it generally takes longer than 2 months.[18] Monthly radiographs should be taken to follow the progression of the disease, and immobilization of the limb continued until complete resolution of the radiolucent areas. In a retrospective report of dogs diagnosed with LCP disease that were treated nonsurgically, only 25% had resolution of their lameness.[18] It is important to note that, even though the prognosis with nonsurgical management is guarded, it remains a reasonable first option (when the radiographic progression of the disease shows no loss of the spherical nature of the femoral head) because surgical management is via a salvage procedure.

A patient that presents with collapse of the femoral head and incongruency of the coxofemoral joint should be treated surgically by femoral head and neck excision. This salvage procedure can be performed simply, is relatively[18] inexpensive, and provides for an improved prognosis. Junggren reported that 30 of 36 dogs that had LCP disease treated with femoral head and neck excision had complete resolution of their clinical signs. In addition, the vast majority of these dogs (80%) had fully recovered within 2 months of surgery. Following femoral head and neck excision, the patient should have exercise restriction until suture removal (7-14 days). After this period, the dog can return to its regular activities. Postoperative rehabilitation including cold and hot packing of the area, passive range of motion, and swimming may further improve the number of dogs that respond favorably to treatment. Several commercially available total hip replacement systems now offer miniature implants. This is no longer true. Patients that have bilateral LCP disease can be treated with bilateral, simultaneous femoral head and neck excision. A ventral approach to the hip for bilateral surgery may reduce morbidity if the surgeon is familiar with the technique.

References

1. Legg A: An obscure affection of the hip joint. Boston Med Surg J 162:202, 1910.

2. Calve J: Sur une forme particuliere de pseudocoxalgie greffee sur des deformations characteristiques de l'extremite superieure du femur. Rev Surg 42:54, 1910.

3. Perthes G: Uber arthritis deformans juvenilis. Dtsch Z Chir 101:779, 1910.

4. Waldenstrom H: Der oobere Tuberculose Collumherd. Orthop Chir 24:487, 1909.

5. Tutt JFD: Tuberculosis of the hip joint in a cairn terrier. Vet Rec 47:428, 1935.

6. Nunamaker DM: Legg-Calve-Perthes disease. *In* Textbook of Small Animal Orthopedics. Philadelphia: JB Lippincott, 1985, pp. 949-952.

7. Ponseti IV, Maynard JA, Weinstein SL, et al: Legg-Calve-Perthes' disease. Histochemical and ultrastructural observations of the epiphyseal cartilage and physis. J Bone Joint Surg 65-A:797-807, 1983.

8. Mickelson MR: Legg-Calve-Perthes' disease in dogs: a comparison to human Legg-Calve-Perthes' disease. Clin Orthop 157:287, 1989.

9. Vasseur PB, Foley P, Stevenson S, Heitter D: Mode of inheritance of Perthes' disease in Manchester Terriers. Clin Orthop 244:281-92, 1989.

10. Fujikawa K: Comparative vascular anatomy of the hip of the miniature dog and of the normal-size mongrel. Kurume Med J 38(3):159-65, 1991.

11. Kemp HBS: Perthes' disease in rabbits and puppies. Clin Orthop 209:139-59, 1986.

12. Calvert PT, Kernohan JG, Sayers DCJ, et al: Effects of vascular occlusion on the femoral head in growing rabbits. Acta Orthop Scand 55:526-30, 1984.

13. Kealey WDC, Mayne EE, Mcdonald W, et al: The role of coagulation abnormalities in the development of Perthes' disease. J Bone Joint Surg (Br) 82-B:744-746, 2000.

14. Glueck CJ, Glueck DG, Freiberg R, et al: Protein C and S deficiency, thrombophilia, and hypofibrinolysis: Pathophysiologic causes of Legg-Perthes disease. Pediatr Res 35:383-8, 1994.

15. Brenig B, Leeb T, Jansen S, Kopp T: Analysis of blood clotting factor activities in canine Legg-Calve-Perthes' disease. J Vet Intern Med 13:570-3, 1999.

16. Leeb T, Kopp T, Deppe A, et al: Molecular characterization and chromosomal assignment of the canine protein C gene. Mamm Genome 10(2):134-9, 1999.

17. LaFond E, Breur GJ, Austin CC: Breed susceptibility for developmental orthopedic diseases in dogs. JAAHA 38:467-77, 2002.

18. Junggren GL: A comparative study of conservative and surgical treatment of Legg Perthes disease in the dog. JAAHA 2(1):6-10, 1966.

19. Lee R, Fry PD: Some observations on the occurrence of Legg-Calve-Perthes disease (coxa plana) in the dog, and an evaluation of excision arthroplasty as a method of treatment. J Small Anim Pract 10(5):309-317, 1969.

20. Gibson KL, Lewis DD, Pechman RD: Use of external coaptation for the treatment of avascular necrosis of the femoral head in a dog. JAVMA 198(7):868-70, 1990.

Chapter 104

Pathogenesis of Hip Dysplasia

Dr. U. Krotscheck
Dr. T. Tohundter

Canine hip dysplasia (CHD) is one of the most common orthopedic complaints in dogs. The severity of clinical signs can vary from occasional lameness to severe dysfunction. It is a complex, polygenic or multifactorial disease which results in osteoarthritis (OA) of the hip joint. This developmental trait is inherited quantitatively and is expressed clinically and morphologically in response to heritable and environmental influences.[1-3]

Dogs affected with hip dysplasia seem to have normal hip joints at birth, but joint laxity accompanied by incongruity develops as early as the first few weeks of life.[2,4-6] It is postulated that initial joint laxity leads to subsequent subluxation of the hip joint during weight-bearing, causing tension on the joint capsule. This trauma is followed by joint capsule thickening, osteophytosis, and enthesiophyte formation.[7] The underlying etiology of joint laxity unknown.

In this chapter we provide an overview of the etiology and pathogenesis of canine hip dysplasia, discuss the proposed genetic and environmental causes of the disease, and discuss hip screening by means of radiography.

Etiology

Historically, CHD has been characterized by the following factors: joint laxity,[8-11] abnormalities of pelvic musculature,[12] chondrosseous factors such as delayed onset of capital femoral ossification,[13-15] altered composition of the chondroepiphysis,[16] and incongruity between the acetabulum and femoral head resulting in dorsolateral subluxation.[17,18] Which of these is the initiating factor is still unknown. Today, two broad etiologies are proposed: hip laxity and abnormal progression of endochondral ossification in multiple joints. These are not mutually exclusive as both could result in an abnormal mechanical environment in the hip that results in OA.

Both the hip joint capsule and the chondrosseous conformation of the hip are major contributors toward the stability of the hip joint during loading and, therefore, must be taken into account when considering an underlying etiology of joint laxity. The round ligament of the femoral head may be the main supporting structure of the hip joint in dogs up to 1 month of age,[7] after which the joint capsule assumes this function. The joint capsule originates in the lateral acetabular rim and inserts into the femoral neck. The strength of the capsule is predominantly due to its fibrillar collagen content and organization, whereas its compliance is due to the extracellular matrix composite of collagen, proteoglycan, water, and elastin.[19-23] As age increases, collagen cross-linking and content increase,[24] contributing to the strength and stiffness of the joint capsule. When load is applied to a normal hip joint capsule, it returns to its original configuration when the load is removed. In the lax capsule, the stress-strain curve is shifted to the right compared with the tight capsule, resulting in further deformation for an equivalent stress than in a tight hip capsule.[25] As a result, the femoral head can undergo lateral translation relative to the acetabulum, a movement that jeopardizes the structural integrity of articular cartilage. This lateral and dorsal translation can be observed in the passive state in the dorsolateral subluxation position. Joint effusion can also cause hip laxity.[17,26]

The joint capsules of dysplastic hips contain a higher ratio of type III to type I collagen in comparison with those of normal greyhounds.[27,28] Whether this is because of tissue immaturity, injury,[29,30] endocrine imbalance,[31] or a genetic abnormality is unknown. These results could be explained by capsular injury;[32] type III collagen is expressed after tissue injury and the dogs in this report were mature and some had been referred for total hip replacement, indicating that OA was advanced.[28] Transmission electron microscopy was used to compare the joint capsules of a dog with hip instability (distraction index 0.8) to one without instability (distraction index 0.4). A heterogeneous group of collagen fibrils was found in the dog with hip laxity and homogeneous collagen fibrils in the capsule of the dog without hip laxity. These same structural differences in collagen fibrils of the ligament of the femoral head were observed in the same loose-hipped and tight-hipped Labrador retrievers. It was not ascertained whether the capsular laxity preceeded or was coincident with synovitis, but it is considered a precursor and risk factor for the development for OA.[6,20,33] Dorsolateral hip luxation cannot develop without passive hip laxity.[17] Dysplastic dogs have abnormal round ligaments of the femoral head. It was shown initially that, in young pups with moderate to severe OA, the volume of this ligament increases.[34] A more recent study comparing the volume of the round ligament of the femoral head and the degree of radiographic OA in adult German shepherds demonstrated that no difference exists between the volume of the ligament of the femoral head in normal joints and those with only "mild" OA (shallow acetabulum/marked dorsal rim attenuation, moderately osteophytic acetabular margin, rounded femoral head, and minimal osteophytes on the femoral neck).[35] An inverse correlation exists between the severity of radiographic OA and the volume of the round ligament of the femoral head.[35]

The second broad etiologic category of CHD is an abnormality in endochondral ossification. The developing hip is composed of two articulating surfaces: the proximal femoral capital chondroepiphysis (including the articular epiphyseal complex, the region where the secondary center of ossification appears and the growth plate) and the acetabulum (Figure 104-1).

In the developing acetabulum are four anlagen that give rise to the ilium, ischium, pubis, and acetabular bone, all contributing to the mature acetabulum. Each anlage has a primary center of ossification and a growth plate that results in growth of each anlage away from the center of the acetabulum. The ilium, ischium, and pubis all have a common epiphysis within which the primary center of ossification of the acetabulum appears. As mineralization proceeds, the growth centers localize in the acetabular cup. This creates the inverted Y shape on a lateral view termed the triradiate growth plate. The acetabular anlage ossifies between the two ventral arms of this growth plate and a secondary center of ossification develops in the common epiphysis prior to closure of the triradiate growth plate. This growth plate closes radiographically at 4 to 5 months of age in medium- to large-breed dogs, whereas the capital physeal growth plate closes between 9 to 11 months of age. This closure is delayed in dysplastic hips.[15] For normal hip joint formation and conformation to occur, proper contact, load, and congruency between the femoral head and the acetabulum are required. This is demonstrated by the success of pelvic harnesses for the treatment of dysplastic human hips. In CHD, this contact is interrupted.

Dogs with the genetic predisposition to CHD have grossly normal hips at birth, but this changes within the first few weeks of life. Whether laxity precedes osseous disconformity or vice versa is unknown. As the hip joint matures, the secondary centers of ossification and the femoral head and acetabular growth plates become histologically apparent and can be seen by diagnostic ultrasound, with radiographs, with computed tomography, and with magnetic resonance imaging (Figure 104-1). Any femoral head dislocation affects the direction, magnitude, and distribution of the resultant femoral head force,[36] leading to a lag in development of the craniodorsal acetabular rim.[37] Additionally, femoral capital chondroepiphyseal ossification is detected later in dysplastic hips than in normal hips.[13,15] It is likely that this early neonatal stage of development is the critical time in hip development when even small perturbations in the mechanical environment and gene expression sequence result in long-term detrimental effects.[38] Serial imaging in this early stage of development may hold the key to early diagnosis of CHD.

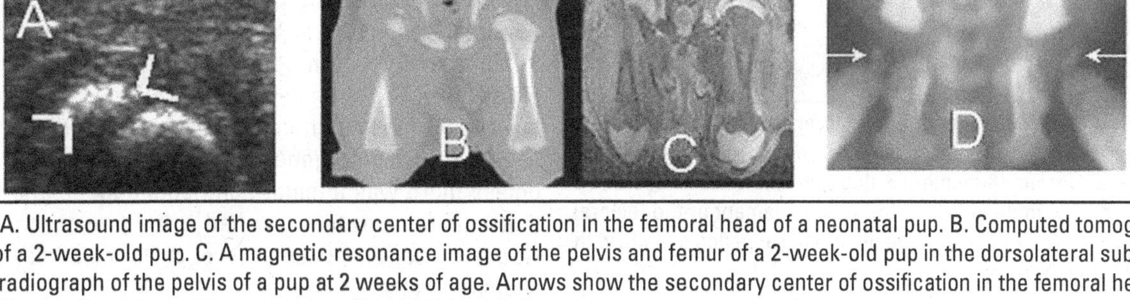

Figure 104-1. A. Ultrasound image of the secondary center of ossification in the femoral head of a neonatal pup. B. Computed tomographic image of the pelvis of a 2-week-old pup. C. A magnetic resonance image of the pelvis and femur of a 2-week-old pup in the dorsolateral subluxation. D. A ventrodorsal radiograph of the pelvis of a pup at 2 weeks of age. Arrows show the secondary center of ossification in the femoral heads. (Compliments of WS Vanden Burg Foels, Bioengineering, Cornell University.)

Epidemiology and Pathogenesis

The prevalence of canine hip dysplasia in one teaching hospital in the United States was 19.7% in purebreds and 17.7% in mixed breed dogs. There was no significant difference in the prevalence of CHD between sexes or between purebreds and mixed breed dogs.[39] The top four breeds presented to teaching hospitals that have been reported to be at increased risk for CHD in comparison with mixed breeds are the Bernese mountain dog, German wirehaired pointer, the kuvasz, and Newfoundland.[40] Hip dysplasia affects dogs of all breeds but is clinically more common in large-breed dogs.[41-46] The prevalence of CHD within breeds is 1% to 75%, as estimated by the OFA (http://www.offa.org/hipstat-breed.html). The estimate may be low because radiographs of normal dogs are more likely to be submitted for certification than are those of dysplastic dogs, thus biasing the data base.

The age of the dog at clinical detection of CHD varies depending on the severity of the disease and owner acuity. Dysplastic dogs often develop gait abnormalities and/or lameness during growth (between 3 and 8 months of age). Examination by palpation and radiographs may reveal subluxation of the hip joint(s). Synovitis, joint capsule thickening, and articular cartilage injury are uniformly present if subluxation is detected. The cartilage and soft-tissue changes characteristic of OA in dysplastic hips have been defined.[47,48] The initial cartilaginous lesion occurs perifoveally, suggesting that abnormal direction or magnitude of load results in increased focal stress in this area.[47,49] The result is joint pain, articular cartilage degeneration, and bony remodeling characteristic of OA (Figure 104-2). As abnormal weight-bearing continues to cause excess articular cartilage wear, the underlying bone is also damaged, possibly causing painful microfractures and sclerosis. In young dogs, perifoveal articular cartilage lesions are accompanied by increased subchondral and femoral head bone density.[50] As the animal ages, the hip laxity decreases as the capsule undergoes fibrosis and the synovial effusion resolves.

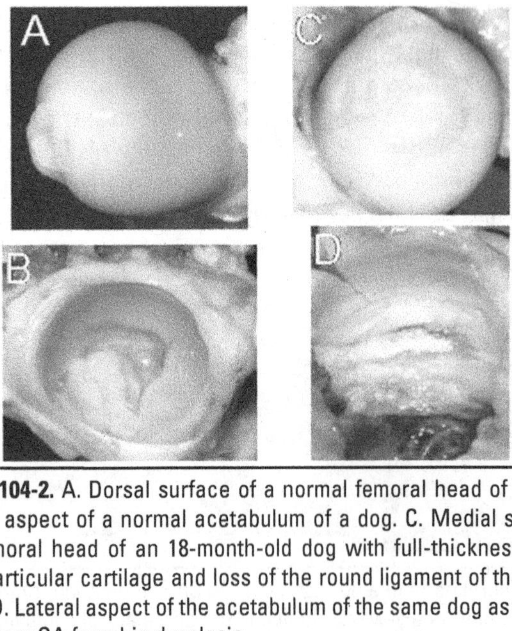

Figure 104-2. A. Dorsal surface of a normal femoral head of a dog. B. Lateral aspect of a normal acetabulum of a dog. C. Medial surface of the femoral head of an 18-month-old dog with full-thickness erosion of the articular cartilage and loss of the round ligament of the femoral head. D. Lateral aspect of the acetabulum of the same dog as in C, with secondary OA from hip dysplasia.

Osteoarthritis remains and is a debilitating chronic condition characterized by loss of articular cartilage, fibrosis, bony remodeling, and eventual loss of function. Radiographic evidence of OA can be clinically apparent as early as 5 to 9 months of age in some dogs, whereas in other dogs it is not evident until 2 years of age or later.[51] Early OA changes such as synovitis, partial or complete tears of the ligament of the femoral head, and partial- to full-thickness articular cartilage abnormalities cannot be radiographically detected (Figure 104-2).[5,52,53] Using arthroscopy to directly evaluate the hip joint grossly in dogs undergoing a triple pelvic osteotomy, only 50% of dogs with Grade 2 to 3 arthroscopic lesions (articular cartilage surface fibrillation and deep fissuring, respectively) had radiographic evidence of OA in the extended hip view.[52]

Genetics

Two main factors are associated with development of CHD: genetics and environment. A dog's phenotype is the result of a complex interaction of its genotype and the environment to which it is exposed.[18,37,54-56]

Canine hip dysplasia is considered a quantitatively inherited, complex, polygenic, or multifactorial disease that results in OA of the hip. Quantitatively inherited genetic traits vary along a continuum from one individual to the next and are influenced by two or more genes in addition to environmental factors.[18] The phenotypic and population genetic correlation is moderate and positive (0.24)[57] and the signs of subluxation reveal the highest heritability estimates.[58] Larger breeds share a heritable tendency to CHD and hip OA, yet many dogs with the genetic susceptibility do not show the clinical phenotype.[46] The heritability estimates (h^2) of CHD vary among authors and study population. Based on radiographic screening studies, the heritability estimates for CHD range from 0.1 - 0.68.[41,45,46,55,57-62] The maternal effect is additive (h_m^2 (additive genetic maternal effect) = 0.1 +/- 0.02),[60] dam and sire hip scores have a significant effect on progeny conformation scores.[63] No significant difference exists in progeny hip conformation scores between the sexes,[63] nor between mixed and purebred dogs.[39] The higher the heritability estimate, the more likely we are to make phenotypic improvements using selective breeding programs.

Using genetic selection to improve the phenotype has been achieved in controlled populations such as the Seeing Eye Inc., Morristown, NJ, by combining individual phenotypic information with parental and offspring information to obtain estimated breeding values.[55] One of the best genetic improvements reported is that of one standard deviation during 10-year period in Finland.[57] Screening programs through open registries such as those conducted in Sweden have resulted in improvement in hip quality,[62] but in other countries[44,64-66] the improvement in phenotypes has been minimal. As CHD has a polygenic mode of inheritance, future attempts to control the disease using tests based on a single genetic marker would not be immediate,[67] unless there was a major contributing locus and it was shown that mutations at that loci had to be present to express CHD. At our present knowledge level of its molecular genetics, this seems unlikely.

The pattern of inheritance indicates that CHD is controlled by several genes located at quantitative trait loci (QTLs) and the expression of which is influenced by environmental factors. Inductive or protective QTLs that control expression of hip OA may exist independent of those controlling the dysplastic phenotype.[68,69] Some dog breeds appear to display different susceptibilities to CHD based on their distraction indices and may tolerate more passive hip laxity than do other breeds.[70,71] Other breeds may develop radiographically detectable hip OA as a result of antecedent CHD faster than others.[70] A major locus contributing to CHD has been implicated in German shepherds, golden retrievers, Labrador retrievers, Rottweilers, and greyhound-dysplastic Labrador retriever crosses based on statistical models.[55,72,73] Using Portuguese water dogs to identify the QTL that regulates CHD, two separate QTLs were found, both on chromosome 1 separated by about 95 Mb, one associated with the Norberg angle of each hip and contributing up to 16% of the phenotypic variance. A major locus is thought to contribute 20% of the phenotypic variance so that molecular genetic results and population genetics are currently at odds.[74] It is interesting to note that any asymmetry in subluxation during extended hip radiographs was not heritable.[74] Alleles contributing to a complex trait such as CHD may be dominant or additive. The magnitude of their effect is independent of its mode of inheritance.[75]

Environment

Many nongenetic and/or environmental factors influence the development and severity of hip dysplasia in genetically predisposed dogs. Not one of these has been shown to cause CHD in dogs that do not have the genetic predisposition. Factors such as body size, growth rate, the season of birth, nutrition, dietary anion gap, in utero endocrine influences, and muscle mass are considered to influence the development and clinical signs of CHD.[18,33] High caloric intake, excess protein intake, excess calcium intake, rapid growth rate, lack of or excessive exercise all result in increased severity of CHD.[18,37,54,55]

Maternal/Litter Effects

Hormones and growth-promoting peptides such as insulin, cortisol, epidermal growth factor, insulin-like growth factors (IGFs), parathyroid-hormone-related peptide, relaxin, estrogen, and estrogen precursors are present in canine colostrum and milk.[76,77] These peptides, absorbed through the gastrointestinal tract particularly in the early postnatal period,[78] have the ability to influence the connective tissue metabolism, especially that of genetically susceptible tissues. Relaxin, estrogen, and estrogen precursors are abundant in the milk of Labrador retrievers.[31] Relaxin persists in the serum of dysplastic Labrador retriever bitches throughout lactation but is detectable for only the first 1 to 2 weeks of lactation in nondysplastic bitches. Relaxin is a potent inducer of neutral matrix metalloproteinase 1 (collagenase 1) and 3 (stromelysin 1) and plasminogen-activator expression. These activated enzymes degrade the extracellular matrix and, therefore, affect the structure and metabolism of joint capsule and ligaments. Local relaxin activity on estrogen-primed tissues may contribute to the capsular and ligamentous laxity associated with CHD. The total serum estrogen is similar in pups born of dysplastic and normal matings, but testosterone was detected only in the milk of dysplastic Labrador retriever bitches, and estradiol-17β appeared only in the serum of pups born to dysplastic matings. Injection of an aromatase inhibitor (preventing the conversion of testosterone to 17β-estradiol) into pups from birth throughout lactation significantly reduced hip joint laxity at maturity in dysplastic-bred Labrador retrievers.[79] Dosing estrogen repetitively during the growing period can induce CHD.[2,80]

The litter effect has been reported to contribute 4% of phenotype variation; this percentage includes all environmental and genetic effects common to members of same litter, but also contains the breed effect.[57] Therefore, it appears that the maternal effect is almost negligible (1.5%).[57,61]

Abundant food consumption shortens the time to first appearance and increases the severity of CHD.[34] Whereas overfeeding itself does not cause CHD, it does maximize trait expression in genetically susceptible individuals. The frequency and severity of CHD and concomitant OA in affected hips were greatly reduced in Labrador retrievers by limiting food consumption to 25% of ad libitum-fed control litter mates.[81-83] Reduction of food resulted in a 67% reduction of CHD at 2 years of age 83 and substantially reduced the prevalence and severity of hip joint OA at 5 years of age.[82] The dogs on the restricted diet had significantly less OA in their hips, shoulders, and lumbar vertebrae when maintained on this diet.[81] One study showed that a dog's body mass at birth is an important factor in determining the age of onset of femoral head ossification as well as the laxity of the immature joint, with dogs of greater body mass having reduced femoral head coverage.[38] The mechanism of operation of these nutritional effects remains unknown, but may be explained by mechanics (maximizing growth allows maximum load to be placed on genetically susceptible hips), or by the effect of nutritional components on local gene expression. Lower body weight (i.e., restricted feeding) delays onset and limits severity of radiographic signs of OA.[81-83] Perinatal nutrition can have long-term effects on metabolism. Bottle-feeding, compared with breast feeding, of puppies predisposed to CHD after caesarean section resulted in reduced growth rate and a low incidence of the trait. Ad libitum feeding of Great Danes induced the expression of several unwanted orthopedic traits including CHD when compared with dogs on restricted feeding.[43] It has also been suggested that excessive exercise in dogs with much joint laxity is likely to cause or worsen CHD, but there is no scientific evidence to support this impression.[84]

Besides reduced food intake, systemic polysulfated glycosaminoglycan (Adequan) is the only treatment that has been shown to significantly reduce the expression of hip OA in CHD when administered to dysplasia-prone Labrador retrievers from 6 weeks to 8 months of age.[85] Polysulfated glycosaminoglycans are inhibitors of neutral matrix metalloproteinase activity and also significantly reduce pubic symphyseal relaxation in estrogen-primed guinea pigs.[86]

Many large-scale studies have attempted to evaluate the environmental factors that affect the incidence of CHD expression. In one study of Rottweilers in Finland (n=2764), the environmental effects influencing CHD were age (the older the dogs, the worse the condition), birth year (1998 best, 1995 worst), birth year x season interaction (season by itself was not a factor as in other studies,[45,59,61] and the experience of veterinarian radiographing the dog (but with no clear trend and small differences between classes).[57] In a more recent study of British Labrador retrievers and gordon setters, the mean hip scores of dogs born between June and October were lower than those of dogs born during the rest of the year. These results are similar to those of Hanssen 1991 and Olerth et al 2001.[87] One hypothesis for this effect is that dogs born during the warmer season can exercise on soft ground, creating a supportive musculature and preventing HD.[88] Many other factors probably influence the results regarding season of birth. Body mass at birth was a significant predictor of age at onset of proximal capital ossification (the greater the mass, the earlier the onset) and of 4-month-old femoral head subluxation (the greater the birth weight, the more reduced coverage in the dorsolateral subluxation position).[38]

Results of studies conflict when trying to determine whether gender influences the expression of CHD. Increased frequency in females,[1,62] males,[59] and equal sex distribution,[71,89] have all been reported. Therefore, it is unknown if the influence of sex is a direct expression of genes on the sex chromosomes or a result of the secondary effects of sex (hormones, weight).[62] The estrus cycle of a dog had no significant effect on hip laxity as measured by the distraction index.[90]

Diagnostics

Dogs with CHD present most commonly at two different ages: as pups at 5 to 9 months of age and as mature adults. Dogs as young as 16 weeks of age with hip joint laxity as measured by the distraction index are at risk for OA.[71] The most common findings on physical examination in young dogs with CHD are discomfort on extension or abduction of the hip and/or a positive Ortolani sign. In 6-month-old dogs, the angle of reduction is repeatable, suggesting that it may be used by multiple examiners with comparable and consistent results.[91] A positive Ortolani sign is thought to be a risk factor for development of OA later in life, but the significance of its presence or absence has not been evaluated long-term.[49] As dogs age, those with subclinical lameness secondary to hip OA will compensate by shifting their weight between trotting pairs rather than within them.[92] As the pain of chronic OA increases, the effects are best judged by an owner or a person familiar with the dog after receiving training regarding the clinical signs of this disease.[93]

Prevention and Radiographs

Radiography is the most common tool used in the diagnosis of CHD, but it also has great utility in determining the likelihood the development of CHD in pups. Several radiographic techniques have been researched extensively to determine their sensitivity and specificity in determining which dog will develop radiographic, clinical, or histopathologic evidence of CHD. The problem with all radiographic techniques is that a dog's phenotype is no guarantee of its genotype. Much of the information published is conflicting or not comparable owing to different study scenarios and end-points. We will give an overview of the different radiographic techniques and the indications for them.

Several radiographic signs have been reported to occur first in CHD. Femoral head subluxation and a lag in the development of the acetabular rim seen as early as 2 to 9 months of age was reported in 1973,[37] and delayed ossification of the femoral head was reported to be the earliest radiographic predictor of CHD on a population basis.[13,15] Later OA changes secondary to CHD include subchondral sclerosis, osteophytosis, joint deformity, proliferative and lytic changes at attachments of joint capsule and supporting ligaments, and intra-articular bodies.[94-96] Radiographic OA can be apparent at 5 to 9 months of age, but some are not evident until at least 24 months of age or later.[51]

All of the available radiographic tests are considered to be inaccurate at 4 months of age or earlier, most likely owing to ongoing endochondral ossification and the inherent difficulty of imaging cartilage with standard radiographic techniques.[9,11,15,97] Diagnostic methods are more accurate at 8 months of age or later;[9,11,15,97,98] once the hip joints are fully mature after the period of rapid growth is complete.[99] When evaluating any dog radiographically for CHD, one must keep in mind that not all dogs with radiographic subluxation develop radiographic evidence of OA by 2 years of age.[97]

Extended-Hip Radiograph

The extended-hip radiograph (EHR) is frequently used for CHD screening purposes.(Figure 104-3) It is performed with the dog in dorsal recumbency, usually heavily sedated. The femurs are

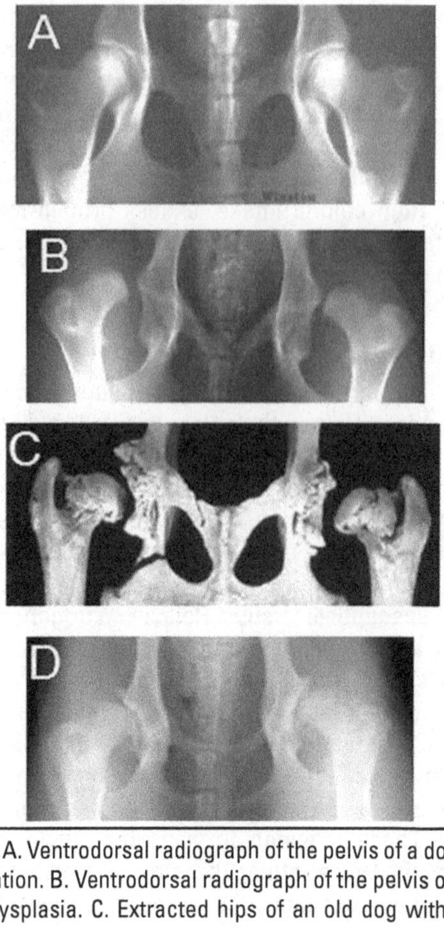

Figure 104-3. A. Ventrodorsal radiograph of the pelvis of a dog with good hip conformation. B. Ventrodorsal radiograph of the pelvis of a dog with severe hip dysplasia. C. Extracted hips of an old dog with severe hip remodeling characteristic of the OA that progresses in a dysplastic hip. D. Ventrodorsal radiograph of the pelvis of a dog with hip OA secondary to hip dysplasia.

pulled parallel to the table top and each other, and the knees extended and rotated such that the patellae are centered in the trochlear grooves. The Orthopedic Foundation for Animals (OFA, www.offa.org) uses this view to grade CHD. (The radiographic view allows determination of the presence of OA, its severity, and of certain degrees of subluxation. Using the EHR, evaluations earlier than 2 years of age are considered preliminary because younger widely affected dogs may not have evidence of subluxation when radiographed in the extended position.[11,33] Findings suggest that the strength of the EHR at 8 months of age is its specificity.[98] It is commonly accepted that the OFA-type hip scoring method is the most specific (96%),[53] but it underestimates the susceptibility to CHD.[100] Smith et al (1995) found that the Norberg angle, obtained from EHR, is not a significant risk factor for subsequent radiographic hip OA.[71]

One finding on the EHR that has shown predictive value in later OA development is the caudolateral curvilinear osteophyte (CCO). First identified in 1961, it appears at the insertion of the joint capsule into the femoral neck.[101] The importance of its appearance has been questioned,[7,96,102-104] as it is often present without any other evidence of OA, and has prompted questioning of its use as an early sign indicating that OA will develop later.[84] It must be differentiated from what has been termed the "puppy line," which resembles the CCO but is thought to be nonpathologic.[84] The puppy line is found in dogs up t oabout 18 months of age and either disappears or transforms into a CCO.[105] No statistical relationship exists between the puppy line and later development of OA. The original hypothesis was that the CCO develops secondary to increases in stress on the joint capsule insertion in dogs with excessive laxity.[96] Other studies have shown that, in Labrador retrievers, a relationship exists between the CCO and subsequent OA development. Dogs with a CCO are 3.7 times more likely to develop radiographically evident OA than are those without a CCO.[105] The CCO was the first radiographic sign in 76% of dogs that later developed radiographic OA and 95% of dogs with histopathologic OA had a CCO.[105] Another study showed that dogs with a CCO are 7.9 times more likely to have radiographic OA than are those without a CCO. The animal's distraction index, weight, and age are significant risk factors for the CCO,[84] but this contemporaneous relationship does not predict ultimate OA development. When evaluating the CCO in relation to feeding group (ad libitum contol group or restricted-fed group), it was found that 100% of control dogs with a CCO and 55% of restricted-fed dogs with a CCO developed later radiographic OA.[105] Regardless of the feeding group, dogs with a puppy line were not more likely to develop OA or a CCO compared with dogs without a puppy line. Diet did not influence the frequency of the CCO, only the time of onset of CCO. This may suggest that the CCO is a more sensitive radiographic marker for susceptibility for OA that is not confounded by environmental factors such as restricted feeding.[105]

Distraction Index (PennHip) and Dorsolateral Subluxation Score

The distraction index (DI) (Figure 104-4A) and the dorsolateral subluxation score (DLS) (Figure 104-4B) assess the laxity of the hip joint. The DI is also measured in dorsal recumbency. For the DI radiograph, the hips are flexed so that the patellae point to the ceiling. A custom-made levering device is placed over the coxofemoral joints between the femurs and an inward force is applied to the stifles to determine the amount of laxity present in the hip joint. The DI is calculated between these views and is used to predict the likelihood of the development of CHD. Individual logistic regression curves can be established for each breed to relate DI to the presence of hip OA secondary to CHD. The operator must have received special training to perform this technique and submit the radiographs for evaluation. However, this ensures a complete unbiased registry. Additionally, the DI can be artificially increased by increasing intra-articular volume, as well as cavitation, without affecting DLS score.[17,106] The DLS view is also performed under heavy sedation or general anesthesia. The animal is placed in sternal recumbency on a pad with a cutout for the rear legs, such that the knees are flexed and weight-bearing. The radiograph is centered over the hip joints and shows the conformation of the hip joints as the animal bears weight. The advantages of the DLS are that it is easy to perform, requires only one radiograph, can be done with the animal anesthetized or sedated, and does not require the operator to hold the dog during radiography. The method and measurements are reproducible.[49] External factors such as dorsal hip loading and whether the test is performed under general anesthesia or heavy sedation do not have marked clinical effects on the DLS score, although loading the hips does increase the DLS score in some cross-breeds.[107] The 6% change between loaded and unloaded DLS scores overall is statistically significant but is unlikely to be clinically significant.[107] The DLS score is an objective measurement of coxofemoral subluxation, whereas the OFA score is subjective.

The DI and DLS scores are associated, but likely represent distinct features of hip joint structure and evaluate different

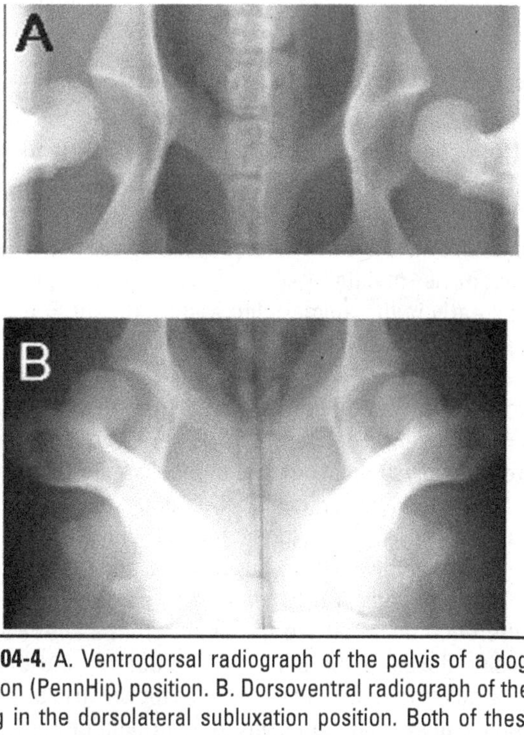

Figure 104-4. A. Ventrodorsal radiograph of the pelvis of a dog in the distraction (PennHip) position. B. Dorsoventral radiograph of the pelvis of a dog in the dorsolateral subluxation position. Both of these dogs have hip laxity, and the dog in 4B has hip dysplasia and subluxation.

components of joint stability.[17] Several studies have suggested that both the DI and DLS scores remain constant after 8 months of age.[9,18,98] In a mature hip, the laxity (DI) can change independently of the DLS score.[17] The use of either the DI or the DLS score improves the detection of subtle cases of CHD compared to the EHR. The specificity of the DLS score for prediction of hip OA at 8 months of age is similar (84%, DLS score < 55%) to the DI (89%, DI > 0.7) in dysplastic Labrador retrievers, greyhounds, and their cross-bred offspring.[73] The sensitivity appears to be better for the DLS score than the DI: depending on the cut-off used for the DI (> 0.7) and the DLS score (< 55%), the former had a sensitivity of 50% and the latter a sensitivity of 83%. At 8 months of age, dogs with DLS scores less than 42% suffered from hip OA at early maturity, whereas those with DLS scores over 55% were highly likely to have normal hips. We have argued that the DLS score represents a component of hip joint conformation independent of passive laxity, yet both are important to subsequent OA development.[49,108]

Several studies have compared a multitude of radiographic techniques with different endpoints – radiographic evidence of OA, gross necropsy findings, and histopathologic OA. One such study compared the EHR, DI, and DLS in 8-month-old dogs and used gross necropsy findings as the endpoint. All radiographic findings were significantly correlated with the gross findings. Specificities were similar for all 3 methods, but the DLS score had higher sensitivity and, therefore, fewer false negatives.[96] Another more recent study also compared the radiographic findings in 8-month-old dogs with gross necropsy findings. Specifically evaluated were the EHR, DI, DLS score, and the Norberg angle (NA). The DLS score and the NA together were best at determining normal joints versus joints with OA, and all models excluding the DLS score were worse than those that included it. The conclusion of this study suggested that two tests were better than one, especially if one was the DLS score, with no improvement if a third test was added for detection of CHD.[109]

Treatment and Prognosis

Two different treatment options are commonly recommended for CHD: medical management and surgical management. Surgical management consists of juvenile pubic symphysiodesis, triple pelvic osteotomy, excision arthroplasty, and total hip replacement. These are discussed elsewhere. Medical management is multifaceted and consists of preventative measures early in the animal's life and treatment to ameliorate the progression and clinical signs of OA later in life.

The two main preventative measures that can be taken in a dog genetically predisposed to CHD are the administration of systemic polysulfated glycosaminoglycans (PSGAG) and limiting the food intake. Administration of systemic PSGAG at 5 mg/kg during growth can significantly ameliorate progression of CHD and secondary OA in susceptible dogs.[85] In dogs with severe OA secondary to CHD, there was no statistically significant difference between the treatment groups with PSGAG at 3 increasing doses or the placebo. The authors attributed this either to a lack of response or a response too small to be detected by the physical examination used to determine effectiveness.[110] PSGAG have chondroprotective effects when used prophylactically or therapeutically.[111-118] Polysulfated glycosaminoglycan (Adequan®) is derived from bovine lung and tracheal tissue, which is structurally similar to the glycosaminoglycans found in hyaline cartilage.[119,120] In vitro, PSGAG can inhibit the rate of collagen and glycosaminoglycan degradation.[121-123] Other in vitro studies suggest that PSGAG treatment may modify the progression of OA in articular cartilage by maintaining chondrocyte viability as well as protecting against extracellular matrix degradation.[124] Similar serum and joint concentrations of PSGAG are achieved after intramuscular and intra-articular administration.[125]

Another method of decreasing the severity of CHD is by limiting food consumption starting at 8 weeks of age. Reduction of food intake by 25% compared with ad libitum-fed controls resulted in a 67% reduction of CHD at 2 years of age 83 and substantially reduced the prevalence and severity of hip-joint OA at 5 years of age.[82] Osteoarthritis also affected multiple joints significantly less commonly in limit-fed dogs.[81] Once a dog is suffering from CHD-induced OA, several recommendations to the owner are suggested: weight reduction to the breed's ideal bodyweight if the animal is overweight; moderate exercise, which increases the supporting muscle mass of the hip joints; and the addition of nonsteroidal anti-inflammatory medications if they can be tolerated by the animal. The addition of a supplement containing glucosamine and chondroitin sulfate or injection of PSGAG is also recommended, especially in younger dogs.

Rigorous application of any detection method for CHD combined with progeny testing seems to be as important as the method of hip evaluation itself in reduction of trait incidence. Simply breeding animals with better hips than the average for the breed will not eliminate the trait.[65] Until genetic screening is available, the best indication of a dog's genetic makeup is the phenotype of its parents and grandparents, its offspring, and its siblings and half siblings. Prospective purchasers of puppies should request from breeders phenotypic information on the puppies' relatives. In the end, the best solution to eliminating the trait from a breed is to know the linked genetic markers and ultimately the mutations at the major contributing loci in that breed. That could lead to genetic screening of pups before purchase and breeding and informed decisions regarding breeding programs.

References

1. Hedhammar A, Olsson SE, Andersson SA, et al: Canine hip dysplasia: Study of heritability in 401 litters of German shepherd dogs. J Am Vet Med Assoc 174:1012, 1979.

2. Henricson B, Norberg I, Olsson SE: On the etiology and pathogenesis of hip dysplasia: A comparative review. J Small Anim Pract 7:673, 1966.

3. Hutt FB: Genetic selection to reduce the incidence of hip dysplasia in dogs. J Am Vet Med Assoc 151:1041, 1967.

4. Mansson J, Norberg I: Dysplasia of the hip in dogs. Hormonally induced flaccidity of the ligaments followed by dysplasia of the acetabulum in puppies. Medlemsbl Sverig Vet Forb 13:330, 1961.

5. Riser WH: The dysplastic hip joint: Its radiographic and histologic development. J Am Vet Radiol Soc 14:35, 1973.

6. Smith GK, Biery DN, Kapatkin AS, et al: Question diagnostic technique for hip dysplasia. J Am Vet Med Assoc 220:20, 2002.

7. Riser WH: The dog as a model for the study of hip dysplasia. Growth,

form, and development of the normal and dysplastic hip joint. Vet Pathol 12:234, 1975.

8. Alexander JW: The pathogenesis of canine hip dysplasia. Vet Clin North Am Small Anim Pract 22:503, 1992.

9. Lust G, Williams AJ, Burton-Wurster N, et al: Joint laxity and its association with hip dysplasia in Labrador retrievers. Am J Vet Res 54:1990, 1993.

10. Smith GK, Biery DN, Gregor TP: New concepts of coxofemoral joint stability and the development of a clinical stress-radiographic method for quantitating hip joint laxity in the dog. J Am Vet Med Assoc 196:59, 1990.

11. Smith GK, Gregor TP, Rhodes WH, et al: Coxofemoral joint laxity from distraction radiography and its contemporaneous and prospective correlation with laxity, subjective score, and evidence of degenerative joint disease from conventional hip-extended radiography in dogs. Am J Vet Res 54:1021, 1993.

12. Cardinet GH 3rd, Kass PH, Wallace LJ, et al: Association between pelvic muscle mass and canine hip dysplasia. J Am Vet Med Assoc 210:1466, 1997.

13. Madsen JS, Reimann I, Svalastoga E: Delayed ossification of the femoral head in dogs with hip dysplasia. J Small Anim Pract 32:351, 1991.

14. Todhunter RJ, Acland GM, Olivier M, et al: An outcrossed canine pedigree for linkage analysis of hip dysplasia. J Hered 90:83, 1999.

15. Todhunter RJ, Zachos TA, Gilbert RO, et al: Onset of epiphyseal mineralization and growth plate closure in radiographically normal and dysplastic Labrador retrievers. J Am Vet Med Assoc 210:1458, 1997.

16. Todhunter RJ, Burton-Wurster N, Vernier-Singer M, et al. Composition of Labrador retriever chondroepiphyses. Proceedings Annual Meeting American College of Veterinary Surgeons, 1998.

17. Farese JP, Lust G, Williams AJ, et al: Comparison of measurements of dorsolateral subluxation of the femoral head and maximal passive laxity for evaluation of the coxofemoral joint in dogs. Am J Vet Res 60:1571, 1999.

18. Lust G: An overview of the pathogenesis of canine hip dysplasia. J Am Vet Med Assoc 210:1443, 1997.

19. Kleftogiannis F, Handley CJ, Campbell MA: Characterization of extracellular matrix macromolecules from bovine synovial capsule. J Orthop Res 12:365, 1994.

20. Parry DA, Flint MH, Gillard GC, et al: A role for glycosaminoglycans in the development of collagen fibrils. FEBS Lett 149:1, 1982.

21. Rosenbloom J: Elastin: An overview. Methods Enzymol 144:172, 1987.

22. Scott JE, Orford CR, Hughes EW: Proteoglycan-collagen arrangements in developing rat tail tendon. An electron microscopical and biochemical investigation. Biochem J 195:573, 1981.

23. Watanabe M, Nojima M, Shibata T, et al: Maturation-related biochemical changes in swine anterior cruciate ligament and tibialis posterior tendon. J Orthop Res 12:672, 1994.

24. Eyre DR, et al: Extraction, separation, and analysis of matirix constituents.In Methods in Cartilage Research. Maroudas M, Kuettner K (eds). New York: Academic Press, 1990, p. 28.

25. Smith GK. PennHip™ training course. Philadelphia, 1994.

26. Lust G, Geary JC, Sheffy BE: Development of hip dysplasia in dogs. Am J Vet Res 34:87, 1973.

27. Madsen JS: The joint capsule and joint laxity in dogs with hip dysplasia. J Am Vet Med Assoc 210:1463, 1997.

28. Madsen JS, Svalastoga E: Inclination and anteversion of collum femoris in hip dysplasia and coxarthritis. Acta Vet Scand 35:115, 1994.

29. Bornstein P, Sage H: Structurally distinct collagen types. Annu Rev Biochem 49:957, 1980.

30. Epstein EH Jr: (Alpha1(3))3 human skin collagen. release by pepsin digestion and preponderance in fetal life. J Biol Chem 249:3225, 1974.

31. Goldsmith LT, Lust G, Steinetz BG: Transmission of relaxin from lactating bitches to their offspring via suckling. Biol Reprod 50:258, 1994.

32. Wiltberger H, Lust G: Ultrastructure of canine articular cartilage: Comparison of normal and degenerative (osteoarthritic) hip joints. Am J Vet Res 36:727, 1975.

33. Smith GK, LaFond E, Gregor TP, et al: Within- and between-examiner repeatability of distraction indices of the hip joints in dogs. Am J Vet Res 58:1076, 1997.

34. Lust G, Beilman WT, Rendano VT: A relationship between degree of laxity and synovial fluid volume in coxofemoral joints of dogs predisposed for hip dysplasia. Am J Vet Res 41:55, 1980.

35. Mande JD, Mbithi PMF, Mbugua SW, et al: Volume of the ligamentum capitis femoris in osteoarthritic hip joints of adult dogs. J S Afr Vet Assoc 74:11, 2003.

36. Weigel JP, Wasserman JF: Biomechanics of the normal and abnormal hip joint. Vet Clin North Am Small Anim Pract 22:513, 1992.

37. Riser WH: Canine hip dysplasia: Cause and control. J Am Vet Med Assoc 165:360, 1974.

38. Vanden Berg-Foels WS, Todhunter RJ, Schwager SJ, Reeves AP: Effect of early postnatal body weight on adult hip joint degeneration in canine developmental dysplasia of the hip. Pediatr Res 60(5):549-554, 2006.

39. Rettenmaier JL, Keller GG, Lattimer JC, et al: Prevalence of canine hip dysplasia in a veterinary teaching hospital population. Vet Radiol Ultrasound 43:313, 2002.

40. LaFond E, Breur GJ, Austin CC: Breed susceptibility for developmental orthopedic diseases in dogs. J Am Anim Hosp Assoc 38:467, 2002.

41. Breur GJ, Lust G, Todhunter RJ: Genetics of canine hip dysplasia and other orthopaedic traits. *In* The Genetics of the Dog. Ruvinsky A, Sampson J (eds). Wallingford,: CABI Publishing, 2001.

42. Cardinet GH 3rd, Guffy MM, Wallace LJ, et al: Canine hip dysplasia in German shepherd dog-greyhound crossbreeds. J Am Vet Med Assoc 182:393, 1983.

43. Hedhammar A, Wu FM, Krook L, et al: Overnutrition and skeletal disease. an experimental study in growing great dane dogs. Cornell Vet 64:Suppl 5:5, 1974.

44. Kaneene JB, Mostosky UV, Padgett GA: Retrospective cohort study of changes in hip joint phenotype of dogs in the United States. J Am Vet Med Assoc 211:1542, 1997.

45. Leighton EA, Linn JM, Willham RL, et al: A genetic study of canine hip dysplasia. Am J Vet Res 38:241, 1977.

46. Willis MB: Hip dysplasia. *In* Genetics of the Dog. Willis MB (ed). New York: Howell Book House, 1989, p. 144.

47. Burton-Wurster N, Farese JP, Todhunter RJ, et al: Site-specific variation in femoral head cartilage composition in dogs at high and low risk for development of osteoarthritis: Insights into cartilage degeneration. Osteoarthr Cartilage 7:486, 1999.

48. Lingaas F, Klemetsdal G: Breeding values and genetic trend for hip dysplasia in the Norwegian golden retriever population. J Anim Breed Genet 107:437, 1990.

49. Farese JP, Todhunter RJ, Lust G, et al: Dorsolateral subluxation of hip joints in dogs measured in a weight-bearing position with radiography and computed tomography. Vet Surg 27:393, 1998.

50. Chalmers HJ, Dykes NL, Lust G, et al: Assessment of bone mineral density of the femoral head in dogs with early osteoarthritis. Am J Vet Res 67(5):796-800, 2005.

51. Corley EA: Role of the orthopedic foundation for animals in the control of canine hip dysplasia. Vet Clin North Am Small Anim Pract 22:579, 1992.

52. Holsworth IG, Schulz KS, Kass PH, et al: Comparison of arthroscopic and radiographic abnormalities in the hip joints of juvenile dogs with hip dysplasia. J Am Vet Med Assoc 227:1087, 2005.

53. Lust G, Summers BA: Early, asymptomatic stage of degenerative joint disease in canine hip joints. Am J Vet Res 42:1849, 1981.

54. Brass W: Hip dysplasia in dogs. J Small Anim Pract 30:166, 1989.

55. Leighton EA: Genetics of canine hip dysplasia. J Am Vet Med Assoc 210:1474, 1997.

56. Mackenzie SA, Oltenacu EA, Leighton E: Heritability estimate for temperament scores in German shepherd dogs and its genetic correlation with hip dysplasia. Behav Genet 15:475, 1985.

57. Maki K, Liinamo AE, Ojala M: Estimates of genetic parameters for hip and elbow dysplasia in Finnish rottweilers. J Anim Sci 78:1141, 2000.

58. Ohlerth S, Lang J, Busato A, et al: Estimation of genetic population variables for six radiographic criteria of hip dysplasia in a colony of Labrador retrievers. Am J Vet Res 62:846, 2001.

59. Distl O, Grussler W, Schwarz J, et al: Analysis of environmentally-conditioned and genetic influences on the frequency of hip joint dysplasia in German shepherd dogs. Zentralbl Veterinarmed A 38:460, 1991.

60. Hamann H, Kirchhoff T, Distl O: Bayesian analysis of heritability of canine hip dysplasia in German shepherd dogs. J Anim Breed Genet 120:258, 2003.

61. Lingaas F, Heim P: En genetisk undersokelse av hofteleddsdysplasi i norske hunderaser. Norsk Veterinaertidsskrift 99:617, 1987.

62. Swenson L, Audell L, Hedhammar A: Prevalence and inheritance of and selection for hip dysplasia in seven breeds of dogs in Sweden and benefit:cost analysis of a screening and control program. J Am Vet Med Assoc 210:207, 1997.

63. Reed AL, Keller GG, Vogt DW, et al: Effect of dam and sire qualitative hip conformation scores on progeny hip conformation. J Am Vet Med Assoc 217:675, 2000.

64. Leppanen M, Maki K, Juga J, et al: Factors affecting hip dysplasia in German shepherd dogs in Finland: Efficacy of the current improvement programme. J Small Anim Pract 41:19, 2000.

65. Leppanen M, Saloniemi H: Controlling canine hip dysplasia in Finland. Prev Vet Med 42:121, 1999.

66. Willis MB: A review of the progress in canine hip dysplasia control in Britain. J Am Vet Med Assoc 210:1480, 1997.

67. Wood JL, Lakhani KH, Henley WE: An epidemiological approach to prevention and control of three common heritable diseases in canine pedigree breeds in the United Kingdom. Vet J 168:14, 2004.

68. Chapman K, Mustafa Z, Irven C, et al: Osteoarthritis-susceptibility locus on chromosome 11q, detected by linkage. Am J Hum Genet 65:167, 1999.

69. Vingsbo-Lundberg C, Nordquist N, Olofsson P, et al: Genetic control of arthritis onset, severity and chronicity in a model for rheumatoid arthritis in rats. Nat Genet 20:401, 1998.

70. Popovitch CA, Smith GK, Gregor TP, et al: Comparison of susceptibility for hip dysplasia between rottweilers and German shepherd dogs. J Am Vet Med Assoc 206:648, 1995.

71. Smith GK, Popovitch CA, Gregor TP, et al: Evaluation of risk factors for degenerative joint disease associated with hip dysplasia in dogs. J Am Vet Med Assoc 206:642, 1995.

72. Maki K, Janss LL, Groen AF, et al: An indication of major genes affecting hip and elbow dysplasia in four Finnish dog populations. Heredity 92:402, 2004.

73. Todhunter RJ, Bliss SP, Casella G, et al: Genetic structure of susceptibility traits for hip dysplasia and microsatellite informativeness of an outcrossed canine pedigree. J Hered 94:39, 2003.

74. Chase K, Lawler DF, Adler FR, et al: Bilaterally asymmetric effects of quantitative trait loci (QTLs): QTLs that affect laxity in the right versus left coxofemoral (hip) joints of the dog (canis familiaris). Am J Med Genet A 124:239, 2004.

75. Bliss S, Todhunter RJ, Quaas R, et al: Quantitative genetics of traits associated with hip dysplasia in a canine pedigree constructed by mating dysplastic Labrador retrievers with unaffected greyhounds. Am J Vet Res 63:1029, 2002.

76. Ballard FJ, Grbovac S, Nicholas KR, et al: Differential changes in the milk concentrations of epidermal growth factor and insulin-like growth factor-I during lactation in the tammar wallaby, macropus eugenii. Gen Comp Endocrinol 98:262, 1995.

77. Xu RJ: Development of the newborn GI tract and its relation to colostrum/milk intake: A review. Reprod Fertil Dev 8:35, 1996.

78. Xu RJ, Wang T: Gastrointestinal absorption of insulinlike growth factor-I in neonatal pigs. J Pediatr Gastroenterol Nutr 23:430, 1996.

79. Steinetz BG, Goldsmith LT, Lust G: Transmission of estrogen and relaxin to suckling pups via milk: a possible role of hormones in canine hip dysplasia. Proceedings of Meeting of the Endocrinology Society, 1997.

80. Beling CG, Gustafsson PO, Kasstrom H: Metabolism of estradiol in greyhounds and German shepherd dogs. an investigation with special reference to hip dysplasia. Acta Radiol Suppl 344:109, 1975.

81. Kealy RD, Lawler DF, Ballam JM, et al: Evaluation of the effect of limited food consumption on radiographic evidence of osteoarthritis in dogs. J Am Vet Med Assoc 217:1678, 2000.

82. Kealy RD, Lawler DF, Ballam JM, et al: Five-year longitudinal study on limited food consumption and development of osteoarthritis in coxofemoral joints of dogs. J Am Vet Med Assoc 210:222, 1997.

83. Kealy RD, Olsson SE, Monti KL, et al: Effects of limited food consumption on the incidence of hip dysplasia in growing dogs. J Am Vet Med Assoc 201:857, 1992.

84. Mayhew PD, McKelvie PJ, Biery DN, et al: Evaluation of a radiographic caudolateral curvilinear osteophyte on the femoral neck and its relationship to degenerative joint disease and distraction index in dogs. J Am Vet Med Assoc 220:472, 2002.

85. Lust G, Williams AJ, Burton-Wurster N, et al: Effects of intramuscular administration of glycosaminoglycan polysulfates on signs of incipient hip dysplasia in growing pups. Am J Vet Res 53:1836, 1992.

86. Steinetz BG, Lust G: Inhibition of relaxin-induced pubic symphyseal "relaxation" in guinea pigs by glycosaminoglycan polysulfates and pentosan polysulfate. Agents Actions 42:74, 1994.

87. Wood JL, Lakhani KH: Effect of month of birth on hip dysplasia in Labrador retrievers and gordon setters. Vet Rec 152:69, 2003.

88. Hanssen I: Hip dysplasia in dogs in relation to their month of birth. Vet Rec 128:425, 1991.

89. Priester WA, Mulvihill JJ: Canine hip dysplasia: Relative risk by sex, size, and breed, and comparative aspects. J Am Vet Med Assoc 160:735, 1972.

90. Hassinger KA, Smith GK, Conzemius MC, et al: Effect of the estrus cycle on coxofemoral joint laxity. Vet Compar Orthop Traumatol 10:77, 1997.

91. Charette B, Dupuis J, Beauregard G, et al: Palpation and dorsal acetabular rim radiographic view for early detection of canine hip dysplasia. Part 1: Standardization and measurement repeatability on six-month-old dogs. Vet Compar Orthop Traumatol 14:125, 2001.

92. Kennedy S, Lee DV, Bertram JEA, et al: Gait evaluation in hip osteoarthritic and normal dogs using a serial force plate system. Vet Compar Orthop Traumatol 16:170, 2003.

93. Hielm-Bjorkman AK, Kuusela E, Liman A, et al: Evaluation of methods for assessment of pain associated with chronic osteoarthritis in dogs. J Am Vet Med Assoc 222:1552, 2003.

94. Carrig CB: Diagnostic imaging of osteoarthritis. Vet Clin North Am Small Anim Pract 27:777, 1997.

95. Martinez SA: Congenital conditions that lead to osteoarthritis in the dog. Vet Clin North Am Small Anim Pract 27:735, 1997.

96. Morgan JP: Canine hip dysplasia. Significance of early bony spurring. Vet Radiol 28:2, 1987.

97. Corley EA, Keller GG, Lattimer JC, et al: Reliability of early radiographic evaluations for canine hip dysplasia obtained from the standard ventrodorsal radiographic projection. J Am Vet Med Assoc 211:1142, 1997.

98. Lust G, Todhunter RJ, Erb HN, et al: Comparison of three radiographic methods for diagnosis of hip dysplasia in eight-month-old dogs. J Am Vet Med Assoc 219:1242, 2001.

99. Adams WM, Dueland RT, Meinen J, et al: Early detection of canine hip dysplasia: Comparison of two palpation and five radiographic methods. J Am Anim Hosp Assoc 34:339, 1998.

100. Kapatkin AS, Gregor TP, Hearon K, et al: Comparison of two radiographic techniques for evaluation of hip joint laxity in 10 breeds of dogs. J Am Vet Med Assoc 224:542, 2004.

101. Whittington K, Banks WC, Carlson WD: Report of panel on canine hip dysplasia. J Am Vet Assoc 139:791, 1961.

102. Ackerman N: Hip dysplasia in the afghan hound. Vet Radiol 23:88, 1982.

103. Klimt U, Tellhelm B, Fritsch R: Importance of morgan's line in the radiographic examination of dogs for hip dysplasia. Kleintierpraxis 37:211, 1992.

104. Torres RCS, Ferreira PM, Araujo RB, et al: Presence of morgan's line as an indicator of canine hip dysplasia in German shepherd dogs. Arq Bras Med Vet Zootec 51:157, 1999.

105. Powers MY, Biery DN, Lawler DE, et al: Use of the caudolateral curvilinear osteophyte as an early marker for future development of osteoarthritis associated with hip dysplasia in dogs. J Am Vet Med Assoc 225:233, 2004.

106. LaFond E, Smith GK, Gregor TP, et al: Synovial fluid cavitation during distraction radiography of the coxofemoral joint in dogs. J Am Vet Med Assoc 210:1294, 1997.

107. Todhunter RJ, Bertram JE, Smith S, et al: Effect of dorsal hip loading, sedation, and general anesthesia on the dorsolateral subluxation score in dogs. Vet Surg 32:196, 2003.

108. Lust G, Todhunter RJ, Erb HN, et al: Repeatability of dorsolateral subluxation scores in dogs and correlation with macroscopic appearance of hip osteoarthritis. Am J Vet Res 62:1711, 2001.

109. Todhunter RJ, Grohn YT, Bliss SP, et al: Evaluation of multiple radiographic predictors of cartilage lesions in the hip joints of eight-month-old dogs. Am J Vet Res 64:1472, 2003.

110. de Haan JJ, Goring RL, Beale BS: Evaluation of polysulfated glycosaminoglycan for the treatment of hip dysplasia in dogs. Vet Surg 23:177, 1994.

111. Altman RD, Dean DD, Muniz OE, et al: Prophylactic treatment of canine osteoarthritis with glycosaminoglycan polysulfuric acid ester. Arthr Rheum 32:759, 1989.

112. Altman RD, Dean DD, Muniz OE, et al: Therapeutic treatment of canine osteoarthritis with glycosaminoglycan polysulfuric acid ester. Arthr Rheum 32:1300, 1989.

113. Carreno MR, Muniz OE, Howell DS: The effect of glycosaminoglycan polysulfuric acid ester on articular cartilage in experimental osteoarthritis: Effects on morphological variables of disease severity. J Rheumatol 13:490, 1986.

114. Golding J, Ghosh P: Drugs for osteoarthrosis II: The effects of a glycosaminoglycan polysulphate ester (arteparon) on proteoglycan aggregation and loss from articular cartilage of immobilized rabbit knee joints. Curr Ther Res 34:67, 1983.

115. Hannan N, Ghosh P, Bellenger C, et al: Systemic administration of glycosaminoglycan polysulphate (arteparon) provides partial protection of articular cartilage from damage produced by meniscectomy in the canine. J Orthop Res 5:47, 1987.

116. Howell DS, Carreno MR, Pelletier JP, et al: Articular cartilage breakdown in a lapine model of osteoarthritis. action of glycosaminoglycan polysulfate ester (GAGPS) on proteoglycan degrading enzyme activity, hexuronate, and cell counts. Clin Orthop Relat Res (213):69, 1986.

117. Ueno R: Results of intramuscular injection of glycosamino-glycan-polysulfate (GAGPS) in experimental arthrosis of the knee in dogs (author's transl). Z Orthop Ihre Grenzgeb 114:108, 1976.

118. Vanharanta H: Glycosaminoglycan polysulphate treatment in experimental osteoarthritis in rabbits. Scand J Rheumatol 12:225, 1983.

119. Burkhardt D, Ghosh P: Labratory evaluation of glycosaminoglycan polysulphate ester for chondroprotective activity: A review. Curr Ther Res 40:1034, 1986.

120. Hamm D, Goldman L, Jones E: Polysulfated glycosaminoglycan: A new intra-articular treatment for equine lameness. Vet Med 79:811, 1984.

121. Glade MJ: Polysulfated glycosaminoglycan accelerates net synthesis of collagen and glycosaminoglycans by arthritic equine cartilage tissues and chondrocytes. Am J Vet Res 51:779, 1990.

122. Halverson PB, Cheung HS, Struve J, et al: Suppression of active collagenase from calcified lapine synovium by arteparon. J Rheumatol 14:1013, 1987.

123. Steinmeyer J, Burton-Wurster N, Lust G: Effects of three antiarthritic drugs on fibronectin and keratan sulfate synthesis by cultured canine articular cartilage chondrocytes. Am J Vet Res 53:2077, 1992.

124. Sevalla K, Todhunter RJ, Vernier-Singer M, et al: Effect of polysulfated glycosaminoglycan on DNA content and proteoglycan metabolism in normal and osteoarthritic canine articular cartilage explants. Vet Surg 29:407, 2000.

125. Muller W, Panse P, Brand S, et al: In vivo study of the distribution, affinity for cartilage and metabolism of glycosaminoglycan polysulphate (GAGPS, arteparon). Z Rheumatol 42:355, 1983.

Chapter 105

Cranial Cruciate Ligament and Meniscal Injuries in Dogs

Kei Hayashi
Jennifer L. Lansdowne
Loïc Déjardin

Cranial cruciate ligament (CCL) rupture is one of the most common causes of lameness in adult dogs. The CCL plays a crucial role in limb function by maintaining stability of the stifle joint throughout the range of motion, thus injury to the CCL will result in joint instability and predispose the joint to degenerative changes. In dogs, the majority of CCL ruptures occurs under normal activity, likely owing to structural deterioration of the ligament and not because of a traumatic injury. Rupture of the CCL owing to degeneration can manifest acutely even in young dogs and eventually is often bilateral. Osteoarthritis, meniscal injury, and persistent lameness commonly occur with CCL rupture. Therefore, the debilitating pathologic condition related to CCL rupture is often referred to as "cruciate disease." Cranial cruciate ligament rupture is particularly common in large and giant breed dogs; however, any breed, size, or age of dog may be affected. Although clinical features and treatment options have been well discussed in the veterinary literature, the disease mechanisms for CCL rupture are poorly understood.

Cranial Cruciate Ligament

Anatomy

The cranial cruciate ligament is a dynamic structure and its anatomy and spatial arrangement are directly related to its function as a constraint of joint motion.[1] The CCL attaches proximally to the caudomedial part of the lateral condyle of the femur, within the intercondylar fossa of the femur, and courses cranially, medially, and distally across the joint as it passes from femur to tibia, and turns on itself in an outward lateral spiral of approximately 90° (Figure 105-1). The CCL extends distally to attach to the cranial intercondylar area of the tibia, beneath the transverse intermeniscal ligament. The caudal cruciate ligament crosses the CCL medially in the middle of the joint. The CCL fans out proximally and distally at its attachments and is narrowest in the middle.[2]

The cranial cruciate ligament is a collection of parallel and twisted collagenous bundles, or fascicles (Figure 105-1). These fascicles have been divided into two groups: the relatively thin craniomedial band that is rotated into an outward spiral (craniomedial spiral), and the caudolateral band that forms the bulk of the CCL (caudolateral bulk) (Figure 105-1). The craniomedial band arises more proximally in the intercondylar fossa of the femur and inserts more cranially in the cranial intercondylar area of the tibia.[1,2] The caudolateral band is shorter and straighter.

When the stifle is extended, both craniomedial and caudolateral

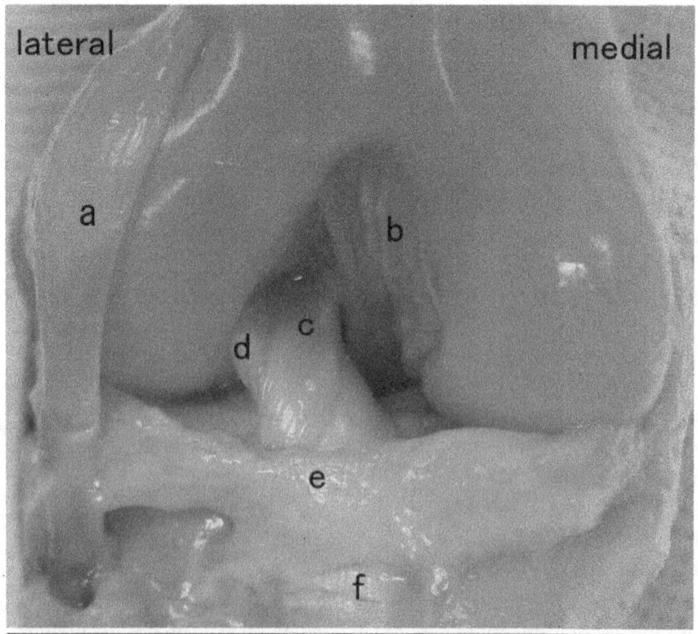

Figure 105-1. Normal anatomy of the canine stifle in flexion. A. long digital extensor tendon, B..caudal cruciate ligament, C. craniomedial band of CCL, D. caudolateral band of CCL, E. intermeniscal transverse ligament, F. distal part of tibial attachment of CCL.

bands are tight, and when the stifle is flexed, the craniomedial band is tight and caudolateral band is relatively lax. However, the CCL is actually a continuum of collagenous fascicles, and a different portion of the CCL is taut throughout the range of motion; therefore, this grouping scheme may oversimplify the structure and function of the CCL.[1]

Mechanics

Stifle mechanics are governed by muscular force and constrained by ligaments and joint capsule as well as by the geometry of the menisci and condyles.[1] The stifle is classified as a hinge joint with a combined motion primarily in two planes. Flexion and extension take place about the transverse axis, whereas rotary movement of the tibia on the femur occurs about the longitudinal axis. Slight craniocaudal and mediolateral movements also occur. The rotary motion is controlled by the condylar geometry and ligamentous constraints; internal rotation of the tibia is mainly limited by the anatomic relationship of cranial and caudal cruciate ligaments. The primary function of the CCL is to prevent cranial displacement of the tibia on the femur (cranial drawer), internal rotation of the tibia, and hyperextension of the stifle. Because the craniomedial band of the CCL is taut in both flexion and extension, it provides the primary check against cranial drawer motion, and because the entire CCL is taut in extension, it serves as the primary check against hyperextension of the stifle.[1] Together the cranial and caudal cruciate ligaments are responsible for craniocaudal stability of the stifle; the CCL prevents cranial drawer motion, and the caudal cruciate ligament prevents caudal displacement of the tibia on the femur (caudal drawer motion).

It has been suggested that the cranial cruciate ligament also functions to resist a force called "cranial tibial thrust".[3] Cranial tibial thrust is hypothesized to occur during weight bearing by compression of the femoral condyles against the tibial plateau.

The magnitude of cranial tibial thrust is dependent on both the degree of compression during weight bearing and the slope of the tibial plateau. The amount of tibial compression is variable and depends on the size, muscular force, and activity level of the dog. The tibial plateau slopes caudodistally and varies among dogs owing to anatomic and conformational differences. The CCL, together with the caudal horn of the medial meniscus and flexor muscle groups of the stifle, balances this force, preventing cranial translation of the tibia.

Histology

The cranial cruciate ligament is a complex structure consisting of an extracellular matrix and a diverse population of cells. The CCL has two histologically distinct regions: an epiligamentous region, composed of cellular synovial intima and loose connective tissue, and a core region, which is the major axial tissue component composed of collagen fiber bundles.[4,5] The collagen fibers are primarily composed of type I collagen and a smaller amount of type III collagen. Bundles of collagen fibers are longitudinally oriented, mostly running parallel to one another. Normal CCL collagen fibers have a recurrent undulating wave or crimped structure. During tensile loading of the ligament's collagen fibers, the crimp is lost before the fiber ruptures. Crimping is a distinct structural feature of organized collagen fibers in dense connective tissue and is an important determinant of the biomechanical properties of the tissue. From a biomechanical standpoint, the loss of crimping reflects the viscoelastic properties of the cruciate ligament and corresponds to the "toe region" on a load/deformation curve.

The predominant cell type in the CCL is the fibroblast. Ligament fibroblasts are arranged in long parallel rows between collagenous fiber bundles. Three different types of fibroblasts have been described: fusiform or spindle-shaped, ovoid, and spheroid.[5] The cytoplasm of fusiform fibroblasts is intimately attached to the extracellular collagen and follows the crimped waveform of the fibers. Ovoid and spheroid fibroblasts are situated in the loose connective tissue between collagen fibers. It is currently unclear whether these cells represent differing metabolic states of the same cells or whether they are distinctly different fibroblasts.

The CCL has a relatively tenuous microvasculature, which arises predominantly from the infrapatellar fat pad and periligamentous tissue, as opposed to the proximal and distal attachment sites.[1] The CCL receives its blood supply from branches of the middle genicular artery, which forms a vascular synovial envelope around the ligament. The innervation of the CCL regulates vasomotor tone and proprioception. The greatest density of mechanoreceptors is found in the proximal region of the CCL. These may function to send impulses during flexion/extension and rotation. The role of these receptors in proprioception is unknown.

Histopathology

The cranial cruciate ligament appears to experience chronic and irreversible degeneration with aging.[4] Idiopathic degeneration is a common histologic finding of the intact CCL, despite its grossly normal appearance. Degenerative changes are generally characterized by a decreased number of normal ligament fibroblasts, chondroid metaplasia of ligament fibroblasts, and loss of the normal fibrous architecture of the extracellular matrix.[4,5] These changes result in a partial transformation of ligamentous tissue into fibrocartilage (Figure 105-2). More severe changes such as hyalinization, mineralization, and cloning of chondrocyte-like cells can also occur; however, inflammatory or reparative responses are not observed. The degenerative changes can occur at a young age, particularly in large dogs, and progresses with aging. The severity of changes is usually similar in both stifle joints and affects the mechanical properties of the CCL.

The interior "core region" of the CCL deteriorates earlier than the surface epiligamentous region, and the midportion of the CCL deteriorates earlier than areas close to bony attachments.[4] These findings may be related to the hypovascularity and ischemic environment of the core region of CCL. Histopathologic changes of CCL degeneration are more prominent in larger dogs weighing more than 15 kg; the onset of the degenerative changes occurs at an earlier age in these large dogs. Increasing body size may also exacerbate the rate and severity of the degenerative process.

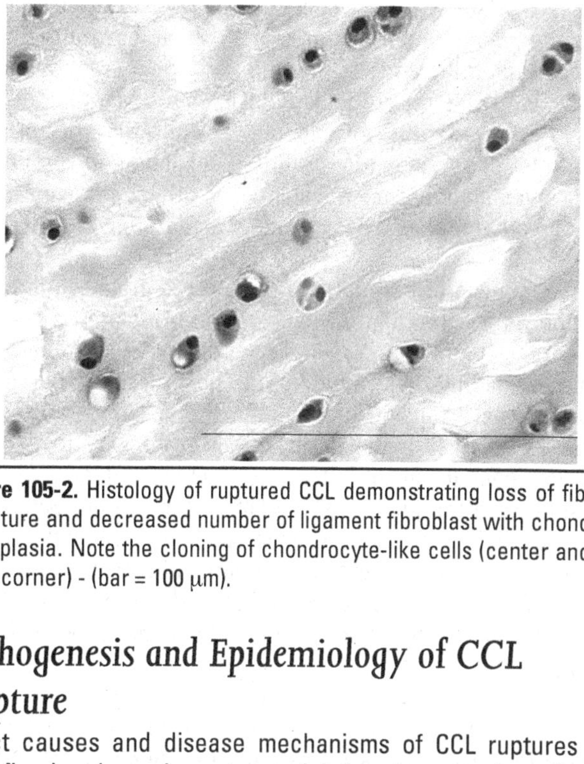

Figure 105-2. Histology of ruptured CCL demonstrating loss of fibrous structure and decreased number of ligament fibroblast with chondroid metaplasia. Note the cloning of chondrocyte-like cells (center and top right corner) - (bar = 100 μm).

Pathogenesis and Epidemiology of CCL Rupture

Exact causes and disease mechanisms of CCL ruptures are undefined and remain controversial; therefore, cruciate disease has been referred to as the "enigma of the canine stifle."[1] Although acute CCL rupture does occur with trauma, it is generally accepted that the majority of CCL lesions are the result of chronic degenerative changes in the ligaments themselves. Rupture of the CCL associated with major traumatic injury is usually unilateral and often involves multiple ligamentous injuries of the stifle and can lead to joint luxation. Isolated traumatic injury to the CCL is rare in dogs, is seen most often in puppies, and typically is associated with avulsion of the ligament at the tibial attachment site distally. In contrast, most pathologic cranial cruciate ligament ruptures are bilateral, midsubstance, incomplete or complete tears. Evidence is conflicting as to whether the degenerative changes seen in CCL are primary or secondary or a combination of multiple factors. Several risk factors have been proposed for CCL rupture; **Table 105-1** summarizes the findings of recent epidemiologic studies.[6-10] Rupture of the CCL has significant association with breed, body weight, and neutering. Other factors, such as aging, gender, conformational variation, medial patellar luxation, inactivity, and obesity have also been associated with CCL rupture. Although the effect of the tibial plateau angle (TPA) on cruciate ligament stresses has been recognized in people, the effect of TPA on CCL rupture in dogs has yet to be established. The risk of CCL rupture is higher in certain breeds, such as the Rottweiler, Labrador and Chesapeake Bay retrievers, Newfoundland, Akita, Neapolitan mastiff, Saint Bernard, and Staffordshire bull terrier. Dog phenotype may have a significant effect on the structural properties of the CCL, as the CCL of certain breeds (e.g., Rottweiler) appears more vulnerable to mechanical overload. Material properties of the CCL from Rottweilers are inferior to those of rarely affected breed dogs (greyhounds), although craniocaudal laxity is similar in both breeds throughout the range of motion. Commonly affected breeds tend to have abnormal posture such as straight stifle, genu varum (bow-leg), or genu valgum (knock-knee). Larger dogs weighing more than 22 kg are at greater risk of cruciate disease and tend to develop CCL rupture at younger ages. It remains unclear whether obesity is a risk factor for the disease independent of the dog's size. Neutering also increases the risk for cruciate rupture, particularly in female dogs, although the cause of this effect is not understood. The effect of hormonal status and endocrinopathy on CCL weakness and rupture are being investigated. The prevalence of CCL rupture increases with age and reaches a peak incidence at around 7 years.

The mechanism of traumatic CCL rupture can be related to its function as a constraint for joint motion. As stated above, the CCL serves to prevent cranial displacement of the tibia on the femur, to limit internal rotation of the tibia on the femur, and to prevent hyperextension of the stifle. Excessive forces during extremes of these motions can result in damage to the CCL. Common mechanisms of CCL injuries include sudden rotation of the stifle with the joint in 20° to 50° of the flexion, which can occur when the dog makes a sudden outward turn on the weight bearing limb, and hyperextension of the stifle, which can occur when a dog steps into a hole while running. Direct trauma to the stifle in any direction may cause damage to the CCL as well as to other joint structures.

Chronic degeneration and progressive weakening of the CCL appear to make it more susceptible to damage from minimal trauma, thereby predisposing the CCL to rupture. Despite extensive efforts in epidemiologic and clinical investigation, instigating causes of CCL degeneration and structural deterioration are not fully understood. Aging, hypovascularity of the CCL, abnormal conformation of the stifle, immune-mediated joint disease, and inflammatory joint disease have been proposed as contributing causes of CCL degeneration and rupture.[11-13] The degenerative changes in cellular and matrix components that develop in a ruptured CCL may result from the effects of remodeling and adaptation to various factors, such as ischemia, mechanical loading, and ligament microinjury.

Idiopathic degeneration of the CCL appears to begin within the central core portion and may be related to the ischemic nature of the tissue, complex mechanical environment (tension, compression, and shear) within the CCL, or both.

In degenerate ligament, the numbers of typical fibroblasts (i.e., fusiform and ovoid cells) are decreased, and the numbers of cells exhibiting chondroid transformation (i.e., spheroid cells) are increased.[5] These cellular changes are associated with extensive disruption of the ligamentous matrix, transforming the ligament into cartilage-like structure. This type of tissue transformation is often attributed to altered oxygenation status and mechanical environment. Inadequate blood supply of the central region of the CCL may be exacerbated by the twisting of the cruciate ligaments on themselves during flexion. This, in turn, may reduce blood flow and may account for the CCL transformation. For ligament fibroblasts to persist under increasingly ischemic conditions, these cells may be undergoing metaplasia to form chondrocytes, which can survive by using anaerobic metabolic pathway. The complex mechanical environment within the CCL, which includes compression and shear, as opposed to simple tension, can also contribute to the tissue transformation. Cartilage-like tissue is more vulnerable to disruption under normal tensile forces; therefore, the degeneration with fibrocartilaginous transformation may predispose CCL to pathologic rupture. However, areas of fibrocartilage are observed in grossly normal CCL in rarely affected breeds (greyhounds), which may represent successful physiologic adaptation to ischemic environment.[11] It is currently unclear whether CCL degeneration and transformation into fibrocartilage constitute a pathognomonic condition causing CCL rupture.

Conformational variation such as straight stifle, narrow intercondylar notch, steep tibial plateau slope, MPL, valgus and varus deformities of the stifle, and repeated stress and microinjury can result in progressive degenerative joint disease and CCL rupture. These changes are frequently bilateral and have been referred to as "postural arthrosis." Postural abnormalities may also be a result of other orthopedic conditions. Straight stifle and narrow intercondylar notch, together with excessive rotation of the tibia and extension of the stifle, may cause constant impingement and abnormal compression of CCL against the cranial aspect of the intercondylar notch. Medial patellar luxation, genu varum, and excessive internal rotation of the tibia, or a steep tibial plateau slope may cause increased stress, micro injury, and degeneration of the CCL. These conformational variations and abnormalities may predispose the CCL to rupture. Although anatomic differences in the shape of the proximal tibia have been documented in dogs with cruciate disease, their role in cruciate disease is unclear because many dogs with a steep tibial plateau angle do not develop cruciate disease. Indeed, although the mean TPA in dogs varies between 23° and 25°, a wide range of TPA has been reported (13° to 34°) in normal dogs. Furthermore, because the functional TPA is approximately parallel to the ground in most dogs, the true effect of TPA on CCL stresses in vivo is unknown. Finally, although the correlation between CCL rupture and pathologic increases in TPA (> 55°), possibly secondary to gross plate injuries, seems established, the association between TPA and CCL rupture in a normal canine population remains controversial. Muscular force, body size, obesity, rapid weight gain,

Table 105-1. Epidemiologic and Clinical Features of CCL Rupture

Benett et al (1988), UK[6]

- 50% < 4 years old (mean 1.8 years)
  - Mostly large dogs (mean body weight 34.1kg), 25% Rottweiler
  - 42% female, 18% spayed female, 38% male, 2% neutered male
  - 53% sudden onset, 47% gradual onset
  - 31% bilateral
- 50% > 4 years old (mean 6.8 years)
  - Variety of breeds (mean body weight 25.8 kg)
  - 36% female, 21% spayed female, 41% male, 2% neutered male
  - 64% sudden onset, 36% gradual onset
  - 26% bilateral

Whitehair et al (1993), USA[7]

- High prevalence associated with age, breed, sex, neutering, and body weight
  - Age: 7-9 years
  - Breed: Rottweiler, Newfoundland, Staffordshire terrier
  - Female
  - Neutered female or male
  - Body weight > 22kg

Duval et al (1999), USA[8]

- Risk factors in young dogs (< 2 years)
  - Breed: Neapolitan Mastiff, Akita, Saint Bernard, Rottweiler, Mastiff, Newfoundland, Chesapeake Bay retriever, Labrador retriever, America Stafford terrier, Chow Chow, English Bulldog
  - Neutered female or male
  - Mean body weight 35.4 kg
  - 37% bilateral
  - 33% partial rupture, 66% complete rupture, 42% meniscal tear

Harasen (2003), Canada[9]

- Comparison between 1983-1994 and 1997-2002
  - Sex: 65% female/35% male vs. 53% female/47% male
  - Body weight: 35% large dogs (> 15 kg) vs. 61% large dogs (> 15 kg)
  - Mean age: 7.7 years vs. 7.3 years
    - (small dogs: 8.7 years vs. 8.0 years)
    - (large dogs: 5.8 years vs. 7.0 years)
  - 30% bilateral vs. 27% bilateral
  - 15% meniscal tear vs. 48% meniscal tear

Jerram and Walker (2003), New Zealand[10]

- Proposed grouping of dogs based on clinical observation
  - Small dogs with medial patellar luxation
  - Large to medium-sized active dogs with trauma (hyperextension or excessive internal rotation)
  - Young large dogs with conformational abnormalities (impingement of CCL owing to hyperextended stifle and narrow intercondylar notch, increased strain on CCL owing to steep tibial plateau slope)
  - Middle-aged, medium to large dogs with chronic inflammatory joint disease

relative inactivity, and exercise can also modify the amount of stress sustained by the CCL. The beneficial effect of activity on ligament strength in dogs is well documented, although the roles of activity and inactivity in CCL rupture are not well understood.

Inflammatory disease may be involved in the initiation of CCL rupture.[13,14] Cruciate disease in dogs is often associated with infiltration of leukocytes into the synovial membrane of the stifle joint and the development of inflammatory changes in the synovial fluid. Anti-collagen antibodies, immune complex, and rheumatoid factors have been identified in synovial fluid of the joint with CCL rupture; therefore, involvement of immune-mediated disease has been proposed as a cause of CCL degeneration. However, anti-collagen antibodies are not likely the major factor of CCL degeneration and rupture, because the increase of anti-collagen antibodies is not specific for the type of joint disorder. More recently, collagenolytic enzyme expression has been found in the ruptured CCL and synovial fluid, and synovial macrophage-like cells that produce matrix-degrading enzymes have been identified. These findings suggest that inflammatory arthropathy predisposes the CCL to rupture, by release of proteolytic enzymes during inflammatory process. Release of collagenolytic proteases from the synovium into the stifle synovial fluid can significantly degrade the structural properties of the CCL and increase the likelihood of a pathologic midsubstance rupture. However, these inflammatory changes could be a secondary phenomenon, in response to the tissue damage during CCL rupture and osteoarthritis.

Genetic and breed predisposition have recently been implicated in the pathogenesis of CCL rupture.[15,16] Early studies suggest that 1) collagen turnover may be increased in dogs predisposed to CCL rupture (Labrador retrievers) compared with dogs not predisposed to CCL rupture (greyhounds); 2) collagen fibril of greyhounds are larger than those of Labrador retrievers; and 3) craniocaudal joint laxity is greater in Labrador retrievers compared with greyhounds. Whether cranial cruciate ligament weakness could be part of generalized collagen abnormality remains uncertain because weakness in other ligaments and joints is not commonly seen in dogs with CCL rupture. These differences may be influenced by genetics and may account for the differential predisposition of the two breeds to CCL rupture. Further studies have revealed the high incidence of CCL rupture in Newfoundlands (22%) and suggested that CCL rupture has a potential recessive mode of inheritance with 51% penetrance in a population of Newfoundlands. A genetic association was also determined between CCL rupture status and a large number of statistically significant microsatellite markers on canine chromosomes 3, 10 and 23 in this population.

Cruciate Ligament Pathology

Pathology of CCL disease appears to involve a gradual degeneration of the CCL itself, inflammatory disease in the stifle joint, partial rupture, progressive rupturing, complete rupture, and secondary disease such as progressive osteoarthritis and meniscal injury. Partial ruptures can occur at any part of the CCL, although it has been suggested that the relatively thinner craniomedial band of the CCL is more susceptible to rupture. Complete ruptures appear to occur near the tibial attachment, although location of the rupture is often indeterminable.

An initial pathology with slight weakening or stretching of the CCL may not cause lameness, but can produce mild instability within the joint and, therefore, initiate the osteoarthritis process. Dogs with early cruciate disease (i.e., minor partial CCL rupture) may have little or no palpable instability, but they are often presented with lameness, effusion of the stifle joint, and mild osteoarthritis. Major partial or complete CCL ruptures produce marked instability of the stifle joint, resulting in pain, lameness, and progressive degenerative changes within the joint. Clinical observations have demonstrated that these changes consist of periarticular osteophyte formation, capsular thickening, and meniscal degeneration. As these changes progress, the joints become less unstable. Advanced or end-stage cruciate disease may have little palpable stifle instability because of extensive periarticular fibrosis.

After a partial or complete CCL rupture, some degree of tissue repair responses arise in the periligamentous region of the ligament. Distinct phases of tissue repair, including an inflammatory phase, a periligamentous repair phase, a proliferative phase, and a remodeling phase, occur after rupture of the anterior cruciate ligament in humans. Whether similar phases exist in dogs is unknown. Expansion of the volume of the periligamentous tissue does occur in the dog during a repair phase that lasts many weeks; however, a bridging scar does not form in the rupture site. Eventually, synovial tissue covers the ruptured ends of the CCL. The extracellular matrix of ruptured CCL has an increased turnover indicated by increased collagen and glycosaminoglycan synthesis, and increased levels of proteolytic enzymes. This response may represent a degrading and remodeling phase of the CCL after rupture.

Rupture of the CCL causes various degrees of inflammation in the stifle. The inflammatory changes within synovium are variable even within the same joint. Plasma cells, lymphocytes, and macrophages are commonly seen in the synovium, although the infiltrate is not noticeable in some cases. Although partial CCL rupture has been associated with moderate synovial fluid inflammatory changes, synovial fluid analysis in dogs with CCL rupture generally shows a non-inflammatory process. This suggests that CCL rupture is a progressive condition with an early inflammatory component. Several studies have investigated osteoarthritic parameters associated with CCL rupture.[17] Proinflammatory factors, cytokines, nitric oxide, degradation products of matrix, epitopes of cartilage matrix, and degrading enzymes have been shown to increase with osteoarthritis in the stifle with CCL rupture; however, no specific marker for CCL rupture is known.

Meniscal Injury

Pathophysiology

Primary lesions of the meniscus are rare in dogs, however meniscal injuries secondary to rupture of the cruciate or collateral ligaments are common. Most frequently the medial meniscus is affected following cranial cruciate ligament rupture. Damage to the menisci can be either acute or degenerative and usually involves the caudal and medial portions of the medial meniscus.[18] A general understanding of the anatomy and biomechanics of the menisci is important in understanding the pathophysiology of injury.

Anatomy

Each stifle contains a medial and lateral meniscus, which are C-shaped fibrocartilaginous disks interposed between the articulating surfaces of the femur and tibia. In cross section, menisci are wedge shaped with a thin, concave central edge and a thick periphery. The lateral meniscus forms a slightly greater arc and is more concave than the medial meniscus, corresponding to the articular surfaces of the femur and tibia. The menisci are anchored to the tibia and femur via five meniscal ligaments and to each other by the intermeniscal ligament (Figure 105-3). The lateral and medial menisci are each firmly anchored to the tibia by a cranial and caudal meniscotibial ligament. The caudal horn of the lateral meniscus is also attached to the lateral aspect of the medial femoral condyle by the meniscofemoral ligament. The medial meniscus is not directly linked to the femur, however. Because of extensive fibrous attachments to the joint capsule and medial collateral ligament, it is intimately attached to the tibia. In contrast, the lateral meniscus is more mobile in part because of the popliteal hiatus (imprint of the popliteal tendon and bursa on the lateral edge of the lateral meniscus) and subsequent lack of peripheral connection with the lateral joint capsule and/or collateral ligament. The intermeniscal ligament lies just cranial to the tibial attachment of the cranial cruciate ligament and joins together the cranial portions of the lateral and medial meniscus.[19,20]

The meniscus is a fibrocartilage that is composed of 60 to 70% water. Collagen accounts for 60 to 70% of the dry weight (15-25% wet weight), with type I collagen predominating (> 90%). Type II collagen, proteoglycans, matrix glycoproteins and small amounts of elastin make up the rest of the dry weight.[21] The articulating surface of the meniscus is composed of fine fibrils arranged in a random mesh-like woven matrix. This random distribution is effective against shear stresses. Immediately below the meniscal surface, large collagen fiber bundles are arranged circumferentially, which optimizes meniscal resistance against hoop stresses. Finally, smaller radially oriented fibers are found throughout the meniscal tissue, tying the large circumferential bundles together. This fibrillar orientation provides the structure to the meniscus and predominates throughout the peripheral two thirds of the tissue. In contrast, the inner third of the region resembles hyaline cartilage in that it contains smaller collagen fibers arranged in a more random pattern.[22] Unlike the meniscal body, which is relatively avascular, the meniscal horns have an abundant blood supply, which arises from branches of the medial and lateral genicular arteries. Further branching supplies the joint capsule, which provides vessels to the periphery of the meniscus. However, vessels penetrate the menisci for only 10 to 25% of their width, the remainder of the meniscus being totally avascular.[21,23] The clinical relevance of this vascular distribution has lead to the recognition of three zones with decreasing healing potential, namely - from the periphery to the center - the red, red-white, and white zones.[23] Owing to the meager blood supply, meniscal injuries occurring axial to the peripheral rim rarely heal. In addition, a layer of vascular synovial tissue, apparently continuous with the sheath that surrounds the cranial cruciate ligament, covers the cranial and caudal horn attachments of both menisci. The caudolateral portion of the lateral meniscus,

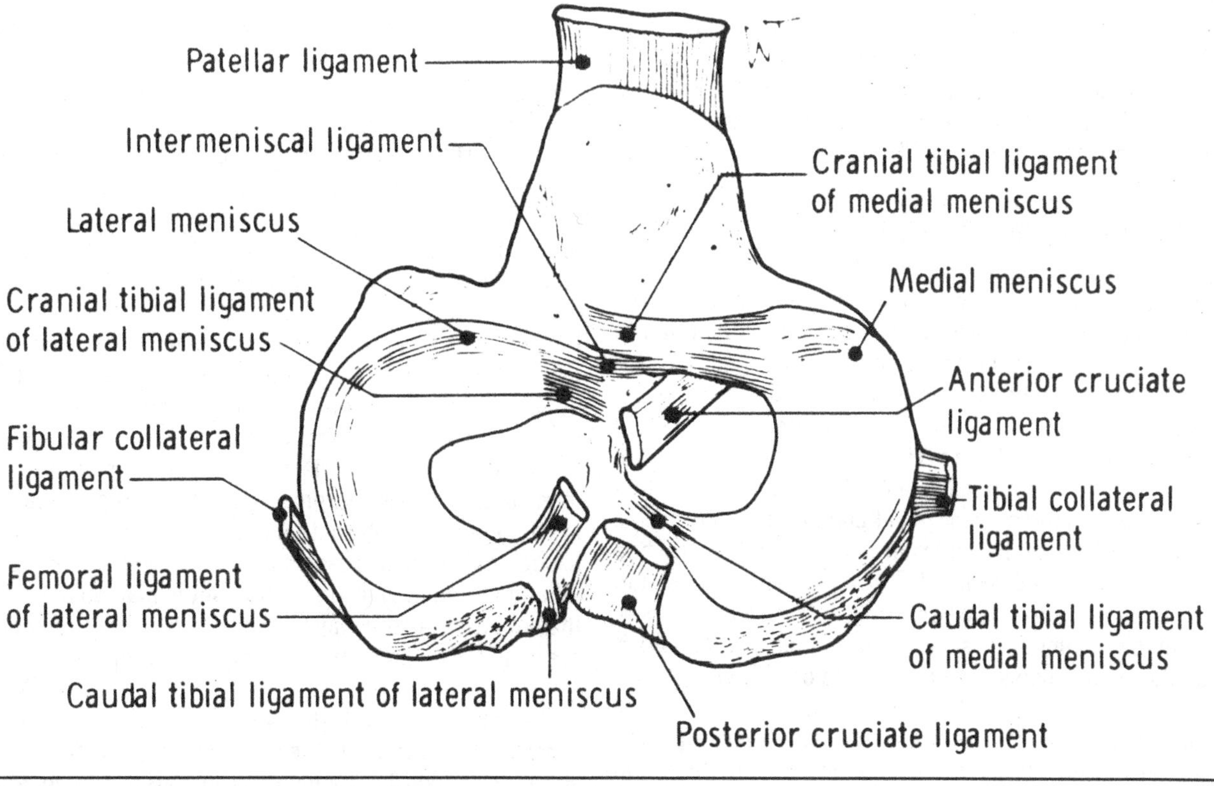

Figure 105-3. Drawing of the dorsal aspect of the tibia showing the menisci and their attachments.

adjacent to the popliteal tendon and the inner aspects of both menisci, lacks vessels and relies on diffusion of synovial fluid for nutrition. The innervation of the menisci follows the vascularization pattern, with the meniscal horns being more richly innervated with mechanoreceptors and free nerve endings than the body of the menisci.

Function

The menisci are thought to participate in four main functions: namely shock absorption, joint stability, sensation, and hydrostatic lubrication.[19,20] The menisci distribute approximately 65% of the joint force through load transmission (shock absorption). The circumferential arrangement of the collagen fibers and the strong ligamentous attachments of the menisci help convert compressive loads across the joint into hoop stresses, thus absorbing most of the energy generated during weight bearing. The viscoelastic behavior of the meniscal tissue further contributes to the shock absorption function of the menisci, thereby sparing the articular cartilage of the tibia and femur from excessive stresses. The menisci also act as elastic movable washers and contribute to joint stability by improving congruity between the femur and tibia. Because of their firm attachment to the tibia and/or femur, the menisci further contribute to limiting the relative motion of the femur with regard to the tibia. The sensory function of the meniscus is achieved via an abundant nerve supply to its periphery. In addition, because mechanoreceptors located in the cranial and caudal horns can detect pressure changes within the joint, it is believed that the menisci can receive and transmit proprioceptive information. Additionally, due to a feedback mechanism to myotactic receptors, the menisci allow specific muscle actions to occur in response to acute changes in intra-articular stresses, which in turn contribute to the protection of intra-articular structures during extreme range of motion. The menisci are also thought to provide hydrostatic lubrication of the articular cartilage. It has been shown that following meniscectomy the intraarticular friction coefficient is increased by up to 20%. As a minor function, the menisci act as space fillers, preventing synovial entrapment between the weight-bearing articular surfaces of the femur and tibia.[19]

Mechanism of Meniscal Injury

The stifle functions as a hinge joint with axial rotation of the tibia on the femur through the range of motion. During range of motion, the displacement of the menisci within the joint is dictated in part by their specific attachment to the tibial plateau and (for the lateral meniscus) to the femur. During extension, the menisci slide cranially on the tibial plateau then return to a more caudal position as the stifle flexes. With extreme flexion the excursion of the medial meniscus is such that the caudal horn may protrude beyond the caudal aspect of the tibial plateau. In such cases, the caudal horn of the medial meniscus may be acutely crushed between the femoral condyle and the tibial plateau. Because the lateral meniscus is more mobile (less firmly attached to the tibia), the lateral meniscus undergoes considerably more displacement than does the medial meniscus during range of motion.

Excessive compressive and/or shear stresses, resulting from stifle instability, whether acute or chronic, lead to meniscal degeneration.[24,25] The degenerative process is associated with structural alteration of the meniscal tissue such as mucoid degeneration of the cartilage matrix, fragmentation of the collagen bundles, and fibrillation. This alteration in fibrocartilage microstructure makes the menisci more vulnerable to injury and tear after minimal trauma. In chronic cases, calcification within the fibrocartilage can also occur secondary to degenerative change. In addition, modification of the biochemical composition of the meniscal tissue characterized by an increase in water content and a decrease in collagen content has also been reported and seems to correlate with the degradation of its biomechanical properties, including a decrease in compressive stiffness to ~ 60% of normal. It has been suggested that the extent of theses changes correlates with the loading of the meniscal tissue and, therefore, varies between the cranial, central, and caudal regions of the meniscus. Interestingly, shifts in weight bearing following CCL rupture also affect the mechanical properties on the contralateral normal medial meniscus. As the weight-bearing forces increase on the sound limb, so do loads to which the healthy meniscus is subjected. Adaptative remodeling is reflected by an increased compressive stiffness of the normal meniscus.

Most commonly, meniscal injuries occur secondary to stifle instability resulting from CCL rupture, with injury to the medial meniscus being reported in at least 50% of cases.[24-26] Although acute meniscal injuries can happen, delayed lesions occurring weeks to months after cruciate rupture are far more typical. Instability in the cruciate-deficient stifle results in a combination of excessive internal tibial rotation and cranial tibial translation. This combined motion induces disproportionately high compressive and shear stresses on the relatively immobile medial meniscus. With cranial displacement of the tibia/medial meniscus complex, the concave inner border of the meniscus may be stretched to the point of creating a transverse tear. It has been estimated that normal meniscal tissue fails at strain levels exceeding 5% and that degenerative menisci could likely tear at lower strain levels. Eventually, shear stresses generated at the surface of the meniscus by the repetitive sliding of the tibia are transmitted to the meniscal stroma, creating a deep horizontal cleavage. Ultimately, this pathologic cleavage plane propagates toward either surface of the meniscus, creating a grossly visible longitudinal tear (Figure 105-4). The term bucket-handle tear has been used to describe the displaced medial portion of a longitudinal tear. Alternatively, the caudal horn of the medial meniscus may become crushed or pushed cranially between the medial femoral and tibial condyles as cranial translation of the tibia occurs during weight bearing. In such cases, the caudal meniscotibial ligament may be severed, which in turn allows the caudal horn of the medial meniscus to move freely between the caudal and cranial compartments of the joint. In some cases, the caudal meniscotibial ligament remains intact and the caudal horn alone is damaged. The alternate motion of the caudal horn is initially associated with a characteristic clicking or snapping sound when the dog is walking or the joint is manipulated. Eventually, the degenerate horn may become fibrotic and even calcified and may interfere with complete range of motion.

In contrast, damage to the lateral meniscus has seldom been reported. However, with the increased popularity of arthroscopic stifle exploration, lateral meniscal lesions are being recognized.[26]

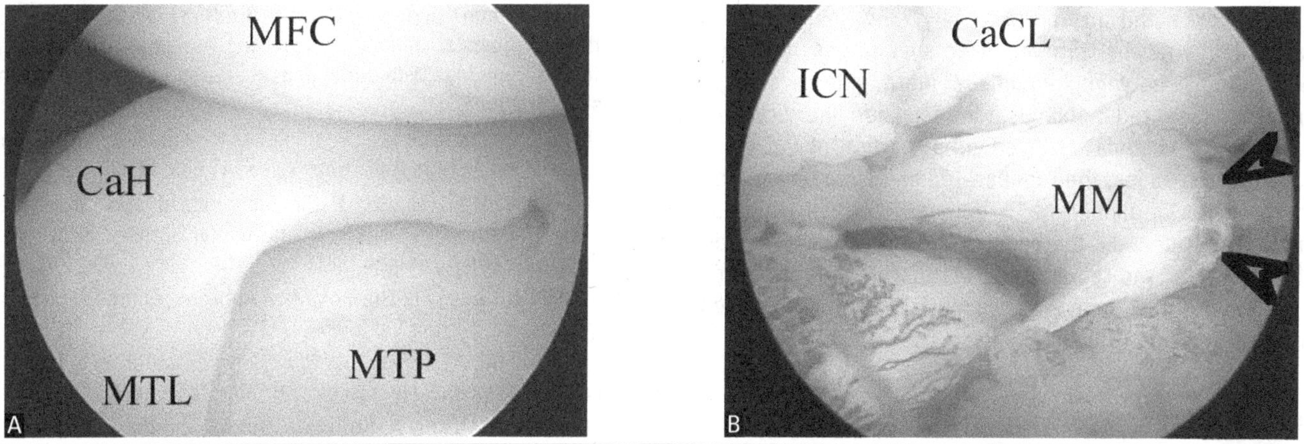

Figure 105-4. Arthroscopic views of a normal medial meniscus immediately following experimental transection of the cranial cruciate ligament (left) and 8 months postoperatively (right). The normal meniscus is viewed from the tibial plateau eminences toward the medial aspect of the joint (along the transverse plane). The torn meniscus is viewed in a cranial to caudal direction (along the sagittal plane). Note the circumferential tear at the limit of the "red-white" zone (arrow heads). Also note the extent of the synovial reaction compared with a normal stifle. MFC: medial femoral condyle, CaH: caudal horn, MTL: meniscotibial ligament, MTP, medial tibial plateau, CaCL: caudal cruciate ligament, ICN: intercondylar notch, MM: medial meniscus.

In a retrospective evaluation of 100 cruciate-deficient stifles, 77% of the joints had gross structural alteration of the lateral meniscal structure, generally observed as a series of small radial tears of the cranial horn (Figure 105-5). The clinical significance of these minor tears is unknown. Because of the lack of connection between the lateral meniscus and the joint capsule or collateral ligament, severe lesions of the lateral meniscus seem unlikely and have yet to be reported. Isolated injuries to either meniscus, in the absence of a cruciate rupture, are rare although theoretically possible following sudden compressive force directly on the meniscus, such as jumping from a height and landing with the stifle in full extension.

Menisectomy

The relative benefit of partial versus total removal of either meniscus remains controversial because both result in gross and microscopic degenerative changes of the articular surfaces of the femur and tibia.[27-29] Although a partial meniscectomy may have a protective effect on articular surfaces, it has been associated with limited tissue regeneration, particularly if the resected segment is entirely located within the avascular center (white zone) of the meniscus. Furthermore, experimental studies in humans have demonstrated that, after partial meniscectomy, the femorotibial articular contact area decreased by approximately 10%, while peak local contact stresses increased by 65%. Conversely, total meniscectomy lead to a 75% decrease

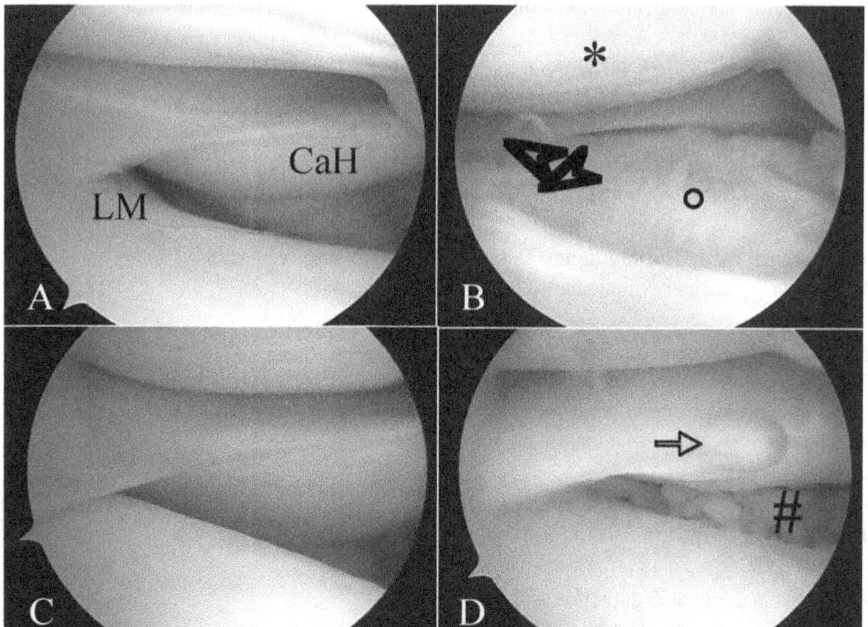

Figure 105-5. Arthroscopic view of normal lateral menisci (A & C) and 8 months following experimental transection of the CCL (B & D). Note (B) the series of small radial tears at the free edge of the meniscus (arrow heads) and the damage to the articular cartilage of the femoral condyle (chondromalacia*) and of the tibial plateau (fibrillation °). Also note (D) the presence of a cartilaginous nodule (open arrow) at the level of the caudal horn and the severe synovial proliferation (#). CaH: caudal horn, LM, lateral meniscus.

in contact area and an approximately 235% increase in peak local contact stresses.[25] The reported advantages of a complete meniscectomy, however, include a more extensive regeneration of the resected meniscus if the excision line runs through the peripheral vascularized (red zone) portion of the meniscal tissue. In such cases, the regenerated meniscal tissue, derived from the synovial membrane, is generally formed within 3 to 6 months. Unfortunately, the regeneration process is somewhat inconsistent and the regenerated fibrocartilage is ineffective in preventing the development of secondary osteoarthritis, which will occur in almost 100% of cases.

References

1. Arnoczky SP, Marshall JL: The cruciate ligaments of the canine stifle: An anatomical and functional analysis. Am J Vet Res 38:1809 1814, 1977.

2. Heffron LE, Campbell JR: Morphology, histology and functional anatomy of the canine cranial cruciate ligament. Vet Rec 102:280 283, 1978.

3. Slocum B, Devine T: Cranial tibial thrust: A primary force in the canine stifle. J Am Vet Med Assoc 183:456 459, 1983.

4. Vasseur PB, Pool RR, Arnoczky SP, et al: Correlative biomechanical and histologic study of the cranial cruciate ligament in dogs. Am J Vet Res 49:1842 1854, 1985.

5. Hayashi K, Frank JD, Hao Z, et al: Histological changes in the canine cranial cruciate ligament after rupture. Vet Surg 32:269 277, 2003.

6. Bennett D, Tennant B, Lewis DG, et al: A reappraisal of anterior cruciate ligament disease in the dog. J Small Anim Pract 29:275 297, 1988.

7. Whitehair JG, Vasseur PB, Willits NH: Epidemiology of cranial cruciate ligament rupture in dogs. J Am Vet Med Assoc 203:1016 1019, 1993.

8. Duval JM, Budsberg SC, Flo GL, et al: Breed, sex, and body weight as risk factors for rupture of the cranial cruciate ligament in young dogs. J Am Vet Med Assoc 215:811 814, 1999.

9. Harasen G: Canine cranial cruciate ligament rupture in profile: Can Vet J 44:845 846, 2003.

10. Jerram RM, Walker AM: Cranial cruciate ligament injury in the dog: Pathophysiology, diagnosis and treatment. NZ Vet J 51:149 158, 2003.

11. Comerford EJ, Tarlton JF, Innes JF, et al: Metabolism and composition of the canine anterior cruciate ligament relate to differences in knee joint mechanics and predisposition to ligament rupture. J Orthop Res 23:61 66, 2005.

12. Fitch RB, Montgomery RD, Milton JL, et al: The intercondylar fossa of the normal canine stifle: An anatomic and radiographic study. Vet Surg 24:148 155, 1995.

13. Lemburg AK, Meyer Lindenberg A, Hewicker Trautwein M: Immunohistochemical characterization of inflammatory cell populations and adhesion molecule expression in synovial membranes from dogs with spontaneous cranial cruciate ligament rupture. Vet Immunol Immunopathol 97:231 240, 2004.

14. Muir P, Hayashi K, Manley PA, et al: Evaluation of tartrate resistant acid phosphatase and cathepsin K in ruptured cranial cruciate ligament in dogs. Am J Vet Res 63:1279 1284, 2002.

15. Wilke VL, Conzemius MC, Rothschild MF: SNP detection and association analysis of candidate genes for rupture of the cranial cruciate ligament in the dog. Anim Genet 36:511 542, 2005.

16. Wilke VL, Conzemius MG, Kinghorn BP, et al: Inheritance of rupture of the cranial cruciate ligament in Newfoundlands. J Am Vet Med Assoc 228(1):61-64, 2006.

17. Innes JF, Little CB, Hughes CE, et al: Products resulting from cleavage of the interglobular domain of aggrecan in samples of synovial fluid collected from dogs with early and late stage osteoarthritis. Am J Vet Res 66:1679-1685, 2005.

18. Flo GL, DeYoung D: Meniscal injuries and medial meniscectomy in the canine stifle. J Am Anim Hosp Assoc 14:683, 1978.

19. Arnoczky SP, Marshall JL: Pathomechanics of cruciate and meniscal injuries. *In* Pathophysiology in Small Animal Surgery. Bojrab MJ (ed). Philadelphia:Lea & Febiger, 1981.

20. Hulse DA, Shires PK: The meniscus: Anatomy, function and treatment. Comp Cont Educ Pract Vet 5:765-777, 1983.

21. Kambic HE, McDevitt CA: Spatial organization of types I and II collagen in the canine meniscus. J Orthop Res 23:142, 2005.

22. Mow VC, Ratcliffe A: Structure and function of articular cartilage and meniscus. *In* Basic Orthopedic Biomechanics, 2nd ed. Mow VC and Hayes C (eds). Philadelphia: Lippincott-Raven, 1997, p. 113.

23. Arnoczky SP, Warren RF: The microvasculature of the meniscus and its response to injury. Am J Sports Med 11:131, 1983.

24. Noone TJ, Millis DL, Korvick DL, et al: Influence of canine recombinant somatotrophin hormone on biomechanical and biochemical properties of the medial meniscus in stifles with altered stability. Am J Vet Res 63(3):419, 2002.

25. Jackson J, Vasseur PB, Griffey S, et al: Pathologic changes in grossly normal menisci in dogs with rupture of the cranial cruciate ligament. J Am Vet Med Assoc 218(8):1281, 2001.

26. Ralphs SC, Whitney WO: Arthroscopic evaluation of menisci in dogs with cranial cruciate ligament injuries: 100 cases (1999-2000). J Am Vet Med Assoc 221(11):1601, 2002.

27. Johnson KA, Francis DJ, Manley PA, et al: Comparison of the effects of caudal pole hemi-menisectomy and complete medial menisectomy in the canine stifle joint. Am J Vet
Res 65(8):1053, 2004

28. Berjon JJ, Munuera L, Calvo M: Degenerative lesions in the articular cartilage after menisectomy: preliminary experimental study in dogs. J Trauma 31:342-350, 1991.

29. Baratz ME, Fu FH, Mengato R: Meniscal tears: The effect of meniscectomy and of repair on intra-articular contact areas and stress in the human knee. Am J Sports Med. 14:270-274, 1986.

Chapter 106

Patellar Luxation in Dogs

Kei Hayashi
Jennifer Lansdowne
Loïc Déjardin

Patellar luxation, defined as the displacement of the patella out of the trochlear groove of the femur, is a common problem in both small and large dogs. The condition may be congenital, developmental, traumatic, or iatrogenic in origin. The pathology can vary from mild instability of the patella within the trochlear groove to severe permanent luxation of the patella, either medially or laterally, with skeletal deformities. Medial patellar luxation (MPL) is more common in all sizes and breeds of dogs. Anatomic deviation of the patella interferes with its normal function, resulting in skeletal deformities of the pelvic limb, contracture of pelvic muscles, loss of normal mechanics of the stifle, degenerative changes of the joints, and impairment of limb function. Clinical signs vary with many factors, including degree of luxation, age of patient, degree of musculoskeletal abnormalities, and degree of degenerative joint disease. The majority of patellar luxations likely have a hereditary basis and genetic predisposition; however, the exact disease mechanisms have not been defined.

Anatomy

The patella is an ossification in the tendon of insertion of the quadriceps muscle group and the largest sesamoid bone in the body.[1] The patella is ovate: the proximal blunt surface is the base and may extend beyond the articular surface, whereas the distal pointed end, the apex, does not (Figure 106-1). The articular surface of the patella is smooth and convex in all directions, and articulates with a wide concave articular groove on the cranial surface of the distal femur called the femoral trochlea. The medial and lateral trochlear ridges, with the medial ridge usually being thicker than the lateral, bound the femoral trochlea.

The patella is held in the trochlea of the femur primarily by the joint capsule, thick lateral femoral fascia (fascia lata), and thinner medial femoral fascia (Figure 106-1). The cranial part of the sartorius and biceps femoris blend into the femoral fascia at the stifle and may contribute to the medial and lateral stability of the patella. The medial and lateral femoropatellar ligaments also aid in stability of the patella within the trochlea. The lateral femoropatellar ligament can be traced from the lateral side of the patella to the lateral fabella. The medial ligament is weaker than the lateral and blends with the periosteum of the medial epicondyle of the femur. The edges of the patella are connected to the femoral fascia via the medial and lateral parapatellar fibrocartilages (Figure 106-1). The parapatellar fibrocartilages ride on the ridges of the femoral trochlea and aid in patellar stability through contact with the ridges of the femoral trochlea. The vastus medialis muscle and vastus lateralis muscle of the quadriceps muscle group are fixed to the patella by the medial and lateral parapatellar fibrocartilages, respectively. A suprapatellar fibrocartilage may also be present in the tendon of the rectus femoris.

The quadriceps muscle group is formed by the rectus femoris, vastus lateralis, vastus intermedius, and vastus medialis. The rectus femoris arises from the ilium cranial to the acetabulum, the vastus lateralis and intermedius arise from the proximal part of the lateral lip of the caudal rough surface of the femur, and the vastus medialis arises from the medial side of the proximal femur. This muscle group converges on the patella and continues as the patellar ligament to insert on the tibial tuberosity distally.

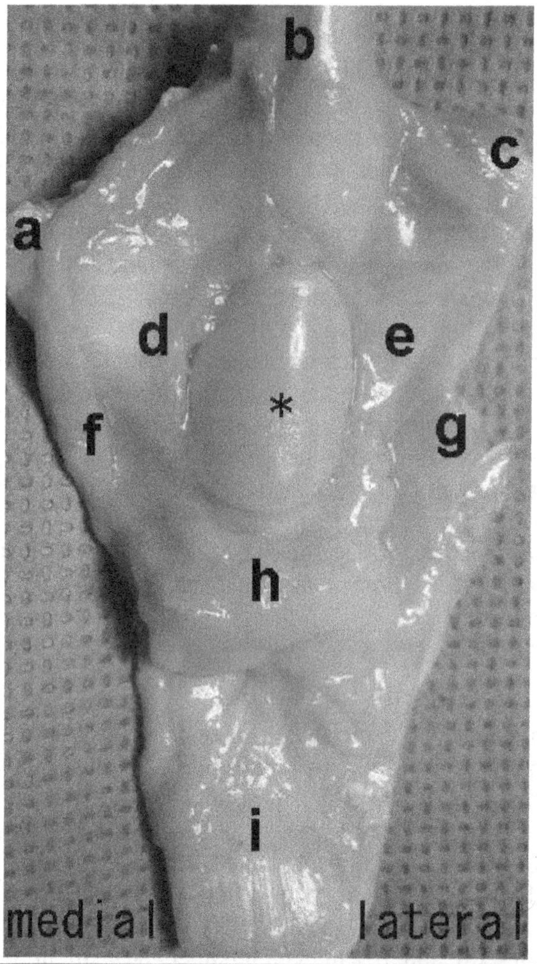

Figure 106-1. Normal anatomy of the articular aspect of canine patella. a: vastus medialis, b: rectus femoris, c: vastus lateralis, d: medial parapatellar fibrocartilage, e: lateral parapatellar fibrocartilage, f: medial retinaculum, joint capsule, femoropatellar ligament, and femoral fascia, g: lateral retinaculum, joint capsule, femoropatellar ligament, and femoral fascia, h: infrapatellar fat pad, i: patellar ligament.

Function

The extensor mechanism is composed of the quadriceps muscle group, patella, trochlear groove, patellar ligament, and tibial tuberosity. Physiologic (near straight) alignment of these structures, together with normal gliding articulation of the patella and trochlea, are essential for smooth and efficient movement of the stifle during its extension.[2] Muscular forces of the vastus medialis and vastus lateralis control medial and lateral movement and stability of the patella. The patella is an essential component of the extensor mechanism, serving to alter the direction of the pull of the quadriceps mechanism, preserving even tension of the extensor mechanism during stifle extension, and acting as a lever arm, increasing the mechanical advantage of the quadriceps muscle group. The patella also protects the tendon of the quadriceps muscle group during movement, provides a greater surface area for the tendon to engage the trochlea of the femur, and provides cranial and rotary stability to the stifle joint in the extensor mechanism. The location and prominence of the tibial tuberosity are important for the mechanical advantage of the extensor mechanism.

Epidemiology

Patellar luxation can be congenital, developmental, iatrogenic, or traumatic, although the majority of luxations are congenital and are often related to other musculoskeletal abnormalities.[3,4] It is a common problem of both small and large dogs and is the most common congenital abnormality in dogs.[5] In a study that examined 1679 pet store puppies, 253 had at least one congenital effect (15%) among which 121 were patellar luxation (7.2%).[6] These puppies were mostly small breeds: 48.8% would likely weigh less than 7 kg when mature. Patellar luxation is diagnosed most commonly in small breed dogs as a congenital or developmental problem within 6 months of age. However, as many as 32 breeds, including large breeds such as Akita, Great Pyrenees, and Labradors have been identified as at increased risk for patellar luxation.[7] Toy and miniature breeds are affected approximately 12 times more frequently than are large breed dogs, with toy poodles, Yorkshire terriers, Pomeranians, Pekingese, Chihuahuas, and Boston terriers being at increased risk for medial luxation.[4]

Medial Patellar Luxation

Medial patellar luxation is more common in all sizes and breeds of dogs than is lateral patellar luxation (LPL). In a study of 124 dogs that were referred for patellar luxation, the majority of dogs had a congenital form (82%), as opposed to acquired patellar luxation (15%), and the majority (89%) had MPL, as opposed to lateral luxation.[3] MPL accounted for 98% in small breeds (< 9.1 kg), 81% in medium breeds (9.1-18.2 kg), 83% in large breeds (18.2-36.4 kg), and 67% in giant breeds (> 36.4 kg). In one study of 70 referred large breed dogs, MPL accounted for 97% and LPL accounted for 2.8%.[8] That study also suggested that in large breed dogs MPL occurs more frequently in males (male:female sex ratio of 1.8:1). In contrast, other studies have shown that in small breed dogs females are more frequently affected (male:female sex ratio of 1:1.5).[4] Although females are more likely to be affected than males, prevalence is similar among spayed females, neutered males, and intact females, with intact males being at a lower risk. Bilateral luxations are significantly more common (65%) than unilateral luxations (35%).[3,8]

Three groups of patients were identified based on clinical pattern by Brinker, Piermattei, and Flo: 1) neonates and older puppies with abnormal hind-leg carriage and function from the time of ambulation; 2) young to mature dogs with intermittent and/or progressively abnormal gait; and 3) older dogs with an acute onset of lameness associated with degenerative changes and cranial cruciate ligament rupture.[9]

Lateral Patellar Luxation

Lateral patellar luxation occurs infrequently in dogs. Although LPL can occur in any size breed, it is proportionally seen more frequently in large breed dogs. The reported incidence of LPL varies widely between studies from 3%[8] to 8.9% of patellar luxations in large breed dogs[4] to 38.7% of patellar luxations when all small and large dogs are included.[3] The male to female ratio of patellar luxation is 1.5:1, with intact males being at lowest risk.[3,4]

Pathophysiology

Medial Patellar Luxation

The cause of MPL remains unclear. Because toy and miniature breeds are affected with MPL approximately 12 times more than large breeds, a hereditary basis and genetic predisposition of this condition is likely. In addition, because many affected dogs are presented at 3 to 6 months of age, in absence of trauma, often with a bilateral condition, a congenital or developmental disorder rather than an acquired disorder is likely. It is also possible that congenital patellar instability predisposes an animal to traumatic luxation.

It is generally accepted that MPL is a multifactorial anatomic anomaly, not only of the stifle but of the entire pelvic limb. Although the sequence of structural remodeling and variety of deformities of the pelvic limb have been well described, information regarding cause and effect relationships in MPL is limited in the veterinary literature. Specific musculoskeletal abnormalities such as coxofemoral anomalies, malalignment of the extensor mechanism, muscular pathology in the quadriceps, and shallow trochlear groove have been proposed as underlying causes of MPL.

Coxofemoral abnormality may cause MPL and related limb deformities, however no correlation has been found between hip dysplasia and MPL. Based on Putnam's hypothesis, it has been proposed that primary changes in the coxofemoral joint and resultant postural abnormalities lead to compensatory mechanisms more distally, resulting in the eventual malformation in the distal part of the limb and patellar luxation.[10] Development of MPL has been linked to the radiographic appearance of coxa vara (decreased angle of inclination of the femoral neck) and decrease in femoral anteversion (relative retroversion), which in turn leads to genu varum, medial displacement of the extensor mechanism, and further anatomic changes during growth by abnormal medial tension of the extensor mechanism (Figure 106-2). In a theory extrapolated from human literature, it was hypothesized that the reduced anteversion causes external rotation of the coxofemoral joint, which requires compensatory internal rotation of the distal limb to place the foot properly. As a result, the lateral soft tissues supporting the stifle joint are stretched and a lateral torsion force is exerted on the distal femoral growth plate, causing lateral torsion of the distal femur. This lateral rotation of the distal femur displaces the femoral trochlea lateral to the line of contraction of the quadriceps.

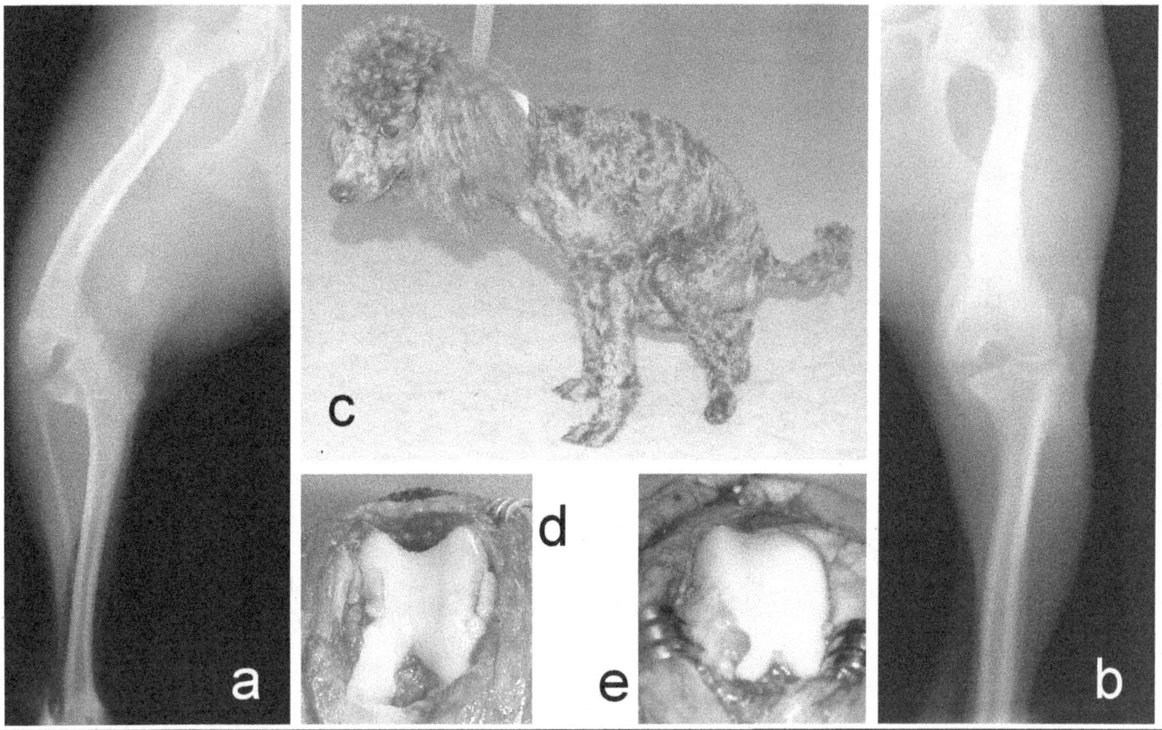

Figure 106-2. Radiographic appearance of grade 4 medial (a) and lateral (b) patellar luxation. Note the extreme internal (a) and external (b) rotation of the tibia as well as the ectopic position of the patella. Clinical signs associated with bilateral grade 4 LPL (c). In such an advanced case, stifle extension is prevented in part because of periarticular adhesions and fibrosis of the periarticular tissues. Permanent stifle flexion may be seen with severe grade 4 LPL and MPL. Intraoperative skyline views of a normally shaped trochlea (d) and a shallow trochlea (e) secondary to juvenile grade 4 patellar luxation.

The compensatory internal rotation of the limb simultaneously causes displacement of the quadriceps muscle group medially, which in turn results in a medial displacement of the patella.

Contrary to this hypothesis, a study of anteversion angle of the femoral neck using magnetic resonance image (MRI) did not reveal any correlation between patellar luxation and anteversion angle.[11] This study also demonstrated that anteversion angle measurement based on radiographs is not reliable. In another radiographic study of 100 papillons, there were no significant differences in angle of anteversion and inclination of the femoral neck between those with patellar luxation and normal dogs.[12] Interestingly, there were significant differences in weight and size between these groups: dogs with patellar luxation were significantly smaller and lighter. In addition, morphologic analysis of the pelvis showed that the origin of the cranial part of the sartorius muscle lies significantly more medially in dogs with MPL than in normal dogs. Such conformational variation may lead to increased medial traction on the patella and medial displacement of the patella. Various deformities of the pelvic limb can cause deviated direction of force of the quadriceps group. The deviation between the direction of force of the quadriceps group (from origin of the quadriceps to the center of the trochlea or patella) and the patellar ligament is referred to as the quadriceps angle or Q-angle (Figure 106-3).[11] The Q-angle has been measured using MRI in dogs with varying degrees of MPL, and dogs with MPL have significantly greater Q-angle, although the cause and effect relationships have not been established.

Malalignment of one or more structures in the extensor mechanism of the stifle may cause MPL. As indicated above, the location and stability of the patella during range of motion are governed by regional anatomic structures about the patella. Quadriceps muscles and other structures in the extensor mechanism, soft-tissue constraints of the patella, and conformation of femoropatellar articulation dictate patellar tracking on the stifle, which is influenced by anatomic relationships among the pelvis, hip joint, femur, tibia, and tarsal joint. Proper anatomic alignment of the extensor mechanism with the underlying skeleton is the primary component of patellar stability.[2] During stifle extension, strong tensile forces within the quadriceps seek to align the patella between the muscular origin and insertion. If the long axis of the quadriceps muscle is not centered over the trochlea, there is an imbalance in muscular force favoring patellar luxation.

Muscular imbalance among the quadriceps may be a primary cause of malalignment of the extensor mechanism and MPL. A clinical study reported grossly evident atrophy and fibrosis of vastus medialis (tight band-like appearance) in puppies with severe MPL.[13] As puppies grow, medial displacement of the patella and the quadriceps muscle group, and underdevelopment of the patella and trochlear groove occur. Abnormal tension from the pathologic vastus medialis and medially displaced extensor mechanism may produce a "bowstring effect," causing lateral bowing of femur and internal rotation of tibia. Clinical observation that skeletal deformities can be completely reversed in young puppies (less than 2 months of age) by the release of tight vastus medialis suggests that muscular pathology is the primary cause of MPL and related deformities of the pelvic limb.

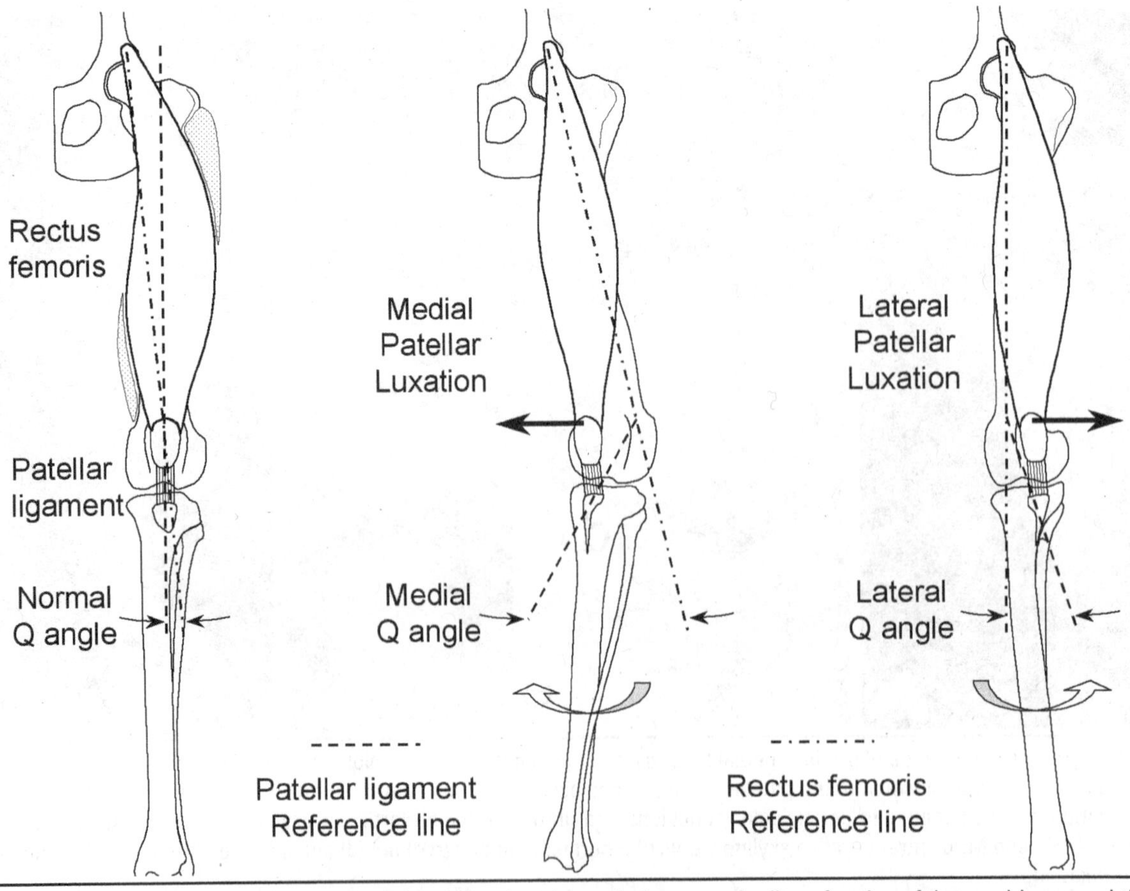

Figure 106-3. In humans, the quadriceps angle (Q-angle) is defined as the angle between the line of action of the quadriceps and the line formed by the patellar ligament and patella in normal limbs. Similarly, the Q-angle in dogs with PL has been defined as the line from the origin of the rectus femoris muscle to the center of the trochlea and the line between the center of the trochlea and the tibial tuberosity. Deviation of the course of the patellar ligament in one direction generates a resultant force (arrow) that pulls the patella in the same direction, resulting in patellar luxation (the greater the Q-angle, the greater the risk of luxation). The average Q-angle increases with the severity of the luxation from ~11° (normal dogs) to ~12° (grade I), ~24° (grade II) and ~37° (grade III). (Adapted from: Kaiser S, Cornely D, Golder W, et al: Magnetic resonance measurements of the deviation of the angle of force generated by contraction of the quadriceps muscle in dogs with congenital patellar luxation. Vet Surg 30(6):552-558, 2001.)

Regardless of primary etiology, medial displacement of the extensor mechanism causes increased pressure on the medial femoral cortex, and thus unequal growth between the medial and lateral aspects of the distal femoral growth plate. Subsequent to this asymmetrical stress distribution, the growth rate on the lateral side of the distal femoral physis is relatively greater than on its medial side. This results in more growth on the lateral side of the bone, and thus lateral bowing of the distal femur (bowstring). Similarly, this increased pressure on the medial part of the distal femur slows the growth of the medial femoral condyle, causing dysplasia of the femoral epiphysis. The proximal tibia compensates with greater bone growth medially, which causes medial bowing of the proximal tibia.

Formation of a shallow femoral trochlea has also been proposed as a primary cause for subsequent dislocation of the patella and extensor mechanism. However, because the femoral trochlea does not develop normally in the absence of normal patellofemoral compression, underdevelopment of the trochlear groove is believed to be a secondary deformity.

The degree of musculoskeletal pathology depends on age and the degree and duration of patellar luxation. Medial patellar luxation often causes progressive deformation of both bony and soft tissues (Table 106-1). Skeletally immature animals develop angular and torsional deformity secondary to abnormal forces directed against open physes, and older animals with MPL may develop degenerative joint disease. Both hip and tarsal joints are also affected. Dogs may show bowlegged appearance with the feet turned inward, with severely decreased range of motion of the stifle and extended tarsal joints (Figure 106-2). Increased rotational laxity of the stifle joint, bidirectional (medial and lateral) instability of the patella, and extensive cartilaginous erosion on the medial trochlear ridge may also be present. In addition to these abnormalities, the stifle joint may have concurrent problems of instability such as rupture of the cranial cruciate ligament. Because one of the functions of the cranial cruciate ligament is to limit tibial internal rotation during flexion, it has been suggested that MPL and subsequent increased tibial internal rotation amplify the stress on the cranial cruciate ligament, predisposing to stretching and rupture. In addition, one can speculate that the loss of the quadriceps support cranially (a secondary constraint against tibial cranial translation) further increases cranial cruciate ligament stresses. The association between MPL and cranial cruciate ligament rupture remains uncertain. Although some studies have reported concomitant cruciate ligament rupture in up to 20% of MLP cases, others found that the prevalence of cranial cruciate ligament injury in dogs with patellar luxation was similar to that of dogs with other orthopedic conditions.[14]

Table 106-1. Musculoskeletal Abnormalities Associated with Medial Patellar Luxation

Femur/Tibia
External rotation of the distal third of the femur
Lateral bowing of the distal femur
Internal rotation of the proximal tibia (medial displacement of the tibial tuberosity)
Shallow or absent femoral trochlea
Formation of pseudotrochlea on the medial condyle of the femur
Hip Joint
Decreased anteversion
Coxa vara
Posture
Genu varum (bow-legged stance)
Stifle Joint
Hypoplastic medial trochlear ridge
Rotational instability of the stifle joint
Femoral and tibial condylar asymmetry
Dysplasia of the distal femoral epiphysis (hypoplastic medial condyle)
Contracture/scarring of medial joint capsule and muscular tissues
Stretching of lateral joint capsule and retinacular tissues
Varying degrees of hyaline cartilage erosion and degenerative joint disease
Tarsal Joint
Compensatory hyperextension

Lateral Patellar Luxation

Owing to the paucity of scientific and clinical studies of LPL in veterinary orthopedics, the proposed pathophysiology of LPL in dogs has often been extrapolated from the human literature where LPL is the most frequent form of patellar luxation. Although several pathologic factors have been associated with LPL, whether these are causative or result from the luxation remains unclear (Table 106-2). Although in rare cases, no apparent factor other than LPL is identified, in most instances (95%) LPL is associated with one or more structural defects.[1,15,16]

As seen with MPL, the normal development of the femoral condyles and trochlear groove depends on the balance between gravity and muscle forces during normal weight bearing.

Table 106-2. Possible Pathologic Factors Leading to Lateral Patellar Luxation.
See text for more information.

1) Increased anteversion angle
2) Coxa valga
3) Femoral deformity with torsion
4) Genu valgum
5) Lateral condylar dysplasia
6) Shallow trochlear groove
7) Lateral rotation of the tibia
8) Lateral displacement of the tibial tuberosity
9) Vastus medialis hypoplasia
10) Pes varus

Anatomic alterations such as angular and torsional malalignment of the femur and tibia may result from an abnormal distribution of growth-plate stresses during growth. Similarly, alteration of the normal anatomy such as coxa valga and excessive anteversion of the femoral neck may induce relative medialization and internal torsion of the distal femur, respectively. An increased anteversion angle either can be compensatory as the dog adjusts the position of the hip, or fixed because of a femoral deformity. Both neck anteversion and coxa valga may contribute to medialization of the trochlea with regard to the line of action of the quadriceps (lateral Q-angle) and, therefore, to lateral luxation of the patella (Figure 106-3). Subsequently, the lateral aspect of the distal femoral growth plate may become overloaded, thus contributing to a slower rate of growth of the lateral femoral cortex compared with the medial one and, over time, to lateral bowing of the distal third of the femur. The lateralization of the compressive loads across the joint may also constrain the development of the tibia, leading to a lateral deviation of the limb at the stifle, a condition known as genu valgum. With genu valgum, although the medial condyles and tibial plateau develop normally, increased forces through the lateral aspect of the distal femoral physis can lead to lateral condylar dysplasia and luxation of the patella. In turn, the absence of patellar pressure during growth interferes with the development of the trochlea, which becomes shallow. Under contraction of the quadriceps, the unconstrained patella is able to move laterally, leading to wear and erosion of the lateral trochanteric ridge, thus exacerbating the problem.

It has been theorized that, in humans, LPL may be initiated by hypoplasia of the vastus medialis muscle.[17] As the vastus medialis becomes hypoplastic, it cannot counteract the antagonist vastus lateralis, resulting in lateral patellar luxation. Phylogenetically, the vastus medialis is the last muscle to develop in humans.[18] It is also the first to undergo atrophy if it is injured or immobilized, and the last to respond to rehabilitation. Although hypoplasia of the vastus medialis may be present in dogs with LPL, this theory is currently unproven.

As with any developmental condition, the anatomic malformations will be more severe if initiated in a younger animal. It has been shown experimentally that alterations in the lines of force produced by soft-tissue restraints in young animals can lead to permanent recognizable bone deformities within 2 weeks.[19] These conformational alterations, including lateral displacement of the tibial tuberosity, are fixed after 4 weeks in 6- to 8-week-old puppies.[19] The permanent lateralization of the quadriceps results in unbalanced strain on the lateral condyle, medial retinaculum, and joint capsule. The lateral retinaculum tightens, and the medial retinaculum stretches further, exacerbating lateral patellar luxation.[19]

Three cases of pes varus resulting in LPL and lameness in miniature dachshunds have been reported.[20,21] Pes varus describes the inward rotation of the distal tibia secondary to the asymmetrical premature closure of the medial aspect of the distal tibial growth plate.[21] As pes varus progresses, compensatory righting of the tarsus and paw placement lead to lateralization of the limb, laxity of the stifle, and eventually, LPL. In two cases, pes varus was thought to be the result of autosomal recessive inheritance;[21] in the third case, it was thought to result from an injury to a distal tibial growth plate.[20] Although the distal tibial physis is affected in 3% of all traumatic physeal injuries,[22] resultant pes varus does not occur in all cases.

Clinical Signs

Clinical signs associated with MPL vary with degree of the pathology of the pelvic limb. A classification of MPL was designed by Putnam and adapted by Singleton.[10,16] Grades I and 2 represent reducible luxations, whereas grades 3 and 4 represent the permanent luxations.

Grade I: Patella can be manually luxated on full extension, with spontaneous reduction on release. Minimal skeletal deformity.
Grade 2: Patella luxates on stifle flexion or manual manipulation, and remains luxated until stifle extension or manual reduction. As much as 30° of medial tibial rotation.
Grade 3: Patella remains luxated continuously but can be reduced manually; 30° to 60° of medial tibial rotation.
Grade 4: Patella luxated permanently and cannot be reduced; 60° to 90° of medial tibial rotation.

Conclusion

The patella/trochlea arrangement acts as a pulley system that optimizes the function of the quadriceps during stifle extension. By moving the patella away from the axis of flexion/extension of the stifle, the trochlea provides a lever arm to the quadriceps muscle, thus minimizing muscle contraction during extension. Any reduction of the trochlear leverage owing to patellar luxation results in a relative increase in the magnitude of the contractile force necessary to produce stifle extension. In extreme cases, such as severe grade IV MLP or LPL, the line of action of the quadriceps may become caudal to the stifle axis of flexion/extension. The net result is flexion rather than extension of the stifle during quadriceps contraction (Figure 106-4). This severe

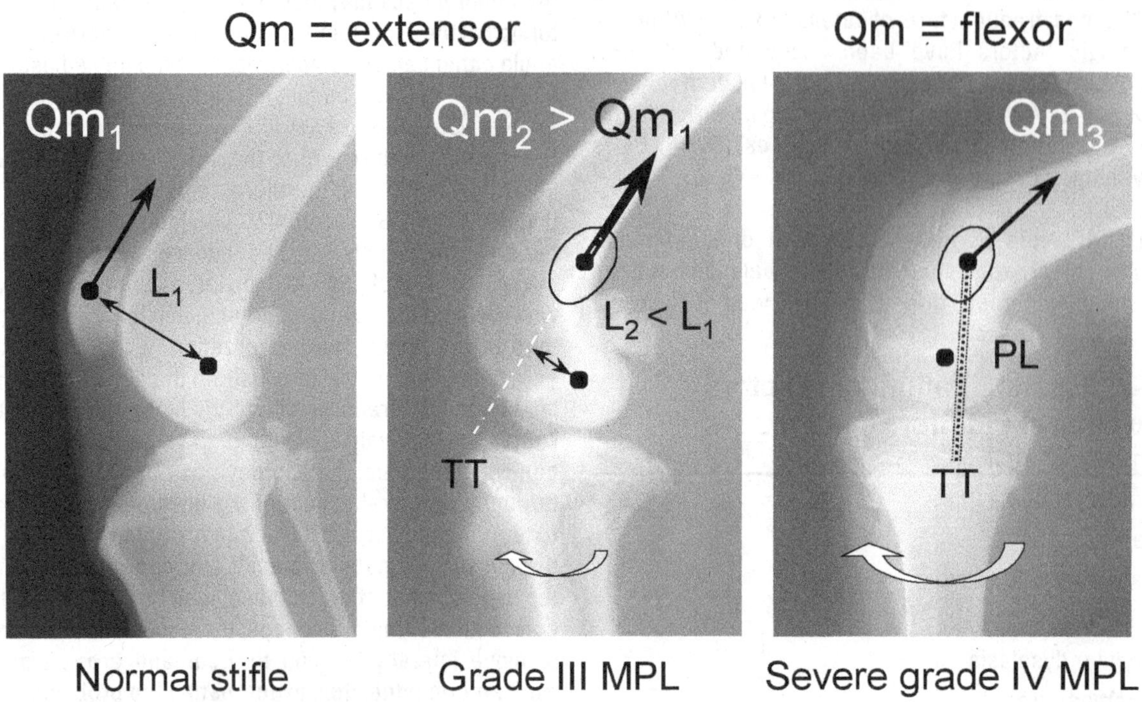

Figure 106-4. The patella and trochlea form a pulley system that optimizes the function of the extensor mechanism by providing a lever arm to the quadriceps muscle (Qm). Patellar luxation reduces the trochlear leverage (L), which in turn induces a relative increase in the quadriceps muscle force needed to achieve stifle extension. Similarly, the quadriceps muscle force has been shown to increase by 15% to 30% following patellectomy in people. In extreme cases, such as severe grade IV luxations, the quadriceps line of action moves caudally to the stifle axis of flexion/extension, thus transforming the quadriceps into a flexor muscle.

alteration of the stifle biomechanics along with the development of fibrous adhesions between the patella and the retinaculum precludes stifle extension and clinically results in dogs walking in a permanently crouched position (Figure 106-2).

Various surgical procedures have been proposed to treat patellar luxations with the common objective of restoring the alignment of the extensor mechanism through a combination of corrective osteotomies and soft-tissue procedures. Until the pathophysiology of patellar luxation is more completely understood, surgeons must be content to repair the apparent structural abnormalities of their patients.

References

1. Roush JK: Canine patellar luxation. Vet Clin North Am Small Anim Pract 23:855-868, 1993.

2. Palmer R: Patellar luxation in large breed dogs. ACVS Veterinary Symposium, p. 364

3. Hayes AG, Boudrieau RJ, Hungerford LL: Frequency and distribution of medial and lateral patellar luxation in dogs - 124 cases (1982-1992). J Am Vet Med Assoc 205:716-720, 1994.

4. Priester WA: Sex, size, and breed as risk factors in canine patellar dislocation. J Am Vet Med Assoc 160:740-742, 1972.

5. Johnson JA, Austin C, Breur GJ: Incidence of canine appendicular musculoskeletal disorders in 16 Veterinary Teaching Hospitals from 1980 through 1989. VCOT 7:56-69, 1994.

6. Ruble RP, Hird DW: Congenital abnormalities in immature dogs from a pet store: 253 cases (1987-1988). J Am Vet Med Assoc 202:633-636, 1993.

7. LaFond E, Breur GJ, Austin CC: Breed susceptibility for developmental orthopedic diseases in dogs. J Am Anim Hosp Assoc 38:467-477, 2002.

8. Gibbons SE, Macias C, Tonzing MA, et al: Patellar luxation in 70 large breed dogs. J Small Anim Pract 47:3-9, 2006.

9. Piermattei D, Flo G (eds): Brinker, Piermattei, and Flo's Handbook of Small Animal Orthopedics and Fracture Repair. Philadelphia: WB Saunders, 1997.

10. Putman RW: Patellar Luxation in Dogs. Guelph: University of Guelph, 1968.

11. Kaiser S, Cornely D, Golder W, et al: The correlation of canine patellar luxation and the anteversion angle as measured using magnetic resonance images. Vet Radiol Ultrasound 42:113-118, 2001.

12. L'Eplattenier H, Montavon P: Patellar luxation in dogs and cats: Pathogenesis and diagnosis. Comp Cont Educ Pract Vet 24:234-240, 2002.

13. Nagaoka K, Orima H, Fujita M, et al: A new surgical method for canine congenital patellar luxation. J Vet Med Sci 57:105-109, 1995.

14. Willauer CC, Vasseur PB: Clinical results of surgical correction of medial luxation of the patella in dogs. Vet Surg 16:31-36, 1987.

15. Rudy RL: Stifle joint. *In* Canine Stifle, 2nd ed. Archibald J (ed). Santa Barbara: American Veterinary Publications, 1974.

16. Singleton WB: Stifle joint surgery in the dog. Can Vet J-Revue Veterinaire Canadienne 4:142, 1963.

17. Fox TA: Dysplasia of the quadriceps mechanism: hypoplasia of the vastus medialis muscle as related to the hypermobile patella syndrome. Surg Clin North Am 55:199-226, 1975.

18. Stokes M, Young A: Investigations of quadriceps inhibition: implications for clinical practice. Physiotherapy 70:425-428, 1984.

19. Stanisavljevic S, Zemenick G, Miller D: Congenital, irreducible, permanent lateral dislocation of the patella. Clin Orthop Relat Res :190-199, 1976.

20. Johnson SG, Hulse DA, Vangundy TE, et al: Corrective osteotomy for pes varus in the dachshund. Vet Surg 18:373-379, 1989.

21. Izumisawa Y, Seno T, Abe R, et al: Axial correction of pes varus by transverse-opening wedge osteotomy and T-plate fixation with beta-tricalcium phosphate (beta-TCP) transplantation in dachshunds. J Vet Med Sci 67:437-440, 2005.

22. Marretta SM, Schrader SC: Physeal injuries in the dog: a review of 135 cases. J Am Vet Med Assoc 182:708-710, 1983.

Chapter 107

Spinal Fractures and Luxations

Brigitte A. Brisson

Fractures and luxations are classified as traumatic or pathologic. Spinal injury in small animals is most commonly associated with blunt force trauma from vehicular accidents.[1-4] Other traumatic causes include gunshot injuries, encounters with other animals, falling from a height and injuries caused by falling objects.[1,3,4] Pathologic fractures and luxations are often associated with congenital vertebral anomalies, metabolic disorders, and neoplasia. In this chapter we discuss traumatic vertebral fractures and luxations. Secondary spinal cord injury and its treatment are discussed in a separate chapter. Conditions such as atlantoaxial luxation, "wobblers" (caudal cervical spondylomyelopathy), and traumatic disc extrusion are not included. Surgical repair of spinal fractures is discussed with regard to biomechanical properties but techniques are not presented in detail.

Anatomy and Biomechanics of the Normal Spine

The spine is composed of bony structures (the vertebrae) and soft tissues (all associated ligaments, muscles, etc.). Normal spinal motion includes flexion and extension (most important) as well as lateral bending and rotation. Violent forces applied to the spine can lead to fracture or luxation.

Models that divide the spine into bony and soft-tissue compartments have been developed to help predict the stability of various fracture configurations and guide surgeons with respect to treatment. Using a two-compartment theory,[5] ventral and dorsal compartments were described. In this model, the ventral compartment consists of the vertebral body, the intervertebral disc (annulus and nucleus pulposus), and the ventral and dorsal longitudinal ligaments. The dorsal compartment contains the dorsal lamina (pedicles and lamina), the articular facets, the joint capsules, the dorsal spinous process, the interspinous and supraspinous ligaments, and the ligamentum flavum. The paraspinal musculature adds stability to both compartments. Lesions that affect both compartments occur most commonly and are generally considered unstable.[6] Traumatic lesions to a single compartment (dorsal or ventral) are rare. When they occur, lesions involving the ventral compartment only are considered more stable than those that involve only the dorsal compartment.

A three-compartment model (three-column) modified from the human literature has also been described.[7,8] In this model, the dorsal compartment remains the same while the structures contained in the ventral compartment are further divided into the following: a middle compartment that contains the dorsal longitudinal ligament, the dorsal half of the disc, and the dorsal half of the vertebral body (basically the floor of the spinal canal), and a ventral compartment that contains the ventral longitudinal ligament, the ventral half of the disc, and the ventral half of the vertebral body.[7] Using the three-compartment model, injuries involving two or more compartments are considered unstable.[8]

Biomechanics of Fracture

During trauma, forces are exerted onto the spinal column that can lead to vertebral subluxation, luxation, fracture, or fracture-luxation. Forces associated with specific fracture-luxation patterns include: compression (axial loading), bending (flexion or extension), torsion (rotation), and shear.[9] Although a traumatic event can result in a single force being applied to the spinal column, most fractures result from a combination of forces; flexion and rotational forces are most common.[6,8]

Axial loading (or compression) develops when a force is applied along the axis of the spine. Pure axial loading is rare but can occur when a standing dog is struck straight from behind or head-on, creating high compression forces across the intervertebral discs and vertebral bodies. Experimental studies performed in human spinal segments show that increased compression across the vertebral segments leads to increased pressure within the normal intervertebral disc and the vertebral endplates.[9] As the pressure increases, blood is squeezed out of the vertebral endplates, which bulge and eventually crack, allowing nucleus pulposus to be displaced within the vertebral body.[9] The intervertebral discs and vertebral endplates are considered important shock-absorbers of the spine.[9]

True compression injuries can occur only in portions of the spine that are in a straight line with the force of trauma at the time of impact. This generally results in a "burst" compression fracture of the vertebral body with or without disruption of the intervertebral disc (Figure 107-1).[20] If damaged, the intervertebral disc can extrude dorsally or into the adjacent vertebral body.[11] If the dorsal compartment remains intact, fractures of this configuration are considered relatively stable.[10] However, bony fragments (from the floor of the spinal canal), disc material, and redundant annulus fibrosus can be driven into the spinal canal, causing spinal cord compression. Studies using segments of spine with normal and degenerate intervertebral discs suggest that compression by extrusion of nucleus pulposus occurs only when the disc is abnormal to begin with.[9]

Pure hyperflexion and hyperextension injuries are rare. Hyperextension injuries occur when a force is applied directly onto the dorsal aspect of the spine, creating compression forces on the structures of the dorsal compartment and tensile forces on the structures of the ventral compartment.[10] With enough force, the ventral longitudinal ligament and the ventral portion of the annulus fibrosus may rupture, leaving the dorsal ligamentous structures intact. These lesions are stable and often reduce spontaneously, making them difficult to diagnose.[10,11]

Pure hyperflexion injuries are rare.[10] Excessive hyperflexion results in a wedge fracture whereby the ventral portion of the vertebral body is crushed, often sparing the ligamentous structures of the spine (Figure 107-2).[20] When referring to the three-compartment model, this type of fracture tends to affect only the

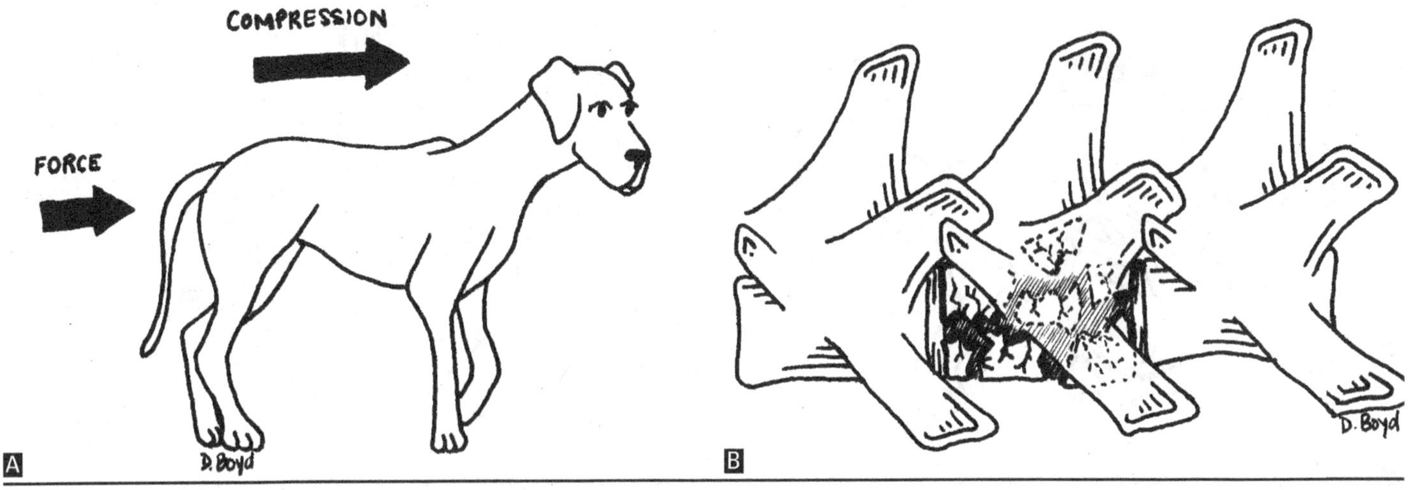

Figure 107-1. Compression injuries occur when the affected vertebrae are in a straight line with the force of trauma at the time of impact. This generally results in a "burst" compression fracture of the vertebral body with or without disruption of the intervertebral disc. Pure compression injuries are rare.

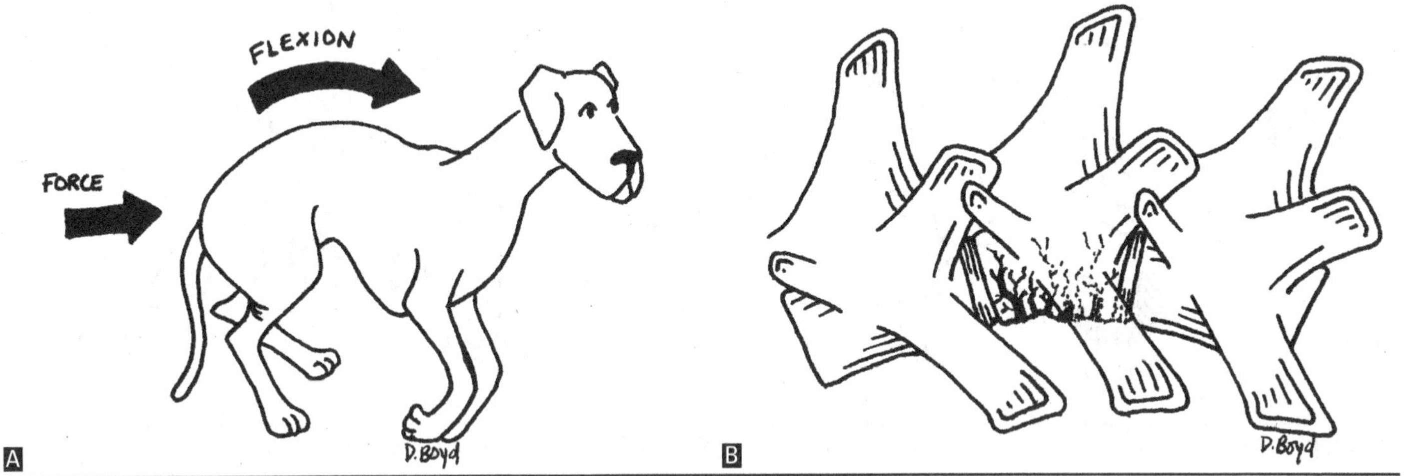

Figure 107-2. Excessive hyperflexion of the spine results in a wedge fracture whereby the ventral portion of the vertebral body is crushed, often sparing the ligamentous structures of the spine. Pure hyperflexion forces are rare.

ventral compartment, leaving the dorsal portion of the disc and vertebral body intact.[7] Sparing of the middle and dorsal compartments prevents subluxation and compression of the spinal cord by bony fragments.[7] These fractures are considered relatively stable.[7,10]

Torsional forces are typically accompanied by flexion of the spine. These forces often cause trauma to bony and ligamentous structures of the ventral and dorsal compartments (two compartment model) and result in unstable fracture-luxations of the spine. When flexion is the primary force applied to the spine and simultaneous rotation occurs, luxation is the typical outcome (Figure 107-3).[8,11,12] When rotation is the primary force applied to the spine with concurrent flexion, fracture-luxation generally occurs (Figure 107-4). Owing to their inherent instability, these lesions are often treated with surgical stabilization.[11,13]

Spinal Cord Trauma

Spinal trauma leads to primary spinal cord injury (concussion, compression, and distraction) caused by the initial impact and by repeated motion at the fracture site. Secondary spinal cord injury involves a series of events that begin soon after the initial injury and include complex vascular, biochemical, and inflammatory processes.[8,14] Because the clinician has no control over the initial spinal cord trauma (primary injury), therapeutic efforts must be aimed at decreasing repeated injury owing to instability and halting or attenuating the secondary processes that begin at the time of injury. The pathophysiology of spinal cord injury and its treatment are discussed in a separate chapter.

Diagnosis

If spinal injury is suspected, patient manipulation should be limited; compliant patients should be strapped to a board to prevent further displacement of an unstable fracture and repeated spinal cord trauma during patient evaluation. A depression or vertebral malalignment along the spine and possible crepitation may be noted on physical examination. A cursory neurologic examination is performed in an attempt to localize the lesion and determine the severity of the spinal cord injury. Sedation of non-compliant patients and administration of analgesics is considered after a rapid assessment of

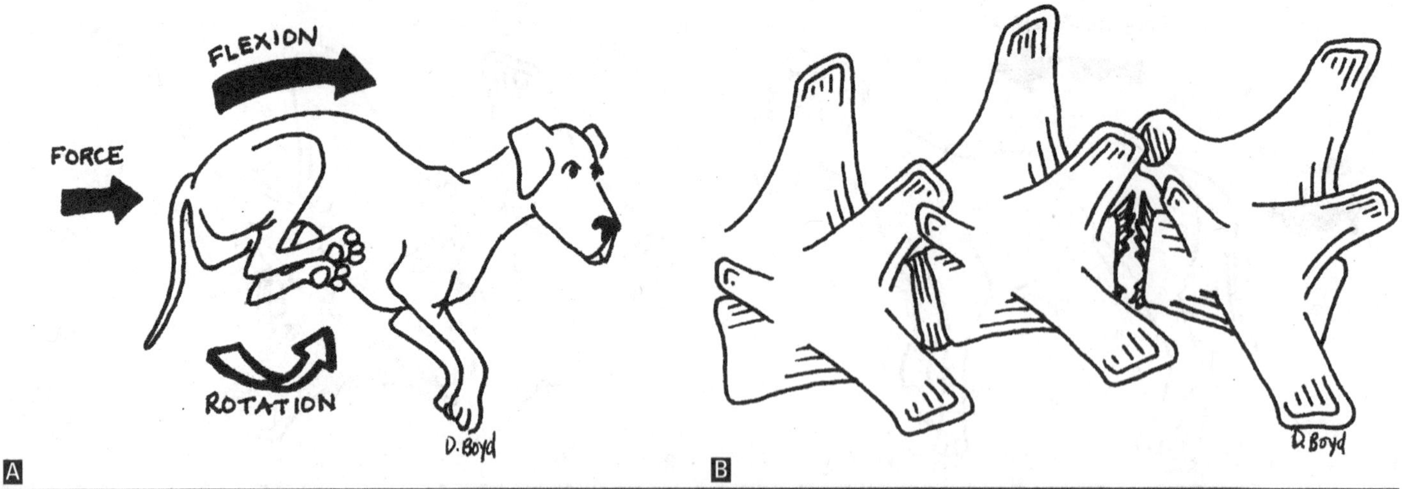

Figure 107-3. When flexion is the primary force applied to the spine and simultaneous rotation occurs, luxation is the typical outcome.

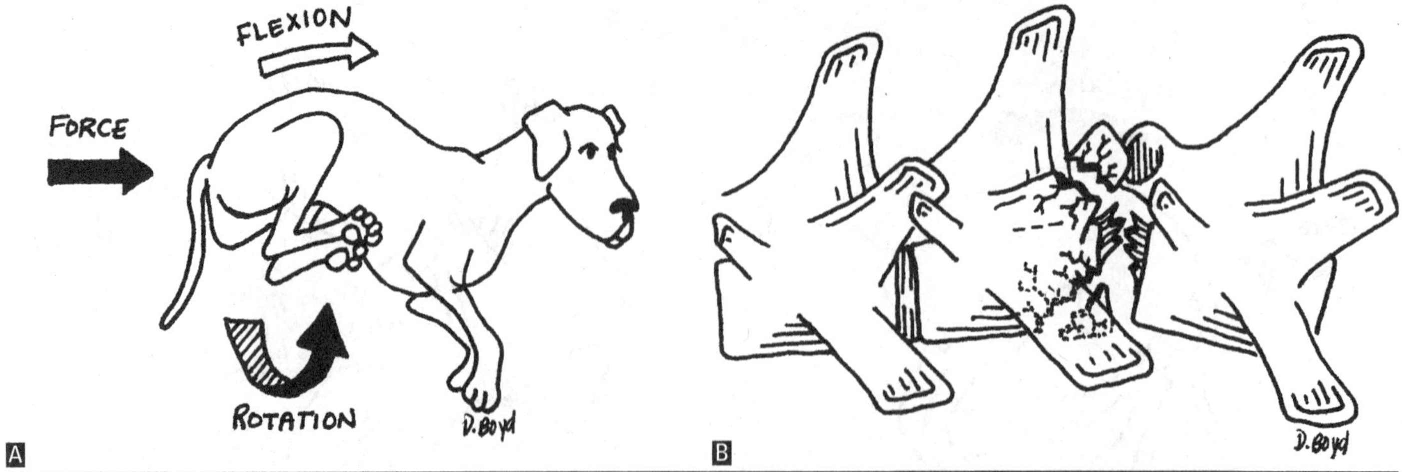

Figure 107-4. When rotation is the primary force applied to the spine with concurrent flexion, fracture-luxation generally occurs.

the neurologic status. Concurrent injuries should be taken into consideration when interpreting the neurologic examination to prevent overstating the neurologic dysfunction and prognosis.[4,15] If possible, survey radiographs should be performed with the patient awake or under light sedation in order to maintain paraspinal muscle tone and decrease the risk of further fracture displacement. It is important to remember that radiographs may not necessarily reflect the maximal displacement that occurred at the time of trauma.[16,17] This helps to explain why correlation is poor between radiographic displacement and neurologic deficits.[2] Lateral radiographic views are recommended first and, if available, horizontal-beam ventrodorsal views should also be performed. Survey radiographs of the entire spine are recommended to rule out multiple spinal lesions.[1-4,18] The benefits of performing more thorough radiographic views once the patient is under general anesthesia must be weighed against the potential risks associated with spinal manipulation. Myelography is recommended when no radiographic evidence exists of vertebral displacement and when the neurologic signs do not correlate with the radiographic lesion. In such cases, myelography can help localize the injury by outlining an edematous section of spinal cord or slight vertebral canal subluxation. In addition, myelography can provide information on the degree of spinal cord compression caused by fracture fragments or hematoma. Some authors recommend myelography for all spinal trauma patients.[19] Advanced diagnostic imaging (CT and MRI) is also useful in cases where vertebral displacement is not evident on survey radiographs. Compared with survey radiography, CT provides an accurate assessment of spinal canal compromise[20] as well as superior detail of the fracture lines and bone fragments. This is especially true for fractures that involve the pedicles and articular facets and for displaced bone fragments that may compress the spinal cord. MRI provides good soft-tissue imaging and may help to determine the severity of spinal cord injury, the presence of spinal cord hemorrhage or edema, and whether disc herniation and spinal cord compression are present.[21] As with survey radiography, the risks associated with patient manipulation and positioning under general anesthesia as well as the additional anesthetic time must be weighed against the potential diagnostic value.

All trauma patients, especially those with spinal pain or neurologic dysfunction should be evaluated for possible vertebral fracture or luxation. Patients should be assessed and appropriately treated for other concurrent injuries such as pneumothorax, pulmonary contusions, diaphragmatic hernia, and fractures of the pelvis, ribs, and apendicular skeleton. Previous reports indicate that approximately 50% of patients with spinal trauma have injuries to other systems,[1-4] and that approximately 48% of patients with a lumbar fracture or luxation have a fracture elsewhere in the body; most frequently a pelvic fracture.[4] Owing to a high rate of concurrent pulmonary injuries, thoracic radiographs are recommended for all patients that are to undergo general anesthesia for fracture fixation.[4]

Incidence and Distribution of Spinal Fractures

Spinal fracture-luxations in dogs have been reported to affect the lumbar vertebrae most commonly, followed by sacrococcygeal, thoracic, and cervical vertebrae.[2,3,18] In cats, the sacrococcygeal region is the most common site for vertebral fracture and/or luxation.[18] Stress concentration at or near the junction between mobile and relatively immobile regions of the spine is thought to result in an increased rate of fracture-luxations at the thoracolumbar and lumbosacral junctions;[18] however, studies have also described a relatively even distribution of fractures along the lumbar spine.[4,22]

The vertebral body has been identified as the most commonly fractured portion of the vertebrae.[2,18] Disc herniation associated with fractures or luxations is fairly uncommon and was reported in fewer than 12% of cases in one study.[18] The presence of more than one spinal lesion has been reported, but this is rare and tends to involve two adjacent vertebrae.[18] These lesions most commonly involve the lumbosacral and sacrococcygeal junctions.[18] Despite their rare occurrence, radiographic evaluation of the entire spine is recommended to rule out multiple lesions.[1-4,18]

Cervical Fractures

Cervical fractures and luxations are associated with various degrees of neurologic dysfunction but do not typically lead to loss of pain perception caudal to the lesion. The main reasons for this may be that: 1) the larger cervical spinal-canal to spinal-cord ratio allows for more displacement without severely damaging the spinal cord, and 2) cervical trauma severe enough to cause loss of pain perception generally causes respiratory failure and death at the time of injury.[12,23] Although some have reported that most dogs with cervical fractures present with mild neurologic deficits and often only neck pain,[23] a study reviewing 56 cases of cervical fracture-luxation revealed that 57% of cases presented with non-ambulatory tetraparesis.[1]

The axis (C2) is most frequently fractured (50-78% of cases) followed by the atlas (C1) (approximately 25% of cases).[1,2,23] The higher incidence of C2 fractures in dogs is thought to relate to the anatomy of the proximal cervical region. It has been hypothesized that the axis acts as a point of leverage between the cranial and caudal cervical regions. This is thought to be due to the close relationship of the vertebral body of the axis with the atlas and the intimate soft-tissue attachment of the dorsal spinous process and caudal articular facets of the axis with the caudal cervical vertebrae.[12,23] One study reports that fractures of C3-7 are more common after dog fights or unknown trauma than after being hit by a car and that fractures involving the caudal cervical vertebrae typically affect more than one vertebra.[1]

High perioperative mortality (36%) has been reported with surgically treated cervical fracture-luxations.[1] However, most patients that survive through surgery and the immediate postoperative period achieve functional recovery.[1] In addition, almost 90% of patients treated conservatively obtain a functional outcome, suggesting that many cervical fractures are amenable to conservative therapy.[1] Negative predictors for recovery include a non-ambulatory status at presentation and being referred more than 5 days after the initial trauma.[1]

Thoracic and Lumbar Fractures

The lumbar and thoracic regions of the spine are common sites for vertebral fracture and/or luxation in dogs and cats.[2,3,18] Although fractures reportedly occur more commonly at the thoracolumbar and lumbosacral junctions,[18] a study by Turner and others revealed that fractures of L2, L4, and L7 were more common than fractures of the other lumbar vertebrae; no statistical difference was found when all lumbar vertebral segments were compared.[4] Fractures between T1 and T9 are less common, typically minimally displaced, and relatively stable. The inherent stability of this section of the spine is thought to be due to the additional support provided by the ribs and their attachments. Neurologic dysfunction varying from alterations in conscious proprioception to loss of pain perception has been reported in as many as 85% of patients with lumbar fractures.[4] Based on previous reports, 45% of patients with lesions between T1 and S1 and as many as 62% of patients with lumbar injuries were euthanized without treatment.[3,4] The decision to euthanize was often based on the severity of the neurologic dysfunction or on surgical confirmation of severe spinal cord injury.[3,4] The high rate of neurologic dysfunction associated with thoracolumbar injuries compared with cervical injuries is likely related to the relatively small spinal-canal to spinal-cord ratio of the thoracolumbar spine.[15] In contrast, fracture-luxations of L6 and L7 only affect nerve roots (cauda equina); these can tolerate a greater amount of displacement without severe neurologic dysfunction.[24] Unlike fractures of the lower thoracic and lumbar regions, which often require surgical fixation, fractures of L6, L7, and the lumbosacral region often heal satisfactorily without surgical intervention.[15]

Sacrococcygeal Fractures

Sacrococcygeal fractures are the most common spinal fracture diagnosed in cats,[18,25] and they occur relatively frequently in dogs.[18,26] Clinical signs associated with these fractures range from sacral pain to loss of sensation and motor function to the tail and perineal area, along with urinary and fecal dysfunction. Although neurologic deficits to one or both hind limbs are possible with traction lesions (tethering) of the cauda equina and spinal cord, these lesions are rare and difficult to differentiate from those associated with concurrent pelvic fractures.[26,27] In dogs, sacral fractures that occur medial to the foramina (axial) are more frequently associated with urinary or fecal incontinence, loss of perineal sensation, and tail analgesia than are sacral fractures that occur lateral to the foramina (abaxial).[26] In addition, dogs with axial fractures have more severe neurologic dysfunction at presentation and discharge than do dogs with abaxial fractures.[26] Additional orthopedic injuries are reported in 76 to 88% of cats and 74 to 97% of dogs, which emphasizes the need for a complete assessment in order to provide an accurate prognosis.[25-27] In cats, sacral fractures are often associated with sacroiliac luxation, whereas in dogs, they are more commonly associated with ilial fracture.[27] More than 70% of cats in one study had temporary or permanent urinary incontinence, but the prognosis for recovery of normal urinary function was good when cats retained anal tone and perineal sensation at presentation.[25] Return of neurologic function to the hind limbs, bladder, and rectum reportedly occurs within 1 month; cats that have not recovered urinary function 1 month after trauma are unlikely to recover.[25] In a canine study, patients with abaxial fractures had a better prognosis for recovery than those with axial fractures.[26] Based on the results of this study, little neurologic improvement should be expected during hospitalization.[26] Surgical treatment of sacrococcygeal fractures has been associated with worsening of the neurologic status in approximately 40% of dogs; this is likely owing to iatrogenic injury.[26]

Principles of Fracture Fixation

Whether to treat spinal fractures conservatively or surgically is a topic of great controversy. Surgical intervention aims toreduce and realign vertebral bone fragments, which in most cases will effectively decompress the spinal cord; and to provide rigid fixation of the affected vertebral segments to prevent continued instability. In some cases, laminectomy is necessary to assess the spinal cord for visible damage and to relieve compression caused by hematoma, disc material, or bony fragments. Because decompressive procedures have the disadvantage of potentially destabilizing the spine, pediculectomy and hemilaminectomy are preferred over dorsal laminectomy because they produce less instability.[2,28] Although the general consensus is that fractures that involve both the dorsal and ventral compartments (two-compartment model) are unstable and should be stabilized surgically, some studies have demonstrated up to 94.4% functional recovery (walking) with non-surgical management.[1,2,22] Although patients with a range of neurologic dysfunction were included in published retrospective studies, reported recovery rates should be interpreted with caution because patients with severe neurologic dysfunction are more likely to have undergone surgical stabilization, whereas patients with less severe neurologic dysfunction are more likely to have been treated conservatively. Despite this, patients retaining even minimal neurologic function should be given the benefit of conservative management if surgery is not an option and the owners are willing to perform supportive care and rehabilitation.[3,22]

Conservative management and external splinting have demonstrated good success in the treatment of some cervical and thoracolumbar injuries.[3,22,29] Because it provides relatively limited immobilization of the fracture site, this treatment option has typically been recommended for patients with relatively stable fractures causing mild neurologic dysfunction or when financial constraints limit treatment options.[5] Experimental bending of a back splint designed for the treatment of lower thoracic and lumbar fractures revealed it could withstand bending moments in excess of those shown to cause failure of commonly used internal fixation techniques and those experienced by large paralyzed veterinary patients undergoing nursing care.[29] This splinting technique is considered suitable for patients that retain some degree of voluntary motor function and have lesions that affect mostly the dorsal compartment; lesions with loss of ventral buttress are not considered ideal for this technique.[29] External splints should extend well beyond the fracture site on either side of the affected vertebral segments to prevent a fulcrum effect at the level of the fracture. Patients should be monitored daily for slippage of the splint and other related complications such as urine scalding, skin abrasion, ulceration or abscessation, and overheating.[22,29] Although conservative management requires significantly more supportive care and generally leads to a longer recovery period, the cost of treatment is often lower and the duration of hospitalization shorter than for surgical stabilization.[3]

Surgical management should be considered for exploratory purposes in patients that have lost pain sensation, and in order to provide stable fixation across the fracture site in all patients with severe neurologic deficits (non-ambulatory patients).[25,30] Surgical stabilization is also recommended for patients with unstable fractures (determined radiographically or by palpation of a "click" during ambulation or patient movement), those that fail to improve or continue to deteriorate neurologically despite conservative therapy, and patients with severe pain beyond the first 48 to 72 hours after injury.[25,30]

Various surgical techniques have been described for fracture stabilization in all regions of the spine. Vertebral body cross-pinning was described for stabilizing fractures of the articular facets, epiphyseal body fractures, and spinal luxations. This technique is considered inadequate for fixation of severe compression or multifragmented fractures[31] and is no longer recommended. Spinal stapling involves applying parallel stainless steel pins through and along the dorsal spinous processes on either side of the fracture, with additional wire stabilization through the dorsal spinous processes spanned by the repair.[32] This technique is only applicable for patients weighing less than 10 kg and requires intact dorsal spinous processes.[5,32] Similarly, modified segmental spinal instrumentation involves placing Steinman pins around and along the dorsal spinous processes of several vertebrae and wiring these pins to the dorsal spinous processes and the cranial articular facets of the vertebrae spanned by the repair.[33] This technique is reportedly applicable for all sizes of dogs but should be reserved for fractures that do not involve the ventral compartment. Modified segmental spinal instrumentation and spinal stapling frequently fail by tearing through the spinous processes and are rarely used. Application of a metal bone plate to the dorsolateral aspect of two or three consecutive vertebral bodies is referred to as vertebral body plating. This technique is limited to the caudal thoracic and cranial lumbar vertebrae because application may require dislocation or removal of any associated rib head and transection of nerve roots (rhizotomy) exiting below the bone plate, precluding its use in the lower lumbar spine.[34]

Dorsal spinous-process plating using plastic (Lubra plate, Lubra Co., Fort Collins CO 80521) or metal (Auburn spinal plate, Richard

Manufacturing Co., Memphis, TN 38101) spinal plates has been described as an option to stabilize dorsal compartment instability in regions with prominent dorsal spinous processes.[30,35,36] This technique has been used extensively but appears to be of limited use on its own. Dorsal spinal plating is most commonly applied in combination with other methods such as transilial pinning and vertebral-body plating to stabilize fractures of the lumbar vertebrae that do not involve the dorsal spinous process or lamina.[30,35,37] Reported complications include fracture of the dorsal spinous processes, ischemia of the dorsal spinous processes as a result of over-tightening, and plate slippage owing to insufficient tightening of the bolts.[30,38] The use of screws or pins plus polymethylmethacrylate (PMMA) has been described for stabilization of spinal fractures in all locations, including those that are less amenable to ventral compartment fixation such as the thoracic and lower lumbar region.[39-42] This procedure requires minimal instrumentation, however, an excellent knowledge of vertebral anatomy is essential to ensure accurate implant positioning. This technique is compatible with decompressive techniques as long as the surgeon carefully applies and irrigates the PMMA during polymerization. Pins and PMMA, unlike several other stabilization techniques, can be applied even when perfect alignment is not achieved.[2] Stabilization using pins and PMMA is currently the most popular technique used to stabilize vertebral fractures. External skeletal fixation has been reported for stabilization of lumbar fractures.[43,44] Advantages include that implants are inserted away from the fracture site and that removal of all implants is possible once healing has occurred.[43,44] Again, excellent knowledge of vertebral anatomy is essential to ensure accurate placement of pins into the vertebral bodies; this can be facilitated by fluoroscopic guidance.[45]

Experimental comparison of the biomechanical characteristics of various surgical techniques used to stabilize spinal fractures has been performed. A drawback of these studies is that they typically evaluate a small number of fixation techniques and cannot be compared with each other because differing methods are used for each evaluation.

It is well accepted that techniques providing stability to both the ventral and dorsal compartments are superior to those that stabilize only a single compartment. When the stability and strength of five internal fixation methods used for lumbar fracture stabilization were compared, vertebral body plating was found to be stronger than all other methods including dorsal spinal plating, pins and methylmethacrylate, and crossed pins.[46] The combination of dorsal spinous-process plating and dorsolateral vertebral-body plating provides the most rigid and strong repair.[46] Similarly, a more recent study comparing five methods of fixation for thoracolumbar instability reported that the application of vertebral body plates or the combination of pins and PMMA was strongest.[47] A biomechanical study comparing five configurations of pins or bone screws with PMMA for internal stabilization of lumbar instability revealed that 8 pin fixations were more rigid and stronger than 4 pin fixations and that the orientation of the pins impacted on rigidity depending on the number of pins used.[48] Furthermore, this study revealed that pins were more rigid and less likely to fail than screws.[48] Finally, a study showed that external skeletal fixation has mechanical properties comparable to internal fixation techniques that use a combination of pins and PMMA.[44]

Prognosis and Recovery

Similar to other spinal disorders, the loss of pain perception caudal to the lesion is the single most accurate prognostic indicator when evaluating patients with spinal fracture and/or luxations.[5,16,49] Patients that have no deep pain have less than 50% chance of recovery, and the rate of recovery decreases to less than 5% if pain sensation has been lost for more than 48 hours.[50] Despite having a positive impact on the prognosis, the presence of pain perception does not guarantee complete neurologic recovery.

Based on previous reports, it appears that the degree of radiographic vertebral displacement does not correlate well with the neurologic status.[2,16] Although survey radiographs are of limited use when trying to determine prognosis in patients with little vertebral displacement, correlations have been made between the degree of radiographic vertebral malalignment and the loss of pain perception caudal to the injury.[16,22] Patients with 80% vertebral displacement in the thoracic spine and 60% displacement between L1 and L5 do not typically maintain pain perception caudal to the lesion.[16] Caudal to L5, survey radiographs are less helpful in determining outcome because the nerve roots at this level can tolerate significant displacement without severe neurologic dysfunction.[16] In general, vertebral displacement of greater than 80% caudal to L5 is associated with LMN signs.[16] Unlike the cervical and thoracolumbar regions, full recovery is possible in patients with severe vertebral displacement if the lesion is caudal to L5.[16]

Patient recovery is difficult to predict, although patients that retain pain perception and purposeful movement are likely to recover functional neurologic status. Based on previous reports, the hospitalization time for surgically treated cases tends to be longer than for cases treated conservatively.[3] However, the overall rate of return to a functional neurologic status is similar for both treatment regimens.[2,3]

References

1. Hawthorne JC, Blevins WE, Wallace LJ, et al: Cervical vertebral fractures in 56 dogs: a retrospective study. J Am Anim Hosp Assoc 35:135, 1999.

2. McKee WM: Spinal trauma in dogs and cats: review of 51 cases. Vet Rec 126:285, 1990.

3. Selcer RR, Bubb WJ, Walker TL: Management of vertebral column fractures in dogs and cats: 211 cases (1977-1985). J Am Vet Med Assoc 198:1965, 1991.

4. Turner DW: Fractures and fracture-luxations of the lumbar spine: a retrospective study in the dog. J Am Anim Hosp Assoc 23:459, 1987.

5. Matthiesen DT: Thoracolumbar spinal fractures/luxations: surgical management. Comp Cont Educ Small Anim Pract 5:867, 1983.

6. Bruecker KA, Seim III HB: Principles of spinal fracture management. Semin Vet Med Surg (Small Anim) 7:71, 1992.

7. Denis F: Spinal instability as defined by the three-column spine concept in acute spinal trauma. Clin Orthop Relat Res 189:65, 1984.

8. Shores A: Spinal trauma. Vet Clin North Am Small Anim Pract 22:859, 1992.b

9. Roaf R: A study of the mechanics of spinal injuries. J Bone Joint Surg 42:810, 1960.

10. Holdsworth FW: Fracture, dislocations and fracture-dislocations of the spine. J Bone Joint Surg 52:1534, 1970.

11. Walker TL, Tomlinson J Jr, Sorjonen DC, Kornegay JN: Diseases of the Spinal Column. *In* Textbook of Small Animal Surgery. Slatter D (ed). Philadelphia: WB Saunders, 1985, p. 1367.

12. Tatcher C: Biomechanics of cranial fractures, spinal fractures and luxations. *In* Pathophysiology in Small Animal Surgery. Bojrab M (ed). Philadelphia: Lea & Febiger, 1993, p. 999.

13. Schwarz PD: Biomechanics of fracture, dislocations, and fractures/ dislocations of the spine: characteristics of stable versus unstable injuries. Proceedings of the Annual Surgical Forum of the American College of Veterinary Surgeons, 1986; 76.

14. Olby N: Current concepts in the management of acute spinal cord injury. J Vet Intern Med 13:399, 1999.

15. Sharp NJH, Wheeler S: Trauma. *In* Small Animal Spinal Disorders Diagnosis and Surgery. Sharp NJH, Wheeler S (eds). Philadelphia: Elsevier Mosby, 2005, p. 281.

16. Feeney DA, Oliver JE: Blunt spinal trauma in the dog and cat: neurological, radiological and therapeutic correlations. J Am Anim Hosp Assoc 16:664, 1980.a

17. Swaim SF: Biomechanics of cranial fractures, spinal fractures and luxations. *In* Pathophysiology in Small Animal Surgery. Bojrab M (ed). Philadelphia: Lea & Febiger, 1981, p. 774.

18. Feeney DA, Oliver JE: Blunt spinal trauma in the dog and cat: insight into radiographic lesions. J Am Anim Hosp Assoc 16:885, 1980.b

19. Sturges BK, LeCouter RA: Vertebral fractures and luxations. *In* Textbook of Small Animal Surgery. Slatter D (ed). Philadelphia: WB Saunders, 2003, p. 1244.

20. Fehlings MG, Rao SC, Tator CH, et al: The optimal radiologic method for assessing spinal canal compromise and cord compression in patients with cervical spinal cord injury. Part II: Results of a multicenter study. Spine 24:605, 1999.

21. Gopal MS, Jeffery ND: Magnetic resonance imaging in the diagnosis and treament of a canine spinal cord injury. J Small Anim Pract 42:29, 2001.

22. Carberry CA, Flanders JA, Dietze AE, et al: Nonsurgical management of thoracic and lumbar spinal fractures and fracture / luxations in the dog and cat: a review of 17 cases. J Am Anim Hosp Assoc 25:43, 1989.

23. Stone EA, Betts CW, Chambers JN: Cervical fractures in the dog: a literature and case review. J Am Anim Hosp Assoc 15:463, 1979.

24. Fletcher TF: Spinal cord and meninges. *In* Miller's Anatomy of the Dog, 3rd ed. Evans HE, Christensen GC (eds). Philadelphia: WB Saunders, 1993, p. 805.

25. Smeak DD, Olmstead ML: Fracture / luxations or sacrococcygeal area in the cat; a retrospective study of 51 cases. Vet Surg 14:319, 1985.

26. Kuntz CA, Waldron D, Martin RA, et al: Sacral fractures in dogs: a review of 32 cases. J Am Anim Hosp Assoc 31:142, 1995.

27. Anderson A, Coughlan AR: Sacral fractures in dogs and cats: a classification scheme and review of 51 cases. J Small Anim Pract 38:404, 1997.

28. Smith GK, Walter MC: Spinal decompressive procedures and dorsal compartment injuries: comparative biomechanical study in canine cadavers. Am J Vet Res 49:266, 1988.

29. Patterson RH, Smith GK: Backsplinting for treatment of thoracic and lumbar fracture / luxation in the dog: principles of application and case series. Vet Comp Orthop Traum 5:179, 1992.

30. Dulisch ML, Withrow SJ: The use of plastic plates for fixation of spinal fractures in the dog. Can Vet J 20:326, 1979.

31. Gage ED: A new method of spinal fixation in the dog (a preliminary report). Vet Med Small Anim Clin 64:295, 1969.

32. Gage ED: Surgical repair of spinal fractures in small-breed dogs. Vet Med Small Anim Clin 66:1095, 1971.

33. McAnulty JF, Lenehan TM, Maletz LM: Modified segmental spinal instrumentation in repair of spinal fractures and luxations in dogs. Vet Surg 15:143, 1986.

34. Swaim SF: Vertebral body plating for spinal immobilization. J Am Vet Med Assoc 158:1683, 1971.

35. Shores A, Nichols C, Rochat M, et al: Combined kirschner-ehmer device and dorsal spinal plate fixation technique for caudal lumbar vertebral fractures in dogs. J Am Vet Med Assoc 195:335, 1989.

36. Yturraspe DJ, Lumb WV: The use of plastic spinal plates for internal fixation of the canine spine. J Am Vet Med Assoc 161:1651, 1972.

37. Lewis DD, Stampley A, Bellah JR, et al: Repair of sixth lumbar vertebral fracture-luxations, using transilial pins and plastic spinous-process plates in six dogs. J Am Vet Med Assoc 194:538, 1989.

38. Trotter EJ: Fixation of vertebral column fractures and luxations by means of flexible spinal plates (Lubra plating). Proceedings of the Third Annual Surgical Forum of the American College of Veterinary Surgeons, 1975.

39. Beaver DP, MacPherson GC, Muir P, Johnson KA: Methylmethacrylate and bone screw repair of seventh lumbar vertebral fracture-luxations in dogs. J Small Anim Pract 37:381, 1996.

40. Blass CE, Seim III HB: Spinal fixation in dogs using steinmann pins and methylmethacrylate. Vet Surg 13:203, 1984.

41. Blass CE, Waldron DR, van Ee RT: Cervical stabilization in three dogs using steinmann pins and methylmethacrylate. J Am Anim Hosp Assoc 24:61, 1986.

42. Rouse GP, Miller JI: The use of methylmethacrylate for spinal stabilization. J Am Anim Hosp Assoc 11:418, 1975.

43. Shores A: Fractures and luxations of the vertebral column. Vet Clin North Am Small Anim Pract 22:171, 1992.

44. Walker TM, Pierce WA, Welch RD: External fixation of the lumbar spine in a canine model. Vet Surg 31:181, 2002.

45. Wheeler JL, Cross AR, Rapoff AJ: A comparison of the accuracy and safety of vertebral body pin placement using a fluoroscopically guided versus an open surgical approach and in vitro study. Vet Surg 31:468, 2002.

46. Walter MC, Smith GK, Newton CD: Canine lumbar spinal internal fixation techniques; a comparative biomechanical study. Vet Surg 15:191, 1986.

47. Viguier E, Petit-Etienne G, Magnier J, Lavaste F: In vitro biomechanical evaluation of unstable T13-L1 stabilization procedures in dogs. Vet Surg 31:288, 2002.

48. Garcia JNP, Milthorpe BK, Russell D, Johnson KA: Biomechanical study of canine spinal fracture fixation using pins or bone screws with polymethylmethacrylate. Vet Surg 23:322, 1994.

49. Griffiths IR: Trauma of the spinal cord. Vet Clin North Am Small Anim Pract 10:131, 1980.

50. Bagley RS: Spinal fracture and luxation. Vet Clin North Am Small Anim Pract 30:133, 2000.

Chapter 108

Fracture Biomechanics of the Appendicular Skeleton

Ross H. Palmer
Susan P. James

Bone Structure and Function

The purpose of the skeletal system is to protect internal organs, and to provide rigid kinematic links and muscle attachment sites to facilitate body movement. These functions are supported by the unique structural and mechanical properties of bone. Bone is a hard, tough material, metabolically active, capable of self-repair, and adaptive to the mechanical demands placed upon it.

Like other connective tissues, bone consists of cells and an organic extracellular matrix. Bone is unique among mammalian tissues because of its high content of inorganic mineral salts, primarily calcium and phosphorus. This inorganic mineral accounts for 65 to 70% of bone's dry weight and gives bone its solid consistency and rigidity. The organic extracellular matrix, composed primarily of collagen and, to a lesser extent, proteoglycans, gives bone its flexibility and resiliency. Abundant amounts of water, which also contribute to bone's flexibility and resiliency, are also present in bone, mostly in the extracellular matrix, but also in the canals and cavities of bone.

Microscopically, bone is composed of multiple osteons or haversian systems (Figure 108-1). In the center of the osteons are haversian canals that form the primary circulatory network in bone. Each osteon consists of concentric layers of mineralized matrix called lamellae that surround the haversian canal. Each osteon is separated from, yet bonded to, surrounding osteons by a cement line composed of a cementing ground substance consisting predominantly of glycosaminoglycans. Collagen connects one lamella to the next within an osteon, but does not cross from one osteon to the next. Interstitial lamellae, which are of the same material as the osteons but oriented differently, are continuous with the osteons and span regions between complete osteons. In long bones, osteons usually run longitudinally.

Biomechanical Properties of Bone

The fracture behavior of whole bones is influenced by both their material and structural properties. Mechanically, bone behaves as a biphasic, composite material with mineral (hydroxyapatite) as one phase and the collagen and ground substance as another.[1] Collagen toughens the bone, preventing the stiff mineral from undergoing brittle fracture, and the hydroxyapatite mineral prevents flexible collagen from excessive deformation and increases the bone's elastic modulus (~stiffness) beyond

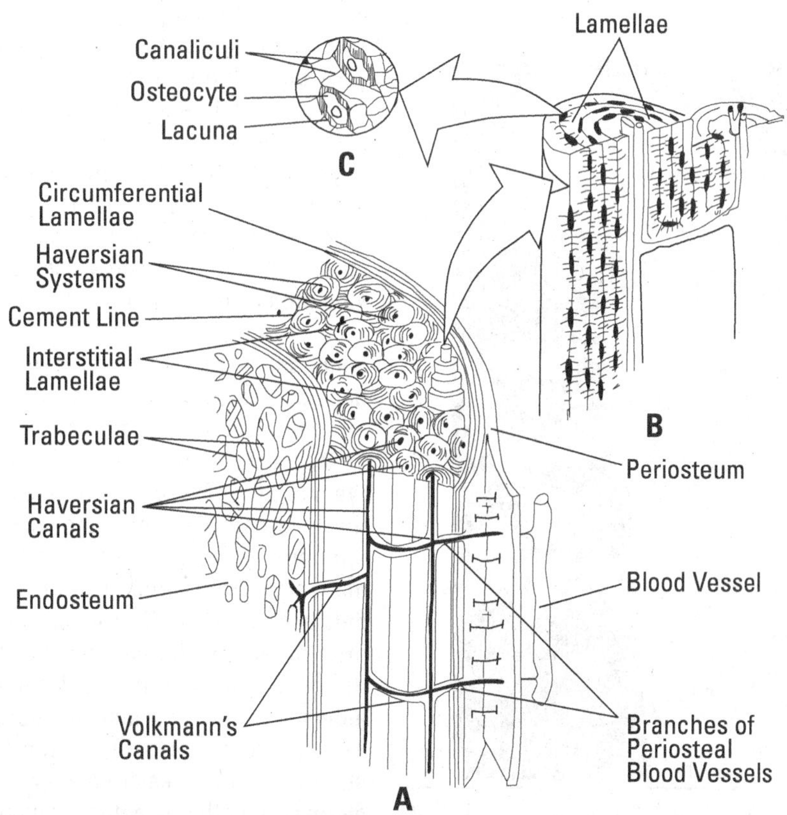

Figure 108-1. Schematic illustration of the fine structure of a section of long bone depicting multiple osteons (also called haversian systems) as the structural units. Haversian canals at the center of each osteon form the primary circulatory network. Each osteon consists of concentric lamellae interconnected by collagen. Each osteon is distinct from, yet bonded to surrounding osteons, by a cementing ground substance. Note the longitudinal orientation of the osteons.

that of collagen alone. Except for minor differences, all bone is formed of identical material. Two distinct macroscopic bone structures observed are cortical (compact) and cancellous (trabecular) bone. The major differences in these two structures of bone are their porosity and structural dimensions. The dense outer shell, or cortex, is made of cortical bone with 5% to 30% porosity. Inside this outer shell, cancellous bone is a fine lattice of thin bony plates with a porosity of 30% to 90% (Figure 108-2).[1] In either case, the hierarchical structure of bone is key to its mechanical performance and multifunctionality.[2] For example, bone's excellent toughness (energy-absorbing capability) is due in part to its hierarchy from the level of the amino acid sequence in collagen and the coiled-coil structure of collagen up through the various haversian, lamellar, and other intermediate-sized structures, to the more macroscopic cortical shell around cancellous bone structures. The large surface area resulting from all the interfaces and levels of hierarchy enable bone to absorb energy as these interfaces, which are widely distributed throughout the structure, fail.

The mechanical performance of whole bones, as for any structure, is understood by measuring its deformation under the influence of externally applied forces. As increasing loads are applied to a bone, it begins to deform until finally, failure occurs. Deformation is the measured change in dimensions of the structure under conditions of known loads and can be plotted on a load-deformation curve (Figure 108-3).[1,3-5] Much can be revealed about a structure (such as a whole bone) by study of its load-deformation curve. Under conditions of low-level loading, a structure typically deforms in direct relation to the load applied.

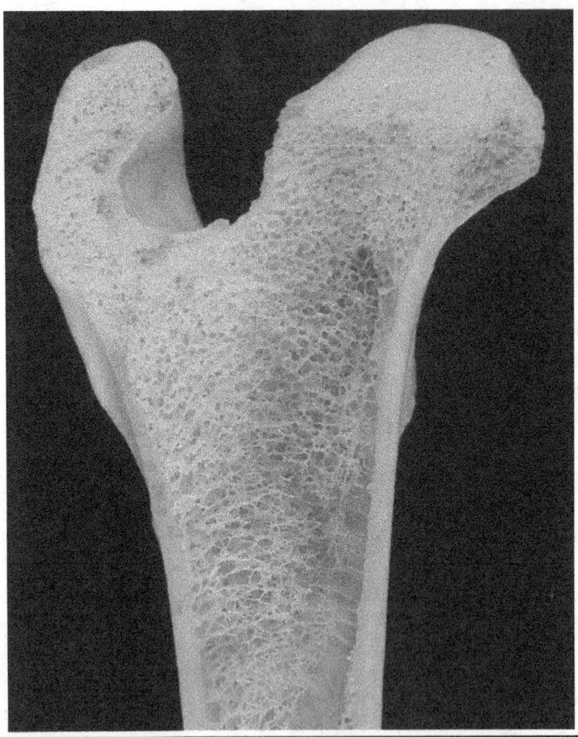

Figure 108-2. Longitudinal section through the proximal end of an adult canine femur. A shell of cortical bone surrounds a fine lattice of cancellous bone. Note how cancellous bone is concentrated in the irregularly shaped epiphyseal and metaphyseal segments and diminishes in the more regularly, cylindrical, thick-cortical diaphyseal segment.

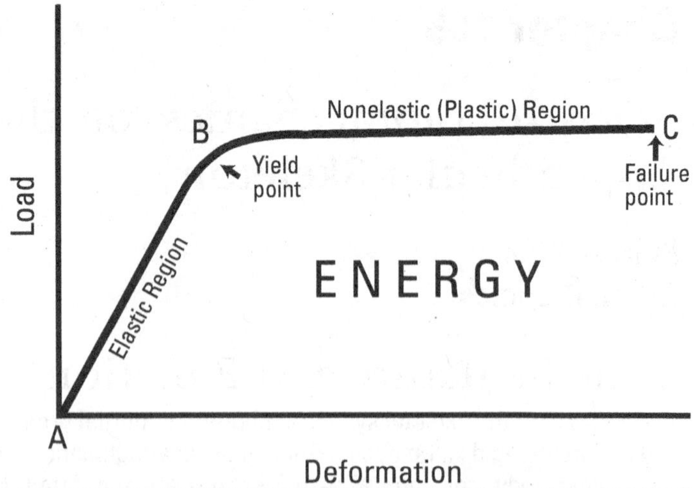

Figure 108-3. A theoretical load-deformation curve for a whole bone. Under conditions of low-level loading (elastic region, A-B), the structure deforms in direct relation to the applied load and returns to its original shape when the load is removed. Loading past the yield point (B) induces permanent deformation of shape (plastic region, B-C) even when the load is removed. If loading is progressively increased, the bone will grossly fail (fracture) at the ultimate failure point (C). The slope of the elastic region of the load-deformation curve indicates the stiffness of the studied bone. The area under the curve indicates the amount of energy absorbed by the bone prior to failure.

This linear portion of the curve is called the elastic region and reveals the elasticity of the structure, because when the load is removed the structure returns to its original shape. The point at which the applied load causes permanent deformation of shape is called the yield point. Living bone loaded to this degree will sustain microstructural damage. As applied load exceeds the yield point, the structure exhibits plastic behavior, revealed in the load-deformation curve between the yield point and the ultimate failure point. This region of the curve is called the plastic region and removal of applied loads at this point will no longer allow the structure to return to its original dimensions (structural damage has occurred). If loading is progressively increased, the structure will fail at some point (gross bony fracture), which is indicated by the ultimate failure point on the curve.

Functionally, two of the most important structural properties of bone are its stiffness and its load-bearing capacity. The stiffness of a structure is indicated by the slope of the elastic region of its load-deformation curve. The steeper the slope is, the stiffer the structure. Three parameters are typically used to determine the load-bearing capacity of a structure: (1) the load that the structure can sustain before failing (ultimate load), (2) the deformation that the structure can sustain before failing (ultimate deformation), and (3) the energy absorbed by the structure prior to failure. The energy-absorbed-to-failure is measured as the area under the load-deformation curve and, because it is indicative of both the load and deformation-to-failure, it provides an approximate measure of the toughness of the bone. These structural properties, from analysis of a load-deformation curve, depend on both the material composition and the dimensions of the tested bones. As an example, a large femur from a Rottweiler and a small femur from a Chihuahua are loaded in torsion to the point of gross fracture (Figure 108-4). The larger Rottweiler

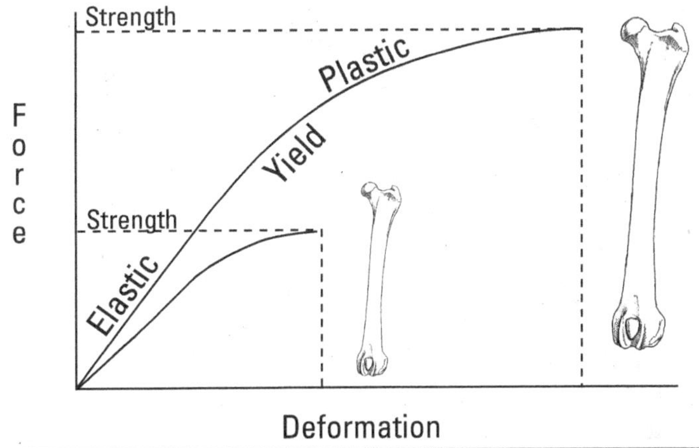

Figure 108-4. Idealized load-deformation curves for femora from a Rottweiler and a Chihuahua tested under torsion. The larger Rottweiler femur deforms less at given load (is stiffer) and fractures at a larger ultimate load (is stronger) than the smaller Chihuahua femur. Since both bones were from mature, healthy, non-osteoporotic animals, one can assume that the material composition of each bone is similar. Thus, the observed differences in mechanical behavior of each bone are attributed to structural differences (outer diameter, cortical thickness, etc).

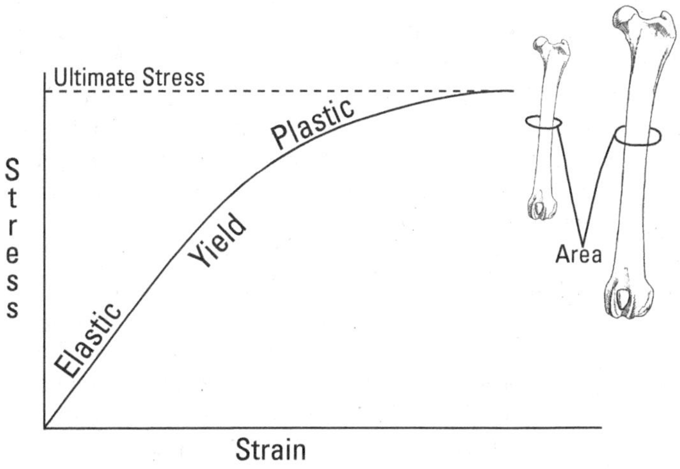

Figure 108-5. Idealized stress-strain curves for simple normalized samples harvested from femora from a Rottweiler and a Chihuahua tested under torsion reveal biomechanical properties of the bones' material (independent of geometry). Stress is the load divided by the cross-sectional area of the specimen. Strain is the measured change in dimension under the externally applied load, divided by its original dimension.

femur deforms less at a given load and fractures at a larger ultimate load than does the smaller Chihuahua femur. Since both bones were from mature, healthy, nonosteoporotic animals, one can assume that the material composition of both bones is then similar. Thus, the observed differences in structural properties can be attributed to the larger size (larger outer diameter and thicker cortical wall) of the Rottweiler femur.

The length of the bone, the cross-sectional area, and the distribution of bone about the neutral axis (cross-sectional shape) are important geometric dimensions that influence these whole bones' biomechanical behavior under various loading conditions. When the geometric dimensions of these whole bones are normalized, most often by testing simple-geometry samples of material cut from the bone, the load-deformation curve from mechanical testing can be converted to a stress-strain curve.[1,3-5] Bones of similar composition, like the Rottweiler and Chihuahua femurs above, have similar biomechanical characteristics as expressed in a stress-strain curve (Figure 108-5). Thus, whereas a load-deformation curve reveals properties of structure and material composition, a stress-strain curve reveals the biomechanical properties of a material (independent of geometric dimensions). Stress is defined as load (or force) divided by cross-sectional area, and the units most commonly used for measuring stress in standardized samples of bone are Newtons per centimeter squared (N/cm^2) or Newtons per meter squared (N/m^2). One N/m^2 is equivalent to one Pascal (Pa). Because Pascals are a small unit of measure with regard to bone testing, multiples of this unit are often employed including the kilopascal (1kPa = 1 $\times 10^3$ Pa), the megapascal (1mPa = 1 $\times 10^6$ Pa), and the gigapascal (1gPa = 1 $\times 10^9$ Pa). Bone typically fails at stresses in the megapascal range.[6]

Strain is the deformation (change in dimension) that develops in response to externally applied loads, divided by its original dimension. The two basic types of strain are linear (or normal) strain, in which a stress that is applied perpendicular to the test axis of an object causes a change in length of the specimen, and shear strain in which a stress applied parallel to the test axis of an object causes a change in angular dimension within it (Figure 108-6).[1,3-5] Linear strain is measured as the amount of linear

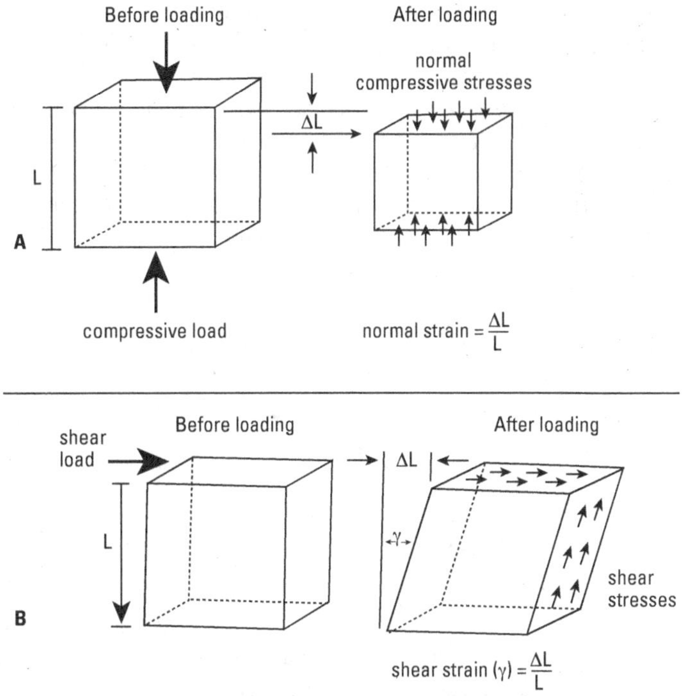

Figure108-6. A. Loading of bone perpendicular to a surface (compressive or tensile force) induces normal stress and strain within the sample. Linear strain is measured as the linear deformation (shortening or lengthening) of the specimen divided by its original length, often expressed as a percentage. B. Loading of bone parallel to a surface causes one part of the bone to slide past an adjacent part, resulting in shear stress and strain within the sample. Shear strain is measured as the amount of angular change in a right angle lying in the plane of interest within the specimen, and is expressed in radians.

deformation (lengthening or shortening) of the specimen divided by its original length and is, therefore, expressed as a dimensionless number or percentage (e.g., 1cm/10cm = 0.1 strain or 10% strain). Often, although not necessarily, the units are listed (e.g., cm/cm) for clarification. Shear strain is measured as the amount of angular change in a right angle lying in the plane of interest within a specimen and is expressed in radians (1 radian equals approximately 57.3 degrees).

A stress-strain curve can be produced by placing a standardized specimen of bone tissue into a testing jig and then loading it to failure in tension, compression, shear, or bending (see Biomechanics of Bone Fracture section further in the chapter for definitions of these loading regimens). The regions of this curve are similar to those of a load-deformation curve in that the curve has elastic and plastic regions, a yield point, and an ultimate failure point. The slope of the linear elastic region of a stress-strain curve is referred to as the elastic modulus or Young's modulus of elasticity. Stiffer materials have a higher Young's modulus.

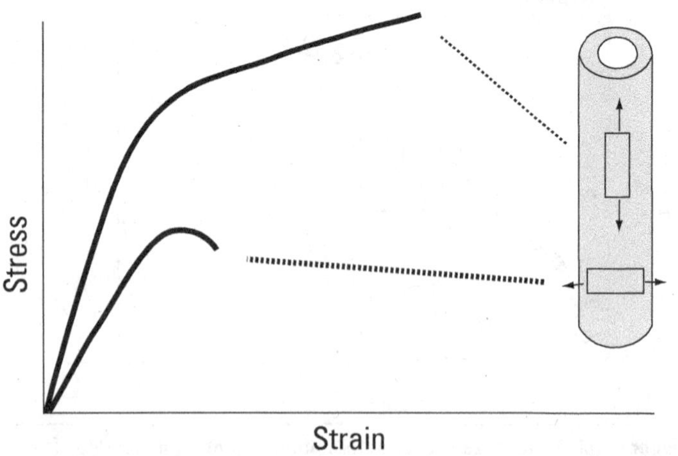

Figure 108-8. Idealized stress-strain curve depicting the anisotropic behavior of bone. Harvested samples are tested in tension in two different orientations: (a) with the longitudinal axis (parallel to the osteonal orientation) and (b) perpendicular to the longitudinal axis.

Mechanical Behavior of Bone

The fracture behavior of bone is influenced by its viscoelastic, anisotropic, and heterogeneous properties. Materials such as bone, the stress-strain behavior of which is dependent on the rate of loading, are viscoelastic.[1,3-5] If bone is loaded at a high rate, such as occurs with vehicular trauma or gunshot injury, its stiffness (Young's modulus), ultimate strain, and energy-to-failure increases (Figure 108-7). The clinical significance of the high toughness of healthy bone is that, if a high-rate loading actually causes macroscopic failure or fracture, as opposed to just distributed microscopic interfacial failures, the large release of the absorbed energy will cause marked comminution and injury to surrounding soft tissues.[7] Bone is also an anisotropic material, meaning that its strength and stiffness are dependent on the orientation of the applied load relative to the bone's microstructure and macrostructure (Figure 108-8).[1,3-5]

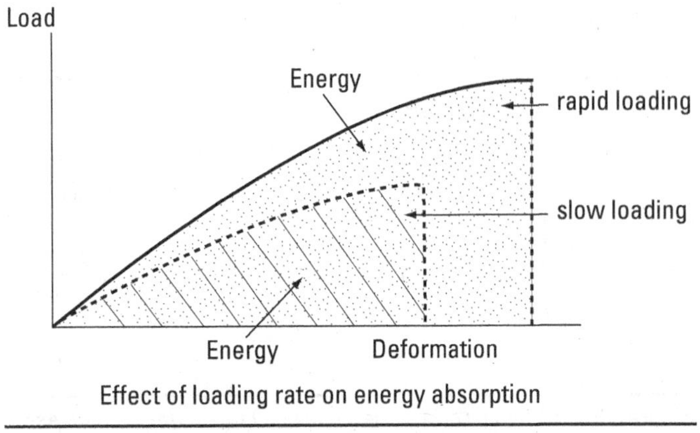

Figure 108-7. Viscoelasticity of bone. Idealized stress-strain curves depicting the effect of rate of load application on bone's stiffness and ultimate strength. The energy absorbed by the bone prior to fracture (area under the curve) is greater when it is rapidly loaded. Much of this absorbed energy is released to the surrounding soft tissues on gross fracture.

Cortical bone is stiffest and strongest when loaded parallel to osteon long axis, rather than perpendicular to the osteon long axis. Thus, long bones are better able to resist loads applied parallel to their long axis (compression and tension) than loads applied perpendicular to their long axis (shear). As predicted by Wolff's law, bone is generally stronger and stiffer in the direction in which the greatest loads are most commonly imposed (e.g., the long axis of the femur).[8,9] Being a heterogenous structure, the mechanical properties vary within a given bone. Porosity has a profound effect on the compressive stress-strain behavior of bone (Figure 108-9). Porosity is the volume of bone occupied by nonmineralized tissue.[4,5] Apparent density, a related measurement, is the mass of bone tissue divided by the bulk unit volume of bone tissue including mineralized bone and marrow space. Apparent density of bone is directly related to its inorganic mineral content. Cortical bone is composed predominantly of inorganic mineralized matrix and, therefore, has a higher apparent density and a lower porosity (varying from 5 to 30%) than cancellous bone.[1,4,5] In contrast, cancellous bone has a lower apparent density and a higher porosity (ranging from 30 to 90%) than does cortical bone.[1,4,5] Under compressive stress, cancellous bone behaves similarly to other porous materials. Under low levels of stress, cancellous bone exhibits elastic behavior. Then, after its yield point is reached, progressive collapse of trabeculae produces a long plateau in the plastic region of the curve. With continued compression, compaction of the compressed trabeculae causes an increase in material stiffness until its ultimate failure point is reached. Under compression, highly porous cancellous bone is capable of absorbing significant amounts of energy and tolerating up to 7% strain prior to failure.[4,10] Conversely, cortical bone with its low porosity, has a more brittle behavior under compressive stress, similar to glass. Cortical bone, which undergoes little plastic deformation prior to failure, absorbs less energy and tolerates little strain (< 2%) before fracture as compared with cancellous bone. However, cortical bone has greater ultimate strength and increased stiffness and can tolerate more stress prior to fracture than can cancellous bone.[4,10,11]

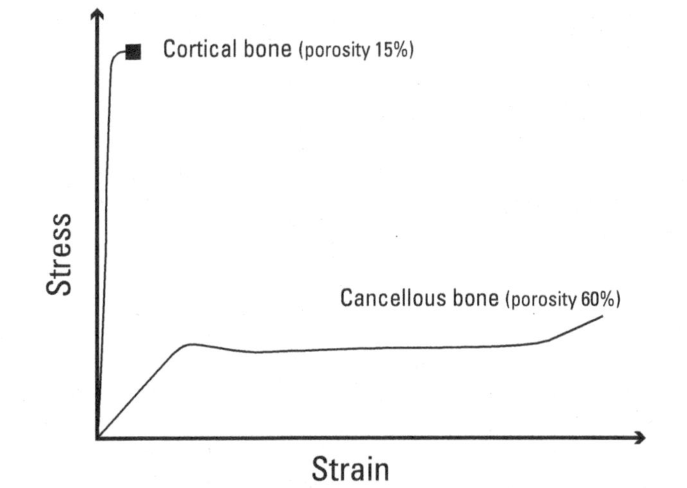

Figure 108-9. Idealized compressive stress-strain curve of cortical and cancellous bone samples depicting the effect of bone porosity on bone's mechanical behavior. Note that porous cancellous bone exhibits elastic behavior prior to its yield point. Following yield, progressive collapse of the bony trabeculae produces a long plateau of plastic deformation followed by a region of increased stiffness as the fractured trabeculae are compressed. This behavior allows cancellous bone to absorb great amounts of energy and tolerate significant strain prior to failure. Conversely, cortical bone, with its low porosity, displays brittle behavior where it is capable of tolerating great amounts of stress in the elastic region of the curve, but then fails abruptly.

There are many clinical implications of the relationship between bone's apparent density and its mechanical behavior. Large changes in tissue strength and modulus of bone can result from small changes in its apparent density. In the clinical setting this is important because changes in apparent density may not be evident on radiographs until it is altered by 30% to 50%.[4,5] Thus, minor reduction in bone density detected on radiographs is associated with greatly reduced stiffness and strength. Conversely, greatly enhanced fracture zone stiffness and strength may be present when even the most minor increases in fracture zone density are detected on radiographs.

Functional Structural Design of Long Bones

Another clinical implication of the relationship between bone porosity and its mechanical behavior is that it allows the clinician to better understand the functional design of long bones. Long bones are supremely designed structures well suited to their function as rigid kinematic links. The distinction between the mechanical behaviors of cancellous and cortical bone comes into play during weight bearing, as the ends of long bones must be able to absorb the tremendous compressive stresses and energy of weight bearing and distribute these to the diaphysis. The relatively high content of porous cancellous bone in the epiphyseal/metaphyseal regions provides bone with this unique capability. Further, the expanded cross-section of many bone ends provides additional strength and stiffness in compression because these properties are proportional to the cross-sectional area of bone. In contrast, both the cross-sectional area and the distribution of bone tissue about the neutral axis affect a structure's resistance to bending and are quantified in the structural parameter called the *area moment of inertia* (AMI). In bending, one side of the bone experiences tension and the other side compression. No stresses or strains are produced at the neutral axis (Figure 108-10).

Bone oriented further from the neutral axis is better able to resist bending loads. This is why an I-beam is an efficient structure for resisting bending forces applied in one direction (within the plane of the height of the beam). When bending is applied within the opposite plane, however, the AMI (and thus bending stiffness) of the I-beam decreases dramatically. Diaphyseal bone, on the other hand, must endure a complex array of bending moments in many directions as a consequence of varied activities, terrains, and muscular contraction. Thus, the cylindrical shape of the diaphysis of most long bones affords resistance to bending moments in all directions (the AMI of a cylinder is proportional to the radius raised to the 4th power). The tubular shape (versus a solid cylinder) of diaphyseal bone distributes much of the bone

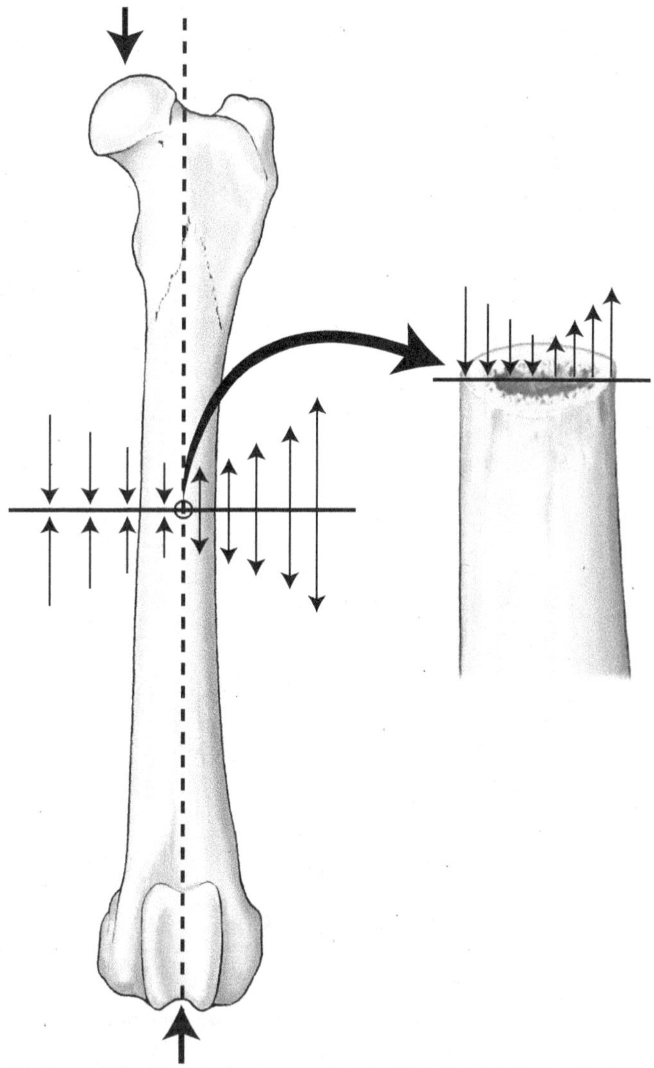

Figure 108-10. During weight-bearing, load applied to the femoral head produces bending forces at the femoral diaphysis. Here, the concave medial side experiences compressive stresses and strains while the convex lateral side experiences tensile stresses and strains. Because the magnitude of these stresses is proportional to their distance from the neutral axis of the bone, the neutral axis is subjected to neither tensile nor compressive stresses and strains.

tissue at a distance from the neutral axis, thus providing considerable resistance to bending (and torsion) with a minimum of bony mass. The factors that affect bone strength and stiffness in torsion are the same as for bending, the cross-sectional area, and the distribution of bone around the neutral axis. The polar moment of inertia (PMI) is used to calculate a structure's resistance to torsion. The larger the PMI is (which for a cylinder is also proportional to the radius raised to the 4th power), the stronger and stiffer the bone is against torsional moments.

Biomechanics of Bone Fracture

Bones are subject to physiologic and non-physiologic forces. Physiologic forces are generated through weight-bearing and muscular contraction. Physiologic forces that are applied in a uniaxial direction (compression or tension) can give rise to torsional or bending moments in bone. Physiologic forces rarely exceed the yield point of healthy bone, or in other words they do not cause plastic (permanent) deformation of bone. On the other hand, non-physiologic forces are the result of some externally applied load (vehicular trauma, horse kick, fall from deck or pickup truck bed, gunshot) and may easily exceed the yield point and load-bearing capacity of bone, creating a fracture. Forces and moments applied to bone in various directions can produce tension, compression, bending, shear, and torsion (Figure 108-11). Bone in vivo is subjected to all these loading modes.

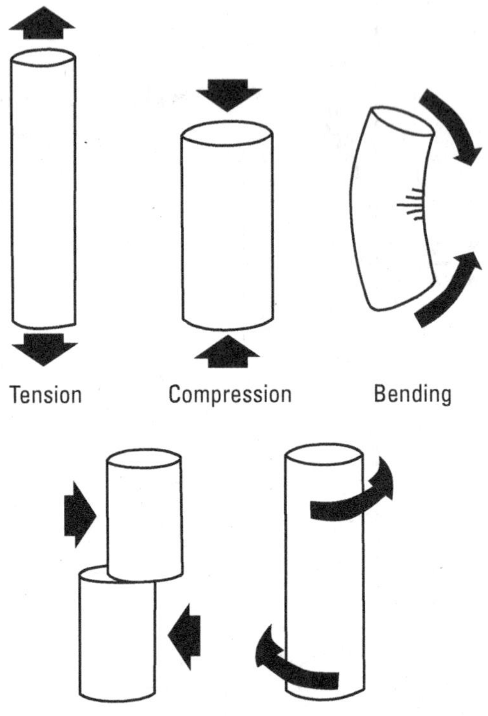

Figure 108-11. Schematic illustration of tensile, compressive, bending, shear, and torsional loading modes.

Compression

During compressive loading, equal and opposite loads are applied toward the center of the structure and parallel to the axis of the structure, causing compressive stress and strain within the bone (Figure 108-12A). Compressive loads cause most structures to shorten and widen. Maximal compressive stress occurs on a plane perpendicular to the applied load and can be thought of as many small forces directed toward the center of the bone that could potentially compact or crush the bone. Intuitively, one might expect compression fractures to develop perpendicularly to the applied compressive load and to crush or buckle the bone much like an empty soda can that is stepped on. However, compression loading also produces internal shear stresses and strains that develop oblique to the longitudinal axis and are maximal on a plane 45° from the axis of compressive loading.[1,3-5] Microscopically, the failure of bone loaded under compression is usually oblique cracking of the osteons created by these internal shear stresses, generated partly because of the bone's anisotropy and the fact that bone is weaker in shear than in compression. These oblique fracture configurations produced by compressive loading are commonly seen clinically with jump-down injuries of the tibia and radius (bones that are loaded along their central axis).[3,4]

Tension

During tensile loading, equal and opposite loads are applied away from the center of the structure, causing tensile stress and strain within the bone. Under tensile loading, most structures lengthen and narrow (Figure 108-12B). Maximal tensile stress occurs on a plane perpendicular to the applied load and can be thought of as many small forces directed away from the center of the bone that could potentially distract or pull apart the bone. Microscopically, the failure mechanism of bone loaded in tension is mainly debonding at the cement lines and other interfaces and pulling out of the osteons.[1,3-5] Grossly, bone tends to fail within a plane that is oriented perpendicularly to the applied tensile force. Clinically, fractures produced by tensile forces are typically at traction apophyses such as the tibial tuberosity, olecranon, tuber calcis, and attachment sites for ligaments.

Shear

During shear loading, equal and opposite loads are applied parallel to the surface of the bone, with the shear forces acting in opposite directions on opposing surfaces, causing shear stress and strain within the bone (Figure 108-12C). Under shear loading, a structure deforms in an angular manner (right angles within the structure are deformed to acute or obtuse angles). Shear stress can be thought of as many small forces acting on the surface of the bone on a plane parallel to the applied load. Not so intuitive is the observation that a geometrically complex and microscopically heterogenous structure loaded in compression or tension experiences internal shear stress (Figure 108-12A and B). Bone is weakest when subjected to shear stresses and tends to fracture in metaphyseal regions rich in cancellous bone along the lines of maximal shear stress.[1,4,5] A clinical example is the fracture of the lateral aspect of the humeral condyle that develops when a cocker spaniel falls from a height and lands on his thoracic limbs. The compressive load applied from the radial head to the lateral aspect of the humeral condyle produces shear stress in excess of the ultimate shear strength of the humeral condyle and lateral epicondylar crest, creating fracture in these structures.

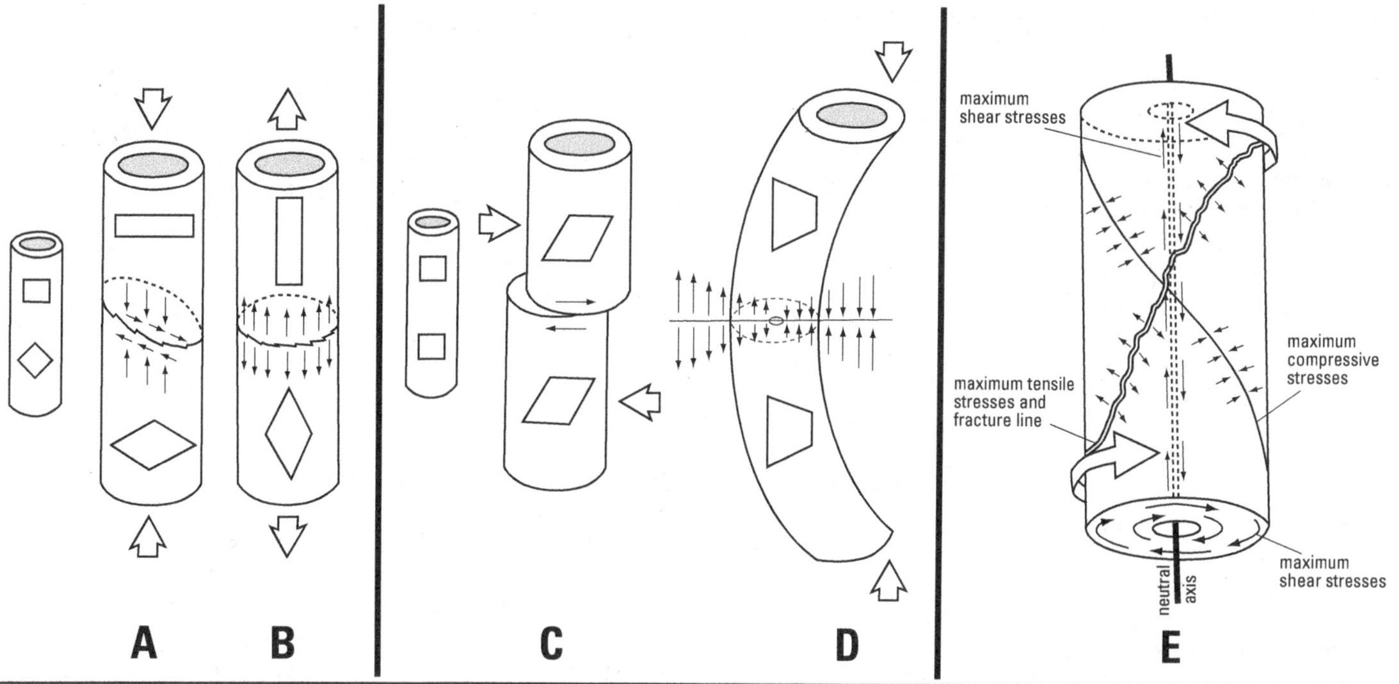

Figure 108-12. Illustration depicting stresses and strains produced by various loading modes on a cylindrical long bone. A, Compressive loading induces compressive and shear stresses and strains that, if excessive, may induce a short oblique fracture. B, Tensile loading induces tensile stresses and strains, which if excessive, induce a transverse fracture. C, Shear loading induces internal shear stresses and strains causing angular deformations. D, Bending loading induces tensile stresses and strains along the convex surface and compressive stresses and strains along the concave surface. There is a continuous gradient from maximal tensile stress, to neutral, to maximal compression. E, Torsional loading induces shear, tensile, and compressive stresses and strains, which if excessive, produce a typical spiral fracture configuration.

Bending

In bending, loads are applied to the surface of the bone in a manner that causes it to bend about an axis (usually the long axis of the bone). Under bending loads compression is generated on one side of the neutral axis and tension is produced on the opposite side (Figure 108-12D). During weight bearing, eccentrically loaded bones such as the femur and humerus experience physiologic bending forces that typically produce internal compressive stresses on the concave surface of the bone and tensile stresses on the convex surface.[1,3-5] No stresses or strains are produced at the neutral axis. The magnitudes of the stresses are proportional to their distance from the neutral axis such that the gradation is continuous from maximal compressive stress down to no stress at the neutral axis and then increases to maximal tensile stress at the opposite bony surface. Because bone is weaker in tension than in compression, the fracture plane generally begins on the tensile surface and transversely migrates toward the compressive surface.[1,3-5] Clinically, these fractures tend to be transverse or short oblique configurations. The obliquity is the result of accumulated internally generated shear stresses causing fracture along the line of maximal shear stress. A large wedge-shaped "butterfly" fragment is often produced when compression is combined with bending because two oblique divergent planes of maximal shear stress cause fracture on the compression side.[1,3-5]

Torsion

In torsion, loads are applied to the surface of the bone in a manner that causes it to twist about an axis (usually the long axis of the bone). Torsion results in shear stresses that are distributed throughout the bone (Figure 108-12E). As in bending, the magnitude of these stresses is proportional to their distance from the central (long) axis. Under torsional loading, maximal shear stresses act on planes perpendicular and parallel to the central axis. Furthermore, the maximal tensile and compressive (normal) stresses resulting from the torsion/shear act on a plane diagonal to the central axis. The spiral fracture pattern seen under torsional loading suggests that bone fails first in shear, with formation of an initial fracture line parallel to the neutral axis. A second crack usually forms along the plane of maximal tensile stress.[1,3-5] Clinically, spiral fractures are commonly seen in the narrow diameters of the distal tibial and distal humeral diaphyses where the polar moment of inertia is relatively small (thus the resultant shear strain from torsional stress is relatively high).

Combined Loads

Although we have considered each mode of loading individually, non-physiologic loads-to-failure in living bone are seldom so pure. In vivo, loading of bones is complex owing to their irregular shape and the constant barrage of multiple, coincident loads. Further, the hierarchical structure of bone allows it to absorb considerable energy prior to failure, particularly under rapidly applied loads. Thus, the energy of complex, rapidly applied non-physiologic loads is rapidly dissipated through the formation of multiple fracture lines (comminution).

Stress Concentration

Alterations and defects in bony structure or density owing to such conditions as drilled holes (biopsy tract, bone graft collection, or screw removal) or neoplasia cause stress concentrations in bone that can initiate failures.[12-14] These stress concentrations can lead to local stresses in the bone near the defect that are many times higher than the nominal applied stress on the bone. One way to think of the stress concentration effect is that the applied force must "flow" through the bone and, in a defect-free, homogenous bone, it can flow equally through all regions, creating equal stress throughout. However, in bone with defects (e.g., holes from removed screws), the force cannot flow through the areas with the holes and thus must flow around the holes. This leads to a build up of force flow (or higher stress) in the regions adjacent to defects and heterogeneities. The result is that a bone with stress concentrations fails at much lower loads or appears weaker than defect-free bones. The weakening effect of a stress concentrator is particularly marked under torsional loading where the decrease in strength may approach 90% and is proportional to the defect size.[13] Although defects smaller than 10% of the bone diameter may be of negligible significance in torsional resistance, larger holes are more problematic and remain so for an extended period of time.[13,15,16] This may be of particular concern in regions such as the distal humeral and distal tibial diaphyses where a relatively small polar moment of inertia already places these regions at risk of torsional failure (spiral fracture).

Another form of stress concentration comes from a mismatch in the elastic moduli (stiffness) of two materials (e.g., stainless steel and bone) placed in close proximity to one another and under load. The stress concentration results from the mismatch because the modulus of a material determines its response to an applied force: high moduli materials deform (strain) much less than do low moduli materials under the same load. The mismatch interrupts homogenous force flow and results in stress concentrations. Common clinical examples are cemented total joint replacement or stainless steel bone plating. As the materials are loaded, the bone exhibits greater elastic deformation, creating a shear stress at the bone-implant interface (Figure 108-13).

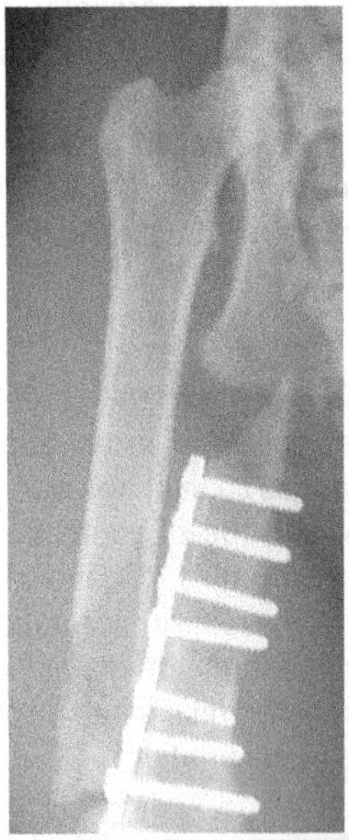

Figure 108-13. Craniocaudal radiograph of a feline femur 7 days following plate fixation of a distal metaphyseal fracture. The new fracture has occurred at the junction of the proximal end of the stainless steel plate with healthy bone and is attributed to stress concentration resulting from modulus mismatch.

Biomechanics of Callus Bone Healing (Indirect Healing)

Bone union can occur by one of two different repair mechanisms, direct healing (osteonal reconstruction) or indirect healing (intermediate callus formation).[3] Direct healing occurs primarily under conditions of anatomic alignment and rigid stability. Fracture line strain is less than 2%, and cutting cones are formed at the ends of the osteons nearest the fracture. Osteoclasts line the tip of the cutting cones for bone resorption and osteoblasts line the sides for bone formation. Resorption and formation of bone occur simultaneously as the cutting cones advance directly from one osteon to the next across the fracture line.

Indirect bone healing occurs through transformation of fibrous tissue or cartilage into osseous tissue in instances when impaired blood supply, fracture instability (deformation), or fracture-gap width do not allow direct formation of lamellar bone. Early events of indirect healing include the formation of granulation tissue in the fracture zone. This loose fibrous and vascular tissue tolerates strain as high 40%. Bone resorption at the fracture ends may be seen early in healing as this increased fracture-gap width effectively decreases fracture-gap strain (strain = change in gap dimension under load/original gap dimension). Fibrous tissue forms at the periphery of the fracture gap where blood supply is adequate, and fibrocartilage forms toward the center of the callus where blood supply is limited. Greater fracture-zone instability stimulates more abundant callus production extending further from the bone's neutral axis. Profound increases in resistance to bending and torsional moments accompany modest increases in external callus deposition because the AMI and the polar moment of inertia are both exponentially related to the radius of a cylindrical structure. Resistance to compression and tension are also related to the cross-sectional area of the filling fracture gap.

This soft callus is able to bridge the fracture gap, but cannot decrease deformation to a level conducive to osteoblast survival. This fibrous and fibrocartilage tissue is stiffer than granulation tissue, but is also less tolerant of strain. Once the soft callus deposition is sufficient to adequately reduce fracture-gap strain, mineralization and woven bone formation begin, starting from the regions with the least motion. Once this stiffer mineralized cartilage and woven bone adequately reduce fracture-gap strain, these tissues are replaced by cancellous bone. After complete bridging by abundant cancellous bone has occurred, the fracture zone can enter into a stage of remodeling where longitudinally oriented lamellar bone and more normal bony contour are restored. In general, during callus healing, the extensive circumferential distribution of the soft callus provides structural strength and stiffness to the fracture to compensate for the relatively weak material properties of the soft callus. As the material properties of the callus strengthen and stiffen, the structural properties of callus become progressively weaker through remodeling.

Appendicular Fractures±

Fractures of the Scapula

The scapula is a thin, flat bone shaped like an I-beam through much of its body. The shape of the scapular body combined with its support by extensive musculature protect it from fracture except in the case of high-energy trauma such as vehicular and gunshot injury.[15] Many of these fractures are effectively treated nonsurgically as a function of both the mechanical and biologic support afforded by the surrounding musculature. In selected scapular-body fractures with excessive displacement (folding), fixation with 1 or 2 inverted semitubular plates and screws placed adjacent to the scapular spine allows for restored alignment and maximal screw purchase in the thin bone without the need for supplemental coaptation.[16] Fractures of the acromion process and supraglenoid tuberosity are subject to pure tensile forces resulting from their musculotendinous attachments. Treatment of acute fractures in these locations should usually incorporate tension-band fixation to counter these tensile forces.[17] Fractures of the glenoid cavity are typically treated with internal fixation because rigid fixation and anatomic reduction are prerequisites for mitigation of osteoarthritis following articular fracture.[17]

Fractures of the Humerus

Fractures of the humerus represent approximately 12% of long-bone fractures and most often involve the distal half of the bone.[15,17-19] Fractures of the proximal humerus, which is larger in diameter than the distal end, are relatively uncommon and are typically the result of high-energy trauma or elastic modulus mismatch inherent to physeal fractures. Low-energy trauma associated with jumping down from an elevation often causes spiral fracture configurations in the narrow distal diaphyseal region. Another common "jump down" fracture of the distal humerus is the fracture of the lateral aspect of the humeral condyle frequently seen in cocker spaniels.[20-26] On landing, axial compressive loads are transmitted from the radial head to the lateral aspect of the humeral condyle (capitulum) and the lateral epicondylar crest. The resultant shear forces in the condylar and epicondylar bone may be excessive, particularly in conditions of incomplete humeral condyle ossification, and result in fracture.[24,25] Simple supracondylar fractures and more complex "Y" fracture configurations are also relatively common and are the result of excessive compression and/or shear stresses within the narrow dimensions of the humeral condyle and epicondylar crest regions.

Fractures of the humerus can, potentially, be treated with most any surgically applied fixation system, depending on fracture location, configuration, disruptive forces, and other factors. The extensive envelope of musculature surrounding the humerus complicates application of external skeletal fixation (ESF) by itself because the connecting elements are placed extremely eccentric to the neutral axis. However, when ESF can be "tied-in" to intramedullary pin fixation, the bending resistance is dramatically increased by virtue of increased AMI.[27,28]

Fractures of the Antebrachium

Fractures of the radius and/or ulna comprised 22% of all long-bone fractures in dogs and cats in one study.[18] Fractures of the diaphyseal segments of these bones are most common. As with any bone, fractures of the physes of immature dogs and cats is relatively frequent owing to the modulus mismatch at these locations. Further, the unique conical shape of the distal ulnar physis appears to predispose it to crushing injury of the resting cells of the physis. "Jump down" injury may disrupt the resting cells along the margins of the conical physis by shear forces, and compression may be focused on the resting cells at the tip of the conical distal ulnar physis. Fractures of the radius and ulna are more common in the distal diaphyseal region where the smaller diameter and lateral position of the ulna combined with the craniocaudally flattened shape of the radius (decreased AMI) may predispose it to fracture from excessive craniocaudal bending moments associated with falls, being stepped on, etc. The cross-sectional geometry of these bones may be disproportionately small in toy breeds of dogs, thereby predisposing them to distal-third antebrachial fracture.[29] Of course, high-energy trauma associated with gunshots and vehicular trauma may be more extensively distributed throughout the two bones. The olecranon is the most common location of fractures involving the proximal antebrachium.[18] Olecranon fractures should usually be stabilized using the tension-band principle because of the pure tensile load applied by the triceps muscle group insertion on the olecranon.[17] Application of a bone plate to the caudal surface of the ulna, using the tension-band principle, may be advantageous in complex olecranon fracture scenarios.[30]

Fractures of the Pelvis

The pelvis (os coxae, sacrum, and first coccygeal vertebra) protects intrapelvic structures from trauma while allowing for load transmission from the pelvic limbs to the spine. Although protected by extensive surrounding musculature, fractures of the pelvis are common, representing 20% to 30% of all fractures in dogs.[17] The pelvis' box-like shape predisposes it to fracture, most often multiple fractures. Displacement of one side of the rectangular box places stress on another side of the box. Although the blood supply provided by the surrounding musculature aids healing for most pelvic fractures even when treated nonsurgically, surgical treatment is often indicated to hasten restoration of locomotor function and to ensure adequate pelvic canal dimensions when healing is complete.

Surgical stabilization is indicated for fractures involving the acetabulum, fractures causing excessive pelvic canal collapse, and many fractures in which load transmission from the pelvic limb to the lumbar spine is interrupted.[17] Anatomic reduction and stabilization of the acetabulum are paramount and can be achieved with bone plate/screw (with or without plate luting) or with screw/wire/polymethylmethacrylate fixation along the dorsal acetabular rim.[31-33] This implant placement creates a tension-band effect because the impact of the femoral head into the acetabulum creates tension along the dorsal acetabular rim. Fractures of the ilium are also commonly treated surgically. The tension surface of the canine ilium is dynamic through the gait cycle, shifting from ventromedial to neutral.[34] Standard lateral plate/screw placement for fixation of longitudinal fractures

± The incidence of fractures involving specific bones, expressed as a percentage, in this section are approximate and taken from several sources, thus, do not sum to 100%.

(relatively parallel to the spinal axis) of the ilium may ignore the tensile stress on the bone's ventromedial aspect.[34-36] Use of ventral-to-dorsally oriented screws alone or in combination with bone plate fixation has been advocated to address this concern. The effects of lateral-to-medial screw purchase in the body of the sacrum are debated.[34-36] Some studies of triple pelvic osteotomies show that screw migration was reduced when substantial sacral screw purchase was achieved.[37,38] Other studies suggested that sacral body screw purchase should be avoided as low-level sacroiliac joint movement may induce screw migration.[35,39] The authors of one study suggested that addition of ventral screws is a better way to increase overall screw purchase and avoids patient morbidity that may be associated with iatrogenic immobilization of the sacroiliac joint.[35]

Fractures of the Femur

Fractures of the femur represent approximately 45% of all long-bone fractures in the dog and cat.[18] Approximately half of these involve the diaphysis, and the other half are evenly divided between the proximal and distal epiphyseal/metaphyseal regions.[18,40] In the proximal region, fractures of the femoral neck are most common. Weight bearing likely generates significant shear stress within the narrow diameter of the femoral neck. These shear stresses may be particularly problematic when transmitted across the physis of the femoral head and neck. Indeed, delayed closure of this physis associated with early neutering has been hypothesized as a predisposing cause of excessive and repetitive shear stress leading to physeal disruption in overweight cats.[41]

Fractures of the femoral diaphysis may be of most any configuration, thus reflecting the wide array of loading leading to fracture. External rotators of the hip (gemelli, internal obturator, quadratus femoris, and iliopsoas muscles) typically produce profound external rotation of the proximal femoral segment that must be corrected during surgical stabilization. Owing to eccentric loading of the femur during weight bearing, the medial surface is the compression side and the lateral surface is the tension side. Indeed, diaphyseal fractures producing medial "butterfly" fragments are relatively common, and this fracture configuration is predictable when strong mediolateral bending forces are generated with compression loads along the medial surface. Further, surgeons must be especially aware of the impact of eccentric loading when surgically stabilizing femoral fractures, particularly with bone plates. With traditional bone-plate application on the lateral surface of the femur, defects present on the medial surface drastically reduce the AMI of the bone/plate construct, thus increasing the likelihood of fixation failure.[28,42] Simple combination of an IM pin to the plate fixation dramatically increases the fatigue life of the fixation by profoundly increasing the AMI of the composite fixation.[43,44] Common fixation methods used for femoral diaphyseal fractures include intramedullary pin plus cerclage wires, IM pin plus ESF, interlocking nail, bone plate, and plate/pin systems. The most appropriate fixation depends on a comprehensive assessment of pertinent biomechanical, biologic, and clinical factors that influence bone healing and return of locomotor function. External skeletal fixation of the femur is complicated by the extensive surrounding musculature (that shifts the ESF's connecting elements far eccentric to the neutral axis) and adjacent body wall (that prevents utilization of many traditional frame configurations). Innovative ESF frame configurations, often in combination with an intramedullary pin "tie-in", are often advisable when applied to the femur.[27,45] Distal femoral physeal fractures are relatively common.[46] This physis has a unique "4 pegs in 4 cups" configuration. Three or 4 of these metaphyseal pegs are often intact (Salter I or II fractures) in dogs and cats. Reduction of 3 or more pegs into their respective cups provides some inherent stability, particularly against torsional moments.[47] These fractures are often surgically stabilized with relatively simple single IM pin, cross-pin, or dynamic pin ("Rush-fashion") fixation.

Tibia/Fibular Fractures

Fractures of the tibia and fibula consist of 22% of all long-bone fractures in the dog and cat.[18] The majority of these fractures are located in the diaphyseal region. The smaller diameter of the distal diaphysis reduces the bones' AMI and polar moment of inertia. Clinically, low-energy bending injury often produces short, oblique fractures or fractures with a small butterfly fragment. On occasion, in young, skeletally immature animals, the traumatic injury produces only a greenstick (incomplete) line in the tibia or a complete fracture of the tibia, but leaves the fibula intact (but sometimes plastically deformed). Low-energy trauma and torsional injury commonly produce spiral fractures in the narrow diameter of the distal tibial diaphysis where the polar moment of inertia is relatively small (thus the resultant shear strain from torsional stress is relatively high). Higher energy trauma, such as vehicular accidents, commonly produces highly comminuted fracture patterns that may extend more proximally than is typical for the lower energy fractures. Simple fractures in the distal tibial physeal region are also common and may reflect the stress-concentrating effect of modulus mismatch. Fractures of the tibial crest are subject to pure tensile loading from the patellar ligament and are best treated with tension band fixation.

Fracture Assessment

The mechanical goal of fracture fixation is to provide appropriate spatial limb alignment and sufficient fracture gap stability to allow for bone healing and full restoration of limb function. In order to achieve this goal, the fixation must effectively neutralize the disruptive forces acting on the fracture. Clinically, this mechanical goal must be tempered against the biologic requirements for bone healing and inherent patient- and client-related factors.

Compression, generated by weight bearing and muscular contraction, must be neutralized in the treatment of diaphyseal fractures of all long bones. In instances in which reconstruction of the bony column is advisable, the reconstructed bony column will provide some resistance to collapse of the fracture zone. When transverse or interdigitating short, oblique fractures are purposefully compressed, the end-to-end bone contact may improve fracture stability and actually aid bone healing. In other instances, however, open anatomic reconstruction of the bony column is not advisable. In these instances, the fixation itself must resist all of the compression forces that tend to cause axial collapse via adequate purchase of the main proximal and distal fracture segments.

Tensile forces result in distraction of fracture fragments and are primarily the result of musculotendinous or ligamentous insertions on the ends of long bones. Tensile forces are best neutralized by application of the tension-band principle using a tension-band wire or tension-band plate. Tension band implants are applied opposite the direction of pull on the fragment. As an example, tensile forces from the triceps insertion on the olecranon tend to pull the proximal segment cranially and proximally. A tension-band wire is placed by initially reducing the olecranon with paired Kirschner wires. The bending force on these wires is neutralized by addition of a taut figure-of-8 tension-band wire placed on the caudal aspect of the olecranon (opposite the direction of pull). Alternatively, a plate applied on the caudal aspect of the olecranon can exert the same tension-band effect.

Bending is inherent to diaphyseal fractures of all long bones and must be neutralized if predictable, low-morbidity healing is to be realized. Bending forces in long bones result from combinations of their curvature, eccentric loading, and contraction of surrounding muscles in addition to a variety of extrinsically applied loads. Bending forces tend to cause collapse on the concave (compression) side of the bone. Loss of cortical contact on the compression side exaggerates the bending forces acting on the fracture fixation system. Neutralizing bending forces must always be a consideration in treating diaphyseal fractures of long bones.

Torsion is induced by muscular contractions, by changes in direction of the body while the foot is planted, and by extrinsic sources. Failure to neutralize torsional forces is a relatively common cause of delayed or nonunions and malunions when intramedullary pinning is used without supplementary fixation. Torsional forces are most predictably neutralized by fixation that purposefully achieves implant-bone purchase on both the proximal and distal main fracture segments. Torsional forces can seldom be adequately resisted by interdigitation of the fractured bone ends and this is only feasible in the smallest and fastest healing of patients.

Fracture Treatment

Fracture treatment must effectively address the mechanical goals stated earlier, the biologic requirements for bone healing, and the inherent clinical concerns such as patient temperament, client compliance, cost, and surgeon expertise. The following description is an overview of the inherent mechanical strengths and weaknesses of various fracture treatment methods.

Full-Cylinder Cast

External coaptation includes soft padded bandages, slings, splints, and casts. The full-cylinder cast is the most rigid form of external coaptation and is capable of effectively neutralizing bending and rotational forces when applied correctly and in the proper situations. A full-cylinder cast must span the joints above and below the fracture (note: this is not feasible for fractures of the humerus and femur), must conform to the limb, and must be sufficiently thick to withstand weight bearing. A full-cylinder cast is not capable of neutralizing axial collapse (compression) or tension. Thus, casting is not ideally indicated for fractures in which end-to-end contact of transverse diaphyseal fractures cannot be accomplished. Likewise, casts do not neutralize the pure tensile forces acting on traction apophyses.

Splints and casts encase the limb, but do not directly interact with the bony segments. Thus, an interface of soft tissue and cast padding exists between the fixation and the bony segments. More stability is provided when there is less soft interface between the cast and the bone(s) being stabilized. Clinical practicality, however, dictates that some soft interface must be present to minimize the risk and severity of cast sores. Increasing cast thickness is the easiest way to increase resistance to bending (by virtue of increased AMI), but this also increases its weight substantially. Alternatively, reinforcement of the cast in one region can be used (i.e., the I-beam effect) if unidirectional bending is anticipated.

Intramedullary Pin Fixation

Intramedullary (IM) pinning, when properly performed, effectively neutralizes bending forces because of their large AMI. Since AMI is a function of radius raised to the 4th power, the diameter of the pin greatly influences its bending strength. Furthermore, theoretically, complete fill of the intramedullary canal with an IM pin would effectively neutralize shear forces resulting from weight bearing on noninterdigitating oblique fractures. Complete (100%) filling of the intramedullary canal with an IM pin is neither realistic (because of the irregular shape of bones) nor desirable (because complete canal filling prevents intramedullary blood supply from redeveloping).[48,49] Instead, filling of 60% to 70% of the intramedullary canal by the IM pin is frequently recommended. Pinning of the radius is seldom recommended; one reason is that the intramedullary canal is so narrow that an appropriately sized IM pin provides neglible bending strength such that the fixation must be supported with coaptation anyway. In selected instances, intramedullary pinning of small bones such as metacarpals or metatarsals is recommended, but these fixations must always be protected with suitable coaptation owing to the small diameter of the pins. Proper pinning technique also requires the IM pin to be well seated into the proximal and distal metaphyses. Unfortunately, IM pin fixation alone lacks the ability to effectively neutralize axial compression or torsion because each of these requires a system that gains purchase of the bone and the connecting element(s) of the fixation system on each side of the fracture (i.e., interlocking nails, bone plates, or external skeletal fixation). Frictional hold between the smooth surface of the IM pin and the endosteal surface of the bone is insufficient to resist torsional moments. Increasing the IM pin diameter or addition of threads does not improve torsional resistance.[50] A trilaminar fluted nail in which the flutes engage the endosteal surface to resist torsion forces has been described in the veterinary literature but has not found widespread clinical application.[51] Use of multiple, smaller diameter pins ("stack pinning") only slightly increases rotational stability and should not be relied on in fractures that are not inherently stable.[52] Supplementing the IM pin with a bone plate or an external skeletal fixator is a common strategy to complement the pin's inherent ability to resist bending forces, with the latter systems' abilities to resist axial collapse and rotation. Fracture fixation with only a single IM pin is seldom recommended – only in instances of interdigitating transverse fractures of very small and rapidly healing patients.

Techniques of cross pinning or dynamic pinning are commonly used for fixation of metaphyseal and epiphyseal fractures where rapidly healing, interdigitating transverse fractures are frequently encountered.[47] These fractures are inherently resistant to collapse. With each of these paired pinning methods, the pins are typically angled such that they cross on the diaphyseal side of the fracture. In this manner, the 2 pins cross the fracture in different pathways, thereby imparting some resistance to rotational moments. With cross pinning, each of the pins passes from one side of the bone and penetrates the far-cortical surface. In contrast, dynamic pins (pins placed in "Rush fashion") are placed such that they deflect off the far endosteal surface rather than penetrate it. The pins are then advanced to seat in the distant metaphyseal region. The interaction of these dynamically placed pins helps resist rotation moments, but not to the same degree as the cross-pinning technique.[47]

Interlocking Nails

Interlocking nailing is an intramedullary system that addresses the axial collapse and rotational instability weaknesses of IM pin fixation while utilizing its inherent ability to resist multidirectional bending loads. By virtue of the interlock between the bone and intramedullary nail on each side of the fracture, the interlocking nail system is capable of resisting axial collapse and torsional moments.[53-56] Interlocking nails, themselves, are weakest at their screw holes (lowest AMI and a stress concentrator).[28] Unlike bone plates, a locking screw through a nail does not reduce the stress-concentrating effects of the hole because the locking screw does not interact rigidly with the nail.[56] Therefore, these screw holes should not be placed in close proximity to the fracture zone with or without an interlocking screw. When used to span nonreconstructed fractures, the interlocking screws resist axial collapse by "tethering" the main bone segments to the level of the nail holes. As nail diameter decreases, the AMI decreases of both the nail and of the corresponding interlocking screws that can be used. When one manufacturer used a relatively large 3.5-mm screw diameter in their 6-mm nail, breakage of nails was the most common mode of clinical failure.[57] As they reduced the size of the screw hole to accept 2.7-mm screws (thus increasing the AMI of the nail), nail breakage became less common but screw failure was noted.[58]

As an alternative to the use of interlocking screws, bolts are now manufactured such that positive-profile threads engage only the near-cortical surface during insertion, and the core diameter of the "tethering" portion of the bolt is maximized (Table 108-1). One does not have to be overly concerned about premature "backing out" of the bolts because they are not subjected to pull-out forces as are screws placed through a bone plate. Whereas unicortical thread engagement of the bolt is sufficient, bicortical penetration

Table 108-1. Area Moment of Inertia of Screws and Locking Bolts of Varying Size. (Area moment of inertia = $\pi r^4/4$ where r = radius = 0.5 x core diameter).

Implant	Core diameter (mm)	Area moment of inertia (mm⁴)
2.0 screw	1.5	0.25
2.0 bolt	2.0	0.79
2.7 screw	2.0	0.79
2.7 bolt	2.7	2.61
3.5 screw	2.5	1.91
3.5 bolt	3.5	7.37
4.0 screw (cancel.)	2.0	0.79
4.5 screw	3.2	5.15
4.5 bolt	4.5	20.13

of the interlocking screws or bolts is important, particularly when functioning as a tether in nonload-sharing situations. Further, in such instances, the longer screw lengths required for use in metaphyseal regions increases their susceptibility to bending or breaking.[59] Eccentric loading of these screws, such as occurs when the nail is not centralized within the metaphyseal region, appears to improve screw fatigue life.[59] Interlocking nail systems compare favorably with bone plate and plate-pin combinations when used to stabilize gap models except with regard to torsional resistance.[53,54] The lack of a rigid interlock between the locking screw and/or bolt and the nail permits slight rotational movement.[54] One way to augment the interlocking nail system's resistance to rotation is to use it in conjunction with external skeletal fixation.[60-62] This can be done by virtue of a connecting bar "tie-in" between the proximal extension of the interlocking nail and the ESF frame or by use of special external fixation pins designed for dual use as an ESF pin and the interlocking bolt.[60,61] One would expect such fixation to dramatically increase both bending resistance (in the plane of the frame by increasing AMI) and torsional resistance (by increasing PMI). Interlocking nails can be dynamized, if desired, by removing the interlocking devices on one side of the fracture, thus exposing the fracture zone to both axial compression and torsional stresses.[60-62]

Orthopedic Wire and Cerclage

Orthopedic wire is malleable stainless steel that is formed into monofilament wire of varying dimensions. Applications in small animals typically vary from as large as 16-gauge to as little as 24-gauge wire. Full-cerclage wire is placed around the full circumference of a completely and anatomically reconstructed bony column. As the wire is tightened, the fracture lines are compressed (much like the staves of an oak barrel are compressed as the band surrounding them is tightened). If perfect anatomic reduction is not achieved, wire tightening will tend to collapse fragments into the intramedullary canal and the wire will be prone to premature loosening. Stabilization of two main fracture segments requires that the fracture line be a long oblique configuration in which the length of the fracture line is at least 2.5 times greater than the bone diameter in that location. When sufficient obliquity is present, a minimum of two properly applied wires is capable of providing excellent compression of the fracture surfaces (interfragmentary compression). When improperly applied to a short oblique fracture, full-cerclage wire creates shear stress at the fracture and, because there is only room for one wire, concentration of bending stresses. Although one should avoid the use of cerclage wire in short oblique fractures, the following "escape strategy" can be employed if alternatives are not available: use of 1 or 2 K-wires oriented perpendicularly to the plane of the fracture can minimize the shear forces created by tightening of the full-cerclage wire. The cerclage wire is placed so that, as it is tightened, the K-wire prevents its orientation perpendicular to the long axis of the bone and directs compression across the fracture line.[63]

Cerclage wires can be tightened and secured in a number of ways and their relative mechanical merits are measured by comparisons of the compression achieved and the resistance to knot loosening.

Twist-knots are properly formed when each of the two ends of the wire wrap evenly around the other (improper formation is one wire wrapped around the core of the other – like a snake wrapped around a stick). Tensioning and securing the wire occur simultaneously with this method. In most instances, it is advisable to cut the knot short rather than bending it over because any manipulation of the knot decreases tension in the wire.[64,65] Resistance to knot failure under loading is determined by the frictional interface between the two wires. The number of twists to leave in the knot has not been clearly established, but cutting the knot with three twists remaining is common. If the twist-knot must be flattened, the flattening process and the final twisting should be simultaneous to minimize loss of loop tension.[64,66] Twist knots untwist when loaded past the yield point and do not exert as much loop tension as other methods.[64,67] Twist-knots sustain greater load to failure than single-loop knots, but similar load to loosening.[63,64]

Single-loop knots are formed using a wire with a loop on one end. After passing the free end of the wire around the bone, it is passed through the loop. The free end is then passed into the end of a purpose-specific tightening instrument. The wire is tensioned by rotating a crank on the tightening instrument. The wire is tightened in the first phase of application; then the knot is locked in the second phase by bending the free end over the loop. This method achieves greater initial loop tension than the twist-knot, but has a similar load resistance before loosening.[66] The single-loop knot fails by unbending of the free end.[67]

Double-loop cerclage is formed from a segment of wire bent 180° in the middle. The bent end is passed around the bone and the 2 free ends are passed through the loop created by the bend. The free ends are tightened with a 2-crank wire tightener. The knot is locked in a similar manner as the single-loop method. The double-strand and double-knot increase the loop tension and knot security. The double-loop knot generates 3 times as much tension as the single loop and resists twice the distracting load prior to wire loosening.[64]

Bone Plates and Screws System (DCP, LC-DCP, Locking-Plate Systems)

Screws convert insertion torque into compression along their shaft such that any structures bone plate, washer, or bone fragment underlying the screw head are compressed during tightening (provided the hole diameter in that underlying structure exceeds the screw-thread diameter such that it may glide freely along the screw shaft). Individual screws may be used in positional or lag fashion. When screws are used as positional screws, their threads engage both the near and the far segments such that the position of each fragment is held in a specific location, and compression of the fracture line is not achieved. When screws are used as lag screws, their threads engage only the far bone segment. Screw tightening compresses the near segment against the far segment because the near bone segment is free to slide along the screw shaft. The amount of interfragmentary compression achieved with the lag screw method is primarily a function of the bone strength, outer-thread diameter, and insertional torque. Screws must often resist significant bending forces. The bending strength of a screw is determined by its AMI which is related to its core radius raised to the fourth power.[28] Therefore, small increases in screw core-diameter profoundly increase its bending strength. For example, a 3.5-mm cortical screw (2.5-mm core diameter) is nearly 2.5 times stronger than a 2.7-mm cortical screw (2.0-mm core diameter) (Table 108-1).

The most common use of screws is to fasten a bone plate to the bone. Unlike an ESF connecting bar, traditional bone plates are not mechanically linked to fixation screws. With traditional plating, the fixation only becomes stable when the screw is firmly tightened, thereby compressing the plate against the underlying bone. Properly applied bone plates resist compression, tension, bending, and torsional and shear forces especially when used to compress a two-piece transverse fracture of a long bone. In this instance, a dynamic compression plate (DCP) is desirable. The DCP screw hole is designed such that tightening of the screws compresses the fractured bone ends together. The DCP screw holes are oval and the surface that comes into contact with the underneath side of the screw head slopes downward and toward the fracture line (much like a playground slide). When the screw is inserted on the "high" side of the oval sloped DCP hole, the screw head comes into contact with the sloped hole as the screw is tightened. The screw is fixed in the bone and is not free to slide down the slope. Instead, the interaction between the screw head and the oval sloped DCP hole draws the plate toward the screw. Using the playground slide analogy, rather than a child sliding down a fixed playground slide, the slide is free to move and is drawn backward as the child descends. Once a traditional bone plate is secured with screws, the plate acts as the connecting element that spans the fracture.

Bone plates are most susceptible to bending forces because of their eccentric position relative to the bone's neutral axis. Their mode of placement determines the likelihood of fixation failure. If a transverse fracture is anatomically reduced and the plate compresses the fracture segments, the plate and the bony column share the loads and their large combined AMI creates a highly rigid construct. If the bone, especially the cortex opposite the plate, is not reconstructed, the plate alone must resist considerable bending forces. The bone plate is weakest at its screw holes (lowest AMI). Further, an open screw hole centered over the fracture functions as a stress concentrator and dramatically increases the risk of failure under bending loads. Several methods can be used to increase the AMI of the fixation. Lengthening plates are available where the middle section of the plate is solid (without screw holes). Another method is to combine an intramedullary pin with bone-plate fixation.[43] The bone plate constrains axial collapse and rotational forces, while the IM pin resists bending forces. By adding the pin, the AMI of the combined fixation is greatly increased and the fatigue life of the plate is greatly extended.

The limited-contact dynamic compression plate (LC-DCP) was designed with a scalloped profile to the underneath side of the plate that contacts the bone.[68] One effect of this scalloped contour is minimized stress-concentrating effect of an open screw hole because the AMI is similar over the length of the plate.[68] Granted, the solid section (between screw holes) of the LC-DCP is significantly weaker than the solid section of a traditional DCP, however, when screw holes are left unfilled the plate is only as strong as its weakest point.[69] Another advantage of the LC-DCP is that the scalloped "footprint" of the plate against the bone may allow for improved vascular supply to the healing bone, but other factors such as bone-surface topography also influence the relative significance of this feature.[70]

Whereas traditional plating depends on firm screw-insertion torque to compress the plate against the bone to ensure rigid fixation, newer locking-plate technology utilizes a locking screw mechanism to link the plate firmly to the fixation screw.[71] These locked screw-plate systems can be thought of as internal skeletal fixators. Because traditional plating does not link the plate and the screw, the screw is free to microtoggle within the plate hole. Bicortical purchase of traditional screws helps to reduce this microtoggling, which among other things, can lead to fretting failure of the plate or screw. Locking screws are rigidly fixed between the bone on one end and the plate on the other. For this reason, bicortical screw purchase is theoretically less important with locking screw-plate- systems. This may be a function of cortical bone thickness that is relatively thin in small animal patients. Pullout of locked screws is not just a function of the strength of their thread interlock in the bone, because the screw is also locked in the plate. Thus, premature screw loosening of a single locking screw is not likely. Further, the linkage between the fixation screw and the plate as a connecting element eliminates the mechanical need for compression of the plate against the bone surface. Because the threads on the screw head correspond to those in the screw hole of the plate, angling of screws is not possible and locking screw-plate systems are fixed-angle constructs. Further, dynamic compression cannot be achieved when only locking screws are used. Combined conventional and locking-screw techniques can be used, but require plate contouring on the end(s) of the plate where conventional screws are used. When conventional and locking screws are combined within a bone segment, the conventional screws are applied first to compress the contoured plate to the bone segment and to achieve the DCP effect (if desired). Locking screws are subsequently applied. If locking screws have been used to fix a plate to a fragment, subsequent insertion of conventional screws should not be performed without first loosening the locking screw (it can be retightened after insertion of all the traditional screws are in place). Dynamic compression can be achieved after one segment has been fixed with locking screws by using conventional screws in the dynamic compression portions of the plate hole.

External Skeletal Fixator

Linear ESF

The external skeletal fixation (ESF) system makes use of fixation pins, connecting bars, and pin-bar linkages. Each component of the system represents a mechanical variable that can be adjusted to the mechanical needs of the patient. Long-term stability of the pin-bone interface is foundational to success with ESF. Threaded pins provide much greater resistance to pin pullout than do nonthreaded pins.[72,73] Pins with a negative-thread profile have less pullout resistance than positive-profile pins in some but not all implantation sites.[74] Negative-thread profile pins are also more prone to breakage as a result of their decreased AMI and the stress concentration at the threaded-nonthreaded junction. Pin rigidity is also a function of pin diameter. As pin diameter increases, so does its AMI and flexural rigidity, but the impact of pin size on bone strength must also be considered. Proportionate loss of bone strength occurs with each increase in circular cortical defect size greater than 20% of the bone diameter.[13] ESF fixation strength and stiffness are increased by increasing the number of fixation pins in each fracture segment (unless the connecting column is the weakest component) up to a maximum of 4 pins per bone segment.[75,76] Evenly distributing pins throughout each main bone segment maximizes resistance to bending in the plane orthogonal to uniplanar ESFs.[75,77] Angling pins closest to the fracture zone in order to decrease the working length of the connecting bars may be advisable for highly comminuted, nonreconstructable fractures because the bending stiffness of the connecting bar is inversely related to its working length raised to the third power. The concept of working length and stiffness also applies to pin length. The connecting bar should be linked to the fixation pins as close as possible to the skin without causing skin irritation (usually a finger's width).[75,76] Linkage clamps should be oriented such that the working length of the pin is minimized.[75]

The rigidity of the connecting bar(s) significantly influences the strength and stiffness of the ESF-bone construct.[78-80] Elastic deformation of the connecting bar of unilateral-uniplanar (type Ia) frames places "to and fro" axial loads on the fixation pins.[80] Elastic deformation of the connecting bar can be minimized by using more rigid materials, increasing bar diameter, adding supplemental bars or plates, or utilizing more complex frame configurations.[78,79] Static strength evaluation of different configurations showed that unilateral-uniplanar (type Ia), unilateral-biplanar (type Ib), bilateral-uniplanar (type II), and bilateral-biplanar (type III) frames to be successively stronger in resisting axial compression and torsion, and bending in the plane of the ESF.[78,81] The ability of the pin-connecting bar linkage to rigidly maintain this interface is essential. In addition to clinical factors such as proper clamp assembly and tightening, clamp design also must be considered.[82,83]

Circular ESF

Circular ESF (CESF), like linear ESF, consists of fasteners (tensioned wires), connecting rods and wire-connecting rod linkages. Variations in these components can be manipulated to alter the mechanical properties of the CESF-bone construct. Unlike linear ESFs, CESFs utilize small-diameter wires tensioned between clamps positioned on rings rather than using traditional fixation pins to fasten the device to the bone. This design feature accounts for a fundamental difference between the load-deformation behavior of linear ESFs and CESFs.[84] Linear ESFs using half-pins loaded in cantilever bending have a linear elastic region of their load-deformation curve followed by plastic deformation to failure with progressive loading.[84,85] CESFs using small-diameter tensioned wires loaded in three- or four-point bending show initial nonlinear elasticity with increasing rigidity followed by linear progression to yield.[84,85] This characteristic difference reveals how CESF devices allow axial micromotion of the bone segments.

Ring diameter, which dictates wire length, profoundly influences the mechanical properties of CESF. As ring diameter increases, so does the length of the tensioned fastening wires, thereby decreasing fixation rigidity.[84-87] Although ring diameter affects stability in all loading modes, its most profound influence is on axial stability.[84,86] This influence is most evident at lower axial loads because self-tensioning of the wires develops during loading, resulting in a progressive increase in stiffness.[84] The smallest diameter ring possible should be used allowing about 2 cm between the skin and the ring for pin-tract care, soft-tissue swelling, etc. Ring diameter has a greater effect on gap stiffness and gap displacement than does wire tension, and the effect of increasing wire tension decreases for larger rings.[87] Complete rings are stiffer than incomplete rings.[88]

As for linear ESF, the bone fasteners (tensioned wires) should be spread over the length of each major bone segment; increasing the number of fasteners up to four per segment is advisable.[85,86,89] In CESF, tensioned wires are distributed over the bone using rings. Where possible, blocks of two rings distributed over the bone-segment length significantly increases the stability of the fixation when compared with configurations that secure individual bone segments at only one level (using a single ring).[85,86,89] Typically, one tensioned wire is placed above each ring and another below each ring for a total of two tensioned wires per ring. When only one ring can be used owing to a short bone-segment length, "drop wires" spanned from posts extending from the ring can be used to increase the number of fasteners and increase resistance to bending.[90]

Whereas much of the wire stiffness is a function of tensioning, wire stiffness is greater in larger diameter wires than in similarly tensioned smaller diameter wires. Wire diameter also influences how much a wire can be tensioned. Wire tension should not exceed 50% of its yield strength to minimize the possibility of breakage.[85] Wire tension affects the overall rigidity of the fixator construct, most notably axial stiffness during low load application. The relationship between wire tension and construct stiffness is nonlinear because of the self-tensioning effect of the wire.[84,85] Tensioning wires before loading increases the axial stiffness of a CESF at low loads, mitigating much of the displacement during physiologic loading. The practical limits of wire tensioning are associated with wire breakage, ring deformation, slippage of the wire within the clamp, and a "ceiling effect" beyond which the gain in axial stiffness is nominal.[84,85] During fixator application, sequential tensioning of wires on the same ring can cause loss of tension in the first wire owing to ring deformation. Simultaneous tensioning of wires on the same ring mitigates this effect, especially for large rings.[85] Subsequent study using 84 mm diameter rings faied to detect any, differences in wire strains or construct stiffness when compairing simultaneous and sequential wire tensioning methods.[91]

Ideally, tensioned wires are placed at 90° angles to one another to maximize stability and shear, but regional anatomy seldom allows this. Reducing the separation from 90° down to 45° particularly reduces the CESF's resistance to bending in the orthogonal plane.[90,91] Reducing this separation further can also lead to plastic deformation of the ring during wire tensioning.[90,92]

Hybrid linear and CESF has been used for stabilization of juxtaarticular fractures. Clinically, a linear ESF is utilized on the larger main fracture segment, and the tensioned wires and ring block are used on the small juxtaarticular segment. Combining fixation pins and tensioned wires within a segment is not advised because the axial motion permitted by the tensioned wires can place excessive stress on the pin-bone interfaces when few pins are used.[85]

Conclusion

A basic understanding of the biomechanics of the appendicular skeleton should include the material and structural properties of bone, the generation of internal stresses caused by applied loads, and common modes of failure under these applied loads. These understandings combined with knowledge of basic biomechanics of various fixation systems enhance the surgeon's ability to create an appropriately stable fracture zone that is conducive to rapid bone healing and restoration of patient function.

References

1. Nordin M, Frankel, VH: Biomechanics of Bone. *In* Basic Biomechanics of the Musculoskeletal System, 2 ed. Nordin M, Frankel VH (eds).Philadelphia: Lea & Febiger, 1989, pp. 3-30.

2. Paris O, Zizak I, Lichtenegger H, et al: Analysis of the hierarchical structure of biological tissues by scanning X-ray scattering using a micro-beam. Cell Mol Biol 46:993-1004, 2000.

3. Hulse D, Hyman, B: Fracture biology and biomechanics *In* Textbook of Small Animal Surgery, 3 ed. Slatter D (ed). Philadelphia: WB Saunders, 1993, pp. 1785-1792.

4. Radasch RM: Biomechanics of bone and fractures. Vet Clin North Am Small Anim Pract 29:1045-1082, 1999.

5. Schwarz PD: Fracture biomechanics of the appendicular skeleton: causes and assessment *In* Disease Mechanisms in in Small Animal

Surgery, 2nd ed. Bojrab M (ed). Philadelphia: Lea & Febiger, 1993, pp.1009-1026.

6. Hara Y, Nakamura T, Fukuda H, et al: Changes of biomechanical characteristics of the bone in experimental tibial osteotomy model in the dog. J Vet Med Sci 65:103-107, 2003.

7. Frank JD, Ryan M, Kalscheur VL, et al: Aging and accumulation of microdamage in canine bone. Bone 30:201-206, 2002.

8. Frost HM: Wolff's Law and bone's structural adaptations to mechanical usage: an overview for clinicians. Angle Orthod 64:175-188, 1994.

9. Frost HM: A 2003 update of bone physiology and Wolff's Law for clinicians. Angle Orthod 74:3-15, 2004.

10. Cowin SC: The mechanical properties of cancellous bone. Bone Mechanics. Boca Raton: CRC Press, 1989, pp. 130-155.

11. Cowin SC: The mechanical properties of cortical bone tissue. Bone Mechanics. Boca Raton: CRC Press, 1989, pp. 98-125.

12. Burstein AH, Currey J, Frankel VH, et al: Bone strength. The effect of screw holes. J Bone Joint Surg Am 54:1143-1156, 1972.

13. Edgerton BC, An KN, Morrey BF: Torsional strength reduction due to cortical defects in bone. J Orthop Res 8:851-855, 1990.

14. Ferguson JF: Fracture of the humerus after cancellous bone graft harvesting in a dog. J Small Anim Pract 37:232-234, 1996.

15. Rani R, Vairavasamy K, Kathiresan D: A retrospective study on bone fractures in canines. Indian Vet J 81:1048-1050, 2004.

16. Mair JJ, Belkoff SM, Boudrieau RJ: An ex vivo mechanical evaluation of single versus double semitubular plate fixation of a transverse distal-third scapular osteotomy in the dog. Vet Surg 32:580-584, 2003.

17. Piermattei D, Flo, GL: Handbook of Small Animal Orthopedics and Fracture Repair, 3 ed. Philadelphia: WB Saunders, 1997.

18. Unger M, Montavon PM, Heim UFA: Classification of fractures of long bones in the dog and cat: introduction and clinical application. Vet Compar Orthop Traumatol 3:41-50, 1990.

19. Bardet J, Hohn RB, Olmstead ML: Fractures of the humerus in dogs and cats: A retrospective study of 130 cases. Vet Surg 12:73-77, 1983.

20. Butterworth SJ, Innes JF: Incomplete humeral condylar fractures in the dog. J Small Anim Pract 42:394-398, 2001.

21. McKee WM, Macias C, Innes JF: Bilateral fixation of Y-T humeral condyle fractures via medial and lateral approaches in 29 dogs. J Small Anim Pract 46:217-226, 2005.

22. Cook JL, Tomlinson JL, Reed AL: Fluoroscopically guided closed reduction and internal fixation of fractures of the lateral portion of the humeral condyle: prospective clinical study of the technique and results in ten dogs. Vet Surg 28:315-321, 1999.

23. Miller A: Incomplete ossification of the humeral condyle in spaniels. Vet Surg 24:176, 1995.

24. Marcellin-Little DJ, DeYoung DJ, Ferris KK, et al: Incomplete ossification of the humeral condyle in spaniels. Vet Surg 23:475-487, 1994.

25. Larsen L, Roush JK, McLaughlin RM, Cash WC: Microangiography of the humeral condyle in cocker spaniel and non-cocker spaniel dogs. Vet Compar Orthop Traumatol 12(1-4); 134-137, 1999.

26. Meyer-Lindenberg A, Heinen V, Fehr M, Nolte I: Incomplete ossification of the humeral condyle as the cause of lameness in dogs. Vet Compar Orthop Traumatol 15:187-194, 2002.

27. Aron D, Foutz TL., Keller WG., Brown J: Experimental and clinical experience with an IM pin external skeletal fixator tie-in configuration. Vet Compar Orthop Traumatol 4:86-94, 1991.

28. Muir P, et al: Area moment of inertia for comparison of implant cross-sectional geometry and bending stiffness. Vet Compar Orthop Traumatol 8:146, 1995.

29. Brianza SZM, Delise M, Ferraris MM, et al: Cross-sectional geometrical properties of distal radius and ulna in large, medium and toy breed dogs. J Biomech 39:302-311, 2006.

30. Muir P, Johnson KA: Fractures of the proximal ulna in dogs. Vet Compar Orthop Traumatol 9:51-57, 1996.

31. Anderson GM, Cross AR, Lewis DD, et al: The effect of plate luting on reduction accuracy and biomechanics of acetabular osteotomies stabilized with 2.7-mm reconstruction plates. Vet Surg 31:3-9, 2002.

32. Stubbs WP, Lewis DD, Miller GJ, et al: A biomechanical evaluation and assessment of the accuracy of reduction of two methods of acetabular osteotomy fixation in dogs. Vet Surg 27:429-437, 1998.

33. Hardie RJ, Bertram JE, Todhunter RJ, et al: Biomechanical comparison of two plating techniques for fixation of acetabular osteotomies in dogs. Vet Surg 28:148-153, 1999.

34. VanGundy TE, Hulse DA, Nelson JK: Mechanical analysis of pelvic fractures. Proc. Vet Orthop Soc 1988; p.40.

35. Fitch R, Kerwin S, Hosgood G, et al: Radiographic evaluation and comparison of triple pelvic osteotomy with and without additional ventral plate stabilization in forty dogs - part 1. Vet Compar Orthop Traumatol 15:164-171, 2002.

36. Fitch R, Hosgood., Staatz A: Biomechanical evaluation of triple pelvic osteotomy with and without additional ventral plate stabilization. Vet Compar Orthop Traumatol 15:145-149, 2002.

37. Whelan MF, McCarthy RJ, Boudrieau RJ, et al: Increased sacral screw purchase minimizes screw loosening in canine triple pelvic osteotomy. Vet Surg 33:609-614, 2004.

38. Simmons S, Johnson AL, Schaeffer DJ: Risk factors for screw migration after triple pelvic osteotomy. J Am Anim Hosp Assoc 37:269-273, 2001.

39. Hosgood G, Lewis D: Retrospective evaluation of fixation complications of 49 pelvic osteotomies in 36 dogs. J Small Anim Pract 34:123-130, 1993.

40. Braden TD, Brinker WO, Little RW, et al: Comparative biomechanical evaluation of bone healing in the dog. J Am Vet Med Assoc 163:65-69, 1973.

41. McNicholas WT Jr, Wilkens BE, Blevins WE, et al: Spontaneous femoral capital physeal fractures in adult cats: 26 cases (1996-2001). J Am Vet Med Assoc 221:1731-1736, 2002.

42. Beaupre GS, Carter DR, Dueland RT, et al: A biomechanical assessment of plate fixation, with insufficient bony support. J Orthop Res 6:721-729, 1988.

43. Hulse D, Hyman W, Nori M, et al: Reduction in plate strain by addition of an intramedullary pin. Vet Surg 26:451-459, 1997.

44. Hulse D, Ferry K, Fawcett A, et al: Effect of intramedullary pin size on reducing bone plate strain. Vet Compar Orthop Traumatol 13:185-190, 2000.

45. Dewey C, Aron, DN, Foutz TL, et al: Static strength evaluation of the two modified unilateral external skeletal fixators. J Small Anim Pract 35:211-216, 1994.

46. Braden T, Eicker SW, Abdinoor D, Prieur WD: Characteristics of 1000 femur fractures in the dog and cat. Vet Compar Orthop Traumatol 8:203-209, 1995.

47. Sukhiani HR, Holmberg DL: Ex vivo biomechanical comparison of pin fixation techniques for canine distal femoral physeal fractures. Vet Surg 26:398-407, 1997.

48. Hupel TM, Aksenov SA, Schemitsch EH: Cortical bone blood flow in loose and tight fitting locked unreamed intramedullary nailing: a canine segmental tibia fracture model. J Orthop Trauma 12:127-135, 1998.

49. Klein MP, Rahn BA, Frigg R, et al: Reaming versus non-reaming in medullary nailing: interference with cortical circulation of the canine tibia. Arch Orthop Trauma Surg 109:314-316, 1990.

50. Rudy RL: Principles of intramedullary pinning. Vet Clin North Am Small Anim Pract 5:209, 1975.

51. Hatch V: Initial experience with a newly developed medullary stabilization nail (Trilam nail). Vet Compar Orthop Traumatol 13:109-114, 2000.

52. Vasseur PB, Paul HA, Crumley L: Evaluation of fixation devices for prevention of rotation in transverse fractures of the canine femoral shaft: an in vitro study. Am J Vet Res 45:1504-1507, 1984.

53. Bernarde A, Diop A, Maurel N, et al: An in vitro biomechanical study of bone plate and interlocking nail in a canine diaphyseal femoral fracture model. Vet Surg 30:397-408, 2001.

54. von Pfeil DJ, Dejardin LM, DeCamp CE, et al: In vitro biomechanical comparison of a plate-rod combination-construct and an interlocking nail-construct for experimentally induced gap fractures in canine tibiae. Am J Vet Res 66:1536-1543, 2005.

55. Horstman CL, Beale BS, Conzemius MG, et al: Biological osteosynthesis versus traditional anatomic reconstruction of 20 long-bone fractures using an interlocking nail: 1994-2001. Vet Surg 33:232-237, 2004.

56. Dueland RT, Berglund L, Vanderby R Jr, et al: Structural properties of interlocking nails, canine femora, and femur-interlocking nail constructs. Vet Surg 25:386-396, 1996.

57. Dueland RT, Johnson KA, Roe SC, et al: Interlocking nail treatment of diaphyseal long-bone fractures in dogs. J Am Vet Med Assoc 214:59-66, 1999.

58. Dueland RT, Vanderby R, McCabe RP: Fatigue study of 6 and 8mm diameter interlocking nails with screw holes of variable size and number. Vet Compar Orthop Traumatol 10:194-199, 1997.

59. Aper RL, Litsky AS, Roe SC, et al: Effect of bone diameter and eccentric loading on fatigue life of cortical screws used with interlocking nails. Am J Vet Res 64:569-573, 2003.

60. Nanai B, Basinger RR: Use of a new investigational interlocking nail supplement in the repair of comminuted diaphyseal tibia fractures in two dogs. J Am Anim Hosp Assoc 41:203-208, 2005.

61. Basinger RR, Suber JT: Two techniques for supplementing interlocking nail repair of fractures of the humerus, femur, and tibia: results in 12 dogs and cats. Vet Surg 33:673-680, 2004.

62. Durall I, Falcon C, Diaz-Bertrana MC, et al: Effects of static fixation and dynamization after interlocking femoral nailing locked with an external fixator: an experimental study in dogs. Vet Surg 33:323-332, 2004.

63. Roe SC: Internal fracture fixation. *In* Textbook of Small Animal Surgery, 3 ed. Slatter D (ed). Philadelphia: Saunders, 2003, p. 1798.

64. Roe SC: Mechanical characteristics and comparisons of cerclage wires: introduction of the double-wrap and loop/twist tying methods. Vet Surg 26:310-316, 1997.

65. Rooks RL, et al: In vitro cerclage wire analysis. Vet Surg 11:39-43, 1982.

66. Roe SC: Evaluation of tension obtained by use of three knots for tying cerclage wires by surgeons of various abilities and experience. J Am Vet Med Assoc 220:334-336, 2002.

67. Wilson JW, Belloli DM, Robbins T: Resistance of cerclage to knot failure. J Am Vet Med Assoc 187:389-391, 1985.

68. Perren SM, Allgower M, Brunner H, et al: The concept of biological plating using the limited contact-dynamic compression plate (LC-DCP): Scientific background, design and application. Injury 222 (Suppl. 1):1-41, 1991.

69. Little FM, Hill CM, Kageyama T, et al: Bending properties of stainless steel dynamic compression plates and limited contact dynamic compression plates. Vet Compar Orthop Traumatol 14:64-68, 2001.

70. Jain R, Podworny N, Hupel TM, et al: Influence of plate design on cortical bone perfusion and fracture healing in canine segmental tibial fractures. J Orthop Trauma 13:178-186, 1999.

71. Egol KA, Kubiak EN, Fulkerson E, et al: Biomechanics of locked plates and screws. J Orthop Trauma 18:488-493, 2004.

72. Anderson MA, Mann FA, Wagner-Mann C, et al: A comparison of nonthreaded, enhanced threaded, and Ellis fixation pins used in type I external skeletal fixators in dogs. Vet Surg 22:482-489, 1993.

73. Bennett RA, Egger EL, Histand M, et al: Comparison of the strength and holding power of 4 pin designs for use with half pin (type I) external skeletal fixation. Vet Surg 16:207-211, 1987.

74. Palmer R, Hulse DA, Pollo FE, et al: Pin loosening in external skeletal fixation: the effects of pin design and implantation site. Vet Surg (abstr) 20:343, 1991.

75. Bouvy BM, Markel MD, Chelikani S, et al: Ex vivo biomechanics of Kirschner-Ehmer external skeletal fixation applied to canine tibiae. Vet Surg 22:194-207, 1993.

76. Palmer RH, Hulse DA, Hyman WA, Palmer DR: Principles of bone healing and biomechanics of external skeletal fixation. Vet Clin North Am Small Anim Pract 22:45-68, 1992.

77. Behrens F, Johnson W: Methods to increase and reduce frame stiffness. Clin Orthop Relat Res 241:48-56, 1989.

78. White DT, Bronson DG, Welch RD: A mechanical comparison of veterinary linear external fixation systems. Vet Surg 32:507-514, 2003.

79. Norris JL, Kraus KH, O'Leary JP: Effect of a supplemental plate on the stiffness of a type I external fixator. Vet Surg 31:133-137, 2002.

80. Pollo F, Hyman WA, Hulse DA: The role of the external bar in a 6-pin type 1 external skeletal fixation device. Vet Compar Orthop Traumatol 6:75-79, 1993.

81. Egger EL: Static strength evaluation of six external skeletal fixation configurations. Vet Surg 12:130-136, 1983.

82. Gilley RS, Bourgeault CA, Wallace LJ, et al: A comparative mechanical study of 3 external fixator clamps. Vet Surg 30:341-350, 2001.

83. Kraus KH, Wotton HM, Rand WM: Mechanical comparison of two external fixator clamp designs. Vet Surg 27:224-230, 1998.

84. Gasser B, Boman B, Wyder D, et al: Stiffness characteristics of the circular Ilizarov device as opposed to conventional external fixators. J Biomech Eng 112:15-21, 1990.

85. Lewis DD, Bronson DG, Samchukov ML, et al: Biomechanics of circular external skeletal fixation. Vet Surg 27:454-464, 1998.

86. Bronson DG: Effect of individual components on the mechanical stability of the Ilizarov external fixation device. Dallas: University of Texas Southwestern Medical Center, 1995.

87. Cross AR, Lewis DD, Murphy ST, et al: Effects of ring diameter and wire tension on the axial biomechanics of four-ring circular external skeletal fixator constructs. Am J Vet Res 62:1025-1030, 2001.

88. Cross AR, Lewis DD, Rigaud S, et al: Effect of various distal ring-block configurations on the biomechanical properties of circular external skeletal fixators for use in dogs and cats. Am J Vet Res 65:393-398, 2004.

89. Calhoun JH, Li F, Ledbetter BR, et al: Biomechanics of the Ilizarov fixator for fracture fixation. Clin Orthop 280:15-22, 1992.

90. Orbay GL, Frankel VH, Kummer FJ: The effect of wire configuration on the stability of the Ilizarov external fixator. Clin Orthop Relat Res 279:299-302, 1992.

91. Ryan S, Ehrhart N, Zuehlsdorff K, James S. Comparison of a alternate and simultaneous tensioning of wire in a single-ring fixator construct. Vet Surg 38:96-103, 2009.

92. Kummer FJ. Biomechanics of the Ilizarov external fixator. Clin Orthop Relat Res 280:11-14, 1992.

Chapter 109

Growth Plate Injuries

Derek B. Fox

Growth plates, or physes, are composed of several merged layers that produce longitudinal growth of the long bones by the method of endochondral ossification. Physeal damage is not uncommon in the small animal and can result from trauma, genetic disorders, nutritional imbalances, or other medical disturbances. The physis can be either completely or partially damaged and injuries can vary in their subsequent extensiveness from total growth arrest to retardation. Common sequelae of physeal injury include shortened limbs, angular limb deformation, and adjacent joint subluxation. Angulations can occur in multiple planes depending on the location of the growth plate damage and whether the affected bone is anatomically paired with another long bone, as with the radius and ulna. Malalignment can be in the frontal plane, resulting in varus and/or valgus deformities, or in the sagittal plane, causing pro- or recurvatum and rotationally causing internal or external bone torsion. A thorough understanding of the resulting pathology from physeal injury necessitates a discussion of the anatomy and physiology of the growth plate.

Growth Plate Anatomy

Although the physiology of the individual layers of the growth plate is unique, the functional unit of the physis can be summarized as a column of chondrocytes that proliferate, hypertrophy, and synthesize matrix before ultimately undergoing apoptosis.[1] These functions are intimately regulated intrinsically by growth factors and mechanical forces and extrinsically both hormonally and mechanically. The growth plate can be divided into its various layers both morphologically and functionally. As such, a standard set of descriptive terms for the layers does not exist and will vary widely depending on the author. For purposes of this discussion, a functional scheme of evaluation is presented including the 1) germinal zone; 2) columnar zone with upper proliferating area and lower maturation area; 3) hypertrophic zone with an upper four fifths possessing nonmineralized matrix and lower one fifth with mineralized matrix; and 4) outer metaphysis (Figure 109-1). The cells within the germinal zone are also frequently referred to as resting cells because they do not proliferate.[2] The small, irregularly spaced cells in the germinal zone contain a high concentration of lipid within their vacuolar contents, suggesting their important role in nutrient storage.[3]

The upper portion of the columnar zone represents the only aspect of the growth plate in which chondrocytes undergo division. The active division in this area results in the stacking of flattened cells into columns that are separated from each other by large conglomerations of type II collagen. This proliferating portion of the columnar zone is high in oxygen content and undergoes active glycogen storage by the chondrocytes.[4,5] The high concentration of rough endoplasmic reticulum within chondrocytes in the lower half of the columnar zone dictates their role in extensive matrix synthesis.[1]

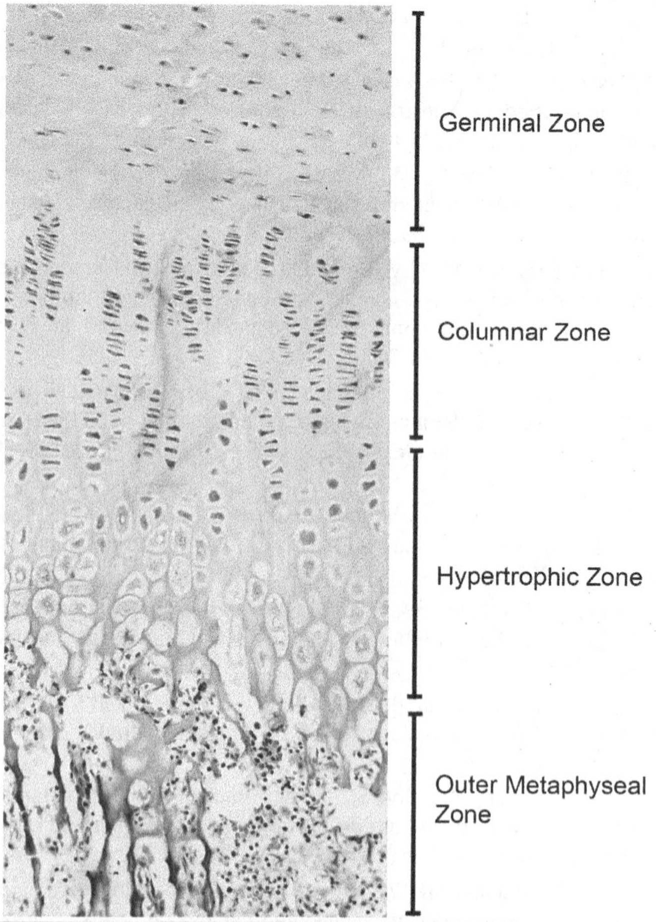

Figure 109-1. Photomicrograph of a normal canine growth plate stained with hematoxylin and eosin and labeled for the four primary functional zones: germinal zone, columnar zone, hypertrophic zone, and outer metaphyseal zone. The proximal aspect of the bone is at the top of the photograph. (Courtesy of Dr. Keiichi Kuroki.)

The hypertrophic zone of the physis is the driving force of longitudinal bone growth through cell expansion. The chondrocytes of this zone increase their intracellular volume anywhere from 5- to 10-fold. Variation in the rate of chondrocyte hypertrophy is now thought to be the main reason for different anatomically located physes to grow at different rates.[6] Like the lower half of the columnar zone, the cells of the hypertrophic zone also possess a highly active metabolism that is responsible for large quantities of matrix synthesis. In addition to abundant type II collagen, both type X collagen and vascular endothelial growth factor (VEGF) are produced in the hypertrophic zone. The production of these elements is a hallmark for cellular differentiation and the ceasing of cellular division. These processes occur in an environment that is lower in oxygen tension and in which glycogen is consumed by the chondrocytes until depleted.[4,5] In the lower one fifth of this zone, the matrix is modified for calcification and vascularization. Whereas recruitment for vessel ingrowth is signaled by the release of VEGF, matrix mineralization is mediated by budding vesicles formed from the chondrocyte plasma membrane.[7] The vesicles contain calcium and enzymes, including both alkaline phosphatase and matrix metalloproteinase (MMP).[1] Newly deposited matrix then forms in longitudinal septa between the columns of chondrocytes and primarily consists of crystalline hydroxyapatite. The septa eventually become primary trabeculae as the upper two thirds are resorbed by chondroclasts and the distal third acts as a scaffolding for osteoid deposition from osteoblasts.[7] Within the mineralized cartilage, matrix forms a transverse septum that is invaded by capillary loops from the metaphysis as they penetrate the distal hypertrophic chondrocyte lacunae. The differentiated chondrocytes then undergo caspase-mediated programmed apoptosis.[8]

Finally, the zone of the outer metaphysis is the area where the endochondral ossification process yields true bone tissue through remodeling of the primary trabeculae into trabeculae of lamellar bone, or secondary trabeculae.[7] This remodeling is mediated by a variety of cells, including undifferentiated mesenchymal cells, preosteoblasts, and osteoblasts in addition to the metaphyseal vascular system.[1] The combined areas of the distal hypertrophic zone and proximal metaphysis are also often referred to as the zone of provisional calcification.

Whereas the layers described above provide for longitudinal growth, they do not account for the necessary increasing width of the physis during bone development. The growth plate zones are thus circumscribed by a wedge-shaped area of chondrocyte progenitor cells known as the perichondrial ossification groove of Ranvier, which contributes germinal cells to allow expansion of the bone's width at the physis. Within this groove is the fibrous ring of LaCroix, which contains fibers arranged vertically, circumferentially, and obliquely to provide mechanical support in response to compression, tension, and shear loads on the physis.[1,7]

During the late embryonic phase of development, the epiphyseal cartilages of the long bones are well vascularized, with vessels frequently crossing the physes either partially or completely.[1] Following birth, the transphyseal vascular bridging is eliminated resulting in the physeal vasculature arising from two separate sources. Epiphyseal vessels supply the germinating, proliferating, and upper hypertrophic zones through diffusion, and separate metaphyseal vessels permeate to the level of the distal hypertrophic zone. The epiphyseal and metaphyseal vessels normally only anastomose once the physis has closed, marking the onset of skeletal maturity.[9] Premature vascular anastomosis across the physis results in pathologic closure of the growth plate. Alteration in this specific vascular pattern can result in aberrant long-bone development at the level of the physis. Disruption of the epiphyseal blood supply is the most devastating injury to the physeal growth plate vasculature. Epiphyseal vessel damage can cause avascular necrosis of both the germinal chondrocytes and secondary ossification center of the epiphysis, resulting in ossification of the growth plate and premature cessation of growth. To the contrary, injury of the metaphyseal vasculature can result in transitory increases in physeal growth.[1,7]

Growth Plate Physiology

A complex and multifactorial array of factors regulate control over a variety of growth-plate functions including cell proliferation, maturation, hypertrophy and apoptosis, matrix synthesis and mineralization, vascular infiltration, and ultimately physeal closure. Ongoing studies elucidating many of these processes are shedding new light on the disease processes that result in growth-plate dysfunction. Major regulating factors are hormones, growth factors, vitamins, and biomechanical forces.

Chondrocyte proliferation within the growth plate is believed to be under the primary control of a local negative feedback loop involving three signaling molecules synthesized by growth-plate chondrocytes: parathyroid hormone-related peptide (PTHrP), Indian hedgehog (Ihh), and transforming growth factor-beta (TGF-β).[5,7,10] The release of Ihh by cells newly undergoing hypertrophic differentiation triggers the release of TGF-β by the perichondrium, which in turn stimulates perichondrial and juxtaarticular cells to increase synthesis of PTHrP, thus slowing the progression of proliferating cells expressing the PTHrP receptor from advancing into the hypertrophic stage.[10] This feedback loop is not exclusive in its control of cell proliferation within the growth plate and is greatly modulated by a number of other systemic and local signaling molecules including the fibroblast growth factor (FGF) family and its receptors.[11] In addition, growth hormone (GH) produced in the anterior pituitary, and its mediator, insulin-like growth factor (IGF), play important roles in physeal chondrocyte proliferation. Chondrocyte maturation and hypertrophy appear to occur spontaneously largely through the actions of the bone morphogenic proteins (BMPs) and their receptors.[12] The peptide hormone thyroxine (T4) can only induce chondrocyte maturation and production of type X collagen through induction of BMP-2.[13] Because hypertrophy can occur spontaneously, negative inhibitors are likely to be crucially important in the regulation of growth-plate kinetics. Once the chondrocytes have terminally differentiated, their purpose is to foster matrix calcification in preparation for osteoblastic bone formation.[7] Subsequent death and removal of the chondrocyte then allows space for infiltrating vasculature and bone marrow stromal cells.[14] It is now accepted that the death of terminally differentiated chondrocytes occurs through highly regulated apoptosis, or programmed cell death. Alteration in the normal caspase-mediated apoptotic process through mutation of regulating FGF receptors is now suspected to be the cause of achondroplasia, or dwarfism.[15] The administration of both glucocorticoids and radiation to juvenile animals has been shown to increase the rates of hypertrophic chondrocyte apoptosis, and can alter the shape and normal activity of the growth plate.[16,17,18]

Matrix synthesis in the growth plate is thought to be regulated by many of the same factors that direct the development and differentiation of physeal chondrocytes. One transcription factor in particular, Sox 9, binds with various related proteins to specific enhancer regions in the promoter regions of genes expressing types II, IX, and XI collagen and aggrecan.[19] Mineralization of the secreted matrix is an essential precursor to the conversion of the chondroid nature of the growth plate to bone. As previously stated, matrix vesicles serve as the principal site for matrix mineralization within the lower hypertrophic zone largely through their accumulation of calcium and alkaline phosphatase. The accretion of calcium is dependent on the calcium channel molecule family of annexins.[20] An interesting relationship exists between type X collagen and annexin V. Type X collagen, present exclusively within the hypertrophic zone of the physis, is able to bind to matrix vesicles with the assistance of annexin V and subsequently stimulates its activity, thus facilitating calcium deposition.[7,21] Although still incompletely characterized, the likely function of the vesicular alkaline phosphatase is the hydrolysis of pyrophosphate, an inhibitor of hydroxyapatite crystal formation, into two molecules of orthophosphate.[22] Vitamin D is well known for its critical influence on increasing both alkaline phosphatase and MMPs within the chondrocyte. In particular, MMP-13, present within matrix vesicles, is important for the cleavage of type II collagen and the activation of latent TGF-β, both of which are associated with the onset of matrix mineralization.[23,24]

Following matrix mineralization, vascular invasion from the metaphyseal side of the physis is an essential precursor to ossification. The process of vascularization is multifactorial but is largely mediated through the actions of VEGF expressed by hypertrophic chondrocytes and targeting vascular endothelial cells, stimulating their proliferation and migration.[25] Another growth factor that has been shown to possess pro-angiogenic characteristics is basic FGF.[26] Failure of appropriate vascularization results in disruption of normal physeal architecture and widening of the hypertrophic zone with diminished trabecular bone formation.[7] Physeal closure is associated with a decrease in chondrocyte proliferation, resulting in a diminished height of both proliferative and hypertrophic zones. In most mammals, the epiphysis and metaphysis become fused with resorption of the growth plate following sexual maturity. Some evidence suggests that physeal closure is estrogen-mediated through promotion of chondrocyte-replicative senescence and not through vascular invasion or ossification.[27]

Fractures of the Growth Plate

A thorough understanding of the mechanical properties of the growth plate has yet to be achieved. Large variation exists among studies, attributable to differences in animal models and their respective ages, test parameters, and the anatomic locations tested. Because the physes represent both the sole source of skeletal longitudinal growth as well as the weakest point of the juvenile skeleton, an understanding of growth-plate biomechanics and modes of failure is essential. Growth-plate fractures are common and can result in significant alteration of physiologic growth function. A close relationship exists between the ultrastructural properties of the physeal extracellular matrix and its mechanical behavior. In cadaveric testing, the germinal and proliferating portion of the columnar zones are somewhat protected from excessive external force owing to a more random organization of collagen fibers and overall higher concentration of collagen.[28] Experimentally, the hypertrophic zone may represent the weakest region within the growth plate during tensile loading owing to the lower concentration and more regular organization of collagen in addition to the parallel chondrocyte orientation with respect to the longitudinal axis of the bone.[5] The clinical situation may differ greatly, however, with differences in anatomic sites and complexity of offending forces.

A commonly used classification system of growth-plate fractures intended to correlate the characteristics and prognoses of each fracture configuration was proposed by Salter and Harris.[29] Salter-Harris fractures have been covered in more detail previously within this text but are briefly discussed here in the context of physeal injuries. Using this classification system, physeal fractures can be categorized into one of five types. Type I fractures represent a displacement of the epiphysis from the metaphysis with no associated bone fracture as a result of shearing and tensile forces. Type I fractures are more common in younger animals (< 6 months of age) and were classically thought to carry more favorable prognoses owing to the larger thickness of the physis at this age and limitations of the fractures to the hypertrophic zone.[30] Several clinical reports now contradict this, however, and important exceptions should be noted. A high incidence of damage to the proliferating portion of the columnar physeal zone has been reported in naturally occurring type I fractures in the dog, explaining the common clinical observation of growth retardation.[31] Additional exceptions occur with specific anatomic sites including the femoral capital physis, which may see direct disruption of ascending epiphyseal vasculature along the femoral neck, resulting in secondary femoral neck resorption. This has been documented to occur in as many as 70% of affected patients following surgery and ultimately necessitated femoral head and neck excision in 20% of cases in one report.[32,33]

Salter-Harris type II fractures occur along the length of the growth plate but extend into the metaphysis, resulting in a wedge-shaped metaphyseal fragment that remains attached to the epiphysis. The side on which the metaphyseal fragment occurs is related to the direction of the impacting force and subsequent bending of the bone. Most metaphyseal fragments remain adhered to the epiphyseal component on the concave aspect of the deformed bone during impact.

Type III fractures are intraarticular in that an epiphyseal fracture communicates with the fissure extending along the growth plate. With disruption of the articular cartilage and subchondral bone, a higher likelihood exists for postoperative osteoarthritis. Goals for surgical treatment include accurate reduction and fixation of the articular components to reestablish the joint surface.

Type IV fractures consist of type III fractures with the addition of a metaphyseal extension of the epiphyseal injury. Like type III fractures, type IV fractures are intraarticular and thus require perfect anatomic reduction to reduce the risk of secondary osteoarthritis. Displaced type IV fractures must also be accurately reduced to minimize the risk of formation of a bone bridge along the fracture line that extends from the joint across the physis and into metaphysis, resulting in subsequent growth retardation.[5]

Type V Salter-Harris fractures are classically described as compression fractures of the growth plate. The offending compression is theorized to result in necrosis of proliferating chondrocytes of the growth plate, resulting in overall growth arrest of the bone if the entire physis is affected or angular limb deformities if only a portion of the physis is involved. The most commonly affected location in the dog is the distal ulnar physis because of its unique conical shape. In cases in which the distal ulna is affected without concomitant involvement of the distal radius, antebrachial deformation ensues in the form of excessive procurvatum, external rotation, and carpal valgus.

Again, caution should be used in extrapolating prognosis based on radiographic interpretations of fracture configurations. Numerous other factors that are difficult or impossible to assess radiographically have a tremendous impact on the response of the bone as it heals, including the post-traumatic status of epiphyseal vasculature, the physeal zone affected, and the nature of insulting forces creating the fracture.

Pathologic States Affecting the Growth Plate

Irradiation

Although much more frequently diagnosed in people, juvenile osteosarcoma has been reported in dogs.[34] Palliative treatment of bone tumors with various forms of radiation has been investigated in several juvenile animal models, elucidating the negative impact radiation has on growth-plate physiology. It has been determined that the proliferating cells of the upper portion of the columnar zone and epithelial cells of the metaphyseal vasculature are the most radiosensitive cellular populations of the growth plate.[35,36] Studies investigating the effects of a β-particle-emitting radionuclide on physeal growth and development in skeletally immature rabbits revealed decreased production of type X collagen and MMP-13 in hypertrophic chondrocytes with subsequent limb shortening in treated animals.[18]

Bacterial

Bacteria are capable of invading the metaphyseal portion of the growth plate causing microabcessation through vascular sinusoids. Although it is not clearly understood why these infections occur, theories include reduced blood velocity through the torturous vascular system, low oxygen tension, and deficiencies in the reticuloendothelial system.[5] Likely to be more common in the horse and human, bacterial physitis has been reported to occur in the dog most frequently in the lumbar vertebra, where it causes lucent widening of the growth plate and loss of definition of the physeal margins.[37] Although collapse of the physis and subsequent sclerosis typically ensues, secondary sequestration has been reported requiring sequestrectomy and long-term antimicrobial therapy.[38]

Endocrine

As previously described, the physes function under intimate guidance by the various components of the endocrine system. Endocrine diseases, therefore, can result in alteration of normal growth-plate physiology and secondary skeletal deformities. It is important to note that some features typical of endocrine disorders are often accepted as breed characteristics in the dog.[39] Increases (gigantism) or decreases (dwarfism) in body size can be considered normal and classified as constitutional, as the result of complex genetic effects, or abnormal, as the result of endocrinopathies or other complex disorders. Each condition can exist either proportionately or disproportionately, depending on whether the appendicular and axial skeletal components are altered in synchrony.

The anterior pituitary gland, under the stimulation of the hypothalamus, releases growth hormone, which plays an important role in chondrocyte proliferation, physeal development, and bone growth. Alterations in available concentrations of growth hormone result in developmental skeletal disorders. Reduction in levels of growth hormone production by the anterior pituitary gland typically results in proportionate dwarfism, which is a rare but well documented disorder in the dog, most frequently affecting the German shepherd dog (Figure 109-2). In this breed, hypopituitary dwarfism is known to be an autosomal inherited disorder.[40] In most of these cases, intrapituitary cysts exist and enlarge with age; suprapituitary stimulation does not increase the release of GH or thyroid stimulating hormone (TSH).[41] Hypopituitary dwarfs demonstrate retarded bone development and delayed epiphyseal fusion.[42] The growth plates may remain open for years, and possess architectural derangement of the proliferating chondrocyte arrangement and intercellular matrix.[42]

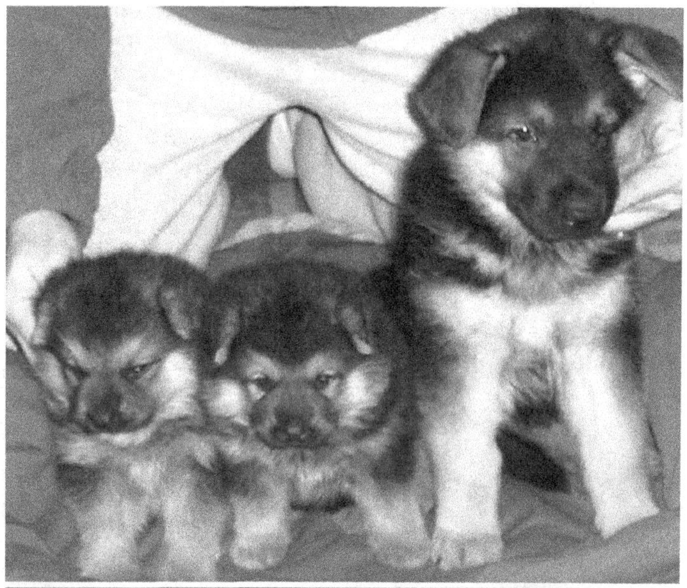

Figure 109-2. Photograph of three German shepherd dog littermates, aged 6.5 weeks. The two puppies on the left represent proportional hypopituitary dwarfs. (Courtesy of Ms. Susie Zeiner and Mr. John Walker.)

True hyperpituitary gigantism (acromegaly) is rare in small animals. Normal giant breeds of dogs represent proportional constitutional gigantism, and may possess the features frequently associated with acromegaly in humans, including bone thickening of the supraoribtal frontal bones and enlarged paws manus and pedes. Interestingly, GH levels are normal in these dogs, but concentrations of IGF-1 may be elevated.[43] An acromegalic syndrome in cats is documented, which occurs in middle-aged to older animals, associated with GH-secreting tumors of the pituitary gland with many clinical sequelae; however, the age of onset obviates growth-plate involvement.

Congenital or juvenile-onset hypothyroidism has been frequently documented in the dog. The skeletal manifestations of this disorder include delay in time of ossification of the epiphyseal centers (epiphyseal dysgenesis) and physeal closure, stunted growth, and disproportionate dwarfism (Figure109-3).[42,44] Familial congenital hypothyroidism has been documented in Scottish deerhounds,[45] giant schnauzers,[46] boxers,[47] and toy fox terriers.[48] Some evidence suggests that, if a diagnosis can be made at an early age (< 4 months), appropriate treatment can result in remission.[46]

A close association exists between the sex steroids, estrogen and testosterone, and the onset of skeletal maturity. Whereas androgen alone does not affect growth-plate closure, estrogen accelerates physeal fusion and terminates linear growth.[49] Androgens are converted to estrogens via aromatization in the male, such that estrogen mediates growth termination in both genders. Thus, prepubertal surgical gonadectomy can affect bone development. Salmeri et al determined that radial and ulnar growth-plate closure was delayed in dogs by 4 months if surgical gonadectomy was completed at 7 weeks of age, and by 3 months if gonadectomy was completed at 7 months of age.[50] Although not examined in this study, it was suspected that animals neutered prior to skeletal maturity might be more susceptible to sustaining traumatic Salter-Harris fractures for a longer time.[50] Subsequently, spontaneous, atraumatic fractures of the capital physis in male cats have now been shown to be linked with prepubertal gonadectomy.[51] This population of cats still possessed open growth plates at a mean age of 94.5 weeks, suggesting that the diminished presence of androgens could have resulted in delayed growth-plate closure and thus posed a higher risk for fractures.[51]

Chondrodysplasias

Chondrodysplasia is a general term referring to any number of disturbances in the development of the cartilaginous growth plates, primarily of the long bones. It frequently results in achondroplasia, which is disproportionate dwarfism, where the long bones of the appendicular skeleton are shortened but the axial components, including skull and vertebral column, are of normal size. Many types of chondrodysplasia have been documented and are cited as specific entities particular to certain breeds. Again, these disorders are distinguished from constitutional dwarfism owing to chondrodystrophy, which is accepted as a nonpathologic breed standard in many types of dog (e.g., Basset hounds, Welsh corgis, and beagles). Brief descriptions of various reported chondrodysplasias are discussed; however the reader is referred to pathology texts and listed references for more detailed descriptions of each.

Pseudoachondroplastic dysplasia has been documented in both miniature poodles and Scottish deerhounds, although the disease has characteristics unique to each breed.[52,53] However, the condition is likely to be autosomal recessive in both breeds and is first recognized when the animals are several weeks old. Although histologic changes of the physeal derangements are specific and well described for the different breeds, linear growth of the long bones only reaches approximately 65% of that of normal dogs of like breed.[52,53,54] By the time the animals achieve skeletal maturity, severe angular limb deformities are noted, with subsequent marked joint laxity.

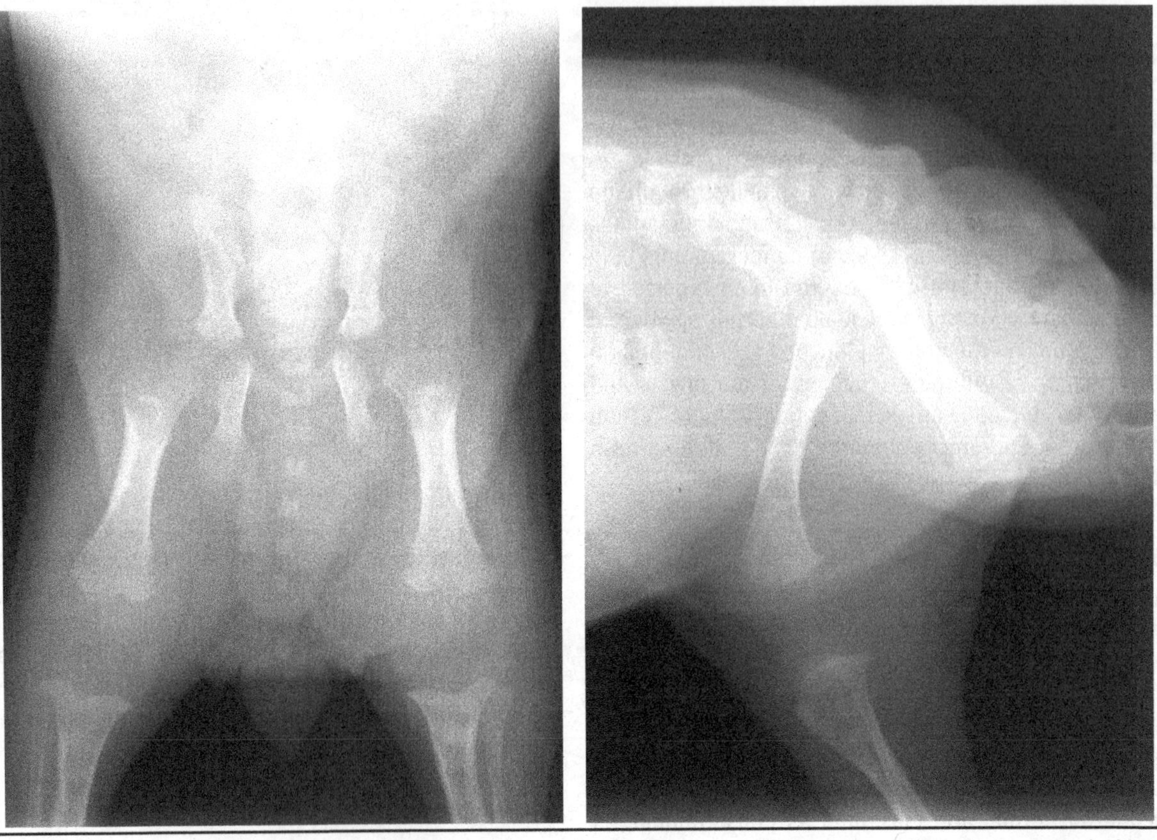

Figure 109-3. Orthogonal radiographs of the pelvis of a 5-month-old intact female miniature schnauzer puppy that was presented with a nonspecific history of chronic lethargy. The animal was diagnosed with congenital hypothyroidism. Note the complete lack of ossification of the epiphyseal centers (epiphyseal dysgenesis). (Courtesy of Dr. Valerie Samii.)

A condition has been documented to affect young beagle dogs called *multiple epiphyseal dysplasia*, in which stippled mineralizations can be radiographically detected in the epiphyses of the femur, humerus, and carpal and tarsal bones.[55,56] Clinical and radiographic signs are first detected at 3 to 4 weeks of age; however, they typically resolve with development and are no longer apparent by 5 months of age.[42] Affected dogs may possess osteoarthritis as adults, attributable to the abnormal epiphyseal development.

Specific chondrodysplasias have now been documented for several canine breeds. The condition is well documented in the Alaskan malamute, in which a disproportionate dwarfism with concurrent macrocytic hemolytic anemia results from the autosomal recessive disorder. Among other clinical sequelae, hallmarks of the disease include derangement of the proliferative zone of the physes and abnormal endochondral ossification that is radiographically most apparent as flattened distal ulnar physes and retarded ossification of cuboid bones detected between 4 and 12 weeks.[42,57] A similar chondrodysplasia causing disproportionate dwarfism in Norwegian elkhounds has been documented, with a distinguishing characteristic being shortened vertebral bodies.[58] Chondrodysplastic dwarfism with vertebral malformation has been described in great Pyrenees, which also exhibit concurrent deafness.[59] Dwarfism has also been reported as autosomal rececssive traits owing to chondrodysplasia in the English pointer and Irish setter breeds.[42,60]

Oculo-skeletal dysplasia has been reported in both the Labrador retriever and Samoyed breeds.[61,62] Aside from the ocular pathology, which includes cataracts and retinal dysplasia, affected animals may also be chondrodysplastic dwarfs with more severely affected forelimbs. Secondary changes can include fragmented coronoid processes, ununited anconeal processes, and hip dysplasia. In the Labrador, the severity of dwarfism is positively correlated with the extent of microscopic degeneration of the physeal chondrocytes, detected in part by the presence of cytoplasmic inclusions.[63]

Nutritional

Many nutritional disorders can affect bone physiology, and with respect to the growth plate specifically, it is well documented that certain dietary alterations can cause pathologic changes to physeal architecture and development. Diets low in vitamin D and phosphorus can result in rickets, causing derangement of the normal chondrocyte columns within the physes, an inability to appropriately calcify the matrix surrounding the hypertrophied cells, and diminished vascular invasion from the metaphysis necessary for physeal closure.[39] Large projections of uncalcified cartilage subsequently protrude into the metaphysis and are occasionally bypassed by the irregular ingrowth of vascularized, ossifying tissue, resulting in a tortuous metaphyseal junction.[42] Angular limb deformities can occur secondary to the growth-plate disturbances. Hypervitaminosis A has been reported to cause exuberant and premature calcification of growth-plate cartilage, resulting in early physeal closure.[64]

Idiopathic

Retardation of endochondral ossification and the formation of apparent retained cartilage cores have been reported to affect most frequently the distal canine ulnar growth plate (Figure 109-4).[65] These lesions consist of a cone of unmineralized hypertrophic cartilage projecting from the growth plate into the metaphysis. Although the etiology is unknown, it is speculated that they arise either from a process similar to osteochondrosis or an interruption to the metaphyseal blood supply.[42] They typically occur bilaterally and can be associated with premature closure of the distal ulnar physis with secondary antebrachial angular limb deformities.

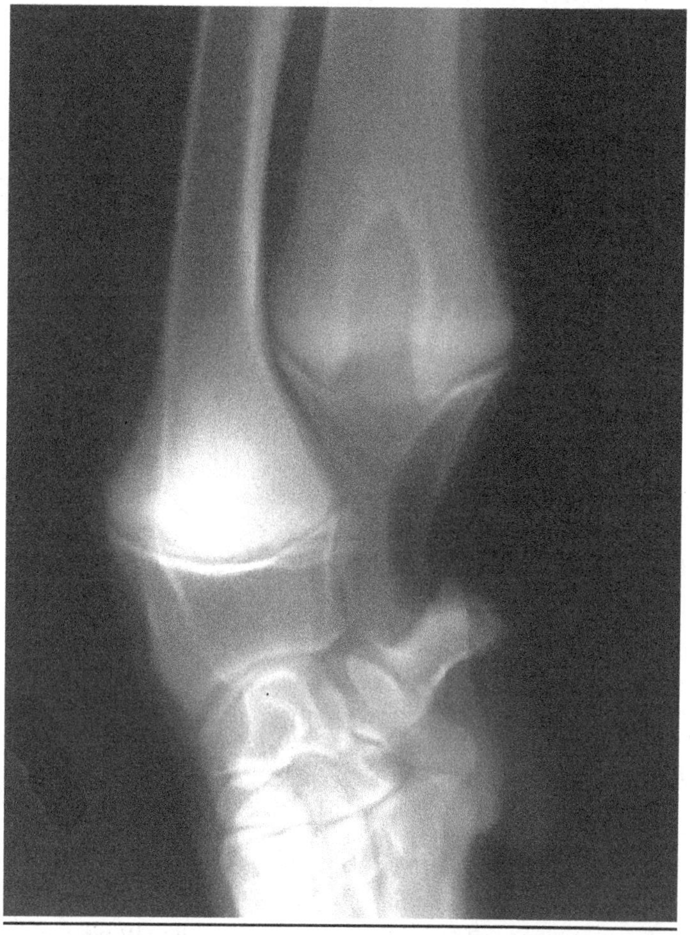

Figure 109-4. Lateral radiograph of a distal canine radius and ulna exhibiting a retained cartilage core apparent as a longitudinal radiolucent projection extending from the open physis proximally into the metaphysis.

References

1. Farriol F, Shapiro F: Bone development: Interaction of molecular components and biophysical forces. Clin Orthop Rel Res 432:14, 2005.

2. Iannotti JP: Growth plate physiology and pathology. Orthop Clin North Am 21:1, 1990.

3. Robertson WW: Newest knowledge of the growth plate. Clin Orthop 253:270. 1990.

4. Brighton CT, Heppenstall RB: Oxygen tension in zones of the epiphyseal plate, the metaphysis and diaphysis. J Bone Joint Surg 53A:719. 1971.

5. Ianotti JP, Goldstein S, Kuhn J, et al: The formation and growth of

skeletal tissues. *In* Orthopaedic Basic Science, Biology and Biomechanics of the Musculokeletal System, 2nd ed. Buckwalter JA, Einhorn TA, Simon SR (eds). Rosemont, IL: American Academy of Orthopaedic Surgeons, 2000, p. 77.

6. Wilsman NJ, Farnum CE, Leiferman EM, et al: Differential growth by growth plates as a function of multiple parameters of chondrocyte kinetics. J Orthop Res 14:927, 1996.

7. Ballock RT, O'Keefe RJ: The biology of the growth plate. J Bone Joint Surg 85A:715, 2003.

8. Salvesen GS, Dixit VM: Caspases: intracellular signaling by proteolysis. Cell 91:443, 1997.

9. Shapiro F: Epiphyseal and physeal cartilage vascularization: A light microscope and tritiated thymidine autoradiographic study of cartilage canals in newborn and young postnatal rabbit. Anat Rec 252:140, 1998.

10. Kronenberg HM, Lee K, Lanske BMK, Segre GV: Parathyroid hormone-related protein and Indian hedgehog control the pace of cartilage differentiation. J Endocrinol 154:S39, 1997.

11. Deng C, Wynshaw-Boris A, Zhou F, et al: Fibroblast growth factor receptor 3 is a negative regulator of bone growth. Cell 84:911, 1996.

12. Volk SW, Leboy PS: Regulating the regulators of chondrocyte hypertrophy. J Bone Miner Res 14:483, 1999.

13. Ballock RT, Mink LM, Chen DHC, et al: Thyroid hormone regulates terminal differentiation of growth plate chondrocytes through local induction of bone morphogenic proteins. Trans Orthop Res Soc 25:160, 2000.

14. Shapiro IM, Hatori M, Rajpurohit R, et al: Studies of fragmented DNA in the avian growth plate: evidence of apoptosis in terminally differentiated chondrocytes. J Bone Miner Res 10(SI):S351, 1995.

15. Sahni M, Raz R, Coffin JD, et al: STAT 1 mediates the increased apoptosis and reduced chondrocyte proliferation in mice overexpressing FGF2. Development 128:2119, 2001.

16. Silvestrini G, Ballanti P, Patacchioli FR, et al: Evaluation of apoptosis and the glucocorticoid receptor in the cartilage growth plate and metaphyseal bone cells of rats after high-dose treatment with corticosterone. Bone 26:33, 2000.

17. Pateder DB, Eliseev RA, O'Keefe RJ, et al: The role of autocrine growth factors in radiation damage to the epiphyseal growth plate. Radiat Res 155:847, 2001.

18. Essman SC, Lattimer J, Cook JL, et al: Effects of 153Sm-ethylenediaminetetramethylene phosphonate on physeal and articular cartilage in juvenile rabbits. J Nucl Med 44:1510, 2003.

19. de Crombrugghe B, Lefebvre V, Behringer RR, et al: Transcriptional mechanisms of chondrocyte differentiation. Matrix Biol 19:389, 2000.

20. Kirsch T, Swoboda B, Nah H: Activation of annexin II and V expression terminal differentiation, mineralization and apoptosis in human osteoarthritic cartilage. Osteoarthr Cart 8:294, 2000.

21. Kirsch T, Harrison G, Golub EE, et al: The roles of annexins and types II and X collagen in matrix vesicle-mediated mineralization of growth plate cartilage. J Biol Chem 275:35577, 2000.

22. Grimsrud CD, Romano PR, D'Souza M, et al: BMP-6 is an autocrine stimulator of chondrocyte differentiation. J Bone Miner Res 14:475, 1999.

23. D'Angelo M, Billings PC, Pacifici M, et al: Authentic matrix vesicles contain active metalloproteinases (MMP). A role for matrix vesicle associated MMP-13 in activation of transforming growth factor-beta. J Biol Chem 276:11347, 2001.

24. Mwale F, Tchetina E, Wu CW, et al: The assembly and remodeling of the extracellular matrix in the growth plate in relationship to mineral deposition and cellular hypertrophy: an in situ study of collagens II and IX and proteoglycan. J Bone Miner Res 17:275, 2002.

25. Carlevaro MF, Cermelli S, Cancedda R, et al: Vascular endothelial growth factor (VEGF) in cartilage neovascularization and chondrocyte differentiation: auto-paracrine role during endochondral bone formation. J Cell Sci 113:59, 2000.

26. Baron J, Klein KO, Yanovski JA, et al: Induction of growth plate cartilage ossification by basic fibroblast growth factor. Endocrinology 135:2790, 1994.

27. Weise M, De-Levi S, Brnes KM, et al: Effects of estrogen on growth plate senescence and epiphyseal fusion. Proc Natl Acad Sci USA 98:6871, 2001.

28. Fujii T, Takai S, Arai Y, et al: Microstructural properties of the distal growth plate of the rabbit radius and ulna: biomechanical, biochemical, and morphological studies. J Orthop Res 18:87. 2000.

29. Salter RB, Harris WR: Injuries involving the epiphyseal plate. J Bone Joint Surg 45A:587. 1963.

30. Braden TD. Histophysiology of the growth plate and growth plate injuries. *In* Bojrab MJ, Sneak DD, Bloomberg MS (eds). Disease Mechanisms in Small Animal Surgery, 2nd ed. Philadelphia: Lea & Febiger, 1993, p. 1027.

31. Johnson JM, Johnson AL, Eurell JA: Histologic appearance of naturally occuring canine physeal fractures. Vet Surg 23:81, 1994.

32. DeCamp CE, Probst CW, Tomas MW: Internal fixation of femoral capital physeal injuries in dogs: 40 cases (1979-1987). J Am Vet Med Assoc 194:1750. 1989.

33. Gibson KL, vanEe RT, Pechman RD: Femoral capital physeal fractures in dogs: 34 cases (1979-1989). J Am Vet Med Assoc 198:886. 1991.

34. Evans LB: Osteosarcoma in a young Great Dane dog. J S Afr Vet Assoc 54:271, 1983.

35. Probert JC, Parker BR: The effects of radiation therapy on bone growth. Radiology 114:155. 1975.

36. Gonzalez DR, Van Dijk DP: Experimental studies on the response of growing bones to x ray and neutron irradiation. Int J Radiat Oncol Phys 9:671, 1983.

37. Jimenez MM, O'Callaghan WO: Vertebral physitis: A radiographic diagnosis to be separated from discospondylitis. Vet Radiol Ultrasound 36:1188, 1995.

38. Walker MC, Platt SR, Graham JP, et al: Vertebral physitis with epiphyseal sequestration and a portosystemic shunt in a Pekingese dog. J Small Anim Pract 40:525, 1999.

39. Olsson SE, Ekman S: Morphology and physiology of the growth cartilage under normal and pathologic conditions. *In* Bone in Clinical Orthopedics, 2nd ed. Sumner-Smith G (ed). Stuttgart: AO Publishing, 2002, p. 139.

40. Andersen E, Willeberg P: Pituitary dwarfism in German shepherd dogs: additional evidence of simple, autosomal recessive inheritance. Nord Vet Med 28:481, 1976.

41. Kooistra HS, Voorhout G, Mol JA, et al: Combined pituitary hormone deficiency in German Shepherd dogs with dwarfism. Domest Anim Endocrinol 19:177, 2000.

42. Palmer N: Bones and joints. *In* Pathology of Domestic Animals, 4th ed. Jubb KVF, Kennedy PC, Palmer N (eds). San Diego: Academic Press, 1993, p. 56.

43. Eigenmann JE, Amador A, Patterson DF: Insulin-like growth factor I levels in proportionate dogs, chondrodystrophic dogs and in giant dogs. Acta Endocrinol (Copenh) 118:105: 1988.

44. Greco DS, Peterson ME, Cho DY, et al: Juvenile-onset hypothyroidism in a dog. J Am Vet Med Assoc 187:948, 1985.

45. Robinson WF, Shaw SE, Stanley B, et al: Congenital hypothyroidism in Scottish Deerhound puppies. Aust Vet J 65:386, 1988.

46. Greco DS, Feldman EC, Petterson ME, et al: Congenital hypothyroid

dwarfism in a family of Giant Schnauzers. J Vet Intern Med 5:57, 1991.

47. Mooney CT, Anderson TJ: Congenital hypothyroidism in a Boxer Dog. J Small Anim Pract 34:31, 1993.

48. Fyfe JC, Kampschmidt K, Dang V, et al: Congenital hypothyroidism with goiter in toy fox terriers. J Vet Intern Med 17:50, 2003.

49. Eshet R, Maor G, Ari BT, et al: The aromatase inhibitor letrozole increases epiphyseal growth plate height and tibial length in peripubertal male mice. J Endocrinol 182:165, 2004.

50. Salmeri KR, Bloomberg MS, Scruggs SL, et al: Gonadectomy in immature dogs: Effects on skeletal, physical, and behavior development. J Am Vet Med Assoc 198:1193, 1991.

51. McNicholas WT, Wilkens BE, Blevins WE, et al: Spontaneous femoral capital physeal fractures in adult cats: 26 cases (1996-2001). J Am Vet Med Assoc 221:1731, 2002.

52. Riser WH, Haskins ME, Jezyk PF, et al: Psuedoachondroplastic dysplasia in miniature poodles: clinical radiologic, and pathologic features. J Am Vet Med Assoc 176:335, 1980.

53. Breur GJ, Zerbe CA, Slocombe RF, et al: Clinical, radiographic, pathologic, and genetic features of osteochondrodysplasia in Scottish deerhounds. J Am Vet Med Assoc 195:606, 1989.

54. Breur GJ, Farnum CE, Padgett GA, et al: Cellular basis of decreased rate of longitudinal growth of bone in psuedoachondroplastic dogs. J Bone Joint Surg 74:516, 1992.

55. Rasmussen PG: Multiple epiphyseal dysplasia in beagle puppies. Acta Radiol Suppl 319:251, 1972

56. Rasmussen PG: Multiple epiphyseal dysplasia in a litter of Beagle puppies. J Small Anim Pract 12:91, 1971.

57. Bingel SA, Sande RD, Wight TN: Chondrodysplasia in the Alaskan malamute. Characterization of proteglycans dissociatively extracted from dwarf growth plates. Lab Invest 53:479, 1985.

58. Bingel SA, Sande RD: Chondrodysplasia in the Norwegian elkhound. Am J Pathol 197:219, 1982.

59. Bingel SA, Sande RD: Chondrodysplasia in five Great Pyrenees. J Am Vet Med Assoc 205:845, 1994.

60. Hanssen I, Falck G, Grammelvedt AT, et al: Hypochondroplastic dwarfism in the Irish setter. J Small Anim Pract 39:10, 1998.

61. Carrig CB, Sponenberg DP, Schmidt GM, et al: Inheritance of associated ocular and skeletal dysplasia in Labrador retrievers. J Am Vet Med Assoc 193:1269, 1988.

62. Aroch I, Ofri R, Aizenberg I: Haematological, ocular and skeletal abnormalities in a Samoyed family. J Small Anim Pract 37:333, 1996.

63. Farnum CE, Jones K, Riis R, et al: Ocular-chondrodysplasia in Labrador retriever dogs: a morphometric and electron microscopical analysis. Calcif Tissue Int 50:564, 1992.

64. Kodaka T, Takaki H, Soeta S, et al: Local disappearance of epiphyseal growth plates in rats with hypervitaminosis A. J Vet Med Sci 60:815, 1998.

65. Johnson KA: Retardation of endochondral ossification at the distal ulnar growth plate in dogs. Aust Vet J 57:474, 1981.

Chapter 110

Biomechanics of Luxation

Dr DA Hulse

Luxations are a common occurrence in small animal veterinary medicine. Decisions on appropriate treatment strategies are based on many factors. One of the most important of these factors is an understanding of the biomechanics of joints. Armed with this knowledge, mechanisms of injury can be understood and sound decisions relative to treatment methods can be made to restore normal function. In this section, we address biomechanics, which is the science of the action of forces, internal and external, on the living body, an unfamiliar topic for many veterinarians.

Diarthrodial or synovial joints are complex structures loacated at the ends of long bones. Each joint is a composite made of hyaline ar¬ticular cartilage, synovial lining tissue, joint capsule, and ligaments. Tendons and muscles cross joint articulations, lending substantial support to the joint. The sequence of events encountered by the joint during trauma and the sequelae of these events are discussed in this chapter. It is important to realize, however, that most forces are exerted indirectly on the joint, and the resultant deformation of anatomic structures depends on many factors, such as (1) the direction of the force, (2) the speed of the force, (3) the attitude (position) of the animal, (4) the age of the animal (e.g., open or closed physes), (5) the configuration of the bones and joints (e.g., bones of basset hounds versus those of a greyhound), and (6) preexisting joint disease (e.g., laxity, hip dysplasia).

Forces singularly or coupled (e.g., rotation and bending) directed at the appendicular skeleton of the animal are transmitted along the limb and may result in a joint subluxation or complete joint luxation. Additional injuries may combine with joint trauma; these may include: bone fracture, tendon tear, capsular tissue avulsion, or physis separation in young animals. The veterinarian should maintain a high degree of suspicion when examining animals subjected to trauma. A clearly evident fracture in a limb may be associated with a less noticeable luxation in the same limb. An example would be a fractured distal tibia with dislocation of the hip in the same limb. The shoulder, elbow, carpal, hip, stifle, and tarsal joints are discussed here, and a set of events that may lead to luxation of the particular joint is outlined. Surgical considerations that deal with the damage done by luxation are discussed when applicable.

Shoulder Joint

Anatomy

Being a ball and socket joint, the shoulder joint is well suited for movement in all directions. Although capable of movement in all directions, the shoulder primarily moves in flexion and extension. Joint stability is provided through a combination of passive and active mechanisms (Figure 110-1). Passive mechanisms include

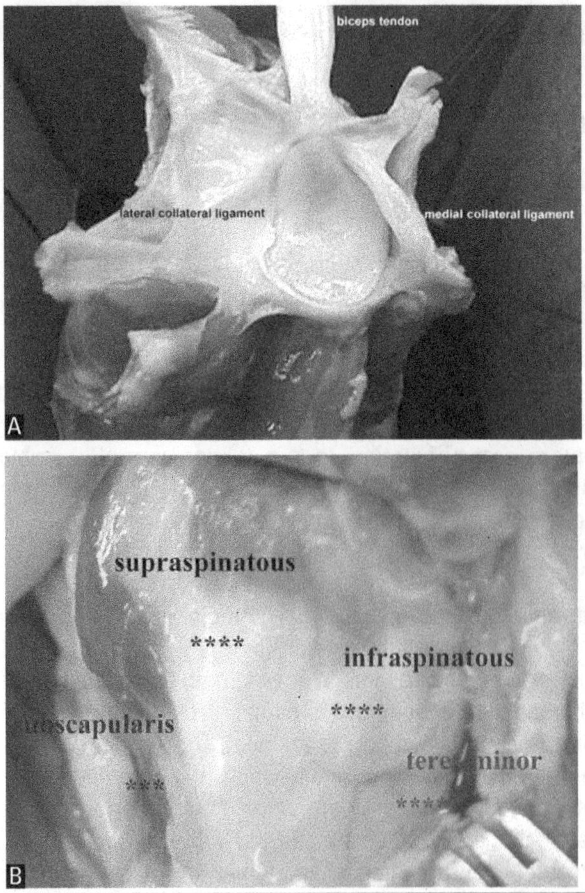

Figure 110-1. Photograph of the passive and active restraints of the shoulder joint. Passive restraints are the medial collateral ligament, lateral collateral ligament, and surrounding joint capsule. Active restraints are the surrounding cuff muscles, which include the biceps, supraspinatus, infraspinatus, and supscapularis muscles.

the medial and lateral glenohumeral ligaments, surrounding joint capsule, joint conformation, and synovial fluid cohesion. The medial collateral ligament (MCL) commonly appears as "Y" shaped with the cranial arm coursing caudally from its origin at the medial surface of the supraglenoid tubercle. The caudal arm of the MCL originates from the medial surface of the scapular neck and joins the cranial arm to insert onto the humeral neck. The MCL and associated joint capsule are major factors in providing joint stability. Complete medial luxation occurs following transection of the medial glenohumeral ligament (MGHL). (1) The lateral collateral ligament (LCL) originates from the lateral rim of the glenoid and extends ventrally to insert onto the humerus at the caudal region of the greater tubercle. The joint capsule originates from the periphery of the glenoid cavity. Medially, the joint capsule forms a synovial recess owing to its attachment several millimeters proximal to the glenoid rim. The concavity of the glenoid and the fit of the humeral head into the glenoid provide joint stability. This is particularly true when compression across the joint is enhanced by active muscle contraction. Dynamic active glenohumeral stability is provided by contraction of the surrounding cuff muscles. These include the biceps brachii, subscapularis, teres minor, supraspinatous, and infraspinatous muscles. Active contraction of all or selective cuff muscles induces compression across the shoulder joint as well as increasing tension in the joint capsule. When tested in a neutral position, the cranial, lateral, and medial translation of the humerus was significantly increased after biceps tendon transection. In the flexed position, translation of the humerus in the cranial and lateral directions was significantly increased after biceps tendon transection. In the extended position, the medial translation of the humerus was significantly increased after biceps tendon transaction.[1]

Examination of the shoulder for stability should be done under anesthesia. Flexion, extension, abduction, adduction, and rotational stability of the shoulder joint should be assessed. Normal ranges of flexion and extension are 40° for flexion and 165° for extension. A normal abduction test is approximately 25°; abnormal abduction is considered present when abduction exceeds this degree and there is a difference in the abduction angle between the injured side and the normal side. Note that dogs with long-standing forelimb lameness often present with laxity. In the majority of these cases, approximately 45° of abduction exists on the affected side with a normal abduction on the sound limb (25°).

Biomechanics

A fall or jump from a height may produce a shoulder subluxation or luxation. An example in a toy breed would be the dog jumping from an owner's arms. Another mechanism of injury causing subluxation/luxation of the shoulder would be if the animal is bearing weight at the time that a blunt force is applied to the proximal area of the humerus. The direction of subluxation/luxation is dependent on the direction of force application (i.e., anterior to posterior, medial to lateral). Because the limb is bearing weight, it forces the proximal humerus to accept most of the blow. If the foot is off the ground, the leg is able to swing in the direction of the force, diminishing the chance of a subluxation or luxation. In addition, when the limb is bearing weight, the humerus is down and away from the chest wall, and no medial, shock-absorbing protection is available from the chest wall. With a laterally to medially directed force, the humeral head can be driven medially, rupturing the medial restraints (MCL, subscapularis tendon, and joint capsule). The humeral head lies medial to the glenoid of the scapula, resulting in a medial luxation (Figure 110-2).

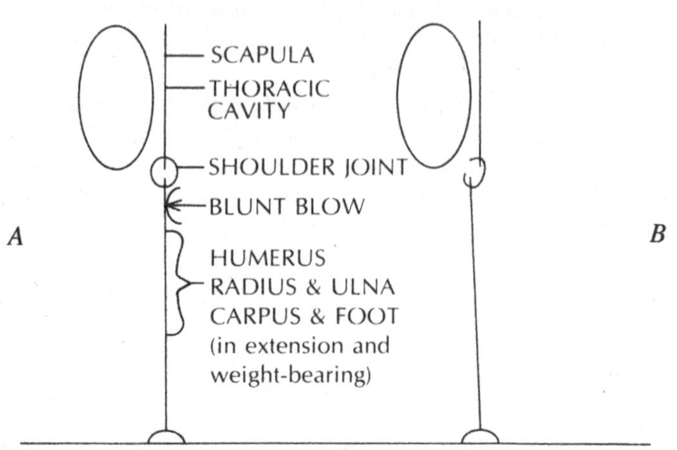

Figure 110-2. A and B, Schematic drawings of an animal seen in an anteroposterior view. A medial luxation of the humeral head is due to a blunt blow to the proximal lateral surface of the humerus.

Medial Luxation

A medial to lateral force directed against the body may result in a medial subluxation or luxation if, when the force is applied, the foot is in contact with the ground. In this position, the leg starts to abduct as the body moves toward the ground. This action may be caused by a blow from a moving vehicle or a fall from a height. As the extended limb starts to abduct, a long lever arm is created from the foot to the shoulder. The greatest stress occurs on the medial side of the shoulder joint, rupturing the medial restraints (Figure 110-3).

Another mechanism for injury is a blow to the proximal end of the humerus. The blow is directed from cranial to caudal. Because the joint is in midflexion, the humeral head is more easily driven out of the glenoid cavity. The tendons surrounding the joint are fairly relaxed, and the greater tubercle is below the scapular tuberosity and glenoid. If the force of the blow is sufficient, the humeral head is driven out of the glenoid cavity. Depending on which tendons rupture first (subscapularis or infraspinatus), the humeral head eventually lies on either the medial or lateral side of the glenoid.

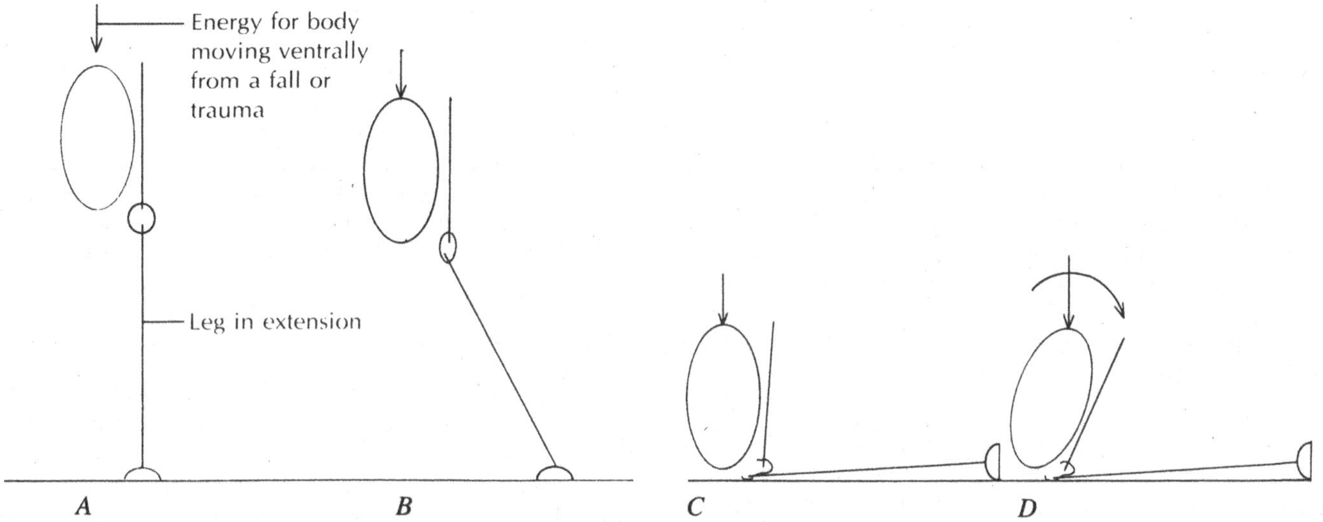

Figure 110-3. A, The animal's body is moving ventrally while the forelimb is in extension and weight-bearing. B, As the chest continues ventrally, the limb begins to abduct, putting stress on the medial side of the shoulder joint. C, As the chest nears the ground, the medial side of the joint ruptures, allowing the humeral head to luxate medially. D, The stress on the medial side of the joint can be greatly exaggerated if at the same time the body is moving ventrally it is also rotating toward the affected limb.

Treatment Strategies

CLOSED REDUCTION: If, following reduction, the shoulder joint maintains the correct position, reduction can be maintained with a Valpeau sling. The elbow should be taped to the chest wall, producing a lateral force at the shoulder joint. A Valpeau sling should remain in place for 3 weeks. Once the splint is removed, the attending veterinarian should radiograph the shoulder and examine the joint under anesthesia. Either palpation to detect subtle subluxation with rotation or the abduction test is performed.

OPEN REDUCTION: A medial approach with careful identification of all injured tissue is required. Placement of suture anchors at the origin and insertion of the Y-shaped medial collateral ligament is achieved. Nonabsorbable suture is used to reconstruct the MCL.

Lateral Luxation

Lateral luxation occurs when the limb is in full extension and is forced into adduction during weight bearing. This action can be caused by a blow from a moving vehicle or a fall. The force is applied principally to the lateral surface of the shoulder. The force injures the lateral cuff muscles and collateral ligament, allowing the humeral head to luxate laterally to the glenoid (Figure 110-4).

Treatment Strategies

CLOSED REDUCTION: Measures are the same as for medial luxation, except that padding is placed between the elbow and chest wall, producing a medial force at the shoulder joint.

OPEN REDUCTION: A lateral approach with careful identification of all injured tissue is required. Placement of suture anchors at the origin and insertion of the lateral collateral ligament is achieved. Nonabsorbable suture is used to reconstruct the LCL.

Elbow

Anatomy

The elbow is a composite ginglymoid (hinge) joint formed by the humeral condyle, the head of the radius and the semilunar notch of the ulna. The entire joint consists of three separate articulations enclosed within a single joint capsule. The humeroradial joint occurs between the humeral capitulum and the radial head and is thought to transmit the majority of weight through the elbow. The humeroulnar joint occurs between the humeral trochlea and olecranon fossa of the humerus and the articulating surface of the semilunar notch and anconeal process of the ulna. The humeroulnar joint, along with the collateral ligaments, provides stability to the elbow, particularly in extension. The proximal radial head fits into the coronoid processes of the

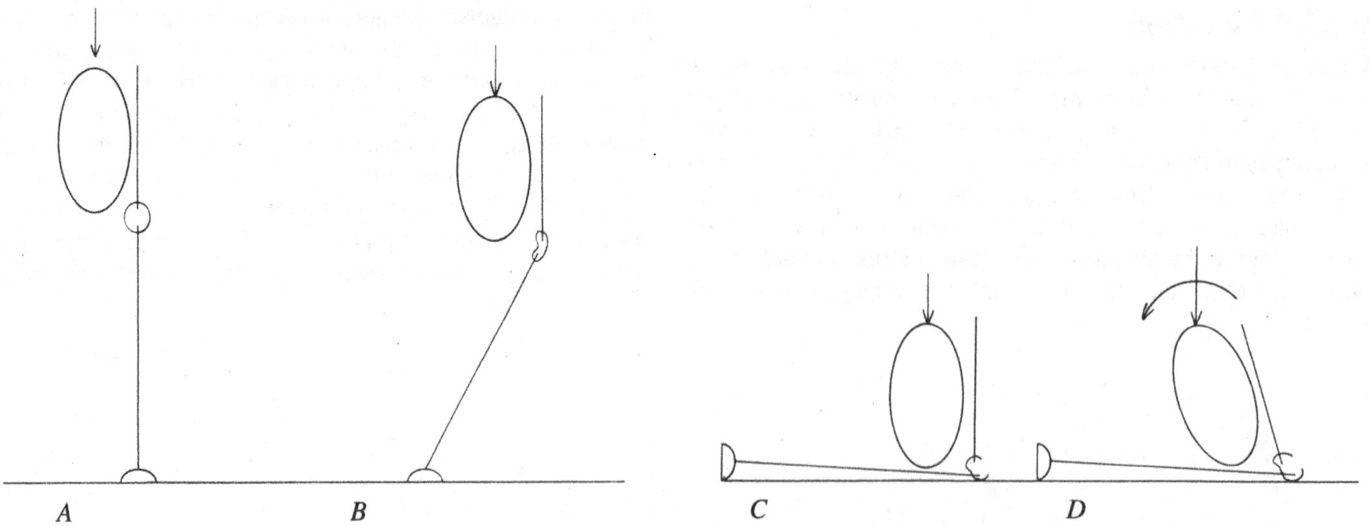

Figure 110-4. A, The animal's body is moving ventrally. The forelimb is in extension and is weight bearing. B, As the body continues ventrally, the limb moves into abduction causing stress on the lateral side of the shoulder joint. C, As the chest nears the ground, the lateral side of the joint ruptures, allowing the humeral head to luxate laterally. D, The stress on the lateral side of the joint can be greatly exaggerated if at the same time the body is moving ventrally it is also rotating away from the side of the affected limb.

ulna and allows some supination and pronation. In the normal Labrador retriever, the elbow joint functions primarily in flexion and extension, allowing up to 36° of flexion and 166° of extension.[2] It has been reported that, with the elbow and carpus flexed to 90°, the collateral ligaments limit internal rotation to 60° and external rotation to 40°.[3] The collateral ligaments originate from the medial and lateral humeral epicondyles and split into cranial and caudal crura as they course distally to insert on the proximal radius (cranially) and the lateral ulna or the caudal radius, annular ligament, and medial interosseous space.

Acquired Elbow Joint Luxation

Elbow luxation is much less common than fractures involving the elbow, likely because of the inherent stability of the anatomy of the joint. When elbow luxation occurs in the dog, it is thought to be caused primarily by rotation of the body around a flexed, weight-bearing limb rather than by a direct blow to the elbow or by landing on an extended forelimb (Figure 110-5). In the dog, lateral luxation occurs in over 90% of cases, although medial and caudal luxation have been reported.[4] The larger shape and orientation of the medial condyle make medial luxation much more unlikely. The one reported case in a cat was a medial elbow luxation.[5] The diagnosis of elbow luxation is almost always associated with significant impact, such as being hit by a car, although luxation has been reported after fighting or rough play. The animal will be severely lame, usually unable to bear weight, will have a swollen elbow with limited range of motion, and painl on attempted manipulation of the joint. Although luxation of both the radial head and the anconeal process laterally are most commonly seen, in about 20% of cases the ulna is not completely luxated. In addition, the clinician should be aware that a caudal blow to the ulna may result in radial head luxation and concurrent ulnar fracture (Monteggia fracture). Monteggia fractures, discussed elsewhere in this text, can be challenging to repair and are handled differently from a straightforward traumatic elbow luxation.

Treatment Strategies

ACUTE LUXATION: A complete physical examination should focus on other major orthopedic or thoracic injuries, which can be present in up to 30% of cases. The affected forelimb should be assessed carefully to assure intact innervation and vascular supply. Radiographs of the antebrachium should be carefully examined for ulnar fracture (which may be very distal) and fractures of the anconeal process, fragmented coronoid process, and avulsions of the epicondyles where the collateral ligaments attach. Once the animal is stable, closed reduction should be performed under general anesthesia. Reduction should be radiographically confirmed, and the elbow should be fairly stable once reduced. Post-reduction coaptation is controversial; a variety of recommendations can be found in the literature, from no bandaging at all to 4 weeks in a Spica splint, incorporating the shoulder joint. At a minimum, bandaging in flexion (for example, a Valpeau sling) should be avoided as the elbow is more likely to reluxate in that position. The animal should be confined to leash walks and crate rest for a minimum of 2 weeks. If malalignment or instability are present after reduction, or if reluxation occurs, open reduction is recommended. Some authors also recommend surgical repair of collateral ligaments even after closed reduction if it is radiographically apparent that one or both epicondyles have avulsed. Although the majority of reductions performed early after luxation give good to excellent results, the owners should be warned that degenerative joint disease and lameness can be the end result.

CHRONIC LUXATION: Luxations of over 1 to 2 weeks' duration are generally considered chronic. All chronic luxations require open reduction. The amount of cartilage damage, muscle contracture, and fibrosis present will dictate whether the luxation can be reduced and also correlate with decreasing prognosis for normal use of the limb. In all cases of chronic elbow luxation, the surgeon should warn the owner that arthrodesis or amputation may be an option.

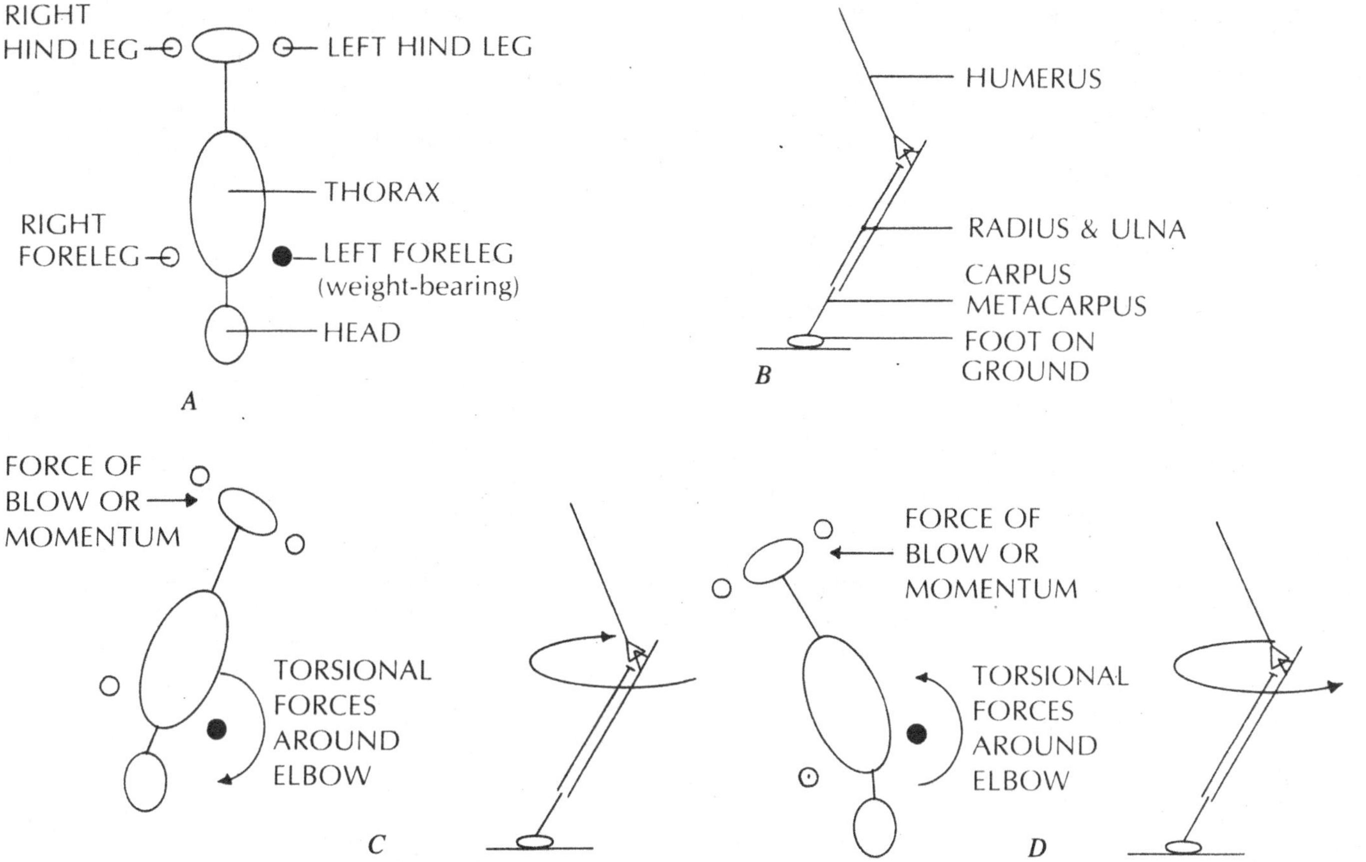

Figure 110-5. Schematic drawings show the animal from two views. A, A top view shows the left foreleg circled in solid black because that will be the weight-bearing limb. B, A lateral view of the forelimb. C, The forces acting on the animal cause the rotational forces to be in a clockwise direction as viewed from above. D, The force acting on the animal's body causes the rotational forces to be in a counterclockwise direction as viewed from above.

Carpus

Anatomy

The carpus consists of seven bones arranged in two rows. The radial carpal and ulnar carpal bones make up the proximal row, while the first, second, third, and fourth carpal bones make up the distal row. The accessory carpal bone lies caudally and articulates with the ulnar carpal bone. The radial carpal bone and ulnar carpal bone articulate with the radius and styloid process of the ulna to form the radiocarpal joint. This joint has the greatest amount of movement. The middle carpal joint, formed by the articulation of the proximal and distal rows of carpal bones, accounts for 10% to 15% of carpal motion. Little motion occurs in the carpometacarpal and intercarpal joints. Collateral ligamentous support arises from the short radial collateral ligament medially and from the short ulnar collateral ligament laterally. Additionally, sleeves of collagenous tissue that house tendons provide medial and lateral collateral support. Palmar support is from the flexor retinaculum proximally and palmar fibrocartilage distally. Multiple small ligaments cross the intercarpal articulations between carpal bones to provide additional collateral and palmar support. Two of these, the palmar radiocarpal ligament and the palmar ulnar carpal ligament are important structures in providing palmar support for the radiocarpal joint (Figure 110-6). Two accessory ligaments originate from the free end of the accessory carpal bone and insert onto the palmar surface of the fourth and fifth metacarpal bones. The caudal position of the free end of the accessory carpal bone, in conjunction with the accessory carpal ligaments, serves to act as a moment arm to balance the vertical force produced when the paw strikes the ground.

Carpal hyperextension injuries are divided into the following three categories. Type I injury is a subluxation or luxation of the radiocarpal joint (may include damage to the middle carpal and

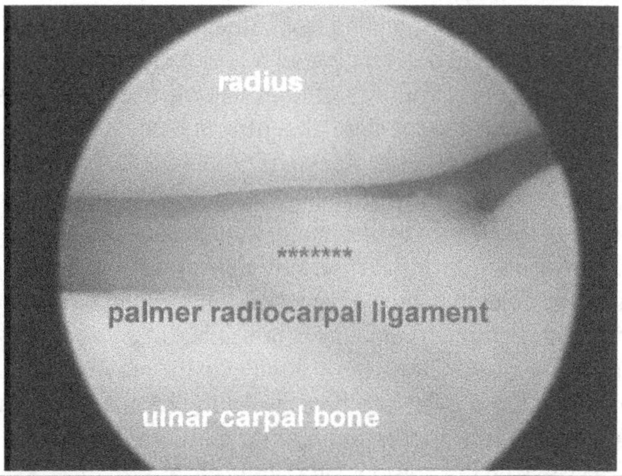

Figure 110-6. Photograph showing the palmar radiocarpal ligament and the palmar ulnar carpal ligament. These ligaments are important in providing craniocaudal and rotational support for the radiocarpal joint.

carpometacarpal joints). A Type II injury is a disruption of the accessory carpal ligaments, palmar fibrocartilage and palmar ligaments of the middle carpal and carpometacarpal joints. The result is a subluxation of the middle carpal and/or carpometacarpal joints with dorsal displacement of the free end of the accessory carpal bone and ulnar carpal bone. A Type III injury is a disruption of the accessory carpal ligaments, carpometacarpal ligaments, and the palmar fibrocartilage. In these injuries, a subluxation of the carpometacarpal joint occurs without disruption and displacement of the accessory carpal and ulnar carpal bones.

With an acute injury, ligamentous disruption is complete and the patient presents with a nonweight-bearing lameness. Swelling, pain, and instability are evident on examination. In Type I injuries, the patient generally remains nonweight bearing until definitive treatment is achieved; in Type II or Type III injuries, the patient may begin to bear minimal weight with the limb after the injury. However, as the patient increases the amount of weight placed on the limb, collapse and hyperextension of the carpus are evident. Standard craniocaudal and medial-to-lateral radiographs are indicated to determine the presence of bone fractures and/or joint malalignment. To accurately assess the integrity of the carpus, however, stress radiographs should be taken. The purpose of stress radiography is to assess the point of injury and to determine if the integrity of the radiocarpal joint is intact. If the integrity of the radiocarpal joint is intact, then a partial arthrodesis is indicated; if the integrity is lost, a pancarpal arthrodesis is preferred. Although stress radiographic evaluation is a valuable tool, false positives (i.e., radiocarpal joint not intact) are possible. Another valuable tool to assess the integrity of the radiocarpal posterior ligamentous support is arthroscopic examination prior to deciding on a partial carpal or pancarpal arthrodesis.

Biomechanics

The carpus is a complex structure. Type I luxations of the carpus are uncommon, and when they occur they usually involve the antebrachiocarpal joint. Luxations can be found with severe shearing injuries involving the carpus. Subluxation associated with hyperextension is the most common form of luxation in the carpus. The energy needed to cause luxation often comes from the animal's falling or jumping from a height or jumping out of a fast-moving vehicle and landing on a fully extended limb. As the foot makes contact with the ground, the carpus hyperextends, allowing the volar aspect of the proximal metacarpal bones to strike the ground. This transmits a violent force proximally through the carpal bones toward the radius. At the same time, the force of the weight of the animal travels ventrally through the radius toward the carpus. When sufficient opposing forces travel through the column of bones held together by ligaments, luxation of one or more the carpal joints is possible. On some occasions, when an animal is falling to the ground as in the previous situation, the foot knuckles over into flexion. As the radius continues to drive ventrally, the foot is forced into extreme flexion, causing severe stress on the anterior side of the carpus. In this case, any or all of the joints of the carpus may open anteriorly, rupturing the joint capsule and interosseous ligaments. When an animal is struck by a vehicle, the carpus may be dragged along the road, causing severe shearing injury to the medial or lateral side. Generally, all the collateral support structures (skin, ligaments, tendons, joint capsule, and sometimes a considerable amount of bone) are lost. Again, the antebrachiocarpal joint is the most susceptible to luxation.

Treatment Strategies

CLOSED REDUCTION: If the damage is not too severe, it is possible to obtain healing and stability with the use of splints or casts. External coaptation must be rigid for the initial 4 weeks and then gradually stabilized over the next 4 weeks. The carpus is originally placed in mild flexion and gradually extended to a normal standing position. External coaptation is more successful with injuries to the anterior (dorsal) restraints as compared with injuries of the caudal restraints.

OPEN REDUCTION: Primary ligamentous repair, i.e., suturing the ligament ends is not successful. Likewise, reconstruction with autogenous or autologous tissue has not been rewarding. The common method for surgical repair is fusion of the injured joint(s). The method of surgical intervention depends on the classification of injury. Type I carpal injury requires a pancarpal arthrodesis; Type II injury can be repaired with a pancarpal or partial carpal fusion, whereas Type III injury requires a partial fusion. Good to excellent results can be expected when this procedure is done correctly.

Hip Joint

The hip is by far the most common site of traumatic luxation in dogs and cats. No collateral ligaments exist, and the muscles that attach to the proximal end of the femur allow a great deal of motion in the joint. The major stabilizing feature of this joint is the ball-and-socket configuration itself. Contraction of the surrounding muscles is of primary importance in lending stability to the hip joint as is the anticavitational effect of synovial fluid. The round ligament and the joint capsule are the major soft-tissue structures providing passive stability and are not of primary importance in preventing subluxation of the hip joint. These structures may become stretched, as with hip dysplasia, allowing subluxation and predisposing the hip to complete luxation. The different classifications of hip luxations are named by the location of the femoral head relative to the acetabulum. For example, with a craniodorsal luxation, the femoral head lies cranial and dorsal to the acetabulum, whereas with a ventral luxation, the femoral head lies beneath the acetablum (often lodged in the obturator foramen).

Craniodorsal Luxation

One of the most common causes of luxation of the hip is a strong blow delivered from the rear or side of the dog or cat. As the animal starts to fall toward the hip to be luxated, the center of gravity moves lateral to the hip joint. Simultaneously, with the foot on the ground, the rear leg moves into adduction. As the hip moves ventral and laterally toward the ground, the lever action of the adducted femoral shaft subluxates the femoral head out of the acetablum (Figure 110-7). The center of gravity of the

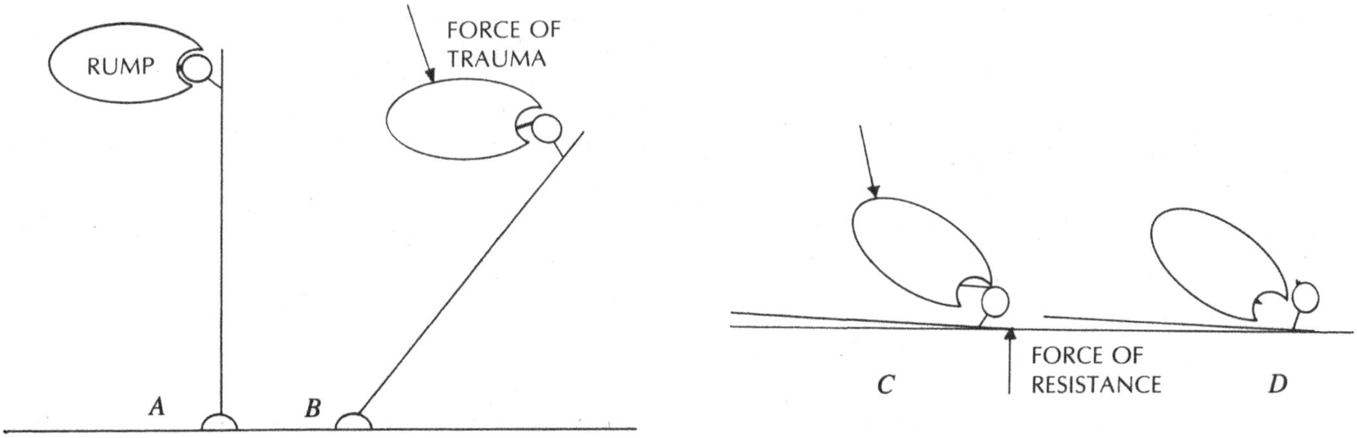

Figure 110-7. A, The hip joint and hind limb viewed from the front. The leg is in extension and is weight bearing. B, A blow is struck to the rump causing the limb to go into adduction. C, Just as the greater trochanter is about to hit the ground, the femoral head is subluxated against the dorsal rim of the acetabulum. D, As the hip hits the ground, the teres ligament ruptures and the femoral head luxates to a dorsoanterior position.

animal moves lateral to the hip joint. This position is exaggerated in dysplastic animals, where the hip joint conformation is poor and the passive restraints (round ligament and joint capsule) are already stretched. The dorsal rim is remodeled, further contributing to instability. When the greater trochanter strikes the ground, the energy of the blow is transmitted through the femoral neck to the femoral head. The femoral head is driven over the dorsal rim, shearing the joint capsule or teres ligament. Sometimes the teres ligament avulses from the femoral head, causing a small fragment to pull from the femoral head. Rarely, a piece of bone is chipped off the dorsal rim of the acetabulum. The femoral head comes to rest in its most common position of luxation craniodorsal to the acetabulum. The strong pull of the gluteal muscles also helps to pull the femoral head to this position. Muscular force and passive restraints (capsule and round ligament) are unable to maintain the reduced state of the joint.

Another way in which hip luxation may occur is when the body is driven ventrally toward the ground. The hind leg is extended and the foot is bearing weight. As the pelvis is forced ventrally, the knee and hip begin to flex. At some point before the pelvis strikes the ground, the knee makes contact with the ground. As the pelvis continues to move ventrally, the hip begins to rotate externally. If the force is sufficient, the teres ligament and joint capsule rupture, allowing the femoral head to luxate. The strong pull of the gluteals causes the femoral head to luxate in a craniodorsal position.

Treatment Strategies

CLOSED REDUCTION: Several techniques are used to reduce hip luxations. The longer the hip is dislocated, the more difficult it is to reduce, owing to muscle contraction and local fibrosis. Generally, the leg must be put into a sling to prevent reluxation. Reported success rates vary from 30% to 85%. Animals with hip dysplasia, severe degenerative joint disease, or avulsion fractures in the hip joint are poor candidates for closed reduction.

OPEN REDUCTION: If the luxation cannot be reduced or if the joint repeatedly reluxates, surgery is indicated. Many techniques are available to the surgeon. Procedures include capsulorrhaphy, iliofemoral suture, trochanteric transposition, transarticular pinning, teres ligament replacement (including a toggle), and triple pelvic osteotomy. Alternatives to preserving the in situ hip joint are excision arthroplasty and total hip replacement.

Ventral Luxation

A distinction may be made between cranial and caudal ventral luxation. The biomechanics are the same for both, except for the position of the femoral head as it is being forced ventrally under the acetabulum. If the leg rotates inward as the hip is luxating ventrally, the femoral head ends up in the obturator foramen. If the leg rotates outward, the femoral head ends up in front of the pubis. It has been reported that a ventral luxation can be created by overzealous reduction of a craniodorsal luxation. Those that occur naturally are usually associated with the trauma of jumping or falling and landing with the leg abducted. As the leg contin¬ues to abduct during the fall, eventually the femoral neck and greater trochanter strike the dorsal aspect of the acetabulum. This forces the femoral head out of the acetabulum, rupturing the teres ligament and ventral joint capsule. An animal with a ventral luxation carries the leg abducted and inwardly rotated and is unable to put the foot on the ground.

Treatment Strategies

CLOSED REDUCTION: Not many cases of ventral luxation have been reported, but they do appear to respond well to closed reduction. If reduction alone leaves the joint unstable, hobbles or an adduction sling may be used to prevent abduction.

OPEN REDUCTION: Any of the techniques mentioned for craniodorsal luxation that prevent luxation in any direction (e.g., transarticular pinning) could be considered. The ventral restraints may be reconstructed by advancement of surrounding soft tissue. If none of these methods works, femoral head and neck excision arthroplasty or total hip replacement should be considered.

Stifle Joint

Anatomy

The stifle joint is a complex diarthrodial (synovial) joint that allows movement in three planes. The stifle consists of three intimately associated joint spaces: the femorotibial (between the femoral and tibial condyles), the femoropatellar (between the patella and the femoral trochlea), and the proximal tibiofibular joints.

The primary motion of the joint is flexion and extension; however, the articulation of the femoral condyles with the surrounding supportive structures, menisci, and proximal tibial surface allows cranial and caudal translation, internal and external rotation, varus and valgus angulation, and medial and lateral movement of the femur in relation to the tibia. The medial and lateral menisci are C-shaped, fibrocartilagenous structures interposed between the articular surfaces of the femur and tibia (Figure 110-8). They perform a load-transmitting function, improve joint stability by providing congruity between the femur and tibia, assist in lubrication of the joint, and are thought to provide a sensory function so they may aid in joint proprioception. The menisci are firmly attached to the femur, tibia, and joint capsule by six ligaments.

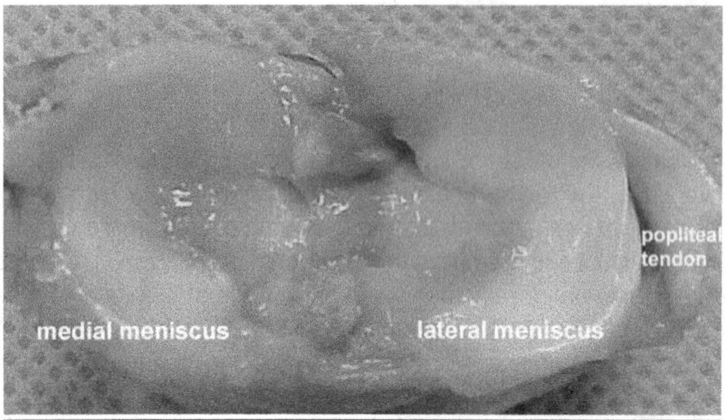

Figure 110-8. Photograph of the medial and lateral meniscal ligament. Both are important intra-articular structures providing joint stability and load transmission.

Primary ligamentous support of the stifle is provided by medial and lateral collateral ligaments, as well as cranial and caudal cruciate ligments. The lateral collateral ligament originates proximal to the origin of the popliteal muscle on the lateral femoral epicondyle and inserts on the fibular head. The medial collateral ligament originates from an oval area on the medial femoral epicondyle and forms a distal attachment to the medial meniscus and surrounding joint capsule. Collateral ligaments are responsible for preventing varus (lateral collateral) and valgus (medial collateral) motion of the tibia and as a secondary stabilizer against rotational forces of the stifle. The cranial cruciate ligament originates on the caudomedial portion of the lateral condyle of the femur and courses in a spiral orientation cranially, medially, and distally through the intercondylar fossa to the cranial intercondyloid area of the tibia. It functions primarily to prevent cranial and caudal translation of the tibia in relation to the femur, to provide rotational stability by preventing internal rotation of the stifle, and also to assist in preventing hyperextension of the stifle. The caudal cruciate ligament begins at the lateral aspect of the medial femoral condyle and extends caudally and distally to the lateral edge of the popliteal notch of the tibia. The caudal cruciate ligament prevents excessive cranial and caudal translation of the tibia in relation to the femur and provides assistance in prevention of hyperextension of the stifle.

Other soft tissues that lend themselves to the stability of the stifle joint include the popliteal muscle, the semitendinosus and semimembranosus muscles, quadriceps femoris, straight patellar ligament, and joint capsule.

Biomechanics

Because of the dynamic variety of muscular and ligamentous structures and the articulation of the femur, tibia, and menisci, movement of the stifle is complex and does not limit itself to a single plane. During flexion of the stifle, the tibia internally rotates slightly because of the relaxation of the lateral collateral ligament and subsequent caudal displacement of the lateral femoral condyle. During extension, the tibia externally rotates because of the cranial displacement of the lateral femoral condyle as the lateral collateral ligament tightens. Cranial and caudal movement of the femur in relation to the tibia is seen in a sagittal plane during flexion and extension; a slight varus and valgus movement of the tibia is also seen but is limited by the ligamentous structures of the stifle.

The most common cause of stifle subluxation is associated with the rupture of the cranial cruciate ligament. Stifle luxation or total derangement of the knee is an uncommon injury in dogs and cats, but has been documented to have a higher incidence in cats.[6] Significant damage to multiple ligaments of the stifle is typically associated with high-energy injury, such as with a fall or vehicular truama. Rupturing of the articular structures is most likely associated with a direct blow to a weight-bearing limb, resulting in a cranial and lateral luxation of the stifle and subsequent rupture of the cranial cruciate, caudal cruciate, and medial collateral ligaments.[7] Also, it is common to see damage to the secondary structures of the joint, such as the joint capsule, menisci, and patellar ligmament. Ipsilateral fractures of the femur and pelvis were also cited as having been seen in 8 of 27 cases (30%).[7]

Damage to the cruciate ligaments and medial collateral ligament is theorized to occur because of the vulnerability of the lateral portion of the limb to blunt trauma or perhaps owing to the resistance of medial and caudal luxation by the quadriceps, hamstring, gastrocnemius, and popliteal muscles.[8] Because of the magnitude of the blow that is necessary to luxate the stifle joint, vascular and nerve complications are a consideration, especially with cranial luxations.

Treatment Strategies

CLOSED REDUCTION: Nonsurgical reduction of a stifle luxation is not recommended. The prognosis for return to function is poor.

OPEN REDUCTION: Return to good function can be expected if primary and secondary joint restraints can be restored. Multiple techniques for open reduction and repair of articular and periarticular structures have been described.[9] Even under general anesthesia, it is difficult to assess the extent of damage without direct visualization of the ligamentous and soft-tissue structures. Consequently, complete exposure and exploration of the joint is recommended.[10] Thorough examination of articular structures is important. Repair or debridement of damaged menisci and repair of the joint capsule should be the first steps in the surgical therapy.

Repair of the stifle depends on immediate repair and stabilization and long-term periarticular fibrosis. Reconstruction of collateral ligaments or placement of prosthetic ligaments using screws and spiked washers is suggested to maintain stability so that stabilizing sutures can be placed. Both intra- and extra-articular repair for the cranial and caudal cruciate ligaments have been used to provide immediate stifle stability. Reconstruction of the caudal cruciate ligament was not found to be necessary in a review of 12 cases of multiple ligamentous injuries of the feline stifle of working dogs, but methods of stabilization must be addressed on a case by case basis.[11] With extensive soft-tissue damage, it is proposed that a strong inflammatory reaction incites significant collagen-repair stages of healing, leading to long-term stability of the joint.

External skeletal fixation has been used as an adjunct therapy to support extra-articular techniques used for the repair of collateral and cruciate ligament damage. The use of a transarticular external fixator provided joint stability and return to function during the period of periarticular fibrous tissue formation. Complications seen with the external fixator are associated with pin loosening, fracture through pin sites, and severe breakdown of repair as was seen with animals that escaped from confinement. Lateral splints may also be used to provide support to surgical procedures. Use of a temporary transarticular pin without reconstruction of the damaged soft tissues has also been successfully used in small dogs and cats to provide support and allow periarticular fibrosis to form and stabilize the stifle.

Regardless of the surgical method used, mild to moderate stifle osteoarthritis is expected and can be attributed to the initial injury, as well as resultant altered biomechanical forces. Lastly, arthrodesis or amputation can be used as an option for acute severe trauma, chronic instability, or a painful joint.

Luxations involving the Tarsus and Metatarsus

The tarsal joints are composite articulations, in which more than two joint surfaces are enclosed within the same joint capsule. The tarsus and metatarsus are frequently involved in trauma and subluxations, and complete luxations are common. The regional anatomy is complex, and most surgeons consider instability at four different horizontal levels from proximal to distal: the talocrural joint, the proximal intertarsal joint, the distal intertarsal joint, and the tarsometatarsal joint. In addition, a multitude of vertically oriented intratarsal joints are considered to be more rigid than the horizontally oriented joints, although instability can occur in these joints as well.[12]

Talocrural Joint Subluxation and Luxation

This joint permits the largest degree of movement (maximum flexion in normal Labrador retrievers is 38°, with maximal extension measured at 165°).[2] The trochlea of the talus (or tibial tarsal bone), with two distinct articular ridges, fits into reciprocal grooves found in the cochlea of the tibia, providing some stability; however, the rest of the stability relies on the medial and lateral collateral ligaments and the plantar ligaments.

In dogs and cats, luxations of the talocrural joint are most commonly associated with trauma, and injuries can be classified as either closed (without soft-tissue injury) and open or as shearing injuries. Most of these injuries are presumably caused by trauma, although in many cases the actual event is not observed. The type of trauma is thought to be forced rotation around the long axis of the joint or a severe blow directly to the joint, most often to the medial aspect. If luxation of the talocrural joint results, either the medial or lateral malleoli (or both) may fracture. In our experience, the lateral malleolus is more likely to fracture and the medial collateral ligament complex is more likely to tear without fracture. Although most injuries to the collateral ligaments involve both the short and long components, injuries to the short collateral (fibulocalcanear and fibulotalar or distal and proximal short lateral collateral ligaments, respectively) can occur and may be difficult to diagnose without careful palpation under anesthesia. Radiographic changes associated with these injuries may be confused with osteochondrosis dissecans.[13,14] Damage to the lateral collateral ligaments may be more likely when the animal rotates at speed around the hindlimb in a flexed, weight-bearing position.[13] In adult cats, a torn medial collateral ligament complex is frequently associated with lateral instability caused by fracture of the fibula at the origin of the lateral collateral ligament;[15] whereas a Salter-Harris 2 fracture of the distal tibia will result in the appearance of a complete luxation of the tibiotarsal joint in the immature cat.

Treatment Strategies

CLOSED INJURY: Using a combination of traditional orthogonal and stressed-view radiography, in addition to careful palpation, the surgeon should identify whether the medial collateral, lateral collateral, or palmar ligamentous support to the talocrural joint has been damaged. For complex injuries, computed tomography should be considered as well.[16] Although closed reduction and coaptation can be attempted, the forces applied to the joint usually exceed the ability of the scar tissue to stabilize the joint, and the joint will not become stable enough for the animal to bear weight.

Surgical repair usually involves reconstruction of the collateral ligaments. It has been shown that reconstruction of both the long and short parts (double prosthetic repair) will give a much better clinical outcome than single prosthetic repair.[17] Although the traditional method of screws and washers using nonabsorbable suture gives good results, alternative methods using bone tunnels[18] and bone anchors can also be used. Regardless of the method used, it is important to support primary repair of the collateral ligaments with either a transarticular external fixator or cast/splint for up to 6 weeks. If excessive damage to the articular surface of the tibiotarsal joint is found during surgical exploration, pantarsal arthrodesis should be done, typically by application of a dorsal plate combined with an intramedullary pin.[19]

SHEARING INJURY: Shearing injury of the hock involves the medial aspect in two thirds or more of cases.[20] Treatment is somewhat controversial and can include immediate or delayed prosthetic reconstruction of the damaged ligaments, immediate or delayed pantarsal arthrodesis, or primary management of the wound with support from either an external fixator or cast alone.[20] If immediate arthrodesis is performed, an external fixator may be preferable to a plate, which may have to be removed owing to chronic infection that cannot be avoided when a large open wound is present.[21]

Proximal Intertarsal Subluxation and Luxation

The proximal intertarsal joint is composed of the talocentral and calcaneoquartal joints, which do not allow noticeable motion in the normal dog and cat. This joint can fail in either hyperextension, which may result in damage to the dorsal ligaments, or more commonly, from failure of the plantar ligaments with or without fractures and luxations of the associated tarsal and metatarsal bones. The Shetland sheepdog appears to be predisposed to proximal intertarsal joint luxation, presumably caused by chronic degeneration of the plantar ligaments of unknown cause.[22] The condition may be bilateral.

Treatment Strategies

HYPEREXTENSION: Because during normal weight-bearing hyperextension injuries tend to be held in reduction, and because most of the support to the joint comes from the plantar ligaments, these injuries can generally be treated with a cast.

HYPERFLEXION: Calcaneoquartal arthrodesis is recommended for hyperflexion injuries, as external coaptation has been shown to be ineffective. Arthrodesis may be effective in a variety of ways (e.g., lateral plate, Steinmann pin, and tension band), use of a tension band in combination with the primary repair and external coaptation until radiographic evidence of arthrodesis is achieved is recommended.[22]

Tarsometatarsal Luxation and Subluxation

The four distal tarsal bones, numbered from medial to lateral first through fourth, articulate with the metatarsals I through V, forming the tarsometatarsal joints. These joints are considered to be low-motion joints in the normal dog and cat. Subluxation and luxation of the tarsometarsal joints usually occur as a result of trauma and may be associated with concurrent fractures of the proximal metatarsal bones.

Treatment Strategies

External coaptation may be appropriate for minor injuries involving only one or two metatarsal bones with minimal displacement. However, if the entire tarsometarsal articulation is luxated, or if significant displacement is present even if only a lateral or medial injury is noted, arthrodesis is recommended. Although many forms of arthrodesis have been reported, plate fixation is likely to be the most successful. Usually the plate is applied laterally,[23] and a hybrid (either 2.0/2.7 or 2.7/3.5 mm) dynamic compression plate may be advantageous.[24]

Talocalcaneal Luxation

The talocalcaneal joint is maintained by two ligaments crossing the tarsal sinus between the two bones, and is considered to be a low-motion joint. Luxation has been reported in the dog after trauma, and may be difficult to see on standard radiographic views.

Treatment Strategies

The reports of this injury are limited, but success has been observed both with reduction and external coaptation and lag screw fixation.[25]

References

1. Sidaway BK, McLaughlin RM, Elder SH, et al: Role of the tendons of the biceps brachii and infraspinatus muscles and the medial glenohumeral ligament in the maintenance of passive shoulder joint stability in dogs. Am J Vet Res 65(9):1216-1222, 2004.

2. Jaegger G, Marcellin-Little J, Levine D: Reliability of goniometry in Labrador Retrievers. Am J Vet Res 63:979-986, 2002.

3. Dassler C, Vasseur PB: Elbow luxation. *In* Textbook of Small Animal Surgery, 3rd ed. Slatter D (ed). Philadelphia: Saunders, 2003, pp. 1923-1927.

4. O'Brien MH, Boudrieau RJ, Clark DN: Traumatic luxation of the cubital joint (elbow) in dogs: 44 cases (1978-1988). J Am Vet Med Assoc 201:1760-1765, 1992.

5. Billings LA, Vasseur PB, Todoroff RJ, Johnson W: Clinical results after reduction of traumatic elbow luxations in nine dogs and one cat. J Am Anim Hosp Assoc 28:137-142, 1992.

6. Piermattei DL, Flo GL, DeCamp CE: Handbook of Small Animal Orthopedics and Fracture Repair, 4th ed. St. Louis: Saunders Elsevier, 2006.

7. Aron DN: Traumatic dislocation of the stifle joint: Treatment of 12 dogs and one cat. J Am Anim Hosp Assoc 24:333, 1988.

8. Hulse DA, Shires P: Multiple ligament injury of the stifle joint in the dog. J Am Anim Assoc 22:105, 1986.

9. Payne JT: Stifle luxation. Stifle joint anatomy and surgical approaches in the dog. Vet Clin North Am 23:850, 1993.

10. Bruce WJ: Multiple ligamentous injuries of the canine stifle joint: a study of 12 cases. J Small Anim Pract 39:333, 1998.

11. Bruce WJ: Stifle luxation in the cat: treatment using transarticular external skeletal fixation. J Small Anim Pract 40:482, 1999.

12. Evans EE (ed): Miller's Anatomy of the Dog, 3rd ed. Philadelphia: WB Saunders, 1993, pp. 222, 252-257.

13. Sjostrom L, Hakanson N: Traumatic injuries associated with the short lateral collateral ligaments of the talocrural joint of the dog. J Small Anim Pract 35:163-168, 1994.

14. Matushek KJ, Dueland RT: Partial rupture of the calcaneofibular ligament of the hock in a dog. Vet Comp Orthop Traum 4:46-47, 1991.

15. Schmokel HG, Ehrismann G: The surgical treatment of talocrural luxation in nine cats. Vet Comp Orthop Traumatol 14:46-50, 2001.

16. Gielen IM, De Rycke LM, van Bree HJ, Simoens PJ: Computed tomography of the tarsal joint in clinically normal dogs. Am J Vet Res 62:1911-1915, 2001.

17. Aron DN: Prosthetic ligament replacement for severe tarsocrural joint instability. J Am Anim Hosp Assoc 23:41-55, 1987.

18. Fox SM, Guerin SR, Burbridge HM: Reconstruction of the medial collateral ligament for tarsocrural luxation.

19. Kirsch JA, Dejardin LM, DeCamp CE, et al: In vitro mechanical evaluation on the use of an intramedullary pin-plate combination for pantarsal arthrodesis in dogs. Am J Vet Res 66:125-131, 2005.

20. Beardsley SL, Schrader SC: Treatment of dogs with wounds of the limbs caused by shearing forces: 98 cases (1975-1993). J Am Vet Med Assoc 207:1071-1075, 1995.

21. Benson JA, Boudrieau RJ: Severe carpal and tarsal shearing injuries treated with an immediate arthrodesis in seven dogs. J Am Anim Hosp Assoc 38:370-380, 2002.

22. Allen MJ, Dyce J, Houlton JEF: Calcaneoquartal arthrodesis in the dog. J Small Anim Pract 34:205-210, 1993.

23. Dyce J, Whitelock RG, Robinson RA, et al: Arthrodesis of the tarsometatarsal joint using a laterally applied plate in 10 dogs. J Small Anim Pract 39:19-22, 1998.

24. Fettig AA, McCarthy RJ, Kowaleski MP: Intertarsal and tarsometatarsal arthrodesis using 2.0/2.7-mm or 2.7/3.5-mm hybrid dynamic compression plates. J Am Anim Hosp Assoc;38:364-369, 2002.

25. Gorse MJ, Purinton PT, Penwick RC, et al: Talocalcaneal luxation: an anatomic and clinical study. Vet Surg 19:429-434, 1990.

Chapter 111

Tendon Injury and Repair

Simon Timothy Kudnig

Function of Tendons

Tendons are a vital component of the locomotor system and are a vital link between muscle and bone. Tendon function includes the transfer of force developed by muscles, joint movement, limb support, gliding motion, and the storage and release of energy. Tendons do not possess contractile elements; however, their elasticity may serve to attenuate sudden forces, thereby protecting the associated muscle, and to enable a final velocity of movement to be attained that is greater than that of the contracting muscle.[1] Muscles possess a tendon attachment whenever their point of insertion is distant or when the muscle must exert its forces of contraction across a joint. Tendons are highly resistant to extension but are relatively flexible and, therefore, can be angulated around bones or a joint.

Tendon Anatomy

The tendon is a complex composite material consisting of collagen fibrils embedded in a matrix of proteoglycans.[2] Collagen fascicles are oriented parallel to the long axis of the tendon, with type I collagen being the major constituent.[2] Fibroblasts are the predominant cell type within the tendon and are arranged in parallel rows in the spaces between the parallel collagen bundles. Collagen chains are arranged in a left-handed configuration, with three collagen chains combined into a collagen molecule. The tertiary structure of type I collagen consists of three collagen chains coiled together in a right-handed triple helix held together by hydrogen and covalent bonds.[2] Collagen molecules are then arranged in a quarter stagger, forming the quaternary structure with the alignment of oppositely charged amino acids providing a great part of the strength of the structure.[2] Five collagen molecules combine to form ordered units of microfibrils, which are arranged to form subfibrils, and these in turn are combined to form fibrils. Collagen fibrils are bound together by a matrix consisting of proteoglycans and glycoproteins in combination with water to form fascicles. A loose connective tissue called the endotendon binds the fascicles within the tendon together and permits longitudinal movement of collagen fascicles as well as support for blood vessels, lymphatics, and nerves. The epitenon covers the surface of a tendon; with tendons that are enclosed by a tendon sheath, a mesotenon originates on the side opposite the pulley friction surface and joins the epitenon. Tendons that are not enclosed within a synovial sheath are surrounded by a looser areolar connective tissue called the paratenon. A tendon sheath surrounds a tendon in areas where there is a marked change in direction, when tendons pass under ligamentous bands or through fascial slings, or when tendons pass across a joint. The tendon sheath consists of a visceral (inner) layer and a parietal (outer) layer and is lined by a secretory endothelium. Sesamoid bones are osseous or cartilaginous structures that protect the tendon as it passes over a bony surface, and the opposed surfaces of the sesamoid and underlying bone are covered by cartilage. This entire structure is enveloped in a bursa or sheath. Tendons receive their blood supply from surrounding tissues via vessels in the paratenon or mesotenon. Tendons surrounded by paratenon have been described as "vascular tendons," with multiple points of vessel entry from the periphery; these vessels anastomose with a longitudinal system of capillaries. Tendons surrounded by a tendon sheath have been described as "avascular tendons" in which the blood supply in the mesotenon is reduced to vessels in the vincula, which divide into dorsal, proximal, and distal branches and vascular loops into the tendon substance.

Pathophysiology of Tendon Injury

Tendon injury results from both direct and indirect trauma. Direct trauma includes lacerations and contusions; indirect trauma results from tensile overload resulting in sprains, rupture, avulsions, and displacements. Most tendons can withstand larger tensile forces exerted by their muscles or sustained by bones, resulting in avulsion fractures of the bone to which the tendon is attached, avulsions of the tendon attachment to bone, or ruptures at the muscle-tendon junction. Preexisting pathology in the tendon can result in midsubstance tears from mechanical overload. Underlying conditions that can predispose to tendon injury include hyperadrenocorticism, excessive administration of corticosteroids, and intratendinous injection of corticosteroids.[3,4] Repeated microstrains and mechanical overload with hyperthermia, free-radical production, and hypoxia are pathophysiologic mechanisms important in the development of tendinitis. Tendon sprains are more commonly diagnosed in horses; however, it is likely that many tendon injuries are unrecognized in small animals. Tendon sprains seen in dogs include the insertion of the flexor carpi ulnaris in racing greyhounds, the deep digital flexor tendon to the digits, and various components of the Achilles mechanism. Tendons commonly undergoing displacements include the biceps tendon, the superficial digital flexor tendon, and the long digital extensor tendon. Tendon avulsions commonly involve the long digital extensor tendon and the gastrocnemius tendon.

Tendon Biomechanics

The presence of collagen and the arrangement of collagen fibers parallel to the direction of the tensile forces provide tendons with considerable tensile strength. As with other collagenous soft tissues such as ligaments, the load-deformation curve of tendons is characterized by a toe region, which corresponds to the straightening of the crimped fibrils and orienting of the fibers in the direction of loading. The toe region for tendons, however, is relatively small owing to the preexistence of collagen fibers nearly parallel with the long axis of the tendon. The toe region is followed by a linear region, and the slope of this region represents the elastic modulus of the tendon. The yield point is the point of the load deformation curve that is followed by the failure region in which plastic deformation leads to irreversible changes in the tendon. Tendons do have viscoelastic properties, with the elongation depending not only on the amount of force applied but also on the rate of force application.[2]

Tendon Healing

Tendon healing is an important area of orthopedic research to maximize strength and rate of repair to facilitate early and complete return to athletic function. Tendon healing is important to enable both sufficient tendon strength and to maintain appropriate tendon length to ensure appropriate function. A healing tendon must also maintain the ability to glide, which is the most difficult aspect of tendon repair to preserve. Healing tendons, as other tissues, undergo four overlapping phases of wound healing, which are inflammation, debridement, repair, and maturation. Immediately after injury, the wounded tendon fills with inflammatory products, neutrophils, and fibrin. The remnants of disrupted tendon are removed during the inflammatory phase, resulting in demarcation of the lesion.[5] The inflammatory and debridement phases of healing delay the onset of the repair phases, necessitating gentle tissue handling, wound lavage, surgical debridement, and resolution of infection to shorten the duration of the inflammatory phase. During the repair phase, undifferentiated mesenchymal cells from the surrounding connective tissues migrate into the wound and differentiate into fibroblasts. The fibroblasts secrete ground substance and collagen, which together with capillary buds, form granulation tissue between the tendon ends. The growth and migration of collagen fibers between the tendon ends are oriented perpendicularly to the long axis of the tendon; however, by the third and fourth weeks, the fibroblasts and collagen fibers orient themselves along the lines of stress.[2] The reorganization of collagen fibers is part of the maturation phase and is partly responsible for the increase in tensile strength. An increase in intermolecular bonds between collagen fibers also contributes to an increase in tensile strength, and this, as well as fiber orientation and collagen production, depends on the application of stresses to the healing tendon.[2] As the maturation phase ensues, the fibroblasts switch from type III collagen to type I collagen.

A distinction has been made with regard to the healing of unsheathed, vascular tendons versus sheathed, avascular tendons. With unsheathed tendons, the undifferentiated mesenchymal cells and capillary buds migrate from the paratenon and blend with the epitenon. With sheathed tendons, contrary to previous investigations indicating that the fibroblasts were derived only from the tendon sheath, tendon cells themselves do have some intrinsic capabilities of repair. The intrinsic response originates from the epitenon and is stimulated by passive range of motion, which results in less adhesion formation and an improvement in healing over the traditional "one wound one scar" theory of avascular tendon healing. Revascularization of ensheathed canine flexor tendons in conjunction with passive range of motion has been shown to occur from vessels in the epitenon, in the absence of ingrowth of peripheral adhesions.[6] Thus repair of sheathed tendons in the correct environment can occur with minimal contribution from cells of the tendon sheath or surrounding connective tissue, thereby avoiding restrictive adhesion formation.

More recent research, particularly in the human and equine fields, has focused on molecular techniques for the improvement in tendon healing. Important growth factors that are involved in tendon healing include insulin-like growth factor-1, transforming growth factor- beta1, growth and differentiation factors (GDFs), epidermal growth factor, platelet-derived growth factor, vascular endothelial growth factor, and bone morphogenic proteins 2 and 7.[7-10] These growth factors form the basis of molecular techniques and gene manipulation techniques to enhance tendon healing.[11] Mesenchymal stem cells found in the bone marrow have been shown to stimulate healing and have additive effects with growth factors.[12] Other therapies to optimize tendon repair have included tissue engineering, extracorporeal shock-wave therapy, therapeutic ultrasound, low-level laser therapy, hyperbaric oxygen therapy, and nitric oxide.[13-17]

Tendon Repair

Tendon repair techniques must follow certain principles to ensure a successful outcome. These include the apposition of the severed ends with minimal disruption of blood supply, minimum amount of suture material for repair, elimination of gap formation, and use of suture techniques with maximum mechanical strength. Gap formation of greater than 3 mm at the site of tendon repair has been shown to delay healing and significantly increase the risk of rupture during the first 6 weeks of rehabilitation.[18] A gap of less than 1 mm is required for a tendon to heal without scar and adhesion formation.[19] Tendon suturing techniques have followed the principle that sutures passed between the fascicles are easily pulled out of the tendon, whereas maximum mechanical strength has been achieved with the placement of sutures perpendicular to the tendon before passing across the site of injury. The optimum rehabilitation of tendon injuries is difficult to achieve in small animals. Excessive activity early in the repair process will result in gap formation and failure of the repair, whereas controlled early passive mobilization stimulates repair and increases the strength of the tendon in the first few months following repair. Early motion also limits adhesion formation and, therefore, enhances the gliding function of the tendon. Vascular tendons achieve 56% and 79% of the original strength at 6 weeks and 1 year, respectively, following repair.[20] Normal forces associated with muscle contraction stress the tendon to approximately 25 to 33% of maximum strength, indicating that by 6 weeks postoperatively the repair should be able to withstand limited exercise.[1,21,22] Numerous suture patterns for the repair of tendons have been developed. The Bunnel-Mayer technique is limited by compromise of the blood supply and a resultant decrease in tensile strength.[23] The Kessler technique was developed to maximize strength by the placement of suture bites perpendicular to the tendon, and the modified Kessler or locking-loop technique allows the knot to be placed at one end of the tendon rather than between the tendon ends. Superior tensile strength has been demonstrated by the three-loop pulley technique over a single and double locking-loop technique.[24] The three-loop pulley technique, owing to its superior tensile strength, is recommended for larger weight-bearing tendons and round tendons, and also for collateral ligament repair. The locking-loop technique is useful for flat tendons, although a continuous cruciate pattern has been shown to be superior to the locking-loop technique for tenorraphy of canine deep gluteal tendons.[25]

Specific Tendon Injuries

Luxation of the Tendon of the Biceps Brachii Muscle

Luxation of the tendon of the biceps muscle occurs because of a displacement of the tendon out of the intertubercular groove as a result of rupture of the transverse humeral ligament.[26] Affected dogs present with forelimb lameness; flexion of the shoulder with external rotation can promote luxation of the tendon. Surgical treatment involves placement of sutures between the remnants of the transverse humeral ligament to the insertion of the supraspinatus muscle, or it involves using a prosthetic suture to replace the transverse humeral ligament.[26]

Severed Superficial and Deep Digital Flexor Tendons

Severance of the digital flexor tendons commonly occurs on the palmar or plantar aspect of the distal extremity where the tendons are superficial; the injury is commonly the result of a penetrating wound. Severance of the deep digital flexor tendon(s) causes hyperextension of one or more digits with hyperextension of the distal interphalangeal joint and dorsal elevation of the claw from the ground during weight bearing. Surgical apposition of the transected tendon ends with a monofilament nonabsorbable locking-loop suture or three-loop pulley suture; an appositional pattern in the tendon sheath has been recommended.[27] Postoperative management should involve a cast or splint designed to maintain the digits in flexion for 6 weeks.[27] Although early passive range of motion is recommended for human tendon repair, such controlled activity is difficult to achieve in canine patients.

Avulsion of Proximal Tendon of the Long Digital Extensor Muscle

Avulsion of the long digital extensor muscle from the lateral femoral condyle commonly affects young, large and giant breeds. Affected dogs present with a weight-bearing pelvic limb lameness with pain and crepitus palpated in the stifle.[28,29] Diagnosis can be made via radiography, computed tomography, or magnetic resonance imaging.[28,29] The avulsion is repaired by reattaching the avulsed bone to the origin on lateral femoral condyle.[28,29] If no bone remains for fixation, the tendon can be sutured to the stifle joint capsule near its point of penetration.

Achilles Mechanism Injury

The Achilles tendon is composed of the gastrocnemius tendon, the common tendon of the biceps femoris, gracilis and semitendinosus muscles, and the superficial digital flexor tendon. Injuries to the Achilles mechanism result in tarsal hyperflexion and a flaccidity of the Achilles tendon when the tarsus is flexed. Flexion of the digits with tarsal hyperflexion resulting in a "claw" appearance occurs when the superficial digital flexor tendon is intact. Ruptures of the Achilles mechanism commonly occur at the musculocutaneous junction rather than the muscle belly. Primary tenorrhaphy of each of the three tendon components is recommended, with additional support provided by a fascia lata autograft or polypropylene mesh. A modified three-loop pulley suture pattern has been shown to be a superior technique for reattachment of the tendon to bone than the lockingloop suture.[30] Postoperative immobilization is important to protect the repair from excessive weight-bearing forces and can be achieved with external coaptation using a cast, orthotics, linear external fixator, or a circular fixator.

Luxation of Superficial Digital Flexor Tendon

The superficial digital flexor tendon can become luxated as it crosses the tuber calcanei. Lateral luxation owing to breakdown of the medial retinaculum is more common. It appears that Shetland sheepdogs[31] are predisposed. Possible contributing factors include exercise, trauma, obesity, rotation around the joint with the tarsus in a flexed position, structural deformities of the calcaneus, and a weaker medial attachment of the tendon to the calcaneus.[31,32] Palpation of instability of the superficial digital flexor tendon during talocrural manipulation is pathognomic for the injury.[32] The injury is repaired by suturing the retinaculum opposite the side of luxation. With lateral luxations, appositional sutures are placed in the medial retinaculum, and bone tunnels can be placed in the calcaneus for additional purchase if required. Polypropylene mesh has been used for failed repairs to reinforce the medial calcaneal retinaculum.[33]

References

1. Elliot DH: Structure and function of mammalian tendon. Biol Rev 40:392, 1965.

2. Woo SL, An K, Arnoczky SP, et al: Anatomy, biology and biomechanics of tendon, ligament, and meniscus. *In* Orthopaedic Basic Science. Simon SR (ed). American Academy of Orthopaedic Surgeons, 1994, p. 45.

3. Kleinmann M, Gross AE: Achilles tendon rupture following steroid injection. J Bone Joint Surg Am 65:1345, 1983.

4. Unverferth LJ, Olix ML: The effect of local steroid injections on tendons. J Sports Med 1:31, 1973.

5. van Schie HT, Bakker EM, Jonker AM, et al: Computerized ultrasonographic tissue characterization of equine superficial digital flexor tendons by means of stability quantification of echo patterns in contiguous transverse ultrasonographic images. Am J Vet Res 64:366, 2003.

6. Gelberman RH, Khabie V, Cahill CJ: The revascularization of healing flexor tendons in the digital sheath. A vascular injection study in dogs. J Bone Joint Surg Am 73(6):868-881, 1991.

7. Dahlgren LA, van der Meulen MC, Bertram JE, et al: Insulin-like growth factor-I improves cellular and molecular aspects of healing in a collagenase-induced model of flexor tendinitis. J Orthop Res 20:910, 2002.

8. Jann HW, Stein LE, Slater DA: In vitro effects of epidermal growth factor or insulin-like growth factor on tenoblast migration on absorbable suture material. Vet Surg 28:268, 1999.

9. Aspenberg P, Forslund C: Enhanced tendon healing with GDF 5 and 6. Acta Orthop Scand 70:51, 1999.

10. Mihelic R, Pecina M, Jelic M, et al: Bone morphpogenetic protein-7 (osteogenic protein-1) promotes tendon graft integration in anterior cruciate ligament reconstruction in sheep. Am J Sports Med 32:1619, 2004.

11. Hildebrand KA, Jia F, Woo SL: Response of donor and recipient cells after transplantation of cells to the ligament and tendon. Microsc Res Tech 58:34, 2002.

12. Caplan AI, Bruder SP: Mesenchymal stem cells: building blocks for molecular medicine in the 21st century. Trends Mol Med 7:259, 2001.

13. Dejardin LM, Arnoczky SP, Ewers BJ, et al: Tissue-engineered rotator cuff tendon using porcine small intestine submucosa. Histologic and mechanical evaluation in dogs. Am J Sports Med 29:175, 2001.

14. Orhan Z, Alper M, Akman Y, et al: An experimental study on the application of extracorporeal shock waves in the treatment of tendon injuries: preliminary report. J Orthop Sci 6:566, 2001.

15. Saini NS, Roy KS, Bansal PS, et al: A preliminary study on the effect of ultrasound therapy on the healing of surgically severed achilles tendons in five dogs. J Vet Med A Physiol Pathol Clin Med 49:321, 2002.

16. Reddy GK, Stehno-Bittel L, Enwemeka CS: Laser photostimulation of collagen production in healing rabbit Achilles tendons. Lasers Surg Med 22:281, 1998.

17. Ishii Y, Ushida T, Tateishi T, et al: Effects of different exposures of hyperbaric oxygen on ligament healing in rats. J Orthop Res 20:353, 2002.

18. Gelberman RH, Boyer MI, Brodt MD, et al: The effect of gap formation at the repair site on the strength and excursion of intrasynovial flexor tendons. J Bone Joint Surg 81:975, 1999.

19. Ketchum LD, Martin NL, Kappel DA: Experimental evaluation of factors affecting the strength of tendon repairs. Plast Reconstr Surg 59:708, 1977.

20. Dueland R, Quenin J: Triceps tenotomy: Biomechanical assessment of healing strength. J Am Anim Hosp Assoc 16:507, 1980.

21. Hirsch G: Tensile properties during tendon healing. Acta Orthop Scand Suppl 153:1, 1974.

22. Walker LB, Harris EH, Benedict JV: Stress-strain relationship in human cadaveric plantaris tendon. Med Electron Biol Eng 2:31, 1964.

23. Pjanowski GJ, Stein LE, Turner TA: Strength characteristics and failure modes of suture patterns in severed goat tendons. Vet Surg 18:335, 1989.

24. Berg RJ, Egger EL: In vitro comparison of the three loop pulley and locking loop suture patterns for repair of canine weightbearing tendons and collateral ligaments. Vet Surg 15:107, 1986.

25. Renberg WC, Radlinsky MG: In vitro comparison of the locking loop and continuous cruciate suture patterns. Vet Compar Orthop Traumatol 14:15, 2001.

26. Boemo CM, Eaton-Wells RD: Medial displacement of the tendon of origin of the biceps brachii muscle in 10 greyhounds. J Small Anim Pract 36:69, 1995.

27. Williams N, Payne JT, Tomlinson JL, et al: Deep digital flexor tendon injuries in dogs. Comp Cont Educ Pract Vet 19:853, 1997.

28. Fitch RB, Wilson ER, Hathcock JT, et al: Radiographic, computed tomographic and magnetic resonance imaging evaluation of a chronic long digital extensor tendon avulsion in a dog. Vet Radiol Ultrasound 38:177, 1997.

29. Pond MJ: Avulsion of the extensor digitorum longus muscle in the dog: a report of four cases. J Small Anim Pract 14:785, 1973.

30. Moores AP, Comerford EJ, Tarlton JF, et al: Biomechanical and clinical evaluation of a modified 3-loop pulley suture pattern for reattachment of canine tendons to bone. Vet Surg 33:391, 2004.

31. Mauterer JV Jr, Prata RG, Carberry CA, et al: Displacement of the tendon of the superficial digital flexor muscle in dogs: 10 cases (1983-1991). J Am Vet Med Assoc 203:1162, 1993.

32. Reinke JD, Mughannam AJ: Lateral luxation of the superficial digital flexor tendon in 12 dogs. J Am Anim Hosp Assoc 29:303, 1993.

33. Houlton JEF, Dyce J: The use of polypropylene mesh for revision of failed repair of superficial digital flexor tendon luxation in three dogs. Vet Compar Orthop Traumatol 6:129, 1993.

Chapter 112

Tendinitis and Bursitis

Simon Timothy Kudnig

Tendinitis

Lower intensity trauma can result in tendon sprains or tendinitis rather than complete rupture. Such injuries are more commonly diagnosed in horses; however, they are recognized in canine athletes and are probably under-diagnosed in active dogs. Tendinitis refers to inflammation of the tendon with a few or many tendon fibers being torn; however, total discontinuity of the tendon is not produced. Hypoxic tendon injury can result in fibrocartilaginous metaplasia, which can interfere with tendon function and be a source of pain. Repeated microstrains and mechanical overload with hyperthermia, free-radical production, and hypoxia are pathophysiologic mechanisms important in the development of tendinitis. Goals of treatment of tendinitis are to increase the number of fibroblasts, increase matrix production, increase the proportion of type I collagen versus type III collagen, and increase the organization of collagen fibers. This will allow an increase in tensile strength, a decreased incidence of reinjury, and a decreased rehabilitation time. Restoration of structurally normal tendinous tissue with normal tensile strength and elasticity is the goal of tendon repair rather than promoting a connective tissue scar.

Mineralization of the Tendon of Insertion of the Supraspinatus Muscle

Mineralization of the tendon of insertion of the supraspinatus muscle or calcifying tendinopathy of the supraspinatus tendon can result in a chronic, intermittent, or progressive weight-bearing lameness that worsens after exercise. Pain is elicited on shoulder extension. Mineralization of soft tissues to the level of the greater tubercle of the humerus cranial to the scapulohumeral joint on a cranioproximal-craniodistal radiographic view is suggestive of the disease. A poor correlation between the size of the lesion and lameness has been identified.[1] Hypoxia of the tendon is considered the primary initiating factor in the deposition of calcium. The tendon undergoes fibrocartilaginous transformation; calcium crystals are then deposited in the matrix and coalesce to form deposits. The location of the injury may be related to a hypovascular area of the tendon adjacent to the major tubercle that may be predisposed to hypoxic injury. Treatment options include rest, nonsteroidal anti-inflammatory therapy, intralesional steroid injections, surgical excision, and extracorporeal shock-wave therapy. The mineral deposits commonly reform; however this is poorly correlated to a recurrence of lameness.[1]

Bicipital Tenosynovitis

Biceps tendon injury is a common cause of forelimb lameness and shoulder pain in dogs. Biceps tears commonly occur within the glenohumeral joint, outside the bicipital groove and adjacent to the supraglenoid tubercle, as this is a relatively avascular zone.[2] Inflammation of the biceps tendon can occur as a primary lesion or secondary to intraarticular disease such as glenohumeral instability. The cause of primary bicipital tenosynovitis is unknown and may include overuse or chronic repetitive trauma resulting in an inflammatory response. Gross pathologic changes include hyperemia of the bursa, leading to joint effusion; chronic synovitis, causing synovial hyperplasia of the bursa; chondromalacia of the intertubercular groove with osteophyte formation at its margins; and metastatic calcification of the biceps tendon. Adhesions between the tendon and the tendon sheath may develop. Hypoxia of the tendon as a result of damaged blood supply promotes chondroid metaplasia and calcification, with the normal synovial space and smooth gliding surface of the intertubercular groove typically being replaced by proliferative synovium and fibrotic adhesions. Fibrocartilaginous metaplasia, however, can be seen in normal dogs,[3] and the relationship between histopathologic findings and clinical findings is inconsistent.[4] Diagnosis of bicipital tenosynovitis can be made via an orthopedic examination, by eliciting a positive "biceps test" (pain on palpation of the biceps tendon with the shoulder in a flexed position), and with plain radiographs including a skyline view of the bicipital groove, contrast arthrography, ultrasonography, or MRI. Treatment includes rest and nonsteroidal anti-inflammatory treatment, intraarticular or intralesional steroid injections, open tenodesis, arthroscopic tenodesis, and arthroscopic biceps tenotomy. Results of tenodesis are excellent,[5,6] however, arthroscopic tenotomy offers a less demanding approach with apparently good results.[7] The indications and long-term results for tenodesis versus tenotomy in dogs has not been established.[6]

Calcaneal Tendinitis

Inflammation of the area of the insertion of the calcaneal tendon onto the calcaneus may progress to avulsion and failure of the Achilles mechanism. It is recommended that evaluation of the opposite calcaneal tendon be performed in cases of a unilateral injury to ensure that calcaneal tendinitis is not present in the contralateral limb. Ultrasonography has been shown to be a useful tool for imaging lesions of the Achilles tendon.[8]

Stenosing Tenosynovitis of the Abductor Pollicis Longus Muscle

The abductor pollicis longus muscle abducts the first digit. Injury of this tendon can result in forelimb lameness, a swelling on the medial aspect of the carpus, and pain on carpal flexion.[9] Connective tissue proliferation leads to stenosis of the synovial sheath and pain associated with constriction of the tendon within the tendon sheath. Radiographically, proliferative bone reactions at the distal radius in the area of the fibro-osseus canal of the abductor pollicis longus can be found in advanced cases of the disease.[9] Conservative treatment involves injection of corticosteroids in the area of the synovial sheath; however, nonresponding cases benefit from surgical release of the tendon rather than tenotomy.[9]

Tendinitis of the Insertion of the Flexor Carpi Ulnaris

This injury commonly occurs in the tendon of insertion of the flexor carpi ulnaris muscle to the accessory carpal bone in racing greyhounds. Chronic inflammation with repeated bouts of lameness is common.[10]

Bursitis

Bursae are connective tissue sacs that are lined by a synovial epithelium and contain synovial fluid. A bursa serves to reduce friction between moving parts such as tendons, ligaments, or muscles or to cushion the effects of excess pressure between these movable structures and bony prominences. True bursae are normal anatomic structures and can be described as subtendinous, submuscular, subfascial, or interligamentous. Bursae are abundantly supplied with vessels and nerves and tendon injuries involving a bursa, therefore, are extremely painful. False bursae are acquired structures secondary to repeated trauma over pressure points and consist of a nonepithelial-lined sac full of fluid, also known as a hygroma.

Many anatomic bursae have been described in the dog.[11] In the forelimb are located bursae associated with the infraspinatus muscle and the caudal part of the greater tubercle of the humerus, where the tendon of the triceps brachii muscle crosses the proximal end of the olecranon (bursa subtendinea olecrani), under the tendon of the extensor carpi radialis tendon at the carpus, under the tendon of origin of the extensor carpi ulnaris muscle, and also between its tendon of insertion and the distal ulna and where the abductor pollicis longus passes over the extensor carpi radialis muscle. A bursa also exists between the tendon of origin of the superficial digital flexor muscle and the underlying medial epicondyle of the humerus and beneath the tendon of origin of the deep digital flexor muscle. In the hindlimb, bursae are located under the tendon of origin of the rectus femoris muscle, between the distal third of the rectus femoris muscle and the femur, under the insertion of the vastus lateralis and medialis muscles, under the superficial digital flexor tendon as it passes over the tuber calcanei, between the internal obturator muscle and the ischial ramus, and at the insertion of the internal obturator muscle in the trochanteric fossa. Many dogs also have bursae beneath the deep and superficial gluteal muscles at the insertion on the greater trochanter of the femur. Projections of joint capsules can also function in a similar manner as bursae, some examples include the projection of the glenohumeral joint capsule beneath the tendon of origin of the biceps brachii muscle, the projection of the elbow joint capsule beneath the origin of the flexor carpi radialis muscle, the projection of the patellar joint capsule under the tendon of the quadriceps muscle, the projection of the stifle joint capsule under the origin of the long digital extensor muscle, and a communication between the joint capsule between the third and fourth tarsal bones and the bursa of the tendon of insertion of the peroneus longus muscle.

Acquired bursae occur as a result of trauma to the skin and subcutaneous tissue over bony prominences. The pressure on bony prominences is transmitted from the surface to the underlying dense bone, compressing all intervening tissues, and this in turn, can obstruct blood flow, leading to cell death. A spectrum of injury exists from a pressure sore, which is a dilatation of blood vessels, inflammatory edema in the skin and subcutaneous tissue over bone, to a false bursa where a hematoma has formed in the subcutaneous tissues and has become enclosed in a well delineated sac. The progression to a false bursa is dependent on the persistence of the underlying trauma and failure of a protective skin callus to protect the underlying tissues.

Specific Injuries of Anatomic Bursae

Bursitis of the Bursa Associated with the Extensor Carpi Radialis

This injury occurs in racing greyhounds and causes lameness after racing and a palpable fluid swelling.[12]

Bicipital Tenosynovitis (Bursitis)

This condition is described above under specific tendon sprains.

Chronic Calcification of the Bursa over the Greater Trochanter of the Femur

This is commonly seen as an incidental finding on radiographs, and lameness is not evident.

Specific Injuries of Acquired Bursae

Acquired bursa have been described over the olecranon (elbow hygroma) and other pressure points including the acromion of the scapula, tuber ischii, tuber coxa, greater trochanter of the femur, lateral malleolus of the tibia, tuber calcanei, and over the fifth digits and the sternum. Acquired bursae are generally sterile unless organisms are introduced via centesis or corticosteroid injection.[13] Treatment of hygromas involves removal of the inciting trauma by providing soft bedding and protective padding. Drainage followed by protective padding is considered for persistent swelling or when the bursa has become infected.

References

1. Laitinen OM, Flo GL: Mineralization of the supraspinatus tendon in dogs: a long-term follow-up. J Am Anim Hosp Assoc 36:262, 2000.

2. Bardet JF: Lesions of the biceps tendon. Diagnosis and classification. A retrospective study of 25 cases in 23 dogs and one cat. Vet Compar Orthop Traumatol 12:188, 1999.

3. Davidson EB, Griffey SM, Vasseur PB, et al: Histopathological, radiographic, and arthrographic comparison of the biceps tendon in normal dogs and dogs with biceps tenosynovitis. J Am Anim Hosp Assoc 36:522, 2000.

4. Gilley RS, Wallace LJ, Hayden DW: Clinical and pathologic analyses of bicipital tenosynovitis in dogs. Am J Vet Res 63:402, 2002.

5. Stobie D, Wallace LJ, Lipowitz AJ, et al: Chronic bicipital tenosynovitis in dogs: 29 cases (1985-1992). J Am Vet Med Assoc 207:201, 1995.

6. Cook JL, Kenter KK, Fox DB: Arthroscopic biceps tenodesis: technique and results in six dogs. J Am Anim Hosp Assoc 41:121, 2005.

7. Wall CR, Taylor R: Arthroscopic biceps brachii tenotomy as a treatment for canine bicipital tenosynovitis. J Am Anim Hosp Assoc 38:169, 2002.

8. Kramer M, Gerwing M, Michele U, et al: Ultrasonographic examination of injuries to the achilles tendon in dogs and cats. J Small Anim Pract 42:531, 2001.

9. Grundmann S, Montavon PM: Stenosing tenosynovitis of the abductor pollicis longus muscle in dogs. Vet Compar Orthop Traumatol 14:95, 2001.

10. Saunders N: Lameness and allied conditions in the greyhound. Aust Vet J 38:239, 1962.

11. Evans HE, Christensen GC: Miller's Anatomy of the Dog. Philadelphia: WB Saunders, 1979.

12. Prole JHB: A survey of racing injuries in the greyhound. J Small Anim Pract 17:207, 1976.

13. Johnston DE.: Hygroma of the elbow in dogs: J Am Vet Med Assoc 167:213, 1975.

Chapter 113

Gait Analysis

Michael Conzemius
Richard Evans

Quantitative analysis of animal motion can provide unique insight into normal and abnormal limb function. This information is useful clinically for the diagnosis of disease and as a measure of outcome following treatment intervention. In addition, gait analysis is commonly used in the development and subsequent use of animal models of disease. Historically, gait analysis has been extremely cumbersome and time-consuming. Routine clinical use was impractical because of the time required for set-up, data collection, and evaluation as well as using bulky and/or awkward equipment. Dramatic computational and equipment improvements over the past 10 years, however, have made these techniques readily available and now allow for routine assessment of gait in a modern-day laboratory or hospital. Perhaps the most attractive draw to gait analysis is that it produces objective, reproducible data of limb function.

Several techniques are available for the analysis of gait. The most common method in veterinary medicine is visual observation of gait. Objective measures of ground reaction forces (GRF) using a force platform, however, is an attractive alternative that is also commonly utilized. Publications of analysis of joint and body movements using two- and three-dimensional stereometric methods and visible markers also exist. These techniques attach markers to the skin on rigid segments of the body structure and track their motion using imaging equipment. Less frequently used methods of analyzing gait in animals include accelerometers, electromyography, electrogoniometry, and roentgenographic and magnetic coupling. Simultaneous use of a combination of evaluation methods should be considered.

Visual Observation of Gait

For most species the entire gait cycle lasts for only one second; thus, a systematic and disciplined approach must be used to clinically evaluate a patient's gait. The animal should be viewed from the front, side, and back. The observation of gait begins with a general assessment, noting symmetry and smoothness of movements of the various body parts. During stance, the clinician should take note of the position of the patient's center of mass, as the center of mass will shift toward a normal or less affected side to reduce the force applied to more painful joints or muscles. In addition, it is important to look at the base width. In general, if the forelimbs are apart and the rear limbs near each other, the animal is shifting its weight to the front; the opposite is also true. Finally, as the patient stands, one should observe for excessive internal or external rotation of a limb. In my experience, external rotation of a limb is associated with an abnormality in that limb, and internal rotation of a limb is associated with an abnormality in a different limb. Of course, disorders that have caused a permanent rotation of the skeleton make this point moot. Watching a patient sit and move from a sitting to standing position is also helpful. The "sit-test" is sometimes advocated. When a dog sits, it is considered abnormal for a foot to be pointed outward. In fact, some consider that position pathognomonic for knee pain. Although this concept frequently holds true, many normal dogs also sit with a foot or feet externally rotated. When a dog rises from a sitting position, the focus should be on the shift of weight onto the front limbs. With experience, one will notice excessive shifts.

As the animal walks, attention to the stance phase of gait is helpful. If lameness is present because of pain, the animal will avoid placing weight on the affected limb. When this occurs, the stance phase of gait will be shorter. For example, if a dog is suspected of having a unilateral forelimb lameness, the observer should watch how much time the dog spends with each of the front feet in contact with ground. The foot that is on the ground for the shortest period of time may be more painful. Some clinicians prefer to observe the position of the head when observing for a forelimb lameness. The concept is similar; the patient will place more weight on the less painful side; as the foot on this side is positioned firmly on the ground, the shoulder and head will drop. Alternatively, the foot on the more painful side will not be in contact with the ground as much and the shoulder and head will be elevated. Circumduction of a limb is abnormal. It is most likely present because of a painful joint; the patient resists flexion because of this pain and swings the limb instead. A preference for observing a patient's gait at several different velocities is common. In addition, some gait abnormalities may be observable only after the patient has been exercised.

The largest concern with the use of visual observation of gait is its subjective nature. Clinical and personal experiences can influence interpretation, thus introducing opinion, which, in the author's point of view, reduces precision, accuracy, and reproducibility. For example, in one publication when the sensitivity of visual observation of gait was compared with that of force platform gait analysis, visual observation was found to be vastly inferior.[1] In this comparison, they evaluated 148 adult Labrador retrievers; 17 were free of orthopedic and neurologic abnormalities, and 131 were 6 months after surgery for unilateral CCL injury. The observer was blinded to the dog's group assignment. Of the 17 normal dogs, the observer correctly identified all as having no gait abnormality, as did the force platform. However, the observer identified only 15 of the 131 dogs that were 6 months after knee surgery as not being normal. Using ground reaction forces from force platform gait analysis, 75% of the 131 dogs failed to achieve GRFs consistent with sound Labradors. In effect, if a dog looked lame it was lame; but if it looked normal to the observer, it may in fact have been abnormal. It should not be surprising that a computational gait analysis is more sensitive than our powers of observation. This fact should be remembered when we inform an owner that a dog "has returned to normal" after a clinical examination.

Force Platforms

A force platform measures the ground reaction forces (GRFs) exerted when it is stepped on during the stance phase. It consists of a metal plate that is mounted level with the surrounding floor or walkway that is separated from a bottom frame by force transducers near each corner. Forces in an X, Y, or Z direction that are exerted on the top surface are transmitted through the force transducers. Commercially available force plates are frequently grouped into either piezoelectric or strain gauge. Although subtle differences exist in the capabilities and cost of the two types, for clinical gait applications, the type used probably has little influence on the data generated. Piezoelectric force plates utilize quartz transducers, which generate an electric charge when stressed. Strain-gauge force plates utilize strain gauges to measure the stress in load cells when a force is applied. Piezoelectric force plates are a bit more sensitive, have a built-in amplifier, and allow for a greater force range than do strain-gauge types. However, they may have some drift, which requires resetting of the charge amplifiers just prior to data acquisition, and they are usually more expensive. There are several different manufacturers to choose from and aside from cost, the potential for customization of a system is something that should be factored into the decision-making process. The size of the force platform, transparency (if photography under the platform is desired), portability, and use with a treadmill (only z direction forces can be measured) are all potential options. Although all of the manufacturers offer compatible software, for veterinary use most clinicians and researchers use commercially available veterinary-specific software. A final consideration is professional installation in an area that encourages frequent clinical and research use but avoids abuse from general hallway traffic.

Pressure Platforms and Walkways

Pressure platforms are comparatively new systems that allow investigators to measure both temporal and spatial gait parameters. In general, pressure platforms are a bit larger (2 square feet) than a traditional force platform. Pressure walkways, which consist of multiple platforms in series, can be customized to virtually any length. These platforms function using a sensor pad that is an ultra thin (~0.1mm), flexible printed circuit. Contained within the circuit are thousands of pressure-sensing locations, or elements, arranged in rows and columns along the length and width of the platform or walkway. The sensing elements act as variable resistors within an electrical circuit. When the sensors are loaded, their resistance is low; when the force is reduced, resistance increases. The output resistance created is then converted to a raw sum for use in analysis. In effect, this allows one to measure ground reaction forces in the z-force direction. Sensors can be produced with pressure ranges from as low as 0-5 psi to as high as 0-25,000 psi. Perhaps it is important to note that ground reaction forces generated from normal dogs on pressure walkways have been shown to be nearly identical to those of force platforms.[2]

Several advantages exist to using a pressure walkway. First, because of its extended length, multiple readings and simultaneous, consecutive, and contralateral foot-strikes can be recorded with a single pass over the walkway. Some of this advantage can be attenuated if a laboratory is equipped with multiple force platforms. A single force platform, however, can only measure on half of a gait cycle in a single pass or trial.

Thus, by increasing the length of the measuring field, one not only gathers data that are more reflective of the patient's gait but fewer trials are needed to generate an adequate amount of data for statistical comparison. Reducing trial repetition is important because it saves time, because some weak or lame patients may not be able to physically perform many trials, and because the majority of variance in force platform data is attributable to trial repetition.[3] Second, because the geometry of the mat is known, spatial parameters of gait can be calculated. Patient stride length and width for each limb can be measured for consecutive steps, allowing the clinician to look for inconsistencies, improvements, or disease progression. Limb velocity and acceleration can be calculated using these data or they can be measured using a speed gun or photoelectric cells. Third, the distribution of pressure from the entire foot can be investigated.[4] Both types of platforms measure cumulative force(s) over the cell. For pressure platforms the cell is usually 0.25-square centimeters and for a traditional force platform the cell is 3-square feet. This difference allows for clinicians to estimate changes in load over the patient's foot (e.g. is load being shifted to the left side of the foot because of an injury on the right). Fourth, because of the small size of the cell in pressure platforms, there are few limitations to the size of the animal for which data can be accurately collected. Using a traditional force platform, a dog's stride length must be long enough that it place only one foot on the platform at a time. In general, dogs weighing less than 20 kg have a difficult time accomplishing this. Likewise, an extremely tall dog with a long stride may step over a traditional force platform. Increasing the animal's velocity through the gaited area will increase its stride length but this methodology creates other limitations. Because pressure platforms allow for data collection in animals with a very short stride length they provide the opportunity to measure limb function in small dogs and cats,[5,6] or in large dogs that have a short stride length because of disease or because they are recovering from surgery.[7] An added benefit to this advantage is that pressure platforms allow users to create, view, and save data in the form of a "continuous framed movie." Movies are recorded over a specified time period, at a specified frame per second speed. These gait movies allow for clinicians to measure load-bearing while the animal stands still.[7] Finally, pressure platforms are easy to set up, break down, and move to a different location. This portability provides opportunities to measure limb function that would otherwise be impossible with a traditional force platform.

Unfortunately, pressure platforms have some disadvantages. One drawback is that they can only measure total ground reaction force. Forces are not deciphered between the x-, y-, and z-direction. Second, our experiences with the software are that it is easy to work with but requires the user to invest much more time to extrude the data from each trial. For example, when using a traditional force platform, the software immediately provides peak vertical force and vertical impulse numbers. The pressure platform would require approximately one minute of additional work to gather that data. In effect, data are not automatically tabulated and summarized; this must be done manually. Furthermore, although some platform systems have components that incorporate velocity and acceleration data for each trial, most pressure platform systems do not. Again, these values, to date, must be manually calculated and added to the database. Pressure platforms are also not nearly as durable as a metal force platform and would not last long if used to measure limb function in a horse. Finally, the many advantages of pressure platforms come with a significant cost.

Technical Aspects of Force Platform Gait Analysis

Documentation of patient kinetics generates an enormous amount of data. Forces in the x-, y-, and z-direction are expressed in both peak and impulse forms, and average rising and falling slope are just a few of the points available. One obvious question is what data the clinician or investigator should focus on. Forces in the z-direction are generated by a vertical compression of the platform, and these forces are dramatically larger than those of the other two directions. Forces in the y-direction (second largest) are generated by cranial-caudal tipping of the platform and are closely related to acceleration or deceleration, which can be measured or controlled in other ways. Forces in the x-direction are generated by medial-lateral tipping and are extremely small in the quadruped. Peak vertical force (PVF) is the single largest force during the stance phase and represents only a single data point. Vertical impulse (VI) is the total area under the stance-phase curve. The results of these facts are that most veterinary publications have focused on z-direction PVF and VI forces. Although this method of expressing the data is reasonable and common, it may not be ideal. Evaluation of the force-time curves that are provided by the software is likely the best representation of limb function. Unfortunately, the statistical methods associated with this can be complicated. A simple method to mathematically explore gait analysis is to use a multivariate, as opposed to a univariate, statistical approach. In one report, the optimal set of GRFs was selected using logistic regression, with normal or not normal as the binary dependent variable and GRFs as candidate explanatory variables.[8] This method built a descriptive yet economical model that evaluated most candidate combinations of GRFs that best discriminated between the GRFs of normal Labrador retrievers and those of Labrador retrievers that had unilateral lameness from a torn cranial cruciate ligament. A cutoff that maximized Youden's index (sensitivity + specificity -1) was established and then a receiver operating curve (an ROC is a plot that represents the relationship between sensitivity and specificity of a diagnostic test) was used to assess the diagnostic properties of GRFs obtained from the force platform. These values were then applied to a group of Labrador retrievers that were 6 months after unilateral CCL-rupture surgery. The probability that an individual Labrador could be discriminated from the normal population of Labradors was calculated from data collected from visual observation of gait and from GRFs generated by force platform gait analysis. There are several advantages to this methodology. Limb function is determined by evaluating all GRFs. In comparison, if clinicians use z-direction PVF, they truly are looking at only 1/1200 (this assumes a sampling frequency of 1200 samples per second and a stance phase of 1second) of the data. In addition, this technique allows clinicians to estimate the probability of normal function after gait analysis and communicate that to an owner. For example, we now know that 6 months after some surgical procedures the probability of normal limb function is only 20%.[9] This does not mean that function after surgery is not improved or that surgery wasn't successful, only that function is not normal. This is an important step toward differentiating outcomes between treatment options.

Subject velocity influences most GFR measurements. For example, as patient velocity increases, z-force PVF increases because the patient hits the platform harder, and z-force VI decreases because the patient spends less time on the platform. Historically, for force platform gait analysis, patient velocity has been recorded via the use of photoelectric cells that project a beam of light across the runway and are set up at a known distance apart from one another with the center photoelectric cell centered at the center of the platform. When a subject interrupts the first photoelectric cell's beam of light, the system is triggered to begin recording time as the subject passes across the force platform. When the last cell's beam of light has been interrupted, the recording system stops. The patient's average velocity through the runway is then calculated. If three or more photoelectric cells are used in the system, patient acceleration can also be calculated. Velocity can also be measured using a speed gun. One limitation of the photoelectric cell system is that the cells are often aligned so that the subject's torso is the trigger of the system. Thus, photoelectric cells measure average torso velocity rather than limb velocity. The significance of this can be envisioned if one were to compare velocities of a Great Dane to that of toy poodle. If both dogs have similar torso velocities, the limb velocity of the smaller dog would have to proportionally increase relative to its shortened stride length. This limitation can be averted by comparing data from dogs of similar stature. The other, perhaps easier, method for controlling for this problem is to standardize stance time on the platform.[10]

Given the importance of subject velocity, it is common for investigators to control this parameter when evaluating and comparing a group of dogs. For walking trials, 1.0 to 1.3 meters per second, and for trotting, 1.7 to 2.0 meters per second, are used. It has been suggested by some that a trotting velocity should be used because it is more of a challenge to the dog and thus more lameness will be detected. This argument may have merit if the patient population being studied has only a subtle limp. However, in one study the effect of patient velocity on GRFs was studied and a walking velocity was clearly superior.[8] Several important messages came from that study. First, GRFs collected at a walk were linearly related and highly correlated to those collected at a trot. Second, in this investigation of dogs with lameness from a torn cranial cruciate ligament, data could be collected from all dogs at a walking velocity but only 62% of the dogs at a trotting velocity. The large proportion of dogs that failed to obtain acceptable trotting trials would dramatically impact a study. Ground reaction forces at a walk were significantly different among dogs that could and could not successfully trot; this occurred because the dogs that were the most severely lame failed to trot (most likely because as velocity increased, force increased, and thus pain increased). These dogs would be eliminated from a clinical study, and the study would be biased toward dogs that were less lame. This may make a study group that received a certain treatment appear less lame than if they were studied at a walking velocity. Use of trotting velocity would affect subject accrual because more candidate dogs would be necessary to reach the sample size required for the study. For example, for a study in which 50 dogs are required, 81 candidate dogs would be needed to perform the study by use of trot velocity (assuming the 38% failure rate reported). In contrast, a similar study to evaluate 50 dogs at a walk would likely require only 50 candidate dogs. Third, among dogs that could walk and trot, fewer trials were required to obtain acceptable walking data than trotting data and walking data had a smaller coefficient of variation, suggesting that walking has less inherent variation than trotting.

Interestingly, the ideal velocity should probably not be determined by the investigator but the subject. If one dog is most comfortable walking through the runway at 1.1 meters per second then that is arguably the speed that you will gather data that is most reflective of that dog's normal gait. If a second dog in the study wants to go 1.8 meters per second that also should be allowed. The velocity of these dogs for subsequent trials should remain the same. The velocity, and/or stance time of these dogs can vary and their influence on GRFs can be calculated and adjusted mathematically.

Kinematic Analysis of Gait

A trained observer may be able to make critical judgments about a patient's gait, but by viewing a video recording, especially if viewed in slow motion, more subtle abnormalities may be detected. Thus, one of the simplest pieces of gait instrumentation, a picture video system, also is one of the most useful. It is also useful to document gait prior to applying any instrumentation so that differences can be resolved if, after equipment has been attached to the animal, motion data do not correspond to the clinician's initial visual image of the subject. In addition to motion photography, automated stereometric systems are commonly used. Other technologies, such as electromechanical linkage and electrogoniometry, which use an exoskeleton that is applied to the patient, are too cumbersome for most animals.

The stereometric method employs visible markers that are attached to the skin on rigid segments of the body (e.g., joints, centers of rotation, or bony prominences) and tracks their motion using imaging equipment. The markers are either infrared light-emitting diodes for active marker systems or solid shapes covered with retroreflective tape for passive marker systems. Digital image analysis allows the horizontal and vertical coordinates of each marker to be computed as the subject moves within the field of view. Using triangulation of the views from an array of cameras and the known location of each camera, computer software computes the coordinates for each marker. This technique has minimal impact on the natural motion of the subject and two- or three-dimensional methods can be employed. Two-dimensional methods have a diminished time and financial investment for the laboratory or clinic that will only perform this method occasionally, but joint motions can only be determined in one plane. Three-dimensional methods generally employ the use of 3 to 8 cameras that are mounted to the ceiling or wall and create a semi-permanent field of view. It is important to note that, in order to document three-dimensional kinematics, each body segment must be defined by at least three markers, each joint center must be defined, and Euler angles calculated. Although these systems allow for collection of state-of-the-art motion data, they are relatively expensive and, if the methods are not well understood, they can be intimidating.

Motion data allows for calculation of time/distance parameters (velocity, cadence, stance, and swing times, etc.) and the angular position of the joints (hips, knees, and ankles) during the different phases of gait. These methods have been well described and demonstrated in normal dogs at a trot, in dogs with orthopedic disease, and in dogs that are swimming.[11-13] Although historically these methods have been used more in the field of veterinary orthopedics, applications for patients with a neurologic disorder that quantify deviation from normal may offer the greatest clinical treatment potential for this technology. Three-dimensional kinematics, when collected simultaneously with force (kinetic) data can provide useful information about the force around a joint.

Electromyography (EMG)

EMG provides a representation of the contribution from muscles during gait. EMG can be useful to the clinician, but detailed attention to the instrumentation and techniques must be made to provide high-quality EMG signals. Surface electrodes have gained widespread use owing to their ease of application and because skin penetration is not required. However, results for deep muscles can be reliably obtained only with intramuscular wire electrodes. As with many of the other techniques described in this chapter, collaboration with an experienced group early on will pay long-term dividends.

References

1. Evans R, Horstman C, and Conzemius M: Accuracy and optimization of force platform gait analysis in Labradors with cranial cruciate disease evaluated at the walking gait. Vet Surg 34:42-46, 2005.

2. Besancon MF, Conzemius MG, Derrick TR, et al. Comparison of vertical forces in normal dogs between the AMTI Model OR6-5 force platform and the Tekscan (industrial sensing pressure measurement system) pressure walkway. Vet Compar Orthop Traumatol 16:153-7, 2003.

3. Budsberg SC, Jevens DJ, Brown J, et al: Evaluation of limb symmetry indices, using ground reaction forces in healthy dogs. Am J Vet Res 54(10):1569-74, 1993.

4. Besancon MF, Conzemius MG, Evans RB, et al: Distribution of vertical forces in the pads of Greyhounds and Labrador Retrievers during walking. Am J Vet Res 65:1497-1501, 2004.

5. Romans CW, Gordon WJ, Robinson DA, et al: Effect of postoperative analgesic protocol on limb function following onychectomy in cats. JAVMA 227(1): 89-93, 2005.

6. Romans CW, Conzemius MG, Horstman CL, et al: Use of pressure platform gait analysis in cats with and without bilateral onychectomy. Am J Vet Res 65:1276-78, 2004.

7. Horstman CL, Conzemius MG, Evans R, et al: Assessing the efficacy of perioperative oral carprofen after cranial cruciate surgery using noninvasive, objective pressure platform gait analysis. Vet Surg 33:286-92, 2004.

8. Evans RB, Gordon W, Conzemius M: The effect of velocity on ground reaction forces in dogs with lameness attributable to tearing of the cranial cruciate ligament. Am J Vet Res 64(12):1479-81, 2003.

9. Conzemius MG, Evans RJ, Besancon MF, et al: Effect of surgical technique on limb function after surgery for rupture of the cranial cruciate ligament in dogs. JAVMA 226(2):232-9, 2005.

10. Renberg WC, Johnston SA, Ye K, et al: Comparison of stance time and velocity as control variables in force plate analysis of dogs. Am J Vet Res 60:814-819, 1999.

11. DeCamp CE, Soutas-Little RW, Hauptman J, et al: Kinematic gait analysis of the trot in healthy Greyhounds. Am J Vet Res 54:627-34, 1993.

12. DeCamp CE, Riggs CM, Olivier NB, et al: Kinematic evaluation of gait in dogs with cranial cruciate ligament rupture. Am J Vet Res 57:120-6, 1996.

13. Marsolais GS, McLean S, Derrick T, Conzemius MG: Kinematic analysis of the hind limb during swimming and walking in healthy dogs and dogs with surgically corrected cranial cruciate ligament rupture. J Am Vet Med Assoc 222(6):739-43, 2003.

Chapter 114

Nutrition in Orthopedics

Herman AW Hazewinkel

Bone is a specialized form of connective tissue with a complex chemical and physical composition. Apart from its cellular fraction and the water phase (10%), it is composed of an organic matrix and a mineral phase. The cellular fraction includes osteoblasts (organic-matrix forming cells), osteoclasts (calcified-matrix resorbing cells), and osteocytes (embedded osteoblasts with bone-resorbing capacity). The organic matrix, which is about 20% of the bone volume, is composed of 90% collagen fibers with a high content of hydroxyproline and 10% aminopolysaccharides, noncollagen proteins, and a small quantity of lipids. The mineral phase encompasses about 70% of the bone volume, mainly in the form of hydroxyapatite crystals and amorphous calcium phosphate, as well as small quantities of other elements. The total amounts of body calcium and phosphorus, 99% and 80%, respectively, are present in the skeleton. Although zinc, copper, manganese, and other elements may influence the development of skeletal abnormalities,[1] they seem of minor significance in small animal practice. The availability of calcium, phosphate, and vitamins A and D has direct and indirect influences on skeletal mineralization. This will be discussed later in the chapter.

This chapter is limited to the recognition and management of orthopedic problems that are significant in small animal practice in which nutritional management is either a causative or a therapeutic factor. The quantity and quality of the food (including the main minerals and vitamins) are discussed in relation to skeletal diseases in growing, and in adult dogs and cats. In addition, nutrition is reviewed in relation to osteoarthrosis and fractures.

Nutrition and Skeletal Growth

Skeletal growth includes cartilage maturation as part of enchondral ossification and osteoid formation and mineralization, as well as bone modeling influenced by skeletal homeostasis and calcium homeostasis. The latter is under the influence of parathyroid hormone (PTH), calcitonin, and vitamin D metabolites.

A food of good quality and palatability that has been shown to be nutritionally adequate for growth should be given. Requirements for a number of nutrients are listed in Table 114-1. Young dogs and cats should have sufficient food during the growth phase to meet their needs, which can be two-and-one half to three times the adult maintenance value.[1] Optimal nutrition in an otherwise satisfactory environment permits optimal growth as ordained by the genotype.

In the following sections the orthopedic consequences of deficient or excessive intake of protein, energy, minerals, and vitamins for young dogs and cats are described.

Restricted Caloric Intake

Slight underfeeding may slow the growth of puppies but will not influence the adult size of the dog. In a controlled study of Great Dane dogs raised on a mixture of balanced complete commercial diets, the animals fed ad libitum had early skeletal maturation and advanced growth, but at 7 months of age the length of long bones of litter-mates fed a restricted diet (two-thirds of the caloric intake) was identical.[2] After a period of inhibited growth owing to malnutrition or illness of short duration, the animal will grow at a greater rate than average for its age (i.e., catch-up growth). Influences of growth factors other than nutrition must be considered when judging an animal that is small for its age,[3] including the extent of variation in growth patterns of normal healthy animals. From different studies of young dogs raised on food with carbohydrate content of 0 to 62%, protein 20% to 48%, and fat 13% to 76% as percentage of metabolizable energy, it was concluded that, so long as adequate protein and essential fatty acids exist

Table 114-1. Nutrient Requirements for Growing Dogs and Cats Expressed as Amount of each Nutrient per 1000 kJ or 100 kcal of Metabolizable Energy (ME)

	Dogs		Cats	
	Per 1000 kJ	Per 100 kcal	Per 1000 kJ	Per 100 kcal
Protein (g)	14	5.8	17	7.0
Fat (g)	4	1.7	5	2.1
Linoleic acid (g)	0.7	0.3	0.7	0.3
Calcium (g)	0.7	0.3	0.	0.25
Phosphorous (g)	0.5	0.2	0.5	0.2
Vitamin A (IU)	300	125	300	125
Vitamin D (IU)	30	12.5	30	12.5

Expression of nutrients per 1000 kJ ME or per 100 kcal ME allows for comparison of different product labels. ME can be calculated from the label as follows1: (g protein x 14.64 kJ) + (g fat x 35.56 kJ) + (g carbohydrates x 14.54 kJ) or (g protein x 3.5 kcal) + (g fat x 8.5 kcal) + (g carbohydrates x 3.5 kcal).

Example: product label states that diet has a calcium content of 2.5% on dmb with a calculated ME=1500 kJ per 100 g diet. Is this enough calcium? 1000/1500 x 2.5=1.7 g/1000 kJ; this is too much calcium. It should have been 1500/1000 x 0.7=1.05% on dmb.

in a palatable diet, it does not appear to matter in growing dogs what proportion of energy comes from carbohydrate, fat, or protein.[1] A study revealed that in 3 groups of Great Danes each fed iso-energetic diets only differing in their dietary protein levels (i.e., 15%, 23%, or 32% protein on dry matter base[dmb]), with carbohydrates exchanged for proteins, and diets fed in equal energetic amounts to all dogs, the 32%-protein-fed dogs had significantly higher body weight without a difference in length of the antebrachial bones than the dogs fed the 15%-protein diet at half a year of age. This lead to the conclusion that a high quality and quantity content of proteins in the diet stimulates soft tissue growth in young dogs, but does not increase skeletal growth or increase the risk for developmental orthopedic diseases.[4]

Low Calcium Intake

Young animals have a great need for calcium to mineralize newly formed cartilage and osteoid. Depending on the dietary regimen and hormonal status, 225 to 900 mg/kg body weight (bw) per day is deposited in the growing skeleton of young dogs, of which 100 to 225 mg/kg per day should be absorbed from the intestine.[1,5,6] The minimal requirement for dietary calcium in growing dogs is 0.4 to 0.6% on dmb in small breed dogs, 0.5% on dmb for growing kittens, and 0.7 to 1.2% for fast-growing dogs of large breeds.[1] Low calcium absorption, either from low calcium content of the food or poorly available calcium (complexes with phytic acid or oxalate, high phosphate content of the food, inadequate vitamin D status), can cause a decrease in the circulating calcium concentration. This situation can be created by feeding an all-meat diet. The decrease in circulating calcium concentration will be counteracted by the increase in PTH secretion, with eventually increased osteoclasia and increased synthesis of the active vitamin D metabolite 1,25-dihydroxycholecalciferol (or 1,25$(OH)_2$ vitamin D_3). The latter stimulates calcium (and phosphate) absorption with a total efficiency of up to approximately 80 to 90% of the digested amount in puppies and kittens.[5-7] Subsequently, the high PTH and vitamin D metabolite levels will stimulate calcium and phosphate resorption from bone. When this situation continues for weeks, massive osteoclasia will weaken the skeleton to such an extent that it can withstand neither body weight nor muscle forces. The result is the development of skeletal deformities, which include bowing of long bones and calcaneus, compression fractures in cancellous bone (metaphyseal and epiphyseal areas), deformation of the pelvis and vertebrae, and greenstick fractures of long bones (Figure 114-1B and Figure 114-2). No changes occur at the growth plates (Figure 114-1B). Compression fractures of the vertebrae can result in compression of the spinal cord that may be severe enough to cause posterior paresis or paralysis in the acute phase.

The bones cannot withstand the stress or load of a splint or cast, and additional greenstick fractures may result proximal to the cast or splint. Therefore, therapy is limited to good nursing care and a diet that fulfills the requirements according to the nutrient requirements of dogs[1] without any injections of vitamin D. This allows the skeleton to become sufficiently mineralized within 3 weeks. Corrective osteotomies of long bones or symphysis pelvis can be considered once the skeleton has become mineralized to acceptable levels. For example, narrowing of the pelvic canal by deformation may result in chronic constipation (Figure 114-2). Failure of the obstipation to respond to medical management may require pelvic osteotomy at a later date.

Low Vitamin D Intake

Vitamin D metabolites stimulate increased plasma levels of calcium and phosphate to mineralize newly formed osteoid and cartilage. Vitamin D is absorbed by the intestine, hydroxylated in the liver to 25OH vitamin D, and then further hydroxylated in the kidney to 24,25$(OH)_2$vitamin D_3 or to the most active metabolite, 1,25$(OH)_2$vitamin D_3. Puppies fed a semipurified balanced dry dog food without added vitamin D did not synthesize sufficient vitamin D when they were irradiated daily with ultraviolet (sun) light under con¬trolled circumstances. This is in contrast to other species, including herbivores and omnivores.[8] Biochemical, radiographic, and histologic evidence showed that these dogs developed rickets within 3 months. Thin cortices and broad physeal growth plates (Figure 114-1C) returned to normal when a commercial dog food was given.

Clinical cases of rickets in dogs and cats are exceedingly uncommon and can be diagnosed by measuring circulating vitamin D_3 metabolites,[8] or by determining the width of the growth plates as seen radiologically and histologically. An increase in width is not seen with low-calcium-high-phosphate diets, but is a strong indication of rickets. In rickets, the bowing of the legs predominates over the number of pathologic fractures.

Dietary therapy consists of commercial food with adequate amounts of calcium, phosphate, and vitamin D_3. No injections of vitamin D_3 are indicated, especially because commercial pet foods may contain more than the minimal recommended amounts.[9] When indicated, corrective surgery can be considered later.

High Energy Intake

Young animals have less tendency to become obese with excessive energy intake before 30 weeks of age than do older animals. Free-choice feeding of young dogs coincides with higher plasma levels of thyroid hormone, and thus stimulation of metabolic processes including heat production.[10] Young Great Danes overfed with a palatable, balanced, complete commercial diet did not show evidence of obesity, but rather advanced increases in weight and height when compared with their littermates fed a restricted diet. The dogs fed restricted diets reached the identical length of long bones at 7 months of age.[2] In another study, Great Danes had an even higher energy intake and a greater growth rate, but again without signs of obesity.[11] These Great Danes, as well as German shepherd dogs and retrievers, suffered from more severe developmental orthopedic diseases (including osteochondrosis, panosteitis, and hip dysplasia) when raised on a high caloric intake, in comparison with littermates raised on a restricted energy intake.[11-13] Dogs grow slower and have less fat deposition when fed a low density food with 8% instead of 24% fat, both offered free of choice.[10] Overweight owing to high energy intake may cause biomechanical stress, which, preceeding or following cartilaginous lesions, may be held responsible for these orthopedic diseases.[10]

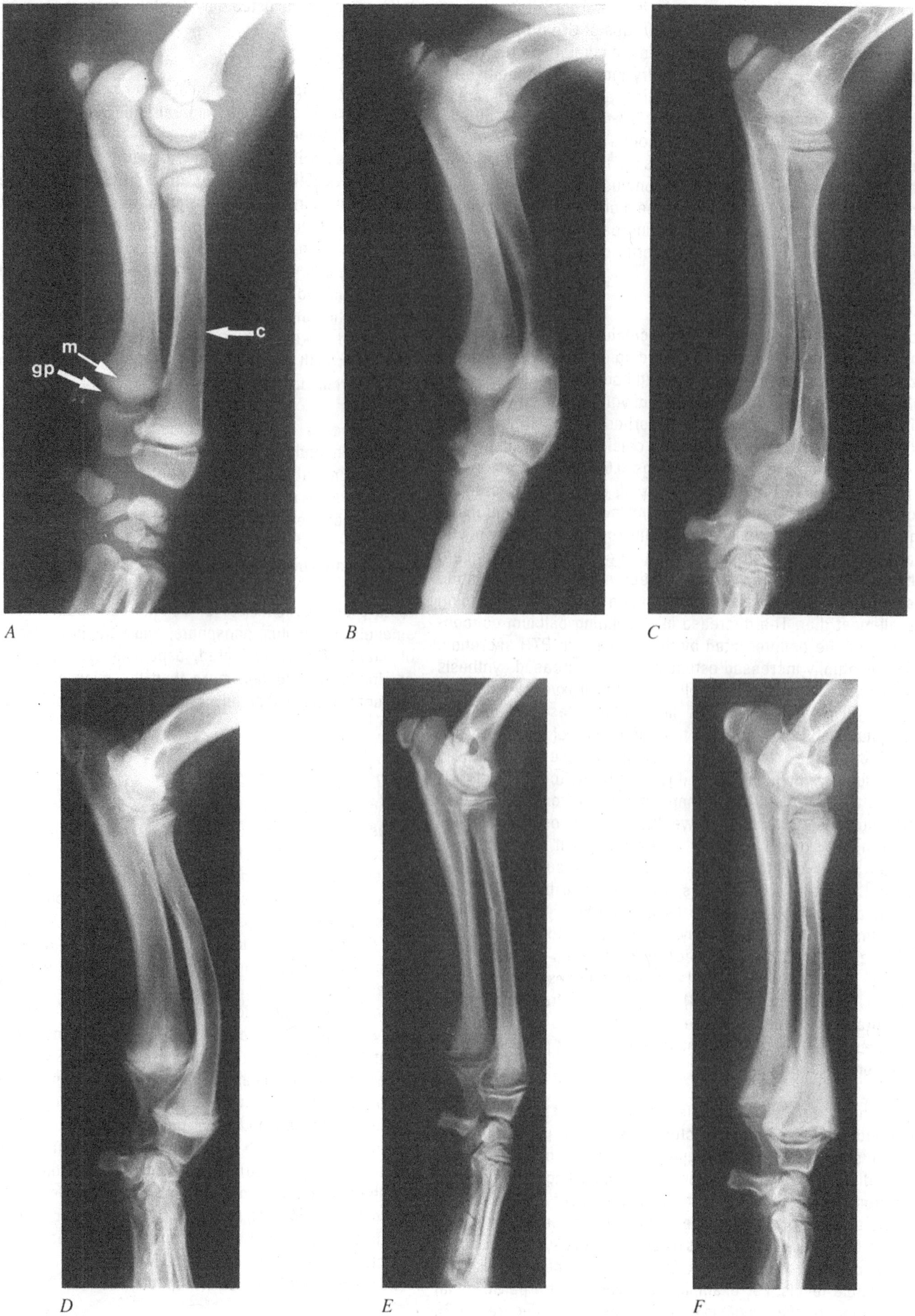
c
m
gp
A
B
C
D
E
F

Figure 114-1. Radiographs of the left radius and ulna of five different young dogs used as a diagnostic aid for nutritionally induced skeletal abnormalities by evaluation of the growth plate (gp) width, the metaphyseal (m) aspect, cortical (c) thickness, and length of ulna when compared with the radius (position of styloid process (sp)).

Age & Breed	Growth plate width	Metaphyseal aspect	Cortical thickness	Length of ulna vs. radius	Nutritional history
A 8 weeks, Rottweiler	normal	normal	normal	normal	normal
B 16 weeks. Great Dane	normal	relatively dense	thin greenstick fracture	normal	low Ca, normal P
C 22 weeks, mongrel	enlarged	mushroom-shaped	thin	normal	low vitamin D
D 24 weeks. Great Dane	central enlarged	retained cartilage in ulna	normal to thick	short ulna radius curvus	high Ca, normal P
E 24 weeks, boxer	normal	lucent line parallel to gp	normal	normal	high Ca, high P
F 28 weeks, boxer	normal	subperiosteal thickening	normal	normal	hypertrophic osteodystrophy, healed by rest and corrected diet

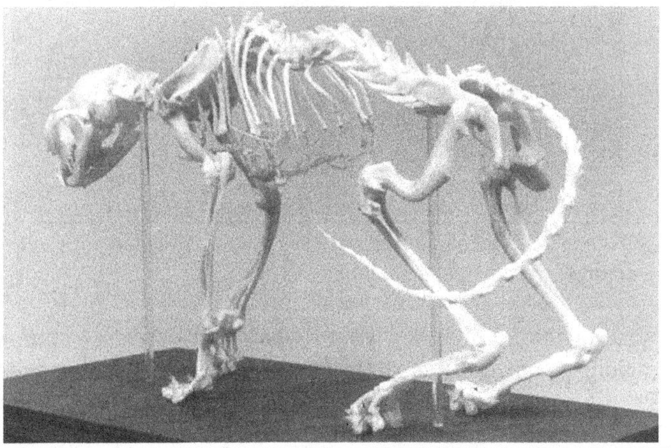

Figure 114-2. Low-calcium diet. Skeleton of a cat fed an all-meat food on a long-term basis. The cat has had severe skeletal abnormalities and recurrent constipation. Note the abnormal alignment of the long bones (especially the femurs), the calcanei, the vertebral column, and pelvis.

The owner of a young dog should monitor growth rate rather than body fat deposition and compare this with the average for that breed. The owner should realize that rapid growth will not lead to a larger adult dog, but will probably increase the risk of orthopedic problems, including hip dysplasia.

High Mineral Intake

To avoid the classic skeletal diseases that are a result of lack of calcium, too much phosphate, or too little vitamin D (as described previously), some owners, as well as some dog food manufacturers, tend to over-supplement with calcium, with or without a proportional addition of phosphate.[9] A high calcium content increases the circulating calcium concentration and eventually increases calcitonin secretion and decreases PTH secretion (for details see Chapter 99). A chronic hypercalcitoninemic state causes decreased activity of osteoclasts, which are of utmost importance for skeletal modeling during growth. Bony foramina should be widened by the osteoclasts in proportion to growth of soft tissues, such as the spinal cord and nutritional vessels of bones. In several studies, Great Danes fed a diet with a high calcium content (2 g/1000 kJ), with or without excess of other constituents such as protein or phosphate) developed an inadequately expanded cervical vertebral canal in proportion to the growth of the cervical cord.[5,11] This causes compression of the cord with clinical, radiographic, and pathologic signs of canine wobbler syndrome.

Decreased diameter and alteration in the course of the nutritional foramina in the diaphyses restrict venous return, leading to edema in the medullary cavity and subperiosteal. Ultimately, this edema leads to intramedullary fibrosis and bone formation, as well as subperiosteal edema and new bone formation. This entity is known as panosteitis.

Disturbance in enchondral ossification, termed osteochondrosis, was more frequent and more severe in young Great Danes receiving a supplementation of calcium when compared with Great Danes with a calcium intake of 0.8 to 1.1% on dmb.[5,11,14] Not only was the weight-bearing cartilage affected, but also the non-weight-bearing growth plates of ribs; therefore, microtrauma owing to overweight could be excluded. Severe signs of osteochondritis dissecans in the proximal humeral head and retained cartilage cones in metaphyseal growth plates (Figure 114-1D), with eventual radius curvus syndrome (Figure 114-3) and deviation of the hind legs[8,11,14] were observed in the dogs whose calcium intake was high. In less severe cases, nutritional correction may restore normal position of the legs (Figure 114-3); more severe cases may have to be treated surgically.

Hypertrophic osteodystrophy (HOD) can be characterized as a massive disturbance of enchondral ossification of growth plates. Typical is the osseous discontinuity in the metaphyseal area of many long bones, close to and parallel with the growth plates. This zone is composed of remnants of cartilage and bone trabeculae, blood, fibrin, and debris. This area becomes visible on radiographs when it is surrounded by mineralized tissue (Figure 114-1E). At a later stage, a superfluous periosteal reaction

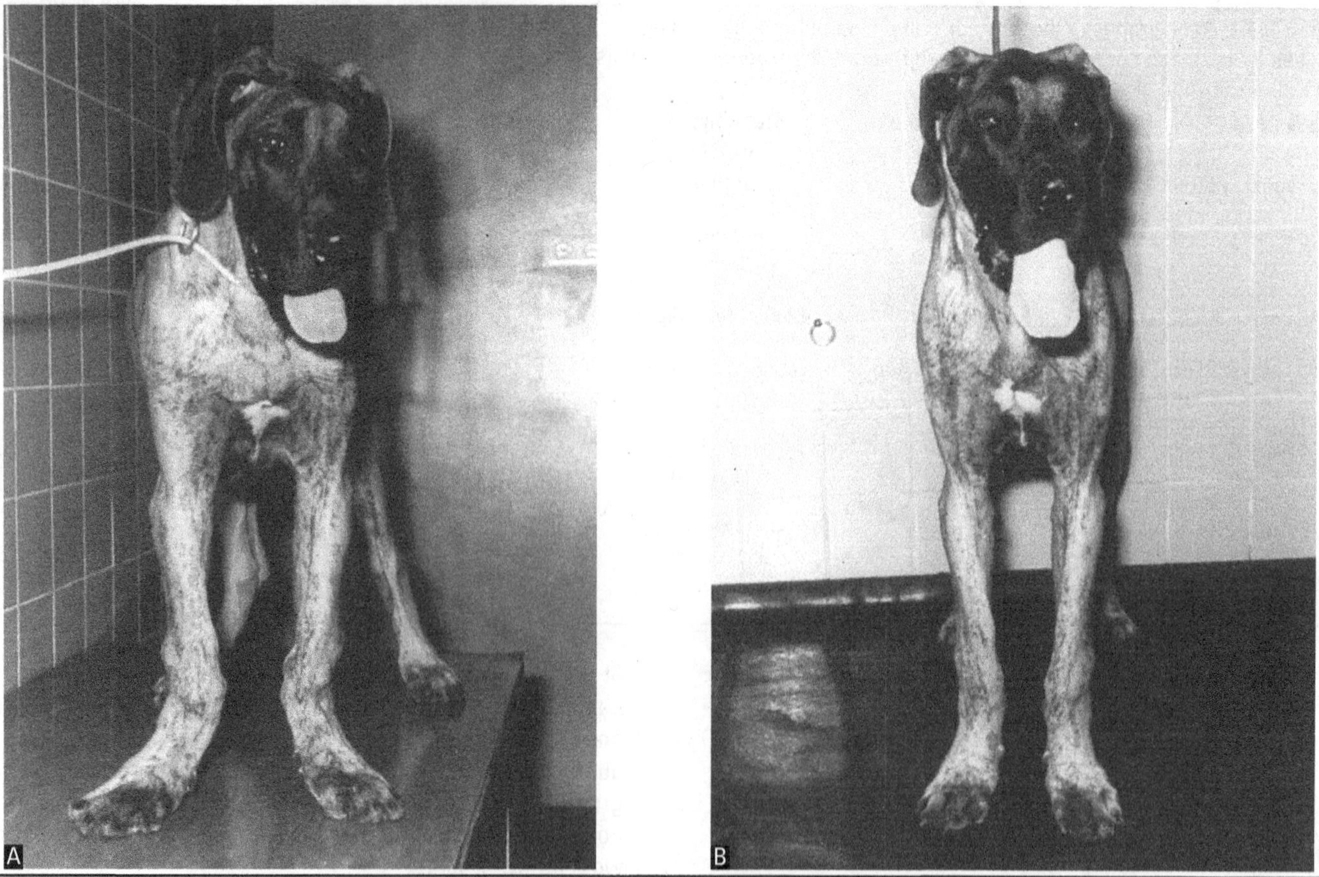

Figure 114-3. A, A 25-week-old Great Dane with both front legs in valgus position and with radiologic evidence of retained cartilage cones. B, The position of both front legs at age 1 year is normalized after the dog was fed a controlled amount of a balanced diet.

becomes visible on clinical and radiographic evaluation, as evidenced by bulging (Figure 114-1F). Pathologic signs of this disease were found in different controlled studies in well vaccinated Great Danes (a breed with a high prevalence for HOD) but all raised on food with a high mineral content.[5,11,15] Vitamin C supplementation may be expected to aggravate HOD more than to cure it.[16] Owners of young, fast-growing dogs should be aware of the severe consequences of high mineral intake on skeletal development.

Vitamin D Excess

The first hydroxylation of vitamin D_3 to 25OHvitamin D_3 in the liver is relatively poorly controlled, whereas the second hydroxylation to $1,25(OH)_2$vitamin D_3 in the kidney is under exquisite control. The allowance for vitamin D_3 is 500 IU/kg food on dmb for dogs (growth and maintenance alike) and 750 IU/kg food for kittens (but possibly as low as 250 IU/ kg food) and 500 IU/kg food for adult cats for maintenance.[1] In case of over supplementation of vitamin D_3, 25OHvitamin D_3 will be metabolized into the less biologically effective $24,25(OH)_2$vitamin D_3 and is the formed $1,25(OH)_2$vitamin D_3 quickly hydroxylated into the non-effective $1,24,25(OH)_3$ vitamin D_3.[17] In a controlled study in Great Danes, vitamin D excess of 100 times the recommended level of 500 IU per kg food, given during a 5-month period, caused plasma concentrations of $1,25(OH)_2$vitamin D_3 lower than controls, coinciding with severe osteochondrosis with radius curvus syndrome[17] with a similar radiologic appearance as in Figure 114-1D. Massive intakes of vitamin D_3 (or even more so of its metab¬olites) can cause hypercalcemia together with hyperphosphatemia, anorexia, polydipsia, polyuria, vomiting, muscle weakness, and lameness.[1] The circulating high levels of calcium and phosphate are a result of increased bone resorption, increased absorption from the gastrointestinal tract, and eventually, tubular mineralization. Vitamin D intoxication in dogs and cats is marked by mineralization of soft tissues, including blood vessels, alveoli, and renal tubules, together with pathologic changes in the gastrointestinal tract and the heart.[1]

Pet foods can contain from 2 to more than 10 times the NRC-recommended amount of vitamin D.[9] Extra supplementation with vitamin D can cause increased calcium and phosphate absorption with *deleterious effects on skeletal development* (see Chapter 99) and probably on kidney function.[9] Owners of young dogs and cats should be aware of the severe effects of clinical and subclinical vitamin D_3 intoxication with cumulative effects owing to vitamin over-supplementation.

Excessive Vitamin A Intake

Because development of hypervitaminosis A demands prolonged intake of vitamin A-rich food stuffs such as raw liver, intoxication is rarely seen clinically in young animals. Metabolism of an excess of vitamin A is more complete in cats than in dogs, so hypervitaminosis A is more likely to occur in kittens than in puppies (see Chapter 99).

Experimentally, massive doses of vitamin A given for several weeks caused profound depression of bone growth, owing to degenerative changes of the growth plates, in addition to decreased osteoblast activity and osteoporosis in both kittens and puppies.[9] Osteophyte formation and periosteal reactions are present but of minor importance in these young animals.[9] The recommendation for vitamin A is 5000 IU/kg of food dmb for dogs (both for growth and for maintenance) and 3333 IU/kg food dmb for kittens and 6000 IU/ kg food for adult cats;[1] supplementation of commercial pet food with a vitamin additive can result in giving 100 times the normal requirement.[9] Owners of young companion animals, especially kittens, should be aware of the severe skeletal abnormalities that can result from over-supplementation with vitamin A.

Nutrition and Skeletal Maintenance

Permanent bone turnover occurs in the adult dog and cat and consists of bone resorption as well as new bone formation. In the adult dog, calcium deposition and resorption are equal in magnitude: approximately 4 to 8 mg/kg bw per day. Daily losses of calcium by endogenous fecal and urinary excretion (i.e., 10 to 30 and 1 to 7 mg/kg bw per day, respectively) can easily be compensated for by a balanced diet.

Natural menopause and other causes of estrogen deficiency in women are characterized by bone loss leading to pathologic fractures of the vertebrae, proximal femur, and wrist. This explains the extensive concern for nutrition in elderly women. Although ovariectomy is a common practice in female cats and dogs, and some osteoporotic changes are noticeable 17 to 36 weeks after surgery,[17,18] this practice does not result in a problem of practical significance in companion animal orthopedics (see Chapter 99).

Feeding adult animals a diet based on some variation of the dietary requirements prescribed for growing animals usually does not result in serious problems. The major clinical problems in relation to orthopedics in adult companion animals are excessive energy intake, low vitamin D or excessive phosphorus intake together with decreased renal function, and excessive vitamin A intake, especially in cats.

Excessive Energy Intake

Superfluous energy content will increase the risk of obesity for the normally active companion animal. In addition to high energy intake, the following factors may underlie an abnormal gain in body weight: the dietary composition (protein-energy ratio), breed and strain differences, hormonal status, the number of adipocytes present, and changes in household circumstances. Between 24% and 44% of dogs and at least 9% and 25% of cats are said to be overtly obese.[1] The females of the species are more frequently obese. About 25% of obese dogs have orthopedic problems, whereas only 10% of all dogs seen in 11 veterinary practices had orthopedic problems.[19] These problems included arthritis, herniated intervertebral disks, and ruptured anterior cruciate ligaments. In a risk assessment study for hip dysplasia in German shepherd dogs, golden retrievers, Labrador retrievers, and Rottweilers, high body weight was shown to be an important risk factor.[20] (see "Osteoarthrosis" later in this chapter). No known dietary aberration is responsible for these diseases, but rather the mechanical effect of the increased weight on the skeleton.[19]

Excessive Mineral Intake

The calcium and phosphate content of ordinary commercial pet foods can significantly exceed the recommended levels, and although this may not have deleterious effects on healthy adults, it is certainly unneccessary.[9] In dogs and cats with severe loss of kidney function, phosphate will accumulate and thereby decrease circulating calcium concentrations. Hyperphosphatemia can go together with decreased 1-α hydroxylation of 25OHvitamin D, resulting in diminished production of 1,25(OH)$_2$vitamin D$_3$ and thus in decreased active calcium absorption. As a result, the parathyroid glands will secrete more PTH (renal secondary hyperparathyroidism), causing an increase in osteoclastic activity to normalize circulating calcium concentrations, with eventual development of osteodystrophy and loosening of teeth in the mandible and maxilla. Of greater clinical significance are the systemic effects of renal failure. Renal osteodystrophy is characterized microscopically by increased osteoclast and osteocyte activity and inadequate mineralization of normal osteoid. High phosphate intake will aggravate the situation by (1) promoting mineral depositions in soft tissues, not only the kidney but also periarticular tissue, tendon sheaths, and foot pads; and (2) decreasing circulating calcium concentrations and subsequently boosting hyperparathyroidism.[21]

Low Vitamin D Intake

Because young dogs are not able to fulfill their need for vitamin D by biosynthesis in the skin via stimulation by ultraviolet light, it seems reasonable to suggest that adults also need dietary vitamin D. Hypovitaminosis D, causing osteomalacia in adult dogs and cats and characterized by increased osteoclasia and unmineralized osteoid layers, is seldom recognized clinically. The deleterious effects of vitamin D intoxication are the same as those previously described for young animals.

Excessive Vitamin A Intake

Hypervitaminosis A is seen more frequently in cats than in dogs, especially at an older age (2 to 9 years). Radiologically, hypervitaminosis A is characterized by new bone formation rather than by osteoporosis or bone loss. New bone formation starts at the points of insertion of ligaments, muscles, and joint capsules, causing narrowing of intervertebral foramina in the cervical area and ankylosis of vertebral, shoulder, elbow, hip, and stifle joints (rarely carpal and tarsal joints). In addition to lethargy, pain on palpation, and changes in character, such changes as stiffness of the neck or of one or more large joints can be the first clinical signs. For further details and treatment see Chapter 99.

Nutrition and Osteoarthrosis

Cartilage contains chondroblasts, proteoglycans, and collagen. Proteoglycans are build out of glycosaminoglycans (GAGs) and a core protein. Aggrecan is an important proteoglycan in joint cartilage, with keratin sulphate and chondroitin sulphate as GAGs. About 200 aggrecan molecules are bound via a glycoprotein to a hyaluran molecule, binding a large quantity of extracellular water, determining the compressability of cartilage. Collagen molecules in cartilage contain large amounts of hydroxyl proline and hydroxyl lysine. The molecules form a triple helix structure, bound to fibrils and these to fibers, with great strength against pull and which form a labyrinth holding proteoglycans in its place. During aging, the length of GAGs decrease, the proteoglycan content decreases, and thus the water content and the flexibility to withstand loading decrease. GAGs may be damaged by reactive oxygen species (ROS), i.e., free radicals formed during different metabolic processes, trauma, infection, and irradiation.

Regeneration of cartilage can occur after microtrauma by proliferation of undamaged chondrocytes and by de novo synthesis of proteoglycans and collagen. Severe cellular damage will lead to a scar without cells, a fibrotic cartilage scar with a low content of proteoglycans.

Under normal circumstances proteolytic enzymes, mainly matrix metalloproteinases (MMPs), will be suppressed by tissue inhibitors of MMPs (TIMPs). In osteoarthrosis (OA), however, MMPs will be formed under the influence of cytokines interleukin-I (IL-I) and tumor necrosis factor-α, released by synovial membrane cells, monocytes, macrophages, and T-cells. These cytokines also stimulate chondrocytes and osteoclasts to produce MMPs as soon as their surrounding cartilage has been destroyed. In addition, IL-I stimulates the release of arachidonic acid (AA) metabolites including prostaglandin PGE_2 from chondrocytes and synovial membrane as well as leukotriene B_4 (LTB_4).[5]

Causative Role of Nutrition

Osteoarthrosis (OA) can be divided into primary OA, i.e., without any other cause than aging, and secondary OA, which has a variety of causes, including incongruency or loose bodies in the joint, joint instability, and infection, immune disease, or hemarthrosis. This wide variety of diseases will eventually result in clinical OA. The age of onset and severity of occurrence of primary OA may depend on the breed (Patronek et al, 1997). Many orthopedic developmental diseases have a low h^2 (as in elbow dysplasia, h^2 = 0.4-0.7), leaving a large influence on the environment. Fragmented coronoid process (FCP) and osteochondrosis of the elbow joint have been explained by Olsson[22] as a disturbance of endochondral ossification and, as such, expressions of the same disease. Osteochondrosis is seen more frequently in certain breeds and subpopulations and can be aggravated by high food intake and excessive calcium intake,[5,8] as well as by over-supplementation of balanced food with vitamin D.[23] Rations rich in protein will not have a disturbing influence on skeletal development;[4] however, Great Danes raised on food with an increased calcium and phosphorous intake but with the same Ca:P ratio (3.3 Ca and 3.0% P versus controls on 1.1% Ca and 0.9% P) also developed disturbances in endochondral ossification in the growth plates of the distal radius or ulna (Figure 114-1D).[14] As a consequence, elbow incongruity developed, owing either to a severe disturbance of growth in length of the radius or to a severe radius curvus syndrome with disturbed growth in length of the ulna (Figure 114-3).[8,14] The latter may coincide with an ununited anconeal process or the painful distraction cubiti; both will lead to OA of the elbow joint. In studies in Labradors,[2,13] Great Danes,[11] and German shepherds[12] it has been demonstrated that OA develops in hip joints in overweight dogs and less frequently in restricted-fed dogs. The frequency and severity of the occurrence of OA can thus be prevented by dietary management, including a food with a lowered calcium-to-energy ratio, or a quantitative restriction of food intake, and without adding minerals or vitamin D to a balanced diet.

Therapeutic Role of Nutrition

The nonsurgical therapy of OA includes adaptations and medicaments. First the body weight of the patient should be adapted. Decrease of weight, gained during the period of decreased mobilization but not with a simultaneous adaptation of energy intake, will be the primary goal. A significant improvement was recorded by Impellieri et al in dogs with HD, following a decrease in body weight by 11 to18%.[24] This clinical finding was supported by the objective score by force-plate analysis by Burkholder et al.[25] Adaptation to the amount and the kind of activity that does the least possible harm to the joint, preferably hydrotherapy (i.e., swimming), should coincide with the weight reduction program.

Corticosteroids suppress phospholipase activity, consequentially with stabilization of blood vessel walls and lysosomes. The joints will be less painful and less synovia is produced. Because regeneration of cartilage will be decreased under the influence of corticosteroids, long-lasting or repetitive use of corticosteroids, especially intraarticular and at higher doses, is contraindicated. Nonsteroidal anti-inflammatory drugs (NSAIDs) have actions against cyclooxygenase (COX) enzymes; COX1 stimulates the production of prostaglandins (PGs), which protect the body, whereas COX2 stimulates the production of PGE_2, which is responsible for clinical signs such as pain and hyperemia (with resultant warm joint and overproduction of joint fluid). Selective COX2 inhibitors with or without suppressive action on lipoxygenase are claimed to be available for dogs, with fewer side effects than most inhibitors of COX1 and COX2. NSAIDs with low incidence of side effects will be prescribed for a prolonged period, not to mask pain but to improve the metabolic condition of the diseased joint.[26]

In order to support regeneration of joint cartilage and to shorten or lower the dosage of NSAIDs, a search continues for nutritional support of patients with OA. These supplements or diseases-modifying osteoarthritis agents (DMOAs) include chondroitin sulphate, glucosamines, polyunsaturated fatty acids, and antioxidants.

Chondroitin sulphate increases in vitro the production of proteoglycans and, therefore, the regeneration of cartilage.[27] When given prophylactically in rabbits, it prevents synthesis of MMPs by IL-3 and thus cartilage damage.

Glucosamines, precursors of GAGs, will stimulate synthesis of GAGs, prostaglandins, and collagen by chondrocytes in vitro.[27] In case of substitution of glucosamines in the medium of chondrocytes, mRNA content for aggrecan increased, and for MMPs decreased and synthesis of proteoglycan increased.[28] In rabbits with a cranial cruciate ligament (CCL) rupture, 120 mg/kg body weight of prophylactic glucosamine decreased the amount of chondropathy in comparison with controls.[29] In a study in dogs with CCL rupture as a model, it has been demonstrated that these dogs had less cartilage swelling, less total and active metalloproteinase (MMP), and lower pathologic scores when injected with 4 mg/kg bw glucosaminoglycan polysulfuric acid (GAGPS) twice weekly for 4 to 8 weeks, starting 4 weeks after the CCL rupture.[30] It is suggested by Altman et al that GAGPS suppress proteoglycan breakdown by MMPs or by directly inhibiting MMP in cartilage, rather than by increasing synthesis of proteoglycans by chondrocytes.[30] De Haan et al demonstrated in a clinical double-blind, placebo-controlled trial that, in dogs with hip dysplasia, 4.4 mg GAGPS per kg bw (IM for 3 to 5 days) revealed an improvement in lameness score, range of motion, and joint pain and no side effects after 8 injections, with only small improvement in the placebo group of dogs.[31]

Combinations of chondroitin sulphate and glucosamines given to dogs with OA subjectively allowed for more normal locomotion and joint movement than in untreated controls.[32] Prophylactically provided, this combination decreased inflammation in dogs with induced arthritis,[33] possibly owing to a modulated metabolism of the articular cartilage. The latter was suggested to occur in dogs with CCL ruptures, supplemented with a mixture of chondroitin sulphate, glucosamine hydrochloride, and manganese ascorbate.[34]

The polyunsaturated free fatty acid (PUFA) component of mussels or plant seeds has a potentially beneficial role in immune-related disorders and OA.[35] Leukotrienes are formed out of arachidonic acid (AA; 20:4Ω -6) and eicosapentaenoic acid (EPA; 20:6Ω-3), originating from cellular membranes, under the influence of the enzyme 5-lipogenase. Pro-inflammatory LTB4 originates from AA, anti-inflammatory LTB5 originates from EPA. The amount and type of these eicosanoids are determined by the availability of the PUFA precursor. A higher Ω–3 intake results in decreased membrane AA levels and thus a decreased synthesis of eicosanoids from AA and an increase in eiconoids derived from EPA. In joints with OA, the LTB4 content is increased.[36] In 36 dogs with elbow OA owing to elbow dysplasia, a double-blind efficacy study was performed by feeding balanced foods with increased Ω-3 content (Ω-3 of 4%, and Ω-6 of 20%) versus a high Ω-6 content (Ω-3 of 0.8%, and Ω-6 of 38%) revealed significant increase in plasma LTB5 concentrations in the former group, although ground reaction forces did not differ between the two groups of dogs.[37] A clinical trial including force-plate analysis performed in two groups of dogs fed either a control food or an EPA-supplemented diet for a 90-day period revealed that 31% of the controls and 82% of the EPA-supplemented group improved their weight-bearing ability.[38] In addition, in vitro studies of canine cartilage indicated that cartilage exposed to EPA stopped further degradation.[39]

Antioxidants may decrease the damage of synovial cells by reactive oxygen species (ROS). For this purpose, vitamins A, C, and E and β-carotene content in the diet can be increased.[40]

Combinations of chondroitin, glucosamine and PUFAs are present in green-lipped mussels (GLM). The flesh part of the GLM, separated from the shell, contains saturated, monounsaturated, and polyunsaturated fatty acids. Of the latter, a large amount is Ω-3 fatty acid, mainly EPA, and docosahexaenoic acid (DHA), with a final ratio of Ω-6: Ω-3= 1: 10. GLM powder is claimed to be a 5-lipoxygenase-pathway inhibitor. Freeze-dried GLM powder contains in addition a variety of nutrients that may have a beneficial effect on joint health, including amino acids (glutamine, methionine), vitamins C and E, and minerals (zinc, copper, and manganese). The combination of Ω-3, PUFA, and other ingredients may have the synergistic potential to limit the progression of OA. In a double-blind, randomized, controlled trial in dogs with OA, 17 dogs were given GLM supplement powder and 15 dogs were given GLM supplement oil (both in a daily dosage of 1000 mg when bw was more than 34 kg; 750 mg when bw was 34 to 25 kg; 450 mg when bw was less than 25 kg) and both groups were compared with 15 controls. A nonobjectivated score of arthritic signs grading from no signs to severe was given for mobility and for all major joints individually before the start of the study and at 6 weeks. Joint swelling, pain, and crepitus were reported to improve in only the GLM-powder supplemented group in comparison with the controls.[41] In addition, Bierer and Bui reported on a dose-response in alleviating arthritis score in 4 groups of dogs: 3 dosage groups (1:2:4) receiving GLM-power and 1 control group.[41] All 3 dosages resulted in a similar improvement in total arthritic score and all significantly different from the controls. However, no significant effects were observed with regard to mobility and range of joint movement with the addition of GLM in any of the groups. Longer study period and more sensitive assessment methods may be helpful in detecting any possible effects in these parameters.[41]

There is great interest in the discovery of natural products to be used as DMOAs, based on the aversion to "chemical substances" (i.e., NSAIDs) that exist among many dog owners, as well as on the less restricted efficacy-control of supplements in terms of dosage and purity, and the approval to add these substances to dog food. There is a growing need to double-blind clinical-efficacy studies with objectivated criteria to demonstrate the evidence gathered in vitro that these DMOAs, "neutraceuticals" and "supplements" may be beneficial to patients suffering from OA. Meta-analyses of the efficacy of glucosamine and chondroitin sulphate for treatment of OA in humans, led to different conclusions: supplementation with glucosamine or chondroitin sulphate demonstrated some efficacy in some symptom-relieving parameters, but the ability to modify the structure of articular cartilage was not confirmed.[42] Research is scarcely available to demonstrate a direct therapeutic effect in support of the treatment of OA in dogs at the level these substances are included in most pet foods.[32,38] Claims for different levels or different combinations of neutraceuticals, or the period before efficacy can be expected, the use in particular breeds or sizes of dogs, or the indication for their use in different joints with OA or at certain stages of OA will be a matter of debate until the onus of proof is laid in the hands of those who claim the efficacy.

Nutrition and Fractures

The skeleton is under the influence of calcium homeostasis. Low calcium or high phosphate intake or low vitamin D intake can cause pathologic fractures owing to poor mineralization of the skeleton (Figure 114-1). These pathologic fractures include compression fractures of cancellous bone and greenstick fractures of cortical bone. In the latter, the abnormal alignment (Figure 114-2) can be corrected only after the bone has achieved normal mineralization. Therefore, the first phase should consist of good nursing and feeding of a balanced diet. Because a great deal of osteoid (and cartilage, in the case of hypovitaminosis D) has to be mineralized in this first phase of treatment, this "bone hunger" can be compensated for by supporting the balanced food with calcium salts (i.e., bone meal) up to 0.7 g calcium and 0.5 g phosphorus per 1000 kJ. Radiographic evaluation (Figure 114-3) will demonstrate dramatic improvement. If the improvement does not occur, other rarer causes of abnormal skeletal development, including osteogenesis imperfecta (see Chapter 99), should be considered. When posterior paralysis or paresis occurs, the prognosis for improvement is guarded.

Spontaneous fractures, especially of the mandibles, in old dogs can be the first sign of severe renal dysfunction and they require treatment.

When properly treated in a healthy animal, traumatic fractures heal via the process of primary or secondary bone healing. The latter has much in common with enchondral ossification and thus needs the same nutritional support. Optimal circumstances can be reached with a balanced commercial pet food containing optimal levels of calcium, phosphate, vitamin A, and vitamin D. Excessively high doses of these nutrients have been demonstrated to retard enchondral ossification[39] and bone healing.[40] Pain owing to trauma or surgery may cause distress, which depletes reserves of protein and diminishes immune competence. In addition, the dietary requirements of ascorbic acid and probably of other nutrients are increased.[1] In surgical patients, the fasting period before and after anesthesia may be detrimental. Therefore, a palatable food formulated to meet the needs of young, growing animals must be considered. Even obese patients should be kept in a positive energy balance, although this demands special management of fracture treatment and postoperative mobilization.

References

1. Hand MS, Thatcher CD, Remillard RL, et al: Small Animal Clinical Nutrition, 4th ed. Marcelin: Walsworth Publishing, 2000.

2. Lavelle, RB: The effect of the overfeeding of a balanced complete commercial diet to a group of growing Great Danes. *In* Nutrition of the Dog and Cat. Burger IH, Rivers JPW (eds). Cambridge: Cambridge University Press, 1989, p. 303.

3. Gelens HC, Ihle SL: Failure to grow. Vet Clin North Am Small Anim Pract 29:989, 1999.

4. Nap RC, Hazewinkel HAW, Voorhout G: Growth and skeletal development in Great Dane pups fed different levels of protein intake. J Nutr 121:S107, 1991

5. Hazewinkel HAW, Mott J: Osteoarticular affections in puppies and adult dogs; nutritional approach. *In* Royal Canine Health Nutrition Encyclopaedia. Paris: Diffomedia, 2005.

6. Hedhammar A, Krook L, Schryver H, et al: Calcium balance in the dog. *In* Nutrition of the Dog and Cat. Anderson RS (ed). Oxford: Pergamon Press, 1980, p. 119.

7. O'Donnell JA, Hayes KC: Nutrition and nutritional disorders. *In* Diseases of the Cat. Vol. I. Holzworth J (ed). Philadelphia: WB Saunders, 1987.

8. Hazewinkel HAW: Nutrition in relation to skeletal growth deformities J Small Anim Pract 30:625, 1989.

9. Kallfelz, FA, Dzanis DA: Overnutrition: an epidemic problem in pet animal practice? Vet Clin North Am Small Anim Pract 19:433, 1989.

10. Richardson DC, Zentek J, Hazewinkel HAW, et al: Developmental orthopaedic disease of dogs. *In* Hand MS, Thatcher CD, Remillard RL, Roudebush P (eds). Small Animal Clinical Nutrition, 4th ed. Marcelin: Walsworth Publishing, 2000, p. 505.

11. Hedhammar A, Wu FM, Krook L, et al: Over nutrition and skeletal disease; an experimental study in growing Great Dane dogs. Cornell Vet 64 (Suppl 5):5, 1974.

12. Kasstrom H: Nutrition, weight gain and development of hip dysplasia; an experimental investigation in growing dogs with special reference to the effect of feeding intensity. Acta Radiol Suppl 344:135, 1975.

13. Kealy RD, Lawler DF, Ballam JM, et al: Evaluation of the effect of limited food consumption on radiographic evidence of osteoarthritis in dogs. J Am Vet Med Assoc 217:1678, 2000.

14. Schoenmakers I, Hazewinkel HAW, Voorhout G, et al: Effect of diets with different calcium and phosphorous contents on the skeletal development and blood chemistry of growing Great Danes. Vet Rec 147:652, 2000.

15. Lauten SD, Cox NR, Brawner WR, et al: Influence of dietary calcium and phosphorus content in a fixed ratio on growth and development in Great Danes. Am J Vet Res 63:1036, 2002.

16. Teare JA, Krook L, Kallfelz FA, et al: Ascorbic acid deficiency and hypertrophic osteodystrophy in the dog: a rebuttal. Cornell Vet 69:384, 1979.

17. Tryfonidou MA, Oosterlaken-Dijksterhuis MA, Mol JA, et al: 24-hydroxylase: potential key regulator in hypervitaminosis D3 in growing dogs. Am J Physiol Endocrinol Metab 284:E505, 2003.

17. Ferguson, HW, Hartles RL: The combined effects of calcium deficiency and ovariectomy on the bones of young adult cats. Calc Tiss Res 4(Suppl):140, 1970.

18. Malluche HH, Faugere MC, Friedler RM,Fanti P: 1,25-Dihydroxyvitamin D corrects bone loss but suppresses bone remodeling in ovariohysterectomized bea¬gle dogs. Endocrinol 122(5):1998-2006, 1988.

19. Edney ATB, Smith PB: Study of obesity in dogs visiting veterinary practices in the United Kingdom. Vet Rec 118:391, 1986.

20. Smith GK, Mayhew PD, Kapathin AS: Evaluation of risk factors for degenerative joint disease associated with hip dysplasia in German Shepherd Dogs, Golden Retrievers, Labrador Retrievers, and Rottweilers. J Am Vet Med Assoc 219:1719, 2001.

21. Polzin DJ, Osborne CA, Ludwig LL: Chronic kidney disease. *In* Ettinger SJ, Feldman EC (eds). Textbook of Veterinary Internal Medicine, 6th ed. St. Louis: Elsevier, 2000, p. 1756.

22. Olsson S-E: Pathophysiology, morphology, and clinical signs of osteochondrosis in the dog. *In* Disease Mechanisms in Small Animal Surgery, 2nd ed. Bojrab MJ, Smeak DD, Bloomberg MS (eds). Philadelphia:Lea & Febiger, 1993, p. 777.

23. Tryfonidou MA, Holl MS, Stevenhagen JJ, et al: 135-fold vitamin D_3 supplementation severely disturbs the endochondral ossification in growing dogs. Domest Anim Endocrinol 24:265, 2003.

24. Impellieri JA, Tetrick MA, Muir P: Effect of weight reduction on

clinical signs of lameness in dogs with hip osteoarthritis. J Am Vet Med Assoc 216:1089, 2000.

25. Burkholder WJ, Taylor L, Hulse DA: Weight loss to optimal body condition increases ground reactive force in dogs with osteoarthritis. Purina Nutrition Forum 2000; 131.

26. Pelletier JP, Lajeunesse D, Jovanovic DV, et al: Carprofen simultaneously reduces progression of morphological changes in cartilage and subchondral bone in experimental dog osteoarthritis. J Rheumatol 27:2893, 2000.

27. Bassleer CT, Combain JPA, Bougaret S, et al: Effects of chondroitin sulfate and interleukin-beta on human articular chondrocytes cultivated in clusters. Osteoarthritis Cartilage 6:196, 1998.

28. Henrotin Y: Influence of neutraceuticals on cartilage health and integrity. *In* Nutrition and Health Care in Large Breed Dogs. Iams Symposium, 2001; 34.

29. Conrozier T, Mathieu P, Piperno M, et al : Glucosamine sulphate significantly reduced cartilage destruction in a rabbit model of osteoarthritis. Arthr Rheum 41S:147, 1998.

30. Altman RD, Dean DD, Muniz OE, et al: Therapeutic treatment of canine OA with glucosaminoglycan polysulfuric acid ester. Arthr Rheum 32:179, 1989.

31. De Haan JJ, Goring RL, Beale BS: Evaluation of polysulfated glycosaminoglycan for the treatment of hip dysplasia in dogs. Vet Surg 23:177, 1994.

32. Beale BS: Use of neutraceuticals and chondroprotectants in osteoarthritic dogs and cats. Vet Clin North Am Small Anim Pract 34:271, 2004.

33. Canapp SO, McLaughlin RM, Hoskinson JJ, et al: Scintigraphic evaluation of glucosamine HCl and chondroitin sulfate for acute synovitis in dogs Am J Vet Res 60:1552, 1999.

34. Johnson KA, Hulse DA, Hart RC, et al: Effects of an orally administered mixture of chondroitin sulphate, glucosamine hydrochloride and manganese ascorbate on synovial fluid chondroitin sulphate 3B3 and 7D4 epitope in a canine cruciate ligament transaction model of osteoarthritis. Osteoarthritis Cartilage 9:14, 2001.

35. Bauer JE: The potential for dietary polyunsaturated fatty acids in domestic animals. Aust Vet J 71:342, 1994.

36. Herlin T, Fogh K, Hansen ES, et al: 15-HETE inhibits leukotriene B4 formation and synovial cell proliferation in experimental arthritis. Agents Actions 29:52, 1990.

37. Hazewinkel HAW, Theyse LFH, Wolvekamp WTH, et al: The influence of dietary omega-6:omega-3 ratio on lameness in dogs with osteoarthrosis of the elbow joint. *In* Reinhart GA, Carey DP (eds). Recent Advances in Canine and Feline Nutrition. Vol. II. Wilmington: Orange Frazer, 1998, p. 325.

38. Schoenherr WD: Fatty acids and evidence-based dietary management of canine osteoarthritis. *In* Proceedings Hill's European Symposium on Osteoarthritis and Joint Health, Genova (Italy), 2005; 54.

39. Caterson B, Little CB, Cramp J, et al:. Eicosapentaenoate supplementation abrogates canine articular cartilage degeneration in *in vitro* explant culture systems. *In* Proceedings Hill's European Symposium on Osteoarthritis and Joint Health, Genova (Italy), 2005; 14.

40. Greenwald RA: Oxygen radicals, inflammation and arthritis: pathophysiological considerations and implications for treatment. Rheum 20:219, 1991.

41. Bierer TL, Bui LM: Improvement of arthritic signs in dogs fed green-lipped mussels (*Perna canaliculus*). J Nutr 132:1634S, 2002.

42. McAlindon TE, LaValley MP, Felson DT: Efficacy of glucosamine and chondroitin for treatment of osteoarthritis. JAMA 284:1241, 2000.

43. Voorhout G, Hazewinkel HAW: A radiographic study on the development of the antebrachium in Great Dane pups on different calcium intakes. Vet Radiol 28:152, 1987.

Chapter 115

Articular Cartilage Healing

C. Wayne McIlwraith

General Concepts

Healing refers to restoration of the structural integrity and function of the tissue after injury or disease. Repair refers to the replacement of damaged or lost cells and matrix with new cells and matrix, a process that does not necessarily restore the original structure or function of a tissue.[1] Regeneration may be considered a special form of repair in which the cells replace lost or damaged tissue with a tissue identical to the original tissue. It has been suggested that, with exception of bone fractures, most injuries and diseases of musculoskeletal tissues do not stimulate regeneration of the original tissue. The limited potential of articular cartilage for regeneration and healing has been appreciated for over 2 centuries. In 1743, Hunter stated "From Hippocrates to the present age, it is universally allowed that ulcerated cartilage is a troublesome thing and that when once destroyed it is not repaired". The response of cartilage to tissue damage is limited, and natural repair responses from adjacent tissues are unable to produce tissue with the same morphologic, biochemical, and biomechanical properties of articular cartilage.

Some of the earlier experimental work provided us with classic concepts. Bennett, Bauer, and Maddock studied the repair of articular cartilage defects, as well as the reaction of normal joints of adult dogs to surgically created defects of articular cartilage and implantation of joint mice. No defects completely healed in the 28-week period. Calandruccio and Gilmer studied the healing of defects in immature dogs.

They recognized the phenomena of matrix flow, proliferation of superficial cartilage cells, proliferation of connective tissue from the base of the defect, and formation of new chondrones as phenomena in the healing process. Using radioactive labeling, other research has recognized increased collagen synthesis, as well as increased proteoglycan synthesis adjacent to the area of cartilage injury. However, despite this evidence for increased proteoglycan and collagen synthesis, no significant contribution was made to the healing of lacerated defects in mature rabbit cartilage. Biochemical studies have been directed at characterization of the collagen types in the repair tissue. Furukawa et al were the first to recognize the early formation of type I collagen with later increases in type II collagen content (the characteristic collagen for articular cartilage). Although type II later predominated, type I collagen always persisted significantly. It addition, there was less hexosamine in the repair tissue, suggesting that the fibrous nature that usually developed in the healing tissue was due to a lack of proteoglycans rather than a change in the type of collagen.[7]

Natural Healing of Articular Cartilage Defects

The major limiting factor in the successful rehabilitation of any joint after injury and disease is the failure of osteochondral defects to heal. Three mechanisms have been recognized as possible contributors to articular cartilage repair. Intrinsic repair (from within the cartilage) relies on the limited mitotic capability of the chondrocyte and a somewhat ineffective increase in collagen and proteoglycan production. Extrinsic repair comes from mesenchymal elements from the subchondral bone participating in the formation of new connective tissue that may undergo some metaplastic change to form cartilage elements. The third phenomenon known as "matrix flow" may contribute to equine articular cartilage repair by forming lips of cartilage from the perimeter of the lesion that migrate toward the center of the defect.[9,10] A publication has suggested that it is possible for synovial membrane (and the subsynovial tissue) to act a source of repair.[11] This experimental study was done with partial-thickness defects in rabbits. With the use of chondroitinase ABC to digest the GAG chains of cartilage proteoglycans (which enhances adhesions) an addition of growth factors and mesenchymal cells that were considered synovial in origin came into the defect. There was no transformation of these cells into chondrocytic elements and at this stage it would seem, although synovial membrane could be a potential source of cells, effective healing is not going to be achieved.

The depth of the injury (full or partial thickness), size of defect, location and relation to weight-bearing or non-weight-bearing areas, and the age of the animal influence the repair and remodeling of an injured joint surface.[4,6,12]

With a partial-thickness defect, some degree of repair with increased glycosaminoglycan synthesis and increased collagen synthesis occurs.[6] However, the repair process is never completely effective. It has been reported in humans that complete repair of chondromalacia of the patella is thought to occur if matrical depletion and surface breakdown are minimal.[13] However, more recent work with arthroscopic debridement of partial-thickness defects in humans questions any actual regeneration.[14] It should also be recognized that superficial defects are not necessarily progressive and do not necessarily compromise joint function.

With full-thickness defects, the response from the adjacent articular cartilage varies little from that of superficial lesions and provides only limited repair necessary to replace dead cells and damaged matrix at the margins of the wound. These defects heal by in-growth of subchondral fibrous tissue that may or may not undergo metaplasia to fibrocartilage.[9,12,15-17] Subchondral bone defects either heal with bone that grows up into the defect or fill in with fibrocartilagenous in-growth. Duplication of the tide mark in the calcified cartilage layer is rare, and adherence of the repair tissue to surrounding non-injured cartilage is often incomplete.

The size and location of articular defects have a significant effect on the degree of healing achieved; several studies in the horse demonstrate this. Convery et al first reported that large defects were less likely to heal.[12] A more recent study distinguished between large (15 mm^2) and small (5mm^2) full-thickness lesions in weight-bearing and non-weight-bearing areas of the radiocarpal, intercarpal and femoropatellar joints.[9] At 1 month, small defects were filled with poorly organized fibrovascular repair tissue; by 4 months, repair was limited to an increase in the amount of organization of this fibrous tissue; and by 5 months, small radiocarpal and femoropatellar lesions were hardly detectable because of the combinations of matrix flow and extrinsic repair mechanisms. Large lesions showed good initial repair but at 5 months perilesional and intralesional subchondral clefts developed.

It has also been demonstrated that induced osteochondral defects (6.5 mm) on the non-weight-bearing aspect of the distal lateral trochlea in the horse healed with fibrocartilagenous tissue at a faster rate, and more completely, than those on the weight-bearing proximomedial trochlear ridge of the talus.[18]

The repair tissue that forms after full-thickness injury to hyaline cartilage, or as a natural repair process in joints with OA, is primarily composed of type I compared to type II collagen at least at 4 months.[19,20] Identification of type II collagen is a critical biochemical factor distinguishing hyaline cartilage from repair fibrous tissue and fibrocartilage. It is believed that the presence of an abnormal subchondral bone plate and the absence of a tide mark reforming may create a stiffness gradient, and that shear stresses of the junction of the repair tissue and underlying bone develop. The propagation of such shear stresses would lead to the degradation of repair fibrocartilage and exposure of the bone. This mechanical failure has been observed experimentally and clinically.[9,21] Of some interest are data from the author's laboratory on the analysis of tissue 12 months after creation of full-thickness articular cartilage defects in a weight-bearing area. In a study looking at the effectiveness of sternal cartilage grafting long-term, the repair tissue in the non-grafted defects at 12 months consisted of fibrocartilaginous tissue with fibrous tissue in the surface layers, as had been seen in control defects at 4 months (Figure 115-1). On biochemical analysis, the repair tissue of the non-grafted defects had a mean type II collagen percentage of 79% compared with being non-detectable at 4 months.[20] On the other hand, the glycosaminoglycan content expressed as milligrams of total hexosamine per gram of dried tissue was 20.6 +/- 1.85 mg/gm compared with 26.4 +/- 3.1 mg/gm at 4 months and 41.8 +/- 4.3 mg/gm DW in normal equine articular cartilage.[20,22]

The fibrocartilaginous repair seen in normal full-thickness defects, therefore, is biomechanically unsuitable as a replacement-bearing surface and has been shown to undergo mechanical failure with use. The lack of durability may be related to faulty biochemical composition of the old matrix and incomplete remodeling of the interface between old and repaired cartilage or to increased stress in the regenerated cartilage because of abnormal remodeling of the subchondral bone plate and calcified cartilage layer. Although some work implies that it may be possible to reconstitute the normal collagen type in articular repair,[22] it is clear that low levels of glycosaminoglycan

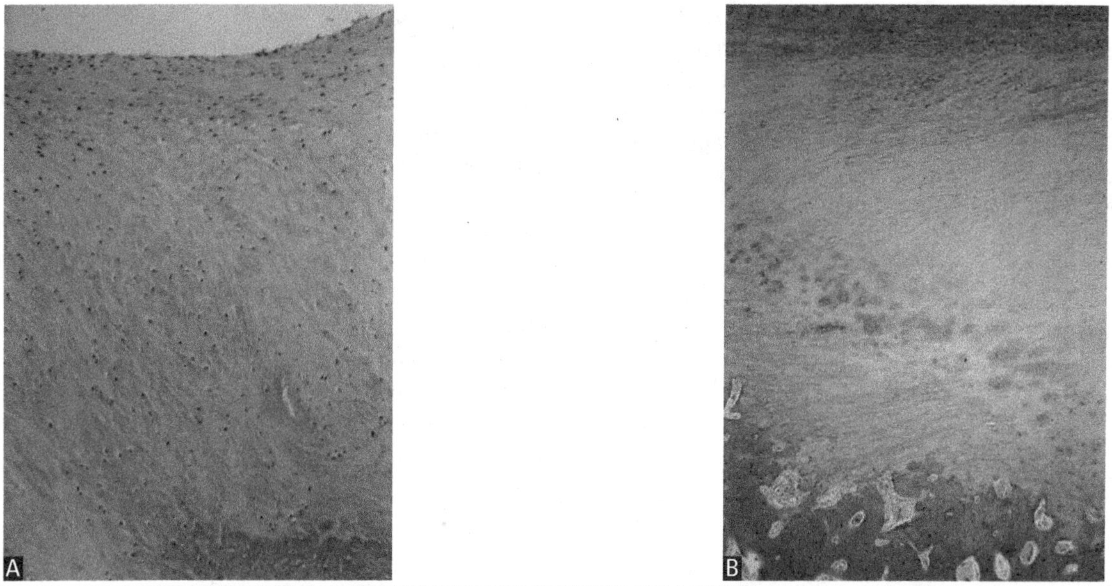

Figure 115-1. Photomicrographs of repair tissue in full-thickness articular cartilage defects in equine radial carpal bone. (A) at 4 months, (B) at 12 months. There is a mixture of fibrous (superficially) and fibrocartilagenous (deeper) tissue in the defect.

persist and these are important components in the overall composition of the cartilage matrix.

It does need to be recognized that the presence of a cartilage defect may not represent clinical compromise. In the equine carpus, it has been shown that up to 30% of articular surface loss of an individual bone may not compromise the successful return of a horse to racing.[21] However, a loss of 50% of the articular surface or severe loss of subchondral bone leads to a significantly decreased prognosis.

It is also to be recognized that the inadequate healing response may not necessarily apply to immature animals nor to non-weight bearing defects. An example is the young patient after surgery for osteochondritis dissecans (OCD) in which impressive healing responses or at least functional responses are obtained. This may be related to increased chondrocytic capacity for mitosis and matrix synthesis and the presence of intracartilaginous vascularity. Complete restoration of the ultrastructure and surface configuration in a hinge-like gliding joint surface such as the femoropatellar joint may be unnecessary for clinical soundness compared with the more severe loading on an osteochondral defect located on the weight-bearing portion of the medial condyle of the femur, for instance. It has been suggested that increasing age may affect the response of cartilage to injury in humans because the ability of the chondrocytes to synthesize and assemble matrix micromolecules could decline with age.[1] Buckwalter and Mow cite a study of transplanted chondrocytes, suggesting that older chondrocytes produce a more poorly organized matrix than do younger chondrocytes,[1] and other studies demonstrate that the proteoglycan synthesized by the chondrocytes change with age.[5,23]

Techniques Attempted for Modulation of Articular Cartilage Healing

Defect Debridement

An old clinical generalization is that superficial defects in articular cartilage do not heal and that full-thickness defects heal through metaplasia of granulation tissue arising at either the articular margin or from the subchondral marrow spaces below.[16] This led to the common practice of clinicians curetting partial-thickness defects into full-thickness ones to stimulate "healing." As mentioned previously, the importance of small partial-thickness defects has been questioned and the quality of the new replacement tissue after full-thickness curettage is now recognized as uncertain and commonly defective.[8] In addition to experimental work, arthroscopic observations (follow-up examinations) by the author of the healing of clinical articular defects confirm the failure of these defects to heal effectively in weight-bearing areas. Because of this inadequate healing response, it is suggested that debridement of partial-thickness defects to full-thickness defects in aggressive debridement to bone is contraindicated.[24] This opinion is also influenced by the observation that superficial defects are not necessarily progressive and do not necessarily compromise joint function.

Having said that, cartilage and bone debridement are common during arthroscopic surgery. As a simple rule, loose fibrous tissue or exposed loose bone should be removed from full-thickness defects. If cartilage is elevated or separated from the bone, it should be debrided back to where it attaches. Debridement should continue down to firm, normal-appearing subchondral bone. Maintaining as much subchondral bone as possible keeps the bone plate and overlying cartilage repair tissue contoured to the normal congruency of the opposing joint surface, thereby enhancing the chance of healing cartilage tissue persisting. It is important, however, that the remaining bone is viable. Crumbly, brownish bone should also be removed by debridement, either using hand instruments or motorized equipment. As has been mentioned, consensus appears to favor not debriding partial-thickness fibrillated cartilage. An argument exists that chondroplasty reduces the possibility of damaged cartilage leaching degraded cartilage-matrix fragments, including collagen, proteoglycan, and cellular components, to the synovial fluid where they increase synovitis and concurrent lameness.[25]

Full-thickness cartilage lesions are debrided to remove residual portions of the calcified cartilage layer. Research has confirmed that persistence of calcified cartilage retards the development of well attached cartilage repair tissue from the subchondral bone and surrounding cartilage (Figure 115-2).[26]

Spongialization

Removal of sclerotic subchondral bone from the base of full-thickness defects has been advocated to achieve the formation of new tissue in the defect.[31] In defects associated with OA, the subchondral plate is often sclerotic and ischemic, and complete removal of the subchondral plate (spongialization) could potentially provide an increased opportunity for tissue filling of cartilage defects. However, long-term follow-up of experimental defects in horses with significant debridement of subchondral bone implies that the biomechanical changes result in stresses that disrupt the new repair tissue.[22] Spongialization has been replaced by less invasive techniques, particularly microfracture.

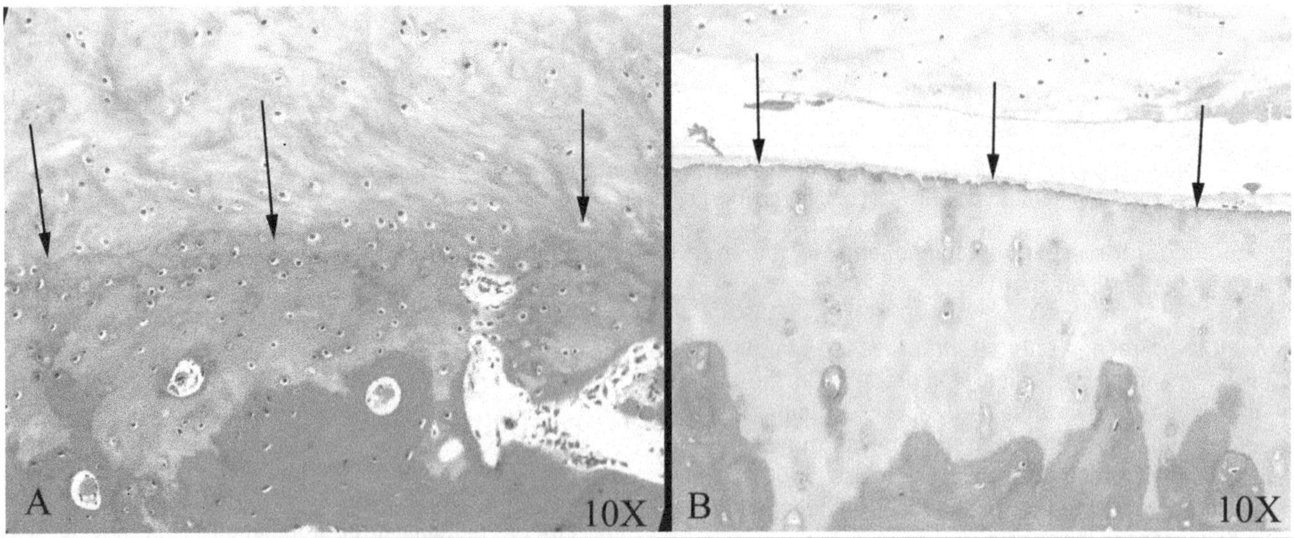

Figure 115-2. Photomicrographs of repair tissue at 12 months in full-thickness articular cartilage defects on the medial femoral condyle where (A) the calcified cartilage layer has been completely removed, and (B) the calcified cartilage layer has not been removed.

Chondroplasty

Resection of the protruding surface strands of partial-thickness cartilage fibrillation has been promoted as a mechanism to reduce cartilage-derived debris entering the synovial environment.[25,27-29] Motorized synovial abraders are used smooth the surface of the more seriously damaged cartilage. The residual cartilage then presents a more uniform non-clefted surface, which may be more durable and incite less synovitis than the large surface area presented by multiple strands of fibrillated cartilage. Although this seems a simple concept, a paucity of evidence exists documenting any discrete benefit, either in reducing synovial levels of fragmented proteoglycan and collagen or in decreasing the symptoms of synovitis. Clinically, chondroplasty to smooth articular cartilage in areas of fibrillation seems to reduce the evidence of persistent effusion when patients go back into exercise, but because of a lack of controlled experimental data, the technique is controversial. It is important that, if done, resection should only involve the fibrillated surface and not be aggressively pursued down to the subchondral bone for reasons previously discussed. Articular cartilage was shaved on the underside of the rabbit patella with no evidence for repair (and no evidence of degenerative changes) in either the superficially or deeply shaved areas.[23,30] Ultrastructural studies after arthroscopic cartilage shaving however, question any regeneration and suggest deleterious effects.[14]

Subchondral Bone Drilling

Subchondral bone drilling has been used with rationale similar to spongialization (access to cancellous bone through a sclerotic or ischemic subchondral bone plate). Controlled studies have been done with experimentally created full-thickness and partial-thickness defects in horses.[32,33] Subchondral bone drilling of full-thickness cartilage defects of the equine third carpal bone was followed by fibrocartilagenous repair tissue of quality and quantity superior to the fibrous tissue of non-drilled defects, but satisfactory functional healing was not achieved.[32] Subchondral drilling did not significantly improve partial-thickness cartilage healing.[33]

Abrasion Arthroplasty

The use of superficial intracortical debridement (arthroscopic abrasion arthroplasty), as opposed to deep cancellous debridement, for sclerotic degenerative lesions has been advocated in humans.[34] The concept is somewhat controversial and argues the necessity to expose cancellous bone to reach both bone supply and pluripotential cells. Abrasion arthroplasty is an arthroscopic technique used to remove eburnated bone by exposing intracortical vessels in the tibial and femoral surfaces of the knee. The organizing hematoma forms over these abraded surfaces and then differentiates into fibrocartilage. The abrasion goes approximately 2 mm into cortical bone. Deep exposure into cancellous bone with removal of subchondral bone is considered counter-productive as it causes a fibrous repair without cartilage.[35] Microfracture is the favored technique for gaining access to cancellous bone elements now.

Subchondral Bone Microfracture

The use of microfracture, or micropicking, as it has been referred to in equine arthroscopy, has many of the advantages associated with subchondral drilling, including focal penetration of the dense subchondral plate to expose cartilage defects to the benefits of cellular and growth-factor influx, as well as improving anchorage of the new tissue to the underlying subchondral bone and, to some extent, surrounding cartilage.[36-38] The simplicity of microfracture comes from the use of a tapered awl (Linvatec, Largo, FL; Arthrex, Naples, FL) instead of a parallel-sided twist drill. Using the awl eliminates the need for powered instrumentation and gives accurate control. A tapered entry into the subchondral marrow space is achieved. The microfracture awl should penetrate the subchondral bone deeply enough to provide ready access to the marrow spaces, thereby maximizing cellular and anabolic growth-factor delivery (Figure 115-3). The microfracture awl also tends to make a crater in the subchondral bone, which may play a role in better attachment of the cartilage repair tissue.[39] Microfracture holes are generally placed 3 to 5 mm apart and cover the entire debrided area in a cartilage lesion. It is also important to microfracture the subchondral bone on the perimeter of the cartilage lesion to encourage new tissue at the junction of repair tissue and residual cartilage. The technique has become popular in human arthroscopy and is now frequently compared to chondrocyte transplantation as one of the two most frequently employed techniques to improve cartilage healing.[36,40,41] One study compared use of microfracture to autologous chondrocyte implantation in a randomized trial. At 2 years' follow-up, both groups had significant clinical improvement, but according to the SF-36 physical component score, the improvement in the microfracture group was significantly better than that in the autologous implantation group.[42]

An experimental study in the horse documented improvement in the quantity of tissue and the type II collagen content at 4 and 12 months after microfracture of full-thickness cartilage defects (Figure 115-4).[37] Improvements in early gene expression of type II collagen and mRNA at 8 weeks have also been demonstrated.[43]

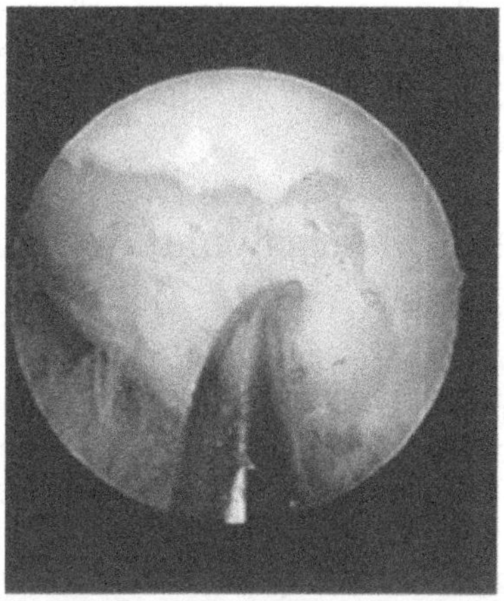

Figure 115-3. Arthroscopic view of a microfractured articular defect.

The technique clearly has advantages over forage and transplantation methods, including ease of application using arthroscopy, use of a simple hand tool, the relative economics of the equipment required, and the apparent increase of cartilage repair tissue that develops after the procedure.

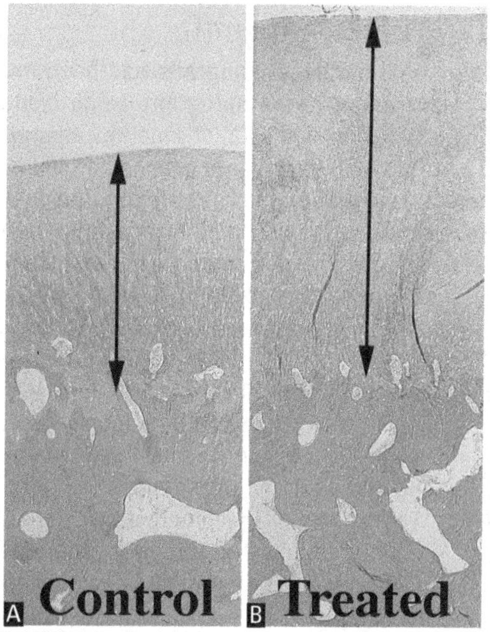

Figure 115-4. Photomicrographs (same level of magnification) of full-thickness defects on the medial femoral condyle that have been (A) simply debrided and (B) debrided and microfractured, demonstrating signficiantly more filling of articular defect that has been microfractured.

Transplantation Procedures

It is generally accepted that most debriding and marrow-stimulating techniques result in fibrocartilage formation with modest biomechanical capabilities. The use of supplemental free cells, various vehicles containing cells or entire tissue such as periosteum or cartilage grafts have been advocated to improve on the modest impact that local manipulative procedures have on both the quality and quantity of cartilage repair tissue. Transplantation procedures can be classified according to the origin of the transplanted tissue: 1) periosteal grafting; 2) periochondral grafting; 3) autogenous cartilage (articular, sternal, or auricular transplantation); 4) osteochondral transplantation; 5) chondrocyte transplantation; and 6) pluripotential stem cell transplantation. These transplantation techniques have practical limitations. Arthrotomy is required for insertion of periosteum, perichondrium, intact cartilage, and osteochondral grafts. Similarly, tissue-engineered analogs such as chondrocytes cultured on collagen, PGA or PGA/PLA, or other synthetic materials such as hyaluronan membranes are also difficult or impossible to implant arthroscopically.

Periosteum

The chondrogenic potentials of perichondrium and periosteum have been used experimentally to restore large osteochondral defects in the rabbit and dog.[44-47] Work in the horse showed that chondroid tissue could be produced after implantation of free periosteal autografts (but not perichondreal autografts).[48] However, when periosteal autografts were placed into osteochondral defects and fixed with fibrin glue, results were unsatisfactory, with the predominant tissue in most defects being fibrous tissue. The poor results and high type I collagen content were related to the formation of adhesions.[17]

Sternal Cartilage Autografts

The use of sternal cartilage autografts has been investigated in horses with fixation of the autografts using biodegradable pins.[20,22] On histologic examination at 4 months, the repair tissue appeared morphologically similar to hyaline cartilage compared with the non-grafted tissue, which was fibrocartilage tissue with fibrous tissue on the surface. On biochemical analysis, the repair tissue with sternal grafting was composed predominantly of type II collagen (non-grafted predominantly type I collagen) and the total GAG content of repair tissue (42.6 =/- 5.9 mg/g DW) was not significantly different from that of normal articular cartilage and was significantly greater than that of non-grafted defects (26.4 +/- 3.1 mg/g DW). Unfortunately, a long-term (12-month) study (together with high-speed treadmill exercise) resulted in repair tissue degenerating and the formation of horizontal and vertical clefts. The type II collagen content was not significantly different from control defects and the mean total GAG content had dropped to 29.1 mg/g DW in grafted defects compared with 19.1 mg/g DW in controls.

Osteochondral Grafts

The use of osteochondral autografts and allografts has cycled through several periods of clinical interest. Originally, autogenous osteochondral shell allografts were used, but there were major problems of limited availability of autogenous osteochondral graft tissue and donor site morbidity. Few locations in humans or animals can sacrifice considerable areas of a joint as osteochondral grafts. The use of osteochondral shell allografts overcomes the limitations of donor site morbidity, and fresh osteochondral hemiarthroplasty shell allografts have been used for advanced degenerative osteoarthritis in humans.[49] These are entire femoral condylar grafts and immunogenicity is always of concern.

Mosaicplasty using autogenous osteochondral dowel grafts has become popular. Osteochondral dowels are harvested arthroscopically from less weight-bearing regions of the same joint, and these dowels are inserted to reconstruct a relatively congruous joint surface with articular cartilage.[50-53]

Several instrument systems are available for the harvest and implantation of osteochondral dowels in humans and animals, including the mosaicplasty system (ACUFEX-Smith and Nephew, Andover, MA); the osteochondral autografts transfer system (OATS-Arthrex, Naples, FL); and the consistent osteochondral repair system (COR-Innovasif BE). Frequently "mosaicplasty" is used as an umbrella term when it is specific to the Smith and Nephew instrumentation. The benefits of this technique include immediate weight-bearing capabilities, relatively good integration of the bony portion of the dowel, and the long-term data available from clinical trials.[52,53]

The mosaicplasty technique has been used in the horse and it has also been shown that age influences the outcome.[54] A case report has been published of the use of mosaicplasty for the repair of a subchondral bone cyst in the medial femoral condyle in the horse.[55] The technical difficulties associated with careful graft harvesting and the precision and crafting needed for heterotopic graft insertion in the recipient bed will probably detract from wider clinical application.[56] Also empty spaces that naturally form between inserted osteochondral dowels heal poorly and allow synovial fluid entry into the bony tunnels of adjacent dowels.

Chondrocyte Transplantation

Autogenous chondrocyte implantation is one of the few FDA-approved tissue engineering techniques to treat articular cartilage injury in humans. It is a two-stage procedure in which articular cartilage biopsies are harvested arthroscopically from minimally weight-bearing regions of the injured knee, propagated ex vivo in cell culture, and later implanted under an autogenous periosteal tissue flap.[57] The indications include focal defects and osteochondritis dissecans.[58,59] The delivery of cells requires an arthrotomy and the harvest and suture attachment of a periosteal flap, which is tedious and technically demanding. One study compared chondrocyte transplantations secured with a periosteal patch to defects treated with periosteal patches without chondrocyte implantation and found no difference between the healing tissues after 1 year.[60] Long-term studies for patients treated with autogenous chondrocyte repair have reported good outcomes.[61-63]

In horses, chondrocyte implantation techniques have been examined in a variety of matrix carrier vehicles.[64-66] Initial research trials indicated enhancement of healing with chondrocyte implantation using a fibrin vehicle,[64] but further tissue engineering approaches with collagen matrix scaffolds did not provide a satisfactory improvement in repair.[65]

Experimental work in the horse with a modified ACI technique (culturing of chondrocytes on a collagen membrane) has yielded positive results at 12 and 18 months.[67] However, more recently, even better results have been obtained with re-implantation of morselized autogenous articular cartilage particles in a one-step procedure.[68] Such techniques have real potential application in dogs and horses.

Pluripotential Mesenchymal Stem Cell Transplantation

The use of pluripotent cells to enhance cartilage repair has been investigated for several years. Initial studies in the rabbit indicated mesenchymal stem cells (MSCs) could enhance cartilage repair.[69] Follow-up work in small animals demonstrated that MSCs can be partially induced down chondrocyte lineages.[70] Studies in the horse indicate bone marrow-derived MSCs can be harvested and cultured for sufficient time and defined media to differentiate toward a chondrocytic lineage,[71] but in vivo studies in the horse report little advantage in the healing at 8 months in a femoral trochlear ridge cartilage defect model.[72] Further work is being done in this area.

Growth Factors

Several naturally occurring polypeptide growth factors play an important role in cartilage homeostasis. The differentiating and matrix anabolic-promoting activity of IGF-1 and TGF-beta are particularly important in counteracting the degradatory and catabolic activities of cytokines, serine proteases, and neutral proteinases. Studies in the horse have largely focused on IGF-1 as TGF-beta has shown synovitis and osteophyte development in animal studies. Slow release of IGF-1 from fibrin composites has been shown to allow for enhanced cartilage repair;[73] however, ideal repair tissue is not obtained and it has been suggested that IGF-1 seems to have better application in combination chondrocyte implantation where more complete cartilage repair develops.[74]

Conclusion

At the present time most cartilage repair techniques in small animals would revolve around endogenous manipulation of healing, such as the use of debridement and microfracture. More advanced techniques including cartilage transplantation and autogenous chondrocyte implantation, as well as autogenous osteochondral grafting techniques, show promise.

References

1. Buckwalter JA, Mow DC: Cartilage repair in osteoarthritis. *In* Osteoarthritis. Diagnosis and Medical/Surgical Management, 2nd ed. Moskowitz RW, Howell DS, Goldberg VM, et al (eds). Philadelphia: WB Saunders, 1992, p. 71.

2. Hunter W: On the structure and diseases of articulating cartilage. Philos Trans R Soc Lond:9:267, 1743.

3. Bennett GA, Bauer W, Maddock SJ: A study of the repair of articular cartilage and the reaction of normal joints of adult dogs to surgically created defects of articular cartilage (joint mice) and patella displacement. Am J Pathol 8:499, 1932.

4. Calandruccio RA, Gilmer S: Proliferation, regeneration and repair of articular cartilage of immature animals. J Bone Joint Surg 44A:431, 1962.

5. Repo RB, Mitchell N: Collagen synthesis of mature articular cartilage of the rabbit. J Bone Surg 53B:541, 1971.

6. Meachim G: The effect of scarification on articular cartilage in the rabbit. J Bone Joint Surg 45B:150, 1963.

7. Furukawa T, Eyre D, Koide S: Biochemical studies on repair cartilage resurfacing of experimental defects in the rabbit knee. J Bone Joint Surg 62A:79, 1980.

8. McIlwraith CW, Vachon AM: Review of pathogenesis and treatment of degenerative joint disease. Equine Vet J S6:3, 1988.

9. Hurtig MB, Fretz PB, Doige CE, Schnurr DL: Effective lesion size and location of equine articular cartilage. Can J Vet Res 52:137, 1988.

10. McIlwraith CW: General pathobiology of the joint and response to injury. *In* Joint Disease in the Horse. McIlwraith CW, Trotter GW (eds). Philadelphia: WB Saunders, ,1996, p. 61.

11. Hunziker EB, Rosenberg LC: Repair of partial-thickness defects in articular cartilage: Cell recruitment from the synovial membrane. J Bone Joint Surg 78-A,:721, 1996.

12. Convery FR, Akeson WH, Keown GH: Repair of large osteochondral defects. An experimental study in horses. Clin Orthop 82:253, 1972.

13. Bentley G: Articular cartilage changes in chondromalacia patellae. J Bone Joint Surg 67B:769, 1985.

14. Schmidt F: Ultrastructural studies after arthroscopical cartilage shaving (abstract). Arthroscopy 3:137, 1987.

15. Mankin HJ: The reactions of articular cartilage to injury and osteoarthritis: I. N Engl J Med 191:1285, 1974.

16. Riddle WE: Healing of articular cartilage in the horse. J Am Vet Med Assoc 157:1471, 1970.

17. Vachon AM, McIlwraith CW, Trotter GW, et al: Morphologic study of induced osteochondral defects of the distal portion of the radial carpal bone in horses by use of glued periosteal autografts. Am J Vet Res 52:317, 1991.

18. Fischer TA, Stover SM, Poole RR: Healing of full thickness articular cartilage defects of the horse. A comparison of weight-bearing to non weight-bearing area. Abstr Vet Surg 15:120, 1986.

19. Vachon AM, McIlwraith CW, Keeley FW: Biochemical study of repair of induced osteochondral defects of the distal portion of the radial carpal bone in horses by use of periosteal autografts. Am J Vet Res 52:328, 1991.

20. Vachon AM, McIlwraith CW, Powers BE, et al: Morphologic and biochemical study of sternal cartilage autografts for resurfacing induced osteochondral defects in horses. Am J Vet Res 53:1038, 1992.

21. McIlwraith CW, Yovich JV, Martin JS: Arthroscopic surgery for the treatment of osteochondral chip fractures in equine carpus. J Am Vet Med Assoc 191:531, 1987.

22. Howard RD, McIlwraith CW, Trotter GW, et al: Sternabral autografts in the repair osteochondral defects in horses: A long term fate and effective exercise. Am J Vet Res 55:1158, 1994.

23. Mitchell N, Shepherd N: Resurfacing of adult rabbit articular cartilage by multiple perforations through the subchondral bone. J Bone Joint Surg 58A:230, 1976.

24. McIlwraith CW: Diagnostic and Surgical Arthroscopy in the Horse. Philadelphia: Lea & Febiger, 1990.

25. Thompson RC: An experimental study of surface injury to articular cartilage and enzyme responses within the joint. Clin Orthop 107:239, 1975.

26. McIlwraith CW, Frisbie DD, Park RD, et al: Effects of calcified cartilage on healing of chondral defects treated with microfracture in horses. Proceedings American Orthopedic Sports Medicine Society, 2005.

27. Childers JC, Ellwood SC: Partial chondrectomy and subchondral bone drilling for chondromalacia. Clin Orthop 144:114, 1979.

28. Kim HKW, Moran ME, Salter RB: The potential for regeneration of articular cartilage in defects created by chondral shaving and subchondral abrasions. J Bone Joint Surg 73A: 1301, 1991.

29. Altman RD, Kates J, Chun LE, et al: Preliminary observations of chondral abrasion in a canine model. Ann Rheum Dis 51:1056, 1992.

30. Mitchell N, Shepherd N: Effective patella shaving in the rabbit. J Orthop Res 5:388, 1987.

31. Ficat RP, Ficat C, Gideon P, Toussant JB: Spongialization: A new treatment for diseased patellae. Clin Orthop 144:74, 1979.

32. Vachon A, Bramlage L, Gabel A, Weisbrode S: Evaluation of the repair process of cartilage defects in equine third carpal bone with and without subchondral bone proliferation. Am J Vet Res 47:2637, 1986.

33. Shamis LD, Bramlage LR, Gabel AA, Weisbrode S: Effective subchondral drilling on repair of partial thickness cartilage defects of third carpal bone in horses. Am J Vet Res 50:290, 1989.

34. Johnson L: Arthroscopic abrasion arthroplasty: Historical and pathologic perspective- present status. Arthroscopy 2:54, 1986.

35. Johnson LL: Arthroscopic abrasion arthroplasty. *In* Operative Arthroscopy. McGinty JB (ed). New York: Raven Press, 1991, p. 341.

36. Rodrigo JJ, Steadman JR, Silliman JF, Fulstone HA: Improvement of full-thickness chondral defect healing in the human knee after debridement and microfracture using continuous passive motion. Am J Knee Surg 7:109, 1994.

37. Frisbie DD, Trotter GW, Powers BE, et al: Arthroscopic bone plate microfracture technique augments healing of large chondral defects in the radial carpal bone and medial femoral condyle of horses. Vet Surg 28:242, 1999.

38. Breinan HA, Minas T, Hsu HB, et al: Effects of cultured autologous chondrocytes on repair of chondral defects in a canine model. J Bone Joint Surg 79A:1439-1451, 1997.

39. Lee CR, Grodzinsky AJ, Hsu HP, Martin SD, et al: Effects of harvest and selected cartilage repair procedures on the physical and biochemical properties of articular cartilage in the canine knee. J Orthop Res 18:790, 2000.

40. Steadman JR, Rodkey WG, Briggs KK: Microfracture to treat full-thickness chondral defects: Surgical technique, rehabilitation, and outcomes. J Knee Surg 15:170, 2002.

41. Steadman JR, Rodkey WG, Rodrigo JJ: Microfracture: Surgical technique and rehabilitation to treat chondral defects. Clin Orthop 391(Suppl):S362, 2001.

42. Knutsen G, Engbretsen L, Ludvigsen TC: Autologous chondrocyte implantation compared with microfracture in the knee. A randomized trial. J Bone Joint Surg 86-A:455, 2004.

43. Frisbie DD, Oxford JT, Southwood L, et al: Early events in cartilage repair after subchondral bone microfracture. Clin Orthop 407:215, 2003.

44. Enkvist O: Reconstruction of patella articular cartilage with free autologous periochondreal grafts. Scand J Plast Reconstr Surg 13:361, 1979.

45. Enkvist O, Valderman S, Pastacaldi P: The cartilaginous potential of the perichondrium in rabbit ear and ribs. Scand J Plast Reconstr Surg 13:275, 1979.

46. Ohlsen L, Widenfalk K: The early development of articular cartilage after perichondral grafting. Scand J Plast Reconstr Surg 17:163, 1983.

47. Rubak JM: Reconstruction of articular cartilage defects with free periosteal grafts. An experimental study. Acta Orthop Scand 53:175, 1982.

48. Vachon A, McIlwraith CW, Trotter GW, et al: Neochondrogenesis in free intra-articular periosteal and periochondreal autografts in horses. Am J Vet Res 50:1787, 1989.

49. Gross AE, Aubin P, Chea HK, et al: A fresh osteochondral allograft alternative. J Arthroplasty 17:50, 2002.

50. Hangody L, Kish G, Karpati Z: Arthroscopic autogenous osteochondral mosaicplasty for the treatment of femoral condylar articular defects. Knee Surg Sports Traumatol Arthrosc 5:262, 1997.

51. Hangody L, Kish G, Karpati Z, et al: Mosiacplasty for the treatment of articular cartilage defects: Application and clinical practice. Orthopedics 21:751, 1998.

52. Hangody L, Feczko P, Bartha L, et al: Mosiacplasty for the treatment of articular defects of the knee and ankle. Clin Orthop 391:S328, 2001.

53. Jakob RP, Franz T, Gautier E, et al: Autologous osteochondral grafting in the knee: Indication, results, and reflections. Clin Orthop 401:170, 2002.

54. Bodo G, Kaposi AD, Hangody L, et al: The surgical technique and the age of the horse both influence the outcome of mosaicplasty in a cadaver equine stifle model. Acta Vet Hung 49:111, 2001.

55. Bodo G, Hangody L, Szabo Z, et al: Arthroscopic autologous osteochondral mosaicplasty for the treatment of subchondral cystic lesion in the medial femoral condyle of the horse. Acta Vet Hung 48:343, 2000.

56. Pearce SG, Hurtig MB, Clarnette R, et al: An investigation of two techniques for optimizing joint surface congruency using multiple cylindrical osteochondral autografts. Arthroscopy 17:50, 2001.

57. Brittberg M, Lindahal A, Nilsson A, et al: Treatment of deep cartilage defects in the knee with autologous chondrocyte transplantation. N Engl J Med 331:889, 1994.

58. Robert H, Bahaud J: Autologous chondrocyte implantation: A review of techniques and preliminary results. Rev Rheum Engl Ed 66:724, 1999.

59. Peterson L, Minas T, Brittberg M, et al: Two 9-year outcomes after autologous chondrocyte transplantation of the knee. Clin Orthop 374:212, 2000.

60. Breinan HA, Minas T, Hsu HP: Effects of cultured autologous chondrocytes on repair of chondral defects in a canine model. J Bone Joint Surg 79A:1439-1451, 1997.

61. Richardson JB, Caterson B, Evans EH, et al: Repair of human articular cartilage after implantation of autologous chondrocytes. J Bone Joint Surg Br 81:1064, 1999.

62. Peterson L, Brittberg M, Kiviranta I, et al: Autologous chondrocyte transplantation. Biomechanics and long-term durability. Am J Sports Med 30:2, 2002.

63. Minas T: Autologous chondrocyte implantation for focal chondral defects of the knee. Clin Orthop 391(Suppl):S349, 2001.

64. Hendrickson DA, Nixon AJ, Grande DA, et al: Chondrocyte-fibrin matrix transplants for resurfacing extensive articular cartilage defects. J Orthop Res 12:485, 1994.

65. Sams AE, Nixon AJ: Chondrocyte-laden collagen scaffolds for resurfacing extensive articular cartilage defects. Osteoarthritis Cartilage 3:47, 1995.

66. Fortier LA, Lust G, Mohammed HO, et al: Insulin-like growth factor-1 enhances cell-based articular cartilage repair. J Bone Joint Surg 84B:276, 2000.

67. Frisbie DD, Calhoun HA, Bowman S, Kawcak CE, et al: Autologous chondrocyte transplantation via a collagen membrane: A long-term study. Proceedings 50th Annual Meeting Orthopedic Research Society, 2003.

68. Lu Y, Colhoun HA, et al: In vivo evaluation of a one step autologous cartilage resurfacing technique in a long term equine model. Proceedings 51st Annual Meeting Orthopedic Research Society 1355, 2004.

69. Grande DA, Southerland SS, Manji R, et al: Repair of articular cartilage defects using mesenchymal stem cells. Tissue Eng 1:345, 1995.

70. Butnariu-Ephrat M, Robinson D, Mendes DG, et al: Resurfacing of goat articular cartilage by chondrocyte derived from bone marrow. Clin Orthop 330:234, 1996.

71. Fortier LA, Nixon AJ, Williams J, et al: Isolation and chondrocytic differentiation of equine bone marrow-derived mesenchymal stem cells. Am J Vet Res 59:1182, 1998.

72. Wilke N, Nixon AJ, Adams TA: Enhanced early chondrogenesis in equine cartilage defects using implanted autologous mesenchymal stem cells. Vet Surg 30:508, 2001.

73. Nixon AJ, Fortier LA, Williams J, et al: Enhanced repair of extensive articular defects by insulin-like growth factor-1 laden fibrin composites. J Orthop Res 17:475, 1999.

74. Fortier LA, Lust G, Mohammed HO, et al: Insulin-like growth factor-1 enhances cell-based articular cartilage repair. J Bone Joint Surg 84-B:276, 2002.

Chapter 116

Osteoarthritis

Michele A. Steffey
Rory J. Todhunter

This chapter is dedicated to Dr. Nancy Burton-Wurster, Cornell University, whose intellectual drive and hard work continues to inspire young minds to pursue investigations into the basic science of osteoarthritis in dogs.

Osteoarthritis (OA) is a degenerative process that leads to changes in all components of a synovial joint: articular cartilage, subchondral bone, synovial membrane, synovial fluid, and periarticular soft tissues. Osteoarthritis affects up to 20% of dogs over 1 year of age.[1] Although idiopathic (primary) osteoarthritis is rare in dogs and cats, secondary osteoarthritis is common and usually due to underlying factors such as prior trauma, joint incongruency, joint instability, inflammation, or developmental conditions. Pathologic changes typically consist of variable synovitis, joint capsule thickening, cartilage destruction, subchondral sclerosis, and the production of new bone (osteophytes and enthesiophytes). Because several reviews of OA have been written in veterinary textbooks, this chapter focuses also on information on the subject especially related to biomarkers.

Anatomy and Normal Joint Physiology

Diathrodial joints are an articulation between adjacent bones of the skeleton that are characterized by a surface of articular cartilage, a joint capsule, and synovial fluid secreted into the joint cavity that lubricates the contact surfaces of the joint. Synovial joints can be classified according to the number of articular surfaces they contain (simple or compound joints), the shape or form of the articulating surfaces (plane, ball and socket, ellipsoidal, hinge, condylar, trochoid, or saddle joints) or by the function of the joint.[2]

The fibrous joint capsule of a diarthrodial joint is lined by a synovial membrane. The outer fibrous layer consists primarily of collagen but also contains the vascular and nervous supply to the joint. It attaches peripherally to the articular cartilage and blends with the periosteum of each bone.[2] The synovial membrane is vascular and consists primarily of loose areolar tissue with an inner layer of cells that is one to two synoviocytes thick (Figure 116-1). The two types of synoviocytes are type A, which are primarily phagocytic, and type B, which are primarily secretory. The synovial membrane covers all structures within the joint except the articular cartilage and the contact surfaces of any fibrocartilaginous plates (menisci) and blends with the periosteum as it reflects onto bone.[2]

The primary functions of articular cartilage are to promote motion with minimal friction and to transmit load to the underlying subchondral bone. Hyaline cartilage is composed primarily of matrix and contains relatively few cells (Figure 116-1). Chondrocytes make up less than 5% of the tissue volume.[1] Each chondrocyte, in association with its pericellular capsule and pericellular matrix, forms a unit described as a "chondron."[3] Cartilage is composed of 70% to 80% water by weight, and is avascular, aneural, and alymphatic (Figure 116-2). The primary large molecules comprising articular cartilage matrix are collagen and proteoglycan, and it is these two molecules that give cartilage its unique biochemical and functional properties. Collagen provides tensile strength, whereas proteoglycan provides compressive strength. Both molecules are produced and secreted locally by chondrocytes.

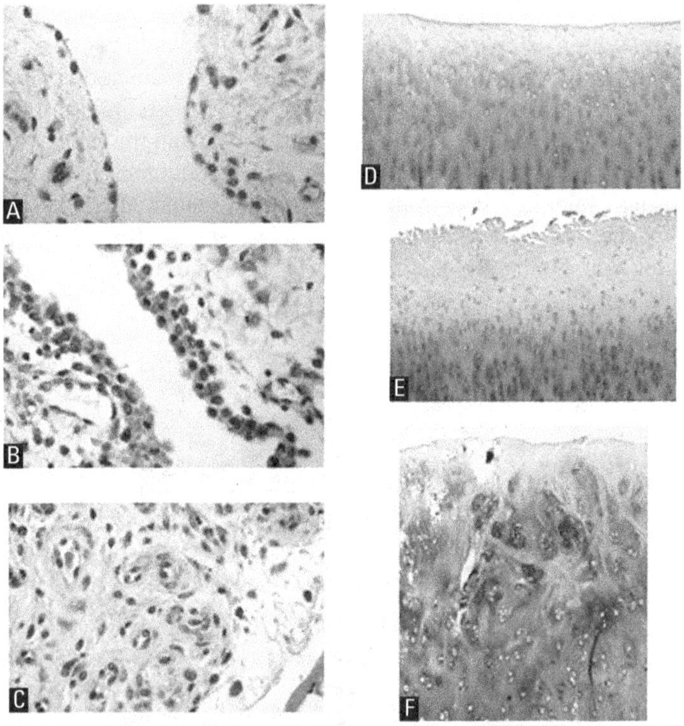

Figure 116-1. A. Photomicrograph of a cross-section of normal synovial membrane. The synovial cavity is between the two pieces of synovial membrane on each side of the photograph. B. Synovial hyperplasia characterized by synovial lining proliferation. C. Chronic synovial hypertrophy characterized by fibroplasia. *(A,B,C: Hematoxylin and eosin, X160.)* D. Photomicrograph of normal articular cartilage showing tissue sparsely populated with chondrocytes that elaborate a profuse extracellular matrix. Chondrocytes in the deep zone tend to align perpendicular to the articular surface (on top). More intense uptake of stain (which binds the sulfated glycosaminoglycan) is seen pericellularly in the deeper layers. E. Photomicrograph of fibrillated articular cartilage showing decreased staining of the extracellular matrix in a dog in the early stages of hip dysplasia. *(D,E: Safranin O/fast green stain, X180.)* E. Cloning of chondrocytes in advanced osteoarthritis. F: Photomicrograph of articular cartilage from a dog with advanced osteoarthritis secondary to hip dysplasia. Surface irregularity, fissures, and chrondrocyte cloning can be seen *(safranin O/fast green stain, X200).*

The classic zonal description of articular cartilage is based on chondrocyte organization, orientation of collagen fibrils, and proteoglycan distribution. Zone one, the tangential zone, is the most superficial region and is characterized by relatively few flattened cells, low proteoglycan content, and collagen fibrils that are oriented tangentially to the articular surface (Figure 116-2). This distribution of collagen and proteoglycan provides the superficial layers of cartilage matrix the greatest ability to withstand tensile forces and resist the swelling pressure exerted by proteoglycan located in the deeper zones.[1] Zones two and three comprise most of the matrix volume. In this region, the density of chondrocytes and proteoglycan content increase with increasing depth in the tissue (Figure 116-1). The cells become more ovoid and in zone two, the transitional zone, are randomly distributed. The direction of the collagen fibrils changes gradually from a tangential orientation to an oblique orientation, and ultimately the fibrils become radially aligned to the articular surface (Figure 116-2). In zone three, the radial zone, the cells line up in vertical columns within the matrix. It is the increased proteoglycan content in these deeper regions that provides most of the ability of cartilage to resist compressive load. A distinct separation, known as the tidemark, exists between zones three and four, at the upper limit of zone four, the calcified zone. It contains radially oriented collagen fibrils, but little proteoglycan. The calcified cartilage is separated from the underlying subchondral bone by a cement line. The osteochondral junction is maintained by the morphology of the interdigitating boundary, the undulating nature of which allows shear stresses to be converted into potentially less damaging compressive forces on the subchondral bone.[4]

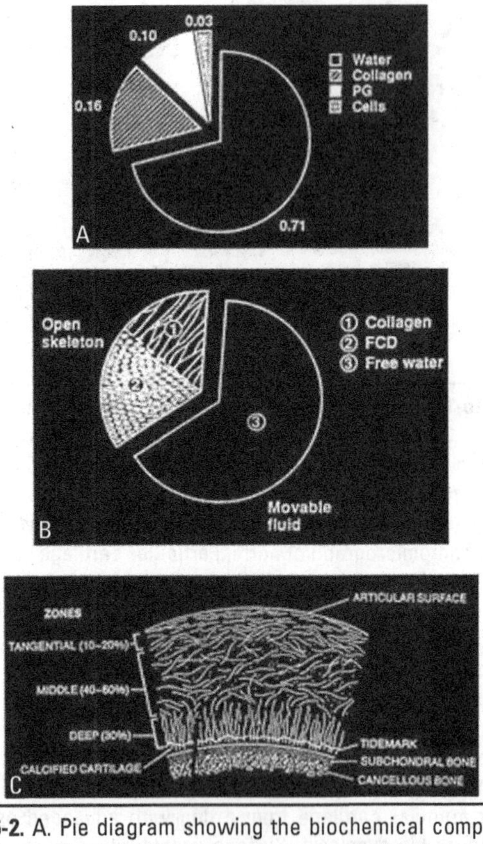

Figure 116-2. A. Pie diagram showing the biochemical composition of the articular cartilage. B. Pie diagram showing the fixed charge density of the proteoglycans, water, and the swelling pressure constrained by the collagen fibrils. C. Diagram of articular cartilage illustrating the selective orientation of the collagen fibrils in normal articular cartilage and the transition through the calcified cartilage to the subchondral bone.

Collagen composes 50% of the dry weight of mature articular cartilage. There are at least 27 different types of collagen.[5] Collagen fibrils are composed of collagen monomers, which in turn are composed of three polypeptide alpha chains arranged in a triple helix. Genetically different alpha chains lead to different types of collagen monomers. Type II collagen is the primary form of collagen in articular cartilage. Other types of collagen that are known to be important in the normal function of articular cartilage are types VI, IX, X, and XI. Type VI collagen is found in the pericellular region of the chondron and may be involved in binding the cell surface to matrix constituents. Type IX links type II fibrils together and is important in the association of collagen and proteoglycan within the matrix. Type X collagen is found during development in the hypertrophic cartilage and in the calcified zone of adult cartilage.[1]

Proteoglycans make up 22% to 28% of the dry weight of adult articular cartilage (Figure 116-2). A proteoglycan molecule is composed of a core protein with glycosaminoglycan side chains. The glycosaminoglycans are chains of repeating disaccharide units of variable length and are negatively charged owing to carboxyl and sulfate groups.[4] This intrinsic ionic charge leads them to repel one another, resulting in the "bottle brush" conformation of the proteoglycan molecule and contributing to its hydrophilic nature. The most common glycosaminoglycans in articular cartilage are chondroitin-6-sulfate (mature articular cartilage), chondroitin-4-sulfate (immature articular cartilage), keratan sulfate, and dermatan sulfate. Proteoglycans may be classified as aggregating or non-aggregating, depending on the ability of the proteoglycan monomer to attach to a hyaluranon backbone by a glycoprotein link. The major aggregating proteoglycan of articular cartilage is aggrecan, whereas the major non-aggregating proteoglycans are decorin and biglycan. Hyaluronan is a non-sulfated glycosaminoglycan that has no core protein. It is found in both the articular cartilage extracellular matrix and the synovial fluid. Hyaluronan is secreted into the extracellular matrix by chondrocytes, where it forms a chain by the noncovalent interaction of hyaluronon monomers, and can aggregate with aggrecan monomers. Hyaluranan is secreted into the synovial fluid by type B synoviocytes where it functions in boundary lubrication, but does not appear to be important in cartilage-on-cartilage lubrication.[1]

The ionic charge of proteoglycan attracts water (Figure 116-2). Proteoglycans can occupy a volume up to 50 times their dry weight volume when hydrated.[1] However, because proteoglycans are trapped in a collagen matrix, their expansion is limited to within 20% of their potential volume, keeping cartilage turgid. It is this relationship between proteoglycan and collagen and the free motion of fluid that allows cartilage to resist deformation and transmit load. When cartilage experiences a compressive load, fluid flows slowly through the collagen meshwork and the pores created by the proteoglycan molecules. The ability of the cartilage to tolerate load is dependent on the interconnections of collagen fibrils (Figure 116-2). If these connections are broken, propagation of fissures through the matrix occurs, leading to morphologic changes characteristic of OA. To a certain extent, articular cartilage adapts to the predominant stress level it experiences and is stiffer in areas of high stress and has increased proteoglycan content.[4] Excessive stress in areas of softer cartilage may result in matrix damage and OA.

Because adult articular cartilage is avascular, it is dependent on the synovial fluid for delivery of nutrition, removal of waste, and circulation of synovial lining cells and leukocytes. Synovial fluid is an ultrafiltrate of plasma, to which large molecules such as hyaluranon have been added by synoviocyte secretion. The viscosity of synovial fluid depends on the molecular weight and concentration of hyaluranon.[4] Joint motion leads to the mechanical compression of cartilage and encourages diffusion of nutrient molecules into the cartilage matrix. In immature animals, nutrients may diffuse into the deep zones of articular cartilage from metaphyseal blood vessels because the calcified cartilage and subchondral plate have not formed. Joint lubrication and the ability of cartilage surfaces to deform under load produces a low coefficient of friction. Under conditions of load, some water is forced out of the matrix, resulting in a weeping of fluid onto the articular surface (hydrostatic lubrication), until an equilibrium is reached between the osmotic force of proteoglycans and the compressive force applied.[1] During weight bearing, articular cartilage lubrication is hydrostatic (squeeze-film) and most important under heavy load whereas boundary lubrication predominates under light load. Load leads to fluid exudation from the matrix, resulting in a thin film of fluid that separates articular surfaces. Boundary lubrication is adherence of a molecular film of lubricant to surfaces of articular cartilage and synovium, which separates opposing surfaces. The boundary lubricant of synovial membrane is hyaluronan. The boundary lubricant of articular cartilage is a glycoprotein called lubricin and its associated protein.

Pathophysiology and Pathology of Osteoarthritis

Osteoarthritis can originate by one of two mechanisms: normal forces acting on an abnormal joint (e.g., in the case of osteochondrosis, hip or elbow dysplasia, or patellar luxation) or abnormal forces acting on a normal joint (e.g., joint trauma resulting in fracture or luxation) (Figure 116-3). Regardless of the specific inciting cause, alterations in the function of the joint lead to specific molecular and cellular changes that result in the ultimate dysfunction of cartilage and periarticular structures that is observed clinically.[1] Changes in cartilage gene expression have been detected as early as 2 weeks after cranial cruciate ligament transaction in a canine model of OA, prior to detectable changes in glycosaminoglycan or collagen content, or evidence of gross or histologic pathology.[6] Joint insult results in release of pro-inflammatory agents such as interleukin 1α (IL-1α) and β and tumor necrosis factor-α (TNF-α) by chondrocytes, synoviocytes, and infiltrating inflammatory cells, resulting in synovitis. The synovitis is marked by synoviocyte proliferation more than neutrophilic infiltration. Synovial lining cells and leukocytes release destructive enzymes, free radicals, cytokines, and prostaglandins. Persistent inflammation alters cartilage metabolism and cartilage degradation follows. At least some of the pain associated with OA has been attributed to the synovitis.[7]

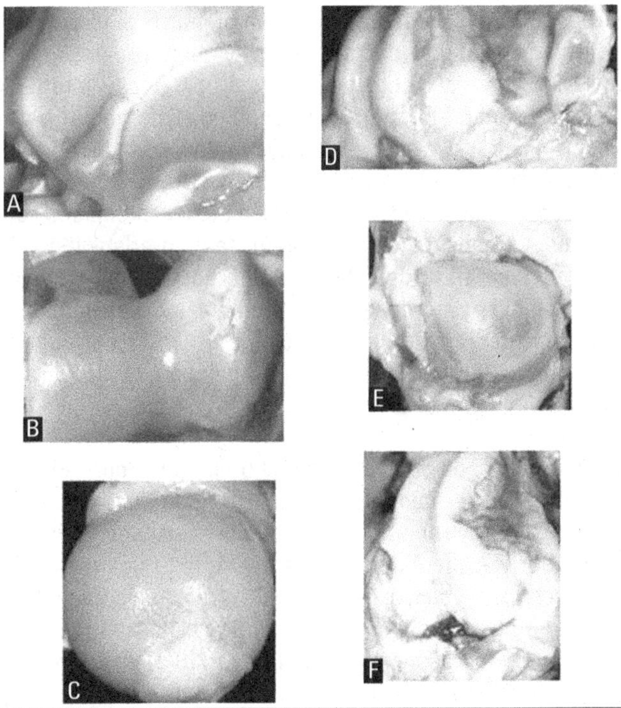

Figure 116-3. Photographs of joint with developmental orthopedic conditions that all result in secondary osteoarthritis owing to surface irregularity or abnormal mechanical loading. A. The proximal radial head and ulnar articular surfaces in the elbow joint showing a slightly elevated triangular-shaped, fragmented medial coronoid process between the medial coronoid of the ulna and the radial head. The full-thickness articular cartilage defect at bottom right is artifact. B. Photograph of an osteochondrosis lesion on the medial humeral condyle in a dog's elbow. C. Photograph of the femoral head of a dog with early hip dysplasia. Notice perifoveal articular cartilage and hypertrophy of the round ligament of the femoral head (bottom center). D. Photograph of the stifle of a dog with medial patellar luxation. Note full-thickness articular cartilage loss along the axial medial trochlea and the articulating surface of the patella (top right). E. Photograph of an osteoarthritic humeral head with full-thickness articular loss (ulcer) caudodorsally. F. Photograph of a stifle joint taken 6 months following experimental transaction of the cranial cruciate ligament. Osteophytes are present along the medial trochlear ridge. (Compliments of Dr. Steven Budsberg, University of Georgia.)

Synovial fluid becomes less viscous as hyaluronan concentration drops and joint lubrication suffers. Release of cartilage fragments and proteinases worsens the inflammatory response and induces further breakdown of collagen cross links.[8] Changes in synovial membrane and synovial fluid may be reversible. Articular cartilage damage is usually irreversible and self-perpetuating. Osteoarthritis is a self-perpetuating destructive cycle involving all components of the joint. The release of leukocytes, prostaglandins, lysozomal enzymes, hyaluronidase, interleukin-1, leukotrienes, and proteinases propagate joint tissue destruction. Synovial fluid viscosity decreases owing to alteration, breakdown, and dilution of hyaluronan and other proteins. Biomechanical properties of synovial fluid are altered with suboptimal lubrication, and decreased diffusion of nutrients into articular cartilage ensues.

Biochemically, OA is characterized by reduction in aggrecan content, alteration in collagen fibril size and structure, and increased synthesis and degradation of matrix macromolecules in cartilage. Proteoglycan synthesis by chondrocytes increases initially but then proteoglycan levels drop.[9] Finally, interleukin-1 and TNF-α induce proteoglycan depletion in articular cartilage by increasing the rate of proteoglycan degradation, decreasing synthesis by chondrocytes, or both. Matrix catabolism is mediated by the effects of matrix metalloproteinases, aggrecanases, cathepsins (acidic proteinases), interleukin-1, TNF-α, hyaluronidase, and prostaglandins. Decreased proteoglycans are accompanied by increased water content, increased compressibility, and decreased stiffness of the articular cartilage. Loss of matrix support that results from collagen fibril degradation permits the matrix to swell.

In the early stages of OA, cartilage fibrillation occurs. Fibrillation (loss of the superficial layer [zone 1]) fundamentally alters the biomechanical properties of articular cartilage.[10] Fibrillation occurs early in the pathogenesis of OA; full-thickness articular cartilage loss follows. Abnormal stresses cause fissures to propagate to deeper layers (Figure 116-1). Chondrocytes cluster and increase in cell size (Figure 116-1). Erosion (uniform surface loss of articular cartilage) follows. Finally, in regions of full-thickness cartilage loss, subchondral bone becomes exposed and eburnated (the polished appearance of sclerotic subchondral bone).

In young dogs with articular cartilage fibrillation owing to hip dysplasia (Figure 116-3), the subchondral and epiphyseal bone mineral content is increased as measured by quantitative computed tomography.[11] In dogs with cranial cruciate ligament deficiency, a marked and sustained rise in urinary excretion of collagen pyridinium cross links was reported, which are thought to derive at least in part from the degradation of mature collagen in bone. Calcitonin, a potent inhibitor of osteoclastic bone resorption, markedly reduced the urinary levels of pyridinium cross links in OA dogs.[12] In canine experimental OA, subcutaneous injection of calcitonin reduced the severity of cartilage osteoarthritis lesions assessed both grossly and histologically.[12] Interestingly, mean bone mineral density of the placebo group was 80% of the calcitonin-treated group.[13]

Periarticular osteophytes can be seen as early as 2 weeks from the onset of osteoarthritis (Figures 116-4 and 116-5). Osteophytes are bony exostoses typically developing at sites of joint capsular attachment. Osteophytes probably represent an attempt by the body to compensate for increased tension on joint capsular attachments owing to chronic synovial effusion, concomitant joint capsular distension, persistent joint instability, and a proliferative repair response. Osteophytes eventually become canalized and the marrow cavity communicates with that of the epiphyseal bone. Enthesiophytes are bone growths or dystrophic mineralization that extends into capsular, ligamentous, and regional soft tissue attachments (Figures 116-4 and 116-5).

Synovial Fluid Analysis

Laboratory evaluation of synovial fluid may be useful in confirming a diagnosis of OA and ruling out other inflammatory or infectious joint diseases. Synovial fluid is evaluated grossly for color, clarity, and viscosity, and microscopically for cell count, cell type, and the presence of infectious agents.[4] The amount of synovial fluid varies according to the joint sampled and the size

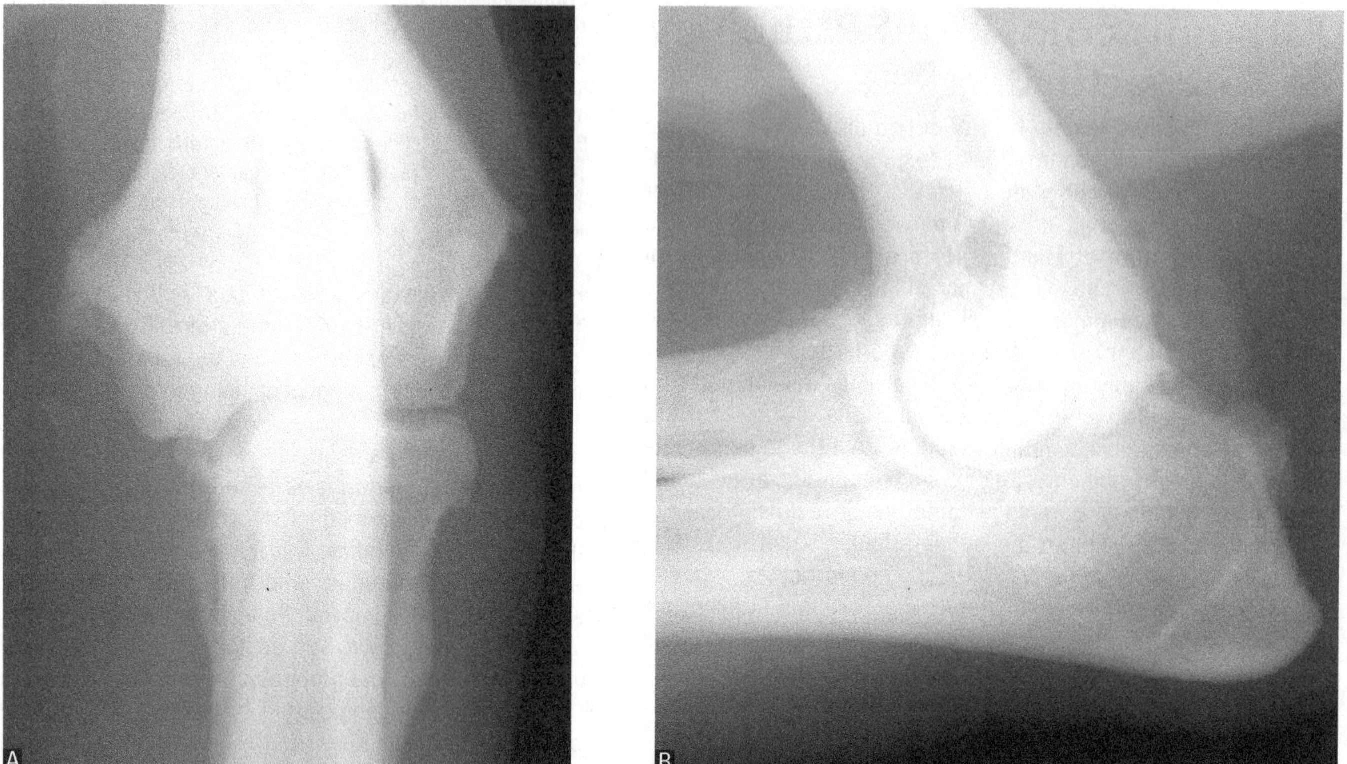

Figure 116-4. A. Cranial-caudal radiograph showing subchondral lucency and osteophyte formation on the medial elbow joint. B. Lateral radiograph of the same elbow, showing osteophyte formation on the proximal anconeal process and cranial proximal radial head. (Compliments of Dr. Peter Scrivani, Cornell University.)

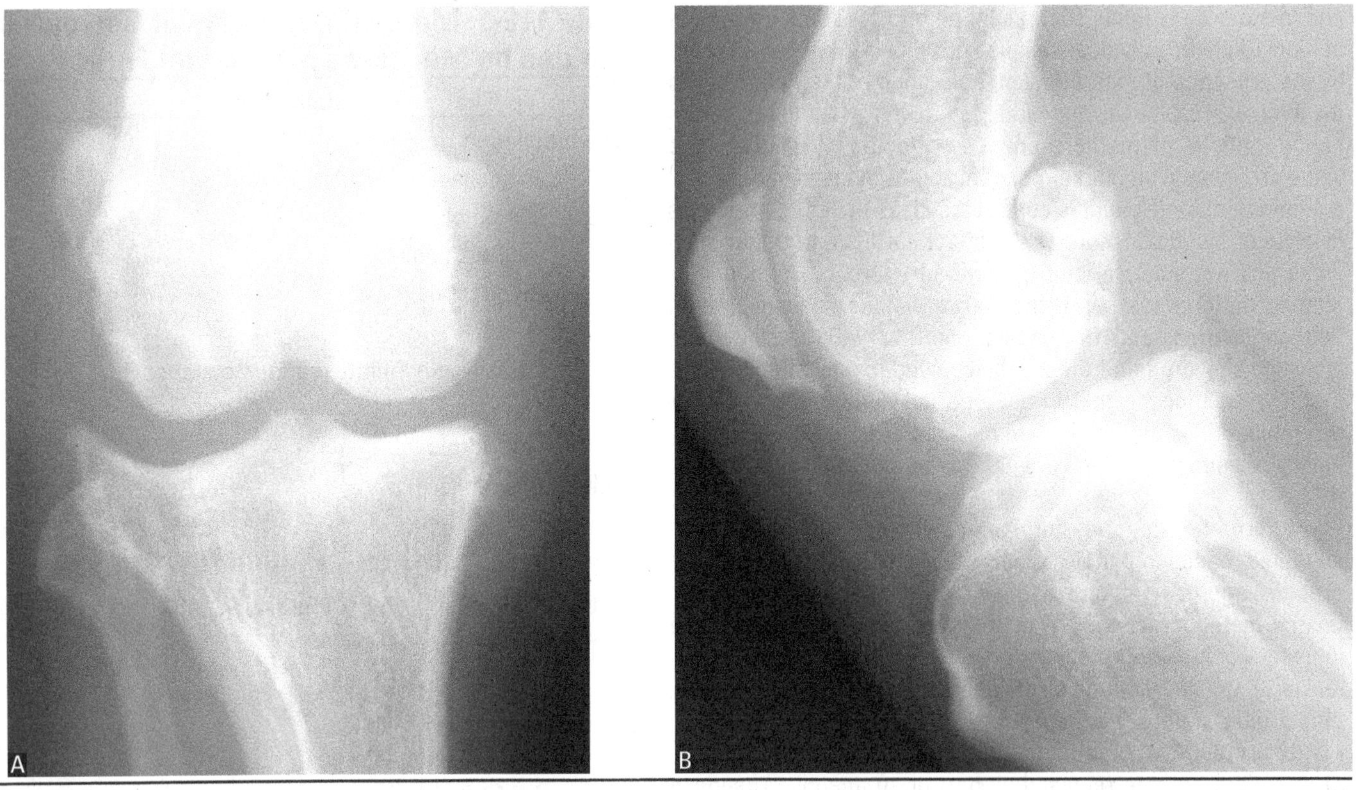

Figure 116-5. A. Photograph of the cranialcaudal view of the stifle showing osteophyte formation on the lateral tibial plates and soft-tissue proliferation on the medial stifle. These findings are consistent with cranial cruciate ligament disruption. B. Lateral radiograph of an osteoarthritic stifle joint of the same dog as in Figure 5A showing increased intra-articular mass and obliteration of fat pad, fabellar remodeling, and osteophytes in the proximal and distal patella and along the nonarticulating surface of the femoral trochlea. (Compliments of Dr. Peter Scrivani, Cornell University.)

of the patient. The average volume of synovial fluid in the normal stifle joint of adult dogs, for example, ranges from 0.2 to 2.0 mL.[2] Synovial fluid volume in OA is generally increased, but may vary according to the chronicity of the condition and the degree of synovitis. Normal synovial fluid is clear, colorless to pale yellow, and contains less than 1000 nucleated cells/μl, whereas synovial fluid from an OA joint may be a clear to hazy pale yellow with nucleated cell counts ranging between 3000 and 5000 cells/μl. The predominant nucleated cell observed in both normal and OA synovial fluid should be the monocyte, and neutrophils should account for less than 10% of the nucleated cells observed (Figure 116-6).[14] Nucleated cell counts in synovial fluid greater than 5000 cells/μl, or cell counts with a higher proportion of neutrophils, indicate arthritis of an infectious or inflammatory etiology that may include an acute exacerbation of a chronic condition. In dogs, the normal synovial fluid cell counts may vary among joints, with the highest cell counts found in synovial fluid from the shoulder and stifle joints.[15] Synovial fluid cell counts from normal and OA stifle and shoulder joints in cats fall within the ranges described above.[16]

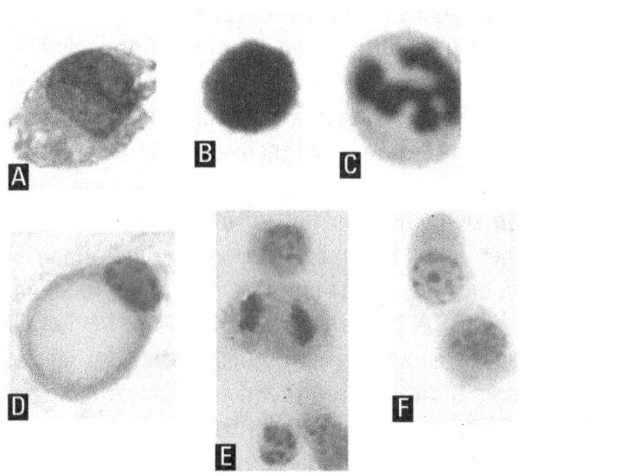

Figure 116-6. Cells found in smears of synovial fluid. A. Polymorphonuclear cells should be less than 10% of the total number. B. Lymphocytes C. Synovial lining cell (probably macrophagic). D. Signet cells indicating joint injury or degeneration. E. Mitotic figure. F. Signet cell indicating joint injury. (Wright Giemsa stain, X160) (Compliments of Dr. Kathleen Freeman, Scotland.)

Biomarkers

Because significant limitations exist in the ability of routine diagnostic methods to detect OA in its early stages or to evaluate subtle changes in progression of the disease in an individual, interest in the identification of endogenous substances as biomarkers for the OA process has arisen. Non- or minimally invasive evaluation of one or more of these substances may eventually allow better identification of individuals in the early stages of the disease, quantification of the severity of the disease and its progression, and objective evaluation of the efficacy of treatment. Biomarkers are typically products of articular cartilage synthesis or degradation. Biomarkers may be anabolic (a product of a synthetic process) or catabolic (a product of degradation) indicators. Alterations in the biomechanics or biochemistry of the joint lead to an imbalance of matrix degradation and synthesis, and the resulting substances that are released may be measured in cartilage, synovial fluid, and in other body fluids such as blood or urine. Concentrations of biomarkers in individual samples of synovial fluid are affected by the presence of joint effusion, clearance of the marker from the joint, exercise level, and circadian rhythms.[4] Although serum concentrations of markers are less affected by dilution, the value of systemic biomarker concentrations in the diagnosis and monitoring of an OA joint is controversial, as the concentrations in urine or blood will more likely reflect cartilage turnover in all joints and not solely a joint or joints of interest.[17] Additionally, although differences exist in the average values of these markers between normal and OA populations, the variation between individuals is large and the extensive overlap limits their use as a solitary diagnostic tool in any one individual patient. Better discrimination is obtained when markers are evaluated longitudinally or multiple markers are used in combination.[18,19]

Three broad categories of molecular markers have been identified based on their origin and function during the OA process: agents related to mechanisms of cartilage degradation (matrix metalloproteinase-1, matrix metalloproteinase-3, tissue inhibitors of metalloproteinase [TIMPs], interleukin-1, and interleukin-6), the degradation products of cartilage (keratan sulfate, chondroitin sulfate, aggrecan fragments, cartilage oligomeric matrix protein, cartilage matrix glycoprotein), and components of articular cartilage released as part of an anabolic response to OA (chondroitin sulfate epitopes 3B3(-) and 7D4, link protein, collagen X, fibronectin) (Table 116-1). Fibronectin is an extracellular matrix glycoprotein through which cells interact with their surrounding matrix. Fibronectin isoforms ED-A and ED-B have previously been described as biomarkers in the rheumatic diseases.[20,21] Total fibronectin concentrations have been demonstrated to be elevated in the cartilage of dogs with OA secondary to hip dysplasia,[22] and in the synovial fluid of dogs with OA secondary to cruciate ligament insufficiency.[23] In the latter study, total fibronectin concentration in synovial fluid was inversely correlated with the duration of clinical signs, suggesting that this marker is an indicator of early repair phase post-injury.[23] Elevation of total fibronectin in the synovial fluid of human patients with OA has also been reported.[24] However, because fibronectins are found in nearly all body tissues, this lack of specificity makes the total fibronectin concentration in serum a poor solitary biomarker for osteoarthritis. (V+C)- fibronectin is a splice variant specific to cartilage so that its presence in bodily fluids implies a cartilage origin.[25] It constitutes 50% to 80% of the total fibronectin present in articular cartilage.[26] A 10-fold elevation of this isoform in OA cartilage has been reported; however, a study of spontaneous OA in the stifles of clinical canine patients failed to demonstrate a significant elevation in synovial fluid (V+C)- concentration as compared with synovial fluid from a control population.[27,23] However, like cartilage oligomeric matrix protein (COMP) evaluated in the same study, (V+C)- fibronectin was elevated in the contralateral stifles, and its elevation could be an indicator of early disease.[23]

Cartilage oligomeric matrix protein (COMP) is a pentameric matrix protein in the thrombospondin family. It is found primarily in cartilage, but has also been identified in ligament, synovium, tendon, and meniscus.[28] Its function is not known, but it may have a role in chondrogenesis and the interaction of the chondrocyte

Table 116-1. Molecular markers of Osteoarthritis that can be Measured in Synovial Fluid.

Biomarker		
Type II Collagen		
	Procollagen Peptides	A
	Pyridinoline	C
	Alpha chains	C
	Telopeptides	C
Aggrecan		
	Chondroitin Sulfate (various epitopes)	A or C
	Keratan Sulfate	C
	Core Protein fragments	C
Type X Collagen		A
Fibronectin		A or C
	(V+C)- Fibronectin	A
Cartilage Oligomeric Matrix Protein (COMP)		C
Matrix Metalloproteinases		R
	MMP-1 (collagenase-1)	R
	MMP-2 (gelatinase)	R
	MMP-3 (stromelysin-1)	R
	MMP-9 (gelatinase)	R
	MMP-13 (collagenase-3)	R
Tissue Inhibitors of Metalloproteinases (TIMPs)		R
Interleukin-1, Interleukin-6		R

A = Anabolic Marker, C = Catabolic Marker, R = Marker related to regulation of cartilage turnover

Adapted from information in Todhunter and Lust[79] and Fox.[17]

with its surrounding matrix.[23] Increases in serum and synovial fluid COMP have been reported in human and canine patients with OA.[29-31] Another canine study found that COMP levels in the synovial fluid of stifles with OA secondary to cranial cruciate ligament insufficiency were not significantly elevated compared with synovial fluid from a control population, but that COMP was elevated in the contralateral (unaffected) stifles of these patients. Given the increased risk of cranial cruciate ligament injury in the contralateral stifle when one stifle is already affected, this elevation may indicate preclinical disease and COMP may be a marker of early cartilage injury.[23] However, within the joint, COMP is also secreted by the synovium and increased concentration of COMP may reflect synovitis. Additionally, owing to its presence in other tissues, serum elevation of COMP is not considered specific for cartilage degradation and individual variation is high; therefore, the utility of COMP as a solitary biomarker is limited.

Chondroitin sulfate is a glycosaminoglycan that is a major constituent of aggrecan. In early OA, newly synthesized aggrecan molecules contain chondroitin sulfate side chains with increased chain length and altered structure that are identifiable utilizing monoclonal antibodies.[32] Two epitopes (3B3(-) and 7D4) have been most thoroughly investigated, but significant difference exists in the timing of elevation in synovial fluid concentration of these epitopes between species. Multiple canine studies have demonstrated significant elevations in the concentration of synovial fluid chondroitin sulfate after experimental induction of OA. Significant increases in the 3B3(-) epitope of chondroitin sulfate have also been demonstrated in the synovial fluid from OA joints in humans.[17] Expression of 7D4 appears to be more prevalent in OA cartilage and synovial fluid from humans, monkeys, and guinea pigs with OA joints and was found to be more elevated in patients with acute injury and early osteoarthritis.[32] In another study, synovial fluid concentrations of 3B3(-), but not 7D4, were elevated in human patients with chronic knee OA.[33] Although the 3B3(-) form of chondroitin sulfate is absent in healthy canine articular cartilage, it has been identified in canine cartilage during early OA.[34,35] A longitudinal study in a canine model found that an increase in 7D4 concentration preceeded the rise in 3B3(-) concentration.[36] A correlation between 3B3(-) and 7D4 epitope concentrations in synovial fluid from a canine model of naturally occurring OA contradicted a study in humans that found that the synovial fluid concentrations of these two epitopes varied independently of each other.[32,37]

Keratan sulfate is a glycosaminoglycan that is a major constituent of aggrecan. Numerous studies with different models of induced and naturally occurring OA have produced a wide variation in results, with synovial fluid concentration of keratan sulfate rising significantly post-injury in some models, a lack of significant change, and even a significant decrease in keratan sulfate concentrations in others.[17]

Matrix metalloproteinases (MMPs) are a family of zinc-dependent endopeptidases. They and their inhibitors, tissue inhibitors of matrix metalloproteinases (TIMPs), play an important role in normal degradation of the extracellular matrix. Once activated, MMPs become susceptible to inhibition by TIMPs, which are secreted by chondrocytes and synoviocytes. Because MMPs appear to play a substantial role in OA, potential treatment strategies include regulation of their activity by control of gene expression and secretion, deactivation of pro-MMPs, and inhibition of active MMPs.[38] Most MMPs are present in articular tissues in an inactive form,[39] but during OA, MMPs are present in higher concentrations than the TIMPs and the latent forms of MMPs become activated.[40] Aggrecanases are members of the ADAMT (a disintegrin and metalloproteinase with thrombospondin motif) family. Several aggrecenases have been described, 6 of which have been associated with aggrecan core protein cleavage. Current thinking is that as many as 11 MMPs are responsible for normal articular cartilage matrix turnover, and the aggrecanases contribute to pathologic degradation.[41]

Stromelysin (MMP-3) degrades collagen II, IX, and X, proteoglycan, and fibronectin. This MMP is released from chondrocytes during OA in response to cytokine stimulation. Stromelysin concentrations have been demonstrated in a number of in vitro and in vivo studies to be elevated in the tissues and synovial fluid of OA joints in dogs, horses, and humans,[39,42-45] so that stromelysin concentration in articular cartilage and/or synovial fluid may be a biomarker for OA.[17] Collagenase (MMP-1) also degrades collagen II, IX, and X. Gelatinases (MMP-2 and MMP-9) were detected in the synovial fluid of healthy joints, while a canine study demonstrated elevated MMP-2 and MMP-9 activity in the synovial fluid of OA joints that paralleled the increase in MMP-9 activity seen in horses with OA.[40,46,47] Although molecular markers of osteoarthritis do not currently have direct clinical application, numerous substances are under investigation as potential biomarkers, and significant advances in understanding the molecular processes of OA have been made. Further identification and understanding of the OA process may ultimately allow for earlier diagnosis and treatment opportunities.

Genetics

Many developmental diseases in dogs are a result of a complex interaction between genetic susceptibility, nutrition, and other environmental factors. Polygenic modes of inheritance have been proposed for hip dysplasia, osteochondritis dissecans, and elbow dysplasia.[4] Osteoarthritis is a secondary disease process that occurs as a result of these joint abnormalities, but these developmental diseases result in variable degrees of OA in a given individual. Heritability of elbow dysplasia has been reported at 10% to 45%, and osteochondrosis of the shoulder joint has been estimated at 55% to 70% in various breeds of dogs. One study showed dogs with hip OA to be predisposed to elbow and stifle osteoarthritis.[48] For further information on the genetics of developmental and acquired orthopedic traits in dogs, see other reviews.[4,49]

Diagnostic Imaging

Radiography

In one study, radiographic evidence of DJD was evident in 90% of older cats evaluated as part of a diagnostic workup for other disease. Other studies of cats of varied ages have reported overall incidences of OA of 20% to 30%.[50] The elbow is the most commonly affected joint in cats.[16,50] In radiographic evaluation of human knee OA, within-observer reproducibility is greater than between observers, and osteophyte score, joint space narrowing, and bony contour are acceptably repeatable, but subchondral sclerosis and subchondral cyst scores suffer from poor reliability.[51] To meaningfully assess joint-space narrowing, a weight-bearing radiograph is required.[52] In assessment of progression of OA in canine stifles, effusion, osteophytosis, and intra-articular mineralization were found to be more reliable than assessment of subchondral sclerosis.[53]

Computed Tomography

When conventional radiography fails to demonstrate changes characteristic of OA, or fails to reveal the underlying etiology when OA is recognized, computerized tomography can be employed to help identify the underlying cause of lameness. Perhaps the most common use of this modality is to identify fragmented medial coronoid process of the elbow. Computed tomography is more sensitive than conventional radiography to early bone changes and three dimensional reconstructions can be useful in evaluating the extent of bone lesions.

Nuclear Scintigraphy

Nuclear Scintigraphy is most useful when the cause of lameness is unknown. A bone-seeking radionuclide compound, such as technecium-99m-labeled methylene diphosphonate, will be taken up in areas of increased bone and periarticular metabolic activity. Therefore, itreflects both the vascular supply to the region and the rate of mineralization as it is adsorbed to the mineralization front. Any process that disturbs the normal balance of bone production and resorption can produce an abnormality on a bone scan. A bone scan is a highly sensitive but relatively nonspecific diagnostic tool. When administered to an animal with a non-localized lameness, areas of increased activity aid in identifying the affected joint(s) and allow for more specific evaluation using conventional radiographic techniques, computerized tomography, or magnetic resonance imaging in order to further identify the underlying etiology.

Magnetic Resonance Imaging

Magnetic resonance imaging (MRI) is infrequently used as an imaging tool for clinical cases of joint disease in veterinary medicine. However, this modality may have its greatest potential use for the evaluation of subtle lesions and assessing cartilage thickness or damage as part of a clinical research protocol. MRI can detect subtle changes in cartilage structure and subchondral bone long before changes in the underlying bone or periarticular structures are detected by conventional radiographic methods. Well hydrated tissues are best imaged with MRI. Changes including cartilage thinning, surface irregularities, and increased signal intensity (called a bone bruise) in subchondral bone have been noted at 4 weeks post-injury in a canine experimental model of OA.[6]

Treatment

Osteoarthritis leads to decreased patient flexibility, increased joint stiffness, and pain; the resultant disuse atrophy of periarticular supporting muscle results in decreased overall strength. As a result, treatment goals include pain relief, reduction of any inflammatory component, improvement of joint function, maintenance of muscle mass, and if possible, preventing or minimizing progression of disease. If an underlying cause of the OA can be identified, treatment is aimed both at correction of the initiating cause and management of the subsequent degenerative cartilage changes.

Surgical management of OA is primarily aimed either at manipulation of joint congruency and stability (e.g., stabilization of a cruciate-deficient stifle or removal of a fragmented coronoid process) early in the disease process in an attempt to minimize progression of OA, or by salvage procedures in end-stage disease (total hip replacement, pancarpal arthrodesis) to reduce pain and improve overall limb function. Medical management of OA may be broadly conceptualized as having four main components: weight management, pharmacologic treatment with analgesics and anti-inflammatories, exercise modification/physical therapy, and slow-acting disease-modifying osteoarthritis agents (SDMOAs). Slow-acting, disease-modifying agents are also described as chondroprotective agents and are purported to have three primary effects: enhancement of chondrocyte and synoviocyte metabolism, inhibition of degradative enzymes within the synovial fluid and matrix, and inhibition of thrombus formation in the small blood vessels supplying the joint.[54]

Obesity is a significant risk factor for the development and progression of OA in people, and may be associated with increased stresses on weight-bearing joints or metabolic alterations.[55] Weight loss in dogs with OA has been demonstrated to have a profound positive effect on the clinical management of the disease.[55] In addition, it has been demonstrated that long-term limitation of caloric intake results in decreased radiographic prevalence and severity of OA in dogs.[48,56] Management recommendations to clients should include long-term efforts to keep patients as lean as possible to reduce force transmission through OA joints. More recently, nutritional supplements and commercial diets with specific ratios of omega-3 and omega-6 fatty acids have been introduced as components of management of the OA patient. By shifting the prostaglandin synthesis pathway from arachidonic acid metabolites to dihydroxyeicosapentanoeic acid metabolites, omega-3 fatty acids are thought to decrease inflammation and decrease the expression and activity of proteoglycan degrading enzymes.[57] The ideal dietary ratio of omega-6:omega-3 fatty acids for dogs is controversial but the current recommendation is between 10:1 and 5:1.[54]

Nonsteroidal Anti-inflammatory Drugs (NSAIDs)

Although the inflammation associated with OA is variable, NSAIDS are used to reduce pain and synovitis as a result of OA. Nonsteroidal anti-inflammatory drugs decrease prostaglandin synthesis by inhibition of cyclooxygenase (Figure 116-7). The two primary isoforms described as cyclooxygenase, COX-1 and COX-2, are simplistically described as the constitutive form and the inducible form, respectively. NSAIDs inhibit sensitization and stimulation of peripheral nociceptors and spinal cyclooxygenase activity. NSAIDs reportedly inhibit nitric oxide-induced apoptosis independent of cyclooxygenase activity. These signalling pathways involve nuclear-factor kappaB and caspase activation. COX-2 and PGE_2 production are affected by the non-COX mechanism.[58]

Nonsteroidal anti-inflammatory drugs can be divided into COX nonspecific, COX-2 preferential, and COX-2 specific. The COX nonspecific drugs include aspirin, phenylbutazone, ibuprofen, and naproxen. Aspirin (acetylsalicylic acid), a first generation NSAID, is a nonspecific COX inhibitor. It has adverse effects on the gastrointestinal tract, inhibits platelet aggregation, can cause renal failure in susceptible patients, and is used at an approximate dose of 1 adult aspirin (375 mg) per 60 lb body weight up to 3 times a day with a little food.

COX-2 preferential drugs are generally well tolerated by dogs, with fewer side effects reported. Their analgesic action is related to inhibition of spinal nociceptive transmission and attenuation of peripheral inflammation. They include carprofen (Rimadyl, Pfizer), which is approved for use in dogs at 2.2 mg/kg twice daily or 4 mg/kg once daily; etodolac (Etogesic, Fort Dodge), which is approved for use in dogs at 10 to15 mg/kg once daily; and meloxicam (Metacam, Merial/Boehringer Ingelheim) used at 0.2 mg/kg as an oral liquid suspension. Carprofen is generally considered to be either COX 2 preferential or nonselective. In cell culture, it has low COX-2 inhibition. It may have an alternative pathway for its analgesic activity. Peak plasma concentration is reached in 1 to 3 hours and plasma elimination half-life is 7 to 9 hours. Carprofen has good analgesic, antipyretic, and anti-inflammatory properties. Idiosyncratic hepatic toxicity has been reported, especially in Labrador retrievers. Minimal gastrointestinal toxicity has been observed in experimental studies. Carprofen probably has no negative impact on articular cartilage metabolism. In the cranial cruciate transaction model of OA in dogs, carprofen was given 4 weeks after induction of disease and continued for 8 weeks at 2.2 and 4.4 mk/kg bid. Carprofen reduced morphologic changes in articular cartilage and subchondral bone normally associated with OA.[59] Carprofen improves limb function in dogs based on both subjective and objective gait evaluation.

Etodolac reaches peak plasma concentration in 1 hour, with an elimination half life of 10 to 14 hours, and is generally considered COX-2 preferential but that is debated. It has been shown to improve hind limb function in dogs with hip OA.[60] Etodolac is reported to spare collagen synthesis by chondrocytes but data conflict on its effect on proteoglycan synthesis. It exhibits minimal gastrointestinal toxicity. Meloxicam exhibits peak plasma concentration at 8 hours and has an elimination half life of 23 hours. It performs comparably to carprofen in clinical trials for lameness in dogs with minimal side effects reported.[61] Derracoxib (Derramax, Novartis) is a COX-2 selective drug which reduced postoperative pain and lameness in dogs given at 1 to 2 mg/kg. Celecoxib (Celebrex) had a positive effect on hyaluronan and proteoglycan synthesis in human OA cartilage explants. Minimal side effects have been so far reported.

In an acute stifle synovitis model in dogs, butorphanol (0.2 mg/kg, IV), etodolac (17 mg/kg, PO), carprofen (4 mg/kg, PO), and meloxicam (0.2 mg/kg, PO) were compared. A Latin cross-over design and 3-week washout was followed. Treatments were given 3 hours after monosodium urate injections into the stifle joint. Ground reaction force (GRF), orthopedic exams, and C-reactive protein were measured.[62] The greatest improvement in vertical GRF was in the carprofen group. Etodolac had the fastest onset of action. Compared with butorphanol, only carprofen and etodolac had decreased stifle pain scores. There were fewer non-responders in the carprofen and meloxicam groups.

Leukotrienes can also be inhibited by combined cyclooxygenase/lipoxygenase inhibitors (Figure 116-7). Leukotriene B_4, for example, induces chemotaxis, aggregation, degranulation, and increased cytokine production by leukocytes, hyperalgesia, and bone resorption. Other leukotrienes affect smooth muscle function, mucus secretion, vascular permeability, and airway inflammation. Cysteinyl leukotrienes may enhance gastric mucosal injury by causing local vasoconstriction. Prostaglandins and leukotrienes have complementary effects but lipoxins can inhibit the inflammatory effects of leukotrienes. Tepoxalin (Zubrin, Schering Plough) inhibits both COX activity and lipoxygenase 5,

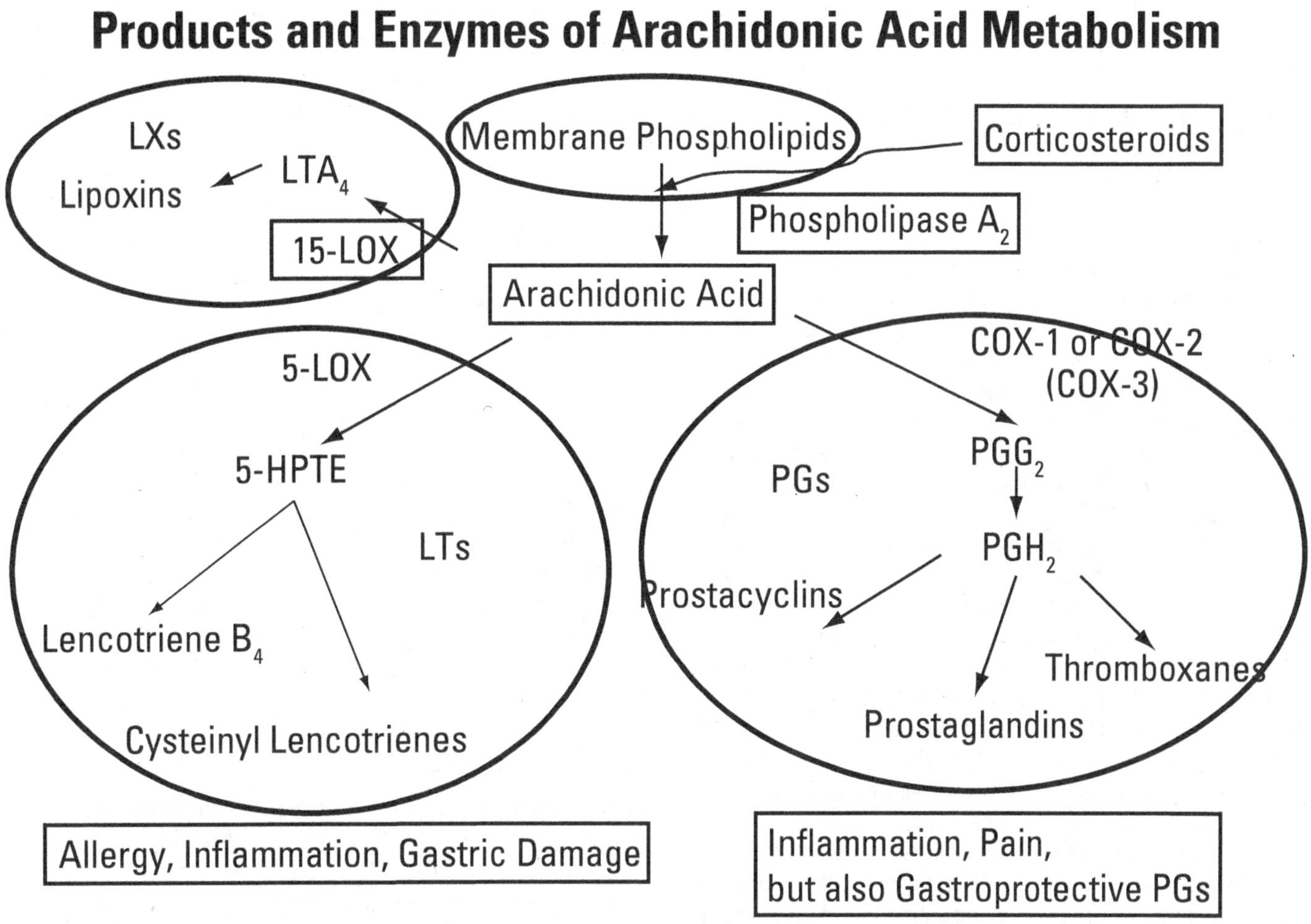

Figure 116-7. Products and enzymes of arachidonic acid metabolism.

the activity of which results in leukotriene synthesis. It has potent anti-inflammatory activity with excellent gastric tolerance. The tables are rapidly disintegrating. A similar drug used in human medicine called licofelone given for 8 weeks beginning the day after surgery in a model of OA induced by cranial cruciate ligament transaction prevented abnormal subchondral bone cell metabolism, reduced PGE2 production in synovial fluid, inhibited collagenase 1 production in articular cartilage, interleukin 1-β, and leukotriene B_4 in synovial membrane, and reduced chondrocyte cell death (decreased caspase 3 activity) probably owing to lower nitric oxide and PGE_2.

Whether NSAIDs can affect the progression of OA is an open question. Prostaglandin inhibition by NSAIDS may have a negative effect on chondrocytes and the cartilage matrix.[63] The detrimental effects of NSAIDs on chondrocytes are partly mediated by inhibition of glycosyltransferase activity, uncoupling of mitochondrial oxidative phosphorylation, activation of cAMP-dependent kinase A, and disruption of protein interactions at the cell surface. The majority of positive effects are due to suppression of inflammation characterized by inhibition of COX-2, which is highly expressed in OA tissues, the inhibitory effects on IL-1 production or IL-1 receptor expression, decreased PGE_2 production, reduced inducible nitric oxide synthase (iNOS) synthesis by interleukin-1, and decreased nitric oxide. Nitric oxide enhances MMP activity, decreases proteoglycan synthesis, and inhibits interleukin 1β receptor antagonists. Inhibition of matrix metalloproteinase activity will encourage maintenance of the extracellular matrix and inhibit chondrocyte apoptosis, a critical feature of OA progression.

Slow-Acting Disease-Modifying Osteoarthritis Agents

Disease-modifying agents of OA comprise a large, diverse group of compounds, many of which are poorly characterized as to their efficacy and/or mechanism of action, and their production and administration are poorly regulated, with varying degrees of quality control. Disease-modifying OA agents are also commonly referred to as "nutraceuticals"; however, the only thing shared in common is that they are neither foods nor drugs recognized by the FDA, and as such undergo no pre-market approval process.[64] The only FDA-approved SDMOA in dogs is injectable Adequan (Luitpold Pharmaceuticals), which is a polysulfated glycosaminoglycan (PSGAG). Because it is a heparin analogue, injectible PSGAG has the potential to affect coagulation. In cats, injectable PSGAG has been demonstrated to produce a prolongation in the activated partial thromboplastin time and should be avoided in animals with bleeding disorders or on concurrent NSAIDs that exhibit antithromboxane effects.[65] The proposed mechanisms of action include inhibition of serine proteases, PGE_2, elastase, stromelysin, MMPs, and hyaluronidases.[66] In one study, dogs treated with an injectable PSGAG from a young age and studied until skeletal maturity had better hip conformation and fewer joint abnormalities than did controls.[67] Pentosan polysulfate is a polysaccharide sulfate ester and is thought to modify disease progression by its antithrombotic and fibrinolytic effects in addition to improving subchondral and synovial membrane blood flow.[4,68] However, a clinical study evaluating the effects of pentosan polysulfate failed to demonstrate a significant clinical improvement over control in the postoperative progression of OA after surgical stabilization of canine stifles with cranial cruciate ligament insufficiency.[68] Glucosamine salt supplements are commonly found in combination products with chondroitin sulfate and manganese ascorbate. Glucosamine is an amino sugar that is a precursor to matrix glycosaminoglycans.[54] Chondroitin sulfate is a glycosaminoglycan found naturally within the extracellular matrix of articular cartilage. It has been proposed that glucosamine supplementation benefits OA articular cartilage by promoting formation and repair of cartilage, whereas chondroitin sulfate is thought to promote water retention and elasticity in cartilage as well as to inhibit degradative enzymes. Clinical and experimental studies support the use of glucosamine-chondroitin-manganese combinations or as individual components.[54] Oral glucosamine-chondroitin sulfate formulations may be obtained over the counter. However, clients should be warned about significant variations among measured concentrations and label claims in both glucosamine and chondroitin sulfate in products on the market.[69,70] In addition, differences in the bioavailability of these substances may be significant between formulations and between species. Oral bioavailability of glucosamine hydrochloride in humans is 84%, but the bioavailability of the sulfate salt is only 47%.[64] The oral bioavailability of glucosamine in dogs was reported to be 10%.[71] The oral bioavailaibility of chondroitin sulfate varies inversely with molecular weight, and molecules of chondroitin sulfate with a molecular weight of 17000 have the most favorable permeability coefficient.[64] In addition to concerns about variations in formulation and bioavailability, accurate pharmacokinetic and pharmacodynamic information for most products is lacking, as are studies on safety and efficacy. Efficacy in veterinary patients is particularly difficult to assess; however, the placebo effect in animals is likely equal or greater than the 30% to 40% placebo effect that is reported in human studies evaluating pain. Recently, it was shown that glucosumine and chondroitin sulfate regulate expression of matrix-degrading enzymes and the inhibitors at the transcriptional level.[72] Products containing glucosamine and chondroitin sulfate have been shown to cause significant decreases in red blood cell and platelet indices in dogs and cats, but these differences stay within clinically normal ranges and are unlikely to be clinically relevant.[73,74]

The use of other nutritional supplements such as elk velvet antler, green-lipped mussels, type-II collagen, and milk protein concentrate have been preliminarily described in veterinary patients for the treatment of OA; however, further evaluation is needed before these substances can be recommended.[75-78] Hyaluronan, methylsulfonylmethane, dimethylsulfoxide, and doxycycline have all been used to treat osteoarthritis, but supporting evidence of their success is lacking.

References

1. Johnston SA: Osteoarthritis. Joint anatomy, physiology, and pathobiology. Vet Clin North Am Small Anim Pract 27:699-723, 1997.

2. Evans H: Miller's Anatomy of the Dog, 3rd ed, 1993.

3. Poole CA, Flint MH, Beaumont BW: Chondrons in cartilage: ultrastructural analysis of the pericellular microenvironment in adult human

articular cartilages. J Orthop Res 5:509-522, 1987.

4. Todhunter RJ, Johnston S: Osteoarthritis. Slatter's Small Animal Surgery, 2003, pp. 2208-2245.

5. Eyre DR: Collagens and cartilage matrix homeostasis. Clin Orthop Relat Res 427:S118-122, 2004

6. Cook.: Proceedings of Veterinary Orthopedic Society, 2005; 41.

7. Todhunter RJ, Yeh LA, Sheldon A, et al: Effects of stromelysin activity on proteoglycan degradation of canine articular cartilage explants. Am J Vet Res 56:1241-1247, 1995.

8. Ghosh P, Smith M: The role of cartilage-derived antigens, pro-coagulant activity and fibrinolysis in the pathogenesis of osteoarthritis. Med Hypotheses 41:190-194, 1993.

9. Mankin HJ, Lippiello L: Biochemical and metabolic abnormalities in articular cartilage from osteo-arthritic human hips. J Bone Joint Surg Am 52:424-434, 1970.

10. Setton LA, Zhu W, Mow VC: The biphasic poroviscoelastic behavior of articular cartilage: role of the surface zone in governing the compressive behavior. J Biomech 26:581-592, 1993.

11. Chalmers HJ, Dykes NL, Lust G, et al: Assessment of bone mineral density of the femoral head in dogs with early osteoarthritis. AJVR 67:796, 2006

12. Manicourt DH, Altman RD, Williams JM, et al: Treatment with calcitonin suppresses the responses of bone, cartilage, and synovium in the early stages of canine experimental osteoarthritis and significantly reduces the severity of the cartilage lesions. Arthritis Rheum 42:1159-1167, 1999.

13. Behets C, Williams JM, Chappard D, et al: Effects of calcitonin on subchondral trabecular bone changes and on osteoarthritic cartilage lesions after acute anterior cruciate ligament deficiency. J Bone Miner Res 19:1821-1826, 2004.

14. Ellison RS: The cytologic examination of synovial fluid. Semin Vet Med Surg (Small Anim) 3:133-139, 1988.

15. Fernandez FR, GC, Lipowitz AJ, et al: Synovial fluid analysis: preparation of smears for cytologic examination of canine synovial fluid. JAAHA 727-734, 1983.

16. Pacchiana PD, Gilley RS, Wallace LJ, et al: Absolute and relative cell counts for synovial fluid from clinically normal shoulder and stifle joints in cats. J Am Vet Med Assoc 225:1866-1870, 2004.

17. Fox DB, Cook JL: Synovial fluid markers of osteoarthritis in dogs. J Am Vet Med Assoc 219:756-761, 2001.

18. Bruyere O, Collette JH, Ethgen O, et al: Biochemical markers of bone and cartilage remodeling in prediction of longterm progression of knee osteoarthritis. J Rheumatol 30:1043-1050, 2003.

19. Otterness IG, Swindell AC, Zimmerer RO, et al: An analysis of 14 molecular markers for monitoring osteoarthritis: segregation of the markers into clusters and distinguishing osteoarthritis at baseline. Osteoarthr Cartilage 8:180-185, 2000.

20. Shiozawa K, Hino K, Shiozawa S: Alternatively spliced EDA-containing fibronectin in synovial fluid as a predictor of rheumatoid joint destruction. Rheumatology (Oxford) 40:739-742, 2001.

21. Claudepierre P, Allanore Y, Belec L, et al: Increased Ed-B fibronectin plasma levels in spondyloarthropathies: comparison with rheumatoid arthritis patients and a healthy population. Rheumatology (Oxford) 38:1099-1103, 1999.

22. Burton-Wurster N, Lust G: Deposition of fibronectin in articular cartilage of canine osteoarthritic joints. Am J Vet Res 46:2542-2545, 1985.

23. Steffey MA, Miura N, Todhunter RJ, et al: The potential and limitations of cartilage-specific (V+C)(-) fibronectin and cartilage oligomeric matrix protein as osteoarthritis biomarkers in canine synovial fluid. Osteoarthritis Cartilage 12:818-825, 2004.

24. Carnemolla B, Cutolo M, Castellani P, et al: Characterization of synovial fluid fibronectin from patients with rheumatic inflammatory diseases and healthy subjects. Arthritis Rheum 27:913-921, 1984.

25. Burton-Wurster N, Borden C, Lust G, et al: Expression of the (V+C)-fibronectin isoform is tightly linked to the presence of a cartilaginous matrix. Matrix Biol 17:193-203, 1998.

26. MacLeod JN, Burton-Wurster N, Gu DN, et al: Fibronectin mRNA splice variant in articular cartilage lacks bases encoding the V, III-15, and I-10 protein segments. J Biol Chem 271:18954-18960, 1996.

27. Burton-Wurster N, Chen H, Gendelman R, et al: Specific immunological detection of the (V+C)(-) fibronectin isoform. Matrix Biol 21:393-398, 2002.

28. Muller G, Michel A, Altenburg E: COMP (cartilage oligomeric matrix protein) is synthesized in ligament, tendon, meniscus, and articular cartilage. Connect Tissue Res 39:233-244, 1998.

29. Clark AG, Jordan JM, Vilim V, et al: Serum cartilage oligomeric matrix protein reflects osteoarthritis presence and severity: The Johnston County Osteoarthritis Project. Arthritis Rheum 42:2356-2364, 1999.

30. Misumi K, Vilim V, Carter SD, et al: Concentrations of cartilage oligomeric matrix protein in dogs with naturally developing and experimentally induced arthropathy. Am J Vet Res 63:598-603, 2002.

31. Neidhart M, Hauser N, Paulsson M, et al: Small fragments of cartilage oligomeric matrix protein in synovial fluid and serum as markers for cartilage degradation. Br J Rheumatol 36:1151-1160, 1997.

32. Johnson KA, Hay CW, Chu Q, et al: Cartilage-derived biomarkers of osteoarthritis in synovial fluid of dogs with naturally acquired rupture of the cranial cruciate ligament. Am J Vet Res 63:775-781, 2002.

33. Belcher C, Yaqub R, Fawthrop F, et al: Synovial fluid chondroitin and keratan sulphate epitopes, glycosaminoglycans, and hyaluronan in arthritic and normal knees. Ann Rheum Dis 56:299-307, 1997.

34. Ratcliffe A, Shurety W, Caterson B: The quantitation of a native chondroitin sulfate epitope in synovial fluid lavages and articular cartilage from canine experimental osteoarthritis and disuse atrophy. Arthritis Rheum 36:543-551, 1993.

35. Visco DM, Johnstone B, Hill MA, et al: Immunohistochemical analysis of 3-B-(-) and 7-D-4 epitope expression in canine osteoarthritis. Arthritis Rheum 36:1718-1725, 1993.

36. Johnson KA, Hart RC, Chu Q, et al: Concentrations of chondroitin sulfate epitopes 3B3 and 7D4 in synovial fluid after intra-articular and extracapsular reconstruction of the cranial cruciate ligament in dogs. Am J Vet Res 62:581-587, 2001.

37. Hazell PK, Dent C, Fairclough JA, et al: Changes in glycosaminoglycan epitope levels in knee joint fluid following injury. Arthritis Rheum 38:953-959, 1995.

38. Kuroki K, Cook JL, Kreeger JM: Effects of tissue inhibitor of metalloproteinases on canine chondrocytes cultured in vitro with tumor necrosis factor-alpha. Am J Vet Res 65:1611-1615, 2004.

39. Brama PA, TeKoppele JM, Beekman B, et al: Influence of development and joint pathology on stromelysin enzyme activity in equine synovial fluid. Ann Rheum Dis 59:155-157, 2000.

40. Trumble TN, Trotter GW, Oxford JR, et al: Synovial fluid gelatinase concentrations and matrix metalloproteinase and cytokine expression in naturally occurring joint disease in horses. Am J Vet Res 62:1467-1477, 2001.

41. Sandy JD: A contentious issue finds some clarity: on the independent and complementary roles of aggrecanase activity and MMP activity in human joint aggrecanolysis. Osteoarthritis Cartilage 14:95-100, 2006.

42. Lohmander LS, Hoerrner LA, Lark MW: Metalloproteinases, tissue inhibitor, and proteoglycan fragments in knee synovial fluid in human osteoarthritis. Arthritis Rheum 36:181-189, 1993.

43. Cook JL, Anderson CC, Kreeger JM, et al: Effects of human recom-

binant interleukin-1beta on canine articular chondrocytes in three-dimensional culture. Am J Vet Res 61:766-770, 2000.

44. Spreng D, Sigrist N, Busato A, et al: Stromelysin activity in canine cranial cruciate ligament rupture. Vet Comp Orthop Traumatol 12:159-165, 1999.

45. Panula HE, Lohmander LS, Ronkko S, et al: Elevated levels of synovial fluid PLA2, stromelysin (MMP-3) and TIMP in early osteoarthrosis after tibial valgus osteotomy in young beagle dogs. Acta Orthop Scand 69:152-158, 1998.

46. Volk SW, Kapatkin AS, Haskins ME, et al: Gelatinase activity in synovial fluid and synovium obtained from healthy and osteoarthritic joints of dogs. Am J Vet Res 64:1225-1233, 2003.

47. Clegg PD, Burke RM, Coughlan AR, et al: Characterisation of equine matrix metalloproteinase 2 and 9; and identification of the cellular sources of these enzymes in joints. Equine Vet J 29:335-342, 1997.

48. Kealy RD, Lawler DF, Ballam JM, et al: Evaluation of the effect of limited food consumption on radiographic evidence of osteoarthritis in dogs. J Am Vet Med Assoc 217:1678-1680, 2000.

49. Breur G, et al: Genetics of hip dysplasia and other orthopedic traits. *In* Ruvinsky and Sampson's The Genetics of the Dog. Oxford: CABI Publishing, 2001, p. 267.

50. Hardie EM: Management of osteoarthritis in cats. Vet Clin North Am Small Anim Pract 27:945-953, 1997.

51. Cooper C, Cushnaghan J, Kirwan JR, et al: Radiographic assessment of the knee joint in osteoarthritis. Ann Rheum Dis 51:80-82, 1992.

52. Morgan JP: Radiological pathology and diagnosis of degenerative joint disease in the stifle joint of the dog. J Small Anim Pract 10:541-544, 1969.

53. Innes JF, Costello M, Barr FJ, et al: Radiographic progression of osteoarthritis of the canine stifle joint: a prospective study. Vet Radiol Ultrasound 45:143-148, 2004.

54. Beale BS: Use of nutraceuticals and chondroprotectants in osteoarthritic dogs and cats. Vet Clin North Am Small Anim Pract 34:271-289, viii, 2004.

55. Impellizeri JA, Tetrick MA, Muir P: Effect of weight reduction on clinical signs of lameness in dogs with hip osteoarthritis. J Am Vet Med Assoc 216:1089-1091, 2000.

56. Kealy RD, Lawler DF, Ballam JM, et al: Five-year longitudinal study on limited food consumption and development of osteoarthritis in coxofemoral joints of dogs. J Am Vet Med Assoc 210:222-225, 1997.

57. Curtis CL, Hughes CE, Flannery CR, et al: n-3 Fatty acids specifically modulate catabolic factors involved in articular cartilage degradation. J Biol Chem 275:721-724, 2000.

58. Yoon JB, Kim SJ, Hwang SG, et al: Non-steroidal anti-inflammatory drugs inhibit nitric oxide-induced apoptosis and dedifferentiation of articular chondrocytes independent of cyclooxygenase activity. J Biol Chem 278:15319-15325, 2003.

59. Pelletier JP, Lajeunesse D, Jovanovic DV, et al: Carprofen simultaneously reduces progression of morphological changes in cartilage and subchondral bone in experimental dog osteoarthritis. J Rheumatol 27:2893-2902, 2000.

60. Budsberg SC, Johnston SA, Schwarz PD, et al: Efficacy of etodolac for the treatment of osteoarthritis of the hip joints in dogs. J Am Vet Med Assoc 214:206-210, 1999.

61. Cross AR, Budsberg SC, Keefe TJ: Kinetic gait analysis assessment of meloxicam efficacy in a sodium urate-induced synovitis model in dogs. Am J Vet Res 58:626-631, 1997.

62. Borer LR, Peel JE, Seewald W, et al: Effect of carprofen, etodolac, meloxicam, or butorphanol in dogs with induced acute synovitis. Am J Vet Res 64:1429-1437, 2003.

63. McLaughlin R: Management of chronic osteoarthritic pain. Vet Clin North Am Small Anim Pract 30:933-949, ix, 2000.

64. Boothe DM: Balancing fact and fiction of novel ingredients: definitions, regulations and evaluation. Vet Clin North Am Small Anim Pract 34:7-38, 2004.

65. de Haan JJ, Goring RL, Beale BS: Evaluation of polysulfated glycosaminoglycan for the treatment of hip dysplasia in dogs. Vet Surg 23:177-181, 1994.

66. Todhunter RJ, Lust G: Polysulfated glycosaminoglycan in the treatment of osteoarthritis. J Am Vet Med Assoc 204:1245-1251, 1994.

67. Lust G, Williams AJ, Burton-Wurster N, et al: Effects of intramuscular administration of glycosaminoglycan polysulfates on signs of incipient hip dysplasia in growing pups. Am J Vet Res 53:1836-1843, 1992.

68. Budsberg S: Proceedings of Veterinary Orthopedic Society Abstract, March 2005.

69. Adabowale A, Cox DS, Liang Z, et al: Analysis of glucosamine and chondrotin sulfate content in marketed products and the caco-2 permeability of chondroitin sulfate raw materials. Am Nutraceut Assoc :37-44, 2000.

70. Russell AS, Aghazadeh-Habashi A, Jamali F: Active ingredient consistency of commercially available glucosamine sulfate products. J Rheumatol 29:2407-2409, 2002.

71. Adebowale A, Du J, Liang Z, et al: The bioavailability and pharmacokinetics of glucosamine hydrochloride and low molecular weight chondroitin sulfate after single and multiple doses to beagle dogs. Biopharm Drug Dispos 23:217-225, 2002.

72. Chan PS, Caron JP, Orth MW: Effect of glucosamine and chondroitin sulfate on regulation of gene expression of proteolytic enzymes and their inhibitors in interleukin-1-challenged bovine articular cartilage explants. Am J Vet Res 66:1870-1876, 2005.

73. McNamara PS, Barr SC, Erb HN: Hematologic, hemostatic, and biochemical effects in dogs receiving an oral chondroprotective agent for thirty days. Am J Vet Res 57:1390-1394, 1996.

74. McNamara PS, Barr SC, Erb HN, Barlow LL: Hematologic, hemostatic, and biochemical effects in cats receiving an oral chondroprotective agent for thirty days. Vet Ther 1:108-117, 2000

75. Moreau M, Dupuis J, Bonneau NH, et al: Clinical evaluation of a powder of quality elk velvet antler for the treatment of osteoarthrosis in dogs. Can Vet J 45:133-139, 2004.

76. Deparle LA, Gupta RC, Canerdy TD, et al: Efficacy and safety of glycosylated undenatured type-II collagen (UC-II) in therapy of arthritic dogs. J Vet Pharmacol Ther 28:385-390, 2005.

77. Gingerich DA, Strobel JD: Use of client-specific outcome measures to assess treatment effects in geriatric, arthritic dogs: controlled clinical evaluation of a nutraceutical. Vet Ther 4:56-66, 2003.

78. Bui LM, Bierer TL: Influence of green lipped mussels *(Perna canaliculus)* in alleviating signs of arthritis in dogs. Vet Ther 4:397-407, 2003.

79. Todhunter RJ, Lust G: Osteoarthritis. *In.* Textbook of Small Animal Surgery. Slatter D (ed). Philadelphia:WB Saunders, 2003.

Chapter 117

Immune Mediated Polyarthritis

Autumn P. Davidson

Immune-mediated polyarthritis (IMPA) is a noninfectious form of inflammatory arthropathy in the dog and cat. IMPA is characterized by inflammation of the synovial membranes reflected by inflammatory cell infiltrate in the synovial fluid and accompanied by systemic signs of illness. Classically these include lethargy, arthralgia, and fever. Accompanying signs of systemic illness can be subtle and vague, making the diagnosis elusive. Polyarticular involvement is reportedly more common than monarticular. Distal joints have been suggested to be more frequently affected; however, proximal joint synovitis is more challenging clinically to document, and may be overlooked.[1-9]

Categorization of IMPA

IMPA is commonly categorized as nonerosive, which is nondeforming and usually proliferative, and erosive, in which a progressive destructive deformation of joints occurs. Nonerosive IMPA occurs more commonly than erosive disease in both the dog and cat. Nonerosive canine IMPA has been further classified into subtypes based on the identification of associated contributory or causative disorders. These subtypes include type I, or idiopathic (no identifiable associated factors); type II, or reactive (associated with systemic infectious or inflammatory disease, most commonly of the respiratory, urinary, and reproductive systems, as well as of the eye and the skin); type III, or enteropathic (associated with gastrointestinal or hepatic disease); and type IV, or paraneoplastic (associated with neoplasia distant from the joints, or with myeloproliferative disease). Additionally, the nonerosive IMPA category includes arthropathy associated with systemic lupus erythematosis (SLE), the polyarthritis/polymyositis syndrome, the polyarthritis/meningitis syndrome, polyarteritis nodosa, Akita juvenile onset polyarthritis, the Shar-Pei fever syndrome, and that associated temporally with the administration of drugs or vaccination.[1-9]

Canine erosive IMPA is characterized by a progressive, refractory, and protracted joint destruction most pronounced in the distal joints. Canine erosive IMPA has been categorized into rheumatoid-like arthritis, idiopathic erosive polyarthritis, and Greyhound polyarthritis.[1-9]

Feline IMPA is classified as progressive polyarthritis (PPA) and has a nonerosive proliferative form and an erosive destructive form. Both generally cause serious systemic illness. The disease most commonly affects young (1 to 5 years of age) male cats and can be associated with feline syncytium-forming viral infection and its associated chronic antigenic stimulation.[1-9]

Pathogenesis

Primary nonerosive polyarticular arthritis, type I, is the most common form of IMPA reported in the dog. Nonerosive types II, III, and IV IMPA are less common. Identification of concurrent significant medical conditions is important for determining prognosis and in therapeutic decision making. Treatment of type I IMPA is directed at immunosuppression and its associated clinical scenarios (opportunistic infection, myelosuppression, and individual side effects of immunosupressant drugs). Treatment of types II, III, and IV IMPA is specifically directed at the associated systemic disorder in anticipation that joint inflammation will improve once the primary disorder is effectively treated or resolves with time.[1-9] Many type II polyarthridities associated with an infectious disease (i.e., coccidioidomycosis) are actually a granulomatous synovitis ("desert rheumatism") or vasculitis (ehrlichiosis, Rocky Mountain spotted fever (RMSF), Lyme disease) rather than a direct extension of the infectious organism into the synovium.[10] Some forms of nonerosive IMPA have been reported to have an underlying genetic predisposition associated with certain histocompatibilty genotypes.[1] Resolution of synovitis in types II to IV IMPA can be delayed when compared with that in type I and is dependent on the degree to which the contributory disorder is resolved.

The pathogenesis of erosive IMPA is better understood than its etiology. As a consequence of either defective immunoregulation (failure of self tolerance) or production of an immunogenic IgG-antigen molecule, the pathogenic autoantibody rheumatoid factor (RF) is formed. Plasma cells and activated B lymphocytes produce RF which circulates into synovial fluid. The synovium functions as a phagocytic tissue; as a consequence, immune complex ingestion occurs, triggering the activation and proliferation of synoviocytes. Activated synoviocytes release inflammatory mediators and enzymes (interleukin 1, collagenases, peptidases, and prostaglandin E_2). Osteoclasts are activated, resorbing subchondral bone. Subchondral bone cysts form as a consequence of this osteolysis. Intraarticular formation of granulation tissue arising from the inflamed synovium forms a pannus. Lymphocytes, plasma cells, neutrophils, and proliferating activated synoviocytes compose the pannus. Fibroblast proliferation promotes fibrosis with scarring and contracture. Joint deformation results.[1-4,11]

Clinical Presentation

IMPA should be part of the differential list for any dog or cat with fever of unknown origin or inexplicable lethargy. Arthralgia can be subtle or obvious, ranging from a simple reluctance to move to a peculiar, stilted, and crouching gait indicative of pain in numerous joints. Fever is common, generally in the range of 103.5 to 104.5° F. Palpation of joints can elicit pain, and the joints can feel effusive and warm, especially later in the course of the disease. With chronicity, the joint capsule may become thickened. Arthralgia can be misinterpreted clinically as myalgia, neuralgia, abdominal discomfort, or even neuropathic or myopathic disorders. Anorexia is variably present, and has been reported to be a poor prognostic sign.[3] Atypical house soiling can occur if the animal is reluctant to move outdoors or to a litter box for defecation or urination. Altered disposition, even aggression, can occur as a result of marked pain. The arthropathic signs of types II to IV IMPA can be completely masked by those of the primary, associated disorder. Incomplete response to therapy for the primary disorders associated with types II to IV IMPA should prompt evaluation of the joints for inflammatory changes. Alternatively, a poor response to immunosuppression for suspected type I IMPA should prompt consideration that the condition could be type II to IV, and clinical evaluation for associated disorders should be pursued.

Some generalizations exist. Type I IMPA is most commonly but not exclusively diagnosed in dogs less than 6 years of age, of either gender. A breed predilection may exist in German shepherds, Doberman pinschers, collies, spaniels, retrievers, terriers, and poodles. Polyarthritis associated with SLE is reported more commonly in German shepherds, collies, Shetland sheepdogs, beagles, and poodles, of any age. Females are more commonly affected.[12,13] Atypical cases of cranial cruciate ligament rupture (young, otherwise fit individuals of large breeds) can belong to a subclass of dogs with plasmacytic-lymphocytic synovitis/tendonitis.[7] Young (less than 3 years), large-breed dogs are more commonly affected with plasmacytic-lymphocyticsynovitis/tendonitis, most frequently diagnosed in the stifle and associated with damage (often bilateral) to the cranial cruciate ligament (ACL). Acute lameness associated with rupture of the ACL occurs and presents as a sudden worsening of lameness and reluctance to ambulate in an individual otherwise successfully under therapy for IMPA. Drug-associated polyarthritis, a vasculitide, has been reported to be associated with Doberman pinschers and Labrador retrievers.[14,15] Vaccine-associated IMPA is suspected clinically if the syndrome occurs within 3 to 4 weeks of vaccination.[7]

Erosive IMPA in the dog typically affects young to middle-aged members of toy and small breeds. A semierosive polyarthritis of greyhounds has been reported, generally in dogs between 3 and 30 months of age. Feline chronic progressive polyarthritis typically affects male cats from 1 to 5 years of age.[1-4]

Diagnostics

Evaluation of veterinary patients with unexplained lethargy, arthralgia, or fever should include arthrocentesis for cytologic evaluation of synovial fluid. Arthrocentesis can be performed in most medium to large dogs with minimal sedation/analgesia. Small dogs and cats usually require sedation or anesthesia to obtain synovial fluid samples without iatrogenic hemorrhage secondary to inadvertent trauma to the synovium during collection. Synovial fluid contaminated with hemorrhage markedly limits conclusive cytology.[8]

Arthrocentesis should be performed on a minimum of four joints. Usually the carpi, stifles, tarsi, and elbows are preferred sites for synovial fluid collection. The site of centesis should be clipped and prepared with aseptic technique. Carpal arthrocentesis is generally performed with a 25-gauge needle and 3-ml syringe. Fluid is aspirated from the joint space between the distal medial radius and the radial carpal bone joint, approached medially (Figure 117-1). Tarsal arthrocentesis is usually performed with a 22-gauge needle and 3-ml syringe, aspirating fluid from the joint space between the fibula and the calcaneus bone of the tarsus, approached laterally (Figure 117-2). Stifle arthrocentesis usually requires a longer needle to penetrate the patellar fat pad; a 20-gauge needle and a 3-ml syringe are typically used, aspirating the joint space between the lateral femoral epicondyle and the lateral tibial intercondylar area (Figure 117-3). Elbow arthrocentesis is technically more difficult. A 22-gauge needle and a 3-ml syringe are used to aspirate the joint space between the radial articular fovea and the ulnar lateral coronoid process (Figure 117-4). Synovial fluid should be immediately evaluated for color and clarity, as well as viscosity. Normal synovial fluid is clear, with viscosity producing a strand when dabbed with a gloved finger or needle. Abnormal synovial fluid is opaque to hemorrhagic with watery consistency.[8,11]

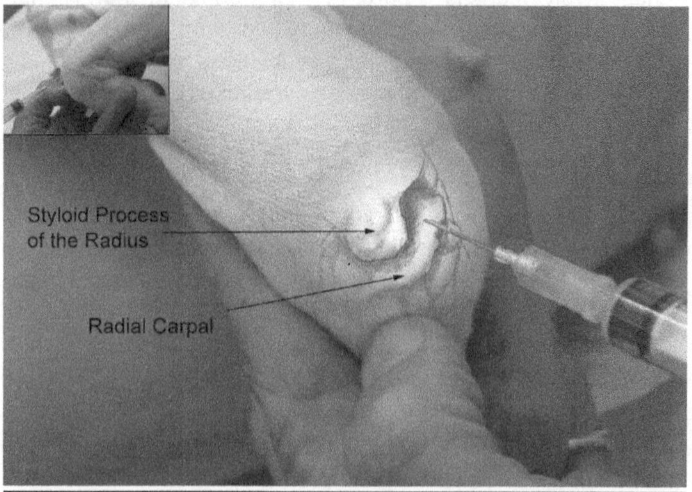

Figure 117-1. Arthrocentesis of the medial proximal radiocarpal joint. (Courtesy of Alexander J. Frederick, University of California School of Veterinary Medicine, Class of 2009.)

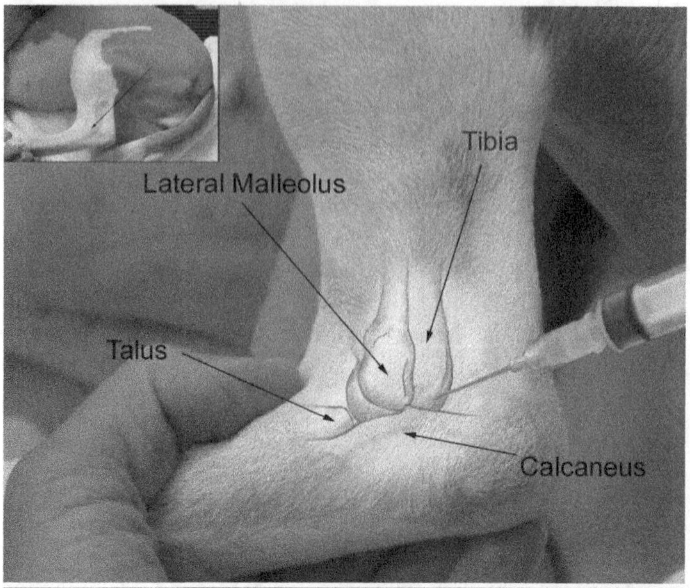

Figure 117-2. Arthrocentesis of the lateral tarsal joint (fibula-calcaneous). (Courtesy of Alexander J. Frederick, University of California School of Veterinary Medicine, Class of 2009.)

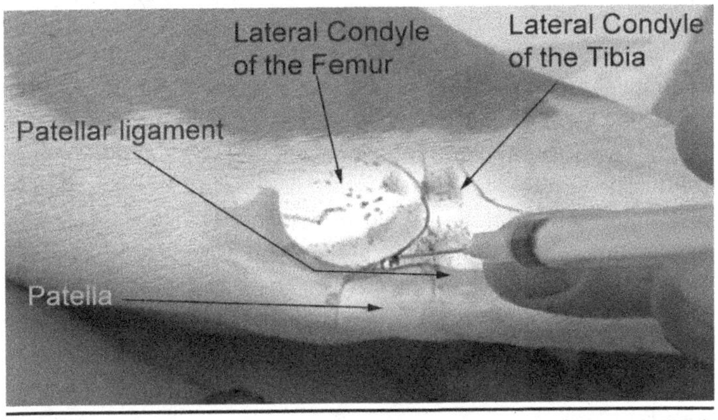

Figure 117-3. Arthrocentesis of the lateral stifle joint (femoral-tibial). (Courtesy of Alexander J. Frederick, University of California School of Veterinary Medicine, Class of 2009.)

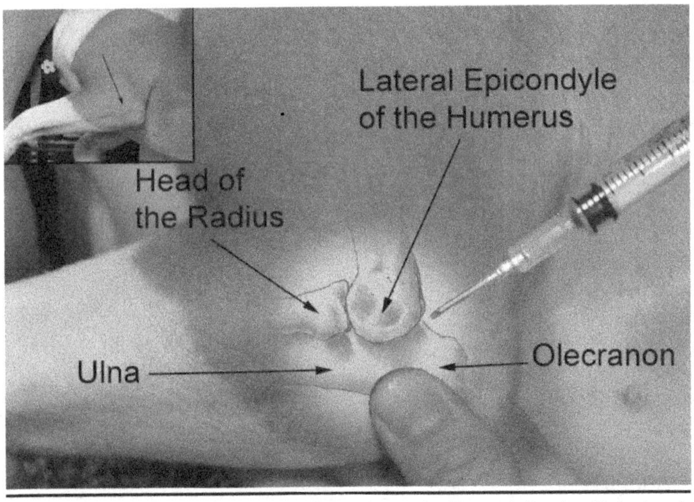

Figure 117-4. Arthrocentesis of the lateral elbow joint (radial-ulnar). (Courtesy of Alexander J. Frederick, University of California School of Veterinary Medicine, Class of 2009.)

Cytology of synovial fluid can be performed in the clinical setting or submitted to a commercial or academic laboratory for evaluation. Normal synovial fluid is poorly cellular (< 2500 nucleated cells/ml). The majority (> 90%) of cells in normal synovial fluid are large and small mononuclears. Synovitis associated with IMPA is characterized by suppurative cytology, with more than 5000 cells/ml, and with neutrophils accounting for more than 10 to 25% of the total cell count. The white blood cell count of synovial fluid can be estimated by counting the number of cells per high dry field and multiplying by 1000. Synovial fluid contaminated iatrogenically with hemorrhage from a traumatic arthrocentesis will have a white blood cell differential similar to peripheral blood, and synovial neutrophilia cannot be readily determined.[8,16]

Careful history-taking and a thorough review of physical examination findings can assist in the characterization of IMPA. Once inflammatory synovitis has been identified, collection of the minimum data base (complete hemogram, serum chemistries, urinalysis with culture) should be accompanied by specific, appropriate diagnostics to identify contributory and concurrent significant disease. Because immunosuppression is the goal of therapy for type I IMPA, prior evaluation for concurrent infectious disorders is important. Hyperglobulinemia and an inflammatory leukogram can be the only clinicopathologic abnormalities with type I nonerosive IMPA, other than suppurative, sterile synovial fluid.[9]

Survey thoracic and abdominal radiographs, serum titers for tick-borne diseases (ehrlichia, RMSF, and Lyme), abdominal and cardiac ultrasonography, and radiography of the thorax and affected joints can be performed. Culture of synovial fluid is performed if sepsis is suspected, but blood and urine cultures are usually more rewarding.[5,8]

Heartworm infection, pyometra, periodontal disease, chronic bacterial endocarditis, discospondylitis, chronic Actinomyces infections, juvenile cellulitis, chronic salmonellosis, and occult urinary tract infection have all been associated with nonerosive type II arthritis, and should be considered.[5,7,8] Idiopathic arteritis causing meningitis can be accompanied by distal joint inflammation. Enteropathic type III arthritis can be associated with inflammatory bowel disease, and hepatopathic arthropathy can be associated with chronic active hepatitis.[5,8]

Differentiation of nonerosive from erosive forms of IMPA can be made with radiography, and should always be pursued if response to therapy for presumed nonerosive IMPA is less than anticipated. Viral serology for feline leukemia can be positive in 66% of cats with progressive polyarthritis associated with feline syncytium-forming virus, and may exacerbate the disease.[4,8]

Review of the physical examination findings and clinical pathology results should identify criteria of SLE if it is present: cytopenia (hemolytic anemia and/or thrombocytopenia), dermatologic lesions, protein losing nephropathy (urine protein: creatinine ratio), myositis, myocarditis/pericarditis, pleuritis, or glossitis. The presence of antinuclear antibodies and LE cells can help confirm the diagnosis of SLE, but are not specific for it. Similarly, a positive Coomb's test can support the diagnosis of SLE.[12,13]

Rheumatoid factor testing is neither sensitive nor specific for erosive polyarthritis in the dog. Serologic testing for the presence of rheumatoid factor is reported to be positive in 25% to 75% of dogs with erosive polyarthritis when performed using the Rose-Waaler test. Additionally, the mucin clot test may support the diagnosis of erosive arthritis. Mucin levels in synovial fluid are typically lowered in patients with erosive arthritis owing to the action of inflammatory substances. Synovial biopsy can support the diagnosis if histopathologic changes typical of erosive arthritis are found: periarticular fibrosis, synovial hyperplasia and villous hypertrophy, and the formation of pannus.[4,11]

Therapeutics

Type I IMPA and SLE-associated polyarthritis are successfully treated in most cases with immunosuppressive levels of corticosteroids alone. One to 2 weeks after initiation of therapy, repeat arthrocentesis and synovial fluid cytologic evaluation should be performed. Effective control of IMPA is reflected by normalization of gross characteristics of synovial fluid and cell counts with return to a predominance of mononuclear cells, in addition to clinical improvement. Gradual tapering of corticosteroid doses should occur in concert with continued improvement of clinical signs and normalization of synovial fluid. Serial arthrocentesis for cytologic evaluation of synovial fluid is important in assessing response to therapy and maintenance of remission. The typical course of immunosuppression in type I idiopathic IMPA is 6 to 12 weeks. Combination therapy as described for erosive IMPA (see below) can be necessary if the initial response (within 2 weeks) to corticosteroids is incomplete, if tapering results in relapse, or if unacceptable side effects are associated with prednisone administration.

IMPA associated with significant concurrent systemic disease warrants treatment of the primary disorder first and synovitis second. Antimicrobial, antiparasitic, antineoplastic, immunomodulatory, and nutritional therapies should prevail Figure 117-5. Analgesic and anti-inflammatory therapy can accompany treatment of the primary disorder if dictated by the level of discomfort associated with arthritis. The use of nonsteroidal anti-inflammatory drugs in combination with corticosteroids is not advised owing to the risk of gastric ulceration. Combination antimicrobial and immunosuppressive therapy can

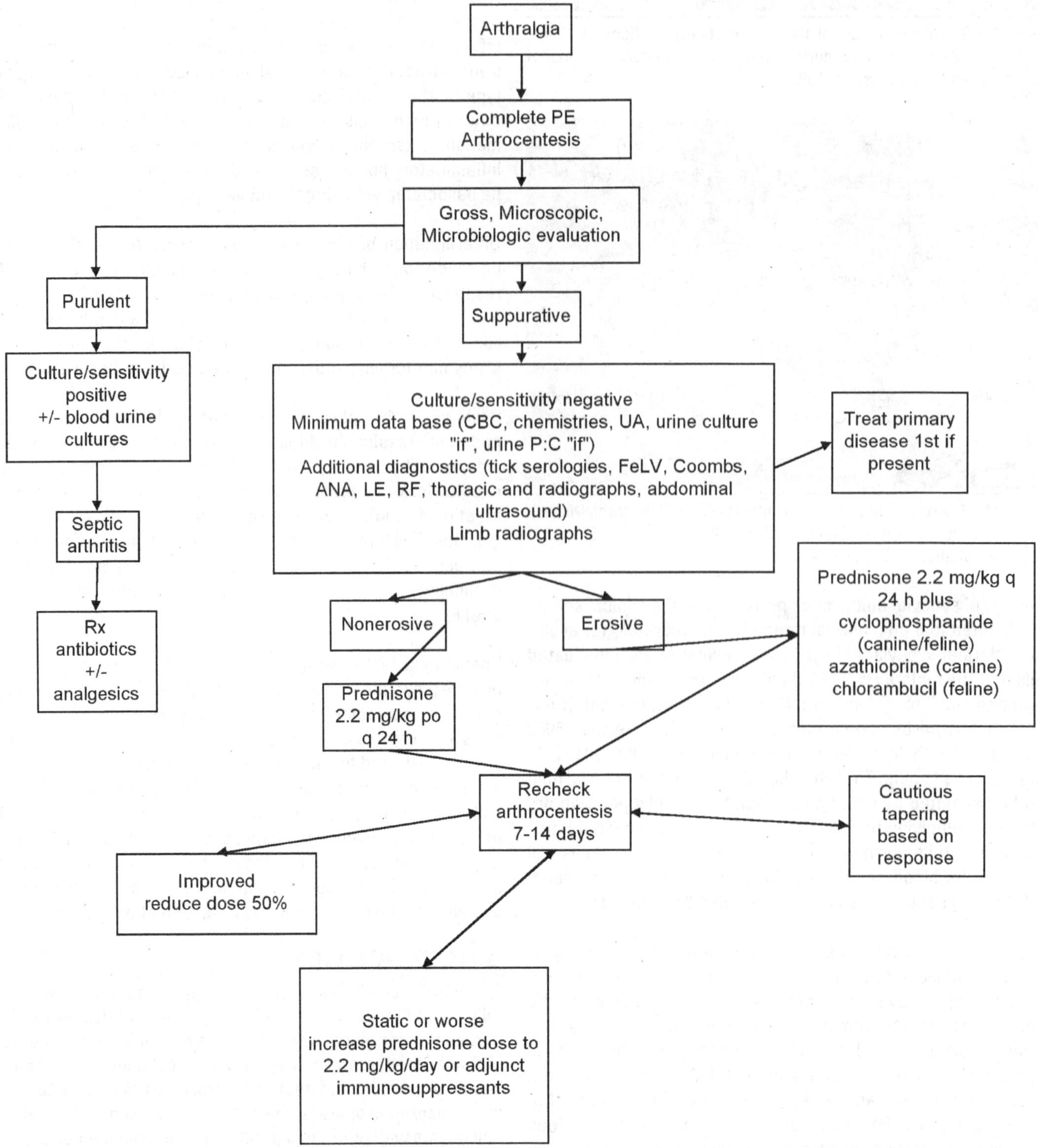

Figure 117-5. Flow chart for clinical evaluation of arthralgia and IMPA.

be cautiously instituted if clinically indicated, while awaiting serologic and microbiologic results, but this demands close patient monitoring.

Current recommendations for therapy of erosive IMPA dictate combination corticosteroid and cytotoxic drug administration. Immunosuppressive doses of prednisone (2.2 mg/kg/day) are combined with cyclophosphamide (Cytoxan, 50 mg/M^2 PO every 24 hours x 4 days each week, or MWF), azathioprine (Imuran, 50mg/M^2 every 24 hours for 7-14 days, then every 48 hours), or cyclosporine (10 mg/kg). Generally, cyclophosphamide is not used for longer that 4 months in dogs owing to its association with sterile hemorrhagic cystitis. Cats are much more susceptible to azathioprine toxicity, and its use is generally not recommended. Chlorambucil (1-2 mg/cat every 24-72 hours) is used as an alternative. Both cyclophosphamide and azathioprine require close monitoring for myelosuppression. Hepatic enzyme elevation can occur with azathioprine. Chlorambucil (Leukeran, 2-6 mg/M^2 every 48 hours canine) can be substituted for cyclophosphamide once remission has been attained, if necessary, in the dog. Side effects of cyclosporine include gastrointestinal upset, anorexia, and gingival hyperplasia. Cyclosporine reversibly inhibits immunocompetent lymphocytes in the G_0 - or G_1 – phase, affecting T-helper cells, T-suppressor cells, and reducing lymphokine production and release. Cyclosporine has variable bioavailability, and the various formulations do not have equal efficacy or dosing. Microemulsified products have improved oral absorption (Neoral, Novartis, Greensboro NC, 5-10 mg/kg/day divided bid). Ketoconazole (10 mg/kg/day divided tid PO with food) can be used concurrently to decrease cytochrome P-450 clearance of cyclosporine, permitting a lower dosage to be effective and saving client expenses. Serum levels should be monitored starting 2 to 3 days after the initiation of therapy; trough levels of 200 to 500 ng/ml are advised.[17] Leflunomide (4mg/kg every 24 hours, with dosage adjustment based on trough plasma levels of 20 μg/ml) is a new immunosuppressive agent showing promise in the treatment of refractory immunologic disease in dogs and cats. Leflunomide can be considered for IMPA unresponsive to conventional therapy. Other than repair of ruptured cranial crucial ligaments, surgical intervention (synovectomy, arthrodesis) for IMPA is unrewarding and uncommon. As with type I IMPA, immunosuppressive drug withdrawal should be performed in concert with clinical signs of remission coupled with synovial fluid evaluation, as improvement in gait does not always correlate with normalization of synovial fluid.

Prognosis

The prognosis for dogs and cats with IMPA varies. The prognosis for nonerosive forms of IMPA is better than that for erosive forms. Early appropriate immunosuppressive therapy, tapered carefully based on clinical and clinicopathologic evaluations, can result in resolution and discontinuation of medication in 1.5 to 3 months.[5,7,8]

The prognosis for polyarthritis associated with concurrent disease (types II-IV) depends on the potential for resolution of the primary, contributory disorder. IMPA associated with infectious/inflammatory diseases responsive to therapy (rickettsial infections, enteropathies) carries a better prognosis than that associated with more refractory disorders (mycoses, viruses, neoplasia).[7]

Erosive forms rarely resolve, but remission with continued medical therapy is possible. Feline erosive progressive polyarthritis carries a poor prognosis. Canine erosive polyarthritis has a fair prognosis if diagnosed and treated early in its course, but is generally considered to be a more aggressive condition than the similar disease in humans (rheumatoid arthritis). Semierosive polyarthritis of greyhounds is reported to have a poor prognosis. Aggressive combination immunosuppressive therapy is indicated to slow progression of erosive IMPA, and postpone joint subluxation, luxation, ankylosis, and collapse, and to minimize periarticular osteophyte production. These changes are irreversible. Caution must be taken that therapy does not result in serious complications such as refractory sterile hemorrhagic cystitis, viral relapse, myelosuppression, or opportunistic bacterial sepsis. Therapy can be expected to continue at high doses for 3 to 6 months, and at maintenance levels for months to years.[4,7]

References

1. Pedersen NC, Morgan JP, Vasseur PB: Joint diseases of dogs and cats. *In* Ettinger SJ, Feldman EC (eds). Textbook of Veterinary Internal Medicine, 5th ed. Philadelphia: WB Saunders, 2000, p. 1862.

2. Pedersen NC, Pool R: Canine joint disease. Vet Clin North Am Small Anim Pract 8:468, 1978.

3. Pedersen NC, Weisner K, Castles JJ, et al: Noninfectious canine arthritis: The inflammatory nonerosive arthritidities. J Am Vet Med Assoc 169:304, 1976.

4. Pedersen NC, Pool R, Castles JJ, et al: Noninfectious canine arthritis: Rheumatoid arthritis. J Am Vet Med Assoc 169:295, 1976.

5. Magne ML: Swollen joints and lameness. *In* Textbook of Veterinary Internal Medicine, 5th ed. Ettinger SJ, Feldman EC (eds). Philadelphia: WB Saunders, 2000, p. 77.

6. Lipowitz AJ: Immune-mediated articular disease. *In* Textbook of Small Animal Surgery. Slatter DH (ed). Philadelphia: WB Saunders, 1985, p. 1302.

7. Rondeau MP, Walton RM, Bisset S, et al: Suppurative, non septic polyarthopathy in dogs. J Vet Intern Med 19:654, 2005.

8. Goldstein R: Swollen joint and lameness. *In* Textbook of Veterinary Internal Medicine, 6th ed. Ettinger SJ, Feldman EC (eds). Philadelphia: Elsevier, 2005, p. 83.

9. Clements DN, Gear RN, Tattersall J, et al: Type I immune-mediated polyarthritis in dogs: 39 cases (1997-2002). JAVMA 224(8):1323, 2004.

10. Davidson AP, Pappagianis D: Canine coccidioidomycosis: 1970-1993. *In* Coccidioidomycosis; Proceedings of the 5th International Conference, Einstein HE, Catanzaro A (eds).: Washington DC: National Foundation for Infectious Diseases, 1996; 155.

11. Lewis RM: Rheumatoid arthritis. Vet Clin North Am Small Anim Pract 24(4):697,1994.

12. Grindem CB, Johnson KH: Systemic lupus erythematosis; Literature review and report of 42 new canine cases. J Am Anim Hosp Assoc 19:489, 1983.

13. Scott DW, Walton DK, Manning TO, et al: Canine lupus erythematosis. J Am Anim Hosp Assoc 19:461, 1983.

14. Giger U, Werner LL, Millichamp NJ, et al: Sulfadiazine-induced allergy in six Doberman pinschers. JAVMA 186:479, 1986.

15. Lees GE, Rogers KS, Troy GC.: Polyarthritis associated with sulfadiazine administration in a Labrador retriever dog. The Southwest Vet 37(1):14, 1986.

16. Fernandez FR, Grindem CB, Lipowitz AJ, et al: Synovial fluid analysis: Preparation of smears for cytological examination of canine synovial fluid. J Am Anim Hosp Assoc 19:727, 1983.

17. Plumb DC. Veterinary Drug Handbook, 4th edition. Ames: Iowa State Press, 2005.

Part XIV

Exotics

Chapter 118

Surgical Diseases of the Ferret

SJ Mehler
RA Bennett

It is estimated that 7 to 10 million ferrets are owned as pets in the United States.[1] Besides traumatic injuries and gastrointestinal foreign bodies, the majority of surgical diseases in ferrets are neoplastic conditions. A group of black-footed ferrets that spent their entire lives in a captive setting had a 100% incidence of cancer at necropsy.[2] It is also common for more than one type of tumor to be present simultaneously in a ferret, with one type usually diagnosed as an incidental finding at surgery.[3-8] The most commonly reported tumors in ferrets are endocrine tumors, with an incidence of 39.7% to 53%.[6,7,9,10] Pancreatic beta-cell tumors or insulinomas are the most common endocrine tumors, and adrenal tumors are the second most common.[8-10]

Surgical procedures in ferrets are similar to those performed in dogs and cats. Because of the small body size of ferrets, microsurgical instruments, magnifying loupes, smaller suture sizes, body-temperature support devices, and smaller retractors (Lone Star retractor, Lone Star Medical Products, Stafford, TX) are important (Figure 118-1). For a majority of the surgical diseases described in this chapter, a ventral midline laparotomy is indicated. Ferrets have relatively thick skin, little subcutaneous tissue, and a wide, thin linea alba.[11]

In the United States, 2 years represents 25% of the average lifespan of ferrets.[8] If the goal of treatment is to prolong life and improve the quality of life of the ferret, then a 1- to 2-year survival with a good quality of life is considered a success.

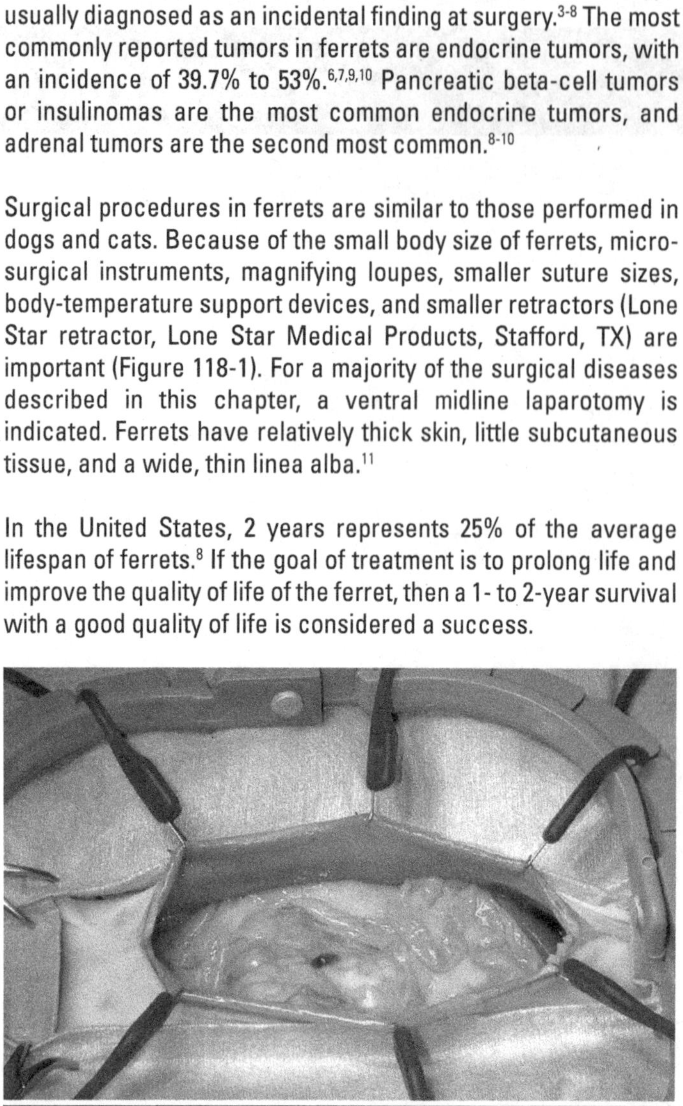

Figure 118-1. Lone Star retractor being used in the abdomen of a ferret.

Insulinoma

Pancreatic beta-cell tumors are the most commonly reported endocrine tumors in ferrets, with a reported incidence of 21.7% to 25%.[6,7,10,12-16] The median age of ferrets with insulinomas is 5 years (range 2-7 years), with males being diagnosed more frequently than females.[7,17,18]

Disease Mechanism

The four types of islet cells are beta cells (insulin secretion), alpha cells (glucagon secretion), delta cells (somatostatin secretion), and F cells (pancreatic polypeptide secretion).[19] Islet cell tumors in ferrets arise from the beta cells and produce insulin, which, when present in excess amounts, leads to hypoglycemia.[6,8,9,19,20] Functional insulin-secreting conditions in ferrets include pancreatic hyperplasia, adenoma, and adenocarcinoma.[6,7,17,21] Neuroglucopenic signs occur because cells in the central nervous system have a higher metabolic rate and glucose is their primary energy source.[19,22] Prolonged and severe hypoglycemia can cause brain damage and, clinically, patients present with neurologic dysfunction.[9,19,22]

Clinical Signs

Clinical signs may not be apparent and the tumor is sometimes diagnosed on health screen biochemical examination or at exploratory laparotomy for another reason. Clinical signs are related to the systemic effects of hypoglycemia, the rate of decline of the blood glucose concentration, and the duration and degree of hypoglycemia.[19] Clinical signs in ferrets with hypoglycemia include hind limb ataxia, paresis or paralysis, seizures, weight loss, ptyalism, gagging, vomiting, and pawing at the mouth.[6,7,12,14,17,21,23,24] Pawing at the mouth is thought to be associated with nausea, but may lead owners and clinicians to believe there is a foreign object in the mouth or throat.[8,25] Owners may report a prolonged waxing and waning history of lethargy and episodes of collapse. They often describe the ferret as having a "glazed" eye appearance.[19] Physical examination of ferrets with an insulinoma may be unremarkable as the hypoglycemia can be episodic.

Diagnostics

The reference range for resting blood glucose concentration in ferrets is 94 to 207 mg/dL and normal fasting blood glucose levels are 90 to 125 mg/dL.[19] Insulin levels can be run concurrently but will only be diagnostic if the patient is hypoglycemic at the time of sampling.[19,26,27] If serum glucose levels are normal and a high clinical suspicion for insulinoma exists, a controlled fast can be performed for no more than 4 hours to better establish hypoglycemia. It is best to fast the ferret in the hospital in case a hypoglycemic crisis occurs. Because ferrets have a rapid gastrointestinal transit time (3-4 hours), a shorter fast than in dogs and cats is diagnostic. A 4-hour fasting glucose concentration less than 60 mg/dL is consistent with a pancreatic islet cell tumor in a ferret.[20,21,27] Typically, abdominal radiography and ultrasonography are not helpful in detecting these masses as they are usually only millimeters in diameter.[8,19]

Treatment

Treatment is aimed at increasing blood glucose levels by both medical and surgical means. It is common (> 50% of surgical cases) that after surgical excision, medical management is still indicated.[17] Only 14% to 15% of ferrets with insulinoma are cured long-term with surgery.[7,17,19,28] This may be due to the high recurrence rate or micrometastatic rate of ferret insulinoma to other regions of the pancreas, regional lymph node, spleen, or liver; however, some have found the metastatic potential to be low.[17,24]

Surgical excision is the treatment of choice for ferrets under 6 years of age or for those suspected of having concurrent adrenal disease.[19] Surgery is indicated for confirmation of insulinoma, for decreasing the tumor burden, and to better evaluate for metastatic and concurrent disease (Figure 118-2).[27] Removal of the left lobe of the pancreas is technically less challenging than removal of the right lobe because of the close proximity of the right lobe to the pancreatic ducts, duodenum, and adjacent blood vessels.[21,29]

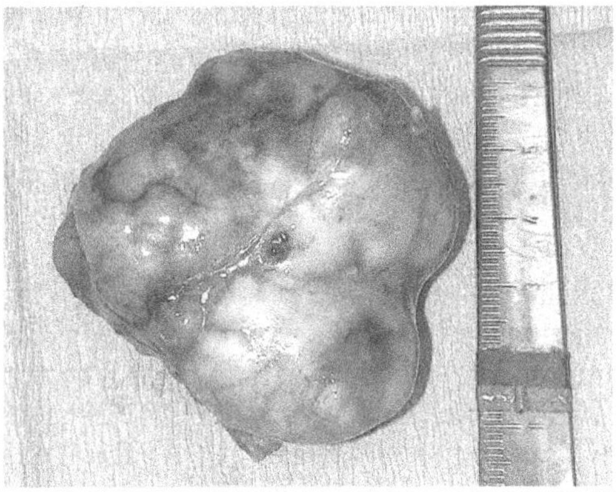

Figure 118-2. An insulinoma removed from the left limb of the pancreas of a ferret. This was an unusually large tumor. Most insulinomas in ferrets are less than a centimeter in diameter.

The pancreas of ferrets is similar to that of cats in that there is typically a common pancreatic duct that joins with the common bile duct and enters the duodenum at the major duodenal papilla. An accessory pancreatic duct is present in about 2.5% of ferrets.[11,13] Medical management can be used concurrently with surgery or as the sole modality for treatment. Ferrets with insulinomas managed medically without surgery have a shorter survival than those treated with surgery or a combination.[17] Medical management is aimed at increasing blood glucose levels. Glucocorticoids increase hepatic gluconeogenesis and decrease glycogenolysis.[19,27,30] Liquid formulations of prednisone or prednisolone are available for more accurate dosing. It is important that the solution does not contain sugar or alcohol that can exacerbate the hypoglycemia.[8,19]

Diazoxide is a nondiuretic benzothiadiazide that effectively increases serum glucose levels by different mechanisms. It inhibits pancreatic islet cell insulin secretion and enhances hyperglycemia by stimulating the beta-adrenergic system and inhibiting the uptake of glucose by cells.[15,31,32] Diazoxide has no antineoplastic activity nor does it affect the synthesis of insulin.[31,32] Glucocorticoids and diazoxide can be given alone or in combination as needed to combat the effects of systemic hypoglycemia. Streptozotocin is a chemotherapeutic agent that exhibits a diabetogenic effect on pancreatic beta cells in dogs but not in humans and has not been evaluated in ferrets.[8,32]

Diet is also important in the medical management of insulinomas in ferrets. Feeding a high-protein, low-carbohydrate diet at frequent intervals is necessary. Treats and snacks, especially those containing sugar, should be avoided.[8,19,27] It has been recommended that serial blood glucose concentrations be taken at 2 weeks post surgery and at 1-4-month intervals for the life of the ferret.[11,19]

Prognosis

The prognosis for ferrets with insulinomas varies but is generally better than for that of dogs with insulinomas.[7,12,21,23,24,26] Young ferrets without metastatic disease that are diagnosed early in the disease process have the best prognosis.[27] With partial pancreatectomy, mean survival time is 668 days; multiple surgeries are sometimes needed to achieve longer survival times.[7,8] The duration of clinical signs before diagnosis may negatively affect survival time and disease-free interval after surgery.[14] No difference in survival time has been identified between ferrets with benign versus metastatic disease.[12,17]

Adrenal Disease

Adrenocortical cell tumors are the second most common tumors in ferrets.[3,6,10,18,30,33-36] The occurrence of hyperadrenocorticism in domestic ferrets in the United States is common and may be present in up to 25% of all ferrets.[3,6,37] The first report of hyperadrenocorticism in a domestic ferret was in 1987.[38] Since then several reports identifying the hormones elevated in ferret hyperadrenocorticism and the pathophysiology of the disease have been published.[3,33,34,39] The mean age of affected ferrets is 3.4 to 4.8 years, with females having a predilection for the disease,[3,30,35] although one study refutes this finding.[37]

Disease Mechanism

These are adrenal cortical reticularis tumors, which produce excessive levels of androgenic hormone precursor and estrogenic hormones. Increases in serum cortisol levels are typically not a feature of this disease in ferrets, nor is primary pituitary disease likely.[8,19,27,35,40-42] These tumors histologically are characterized as adrenal cortical hyperplasia, adenomas, or adenocarcinomas, and it is possible that this is a continuum of a disease process.[3,43] The clinical signs and prognosis are the same regardless of the histopathologic diagnosis.[2,3,8,30,37] Adrenocortical spindle-cell tumors and pheochromocytomas have also been reported alone and concurrently with functional adrenocortical cell neoplasms in ferrets.[9,18,19,30,44] The incidence of adrenal disease in ferrets in Europe and Australia appears to be much lower than in the United States. It has been speculated that adrenal gland hyperplasia and tumor development are due to the early neutering of ferrets.[27,45,46] This has been shown to occur in mice.[45] Other suggested causes include feeding a commercial brand ferret food (instead of whole prey items), inbreeding, and the lack of a natural light cycle for ferrets in the United States.[19]

Clinical Signs

Clinical signs in ferrets with functional adrenocortical tumors are primarily a result of the hypersecretion of estrogenic and other steroid hormones by tumor cells.[9] Clinical signs are variable in affected animals and may include a bilaterally symmetrical endocrine alopecia which may be seasonal, pruritis (sometimes the only clinical sign), vulvar enlargement in females, prostatic enlargement in males, aggressive sexual behavior, comedones on the tail, and mammary gland enlargement (Figure 118-3).[3,19,20,28,33,37,39,47] Males with prostatic disease secondary to hyperadrenocorticism may present with dribbling urine or straining to urinate and defecate. Prostatic abscessation, paraurethral cysts, and urinary obstruction can also accompany the disease in males. Large tumors can be palpated in the cranial abdomen.

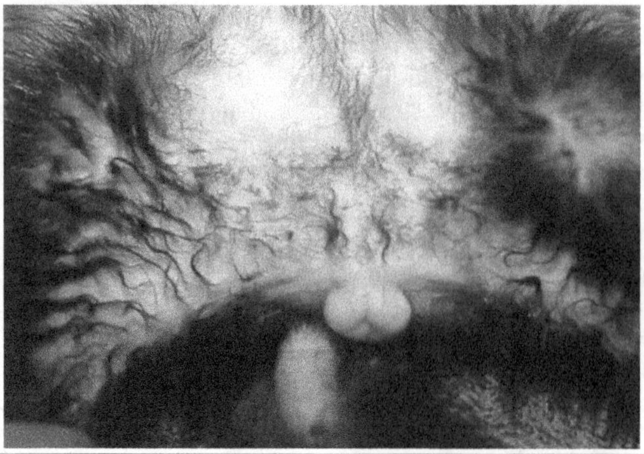

Figure 118-3. The ventral abdomen of a female ferret diagnosed with hyperadrenocorticism. Notice the alopecia of the ventral tail and abdomen. Moderate swelling of the vulva is secondary to an increase in circulating estrogens and androgens.

Diagnostics

Hyperadrenocorticism in ferrets is diagnosed based on a combination of clinical signs, abdominal ultrasound, and plasma concentrations of estrogens and androgens.[19,34,35,40,41] Serum chemistry and hematologic profiles are usually normal except for the occasional thrombocytopenia and anemia, thought to occur owing to estrogen-induced bone marrow suppression.[3] In ferrets with anemia and pancytopenia, a packed cell volume less than 15% is associated with a grave prognosis.[19] A serum androgen profile has been established and is commercially available at the University of Tennessee. The assay measures levels of 17-hydroxyprogesterone, androstenedione, and estradiol. An elevation of any one of these hormones is considered diagnostic for hyperadrenocorticism in ferrets.[19,33,34] Elevations in dehydroepiandrosterone may also be detected in ferrets with adrenal disease.[40] Urine cortisol:creatine ratios are not useful in diagnosing hyperadrenocorticism in ferrets because serum cortisol is not elevated in these patients,[3,41] although one study disagrees with this.[35]

History and physical examination appear to be the most useful in diagnosing the disease. Abdominal radiographs are usually unremarkable unless the mass is large or if mineralization of the affected adrenal gland has occurred.[3] Adrenal lesions are the most commonly found ultrasonographic abnormalities in ferrets.[8,48,49] Ultrasound has been reported to have an 84% sensitivity for detecting adrenal disease in ferrets, with histopathology being the gold standard.[43] Ultrasound findings in ferrets with hyperadrenocorticism may also include a prominent uterus or uterine stump, or a prominent prostate with or without prostatic cysts.[43] The authors have also observed ultrasonographic evidence of urinary tract dilation (urethra, bladder, and ureters) owing to an enlarged prostate obstructing the prostatic urethra.

Treatment

Currently, medical management of adrenal disease in ferrets is focused on controlling abnormal hormone levels and their effects. These treatments do not cure the condition but may help alleviate clinical signs. Medical management is recommended if the owner is unable to afford surgery, if the ferret is a poor surgical candidate, or if the ferret has bilateral adrenal tumors that cannot be resected.[19] The use of leuprolide acetate, a repositol gonadotropin releasing hormone (GnRH) analog, causes a transient increase and then a rapid decrease in luteinizing hormone, follicle-stimulating hormone, and testosterone levels.[19,50] It is rare that patients become refractory to leuprolide acetate treatments.[8] Other hormone therapies include bicalutamide, anastrazole, and melatonin.[8,19,51]

A ventral midline and a lateral celiotomy have been described for adrenalectomy in ferrets (Figure 118-4).[20,52-59] In 85% of ferrets with hyperadrenocorticism, one adrenal gland is enlarged and the other is small to normal. In the remaining 15% of cases, bilateral adrenal enlargement is identified.[3,37] In unilateral enlargement, disease may occur in the contralateral gland after the affected adrenal is removed.[37] In some cases, both adrenal glands will appear grossly normal and direct visualization of the entire gland via careful dissection of surrounding retroperitoneal fat is necessary. Historically, the recommended surgical treatment for bilateral adrenal disease in ferrets has been total adrenalectomy of the one side and partial resection of the contralateral side.[40,57] This will ultimately lead to recurrence of the disease as the remaining adrenal tissue proliferates, and it may not even temporarily relieve clinical signs.

The prostate is not grossly visible in a normal male ferret. If the ferret presented with a urinary obstruction from prostatic disease, a urinary catheter should be left in place for a couple of days until voluntary urinary function returns.

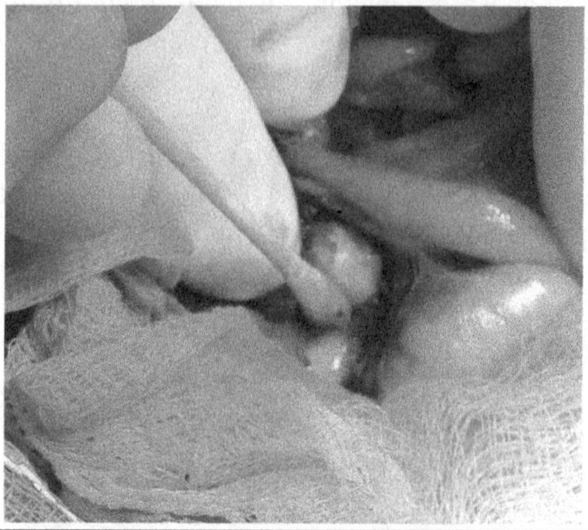

Figure 118-4. A 2 cm x 1.5 cm right adrenal mass is being removed from the caudal vena cava and liver. A combination of blunt dissection with sterile cotton tip applicators, hemoclips, and bipolar electrocautery facilitate removal of these tumors.

If both glands are abnormal, bilateral adrenalectomy is achievable and preferred. Removing both adrenal glands can lead to iatrogenic hypoadrenocorticism (Addison's disease); however, most ferrets do well on glucocorticoid supplementation only and do not need long-term mineralocorticoid therapy. Most ferrets will not require long-term steroid administration.[20] Many ferrets are concurrently diagnosed with insulinoma and already on glucocorticoid therapy for that disease process. Periodic electrolyte analysis of ferrets having had a bilateral adrenalectomy is recommended because some patients will require mineralocorticoid therapy.

Prognosis

Following complete surgical removal of the affected gland or glands, prostatic and vulvar enlargement decreases within days and hair regrowth occurs within 3 months.[8] The prognosis for adrenal gland disease in ferrets is good, if the gland is completely excised, owing to a low metastatic potential.[3,8,27,30]

Splenomegaly

Splenomegaly is a common finding in adult ferrets but is poorly understood.[11,60,61] The spleen in ferrets increases gradually and slightly in size with increasing age[30] but can also enlarge owing to proliferative lesions, reactive processes, compensatory mechanisms, or certain anesthetics.[29,60] The most common cause of splenomegaly is extramedullary hematopoesis (EMH) in the presence or absence of anemia or other hematologic dyscasias.[60-62] Other causes include lymphoma, insulinoma, cardiomyopathy, adrenal disease, systemic mast cell tumors, Aleutian disease, eosinophilic gastritis, hemangiosarcoma, primary splenic neoplasia, hypersplenism, and splenitis.[54] Most causes of splenomegaly are not surgical diseases and should be evaluated with clinicopathologic data and imaging modalities before splenectomy is considered. Percutaneous splenic biopsy is contraindicated in ferrets suspected of having splenic hemangiosarcoma, although this condition is rare in ferrets.[54] Ultrasound is useful in determining the safety of percutaneous biopsy. Ultrasound is also useful in guiding biopsy needles or smaller gauge needles for obtaining a sample of the spleen. Fine-needle aspiration is simple, carries little risk, is associated with low morbidity, and provides useful samples.

Indications for splenectomy in ferrets include splenic neoplasia, splenomegaly or hypersplenism causing compression of abdominal viscera, splenic torsion, and non-self-limiting traumatic fractures of the spleen. Splenectomy is contraindicated in ferrets with bone marrow hypoplasia because the spleen is the primary site of hematopoiesis in these patients.[54] Ferrets with splenic extramedullary hematopoiesis may develop chronic anemia after splenectomy because of the absence of splenic production of erythrocytes.

Gastrointestinal (GI) Foreign Body

In pet ferrets, foreign body ingestion is common.[11,63] Ferrets are inquisitive and have a propensity to chew on rubber and plastic.[64,65] Ingestion of foreign objects usually occurs in ferrets under the age of 2 years, whereas trichobezoars are more commonly observed in older ferrets.[64] Linear foreign bodies are rarely seen in ferrets.

Disease Mechanism

Ferrets have a rapid GI transit time compared with other carnivores.[25] This is likely owing to a lack of the proximal-to-distal digestive-enzyme gradient seen in other carnivores, resulting in a continuous exposure of nutrients to digestive enzymes during GI transit.[25] Most GI foreign bodies lodge in the stomach or jejunum.[64]

Clinical Signs

Clinical signs of gastrointestinal foreign bodies in ferrets include anorexia or inappetance, diarrhea, ptyalism, facial rubbing, and vomiting (although this is not commonly reported by the owners).[63-65] Abdominal palpation may elicit discomfort. Palpation of the foreign body is usually possible, especially if it is in the intestinal tract.[10,63,65]

Diagnostics

Diagnosis is based on signalment, history, and physical examination. Ferrets have an abdomen that is easy to palpate, making most foreign bodies readily palpable within the gastrointestinal tract.[54] A complete blood count, serum biochemistry panel, and urinalysis should be performed. Abdominal radiographs and ultrasonography are useful in confirming the diagnosis and determining the location of the obstruction (Figure 118-5). The ferret should be stabilized with intravenous fluids before surgical removal is pursued.

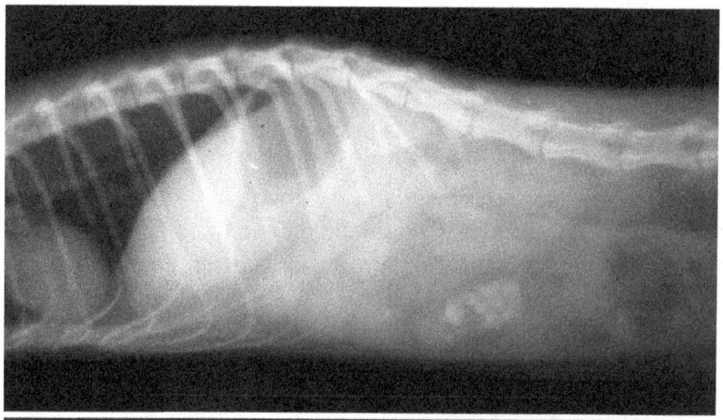

Figure 118-5. A right lateral abdominal radiograph of a 1-year-old ferret with decreased appetite and lethargy. Notice the numerous, circular, soft-tissue opacities in the jejunum. Fluid and gas dilation of the small intestine is present. This ferret had a jejunal foreign body obstruction.

Treatment

Most GI foreign bodies in ferrets must be removed surgically. Gastrointestinal foreign bodies in ferrets rarely pass on their own. The use of gastrointestinal lubricants and fluid replacement therapy may allow smaller nonobstructive materials to pass, especially hairballs.[65]

A ventral midline abdominal exploratory surgery should be performed in any ferret with a GI foreign body. Ferrets lack a grossly obvious ileum, and the jejunoileum extends from the duodenojejunal flexure to the ascending colon.[11,13] A gastrotomy and/or enterotomy are usually indicated, with intestinal resection and anastamosis less frequently necessary.

Prognosis

In general, ferrets have an excellent prognosis after surgery for foreign body removal as long as a perforation and septic peritonitis are not present. Intestinal necrosis or perforation seem to occur less frequently in ferrets compared with dogs and cats with foreign body obstruction. Preventing foreign body ingestion can be difficult in ferrets. Usually by 2 years of age, ferrets ingest foreign bodies less frequently. The routine use of GI lubricants to prevent trichobezoars is helpful.

Gastrointestinal Neoplasia

GI neoplasia has been reported in ferrets,[6,10,18,30,66-69] but it is not a common site for primary neoplasia.[65] Pyloric adenocarcinoma has been described in ferrets and clinical signs include those associated with an upper GI obstruction: vomiting, weight loss, anorexia, and lethargy.[6,67,68]

The anatomy of the ferret stomach is similar to that of dogs, but is physiologically more like the human stomach.[13,25] Blood gas analysis commonly reflects a hypochloremic metabolic alkalosis. Ultrasound is useful in diagnosing the presence and location of the mass. Attempts at surgical resection with a Bilroth have been made but were unsuccessful.[67,68] Palliative stenting across the pylorus of a ferret with adenocarcinoma was successfully performed and alleviated clinical signs.[69]

Obstructive Urolithiasis

Urolithiasis in ferrets can be characterized by solitary or multiple renal or cystic calculi or by the presence of sandy material in the urinary bladder and urethra.[70] Clinically, obstructive urolithiasis tends to be less common now than it was 10 years ago.[70] Obstructive urolithiasis is more common in male ferrets than in female ferrets owing to the narrow diameter of the urethra as it passes through the os penis in males. The most common type of stone identified in ferrets is magnesium ammonium phosphate (struvite).[70]

Disease Mechanism

Although not studied as extensively as in dogs and cats, the pathogenesis of struvite urolithiasis in ferrets is probably related to diet.[70] Ferrets are carnivores with a normal urine pH of about 6.0.[71] Struvite crystallizes when the urine pH rises above 6.4. Although the mineral content of the food was once thought to be the cause of urolithiasis in ferrets, it is now thought to be caused by ingestion of plant proteins.[70] The metabolism of organic acids in plant protein produces an alkaline urine that results in the formation of struvite crystals.[71] This was demonstrated in a group of pregnant jills fed a diet high in plant protein (mainly corn) and in a group of ferrets fed a commercial dog food.[71,72] Historically, the prevalence of the disease in the American ferret population was probably related to feeding poor quality dog and cat diets that contained a high percentage of plant-based protein. In recent years, many commercial ferret diets have become available and ferrets are not commonly fed dog and cat foods with plant proteins.

Clinical Signs

The systemic effects of obstructive urolithiasis in ferrets are the same as those in dogs and cats. Dysuria, hematuria, stranguria, frequent licking of the perineum, and urine dribbling are reported clinical signs in ferrets with urolithiasis.[70] Ferrets with obstructive urolithiasis may strain violently or cry when attempting to urinate, or they may present depressed, moribund, or comatose. Rarely, ferrets present with lethargy and inappetance without lower urinary tract signs.

Diagnostics

The presence of lower urinary tract signs and palpation of a firm, distended, unexpressable urinary bladder confirms an obstruction. Obstructive urolithiasis can be identified with abdominal radiographs because struvite stones are radioopaque. However, sand is not always visible radiographically. Abdominal ultrasound is often useful as the fine sand-like crystals are easily identified. It is also helpful if another cause is suspected (prostate disease secondary to adrenal neoplasia) and to identify radiolucent urinary calculi. Serum chemistry and hematologic profiles should be run to determine the extent of azotemia and electrolyte abnormalities, as well as to look for concurrent disease.

Treatment

If severe cardiac arrhythmias and electrolyte abnormalities are present, they are treated before attempting to unobstruct the urethra. Once intravenous fluids and supportive care have been initiated, the urethra should be unblocked. The treatment of obstructive urolithiasis in male ferrets is challenging because it is difficult to pass a urinary catheter in males. Males have an operculum covering the distal urethra and a hook directed dorsally at the tip of the os penis, making it difficult to identify the urethral opening.[58] The technique for urinary catheterization in ferrets has been described.[54,73]

If the distal urethra cannot be cleared of stones or if the ferret has recurrence of obstruction, an emergency cystotomy, percutaneous tube cystostomy, or perineal urethrostomy (PU) can be performed if the ferret is stable.

The anatomy of a ferret penis is similar to that of a dog.[58] The penis exits the pelvic canal, runs subcutaneously along the ventral pelvis, and lies along the caudal ventral abdominal body wall.[58] The opening of the prepuce is just caudal to the umbilicus. The PU site should be between the caudal portion of the os penis and the pelvic urethra. The stoma should be perineal and not ventral to avoid trauma to the site during normal ambulation. The penis is not resected as is done in cats. A 3.5 to 5.0 Fr red rubber catheter is then placed in the proximal urethrostomy site to assess the diameter of the urethra and make sure it is patent. Fine monofilament suture (6-0 to 8-0) is used to appose the mucosa of the urethra to the skin. The urethral drain board should be at least 1 cm. This technique works well in ferrets and is well tolerated long term.

Prognosis

If the ferret is on an inappropriate diet it should be changed to a commercial ferret diet with no plant protein source. The ferret should be monitored for struvite urolithiasis every 3 to 6 months with a urinalysis and abdominal radiographs. The prognosis is good for ferrets with obstructive urolithiasis if they are stabilized before general anesthesia. Recurrence can happen but is uncommon when dietary changes are made.

Blood Products

Many of the surgical diseases presented in this chapter require aggressive and challenging operative procedures. The use of perioperative blood products may be needed in some cases. Whole blood or packed red blood cell transfusions have been used in clinical patients. Ferrets have only one blood type and transfusion reactions have not been reported in ferrets, but minor cross-matches are still recommended by some.[8,25,74] Oxyglobin (Biopure, Cambridge, Massachusetts) is a hemoglobin replacement product that increases the oxygen carrying capacity of the blood and has been used in ferrets with no reports of adverse reactions. The beneficial effects are still speculative.

References

1. Jurek RM: A review of national and California population estimates of pet ferrets. California Department of Fish and Game, Wildlife Management Division, Bird and Mammal Conservation Program Report. Sacramento, 1998.

2. Carpenter JW, Novill MN, Kaiser HL: Neoplasia and other disease problems in black footed ferrets; implications for an endangered species. *In* Neoplasms-Comparative Pathology of Growth in Animals, Plants, and Man. Kraiser HE (ed). Baltimore: Williams & Wilkins, 1981, pp. 739-746.

3. Rosenthal KL, Peterson ME, Quesenberry KE, et al: Hyperadrenocorticism associated with adrenocortical tumor or nodular hyperplasia of the adrenal gland in ferrets: 50 cases (1987-1991). J Am Vet Med Assoc 203:271-275, 1993.

4. Stauber E, Kraft S, Robinette J: Multiple tumors in a ferret. J Small Exotic Anim Med 1:87-88, 1991.

5. Jenkins JR: Multiple concurrent neoplasia and metabolic diseases in the ferret: selected cases. J Small Exotic Anim Med 1:118-121, 1991.

6. Li X, Fox JG, Padrid PA: Neoplastic diseases in ferrets: 574 cases (1968-1997). J Am Vet Med Assoc 212:1402-1406, 1998.

7. Weiss CA, Williams BH, Scott MV: Insulinoma in the ferret: clinical findings and treatment comparison of 66 cases. J Am Anim Hosp Assoc 34:471-475, 1998.

8. Antinoff N, Hahn K: Ferret oncology: diseases, diagnostics, and therapeutics. Vet Clin North Am: Exotic Anim Pract 7:579-625, 2004.

9. Li X, Fox JG: Neoplastic diseases. *In* Biology and Diseases of the Ferret, 2nd ed. Fox JG (ed). Baltimore:Williams & Wilkins, 1998, pp. 405-447.

10. Williams BH, Weiss CA: Neoplasia. *In* Ferrets, Rabbits, and Rodents: Clinical Medicine and Surgery, 2nd ed. Quesenberry KE, Carpenter JW (eds). Philadelphia:WB Saunders, 2004, pp. 91-106.

11. Ludwig L, Aiken S: Soft tissue surgery. *In* Ferrets, Rabbits, and Rodents: Clinical Medicine and Surgery, 2nd ed. Quesenberry KE, Carpenter JW (eds). Philadelphia:WB Saunders, 2004, pp. 121-134.

12. Jergens AR, Shaw DP: Hyperinsulinism and hypoglycemia associated with pancreatic islet cell tumor in a ferret. J Am Vet Med Assoc 194:269-270, 1989.

13. Evans HE, An NQ: Anatomy of the ferret. *In* Biology and Disease of the Ferret, 2nd ed. Fox JG (ed). Baltimore:Williams & Wilkins, 1998, pp. 19-69.

14. Ehrhart N, Withrow SJ, Ehrhart EJ, et al: Pancreatic beta cell tumors in ferrets: 20 cases (1986-1994). J Am Vet Med Assoc 209:1737-1740, 1996.

15. Hillyer EV: Ferret endocrinology. *In* Kirk's Current Veterinary Therapy, 11th ed. Kirk RW, Bonagura JD (eds). Philadelphia:WB Saunders, 1992, pp. 1185-1189.

16. Kauffman J, Schwarz P, Mero K: Pancreatic beta cell tumor in a ferret. J Am Vet Med Assoc 185:998-1000, 1984.

17. Caplan ER, Peterson ME, Mullen HS, et al: Diagnosis and treatment of insulin-secreting pancreatic islet cell tumors in ferrets: 57 cases (1986-1994). J Am Vet Med Assoc 209:1741-1745, 1996.

18. Li X, Fox JG, Padrid PA. Neoplastic diseases in ferrets (*Mustela putorius furo*): a review of Veterinary Medical Data Base (1968-1997). J Am Vet Med Assoc 1402:212, 1998.

19. Quesenberry KE, Rosenthal KL. Endocrine diseases. *In* Ferrets, Rabbits, and Rodents: Clinical Medicine and Surgery, 2nd ed. Quesenberry KE, Carpenter JW (eds). Philadelphia:WB Saunders, 2004, pp. 79-90.

20. Wheeler J, Bennett RA: Ferret abdominal surgical procedures. Part 1. Adrenal gland and pancreatic beta-cell tumors. Compendium 21:815-822, 1999.

21. Marini RP, Ryden EB, Rosenblad KS, et al: Functional islet cell tumor in six ferrets. J Am Vet Med Assoc 202:430-433, 1993.

22. Nelson RW: Insulin-secreting islet cell neoplasia. *In* Textbook of Veterinary Internal Medicine, 4th ed. Ettinger SJ, Feldman EC (eds). Philadelphia:WB Saunders, 1995, pp. 1501-1509.

23. Lumeij JT, van der Hage MG, Dorrestein GM, can Sluijs FJ: Hypoglycemia due to a functional pancreatic islet cell tumor (insulinoma) in a ferret. Vet Rec 120:129-130, 1987.

24. Luttgen PJ, Storts RW, Rogers KS, Morton LD: Insulinoma in a ferret. J Am Vet Med Assoc 189:920-921, 1986.

25. Whary MT, Andrews PL: Physiology of the ferret. *In* Biology and Diseases of the Ferret, 2nd ed. Fox JG (ed). Baltimore:Williams & Wilkins, 1998, pp. 103-148.

26. Mann FA, Stockham SL, Freeman MB, et al: Reference intervals for insulin concentrations and insulin:glucose ratios in the serum of ferrets. J Small Exotic Anim Med 2:79-83, 1993.

27. Fox JG, Marini RP: Diseases of the endocrine system. *In* Biology and Diseases of the Ferret, 2nd ed. Fox JG (ed). Baltimore:Williams & Wilkins, 1998, pp. 291-305.

28. Mehler SJ, Bennett RA: Surgical oncology of exotic animals. Vet Clin North Am Exotic Anim Pract 7:783-805, 2004.

29. Marini RP, Fox JG: Anesthesia, surgery, and biomethodology. *In* Biology and Diseases of the Ferret, 2nd ed. Fox JG (ed). Baltimore:Williams & Wilkins, 1998, pp. 449-484.

30. Brown SA: Neoplasia. *In* Ferrets, Rabbits, Rodents: Clinical Medicine and Surgery. Hillyer EV, Quesenberry KE (eds). Philadelphia:WB Saunders, 1997, pp. 91-114.

31. Plumb DC: Veterinary Drug Handbook, 4th ed. Ames:Iowa State Press, 2002, pp. 249-251.

32. Meleo KA, Caplan ER: Treatment of insulinoma in the dog, cat, and ferret. *In* Kirk's Current Veterinary Therapy, 13th ed. Bonagura JD (ed). Philadelphia:WB Saunders, 2000, pp. 357-361.

33. Lipman NS, Marini RP, Murphy JC, et al: Estradiol-17-secreting adrenocorticol tumor in a ferret. J Am Vet Med Assoc 203:1552-1555, 1993.

34. Rosenthal KL, Peterson ME: Evaluation of plasma androgen and estrogen concentrations in ferrets with hyperadrenocorticism. J Am Vet Med Assoc 209:1097-1102, 1996.

35. Gould WJ, Reimers TJ, Bell JA, et al: Evaluation of urinary cortisol:creatinine ratios for the diagnosis of hyperadrenocorticism associated with adrenal gland tumors in ferrets. J Am Vet Med Assoc 206:42-46, 1995.

36. Neuwirth L, Isaza R, Bellah J, et al: Adrenal neoplasia in seven ferrets. Vet Radiol Ultrasound 34:340-343, 1993.

37. Weiss CA, Scott MV: Clinical aspects and surgical treatment of hyperadrenocorticism in the domestic ferret: 94 cases (1994-1996). J Am Anim Hosp Assoc 33:488-93, 1997.

38. Fox JG, Pequet-Goad ME, Garihaldi BA, Wiest LM: Hyperadrenocorticism in a ferret. J Am Vet Med Assoc 191:343-344, 1987.

39. Wagner RA, Dorn DP: Evaluation of serum estradiol concentrations in alopecic ferrets with adrenal gland tumors. J Am Vet Med Assoc 205:703-707, 1994.

40. Rosenthal KL: Adrenal disease in ferrets. *In* Veterinary Clinics of North America, Small Animal Practice. Kintzer PP (ed). Philadelphia:WB Saunders, 1997, pp. 401-418.

41. Schoemaker NJ, Wolfswinkel J, Mol JA, et al: Urinary corticoid/creatinine ratios in healthy ferrets and ferrets with hyperadrenocorticism. *In* Hyperadrenocorticism in Ferrets. Schoemaker NJ (ed). PhD thesis, 2003.

42. Schoemaker NJ, van der Hage MH, Lumeij JT, Rijnberk A: Morphology of the pituitary gland in ferrets (*Mustela putorius furo*) with hyperadrenocorticism. *In* Hyperadrenocorticism in Ferrets. Schoemaker NJ (ed). PhD thesis, 2003.

43. Besso JG, Tidwell AS, Gliatto JM. Retrospective review of the ultrasonographic features of adrenal lesions in 21 ferrets. Vet Radiol Ultrasound 41:345-52, 2000.

44. Gliatto JM, Alroy J, Schelling SH, et al: A light microscopical, ultrastructural and immunohistochemical study of spindle-cell adrenocortical tumors of ferrets. J Comp Pathol 113: 175-178, 1995.

45. Murthy AS, Brezak MA, Baez AG: Postcastrational adrenal tumors in two strains of mice: morphological, histochemical, and chromatographic studies. J Natl Cancer Inst 25:2111-2115, 1970.

46. Schoemaker NJ, Schuurmans M, Moorman H, Lemeij JT: Correlation between age at neutering and age at onset of hyperadrenocorticism in ferrets. *In* Hyperadrenocorticism in Ferrets. Schoemaker NJ (ed). PhD thesis, 2003.

47. Rosenthal KL, Peterson ME, Quesenberry KE, et al: Evaluation of plasma cortisol and corticosterone responses to synthetic adrenocorticotropic hormone administration in ferrets. Am J Vet Res 54:29-31, 1993.

48. O'Brien R, Paul-Murphy J, Dubielzig RR: Ultrasonography of adrenal glands in normal ferrets. Vet Radiol Ultrasound 37:445-448, 1996.

49. Neuwirth L, Collins B, Calderwood-Mays M, et al: Adrenal ultrasonography correlated with histopathology in ferrets. Vet Radiol Ultrasound 38:69-74, 1997.

50. Wagner RA, Bailey EM, Schneider JF, et al: Leuprolide acetate treatment of adrenocorticol disease of ferrets. J Am Vet Med Assoc 218:1272-1274, 2001.

51. Weiss CA: Medical management of ferret adrenal tumors and hyperplasia. Exotic DVM Magazine 1:38-39, 1999.

52. Beeber NL: Abdominal surgery in ferrets. Vet Clin North Am Exotic Anim Pract 3:647-662, 2000.

53. Mullen HS, Beeber NL: Miscellaneous surgery in ferrets. Vet Clin North Am Exotic Anim Pract 3:663-671, 2000.

54. Wheeler J, Bennett RA: Ferret abdominal surgical procedures. Part II. Compendium 21:1049-1057, 1999.

55. Beeber NL: Surgery of pet ferrets. *In* Current Techniques in Small Animal Surgery, 4th ed. Bojrab MJ (ed). Philadelphia: Williams & Wilkins, 1998, pp. 763-769.

56. Filion DL, Hoar DM: Adrenalectomy in the ferret. Lab Anim Sci 35:294-305, 1985.

57. Weiss CA, Williams BH, Scott JB, Scott MV: Surgical treatment and long-term outcome of ferrets with bilateral adrenal tumors or adrenal hyperplasia: 56 cases (1994-1997). J Am Vet Med Assoc 215:820-823, 1999.

58. Mullen H: Soft tissue surgery. *In* Ferrets, Rabbits, Rodents: Clinical Medicine and Surgery. Hillyer EV, Quesenberry KE (eds). Philadelphia: WB Saunders, 1997, pp. 131-144.

59. Laraio L, Weisse C, Zwingerberger A, et al: Collateral circulation during balloon occlusion of the caudal vena cava in ferrets. Proceedings of the Annual Conference of the American College of Veterinary Surgeons, Washington, DC, 2003.

60. Erdman SE, Li X, Fox JG: Hematopoietic diseases. *In* Fox JG (ed). Biology and Diseases of the Ferret, 2nd ed. Baltimore:Williams & Wilkins, 1998, pp. 231-246.

61. Petrie JP, Morrisey JK: Cardiovascular and other diseases. *In* Ferrets, Rabbits, and Rodents: Clinical Medicine and Surgery, 2nd ed. Quesenberry KE, Carpenter JW (eds). Philadelphia:WB Saunders , 2004, pp. 58-71.

62. Brown SA, Rosenthal KL: Causes of splenomegaly in ferrets. Vet Med 95:599, 2000.

63. Mullen HS, Scavelli TD, Quesenberry KE, et al: Gastrointestinal foreign body in ferrets: 25 cases (1986-1990). J Am Anim Hosp Assoc 28:13-15, 1989.

64. Fox JG: Disease of the gastrointestinal system. *In* Biology and Diseases of the Ferret, 2nd ed. Fox JG (ed). Baltimore:Williams & Wilkins, 1998, pp. 273-290.

65. Hoefer HL, Bell JA: Gastrointestinal diseases. *In* Ferrets, Rabbits, and Rodents: Clinical Medicine and Surgery, 2nd ed. Quesenberry KE, Carpenter JW (eds). Philadelphia:WB Saunders, 2004, pp. 25-40.

66. Jones TC, Hunt RD: Veterinary Pathology, 5th ed. Philadelphia:Lea & Febiger, 1983, pp. 116-119.

67. Sleeman JM, Clyde VL, Jones MP, Mason GL: Two cases of pyloric adenocarcinoma in the ferret (*Mustela putorius furo*). Vet Rec 137: 272-273, 1995.

68. Rice LE, Stahl SJ, McLeod CG: Pyloric adenocarcinoma in a ferret. J Am Vet Med Assoc 200:1117-1118, 1992.

69. Weisse C, Hume DZ, Berent A, et al: Palliative stenting for malignant obstructions in a dog, cat, and ferret. Proceedings of the 2004 Annual Meeting of the American College of Veterinary Surgeons. Denver, 2004;23.

70. Pollock CG: Urogenital diseases. *In* Ferrets, Rabbits, and Rodents: Clinical Medicine and Surgery, 2nd ed. Quesenberry KE, Carpenter JW (eds). Philadelphia:WB Saunders, 2004, pp. 41-49.

71. Bell JA: Periparturient and neonatal diseases. *In* Ferrets, Rabbits, and Rodents: Clinical Medicine and Surgery, 2nd ed. Quesenberry KE, Carpenter JW (eds). Philadelphia:WB Saunders, 2004, pp. 50-57.

72. Nguyen HT, Moreland AF, Shields RP: Urolithiasis in ferrets (*Mustela putorius*). Lab Anim Sci 29:243-245, 1979.

73. Marini RP, Esteves MI, Fox JG: A technique for catheterization of the urinary bladder in the ferret. Lab Anim 28:155-157, 1994.

74. Manning DD, Bell JA: Lack of detectable blood groups in domestic ferrets: implications for transfusion. J Am Vet Med Assoc 197:84-86, 1990.

Chapter 119

Surgical Diseases of the Rabbit

SJ Mehler
RA Bennett

Rabbits can be challenging surgical patients. Fear, pain, and stress have a profound effect on survival in the perioperative period. Anorexia, depression, and death can occur following minor surgical procedures. This is believed to be a result of increased catecholamine release.[1]

Rabbits ferment cellulose in their cecum. Stress, antibiotics, anesthetics, and diet can alter gastrointestinal function and physiology, which can lead to serious gastrointestinal (GI) complications, especially gastrointestinal ileus, postoperatively. Rabbits are unable to vomit so fasting to prevent aspiration pneumonia is not necessary. Rabbits have a relatively large GI volume. A fast prior to laparotomy in rabbits is not routinely performed; however, some suggest a fast of 6 to 12 hours prior to laparotomy in order to decrease GI volume, improve surgical visualization and exposure, and improve the ability to manipulate GI structures. Yet, a fast of this duration will have little effect on cecal volume where the majority of ingesta (about 40%) is located.[2,3]

It is important to have airway and venous access during anesthesia in the event of cardiac and/or respiratory arrest. Intubation is recommended for major surgeries in rabbits, and is essential during thoracotomies and procedures lasting greater than 20 minutes. Techniques for intubation are not covered in this chapter but are found elsewhere.[4] Repeated attempts to intubate rabbits can result in swelling and edema of the glottis that can result in fatal upper airway obstruction. If the intubation is not successful after 3 or 4 attempts, the rabbit should be maintained on mask anesthesia or, if appropriate, the procedure should be postponed for 2 to 3 days, allowing the glottis to recover.

Rabbits have a blood volume of 57 ml/kg body weight.[5] Loss of 15 to 20% of total blood volume in a rabbit causes massive cholinergic release. An acute blood loss of 20 to 30% of the total blood volume causes hemodynamic collapse and shock.[5] Fresh whole blood can be collected and prepared from donor rabbits for transfusion. Rabbits do have blood groups and transfusion reactions do occur, because of this a cross match is recommended before a blood transfusion is given. Purified bovine hemoglobin with oxygen-carrying capacity can be used temporarily to restore tissue perfusion and oxygenation while hemorrhage is controlled intraoperatively.

The success of surgery is often dependant on minimizing pain, stress, and fear. The use of analgesics, sedatives, anxieolytics, and shorter hospitalization times will minimize the negative effects of increased catecholamines on the surgical outcome. A positive outcome is also dependant on getting the rabbit to eat within 1 to 2 hours after surgery. If the rabbit is not eating after surgery, it should be force fed every few hours. Intravenous or subcutaneous fluids should be administered and continued until the rabbit is eating and drinking on its own.

Uterine Adenocarcinoma

Endometrial adenocarcinoma is the most common tumor of female rabbits.[6,7] In intact female New Zealand White rabbits that are greater than 3 to 4 years of age, incidence approaches 80%.[6,8]

Disease Mechanism

As the rabbit ages, the endometrium of the uterus undergoes cellular changes, characterized by increases in endometrial collagen content.[9] The increase in collagen and decrease in cells are considered senile changes and are associated with the development of uterine adenocarcinomas.[9,10] An identical process occurs in humans.[11]

Uterine adenocarcinomas in rabbits tend to be slow growing tumors and are slow to metastasize (Figure 119-1A and B). Local invasion of the tumor into the myometrium can occur early in the development of the tumor, and the neoplasm can extend through the uterine wall to invade other visceral structures.[6] Relevant medical history may include reproductive abnormalities such as decreased litter size, abortion, retention of feti, and stillbirth.[8,10]

Clinical Signs

Clinical signs include depression, anorexia, hematuria, and bloody vaginal discharge.[8,10] Hematuria is the most common presenting complaint but the hemorrhage is from the reproductive tract. Owners are usually not able to differentiate between hematuria and a hemorrhagic vaginal discharge. Cystic mammary glands can also develop concurrently with uterine endometrial hyperplasia and adenocarcinoma.[11,12]

Diagnostics

Larger tumors are easily palpated on physical examination. Adenocarcinoma is often present in both horns at the time of diagnosis.[6,9,13] A complete blood count, serum biochemistry panel, and urinalysis should always be performed. Abdominal and thoracic radiographs are useful in detecting primary tumors as well as metastatic disease. Metastatic uterine carcinoma has been reported in the lungs, liver, bone, brain, and throughout the peritoneal cavity (Figure 119-2).[8,13-15] Hypertrophic osteopathy associated with metastasis to the lungs has also been reported in rabbits.[8] Abdominal ultrasonography is useful in differentiating between uterine masses and other causes of reproductive tract enlargement or disease (endometrial hyperplasia, endometrial polyps, pyometra, and endometritis), metastatic disease in the abdomen, or concurrent abdominal disease.

Treatment

Prevention is the best treatment for uterine adenocarcinoma. It is recommended that rabbits undergo ovariohysterectomy (OHE) between the ages of 6 and 12 months.[10] The treatment of

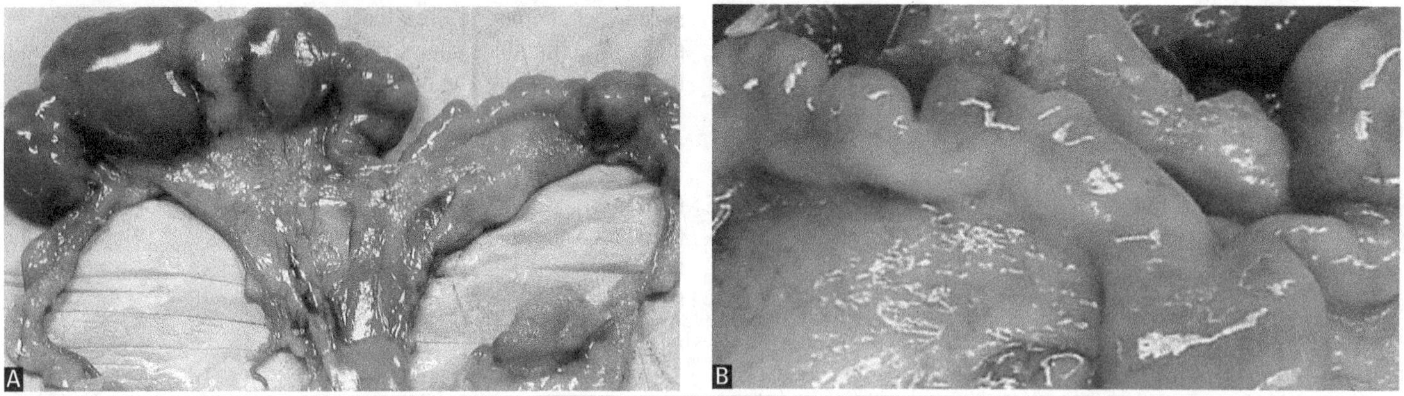

Figure 119-1A and B. Uterine adenocarcinoma in the rabbit. At the time of diagnosis, the tumor is commonly found in both uterine horns. Note the bicornuate uterus in figure B.

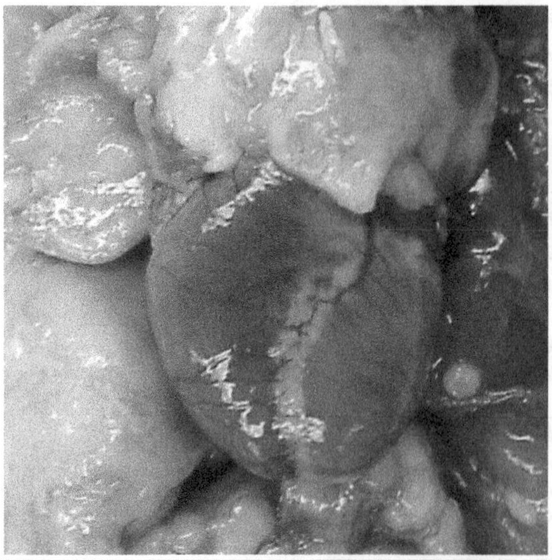

Figure 119-2. Metastatic uterine carcinoma in the rabbit. Note the circular white lesions in the lungs. Although metastatic spread of uterine adenocarcinoma in the rabbit is uncommon, disseminated disease can be found in the lungs, liver, bone, brain, and throughout the peritoneal cavity.

choice for rabbits with uterine adenocarcinoma is OHE.[8,13-15] The uterus of young rabbits is found just dorsal to the bladder, coiled in the caudal abdomen. In older rabbits, the cervix is dorsal to the bladder and the horns extend laterally but not very cranially. The doe reproductive anatomy lacks a uterine body. The uterus is bicornuate and each horn has its own cervix that empties into the relatively large vagina. The mesometrium is a major adipose storage site in rabbits, which makes identification of the ovarian and uterine vessels difficult during OHE. The oviduct in rabbits encircles the ovary and must be removed during OHE. If a remnant of the oviduct is present, it can become cystic.[16] The cranial vagina is ligated caudal to the cervices to avoid the development of cervical aneurysms, which may rupture resulting in fatal hemorrhage.[16]

Prognosis

If no macro/micrometastatic disease is present at the time of surgery, OHE may be curative. If pulmonary metastatic disease is present, the rabbit is given a grave prognosis.[10] It has been suggested that rabbits with uterine adenocarcinoma at the time of OHE be examined for pulmonary and abdominal metastasis every 2 to 3 months after OHE for 1 to 2 years.[10]

Urinary System and Cystic Calculi

The urine of normal rabbits varies in color from yellow, to creamy, to red or brown, which can be linked to pigments in the diet. The reddish hue of some rabbits' urine is normal but will lead rabbit owners to present their rabbit for hematuria.[2] The most common surgical disease of the urinary tract in rabbits is urinary bladder sludge and associated cystic calculi. Both conditions are likely related to the diet of the rabbit. Urinary sludge and calculi are composed mostly of calcium carbonate.

Disease Mechanism

It is reported that the total serum calcium levels in rabbits reflects the level of calcium in the diet and is not regulated within a narrow range;[2] however, recent research has identified that both ionized and total serum calcium concentrations in rabbits are maintained in a narrow reference range regardless of diet, although normal levels are higher than those in dogs and cats (personal communication, KR Rosenthal). Urine is a major route of calcium excretion in rabbits. The fractional excretion of calcium in rabbits is 20 to 30 times that of most mammals.[2] The calcium carbonate excretions may accumulate in the urinary bladder and form a thick sludge or cystic calculi. The color and consistency of rabbit urine can be greatly affected by dietary calcium levels, often appearing thick and white while ingesting high levels of calcium. Prolonged ingestion of a diet high in calcium levels can lead to mineralization of the aorta and kidneys.[2]

Clinical Signs

Clinical signs of cystic calculi may include straining to urinate, decreased appetite with subsequent decreased fecal production, or, if a lower urinary tract obstruction is present, the rabbit may become depressed, anorectic, and recumbent.

Diagnostics

Routine diagnostics should be performed in any rabbit demonstrating signs of lower urinary tract disease. These include a complete blood count, serum biochemistry profile, urinalysis, abdominal radiographs, and abdominal ultrasound. Mineralized calcium excretions (sludge) are commonly detected in the bladder on abdominal radiographs as an incidental finding while another disease process is being investigated. The material in the bladder is usually radiopaque because the composition is mainly calcium carbonate (Figure 119-3). Abdominal ultrasound is also helpful in evaluating the entire urinary tract, especially if a partial or complete urinary tract obstruction is suspected.

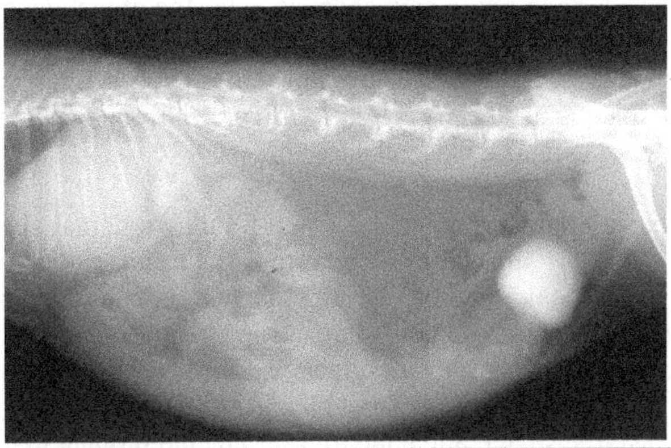

Figure 119-3. A right lateral radiograph of a rabbit with cystic calculi. The material in the bladder is usually radiopaque because the composition is mainly calcium carbonate.

Treatment

In some patients, this sludge-like material can be removed by lavaging the urinary bladder using a urinary catheter, sterile saline, and manual expression. This procedure is performed under general anesthesia. Occasionally, the material becomes thick enough that it will not pass or it forms a stone and causes lower urinary tract obstruction. Cystotomy in rabbits is analogous to that in other species.

Prevention and Prognosis

Some controversy exists as to whether dietary calcium restriction is beneficial in preventing urinary sludge or stone formation in rabbits. Commercial alfalfa pellets and alfalfa hay are relatively high in calcium. They were originally formulated for meat-production rabbits to cause rapid weight gain. As such, they are also high in protein and can predispose to obesity. Reducing the daily intake of pelleted alfalfa diets and feeding rabbits a diet composed mostly of timothy hay and timothy hay pellets, which are lower in calcium, is currently recommended. Additionally, treats high in calcium should be avoided. The prognosis is good after cystotomy but recurrence of sludge and of calculi formation is common.

Dental Abscesses

The dental formula in rabbits is 2 x (I 2/1 C 0/0 PM 3/2 M 3/3), making the total number of teeth 28.[17,18] The rostral incisors of the upper and lower jaw are modified to form a chisel-like cutting tool.[2,3] Rabbits keep these teeth sharp by gnawing on objects in their environment. The thicker enamel on the labial surface of the incisors allows the front surface of the teeth to wear down more slowly, creating the sharp edge.[3] The peg teeth (maxillary I_2) are smaller than the other incisors and are just caudal to the rostral incisors. The points of the lower incisors rest on the peg teeth. Therefore, in a normal rabbit's mouth, the lower incisors rest caudal to the upper incisors. The premolars and molars are often grouped together and called cheek teeth. The diastema is the toothless space between the last incisor and the first cheek tooth.[2]

The rabbit's nasolacrimal duct narrows at the maxilla bone and as it passes over the roots of the upper incisor teeth. The duct opens at a nasal punctum, depositing tears in the nostril as in dogs and cats. Abscessation of the upper incisors can lead to occlusion of the ipsilateral nasolacrimal duct.

All rabbit teeth grow continuously, and the permanent teeth are completely erupted by 3 to 5 weeks of age.[2] The teeth continue to grow from the highly metabolically active apical germinal cells. The cheek teeth of adult rabbits consist mostly of crown. The clinical crown is exposed in the oral cavity.[18] The reserve crown makes up most of the tooth but is within the bone of the mandible or maxilla. In rabbits, the growth of the permanent teeth is never completed, so no tooth roots are formed. The process of continual growth leaves rabbits susceptible to dental disease throughout their lives.

Disease Mechanism

In rabbits eating natural vegetation, the power stroke of chewing, the lingual edges of the mandibular cheek teeth occlude against the food on the buccal edges of the maxillary cheek teeth.[18] This repetitive movement of the cheek teeth during chewing enables even wear. Rabbits being fed a pellet diet have a decreased lateral excursion of the cheek teeth against the pellet and an increase in the vertical movement of the teeth. This altered motion of the jaw leads to abnormal tooth wear. Abnormal tooth wear can lead to erosions or ulcerations of the oral mucosa (maxillary cheek teeth) and tongue (mandibular cheek teeth) from the sharp points that develop. Anorexia, oral pain, arrested tooth development, and infection of the oral cavity occur secondary to abnormal tooth wear and growth. Systemic disease and metabolic abnormalities may also lead to inappropriate tooth growth and development.

The most common cause of periodontal disease in rabbits is the impaction of food debris into the peridontium.[18] This occurs secondary to abnormal or arrested tooth growth from inappropriate diet and systemic disease. The inflamed and infected peridontium, periodontal ligament, and surrounding tissues remodel and reabsorb. Tissue loss leads to deeper periodontal pockets, advanced infection into surrounding tissues, and local spread of bacteria toward the apex and bone of the mandible and maxilla. If not addressed, osteomyelitis and abscessation ensue.

Historically, abscesses in rabbits were thought to be caused by *Pasteurella multocida*; however, a variety of other organisms are routinely cultured. It is actually rare to isolate Pasteurella sp. from abscesses in rabbits. Anaerobic bacteria, Staphylococcus sp. and Streptococcus sp. are most commonly cultured.[19]

Abscesses of the head in rabbits may develop secondary to dental disease, food or foreign body impaction between the gingiva and tooth, periodontal disease, tooth fracture, or tooth root abscess. Abscesses occur in rabbits of all ages and can be soft or firm. When the bone is involved, there is often bony swelling owing to the periosteal reaction. If the maxillary cheek teeth are involved, ocular discharge is observed owing to the involvement of the ipsilateral nasolacrimal duct. The wall of the abscess is commonly thick and contains bacteria. The pus is usually caseous, thick, and creamy-white in appearance. Of all the abscesses occurring in rabbits, retrobulbar and dental abscesses are likely the most difficult to cure.

Diagnostics

Many rabbits with dental abscesses present with a swelling or a mass palpable during a physical examination. During a routine physical examination, the ventral mandible is palpated for any bumps. Bumps or scalloping along the ventral mandible is indicative of mandibular cheek teeth root disease resulting in cortical penetration.

Clinical work up includes a minimum data base including a complete blood count, serum biochemistry panel, and urinalysis. An oral examination is helpful in evaluating the crowns of the teeth for elongation, points, and other structural abnormalities; however, the extent of involvement of the reserve crowns, germinal tissue, and bone cannot be assessed by oral examination alone. Additionally, many attempt to evaluate the crowns in an awake rabbit. This is often difficult because the rabbit's mouth does not open very far, it chews constantly while the oral examination is being attempted, and it is difficult to evaluate all surfaces of the crowns. Because some type of imaging modality (radiography or computed tomography) is essential when evaluating dental abscesses, an oral examination is best conducted under general anesthesia.

Skull radiographs under anesthesia are useful to evaluate for the presence and extent of infection. The four or five views recommended are a ventrodorsal or dorsoventral, a lateral, a left lateral oblique, and a right lateral oblique at a minimum. A rostrocaudal projection allows evaluation of the occlusal surface of the cheek teeth and for any bony proliferation of maxillary bone. Computed tomography (CT scan) has become more available in veterinary medicine and is far more useful for evaluating the extent of dental disease.

Aspirates of the abscess are obtained to confirm the presence of pus and for cytologic and microbiologic evaluation. Cultures of aspirated pus have yielded higher quantities and more species of bacteria than intraoperative cultures of the abscess walls.[19] A positive preoperative culture is useful for starting antibiotic therapy prior to surgery as well as for deciding which antibiotics would be best for local therapy. Cytology, including a Gram's stain, is useful to confirm that the mass is an abscess and define the types of bacteria present. This is useful in deciding on antibiotic therapy prior to receiving culture results. Additionally, some aspirates will fail to grow bacteria and the Gram's stain may be the only objective data on which to base antibiotic therapy.

Treatment

A variety of surgical therapies has been used in treating dental abscesses in rabbits with variable results. The traditional treatment of abscesses in mammals (lancing, draining, and flushing) is not effective in rabbits because the pus is too thick to drain effectively. Also typically fibrous tracts are present that contain bacteria, making recurrence common. As a result, the skin surface usually heals over before the infection has completely been eliminated. This traps infected tissue below the skin surface and a new abscess develops at the same site. Failure to completely remove any teeth that are associated with the abscess will result in recurrence of the abscess regardless of the technique used because bad teeth and surrounding infected bone will serve as a nidus of infection.

The basic principles employed when treating a dental abscess in a rabbit are to remove all infected soft tissue including the abscess capsule, debride all infected bone, remove any teeth involved, minimize contamination of remaining tissues with pus, irrigate extensively, implant antibiotic-impregnated polymethylmethacrylate (AI-PMMA) beads (Figure 119-4A, B, and C), and administer systemic antibiotic to treat any bacteremia that may result from the surgery.

The use of antibiotic impregnated polymethylmethacrylate beads, which release relatively high concentrations of antibiotic locally with little systemic absorption, is currently the recommended surgical option for rabbits with oral cavity abscesses.[20-25] It appears that antibiotics that are not safe when administered systemically in rabbits, such as cefazolin and clindamycin, are safe in AI-PMMA beads. Different antibiotics should not be mixed together in the same bead as this has been shown to unacceptably alter the elution rate.[22] It is also important to refrain from using antibiotics in beads for which the elution rate and appropriate concentration are unknown, for example, enrofloxacin will not mix into PMMA. The rabbit should still be placed on systemic antibiotics for 2 to 3 weeks but long-term therapy is not needed as the beads release antibiotic for many months. The antibiotics chosen are based on culture and sensitivity or Gram's stain results.

Some teeth, even after they are removed, will grow back if the germinal bud remains viable. Because rabbit teeth grow continuously, the question arises, if teeth are removed, is it necessary to remove the opposing teeth? This is not usually necessary. The maxillary teeth tend to grow and erupt at a slower rate than the mandibular teeth. Often, after the mandibular teeth are removed, the maxillary teeth stop erupting.[18] Some removed cheek teeth grow back because the germinal tissue is still healthy. Because of the extensive movement during chewing, even 2 to 3 teeth are often enough to wear the opposing teeth. Sometimes, the opposing teeth overgrow, in which case they either need to be trimmed on a regular basis (every 6 to 8 weeks) or they need to be removed.

Even after aggressive surgical debridement, rabbits recover quickly. Most begin eating within a couple of hours of surgery. It appears that removing the abscess helps resolve the pain associated with the abscess.

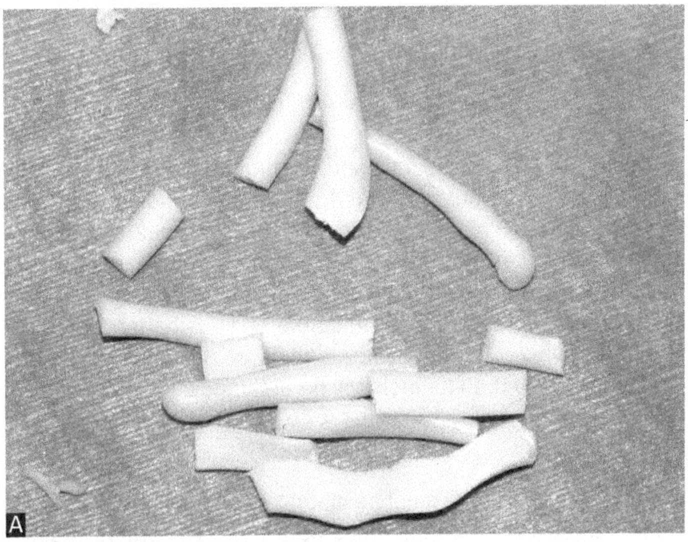

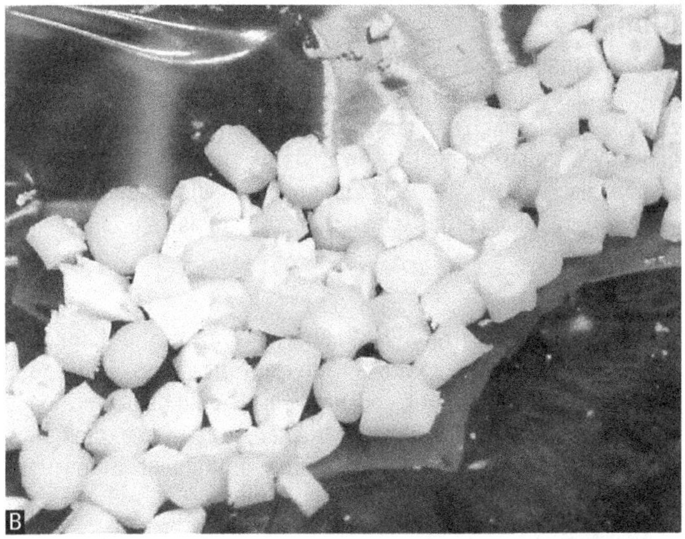

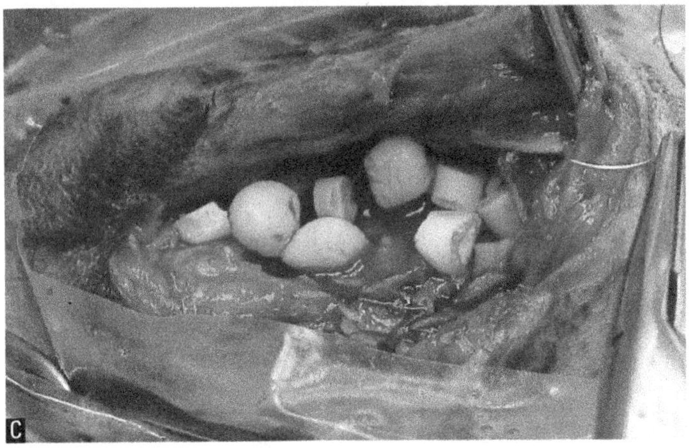

Figure 119-4. A. AI-PMMA is rolled out into fine tubular strips. B. The tubular strips are then cut into appropriate size pieces for the wound. The pieces are cut before the PMMA hardens. A scalpel blade works well for this. Bead makers are also available but are limited to one bead size. C. The beads are then placed in the wound. In this photograph, the beads are being used in a thoroughly debrided mandibular abscess in a rabbit.

Prognosis

In general, the prognosis for complete recovery without recurrence is fair to good using this technique. The best chance for surgical cure is with the use of CT imaging, aggressive removal of all grossly abnormal tissue including teeth and bone based on the CT images, and the implantation of PMMA beads impregnated with an appropriate antibiotic based on preoperative culture and sensitivity results. Even with all of this, dental abscesses in rabbits can be difficult to completely eliminate. Owners should be advised before surgery about the nursing care, frequency of follow-up visits, and financial commitment involved.

Gastric Stasis Syndrome (Ileus), Trichobezoar, and Gastrointestinal Foreign Body

The most common clinical problems in rabbits involve the gastrointestinal tract. Most of these are directly or indirectly related to diet.[26] Rabbits are unable to vomit because of the anatomic arrangement of the cardia and stomach.[26,27] The pylorus is easily compressed by the duodenum because it exits the stomach at a sharp angle.[2] The ileocecal junction is a common site for foreign body obstruction in rabbits.[2] The cecum of rabbits is thin-walled and holds 40% of the total gastrointestinal contents.[2] Rabbits are hindgut cecal fermentors that efficiently ingest large quantities of poorly digestible fiber that is essential for normal peristalsis more than it is important for nutrition.[26,27]

Disease Mechanism of Trichobezoar and Gastric Stasis

It has previously been suggested that, when rabbits are fed a diet deficient in fiber or if gastric stasis occurs for another reason, trichobezoars can become a clinical problem by obstructing the pyloric outflow tract and proximal duodenum.[28,29] Although trichobezoars are described as a clinical problem, it is now accepted that the presence of a trichobezoar is normal in rabbits and the illness is not directly related to the presence of a mass of hair and fiber. Rabbits that present with clinical signs of anorexia, lethargy, and mild abdominal distention that have radiographic evidence of a hairball are commonly ill for other reasons, most likely gastrointestinal ileus. Historically, rabbits with a trichobezoar were treated by gastrotomy to remove the hairball. Most of these rabbits did not survive because the mass of hair was not causing the illness and little attention was paid to managing the underlying ileus and dehydration. It is now accepted that the hairball is an incidental finding and this syndrome is more accurately termed gastric stasis. It is best managed medically, not surgically.

In rabbits with dental disease, the discomfort associated with chewing food will cause rabbits to quickly decrease daily food intake and appears to be a common cause of ileus. Ileus is also commonly associated with a high-carbohydrate/low-fiber diet, stress, pain, and a lack of exercise.

Clinical Signs

Gastric stasis syndrome (ileus) is common in rabbits and is defined clinically by anorexia, decreased or no stool production, and a large stomach typically containing a mass of fiber and hair along with gastric fluid.[26] If an underlying disease is present, clinical signs associated with that condition should be evaluated and treated concurrently with the gastric stasis.

Diagnostics

A detailed dietary history is an important part of the diagnostic investigation in rabbits with GI ileus. A complete blood count, serum biochemistry panel, and urinalysis should be performed to look for the underlying cause for the ileus. A dental examination should also be performed. If indicated, abdominal radiographs and ultrasound should be performed.

Treatment

The most important aspects of medical management for rabbits with gastrointestinal stasis are fluid support, getting fiber into the GI tract to stimulate motility, administering GI motility-enhancing drugs, and providing nutritional support to minimize the risk of secondary hepatic lipidosis. Medical management usually includes intravenous fluid support because rabbits with GI stasis are typically dehydrated. Although most patients have a decreased appetite, many will still eat fresh leafy green vegetables. Eating such materials will provide additional fluids, compared with dry hay or pellets, as well as fiber. If the patient will not eat, nasogastric intubation for alimentation may be necessary. Analgesics are often beneficial to palliate concurrent abdominal discomfort and increase the activity level of the rabbit, which may help stimulate GI motility.

The condition may be complicated by the presence of hepatic lipidosis secondary to the anorexia. Pelleted diets are relatively high in protein and carbohydrates, resulting in obesity and predisposing to hepatic lipidosis. Correcting the nitrogen balance will decrease the acidosis and ketosis, and counter the negative effects of the lipid hepatopathy.

Disease Mechanism of Gastrointestinal Foreign Body

Carpet fiber is a common cause of foreign body obstruction seen in rabbits. Another cause of intestinal foreign body is a piece of gastric hairball that breaks off and migrates into the duodenum. Rabbits with GI foreign body obstruction can present with clinical signs similar to those of ileus, and both conditions can occur simultaneously. The disease process associated with GI foreign body is generally an acute condition that does not allow time for the rabbit to adjust systemically. The acute distention of the stomach with gas and fluid, the inability of rabbits to vomit, and the pain associated with a foreign body obstruction make this disease in rabbits a rapidly life-threatening emergency.

Clinical Signs

Rabbits with gastrointestinal foreign body obstruction commonly present with acute depression and severe and rapid abdominal distention. They are typically much more critically ill than are rabbits with GI ileus alone.

Diagnostics

A complete blood count, serum biochemistry panel, and urinalysis should be performed. Abdominal radiographs and ultrasound are useful in determining the presence of a foreign body obstruction. The presence of a mass of hair in the stomach is considered normal in rabbits and does not confirm a diagnosis of obstruction. Obstruction can cause an ileus pattern on radiographs; however, if the obstruction is at the pylorus or orad duodenum, only the stomach will be distended.

Treatment

Systemically ill rabbits must be stabilized with intravenous fluids and analgesics before definitive surgery is performed. Gastric decompression by nasogastric or orogastric intubation or by trocharization is vital in critically ill patients. Routine exploratory laparotomy and gastrotomy with two-layer closure, as performed in dogs and cats, should be performed in rabbits with a gastric foreign body causing pyloric outflow obstruction. For an intestinal obstruction, enterotomies and intestinal resection and anastamosis are performed as needed. The small intestine of rabbits has a much thinner wall than that of dogs and cats. Surgical magnification and appropriate suture and atraumatic needle sizes are used. Postoperatively, rabbits should be treated with analgesics and for gastrointestinal stasis as previously described.

Prognosis

Rabbits with GI foreign body obstruction do poorly postoperatively and have a high perioperative mortality rate compared with dogs and cats. These patients need to be rapidly stabilized and decompressed on presentation. Short anesthesia and operative times, aggressive analgesia, fluid therapy, and postoperative nutritional and GI motility support are vital.

Thymoma

The thymus in rabbits persists into adult life, lies ventral to the heart, and extends to the thoracic inlet.[2] Thymomas in rabbits are infrequently reported, but make up as much as 8% of all neoplasms.[8,30] Two age groups appear to be affected. Genetically based thymomas occur in rabbits 1 to 4 years of age and have been associated with a systemic immunopathy and hemolytic anemia.[6,8] Older rabbits, 7 to 9 years of age, are affected with primary thymoma. Most of these tumors are diagnosed post mortem.

Disease Mechanism

The thymus is responsible for the normal development and regulation of the immune system.[31] Thymomas are uncommon tumors in rabbits, dogs, and cats.[8,30,32,33] In dogs, cats, and humans, paraneoplastic syndromes associated with thymoma include myasthenia gravis, cytopenia, thyroiditis, hypogammaglobulinemia, and polymyositis.[32,33] Potential paraneoplastic conditions associated with thymoma in rabbits include hypercalcemia, systemic immunopathy, and hemolytic anemia.[6,8]

Clinical Signs

Clinical signs are variable and are related to a space-occupying mass in the cranial mediastinum or to the paraneoplastic processes. Rabbits can present with clinical signs including respiratory distress and precaval syndrome (swelling of the head, exopthalmos, and prolapse of the third eyelids).[34-36]

Diagnostics

Complete blood count, serum biochemistry panel, and urinalysis should be performed. Thoracic radiographs of rabbits with thymoma reveal a cranial mediastinal mass (Figure 119-5). Because the radiographic density of the mass is the same as the heart, it is difficult to distinguish the two structures.[34-36] Ultrasound-guided transthoracic fine-needle aspiration and needle-core biopsy are helpful to evaluate the extent of the mass, and to evaluate the heart and other thoracic structures as well as to rule out other causes of a cranial mediastinal mass. Although cystic and necrotic areas are commonly associated with thymomas, a diagnosis via fine-needle aspiration or needle-core biopsy is usually possible with ultrasound guidance.

CT or MRI is highly useful in evaluating the invasiveness of the mass and its association with vital thoracic structures. This can be valuable in planning the surgery and offering a prognosis.

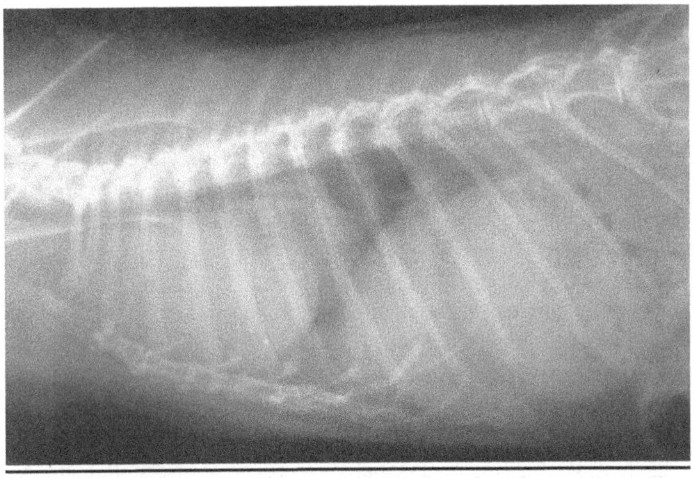

Figure 119-5. A right lateral thoracic radiograph in a rabbit with a thymoma. The cranial borders of the heart are obscured by a soft tissue opacity in the cranial mediastium.

Treatment

Thymomas are surgically resected using a ventral midline approach (Figure 119-6). The sternebrae of rabbits are usually too narrow to be able to split longitudinally. Therefore, it is best to disarticulate the ribs from the sternebrae on one side, allowing the chest to be opened. Invasion of the thymic capsule, vena cava, pericardium, pleura, and lung parenchyma can make complete resection difficult in some cases.[31] Care is taken to avoid important neurologic and vascular structures in the cranial thorax. Complications of thymoma removal include fatal hemorrhage, pneumothorax, and inadvertent damage to vital thoracic structures.[8,34-36]

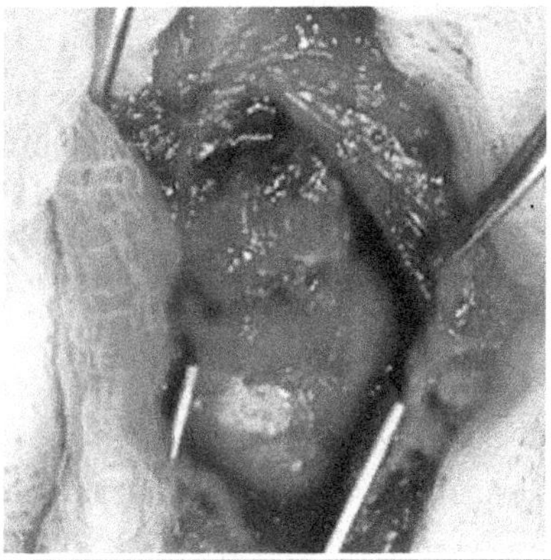

Figure 119-6. A ventral approach to the thoracic cavity has been performed in a rabbit. The sternebrae of rabbits are usually too narrow to be able to split longitudinally. Therefore, it is best to disarticulate the ribs from the sternebrae on one side allowing the chest to be opened. A cranial mediastinal mass is noted with adhesions to the pericardium, aortic root, and cranial aspect of the heart.

Prognosis

If rabbits survive the postoperative period and the mass is completely removed, prognosis is good. Radiographic rechecks are recommended every 3 to 4 months for the first year to assess for evidence of recurrence. Recurrence following complete excision of a thymoma in rabbits has not been reported.

Vertebral Fracture, Subluxation, or Luxation

The most common cause of acute paraparesis or paraplegia in rabbits is vertebral body fracture, subluxation, or luxation.[37] Fractures are more common than luxations, with the most common site of injury being the caudal lumbar vertebral bodies.

Disease Mechanism

Injury results from improper handling, from accidentally stepping on the rabbit, or when a caged rabbit is startled while in its enclosure. The heavily muscled hindquarters are allowed to twist at the lumbosacral junction, which acts as a fulcrum in applying leverage to the caudal lumbar vertebral column.[38] Also, the bones of rabbits are hard and brittle compared with those of dogs and cats. The bones of rabbits comprise only 8% of the total bodyweight, compared with 13% in cats.[39] The spinal cord in rabbits extends all the way to the sacrum so even lower lumbar vertebral fractures in rabbits can results in upper motor neuron signs.

Clinical signs

Clinical signs are dependant on the location and severity of the injury to the spinal cord. In addition to paraparesis or paraplegia, loss of urinary and fecal continence, urine retention, and myelomalacia can occur. Again, it is important to note that, because the spinal cord ends at the sacrum, neurolocalization is dissimilar to that in cats and dogs.

Diagnostics

Diagnosis is based on a thorough neurologic examination and survey spinal radiographs. Magnetic resonance imaging (MRI), myelography, and/or computed tomography (CT scan), are useful for defining the nature of the injury and prognosis for neurologic recovery in preparation for surgery. MRI is preferred if available.

Treatment

Both medical management and surgical intervention have been applied to rabbits with spinal cord injury. Medical management includes strict cage rest, management of urine retention (UMN lesion) or dribbling (LMN lesion), analgesics, nonsteroidal anti-inflammatories, and physical therapy. Surgical options depend on the location of the injury and whether the injury involves a fracture, instability, or both. Fixation of vertebral body fractures or instabilities can be performed with plates, pins and polymethylmethacrylate, screws and polymethylmethacrylate, or spinal stapling.

Prognosis

Prognosis depends on the severity of the neurologic deficits present during the perioperative period and the degree of displacement of the fracture and/or luxation. Owners should be informed that nursing care will be intensive regardless of whether medical or surgical options are pursued. Loss of deep pain perception in the limbs is usually considered a poor prognostic indicator for the return of neurologic function in rabbits suffering from a vertebral body luxation or fracture.

References

1. Jenkins JR: Soft tissue surgery. *In* Ferrets, Rabbits, and Rodents: Clinical Medicine and Surgery, 2nd ed. Quesenberry KE, Carpenter JW (eds). Philadelphia: WB Saunders, 2004, pp. 221-230.

2. Donnelly TM: Basic anatomy, physiology, and husbandry. *In* Ferrets, Rabbits, and Rodents: Clinical Medicine and Surgery, 2nd ed. Quesenberry KE, Carpenter JW (eds). Philadelphia: WB Saunders, 2004, pp. 136-146.

3. Popesko P, Raijtova V, Horak J: A colour atlas of the anatomy of small laboratory animals. Vol. 1. London: Wolfe Publishing, 1992.

4. Mason DE: Anesthesia, analgesia, and sedation for small mammals. *In* Hillyer EV, Quesenberry KE (eds). Ferrets, Rabbits, and Rodents: Clinical Medicine and Surgery. Philadelphia: WB Saunders, 1997, pp. 378-391.

5. Kozma C, Macklin W, Cummins LM, et al: Anatomy, physiology, and biochemistry of the rabbit. In Weisbroth SH, Flatt RE, Kraus AL (eds). The Biology of the Laboratory Rabbit. New York: Academic Press, 1974, pp. 50-72.

6. Weisbroth S: Neoplastic disease. *In* Manning P, Ringler D, Newcomer C (eds). The Biology of the Laboratory Rabbit, 2nd ed. San Diego: Academic Press, 1994, pp. 259-292.

7. Harkness J, Wagner J: The Biology and Medicine of Rabbits and Rodents, 4th ed Philadelphia: Williams & Wilkins, 1995.

8. Heatley JJ, Smith AN: Spontaneous neoplasms of lagamorphs. Vet Clin Exotic Anim 7:561-577, 2004.

9. Baba N, von Haam E: Animal model for human disease: spontaneous adenocarcinoma in aged rabbits. Am J Pathol 68:653-656, 1972.

10. Pare JA, Paul-Murphy J: Disorders of the reproductive and urinary systems. *In* Ferrets, Rabbits, and Rodents: Clinical Medicine and Surgery, 2nd ed. Quesenberry KE, Carpenter JW (eds). Philadelphia: WB Saunders, 2004, pp. 183-193.

11. Kraus AL, Weisbroth SH, Flatt RE, et al: Biology and Disease of Rabbits. *In* Laboratory Animal Medicine. Fox JE, Cohen BJ, Loew FM (eds). New York: Academic Press, 1984, pp. 207-237.

12. Hillyer EV: Pet rabbits. Vet Clin North Am Small Anim Pract 24:25-65, 1994.

13. Sommerville L: Treatment of uterine adenocarcinoma in a domestic rabbit by ovariohysterectomy. Vet Rec 142:550-551, 1998.

14. Flatt R: Pyometra and uterine adenocarcinoma in a rabbit. Lab Anim Care 19:398-401, 1969.

15. Raftery A: Uterine adenocarcinoma in pet rabbits. Vet Rec 142(245):704, 1998.

16. Jenkins JR: Surgical sterilization in small mammals. Vet Clin North Am 3:617-627, 2000.

17. Kertesz PA: Colour atlas of veterinary dentistry and oral surgery. London: Wolfe Publishing, 1993.

18. Crossley DA: Oral biology and disorders of lagomorphs. Vet Clin North Am 6:629-659, 2003.

19. Tyrrell KL, Citron DM, Jenkins JR, Goldstein EJ: Periodontal bacteria in rabbit mandibular and maxillary abscesses. J Clin Micro 40:1044-1047, 2002.

20. Tobias KM, Schneider RK, Besser TE: Use of antimicrobial-impregnated polymethyl methacrylate. J Am Vet Med Assoc 208:841-844, 1996.

21. Ethell MT, Bennett RA, Brown MP, et al: In vitro elution of gentamicin, amikacin, and ceftiofur from polymethylmethacrylate and hydroxyapaptite cement. Vet Surg 29:375-382, 2000.

22. Ramos JR, Howard RD, Pleasant RS, et al: Elution of metronidazole and gentamicin from polymethylmethacrylate beads. Vet Surg 32:251-261, 2003.

23. Adams K, Couch L, Cierny G, et al: In vitro and in vivo evaluation of antibiotic diffusion from antibiotic-impregnated polymethylmethacrylate beads. Clin Orthop Rel Res 278:244-252, 1992.

24. Nelson CL, Hickmon SG, Skinner RA: Treatment of experimental osteomyelitis by surgical debridement and the implantation of bioerodable, polyanhydride-gentamicin beads. J Orthop Res 15:249-255, 1997.

25. Wahlig H, Dingeldein E, Bergmann R, Reuss K: The release of gentamicin from polymethylmethacrylate beads. An experimental and pharmacokinetic study. J Bone Joint Surg 60:270-275, 1978.

26. Jenkins JR: Gastrointestinal diseases. *In* Ferrets, Rabbits, and Rodents: Clinical Medicine and Surgery, 2nd ed. Quesenberry KE, Carpenter JW (eds). Philadelphia: WB Saunders, 2004, pp. 161-171.

27. Brooks DL: Nutrition and gastrointestinal physiology. *In* Ferrets, Rabbits, and Rodents: Clinical Medicine and Surgery, 2nd ed. Quesenberry KE, Carpenter JW (eds). Philadelphia: WB Saunders, 2004, pp. 155-160.

28. Brooks DL: Rabbit gastrointestinal disorders. *In* Kirk's Current Veterinary Therapy VIII. Kirk RW, Bonagura JD (eds). Philadelphia: WB Saunders, 1983, pp. 654-657.

29. Harkness JE, Wagner JE: The Biology and Medicine of Rabbits and Rodents, 3rd ed. Philadelphia: Lea & Febiger, 1989.

30. Greene H, Strauss J: Multiple primary tumors in the rabbit. Cancer 2:673-91, 1949.

31. Aronsohn M. Pathophysiology of the thymus gland. *In* Disease Mechanisms in Small Animal Surgery. Bojrab MJ, Smeak DD, Bloomberg MS (eds). Philadelphia: Lea & Febiger, 1993, 626-629.

32. Aronsohn MG: Clinical and pathologic features of thymoma in 15 dogs. J Am Vet Med Assoc 184:1355, 1984.

33. Carpenter JL, Holzworth J: Thymoma in eleven cats. J Am Vet Med Assoc 181:248, 1982.

34. Clippinger TL, Bennett RA, Alleman R, et al: Removal of a thymoma via median sternotomy in a rabbit with recurrent appendicular neurofibrosarcoma. J Am Vet Med Assoc 213:1140-1143, 1998.

35. Kostolich M, Panciera R: Thymoma in a domestic rabbit. Cornell Vet 82:125-129, 1991.

36. Vernau K, Grahn B, Clarke-Scott H, Sullivan N: Thymoma in a geriatric rabbit with hypercalcemia and periodic exopthalmus. J Am Vet Med Assoc 206:820-822, 1996.

37. Deeb BJ, Carpenter JW: Neurologic and musculoskeletal diseases. *In* Ferrets, Rabbits, and Rodents: Clinical Medicine and Surgery, 2nd ed. Quesenberry KE, Carpenter JW (eds). Philadelphia: WB Saunders, 2004, pp. 203-210.

38. Gentz E, Carpenter JW: Neurologic and musculoskeletal diseases. *In* Hillyer EV, Quesenberry KE (eds). Ferrets, Rabbits, and Rodents: Clinical Medicine and Surgery. Philadelphia: WB Saunders, 1997, pp. 220-226.

39. Redrobe S: Surgical procedures and dental disorders. *In*: Flecknell PA (ed). BSAVA Manual of Rabbit Medicine and Surgery. Quedgeley: BSAVA, 2000, pp. 117-133

Index

G

H

J

K

L